ADVANCES IN NEUROLOGY
VOLUME 44

Advances in Neurology

Advances in Neurology
Volume 44

Basic Mechanisms of the Epilepsies
Molecular and Cellular Approaches

Editors

Antonio V. Delgado-Escueta, M.D.

Professor of Neurology
Director, Comprehensive Epilepsy Program
UCLA School of Medicine and
VA Southwest Regional Epilepsy Center
West Los Angeles VA Medical Center (Wadsworth)
Los Angeles, California

Arthur A. Ward, Jr., M.D.

Professor and Chairman Emeritus
Department of Neurological Surgery
University of Washington School of Medicine
Seattle, Washington

Dixon M. Woodbury, Ph.D.

Professor
Departments of Physiology and Pharmacology
Head of Division of Neuropharmacology and Epileptology
University of Utah College of Medicine
Salt Lake City, Utah

Roger J. Porter, M.D.

Chief, Medical Neurology Branch
Intramural Research Program
National Institute of Neurological
and Communication Disorders and Stroke
National Institutes of Health
Bethesda, Maryland

Raven Press ■ New York

Raven Press, 1140 Avenue of the Americas, New York, New York 10036

Made in the United States of America

Library of Congress Cataloging-in-Publication Data
Main entry under title:

Basic mechanisms of the epilepsies.

(Advances in neurology ; v. 44)
Based on workshops held at the Kroc Foundation headquarters in Calif. in Dec. 1982 and during the International Symposium on Basic Mechanisms of the Epilepsies, held in San Diego, Dec. 1983; both sponsored by the Subcommittee on Basic Research of the Epilepsy Advisory Committee, National Institute of Neurological and Communicative Disorders and Stroke.
Includes bibliographies and index.
1. Epilepsy—Congresses. 2. Pathology, Molecular—Congresses. 3. Pathology, Cellular—Congresses.
I. Delgado-Escueta, Antonio V. II. International Symposium on Basic Mechanisms of the Epilepsies (1983 : San Diego, Calif.) III. National Institute of Neurological and Communicative Disorders and Stroke. Epilepsy Advisory Committee. Subcommittee on Basic Research. IV. Series. [DNLM: 1. Epilepsy—congresses. W1 AD684H v.44 / WL 385 B311 1982-83]
RC321.A276 vol. 44   616.8′53   85-25800
[RC372.5]
ISBN 0-88167-152-5

Advances in Neurology Series

Advances in Neurology, Volume 44

Preface

This volume represents a confluence of information from the neurosciences, molecular genetics, and the clinical epilepsies. This multidisciplinary effort provides the substance of the present volume, which contains seven sections and 53 chapters.

In the first section, an introductory chapter advances a picture of the generalized and partial epilepsies by summarizing the cornucopia of information on molecular and cellular events in the epilepsies. This chapter offers a tabular summary of useful data on experimental and human epilepsies and presents a conceptual blueprint for the priority challenges in epilepsy research for the end of this century. The subsequent four sections cover biochemical genetics as they apply to the epilepsies (Section 2); molecular machinery of the cell and intracellular communication (Section 3: Epileptogenesis I); cell–cell communication: neurotransmitters, neuromodulators, and receptors (Section 4: Epileptogenesis II); ion transport and neuron–glia relations during spread and arrest of seizures (Section 5); modern neuroanatomical methods and mechanisms of epileptic cell damage (Section 6); and basic research in human epilepsies as exemplified by positron emission tomography and *in vivo* and *in vitro* cell recordings in human partial epilepsies and biochemical membrane studies in human temporal lobe epilepsy (Section 7).

Despite the revolutionary transformation of its contents, its conversion to a "cellular and molecular approach," its call for more research on the human epilepsies, and the reaffirmation of our primary goal, namely, the eradication of epilepsy, this volume reflects the intentions of the organizers and editors of a 1969 work, *Basic Mechanisms of the Epilepsies:*

> . . . to bring together the current work considered significant, viable and provocative in the field of epilepsy. . . . by so doing, it will serve as a benchmark which summarizes past scientific accomplishments, against which future progress can be measured. To this end, the monograph has a twofold mission: to make available to clinicians, scientists, and students a body of data and concepts relevant to epilepsy; and to serve as stimulus for an expanded interdisciplinary research effort in the epilepsies (2).

The current volume is designed to provide the student, the clinician, and the research scientist with a critical synthesis of knowledge and a base from which to track developments in the expanding fields of epilepsy research. In fact, its major aim is to serve as a textbook in basic mechanisms of the epilepsies for students in biomedical sciences and for physicians desirous of entering epilepsy research. We have chosen authors who are at the forefront of their fields and who can write chapters with a perspective that extends from the past and into the future. Accordingly, to set a standard for completeness and clarity, we established a format for each chapter. Every chapter is preceded by a detailed summary. The chapter opens with a historical note on the developments and importance of particular aspects of epilepsy research. The ensuing discussion contains a precise description of what is known about the normal condition in a given area as well as how epilepsy and seizures are affected by this area. Each author then considers such questions as the effect of the research area on the development or cessation of seizures, then speculates about what is yet to be learned in the field.

As with the original 1969 volume, this work "does not purport to be an all-inclusive presentation on the present state of the subject. Other material might have been included, but the practical limitations of space required that a selection be made of both subjects and authors" (2).

REFERENCES

1. Delgado-Escueta, A. V., Ferrendelli, J. A., and Prince, D. A. editors (1984): Basic Mechanisms of the Epilepsies. Proceedings of a Workshop at the Kroc Foundation Headquarters, *Ann. Neurol.,* 16(S)2:1–158.
2. Jasper, H. H., Ward, A. A. Jr., and Pope, A. editors (1969): *Basic Mechanisms of the Epilepsies,* Little, Brown and Co., Boston.

Acknowledgments

The editors are grateful for the help of many diligent and capable people. We thank the Department of Continuing Education in Health Sciences, UCLA Extension, for helping to organize the International Symposium on Basic Mechanisms of the Epilepsies in San Diego, California on December 7 to 10, 1983. We thank the Kroc Foundation for supporting a one week conference-workshop on a similar topic in December 1982 at the Kroc Foundation Headquarters in California's Santa Ynez Mountains. These two events formed the foundation for the content of this book.

With appreciation, we also want to mention the editorial assistance of Candace Porter. Word processing assistance was provided by Corey Elias and Susan Pietsch. Bob Mitchell assisted in the design of the Table of Contents and section dividers.

This project was supported by USPHS grant 1 R13 NS17921-01, in part by USPHS contract N01-NS-0-2332 from the National Institute of Neurological and Communicative Disorders and Stroke, and by grants-in-aid from Abbott Laboratories, Burroughs Wellcome, Geigy Pharmaceuticals, Parke-Davis Division of Warner-Lambert Company, Biomedical Monitoring Systems, Inc., and Grass Instrument Company.

We express our appreciation to all our contributors for their adherence to the deadline and to the new publication standards we have set. We also salute our predecessors upon whose contributions we have built.

Finally, credit should be given to the 1980 Subcommittee on Basic Research of the Epilepsy Advisory Committee, National Institute of Neurological and Communicative Disorders and Stroke, who conceived and sponsored the 1982 Workshop and the 1983 International Symposium. Members of this subcommittee were Antonio V. Delgado-Escueta, Chair, Katherine L. Bick, James A. Ferrendelli, Robert Grossman, Roger J. Porter, David A. Prince, Dominick P. Purpura, Dorothy Schottellius, and Arthur A. Ward, Jr.

*   *   *

To arrive at this volume's present format and content, three planning meetings, a closed workshop, and an open international symposium were held. In December 1982, during a week-long workshop at the Kroc Foundation Headquarters in the Santa Ynez Mountains, molecular geneticists, neurochemists, and cellular physiologists gathered to consider strategies for unlocking the mysteries of the epilepsies. They were given opportunities to explore what other disciplines can offer and contribute to epilepsy research. The results of these collaborations among specialties are destined to become the vanguard of research in epilepsy. At the same time, these interactions defined the immediate priority challenges in the field.

The Kroc Foundation workshops covered five major fronts of research that have advanced understanding of how epileptic seizures start and stop. The first front explored recombinant DNA technology, and its use of restriction fragment length polymorphisms and candidate gene markers, as a tool in unraveling genotypes of human epilepsy and as a method of providing a collection of genes involved in the production of epilepsy. The second, third, and fourth fronts addressed the roles of neurotransmitters, neuromodulators, and neuron–glia relations in cell–cell communication. In the process, discussions were focused on how convulsions spontaneously arrest. These research efforts offered as novel explanations for the arrest of seizures the release of endogenous anticonvulsant substances, the recruitment of specific GABAergic inhibitory systems in the substantia nigra, and the stimulation of glial protective mechanisms that regulate ionic and neurotransmitter composition of the extracellular environment of the neuron. The fifth area of research discussed at the workshops considered how neuronal ensembles generate depolarization shifts—the cellular hallmark of the seizure focus.

These workshops at the Kroc Foundation Headquarters held in late 1982 served as a springboard for the December 1983 International Symposium on Basic Mechanisms of the Epilepsies in San Diego. During the international symposium, two additional evening workshops were held on new methods of modern neuroanatomy and basic research in human epilepsies. The organizing committee saw the urgent need for these two latter workshops because accelerated application of other fields of neurosciences continued in experimental epilepsies, whereas modern neuroanatomical methods infrequently found their way into epilepsy research and basic research in the human condition remained neglected.

*   *   *

The strong interest in publishing this volume was expressed in the financial subsidies provided by Mrs. Ellen Grass, CIBA Geigy Pharmaceuticals, and Sanofi. To these friends and supporters of the epilepsy movement and to many other unnamed friends and helpers, our thanks are due.

Foreword

The 1969 volume *Basic Mechanisms of the Epilepsies* was developed by the Basic Research Task Force of the Subcommittee on Research of the Public Health Service Advisory Committee on the Epilepsies. The late Dr. H. Houston Merritt, then Professor of Neurology and Dean, College of Physicians and Surgeons, Columbia University, was Chairman of this committee, which was established in 1966. Dr. Arthur A. Ward, Jr., was Chairman of the Research and Research Training Subcommittee, and I was Chairman of the Subcommittee's Basic Research Task Force, which organized the Colorado Springs symposium on basic mechanisms of the epilepsies, and subsequently developed the first volume on this subject. Presumably, this is why I was asked to write the Foreword for this new work. I am pleased that Arthur A. Ward, Jr., is one of the editors of this volume. Together with Alfred Pope and myself, he made a large contribution to the editing of the earlier volume.

With the exception of some of the old faithful, like Dixon Woodbury, Arthur A. Ward, Jr., David Prince, and myself, most of the authors in this new edition were not contributors to the first volume. This reflects the remarkable advances that have been made in the neurosciences in the past 16 years, particularly at the cellular and molecular level, the major thrust of this edition.

The motivation behind the development of the 1969 work was the conviction that most important advances in our understanding and treatment of the epilepsies might come from basic research into mechanisms for the control of excitatory and inhibitory processes in the brain considered from all points of view: genetic, developmental, anatomical, pathological, and neurochemical or pharmacological. Although kept conveniently in the background, some of us had another equally strong motivation, namely, the insight that the epileptiform disorders of the brain might reveal an exaggerated caricature of normal brain function, as Arthur A. Ward, Jr., suggested in the title of the recent book, *Epilepsy, a Window on the Brain* (Raven Press, 1980).

As neuroscientists in the broadest sense, and in the tradition of Hughlings Jackson and Wilder Penfield, we are not only interested but also obligated to learn the basic mechanism of normal brain function from the brain disorders of our epileptic patients. As members of the medical profession, we are equally obligated to keep abreast of all developments in basic neuroscience, to search for a better understanding of the epilepsies, and to seek more rational methods of prevention and treatment. The remarkable advances in neurosciences during recent years has made this a most challenging task, but one that has opened up many new and unexpected opportunities for understanding and, it is hoped, for improving treatment of patients with epilepsy.

The following discussion highlights some of the most important advances in neurosciences furthering our understanding of the epilepsies. These topics have been given thorough consideration in this volume.

NEUROGENETICS AND DEVELOPMENTAL NEUROBIOLOGY

The revolutionary advances in biochemical genetics and their expression in developmental neurobiology is one of the subjects of this volume. I am continually amazed by the facility with which genetic engineers are able to dissect the amino acid sequences of DNA macromolecules and to determine precise genetic defects underlying hereditary diseases, such as the notable recent discovery of the precise biochemical defect in the chromosomes of Huntington's chorea. Equally amazing is the ability to reconstruct and to clone the genes which determine or predispose to the principal characteristics of development. However, it is also important to realize that there is considerable plasticity in development, the expression of genetic determinants being capable of modification by their biochemical and structural environment, as well as by the function of synaptic circuits during critical stages of growth.

We know that hereditary predisposition more or less plays an important role in all forms of epilepsy. The nature of this predisposition may vary with the various causes of seizures. Developmental and environmental factors are also of critical importance. Understanding of critical genetic and developmental factors may lead us to certain common neurochemical or structural defects in control systems of the brain in all forms of epilepsy.

ADVANCES IN NEUROANATOMY AND HISTOCHEMISTRY

There have been revolutionary advances in neuroanatomical techniques and histochemistry during recent years. Anterograde and retrograde axonal flow radioautographic methods have given us precise and beautiful pictures of neuronal interconnections within the brain at both the light and ultramicroscopic levels of observation. Intracellular staining of individual nerve cells by dye injections through a recording microelectrode has surpassed the Golgi technique for visualization of a single neuron with all of its dendritic and axonal extensions. It also has made possible the visualization of cells whose functional properties have been characterized by intracellular electrophysiological studies, thus linking anatomy and physiology with remarkable precision. Of even greater importance is the precise linking of neurochemistry and anatomy which has developed with almost explosive rapidity.

Little did we realize 16 years ago in Colorado Springs when George Koelle presented methods for the identification of cholinergic neuronal systems in the brain and when Annica Dahlström illustrated the histofluorescent staining of the monoamine cells and circuits in the brain, that the refinement of radioautographic techniques would enable electron microscopic visualization of a bewildering number and variety of neurochemical transmitter substances in cells, fibers, and synaptic terminals throughout the central nervous system. The perfection of immunocytochemistry has made possible the visualization of synthesizing enzymes specific for classical transmitter substances such as acetylcholine, amino acids, and the monoamines. It has revealed a whole new series of transmitter or modulator substances and peptides, such as the endorphins, the enkephalins, substance P, somatostatin, and VIP. There are at least 25 to 30 neurochemical substances of critical importance in the control of excitatory and metabolic states of brain cells and synapses that were unknown 15 years ago. Not only can the cells and synaptic terminals containing and liberating these substances be identified, but their receptor sites can be visualized and measured in a quantitative manner by means of ultrasensitive radioenzymatic neurochemical techniques, offering an entirely new perspective on the functional anatomy of the brain.

CELLULAR MICROPHYSIOLOGY AND MICRONEUROCHEMISTRY

There were good examples of pioneer workers with these powerful techniques in our first volume, *Basic Mechanisms of the Epilepsies*. These pioneer workers included Jack Eccles, David Curtis, Kris Krnjević, Dominick Purpura, Arthur A. Ward, Jr., and David Prince. The refinement of these techniques plus the introduction of ion-specific microelectrodes have provided us with many new concepts of the action of neurochemical substances upon nerve cells and their synaptic membranes.

Although *in vitro* techniques for microphysiological studies of single nerve cells from experimental epileptic brain tissues and brain tissues removed from epileptic patients are still being perfected, they have already provided us with a wealth of important new data on both short- and long-term changes in normal systems regulating the stability of ionic flux and the molecular and metabolic determinants underlying basic mechanisms of epileptic discharge. Of particular importance has been the quantitative demonstration of Ca^{2+} as well as K^+, Na^+, and Cl^- fluxes, and their much slower and longer-lasting effects on second messengers such as cyclic nucleotides.

Of equal importance is the critical role of amino acids in controlling both excitatory and inhibitory synaptic mechanisms in the brain. Glutamic acid and aspartic acid, liberated at synaptic terminals, have strong excitatory effects upon nearly all brain cells, whereas GABA has an equally universal inhibitory action. Taurine may be of importance, although its mode of action is yet obscure. Defects in amino acid metabolism may well prove to be a common denominator in epileptic brain tissue, even though there may be varied causes and many modulating or precipitating factors. Inhibitory mechanisms, mediated largely by GABA, have assumed a major role in the regulation of neuronal excitability and are found defective during many forms of epileptic discharge, as discussed by several researchers in this volume. The inhibitory action of GABA was discovered by K. A. C. Elliott and colleagues in 1956 and reviewed in a most memorable symposium, organized by Eugene Roberts and others, in 1960. The importance of the inhibitory action of GABA for epilepsy and the close relation with receptors for the benzodiazepines have been revealed only during recent years.

The study of single ion-specific ionophores impaled on the tip of a microelectrode has given refined information on the biophysics of nerve membranes. Such patch-clamp techniques are rapidly revealing precise ionic and molecular events during long- and short-term cell depolarizations and hyperpolarizations. However, since single cells do not cause epileptic seizures, we still must improve our understanding of interactions between assemblies of neurons, both local and widely distributed, before the ionic and molecular mechanisms can be brought to bear upon the more general problems of seizures in the epileptic brain.

LOCAL BRAIN METABOLISM AND BLOOD FLOW

Another important new development in neuroscience, one with great promise for our understanding of metabolic and cerebrovascular aspects of epilepsies and one which may help bridge the gap between cellular and areal approaches towards experimental and human epilepsy, is the D-oxyglucose radiographic method of measuring local glucose metabolism introduced by Louis Sokoloff. Also important is the development of computer-assisted radiographic scanning techniques, such as positron emission tomography (the PET scan) especially as applied to the intact human brain, and to human epileptic brains. Interpretation of the results obtained to date represents a great challenge for the future.

I have mentioned only in general terms some of the most important developments in neuroscience since *Basic Mechanisms of the Epilepsies* was first published 16 years ago. These advances have provided us with a wealth of new tools and techniques, new facts, and concepts, all of which have greatly expanded our understanding of brain mechanisms from the ionic and molecular to the behavioral perspectives. We have yet to digest thoroughly all of this new information, its ramifications, and interrelationships, to formulate a more comprehensive, integrated conception of brain mechanisms underlying all aspects of thought and behavior, including the caricatures manifest in epileptic seizures.

In conclusion, I wish to express my personal thanks for the opportunity to write the Foreword to another landmark volume on the basic mechanisms of the epilepsies. Last, let us pay tribute to our epileptic patients who have taught us so much over the years about how the brain works.

Herbert H. Jasper

Contents

Contributors

Section 1

INTRODUCTION

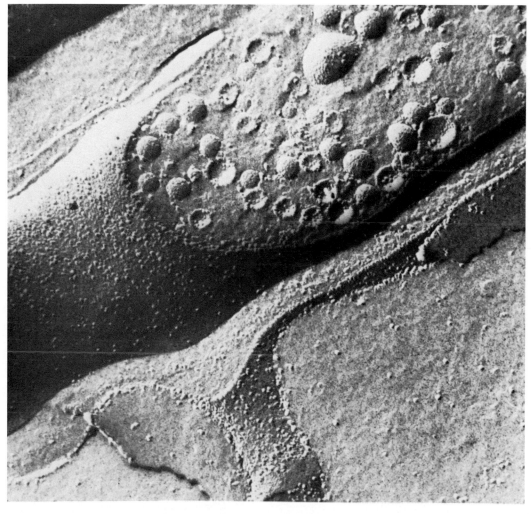

Synapse in the electric organ of the fish *Torpedo marmorata* magnified 76,320 times. The electron micrograph was made by Luis-Miguel Garcia-Segura, Lelio Orci, and Yves Dunant. From Y. Dunant and M. Israel (1985): The release of acetylcholine. *Sci. Am.*, 252(4):59.

Advances in Neurology, Vol. 44, edited by
A. V. Delgado-Escueta, A. A. Ward, Jr.,
D. M. Woodbury, and R. J. Porter.
Raven Press, New York © 1986.

1

New Wave of Research in the Epilepsies

*Antonio V. Delgado-Escueta, **Arthur A. Ward, Jr.,
†Dixon M. Woodbury, and ‡Roger J. Porter

*Comprehensive Epilepsy Program, UCLA Center for the Health Sciences, and VA Southwest Regional
Epilepsy Center, West Los Angeles VA Medical Center (Wadsworth), Los Angeles, California 90073; and
**Department of Neurological Surgery, University of Washington Hospital, Seattle, Washington 98104; and
†Departments of Physiology and Pharmacology and Division of Neuropharmacology and Epileptology,
University of Utah College of Medicine, Salt Lake City, Utah 84132; and ‡Intramural Research Program,
NINCDS, National Institutes of Health, Bethesda, Maryland 20205.*

SUMMARY   The epilepsies affect at least 1 to 2 million people in the United
States and 20 to 40 million people worldwide. Because the causes and basic
mechanisms of the epilepsies have only started to unravel, there is still no cure
for the disease.

The purpose of this chapter is to present the new routes of navigation in epilepsy research, the salient theories on mechanisms of epilepsies, and their cogency to cause (generation of seizures) and effects (epileptic cell damage). In
particular, it advances a comprehensible picture of the major cellular events involved in the generation, arrest, or spread of partial epileptic seizures; it also
questions the major molecular events involved in the transmission and use of
genetic information in the generalized epilepsies. In reviewing the many theories
on mechanisms of epilepsies, this chapter establishes the connections between
neurosciences, molecular genetics, and the epilepsies. The knowledge gained
from such connections will certainly bear on the diagnosis of the subvarieties of
epilepsies and is already promoting new methods of treatment of the disease.
Indeed, it is this fusion between molecular genetics, neurosciences, and the clinical epilepsies that provides the excitement and new ferment in research of the
epilepsies.

This chapter also advances a conceptual blueprint for priority challenges in
epilepsy research. It calls attention to the primary goal, namely, understanding
the mechanisms of human epilepsies. In the most common of human epilepsies,
namely, temporal lobe epilepsy, a priority challenge is to analyze paroxysmal
depolarization shifts in hippocampal slices *in vitro*, slices excised from known
sites of epileptogenicity. Parallel experiments exploring biochemical membrane
abnormalities in neuronal and glial membranes isolated from the hippocampal
seizure focus would be especially valuable. The role of kindling and the mirror
focus in human temporal lobe epilepsy must be resolved. A second important
goal is the search for polymorphisms of restriction endonuclease patterns in monogenic epilepsies in order to localize the abnormal gene to a specific chromosome.
Because of the recent successful applications of positron emission tomography
(PET), single-photon-emission computed tomography, and nuclear magnetic resonance computed tomography (NMR-CT), ion transport pathways, neurotransmitter systems, and metabolic processes may be constructed within the func-

tioning brains of epileptic patients. An ultimate priority challenge is the development of new classes of antiepileptic drugs and novel approaches to treatment, such as the exploration of replacement therapy with endogenous antiepileptic compounds and the testing of aspartate receptor antagonists and calcium channel blockers as agents that prevent epileptic cell damage.

The epilepsies are common disorders of the brain affecting at least 1 to 2 million people in the United States and approximately 20 to 40 million people worldwide. Although highly accurate figures are not available, estimates from various epidemiologic studies indicate that ~0.6% (Rochester, Minnesota) to 2.7% (Chile) of the population is under treatment for recurrent seizures (9,158). Kurland estimates that the annual incidence rate in the United States is 48/100,000 population (158), with the highest incidence under 5 years of age (152/100,000). Incidence is lower (40/100,000) between the ages of 20 and 70 years. The epilepsies are, therefore, a major worldwide public health problem. Because the basic mechanisms of the various epilepsies have only started to unravel, there is still no cure for the disease.

Clinically, the epilepsies (Table 1) (63) are characterized by recurrent convulsive and nonconvulsive seizures, which are caused by partial or generalized epileptogenic discharges in the cerebrum (64). Their ultimate solutions lie in the unraveling of cellular and molecular mechanisms of the ways in which epileptic attacks inherently start, regenerate, arrest spontaneously, or progress to status epilepticus. The mechanisms of the spread of epileptic seizures, their induction of chronic enhanced states of excitability, and eventually production of cell damage must also be understood, if these consequences are to be prevented (49,99,127,155,197,205,227, 228,293,295).

Over the past 15 years, new discoveries in the neurosciences and molecular genetics have caused the development of novel concepts in cell–cell information transfer, cell recognition, and intracellular communication (3,22,32,128, 129,153,157,292,305). Recombinant DNA technologies have revealed the sequence complexities of brain RNA transcriptional control and the processing of secretory products. Furthermore, gene mapping and gene transfer in mammalian cells has now been applied to humans (32,111,261). In the neurosciences, dendodendritic nets of Golgi Type II short axon neurons in Shepherd's microcircuits (288) or Mountcastle's columns (219) have assumed important roles as neuronal ensembles responsible for higher cortical functions. Electrical coupling may be the transductive link between ionic currents and protein subunits (22), emphasizing the importance of gates and regulators of ionic channels in information processing. The recent application of double- and single-microelectrode voltage-clamp methods to hippocampal slices, neuronal and glial cell tissue cultures, and to invertebrate preparations have reignited an old issue: Is cellular hypersynchrony or intrinsic membrane defects the explanation for paroxysmal depolarization shifts? (147,249,250)

Simultaneously with these rapid advances, there was an explosion of data on cellular and molecular mechanisms in experimental epilepsy (Tables 2 and 3). From these data, many theories on how epilepsies start have been proposed and their cogency in seizure generation, effects, spread, and arrest is now being explored (59). In the past, such theories, based on studies of properties of invertebrates or partial systems, have been subject to what F. O. Schmitt calls "the component-system dilemma that bedevils all attempts at biological generalization" (277). However, with the new methods of imaging brain biochemistry, e.g., positron emission tomography (PET), epileptic dysfunctions at various biochemical levels of complexity can now be studied. Finally, recombinant DNA technology allows us finally to study the relevance of animal data to mechanisms of epilepsy in humans (Table 4), and how the regulation of gene expression in the nervous system is transmitted and translated into clinical epilepsies.

HISTORICAL DEVELOPMENT OF THE CONCEPT OF EPILEPSIES

. . . Three lines of inquiry should be pursued. . . . It is an anatomical inquiry to seek the organ or part damaged. . . . It is a physiological inquiry to search into defective working of the nervous tissue of the organ damaged, the functional affection. It is a pathological inquiry to trace the processes by which nutrition of nervous tissue is altered (133).

It is said that the modern era of research in the epilepsies began with the work of Hans

TABLE 1. *Classification of the epilepsies*

Generalized epilepsies

Idiopathic or primary generalized epilepsies: genetically determined with specific age penetrance
  Absence epilepsies
    Childhood absence with diffuse 3-Hz spike-wave complexes.
    Juvenile absence with diffuse 8- to 12-Hz rhythms and/or 3-Hz spike-wave complexes and 3- to 6-Hz multispike wave complexes
    Myoclonic absence with diffuse 3- to 6-Hz multispike-and-wave complexes.
    Myoclonus absence: staring, fragmentary myoclonus, automatisms, and diffuse 12-Hz rhythms.

  Myoclonic epilepsies
    Benign myoclonic epilepsy of infancy
    Benign familial epilepsies of West syndrome
    Benign myoclonic seizures of early childhood, with 3- to 6-Hz multispike-and-wave complexes without mental retardation (idiopathic and familial forms of Lennox-Gastaut syndrome)
    Benign juvenile myoclonic seizures or "impulsiv petit mal" of Janz

  Grand mal epilepsies
    Clonic-tonic-clonic epilepsy (commonly awakening)
    Tonic-clonic epilepsy

Symptomatic or secondary generalized epilepsies: caused by a structural lesion(s)
  Symptomatic or secondary tonic-clonic epilepsies

  Simple partial evolving to tonic-clonic seizures

  Symptomatic neonatal seizures

  Infantile spasms (propulsive petit mal, infantile myoclonic encephalopathy with hysarrhythmia or West syndrome)

  Myoclonic astatic or atonic epilepsies of early childhood (epileptic drop attacks, atypical absence, tonic seizures of Lennox-Gastaut in children with mental retardation)

  Progressive myoclonic epilepsies in adolescents and adults with dementia (myoclonic epilepsies of Unverricht, Lafora, Lundborg-Hartung, Ramsay-Hunt, Kuf, and Zeman)

Partial epilepsies or localization-related epilepsies

Idiopathic or primary partial epilepsies: genetically determined with specific age penetrance
  Benign childhood epilepsy with centrotemporal spikes or Rolandic epilepsy

  Benign childhood epilepsy with occipital spike-wave complexes

Symptomatic or secondary partial epilepsies: caused by a structural lesion(s)
  Epilepsies not involving the limbic system or partial epilepsies without loss or impairment of consciousness:
    Sensorimotor epilepsies
    Partial or focal motor epilepsies
    Kojewnikow's syndrome
    Occipital epilepsies

  Epilepsies involving the limbic system or partial epilepsies with loss or impairment of consciousness:
    Temporal lobe epilepsics
      Hippocampal-amygdalar epilepsy or medial basal limbic epilepsy
      Amygdalar or anterior temporal polar-amygdalar epilepsy
      Lateral posterior temporo-parietal epilepsy
      Opercular-insular or Island of Reil epilepsy
      Lateral temporal neocortical epilepsy
    Frontal lobe epilepsies
      Cingulate or cingular epilepsies
      Supplementary motor epilepsies
      Orbito-frontal and prefrontal epilepsies
      Dorsolateral frontal epilepsies
    Medial occipital-hippocampal epilepsies

Unclassified epilepsies

Undetermined whether focal or generalized

Special epilepsy syndromes

Modified from classification of A. V. Delgado-Escueta and from a simplified version of the classification proposed by the Commission of Classification and Terminology of the International League Against Epilepsy.

TABLE 2. *Partial epilepsies in experimental animals*

Experimental models of partial epilepsies	Some associated cellular and molecular defects				
	Ion transport and membrane-bound proteins and lipids	Catecholamines	Serotonin (5-HT)	Acetylcholine	GABA/glutamate
Kindling	No change in K^+ regulation Probable change in Ca^{2+} regulation: reduction of $[Ca^{2+}]_0$ with altered laminar profiles: particularly in stratum radiatum and stratum moleculare in CA1 area of hippocampus (120) Decreased phosphorylation in synaptic plasma membranes of 50,000–60,000 MW proteins which are subunits of Ca^{2+} calmodulin-stimulated protein kinase (65,341)	Kindling decreases whole brain NA (265) but increases homovanillic acid in amygdala, suggesting hyper-reactive dopaminergic metabolism Kindling depletes amygdala DA at kindled side (78) Kindling is facilitated by pharmacologic reduction of catecholamine function with reserpine, blockade of DA or B-NA receptors, or intracerebral injection of 6-hydroxydopamine (213) or systemic pimozide, haloperidol, and spiroperidol Kindling is suppressed after apomorphine sensitization from chronic pretreatment with cocaine or methamphetamine	5-HT inhibits kindling while (356) lesions of serotonin pathways facilitate kindling (252)	Cholinergic agonist carbachol, muscarine, or ACHE inhibitor, physostigmine, can be used to kindle (329,341) Neuronal supersensitivity to ACh iontophoresis onto hippocampal pyramidal cells followed electrical kindling (38) No change in CHAT or ACHE activities in electrical or carbachol kindling (341) Decreased muscarinic binding sites in hippocampal dentate gyrus and amygdala in electrical kindling (195,196)	No change in GABA receptor binding (11) or high-affinity transport (30) Increase in glutamate receptor binding (267) GABA agonists protect against kindling (196)
Freeze or cold lesion	Decreased synaptosomal Na^+K^+-ATPase activities and Na and K transport (61) Decreased cerebral cortical homogenate, synaptosomal and glial Na^+K^+-ATPase activities interictally (108)	Increased sprouting of NA nerve terminals 1 week after lesion production with accumulation of norepinephrine (34)	—	—	Taurine is decreased, glutamic acid is elevated, but brain GABA does not change (169)

Alumina cream	Increased synaptic Na$^+$K$^+$-ATPase, but decreased glial Na$^+$K$^+$-ATPase during ictus (107,108) Elevations in K$^+_0$ and reductions of [Ca^{2+}]$_0$ but enhanced [Ca^{2+}]$_0$ signals with unpredictable laminar distribution during interictus (120) But stimulation induces similar elevations in K$^+_0$ and reductions of [Ca^{2+}]$_0$ (120) Hence, no disturbances of K$^+_0$ regulation but probable disturbance of Ca^{2+} regulation (120,181,182)	—		Decreased muscarinic and cholinergic binding sites in parafocal area ACHE activity is increased in primary and mirror foci (109) EEG discharges are exacerbated by carbachol (328)	GABA, GAD, GABA receptor binding (15) GAD-containing nerve terminals are all decreased in lesion and epileptogenic area (255)
Cobalt	Reductions of [Ca^{2+}]$_0$ with shift of major sinks for [Ca^{2+}]$_0$ from layers II in normal cortex to layers III and IV in chronic cobalt focus (120) Increased glial carbonic anhydrase, decreased CO$_2$ and increased CO$_2$ fixation in cerebral cortical focus (351) Increased ganglioside sialic acid including mirror focus; decreased total lipids, total phospho-lipids and free cholesterol; increased cholesterol esters and triglycerides and lignoceric acids; decreased proportions of phosphatidyl ethanolamine, oleic acid, arachidonic acid, and nervonic acid (54)	Decreased density of NA-containing synaptic terminals; decreased NA content; decreased tyrosine hydroxylase activities; decreased norepinephrine uptake in perifocal cerebral cortex Pharmacologic reduction of catecholamine function facilitates development of mirror focus (321)	No change in 5-HT levels and turnover (54)	EEG discharges are antagonized by cholinergic agonists (125) CHAT and ACHE are maximally reduced at time of peak seizure activity (101) ACh is maximally reduced at time of peak seizure activity (125)	Glutamic acid is decreased and taurine is unchanged; GAD, GABA, and GABA high-affinity uptake are all decreased (16,326)

TABLE 2—(Continued)

Experimental models of partial epilepsies	Some associated cellular and molecular defects				
	Ion transport and membrane-bound proteins and lipids	Catecholamines	Serotonin (5-HT)	Acetylcholine	GABA/glutamate
Penicillin	Reductions of $[Ca^{2+}]_0$ over 2–4 min after penicillin application to the somatosensory cortex and during interictal discharges, with the sharpest reductions between cerebral cortical layers III and IV (120) Low-threshold (Na^+)-mediated spikes are followed by Ca^{2+}-mediated depolarizing afterpotentials, subthreshold slow depolarizations, and Ca^{2+} spikes (250)	—	—	Atropine is ineffective	GABA, GAD, and GABA uptake and release are all decreased (57,104) GABA agonists protect against seizures (204) Penicillin is most effective in inducing epileptiform paroxysms when injected into neocortical layer 4, suggesting that GABA inhibition across a cortical column is not uniform (72)
Kainic acid	Preferential destruction of CA3 pyramidal cells of hippocampus; loss of calcium-mediated-K^+ induced after hyperpolarizations in CA1 neurons; depolarizing after potentials and burst discharges (120)	DA cell firing and DA synthesis and turnover are increased (18)	—	CHAT activity and the density of muscarinic ACh receptors are decreased (354)	Decreased GABA concentrations and GABA binding GABA agonists protect against seizures (204,354)

NA, norepinephrine or noradrenergic system; DA, dopamine or dopaminergic system; 5-HT, serotonin or 5-hydroxytryptamine; GABA, γ-aminobutyric acid; K^+_0, extracellular K; ACh, acetylcholine; ACHE, acetylcholinesterase; CHAT, cholineacetyltransferase; GAD, glutamine acid decarboxylase; Ca^{2+}_0, extracellular Ca^{2+}; —, no available data.

Modified from Delgado-Escueta, A.V. (1984): Summation of discussion and workshop: The new wave of research in epilepsy, In: *Basic Mechanisms of the Epilepsies*, KROC Foundation Workshop, *Ann. Neurol.*, 16(Suppl.):140–146. Little, Brown and Co.. Boston.

TABLE 3. *Genetic epilepsies in experimental animals*

Experimental models of Genetic epilepsies	Some associated cellular and molecular defects				
	Ion transport and membrane-bound proteins and lipids	Catecholamines	Serotonin (5-HT)	Acetylcholine	GABA/glutamate
Audiogenic seizures mice (DBA/2J)	Higher concentration of G_{MI} gangliosides and cerebroside, glycosphingolipids in cerebrum, cerebellum, and brainstem (285) Decreased cerebral Ca^{2+} ATPase (259,285) Decreased cerebral Na^+K^+-ATPase, increased carbonic anhydrase, HCO_3ATPase, chloride transport, and decreased iodide transport (351) No significant changes in synaptic or glial Na^+K^+-ATPase (108)	Lower turnover rate of DA and NA; lower NA content at age of maximal seizures; resistance to seizures with age appears as DA and NA turnover increases (287) Chronic depletion of catecholamines exacerbates seizures, especially NA depletion (139–142) Lower activity of catechol-O-methyltransferase and tyrosine hydroxylase (276)	Low brain serotonin levels (149,274,275) Slower rate of serotonin synthesis in forebrain and faster in hindbrain (150) Low monoamine oxidase activity and normal 5-hydroxytryptophan decarboxylase activities (149) Intracerebroventricular 5-HTP decreases intensity of seizures (274–276)	Increased brain ACh in seizure-prone mice compared with seizure-resistant mice. Young mice have higher ACh levels than older seizure-prone animals (222) Higher cholinergic receptor density in hippocampus (10)	Low number of GABA receptors (315) versus increased benzodiazepine receptor density (257) GABA-T inhibitors [ethanolamine, O-sulfate (EOS), γ-vinyl GABA (GVG) and valproic acid (VPA)] and taurine protect against seizures (271,272) Audiogenic seizures reduce GABA in basal ganglia, cerebellum, cerebral cortex, hippocampus, and amygdala (47,270)
Genetic epilepsy-prone rats (GEPR) with audiogenic seizures	—	Lower NA levels in most brain areas; normal monoamine oxidase activities but high tyrosine hydroxylase in midbrain (162)	pCPA (p-chlorophenylalanine) depletion of 5-HT increases intensity of seizures (139–142) Elevation of brain serotonin reduces seizure intensity and susceptibility (139–142) Low serotonin content in cerebral hemisphere and midbrain (162)	Reduced ACh levels during audiogenic convulsions (144) Atropine reduces but physostigmine exacerbates audiogenic seizures in rats (130)	Increased number of benzodiazepine binding sites with normal receptor affinity (211) Taurine, GABA, glycine, and aminoisobutyric acid exert anticonvulsant actions but cerebral cortex and inferior colliculi GABA levels are normal; taurine injected into

TABLE 3—(Continued)

		Some associated cellular and molecular defects			
Experimental models of Genetic epilepsies	Ion transport and membrane-bound proteins and lipids	Catecholamines	Serotonin (5-HT)	Acetylcholine	GABA/glutamate
					inferior colliculi elevates intracerebral electroshock threshold (161)
Photic-induced myoclonic and grand mal epilepsies in baboon *Papio papio*	Elevations in K^+_0 and abnormally large reductions in $[Ca^{2+}]_0$ during photic-induced seizures (120)	Chronic depletion of catecholamines (NA) produces photosensitivity in previously insensitive baboons; intracerebroventricular norepinephrine suppresses photic-induced seizures (5); apomorphine blocks photosensitivity	Intracerebroventricular 5-HTP protects against seizures but not intracerebroventricular serotonin (320,330) No change in seizure propensity on intracerebroventricular serotonin or intraperitoneal L-tryptophan (5)	ACh is not involved in regulation of seizures No change in ACh concentrations; atrophine eserine and scopolamine have no effects (203)	Progabide protects against seizures induced by intermittent light stimulation GABA-T inhibitors protect but muscimole exacerbates seizures (199)
Tottering mice with spike-wave seizures	Reduced gangliosides in cerebellum but no change in cerebrum and brainstem (285) No consistent abnormalities in gangliosides (54)	Increased NA content and NA axon terminal density in cerebral cortex, hippocampus, subcortical nuclei, and cerebellum No change in forebrain DA (225)	—	—	—

Animal model					
Mongolian gerbils with myoclonic and grand mal epilepsies	In the interictal state, phosphorylation of cAMP-independent. Ca^{2+}-calmodulin-inhibited. 19,000-stimulated. MW protein is increased but decreases immediately after convulsions (14)	DA agonist apomorphine protects against seizures and DL-threodihydroxy-phenylserine reduces seizure intensity; but whole-brain concentration and striatal uptake of DA is not altered (53)	No change in serotonin content (53)	—	Decreased benzodiazepine/GABA receptors in substantia nigra and periventricular gray matter (230). Increased GAD-containing neurons and axon terminals in septal half of hippocampal dentate gyrus (246)
Photic-induced seizures in epileptic fowl	Alterations in phosphorylation of cAMP, Ca^{2+}-independent, Mg^{2+}-dependent 80,000, 55,000, and 16,000-MW protein fractions (323)	Increased concentration of NA in cerebral hemispheres with decreased brain DA but apparently unrelated to seizure susceptibility (146)	Concentrations of brain 5-HT are decreased but increasing brain level does not alter susceptibility to seizures (146)	Acetylcholinesterase is abnormally high; cholineacetyltransferase activity is decreased (146)	—
Beagle dog with grand mal convulsions	—	No change in NA, DA, or 5-HT (73)	Normal brain serotonin concentration (73)	—	No differences in GABA concentration between seizure-prone and seizure-resistant animals (73)

NA, norepinephrine or noradrenergic system; ACh, acetylcholine; DA, dopamine or dopaminergic system; ACHE, acetylcholinesterase; 5-HT, serotonin or 5-hydroxytryptamine; CHAT, cholineacetyltransferase; GABA, γ-aminobutyric acid; GAD, glutamic acid decarboxylase; 5-HTP, 5-hydroxytryptophan; K^+_o, extracellular K^+; Ca^{2+}_o, extracellular Ca^{2+}; —, no available data.

Modified from Delgado-Escueta, A.V. (1984): Summation of discussion and workshops: The new wave of research in epilepsy, In: *Basic Mechanisms of the Epilepsies*, KROC Foundation Workshop, *Ann. Neurol.*, 16(Suppl.):140–146, Little, Brown and Co., Boston.

TABLE 4. *Some biochemical abnormalities in human partial epilepsies*

Ion transport pathways
  Decreased K uptake in brain slices (317,318)
  Impaired brain Na^+K^+-ATPase (253)
  Decreased glial Na^+K^+-ATPase and synaptic Na^+K^+-ATPase activities and impaired K clearance by glial Na^+K^+-ATPase as indicated by rate reactions with K_0 in the interictal state (107)

GABA systems
  Conflicting reports on GAD activities: decreased GAD activity and GABA binding site (172) and no decrease in GAD activity relative to surrounding nonspiking cortex (289); no change in GABA-T (172,289)
  Decreased CSF GABA due to impaired GABA synthesis (77,350)
  Decreased taurine (327)

Glycine
  Elevated glycine in epileptogenic foci (244,245,326)

Glutamate
  Increased GDH activity and no change in glutamine synthetase (289)
  Conflicting results on glutamic acid and aspartic acid levels: relative diminution in glutamic acid and aspartic acid (326) or no changes (244)

Catecholamines
  Increased tyrosine hydroxylase activities (289)
  Decreased density of α-1 postsynaptic receptor sites (35)

GAD, glutamine acid decarboxylase; GABA, γ-aminobutyric acid; CSF, cerebrospinal fluid; GDH, glutamic acid dehydrogenase.

Modified from Delgado-Escueta, A.V. (1984): Summation of discussion and workshops: The new wave of research in epilepsy, In: *Basic Mechanisms of the Epilepsies*, KROC Foundation Workshop, *Ann. Neurol.* 16(Suppl.):140–146, Little, Brown and Co., Boston.

Berger half a century ago. Through the electroencephalograph (EEG), Berger, and others including Lennox et al., Gibbs, and Penfield and Jasper et al., confirmed the nature of epileptic seizures as abnormal paroxysmal neuronal discharges (24,25,163–167,235–243). However, the concept of the epilepsies as recurrent disorders produced by abnormal neuronal discharges within the central nervous system (CNS), symptomatic of a variety of diseases affecting the brain, began over 100 years ago with J. Hughlings Jackson (133) and W. R. Gowers (105). In 1863, J. Hughlings Jackson distinguished between "symptomatic and genuine forms of the epilepsies." As quoted above, Jackson sought the anatomical, physiological, and pathological

bases of seizures. His three lines of inquiry remain cornerstones in modern diagnostic approaches to epileptic seizures.

Jackson had observed that chronic convulsions could be divided into two groups or classes: "(1) those in which the spasm affects both sides of the body almost simultaneously—usually called epileptic and sometimes cases of 'genuine' or 'idiopathic' epilepsy. (2) those in which the fit begins by deliberate spasm on one side of the body and in which parts of the body are affected one after the other." (133). Today, Jackson's concepts are firmly embedded in the 1980 Classification of Epileptic Seizures of the International League Against Epilepsy (ILAE) (52). This classification distinguishes between seizures that are generalized from the beginning (generalized seizures) and those that are partial at onset (partial seizures) and which may become generalized secondarily.

The ILAE Classification of Epileptic Seizures, as it has evolved since 1970, serves well as a taxonomic scheme for analysis of individual attacks. It is clear, however, that if defects in the structural gene or molecule or systems of the brain are to be defined in specific forms of the epilepsies, investigators must understand and apply in their research a classification of epilepsies or epilepsy syndromes and not a classification of individual epileptic attacks. Such a classification of the epilepsies or epilepsy syndromes should follow the clinical pathologic principles espoused by Jackson and Gowers, refined by the modern experiences of Jasper and Penfield, and the new descriptions of the clinical attack recorded on closed-circuit television (CCTV)-videotape and EEG biotelemetry. It should also consider the age at onset and remission of epileptic seizures, the interictal neurological status, the etiology and trigger mechanisms of epileptic attacks, the interictal and ictal EEG, different responses to antiepileptic medication, remission rates after drug treatment and, if pertinent and available, patterns of hereditary transmission (Table 1) (63,64). Although no satisfactory classification of the epilepsies presently exists, the classification in Table 1 is a simplified and short version being considered by the ILAE Commission on Classification as a new classification of the epilepsies. It distinguishes idiopathic or primary generalized and idiopathic or primary partial or focal epilepsies (both with major genetic contributions) from symptomatic or secondary partial or focal epilepsies (which are caused by structural lesions). As such, this classification of the epilepsies incorporates

Gowers' principles (52). Gowers had maintained a clear distinction between "(1) convulsions which are the result of organic disease such as can be recognized after death and (2) those which are the expression of a condition of the brain which is not evidenced by any visible alteration" (105). The ILAE Classification of Epilepsies, following Gowers' distinction, also recognizes that generalized epileptic seizures consist of two subgroups: (1) primarily generalized seizures without any signs of organic brain disorder (e.g., Calmeil's epileptic absence of 1884 or Esquirol's petit mal of 1815 and Gowers' grand mal clonic-tonic-clonic seizures of 1885); and (2) secondarily generalized seizures caused by a demonstrable or at least presumptive organic brain disease. This proposed ILAE Classification of Epilepsies also recognizes two other groups of epilepsies such as undetermined and unclassified epilepsies and special epilepsy syndromes. Examples of special epilepsy syndromes are reflex epilepsies and rare episodes of spike-wave stupor in adults.

In classifying epilepsies as idiopathic or primary with specific age penetrance, modern clinicians generally assume a monogenic or polygenic basis. Gowers' and Jackson's concept that some forms of epilepsies do not have demonstrable structural lesions and could have a hereditary basis was first espoused by Hippocrates. This concept found support in the 1950 studies of Lennox et al., who found a high degree of concordance (74%) of primarily generalized epilepsy in uniovular twins (163–167). Lennox et al. also found five times the expected incidence of epileptic seizures (2.7%) in near relatives of epileptics. In the 1960s, Metrakos and Metrakos showed a high occurrence of epileptiform discharges in the EEGs of relatives of patients with generalized *or* partial epilepsies and provided further convincing evidence of the importance of heredity not only in generalized epilepsies, but also in some partial epilepsies (207,208). In studies of genetic focal epilepsy and absence attacks in experimental animals, Noebels (225) has provided even stronger arguments that some of these so-called idiopathic epilepsies can be caused by a single gene defect.

In stark contrast, some of the partial epilepsies appear to be due solely to environmental insults, such as are caused by the meningococcal and pneumococcal bacteriae, the herpes simplex virus, or slow measle viruses. After classifying epileptic attacks as symptomatic or secondary, clinicians compulsively look for the presence of a structural lesion, using modern methods of brain imaging. Thus, today, primary generalized epilepsies and primary partial epilepsies (see classification in Table 1) are ripe for experiments on fundamental genetic mechanisms. New information differentiates partial epilepsies that are purely environmental from partial epilepsies that are purely genetic. In the future, we may be able to differentiate between the contributions of genetic lesions and environmental insults in the multifactorial forms of secondary partial epilepsies (60,63,64).

EPILEPTOGENESIS AND SPREAD OR ARREST OF SEIZURES

Continuing Saga of the Paroxysmal Depolarization Shifts (PDSs): Their Spread or Arrest

Of the 2 million Americans with epilepsy, approximately two-thirds have secondary partial epilepsies. Of these, 85% are due to complex partial epilepsies with psychomotor symptomatology. Most of these epilepsies originate either in the hippocampus or in the frontal lobe (Tables 5 and 6). Thirty to 45% of these patients are intractable to conventional antiepileptic drugs, and at least 240,000 to 500,000 have inadequate seizure control. Because of their importance in human terms, early investigators searched for experimental models that simulated the clinical manifestations of partial epilepsies. A variety of physical and chemical methods were used to produce animal models (Table 2). We still have no animal model that truly mimics complex partial epilepsies in humans, and the closest experimental version of psychomotor epilepsies in animals is the kindling phenomenon.

Because secondary partial epilepsies are caused by a variety of etiologies, investigators sought a common denominator. In 1963 and 1964, respectively, Goldensohn and Purpura (102) and Matsumoto and Ajmone-Marsan (188, 189) found a common cellular event during interictal EEG spikes—the PDSs. Since then, there has been continuing controversy, with emphasis either on the synaptic network theorem or endogenous membrane alterations as the fundamental alteration causing PDSs (12). Most authorities now concede that a variety of factors, both intracellular and transcellular, contribute to epileptogenesis. The school of Prince and Connors (250) maintains that three key elements contribute to the development of epileptogenesis: the capacity of membranes in some pacemaker neurons to develop intrinsic burst dis-

TABLE 5. *Temporal lobe epilepsies*[a]

Regional localization	Aura	Clinical seizure patterns	EEG and Stereo EEG	Brain imaging	Psychology[b]	Common etiologies
Hippocampal epilepsy[a] or medial basal, limbic epilepsy	Strange, indescribable feeling, experiential hallucinations, interpretative illusions	Arrest (motionless stare), oral and alimentary automatisms, and amnesia averaging 2 min >60% with secondary TC	Interictal: anterior temporal sharp waves, especially during sleep Ictus: initial unilateral flattening, especially one temporal lobe and background EEG changes; or nonfocal or nonlateralizing surface EEG changes; or focal or lateralized, 4- to 6-Hz sharp waves Stereo EEG: high-frequency 16- to 28-Hz low-voltage spikes building up in one hippocampus propagating to amygdala and cingulate and parietal regions	Skull x-ray study: asymmetry of skull, especially sphenoid fossa CAT scan: usually negative PEG: enlarged one temporal horn Metrizamide CT scan: signs of tentorial herniation NMR: may be useful Bilateral carotid angiography: rule out anterior choroidal aneurysm	Impaired recent memory (verbal—dominant hemisphere; visuospatial—nondominant hemisphere)	More commonly: incisural or hippocampal sclerosis. Less frequently: gangliogliomas, hamartomas, arteriovenous malformation, astrocytoma, oligodendroglioma, focal gliosis, rarely aneurysms (cicatrix)
Amygdalar epilepsy or anterior polaramygdalar epilepsy	Rising epigastric discomfort, nausea, autonomic symptoms, and signs including borborygmi, belching, pallor, fullness of face, flushing of face, arrest of respiration, pupillary dilation. Fear, panic, olfactory–	Gradual onset of unconsciousness, staring, oral and alimentary automatisms, confusion, amnesia Less commonly (30%) with secondary TC. Seizures: REM sleep facilitates partial symptomatology	Scalp EEG: same as above Stereo EEG: high frequency, low-amplitude, 16- to 28-Hz rhythm in amygdala or amygdala and anterior temporal pole with spread to homolateral frontoorbital regions and contralateral homologous areas	Same as above Metrizimide CT scan: may be useful	Reduced autonomic responsivity[c]	Ganglioglioma, focal gliomas, atypical cell layers in amygdala (and hippocampal formation) anterior temporal pole gliosis, arteriovenous malformation, hamartoma, trauma, with focal gliosis

	gustatory hallucinations				
Lateral posterior temporal-partial epilepsy	Auditory hallucinations, visual perceptual hallucinations, language disorder when lateralized to hemisphere dominant for language	Dysphasia, disturbed orientation and prolonged auditory hallucinations; head movement to one side; sometimes staring automatisms and amnesia.	EEG: lateral midtemporal or post temporal spikes. Stereo EEG: low frequency rapid spikes (16–28 Hz) building up in the supramarginal angular gyrus and posterior temporal regions	Normal skull films, but CT, PEG, A/G, PET, and NMR are recommended.	Dominant: anomia (Benson); impaired word-sorting (Hiatt) Nondominant: tonal memory and timbre tests (Seashore), McGill Picture Anomalies. Lateralizing: Dichotic auditory detection.	Most commonly due to trauma with focal gliosis, post infections, glioma, postcerebral infarction.
Opercular or Island of Reil or insular epilepsy	Vestibular hallucinations, followed by borborygmi, belching, autonomic symptoms or olfactory—gustatory hallucinations due to spread to medial temporal structures	Similar to amygdalar epilepsy except for initial vestibular hallucinations	EEG and stereo EEG: isolated opercular rapid spikes (16- to 28-Hz) with minimal spread	Normal skull films, CT, and PEG, but PET and NMR may be useful.	Unknown	Glioma, astrocytoma, arteriovenous malformations, aneurysms, postcerebral infarction

[a] Synonyms: Primary rhinencephalic psychomotor epilepsy of Bancaud, Szikla, and Talaraich et al., 1965; CPS, Type I of hippocampal origin (Delgado-Escueta and Walsh, 1985); Mesial-basal Limbic epilepsy (Wieser, 1983); Comprises 70–80% of temporal lobe epilepsies; Commonly combines with amygdalar epilepsy; Mode of recurrence, random or cluster.

[b] In this column are listed the neuropsychological tests that most specifically indicate functional damage in the region of the focus. However, it is important to note that functional damage and the seizure focus are not necessarily in the same place. In particular, recent memory deficits, suggestive of hippocampal damage, frequently occur in complex partial epilepsy, especially if there is a history of status epilepticus. A discrepancy of 20 or more points between verbal and nonverbal IQ suggests generalized dysfunction of one hemisphere. If confirmed, this helps to lateralize the focus, although it does not indicate the location of the focus within the hemisphere. Psychomotor slowing is a very common, but nonspecific sign of organic brain damage and/or antiepileptic drug side effect.

[c] Hypothesized correlate based on isolated report.

Modified from classification prepared by Delgado-Escueta, Quesney, and Wieser for ILAE commission on classification, 1984 Bethesda, Maryland workshop.

TABLE 6. *Frontal lobe epilepsies*[a]

Regional localization	Clinical seizure patterns	EEG Stereo/EEG	Brain imaging	Psychology[b]	Common etiologies
Supplementary motor	Postural, PMT, vocalization, speech arrest, fencing, PCS, urinary incontinence	Flattening rhythmic polyspike (16–24 Hz) and secondary generalization. Depth electrode exploration	Normal skull x-ray studies and CTs; focal atrophic lesion on PEG. PET and NMR may be useful	Dominant: impaired verbal fluency Nondominant: impaired design fluency	Focal atrophy, tumor, arteriovenous malformations
Cingular	PCS with initial automatisms with sexual features, vegetative signs, urinary incontinence	Depth electrode exploration	Normal skull x-ray studies; CT; PEG. PET and NMR may be useful	Dominant: impaired verbal fluency Nondominant: impaired design fluency	Focal atrophy, tumor, arteriovenous vascular malformation
Orbito-frontal	PCS with intial automatisms; olfactory hallucinations	Flattening rhythmic polyspikes (16–24 Hz) and secondary generalization. Nasoethmoidal and orbital electrodes[c]	Skull: signs of trauma; CT: signs of trauma. PEG: focal atrophy. PET and NMR may be useful.	Lability of mood[e]	Trauma, astrocytoma, oligodendroglioma
Dorso-lateral	PMT, versive, aphasia, PCS with initial automatism	Satisfactory interictal and ictal localization	Normal skull x-ray studies, CT: usually localizes lesion PEG: often not required; PET and NMR may be useful	Perseveration, poor recency judgments, response disinhibition	Trauma, astrocytoma, oligodendroglioma

PMT, partial motor tonic; PCS = partial complex seizure; CT, computed tomography; PEG, pneumoencephalography; PET, positron emission tomography; NMR, nuclear magnetic resonance.

[a] Very frequent short attacks stimulating absence with minimal or no postical confusion can occur in frontal lobe epilepsies. When bizarre behaviors appear as automatisms, longer attacks are frequently mistaken for psychogenic seizures.

[b] In this column are listed the neuropsychological tests that most specifically indicate functional damage in the region of the focus. However, it is important to note that functional damage and the seizure focus are not necessarily in the same place. In particular, recent memory deficits, suggestive of hippocampal damage, frequently occur in complex partial epilepsy, especially if there is a history of status epilepticus. A discrepancy of 20 or more points between verbal and nonverbal IQ suggests generalized dysfunction of one hemisphere. If confirmed, this helps to lateralize the focus, although it does not indicate the location of the focus within the hemisphere. Psychomotor slowing is a very common but completely nonspecific sign of organic brain damage and/or antiepileptic drug side effect.

[c] Often required.

[d] Mandatory.

[e] Hypothesized correlate based on isolated report.

Modified from classification prepared by Delgado-Escueta, Quesney, and Wieser for ILAE commission on classification, 1984 Bethesda, Maryland Workshop.

charges (e.g., pyramidal neurons in the CA3 region of the hippocampus and in layer 4 of the cerebral cortex); the presence of disinhibition; and the proper excitatory synaptic circuits. Johnston and Brown (147) reject a strict reductionist perspective and place more emphasis on the contribution of synaptic transmissions. They conclude that PDSs behave like large excitatory postsynaptic potentials (EPSPs), with synaptic conductances five to 10 times greater than normal spontaneous and evoked EPSPs. They emphasize that the entire envelope of the PDS can be accounted for by the large synaptic conductances and suggest that epileptiform activity can only be understood in terms of interactions between cellular and network properties.

Multicellular Synchronization

Although membrane dysfunctions provide a substrate for epileptogenesis, circuit dynamics are undeniably vital to the expression of paroxysmal tendencies. Multicellular synchronization is necessary for the clinical expression of the epileptogenic process, and cellular synchronization is involved not only in interictal and ictal discharges, but also in the generation of cellular depolarization shifts. Substantial insight into the nature of multicellular coupling was provided earlier by Walsh (339) and subsequently by Ebersole and Chatt (72), who studied cellular behavior in cat neocortex and visual cortex, respectively, during penicillin iontophoresis. Walsh (339) was able to increase the amplitudes of EPSPs in the neocortex by penicillin iontophoresis, but such treatment did not induce high-amplitude, long-duration depolarization shifts. Topical application of penicillin to the cortex, involving a much greater volume of tissue, did elicit EEG discharges and corresponding intracellular PDSs. Ebersole and Chatt (72) used low doses of iontophoresed penicillin to augment monosynaptic geniculocortical responses of visual cells to normally "adequate" stimuli, an effect termed "enhanced physiological response" (EPR). Graded development of a longer latency burst (LR) subsequently developed in response to field-specific and nonspecific stimuli. Further administration of penicillin was accompanied by the appearance of a single stereotyped burst of neuronal PDSs or LR discharge. Occurring in association with EEG spikes, these PDSs could be evoked by previously inadequate visual stimuli. The initial actions of penicillin were attributed to direct effects on the neuronal membrane or synaptic processes, resulting in EPR. Involvement of additional neurons already engaged in recurrent or collateral input in such excitatory processes allowed the hypersynchrony inherent in PDSs. Further analysis revealed layer 4 of striate visual cortex to be most sensitive to penicillin microinjection. Layer 4 recruited pyramidal cells in layers 3 and 2 by propagations of long LR responses. Layers 5 and 6 were then invaded by burst responses of layer 4 and layers 3 and 2. Interestingly, phenytoin disproportionately suppressed epileptiform responses propagated to pyramidal layers 2 and 3, whereas phenobarbital induced a generalized translaminar suppression of evoked epileptiform potentials.

The importance of neuronal synchronization in epileptogenesis is especially apparent in mammalian hippocampus. Neuronal bursting is common in the "normal" hippocampus (147), yet the lack of burst synchrony usually precludes the generation of epileptiform field potentials. Nevertheless, the bursting predisposition of hippocampal cells renders them particularly susceptible to rhythmic discharge, and multicellular synchronization can easily trigger paroxysmal events. Indeed, by applying penicillin to the *in vitro* tissue slice preparation, Schwartzkroin and Prince (282) converted asynchronous bursts of CA1 and CA3 hippocampal neurons into widespread, synchronous depolarization shifts. These PDSs were accompanied by the development of epileptiform field potentials.

Paroxysmal bursting, therefore, must occur simultaneously in a critical number of interrelated neurons in order to generate EEG discharges. Within any natural or artificial focus, variable numbers of cells may be actively involved in epileptiform events. During interictal spikes of chronic seizure foci, depolarization shifts occur in roughly 10–25% of the neurons (102,340). Involvement of cells in acute penicillin foci is much more prevalent, with nearly 90% of cells participating in interictal discharges (188,189).

Wong et al. also recently addressed the important question of how entrainment and synchronization occur in neuronal aggregates (see Chapter 29). Both experiments and network simulation of 400 neurons showed that during the initiation of synchronized burst, neurons are recruited into the activity sequentially; these activities terminate at different times if an absolute refractory period sets in after a fixed period of excitation in a given cell. Afterdischarges could arise as a consequence of residual activity in neurons recruited late in one synchronized event, reexciting neurons activated during the early phase of the event. Dudek et al. (see Chapter 30) added the novel concept of electrical field effects to the mechanisms of epileptiform burst synchronization. Differential recordings during synchronous bursts revealed brief transmembrane depolarizations as prepotentials, implying that electrical interactions are important for synchronization.

Extracellular Ionic Shifts: $[K^+]_o$ Rises and $[Ca^{2+}]_o$ Falls

When applied to cobalt and alumina cream lesions, potassium is extremely effective in producing epileptogenic activity (357). Ouabain can also induce seizure activity, presumably by inhibiting cationic transport and thus elevating extracellular potassium levels (17,233). Speculation arose that the neuronal hyperexcitability of seizure foci depends upon accumulated extracellular potassium, perhaps caused by defective glial or macromolecular buffering. Fertziger and Ranck (87) proposed a mechanism whereby abnormal regulation of K^+_o might result in seizure activity. Sufficient increases in K^+_o, observed after intense neuronal discharges, potentially depolarize local neurons. Depolarization favors excitation and further potassium efflux. This self-sustaining depolarization, allowed by defective ionic regulation enhances transneuronal coupling and leads to seizures. The cycle is terminated when depolarization is sufficient to inactivate membrane conductances.

Despite a clear association between K^+_o and epileptogenesis, potassium-sensitive microelectrode recordings have cast serious doubt upon a causative role of this cation in seizure initiation or termination. During seizures in mammalian cortex, K^+_o increases from a resting level of 2.8–3.5 mM to reach a plateau of 8–12 mM (91,182). Seizures initiation does not correspond to a threshold level of K^+_o; in fact, neurons seem to be more excitable when K^+_o is near or below resting values (182). During repeated interictal discharges of a primary focus, K^+_o can reach levels of 8 mM without resulting in an ictal episode (182). Most important, rises in K^+_o follow rather than anticipate the onset of ictal activity (177,233). Termination of ictal episodes usually occurs long after K^+_o has reached a peak, ruling out the possibility of a potassium-induced conductance block. Restoration of K^+_o begins after the ictal session has terminated (182).

Membrane excitability also varies inversely with calcium levels (Ca_o^{2+}) (92), and calcium conductances may have a role in paroxysmal bursting. With ion-sensitive microelectrodes, Heinemann et al. (121) measured extracellular concentrations of potassium and calcium in normal and epileptogenic cortex. Resting levels of Ca_o^{2+} and K^+_o ranged, respectively, from 1.2 to 1.5 mM and from 2.7 to 3.2 mM. Topical application of penicillin led to the development of periodic interictal discharges. These events were associated with increases in K^+_o of up to 2.5 mM and decreases in Ca_o^{2+} of ~0.1 mM. Repetitive stimulation of the penicillin cortex eventually triggered propagated seizures, during which Ca_o^{2+} dropped to 0.9 mM which K^+_o rose as high as 10 mM. K^+_o recovered quickly after ictal episodes and reached levels below baseline. In contrast, Ca_o^{2+} recovered slowly following seizures. Intravenous (i.v.) injection of pentylenetetrazol (PTZ), at doses that eventually led to seizures, also initiated decreases in Ca_o^{2+} long before the ictal onset. K^+_o did not rise until electrical discharges appeared. The decreases in Ca_o^{2+} accompanying spontaneous seizures are larger and more widespread than those detected by electrical stimulation of normal cortex (Table 2). In the *in vitro* hippocampal slice preparation, Lux et al. (see Chapter 31) also emphasized the importance of spatial K^+ redistribution as an important nonsynaptic factor for the spread of epileptiform discharges. Pressure injections of CSF containing 7 mM K^+ (compared with a resting level of 5 mM K^+) at low Ca_o^{2+} induced spreading epileptiform paroxysms.

In chronic models of focal epilepsies, such as the alumina cream focus, the chronic cobalt focus and photosensitive epilepsies of baboons, studies with ion-sensitive microelectrodes gave little indication that K^+ regulation was involved in the induction of seizures. Rather, the uptake of Ca^{2+} into cells was increased, suggesting that Ca^{2+} and Ca^{2+}-dependent electrogenesis is more important in these chronic epilepsies. Heinemann et al. (see Chapter 32) suggest that these shifts in Ca^{2+} sinks contribute to synchronization, spread, and maintenance of ictal activity.

Glial Protective Mechanisms

The concept of protective role of glial cells in containing seizures was developed by Woodbury et al. in Salt Lake City (351). A number of experiments have now demonstrated that convulsive seizures increase the number of glial cells and their HCO_3-ATPase, Na^+K^+-ATPase, and carbonic anhydrase enzymatic activities. Glial cells thereby increase their ability to regulate cation and anion homeostatis in brain interstitial space and help to contain the spread of seizures. Observations that aging—which causes gliosis and enhanced carbonic anhydrase activity—decreases seizure susceptibility, and that ketogenic diet and phenytoin both promote gliosis (351) are further evidence for a protective role of glial cells.

There is also growing evidence that failure in glial protective mechanisms may signal the ictal transformkation and secondary generalization of a partial discharge. In the freezing lesion, a chronic experimental model for cortical epilepsy, Na^+K^+-ATPase activities increased in response to generalization of focal epileptogenic discharges, whereas glial Na^+K^+-ATPase remained decreased. In this chronic epileptogenic focus, $[K^+]_o$ activation of glial Na^+K^+-ATPase is dramatically decreased and remains decreased even during sustained epileptogenic paroxysms. The reduced capacity of glial membranes actively to control elevated concentrations of $[K^+]_o$ probably plays a key role in ictal transformation (108).

How elevated and sustained $[K^+]_o$ concentrations signal the transcellular interactions between neurons and glia to produce gliosis remains unknown. However, several biochemical events, known to be specific for glial cells, are receiving attention as reactions important in the production of focal gliosis in the epileptogenic focus. Enhanced neuronal firing during seizures elevates concentrations of $[K^+]_o$, and in the process enhances glial O_2 consumption, glutamate and glucose uptake, and their incorporation into a variety of intermediate substances. Elevated $[K^+]$ concentrations also alter ATP concentrations, ATPases and pyruvate kinases, and promote glycogen synthesis of local glial cells. The role of all these events in the production of focal gliosis in the epileptogenic focus is now being investigated intensively (108).

Ectopic Spiking in Dendrites and Axons

Within the primary focus itself, changes in ionic microenvironment may not only amplify neuronal excitation and facilitate transition from interictal to ictal states, but may also contribute to ectopic impulse initiation in local dendrites and axonal terminals. Gutnick and Prince and Schwartzkroin et al. (112,281) postulated such phenomena upon observation of antidromic spiking or "backfiring" in thalamocortical relay cells. Subsequently, similar antidromic spikes have been observed by Gabor and Scobey in the lateral geniculate nucleus after application of penicillin in visual cortex (95,283) and by Schwartzkroin et al. in contralateral projection areas of cortical penicillin foci (281). It should be emphasized that antidromic bursts occur after the onset of interictal discharges, and therefore do not contribute to their initiation. However, ectopic spiking in axons can participate in repetitive interictal events or transition into ictal states. Prince (249) views the role of axonal bursts as one of synchronization and amplification of electrical discharges.

Within primary foci, ectopic spiking may occur in dendrites as well as axons. In freeze lesions (102) and in hippocampal cells exposed to penicillin (282), low-amplitude potentials with abrupt onsets and short durations have been observed. Although hippocampal cells can generate such "fast prepotential" or "d-spikes" under normal circumstances, the frequency of these events increases markedly when penicillin is present. Epileptiform bursts in CA1 neurons often appear to be triggered by d-spikes, and d-spikes frequently accompany late phases of the slow depolarization shifts (282). D-spikes in these cells are suspected to have a dendritic origin, since they strongly resemble the dendritic spikes which occur in various Purkinje cells. Dendritic spiking, and associated depolarization shifts, could amplify and prolong neuronal responses to synchronous synaptic input, and thereby facilitate the process of recruitment.

Inhibitory Control Mechanisms

Powerful mechanisms serve to limit, both temporally and spatially, the seizure process. The most noteworthy of these are postdischarge hyperpolarization and surround inhibition. In virtually all models of epileptogenic tissue, neuronal PDSs are usually followed by long-lasting periods of profound membrane hyperpolarization (247,249,250,288). This inhibitory phase tends to prevent immediate repetition of the paroxysmal event. Postactivation hyperpolarization (PAH) in the penicillin model can last up to 2 sec, and is primarily synaptic in origin. Aside from chloride entry, several mechanisms may participate in PAH, although their relative contributions are uncertain. During repetitive neuronal firing, potassium enters the extracellular fluid compartment, while sodium accumulates within the cell. Redistribution of these ions activates membrane-bound Na^+K^+-ATPase, which functions to restore ionic equilibrium. The electrogenic potential and ionic translocation achieved by this enzyme can contribute significantly to PAH. Calcium influx is another consequence of neuronal activity. In a manner analogous to that of molluscan and spinal neurons (197), calcium could activate a prolonged potassium conductance. Increased potassium conductances would contribute to the hyperpolarization that follows intense neuronal discharges.

Inhibition is a typical consequence of PDSs, but many cells are subjected only to inhibition during interictal discharges. Simple inhibition, or inhibition following brief excitation (not PDSs), occasionally occurs in itself, although such events are extremely common in areas surrounding an active focus (247). Many cells in contralateral projection zones are also inhibited by discharges of the primary focus (55,281). Projection areas and the focal surround therefore appear to receive potent inhibitory drive during interictal discharges through recurrent and/or longer association pathways. These influences may restrict spread of epileptiform events. Nevertheless, evoked inhibition, like phasic excitation, acts to disrupt normal neuronal processing. Hence, the impact of focal epileptiform activity extends well beyond the pathological region itself.

With the onset of ictal episodes, cells in and around a primary seizure focus undergo a progressive increase in excitability, leading to propagated discharges. Perhaps the earliest and most consistent cellular correlate of ictal onset is loss of inhibitory tone. The hyperpolarization that normally follows neuronal PDSs diminishes and is eventually replaced by depolarizing afterpotentials (DAP). This progressive change in afterpotentials has been observed in seizures elicited by penicillin (188,189), strychnine (267), and metrazol (309). DAPs, which develop during penicillin-induced seizures, are often of rhythmic oscillating character. While afterhyperpolarizations (AHPs) are evolving into DAPs, cellular depolarization shifts become larger in amplitude and longer in duration. In areas surrounding the primary focus, prevailing inhibitory postsynaptic potentials (IPSPs) are gradually transformed into EPSPs and later into full PDSs. These cells become coupled to the bursting neurons of the focus, and the rhythmic discharges generate massive epileptiform field potentials.

Several authors (188,189,310,311) have distinguished "active" from "passive" participants of the ictal process. "Active" neurons undergo the initial changes described below, whereas "passive" elements are recruited well after the seizure has begun. Matsumoto and Ajmone-Marsan (188,189) thoroughly documented the behavior of both cell types during penicillin-induced seizures. In active neurons, DAPs that followed PDSs began to summate, and a prolonged state of membrane depolarization developed. Although >95% of cells in these penicillin foci were involved in interictal discharges, only ~40% of the cells should be classified as "active" (i.e., participating from the onset of ictal episodes). The remaining "passive" cells persisted in their interictal behavior until the seizure was already underway. Even after they were recruited, many cells did not display dramatic membrane depolarization and oscillation during the tonic phase of seizures. Their behavior during the clonic phase, however, was comparable to that of "active" cells.

The percentage of cells responsible for initiating seizure episodes varies considerably, depending upon the seizure model and state of arousal. In a recent review of ictal propagation, Ward (340) classified cells of chronic seizure foci into two groups. Group I neurons were defined as those whose output was nearly always in a bursting pattern. Such "pacemaker" cells can constitute up to 25% of the neuronal pool in chronic foci of monkeys and humans. Group II neurons, on the other hand, do not normally generate epileptiform bursts. However, these cells can be recruited into the ictal episode by the synchronous bursting of group I neurons. The most important concept offered by Ward was that of varying degrees of neuronal abnormality. The group II neurons, which might be considered "passive," exhibit differing susceptibilities to epileptiform activity. Thus, they may be classified as "weakly epileptogenic," but not "normal." This pool of group II cells provides the matrix for recruitment and spread of seizure discharges. Under most circumstances, these and other cells do not become involved in sustained paroxysms, and discharges remain brief and localized. Occasionally, however, appropriate conditions favor breakdown of the control mechanism and spread of discharges (340).

The relative roles of all these factors (the PDS, EPRs, laminar pacemakers, entrainment, extracellular ion shifts, glial protective mechanisms, electrical field effects, inhibitory control mechanisms) remain to be defined in the chronic epileptogenic focus of humans (59). Whether PDSs really have a role in partial epilepsies of humans is of immediate concern. It is possible that in the chronic focus of humans, one, or some, of these factors is more important than another. Loss of GABAergic terminals (36,88,255), dendritic pathology, axonal sprouting (36,273), astrocytic proliferation (237), and progressive endothelial cell wall damage (see Chapter 39) have all been described in the chronic focus. Before the relative importance of epileptogenic factors described in the penicillin focus can be understood in the chronic focus, we must first unravel the ways in which the neuropathological changes in the neuropil and the blood–brain barrier have altered the properties of ion channels that are gated directly by voltage, intracellular Ca^{2+}, and chemical transmitters. The slow transmitter modulations of voltage-dependent channels directly or indirectly through activation of an adenylate cyclase must also be understood in the chronic focus (59).

Mechanisms subserving transition from interictal to ictal periods have not been established with any certainty. Clearly, extracellular concentrations of free ions, the integrity of transport system, voltage-dependent and time-dependent ionic conductances, ectopic impulse initiation, and comparative status of excitatory and inhibitory neurotransmission are all potential factors. But the relative importance of these variables is not understood at all. Unfortunately, very little experimental attention has been directed toward the loss of inhibitory control, the process of recruitment, and the spontaneous termination of seizures. These phenomena deserve high priority in future research endeavors (59).

Voltage- and Patch-Clamp Measurements

In the final analysis, chemical and biophysical properties of normal membranes must be defined much more completely before epileptiform pathology can be understood. Voltage-clamp and current-clamp experiments using single-electrode and two-electrode impalements of sympathetic ganglion cells, spinal cord neurons, and hippocampal CA1 and CA3 neurons have recently permitted a detailed picture of membrane and ionic currents within vertebrate neurons. In addition to the Hogkin-Huxley fast transient Na current (I_{Na}), independent investigators, notably Adams (2) and Schwindt and Crill (280), have observed several slow and fast potassium currents (I_k), a persistent inward calcium current (Ca), and an anomalous rectifier (inward-going) current (Ia). I_{Na}, I_k, I_{Ca}, as well as a calcium activated K conductance (I_c), are all activated during the spike potential. Two other currents, namely, I_m and I_a, operate in the subthreshold range and influence the occurrence and timing of spike potentials and cell depolarization. I_m and I_c (via I_{Ca}) are controlled by various transmitters such as acetylcholine, norepinephrine, and leutinizing hormone-releasing hormone (LHRH) (2,280).

Schwindt and Crill suggest that factors that increase depolarizing persistent inward currents, directly or indirectly (e.g., by depressing outward currents), can cause prolonged depolarizations with self-sustained bursting or PDSs (280). In penicillin-induced spinal seizures, a marked enhancement of subthreshold inward Ca^{2+} currents, indirectly caused by a decrease in outward K currents, is present during bursting. Fluctuations in external K concentrations presumably decreased outward K currents. Schwindt and Crill have also shown that neuromodulators and neurotransmitters can also induce bursting. Thus, their theoretical construct is that both fluctuations in extracellular ionic concentrations and the actions of neurotransmitters and neuromodulators could markedly alter neuronal ionic gates and initiate epileptiform activity (280). Further resolution of these voltage and chemically sensitive ion gates, through recordings of their picoamperic currents by the patch-clamp techniques of Neher, can picture for us the open and closed states of ion gates. Such studies can also detail the interactions of neurotransmitters and ion gates as well as the effects of drugs on the Na^+ and Ca^{2+} channels. It is important to determine how the pathological processes in the epileptogenic focus of humans alter these specific membrane conductances and ion gates within neurons. Do alterations in the closed and open states of voltage-sensitive and chemically sensitive [GABA and acetylcholine (Ach)] ion channels produce PDSs in humans (59)?

Ion Transport, Membrane Proteins, and Lipid Matrix

Subunits of the Na^+ Channel and the Na^+K^+-ATPase

Understanding the molecular mechanisms underlying selective ion transport, voltage-dependent gating and chemically sensitive ion channels may reveal the basis for ion shifts observed during PDSs and during generalized seizures. Our first glimpses of the molecular structure of the voltage-sensitive sodium channels has come from its purification from rat brain, rat skeletal muscle, chick cardiac muscle, and eel electroplax. The eel electrophorus Na^+ channel and its avian counterpart consist of a single polypeptide of molecular weights (MW) of 260,000–300,000 and 230,000–270,000, respectively. Its mammalian counterparts contain, in addition to the large polypeptide (α subunit), two or three smaller polypeptides of 37,000–45,000 MW (42,209). The purified eel and rat sodium channel preparations have been shown to be functional when reconstituted into phospholipid vesicles.

Most recently, Noda et al. cloned and sequenced the cDNA for the electrophorus electricus electroplax sodium channel. They showed that it consists of 1,820 amino acid residues and exhibits four internal repeated homology units, which are probably oriented in a pseudosymmetric fashion across the membrane (224). The sodium channel protein, in contrast to many other transmembrane proteins, does not possess an amino-terminal sequence characteristic of the signal peptide. Transmembrane proteins devoid of a cleavable signal peptide have their amino terminus on the cytoplasmic side of the membrane. Available evidence suggests that the activation and inactivation gates of the Na^+ channel are located near the inner membrane surface. Noda et al. hypothesize that each of the four positively charged segments, possibly in conjunction with each of the four negatively charged segments, act as a voltage sensor, thus being involved in an activation gate (224). The availability of cloned and sequenced cDNA for the Na^+ channel should now allow investigators to test whether altered structures of the Na^+ channel gene may be responsible for some forms of epilepsy. The structure and inheritance of this gene can be studied not only in experimental models of genetic epilepsies but also in families of patients with epilepsy.

Substantial progress toward understanding the molecular basis of PDSs should become possible with further discoveries on the biochemical structure of other membrane ionic channels, such as the K^+ and Ca^{2+} channel proteins. Selective purification of Na^+K^+-ATPase and Ca^{2+},Mg^{2+} ATPase and reconstitution experiments of the α, β, and γ subunits of the Na^+K^+-ATPase now are also realities, and are being tested for functional abnormalities in epileptogenic states.

Sweadner resolved two molecular forms of α subunit brain Na^+K^+-ATPase by gel electrophoresis in sodium dodecyl sulfate. One form (called $\alpha-$) was found in glial membranous structures mainly if not alone and the other form (called $\alpha+$) was found alone in axolemma membranes although both ($\alpha-$ and $\alpha+$) were found in synaptosomal and microsomal structures. These two catalytic subunits showed differences in affinity to strophantidin, i.e., to the glycosidic site that is usually considered to be identical to the catalytic site of K^+ ions (308).

Recently, Siegel et al. also verified the presence of these Na^+K^+-ATPase catalytic subunits subspecies. The "doublets" were demonstrated by the immunoblot method with specific polyclonal antisera not only in neural but also in muscle, renal, and secretory tissues. These results question the concept of two separate and distinct molecular forms of Na^+K^+-ATPase in glia and neurons (290).

Matsuda et al., however, also showed that pyrithiamin inhibited the $\alpha+$ molecular form of Na^+K^+-ATPase. Pyrithiamin inhibited neuronal Na^+K^+-ATPase but not nonneuronal Na^+K^+-ATPase (187). From the articles of Matsuda et al. and Sweadner, it seems that $\alpha-$ could be the glial form and $\alpha+$ the neuronal form of Na^+K^+-ATPase catalytic subunits (187,308).

These points clearly must be elucidated, especially in view of the differences in glial Na^+K^+-ATPase and neuronal–synaptosomal Na^+K^+-ATPase dysfunctions observed in the epileptogenic states.

In 1978, Delgado-Escueta and collaborators described a defect in the function of the synaptic Na^+K^+-ATPase system in one experimental model for chronic cortical epilepsy (the cold or freezing lesion) (Table 2). More specifically, the malfunction of the synaptic Na^+K^+-ATPase consisted of a relative insensitivity to both *cis* and *trans* ion. As a result, the pump rates of Na^+ and K^+ decreased. These investigators also described an enhancement in calcium influx within nerve terminals of the chronic seizure foci. The relationship of the enhanced calcium influx to the decreased [Na^+K] pump was not understood, with the exception that the increased calcium influx was apparently not a function of the internal Na concentrations (62).

More recently, Grisar et al. described a defect in K_o activation of glial Na^+K^+-ATPase, highlighting the important role of glial cells in clearing extracellular K_o within the epileptogenic focus (108). Glial Na^+K^+-ATPase decreased reaction velocities between 3 and 18 mM K^+ in the actively firing epileptogenic focus, whereas the catalytic activity was increased in cortical tissues surrounding the focus. Synaptic Na^+K^+-ATPase increased activities during ictus, whereas glial Na^+K^+-ATPase stayed de-

TABLE 7. *Partial list of compounds labeled with positron-emitting radionuclides*

Labeled Compounds	Primary Applications
$H_2{}^{15}O$, $C^{15}O_2$, ^{77}Kr,CH_3-^{18}F, ^{18}F-antipyrine ^{11}C-Alcohols, $^{13}NH_3$, ^{18}F-ethanol	Cerebral blood flow
^{11}CO, $C^{15}O$, ^{68}Ga-EDTA	Cerebral blood volume, transport, and metabolism
$^{15}O_2$	Oxygen
2-(^{18}F)-fluoro-2-deoxy-D-glucose 2-(^{11}C)-deoxy-D-glucose, ^{11}C-glucose ^{11}C-Lactate, ^{11}C-pyruvate	Glucose and metabolites
L-(^{13}N)-Glutamate, α- and ω-glutamine, alanine, aspartate, leucine, valine, isoleucine, methionine, malate, oxaloacetate L(^{11}C)-Aspartate, leucine, glutamate, valine, malate, oxaloacetate D,L(^{11}C)-Alanine, leucine, tryptophan, oxaloacetate 1-Aminocyclopentane and butane Carboxylic acid	Amino acids
3(^{11}C)-O-Methyl-D-glucose ^{68}Ga-EDTA, ^{82}Rb	Ion transport and glucose diffusion
1-(^{11}C)-L-Leucine (^{11}C-Methyl)-L-methionine	Protein synthesis
^{18}F-, ^{11}C-Spiroperidol, ^{75}Br, ^{76}Br-p-bromospiroperidol, ^{18}F-haloperidol, ^{11}C-pimozide ^{18}F-, ^{11}C-L-DOPA	Dopamine receptors
^{11}C-Flunitrazepam	Benzodiazepine receptors
^{11}C-Etorphine	Opiate receptors

From Phelps, M. E., Mazziotta, J. C., and Huang, S. C. (1982): Study of cerebral function with positron computed tomography. *J. Cereb. Blood Flow. Metab.* 2:113–162; and Phelps, M. E., Schelbert, H., and Mazziotta, J. C. (1983): Positron computed tomography in the study of myocardial and cerebral function, *Ann. Intern. Med.* 98:339–359 with permission.

ficient in function even as epileptiform paroxysms secondarily generalized at the height of ictus. These series of experiments suggested that impaired glial Na^+K^+-ATPase functions may be important in ictal transformational discharges, whereas impaired synaptic Na^+K^+-ATPase could be a critical event in initiating interictal discharges (107,108).

In addition to abnormal drops in $[Ca^{2+}]_o$, an enhanced calcium influx and a decreased $[Na^+K]$ pump, the release of endogenous adenosine and its immediate metabolites, inosine and hypoxanthine (170), and elevation of cyclic AMP (cAMP) (337,338) levels have been postulated to play a role in the initial development and propagation of epileptogenic activity in freezing lesions. Cyclic AMP rises in the lesion site during the acute stage (4 hr) and decreases gradually after 8 and 24 hr. Unfortunately, like early studies on Na^+K^+-ATPase activities that showed an activated state of the enzyme 8 hr after lesion production, these reports did not exclude the role of edema and tissue destruction in the acute state of the freezing lesion. The exact relation of decreased $[Na^+K]$ pump and enhanced Ca^{2+} influx to elevated cyclic AMP, inosine, and hypoxanthine levels therefore remains unknown.

Four Major Phosphorylation-dependent Protein Systems May Be Affected by Seizures

Extraction of synaptic membranes with detergent yields an insoluble residue enriched in postsynaptic densities and associated with presynaptic membranes. Polyacrylamide gel electrophoresis reveals an array of 14 protein bands in synaptic plasma membranes and postsynaptic densities ranging in mw from 275,000 daltons to <20,000 daltons (184). The majority of proteins in the plasma membrane are accounted for by bands at 110,000–105,000 daltons (15%), 54,000 daltons (24%), 44,000 daltons (12%), and 37,000 daltons (12%). Identified proteins of the postsynaptic apparatus include actin, α and β tubulin, myelin-associated protein I, neurofilaments, fodrin (α and β) calmodulin, and a 51,000 dalton protein that is highly concentrated in the postsynaptic densities. Among proteins, sugar moieties are observed to be most abundant in bands 4, 5, 6, 8, and 11, having high mw of 110 KD, 130 KD, 145 KD, 180 KD, and 210 KD. These glycoproteins, which are considered to be important in receptor function and Ca^{2+} transport, are located on or in the external face of the membrane (184). Another class of proteins that is of importance in synaptic functions is the fibrous proteins. Tubulin, near band 8, and actin, near band 9, contribute 20% and 10%, respectively, of the total mass of proteins in the synpatic plasma membrane. Actin, tropomyosin, and troponin are found only in the interior face of the membrane, whereas tubulin probably spans the whole membrane (184).

Among these arrays of synaptic proteins, four major phosphorylation-dependent systems that regulate signal processing are receiving attention in the epilepsies:

1. cAMP-dependent protein kinases that phosphorylate protein Ia and b (80,000 and 86,000 daltons); protein IIIa (74,000 daltons); and protein IIIb (55,000 daltons) (151). The phosphoproteins are localized in presynaptic and postsynaptic structures, and their kinase/phosphatase system has been isolated and characterized. Protein I is neuron-specific, being present in both peripheral and central neurons, and its phosphorylation is correlated with ionic fluxes (Ca^{2+} especially), the state of depolarization, and stimulus secretion coupling (151, 334,335).

2. Transmitter release has also been correlated in the presynaptic vesicles with a second major group of phosphoproteins, namely, 52,000 daltons and 61,000 daltons, whose phosphorylation is Ca^{2+}-calmodulin–stimulated. Phenytoin, carbamezepine, and benzodiazepines inhibit the kinases of these phosphoproteins. The 52,000-dalton protein may actually be the catalytic subunits of the kinases, and may act in the brain as a low-affinity benzodiazepine receptor (65).

3. The third major system involves both membrane and cytosolic components: a cytosolic C-kinase stimulated by membrane phospholipids, particularly phosphotidylserine and diacylglycerol (215). Signal transduction in this system is complex. Receptor stimulation activates a phospholipidase C that acts on membrane phosphoinositides, releasing inositol phosphates and diacylglycerol. Diacylglycerol activates the cytosolic C-kinase and promotes Ca^{2+} mobilization from the endoplasmic reticulum or mitochondrial or extracellular space. Analogous to cAMP synthesis, diacylglycerol, inositoltriphosphate, and Ca^{2+} act as second and third messengers to regulate cellular events. Suspected C-kinase substrates are the Ca^{2+} calmodulin kinase, the neuropeptide-sensitive B-50 phosphoprotein from presynaptic endings, glycogen synthetase phosphorylase B, and other uncharacterized neuronal proteins (215).

4. The fourth phosphorylation-dependent system consists of receptors, channel proteins, and enzymes. An excellent example of these phosphoproteins is the GABA receptor modulating protein, GABA-modulin (16,500 MW). It inhibits GABA binding to synaptic membranes and inhibits GABA stimulation of benzodiazepine binding. Phosphorylation of GABA-modulin abolishes this down-regulation effect (110).

Some information is now available on the relationship between the cAMP, Ca^{2+}, and calmodulin-sensitive phosphorylation of membrane proteins and epilepsy. Ehrlich et al. (74), using a foot shock paradigm, increased the phosphorylation of proteins with 47,000 and 18,000 MW. These animals were killed 24 hr after their behavioral test; the *in vitro* phosphorylation was then performed. Stromborn et al. (306) have also shown that the phosphorylated state of synaptosomal membrane proteins (protein 1a and 1b) increased in response to the convulsive agents PTZ and picrotoxin. This was in agreement with the earlier work of Ferrendelli (86), which demonstrated that cyclic AMP, a major regulator of synaptosomal protein kinase activity, was increased in the hippocampus during seizure activity induced by PTZ. A similar result was found for the cyclic nucleotide, cGMP.

Meanwhile, Delgado-Escueta and Horan (61) also observed the elevated phosphorylation of 18,000- to 20,000-MW proteins after electroshock convulsions and metrazol seizures in agreement with Ehrlich's results. The identity of these phosphoproteins has not been established, though Bajorek reports (see Chapter 25) that they are similar to calmodulin-inhibited, cAMP-insensitive proteins whose phosphorylation is increased in the interictal state of Mongolian gerbils and is decreased after grand mal clonic-tonic-clonic convulsions. In the tottering mice with spike-wave paroxysms and in the epileptic fowl, the phosphorylation of 16,000-, 50,000-, and 80,000-dalton proteins are all reported to be decreased *in vitro* (Tables 2 and 3).

Most recently, a decrease in the concentration of a calcium-binding protein in hippocampus of kindled rats was reported (210). An increased permeability of hippocampal slices to $^{45}Ca^{2+}$ has also been observed after long-term potentiation. In addition, in collaboration with Goldenring and DeLorenzo, Wasterlain et al. have observed a reduction in vitro in the calcium- and calmodulin-stimulated phosphorylation of the 50,000-dalton and 58,000- to 60,000-dalton proteins that are subunits of the calmodulin kinase (341). Wasterlain et al. (see Chapter 21) hypothesize that in the *in vivo* state, the resulting rise in Ca^{2+} inside the presynaptic apparatus stimulates calmodulin kinase to autophosphorylate to the point that its activity enhances transmitter release. In the postsynaptic apparatus, a lasting increase in calmodulin kinase activity could alter the response of postsynaptic densities to calcium entry in such tissues as the hippocampus (341).

Disturbances of Cholesterol or Gangliosides Can Initiate Epileptogenesis

In addition to abnormalities of structural proteins within synaptic membranes, accumulating evidence suggests that lipid matrix abnormalities are also present in the epileptogenic focus. In experiment cobalt-induced epileptic foci, significant changes in cerebral cortical lipids are found (29,54) not only in the necrotic center of the lesion but in the adjacent nonnecrotic tissue as well. The lipid changes precede the onset of epileptiform activity (54).

Although the stabilizing effect of cholesterol in membranes has been recognized for some time, changes in membrane cholesterol content have only recently been related to epileptogenesis. Inhibitors of cholesterol synthesis induce seizures in rats and opposums (29,54), whereas hypercholesterolemia protects mice, rats, and monkeys against seizures (54). It is reasonable to suppose that cholesterol inhibitors, as well as dietary changes, ultimately affect membrane lipid composition, and that such membrane changes may mediate important functional changes in seizure activity. The anticonvulsant effects of a high fat ("ketogenic") diet in human epilepsy has long been known. The diet induces a chronic mild acidosis, but whether acidosis or some other effect of the diet is the primary mediator of anticonvulsant activity is not known. Changes in membrane lipid composition can be induced by a ketogenic diet. In this regard, we do not know whether antiepileptic drugs induce changes in neuronal membrane composition. Anesthetics are known to decrease membrane viscosity, and phenytoin has been reported to normalize erythrocyte membrane viscosity in myotonic muscular dystrophy (260). Not only is it important that future experiments directly evaluate viscosity changes and lipid components of the synaptic or glial membrane in epileptogenic states, but their relations to the ion pump and leak systems of the membrane should also be examined.

Gangliosides have also been suspected to play a role in epileptogenesis. Since 1961, a number of investigators have shown that antisera to neuronal tissue is epileptogenic and causes morphologic changes in synaptic membrane (254). The epileptogenic activity of such antisera appears to be largely due to antiganglioside fractions, especially antiGM1, although antisera to a specific protein fraction has also been reported to generate epileptiform activity. Antisera to other brain fractions, such as myelin, or specific proteins, such as S-100 and 14-32, or antisera to other membranes, such as erythrocytes, fail to generate seizures even though some, such as myelin, contain large amounts of gangliosides (254).

A number of bacterial toxins, including cholera toxin, tetanus toxin, and botulinum have a high affinity for gangliosides and are powerfully epileptogenic. Cholera toxin and its subunit, choleragenoid, bind very specifically to GM1. Thus, again, gangliosides appear to play a role, possibly a major one, in epileptogenesis. However, the exact details of how gangliosides influence seizure generation are still unknown. Genetic differences in regional content of brain gangliosides have also been demonstrated in some animals with genetic epilepsies, such as the audiogenic mice. Strains susceptible to audiogenic seizures are found to have the highest content of GM1 in all brain regions studied. Higher ganglioside content is thought to be associated with a higher level of myelination (285), but the manner by which such changes lead to increased susceptibility to seizures is unknown.

Studies of the influence of seizures upon brain gangliosides have yielded variable results. A large reduction in gangliosides after metrazol-induced status epilepticus has been observed in dogs. A large increase of gangliosides in some cerebral cortical layers of cobalt lesions in rats, and small but statistically significant changes in neocortical ganglioside sialic acid levels in acute chemically induced seizures in rats have been reported (54). Subsequent investigations have demonstrated measurable decreases in gangliosides within synaptosomal and microsomal fractions after metrazol-induced convulsions in rats (352). It has been suggested that the decreased gangliosides may result from activation of endogenous membrane-bound neuraminidase by seizure activity (neuronal gangliosides are apparently not susceptible to hydrolysis by exogenous neuraminidase, at least in the absence of proteolytic enzymes) (54).

Although it is increasingly clear that epilepsy is a disorder of membranes, especially synapses and glial membranes, our understanding of the essential membrane changes that initiate epileptogenesis is still very primitive. Many of the most important properties of membranes are mediated by protein element, some of which have been shown to function abnormally in epileptogenic tissue (Tables 2 and 3). However, attempts to isolate abnormalities of composition, as opposed to function, have more often implicated nonprotein elements of the membrane. Although protein malfunction may also lead to secondary changes of lipid matrix composition, it appears that primary disturbances of nonprotein components, such as cholesterol, or gangliosides, may be sufficient to initiate seizure generation.

Cell–Cell Communication: Neurotransmitters and Neuromodulators in Epilepsy

Norepinephrine and Serotonin Suppress but Ach Facilitates Generalized Convulsions and Partial Seizures

Perhaps the best examples of abnormal cell–cell communication and plasticity in neurobiology are the mirror focus and the kindling phenomenon. It is no accident then, that in these particular phenomena, the role of neurotransmitters and neuromodulators are suspected to be of prime importance (Tables 2 and 3). Wada et al. (331,332) summarized pharmacologic studies on amygdaloid kindling and hypothesized that acetylcholine facilitates and norepinephrine inhibits, whereas serotonin and dopamine have no clear-cut effect on kindling. The studies they reviewed, however, were restricted to the intraperitoneal (I.P.) or intraventricular injection of drugs that modify neurotransmitter levels. Dubicka et al. (67) and Zoll et al. (356) showed that medial forebrain bundle (MFB) stimulation retarded development of kindling induced by acetylcholine. These studies suggested that catecholamines or serotonin can suppress kindling.

Reserpine, which depletes catecholamines and serotonin, facilitated kindling, whereas tricyclic antidepressants (which depress uptake of biogenic amines) suppressed kindling. Catecholamine agonists did not consistently affect kindling.

In further support of the notion that norepinephrine is usually inhibitory to the initiation and spread of seizures, Sato and Ogawa (265) and Trottier et al. (321) independently reported a decrease in whole-brain noradrenalin and/or dopamine in kindling or in cobalt epilepsies. Engel and Sharpless (78) also reported a reduction in dopamine levels in the kindled amygdala of the rat (Tables 2 and 3). More recently, however, Sato and Ogawa claimed that amygdala and striatal homovanillic acid increases after kindling, suggesting hyperreactive dopaminergic metabolism (265).

It is not a new concept that the central noradrenergic system, in particular norepinephrine, has inhibitory or suppressing effects in seizures. As early as 1954, a role for the central catecholamines (norepinephrine and dopamine) in modulating seizure activity was suggested by Chen et al. (45). They observed that reserpine enhanced PTZ and electroshock seizures in mice, presumably by depleting the brain of biogenic amines. Depletion of catecholamines not only can increase susceptibility to convulsive seizures, but also can facilitate the development of the mirror focus. Originating in neuronal cell bodies located in the brainstem locus coeruleus (LC) and lateral tegmental nucleus, noradrenergic axons project diffusely throughout the neuraxis in the reticular formation, cerebellum, and cortex. Therefore, they influence overall neuronal activity. The dopaminergic neuronal systems, in contrast, are more localized in their projections. This may explain contradictory dopaminergic influences on seizures in various experimental models of epilepsy.

The importance of differentiating the role of catecholamines as modulators of seizure activity from their role as primary factors in epileptogenesis is best seen in the genetic epilepsy-prone rats, the epileptic fowl, and the tottering mouse (Tables 2 and 3). Jobe et al. (139–144) showed that decreased central noradrenergic function, but not reduced dopaminergic function, increases the severity of audiogenic convulsions. Bourn et al. (33) injected 6-hydroxydopamine (6-OH) into the ventricles of genetically susceptible rats and enhanced their seizures. Selective destruction of noradrenergic neurons with 6-OH dopamine enhanced seizures, whereas destruction of dopaminergic neurons did not affect seizures. These data suggest that a deficit in the noradrenergic system, if coupled with some other genetically determined abnormality, may be responsible for audiogenic seizure susceptibility. However, if deficits in noradrenergic systems contribute to seizure generation, why are noradrenergic synaptic terminals and norepinephrine concentrations increased in the cerebral cortex of the mutant tottering mice and the epileptic fowl (see Chapters 4 and 24)? Are these observations the effects of seizures, or are they involved in seizure generation as well?

Laird and Huxtable (161) showed that the inferior colliculi of audiogenic rats had a low intracerebral electroshock threshold. Electrical stimulation of this area replicated the audiogenic seizure. Taurine elevated the intracerebral electroshock threshold, but this did not stop the spread of seizures, suggesting that taurine primarily affected the inferior colliculi (161).

Acetylcholine, in contrast, seems to be more directly involved in the development of kindled foci. Several investigators independently showed that cholinergic agonists carbachol or physostigmine induced the kindling phenomenon in amygdala. Atropine, a cholinergic blocking agent, decreased the rate of such chemical kindling. Electrical kindling is also associated with a decrease in muscarinic binding sites in dentate and amygdala. These findings must be interpreted in the light of presently known cholinergic pathways. The first forebrain cholinergic pathway identified was that pathway arising from the medial septal and diagonal band nuclei and projecting to the hippocampus and dentate gyrus. The cholinergic projections in the amygdala are both intrinsic and from the lateral presynaptic nuclei, whereas cholinergic neurons are also intrinsic to the cerebral cortex.

Impaired GABA-mediated Inhibition in Substantia Nigra Favors Spread of Partial Seizures and Induction of Myoclonic and Tonic-Clonic Convulsions in Mongolian Gerbil

The kindling phenomenon of Goddard provides further proof that other neurotransmitter systems are operating to contain the generalization and spread of seizures. As outlined in Tables 2 and 3 and discussed above, the catecholamines, particularly norepinephrine, suppress kindling whereas cholinergic mechanisms facilitate the development of stage 5 kindling. Endogenous serotonergic pathways have also been shown to inhibit kindling. Several lines of evidence suggest that muscarinic receptors and β-adrenergic receptors decrease whereas benzodiazepine receptors increase in the dentate gyrus of the hippocampus in an attempt to reduce excitability and spread of kindled seizures (196). More recently, Iadorola and Gale (132) and McNamara (196) independently identified the downstream structure instrumental in suppressing the motor seizure expression of kindling, bicuculline, PTZ, and electroshock seizures. Iadorola and Gale (132) first discovered that intracerebral γ-vinyl-GABA (GVG), an irreversible catalytic inhibitor of GABA transaminase, elevated GABA content of midbrain substantia nigra and suppressed motor seizures induced by electroshock, PTZ, and bicuculline. Microinjection of a 5-mg dose of muscimol, a GABA receptor agonist, bilaterally into the substantia nigra also suppressed seizures induced by bicuculline. McNamara administered n-dipropyl acetate systematically and GVG intracerebrally in rats who had undergone stage 5 kindling. GABA levels in the midbrain substantia nigra increased, and the motor component of kindled seizures was blocked. McNamara (196) also microinjected muscimol into the pars reticulata region of the substantia nigra and again suppressed the motor components of amygdala kindling. These independent but complementary experiments by Gale and Iadorola and McNamara provide a biochemical basis for earlier electrophysiological studies that had emphasized the engagement of caudate nucleus, globus pallidus putamen, and substantia nigra by epileptiform paroxysms in the expression of motor seizures. These structures have always been considered the preferred pathways for seizure propagation, and it is now clear that enhancing GABA-mediating inhibition on nigral efferent neurons in pars reticulata stops the progress of seizure propagation.

At the same time that Iadorola and Gale (132) and McNamara (196) were examining GABA inhibition in the substantia nigra as a "way station" for stopping propagation of seizures, Olsen et al., in collaboration with Wamsley (230), were investigating the benzodiazepine/barbiturate/GABA receptor ionophore complex in different brain regions as a possible molecular defect in Mongolian gerbils with genetically determined generalized epilepsies. Their studies also pointed to the importance of GABA-mediated inhibition in the substantia nigra as one possible defect in generalized myoclonic and grand mal epilepsies (230). GABA receptors assayed *in vitro* by [³H]diazepam binding and by brain-slice autoradiography of [^{3}H]flunitraze-paim revealed 20–30% lower binding in the substantia nigra. Other brain regions studied, including the cerebral cortex and hippocampus, showed normal results. This deficit in benzodiazepine receptor binding has been shown most recently to consist of a decrease in the number of the GABA receptors in the substantia nigra.

In Chapter 15, Roberts presents a physiologic sculpture of GABAergic circuits in the CNS which act as tonic inhibitory command neurons, or as local circuits involved in feed-forward, feedback, surround and presynaptic inhibition, or presynaptic facilitation. He delineates those GABAergic systems that must still be understood in addition to those presently reported in the substantia nigra (256). GABAergic systems in the striatum, hippocampus, and neocortex should now be studied carefully in convulsing and kindled animals, especially their relations to the cholinergic and opiate systems.

Is GABAergic Transmission Increased in Generalized Epilepsies Such as Petit Mal Seizures?

In contrast to the hypothesis of decreased GABA inhibition in experimental partial epilepsies, Fromm and Terrence (94), Snead et al. (298), Fariello et al. (83), and Myslobodsky (220) have independently suggested that hyperfunction or paroxysmal activity of GABAergic or opiate inhibitory pathways may cause petit mal seizures. All evidence to support this contention, however, is circumstantial, and the models of petit mal epilepsy used are quite different from the human condition (Tables 2, 3, 8, and 9). Nonetheless, these models argue for a case of increased cortical GABAergic inhibition in petit mal seizures. An augmentation of GABAergic transmission by GABAergic agonists is reported to exacerbate models of absence seizures, notably, the γ-hydroxybutyrate (GHB) model, flash evoked after discharges, PTZ, and generalized beline penicillin model. Baclofen and muscimole induce absence-like seizures, and GHB, a metabolite of GABA, produces petit mal-like seizures.

GHB-induced seizures are considered to be mainly due to its GABAergic effects, since petit mal-like seizures are potentiated by GABA agonists and are not blocked by bicuculline (297,298). Fromm's arguments are derived from antiepileptic drug experiments in the spinal trigeminal nucleus oralis of cats. Because drugs effective against petit mal (valproate, ethosux-imide, trimethadione, imipramine, and clomipramine), depress descending inhibitory mechanisms in the spinal trigeminal nucleus, he suggested that the latter (inhibitory mechanisms), which are mediated by GABAergic and cholinergic mechanisms, must be increased in petit mal seizures (94). Fariello, using the 2-deoxy-glucose technique during epileptiform paroxysms induced by muscimol, (4,5,6,7 tetrahy-droxyisoxasolo[4,5-c] pyridine 3-ol) (THIP) and progabide, suggests that an excess of inhibitory activity rather than neuronal disinhibition is present in the brain (83). Myslobodsky further contends that the "petit mal" potentiating action of γ-acetylenic and γ-vanylic derivatives of GABA (GAG and GVG) may be related to enhanced potency of postsynaptic inhibition underlying the slow secondary negative wave (220).

Most recently, Peterson and Ribak et al. have shown through immunocytochemical methods that GABAergic neurons are increased in the hippocampus of Mongolian gerbils with grand mal and myoclonic epilepsies (246). Similar findings of increased GABAergic neurons were observed in the inferior colliculus of genetic epilepsy-prone rats with audiogenic seizures (Table 9) (Chapter 37). Patients with generalized epilepsies and their first-degree relatives have recently been shown to have abnormally elevated plasma levels of glutamic acid but have low levels of taurine and aspartic acid (51).

Glutamic Acid, Aspartic Acid, Taurine, and GABA Decrease in the Experimental Seizure Focus

The relationship of amino acid levels to experimental epilepsy has probably been studied best by Van Gelder et al. (327) and Koyama and Jasper (153) in the cobalt model of focal epilepsy (Tables 2 and 3; Chapter 51). Eight to 10 days after cobalt implantation in rats, GABA, glutamic acid, aspartic acid, and taurine levels are 60–70% lower than control levels, the decrease being most pronounced in the epileptic focus. Glycine and glutamine levels remain unchanged. On superfusion of the exposed cortex with artificial cerebrospinal fluid (CSF) *in vivo*, the cobalt focus exhibited three- to fourfold increase in glutamic acid release. The diminution in glutamic acid content and its enhanced efflux exhibited a temporal relationship to the onset of focal spikes (153). Similar observations have been reported in the penicillin epileptic foci. In photoepileptic baboons, however, amino acid

TABLE 8. *Some hypotheses on the generation of partial epilepsies in experimental animals*

1. GABA/glutamate hypothesis
   a. Decreased GABAergic transmission (decreased GABA, GAD, and GABA uptake) in the seizure focus (255,326)
   b. Hypothesis of glutamate–GABA ratio as determinant of excitation or inhibition (327)
   c. Decreased taurine inhibition (326)

2. Na^+K pump hypothesis
   a. Decreased Na^+K pump function within synapses and glial cells with impaired clearance of extracellular K^+ (61,107,108)
   b. Impaired glial protective properties: diminished anion pump and Na^+K^+-ATPase activities in the seizure focus (351)

3. Ca^{2+} influx hypothesis
   a. Marked enhancement of subthreshold inward Ca^{2+} currents during cell bursting in penicillin spinal seizures (280)
   b. Decrease of Ca^{2+} during seizures in alumina cream and cobalt focus (120)

4. Catecholamine hypothesis
   a. Decreased norepinephrine inhibition in the cobalt focus and surround (321) and in the kindled focus (265)

5. Acetylcholine hypothesis
   a. Acetylcholine and agonists can induce the kindling paradigm (329,341); decreased muscarinic binding sites in kindled focus, in alumina cream focus, and kainic acid focus (195,196,355)

6. Ca^{2+} calmodulin protein kinase hypothesis
   a. Decreased Ca^{2+} calmodulin protein kinase autophosphorylation in synaptic terminals of kindled focus (65,341)

7. Membrane lipid matrix hypothesis
   a. Decrease of free cholesterol and unsaturated fatty acid moieties and of phosphotidylethanolamine decrease membrane viscosity and increase membrane permeability (54)
   b. Antiganglioside (anti-GM1) sera is epileptogenic and produces morphologic changes in synapses (254)

GABA, γ-aminobutyric acid; GAD, glutamic acid decarboxylose.

content of the frontal lobe does not change. In PTZ seizures, glutamate concentrations decrease, whereas alanine and ammonia increase, suggesting increased protein catabolism. Picrotoxin-induced seizures decrease aspartic acid (59,198).

Tables 2 and 3 describe the changes in free amino acid concentrations in other experimental foci. Most commonly, GABA, taurine, and glutamate are decreased whereas glycine is elevated. It is hypothesized that low concentrations

of GABA and glutamate result in net depolarization. Van Gelder et al. (327) reported that taurine returns the ratio of glutamate/glutamine and the brain glutamate content to normal. On this basis, Van Gelder et al. theorized that epilepsy was caused by an increased excitability caused by imbalances in taurine, glutamate, and glutamine. Laird and Huxtable (161) question this concept, because genetically susceptible rats did not show any disturbance in amino acid content, and taurine elevated intracerebral elec-

TABLE 9. *Some hypotheses on the genesis of primary generalized epilepsies in experimental animals*

Absence or Petit Mal
1. γ-Hydroxybutyric acid produces seizures similar to petit mal (298)
2. Opiate receptor agonists produce seizures similar to petit mal (296)
3. Increased norepinephrine terminals in cerebral cortex of tottering mice with spike-wave seizures (225)

Myoclonic and clonic-tonic-clonic convulsions
1. Abnormally decreased GABA receptors and increased opiate receptors in substantia nigra and periventricular gray in Mongolian gerbils (230)
2. Abnormally increased number of GABAergic- or GAD-containing neurons and nerve terminals in hippocampus of Mongolian gerbils and inferior coliculi of epilepsy-prone mice with sound-induced convulsions (246)

GABA, γ-aminobutyric acid; GAD, glutamic acid decarboxylase.

troshock thresholds without effects on gluta- mate concentrations. An antiepileptic action for taurine has also been shown against seizures in- duced by penicillin, alumina, estrogens, and light (59).

Aside from measurements of brain-tissue levels, other evidence indicates an involvement of GABAergic systems in both partial and gen- eralized epilepsies in experimental animals. Glu- tamic acid decarboxylase (GAD) activity and/or GABA uptake and release are all decreased in the epileptic foci produced by penicillin, alumina cream, and cobalt (15,16,56,104,327). There is no change in GABA levels or GABA receptor binding in kindling and the epileptogenic freeze lesion (11,169). There is, however, an increase in glutamate receptor binding in kindling.

Morphological and immunocytochemical data also support a role for the GABA system in focal epilepsy. GABAergic neurons are decreased in experimental focal seizures. Fischer (88) and Brown (36) independently showed that symme- tric synaptic junctions (axon terminals of GA- BAergic neurons) on the somata and dendritic shafts of pyramidal neurons are decreased in the seizure foci. Hoover et al. (125) also showed that in rats exhibiting early stages of seizure activity cortical neuronal somata showing a covering of dense, dark staining granules in Fink-Heimer- stained preparations. Ribak et al. (255) have sug- gested that these dark granules may represent degenerating axon terminals of GABAergic cor- tical neurones, since GAD-containing terminals are observed with a similar frequency at the sites where the dark granules appear. These granules in Fink-Heimer preparations appeared at the onset of seizure activity in the cobalt-treated rat cortex, but they were never observed in copper- and glass-treated rat cortices that never exhib- ited seizure activity. More recently, Ribak et al. (255) (see Chapter 37) studied alumina gel sei- zure foci by incubating slices for GAD immu- nocytochemistry. GAD-positive terminals were decreased at sites of the epileptogenic activity.

Other Dicarboxylic Amino Acids May Also Play a Role in Epilepsy

Evidence derived primarily from the anticon- vulsant potencies of excitatory amino acid an- tagonists suggest that N-methyl-D-aspartic acid (NMDA) receptors are involved in the initiation or spread of seizures in focal epilepsy in audio- genic mice and in *Papio papio*. Applied focally in the cortex, hippocampus, or amygdala, dicar- boxylic amino acids or various analogues—in- cluding the excitotoxins, kainic acid and ibo- tenic acid—produce focal epileptogenic parox- ysms. In models of generalized epilepsies, antagonists that specifically block NMDA-sen- sitive receptors, specifically 2-amino-7-phos- phonoheptanoic acid (2-APH), suppressed all phases of audiogenic seizures in DBA/2 mice and photically-induced myoclonus in *Papio papio*. On the basis of these observations, Croucher and Meldrum suggest that NMDA re- ceptor-mediated excitation subserves initiation or spread of seizures in focal epileptogenesis and in generalized epilepsies (56). In addition, 2- APH has been shown to block convulsions in- duced by 3-mercaptopriopionic acid and thio- semicarbazide (294). The 2-APH causes a pro- nounced reduction in aspartate levels in all brain regions along with decreases in brain GABA and glutamate levels and increases in glutamine levels in some regions (43). Antiepileptic drugs, such as phenobarbital, trimethadione, and phe- nytoin, suppress K^+-induced release of $[^3H]D$- aspartate in brain slices (294). Barbiturates and benzodiazepines do not affect brain GABA levels, but they do elevate aspartate levels. Val- proate increases brain GABA level and de- creases brain aspartate levels (43).

Cyclic Nucleotides in Spread and Sustenance of Seizures

Although the up-regulation of benzodiaze- pine, norepinephrine, and serotonin receptors and the down regulation of muscarinic and β- adrenergic receptors contain the spread of sei- zures, the rapid rise of cortical cAMP may con- tribute to the sustenance and spread of seizures. The first indication that cyclic nucleotide-me- diated events may contribute to seizures was provided by Krishna et al. in 1970 (156). They injected the dibutyryl analog of cyclic AMP into the brain ventricles of mice; seizures developed within a few seconds. Subsequently, it was shown that barbiturates antagonized dibutyryl cAMP-induced seizures. Electroshock convul- sions and hexafluorodiethyl ether produced rapid elevations of cAMP and cGMP in the cer- ebellum of mice (179–181,226). More recently, a host of convulsants (isoniazid, picrotoxin, homocysteine, PTZ, and 3-mercaptopropionic acid) have been shown to raise the content of cAMP and cGMP in the cerebellum and cere- brum of experimental animals (27,86,231,262). cAMP levels also increase in the primary focus and to a lesser degree in the mirror focus of freezing lesions (336,337). Penicillin administration to rat cerebrum induced a rise in both cAMP and cGMP (86).

To differentiate between the cause and effect relationship, two groups of investigators studied the temporal relationships of seizures and cyclic nucleotide levels. In PTZ seizures, cAMP did not increase until myoclonic or clonic seizures appeared. cGMP levels gradually rose during myoclonic and clonic seizures (86). Lust et al. conducted similar studies and found that, after electroshock convulsions, cortical cAMP rose rapidly and remained elevated for several minutes, whereas cGMP rose rapidly but declined within 4 min. In contrast, cerebellar cAMP rose within the first few seconds and declined rapidly, whereas cGMP content remained at an elevated level for several minutes (179,180).

Additional evidence supporting an important role for cAMP in the spread and sustenance of seizures is provided by experiments which show that drugs that suppress seizure activity also prevent the elevations in cAMP associated with seizures. The rapid rises seen in *in vitro* levels of cAMP, following PTZ, are prevented by pretreatment with phenytoin, phenobarbital, carbamazepine, diazepam, and lorazepam. In tissue homogenates, however, Palmer et al. (232) have shown that only carbamazepine will inhibit norepinephrine activation of adenylate cyclase, whereas diazepam and clonazepam stimulate adenylate cyclase (basal- and norepinephrine-stimulated levels). Only diazepam and clonazepam act to inhibit cAMP phosphodiesterase.

Benzodiazepines inhibit cAMP-phosphodiasterase (342); their effects on cGMP phosphodiesterase are unknown. Lust et al. (179,180) reported that phenobarbital caused a striking decrease in cAMP and a lesser effect on cAMP in the mouse cerebellum prior to and after electroconvulsive seizures (ECS). Similar data were reported by Ferrendelli (86).

Phenytoin has no direct action on either adenylate cyclase or phosphodiesterase (342). In incubated tissue slices of rat cerebral cortex, phenytoin partially inhibits the rise in cAMP elicited by adenosine and ouabain (171). Phenytoin inhibits the rise in cAMP and cGMP induced by ouabain or veratridine but not the elevation induced by KCl (86). Because phenytoin inhibits both sodium and calcium influx, it may affect cyclic nucleotides through ionic modulation.

In related work, Ferrendelli (86) showed that phenytoin prevented the rise in cerebral cAMP but had little effect on cGMP. PTZ-induced tonic seizures in mice were partially prevented by phenytoin. However, phenytoin had little effect on the resultant elevations cGMP, and it prevented the rise in cerebral cAMP. Lust et al. (179,180) further showed that phenytoin could block the rise in cerebellar and cerebral cAMP as a consequence of electroconvulsive shock (ECS) or decapitation. Lust and collaborators examined further phenytoin effects and found that it decreased the steady state levels of cGMP in the cerebral cortex both prior to and after ECS whereas cAMP levels were only slightly decreased. However, in the cerebellum, cGMP accumulation after ECS was reduced by 50% in phenytoin-treated mice. Pretreated rabbits with phenytoin decreased both the basal levels and the rise of cAMP induced by ECS (220).

In summary, accumulating evidence supports an important role for cyclic nucleotides in neurotransmission and in the spread and sustenance of the seizure process. Drugs that suppress seizure activity also prevent the elevations in cyclic nucleotides associated with seizures.

Opioid-Like Peptides, Especially Leu-enkephalin, Produce Absence-Like Seizures and Modulate Kindling and Convulsions

Recent experimental data indicate that endogenous brain ligands for the opiate receptor such as the pentapeptides, leucine and methionine enkephalin, and β-endorphins may be involved in both generalized and partial seizures. Frenk et al. (93) produced epileptiform activity in rats by single intraventricular injections of high doses (25–100 µg) of Leu-enkephalin and Met-enkephalin. Immobility and myoclonic seizures were blocked by naloxone (a specific opiate antagonist) and anti-petit mal drugs but not by phenytoin. Snead et al. (297,298) also demonstrated that opiate receptor agonists, especially leucine enkephalin, produce seizures, but these investigators interpreted the induced attacks as absence-like behavior. In their experiments, morphine produced both absence and generalized seizures, whereas ethylketocyclazocine (EKZ), SKF 10,047, and β-endorphin all produced hippocampal and amygdaloid spiking. These authors also showed that naloxone effectively suppressed absence in the GHB model of petit mal seizures.

Several lines of evidence now support the concept that opiate receptors have a role in kindling. First, the brain regions that develop kindling most rapidly (amygdala and globus pallidum) show intense enkephalin immunoflorescense and are extremely high in opiate receptors and enkephalinergic terminals (324). Second, Stone et al. (304) have demonstrated that peripherally administered opiates like naloxone or naltrexone reduce kindling whereas morphine potentiates kindling. Third, multiple injections of β-endorphin have now been used to kindle site-specific areas of the amygdala and hippocampus. Permanent increases in dynorphin and enkephalin levels in amygdala following kindling suggest that they may have a role in maintenance of the condition.

Intraventricular injection of β-endorphin in rats has also been shown to produce ECG spikes and is correlated with hippocampal neuronal firing (122). The effects of endogenous opioid peptides on seizure models have also been studied through naloxone administration before seizure induction. Naloxone potentiates biculline-induced seizures and produces ECG spikes and convulsions. It also increases attacks in Mongolian gerbils with grand mal seizures and in mice with audiogenic seizures (279). Naloxone did not have a consistent effect in the photosensitive baboon, *Papio papio* (201). The endorphins and enkephalins have not been thoroughly tested in the maximal electroshock or PTZ seizures.

Vasopressin, TRH, CRF, and Somatostatin Also Enhance Seizures

In addition to the enkephalins, more than 20 peptides have been identified as neurotransmitter candidates in the brain. Of these, ACTH, Arg-vasopressin, thyroid-releasing hormone (TRH), somatostatin, and corticotrophin-releasing factors (CRF), have been shown to modulate seizures. Neuropeptidergic substances, such as ACTH, Arg-vasopressin, dynorphin, and the growth hormone have been shown to be released in significant amounts during repeated convulsions and status epilepticus. CRF, vasopressin, and TRH increase susceptibility to seizures whereas ACTH is useful in the treatment of infantile spasms. Classical endocrine hormones like gonadal steroids, glucocorticoids, thyroid hormones, insulin, and melatonin also have modulating effects in the epileptic system (316). The most extensively studied phenomenon is the increase in seizures induced by glucocorticoids. A role for gastrin and vasoactive intestinal peptide (VIP) in seizures has yet to be shown.

Endogenous Anticonvulsants: β-endorphins, Cholecystokinin (CCK), Adenosine, Inosine, and Hypoxanthine

In the acute management of tonic-clonic seizures, clinicians have traditionally taught their younger colleagues to protect the victim from injuring himself and to wait patiently for the seizure to end. "The convulsion usually stops by itself," they maintain. Similarly, for two decades, neurochemists have noted that a phenomenon of tolerance develops to repeated convulsions. Essig showed that tolerance to convulsions depended on the convulsion itself and not on the stimulus, and that cross-tolerance to PTZ convulsions after electroshock convulsions, can develop (81,82). Some have suggested that endogenous anticonvulsants, such as β-endorphins, CCK, adenosine, inosine, hypoxanthine, and other unknown dipeptides are released during a seizure and stop the convulsive attack, induce a refractory period, and elevate the threshold for a second convulsion. This concept is based on the antiepileptic properties of these modulators when injected intraventricularly, their hyperpolarizing effects on cerebral cortical neurons which evidence that their release during a convulsive attack is associated with the postconvulsive refractory period, and proof that their antiepileptic properties are reversed by pharmacologic antagonists (13).

Brain β-endorphins, adenosine, inosine, and hypoxanthine levels increase dramatically within 10 s of a convulsive seizure (13) and reduce neuronal excitability as part of a neurochemical adaptive process that terminates the convulsive seizure. Recent *in vivo* studies suggest that A_1 receptors mediate the anticonvulsant effects of adenosine analogues (70,71). Dunwiddie and Worth found that L-phenylisopropyladenosine (L-PIA), a ligand for adenosine A_1 receptors, is approximately 20 times more potent than D-phenylisopropyladenosine (D-PIA), a ligand for adenosine A_2 receptors (71). Adenosine, a cotransmitter stored with primary neurotransmitters in synaptic vesicles in the form of adenosine triphosphate (ATP), is synaptically released by calcium to adenine nucleotides and adenosine. Adenosine then acts on specific extracellular recognition sites to modulate further release of neurotransmitters or to modulate the sensitivity of postsynaptic neurotransmitter receptors by interacting with specific adenosine recognition sites. Adenosine and adenine nucleotides depress neuronal excitability in several regions of the CNS, hyperpolarize cerebral cortical neurons, and suppress spontaneous and evoked EPSPs (69). Methylxanthines (caffeine, theophylline, isobutylmethylxanethines) antagonize the effects of adenosine, enhance firing of cortical neurons and reduce PTZ seizure and lethal dose (266).

The purines, inosine, hypoxanthine, and nicotinamide, proposed ligands for the benzodiazepine–GABA receptor complex, mediate the anticonvulsive actions of benzodiazepines (185,186,295). Because inosine and hypoxanthine inhibit seizures produced by PTZ in doses sufficient to raise brain levels that inhibit [³H]diazepam binding (185,186,295), the increased levels of inosine and hypoxanthine during a convulsive attack added one further argument that endogenous antiepileptic substances are released during a convulsion.

Similar proof supporting the role of β-endorphine as an endogenous antiepileptic substance exists. β-Endorphins, the C-terminal of β-lipotropin and containing 31 amino acids, are released during electroshock convulsions, during clonic-tonic-clonic seizures of Mongolian gerbils, and during kindled seizures. Three micrograms of intraventricular β-endorphin reduces the incidence and severity of clinical and electrographic seizures. Opioid peptides, morphine, ketocyclazocine, and *N*-allylmormetazocine mimic β-endorphin anticonvulsant effects. Naloxone reverses the anticonvulsant effects of β-endorphin, morphine, and ketocyclazocine, but not those of *N*-allylmormetazocine. At higher doses (>5 μg), intraventricular β-endorphin produces epileptiform paroxysms and drop attacks. Intraventricular morphine, Leu-enkephalin, and Met-enkephalin also produce epileptiform activity (93,94,122) (see Chapter 25). Prior administration of naloxone also prevents the convulsant effects of high doses of β-endorphins.

These observations suggest that endogenous opioid peptides released during convulsions may arrest seizures and suppress the development of further attacks. They also suggest that if brain levels of opioid peptides reach convulsant levels after repeated seizures, they could cause the transformation of seizures into the fixed and lasting state of status epilepticus.

Another group of potential antiepileptic substances consist of caerulin and the C-terminal octapeptide of CCK. When administered subcutaneously, they delay the development of strychnine, PTZ, bicuculline, and picrotoxin seizures. In addition, screen of peptidergic compounds have revealed anticonvulsant properties for LHRH, TRH, and MSH against audiogenic

seizures. Dipeptides have now been synthesized with specific cell functions and antiepileptic properties. One group antagonizes aspartic acid receptors and protects against audiogenic seizures. Another is a dipeptide analogue of GABA effective against PTZ seizures. As more propeptide precursors are recognized, and as improvements in synthesis and structural analysis of peptides identify more and more endogenous peptides, replacement therapy with these peptides will be considered as a form of epilepsy treatment (see Chapter 25).

NEUROCELLULAR ANATOMY AND THE CONSEQUENCES OF EPILEPSIES

Cellular Ultrastructure and Chemical Neuroanatomy in the Epilepsies Minicolumns or Modules in Neocortex

Over the last two decades, attention has been focused on basic components of the brain and its mode of functioning in terms of structural, electrical, and chemical circuits. Electrophysiologists envision the neocortex as a mosaic of columnar processes containing 10^2 and 10^4 cells about 200–300 mm in diameter (minicolumns or modules), connected with one another and with a number of subcortical sources and targets according to a very highly specific wiring blueprint (312). Modular arrangement of excitatory and inhibitory interneurons provides for specific cells to act as output channels toward other cortical columns. The selection mechanism is based on the interaction of excitatory and inhibitory interneurons arranged in mutually interpenetrating space modules smaller than the main columns (~30 mm). Thus, information on the synaptic relations of pyramidal and nonpyramidal cells, spine-free multipolar stellate cells, basket cells, double bouquet cells, and spiny stellate cells has gradually become available (312). Heinemann et al. (120,121), Goldensohn (Chapter 28), and Ebersole (72) have independently explored the modular function of neocortical columns in acute and chronic epileptogenic focus, and a substantial portion of local interneurons and intracortical connectivity is now being incorporated into existing concepts of epileptogenesis and spread of seizures. These neuronal local circuits which have been defined are composed mainly of short axon, Golgi Type II neurons with interneuronal linkages that are primary dendrodendritic. Specific linkages within these circuits via dendro-somatic, somatic-dendritic, somatic-axonic and even dendro-axonic and axo-axonic synapses must now be fully explored.

"Gap" Junctions

In addition to synaptic circuitry, electromicroscopic examinations of neuronal local circuits revealed the existence of several unconventional modes of synaptic connectivity. These include reciprocal electronical ("gap") junctions, mixed chemical and electrical junctions, and other forms of dendrodendritic (D-D) synapses, including triads and serial synapses. Bullock suggested in 1959 that neuronal interaction may result from non-spike, graded electrotonic currents, and this hypothesis has now received strong experimental support (37). Studies of sensory transduction in the retina, and measurements of energy required to release transmitters in D-D synapses have shown that in some synapses, transmitter release is triggered by a relatively small change in membrane potential, well within the range of electrotonic currents in local circuits (23). Their role in the spread and generation of epileptogenic discharges has been studied well by Dudek's group (see Chapter 30).

Degeneration in Epileptic Brains

As new information develops on the architectonics of the normal brain, a new dynamic picture of cellular ultrastructure and circuitry in the epileptic brain is also emerging, requiring a concentrated multidisciplinary attack. Our classical concepts of progressive degeneration of the neuropil in the epileptic brain are based primarily on the structural studies of Penfield and collaborators (237,239,240) and Alexander and Woodhall (4), which were performed between 1940 and 1942. They described loss of neurons, glial proliferation, increased numbers of blood vessels, and compound granular corpuscles. In 1974, Scheibel et al. (273) first showed progressive pathology of dendrites, namely, dendritic spine loss and nodular changes in dendritic shafts of neurons in the hippocampus of human epileptics. Recently, Scheibel has described abnormalities in the basement membrane of the microvascular tree as a possible reason for the degeneration of dendritic bundles (Scheibel, 1984, *personal communication*). In 1964, Westrum, et al. had reported findings similar to

Scheibel's within the alumina cream-induced epileptic foci of monkeys (344). Harris had also emphasized glial structural changes in addition to neuronal pathology. Degeneration of axons, terminals, and dendrites continued for many years as progressive changes involved an increasing number of filaments in cellular processes, and an increased number of connections, gap junctions, and puncta-adherentia between cells appeared. The significance of these increasing connections is not known, but they may be important for initiation, spread, and arrest of seizures (115,116). Meanwhile, Butler et al. (40) also reported that cobalt preferentially involves pyramidal cell dendrites as well as astrocytes during evolution of epileptiform discharges.

Recently, White has identified axo-axonic synapses on the initial segment of the pyramidal neurons with denuded dendrites. White postulates that these axo-axonic synapses from Golgi Type II cells could be the morphologic explanation for the hyperexcitable state of neurons in the focus (115,116). In contrast, Ribak et al. claim that small multipolar cells in the seizure focus are decreased (255). Ribak et al. examined the distribution of GAD (glutamate decarboxylase) positive axon terminals, which are known to belong to smooth and sparsely spined stellate cells, in the alumina cream epileptogenic focus. Brown reported similar findings in the hippocampus of epileptics with temporal lobe seizures (36).

Fischer et al. studied the number, size, and shape of synaptic vesicles in electron micrographs of the projected cortical epileptic focus (88–90). Fifteen minutes after application of penicillin, synaptic vesicles in the mirror focus increased. Thirty minutes after application of penicillin, thinning of synaptic and glial membranes, changes in synaptic densities, in the distances between the pre- and postsynaptic densities, and in synaptic configurations were found. Fischer and Langmeier emphasized the increase in the number of synaptic vesicles close to the synaptic cleft and suggested that these morphometric changes explained the development of the secondary focus (90).

Glial cells have also received attention lately because reactive astrocyte proliferation is the most consistent abnormal cytological feature in the epileptic focus. Freeze-fracture electronmicroscopic studies of astrocytic plasma membranes have shown that astrocytic membranes are radically altered within 30 min to 3 hr following epileptic freeze lesions. One to 7 months later, intramembraneous protein particle com-

plexes, called assemblies, increase; their configuration changes into large squares and long rectangles. This change in astrocytic membrane
structure has implications not only in astrocyte
membrane transport of ions and proteins but
also in astrocyte neuronal interactions (see
Chapter 38).

Chemical Neuroanatomy

The new methods of neurocytology that examine neurotransmitter function and neuronal
circuitry through immunocytochemistry, receptor autoradiography, and computer-assisted
quantitative morphometry should lead to a
better understanding of the relationships between morphological and biochemical changes
in the epileptic brain. The indirect immunoperoxidase method commonly used for localization
of antigens at both light and electron microscopic level has been well applied to the study
of glutamate decarboxylase containing neurons.
The loss of GABAergic terminals at epileptic
foci of the alumina cream in monkey brains has
already been mentioned. Similar immunocytochemical methods for choline acetyltransferase,
noradrenaline serotonin, and neuroactive peptides (e.g., enkephalins and substance P) should
now find applications in studies of both partial
and generalized epilepsies. Although the cholinergic projection systems of the septum, nucleus
of the diagonal band, and Maynert's basal nucleus and the intrinsic cholinergic systems in the
cerebral cortex and hippocampus are still being
studied, there are early reports of increased noradrenergic axon terminal density in the cerebral
cortex, hippocampus, subcortical nuclei, and
cerebellum of tottering mice with spike-wave
seizures (225), increased sprouting of noradrenergic nerve terminals in the epileptogenic
freezing lesion (59), but decreased noradrenergic
synapse density in the cobalt epileptogenic focus
(321). Although GAD-containing neurons are reported to decrease in the alumina cream focus
(255), GAD-containing neurons and axon terminals have recently been reported to increase
in the septal half of the hippocampal dentate
gyrus of the Mongolian gerbil with grand mal
and myoclonic seizures (see Chapter 37) and in
the inferior caliculus of the genetic epilepsy
prone rate with audiogenic seizures.

Incisural Sclerosis: Epileptic Cell Damage

Excitotoxic Glutamate/Aspartate
Destroys Neurons

Ever since 1880, when Sommer established a
pattern of histological damage in Ammon's horn
("Ammon's horn scleroses") among chronic
epileptics (299), investigators have wondered
whether the damage caused epilepsy or whether
scleroses were effects of sustained seizures.
Neuropathological observations by Corsellis
and Bruton (51) and experimental studies by
Meldrum et al. (205) and subsequently by
Chapman (43) and Seisjo (293) have now clearly
shown that hippocampal sclerosis results from
repeated seizures and convulsive status epilepticus. Corsellis and Bruton showed destruction
of selectively vulnerable nerve cells in the hippocampus, amygdala cerebellum, thalamus, and
the middle cerebral cortical layers occur among
infants, children, and adults who died shortly
after status epilepticus (51). Meldrum et al. (205)
and Siesjo (293) showed that selective cell
damage is related to the duration of convulsive
status epilepticus and continues even in ventilated animals whose metabolic side effects are
corrected (43,51). In these experiments with
bicuculline convulsive status, selective cell
damage appears after 60 min of convulsive
status. Clinical and experimental evidence also
now exists demonstrating that sustained complex partial seizures consistently result in a pattern of cellular damage similar to hippocampal
sclerosis if allowed to continue for more than 1
hr. Most important, the "dendrosomatotoxic
axon-sparing nature of cell damage" suggests
that major excitatory transmitters participate in
the genesis of epileptic cell damage (229,296).
Olney's school from St. Louis proposes that the
cholinergic system contributes to initiation and
maintenance of seizures, whereas the gluta-
mate/aspartate system is responsible for the excitotoxic destruction of neurons (227–229,296).

Enhanced Local Metabolic Rate and Oxygen
Insufficiency Are Partly Responsible for
Cell Death

Meldrum et al. (205) and Siesjo (293) concluded that vulnerable neurons succumb in spite
of adequate oxygenation and an adequate energy
state. Meldrum et al. documented in the first
minute of convulsion a ninefold increase in cerebral blood flow (CBF) and a fourfold increase
in glucose consumption. Subsequently, CBF
dropped to a twofold level after 60–120 min of
convulsion, whereas glucose consumption was
stoichiometrically matched to O_2 consumption
at two to three times control values. The phosphorylation state of the adenine nucleotide pool

was close to normal after 2 hr of status epilepticus. In fact, since neuronal lesions were ameliorated rather than accentuated by a restriction of cerebral oxygen supply, he proposed that cell death resulted purely from excessively increased metabolic demands by the vulnerable cell. In addition, Siesjo (293) contends that histopathological damage is already present after 1 hr of status epilepticus, at a time when a mismatch between metabolic rate and blood flow has not yet developed. Moreover, as mentioned above, ventilation with 100% O_2 does not ameliorate the lesions. Thus, like Meldrum et al., Siesjo concluded that excessive enhancement of local metabolic rate causes selective cell death.

An opposite school contends that oxygen insufficiency is at least partially responsible for the neuronal damage inflicted by repeated depolarizations and status epilepticus (155). Kreisman et al. showed that cortical PO_2 and oxidations of cytochrome α, α^3 transiently increased during initial convulsions, confirming that oxygen provision is sufficient to meet metabolic demand early during status. After seizures had progressed for 20 min, however, a transition took place. Tissue PO_2 and cytochrome α, α^3 reductions decreased, signaling cortical oxygen insufficiency. This transition from oxygen sufficiency to insufficiency was presumably due to inappropriate vascular reactivity, resulting in decreased delivery of oxygen to focal areas of metabolically hyperactive cerebral tissues. These investigators conclude that 20 min of status epilepticus is an important transitional state, after which regional oxygen insufficiency becomes an important factor that adds to further cell damage (155).

What has clearly emerged from these various studies is that selective cell damage is already present after 60 min of convulsive status even in properly ventilated and physiologically maintained animals (197,205,293). During the first 20 min, regulatory homeostatic systems are still operational and intact. Glucose and free fatty acid utilization proceeds rapidly to compensate for the increased metabolic rates due to the hyperexcitable state. Cerebral blood flow increases, and PO_2 levels suffice for prolonged periods of time. However, as the seizure progresses past 20 min, regulatory mechanisms break down and the increase in CBF is somewhat reduced, whereas cerebral metabolic rates (CMR) continue to increase in relation to continuing seizure discharge. Increasing lactate levels and decreasing glucose sources, coupled with the differential in CMR and CBF, lead to a metabolic

and O_2 insufficiency that results in further cell damage. These findings correlate well with the clinical observation that the longer the duration of status epilepticus the more likely complications are to develop (197,205).

Ca^{2+} and Arachidonic Acid Are Also Toxic to Cells

After convulsive status starts, a number of other biochemical events are known to occur that could also contribute to selective cell damage. Meldrum et al. (197,205) and Siesjo (293) attribute cell damage to an abnormal influx of calcium into postsynaptic dendrites and cell bodies and claim that this ionic event starts a cascade of reactions that lead to cell death. Chapman (43), with Siesjo (293) and Bazan et al. (21), independently showed that polyenoic fatty acids, particularly arachidonic acid and arachidonyl diglycerols, accumulate in selectively vulnerable regions during status epilepticus. A burst of oxidative reactions along the fatty acid cyclooxygenase and the lipoxygenase pathways leads to the formation of prostaglandins and leukotrienes, respectively. These compounds are potentially toxic to cells, cause brain edema, and, together with the breakdown of the membrane phospholipid pool, could be responsible for the selective cell death observed in status epilepticus (21).

There are still other biochemical consequences of sustained seizure that may play a role in cell damage. One is the release of cyclic nucleotides even in ventilated animals. There is also a complex release of hormonal factors (increases in plasma prolactin, growth hormone, ACTH, cortisol, insulin, glucagon, epinephrine, and norepinephrine) during seizures that could affect subsequent neuronal metabolism and cause a loss of capability for physiological responsiveness and cell death (99,197).

PRIORITY RESEARCH CHALLENGES IN THE EPILEPSIES

Cell Physiology in Hippocampal Slices and Biochemical Membrane Studies in Human Partial Epilepsies

The 1982 Kroc Foundation Workshops and the 1983 International Symposium on the Basic Mechanisms of the Epilepsies in San Diego, through formal and informal deliberations, developed a conceptual blueprint for priority challenges in epilepsy research (59). In addition,

TABLE 10. *Top priority challenges in epilepsy research for the next decade[a]*

1. Understand molecular mechanisms of partial epilepsies in humans by using electrophysiological recordings of hippocampal and neocortical slices in *in vitro* and molecular biochemical techniques. Understand mechanisms of cell bursting and synchronization in humans; are they heritable traits? Specify cell and membrane mechanisms of interictal to ictal transformation and their relation to genetic predisposition to epilepsy.

2. Assess biochemical functions of chronic epileptic human brains *in situ*, using PET and NMR imaging, to uncover epileptogenic sites in damaged brain areas. The roles of disinhibition, altered ionic conductances, and responses to excitatory neurotransmitters can then be defined *in situ* in these epileptogenic sites.

3. Search for epilepsy genes in human monogenic and polygenic epilepsies, their chromosomal localization and the isolation of their amino acid sequence abnormalities. Study interrelationships between the monogenic and polygenic epilepsies on one hand and the acquired partial epilepsies on the other, in both humans and animals, e.g., *Papio papio* and DBA mice, with and without focal brain lesions with respect to electrophysiology and biochemistry.

4. Understand relations between brain development, kindling, and epileptic cell damage, e.g., ontogenesis of seizure mechanisms, neonatal seizures, brain nutrition, development of epilepsy, and their consequences. Can seizures change neuronal circuits to cause epilepsy? Apply new methods of neurocytology and neuroanatomy in studying the development of epilepsy, in addition to cellular and molecular biochemical studies. Address effects of hypoxia, infarction, and hemorrhage on epilepsy-prone brains. Discover mechanisms of epileptogenic cell death: Are free fatty acids (arachidonic acid) or prostaglandins or leukotrienes or enhanced calcium influx or glutamate–aspartate the triggers for the events leading to epileptic cell damage?

5. Explore new approaches to treatment. Develop new categories of antiepileptic drugs, e.g., calcium channel blockers; assess metabolic and replacement treatment of epilepsy with amino acids, trace metals, phosphates, etc.; and explore so-called endogenous antiepileptic substances as potential drugs for replacement treatment. Can epileptic cell damage be prevented in humans by calcium channel blockers and glutamate–aspartate antagonists?

[a] Most common top priority challenges listed by 64 neuroscientists who participated in the 1982 Kroc Foundation Workshops and the 1983 San Diego International Symposium on Basic Mechanisms of the Epilepsies.

after the Workshop and the International Symposium, all the participants were canvassed for their opinion on the top five priority challenges in epilepsy research (Table 10). All agreed that unraveling mechanisms of human epilepsies remains the ultimate goal and the top priority challenge is to solve human partial epilepsies, which afflict approximately 1.3 million persons in the United States.

In the past 10 years, experimental partial epilepsies have been studied by detailed analysis of simple neuronal model systems, followed by verification of their results in integrated complex systems of vertebrate spinal cords and brains. As we reach the turn of the twentieth century, this approach is more promising than ever for human epilepsy because of the following new technological developments: (1) the availability of human temporal lobe and cerebral cortical specimens from "*en bloc*" resections—e.g., anterior temporal lobectomies and corticectomies—and the popularity of brain tissue slices for *in vitro* electrophysiological studies; (2) the use of single-electrode voltage-clamp and patch-clamp methods in dissociated cell cultures of the hippocampus; (3) the advent of human brain banks as a source of tissue specimens for various studies; and (4) the successful application

of microchemistry, subcellular fractionation, and bulk isolation methods for studying membrane fractions enriched in synaptic terminals, synaptic plasma membranes, synaptic vesicles, postsynaptic densities, neuronal soma, and glial cells.

These technological advances have been applied especially to human temporal lobe epilepsy. Most neuroscientists, attending the Kroc Foundation Workshops and San Diego Symposium, also agreed that a more specific priority challenge in human temporal lobe epilepsy is the search for PDSs in *in vitro* hippocampal slices excised from known sites of epileptogenicity. Understanding how neuronal systems enhance excitability, produce long-term potentiation, and endogenously regenerate epileptiform discharges in human and animal brain slices are some of the more specific challenges enumerated (Table 11).

Several laboratories have taken up these challenges. Schwartzkroin, for example, recently described the necessity of using thick hippocampal slices to detect spontaneous rhythmic postsynaptic potentials (see Chapter 50). Earlier, Wong and Prince had observed stimulus evoked PDS-like events in neocortical cells of human brain slices that contained epileptic foci.

TABLE 11. *Some specific priority challenges in epilepsy research*[a]

1. Clarify the role of the GABA/glutamate system in partial epilepsies in humans. Study cerebrospinal fluid neurotransmitters and metabolites and determine if predictive correlations can be made during drug treatment.

2. Clarify the possible periodic transformation of the GABA inhibitory input to an excitatory system in partial epilepsies and the influence of phenylalanine, ph fluctuations and glucose metabolism, and Ca^{2+}/Zn^{2+} ratios.

3. Develop more accurate animal models for human focal epilepsy (especially complex partial epilepsy) and primary generalized human epilepsy. Study animal models of epileptogenesis that more closely resemble the human condition.

4. Do all animal models of focal epilepsy display a preferential loss of GABAergic synapses? Are similar observations present in human focal epilepsy?

5. Is the increase in GABAergic neurones and axon terminals present in all animal models of generalized epilepsies?

6. What gene or genes regulate the formation of GABAergic neurons? What genes regulate ion channels and transmitter systems? What is their role in epilepsy?

7. Study the development of normal and epilepsy-prone brains: the effects of brain injuries on perinatal development of mitochondrial calcium uptake system and relationship to development of epilepsy.

8. What are the functional and chemical anatomies of primarily generalized epilepsies? Work on the metabolism, localization, and physiological actions of traditional and new transmitters and modulators, particularly those with long-duration actions on voltage-dependent membrane events.

9. Is the release of free fatty acids, particularly arachidonic acid, engaged in a selective receptor-mediated sequence of events in epileptic cell damage? Is protein phosphorylation involved? Why do diglycerides enriched in stearate-arachidonate accumulate in brains during convulsions?

10. What is the role of prostaglandin and lypoxygenase–leukotriene pathways in epilepsy and epileptic cell damage?

11. Document the presence of paroxysmal depolarization shifts in hippocampal slices from human temporal lobe epilepsy. Understand long-term potentiation and regeneration of epileptiform discharges.

[a] Some specific priorities listed by individual participants in the 1982 Kroc Foundation Workshop and 1983 San Diego International Symposium on Basic Mechanisms of the Epilepsies.

Although *in vitro* studies of human brain slices with epileptic foci are in their infancy, the technology of human hippocampal slice unit recordings can now be refined to pave the way for classical voltage, single-electrode voltage-clamp, and patch-clamp studies. Current and voltage-clamp techniques are necessary to detect changes in current/voltage (I/V) relationship and synaptic current events (346,347,349). To explain neuronal burstings and PDSs, the actions of transmitter agonists and antagonists, neuromodulators, as well as the effects of ionic and protein chemistry alterations, can be tested.

Parallel experiments exploring biochemical membrane abnormalities in subcellular neuronal and glial membranes isolated from the epileptogenic cortex of humans are now being performed in Liege, Paris, and Vancouver (244), Montreal (327), Seattle (253), and Los Angeles (107). Defining the precise molecular abnormalities of these focal epilepsies will be especially valuable in explaining the functional abnormalities recorded by the electrophysiologists. Elec-

tron paramagnetic resonance studies of red cell membranes in patients with genetically determined generalized epilepsies had suggested a water permeability defect (22), and similar studies should be done in partial epilepsies. Tower's hypothesis of impaired K^+ transport in human partial epilepsy has recently been confirmed and refined by Grisar and Delgado-Escueta (107). Not only have inefficient synaptic and glial N^+K^+-ATPase enzymes been demonstrated in human temporal lobectomy specimens, but the inability of glial N^+K^+-ATPase to clear $[K^+]_o$ has been blamed for at least part of the biochemical events subserving ictal transformation (107,108).

Reports on GABA/glutamic acid neurotransmitter systems in human epileptic foci continue to be conflicting (244,245,327). And the most recent data from Montreal and Paris show more incongruent results (Table 4). Van Gelder et al. (327) and Sherwin et al. (289) showed a relative diminution in glutamic acid and aspartic acid, whereas glycine concentrations increased in cortical tissues that were active with epileptiform spikes. They noted a significant rise in glutamic acid dehydrogenase (GDH), the enzyme predominantly involved in the reductive amination of 2-oxoglutaric acid to form glutamic acid. In contrast, GAD, glutamine synthetase, and GABA amino transferase did not change significantly (289). The absence of change in GAD (the enzyme responsible for the formation of GABA), was in contrast to the reports of Lloyd in collaboration with Morselli (172) who observed a drop in GAD activity and the number of GABA binding sites in human seizure foci, particularly those secondary to tumors. Changes in amino acid content of CSF have also been found in human epileptics (59). Aspartic acid, glutamic acid, histidine, and lysine levels were elevated, whereas alanine, methionine, and threonine levels were decreased relative to the normal population. Sherwin et al. (289) also observed higher tyrosine hydroxylase activities and a concomitant decrease in β-adrenergic receptor binding sites (B_{max}) in epileptic cortex. These conflicting data over GABA concentrations, GAD activities, and the hypothesis of the glutamate/GABA ratio as a critical determinant of excitation or inhibition in human focal epilepsy, should be resolved by collaborative efforts. Conflicting reports can best be resolved by sharing human tissues excised through the Falconer method of "*en bloc*" anterior temporal lobectomy and the Penfield method of "corticectomy" or anterior temporal lobectomy. The method of Falconer has the advantage of having large materials for collaborative morphological, physiological, and biochemical studies. Most often, however, these tissues are obtained under general anesthesia and optimal antiepileptic drug management. The Penfield method of anterior temporal lobectomy or corticectomy yields smaller amounts of tissue, but is obtained under local anesthesia and after complete withdrawal of antiepileptic drugs (see Chapter 51). Conflicting results may well result from the method of excision and the presence of general anesthesia and/or antiepileptic drugs. Protocol using similar biochemical methods are needed so that data from different laboratories can be integrated.

Biochemistry of the Functioning Epileptic Human Brain *In Situ*

The second top priority challenge listed by the polled neuroscientists consists of developing new biochemical screening methods (such as PET and NMR) to uncover epileptogenic sites in damaged brain areas of patients with chronic epilepsies. In addition to already existing technology in PET, single-photon emission computed tomography (SPECT) (66,84,183), and nuclear magnetic resonance computed tomography (NMR-CT) (193), advances in the radiochemistry of positron-labeled compounds should allow assessment of abnormal neurotransmitter systems, ion pathways, and antiepileptic drug metabolism in living patients. The local CMR for glucose using 2-deoxyglucose labelled with ^{18}F has been measured interictally in over 120 patients and ictally in six psychomotor patients (78,80,193). Reports showed focal areas of decreased cerebral glucose metabolic activity (hypometabolic zones) in the interictal state. Engel and collaborators proved that these hypometabolic zones: (a) reflected structural abnormalities, (b) corresponded to EEG evidence of depressed function, and (c) complemented the EEG in assessing the site of epileptogenicity in candidates for anterior temporal lobectomy (79,80,159). A few patients studied interictally with ^{13}NH$_3$ and FDG demonstrated focal reductions in CBF in the hypometabolic zones (159). Bernardi et al. (26) also showed that mean CBF and CMR for oxygen can be reduced ipsilateral to the temporal lobe seizure focus with maximal reductions in the temporal cortex. Oxygen extraction fractions, on the other hand, were significantly increased in the entire temporal lobe ipsilateral to the seizure focus. A relative increase in glucose utilization at anatomical sites, which are hypometabolic in the interictal state, generally occurs during ictal episodes of partial seizures (79,80,159,314).

PET studies of patients with epilepsy have thus far used only measurements of blood flow and oxygen and glucose utilization. PET approaches have also been developed to measure such variables as protein synthesis, blood–brain barrier, diffusion pH, water content (311); dopamine (96,333), benzodiazepine (50), and opiate receptor binding (192) of ligands (212); and brain metabolism of antiepileptic drugs ([^{11}C]diphenylhydantoin (19), [^{11}C]valproate) (Table 7). This ability of PET to assess regional biochemical functions *in situ* should provide one means of evaluating the basic mechanisms of epilepsy in humans.

A number of tracers have also been developed for the measurement of CBF using SPECT. Although these compounds, which include xenon-133, N-isopropyl-*p*-(^{123}I)-iodoamphetamine (IMP), and ^{123}I-labeled hydroxyiodopropyldiazine (HIPDm) (193), are in an early stage of development, there are now three reports of SPECT in epilepsy. CBF was decreased in some patients with partial seizures; the hypoperfused regions were more extensive than predicted by the EEG focus. NMR scanning will also soon be used to study biochemical processes in human epilepsies, with studies of carbon- and phosphorus-containing compounds (e.g., ATP) as well as ions like K^+. The combined use of PET, SPECT, and NMR should greatly improve our understanding of the *in vivo* ion transport pathways, neurotransmitter systems, and metabolism of the brains of epileptic patients (193).

Gene Mapping in Human Generalized Epilepsies: Candidate Gene Markers

At present, epilepsies come to the attention of clinicians because of disturbances expressed at the level of cells and systems of the brain as manifested by clinical signs and symptoms and electrographic discharges. Understandably, most epilepsy research efforts have addressed the abnormalities of cells and molecules associated with neuronal, glial, and neurotransmitter dysfunctions of the brain. However, to be fully understood, the epilepsies must be explored at all levels of expression—the DNA, protein, and cell-system dysfunctions. This goal was clearly expressed in the poll of neuroscientist-epileptologists (Table 10).

In fact, the third most important priority challenge enumerated by epileptologists is the need for human gene mapping in the generalized epilepsies and for developing candidate gene markers. Epilepsy genes should be sought in monogenic and polygenic epilepsies in humans; their chromosomal location and the isolation of their amino acid sequence abnormalities, using molecular genetics and recombinant DNA technology, should be accomplished. Studies on the interrelationships between genetic and acquired epilepsies was also enumerated as one more specific priority challenge (Table 11). The complete etiological sequence for expression of seizures in genetic epilepsies of animals and humans was also listed as a specific priority challenge.

Genetic variations of a restriction endonuclease site closely linked to specific diseases have now been detected in the sickle mutation (148), Duchenne Dystrophy XP21 (261), and most recently in Huntington's chorea (chromosome 4) (111). Polymorphisms of restriction endonuclease patterns should thus be sought in monogenic forms of epilepsies; all epileptologists were hopeful that the abnormal gene(s) in specific epilepsies will soon be detected. When the chromosomal location of a gene is not known, the principles of classical genetic linkage and protein polymorphisms can be used to map the location of the epilepsy gene in a given chromosome (8,32,111,126,286). Unfortunately, once the location of a specific epilepsy gene is narrowed down to a region of 10^6 base pairs, the problem of identifying the actual molecular defect is difficult, since we have no assay or method to show that a given gene is culpable for epilepsy (111,126,286). A solution, suggested by White (see Chapter 2), is to use, as candidate gene markers, DNA fragments of proteins, abnormalities of which are suspected to cause epileptic attacks in experimental models of genetic epilepsies (60,345). If the protein suspected to cause seizures in an animal model of epilepsy is actually the cause of a human form of epilepsy, the loci or molecular sites of both the suspected protein and the human epilepsy would be the same in a given chromosome and would have 0% recombination (60,345).

Following White's suggestions, several laboratories are now rapidly seeking the amino acid sequences of proteins suspected to be abnormal in experimental epilepsies (Tables 2 and 3) and in human epilepsies (Table 4); their sequenced fragments are to be used as markers (restriction fragment length polymorphisms or RFLPs) for genetic linkage studies in human epilepsies (60). Candidate gene markers such as N^+K^+-ATPase (107,253,302) the Na^+ gating proteins (42,224), the Ca^{2+} gating proteins (248,250), and the GABA receptor (230) are being envisioned as probes. In addition, many other markers may prove as useful (outlined in Tables 2 and 3). The effort is to separate mendelizing phenotypes of epilepsy such as absence, benign juvenile myoclonic and Rolandic epilepsies, and fatal progressive myoclonic epileptic encephalopathies (59,60).

Theoretically, these strategies of research, using recombinant DNA methods, are more easily applied to animal models of genetic epilepsies, such as the seizure-prone Mongolian gerbil, the audiogenic-induced seizures of mice, and the mutant tottering mouse. Perhaps the best model would be the mutant tottering mouse, whose single-gene defect is known to be in chromosome 8 (225). Noebels initially analyzed several forms of inherited seizures using single locus mutations in mice, and described "absence with diffuse 6- to 8-Hz spike-waves and focal motor seizures in the mutant mouse tottering." Noebels showed that a different genotype may be responsible for clinically identical forms of seizures in mice; he linked the increased number of noradrenergic axons in the terminal fields innervated by the nucleus LC to the epileptic trait of the mutant mouse tottering (225). To identify the specific gene (or genes) in the mutant tottering mice, White suggested the use of insertion retroviruses to mutagenize the gene and, hence, to tag it molecularly. If the disorder is recessive, inactivating the homologous gene, in the wild type mouse it may occasionally produce the tottering phenotype, presumably as a result of the insertion of new elements into that gene. Creation of a DNA library from this mouse strain and utilization of their amino acid sequences as radioactive probes for this DNA library should isolate the version of the wild type gene that was inactivated by the retrovirus. The same labeled genome can then be used for studies of expression and regulation of an epileptic gene in brains of normal and seizure-susceptible animals.

A. Tobin recently (*personal communication*, 1984) suggested a novel way to test the role of GAD and GABA receptor (GABA-R) in epilepsy. He proposed to block specifically the expression of the genes for GAD or GABA-R in mice and to see if epilepsy results. This method of genetic engineering should be used to test the role of various proteins in epilepsy.

The pro-opiomelanocortin (POMC) gene recently localized to chromosome 2p is another such protein that has recently acquired prominence as a modulator of epileptic activity (124). It is an excellent example of a model for studying regulation of gene expression (see Chapter 25). Studies of the organization of the POMC gene have revealed the surprise that the entire region coding for active products of POMC resides within a single continuous nucleotide domain of the gene (123,124). At least three different genes code for the opioid peptides. One gene codes for POMC from which β-endorphin, ACTH, and melanocyte-stimulating hormones are derived. A second gene codes for Pro-enkephalin. A third gene codes for the protein precursor of dynorphin and α-neo-endorphin. The products of POMC can be anticonvulsants (β-endorphin) (13) or convulsants (enkephalins) (93,94), and are extremely important in the regulation of epileptic behavior.

Relation of Genetic Epilepsies to Acquired Epilepsies

As mentioned earlier, recombinant DNA technology can also be applied to a more specific priority challenge (Table 11), namely studies that address the interrelationship between the mon-ogenic and polygenic epilepsies on one hand and acquired brain lesions on another. Electrophysiological, biochemical, and modern neuroanatomical methods should be applied in order to understand how such epilepsies are expressed clinically. For instance, recombinant DNA technology has improved our picture of receptor and channel proteins and has raised questions on the synthesis of these protein subunits and on their assembly into functional oligomeric complexes. If abnormalities in ion transport accompany neuronal hyperexcitability in partial epilepsies and the PDS, it is only reasonable to ask if abnormalities exist in the structure of channel proteins in these forms of epilepsies. Are there abnormalities in biogenesis of important membrane channel proteins and other membrane-bound proteins involved in ionic homeostasis? Although the studies of these proteins are in a transition period, the success achieved in defining the ACH receptor as a tightly associated noncovalent complex of four large (50,000 MW) glycoprotein subunits in stoichiometry (7) should encourage epileptologists to pursue the cell biology of membrane protein synthesis that is important in experimental models and human forms of epilepsy.

Neonatal Seizures, Mirror Focus, Kindling, and Epileptic Cell Damage

The fourth top priority challenge listed are studies that explain the molecular basis of neonatal seizures, the effects of neonatal nutrition, how epilepsy subsequently develops, and whether all these events have a role in hippocampal-amygdalar epilepsy with the development of chronic enhanced states of excitability such as the mirror focus and the kindling phenomenon (Table 10). Perhaps the best systems that emphasize how abnormal cell–cell communication can lead to chronic enhanced states of excitability are the two paradigms: the mirror or secondary focus of Morrell et al. (216,217), and the kindling phenomenon of Goddard (100). Physiological investigations in both paradigms have revealed long-lasting alterations and enhancement of evoked potentials; long-term potentiation (LTP) may even involve the same process as kindling. In both models, phenytoin is far less effective than phenobarbital, and for prophylaxis, diazepam or phenobarbital is more effective (100).

In kindling phenomenon, muscarinic cholinergic receptors have been implicated by Wasterlain (341). In both the kindling phenomenon and the mirror focus, depletion of noradrenaline facilitates paroxysms (41,291,332). Reduction of brain dopamine or serotonin (5-HT) also facilitates paroxysms in both models. Although benzodiazepine receptors, GABA, and GABA-Rs have yet to be clearly delineated, some electrophysiologic studies are now available, which suggest that inhibition is not reduced in both models and may even be increased. Hence, excitation is claimed to play a bigger role in both models (100).

Some researchers claim that LTP may involve the same process as kindling and in fact may provide part of the explanation for kindling. There is as yet no clear proof that LTP always remains during kindling. Some studies show kindling outlasting LTP (100). Baudry (20) recently proposed a model for LTP in which calcium influx stimulates a Ca^{2+}-dependent enzyme that specifically degrades cytoskeleton-associated proteins, in particular the spectrin-like protein fodrin. Fodrin regulates cell surface receptors and the shape of dendritic spines. Its degradation unmasks and increases glutamate receptors and eventually leads to structural changes and enhanced cell excitability (20).

Wasterlain (341), in collaboration with DeLorenzo (65), has recently proposed that calcium influx decreases calcium calmodulin-dependent protein kinase (50,000 MW). Diazepam inhibits phosphorylation of this Ca^{2+} calmodulin-dependent protein kinase; this may explain how diazepam prevents kindling. More recently, Baimbridge and Miller (210) have described decreased levels of calcium-binding proteins in granule cells of the dentate gyrus after kindling as afterdischarges appear and inhibition increases. The role of posttranslational processes, such as protein phosphorylation, acetylation, and methylation as modifiers of protein function in epileptogenic processes clearly needs further investigation (65,284).

The pace of experiments on LTP and kindling has indeed been rapid. In all these experiments, the crucial test remains as to whether changes described in protein function or neurotransmitter systems last long enough to explain the durability of kindling. Within this field of abnormal cell–cell and transynaptic communication lies also the central question of its relevance to human epilepsy. We still do not know if the kindling phenomenon has relevance to the generation of human epilepsy. In his 1983 Merritt-Putnam address, Goldensohn questioned the validity of kindling as a clinical concept and whether the "development of a mirror focus" should guide our judgment to early excision of the primary seizure focus (103). Morrell (216)

has provided evidence from 11 humans with mirror foci in intermediate stages and five humans with fully independent autonomous mirror foci. These studies, however, require substantiation; the concept of the mirror focus in primates has been challenged by other independent studies (117). These arguments, plus the rare incidence of clinical seizures produced by mirror areas, continuously nag investigators about whether kindling and the mirror phenomenon have a real role in human epileptogenesis. This question clearly must be resolved.

If the role of kindling and the mirror focus in generation of human epilepsy is uncertain, we can still learn from these models about neuronal plasticity, memory, and the spread of seizures. In humans, one of the devastating effects of prolonged epileptogenic discharges in both temporal lobes is impairment of recent memory. Understanding of how transient and permanent cell dysfunction occurs may be achieved by studies of the kindling phenomenon and the mirror focus. Discovering the mechanisms of temporary or permanent impairment of recent memory after complex partial status epilepticus or convulsive status epilepticus should also help uncover some mechanisms for epileptic cell damage.

New Methods of Epilepsy Treatment

Developing new classes of antiepileptic drugs and new principles of epilepsy treatment is the fifth most important priority challenge; most neuroscientists listed the clarification of methods of cell bursting synchronization, spread of discharges, and the ways in which the brain stops seizures by itself as a prerequisite to this challenge (Table 10).

The spur to develop new categories of antiepileptic drugs has been prompted by new discoveries of how PDSs epileptiform paroxysms and seizures may stop. The new notion of endogenous anticonvulsants such as β-endorphin, CCK, adenosine, inosine, hypoxanthine, and other newly synthesized dipeptides being released during a convulsion to induce a postconvulsive refractory period, compels us to search for more substances that may have similar function (13). These discoveries also prompt us to consider a new principle in epilepsy treatment, namely, replacement therapy with endogenous anticonvulsants. Antiepileptic drugs, such as valproic acid, that act at inhibitory command posts, such as the GABA system in the substantia nigra, should also be sought at the same time that we search for other inhibitory command posts in the basal ganglia and brainstem (132). More GABAergic drugs and antagonists of excitatory amino acids, such as 2-APH, must be developed for trials in human epilepsies. We should also search for antiepileptic drugs that promote glial protective mechanisms (351). Of equal importance are experimental attempts to stop ischemic and epileptic cell damage by calcium channel blockers or aspartate receptor antagonists such as those conducted by Meldrum and his colleages (see Chapter 42).

One issue that looms in the future of epilepsy treatment concerns the advances in techniques for intracerebral grafting using transplantation of embryonic neural tissue to the brain of host animals. This has recently been shown in rats with lesions in the intrinsic forebrain dopamine pathways (68). As more and more neurotransmitter and ion transport systems are found to be deficient in various forms of experimental epilepsies, e.g., if neuronal systems indeed are lacking GABA-Rs in experimental "grand mal" and "myoclonic epilepsy," a bold experiment would be to try grafting normal embryonic neuronal tissue in some genetic forms of epilepsies. Similarly, neuronal tissue, hyperproducing for a specific endogenous anticonvulsant, could also be grafted as a form of treatment in some forms of epilepsies unresponsive to conventional antiepileptic drugs.

REFERENCES

1. Abragam, A. (1961): *The Principles of Nuclear Magnetism.* Oxford University Press, London.
2. Adams, P. (1982): Voltage dependent conductances of vertebrate neurons. In: *TINS,* pp. 116–119, Elsevier Biomedical Press, Amsterdam.
3. Ahlquist, R. P. (1948): Study of adrenotropic receptors. *Am. J. Physiol.,* 153:586–560.
4. Alexander, L., and Woodhall, B. (1942): Calcified epileptogenic lesions as caused by incomplete interference with the blood supply of the diseased areas. *J. Trans. Am. Neurol. Assoc.,* 67:175–176.
5. Altshuler, H. L., Killam, E. K., and Killam, K. F. (1976): Biogenic amines and the photo-myoclonic syndrome in the baboon, *Papio papio. J. Pharmacol. Exp. Ther.,* 196:156–166.
6. Andermann, E. (1982): Multifactorial inheritance of generalized and focal epilepsy. In: *Genetic Basis of the Epilepsies,* edited by V. E. Anderson, W. A. Hauser, J. K. Penry, and C. F. Sing, pp. 355–374. Raven Press, New York.
7. Anderson, D. J. (1983): Acetylcholine receptor biosynthesis: From kinetics to molecular mechanism. *TINS,* 2:169–171. Elsevier Biomedical Press, Amsterdam.
8. Anderson, S., Bankier, A. T., Barrell, B. G., deBruijn, M. H. L., Coulson, A. R., Drovin, J., Eperon, I. C., Nierlich, D. P., Roe, B. A., Sanger, E., Schreier, P. H., Smith, A. J. H., Staden, R., and Young, I. G. (1981): Sequence and organization of the human mitochondrial genome. *Nature,* 290:457–465.
9. Anderson, E. S., and Hauser, W. A. (1984): The genetics of epilepsy. In: *Progress in Medical Genetics,* edited by A. G. Bearn, B. Childs, A. Motulsky.
10. Aronstam, R. S., Kellogg, C., and Abood, L. G. (1979): Development of muscarinic cholinergic receptors in inbred strains of mice: Identification of receptor heterogeneity and relation to audiogenic seizures susceptibility. *Brain Res.,* 162:231–241.
11. Ashton, D., Leysen, J. E., and Wauquier, A. (1980): Neurotransmitters and receptor binding in amygdaloid kindled rats: Serotonergic and noradrenergic modulatory effects. *Life Sci.,* 27(17):1547–1556.
12. Ayala, G. F., Dichter, M., Gumnit, R. J., Matsumoto, H., and Spencer, W. A. (1973): Genesis of epileptic interictal spikes—New knowledge of cortical feedback systems suggests a neurophysiological explanation of brief paroxysms. *Brain Res.,* 52:1–17.
13. Bajorek, J. G., Lee, R. J., and Lomax, P. (1984): Neuropeptides: A role as endogenous mediators or modulators of epileptic phenomena. *Ann. Neurol.,* 16(Suppl.):31–38.
14. Bajorek, J., and Delgado-Escueta, A. V. (1985): Neuronal protein phosphorylation in a seizure sensitive strain of mongolian gerbil. *J. Neurochem.* (in press).
15. Bakay, R. A., and Harris, A. B. (1981): Neurotransmitter, receptor and biochemical changes in monkey cortical epileptic foci. *Brain Res.,* 206(2):387–404.
16. Balcar, V. J., Pumain, R., Mark, J., Borg, J., and Mandel, P. (1978): GABA-mediated inhibition in the epileptogenic focus, a process which may be involved in the mechanism of the cobalt-induced epilepsy. *Brain Res.,* 154:182–185.
17. Baldy-Moulinier, M., Ariea, L. P., and Passonaut, P. (1973): HPC epilepsy produced by ouabain. *Eur. Neurol.,* 9:333–348.
18. Baraszko, J. J., Baanon, M. J., Bunney, B. S., and Roth, R. H. (1981): Intrastriatal kainic acid: Acute effects on electrophysiological and biochemical measures of nigrostriatal dopaminergic activity. *J. Pharmacol. Exp. Ther.,* 216:289–293.
19. Baron, J. C., Comar, D., Crouzel, C., et al. (1983): Brain regional pharmacokinetics of ^{11}C-labeled diphenylhydantoin and pimozide in man. In: *Positron Computed Tomography of the Brain,* edited by W. D. Heiss, and M. E. Phelps, pp. 212–224. Springer-Verlag, New York.
20. Baudry, M., and Lynch, G. (1980): Hypothesis regarding the cellular mechanisms responsible for long term synaptic potentiation in the hippocampus. *J. Exp. Neurol.,* 68:202.

21. Bazan, N. G., Birkle, D. L., Tang, W., and Reddy, T. S. (1986): The accumulation of free arachidonic acid, diglycerides, prostaglandins and lipoxygenase reaction products in the brain during experimental epilepsy. In: *Basic Mechanisms of the Epilepsies*, edited by A. V. Delgado-Escueta, A. A. Ward, Jr., D. Woodbury, and R. J. Porter, Chapter 44. Raven Press, New York (in press).

22. Benga, G., and Morariu, V. V. (1977): Membrane defect affecting water permeability in human epilepsy. *Nature*, 265:636–638.

23. Bennett, M. V. L., and Goodenough, D. (1978): Gap junctions. *Neurosci. Res. Program Bull.*, 16:373–486.

24. Berger, H. (1929): Ueber das elektrendephalogram des meuschen. *I mitteilung Arch. Psychiat. J. Nervenkr.*, 87:527.

25. Berger, H. (1935): Uber die entstehung der erscheinungen des grossen epileptischen anfalls. *Klin. Wochenschr.*, 14:217.

26. Bernardi, S., Trimble, M. R., Frackowiak, R. S., Wise, R. J., and Jones, T. (1983): An interictal study of partial epilepsy using positron emission tomography and the oxygen-15 inhalation technique. *J. Neurol. Neurosurg. Psychiatry*, 46(6):473–477.

27. Berti, F., Bernareggi, V., Folco, G. C., Feimagalli, R., and Paoletti, R. (1976): Prostaglandin E2 and cyclic nucleotides in rat convulsions and tremors. *Adv. Biochem. Psychopharmacol.*, 15:367–377.

28. Bierkamper, C. G., Craig, C. R., and Cenedella, R. J. (1976): Cerebral cortical sterol changes in cobalt induced epilepsy. *J. Fed. Proc.*, 35:544.

29. Bierkamper, C. G., and Cenedella, R. J. (1978): Induction of chronic epileptiform activity in the rat by an inhibitor of cholesterol synthesis, U18666A. *Brain Res.*, 150:343.

30. Bondy, S. C., Tepper, J. M., and Bettis, D. B. (1979): Seizure proneness and neurotransmitter uptake. *Neurochem. Res.*, 4(6):755–761.

31. Bonte, F. J., Stokely, E. M., Devous, M. D., et al. (1983): Single photon tomographic study of regional cerebral blood flow in epilepsy. *Arch. Neurol.*, 40:267–270.

32. Botstein, D., White, R. L., Skolnick, M., and Davis, R. W. (1980): Construction of a genetic linkage map in man using restriction fragment length polymorphisms. *Am. J. Hum. Genet.*, 32:314–331.

33. Bourn, W. M., Chin, L., and Picchioni, A. L. (1977): Effect of neonatal 6-hydroxydopamine treatment on audiogenic seizures. *Life Sci.*, 21(5):701–705.

34. Bowen, F., Karpiak, S. E., Demirjian, C., and Katzman, R. (1975): Sprouting of noradrenergic nerve terminals subsequent to freeze lesions of rat cerebral cortex. *Brain Res.*, 83:1–14.

35. Briere, R., Sherwin, A., Robitaille, Y., Olivier, A., Quesney, F., and Reader, T. (1985): Markers of altered adrenergic receptor function in human focal epilepsy. *Can. J. Neurol. Sci.* (in press).

36. Brown, W. J. (1973): Structural substrates of seizure foci in the human temporal lobe. In: *Epilepsy, Its Phenomena in Man*, edited by M. A. B. Brazier, pp. 339–374. Academic Press, Orlando, Florida.

37. Bullock, T. H. (1959): Neuron doctrine and electrophysiology. *Science*, 129:997.

38. Burchfiel, J. C., Duchoway, M. S., and Duffy, F. H. (1976): Kindling stimulation of the rat hippocampus: Altered neuronal sensitivity to microiontophoresis of acetylcholine. *Science*, 204:1096–1098.

39. Burger, M. M., Burnfir, B. M., Buckenbridge, B. Mch., and Sheppard, J. R. (1972): Growth control and cyclic alterations of cyclic AMP in the cell cycle. *Nature New Biol.*, 239:161–163.

40. Butler, A. B., Willmore, L. J., Fuller, P. M., and Bass, N. H. (1976): Focal alteration of dendrites and astrocytes in rat cerebral cortex during initiation of cobalt-induced epileptiform activity. *Exp. Neurol.*, 51:216–218.

41. Callaghan, D. A., and Schwark, W. S. (1980): Pharmacological modification of amygdaloid kindled seizures. *J. Neuropharmacol.*, 9:1131–1136.

42. Catterall, W. A. (1981): Localization of sodium channels in cultured neural cells. *J. Neurosci.*, 1:777–783.

43. Chapman, A. G. (1977): Effect of anticonvulsant drugs on brain amino acid metabolism and GABA turnover in neurotransmitters, In: *Seizures and Epilepsy II*, edited by R. G. Fariello, P. L. Morselli, K. G. Lloyd, L. F. Quesney, and J. Engel, Jr. Raven Press, New York.

44. Chauvel, P., and Trottier, S. (1986): The role of the noradrenergic ascending system in extinction of epileptic phenomena, In: *Basic Mechanisms of the Epilepsies*, edited by A. V. Delgado-Escueta, A. A. Ward, Jr., D. Woodbury, and R. J. Porter. Raven Press, New York (in press).

45. Chen, G., Ensor, C., and Bohner, B. (1954): Facilitation action of reserpine on central nervous system. *Proc. Soc. Expl. Biol. Med.*, 86:507–510.

46. Chronister, R. B., Sikes, R. W., and White, L. E., Jr. (1977): Axo-axonic synapses on initial segments of hippocampal pyramidal cells. Seventh Annual Meeting of the Society for Neuroscience. *J. Neurosci. Abstr.*, 3:196.

47. Ciesielski, L., Simler, S., and Mandel, P. (1981): Effect of repeated convulsive seizures on brain GABA levels. *Neurochem. Res.*, 6:267–273.

48. Colasanti, B. K., and Craig, C. R. (1973): Brain concentrations and synthesis rates of biogenic amines during chronic cobalt experimental epilepsy in the rat. *Neuropharmacology*, 12:221–232.

49. Collins, R. C., McLean, M., and Olney, J. (1980): Cerebral metabolic responses to systemic kainic acid: ^{14}Cdeoxyglucose studies. *Life Sci.*, 27:855–862.

50. Comar, D., Maziere, M., Gadot, J. M., Berger, G., and Soussaline, F. (1979): Visualization of ^{11}C-flunitrazepam displacement in the brain of the live baboon. *Nature*, 280:329–331.

51. Corsellis, J. A. N., and Bruton, C. J. (1983):

Neuropathology of status epilepticus in humans, In: *Status Epilepticus: Mechanisms of Brain Damage and Treatment, Advances in Neurology*, vol. 34. Edited by A. V. Delgado-Escueta, C. W. Wasterlain, D. M. Treiman, and R. J. Porter, pp. 129–140. Raven Press, New York.

52. Commission on Classification and Terminology of the International League Against Epilepsy (1981): Proposal for revised clinical and electroencephalographic classification of epileptic seizures. *Epilepsia,* 22:489–501.

53. Cox, B., and Lomax, P. (1976): Brain amines and spontaneous epileptic seizures in the Mongolian gerbil. *Pharmacol. Biochem. Behav.,* 4:263–267.

54. Craig, C. R., and Colasanti, B. K. (1986): GABA receptors, lipids and gangliosides in cobalt epileptic focus. In: *Basic Mechanisms of the Epilepsies,* edited by A. V. Delgado-Escueta, A. A. Ward, Jr., D. M. Woodbury, and R. J. Porter. Raven Press, New York (in press).

55. Cromwell, R. M. (1980): Distant effects of local epileptogenic process. *Brain Res.,* 18:137–154.

56. Croucher, M. J., and Meldrum, B. S. (1984): Role of dicarboxylic amino acids in epilepsy and the use of antagonists as antiepileptic agents. In: *Neurotransmitters, Seizures and Epilepsy II,* edited by R. G. Fariello, P. L. Morselli, K. G. Lloyd, L. Felipe Quesney, and J. Engel, Jr. Raven Press, New York.

57. Cutler, R. W. P., and Young, J. (1979): The effect of penicillin on the release of gamma-aminobutyric acid from cerebral cortex slices. *Brain Res.,* 170:157–163.

58. Dam, M., and Kiorboe, E. (1980): *Epilepsy Diagnosis and Treatment.* Scriptor, Copenhagen.

59. Delgado-Escueta, A. V. (1984): Summation of Kroc Foundation workshop and discussion: The new wave of research in the epilepsies. *Ann. Neurol.,* 16(Suppl.):140–148.

60. Delgado-Escueta, A. V., and Greenberg, D. (1984): The search for epilepsies ideal for clinical and molecular genetic studies. *Ann. Neurol.,* 16(Suppl.):1–16.

61. Delgado-Escueta, A. V., and Horan, M. (1983): Effects of seizures on ion transport and membrane protein phosphorylation. In: *Status Epilepticus: Mechanisms of Brain Damage and Treatment, Advances in Neurology,* vol. 34, edited by A. V. Delgado-Escueta, C. W. Wasterlain, D. M. Treiman, and R. J. Porter, pp. 311–325. Raven Press, New York.

62. Delgado-Escueta, A. V., and Horan, M. (1980): Brain synaptosomes in epilepsy: organization of the Na^+K^+ pump. In: *Antiepileptic Drugs: Mechanisms of Action, Advances in Neurology,* vol. 27, edited by G. H. Glaser, J. K. Penry, and D. M. Woodbury, pp. 85–126. Raven Press, New York.

63. Delgado-Escueta, A. V., Treiman, D. M., and Enrile-Bacsal, F. (1982): Phenotypic variations of seizures in adolescents and adults. In: *Genetic Basis of the Epilepsies,* edited by V. E. Anderson, W. A. Hauser, J. K. Penry, and C. F. Sing, pp. 49–81. Raven Press, New York.

64. Delgado-Escueta, A. V., Treiman, D. M., and Walsh, G. O. (1983): The treatable epilepsies: *New Engl. J. Med.,* 308:1508–1514, 1576–1584.

65. DeLorenzo, R. (1984): Calmodulin systems in neuronal excitability: A molecular approach to epilepsy. *Ann. Neurol.,* 16(Suppl.):104–114.

66. Drayer, B., Albright, R., Jaszczak, R., Kung, H., Coleman, E., and Friedman, A. (1983): Quantitative rCBF in man: The SPECT-HIPDm method. *J. Cereb. Blood. Flow. Metab.,* 3(Suppl. 1):56–57.

67. Dubicka, I., Frank, J. M., and McCutcheon, B. (1978): Attenuation of a convulsive syndrome in the rat by lateral hypothalamic stimulation. *J. Physiol. Behav.,* 20:31.

68. Dunnett, S. B., Bjorklund, A., and Stenevi, W. (1983): Dopamine-rich transplants in experimental parkinsonism. *TINS,* Elsevier Biomedical Press, Amsterdam, pp. 266–270.

69. Dunwiddie, T. V. (1980): Endogenously released adenosine regulates excitability in the in vitro hippocampus. *Epilepsia,* 21(5):541–548.

70. Dunwiddie, T. V., Hoffer, B. J., and Fredholm, B. B. (1981): Alkylxanthines elevate hippocampal excitability. Evidence for a role of endogenous adenosines. *Naunyn Schmiedebergs Arch. Pharmacol.,* 316(4):326–330.

71. Dunwiddie, T. V., and Worth, T. (1982): Sedative and anticonvulsant effects of adenosine analogs in mouse and rat. *J. Pharmacol. Exp. Ther.,* 220(1):70–76.

72. Ebersole, J. S., and Chatt, A. B. (1986): Spread and arrest of seizures: The importance of layer 4 in laminar interactions during neocortical epileptogenesis. In: *Basic Mechanisms of the Epilepsies,* edited by A. V. Delgado-Escueta, A. A. Ward, Jr., D. M. Woodbury, and R. Porter, pp. 515–558. Raven Press, New York.

73. Edmonds, H. C., Hegreberg, G. A., van Gelder, N. M., Sylvester, D. M., Clemmons, R. M., and Chatburn, C. B. (1979): Spontaneous convulsions in beagle dogs. *Fed. Proc.,* 38:2424–2427.

74. Ehrlich, Y. H., Reddy, M. V., Keen, P., Davis, L. G., Daugherty, J., and Brunngraber, E. G. (1980): Transient changes in the phosphorylation of cortical membrane proteins after electroconvulsive shock. *J. Neurochem.,* 34(5):1327–1330.

75. Eisner, V., Pauli, L. I., and Livingston, S. (1959): Hereditary aspects of epilepsy. *Johns Hopkins Hosp. Bull.,* 105:245–271.

76. Emson, P. C., Fahran-Krug, J., Schaffalitzky, D. E., Muckadell, O. B., Jessel, T. M., and Iverson, C. C. (1978): Vasoactive intestinal polypeptide (VIP): Vesicular localization and potassium evoked release from rat hypothalamus. *Brain Res.,* 143:174–178.

77. Enna, S. J., Wood, J. H., and Snyder, S. H. (1977): Gamma-aminobutyric acid (GABA) in human cerebrospinal fluid: Radioreceptor assay. *J. Neurochem.,* 28:1121–1124.

78. Engel, J. Jr., and Sharpless, N. S. (1977): Long-lasting depletion of dopamine in the rat amygdala induced by kindling stimulation. *Brain Res.,* 136:381–386.

79. Engel, J., Jr., Brown, W. J., Kuhl, D. E., Phelps, M. E., Mazziotta, J. C., and Crandall, P. H. (1982): Pathological findings underlying focal temporal lobe hypometabolism in partial epilepsy. *Ann. Neurol.*, 12:518–528.

80. Engel, J., Jr., Kuhl, D. E., Phelps, M. E., and Crandall, P. J. (1982): Localization of the epileptic focus in partial epilepsy with PCT and EEG. *Ann. Neurol.*, 12:529–537.

81. Essig, C. F. (1965): Repeated electroconvulsions resulting in elevation of pentylenetrazole seizure threshold. *Int. J. Neuropharmacol.*, 4:201–204.

82. Essig, C. F. (1969): Frequency of repeated electroconvulsions and the acquisition rate of a tolerance-like response. *Exp. Neurol.*, 25:571–574.

83. Fariello, R. G., Golden, G. T., Reyes, P. F., Alexander, G. W., and Schwartzman, R. J. (1984): Metabolic correlates of GABAmimetic-induced EEG abnormalities, In: *Neurotransmitters, Seizures, and Epilepsy II,* edited by R. G. Fariello, P. L. Morselli, K. G. Lloyd, L. F. Quesney, and J. Engel, Jr., pp. 245–252. Raven Press, New York.

84. Fazio, F., Lenzi, G. L., Gerundini, P., Fieschi, C., Collice, M., Pozzilli, C., and Gilardi, M. P. (1983): Regional cerebral perfusion with SPECT and I-123 trimethylpropanediamine (HIPDM). *J. Cereb. Blood Flow Metab.*, 3(Suppl. 1):158–159.

85. Feindel, W., and Penfield, W. (1954): Localization of discharge in temporal lobe automatism. *AMA Arch. Neurol. Psychiatry*, 72:605.

86. Ferrendelli, J. (1984): Role of biogenic amines and cyclic nucleotides in seizure mechanisms. *Ann. Neurol.*, 16(Suppl.):98–103.

87. Fertziger, A. P., and Ranck, J. B. (1970): K^+ accumulation in interstitial space during epileptiform seizures. *Exp. Neurol.*, 26:571–585.

88. Fischer, J. (1969): Electron-microscopic changes in the perikarya and in the processes of ganglion cells in the cobalt-gelatine epileptogenic focus. *Physiol. Bohemoslov.*, 18:387–394.

89. Fischer, J. (1973): Change in the number of vesicles in synapses of a projected epileptic cortical focus in rats. *Physiol. Bohemoslov.*, 22:537–542.

90. Fischer, J., and Langmeier, M. (1980): Changes in the number, size, and shape of synaptic vesicle in an experimental, projected cortical epileptic focus in the rat. *Epilepsia*, 21(6):571–587.

91. Fisher, R. S., Pedley, T. A., Moody, W. J., Jr., and Prince, D. A. (1976): The role of extracellular potassium in hippocampal epilepsy. *Arch. Neurol.*, 33:76–83.

92. Frankenhaeuser, B., and Hodgkin, A. L. (1957): The action of calcium in the electrical properties of squid axons. *J. Physiol.*, 137:218–244.

93. Frenk, H., Urca, G., and Liebeskind, J. C. (1978): Epileptic properties of leucine and methionine enkephalin: Comparison with morphine and reversibility by naloxone. *Brain Res.*, 147:327–337.

94. Fromm, G. H., and Terrence, C. F. (1984): What is the role of GABA in the mechanism of action of anticonvulsant drugs? In: *Neurotransmitters, Seizures and Epilepsy II,* edited by R. G. Fariello, P. L. Morselli, K. G. Lloyd, L. F. Quesney, and J. Engel, Jr., pp. 81–94. Raven Press, New York.

95. Gabor, A. J., and Scobey, R. P. (1975): Spatial limits of epileptogenic cortex: Its relationship to ectopic spike generation. *J. Neurophysiol.*, 38:395–404.

96. Garnett, E. S., Firnau, G., and Nahmias, C. (1983): Dopamine visualized in the basal ganglia of living man. *Nature*, 305:137–138.

97. Gastaut, H., and Tassinari, C. A. (1975): Epilepsies. In: *Handbook of EEG and Clinical Neurophysiology,* vol. 13, edited by A. Remond, 13A:3–104. Elsevier, Amsterdam.

98. Gedda, L., Tatarelli, R. (1971): Essential isochronic epilepsy in MZ twin pairs. *Acta Genet. Med.*, 20:380–383.

99. Glaser, G. H. (1983): Medical complications of status epilepticus. In: *Status Epilepticus: Basic Mechanisms of Brain Damage and Treatment, Advances in Neurology,* vol. 34, edited by A. V. Delgado-Escueta, C. W. Wasterlain, D. M. Treiman, and R. J. Porter. Raven Press, New York.

100. Goddard, G. V. (1983): The kindling model of epilepsy. *TINS.* Elsevier Biomedical Press, Amsterdam, pp. 275–279.

101. Goldberg, A. M., Pollock, J. J., Hartman, E. R., and Craig, C. R. (1972): Alterations in cholinergic enzymes during the development of cobalt-induced epilepsy in the rat. *Neuropharmacology*, 11:253–259.

102. Goldensohn, E. S., and Purpura, D. P. (1963): Intracellular potentials of cortical neurons during focal epileptogenic discharges. *Science*, 139:840–842.

103. Goldensohn, E. S. (1983): The kindling phenomenon: A reappraisal of its role in human epilepsy (abstr.). Merritt-Putnam Symposium, Washington, D.C.

104. Gottesfeld, Z., and Elazar, Z. (1972): GABA and glutamate in different EEG stages of the penicillin focus. *Nature*, 240:478–479.

105. Gowers, W. R. (1901): *Epilepsy and Other Chronic Convulsive Diseases: Their Causes, Symptoms and Treatment,* 2nd ed. J. and A. Church, London.

106. Greaves, M., Belanger, M., and Van Gelder, N. M. (1976): A specific protein abnormality associated with cobalt-induced epilepsy in mice. *Neurochem. Res.*, 1:313–327.

107. Grisar, T., and Delgado-Escueta, A. V. (1985): Glial contribution in human epilepsy: K^+ activation of (Na^+K^+)-ATPase in bulk isolated glial cells and synaptosomes form temporal lobes of patients with intractable complex partial epilepsies. *Brain Res.* (in press).

108. Grisar, T., Franck, G., and Delgado-Escueta, A. V. (1983): Glial contribution to seizures: K^+ activation of (Na^+K^+)-ATPase in bulk isolated glial cells and synaptosomes of epileptogenic cortex. *Brain Res.*, 261:75–84.

109. Guerrero-Figueroa, R., Barros, A., de Balbain Verster, F., and Heath, Z. G. (1963): Experimental "petit mal" in kittens. *Arch. Neurol.*, 9:297–306.

110. Guidotti, A., Konkel, D. R., Ebstein, B., Corda, M. G., Wise, B. C., Krutzsch, H., Meek, J. L., and Costa, E. (1982): Isolation, characterization, and purification to homogeneity of a rat brain protein (GABA-modulin). *Proc. Natl. Acad. Sci. USA*, 79:6084–6088.

111. Gusella, J. F., Tamzo, R., Anderson, M. A., Ottina, K., Wallace, M., and Coneally, P. M. (1984): Linkage analysis of Huntington's disease using RFLPs, in human gene mapping 7. *Seventh International Workshop*, Karger, Switzerland. *Cytogenet. Cell Genet.*, 37:1–4.

112. Gutnick, M. J., and Prince, D. A. (1972): Thalamocortical relay neurons: Antidromic invasion of spikes from a cortical epileptogenic focus. *Science*, 176:424–426.

113. Haldane, J. B. S., and Smith, C. A. B. (1947): A new estimate of the linkage between the genes for color blindness and haemophilia in man. *Ann. Eugen.*, 14:10–31.

114. Hansen, S., Perry, T. L., Wada, J. A., and Sokol, M. (1973): Brain amino acids in baboons with light-induced epilepsy. *Brain Res.*, 50:480.

115. Harris, A. B. (1975): Cortical neuroglia in experimental epilepsy. *Exp. Neurol.*, 49:691–715.

116. Harris, A. B. (1980): Structural and chemical changes in experimental epileptic foci. In: *Epilepsy: A Window to Brain Mechanism*, edited by J. S. Lockard and A. A. Ward, Jr. Raven Press, New York.

117. Harris, A. B., and Lockard, J. S. (1981): Absence of seizures or mirror foci in experimental epilepsy after excision of alumina and astrogliotic scar. *Epilepsia*, 22:107–122.

118. Hartung, E. (1920): Zwei falle van paramyoclonus multiplex mit epilepsie. *Z. Gesamte Neurol. Psychiatr.*, 56:151–153.

119. Harvald, B. (1954): Heredity in epilepsy. An EEG study of relatives of epileptics. *Op. Ex. Dom. Biol. Hered. Hum. Univ. Hafor.*, 35:9–122.

120. Heinemann, U., Konnerth, A., Pumain, R., and Wadman, W. (1986): Changes in extracellular volume, Ca^{2+}, Na^+, and K^+ in chronic epilepsies. In: *Basic Mechanisms of the Epilepsies*, edited by A. V. Delgado-Escueta, A. A. Ward, Jr., D. M. Woodbury, and R. J. Porter, pp. 641–661. Raven Press, New York.

121. Heinemann, U., Lux, H. D., and Gutnick, M. J. (1977): Extracellular free calcium and potassium during paroxysmal activity in the cerebral cortex of the cat. *Exp. Brain Res.*, 27:237–243.

122. Henriksen, S. J., Bloom, F. E., McCoy, F., Ling, N., and Guillemin, R. (1978): Beta-endorphin induces non-convulsive limbic seizures. *Proc. Natl. Acad. Sci. USA*, 75:5221–5225.

123. Herbert, E., Birnberg, N., Lissitsky, J. C., Civelli, O., and Uhler, M. (1981): Pro-opiomelanocortin: A model for the regulation of expression of neuropeptides in pituitary and brain. *Neurosci. Newslett.*, 12:16–27.

124. Herbert, E., Douglass, J., Civelli, O., Burnberg, N., Comb, M., Uhler, M., and Lissitzky, J. (1984): Regulation of expression of opioid peptide genes. *Ann. Neurol.*, 16(Suppl.):22–30.

125. Hoover, D. B., Craig, C. R., and Colasanti, B. K. (1977): Cholinergic involvement in cobalt-induced epilepsy in the rat. *Exp. Brain Res.*, 29:(3–4):501–513.

126. Houseman, D., and Gusella, J. (1982): Molecular genetic approaches to neural degenerative disease. In: *Molecular Genetic Neuroscience*, edited by F. O. Schmitt, S. J. Bird, and F. E. Bloom. Raven Press, New York.

127. Howse, D. A. (1978): Metabolic responses to status epilepticus in the rat, cat and mouse. *Can. J. Physiol. Pharmacol.*, 57:205–212.

128. Hughes, J., Smith, T., Morgan, B., et al. (1975): Purification and properties of enkephalin: The possible endogenous ligand for the morphine receptor. *Life Sci.*, 16:1753–1758.

129. Hughes, J., Smith, T. W., Kosterlitz, H. W., et al. (1975): Identification of two related pentapeptides from the brain with potent opiate agonist activity. *Nature*, 258:577–580.

130. Humphrey, G. (1942): Experiments on physiological mechanism of noise-induced seizures in albino rat; action of parasympathetic drugs. *Comp. Psychol.*, 33:315–323.

131. Hunt, J. R. (1921): Dyssynergia cerebellaris myoclonica—Primary atrophy of the dentate system: A contribution to the pathology and symptomatology of the cerebellum. *Brain*, 44:490–538.

132. Iadorola, M. J., and Gale, K. (1982): Substantia nigra: Site of anticonvulsant activity mediated by gamma-aminobutyric acid. *Science*, 218:1237–1240.

133. Jackson, J. H. (1931): Selected writings of John Hughlings Jackson. In: *On Epilepsy and Epileptiform Convulsions*, vol. 1, edited by J. Taylor. Hodder and Stoughton, London.

134. Jackson, M. (1984): Chemically activated channels in muscle and spinal cord. *Ann. Neurol.*, 16(Suppl.):52–58.

135. Janz, D. (1982): In tema di remissione e di ricomparsa di crisi durante e dopo il trattamento farmacologico dell'epilessia. *Boll. Legal Ital.*, 39:95–100.

136. Janz, D., Dern, A., Mossinger, H. J., and Puhlmann, H. U. (1982): Ruckfall-Prognose warend und nach reduktion der medikamente bei epilepsie begandlung. In: *Epilepsie 1981*, edited by H. Remschmidt, R. Rentz, and J. Jungmann. Georg Thieme, Stuttgart.

137. Jasper, H. H., and Kershman, J. (1941): Electroencephalographic classification of the epilepsies. *Arch. Neurol. Psychiatry*, 45:903.

138. Jasper, H. H., Ward, A., and Pope, A. (1969): *Basic Mechanisms of the Epilepsies*, Little, Brown and Co., Boston.

139. Jobe, P., Picchioni, A., and Chin, L. (1973): Role of brain norepinephrine in audiogenic seizure in rat. *J. Pharmacol. Exp. Ther.*, 184:1–9.

140. Jobe, P. C., Picchioni, A. L., and Chin, L. (1973): Effect of lithium carbonate and alpha-

methyl-*p*-tyrosine on audiogenic seizure intensity. *J. Pharm. Pharmacol.*, 25:830–831.

141. Jobe, P. C., Picchioni, A. L., and Chin, L. (1973): Role of brain 5-hydroxytryptamine in audiogenic seizure in the rat. *Life Sci.*, 13:1–13.

142. Jobe, P. C., Stull, R. E., and Geiger, P. F. (1974): The relative significance of norepinephrine, dopamine and 5-hydroxytryptamine in electroshock seizure in the rat. *Neuropharmacology*, 13:961–968.

143. Jobe, P. C., and Brown, R. D. (1980): Auditory pharmacology. *Trends in Pharmacological Sciences*, 1(8):202–206.

144. Jobe, P. C., and Laird, H. E. (1981): Neurotransmitter abnormalities as determinants of seizure susceptibility and intensity in the genetic models of epilepsy. *Biochem. Pharmacol.*, 30:3137–3144.

145. Johnson, D. D., Davis, H. L., and Crawford, R. D. (1979): Pharmacological and biochemical studies in epileptic fowl. *Fed. Proc.*, 38:2417–2423.

146. Johnson, D. D., Jaju, A. R., Ness, L., Richardson, J. R., and Crawford, R. D. (1981): Brain norepinephrine, dopamine, and 5-hydroxytryptamine concentration abnormalities and their role in the high seizure susceptibility of epileptic chickens. *Can. J. Physiol. Pharmacol.*, 59:144–149.

147. Johnston, D., and Brown, T. (1984): The synaptic nature of the paroxysmal depolarizing shift in hippocampal neurons. *Ann. Neurol.*, 16(Suppl.):65–71.

148. Kan, Y. W., and Dozy, A. M. (1978): Polymorphisms of DNA sequence adjacent to human beta-globin structural gene. Relationship to sickle mutation. *Proc. Natl. Acad. Sci. USA*, 75:5631.

149. Kellogg, C. (1971): Serotonin metabolism in the brains of mice sensitive or resistant to audiogenic seizures. *J. Neurobiol.*, 2:209–219.

150. Kellogg, C. (1976): Audiogenic seizures: Relation to age and mechanisms of monoamine neurotransmission. *Brain Res.*, 106:87–103.

151. Kennedy, M. B., and Greengard, P. (1981): Two calcium/calmodulin dependent protein kinases, which are highly concentrated in brain, phosphorylate protein I at distinct sites. *Proc. Natl. Acad. Sci. USA*, 78:1293–1297.

152. Kosterlitz, H. W., and Hughes, J. (1977): Peptides with morphine-like action in the brain. *Br. J. Psychiatry*, 130:298–304.

153. Koyama, I., and Jasper, H. (1977): Amino acid content of chronic undercut cortex of the cat in relation to electrical after discharge: Comparison with cobalt epileptogenic lesions. *Can. J. Physiol. Pharmacol.*, 55:523–536.

154. Kovacs, D. A., and Zoll, J. G. (1974): Seizure inhibition by median raphe nucleus stimulation in the rat. *Brain Res.*, 70:165.

155. Kreisman, N. R., Rosenthal, M., LaManna, J. C., and Sick, T. J. (1983): Cerebral oxygenation during recurrent seizures. In: *Status Epilepticus: Basic Mechanisms of Brain Damage*

and Treatment, Advances in Neurology, vol. 34, edited by A. V. Delgado-Escueta, C. W. Wasterlain, D. M. Treiman, and R. J. Porter. Raven Press, New York.

156. Krishna, G., Forn, J., Voight, K., Paul, M., and Gessa, G. L. (1970): Dynamic aspects of neurohormonal control of cyclic 3′,5′-AMP synthesis in brain. *J. Adv. Biochem. Psychopharmacol.*, 3:155–172.

157. Kirvoy, W. A., Couch, J. R., Henry, J. L., and Stewart, J. M. (1979): Synaptic modulation by substance P. *Fed. Proc.*, 38(9):2344–2347.

158. Kurland, L. T. (1959): The incidence and prevalence of convulsive disorders in a small urban community. *Epilepsia*, 1:143–161.

159. Kuhl, D. E., Engel, J., Jr., Phelps, M. E., and Selin, C. (1980): Epileptic patterns of local cerebral metabolism and perfusion in humans determined by emission computed tomography of ^{18}FDG and ^{13}NH$_3$. *Ann. Neurol.*, 8:348–360.

160. Lafora, G. R., and Glueck, B. (1911): Contributions to the histopathology and pathogenesis of myoclonic epilepsy. *Bull. Gov. Hosp. Insane*, 3:96.

161. Laird, H. E., and Huxtable, R. J. (1976): Effects of taurine on audiogenic seizure response in rats. In: *Taurine and Neurological Disorders*, edited by A. Barbeau and R. J. Huxtable, pp. 267–274, Raven Press, New York.

162. Laird, H. E., Chin, L., and Picchioni, A. L. (1980): Lower endogenous levels of norepinephrine and serotonin in brains of rats from a genetically seizure susceptible strain. *Soc. Neurosci. Abstr.*, 6:724.

163. Lennox, W. G. (1936): The physiological pathogenesis of epilepsy. *Brain*, 59:113.

164. Lennox, W. G. (1945): The petit mal epilepsies: Their treatment with tridione. *JAMA*, 129:1069.

165. Lennox, W. G. (1951): Phenomena and correlates of the psychomotor triad. *Neurology*, (Minn.) 1:357.

166. Lennox, W. G., and Lennox, M. A. (1960): *Epilepsy and Related Disorders*, Little, Brown and Co., Boston.

167. Lennox, W. G., Gibbs, F. A., and Gibbs, E. L. (1936): Effect on the electroencephalogram of drugs and conditions which influence seizures. *Arch. Neurol. Psychiatry*, 36:1236.

168. Levitt, P., and Noebels, J. L. (1981): Mutant mouse tottering: Selective increase of locus ceruleus axons in a defined single locus mutation. *Proc. Natl. Acad. Sci. USA*, 78(7):4630–4634.

169. Lewin, E. (1972): The freeze lesion, In: *Experimental Models of Epilepsy—A Manual for the Laboratory Worker*, edited by D. P. Purpura, J. K. Penry, D. Tower, D. M. Woodbury, and R. Walter, pp. 13–49. Raven Press, New York.

170. Lewin, E. (1983): Inosine, hypoxanthine, and seizures, In: *Status Epilepticus: Mechanism of Brain Damage and Treatment, Advances in Neurology*, vol. 34, edited by A. V. Delgado-Escueta, C. Wasterlain, D. M. Treiman, and R. J. Porter, pp. 365–368. Raven Press, New York.

171. Lewin, E., and Bleck, V. (1977): Cyclic AMP

accumulation in cerebral cortical slices: Effects of carbamezepine, phenobarbital, and phenytoin. *Epilepsia*, 18:237.

172. Morselli, P. C. (1981): The role of GABA mediated neurotransmission in convulsive states. *Adv. Biochem. Psychopharmacol.*, 26:199–206.

173. Lomax, P., and Bajorek, J. G. (1977): Animal models in epilepsy. In: *Animal Models in Psychiatry and Neurology*, edited by I. Hainin and E. Usdin, pp. 365–370. Pergamon Press, New York.

174. Longo, V. G., Nechmanson, D., Bovet, D. (1960): Electroencephalographic aspects of the antagonism between 2-pyridine aldoxime iodomethylate (PAM) and isopropyl methylfluorophosphate (sarin). *Arch. Int. Pharmacodyn. Ther.*, 123:292–290.

175. Longo, V. G. (1966): Behavioral and electroencephalographic effects of atropine and related compounds. *Pharmacol. Rev.*, 18:965–996.

176. Loskota, W. J., Lomax, P., and Rich, S. T. (1974): The gerbil as a model for the study of the epilepsies: Seizure patterns and ontogenesis. *Epilepsia*, 15:109.

177. Lothman, E. W., and Somjen, G. G. (1976): Functions of primary afferents and responses of extracellular potassium during spinal epileptiform seizures. *EEG Clin. Neurophysiol.*, 41:253–267.

178. Lundborg, H. (1912): Der erbang der progressiven myoklonusepilepsie. *Z. Gesamte. Neurol. Psychiatr.*, 9:353–358.

179. Lust, W. D., and Passoneau, J. V. (1976): Cyclic nucleotides in murine brain: Effects of hypothermia on adenosine 3′ 5′ monophosphate, glycogen phosphorylase, glycogen synthelase and metabolites following electroshock or decapitation. *J. Neurochem.*, 26:11.

180. Lust, W. D., Goldberg, N. D., and Passoneau, V. (1976): Cyclic nucleotides in murine brain: The temporal relationship of changes induced in adenosine 3′ 5′ monophosphate following maximal electroshock convulsions or decapitation. *J. Neurochem.*, 26:5.

181. Lux, D., Heinemann, J., and Dietzel, I. (1985): Ionic changes and alterations in the size of the extracellular space during epileptic activity, In: *Basic Mechanisms of the Epilepsies*, edited by A. V. Delgado-Escueta, A. A. Ward, Jr., D. M. Woodbury, and R. J. Porter, pp. 619–639. Raven Press, New York.

182. Lux, H. D. (1974): Kinetics of EC K⁺-relation to epileptogenesis. *Epilepsia*, 15:375–393.

183. Magistretti, P., Uren, R., Blume, H., et al. (1982): Delineation of epileptic focus by single photon emission tomography. *Eur. J. Nucl. Med.*, 7:484–485.

184. Mahler, H. R. (1977): Proteins of the synaptic membrane. *Neurochemistry*, 2:119–147.

185. Marangos, P. J., Martino, A. M., Paul, S. M., and Skolnick, P. (1981): The benzodiazepines and inosine antagonize caffein induced seizures. *Psychopharmacology*, 72:269–273.

186. Marangos, P. J., Trams, E., Clark-Rosenberg, R. L., Paul, S. M., and Skolnick, P. (1981): Anticonvulsant doses of inosine result in brain levels sufficient to inhibit [³H]-diazepam binding. *Psychopharmacology*, 71:175–178.

187. Matsuda, T., Iwata, H., and Cooper, J. R. (1984): Specific inactivation of a(+) molecular form of (Na⁺K⁺)ATPase by pyrithiamine, *J. Biol. Chem.*, 259:3858–3863.

188. Matsumoto, H., and Ajmone-Marsan, C. (1964): Cortical cellular phenomena in experimental epilepsy: Interictal manifestations. *Exp. Neurol.*, 9:286–304.

189. Matsumoto, H., and Ajmone-Marsan, C. (1964): Cortical cellular phenomena in experimental epilepsy: Ictal manifestations. *Exp. Neurol.*, 9:305–326.

190. Matsumoto, H., Ayala, G. F., and Gumnit, R. J. (1969): Neuronal behavior and triggering mechanism in cortical epileptic focus. *J. Neurophysiol.*, 32:638–703.

191. Mayman, C. I., Manlapaz, J. S., Ballantine, H. T., and Richardson, E. P. (1965): A neuropathological study of experimental epileptogenic lesions in the cat. *J. Neuropathol. Exp. Neurol.*, 24:502–511.

192. Maziere, M., Berger, G., Godot, J. M., Prenant, C., and Comar, D. (1981): Etorphine ¹¹C: A new tool of the "in vivo" study of brain opiate receptors. *J. Label. Compounds Radiopharm.*, 18:15–16.

193. Mazziotta, J. C., and Engel, J., Jr. (1984): Advanced neuro-imaging techniques in the study of human epilepsy. PET, SPECT and NMR-CT, In: *Recent Advances in Epilepsy, Vol. 2*, edited by T. Pedley and B. Meldrum. Churchill Livingston, London.

194. McKusick, V. A. (1978): Mendelian inheritance in man. In: *Catalogs of Autosomal Dominant, Autosomal Recessive and X-linked Phenotypes. 5th ed.*, Johns Hopkins University Press, Baltimore.

195. McNamara, J. O. (1978): Muscarinic cholinergic receptors participating in the kindling model of epilepsy. *Brain Res.*, 154:415–420.

196. McNamara, J. (1984): Kindling, an animal model of complex partial epilepsy. *Ann. Neurol.*, 16(Suppl.):72–76.

197. Meldrum, B. S. (1983): Endocrine consequences of status epilepticus. In: *Status Epilepticus: Basic Mechanisms of Brain Damage and Treatment*, Advances in Neurology, Vol. 34, edited by A. V. Delgado-Escueta, C. W. Wasterlain, D. M. Treiman, and R. J. Porter, pp. 399–404. Raven Press, New York.

198. Meldrum, B. S. (1975): Epilepsy and gamma-aminobutyric acid-mediated inhibition. *Inter. Rev. Neurobiol.*, 17:1–36.

199. Meldrum, B. S. (1981): GABA-antagonist as antiepileptic agents. *Adv. Biochem. Psychopharmacol.*, 26:207–217.

200. Meldrum, B. S., Anlezark, G., and Trimble, M. (1975): Drugs modifying dopaminergic activity and behavior, the EEG and epilepsy in *Papio Papio*. *Eur. J. Pharmacol.*, 32:203–213.

201. Meldrum, B. S., Menini, C., Stutzmann, J. M., and Naquet, R. (1979): Effects of opiate-like

peptides, morphine and naloxone in the photosensitive baboon, *Papio Papio. Brain Res.,* 170:333–348.

202. Meldrum, B. S., and Horton, R. W. (1971): Convulsive effects of 4-deoxypyridoxine and of bicuculline in photosensitive baboons (*Papio Papio*) and in rhesus monkeys (*Macaca mulata*). *Brain Res.,* 35:419–436.

203. Meldrum, B. S., Naquet, R., and Balzano, E. (1970): Effects of atropine and eserine on the electroencephalogram on behavior and on light-induced epilepsy in the adolescent baboon (*Papio Papio*). *EEG Clin. Neurophysiol.,* 28:449–458.

204. Meldrum, B. S., Pedley, T., Horton, R., Anlezark, G., and Franks, A. (1980): Epileptogenic and anticonvulsant effects of GABA agonists and GABA uptake inhibitors. *Brain Res. Bull.,* 5(Suppl 2):685–690.

205. Meldrum, B. S., Vigoroux, R. A., and Brierley, J. B. (1973): Systemic factors and epileptic brain damage: Prolonged seizures in paralyzed artificially ventilated baboons. *Arch. Neurol.,* 29:82–87.

206. Meech, R. W. (1978): Ca^{+2} stimulated potassium conductance. *Annu. Rev. Biophys. Bioengineering,* 7:1–18.

207. Metrakos, K., and Metrakos, J. D. (1961): Genetics of convulsive disorders. II. Genetic and electroencephalographic studies in centrencephalic epilepsy. *Neurology (Minneap)*, 11:474–483.

208. Metrakos, J. D., and Metrakos, K. (1969): Genetic studies in clinical epilepsy in man. In: *Basic Mechanisms of Epilepsies,* edited by H. H. Jasper, A. A. Ward, and A. Pope, pp. 700–708. Little, Brown & Co., Boston.

209. Miller, J. A., Agnew, W. S., and Levison, S. R. (1983): Principal glycopeptide of the tetrodotoxin/saxitoxin binding protein from electrophorus electricus: Isolation and partial chemical and physical characterization. *Biochemistry,* 22:462–470.

210. Baimbridge, K. G., and Miller, J. J. (1984): Hippocampal calcium-binding protein during commissural kindling-induced epileptogenesis: Progressive decline and effects of anticonvulsants. *Brain Res.,* 17:85–90.

211. Mimaki, T., Yubuuchi, H., Laird, H. E., and Yamamura, H. I. (1981): Effects of seizures and antiepileptic drugs on benzodiazepine receptors in rat brain. *Abstracts, Epilepsy International Congress,* Kyoto, Japan. Raven Press, New York.

212. Mintun, M. A., Wooten, F., and Raichle, M. E. (1983): A quantitative model for the in vivo assessment of drug-binding sites with PET. *J. Cereb. Blood Flow Metab.,* 3(Suppl. 1):566–567.

213. Mohr, E., and Corcoran, M. E. (1981): Depletion of noradrenaline and amygdaloid kindling. *Exp. Neurol.,* 72:507–511.

214. Moody, W. J., Jr., Futamachi, K. J., and Prince, D. A. (1974): Extracellular potassium activity during epileptogenesis. *Exp. Neurol.,* 42:248–263.

215. Mori, T., Takai, Y., Minakuchi, R., Yu, B., and Nishizuka, Y. (1980): Inhibitory action of chlorpromazine, dibucaine, and other phospholipid-interacting drugs on calcium-activated phospholipid dependent protein kinase. *J. Biol. Chem.* 255:8378–8380.

216. Morrell, F. (1979): Human secondary epileptogenic lesions. *Neurology,* 29:558.

217. Morrell, F., Tsume, H., Hoeppner, T. J., Morgan, D., and Harrison, W. H. (1975): Secondary epileptogenesis in frog forebrain: Effect of inhibition of protein synthesis. *Can. J. Neurol. Sci.,* 2:407–416.

218. Morton, N. E. (1962): Segregation and linkage. In: *Methodology in Human Genetics,* edited by W. J. Burdette, pp. 17–52. Holden Day, San Francisco.

219. Mountcastle, V. B. (1979): An organizing principle for cerebral function: The unit module and the distributed system. In: *The Neurosciences, Fourth Study Program,* edited by F. O. Schmitt and F. G. Worden. The MIT Press, Boston.

220. Myslobodsky, M. S. (1984): Too little or too much GABA? In: *Neurotransmitters, Seizures and Epilepsy II,* edited by R. G. Fariello, P. L. Morselli, K. G. Lloyd, L. F. Quesney, J. Engel, Jr., pp. 337–347. Raven Press, New York.

221. Narahashi, T. (1984): Drug-ionic channel interactions: Single channel measurements. *Ann. Neurol.,* 16(Suppl.):39–51.

222. Naruse, H., Kato, M., Kurokawa, M., Haba, R., and Yabe, T. (1960): Metabolic defects in a convulsive strain of mouse. *J. Neurochem.,* 5:359–369.

223. Neumann, E., Nachmansohn, D., and Katchalsky, A. (1973): An attempt at an integral interpretation of nerve excitability. *Proc. Natl. Acad. Sci., USA* 70:727–731.

224. Noda, M., Shimizu, S., Tanabe, T., Takai, T., Kayano, T., Ikeda, T., et al. (1984): Primary structure of electorophorus electricus sodium channel deduced from cDNA sequence. *Nature,* 312:121–127.

225. Noebels, J. L. (1984): Isolating single genes of the inherited epilepsies. *Ann. Neurol.,* 16(Suppl.):18–21.

226. Ogata, N. (1977): Effects of cycloheximide on experimental epilepsy induced by daily amygdaloid stimulation in rabbit. *Epilepsia,* 18:202–208.

227. Olney, J. W., deGubareff, T., and Labruyere, J. (1983): Seizure-related brain damage induced by cholinergic agents. *Nature,* 301:520–522.

228. Olney, J. W., deGubareff, T., and Sloviter, R. S. (1983): Epileptic brain damage in rats induced by sustained electrical stimulation of the perforant path. II. Ultrastructural analysis of acute hippocampal pathology. *Brain Res. Bull.,* 10:699–712.

229. Olney, J. W., Fuller, T., and deGubareff, T. (1979): Acute dendrotoxic changes in the hippocampus of kainate treated rats. *Brain Res.,* 176:91–100.

230. Olsen, R. W., Snowmen, A. M., Lee, R.,

Lomax, P., and Wamsley, J. K. (1984): Role of aminobutyric acid receptor/ionophore complex in seizure disorder. *Ann. Neurol.*, 16(Suppl.): 90–97.

231. Opmeer, F. A., Gumulka, S. W., Dinaendahl, V., and Schernhofer, P. S. (1976): Effects of stimulatory and depressant drugs on cyclic guanosine 3' 5' monophosphate and adenosine 3' 5' monophosphate levels in mouse brain. *Naunyn Schmiedebergs Arch. Pharmacol.*, 292:259.

232. Palmer, G. C., Jones, D. C., Medina, M. A., and Stavinoha, W. D. (1979): Anticonvulsant drug actions on *in vitro* and *in vivo* levels of cyclic AMP in the mouse brain. *Epilepsia*, 29:95–104.

233. Pedley, T. A., Fisher, R. S., Futamachi, K. J., and Prince, D. A. (1976): Regulation of extracellular potassium concentration in epileptogenesis. *Fed. Proc.*, 35:1254–1259.

234. Pedley, T. A., Buckerman, E. C., and Glaser, G. H. (1969): Epileptogenic effects of localized ventricular perfusion of ouabain endorsal HPC. *Exp. Neurol.*, 25:207–219.

235. Penfield, W. (1958): *The Excitable Cortex in Conscious Man*. Liverpool University Press, Liverpool.

236. Penfield, W. (1968): Engrams in the human brain. *Proc. Rev. Soc. Med.*, 61:831.

237. Penfield, W., and Bridges, W. H. (1942): Progressive tissue destruction in epileptogenic lesions of the brain. *Trans. Am. Neurol. Assoc.*, 67:158–163.

238. Penfield, W., and Gage, L. (1933): Cerebral localization of epileptic manifestations. *AMA Arch. Neurol. Psychiatry*, 30:709.

239. Penfield, W., and Humphreys, S. (1942): Epileptogenic lesions of the brain. *Arch. Neurol. Psychiatry*, 43:240–261.

240. Penfield, W., and Jasper, H. H. (1954): *Epilepsy and the Functional Anatomy of the Human Brain*, p. 20. Little, Brown and Co., Boston.

241. Penfield, W., and Kristiansen, K. (1951): *Epileptic Seizure Patterns*. Springfield, Ill.

242. Penfield, W., and Perot, P. (1963): The brain's record of auditory and visual experience. *Brain*, 86:595

243. Penfield, W., and Roberts, L. (1959): *Speech and Brain-Mechanisms*. Princeton University Press, Princeton, New Jersey.

244. Perry, T. L., Hansen, S., Kennedy, J., Wada, J. A., and Thompson, G. B. (1975): Amino acids in human epileptogenic foci. *Arch. Neurol.*, 32:752–754.

245. Perry, T. L., and Hansen, S. (1981): Amino acid abnormalities in epileptogenic foci. *Neurology*, 31:871–876.

246. Peterson, G. M., Ribak, C. E., and Oertel, W. H. (1985): Differences in the hippocampal GABAergic system between seizure sensitive and seizure resistant gerbils. *Anat. Rec.* (in press).

247. Prince, D. A. (1968): Inhibition in epileptic neurons. *Exp. Neurol.*, 21:307–321.

248. Prince, D. A., and Wong, R. K. (1976): Cellular activities in focal epilepsy. In: *Brain Dysfunction in Infantile Febrile Convulsions*, edited by M. A. B. Brazier and F. Coceani. Raven Press, New York.

249. Prince, D. A. (1983): Mechanisms underlying interictal-ictal transition. In: *Mechanisms of Brain Damage and Treatment*, Advances in Neurology, Vol. 34, edited by A. V. Delgado-Escueta, C. W. Wasterlain, D. Treiman, and R. Porter. pp. 177–188. Raven Press, New York.

250. Prince, D., and Connors, B. (1984): Mechanisms of epileptogenesis in cortical structures. *Ann. Neurol.*, 16(Suppl.):59–64.

251. Prince, D. A., and Wilder, B. J. (1967): Control mechanisms in cortical epileptogenic foci: Surround inhibition. *Arch. Neurol.*, 16:194–202.

252. Racine, R. J., Burnham, W. M., and Livingston, K. (1979): The effects of atropine and reserpine on cortical kindling in the rat. *Can. J. Neurol. Sci.*, 6:47–51.

253. Rapport, R. L., II, Harris, A. B., Friel, P. N., Ojemann, G. A. (1975): Human epileptic brain Na^+K^+ATPase activity and phenytoin concentrations. *Arch. Neurol.*, 32:549–554.

254. Rapport, M. M., Karpiak, S. E., and Mahadis, S. P. (1979): Biological activities of antibodies injected into the brain. *Fed. Proc.*, 38:2391.

255. Ribak, C. E., Harris, A. B., Vaughn, J. E., and Roberts, E. (1979): Inhibitory GABAergic nerve terminals decrease at sites of focal epilepsy. *Science*, 205:211–214.

256. Roberts, E. (1984): GABA-related phenomena, models of nervous system functions and seizures. *Ann. Neurol.*, 16(Suppl.):77–89.

257. Robertson, H. A. (1980): Audiogenic seizures: Increased benzodiazepine receptor binding in a susceptible strain of mice. *Eu. J. Pharmacol.*, 66:249–252.

258. Rosenblatt, D. E., Lauter, C. J., Baird, H. R., and Trams, E. G. (1977): ATPases in animal models of epilepsy. *J. Mol. Med.*, 2:137–144.

259. Rosenblatt, D. E., Lauter, C. J., and Trams, E. G. (1976): Deficiency of a Ca^{2+}-ATPase in brains of seizure prone mice. *J. Neurochem.*, 27:1299–1304.

260. Roses, A. D., Butterfield, D. A., Appel, S. H., and Chestnut, D. B. (1975): Phenytoin and membrane fluidity in myotonic dystrophy, *Arch. Neurol.*, 32:535.

261. Roses, A. D., Pericak-Vance, M. A., and Yamaoka, L. H. (1983): Recombinant DNA strategies in genetic neurological diseases. In: *Molecular Aspects of Neurological Diseases*, edited by L. Austin and P. L. Jeffrey. Academic Press, Sydney, Australia.

262. Rubin, E. H., and Ferrendelli, J. A. (1977): Distribution and regulation of cyclic nucleotide levels in cerebellum *in vivo*. *J. Neurochem.*, 29:43

263. Sugratella, S., and Massotti, M. (1982): Convulsant and anticonvulsant effects of opioids: Relationship to GABA-mediated transmission. *Neuropharmacol.*, 21:991–1000.

264. Salas, C. E., Ohesson, W. G., and Sellinger, O. Z. (1977): The stimulation of cerebral *N*2 methyl and *N*2-2-dimethyl guanine-specific

52

CHAPTER 1

tRNA methyltransferases by methonine sulfoximine: An *in vivo* study. *Biochem. Biophys.
Res. Commun.*, 76:1107–1115.

265. Sato, M., and Ogawa, T. (1984): Abnormal behavior in epilepsy and catecholamines. In: *Neurotransmitters, Seizures and Epilepsy II*, edited
by R. G. Fariello, P. L. Morselli, K. G. Lloyd,
L. F. Quesney, J. Engel, Jr., pp. 1–10. Raven
Press, New York.

266. Sattin, A. (1971): Increase in the content of
adenosine 3′ 5′ monophosphate in mouse forebrain during seizures and prevention of the increase by methylxanthines. *J. Neurochem.*,
18:1987.

267. Savage, D. D., Werling, L. L., Nadler, J. V.,
and McNamara, J. O. (1982): Selective increase
in L-(^{3}H) glutamate binding to a quisqualate-sensitive site on hippocampal synaptic membranes
after angular bundle kindling, *Eur. J. Pharmacol.*, 85(2):255–256.

268. Schatz, R. A., and Sellinger, O. A. (1975): Effect of methionine and methionine sulfoximine
on rat brain sadenosyl methionine levels. *J.
Neurochem.*, 24:63–66.

269. Schatz, R. A., Frye, K., and Sellinger, O. Z.
(1978): Increased in vivo methylation of [^{3}H]
histamine in the methionine sulfoximine epileptogenic mouse brain. *J. Pharmacol. Exp. Ther.*,
207(3):784–800.

270. Schechter, P. J., and Grove, J. (1980): Biochemical and pharmacological similarities and differences among four irreversible enzyme-activated
GABA-T inhibitors. *Brain Res. Bull.*, 5(Suppl.
2):627–631.

271. Schechter, P. J., Tranier, Y., Jung, M. J., and
Bohlen, P. (1977): Audiogenic seizure protection by elevated brain GABA concentration in
mice: Effects of gamma-acetylenic GABA and
gamma-vinyl GABA, two irreversible GABA-T
inhibitors. *Eur. J. Pharmacol.*, 45:319–328.

272. Schechter, P. J., Tranier, Y., Jung, M., and
Sjoerdsma, A. (1977a): Antiseizure activity of
gamma-acetylenic gamma-aminobutyric acid: A
catalytic irreversible inhibitor of gamma-aminobutyric acid transminase, *J. Pharmacol. Exp.
Ther.*, 201:606–612.

273. Scheibel, M. E., Crandall, P. H., and Scheibel,
A. B. (1974): The hippocampal-dentate com-
plex in temporal lobe epilepsy: A golgi study.
Epilepsia, 15:55–80.

274. Schlesinger, K., Boggan, W., and Freedman,
D. X. (1965): Genetics of audiogenic seizures:
I. Relation to brain serotonin and norepineph-
rine in mice. *Life Sci.*, 4:2345–2351.

275. Schlesinger, W., Boggan, K., and Freedman,
D. X. (1968): Genetics of audiogenic seizures,
II. Effects of pharmacological manipulation on
brain serotonin, norepinephrine and gamma-
aminobutyric acid. *Life Sci.*, 7(part 1): 437–447.

276. Schlesinger, K., Harkins, J., Deckard, B. S.,
and Paden, C. (1975): Catechol-O-methyltrans-
ferase and monoamine oxidase activities in
brains of mice susceptible and resistant to audiogenic seizures. *J. Neurobiol.*, 6:587–596.

277. Schmitt, F. O. (1979): The role of structural,

electrical and chemical circuitry in brain function. In: *The Neurosciences, Fourth Study Program*, edited by F. O. Schmitt and F. G.
Worden, The MIT Press, Boston.

278. Schreiber, R. A. (1979): Sources of energy for
the brain and susceptibility to audiogenic seizures. *Med. Hypotheses*, 5:487–492.

279. Schreiber, R. A. (1979): The effect of nalaxone
on audiogenic seizures. *Psychopharmacology,
Berlin* 66(2):205–206.

280. Schwindt, P. C., and Crill, W. E. (1980): Role
of a persistent inward current in motor neurons
bursting during spinal seizures. *J. Neurophysiol.*, 43:1296–1318.

281. Schwartzkroin, P. A., Mutani, R., and Prince,
D. A. (1975): Orthodromic and antidromic effects of a cortical epileptiform focus on ventrolateral nucleus of the cat. *J. Neurophysiol.*,
38:795–811.

281. Schwartzkroin, P. A., and Prince, D. A. (1978):
Cellular and field potential properties of epileptogenic hippocampal slices. *Brain Res.*,
147:117–130.

283. Scobey, R. P., and Gabor, A. J. (1975): Ectopic
action potential generation in epileptiform
cortex. *J. Neurophysiol.*, 38:383–394.

284. Sellinger, O. Z. (1984): Brain methylation and
epileptogenesis: The case of methionine sulfoximine. *Ann. Neurol.*, 16(Suppl.):115–120.

285. Seyfried, T. N. (1979): Audiogenic seizures in
mice. *Fed. Proc.*, 38:2399–2401.

286. Shaws, T. B., Sakaguchi, A. Y., and Naylor,
S. L. (1982): Mapping the human genome,
cloned genes, DNA polymorphisms and inherited disease., *Adv. Hum. Genet.*, 12:341–353.

287. Shaywitz, B. A., Yager, R. D., and Gordon,
J. W. (1978): Ontogeny of brain catecholamine
turnover and susceptibility to audiogenic seizures in DBA/2J mice. *Dev. Psychobiol.*,
11:243–250.

288. Shepherd, G. M. (1978): Microcircuits in the
nervous system. *Sci. Am.*, 238:93–103.

289. Sherwin, A., Quesney, F., Gauthier, S., Olivier,
A., Robitaille, Y., Harvey, C., and van Gelder,
N. M. (1984): Enzyme changes in actively
spiking areas of human epileptic cerebral
cortex. *Neurology*, (Cleve), 34:927–933.

290. Siegel, G. J., Desmond, T. J., and Ernst, S. A.
(1984): Immunoreactive subspecies of (Na$^+$K$^+$)-
ATPase catalytic subunit. *Abstracts, 15th Annual Meeting of the American Society of Neurochemistry*, Portland, Oregon.

291. Siegel, J., and Murphy, G. J. (1979): Serotonergic inhibition of amygdala-kindled seizures
in cats. *Brain Res.*, 174:337–340.

292. Siegelbaum, S. A., Camardo, J. S., and Kandel,
E. R. (1982): Serotonin and cyclic AMP close
single K$^+$ channels an Aplysia sensory neurons.
Nature, 299:413–415.

293. Siesjo, B. K. (1983): Cell damage in the brain:
A speculative synthesis. *J Cereb. Blood Flow
Metab.*, 1:155–185.

294. Skeritt, J. H., and Johnston, G. A. R. (1984):
Modulation of excitant amino acid release by
convulsant and anticonvulsant drugs, In: *Neu-*

rotransmitters, Seizures and Epilepsy II, edited by R. G. Fariello, P. L. Morselli, K. G. Lloyds, L. F. Quesney, and J. Engel, Jr., Raven Press, New York.

295. Skolnick, P., Syapin, P. J., Paugh, B. A., Moncada, V., Marangos, P. J., and Paul, S. M. (1979): Inosine, an endogenous ligand of brain benzodiazepine receptor, antagonizes pentelenetetrazol-evoked seizures. *Proc. Natl. Acad. Sci. USA*, 76:1515–1518.

296. Sloviter, R. S. (1983): Epileptic brain damage in rats induced by sustained electrical stimulation of the perforant path. I. Acute electrophysiological and light microscopic studies. *Brain Res. Bull.*, 10:675–697.

297. Snead, O. C., III, and Bearden, L. J. (1982): The epileptogenic spectrum of opiate agonists. *Neuropharmacology*, 21:1137–1144.

298. Snead, O. C., III, Yu, R. K., and Huttenlocker, P. R. (1976): Gamma hydroxybutyrate. Correlation of serum and cerebrospinal fluid levels with electroencephalographic and behavioral effects. *Neurology* (Minn), 26(1):51–56.

299. Sommer, W. (1980): Erkrankung des ammonshornes als aetiologisches moment der epilepsie. *Arch. Psychiatr. Nervenkr.*, 10:631–675.

300. Speth, R., and Yammamura, H. (1979): Benzodiazepine receptors; Alterations in mutant mouse cerebellum. *Eur. J. Pharmacol.*, 54:398–399.

301. Squires, R., Naquet, R., Riche, D., and Braestrup, C. (1979): Increased thermolability of benzodiazepine receptors in central cortex of a baboon with spontaneous seizures: A case report. *Epilepsia*, 20:215–221.

302. Stahl, W. (1984): Na$^+$K$^+$ATPase: Function, structure and conformations. *Ann. Neurol.*, 16(5):121–127.

303. Stanbury, J. B., Wyngaarden, J. B., Fredrickson, D. S., Goldstein, J. L., and Brown, M. S. (1983): Inborn errors of metabolism in the 1980s. In: *The Metabolic Basis of Inherited Disease*, edited by J. B. Stanbury, B. J. Wyngaarden, and D. S. Fredrickson, pp. 3–61. McGraw-Hill, New York.

304. Stone, W. S., Eggleton, C., and Berman, R. F. (1980): Modification of amygdaloid kindled seizures in rats by opiates. *Neurosci. Abstr.*, 6:584.

305. Stourke, K., Taube, H. D., and Borowski, E. (1977): Presynaptic receptor systems in catecholamingeric transmission. *Biochem. Pharmacol.*, 26:259–268.

306. Stromborn, U., Form, J., Dolphin, A. C., and Greengaard, P. (1979): Regulation of the state of phosphorylation of specific neuronal proteins in mouse brain by *in vivo* administration of anaesthetic and convulsant agents. *Proc. Natl. Acad. Sci. USA*, 76:4687–4690.

307. Sugaya, E., Goldring, S., and O'Leary, J. L. (1964): Intracellular potentials associated with direct cortical response and seizure discharge in cat. *Handbook EEG Clin. Neurophysiol.*, 17:661–669.

308. Sweadner, K. J. (1979): Two molecular forms of (Na$^+$K$^+$)ATPase in brain. Separation and different affinity for strophantidin. *J. Biol. Chem.*, 254:600.

309. Sypert, G. W., Oakley, J., and Ward, A. A., Jr. (1970): Single unit analysis of propagated seizures in neocortex. *Exp. Neurol.*, 28:308–325.

310. Sypert, G. W., and Ward, A. A., Jr. (1967): The hyperexcitable neuron: Microelectrode studies of the chronic epileptic focus in the intact, awake monkey. *Exp. Neurol.*, 19:104.

311. Syrota, A., Castain, G. M., Rougemount, D., et al. (1983): Tissue acid base balance and oxygen metabolism in human cerebral infarction studied with PET. *Ann. Neurol.*, 14:419–428.

312. Szentagothai, J. (1975): The module concept in cerebral cortex architecture. *Brain Res.*, 95:475–496.

313. Taylor, C. P., and Dudek, F. E. (1982): Synchronous neural after discharges in rat hippocampal slices without active chemical synapses. *Science*, 218:810–812.

314. Theodore, W. H., Newmark, M. E., Sato, S., et al. (1983): [^{18}F] fluorodeoxyglucose positron emission computed tomography in refractory complex partial seizures. *Ann. Neurol.*, 14:429–437.

315. Ticku, M. K. (1979): Differences in gamma-aminobutyric acid receptor sensitivity in inbred strains of mice. *J. Neurochem.*, 33:1135–1138.

316. Timiras, P. S., and Hill, H. F. (1980): Hormones and epilepsy, In: *Antiepileptic Drugs: Mechanisms of Action, Advances in Neurology*, vol. 27, edited by G. H. Glaser, J. K. Penry, and D. M. Woodbury, pp. 655–666. Raven Press, New York.

317. Tower, D. B. (1965): Problems associated with studies of electrolyte metabolism in normal and epileptogenic cerebral cortex. *Epilepsia*, (ser. 3 Amst) 6:183.

318. Tower, D. B. (1969): Neurochemical mechanisms. In: *Basic Mechanisms of the Epilepsies*, edited by H. H. Hasper, A. A. Ward, Jr., and A. Pope, pp. 611–638, Little, Brown and Co., Boston.

319. Traub, R. D., and Wong, R. K. S. (1982): Cellular mechanisms of neuronal synchronization in epilepsy. *Science*, 261:745–747.

320. Trimble, M., Anlezark, G., and Meldrum, B. (1977): Seizure activity in photosensitive baboons following antidepressant drugs and the role of serotoninergic mechanisms. *Psychopharmacology*, 51:159–164.

321. Trottier, S., Claustre, Y., Caboche, J., Dedek, J., Chauvel, P., Nassif, S., and Scatton, B. (1983): Alterations of noradrenaline and serotonin uptake and metabolism in chronic cobalt-induced epilepsy in the rat. *Brain Res.*, 27(2):255–262.

322. Tsuboi, T. (1980): Genetic aspects of epilepsy. *Folia Psychiatr. Neurol. Jpn.*, 34:215–225.

323. Tuchek, J. M., Johnson, D. D., and Crawford, R. D. (1981): Abnormal phosphorylation of brain proteins in epileptic fowl. *Fed. Proc.*, 40:302.

324. Uhl, G. R., Kuhar, M. J., and Snyder, S. H. (1978): Enkaphalin-containing pathway: Amyg-

daloid efferents in the stria terminalis. *Brain Res.,* 149(1):223–228.

325. Unverricht, H. (1891): *Die Myoklonie.* Deutiche, Leipzig.

326. Van Gelder, N. M., and Courtois, A. (1972): Close correlation between changing content of specific amino acids in epileptogenic cortex of cats and severity of epilepsy. *Brain Res.,* 43:477.

327. Van Gelder, N. M., Sherwin, A. L., and Rasmussen, T. (1977): Amino acid content of epileptogenic human brain: Focal versus surrounding regions. *Brain Res.,* 40:385–397.

328. Velasco, M., Velasco, F., Romo, R., and Martinez, A. (1981): Effect of carbachol "push-pull" perfusion in the reticular formation on alumina cream-induced focal motor seizures in cats. *Exp. Neurol.,* 72:332–345.

329. Vosu, H., and Wise, R. A. (1975): Cholinergic seizure kindling in rat: Comparison of caudate, amygdala and hippocampus. *Behav. Biol.,* 13:491–495.

330. Wada, J. A., Balzama, F., Meldrum, B. S., and Naquet, R. (1972): Behavioral and electrographic effects of L-5 hydroxytryptophan and D,L parachlorophenylalanine on epileptic Senegalese baboon (*Papio papio*). *Handbook EEG Clin. Neurophysiol.,* 33:520–526.

331. Wada, J. A., Osawn, T., Wake, A., and Corcoran, M. E. (1975): Effects of taurine on kindled amygdaloid seizures in rats, cats, and photosensitive baboons. *Epilepsia,* 16:229.

332. Wada, J. A. (1977): Pharmacological prophylaxis in the kindling model of epilepsy. *Arch. Neurol.,* 34:389.

333. Wagner, H. N., Burns, H. D., Dunnals, R. F., Wong, D. F., Langstrom, B., Dueffler, T., Frost, J. J., Ravert, H. T., Links, J. M., Rosenbloom, S. B., Lukas, S. E., Kramer, A. V., and Kuhar, M. J. (1983): Imaging dopamine receptors in the human brain by positron tomography. *Science,* 22:1264–1266.

334. Walaas, S. I., Nairn, A. C., and Greengard, P. (1983a): Regional distribution of calcium- and cyclic adenosine 3′:5′-monophosphate-regulated protein phosphorylation systems in mammalian brain. I. Particulate systems. *J. Neurosci.,* 3:291–301.

335. Walaas, S. I., Nairn, A. C., and Greengard, P. (1983b): Regional distribution of calcium- and cyclic adenosine 3′5′-monophosphate-regulated protein phosphorylation systems in mammalian brain. II. Soluble systems. *J. Neurosci.,* 3:302–311.

336. Walker, J. E., Lewin, E., Sheppard, J. R., and Cromwell, R. (1973): Enzymatic regulation of adenosine 3′,5′-monophosphate in the freezing epileptogenic lesion of rat brain and homologous contralateral cortex. *J. Neurochem.,* 21:79.

337. Walker, J. E., Lewin, E., and Moffitt, B. C. (1974): Production of epileptiform discharges by application of agents which increase cyclic AMP levels in rat cortex. In: *Epilepsy,* pp. 30–36. *Proceedings of the Hans Berger Centenary Symposium,* edited by P. Harris, and C. Mawdsley, Churchill-Livingstone, New York.

338. Walker, J. E., Goodman, P., Jacobs, D., and Lewin, E. (1978): Uptake and release of norepinephrine by slices of rat cerebral cortex: Effect of agents which increase cyclic AMP levels. *Neurology,* 28:900–904.

339. Walsh, G. O. (1971): Penicillin iontophoresis in neocortex of cat. Effects on the spontaneous and induced activity of single neurons. *Epilepsia,* 12:1–11.

340. Ward, A. A., Jr. (1983): Physiological basis of chronic epilepsy and mechanisms of spread. In: *Status Epilepticus: Mechanisms of Brain Damage and Treatment, Advances in Neurology,* vol. 34, edited by A. V. Delgado-Escueta, C. G. Wasterlain, D. M. Treiman, and R. J. Porter, pp. 189–199. Raven Press, New York.

341. Wasterlain, C. G., Farber, D. B., Morin, A. M., Fando, J. M., and Fairchild, M. D. (1986): Synaptic mechanisms in the kindled epileptic focus. In: *Basic Mechanisms of the Epilepsies,* edited by A. V. Delgado-Escueta, A. A. Ward, Jr., and D. M. Woodbury, pp. 411–433. Raven Press, New York.

342. Weinryb, I., Chasin, M., Free, C. A., Harris, D. N., Goldberg, H., Michel, I. M., Park, V. S., Phillips, M., Sermaniego, S., and Hess, S. M. (1972): Effects of therapeutic agents on cyclic AMP metabolism in vitro. *J. Pharm. Sci.,* 61:1556–1567.

343. Westmoreland, B. F., Hanna, G. R., and Bass, N. H. (1972): Cortical alterations in zones of secondary epileptogenesis. *Brain Res.,* 43:485.

344. Westrum, L. E., White, L. E., Jr., Ward, A. A., Jr. (1964): Morphology of the experimental epileptic focus. *J. Neurosurg.,* 21:1033–1046.

345. White, R. (1984): Looking for epilepsy genes. *Ann. Neurol.,* 16(Suppl.):12–17.

346. Wilson, W. A., and Delgado-Escueta, A. V. (1974): Common synaptic events of pentelenetetrazol and penicillin. *Brain Res.,* 72:168–172.

347. Wilson, W. A., and Goldner, M. (1975): Voltage clamping with a single microelectrode. *J. Neurobiol.,* 6:411–422.

348. Winn, H. R., Welsh, J. E., Rubio, R., and Berne, R. M. (1980): Changes in brain adenosine during bicuculline-induced seizures in rats. Effects of hypoxia and altered systemic blood pressure. *Circ. Res.,* 47(4):568–577.

349. Wong, R. K., and Prince, D. A. (1978): Participation of calcium spikes during intrinsic burst firing in hippocampal neurons. *Brain Res.,* 159:385–390.

350. Wood, J. D., Russell, M. P., Kurylo, E., and Newstead, J. D. (1979): Stability of synaptosomal GABA levels and their use in determining the in vivo effects of drugs: Convulsant agents. *J. Neurochem.,* 33:61–68.

351. Woodbury, D. M., Engstrom, F. L., White, H. S., Chen, C. F., Kemp, J. W., and Chow, S. Y. (1984): Ionic and acid base regulation of neurons and glia during seizures. *Ann. Neurol.,* 16(Suppl.):135–144.

352. Yohe, H. E., Ueno, K., Chang, H., Glaser, G. H., and Yu, R. K. (1980): Incorporation of *N*-acetylmannosine into rat brain subcellular

gangliosides and effects of pentylentetrazol-induced convulsions on brain gangliosides. *J. Neurochem.*, 34:560.

353. Young, I. R., Burl, M., Clarke, G. J., Hall, A. S., Pasmore, T., Collins, A. G., Smith, D. T., Orr, J. S., Bydder, G. M., Doyle, F. H., Greenspan, R. H., and Steiner, R. E. (1981): Magnetic resonance properties of hydrogen: Imaging the posterior fossa. *AJR*, 137(5):895–901.

354. Zaczek, R., Nelson, M. F., and Coyle, J. T. (1978): Effects of anaesthetics and anticonvulsants on the action of kainic acid in the rat hippocampus. *Eur. J. Pharmacol.*, 52:323–327.

355. Zeman, W., Donahue, S., Dyken, P., and Green, J. (1970): The neuronal ceroidlipofuscinoses (Batten-Vogt syndrome). In: *Handbook of Clinical Neurology*, vol. 10, edited by P. J. Vinken, and G. W. Bruyn, pp. 588–679. North-Holland, Amsterdam.

356. Zoll, J. G., Kovacs, D. A., and Lineham, D. T. (1976): Effect of lysergic acid diethylamide on kindled seizures. *Soc. Neurosci. Abstr.*, 1:270.

357. Zuckerman, E. C., and Glaser, G. H. (1968): Hippocampal epileptic activity induced by localized ventricular perfusion with high potassium cerebrospinal fluid. *Exp. Neurol.*, 20:87–110.

Section 2
BIOCHEMICAL GENETICS AND THE EPILEPSIES

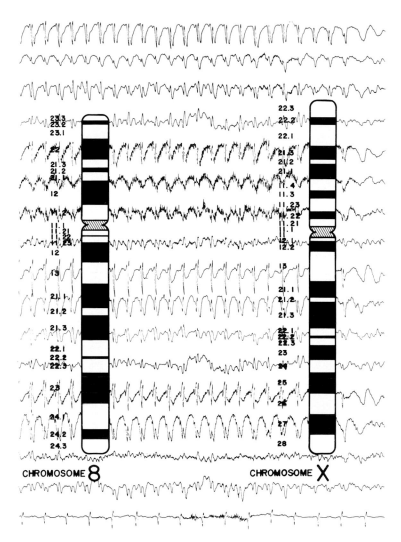

Four commingling streams in gene mapping, namely: family linkage studies, chromosome studies, somatic cell studies, and molecular approaches using restriction fragment length polymorphisms, *in situ* hybridization and restriction enzyme fine mapping are now being used to define the locus or loci of specific genetic epilepsies. The EEG trait of genetic generalized epilepsies—namely, bilaterally symmetrical diffuse spike-wave and multispike-wave complexes—is shown together with cartographies of chromosome 8 and X.

Advances in Neurology, Vol. 44, edited by
A. V. Delgado-Escueta, A. A. Ward, Jr.,
D. M. Woodbury, and R. J. Porter.
Raven Press, New York © 1986.

2

Genetic Heterogeneity in the Epilepsies

*V. Elving Anderson, **W. Allen Hauser, and *Stephen S. Rich

*University of Minnesota, Minneapolis, Minnesota 55455; and **G. H. Sergievsky Center and Faculty of Medicine, Columbia University, New York, New York 10032.

SUMMARY   There is ample evidence for genetic and other heterogeneity in the mechanisms leading to epilepsy. Animal models of epilepsy show that genetic factors can influence the hypersensitivity of neurons. In the human, there are over 140 Mendelian traits (including disorders of amino acids, enzymes, hormones, and vasculature) that increase the risk of seizures. Furthermore, systems with an intermediate optimum (such as blood clotting and blood glucose) involve a number of mechanisms under independent genetic control, and it is reasonable to assume that the same principle applies to neuronal excitability. Finally, genetic variation can be expected in any of the factors that are altered in the origin of seizures: neuronal inhibition, inactivation of excitatory neurotransmitters, feedback control, and seizure generalization.

One goal of future research is to define etiological subtypes on the basis of biochemical data or other factors. Meanwhile, it is possible to analyze currently available indicators of phenotypic variability (age at onset of seizures, family history of seizures, seizure type, EEG pattern, and history of antecedent factors such as fever or trauma) to address the following questions: (a) Do any phenotypic groups have different sibling risks for seizures? (b) How much phenotypic variability is seen among affected siblings of each defined group of probands (index cases)? (c) Do any groups of probands show significant biochemical differences? (d) Within a specific group, do isolated and familial cases show the same phenotype? (e) Within a presumed single entity, will linkage marker studies show further heterogeneity?

With such data in hand, certain strategies can be recommended. Complex segregation analysis of family data will permit a test of alternative models for genetic transmission. Linkage studies of selected large families (using recombinant DNA probes) will establish the genetic map location of any single-locus major factor. Selected samples of multiplex families (with several affected siblings) will concentrate the likelihood of genetic factors and will permit the detection of biochemical factors that might be significant in only a few families. Biochemical and other hypotheses can be tested in a panel of twin pairs concordant or discordant for epilepsy.

The search for genetic heterogeneity clearly has implications for diagnosis, prognosis, therapy, and genetic counseling, as well as for other research studies on the basic mechanisms of the epilepsies. When studies are carried out on human subjects or tissues, it is important that the patient samples be well defined in terms of family seizure history and the other indicators outlined above. Special note should be made of twin-born patients and families with several siblings or multiple generations affected, as possible subjects in collaborative studies.

The title of this volume, *Basic Mechanisms of the Epilepsies,* implies that we cannot expect to find a single etiological mechanism. This assumption of heterogeneity has important implications for diagnosis, therapy, prognosis, and genetic counseling (2,7,44,79).

It is generally accepted that there are a number of environmental mechanisms (head trauma, cerebral vascular accidents, fever, and use of alcohol or drugs) that can precipitate seizures. It may not be fully appreciated, however, that genetic variability adds an extra complexity to the problem. The definition of the sources of heterogeneity, therefore, is a fundamental and common task for those involved in epilepsy research.

The evidences for genetic heterogeneity can be assessed at any of three levels: (1) the phenotype itself (the observed features of the seizures together with electroencephalographic and other laboratory data); (2) the level of primary gene action (a developmental process, an enzyme, or a structural component of cells or membranes); and (3) the level of the genetic code. A definition of heterogeneity at one of the first two levels does not resolve the question, but simply opens the door to further investigation in finer detail.

An alternative approach is to consider the transmission of genetic factors, whether or not the phenotype is well understood. Here one seeks to determine if a single locus (Mendelian) pattern of inheritance is involved (autosomal dominant, autosomal recessive, or X-linked recessive). If a single locus pattern is not detected, we would then test for multifactorial inheritance. This implies that a number of genetic determinants are inherited independently, and that other nongenetic (or environmental) factors may be involved in shaping the final phenotype. There is the further option that a single genetic locus may have a major effect that is modified by a multifactorial genetic background. It is possible that two or more multifactorial systems may be involved (for example, one affecting brain development and another affecting the level of a neurotransmitter). Finally, it should be noted that a complex mixture of several multifactorial and single-locus determinants may be very hard to distinguish from a single multifactorial system.

EVIDENCE FOR GENETIC HETEROGENEITY IN EPILEPSY

The editors of this volume have summarized

the types of genetic variation that have been observed for animal models of seizures (see Table 3 in Chapter 1). Although none of these is an exact parallel of a human epilepsy state, these animal models present firm evidence that genetic factors can influence the hypersensitivity of neurons. Furthermore, Appendix A in this chapter lists over 140 Mendelian traits in the human which increase the risk of seizures. These conditions include disturbances of amino acids, enzymes, hormones, vascular changes, and neoplasms in the brain, as well as other syndromes for which the etiological mechanism is not yet apparent.

A third argument for genetic heterogeneity in the epilepsies comes from the observation that the optimum for neuronal excitability is intermediate between two extremes. It is generally observed that systems with an intermediate optimum (such as blood clotting and blood glucose) are complex and involve a number of mechanisms under independent genetic control. Thus, we expect to find heterogeneity in the epilepsies and would require strong evidence to accept the contrary opinion.

Many of the other chapters in this volume have made a significant contribution to our understanding of the causal factors involved in seizures. Seizures may result if there are defects in any of the following steps: neuronal inhibition, inactivation of excitatory neurotransmitters, feedback control, and the generalization or spread of the seizure state. Each of these can be expected to reflect genetic variation.

GENETIC HETEROGENEITY IN OTHER CONDITIONS

The topic of heterogeneity has been important in genetic journals for a number of decades and is even more obvious currently. A brief review of some selected conditions will illustrate the methods used to detect heterogeneity.

Gargoylism was the term applied earlier to a complex set of physical malformations. Careful comparison of clinical findings with family history data showed that affected individuals in families showing an X-linked mode of inheritance had a different set of phenotypic features than did the remainder. The X-linked cases became known as Hunter syndrome, and the autosomal recessive cases became known as the Hurler syndrome; other related conditions were identified. Some of the mucopolysaccharidoses were shown to be genetically distinct because the mixing of two cell lines in tissue culture corrected the metabolic error (62). Currently, 15 distinguishable conditions are recognized (52).

Congenital hydrocephalus can occur as one manifestation of a multifactorial liability to central nervous system (CNS) malformations, as part of other malformation syndromes, or as a rare X-linked condition involving occlusion of the aqueduct of Sylvius. Further subtypes have been defined by the presence or absence of anomalies in the CNS or in other parts of the body (95).

Cases of osteogenesis imperfecta (OI) can be subdivided into three groups on the basis of small differences in clinical and radiographical findings (78). Biochemical evidence was interpreted as suggesting that further subdivision may become necessary. Recent studies of collagen (which is defective in OI) have provided clear evidence for phenotypic heterogeneity among the collagen disorders, together with a surprising unity in molecular mechanisms (70).

An earlier study of the muscular dystrophies by Morton and Chung (59) used segregation analysis to evaluate the clinical findings of cases assessed with families. Currently, there is good evidence for three different X-linked recessive forms, five different autosomal dominant forms, and three autosomal recessive forms, as well as case reports that may represent additional entities (51).

Studies of linkage in Duchenne muscular dystrophy (DMD) have been facilitated by the use of restriction fragment length polymorphisms (RFLPs). O'Brien et al. (66) found that all informative families showed linkage to the same marker on the X chromosome. These results are of practical importance, since the existence of several loci causing DMD would have made it much more difficult to use linkage data for prediction of genotype.

Parkinsonism is observed with a small but significant increase among parents and siblings of probands. Martin et al. (50) found that the cumulative risk for siblings approached 30% when there was an affected parent, but was not significantly elevated above control values when no parent was affected. [Parallel findings were observed for Alzheimer disease by Heston et al., (37).] The authors could not distinguish between a single multifactorial trait or a heterogeneous mixture of several modes of inheritance. More recently, Barbeau and Roy (8) argued strongly for heterogeneity and presented evidence for several rare forms with a simple mode of inheritance and high sibling risks.

It is well known that there are several Mendelian traits affecting cholesterol metabolism, but most cases do not fit this explanation. Several studies (58,72) have given careful attention to statistical methods that can be used to search for heterogeneity within and between populations. These theoretical articles form part of the recent effort to attack the problem of genetics for common disorders (12,79,80).

Diabetes mellitus has been separated into two broad categories, insulin-dependent and insulin-independent. The former group generally has an earlier age at onset and a lower sibling risk. Rotter (75) summarized the various hypotheses for heterogeneity within the insulin-dependent category. Further tests of heterogeneity were based on data concerning association and linkage with HLA and other genetic markers (13,39). The possibility of two disease loci was explored, and several different tests of linkage heterogeneity were performed.

Even when the biochemical basis for a condition is firmly established, evidence for further heterogeneity may be found. Mutations in different families affected one or more of the following parameters of the enzyme adenosine deaminase: electrophoretic mobility, isoelectric point, heat stability, and enzyme activity (38). Two different mutations in the pyruvate carboxylase gene have been reported (74), one resulting in a relatively inactive protein and the other in no recognizable protein.

This review has included examples of: (a) assessment of clinical findings; (b) statistical analysis of pedigree data; (c) biochemical studies; and (d) the use of linkage markers. Similar methods can be incorporated in the design of more informative studies of epilepsy.

Animal Models

The relevance of animal models is often discounted by the claim that the seizures produced are not precisely the same as those found in the human, but this demand for an exact fit may be misleading. It is more important to ask what each animal model tells us about the etiological mechanisms involved. It then becomes possible for us to search for the possibility that a similar type of mechanism may be involved in human seizure conditions. Thus, the parallelism should be sought at the level of gene action rather than the phenotypic consequences. It is particularly important that the information about animal models be compared carefully with the results from experimental studies at the tissue and cellular levels. The editors of this volume deserve our appreciation for organizing these data in a parallel fashion (see Tables 2 and 3 in Chapter 1).

Mendelian Traits in the Human

In the evaluation of a new patient with seizures, it is essential to consider the possibility of one of the Mendelian traits that increase the risk of seizures (Appendix). The differential diagnosis requires attention to a number of otherwise minor characteristics such as hair form, skin texture, visual or hearing loss, mental retardation, and other manifestations of nervous system dysfunction.

A more important function of the Appendix for our present purpose is the documentation of the wide variety of mechanisms that can lead to seizures. Generally, when a genetic disorder is diagnosed, the medical attention turns toward means of treatment for the underlying condition. As a result, the pathways leading to the seizures are seldom explored, and we lose the opportunity to gain more insight into the etiology of seizures. Thus, information about conditions in the Appendix should be compared with the data in Tables 2 and 3 in Chapter 1 of this volume (16). It is likely that genetic mutations may be as useful in discriminating among various physiological explanations for seizures as they have been for the explication of enzyme pathways.

For each of these conditions we need thoughtful attention to these questions: (a) Why do seizures occur at all in this syndrome? (b) Why do seizures occur in some, but not all, of the affected individuals? (c) What variability is observed within families that might be ascribed to environmental variables, modifying genes, sex, and age.

Some Basic Epidemiology

Before we review the family studies of epilepsy, it is necessary to indicate two areas of epidemiological concern (34,61,92). The first has to do with the selection of samples for study. Clinic samples include an overrepresentation of chronic cases. If the risk of seizure recurrence is correlated with a family history of seizures, samples chosen in this way will give a biased estimate of the role of genetic factors. It is also possible that familial cases of epilepsy will be referred to major medical centers more often than isolated cases are. Therefore, it is essential that the details of case ascertainment be presented in any reports and that the possible effects of bias and ascertainment be considered.

A second problem is the choice of population rates for estimating expected numbers of affected relatives. The age-specific incidence rates for epilepsy (the number of newly diagnosed cases per 100,000 in the population per year) are the highest in the very young, drop to a relatively constant rate between ages 10 and 70 years, and increase again thereafter (Fig. 1). The age-specific prevalence rates (the percentage of the population under treatment at any specific time) increase through age 14 years and are similar in each age group thereafter. (The prevalence at any age reflects the sum of all incidence cases through that age less those who are no longer receiving medical care, presumably due to remission, or who have died. Thus, after age 15 years, the number of incidence cases equals the number of cases withdrawing from the pool.) In family studies, however, we wish to estimate the chance that persons at a given age will have had epilepsy at any point in their lives. For this purpose, the cumulative incidence is the statistic of choice. From Fig. 1, it appears that the cumulative incidence for epilepsy by age 40 years is 1.7%. This estimate can be used (for middle-class Caucasian populations) as the base-rate expectation for comparison with any elevated risk for siblings of epilepsy probands (index cases).

Clinical Variables

There have been several comprehensive reviews of the family studies of epilepsy (4,5,17,44,60,63,86). These family studies can be separated into three general groups based on year of publication.

1. Most of the studies published before 1959 deal with epilepsy as a whole or with subdivisions that are too broad to serve as the basis for studies of heterogeneity. Furthermore, all categories of relatives were commonly grouped together. Other problems were summarized by Newmark and Porter (64).

2. Reports published in 1959–1975 were considerably more informative. Eisner et al. (23) used a more detailed classification of seizures and carefully tabulated the ages of siblings. The series of papers by Metrakos and Metrakos (53–56) outlined the criteria needed for a careful genetic studies and provided benchmark data on probands with a generalized spike-wave EEG.

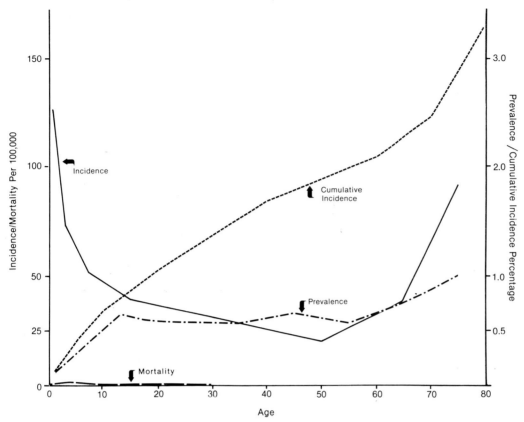

FIG. 1. Incidence, prevalence, and cumulative incidence rates for epilepsy in Rochester, Minnesota, 1935–1974. From J. F. Annegers, *personal communication.*

Another series by Andermann (1) provided data about probands with focal seizures. Other informative reports were published in the 1960s and 1970s.

3. The questions that we are facing currently require finer clinical detail about the probands, explicit information about family history, and the ability to retabulate the data to answer new questions as they emerge. For these purposes, we are dependent mainly upon the ongoing studies that have a sufficient sample size and in which the data are available for reanalysis. Furthermore, it is mainly from these ongoing studies (6,9,18,43) that it is possible to select smaller subsets of probands and relatives to test specific biochemical hypotheses (42,71,91).

In the following review, attention will be given primarily to the second and third groups. Furthermore, particular attention will be given to the following questions, which are designed to detect heterogeneity:

1. Do any phenotypic groups have different sibling risks, particularly when the probands are sorted by presence or absence of seizures in parents?

2. How much phenotypic variability is seen among the affected siblings of defined groups of probands?

3. Do any groups of probands show significant differences on biochemical variables that may be causally related to epilepsy?

4. Within specific subgroups of probands, do isolated and familial cases show the same phenotype?

5. Within specific seizure categories, do all affected families show the same linkage relationship between seizure history and genetic markers?

An illustration of the effect some of the clinical variables have upon offspring risk is shown in the data from the study by Tsuboi and Endo (89) (Table 1). The following points may be noted.

1. Although their probands were selected for epilepsy, the risk of febrile convulsions in offspring is higher than expected. This strongly suggests some genetic connection between a susceptibility to febrile convulsions and to epilepsy in general.

2. The risk of epilepsy and of febrile convulsions in offspring shows a clear relationship to the age of the proband at onset of epilepsy.

3. In the small set of probands with an affected parent or sibling, the risk of seizures in offspring is sharply increased.

4. In the group of probands with symptomatic epilepsy, the risk of seizures in offspring is small, possibly no higher than the rate expected in the general population.

5. The offspring risks (both for epilepsy and for febrile convulsions) are higher when the epileptic proband is a female. The sex-related differences in risks of epilepsy present some genetic problems that have not yet been resolved (67).

6. The final observation deals with value of

EEG tests in the offspring. It seems apparent that persons having epilepsy in a parent and a generalized spike-wave EEG in themselves have a sharply elevated risk of a seizure.

Age at Onset

Seizures involve a number of age-related phenomena (46). Seyfried, for example, has shown in the mouse that susceptibility to audiogenic seizures at 21 days of age is genetically distinct from seizures at 60 days (77). Many of the abnormal EEG patterns in humans show characteristic age patterns rising to a peak at a certain age and falling thereafter.

One of the clearest demonstrations of age at onset effects is shown by the data for major motor seizures by Eisner et al. (Fig. 2). When the onset of major motor seizures in the proband occurred before age 4 years, the cumulative incidence of seizures in siblings rose more sharply than when the onset in the proband was at an older age. The control group had a cumulative incidence of 2.3% by age 40 years, a frequency which compares quite closely with the figure of 1.7% for the Rochester study (Fig. 1).

A similar pattern is seen in the data for siblings of the 1,047 newly diagnosed cases of seizures studied as part of the Minnesota Comprehensive Epilepsy Program (Table 2). The risk of seizures among siblings was highest for probands having onset in the first decade of life, a tendency that is more readily apparent when all seizures are considered.

This effect of age at onset may result from two

TABLE 1. *Risk of seizures among offspring of epileptic probands*

	Offspring			
Category	Total No.	Epilepsy (%)	FC (%)	Total (%)
All probands	506	2.4	6.7	9.1
Age of proband at onset				
0–9 years	99	3.0	11.1	14.1
10–29 years	250	2.8	6.4	9.2
30 or older	157	1.3	4.4	5.7
Sex of proband				
Male	233	1.7	5.2	6.9
Female	273	2.9	8.1	11.0
Proband with affected parent or sibling				
Yes	55			21.8
No	451			7.5
Proband with				
Idiopathic epilepsy	382			11.0
Symptomatic epilepsy	124			3.2
EEG in offspring				
GSW	38			28.9
No specific anomaly	64			4.7

FC, febrile convulsion; GSW, generalized spike-wave.

From Tsuboi and Endo, ref. 89, with permission.

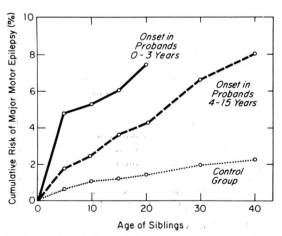

FIG. 2. Cumulative risk for major motor epilepsy in siblings of probands with epilepsy. Based on data from Eisner et al., ref. 23, with permission.

TABLE 2. *Sibling cumulative risk for seizures and epilepsy by age at onset in the proband*

Age at onset in proband	Siblings (total no.)	Risk to age 40 years (%)	
		Epilepsy	Any seizure
0–9	339	3.4	8.0
10–24	772	3.4	4.6
25–49	972	2.3	2.5
50 up	1294	1.5	1.7

factors. First, those etiological subtypes of seizures that have an earlier age at onset may be more influenced by genetic variables (a heterogeneity hypothesis). Second, those probands with early onset of seizures may have a higher genetic liability with a corresponding risk for siblings (a multifactorial hypothesis). Under either hypothesis, it is essential to define carefully the age at onset in the proband and to adjust the sibling data for their age at last report.

Family History of Seizures

In the absence of information about specific etiological pathways, the major source of data about possible genetic factors comes from the reported history of epilepsy and seizures in near relatives. It is important, however, to keep the information about the several types of relatives separate. Siblings of probands, for example, are at increased risk for any of the modes of inheritance, whether autosomal, X-linked, or multifactorial. Affected parents or offspring may represent dominant or multifactorial patterns of inheritance, but seldom recessive.

As a first approximation, we examined the data from the Minnesota Comprehensive Epilepsy Program tabulating the proportion of seizure probands having an affected parent (Table 3). The term "remote symptomatic" refers to cases in which there is a history of an antecedent event felt to increase the risk of epilepsy (such

as head trauma), but in which the first seizure occurred more than 1 week following the insult in question (33). It will be noted that the percentage of probands having an affected parent is consistently higher with onset of seizures at a young age, even in the case of the acute symptomatic category. This would suggest that special attention should be given to cases with presumed acute symptomatic etiology if there is a history of seizures or epilepsy in one or both parents.

It is preferable to examine parental and sibling data simultaneously. Studies of parkinsonism (50) and of Alzheimer disease (37) have shown that sibling risks are sharply higher in those relatively few families in which the proband has a parent affected with the same disorder. A parallel kind of tabulation is shown in Table 4 concerning febrile convulsions in Japan and Minnesota. It will be noted that there is a steady increase in sibling risk depending upon whether neither parent, or one, or both parents had febrile convulsions.

Seizure Type

A system for classifying seizure type must meet several different and sometimes conflicting purposes. For clinical purposes, one needs a system that will help to provide guidance for prescribing treatment and assessing prognosis, but such a system does not necessarily represent discrete etiologic classes. Excellent descriptions of the various seizure types and their relevance for genetic counseling are provided by Blume (11), and by Delgado-Escueta, et al. (15).

In reviewing the currently available genetic studies, it becomes apparent that not all have used the same taxonomic scheme. A more serious limitation is that some studies report the sibling risk for any seizure and others for epilepsy alone, whereas only a few give both kinds of data.

It must also be recognized that some of the presumed unique seizure syndromes discussed

TABLE 3. *Probands with parent affected by antecedent factor and by age at onset*

Antecedent factor	Onset 0–24 years			Onset 25+ years		
	Probands	Parent affected		Probands	Parent affected	
		No.	(%)		No.	(%)
Idiopathic	264	41	(15.5)	219	13	(5.9)
Remote symptomatic	81	11	(13.6)	133	9	(6.8)
Acute symptomatic	150	18	(12.0)	190	8	(4.2)

TABLE 4. *Risk of febrile convulsions (FC) in siblings of probands by parental history of FC*

Parental history	Fukuyama et al. (27)			Tsuboi (87)			Hauser et al. (35)		
	Total siblings	With FC		Total siblings	With FC		Total siblings	With FC	
		No.	(%)		No.	(%)		No.	(%)
Both with FC	3	2	(66.6)	18	7	(38.9)	18	10	(55.6)
One with FC	73	17	(23.3)	210	66	(31.4)	106	23	(21.7)
Neither with FC	211	38	(18.0)	866	154	(17.8)	922	51	(5.5)
Total	287	57	(19.9)	1,094	227	(20.7)	1,046	84	(8.0)

in the literature are not different entities, but instead are age-specific variations in the manifestations of seizure predisposition. Thus, a given individual may show distinct seizure syndromes at different ages. Age-related changes in seizure type appear to reflect the complex interaction of: (a) the nature and likelihood of specific antecedent factors, (b) the developmental maturation of the nervous system, and (c) genetic variation influencing the structure and biochemistry of the developing brain.

The results from some of the larger and more adequately reported studies are shown in Table 5. It will be noted that some of the studies select probands on the basis of seizure type only, whereas others use a combination of seizure type and EEG pattern. In general, the sibling risks are higher when the proband has seizures that would be classified as generalized onset based upon the 1981 revision of the International League Against Epilepsy (ILAE) International Classification of Epileptic Seizures. Only the first, second, and last studies in Table 5 include control or population values for comparison. Age adjustments were made only in the last study.

Some of the rarer forms of seizures appear to be of more interest from the genetic point of view. Progressive myoclonus epilepsy is a type identified first by Unverricht and Lundborg and is also known as Baltic myoclonus epilepsy. Norio and Koskiniemi (65) reviewed the data for 74 Finnish families and calculated the risk to siblings to be 26.0%. Juvenile myoclonic epilepsy (listed in Table 5 as impulsive petit mal) has distinctive phenotypic signs and has been identified as an important category for linkage studies (14).

EEG Pattern

Generalized epilepsies usually are accompanied by an interictal generalized spike-wave pat-

TABLE 5. *Risk of seizures and epilepsy among siblings of probands with epilepsy*

Study/probands	Siblings	Epilepsy (%)	Any seizure (%)
Metrakos and Metrakos (55)			
Centrencephalic epilepsy (GSW)	519	—	12.7
Controls	322	—	4.7
Andermann (1)			
Focal (mostly temporal)	229	—	4.8
Controls	458	—	3.9
Doose et al. (20)			
Absence (GSW)	448	—	6.7
Doose et al. (21)			
Myoclonic-astatic petit mal (GSW)	95	—	12.6
Tsuboi and Christian (88)			
Impulsive petit mal	705	4.4	—
Jensen (45)			
Temporal lobe	171	2.9	7.6
Norio and Koskiniemi (65)			
Progressive myoclonus epilepsy	125	26.0	
Annegers et al. (6)			
Idiopathic epilepsy, onset <15 years	489	3.6[a]	11.6[a]
General population	—	1.7[a]	5.1[a]

GSW, generalized spike and wave.
[a] Cumulative incidence to age 40 years.

tern (GSW). A GSW pattern may occur also in individuals who have other forms of epilepsy or even in symptomatic individuals. Thus, the data reported in Table 5 for centrencephalic epilepsy (55) are based on probands who showed a GSW pattern together with recurrent petit mal or grand mal seizures.

Gloor et al. (29) explained GSW pattern as representing an oscillation between a short period of increased excitation (the spike) and a following longer period of increased inhibition (the wave). They assumed that a 3/s GSW pattern results from the activity of a major gene that may produce a predisposition common to most epileptogenic conditions.

Doose et al. (20) found lower sibling risks for seizures among absence probands than did Metrakos and Metrakos. Furthermore, Doose et al. categorized probands with GSW occurring spontaneously separately from those with GSW occurring only during photoconvulsive response (PCR) (Table 6). The two reports (19,28) are based on the same sample of probands and controls, but the number of siblings tabulated for PCR is considerably smaller because of the authors' stringent requirement of repeated testing over a specific age range before a PCR-negative status was assigned. The frequency of PCR in the general population over the age range studied is higher than a GSW in the EEG at rest or during hyperventilation (line 5). The presence of epilepsy (without GSW or PCR) in the probands increases the frequency of both GSW and PCR in the siblings (lines 4 and 5). The added presence of a GSW in the proband does not further increase the sibling risk for GSW or PCR (lines 2 and 4), whereas the added presence of a PCR is associated with increases in both GSW and PCR in the siblings (lines 1 and 2). These results suggest that a GSW in the EEG at rest or during hyperventilation may be genetically different from GSW occurring only during photic stimulation (18).

The data from the Minnesota Comprehensive Epilepsy Program appear to support a similar type of heterogeneity (36). An increased sibling risk for seizures is found only for those seizure probands who have a GSW pattern together with a PCR and/or multifocal spikes (MF). The seizure risk for siblings of seizure probands with only a GSW is no higher than it is for seizure probands who have none of these EEG patterns.

Antecedent Factors

A distinction can be made between predisposing factors (that increase the general hypersensitivity of neurons without necessarily triggering a seizure) and precipitating factors (that can more directly trigger a seizure episode). In practice, these tend to be lumped together, and those cases of seizures for which an antecedent factor can be identified are often termed symptomatic. We have found it helpful to make a further distinction between those cases in which the antecedent factor is closely related in time with the seizure event (acute symptomatic) and those in which the time relationship is more distant (remote symptomatic).

We already have presented evidence (Table 3) that the question about family history of seizures should be asked even if an antecedent factor can be identified. Furthermore, there are age-specific changes in the relative contribution of various types of antecedent factors. For example, seizures associated with CNS infections are seldom seen after 5 years of age. Nevertheless, the proportion of epilepsies which appear idiopathic (for which no antecedent factors are apparent) appears relatively stable over age.

Febrile convulsions are one of the types of acute symptomatic seizures that have been studied extensively (26,27,32,49,76,87,90). One significant observation (Table 7) is that the population rates are higher in several large Japanese studies than they are in studies from the United

TABLE 6. *Electroencephalographic findings in siblings of probands and in control children*

Probands			Gerken and Doose (28)		Doose and Gerken (19)	
Epilepsy	GSW	PCR	Total siblings	GSW (%)	Total siblings	PCR (%)
1. Yes	Yes	Yes	233	8.6	163	16.6
2. Yes	Yes	No	171	4.7	124	7.3
3. Yes	No	Yes	69	4.4	50	22.0
4. Yes	No	No	68	4.4	49	8.2
5. No	(control children)		685	1.8	662	5.0

GSW, generalized spike-wave at rest or during hyperventilation; PCR, photoconvulsive response.

TABLE 7. *Risk of febrile convulsions (FC) among siblings of probands with FC*

Study	Siblings of probands			Population		
	Total no.	With FC		Total no.	With FC	
		No.	(%)		No.	(%)
Fukuyama et al. (27)	287	57	19.9			
Tsuboi (87)	1,094	227	20.7	16,806	1,123	6.7
Frantzen et al. (26)	303	33	10.9			
Van den Berg (90)	432	37	8.6	6,956	144	2.1
Hauser et al. (35)	1,046	84	8.0			2.4

States and Denmark. The risks to siblings of probands are correspondingly higher in the Japanese studies. These relationships between sibling risks and population values can be analyzed under the assumption of an underlying liability that is multifactorial in nature (Fig. 3). When this is done, it is obvious that the estimates of familial contribution (the heritability of liability) are similar.

It may also be noted (Table 4) that the two Japanese and the one American series have quite different sibling rates when neither parent is affected, whereas the sibling rates are very similar when one or both parents are affected. The implications of this point are not clear and deserve further study.

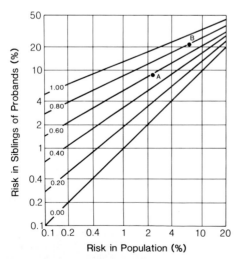

FIG. 3. Estimates of the heritability of liability for febrile convulsions in population samples from Minnesota (A) and Japan (B). Based on data from Fukuyama et al. and Hauser et al., refs. 27 and 35, with permission (see Table 7). Graph adapted from Smith, ref. 81, with permission.

Strategies for Detecting Genetic Heterogeneity in Epilepsy

Segregation Analysis

Few of the presently available genetic studies of epilepsy have taken full advantage of the information about the distribution of seizures within and between families. It is now possible to take advantage of the methods for complex segregation analysis that have been developed to estimate a number of genetic parameters and to test genetic models (30,47,58,73,94). Several issues should be addressed, however, before attempting such analysis.

1. It does not seem appropriate to apply sophisticated analytical procedures to pooled data for all of the epilepsies. Even though our present knowledge is still incomplete, some effort to identify presumed entities in advance will provide more meaningful results.

2. Relatively large sample sizes are advised. In the cases of febrile convulsions, for example, the sample size is now large enough and the category is sufficiently discrete that complex segregation analysis appears appropriate.

3. It is important that the genetic models to be tested be well defined (57). Insofar as possible, this process should include presumed environmental variables, age-specific changes in signs and symptoms, and other possible etiological mechanisms.

4. It is most desirable to provide several genetic models to be tested simultaneously. It is of little interest, for example, to show that epilepsy can be explained by multifactorial inheritance without simultaneous information about the possibility of simple autosomal pattern.

5. The possibility of etiological heterogeneity should be considered in the analysis wherever possible. In our opinion, it is better to start with the possibility of heterogeneity and find evi-

dence to the contrary than it is to start with the assumption of an overall homogeneity.

Linkage

The development of recombinant DNA technology has introduced new dimensions to the study of genetic linkage. The identification of new RFLPs is proceeding at a rapid pace. These new markers are expanding significantly the ability to test various areas of the genome (10,93).

There are some cautions, however, that should be considered before embarking upon large-scale linkage studies.

1. Whenever possible, linkage studies should be applied first to large pedigrees. The pooling of data from smaller families assumes a high degree of homogeneity. If, in fact, several genetic loci are involved, possible evidence for linkage will be obscured. If linkage with a marker can be established for one or two large families, smaller families can be tested using the same marker.

2. The test of autosomal linkage requires that the mode of inheritance (dominant or recessive) be identified. If this distinction cannot be made on other grounds, extreme caution must be used (85).

3. For autosomal recessive modes of inheritance, families with several affected siblings are required. However, the ascertainment of multiplex sibships can introduce biases that must be anticipated in the analysis (69,83,84).

4. For most categories of seizures, age-at-onset corrections will be needed.

Studies of HLA linkage in the case of epilepsy have not yet provided conclusive results (4). The approach used to study linkage in juvenile myoclonic epilepsy appears to be more promising (14).

Multiplex Families

The possibility of etiological heterogeneity greatly reduces the efficiency of the search for biochemical or other causal variables. Anderson et al. (3) suggested that families with several affected siblings will concentrate the likelihood of genetic factors and will permit the detection of biochemical factors that might be significant in only a few families.

This approach has been used for the Minne-

sota Comprehensive Epilepsy Program and has led to the identification of a possible and previously nonrecognized explanation for some seizures. Of the first 14 probands from multisib families that were screened utilizing a two-dimensional electrophoresis approach (68), five were found to have missing or low haptoglobin, a plasma protein that binds free hemoglobin. Further work is required to verify the genetic basis of the low haptoglobin in these families, and to explore the relationship with seizures. The proposed hypothesis is that individuals with a previously existing low haptoglobin will have difficulty in resolving areas of blood in brain tissue that have resulted from hemorrhage or trauma.

Those who are carrying out detailed and sophisticated studies of seizure patients would be encouraged to apply their methodologies first to the multiplex families that may be available to them.

Twins. Many studies of epilepsy in twins have stressed the estimation of concordance rates in monozygotic as compared with dizygotic pairs (31,41,48,76). Meanwhile, in other conditions, twin methods have been used to explore a number of potentially more interesting questions (40). Eaves (22) for example, showed how twin studies can be used to study developmental features and the interaction of multiple variables. A further suggestion is that monozygotic twin pairs concordant for epilepsy would provide an excellent panel for analyzing the effectiveness of anticonvulsants.

Recommendations for Future Studies

The importance of heterogeneity can be highlighted by quotations from two recent papers. Spranger (82) commented on the revised classification of OI proposed by Sillence et al. (78). He recognized that proof for the difference between subtypes will require the help of biochemists. Nevertheless, clinicians must go as far as they can with careful observation.

If we provide the biochemist with heterogeneous material his results will be heterogeneous and hence inconclusive. Only when the clinician learned to differentiate rubella from scarlet fever, we recall, did the microbiologist consistently find streptococci in the latter and thus establish its cause (82).

The importance of this topic for conditions as

well defined as Huntington disease (HD) was stressed by Folstein et al. (25).

Given the current stage of knowledge it is important in conducting HD research that the possibility of genetic heterogeneity not be dismissed. If it is present and results in variability among biological samples, important findings can be masked or "refuted" by large standard errors resulting from a mixture of samples. A failure to replicate can result if a family, or families with different genotypes, is used in the second study.

We have several specific suggestions that should help in the detection and analysis of heterogeneity in studies of epilepsy. Some of these involve relatively simple changes in the way in which publications are prepared. Others involve special samples that may be of interest within clinical centers, whereas others provide a basis for collaboration among institutions. Finally, we have some comments on developments arising in molecular neurobiology.

When studies are carried out on human subjects or tissues, it is important that the samples be well defined. In addition to the description of seizure type and EEG pattern, it will be helpful to have some brief information about family history. For initial analysis, it is sufficient to identify for each case the number of parents with a history of seizures and the number of siblings with a similar history. In biochemical studies, for example, the results might be analyzed separately for four family history groups defined by the presence or absence of a seizure history in parents and in siblings. If any interesting differences appear among these four groups, some further review of the data would be advised.

We urge that epilepsy clinics keep a running record of those families in which two or more siblings have seizures. These multisib families would provide an excellent panel for extensive biochemical, clinical, or other laboratory studies.

A similar record should be maintained for patients who are twin-born. Both concordant and discordant pairs of twins can be very useful, although for different questions. In the near future, we envision that twin studies might focus on specific rare clinical patterns. In such an event, it would be extremely important and necessary to have a basis for collaboration among various institutions.

We also urge that special note be made of families in which a number of individuals have a seizure history. Kindreds with five or more affected persons can be reviewed to determine which persons are likely to be informative for linkage studies.

A number of papers in this book reflect recent advances in molecular genetics. Of particular importance will be those studies that identify polymorphic variation in DNA recognized by probes for genes that produce neurotransmitter substances or other products that may be important in the etiology of seizures. For example, Feder et al. (24) have found a polymorphism for the POMC gene that could be used for linkage studies of epilepsy.

In his book, *First Principles*, Herbert Spencer described evolution as "an integration of matter and concomitant dissipation of motion; during which the matter passes from an indefinite incoherent homogeneity to a definite coherent heterogeneity; and during which the retained motion undergoes a parallel transformation." In a similar manner, we would hope that epilepsy research would pass from "an indefinite incoherent homogeneity to a definite coherent heterogeneity."

REFERENCES

1. Andermann, E. (1982): Multifactorial inheritance of generalized and focal epilepsy. In: *Genetic Basis of the Epilepsies*, edited by V. E. Anderson, W. A. Hauser, J. K. Penry, and C. F. Sing, pp. 355–374. Raven Press, New York.
2. Anderson, V. E. (1977): Genetic counseling for epilepsy. In: *Plan for Nation-wide Action on Epilepsy,* vol. II, part 1, pp. 141–162. DHEW Publication No. (NIH) 78-311.
3. Anderson, V. E., Chern, M. M., and Schwanebeck, E. (1981): Multiplex families and the problem of heterogeneity. In: *Genetic Research Strategies for Psychobiology and Psychiatry,* edited by E. S. Gershon, S. Matthysse, X. O. Breakefield, and R. D. Ciaranello, pp. 341–351. The Boxwood Press, Pacific Grove, California.
4. Anderson, V. E., and Hauser, W. A. (1985): The genetics of epilepsy. *Prog. Med. Genet.,* 6:9–52.
5. Anderson, V. E., Hauser, W. A., Penry, J. K. and Sing, C. F., editors (1982): *Genetic Basis of the Epilepsies.* Raven Press, New York.
6. Annegers, J. F., Hauser, W. A., and Anderson, V. E. (1982): Risk of seizures among relatives of patients with epilepsy: Families in a defined population. In *Genetic Basis of the Epilepsies,* edited by V. E. Anderson, W. A. Hauser, J. K. Penry, and C. F. Sing, pp. 151–159. Raven Press, New York.
7. Baraitser, M. (1983): Recurrence risks in epilepsy. In: *Research Progress in Epilepsy,* edited by F. C. Rose, pp. 71–77. Pitman, London.
8. Barbeau, A., and Roy, M. (1984): Familial subsets in idiopathic Parkinson's disease. *Can. J. Neurol. Sci.,* 11:144–150.

9. Beck-Mannagetta, G., and Janz, D. (1982): Febrile convulsions in offspring of epileptic probands. In: *Genetic Basis of the Epilepsies*, edited by V. E. Anderson, W. A. Hauser, J. K. Penry, and C. F. Sing, pp. 145–150. Raven Press, New York.

10. Bishop, T. D., Williamson, J. A., and Skolnick, M. H. (1983): A model for restriction fragment length distributions. *Am J. Hum. Genet.*, 35:795–815.

11. Blume, W. T. (1982): Some seizure disorders affecting neonates and children. In: *Genetic Basis of the Epilepsies*, edited by V. E. Anderson, W. A. Hauser, J. K. Penry, and C. F. Sing, pp. 35–48. Raven Press, New York.

12. Cloninger, C. R., Rice, J., Reich T., and McGuffin, P. (1982): Genetic analysis of seizure disorders as multidimensional threshold characters. In: *Genetic Basis of the Epilepsies*, edited by V. E. Anderson, W. A. Hauser, J. K. Penry, and C. F. Sing, pp. 291–309. Raven Press, New York.

13. Conte, W. J., and Rotter, J. I. (1984): The use of association data to identify family members at high risk for marker-linked diseases. *Am. J. Hum. Genet.*, 36:152–166.

14. Delgado-Escueta, A. V., and Greenberg, D. (1986): Looking for epilepsy genes: clinical and molecular genetic studies. In: *Basic Mechanisms of the Epilepsies*, edited by A. V. Delgado-Escueta, A. A. Ward, Jr., D. M. Woodbury, and R. Porter, pp. 77–95. Raven Press, New York.

15. Delgado-Escueta, A. V., Treiman, D. M., and Enrile-Bacsal, F. (1982): Phenotypic variations of seizures in adolescents and adults. In: *Genetic Basis of the Epilepsies*, edited by V. E. Anderson, W. A. Hauser, J. K. Penry, and C. F. Sing C. F., pp. 49–81. Raven Press, New York.

16. Delgado-Escueta, A. V., Ward, A. A., Jr., Woodbury, D., and Porter, R. (1986): The new wave of research in experimental and human epilepsies. In: *Basic Mechanisms of the Epilepsies*, edited by A. V. Delgado-Escueta, A. A. Ward, Jr., D. M. Woodbury, and R. Porter, pp. 3–55. Raven Press, New York.

17. Doose, H. (1981): Genetic aspects of the epilepsies. *Folia Psychiatr. Neurol. Jpn.*, 35:231–242.

18. Doose, H. (1982): Photosensitivity: Genetics and significance in the pathogenesis of epilepsy. In: *Genetic Basis of the Epilepsies*, edited by V. E. Anderson, W. A. Hauser, J. K. Penry, and C. F. Sing, pp. 113–121. Raven Press, New York.

19. Doose, H., and Gerken, H. (1973): On the genetics of EEG—Anomalies in childhood. IV. Photoconvulsive reaction. *Neuropadiatrie*, 4:162–171.

20. Doose, H., Gerken H., Horstmann, T., and Völzke, E. (1973): Genetic factors in spike-wave absences. *Epilepsia*, 14:57–75.

21. Doose, H., Gerken, H., Leonhardt, R., Völzke, E., and Völz, C. (1970): Centrencephalic myoclonic-astatic petit mal: Clinical and genetic investigations. *Neuropadiatrie*, 2:59–78.

22. Eaves, L. J. (1982): The utility of twins. In: *Genetic Basis of the Epilepsies*, edited by V. E. Anderson, W. A. Hauser, J. K. Penry, and C. F. Sing, pp. 249–276. Raven Press, New York.

23. Eisner, V., Pauli, L. L., and Livingston, S. (1959): Hereditary aspects of epilepsy. *Johns Hopkins Hosp. Bull.*, 105:245–271.

24. Feder, J., Mignone, N., Chang, A. C. Y., Cochet, M., Cohen, S. N., Cann, H., and Cavalli-Sforza, L. L. (1983): A DNA polymorphism in close physical linkage with the proopiomelanocortin gene. *Am. J. Hum. Genet.*, 35:1090–1096.

25. Folstein, S. E., Abbott, M. H., Franz, M. L., Huang, S., Chase, G. A., and Folstein, M. F. (1984): Phenotypic heterogeneity in Huntington disease. *J. Neurogenet.*, 1:175–184.

26. Frantzen, E., Lennox-Buchthal, M., Nygaard, A., and Stene, J. (1970): A genetic study of febrile convulsions. *Neurology*, 20:909–917.

27. Fukuyama, Y., Kagawa, K., and Tanaka, K. (1979): A genetic study of febrile convulsions. *Eur. Neurol.*, 18:166–182.

28. Gerken, H., and Doose, H. (1973): On the genetics of EEG—Anomalies in childhood. III. Spikes and waves. *Neuropadiatrie*, 4:88–97.

29. Gloor, P., Metrakos, J., Metrakos, K., Andermann, E., and van Gelder, N. (1982): Neurophysiological, genetic and biochemical nature of the epileptic diathesis. In: *Henri Gastaut and the Marseilles School's Contribution to the Neurosciences*, edited by R. J. Broughton, EEG (Suppl. 35) pp. 45–56. Elsevier Biomedical Press, Amsterdam.

30. Greenberg, D. A. (1984): Simulation studies of segregation analysis: Application to two-locus models. *Am. J. Hum. Genet.*, 36:167–176.

31. Harvald, B., and Hauge, M. (1965): Hereditary factors elucidated by twin studies. In: *Genetics and the Epidemiology of Chronic Diseases*, edited by J. V. Neel, M. W. Shaw, and W. J. Schull, pp. 61–76. Public Health Service Publication, No. 1163.

32. Hauser, W. A. (1981): The natural history of febrile seizures. In: *Febrile Seizures*, edited by K. B. Nelson and J. H. Ellenberg, pp. 5–17. Raven Press, New York.

33. Hauser, W. A. (1982): Genetics and the clinical characteristics of seizures. In: *Genetic Basis of the Epilepsies*, edited by V. E. Anderson, W. A. Hauser, J. K. Penry, and C. F. Sing, pp. 3–9. Raven Press, New York.

34. Hauser, W. A., Annegers, J. F., and Anderson, V. E. (1983): Epidemiology and the genetics of epilepsy. In: *Epilepsy*, edited by A. A. Ward, Jr., J. K. Penry, and D. Purpura, pp. 267–292. Raven Press, New York.

35. Hauser, W. A., Annegers, J. F., Anderson, V. E., and Kurland, L. T. (1985). The risk of seizure disorders among relatives of children with febrile convulsions. *Neurology*, 35:1268–1273.

36. Hauser, W. A., Rich, S., and Anderson, V. E. (1983): The electroencephalogram as a predictor of sibling risk for epilepsy. Paper presented at the 15th Epilepsy International Symposium, Washington, D.C.

37. Heston, L. L., Mastri, A. R., Anderson, V. E., and White J. (1981): Dementia of the Alzheimer type. *Arch. Gen. Psychiatry*, 38:1085–1090.

38. Hirschhorn, R., Martiniuk, F., Roegner-Maniscalco, V., Ellenbogen, A., Perignon, J.-L., and Jenkins, T. (1983): Genetic heterogeneity in partial adenosine deaminase deficiency. *J. Clin. Invest.*, 71:1887–1892.

39. Hodge, S. E., Anderson, C. E., Neiswanger, K., Sparkes, R. S., and Rimoin, D. L. (1983): The search for heterogeneity in insulin-dependent diabetes mellitus (IDDM): Linkage studies, two-locus models, and genetic heterogeneity. *Am. J. Hum. Genet.*, 1139–1155.

40. Hrubec, Z., and Robinette, C. D. (1984): The study of human twins in medical research. *New Engl. J. Med.*, 310:435–441.

41. Inouye, E. (1960): Observations on forty twin cases with chronic epilepsy and their co-twins. *J. Nerv. Ment. Dis.*, 13:401–416.

42. Janjua, N. A., Metrakos, J. D., and van Gelder, N. M. (1982): Plasma amino acids in epilepsy. In: *Genetic Basis of the Epilepsies*, edited by V. E. Anderson, W. A. Hauser, J. K. Penry, and C. F. Sing, pp. 181–197. Raven Press, New York.

43. Janz, D., and Beck-Mannagetta, G. (1982): Epilepsy and neonatal seizures in the offspring of parents with epilepsy. In: *Genetic Basis of the Epilepsies*, edited by V. E. Anderson, W. A. Hauser, J. K. Penry, and C. F. Sing, pp. 135–143. Raven Press, New York.

44. Jennings, M. T., and Bird, J. D. (1981): Genetic influences in the epilepsies. Review of the literature with practical implications. *Am. J. Dis. Child.*, 135:450–457.

45. Jensen, I. (1975): Genetic factors in temporal lobe epilepsy. *Acta Neurol. Scand.*, 52:381–394.

46. Kellaway, P. (1982): Maturational and biorhythmic changes in the electroencephalogram. In: *Genetic Basis of the Epilepsies*, edited by V. E. Anderson, W. A. Hauser, J. K. Penry, and C. F. Sing, pp. 21–33. Raven Press, New York.

47. Lalouel, J. M., Rao, D. C., Morton, N. E., and Elston, R. C. (1983): A unified model for complex segregation analysis. *Am. J. Hum. Genet.*, 35:816–826.

48. Lennox-Buchthal, M. (1971): Febrile and nocturnal convulsions in monozygotic twins. *Epilepsia*, 12:147–156.

49. Lennox-Buchthal, M. (1973): Febrile convulsions: A reappraisal. *Electroencephalogr. Clin. Neurophysiol.*, 32 (Suppl.):1–138.

50. Martin, W. E., Young, W. I., and Anderson, V. E. (1973): Parkinson's disease—A genetic study. *Brain*, 96:495–506.

51. McKusick, V. A. (1983): *Mendelian Inheritance in Man. Catalogs of Autosomal Dominant, Autosomal Recessive, and X-Linked Phenotypes*, 6th ed. Johns Hopkins University Press, Baltimore.

52. McKusick, V. A., and Neufeld, E. (1983): The mucopolysaccharide storage diseases. In: *The Metabolic Basis of Inherited Disease*, 5th ed., edited by J. B. Stanbury, J. B. Wyngaarden, S., Fredrickson, J. L. Goldstein, and M. S. Brown, pp. 751–777. McGraw-Hill, New York.

53. Metrakos, J. D., and Metrakos, K. (1960): Genetics of convulsive disorders. I. Introduction, problems, methods, and base lines. *Neurology*, 10:228–240.

54. Metrakos, J. D., and Metrakos, K. (1970): Genetic factors in epilepsy. *Mod. Probl. Pharmacopsychiatry*, 4:71–86.

55. Metrakos, K., and Metrakos, J. D. (1961): Genetics of convulsive disorders II. Genetic and electroencephalographic studies in centrencephalic epilepsy. *Neurology*, 11:474–483.

56. Metrakos, K., and J. D. Metrakos. (1974): Genetics of epilepsy. In: *Handbook of Clinical Neurology, The Epilepsies*, vol. 15, edited by O. Magnus, and A. M. Lorentz de Haas, pp. 429–439. North-Holland, Amsterdam.

57. Moll, P. P. (1982): Alternative genetic models: An application to epilepsy. In: *Genetic Basis of the Epilepsies*, edited by V. E. Anderson, W. A. Hauser, J. K. Penry, and C. F. Sing, pp. 277–289. Raven Press, New York.

58. Moll, P. P., Berry, T. D., Weidman, W. H., Ellefson, R., Gordon, H., and Kottke, B. A. (1983): Detection of genetic heterogeneity among pedigrees through complex segregation analysis: An application to hypercholesterolemia. *Am. J. Hum. Genet.*, 35:197–211.

59. Morton, N. E., and Chung, C. S. (1959): Formal genetics of muscular dystrophy. *Am. J. Hum. Genet.*, 11:360–379.

60. Myrianthopoulos, N. C. (1981): *Neurogenetic Directory, Part I. Vol. 42, Handbook of Clinical Neurology*, edited by P. J. Vinken and G. W. Bruyn, pp. 667–719. North Holland, Amsterdam.

61. Neugebauer, R., and Susser, M. (1979): Epilepsy: Some epidemiological aspects. *Psychol. Med.*, 9:207–215.

62. Neufeld. E. (1983): The William Allan memorial award address: Cell mixing and its sequelae. *Am. J. Hum. Genet.*, 35:1081–1085.

63. Newmark, M. E., and Penry, J. K. (1980): *Genetics of Epilepsy: A Review*. Raven Press, New York.

64. Newmark, M. E., and Porter, R. J. (1982): Clinical research trends in the genetics of epilepsy. In: *Genetic Basis of the Epilepsies*, edited by V. E. Anderson, W. A. Hauser, J. K. Penry, and C. F. Sing, pp. 161–168. Raven Press, New York.

65. Norio, R., and Koskiniemi, M. (1979): Progressive monoclonus epilepsy: Genetic and nosological aspects with special reference to 107 Finnish patients. *Clin. Genet.*, 15:382–398.

66. O'Brien, T., Harper, P. S., Davies, K. E., Murray, J. M., Sarfarozi, M., and Williamson, R. (1983): Absence of genetic heterogeneity in Duchenne muscular dystrophy shown by a linkage study using two cloned DNA sequences. *J. Med. Genet.*, 20:249–251.

67. Ottman, R. (1983): Poor fit of epilepsy to polygenic threshold model. Paper presented at the 15th Epilepsy International Symposium in Washington, D.C.

68. Panter, S. S., Sadrzadeh, S. M. Hallaway, P. E., Haines, J. L., Anderson, V. E., and Eaton, J. W.

(1985): Hypohaptoglobinemia associated with familial epilepsy. *J. Exp. Med.*, 161:748–754.

69. Payami, H., Thomson, G., and Louis, E. J. (1984): The affected sib method. III. Selection and recombination. *Am. J. Hum. Genet.*, 36:352–362.

70. Prockop, D. J. (1984): Osteogenesis imperfecta: Phenotypic heterogeneity, protein suicide, short and long collagen. *Am. J. Hum. Genet.*, 36:499–505.

71. Quesney, L. F., Andermann, F., and Gloor, P. (1981): Dopaminergic mechanism in generalized photosensitive epilepsy. *Neurology*, 31:1542–1544.

72. Rao, D. C., Morton, N. E., Glueck, C. J., Laskarzewski, P. M., and Russell, J. M. (1983): Heterogeneity between populations for multifactorial inheritance of plasma lipids. *Am. J. Hum. Genet.*, 35:468–483.

73. Risch, N. (1984): Segregation analysis incorporating linkage markers. I. Single-locus models with an application to type I diabetes. *Am. J. Hum. Genet.*, 36:363–386.

74. Robinson, B. H., Oei, J., Sherwood, W. G., Applegarth, D., Wong, L., Haworth, J., Goodyer, P., Casey, R., and Zaleski, L. A. (1984): The molecular basis for the two different clinical presentations of classical pyruvate carboxylase deficiency. *Am. J. Hum. Genet.*, 36:283–294.

75. Rotter, J. I. (1981): The modes of inheritance of insulin-dependent diabetes or the genetics of IDDM, no longer a nightmare but still a headache. *Am. J. Hum. Genet.*, 33:835–851.

76. Schiøttz-Christensen, E. (1972): Genetic factors in febrile convulsions. *Acta Neurol. Scand.*, 48:538–546.

77. Seyfried, T. N. (1983): Genetic heterogeneity for the development of audiogenic seizures in mice. *Brain Res.*, 271:325–329.

78. Sillence, D. O., Barlow, K. K., Garber, A. P., Hall, J. G., and Rimoin, D. L. (1984): Osteogenesis imperfecta type II. Delineation of the phenotype with reference to genetic heterogeneity. *Am. J. Med. Genet.*, 17:407–423.

79. Sing, C. F., Boerwinkle, E., and Moll, P. (1985): Strategies for elucidating the phenotypic and genetic heterogeneity of a chronic disease with a complex etiology. In: *Diseases of Complex Etiology in Small Populations: Ethnic Differences and Research Approaches*, edited by R. Chakraborty and E. J. E. Szathmary, pp. 39–66. Alan R. Liss, New York.

80. Sing, C. F., Hanis, C. L., and Moll, P. P. (1982): Questions, measures, and analytical strategies in human genetics. In: *Genetic Basis of the Epilepsies*, edited by V. E. Anderson, W. A. Hauser, J. K. Penry, and C. F. Sing, pp. 239–247. Raven Press, New York.

81. Smith, C. (1970): Heritability of liability and concordance in monozygous twins. *Ann. Hum. Genet.*, 34:85–91.

82. Spranger, J. (1984): Osteogenesis imperfecta: A pasture for splitters and lumpers. *Am. J. Med. Genet.*, 17:425–428.

83. Suarez, B. K., Rice, J. P., Crouse, J., and Reich, T. (1983): HLA and disease: Haplotype sharing in multiplex families. *Clin. Genet.*, 23:267–275.

84. Suarez, B. K., and Van Eerdewegh, P. (1984): A comparison of three affected-sib-pair scoring methods to detect HLA-linked disease susceptibility genes. *Am. J. Med. Genet.*, 18:135–146.

85. Thomson, G. (1984): The genotypic distribution among non-insulin-dependent diabetes mellitus (NIDDM) patients of a restriction fragment length polymorphism. *Am. J. Hum. Genet.*, 36:466–470.

86. Tsuboi, T. (1980): Genetic aspects of epilepsy. *Folia Psychiatr. Neurol. Jpn.*, 34:215–225.

87. Tsuboi, T. (1982): Febrile convulsions. In: *Genetic Basis of the Epilepsies*, edited by V. E. Anderson, W. A. Hauser, J. K. Penry, and C. F. Sing, pp. 123–134. Raven Press, New York.

88. Tsuboi, T., and Christian. W. (1973): On the genetics of the primary generalized epilepsy with sporadic myoclonias of impulsive petit mal type. A clinical and electroencephalographic study of 399 probands. *Humangenetik*, 19–155–182.

89. Tsuboi, T., and Endo, S. (1977): Incidence of seizures and EEG abnormalities among offspring of epileptic patients. *Hum. Genet.*, 36:173–189.

90. van den Berg, B. J. (1974): Studies on convulsive disorders in young children. IV: Incidence of convulsions among siblings, *Develop. Med. Child Neurol.*, 16:457–464.

91. van Gelder, N. M. (1981): The role of taurine and glutamic acid in the epileptic process: A genetic predisposition. *Rev. Pure Appl. Pharmacol. Sci.*, 2:293–316.

92. Ward, R. H. (1982): Genetics and epidemiology: A fruitful interface for the study of epilepsy. In: *Genetic Basis for the Epilepsies*, edited by V. E. Anderson, W. A. Hauser, J. K. Penry, and C. F. Sing, pp. 317–332. Raven Press, New York.

93. White, R., and Skolnick, M. (1982): DNA sequence polymorphism and the genetics of epilepsy. In: *Genetic Basis of the Epilepsies*, edited by V. E. Anderson, W. A. Hauser, J. K. Penry, and C. F. Sing, pp. 311–316. Raven Press, New York.

94. Williams, W. R., Thompson, M. W., and Morton, N. E. (1983): Complex segregation analysis and computer-assisted genetic risk assessment for Duchenne muscular dystrophy. *Am. J. Med. Genet.*, 14:315–333.

95. Williamson, R. A., Schauberger, C. W., Varner, M. W., and Aschenbrener, C. A. (1984): Heterogeneity of prenatal onset hydrocephalus: Management and counseling implications. *Am. J. Med. Genet.*, 17:497–508.

APPENDIX

Genetic Syndromes Associated with Seizures

As listed in McKusick (51). An asterisk preceding an entry indicates that the particular mode of inheritance is considered quite certain.

Autosomal Dominant Phenotypes (N = 25)

*10413   Alopecia, psychomotor epilepsy, pyorrhea, and mental subnormality

*10521 Amyloidosis VII (oculoleptomeningeal type amyloidosis)
*10940 Basal cell nevus syndrome
*11686 Cavernous angioma, familial
*11755 Cerebral gigantism (Sotos syndrome)
*11880 Choreoathetosis, familial paroxysmal
*12120 Convulsions, benign familial neonatal
*12130 Coproporphyria
12247 Cornelia de Lange syndrome
*12300 Craniometaphyseal dysplasia, dominant type
*13110 Endocrine adenomatosis, multiple (Wermer syndrome; multiple endocrine neoplasia, type I)
13230 Epilepsy, reading
*13540 Fibromatosis, gingival, with hypertrichosis
*13630 Flynn-Aird syndrome
14130 Hemifacial atrophy, progressive (Parry-Romberg syndrome)
*14310 Huntington disease
*14940 Kok disease (hyperexplexia)
*15960 Myoclonic epilepsy, Hartung type
16170 Necrotizing encephalomyelopathy, subacute, of adult (adult Leigh syndrome)
*16220 Neurofibromatosis
*16235 Neuronal ceroid-lipofuscinosis, dominant or Parry type
17250 Photomyoclonus, diabetes mellitus, deafness, nephropathy, and cerebral dysfunction
*17600 Porphyria, acute intermittent
*17620 Porphyria variegata
*19110 Tuberous sclerosis

Autosomal Recessive Phenotypes (N = 96)
20237 Adrenoleukodystrophy, autosomal neonatal form
20333 Albright hereditary osteodystrophy (pseudohypoparathyroidism, type II)
20360 Alopecia–epilepsy–oligophrenia syndrome of Moynahan
*20370 Alpers diffuse degeneration of cerebral gray matter with hepatic cirrhosis
*20420 Amaurotic family idiocy, juvenile type (Batten disease, Vogt-Spielmeyer disease, neuronal ceroid-lipofuscinosis)
*20430 Amaurotic idiocy, adult type (Kufs disease)
*20440 Amaurotic idiocy, congenital form
*20460 Amaurotic idiocy, late infantile, with multilamellar cytosomes

*20657 Angiomatosis, diffuse corticomeningeal, of Divry and Van Bogaert
*20780 Argininemia
*20790 Argininosuccinicaciduria
20870 Ataxia with myoclonus epilepsy and presenile dementia
21138 Brachio-skeletal-genital syndrome
*21220 Carnosinemia
21360 Cerebral calcification, nonarteriosclerotic
*21410 Cerebro-hepato-renal syndrome (Zellweger syndrome)
*21450 Chediak-Higashi syndrome
*21570 Citrullinuria (citrullinemia)
21720 Convulsive disorder, familial, with prenatal or early onset
*21800 Corpus callosum, agenesis of, with neuronopathy (Charlevoix disease)
*21830 Craniodiaphyseal dysplasia
21835 Craniofacial dyssynostosis
*21890 Crome syndrome
*21950 Cystathionuria
22030 Deaf-mutism and familial myoclonus epilepsy
*22050 Deafness, congenital and onychodystrophy, recessive form
*22180 Dermochondrocorneal dystrophy (Francois syndrome)
22425 Dysmyelination with jaundice
22675 Epilepsy and yellow teeth
22680 Epilepsy, photogenic, with spastic diplegia and mental retardation
22685 Epilepsy–telangiectasia
*22905 Folic acid, transport defect involving
*22950 Fructose and galactose intolerance
*22960 Fructose intolerance, hereditary (fructosemia)
*22970 Fructose-1,6-diphosphatase deficiency
*23040 Galactosemia
*23050 Gangliosidosis, generalized GM1, type I
*23060 Gangliosidosis, generalized GM1, type II
23100 Gaucher disease type III (juvenile and adult, cerebral)
*23220 Glycogen storage disease I (Von Gierke disease)
*23420 Hallervorden-Spatz disease
23440 Happy Puppet syndrome (Angelman syndrome)
23500 Hemihypertrophy
*23583 Histidinuria due to a renal tubular defect
23610 Holoprosencephaly, familial alobar
*23620 Homocystinuria
*23690 Hydroxylsinuria

23740	Hyper-beta-alaninemia
*23830	Hyperglycinemia, isolated nonketotic
*23870	Hyperlysinemia
*23890	Hyperornithinemia – hyperammonemia–homocitrullinuria syndrome
*23920	Hyperparathyroidism, neonatal severe primary
*23930	Hyperphosphatasia with mental retardation
23935	Hyperphosphatemia, polyuria, and seizures
*23951	Hyperprolinemia, type II
*24030	Hypoadrenocorticism with hypoparathyroidism and superficial moniliasis
*24060	Hypoglycemia with deficiency of glycogen synthetase in the liver
*24080	Hypoglycemia, leucine-induced
24130	Hypomagnesemia, primary
*24350	Isovalericacidemia
24518	Kifafa seizure disorder
*24520	Krabbe disease (globoid cell leukodystrophy)
*24540	Lactic acidosis, congenital infantile
*24680	Lipidosis, juvenile dystonic
*24710	Lipoid proteinosis of Urbach and Wiethe (lipoproteinosis; hyalinosis cutis et mucosae)
*24720	Lissencephaly syndrome
*24860	Maple syrup urine disease (branched-chain ketoaciduria)
*24931	Megalocornea-mental retardation syndrome
*24965	Mercaptolactate-cysteine disulfiduria
*25010	Metachromatic leukodystrophy, late infantile
*25090	Methionine malabsorption syndrome
*25100	Methylmalonicaciduria due to methylmalonic CoA mutase deficiency
*25240	Mucolipidosis I (lipomucopolysaccharidosis)
*25250	Mucolipidosis II (I-cell disease)
*25327	Multiple carboxylase deficiency, biotin-responsive
*25478	Myoclonus epilepsy of Lafora
*25480	Myoclonic epilepsy of Unverricht and Lundborg
*25490	Myoclonus-nephropathy syndrome
*25654	Neuraminidase deficiency with beta-galactosidase deficiency (Goldberg syndrome)
*25655	Neuraminidase deficiency (sialidoses, types I and II)
*25660	Neuroaxonal dystrophy, infantile (Seitelberger disease)

*25671	Neuroectodermal melanolysosomal disease
*25673	Neuronal ceroid-lipofuscinosis, infantile Finnish type
*25720	Niemann-Pick disease (sphingomyelin lipidosis)
*26160	Phenylketonuria
*26470	Pseudovitamin D deficiency rickets (Vitamin-D-dependent rickets, type I)
*26610	Pyridoxine dependency with seizures
*26613	Pyroglutamicaciduria (5-oxoprolinuria)
*26615	Pyruvate carboxylase deficiency
26774	Retinal degeneration and epilepsy
*26880	Sandhoff disease
*27060	Spastic diplegia, infantile type
27255	Tachycardia, hypertension, microphthalmos, hyperglycinuria
*27280	Tay-Sachs disease (GM2-gangliosidosis, type I)
27377	Threoninemia
27890	Xylosidase deficiency

X-linked Phenotypes (N = 20)

*30020	Adrenal hypoplasia
*30025	Adrenal unresponsiveness to ACTH
30080	Albright hereditary osteodystrophy (pseudohypoparathyroidism and pseudopseudohypoparathyroidism, type I)
*30190	Borjeson syndrome (mental deficiency, epilepsy, endocrine disorders)
*30410	Corpus callosum, partial agenesis of, with chorioretinal abnormality (Aicardi syndrome)
*30545	FG syndrome
30696	HHHH syndrome (Hereditary hemihypotrophy hemiparesis hemiathetosis)
30705	Hyperphenylalaninemia, ? X-linked
*30760	Hypomagnesemic tetany
*30770	Hypoparathyroidism, X-linked
*30800	Lesch-Nyhan syndrome
*30830	Incontinentia pigmenti
30835	Infantile spasms, X-linked (West syndrome)
'30940	Menkes syndrome
*30950	Mental deficiency (Martin-Bell, or Renpenning type)
30965	Methylmandelicaciduria
31037	Myoclonus epilepsy, progressive
31140	Paine syndrome (microcephaly with spastic diplegia)
31145	Pallister W syndrome
*31160	Pelizaeus-Merzbacher disease

Advances in Neurology, Vol. 44, edited by
A. V. Delgado-Escueta, A. A. Ward, Jr.,
D. M. Woodbury, and R. J. Porter.
Raven Press, New York © 1986.

3

Looking for Epilepsy Genes: Clinical and Molecular Genetic Studies

**‡Antonio V. Delgado-Escueta, *Ray White, **†‡David A. Greenberg, and **Lucy J. Treiman

*Howard Hughes Medical Institute and Department of Cellular, Viral and Molecular Biology, University of Utah School of Medicine, Salt Lake City, Utah; and **the Comprehensive Epilepsy Program, Departments of Neurology and †Biomathematics, UCLA School of Medicine; and the VA Southwest Regional Epilepsy Center, Neurology and Research Services, West Los Angeles, ‡VA Medical Center (Wadsworth), Los Angeles, California.

SUMMARY   The complexity of the human genome creates special problems in understanding the genetic component of disease processes. An estimated 50,000 genes exist in the human genome, and it is reasonable to assume that mutation in any one of these genes may result in an inherited disorder. Because of the complex pattern of gene expression controlling the development and organization of the central nervous system (CNS), insights into the genetic component, if any, of diseases such as epilepsy are most accessible to analysis by genetic linkage studies.

Advances in the manipulation of DNA have made possible more effective acquisition of genotypic information in humans by studying the inheritance of restriction fragment length polymorphisms (RFLPs) using cloned DNA probes. Two approaches exist to utilize this technology in studying inherited disorders. The first approach consists of genotypic determinations in affected families with cloned genes in which a mutation might result in the phenotype observed. Analysis of these data will show whether the inheritance of an allele of the candidate gene is linked to the disease. The second approach relies upon the construction with these probes of a linkage map for the human genome such that disease families can be screened in order to determine with which of these markers the phenotype is linked, indicating the map position of a gene associated with the inherited disorder. The use of these new approaches enables investigators to screen either specific biochemical defects in disease families or to identify the underlying genetic mechanisms in inherited disorders whose phenotype is expressed only in the intact human (84).

The first step in localizing the chromosomal site of specific epilepsies is to define their pattern of inheritance. This determination is now being carried out for benign juvenile myoclonic epilepsy; 50 multigenerational families are being studied in three separate epilepsy programs in Los Angeles, Winston-Salem, North Carolina, and Berlin. Concurrent with these studies, investigators are combining the principles of classic linkage analysis, using 30 protein markers, with the use of RFLPs to determine the chromosomal location of juvenile myoclonic epilepsy. Two problems appear formidable, however. First, since the chromosomal location of specific epilepsies is unknown, the entire human genome must be screened. Second, once the location of a specific epilepsy gene is narrowed down to a region of 10^6 base pairs, the problem of identifying the actual molecular defect is difficult, especially as we have no assay or method to show that a given gene is culpable of producing epilepsy. An approach more likely to succeed is to use as markers the DNA fragments of proteins that are suspected to cause the disease in experimental models of genetic epilepsies; for example, the γ-aminobutyric acid (GABA) receptor genes, which are suspected to cause myoclonic epilepsy in experimental animals, can be tested in benign juvenile myoclonic epilepsy. At the same time, other marker proteins can be used to locate the chromosomal site of other specific epilepsies. Once the chromosomal site is determined, recombinant DNA technology will permit the measurement of the precise arrangement of the genes for these RFLPs and protein markers at a given locus of a chromosome (17).

ADVANCES IN HUMAN GENETICS

Research in human genetics has entered an era of rapid growth. New approaches are now possible in a number of promising areas, ranging from analysis of the DNA sequences of individual genes and their mutant forms to linkage analysis using new and more effective genetic markers based on DNA sequence polymorphisms (10). These developments are due primarily to new technologies for the manipulation of DNA *in vitro* and for the growth of human cells in culture, which are making possible a number of new approaches to human genetics that do not require experimentation in the intact human system. One result of these advances is that investigators in many fields of human research are now entertaining the possibility that genetic analysis may be useful in their studies. The question is timely. Literally hundreds of genes have been mapped to specific human chromosomes using cell culture methods with rodent–human hybrid cell lines. Furthermore, a large and rapidly growing number of human genes have now been cloned as recombinant DNA strands and can be studied in detail. The recombinants can also be used as DNA probes in individual humans to determine whether a specific genetic disease can be explained by mutations in these genes (4). For example, it has been learned recently that at least some dwarfism can be accounted for by deletion of the gene for growth hormone (63), and inheritance of a mutation at the Rb-1 locus (band q-14, chromosome 13) results in a predisposition to retinoblastoma (12).

It has been estimated that on the order of 50,000 different genes may exist in the human genome. Each gene is expressed in some tissue at some time during human development. Thus, there are many possibilities for mutations that could result in human genetic diseases. Some of these genes, however, are probably responsible for the "housekeeping" functions required to keep all cells alive. For example, because all living cells synthesize RNA, the genes required for the synthesis of the RNA precursors uridine (U), adenosine (A), guanosine (G), and cytosine (C) are likely to be functionally required at some level of expression in almost all cells. However, other genes would be expected to be specific to a certain tissue or stage of development and would be expressed only at certain times and in certain tissues. For example, hemoglobin genes are expressed only in the red blood cells. Furthermore, there is developmental specificity with regard to which hemoglobin genes are expressed at each developmental stage, such that there are specific hemoglobin genes for the embryonic, fetal, and adult stages of development.

It is virtually certain that mutations that can inactivate or change the level of expression of each of these 50,000 genes must occur in the human population. Some mutations are so deleterious that they are lethal at early embryonic stages and are thus not seen in or are quickly eliminated from the population. Other mutations are seen but are present at only very low frequencies in the population. Still other mutant alleles are present at relatively high frequencies, perhaps owing to selection.

Of greatest interest to those concerned with epilepsy, however, is the likelihood that there are genes specific to the nervous system in which mutations could occur that result in epilepsy. For example, mutations in the GABA receptor that alter affinity for the GABA transmitter could have profound effects on neurostasis. What is not clear is whether any such mutant genes have increased in frequency so as to become established in the human population.

EXISTENCE OF EPILEPSY GENES

An important question to be addressed before discussing how to look for epilepsy genes is whether such genes exist. Several lines of evidence suggest that they exist and, furthermore, that they may be important in the etiology of at least some specific forms of this very heterogeneous syndrome. Perhaps the most direct evidence (and also the least promising) is that genetic defects in specific metabolic pathways produce phenotypes in which epileptic seizures are prominent symptoms (72) (Table 1). In cataloguing 2,336 genetically determined diseases, McKusick (49) listed 133 single-gene disorders that were associated with epileptic seizures. Sixty percent of these disorders also involved mental retardation, and a modest list of some of these mendelian disorders is presented in Chapter 2. Because many of these inherited diseases are known to have a defect in a specific enzyme or protein, they are presumed to have a structural gene defect (72). Mapping the normal structural gene has also identified the chromosomal location of some of these disorders (Table 1). Most of the epilepsies described in this chapter, however, do not belong to these neurogenetic disorders catalogued by McKusick. Clearly, these 133 neurogenetic disorders listed in Chapter 2 must be excluded from consideration in the genetic analysis of the epilepsies, because seizures are only one of many neurologic abnormalities produced by the underlying metabolic disorder. Furthermore, it is difficult to establish what the most apparent effect of a specific metabolic defect is or whether a phenotype is due to a metabolic disorder.

The more interesting question is whether mutant alleles of genes specific to functional or developmental neurological pathways exist and whether they are frequent enough in the human population to be detected as important in the causation of some of the epilepsies. The demonstration of such mutations would be of great value in the analysis of the relevant pathways towards phenotypic expression. It is an encouraging development that mice, gerbils, baboons, and chickens with certain mutations and marked epileptic predisposition have been bred specifically to serve as models of genetic epilepsies. Some of these mutant alleles seem to be specific in their effects on the nervous system, producing specific phenotypes of epilepsies, e.g., absence in tottering mice, and myoclonic and grand mal in gerbils (54–56,71) (Table 2). Again, it is a question of the frequency of the mutant alleles in the human population that is important. For two reasons, it is useful to know whether such mutant alleles exist. First, such information could be quite important to the families in which

TABLE 1. *Gene mapping of some neurological diseases associated with epilepsies*[a]

Disorder	Enzyme defect	Locus	Chromosome assignment
	Amino acid metabolism		
Phenylketonuria	Phenylalanine hydroxylase	PKU	1
Arginosuccinic aciduria	Anginosuccinate lysate	ASL	7 pter → q22
	Lipid metabolism		
GM$_1$ gangliosidosis	β-galactosidase	GLB$_1$	3 p21 → q24
GM$_2$ gangliosidosis (Tay-Sachs)	β-hexosaminidase A	HEX A	15 q22 → q23
GM$_2$ gangliosidosis (Sandhoff's)	β-hexosaminidase A and B	HEX B	5 q11 → q13
Metachromatic leukodystrophy	Arylsulfatase A	ARSA	22q
	Monopolysaccharide metabolism		
Hunter's disease	Iduronate sulfatase	IDS	X
β-glucoronidase deficiency (MPS VII)	β-glucoronidase	GUSB	7 cen → q22
	Nucleic acid metabolism		
Lesch-Nyhan syndrome	Hypoxanthine phosphoribase transferase	HPRT	X q26 → q28
	No known metabolic defects		
Spinal cerebellar ataxia		SCAI	6
Herpes virus		HVIS	3 or 11

[a] Modified from Shaws et al, ref. 72, with permission.

TABLE 2. *Some human genetic epilepsies and proposed animal models*

Possible human equivalents	Proposed mode of inheritance	Experimental animals	Proposed mode of inheritance
A. *Generalized epilepsies*	Benign or non-fatal epilepsies		
Absence of childhood Benign juvenile myoclonic epilepsies (myoclonic, clonic-tonic-clonic and absence)	Autosomal dominant Polygenic or two gene loci or autosomal dominant	Tottering mice[a] Mongolian gerbil	Autosomal recessive Unknown; probably autosomal dominant
Traditional grand mal Clonic-tonic-clonic	Polygenic or two gene loci or autosomal dominant	Baboon (*Papio papio*) with light induced myoclonic and tonic-clonic seizures	Unknown; possibly autosomal dominant
—	—	Tonic-clonic convulsions in chicken	Autosomal recessive
—	—	Tonic-clonic convulsions in epileptiform (epf) mice of Hare and Hare	Autosomal recessive
—	—	Spontaneous behavioral arrest and tonic-clonic seizures (SPS) in mice by Maxson et al.	Autosomal recessive
—	—	Tonic-clonic convulsions in mice (epilepsy-prone) by Imaizumi	Autosomal recessive
—	—	Genetic epilepsy prone mice and rats with audiogenic seizures[a]	Multifactorial
B. *Partial epilepsies*			
Musicogenic	Unknown	Audiogenic seizures (mice and rats)[a]	Multifactorial
Complex partial (psychomotor)	Autosomal dominant	None	—
Rolandic epilepsy	Autosomal dominant	Tottering mice with focal motor seizures[a]	Autosomal recessive
	Progressive or fatal epilepsies		
Progressive myoclonus of Unverricht and Lafora	Autosomal recessive	Beagle with Lafora inclusion bodies	Autosomal recessive
Progressive myoclonus of Lundborg and Hartung	Autosomal dominant or sporadic	None	—
Progressive myoclonus of Kuf	Autosomal recessive	None	—
Progressive myoclonus of Zeman	Autosomal recessive	None	—

[a] Some animal models of genetic epilepsies have been proposed to be equivalent to several forms of human epilepsies.

such genes segregate. Second, these mutant alleles would afford a valuable opportunity for the study of the disease process.

Why might these mutant alleles be prevalent in the human population? This is a problematic question, but in fact such apparently deleterious mutant alleles do exist for some genes in the human population. The gene for sickle-cell anemia is an often-used example of a mutant allele that occurs at high frequency in some populations. In this case, it is believed that there has been selection for the heterozygotes, because of their resistance to malaria. Of course, the more rare homozygotes are the only individuals who show the sickle-cell disease. This does constitute at least an example; it is possible that other mutant genes as well may be selected for in the population because of their ability to enrich the heterozygotes while being severely deleterious in the homozygotes. At our present stage of knowledge of the genetic mechanisms of epilepsy, all options are open.

The best evidence available for the existence of such interesting mutant genes in the human population comes from family studies designed to examine familial clustering of specific forms of epilepsy. Current evidence suggests that the genetic hypothesis certainly cannot be discounted for several of the epilepsies. In the idiopathic generalized epilepsies, a major genetic factor is established by studies of twins. The overall concordance rate for epilepsy reported in six major twin studies was 60.2% for monozygotic pairs and 13.2% for dizygotic pairs (78). If twin studies are confined to absence and generalized tonic-clonic convulsions, and if pairs are examined at the peak age of phenotypic expressions (6–18 years of age), concordance rate is 100% (11). Lennox and Lennox (44) noted that when epilepsies without organic brain lesions were identified, concordance was 70.2% (33/47) for monozygotic twins and 5.6% (3/54) for dizygotic pairs. When he confined his analysis to 30 twin pairs with spike-wave traits on the electroencephalograph (EEG), concordance was 74% for the spike-wave trait in monozygotic twins and 27% for dizygotic twins. Gedda and Tatarelli (27) identified 45 pairs of twins with primarily generalized seizures and reported concordance rates of 94.7% in 19 monozygotic twins and 15.4% of 26 dizygotic twins.

The partial epilepsies are usually thought of as acquired forms of epilepsy that are caused by structural cerebral cortical lesions, with the pattern of seizures being determined by the area of cortical involvement. Several studies, however, have demonstrated a greater incidence of epilepsies among first-degee relatives of patients with partial seizures than in relatives of control patients. This suggests that in some patients there may be a genetically determined susceptibility to the development of seizures in response to an environmental insult. Support for this hypothesis is provided by Rimoin and Metrakos (67) who studied the incidence of seizures in families of children with infantile hemiplegia. Seizures occurred more frequently in families of children who had hemiplegia and seizures as compared with control families and as compared with families of those children with hemiplegia who did not develop seizures (67).

APPROACHES TO IDENTIFYING EPILEPSY GENES

Candidate Gene Markers

Two similar but distinct approaches to the problem of determining individual genotypes have recently emerged as potentially useful in the study of such complex disease states as the epilepsies. Both approaches are based on the same technology and share a similar logic but differ markedly in their properties. The first and most powerful of these approaches depends on the identification and isolation of specific cloned genes that are viewed as candidates (candidate gene markers) for carrying a mutation that could result in epilepsy. Table 3 lists proteins that have been linked pathophysiologically to epilepsies in experimental animals. If the protein suspected of causing genetic epilepsy in an experimental animal actually is the cause of the human epilepsy, the locus for the human epilepsy gene and the locus for the suspected protein gene would be the same and would have close to 0% recombination during genetic linkage studies in multiplex and multigeneration families with epilepsy. A specific example of the candidate gene approach was used recently by Barker and associates in studies on the role of oncogenes in inherited predispositions to cancer (4). The hypothesis being examined was that specific genes that are considered to be candidates in the causation of complex diseases can be tested for linkage in family studies of modest scale. Specifically, the Kirsten ras oncogene was isolated from human colon cancers and was shown by DNA transfection experiments to cause transformation of mouse 3T3 cells. Individuals carrying the gene for Gardner's syndrome phenotype show a major predisposition to colon cancer. If the Kirsten gene and the gene for Gardner's syndrome are the same, then no recombination should be seen between the two loci. In fact, as seen in Fig. 1, considerable re-

TABLE 3. *Some biochemical abnormalities in experimental animals with genetic epilepsies*

I. Ion transport and membrane-bound proteins
   A. Glial carbonic anhydrase and HCO_3-adenosine-triphosphatase increase in response to impaired anion transport in audiogenic seizures
   B. Extracellular K^+ increases and Ca^{2+} decreases during photic-induced seizures in *Papio papio*
   C. 18,000 MW synaptic membrane protein-enhanced phosphorylation in photic-induced seizures of epileptic fowl and in grand mal and myoclonic seizures of Mongolian gerbils

II. γ-Aminobutyric acid (GABA) system
   A. Decreased GABA receptors in substantia nigra and periventricular gray matter are linked to grand mal and myoclonic epilepsy in Mongolian gerbils
   B. GABA is decreased in cerebral cortex, hippocampus, amygdala, basal ganglia, and cerebellum of mice with audiogenic seizures
   C. Benzodiazepine-GABA receptor binding, and density and glutamic acid decarboxylase-containing neurons are all increased in audiogenic mice

III. Catecholamines
   A. Number of norepinephrine axon terminals increases in cerebral cortex of tottering mice
   B. Concentrations of norepinephrine increase, while dopamine concentrations decrease, in photic-induced seizures of epileptic fowl

Reproduced with permission from Table 4, A.V. Delgado-Escueta and D. Greenberg (1984): *Ann. Neurol.*, 16(S):8.

combination was seen, even in a relatively small study, establishing that Gardner's syndrome is not due to inheritance of a mutant Kirsten oncogene (4).

It should be noted that the usefulness of such an experiment depends on the sensibleness of the hypothesis. It would probably not be useful to test the hemoglobin gene as a candidate for a role in epilepsy. However, there are genes that

are reasonable candidates for having a role in epilepsy, and experiments designed to isolate relevant cloned DNA segments are under way in many laboratories (Table 3). For example, it would be of interest to determine the role of GABA receptors in suspected familial epilepsy. These receptor proteins which transduce GABA inhibition are one of several proteins (Table 3) that have recently been shown to be abnormal

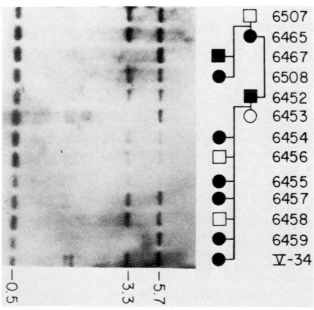

FIG. 1. Genotypes at the Kirsten ras oncogene locus of individuals from a family in which the gene for Gardner's syndrome segregates. Filled symbols represent affected individuals. DNA was obtained from each individual and was digested with the restriction enzyme Taq I, subjected to electrophoresis on an agarose gel, transferred to nitrocellulose paper by the method of Southern (75), and probed with a cloned sequence from the Kirsten ras locus. (Reproduced with permission from Fig. 2, R. White (1984): *Ann. Neurol.*, 16(S):15.)

in an experimental animal model for genetic myoclonic and grand mal clonic-tonic-clonic seizures. The midbrain substantia nigra is apparently the site at which GABAergic drugs act to contain the spread of seizures (38,56). It is also one of the sites at which decreased GABA receptors and loss of GABAergic function has been postulated to lead to myoclonic and tonic-clonic seizures in Mongolian gerbils (56). The GABA receptor protein is therefore a likely site for the molecular pathology of some human myoclonic and tonic-clonic epilepsies. This line of reasoning might be particularly applicable to the benign juvenile myoclonic epilepsy (16). These patients suffer from seizures that are clinically and electrographically simiar to the seizures of Mongolian gerbils. In addition, these epilepsies are extremely sensitive to anticonvulsants, such as valproic acid and γ-vinyl-GABA (GVG), that either elevate GABA levels or act on the same protein complex as the benzodiazepine–GABA receptor complex (17).

Other neurotransmitter receptor genes, as well as the structural and possibly the regulatory genes for the transmitters themselves, should also be considered candidates. Genes that have a role in neural cell development, determination, and maintenance will ultimately be defined and can also be tested in this manner. Because such experiments will usually result in disproving the hypothesis, care must be taken in assessing the realistic likelihood of the proposed candidacy of these genes. Furthermore, an important feature of a successful correlation between gene and disease is the ability to begin to unravel the molecular biological features of the system. With the cloned gene segment as a probe, it is possible to determine the cell type and time in development of the synthesis of the gene product (both messenger RNA and protein). The messenger RNA can then be obtained and used to synthesize protein for the production of specific monoclonal antibodies.

Polymorphic Gene Markers

The second approach, which is more brute force in nature, seeks to determine whether affected individuals within a family with epilepsy share the inheritance of a variation in a specific allele at any locus (genetic polymorphisms). If so, it becomes important to determine whether other families with a similar epilepsy phenotype show the same correlation. With this approach, correlations are sought through the use of a large number of genetic loci, each of which is defined by an arbitrary DNA segment probe (9). It has been estimated that an evenly spaced set of less than 100 genetic markers would completely cover the human genome. The significance of this estimate is that such a set of markers would reliably detect genetic linkage with any unknown genetic disease locus (such as a locus for juvenile myoclonic epilepsy). This approach would establish its map location and confirm the primary role of a genetic component in the disease process. However, the requirements for such a study are somewhat stringent. Over 100 family members from families suspected of harboring a gene for a specific form of epilepsy, distributed over as few different families as possible, would likely be needed (Fig. 2). However, if genes at several loci were to produce the same phenotype, the results would be confounded.

Therefore, genetic linkage studies in multiplex families with epilepsy can determine if the polymorphism is situated on the same chromosome as the epilepsy gene (synteny). This can be done by typing all family members (affected and unaffected) for the polymorphism marker in question. If one finds that the affected members of a family have the same allele at the marker locus more often than chance, this increases the probability of linkage between the marker and the disease. The linkage score (called the lod score, or "log of the odds" for linkage) is then summed over all the families in the study (51,53).[1]

Once linkage and synteny have been established, the next step is to estimate the chromosomal map distances between the marker gene and the epilepsy gene. These distances are expressed in morgans and centimorgans; one centimorgan map unit (cM) or approximately 10^6 base pairs of DNA means 1% recombination. At a distance of 1.0 centimorgan, two genes will be inherited together 99% of the time. With in-

---

[1] The principles of calculation are expressed as follows: The probability (p_2) that the observed family data conform to the behavior of two loci under full recombination without any linkage is calculated. Similarly, a probability (p_2) that the identical family data are the result of two linked loci under a specified recombination fraction (~) is determined. The ratio of these two probabilities is the likelihood ratio and expresses the odds for and against linkage. This ratio must be calculated for each family (51,53); $Z = \log_{10} p$ (family given θ = 0.0 − 0.5)/p (family given θ = 0.5 = free recombinations). Lod scores can be added over families and sums of lod scores > +3 are evidence for 1,000:1 odds for linkage, whereas sums of < −2 are evidence of 100:1 odds against linkage (13).

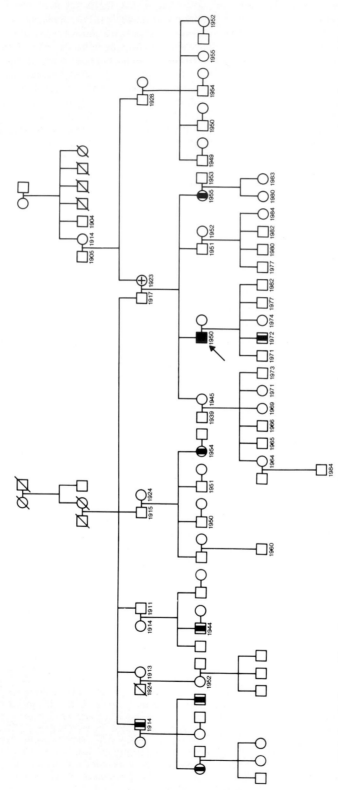

FIG. 2. Pedigree of juvenile myoclonic epilepsy: The propositus (indicated by the arrow) is 35 years of age and has awakening myoclonic jerks and clonic-tonic-clonic convulsions, which started during adolescence. He has a 12-year-old son and a 30-year-old sister with the disorder. The mother of the propositus has paroxysmal theta rhythms and spike-wave formations in the EEG but a paternal uncle and paternal cousins are clinically affected with the disorder. Affected with the trait and examined, ■; reliably reported to have the trait, □; positive for EEG epileptiform paroxysms (spike-wave formation), ⊞; and deceased, ⬚

creasing distance, there is more likelihood that the two characteristics will be inherited separately. Thus, linkage in multiplex epilepsy families will be detected confidently if the locus for the polymorphism marker and the locus for epilepsy are inherited together 90% of the time, or a distance of 10 centimorgans (13).

In the past, genetic linkage analysis could not be undertaken when the mode of inheritance of the disease was not known. Linkage analysis can now be performed without knowledge of the mode of inheritance by performing the analysis assuming different modes of inheritance. Hodge et al. (36), for example, have shown that linkage results for their data remained reasonably stable under the assumption of different modes of inheritance. Morton has attempted to combine linkage analysis and segregation analysis into complimentary methods instead of linkage analysis depending on segregation analysis. The mode of inheritance of the vast majority of epilepsies must be reinvestigated, and the problem of heterogeneity must be addressed. Fortunately, there are now statistically based methods that can sometimes detect heterogeneity in a linkage data set. If candidate gene markers and markers for genetic polymorphisms can be developed to differentiate the various forms of epilepsies, these methods can provide supporting evidence for heterogeneity and identify specific epilepsy phenotypes.

Using linkage, one can therefore examine whether some of these RFLPs markers might be located near the locus or loci influencing epilepsy liabilities. In theory, if a single genomic alteration, e.g., the sequence of nucleotides, is altered by substitution of one base for another, or by insertions or deletions is responsible for the production of the disease, that allele should be present in the DNA of all affected individuals (or gene carriers) but not present in DNA from unaffected (noncarrier) individuals (69).

The identification of the genotypic makeup of at-risk individuals within these families can be greatly aided by finding the EEG trait in phenotypically normal siblings, parents, or children of probands (Figs. 2 and 4). If an easily identifiable polymorphic marker system (e.g., phenotypic blood markers, whose location on a chromosome is well established) could be linked to one of the epilepsies, the marker locus instead of the epilepsy trait could be used in the RFLP

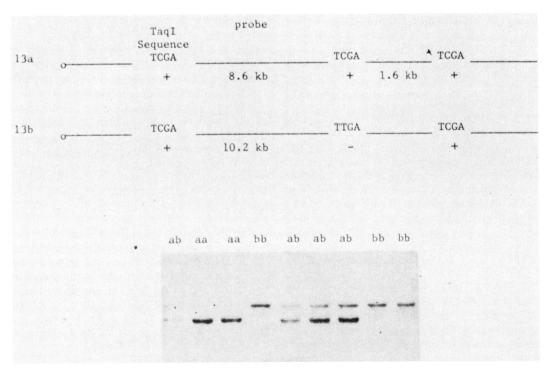

FIG. 3. Method for detecting DNA sequence polymorphism. Recombinant DNA probes define loci, using the method of Southern (75), and Taq I restriction enzymes detect some variation in DNA sequence; kb, kilobases. (Reproduced with permission from Fig. 1, R. White (1984): *Ann. Neurol.*, 16(S):14.

A

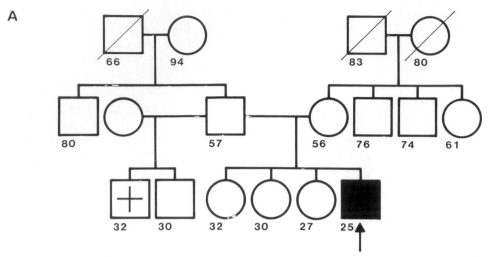

FIG. 4.   **A:** Proband with juvenile myoclonic epilepsy (*indicated by the arrow*) belongs to a family who denied any history of epilepsy. **B:** (*facing page*) But a half brother who is not symptomatic for epilepsy has diffuse 4- to 6-Hz spike-wave and multispike-wave complexes (⊞).

screening process. Once an RFLP linked to a marker locus is discovered, it can be similarly investigated with the epilepsy locus.

CLEAVAGE WITH DNA RESTRICTION ENDONUCLEASES

In order to make feasible approaches such as those just described, several laboratories have been developing the technology to make cloned DNA segments into genetic markers that can be assayed in small blood samples. The cloned DNA segments can be arbitrary (in the sense of not encoding any known gene) or can be specific cloned genes. The underlying principal of this method is illustrated in Fig. 4. It is known that there are many variations in DNA sequence among individuals. Although, for the most part, the DNA sequence at the same locus will be identical among many individuals, there is variation at the level of 1/200 to 1/500 base pairs. These variations are believed to be silent polymorphisms in DNA sequence, having no known deleterious effects. Restriction enzymes or DNA restriction endonucleases recognize specific small sequences in DNA and cleave the DNA strand at the recognition site, yielding fragments of defined length. The restriction enzymes can detect some of these natural variations in DNA sequence, which can arise from either substitution of one or more bases in the DNA resulting in the loss of a cleavage site or

the formation of a new one, or from insertion or deletion of blocks of DNA within a fragment. Figure 4 illustrates a specific example: the enzyme Taq I recognized the DNA sequence TCGA and cut, yielding fragments of a specific length. In chromosome 7a, a Taq site is present and yields a fragment of a length of 8.6 kilobases (kb). In chromosome 7b, the homologous Taq site is no longer present, owing to a variation in the DNA sequence, and the result of Taq digestion is a fragment of a different length, 10.2 kb. DNA fragments of different lengths can be separated according to molecular size by agarose gel electrophoresis and tranferred to a stable matrix, such as nitrocellulose, according to the Southern technique (74). DNA fragments can then be hybridized with highly radioactive DNA sequences (probes). This process enables the investigator to score individuals as being either heterozygous or homozygous for the polymorphic Taq sequence.

The first polymorphic DNA sequence was identified in humans at an arbitrary locus by Wyman and White (85). It was not due to a base pair change at a restriction site (as illustrated in Fig. 3), but rather to a deletion within a fragment defined by the restriction enzyme Eco RI. In fact, a series of restriction fragments of different lengths was observed, reflecting the presence of a number of deletions of different lengths within the fragment and resulting in the ability to identify a number of alleles at the locus. This type of polymorphic series is much more useful as a

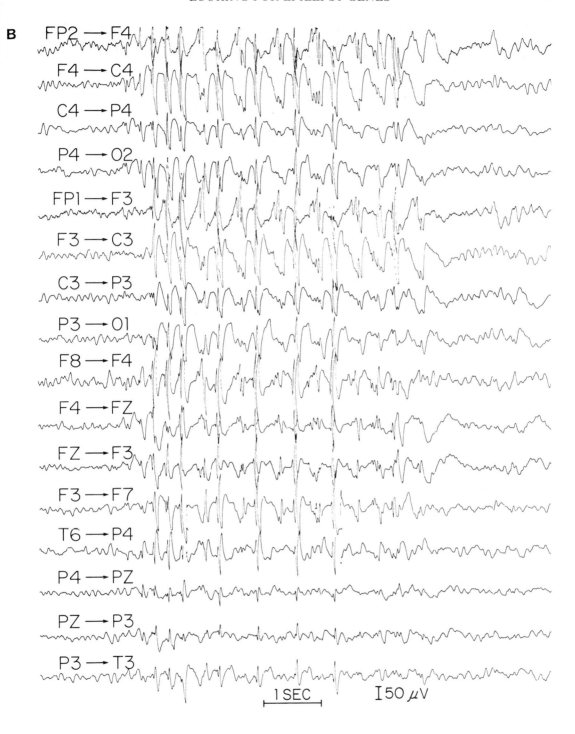

B

FP2 → F4

F4 → C4

C4 → P4

P4 → O2

FP1 → F3

F3 → C3

C3 → P3

P3 → O1

F8 → F4

F4 → FZ

FZ → F3

F3 → F7

T6 → P4

P4 → PZ

PZ → P3

P3 → T3

1 SEC   I 50 µV

genetic marker than a base pair change variant that gives only two alleles, since the likelihood of heterozygosity and for the correct identification of progeny genotypes is much improved.

However, further examinaton by Barker et al. (5) of some 35 additional loci with more than a dozen restriction enzymes failed to reveal another multiallelic deletion locus, even though well over a million base pairs were screened for this type of variation. A result of some interest was obtained, however. Of the 10 polymorphic restriction sites observed at nine loci, nine were polymorphic with either of only two enzymes, Msp I and Taq I. These two restriction enzymes hold in common the dimer sequence CG in their recognition sites (Msp I = CCGG; Taq I = TCGA). Two additional facts were known: the C in CG dimer sequences in mammalian DNA are very frequently methylated, and methyl-C is a "hot spot" for mutation in bacterial systems. From this information, we may hypothesize that methyl-C is also a hot spot for mutation in humans, and consequently that it is a hot spot for population polymorphism. An important result of these studies, however, is the knowledge that the majority of DNA sequence polymorphisms that are detectable by restriction enzymes can be detected by the use of only two such enzymes, Msp I and Taq I. This knowledge results in substantial economies in further screening. Barker and collaborators have extended this approach to a number of other loci and found that approximately one-quarter of arbitrarily selected loci reveal polymorphism with one of these two enzymes. Additional multiallelic loci whose polymorphism is based on a deletion series have been found in the vicinity of several known genes, specifically the insulin gene, β-globin gene, and Harvey ras oncogene. These polymorphisms are apparently due to variations in the number of sets of tandem repeats of short sequences (5).

Roses et al. (69) recently reviewed the genetic strategies of screening unique sequence DNA polymorphisms for linkage with Huntington's disease (HD), Duchenne muscular dystrophy (DMD) and myotonic dystrophy (MD). Myotonic dystrophy was one of the first autosomal dominant disorders for which significant linkage was established (33,61,62,69). The MD gene was closely linked to the secretor (Se) locus and loosely to the Lutheran (Lu) blood group locus, and the three have been provisionally assigned to the chromosome 19. Sex-linked DMD was localized to Xp21 (86) Charcot-Marie-Tooth disease has been localized to chromosome 1. Until recently, the chromosome carrying the abnormal gene for Huntington's chorea was unknown, and screening for unique sequence DNAs was planned for the entire human genome. The amount of data for screening (approximately 300 plates with a cosmid vector carrying DNA pieces of approximately 35-kb length) that would have been needed to establish linkage between

HD and RFLPs would have been tremendously large (30,31). Fortunately, a polymorphic marker system (G8 marker) was recently linked and tentatively localized to chromosome 4. Therefore, the technical aspects of screening each random RFLP with a given chromosome library compared to the whole genome was solved (30,31).

FURTHER STEPS TOWARDS IDENTIFYING THE EPILEPSY LOCUS

If the method utilizing candidate gene markers successfully localizes the site of the epilepsy gene on a given chromosome, the next step is the definition of the abnormal amino acid sequence in epilepsy. While the technology for candidate gene markers is being developed, and while families are being screened for candidate gene markers, linkage to an RFLP marker can also identify the chromosome in which a specific epilepsy resides.

Once the chromosomal location of a specific epilepsy locus is linked to an RFLP marker, the principles of recombinant DNA technology should then determine the precise arrangements of the mutant epilepsy gene at a specific given locus. For example, the arrangement of immunoglobulin genes in humans was determined by cloning overlapping segments of DNA carrying these genes and then aligning their structures by determining the specific positions of restriction endonuclease cleavage sites within each fragment, the so-called "walking the chromosome" method.

Several strategies, aside from "walking the chromosome" method, which is time-consuming, can be used to bridge this gap between flanking DNA linkage markers (probably a few million base pairs away) and an epilepsy locus. Directional cloning of DNA fragments 50–200 kb away from an initial probe using the circularization method can now be used to produce the chromosome "hop." This method allows directional scanning of the genome over relatively large distances without the need to characterize all of the intervening DNA and is thus considerably more efficient than chromosome-walking (13). The pulse field gradient electrophoresis of Schwartz and Cantor (73) can be used to resolve very large restriction fragments (200–5,000 kb) produced by enzymes that cut infrequently in human DNA before chromosome "hopping" (13). These large segments can be digested further with a second enzyme, and the smaller segments can be cloned in an appropriate vector. In addition, somatic cell genetics techniques could construct a cell line with one or more of the successfully linked DNA markers integrated into the vicinity of the disease locus. This region could then be transferred into a rodent cell, after which all human sequences could be recovered by hybridization to human-specific repetitive sequence probes.

After the region containing the epilepsy locus has been cloned, differences in DNA sequences as small as a single base change can be detected by the denaturing gradient gels developed by Fischer and Lerman (25). Alternatively, coding sequences within the region containing the epilepsy locus can be isolated by fusion of "open reading frames" of the human genes into bacterial expression vectors. Antiserums could then be produced to detect the corresponding human proteins (28,83).

SELECTION OF EPILEPSIES FOR LINKAGE ANALYSIS WITH CANDIDATE AND POLYMORPHIC GENE MARKERS

In any consideration of genetics and epilepsy, it is important to recognize the distinction between seizures and epilepsy. The term "seizure" refers to "a sudden and transitory abnormal phenomenon of a motor, sensory, autonomic, or psychic nature resulting from transient dysfunction of all or part of the brain." On the other hand, epilepsy (from the Greek word "epilepsia" meaning "a condition of being overcome, or seized, or attacked") is defined as "a chronic brain disorder characterized by recurrent seizures due to excessive discharges of cerebral neurons" (15,26). Thus, it can be seen that seizures per se are but a symptomatic manifestation of an underlying neurological or systemic disorder. In the case of epilepsy, seizures are the primary manifestation of the disorder, and symptoms or signs of an active neurological disease are usually absent.

Table 1 in Chapter 1 is a classification of the epilepsies presently under consideration by the International League Against Epilepsy (ILAE) and modified from the World Health Organization Classification of the Epilepsies. The more common epilepsies generally afflict humans who are otherwise normal, mentally and neurologically, between seizures, have good to excellent response to antiepileptic drugs and, in specific instances, may have high remission rates after withdrawal of antiepileptic drugs (18). These epilepsies are distinguished from the more progressive and debilitating epileptic encephalopathies, such as the Lennox-Gastaut syndrome,

and the heredofamilial myoclonic epilepsies of Lafora and Glueck (43), Zeman (87), Unverricht (80), Lundborg (46), Hartung (34) and Hunt (37).

Among all these epilepsies, those best suited for linkage analysis with candidate gene markers and polymorphic DNA markers are the epilepsies most likely caused by single mutant genes showing mendelian patterns of inheritance. These include childhood absence, juvenile myoclonic epilepsy and pure grand mal (tonic-clonic, clonic-tonic-clonic), rolandic epilepsies, and the progressive myoclonic epilepsies of Lafora and Kuf. Because the progressive myoclonic encephalopathies are rare disorders, we will discuss the epilepsies that provide the most available and informative pedigrees.

Childhood Absence: Synonyms— Simple Petit Mal, Pure Petit Mal, and Pykno-Epilepsy (3,18,26,60)

Childhood absence, which appears in 3–4% of all patients with epilepsy (18,26,60), is distinguished from four other forms of absence which start during later childhood and adolescence and which may represent phenocopies or a different genetic basis (Fig. 5). Absence attacks in these adolescents are infrequent; however, patients almost always have tonic-clonic seizures, and the electroclinical traits persist into later life (18). The EEG trait is the typical bilaterally synchronous and symmetrical 3 Hz spike-wave complex.

Family studies in the general population show the presence of absence seizures in 3.0% of siblings (47) and of epileptic seizures as a group in 3.9–6.7% (19–21,47,48). The incidence is highest at 9.1% in relatives of female probands with absence. EEG abnormalities are more frequently found than clinical seizures in relatives of absence patients. Generalized EEG abnormalities in siblings range from 24 to 27.7% (20,48) but the specific 3-Hz spike-wave trait is found in 9.2–36.7% of siblings (47,50). The spike-wave EEG abnormalities are even more frequent when siblings and offspring of probands with absence are studied below 16 years of age. Metrakos and Metrakos reported 35% of offspring to have the trait being most common (51%) at ages 4.7–10.5 years (50).

In 1961, Metrakos and Metrakos (50) hypothesized that 3-Hz spike-wave complexes are inherited as an autosomal dominant trait with maximum penetrance at age 10 years (range 4.5–16.5 years), disappearing rapidly in older age groups so that by 40 years of age it is very

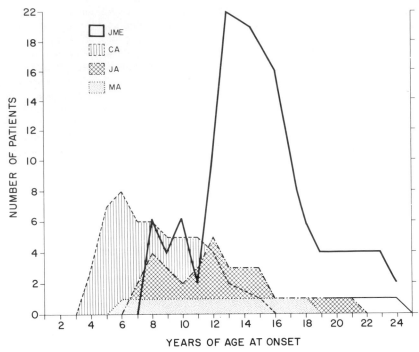

FIG. 5. Age penetrance of classic absence (CA), juvenile absence (JA), myoclonic absence (MA), and juvenile myoclonic epilepsy (JME). (Reproduced with permission from Fig. 2, A.V. Delgado-Escueta and D. Greenberg (1984): *Ann. Neurol.*, 16(S):4.)

seldom present. These investigators suggested that siblings and offspring had a 50% risk of inheriting the spike-wave EEG trait (implying dominant inheritance), a 35% risk of expressing the EEG trait during their lifetime, a 12% risk of having one of the generalized seizures, and an 8% risk of developing absence. More recent interpretation of similar observations have emphasized how the recurrence of risk of absence is much below that expected for a single gene with clear-cut mendelian segregation (1,3,13,82). To explain these observations, Anderman suggests that other genetic and/or environmental factors must interact with whatever is producing the spike-wave EEG trait before clinical absence is produced, e.g., two gene loci may need to interact (1,3,13,82) to produce the phenotype of absence. However, a more likely explanation is that these previous studies used a heterogenous population of absence, and an unknown proportion of cases may have been phenocopies or sporadics. These various hypotheses of modes of transmission are now being restudied in a homogenous population of childhood absence. An important lead is that, contrary to other phenotypes, childhood absence unassociated with tonic-clonic seizures has an excellent prognosis. We now suspect this genotype explains its low remission rates after withdrawal of antiepileptic drugs in contrast to absence combined with tonic-clonic seizures and absence found in juvenile myoclonic epilepsy. Independent investigators report that 80–95% of children with pure childhood absence remain free from attacks when 3 years of successful antiepileptic drug treatment is stopped (18,40). The 5–20% of those with pure absence who relapse may represent sporadics or phenocopies of absence with a different genetic basis.

Two independent reports by Rivas (68) and Fichsel and Kessler (24) suggest that pure absence is associated with alleles of the major histocompatibility complex on chromosome 6p. In 25 of 42 probands with absence, Rivas (68) and Fichsel and Kessler (24) independently found an increased incidence of the A1-B8 haplotype in absence patients. Eeg-Olofsson et al. (22) however, did not find such results. They found a decreased incidence of A1-B8 haplotype in 16 probands with absence.

Juvenile Myoclonic Epilepsy: Synonym—Impulsiv Petit Mal of Janz or Herpin-Lundborg-Janz Syndrome (16,39,40,41)

The Janz school of Berlin and the Comprehensive Epilepsy Program in Los Angeles have been mainly responsible for the identification of juvenile myoclonic epilepsy (JME) as a separate disorder. As the disorder becomes recognized more frequently in different parts of the world, its incidence among all epilepsies has grown from 2.7% in 1957 to 5.4% in 1977 to 11.9% in 1984. Most frequently, the disorder starts undiagnosed as minor irregular jerks of shoulders and arms. After 3.3 years, a major convulsion occurs, prompting a medical consultation. A series of successive myoclonic jerks usually precedes the tonic-clonic convulsion (myoclonic grand mal of Jasper and Kershman, impulsiv grand mal of Janz, or clonic-tonic-clonic seizure of Delgado-Escueta) (16,39–41). Various authors have noted that 52–95% of patients report seizures mainly in the morning hours after awakening, induced by lack of sleep or premature awakening. Ten to 37% of patients also have absence. Rapid 4- to 6-Hz diffuse polyspike-wave complexes characterize the interictal EEG, although 10% have the classical 3-Hz diffuse spike-wave sequences or 3-Hz polyspike-wave complexes mixed with the rapid 4- to 6-Hz polyspike-wave complexes. Some 25–39% of family relatives have epileptic seizures.

Aside from confirming the peak age of onset between 13 and 15 years (Fig. 5), recent analysis of its electroclinical trait show that the disorder persists into the sixth and seventh decades of life regardless of treatment (16,39). This persistence of electroclinical traits during most of the patient's lifetime explains its high recurrence rate (90%) on withdrawal of drug treatment (16,39). Tsuboi and Christian (76) investigated relatives of 319 patients with JME and discovered that 27.3% of patients had either a parent, child, or sibling whose history included epilepsy and that 33.5% of female patients had a positive family history. Tsuboi and Christian suggested a polygenic mode of inheritance, but recent analysis by our group suggests an autosomal dominant pattern of inheritance (Fig. 6), consistent with an abnormality in a single protein molecule. Unlike previous reports of female preponderance, more recent studies show equal sex ratio. Monaghan et al. investigated the genetic association of the HLA haplotype with cryptogenic myoclonic epilepsy in 29 probands and found no significant association (52).

Traditional Grand Mal Epilepsy: Synonyms—Generalized Tonic-Clonic and Clonic-Tonic-Clonic Epilepsies

In addition to the segregation of JME as a phenotype of epilepsy, two forms of traditional and pure "grand mal" epilepsies are now recognized. Grand mal epilepsies are considered pure when they are not associated with absence epilepsies or myoclonic epilepsies or other forms of epileptic attacks. Only convulsive seizures afflict the patient. Four to 10% of all epileptic patients have pure "grand mal" as the only type of attack (15,18,26).

The first subvariety consists of clonic-tonic-clonic seizures ("impulsiv grand mal") which occur often on awakening and are usually triggered by sleep deprivation, excessive fatigue, and alcohol intake. These seizures have an interictal EEG trait of diffuse 4- to 6-Hz multispike-wave complexes. Diffuse 4- to 6-Hz multispike-wave complexes appear during the initial clonic phase and precede the rhythmic fast spikes at 16–18 Hz and tonic contractions. Multi-spike-wave complexes appear again during the last clonic phase. Clonic-tonic-clonic seizures may be one of the phenotypes of the genetic substrate responsible for JME (18). Pure grand mal has an extremely good prognosis since convulsions disappear in 85% of patients on treatment with valproic acid. Our recent experience with these patients show that their electroclinical traits persist into the later years of life, and that most patients relapse on withdrawal of drug treatment (16,18).

The second subvariety of "grand mal" epilepsy consists of tonic-clonic seizures whose interictal EEG trait is the well-formed diffuse 3-Hz spike-wave and multispike-wave complexes. During ictus, epileptic recruiting patterns of 9- to 12-Hz diffuse rhythms herald the tonic phase. Infrequently, these seizures appear only as nocturnal tonic-clonic seizures, characteristically triggered by stage 1 or 2 sleep. More frequently, tonic-clonic seizures occur during both diurnal and nocturnal hours. Sixty-four to 75% of pure "grand mal" tonic-clonic seizures studied by Gastaut and Tassinari (26) and Pedersen and Krogh (59) disappeared with treatment; a further 22% decreased in frequency. The remission rate of pure "grand mal" tonic-clonic seizures is

better than awakening clonic-tonic-clonic seizures, since only 8 to 20% of the former patients
relapse after drug withdrawal.

The mode of transmission of "grand mal"–
tonic-clonic seizures has not been defined; however, a genetic contribution has been documented in family studies by Eisner et al. (23) and
Tsuboi and Endo (77). Eisner et al. examined
siblings and parents of patients with tonic-clonic
convulsions and found a seizure rate of 5.26%
for relatives, a rate considerably higher than the
control rate of 1.75%. Convulsive seizures were
most common in relatives (8.3%) when epilepsies began before the proband reached 4 years
of age (23). Tsuboi and Endo restricted their
studies to offsprings of 30 patients with tonic-
clonic seizures with or without an aura. Probands whose generalized tonic-clonic seizures
had no aura had 4.7% of their offspring with
epileptic seizures and 16.8% of their offspring
with either febrile convulsions or seizures. A
total of 102 offspring had EEGs and 37.3% had
generalized epileptiform patterns (77).

ROLANDIC EPILEPSY

Rolandic epilepsy (also known as benign epilepsy with Rolandic spikes) deserves special
consideration among the partial epilepsies of
childhood, because it is transmitted in an autosomal dominant mode and is self-limiting. It
starts to disappear in midadolescence and is almost always easily controlled by a single antiepileptic drug (18). Complete remission after
withdrawal from 4 years of drug treatment is
probably indicated by the disappearance of the
clinical trait by 20 years of age.

Rolandic epilepsy occurs in otherwise healthy
boys and girls and accounts for 15% of all childhood seizures (21). Seizures begin between 5
and 9 years of age, when a single nocturnal
tonic-clonic seizure with focal onset most commonly occurs. Subsequently, focal seizures implicate the lower Rolandic region. Involuntary
muscular contractions typically involve one side
of the face and occasionally the arm. The seizures may begin with arrested speech due to
motor interference of the tongue and oral function. Less commonly, the pharynx or the leg is
involved in clonic contractions. The characteristic interictal EEG trait is high-voltage spikes
followed by prominent slow waves appearing
singly or in groups at the Rolandic region (18).
A family history of epilepsy is present in 13% of
patients with Rolandic epilepsy. Rolandic spikes
are detectable in 34% of siblings (18).

PENETRANCE AND EXPRESSION OF EPILEPSIES

The genetics of these various forms of epilepsies can be best accomplished by knowing where
the affected gene is located. Subsequently, we
may know what relationship it has to other and
adjacent genes. Hence, isolating epilepsy genes
allows questions on their penetrance and variable expressivity. If a structural gene's function,
expression, or product is dependent on additional modifier genes, such as processing genes,
temporal genes, or architectural genes, a mutation in any of these steps in expression could
possibly result in a phenotype similar to one involving a structural gene defect (9,20).

Why epilepsies are preponderant in females of
all afflicted generations has remained unanswered. The higher incidence of epilepsy in
mothers than in fathers of children with convulsions was reported by Ounsted in 1952 (57).
Harvald found the incidence of "genuine epilepsy" higher in mothers than in fathers, and in
sisters than in brothers (35). Doose et al. found a
higher incidence of seizures in females in three
generations of photosensitive epilepsy (19).
Tsuboi and Christian also found the incidence of
epilepsy to be higher among female relatives,
mothers, and daughters of patients with juvenile
myoclonic epilepsy (76). This higher frequency
of the disease among females and among relatives of female probands does not fit the polygenic mode of inheritance. However, 10% of
penetrance among near relatives of probands is
difficult to explain by autosomal dominant inheritance. An understanding of how the mutations of one gene affect the expression of another gene makes it possible to identify the loci
that function in the final realization of a structural gene product. Thus, if mutant genes involved in a sequence of physiological steps
manifesting as epilepsy can be chromosomally
located, it can be investigated whether epilepsy
is the result of mutations to several genes that
are closely linked, clustered on the same chromosome, or under the same coordinate control.
It may eventually be possible to insert cloned
normal genes or genes that will suppress the effect of the gene mutation.

Through this approach, we may finally understand which specific forms of epilepsies require
one or two or more genes to be expressed clinically, why females have a lower threshold for
clinical manifestation (19,35,57,76), why the fertility of epileptics is 60.4% of that found in the
average population, and why the fertility is lower for male (52.5%) than for female patients (35).

REFERENCES

1. Anderman, E. (1982): Multifactorial inheritance of generalized and focal epilepsy. In: *Genetic Basis of the Epilepsies*, edited by V. E. Anderson, W. A. Hauser, J. K. Penry, and C. F. Sing, pp. 355–374. Raven Press, New York.

2. Anderson, S., Bankier, A. T., Barrell, B. G., deBruijn, M. H. L., Coulson, A. R., Drovin, J., Eperson, I. C., Nierlich, D. P., Roe, B. A., Sanger, E., Schreier, P. H., Smith, A. J. H., Staden, R., and Young, I. G. (1981): Sequence and organization of the human mitochondrial genome. *Nature*, 290:457–465.

3. Anderson, V. E., and Hauser, W. A. (1985): The genetics of epilepsy. In: *Progress in Medical Genetics*, edited by A. G. Bearn, B. Childs, and A. Motulsky (in press).

4. Barker, D., McCoy, M., Weinberg, R., et al. (1983): A test of the role of two oncogenes in inherited predisposition to colon cancer. *Mol. Biol. Med.*, 1:199–206.

5. Barker, D., Schafer, M., and White, R. (1984): Restriction sites containing CpG show a higher frequency of polymorphism in human DNA. *Cell*, 36:131–138.

6. Bajorek, J. (1984): Neuropeptides: A role as endogenous mediators or modulators of epileptic phenomena. *Ann. Neurol.*, 16(Suppl.)2:31–38.

7. Benton, W. D., and Davis, R. W. (1977): Screening lambdgt recombinant clones by hybridization to single plaques in situ. *Science*, 4286:180–182.

8. Bird, T. D., Ott, J., and Giblett, E. R. (1982): Evidence for linkage of Charcot-Marie-Tooth neuropathy to the Duffy locus on chromosome 1. *Am. J. Hum. Genet.*, 34:388–394.

9. Botstein, D., White, R. L., Skolnick, M., and Davis, R. W. (1980): Construction of a genetic linkage map in man using restriction fragment length polymorphisms. *Am. J. Hum. Genet.*, 32:314–331.

10. Caskey, C. T., and White, R. I., editors (1983): *Banbury Report 14: Recombinant DNA Applications to Human Disease*. Cold Spring Harbor, New York, Cold Spring Harbor Laboratory.

11. Catalano, F. (1974): Remarks on the pathogenesis of so-called idiopathic epilepsy. *Acta Neurol.*, 28:183–207.

12. Cavenel, W. K., Dryja, T. P., Phillips, R. A., Benedict, W. F., Godboat, R., Gallie, B. L., Murphree, A. L., Strong, L. C., and White, R. L. (1983): Expression of recessive alleles by chromosomal mechanisms in retinoblastoma. *Nature*, 305(5937):779–784.

13. Collins, F. S., and Weissman, S. M. (1984): Directional cloning of DNA fragments at a large distance from an initial probe: A circulation method. *Proc. Natl. Acad. Sci. Genet. USA*, 81:6812–6816.

14. Conneally, P. M., and Rivas, M. L. (1980): Linkage analysis in man. *Adv. Hum. Genet.*, 10:209–266.

15. Dalby, M. A. (1969): *Epilepsy and 3 per Second Spike and Wave Rhythms*. Munksgaard, Copenhagen.

16. Delgado-Escueta, A. V., and Enrile-Bacsal, F. (1984): Juvenile myoclonic epilepsy of Janz. *Neurology (NY)*, 34:285–294.

17. Delgado-Escueta, A. V., and Greenberg, D. (1984): The search for epilepsies ideal for clinical and molecular genetic studies. *Ann. Neurol.*, 16(Suppl.)2:1–11.

18. Delgado-Escueta, A. V., Treiman, D. M., and Walsh, G. O. (1983): The treatable epilepsies. *New Engl. J. Med.*, 308:1508–1514, 1576–1584.

19. Doose, H., Gerken, H., Hien-Volpel, K. F., and Volzke, E. (1969): Genetics of photosensitive epilepsy. *Neuropadiatrie*, 1:56–73.

20. Doose, H., Gerken, H., Hortzmann, T., and Volzki, E. (1973): Genetic factors in spike wave absence. *Epilepsia*, 14:57–75.

21. Doose, H., and Scheffner, D. (1982): Zur therapie und prognose der absencen. *Med. Welt*, 1763–1767.

22. Eeg-Olofsson, O., Safwenberg, J., and Wigertz, A. (1982): HLA and epilepsy: An investigation of different types of epilepsy in children and their families. *Epilepsia*, 23:27–34.

23. Eisner, V., Pauli, L. L., and Livingston, S. (1959): Hereditary aspects of epilepsy. *Johns Hopkins Hosp. Bull.*, 105:245–271.

24. Fichsel, H., and Kessler, M. (1980): Immunogenetics of 3/s-SW absence epilepsy: Frequency of HLA antigens and haplotypes in patients and relatives. In: *Advances in Epileptology* (XIth Epilepsy International Symposium), edited by R. Canger, F. Angeleri, and J. K. Penry, pp. 475–477. Raven Press, New York.

25. Fischer, S. G., and Lerman, L. S. (1983): DNA fragments differing by single base-pair substitutions are separated in denaturing gradient gels: Correspondence with melting theory. *Proc. Natl. Acad. Sci. USA*, 80(6):1579–1583.

26. Gastaut, H., and Tassinari, C. A. (1975): Epilepsies. In: *Handbook of EEG and Clinical Neurophysiology*, vol. 13(A), pp. 3–104, Elsevier, Amsterdam.

27. Gedda, L., and Tatarelli, R. (1971): Essential isochronic epilepsy in MZ twin pairs. *Acta Genet. Med.*, 20:380–383.

28. Gray, M. R., Colot, H. V., Guarente, L., and Rosbash, M. (1982): Open reading frame cloning: Identification, cloning and expression of open reading frame DNA. *Proc. Natl. Acad. Sci. USA*, 79(21):6598–6602.

29. Grisar, T., Franck, G., and Delgado-Escueta, A. V. (1983): Glial contribution to seizures: K$^+$ activation of (Na$^+$,K$^+$)-ATPase in bulk isolated glial cells and synaptosomes of epileptogenic cortex. *Brain Res.*, 261:75–85.

30. Gusella, J. F., Tanzi, R. E., Anderson, M. A., Hobbs, W., Gibbons, K., Raschtchian, R., Gilliam, T. C., Wallace, M., Wexler, N. S., and Conneally, P. M. (1984): DNA markers for nervous system disease. *Science*, 225:1320–1326.

31. Gusella, J. F., Wexler, N. S., Conneally, P. M., et al. (1983): A polymorphic DNA marker genetically linked to Huntington's Disease. *Nature*, 306:234–238.

32. Haldane, J. B. S., and Smith, C. A. B. (1947): A new estimate of the linkage between the genes

for color blindness and haemophilia in man. *Ann. Engen.*, 14:10–31.

33. Harper, P. S., Rivas, M. L., Bias, W. B., Hutchinson, J. R., Dyken, P. R., and McKusick, V. A. (1972): Genetic linkage confirmed between the locus for myotonic dystrophy and the ABH secretion and Lutheran blood group loci. *Am. J. Hum. Genet.*, 24:310.

34. Hartung, E. (1920): Zwei falle von paramyoclonus multiplex mit epilepsie. *Z. Gesamte Neurol. Psychiatr.*, 56:151–153.

35. Harvald, B. (1954): Heredity in epilepsy. An EEG study of relatives of epileptics. *Op. Ex. Dom. Biol. Hered. Hum Univ. Hafor*, 35:9–122.

36. Hodge, S. E., Anderson, C. E., Neiswanger, K., et al. (1983): The search for heterogeneity in insulin dependent diabetes mellitus (IDDM): Linkage studies, two locus, models, and genetic heterogeneity. *Am. J. Hum. Genet.*, 35:1139–1155.

37. Hunt, J. R. (1921): Dyssynergia cerebellaris myoclonica—Primary atrophy of the dentate system: A contribution to the pathology and symptomatology of the cerebellum. *Brain*, 44:490–538.

38. Iadorola, M. J., and Gale, K. (1982): Substantia nigra: Site of anticonvulsant activity mediated by γ-aminobutyric acid. *Science*, 218:1237–1240.

39. Janz, D., and Christian, W. (1957): Impulsiv-petit mal. *Dtsch. Z. Nervenheilk.*, 19:155–182.

40. Janz, D., Kern, A., Mossinger, H. J., and Puhlmann, H. U. (1982): Ruckfall-prognose warend und nach reduktion der medikamente bei epilepsiebegandlung. In: *Epilepsie 1981*, edited by H. Remschmidt, R. Rentz, and J. Jungmann, pp. 311–318. Georg Thieme, Stuttgart.

41. Janz, D. (1982): In tema di remissione e di ricomparsa di crisi durante e dopo il trattamento farmacologico dell'epilessia. *Boll. Lega Ital. Epil.*, 39:95–100.

42. Kredich, N. M., and Hershfield, M. S. (1983): Immunodeficiency diseases caused by adenosine deaminase deficiency and purine nucleoside phosphorylase deficiency. In: *The Metabolic Basis of Inherited Disease*, edited by J. B. Stanbury, J. B. Wyngaarden, D. S. Frederickson, et al., pp. 1157–1183. McGraw-Hill, New York.

43. Lafora, G. R., and Glueck, B. (1911): Contributions to the histopathology and pathogenesis of myoclonic epilepsy. *Bull. Gov. Hosp. Insane*, 3:96.

44. Lennox, W. G., and Lennox, M. A. (1960): *Epilepsy and Related Disorders*, Little, Brown and Co., Boston.

45. Lewin, E. (1983): Inosine, hypoxanthine, and seizures. In: *Status Epilepticus: Mechanisms of Brain Damage and Treatment, Advances in Neurology*, vol. 34, edited by A. V. Delgado-Escueta, C. Wasterlain, D. M. Treiman, and R. Porter, pp. 365–368. Raven Press, New York.

46. Lundborg, H. (1912): Der erbang der progressiven myoklonusepilepsie, *Z. Gesamte Neurol. Psychiatr.*, 9:353–358.

47. Matthes, A., and Weber, H. (1968): Clinical and electroencephalographic family studies in pyknolepsies, *Dtsch. Med. Wochenschr.*, 93:429–435.

48. Matthes, A. (1969): Genetic studies in epilepsy. In: *The Physiopathogenesis of the Epilepsies*, edited by H. Gastaut, H. Jasper, J. Bancaud, and A. Waltregny, pp. 26–30. Charles C Thomas, Springfield.

49. McKusick, V. A. (1983): Mendelian inheritance in man. In: *Catalogs of Autosomal Dominant, Autosomal Recessive and X-linked Phenotypes*, 5th ed., Johns Hopkins University Press, Baltimore.

50. Metrakos, K., and Metrakos, J. D. (1961): Genetics of convulsive disorders. II. Genetic and electroencephalographic studies in centrencephalic epilepsy. *Neurology (Minn)*, 11:474–483.

51. Mohr, J. (1954): *A Study of Linkage in Man*, Munksgaard, Copenhagen.

52. Monaghan, H. P., O'Sullivan, M., and O'Donohoe, N. V. (1982): HLA antigens and cryptogenic myoclonic epilepsy. *J. Med. Sci.*, 151(6):188–189.

53. Morton, N. E. (1962): Segregation and linkage. In: *Methodology in Human Genetics*, edited by W. J. Burdette, pp. 17–52. Holden Day, San Francisco.

54. Noebels, J. L. (1979): Analysis of inherited epilepsy using single locus mutations in mice. *Fed. Proc.*, 38:2405–2410.

55. Noebels, J. L. (1982): Defined gene models of the inherited epilepsies. In: Anderson VE, *Genetic Basis of the Epilepsies*, edited by W. A. Hauser, J. K. Penry, and C. F. Sing, pp. 211–224. Raven Press, New York.

56. Olsen, R. W., Snowmen, A. M., Lee, R., Lomax, P., and Wamsley, J. K. (1984): Role of the γ-aminobutyric acid receptor/ionophore complex in seizure disorders. *Ann. Neurol.*, 16(S):90–95.

57. Ounsted, C. (1952): The factor of inheritance in convulsive disorders in childhood. *Proc. Soc. Med.*, 45:865–868.

58. Overweg, J., Rowan, A. J., Binnie, C. D., Nagelkerke, N. J. D., and Costing, J. (1981): Prediction of seizure recurrence after withdrawal of antiepileptic drugs. In: *Advances in Epileptology: XIIth Epilepsy International Symposium*, edited by M. Dam, L. Gram, and J. K. Penry, pp. 503–508. Raven Press, New York.

59. Pedersen, H. E., and Krogh, E. (1970): Decentraliseret behaudling og kontrol of patienter med epilepsi. *Nord. Med.*, 83:689–694.

60. Penry, J. K., Porter, R., and Dreifuss, F. E. (1975): Simultaneous recordings of absence seizures with videotape and EEG. *Brain*, 98:427–440.

61. Pericak-Vance, M. A., Conneally, P. M., Merritt, A. D., Roos, R., Vance, J. M., Yu, P. L., Norton, J. A., and Antel, J. P. (1979): In: *Advances in Neurology*, edited by T. N. Chase, N. S. Wexler, and A. Barbeen, p. 59. Raven Press, New York.

62. Pericak-Vance, M. A., Stajich, J. M., Conneally, P. M., Vance, J. M., Herbstreith, M. H., and

Roses, A. D. (1983): Genetic linkage analysis of myotonic dystrophy with the complement component 3 (C_3), secretor (Se), and Lewis (Le) loci on chromosome 19. Program Abstracts, International Human Gene Mapping Workshop VII, UCLA, August 21–26.

63. Phillips, J. A., Hjelle, B. L., Seeburg, P. H., and Zachmann, M. (1981): Molecular basis for familial isolated growth hormone deficiency. *Proc. Natl. Acad. Sci. USA*, 78:6372–6375.

64. Rapport, R. L., II, Harris, A. B., Friel, P. N., and Ojemann, G. A. (1975): Human epileptic brain Na^+K^+-ATPase activity and phenytoin concentrations. *Arch. Neurol.*, 32:549–554.

65. Renwick, J. H., Bundey, S. E., Ferguson-Smith, M. A., and Izatt, M. M. (1971): Confirmation of linkage of the loci for myotonic dystrophy and ABH secretion. *J. Med. Genet.*, 8:407–416.

66. Rigby, P. W., Dieckmann, M., Rhodes, C., and Berg, P. (1977): Labeling deoxyribonucleic acid to high specific activity in vitro by nick translation with DNA polymerase I. *J. Mol. Biol.*, 113(1):237–251.

67. Rimoin, D. L., and Metrakos, J. D. (1964): The genetics of convulsive disorders in the families of hemiplegics. *Proc. 2nd Intl. Congr. Hum. Genet.*, 3:1655–1658.

68. Rivas, M. L. (1983): Genetic analyses of petit mal epilepsy I. Evaluation of HLA, blood groups, serum proteins, and red cell enzymes. *Epilepsia*, 24:115.

69. Roses, A. D., Pericak-Vance, M. A., and Yamaoka, L. H. (1983): Recombinant DNA strategies in genetic neurological diseases. In: *Molecular Aspects of Neurological Diseases*, edited by L. Austin, and P. L. Jeffrey, pp. 3–16. Academic Press, Sydney, Australia.

70. Sarfarazi, M., Ball, S., O'Brien, T., Davies, K., Shaw, D., and Harper, P. S. (1983): Myotonic dystrophy and markers on chromosome 19. Program Abstracts, International Human Gene Mapping Workshop VII, UCLA, August 21–26.

71. Seyfried, T. N. (1982): Developmental genetics of audiogenic seizure susceptibility in mice. In: *Genetic Basis of the Epilepsies*, edited by V. E. Anderson, W. A. Hauser, J. K. Penry, and C. F. Sing, pp. 199–210. Raven Press, New York.

72. Shaws, T. B., Sakaguchi, A. Y., and Naylor, S. L. (1982): Mapping the human genome, cloned genes, DNA polymorphisms and inherited disease. *Adv. Hum. Genet.*, 12:341–353.

73. Schwartz, D. C., and Cantor, C. R. (1984): Separation of yeast chromosome-sized DNAs by pulsed field gradient gel electrophoresis. *Cell*, 37(1):67–75.

74. Southern, E. M. (1975): Detection of specific sequences among DNA fragments separated by gel electrophoresis. *J. Mol. Biol.*, 98:503–517.

75. Tower, D. B. (1965): Problems associated with studies of electrolyte metabolism in normal and epileptogenic cerebral cortex. *Epilepsia*, 6:183.

76. Tsuboi, T., and Christian, W. (1973): On the genetics of primary generalized epilepsy with sporadic myoclonias of the impulsive petit mal type: A clinical and electroencephalographic study of 399 probands. *Humangenetik*, 19:155–182.

77. Tsuboi, T., and Endo, S. (1977): Incidence of seizures and EEG abnormalities among offspring of epileptic patients. *Hum. Genet.*, 36:173–189.

78. Tsuboi, T. (1980): Genetic aspects of epilepsy. *Folia Psychiatr. Neurol. Jpn.*, 34:215–225.

79. Tudor, I., Milea, S., Bicescu, E., and Ivana, D. (1973): Catamnestic study of childhood epilepsy. *Rev. Roum. Neurol.*, 10:341–352.

80. Unverricht, H. (1891): *Die Myoklonie*, Deuticke, Leipzig.

81. Vogel, F., and Motulsky, A. G. (1979): *Human Genetics: Problems and Approaches*, Springer-Verlag, New York.

82. Ward, R. H. (1982): Genetics and epidemiology: A fruitful interface for the study of epilepsy. In: *Genetic Basis of the Epilepsies*, edited by V. E. Anderson, W. A. Hauser, J. K. Penry, and C. F. Sing, pp. 317–332. Raven Press, New York.

83. Weinstock, G. M., Rhys, C., Berman, M. L., Hampar, B., Jackson, D., Silhary, T. J., Weisemann, J., and Zweig, M. (1983): Open reading frame expression vectors: A general method for antigen production in *Escherichia coli* using protein fusions to beta-galactosidase. *Proc. Natl. Acad. Sci. USA*, 80(14):4432–4436.

84. White, R. (1984): Looking for epilepsy genes. *Ann. Neurol.*, 16(Suppl.)2:12–17.

85. Wyman, A. R., and White, R. (1980): A highly polymorphic locus in human DNA. *Proc. Natl. Acad. Sci. USA*, 77:6754–6758.

86. Zatz, M., Vianna-Morgante, A. M., Campos, P., and Diament, A. J. (1981): Translocation (X;6) in a female with Duchenne muscular dystrophy: Implications for the localization of the DMD locus. *J. Med. Genet.*, 19:442.

87. Zeman, W., Donahue, S., Dyken, P., and Green, J. (1970): The neuronal cereoidlipofuscinoses (Batten-Vogt syndrome). In: *Handbook of Neurology*, vol. 10, edited by P. J. Vinken, and G. W. Bruyn, pp. 588–679. North-Holland, Amsterdam.

With permission Ch. 3 has modified and expanded on portions of the text from Chs. 1 and 2, *Ann. Neurol.*, 16(S):1–17 (1984).

Advances in Neurology, Vol. 44, edited by
A. V. Delgado-Escueta, A. A. Ward, Jr.,
D. M. Woodbury, and R. J. Porter.
Raven Press, New York © 1986.

4

Mutational Analysis of Inherited Epilepsies

Jeffrey L. Noebels

Departments of Neurology, Massachusetts General Hospital, and Neuroscience, Children's Hospital, Harvard Medical School, Boston, Massachusetts 02114.

SUMMARY Single-gene mutations in mice initiate specific heritable neuronal diseases featuring different patterns of epilepsy. Thirteen chromosomal loci for convulsive seizures and four loci for spike-wave seizures have been assigned. Within this genetic framework, a few general principles are emerging. Mutations located on different chromosomes may result in identical seizure patterns. Interactions between specific genes, demonstrated by the synthesis of compound heterozygotes, can express intermediate syndromes. Interactions with unknown genes in the background can mask neurological disease expression.

Analysis of the cellular phenotypes of epileptic mutants is a direct strategy to define naturally occurring defects in central synaptic pathways involved in cortical synchronization. In one allele of the *tottering* locus, a pathogenetic lesion linking noradrenergic hyperinnervation with cortical spike-wave discharges has been identified. The tottering gene initiates an overgrowth within all target innervation areas of axon terminals originating from the locus coeruleus (LC). Selective neonatal denervation of the excess noradrenergic axons permanently prevents the subsequent appearance of cortical spike-wave seizures in the adult animal. Partial lesions of central noradrenergic afferent fibers in adults temporarily reverse the seizure disorder. Other criteria defining the relationship between the mutant gene and the electrophysiologic traits and the role of central noradrenergic pathways in neuronal synchronization are reviewed.

Isolating and tracing the developmental expression of epileptic mutations permits a formal classification of gene-linked excitability defects, a derivation of basic rules governing their inheritance, and the design of strategies to correct the gene error. By allowing phenotypic comparisons with over 60 known human inherited neurological diseases associated with seizures, these models may directly contribute to advances in the clinical management of epileptic gene expression.

Nature is nowhere accustomed more openly to display her secret mysteries than in cases where she shows traces of her workings apart from the beaten path; nor is there any better way to advance the proper practice of medicine than to give our minds to the discovery of the usual law of Nature by careful investigation of cases of rarer forms of disease. For it has been found, in almost all things, that what they contain of useful or applicable nature is hardly perceived unless we are deprived of them, or they become deranged in some way.

William Harvey, 1657

Are epilepsies inherited? How many genes need be altered, and what specific excitability properties of the neuronal membrane or synapse do they disturb? Can the defects be isolated and selectively corrected prior to their clinical expression by medicine or other genes? These three questions, raised from the perspective of a patient, a scientist, and a physician, define the primary targets and the descriptive power of a neurogenetic approach to basic mechanisms of epilepsy.

In a Croonian Lecture entitled, "Lessons From Rare Maladies" (27), Archibald Garrod's (1858–1936) quote from Harvey bears eloquent testimony to early perceptions of the inherent advantages of mutational analysis to understand hereditary disease. Garrod was the first to formalize the concept of inborn errors of metabolism and the relationships linking single genes and enzymes that shape the present search to uncover general principles of aberrant gene expression in the nervous system. Other key concepts followed, notably the complex issue of pleiotropism (Plate, 1910) to explain the protean phenotypic alterations following the disturbance of a single gene. The next year, E. B. Wilson (1911) assigned the first gene to a chromosome; a neurological gene for color blindness located on the X chromosome. Continuing interest in mammalian nervous system genes centered on the examination of retinal defects ["rodless retina" (49)], agenesis of the corpus callosum (47), and inherited ataxias in mice, notably the *shaker, circler, pirouette,* and *waltzing* ("souris valseuses") mutations, which were curiosities of naturalists in China as early as 80 B.C. (30,48,134).

The report by Pauling in 1949 of the distinction between hemoglobins A and S (93) clarified the molecular basis of hereditary diseases and established a definitive conceptual framework to analyze the developmental biology of inherited neurological disorders. In the search for natural models, Sidman et al. collected the diverse neuropathological findings of nearly 90 neurological murine mutations characterized by 1964 (110). This systematic overview coincided with the beginning of elegant morphological analyses of the developmental mechanisms directing neuronal migration, synaptogenesis, myelination, and lifespan within the central nervous system (CNS) (6,13,109). Subsequently, electrophysiologic and metabolic traits were added to screen the genome for the subset of mapped genes that exert phenotypic effects on neuronal excitability and synchronization (83).

In parallel with the mouse genome, rapid progress in human gene mapping began with the introduction of murine chromosomes into somatic cell hybrids and of restriction endonuclease analysis. In 1973, Ruddle reported that only two genes had been localized to the human autosomes; in the following decade, over 1400 chromosomal locations have been assigned (66), and restriction fragment length polymorphisms (RFLPs) are now in use as linkage markers for family studies to map neuronal disease (19, 31,130). The accelerating advance in the status of mammalian gene maps, together with new evidence for substantial DNA sequence conservation across species (64,78) (Fig. 1) and the probable structural homology of major gene products such as ion channels and surface antigens (12,69), are good predictors that genetic studies of all nervous systems may directly contribute to the analysis of inherited human neurological disease.

This chapter specifically reviews recent developments in the molecular and cellular characterization of gene errors in the mouse that initiate inherited epilepsies, and several lines of evidence that alterations in central neuromodulatory pathways, rather than intrinsic defects in principal cortical neurons, may comprise one discrete category of the many basic mechanisms underlying abnormal patterns of cortical synchronization.

ISOLATING EPILEPTIC GENES

Two complementary approaches, descriptive (genotype), and functional (phenotype) are central to developmental neurogenetic analysis; potential systems to combine them are under intensive exploration.

Genotype Analysis

The mouse genome is estimated to consist of 1.6 billion base pairs—1,600 centimorgans—less than 100,000 genes located on 40 chromosomes. Coding (exon) regions of these genes direct the synthesis of about 2×10^5 kilobases (kb) of polyribosomal RNA, composed of polyadenylated and nonpolyadenylated RNA molecules of similar complexity in roughly equal proportions (14,125). The end product expression of these genes is multiplied by cleavage of polypeptides into smaller active fragments, and it has been proposed that the gene product number might be exponentially increased by DNA sequence rearrangements, as shown in families of

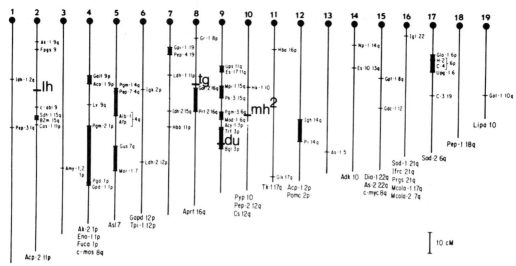

FIG. 1. Linkage map of the mouse showing autosomal loci (initial symbol) whose human homologues have been assigned to specific chromosomes (second symbol). The lengths of the conserved segments (heavy lines) are probably greater than indicated by the identified markers available. Four recessive loci that alter cortical synchronization in a stereotyped spike-wave pattern, *lethargic* (*lh*), *ducky* (*du*), *tottering* (*tg*), and *mocha* 2j (*mh²ʲ*) are indicated by arrows. No locus for this seizure pattern has yet been assigned in humans. Modified from Nadeau and Taylor, ref. 78, with permission.

500 or so exons that code for 10^7 immunoglobulin species (36), although this possibility has not yet been demonstrated in CNS tissue.

A subset of these genes, turned on and off at critical periods by cell–cell interactions within the emerging tissue, control the growth and equilibrium of the membrane excitability properties that regulate neuronal signaling. For the present analysis, genes of interest are divisible into three categories.

Neuronal Genes

Northern (mRNA) blot analysis of a class of polyadenylated mRNA transcripts cross-hybridized with liver and kidney reveals that at most 30,000 genes, identifiable by characteristic noncoding (intron) intervening ID sequences, are actively and perhaps exclusively transcribed within the CNS (70). Approximately half of the brain-specific mRNA sequences in the mouse are not polyadenylated and are unique in being almost entirely expressed postnatally (33). The function of this class of mRNA molecule and its translation products are not yet known.

Nonneuronal Genes

Loci expressed only in tissues outside the nervous system, when mutated, may also alter normal brain development (e.g., thyroid hormone), or allow accumulated metabolites to enter and alter neural excitability, eventually causing seizure disorders. Genes in this category therefore cannot be eliminated from consideration.

Shared Genes

Genes that are not tissue-specific and that alter both neuronal and nonneuronal targets are also candidate epileptic genes, for example, the neuraminidase gene in cherry red spot–myoclonus syndrome (89). These loci are not isolated by purification strategies using differential hybridization.

Recombinant cDNA isolation strategies are now being extended to catalog gene subsets exclusive to specific classes of neurons or regions within the brain by in situ hybridization (132), and can in principle allow the identification of putative gene products and their subcellular fate with immunohistochemical localization (114). The principal drawback of applying this powerful set of techniques *in vacuo* is that there is no method to predetermine which of the purified gene clones might play a pathologic role in neuronal excitability. Induced mutations in these isolated gene sequences, once reintroduced into the organism, can provide this functional information; however, multiple alternative point mutations at the same locus could differentially alter activity in a structural gene. For example, overlapping deletions causing less or no gene product; or frameshift insertions, causing a nonsense mutation affecting the substrate binding (Km variant), turnover rate (Vm variant), and polypeptide length (and hence solubility) of the gene product may all create different phenotypes. Mutations in regulatory genes are less well understood, but might alter temporal expression of the gene, creating alleles with variable degrees of pleiotropism. Nevertheless, once combined with the new techniques of site-directed mutagenesis and transgenic (inserted gene copy) models, sequence-oriented molecular genetics will play a critical role in examining the expression of electrogenic neuronal membrane behavior in a developing nervous system (45).

Phenotype Analysis

A second approach toward dissecting complex CNS gene actions uses the reverse strategy, starting with the desired trait and searching for the genes responsible. Over 1100 assigned single-locus mutations which arise spontaneously (18) or are induced (102) on coisogenic and congenic inbred mouse strains are available to survey for relevant neurological phenotypes.

Experimental Advantages of Single-Gene Mutations

The singular advantage of defined mutations in coisogenic inbred strains of the mouse is that individual epileptic genes can be isolated and analyzed one at a time within a highly reproducible mammalian nervous system, and then compared directly with littermates possessing one-half (+ /a) or none (+ / +) of the mutant gene dose. The remainder of the genome is homozygous at virtually every other allele. The allogenic interactions of additional mutations and background genotypes can be systematically explored. An early expression of the biochemical defect allows assessment of the natural history and spatial profile of the cellular lesion before it is masked by misleading secondary changes, thereby outlining a developmental timetable for intervention prior to irreversible expression of the disease. Finally, mutations disturb neural pathways in unusually precise yet unpredictable ways, that not only allow the study of disease processes thus far not phenocopied, but offer

valuable insight, as Harvey suggested, into the normal workings of the brain.

LESSONS FROM EPILEPTIC GENES

Initially, 13 loci were identified as epileptic mutations based on behavioral criteria (110). This survey has been extended using electrocorticographic and regional metabolic probes (83), which, in combination, can detect abnormal signaling in both superficial cortical and deep central pathways.

Mutational analysis has so far revealed several important general principles governing the genetic transmission of epilepsy.

Single Genes Can Cause Spontaneous Seizure Disorders

At present there are 17 identified loci, located on 10 chromosomes, expressing neurological syndromes with associated seizures of convulsive and nonconvulsive patterns. The extent to which pairing of these epileptic genes with unrelated neurological loci or each other ("double mutants") can alter expression has not yet been systematically examined, although a study of the interaction in a compound heterozygote tg/tg^{la} mutant derived from two alleles at the tottering locus shows overlapping features of both syndromes (67,86,120).

Epileptic Genes Express Specific Neuropathological Lesions

The observation that many gene mutations with mild to severe effects on cerebral development do not initiate seizures provides strong evidence to reject the hypothesis that epilepsy is a "nonspecific" lesion of the nervous system. The list of mutations surveyed for ECoG abnormalities to date is given in Table 1. In this series, the exceptions to the group of genes causing inheritance of a seizure disorder are as interesting to consider as the epileptic loci themselves. For example, the gene error in *reeler* (chromosome 5), with aberrant "inside out" lamination of neocortex and malpositioning of neurons (13), apparently does not constitute a sufficient epileptogenic lesion. *Purkinje cell degeneration* (chromosome 13) and *lurcher* (chromosome 6), both with total degeneration of cerebellar Purkinje cells, do not show spontaneous seizures, despite reports that reduction in Purkinje cell output augments seizures (41).

TABLE 1. *ECoG survey of gene mutations in the mouse*

Locus	Chromosome	Pattern	Genotype	ECoG
Lethargic	2	Rec	*lh/lh* (B6C3/a/A-lh)	PD
Spastic	3	Rec	*spa/spa* (C57B1/6J-spa)	un
Meander	4	Rec	*mea/mea* (non-inbred)	un
Cribriform	4	Rec	*cri/cri* (DBA2J-cri/+)	S
Lurcher	6	Dom	*Lu/+* (B6CBA-Aw-j/A-LcT7CaMi)	un
Leaner	8	Rec	tg^{la}/tg^{la} (C57B1/6J-Os +/+ tg^{la})	PD
Tottering	8	Rec	*tg/tg* (C57B16-tg)	PD
Tottering/leaner	8	Rec	tg/tg^{la} (C57B1/6)	PD
Ducky	9	Rec	*du/du* (a/ad + du/d + k +)	PD
Staggerer	9	Rec	*sg/sg* (C57B1 se/sg)	S
Dystrophia muscularis	10	Rec	*dy/dy* (C57B1/6J-dy)	un
Mocha^{2j}	10	Rec	C3H/HeJ-mh^{2j}/+	PD
Shambling	11	Rec	*shm/shm* (shr/GnEiRe +/+ shm)	un
Teetering	11	Rec	*tn/tn* (B6C3 a/a-tn)	un
Trembler	11	Dom	*Tr/+* (C57B1/6J-Tr)	S
Vibrator	11	Rec	*vb/vb* (C57B1/6J-vb)	un
Purkinje cell degeneration	13	Rec	*pcd/pcd* (C57B1/6J-pcd)	un
Jolting (motor end plate disease)	15	Rec	*med^{jo}/med^{jo}* (B6C3-a/a-med^{jo})	un
Weaver	16	Rec	*wv/wv*	S

Note: in selected cases, abnormalities were also, or only, seen in the heterozygous mouse (*du,mh^{2j},lh,wv*). ECoG, electrocorticogram; un, unremarkable relative to the control genotype; PD, generalized paroxysmal discharges; S, abnormal slowing. (J. L. Noebels, *unpublished observations*.)

Different Gene Loci Cause Similar Phenotypes

A third major principle is that a gene mutation may be only one of several that initiate a specific synchronization abnormality. For example, *du* (chromosome 9), *lh* (chromosome 2), and *mh^{2j}* (chromosome 10) all express spike-wave seizure patterns similar to the *tottering* mutant (88). It is improbable that they represent multiple gene copies with a unique gene sequence in common, since the remainder of the syndromes are dissimilar; however, it will be instructive to ascertain whether the genes act in concert on a specific class of neurotransmitter or whether they share control of a particular synaptic pathway.

TRACING CELLULAR EXPRESSION OF EPILEPTIC GENE SPECIFICITY

If a gene sequence is known, and the copy number is sufficient, it may be possible to search the mutant nervous system directly to define the cell type containing the altered or missing mRNA transcript (99). When no gene information is available, conventional neuropathological and neurophysiological tools suffice, recognizing that serial studies are required to stage the cascade of compensatory reaction to the mu-

tant gene. Although the molecular precision of a single-gene mutation is exquisite, the specificity of the resulting disease cannot be predicted beyond an obvious generalization that alterations confined to a rarely expressed sequence late in development minimize the extent of the lesion. An implicit corollary is that many mutations initiate defects in multiple cell types, and subsequent interactions obscure the initial lesion during ontogeny.

PRIMACY

To ascertain whether a cytologic lesion is the primary expression of a gene error and whether it simultaneously represents a direct and exclusive cause of the disease phenotype, a set of minimal criteria has been derived (44) from the list of Koch's postulates relating to the germ theory of disease.

1. The biochemical abnormality must be genetically determined (one proof would require persistence in cell culture over multiple generations, a difficult test in nontransformed neurons.) If an antibody or sequence can be procured, the neuronal genome can be examined directly with in situ hybridization techniques. To

establish the presence of a gene that alters cells by interfering with normal cell–cell interactions will prove to be the more common, and complex situation.

2. Within a kindred, the defect is inherited in the same pattern as the disease.

3. Variable expression of the mutant cellular phenotype accounts for clinical variability in the neurological signs of the disease.

4. There is a gene dose effect. The lack of absolute correlation of partial enzyme deficiency with severity of disease, however, is still incompletely understood (16).

5. Expression of the defect antedates or coincides with clinical expression of the disease.

6. Experimental recreations (phenocopies) of the defect mimic, or at least produce essential elements of, the disease. Multistage, developmental defects bridging critical trophic periods of organogenesis may not be easily induced in the CNS, and may only be replicable once a gene sequence can be cloned and specific transgenic models created.

7. Treatment that corrects or minimizes the defect also limits the appearance of the disease.

Recent progress toward satisfying these criteria in a genetic model of epilepsy has been made in the *tottering* mutation, an interesting example of an inherited spike-wave seizure disorder.

TOTTERING MUTATION: GENE CONTROL OF CENTRAL NORADRENERGIC PATHWAYS

The *tottering* mouse (chromosome 8, recessive) (29) is a prototype model of inherited epilepsy because it represents the first genetic model of a spontaneous nonconvulsive seizure disorder and is linked to an unusual lesion of terminal neurogenesis in a well-studied neurotransmitter system.

Behavioral Phenotype

The *tg* locus causes a delayed-onset recessive neurological disorder in the mouse, featuring a stereotyped triad of ataxia, intermittent focal myoclonic seizures, and generalized spike-wave arrest seizures (87).

Ataxia in the hindlimbs is easily noted by the fourth postnatal week. *Intermittent myoclonic* seizures are manifest at the same age in 10- to 30-min stereotyped episodes, progressing from spastic jerking in a single hindlimb to alternating clonic movements of all limbs, while the mouse remains behaviorally responsive. The episodes occur spontaneously 1–3 times daily with a prolonged refractory period, and are often precipitated by handling. There is no characteristic cortical discharge accompanying these episodes, although 2-deoxyglucose uptake autoradiograms reveal clear alterations in regional cerebral metabolic activity, including increases in several subcortical nuclei (87). *Arrest seizures* with vibrissal twitching and occasional jerks of head or jaw coincide with 6 to 7/sec spike-wave discharge bursts in the electrocorticogram (ECoG), followed immediately by a return to normal cortical rhythms and behavior (43,87). The morphology of the discharge complex is highly uniform, with only a few variant patterns randomly observed in over 80 homozygotes studied (Fig. 2). The bursts vary from 0.1 to 10 sec in duration, and occur at a rate of 1/hr in the 18-day-old mutant, rising to 40–60/hr in the awake adult without any significant diurnal variation. The

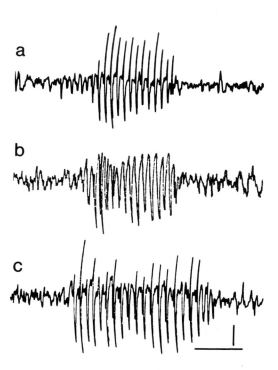

FIG. 2. Burst morphology in awake, adult homozygous tottering mice. Cortical surface recordings reveal separable components of the 6–7/sec synchronous discharge: (a) primarily spike burst; (b) primarily wave burst; (c) mixed spike-wave discharge. The patterns vary in all affected mice. Bar = 1 sec, 100 μV. (J. L. Noebels, *unpublished observations*.)

discharges cannot be evoked by photic stimuli, but can be instantly interrupted by stimuli within any sensory modality.

Cellular Phenotype

Routine histopathologic surveys of the *tg/tg* brain reveal no cytopathological features, and the cerebral weight and nuclear dimensions are reliably similar to unaffected littermates. Two more severely affected alleles at the *tg* locus, *rolling* (90) and *leaner* (120), possess variably hypoplastic granuloprival cerebella with a significant anterior lobe gradient of cell loss (1,35,67,82). In *tg/tg* cerebellar cortex, there is no evidence as yet for granule cell loss, and the presence of irregular purkinje cell plasma membranes (67) is not seen in mice on the B1/6 background (Noebels and Sidman, *unpublished observations*), suggesting fixation artifact. Two-dimensional gel protein electrophoresis of cerebral cortex, brainstem, and cerebellar cortex fails to distinguish any variant polypeptide product (84). Analysis of similar regions for ganglioside or phospholipid abnormalities reveal a <10% alteration in cerebellar ganglioside content in a group of three samples in 70-day-old (but not in 21-day-old) *tg/tg* when compared with nonlittermate controls (108).

The only significant cellular pathology as yet uncovered in the *tg* nervous system is a selective overgrowth of LC axons (57), a small bilateral pontine nucleus containing approximately 1,400–1,600 cells that supply the majority of forebrain norepinephrine (NE) innervation (59). This is reflected in a 100–200% elevation in NE levels within most LC terminal projection fields, including neocortex, hippocampus, thalamus, and cerebellum. The number of parent cell somata in the LC nucleus is unchanged, indicating that the increased numbers of fluorescent axons identified in the target regions represent a proliferation of the terminal axon branches (Fig. 3). The remaining catecholaminergic systems, the lateral tegmental cell group and dopaminergic nuclei, are apparently unaffected by the gene. Levitt et al. (58) have recently shown that both α- and β-receptor populations in target regions hyperinnervated by LC axons in the *tg/tg* mutant are not significantly affected either in receptor number or ligand binding affinity. This finding is especially significant, since it indicates that at least one potential pathologic consequence of NE hyperinnervation, i.e., excess α or β stimulation, is not locally compensated for by postsynaptic receptor down-regulation (97).

A secondary correction in sensitivity might have been expected, since β-receptor decreases have been found in two experimental models of noradrenergic hyperinnervation, although in the methylazoxymethanol acetate model (8,40) there is a substantial loss of postsynaptic target cells, and in the case of 6-hydroxydopamine-induced regenerative hyperinnervation, early evidence (34,122) for down-regulation has not been confirmed despite a 160% increase in NE levels (115). In addition, the C57B1/6 coisogenic strain on which the *tg* locus is maintained possesses at least 36% more LC neurons (e.g., $n = 1,408$ versus 1,030) than the Balb/c strain (9,118); consequently the number of axon terminals, tyrosine hydroxylase (TH) activity, and regional NE levels are significantly higher than those in Balb/c and several other inbred strains (9,80,127). In fact, the relative increase of cortical NE levels in the C57B1/6 strain over Balb/c mice is as large (100–200%) as the ratio of C57B1/6 *tg/tg* to its +/+ littermate. Berger et al. (9) produced regional Scatchard plots of [^{3}H]dihydroalprenolol binding in neocortex, and found that the number of ligand binding sites remained the same, if not slightly greater, in C57B1/6 and Balb/c brains, whereas the binding affinity was unchanged. These data from unaffected inbred strains suggest that developmental NE hyperinnervation does not necessarily induce a persistent change in postsynaptic receptor number, and thus it is not yet clear that the absence of receptor regulation represents a second action of the *tg* gene.

DETERMINING ROLE OF LC INNERVATION IN SPIKE-WAVE SEIZURES

Three relational hypotheses require evaluation once a candidate lesion is uncovered.

1. *Cause.* Even if primarily linked with the pathogenesis of the clinical phenotype, inferences regarding the number of intervening steps between the unidentified mutant gene product, the altered LC neurons, and the abnormal cortical physiology cannot be directly drawn. However, if the altered LC input is simply and not irreversibly linked to abnormal synchronization, lesions should abolish the cortical discharges.

2. *Result.* Abnormal synaptic input and firing patterns related to frequent seizures during development cause extensive cellular restructuring and modification of synaptic release behavior. There is substantial evidence for developmental plasticity within the neonatal and adult LC fiber system following subtotal axon lesions, with hy-

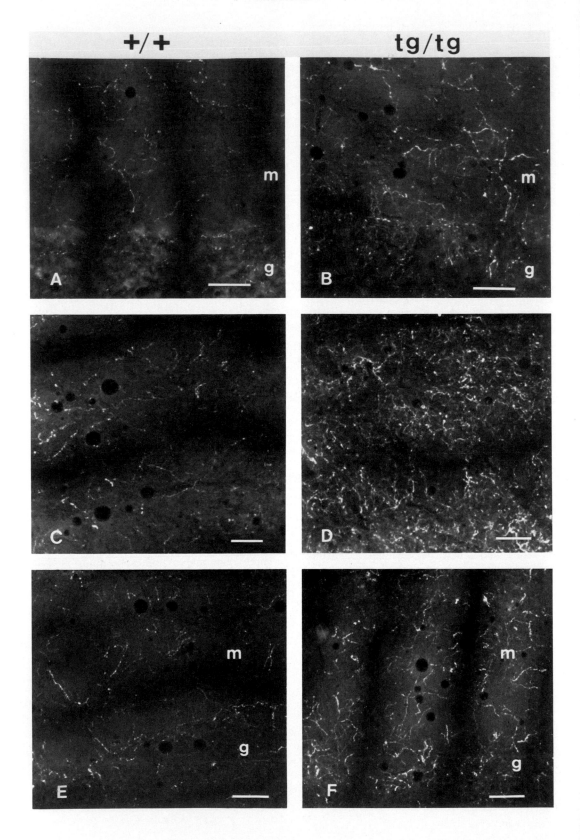

perinnervation occurring in the region of damage and throughout remaining terminal innervation targets (56,96). Impulse activity is also known to raise TH activity, and damage to LC neurons increases the spontaneous firing rate (15), but these are not known to stimulate axon outgrowth. If NE axon proliferation is a compensatory change to inhibit seizure generation, NE axon lesions should enhance the severity of the disorder.

3. *Unrelated.* NE hyperinnervation might be a distant effect of the gene error and an epiphenomenon in relation to the seizure trait. Experimental interference with its expression will have no effect on the clinical phenotype.

To evaluate the phenotypic significance of LC hyperinnervation and distinguish between these relationships, the size of the terminal LC axonal arbor was selectively reduced in *tg/tg* mutants at two stages of maturity.

Neonatal Alteration in LC Innervation Abolishes Spike-Wave Seizures

Selective neonatal denervation of the hypertrophic LC axonal arborization can be reproducibly achieved by a single subcutaneous injection of the neurotoxin 6-hydroxydopamine (6-OHDA) on the first postnatal day (56,103) (Fig. 4). This neurotoxin is only accumulated in neurons with high-affinity catecholamine uptake systems, and initiates an axonal reaction within the initial 24 hr of exposure (112). Neonatal NE denervation by this method in *tg/tg* mutants entirely prevents the later appearance of spikewave absence seizures in the adult animal (85) (Fig. 5); the effect is essentially permanent in the mice that showed 85–95% depletion of NE content and comparable losses of NE axon terminal glyoxilic acid-induced histofluorescence within cortical and hippocampal target fields. Mutants with less complete lesions showed diminished cortical discharges (Fig. 5c).

Adult Lesions in LC Innervation: Temporary Desynchronization

In a second group of adult *tg/tg* animals with fully expressed seizure disorders, verified unilateral injections of 6-OHDA into the LC nucleus rapidly but not permanently altered the frequency and symmetry of the cortical discharges (85) (Fig. 6).

These data show a direct, causal, but not exclusive link between a single-gene error of LC hyperinnervation associated with elevated cerebral NE levels and electrocortical synchronization causing spontaneous arrest seizures in the *tg* mutation. In addition, the evidence suggests that there is no critical period in development beyond which the abnormal bursting in cortical networks cannot be reversed.

The developmental sequence of the cellular and electrographic traits in the *tg/tg* mutant, if comparable to normal mice, appear to coincide: LC cells complete mitosis by embryonic day E13 in the rodent (54), and extend afferents to hippocampus, cerebral, and cerebellar cortex by E19, but do not attain full terminal arborization and transmitter synthesizing capacity until 3–4 weeks postnatal (17,23,55), the stage roughly coincident with the appearance of major clinical abnormalities in the *tg/tg* mutant.

Is NE Hyperinnervation a Sufficient Lesion?

LC hyperinnervation is present in both alleles of the tottering locus [*leaner* (1), *rolling* (77,79)], and *leaner* homozygotes show spike-wave discharges virtually identical to those in *tg/tg*. Other mutations with increased NE-terminal density, *pcd* (28,52,100), *weaver, reeler,* and *staggerer* (52,76), either do not show cortical discharges in the homozygous animal (Table 1), or have not been studied electrophysiologically (*quaking*) (50,117); however, the absolute content (per brain), and relative concentrations (per tissue weight) of NE vary from low to high, and are normal in some brain regions. Because these mutants all express other well-documented cellular disturbances in addition to the variable patterns of forebrain NE innervation, they cannot clarify the issue further. The three identified mutant loci (*du, lh, mh²ʲ*) that also show hypersynchronous discharges similar to *tg* (88) remain to be evaluated for NE-terminal innervation patterns.

NORADRENERGIC NEUROMODULATION AND CELLULAR SYNCHRONIZATION

What are the cellular mechanisms by which excess norepinephrine might initiate intermittent

---

FIG. 3. Fluorescence histochemical patterns of the LC-derived NE innervation in cerebellum (A and B), dorsal lateral geniculate nucleus (C and D), and area dentata of the hippocampus (E and F) in age-matched *tg/tg* and +/+ mice. In each region, there is a striking proliferation of the *tg/tg* terminal NE axonal plexus. (m, molecular layer; g, granular layer; bar = 50 μm). From Levitt and Noebels (57).

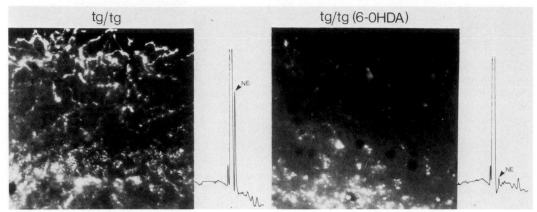

FIG. 4. Regional depletion of cerebral noradrenaline by neonatal exposure to the neurotoxin 6-OHDA in adult *tottering* homozygote. (*Left*) Glyoxilic acid-induced histofluorescence of noradrenaline-containing axons in cerebral cortex of *tg/tg* adult, and the associated chromatographic peak reflecting local noradrenaline content. The terminals all originate from locus coeruleus neurons. (*Right*) Comparable histofluorescence pattern and NE content in age-matched, neonatally injected *tg/tg* littermate. The virtual disappearance of fluorescent cortical NE terminals is mirrored by 85 to 95% decrement in tissue NE content. (From J. L. Noebels (85); and *unpublished observations.*)

synchronous discharges in neocortical and hippocampal neurons? Before addressing this question, certain behavioral observations concerning NE actions within the CNS should be clarified, since it has been generally shown that seizure thresholds decrease with NE denervation. For example, NE depletion lowers the threshold for kindling, metrazol, sound, light, and electrically induced convulsions (2,22,39,63,65,68). This evidence for an anticonvulsant effect does not contradict the results observed in the *tg* mouse for the following reasons:

1. The behavioral and electroencephalographic epileptic patterns differ—spike-wave arrest seizures are not convulsions, nor is there any available evidence that the two seizure types share any neurophysiological or pharmacologic features in common.

2. *tg* seizures are spontaneous, not evoked. In convulsive models of epilepsy, NE depletion lowers the stimulus threshold, but typically does not affect other parameters of the discharge.

3. *tg* expresses an early lesion of NE hyperinnervation; until more is understood of its extended effects on target cell membranes and metabolism, NE lesions in *tg* brain are not directly comparable to NE depletions in normal CNS.

In order to begin formulating testable hypotheses of NE involvement in synchronous neuronal discharges, a few salient characteristics of the cellular neurobiology of central nor-

adrenergic pathways are briefly outlined. Several authors have reviewed LC biology in detail (3,24,72).

ANATOMY

The afferent inputs to locus cells, their internal organization, and the pattern of their projections have been well described (24). Single LC axons branch to innervate widespread target regions (113), and supply 90% of intracortical NE levels. A single LC soma innervates the neocortex with an average of 20,000 NE-terminal branches, with roughly 5% of axonal contacts described as conventional synapses (7). Other major projection areas include cerebellum, hippocampus, insular cortex, septum and amygdala, thalamic–hypothalamic and related diencephalic nuclei, and the spinal cord. Release of NE occurs at varicosities and conventional presynaptic sites, which may vary in distribution according to the nuclear region. The terminal axon innervation pattern within specific target regions is also nonuniform; for example, there are at least five types of NE axonal ramifications identified in diencephalic nuclei (60), whereas in neocortex there is a diffuse tangential laminar distribution of afferents across cortical columns (73). At least 33% of all cortical terminals traverse dendrites of principle neurons in the molecular layer, and the remainder occupy deeper laminae. Because the termination of NE action

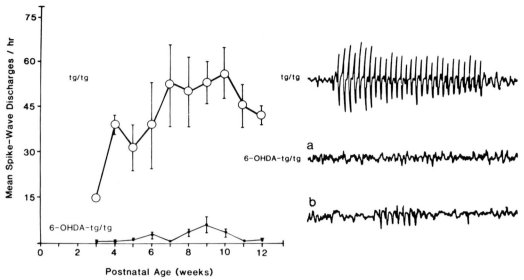

FIG. 5. Effect of neonatal systemic injection of 6-OHDA on spontaneous expression of cortical spike-wave discharges in developing *tg/tg* mice (●, n = 9), compared with saline-injected control *tg/tg* littermates (○, n = 9). Early and permanent suppression of the inherited seizures was absolute in five of nine mutants given a single subcutaneous injection of the neurotoxin on the first postnatal day. In four other mutants with incomplete NE lesions, rare discharges persisted at rates of <1/hr. In the final week, the control group averaged 41.4 discharges/hr (±3.6 SEM) as compared with 0.1 discharges/hr in the treated group. *Right:* (*Upper*) synchronous cortical burst in untreated *tg/tg*. A typical mutant averages 900–1,000 bursts in 24 hr. (*Center*) (a) representative tracing of unaltered ECoG activity in mutant treated at birth with systemic 6-OHDA. This mutant failed to show a single discharge in over 100 hr of daily recording. (b) Rare discharge in a treated mutant with incomplete NE lesion. From J. L. Noebels (85).

depends largely upon presynaptic reuptake, spatial aspects of the innervation pattern play a major role in regulating NE effects. There is evidence for local control of NE release (81,129), partially self-mediated by presynaptic receptors, although their role in neurotransmission remains controversial (42). The distribution of the four known postsynaptic noradrenergic subtypes is heterogeneous (92,116,121) and not confined to neurons (119).

PHYSIOLOGY

NE increases presynaptic axon terminal excitability in both central (61,104) and peripheral (20) fibers. A specific augmentation of posttetanic potentiation by a calcium ion dependent process has been shown to enhance spontaneous (mepp frequency) and evoked transmitter release at the rat neuromuscular junction (10).

The postsynaptic actions of NE within the neuraxis have been frequently oversimplified, despite requisite caution to separate bimodal dose–response and anesthetic effects (116); *in vitro* studies showing effects in some instances

directly opposite to those *in situ* (5) raise further concern over the generality of the findings. The first atypical property noted following NE iontophoresis is the prolonged latency and duration of the response, over 10–100 times greater than for most other neurotransmitter candidates, in some instances outlasting the period of application by over 60 sec. Postsynaptic responses to NE exposure and LC stimulation (see refs. 116 and 124 for detailed references) can be divided into several categories.

Firing Rate

In most neocortical areas, *in situ* studies show a decrease in spontaneous firing rates in central neurons following NE iontophoresis (11,51, 91,95,126); a small percentage of cells (0–30%) show early or late excitation. Superficial cells are uniformly inhibited, and deep neurons are excited for long periods with very low NE concentrations, (10^{-8} M) and inhibited at concentrations 10–100 times higher (4). Subcortical nuclei are predominantly excited by NE iontophoresis or LC stimulation (46,101,123,131). A laminar profile was found in the superior collic-

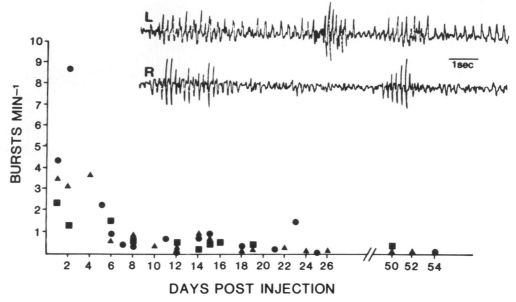

FIG. 6. Biphasic alteration in burst frequency by unilateral ablation of nucleus locus coeruleus (LC) in three adult *tg/tg* mice. The seizure frequency initially increases over 48–72 hr, then rapidly declines during the first week following 6-OHDA injection into the left LC nucleus. Mean preinjection baseline is less than 1 burst/min in all mice. Insert: electrocorticogram recording after 24 hr shows transcortical uncoupling of generalized synchronous bursts with near-continuous left hemisphere discharges and spike broadening in cortex ipsilateral to LC injection. The right hemisphere discharges retain unaltered morphology. Subsequent recordings showed further striking interhemispheric asymmetry and a global reduction of bursts to a frequency averaging 90% below baseline by the third week of monitoring. (J. L. Noebels, *unpublished data*).

ulus, where superficial cells were predominantly inhibited and deeper neurons were excited (105). Intracellular recordings from cortical neurons typically reveal 1–5 mV membrane hyperpolarization, and similar results are obtained in hippocampal and cerebellar cortices (5,53,106). In cerebellar slices *in vitro*, NE superfusion increases and decreases in purkinje cell firing, mediated by β- and α-receptors, respectively (5), directly opposite to excitability changes seen *in vivo* (119) and in the hippocampus *in vitro* (75).

Action Potential Currents

An important effect of norepinephrine, similar to serotonin, on excitable membranes is the demonstrated *modulation of gated ion channels,* through alterations in cAMP levels (98,111). Reductions of calcium currents by NE has also been shown in sympathetic neurons (26,38). A *blockade of membrane accommodation* by NE, resulting in prolonged repolarization and burst firing has been recently ascribed to an effect on á calcium-activated potassium channel in hippocampal neurons (32,62). A potentially related

finding in purkinje cells revealed a conversion of spike-inactivated wave complexes to full-amplitude action potentials during NE application (25); both effects increase axonal output of the cell.

Synaptic Mechanisms

Three main actions of NE on synaptic networks have been described:

1. An *increase in evoked response* amplitude relative to the spontaneous impulse activity during NE application. This increased "*s/n ratio*" follows both excitatory and inhibitory synaptic inputs and iontophoretically applied neurotransmitters (21,107,128,133).

2. A *frequency-dependent synaptic* effect resulting in increases in the magnitude and duration of long-term potentiation at hippocampal mossy fiber-CA3 pyramidal cell synapses (37).

3. A *co-convulsant action* in vitro, mediated by β-receptors, increases penicillin and potassium-induced spontaneous bursting in hippocampal slices (74); α-agonists produced an op-

posite, anticonvulsant response. This may partly explain a convulsant effect of NE in hippocampal slices previously denervated of LC inputs (71) where receptor regulation has occurred; alternatively NE may be involved in the disinhibition of interneurons (71,105).

In summary, the actions of one of the most studied central neurotransmitter systems remain highly individualized and are still incompletely understood at the membrane and network level. Postsynaptic effects are specific according to the population of NE receptor subtypes and location and nature of neighboring co-activated afferents, as well as the nonuniform intrinsic bursting properties of the individual cell (94). These factors are probably sufficient to account for the regional heterogeneity of NE action, but offer no more of a direct explanation of the phenotypic results of inherited increases in NE pathways than their simple portrayal in the tottering mouse.

CONCLUSION

The tottering gene is reversibly linked to the delayed onset of spike-wave cortical discharges through a lesion of central noradrenergic hyper-innervation. The dimensions of a few basic mechanisms of central NE neuromodulation have been extended to the point that a simple outline for a uniform neurobiology of noradrenaline action cannot be drawn independently of the local circuits within the target region. The necessary and sufficient CNS pathways underlying generalized spike-wave discharges remain to be identified. Further detailed physiological analyses of single-gene mutations such as the tottering mouse may be able to define other naturally occurring synaptic mechanisms of inherited epilepsies, isolate the restricted target regions involved, and uncover selective antiepileptic therapies directed specifically at the inherited lesion.

ACKNOWLEDGMENTS

I have been fortunate to work with Richard Sidman and Pat Levitt at different stages of this research. This work was supported by the Lennox Foundation, the Klingenstein Foundation, and the Epilepsy Foundation of America.

REFERENCES

1. Adachi, K., Sobue, I., Tohyama, M., and Shimizu, N. (1975): Changes in the cerebellar noradrenaline nerve terminals of the neurological murine mutant rolling mouse Nagoya: A histofluorescence analysis. *IRSC Med. Sci. (Jpn)*, 3:329–330.
2. Altschuler, H. L., Killam, E. K., and Killam, K. F. (1976): Biogenic amines and the photomyoclonic syndrome in the baboon. *J. Pharmacol. Exp. Ther.*, 196:156–166.
3. Amaral, D. G., and Sinnamon, H. M. (1977): The locus coeruleus: Neurobiology of a central noradrenergic nucleus. *Prog. Neurobiol.*, 9: 147–196.
4. Armstrong-James, M., and Fox, K. (1983): Effects of iontophoresed noradrenaline on the spontaneous activity of neurones in rat primary somatosensory cortex. *J. Physiol.*, 335:427–447.
5. Basile, A. S., and Dunwiddie, T. V. (1984): Norepinephrine elicits both excitatory and inhibitory responses from purkinje cells in the in vitro rat cerebellar slice. *Brain Res.*, 296:15–25.
6. Baumann, N., editor (1980): *Neurological Mutations Affecting Myelination*, Elsevier/North Holland, Amsterdam.
7. Beaudet, A., and Descarries, L. (1978): The monoamine innervation of rat cerebral cortex: Synaptic and non-synaptic axon terminals. *Neuroscience*, 3:851–860.
8. Bealieu, M., and Coyle, J. T. (1982): Fetally-induced noradrenergic hyperinnervation of cerebral cortex results in persistent down regulation of beta-receptors. *Dev. Brain Res.*, 4:491–494.
9. Berger, B., Herve, D., Dolphin, A., Barthelemy, C., Gay, M., and Tassin, J. P. (1979): Genetically determined differences in noradrenergic input to the brain cortex: A histochemical and biochemical study of two inbred strains of mice. *Neuroscience*, 4:877–888.
10. Bergman, H., Glusman, S., Harris-Warwick, R., Kravitz, E. A., Nussinovitch, I., and Rahamimoff, R. (1981): Noradrenaline augments tetanic potentiation of transmitter release by a calcium dependent process. *Brain Res.*, 214:200–204.
11. Bevan, P., Bradshaw, C. M., and Szabadi, E. (1977): The pharmacology of adrenergic neuronal responses in the cerebral cortex: evidence for excitatory α and inhibitory β receptors. *Br. J. Pharmacol.*, 59:635–641.
12. Brown, A. M., Camerer, H., Kunze, D. L., and Lux, H. D. (1982): Similarity of unitary Ca^{2+} currents in three different species. *Nature*, 299:156–158.
13. Caviness, V. S., Jr., and Rakic, P. (1978): Mechanisms of cortical development: A view from mutations in mice. *Ann. Rev. Neurosci.*, 1:297–326.
14. Chaudhari, N., and Hahn, W. E. (1983): Genetic expression in the developing brain. *Science*, 220:924–928.
15. Chiodo, L., Acheson, A. L., Zigmond, M. J., and Stricker, E. M. (1983): Subtotal destruction of central noradrenergic projections increases

the firing rate of locus coeruleus cells. *Brain Res.*, 264:123–126.

16. Conzelman, E., and Sandhoff, K. (1984): Partial enzyme deficiencies: Residual activities and the development of neurological disorders. *Dev. Neurosci.*, 6:58–71.

17. Coyle, J. T., and Molliver, M. E. (1977): Major innervation of newborn rat cortex by monoaminergic neurons. *Science*, 196:444–446.

18. Davisson, M. T., and Roderick, T. H. (1981): In: *Genetic Variants and Strains of the Laboratory Mouse*, edited by M. C. Green. pp. 283–313. Gustav Fischer, Stuttgart.

19. Delgado-Escueta, A. V., and Greenberg, D. (1984): The search for epilepsies ideal for clinical and molecular genetic studies. *Ann. Neurol.* (Suppl.), 16:1–11.

20. Devor, M., and Janig, W. (1981): Activation of myelinated afferents ending in a neuroma by stimulation of the sympathetic supply in the rat. *Neurosci. Lett.*, 24:43–47.

21. Dolphin, A. (1982): Noradrenergic modulation of glutamate release in the cerebellum. *Brain Res.*, 252:111–116.

22. Ehlers, C. L., Clifton, D. K., and Sawyer, C. H. (1980): Facilitation of amygdala kindling in rat by transecting ascending noradrenergic pathways. *Brain Res.*, 189:274–278.

23. Elias, M., Deacon, T., and Caviness, V. S., Jr. (1982): The development of neocortical adrenergic innervation in the mouse: A quantitative radioenzymatic analysis. *Dev. Brain Res.*, 3:652–656.

24. Foote, S. L., Bloom, F. E., and Aston-Jones, G. (1983): Nucleus locus coeruleus: New evidence of anatomical and physiological specificity. *Physiol. Rev.*, 63:844–914.

25. Freedman, R., Hoffer, B. J., Woodward, D. J., and Puro, D. (1977): Interaction of norepinephrine with cerebellar activity evoked by mossy and climbing fibers. *Exp. Neurol.*, 55:269–288.

26. Galvan, M., and Adams, P. R. (1982): Control of calcium current in rat sympathetic neurons by norepinephrine. *Brain Res.*, 244:135–144.

27. Garrod, A. (1928): Lessons from rare maladies. *Lancet*, 1:1055.

28. Ghetti, B., Fuller, R. W., Sawyer, B. D., Hemrick-Lueke, S. K., and Schmidt, M. J. (1981): Purkinje cell loss and the noradrenergic system in the cerebellum of pcd mutant mice. *Brain Res. Bull.*, 7:711–714.

29. Green, M., and Sidman, R. L. (1962): Tottering—A neuromuscular mutation in the mouse. *J. Hered.*, 53:233–237.

30. Gruneberg, H. (1943): *The Genetics of the Mouse*. Cambridge University Press, London.

31. Gusella, J. F., Wexler, N. S., and Conneally, P. M. (1983): A polymorphic marker DNA marker genetically linked to Huntington's disease. *Nature*, 306:234–238.

32. Haas, H. L., and Konnerth, A. (1983): Histamine and noradrenaline decrease calcium-activated potassium conductance in hippocampal pyramidal cells. *Nature*, 302:432–434.

33. Hahn, W. E., Chaudhari, N., Beck, L., Wilber, K., and Peffley, D. (1983): Gene expression and postnatal development of the brain: Some characteristics of nonpolyadenylated mRNAs. *Cold Spring Harbor Laboratory Symposia on Quantitative Biology*, 48:477–484.

34. Harden, T. K., Mailman, R. B., Mueller, R. A., and Breese, G. R. (1979): Noradrenergic hyperinnervation reduces the density of beta-adrenergic receptors in rat cerebellum. *Brain Res.*, 166:194–198.

35. Herrup, K., and Wilczynski, S. L. (1982): Cerebellar cell degeneration in the leaner mutant mouse. *Neuroscience*, 7:2185–2196.

36. Hood, L. (1982): Antibody genes: Arrangements and rearrangements. In: *Molecular Genetic Neuroscience*, edited by F. O. Schmitt, S. J. Bird, and F. E. Bloom. pp. 75–85. Raven Press, New York.

37. Hopkins, W. F., and Johnston, D. (1984): Frequency dependent noradrenergic modulation of long-term potentiation in the hippocampus. *Science*, 226:350–352.

38. Horn, J. P., and McAfee, D. A. (1980): Alpha-adrenergic inhibition of calcium-dependent potentials in rat sympathetic neurones. *J. Physiol.*, 301:191–204.

39. Horton, R., Anlezark, G., and Meldrum, B. (1980): Noradrenergic influences on sound-induced seizures. *J. Pharmacol. Exp. Ther.*, 214:437–442.

40. Jonsson, G., and Hallman, H. (1982): Effects of prenatal methylazoxymethanol treatment on the development of central monoamine neurons. *Dev. Brain Res.*, 2:513–530.

41. Julien, R. M., and Laxer, K. D. (1974): Cerebellar responses to penicillin-induced cortical cerebral epileptiform discharge. *Electroencephalogr. Clin. Neurophysiol.*, 37:123–132.

42. Kalsner, S. (1982): The noradrenergic presynaptic receptor controversy. *Fed. Proc.*, 43:1351.

43. Kaplan, B. J., Seyfried, T. N., and Glaser, G. H. (1979): Spontaneous polyspike discharges in an epileptic mutant mouse (tottering). *Exp. Neurol.*, 66:577–586.

44. Kark, R. A. P., Rosenberg, R. N., and Schut, L. J. (1978): Postscript: Criteria for accepting a biochemical defect as primary. *Adv. Neurol.*, 21:411–412.

45. Kaufman, D. L., and Tobin, A. J. (1984): Prospects for the isolation of genes for receptors and other proteins of pharmacological interest. In: *Molecular and Chemical Characterization of Membrane Receptors*, pp. 241–259. Alan R. Liss, New York.

46. Kayama, Y., Negi, T., Sugitani, M., and Iwama, K. (1982): Effects of locus coeruleus stimulation on neuronal activities of dorsal lateral geniculate nucleus and perigeniculate reticular nucleus of the rat. *Neuroscience*, 7:655–666.

47. Keeler, C. E. (1933): Absence of the corpus callosum as a mendelizing character in the house mouse. *Proc. Natl. Acad. Sci. USA*, 19:609–611.

48. Keeler, C. E., and Fuji, S. (1937): The antiquity of mouse variations in the Orient. *J. Hered.*, 28:93–96.

49. Keeler, C. E., Sutcliffe, E., and Chaffee, E. L.

(1928): A description of the ontogenetic development of retinal action currents in the house mouse. *Proc. Natl. Acad. Sci. USA*, 14:811–815.

50. Kempf, E., Greilsamer, J., Mack, G., and Mandel, P. (1973): Turnover of brain adrenergic transmitters in quaking mice. *J. Neurochem.*, 20:1269–1273.

51. Krnjevic, K., and Phillis, J. W. (1963): Iontophoretic studies of neurones in the mammalian cerebral cortex. *J. Physiol.*, 165:274–304.

52. Landis, S. C., Shoemaker, W. J., Schlumpf, M., and Bloom, F. E. (1975): Catecholamines in mutant mouse cerebellum: Fluorescence microscopic and chemical studies. *Brain Res.*, 93:253–266.

53. Langmoen, I. A., Segal, M., and Andersen, P. (1981): Mechanisms of norepinephrine actions on hippocampal pyramidal cells in vitro. *Brain Res.*, 208:349–362.

54. Lauder, J. and Bloom, F. E. (1974): Ontogeny of monoamine neurons in the locus coeruleus, raphe nuclei, and substantia nigra of the rat. I. Cell differentiation. *J. Comp. Neurol.*, 155:469–482.

55. Levitt, P., and Moore, R. Y. (1979): Development of the noradrenergic innervation of neocortex. *Brain Res.*, 162:243–259.

56. Levitt, P., and Moore, R. Y. (1980): Organization of brainstem noradrenaline hyperinnervation following neonatal 6-hydroxydopamine treatment in rat. *Anat. Embryol.*, 158:133–150.

57. Levitt, P., and Noebels, J. L. (1981): Mutant mouse tottering: Selective increase of locus coeruleus axons in a defined single locus mutation. *Proc. Natl. Acad. Sci. USA*, 78:4630–4634.

58. Levitt, P., Lau, C., Pylypiw, A., and Ross, L. L. (1984): Central adrenergic receptors in the inherited noradrenergic hyperinnervated mutant mouse tottering. *Soc. Neurosci. Abstr.*, 10:672.

59. Lindvall, O., and Bjorklund, A. (1978): Organization of catecholamine neurons in the rat central nervous system. In: *Handbook of Psychopharmacology*, edited by L. L. Iversen, S. D. Iversen, and S. Snyder, pp. 139–231. Plenum Press, New York.

60. Lindvall, O., Bjorklund, A., Nobin, A., and Stenevi, U. (1974): The adrenergic innervation of the rat thalamus as revealed by the glyoxilic acid fluorescence method. *J. Comp. Neurol.*, 154:317–348.

61. Lucier, G. E., and Sessle, B. J. (1981): Presynaptic excitability changes induced in the solitary tract endings of laryngeal primary afferents by stimulation of nucleus raphe magnus and locus coeruleus. *Neurosci. Lett.*, 26:221–226.

62. Madison, D. V., and Nicoll, R. A. (1982): Noradrenaline blocks accommodation of pyramidal cell discharge in the hippocampus. *Nature.*, 299:636–638.

63. Mason, S. T., and Corcoran, M. E. (1979): Catecholamines and convulsions. *Brain Res.*, 170:497–507.

64. McGinnis, W., Hart, C. P., Gehring, W. J., and Ruddle, F. H. (1984): Molecular cloning and chromosome mapping of a mouse DNA sequence homologous to homeotic genes of *Drosophila*. *Cell*, 38:675–680.

65. McIntyre, D. C., and Edson, N. (1981): Facilitation of amygdala kindling after norepinephrine depletion with 6-hydroxydopamine in rats. *Exp. Neurol.*, 74:748–757.

66. McKusick, V. A. (1983): *Mendelian Inheritance in Man*. 6th ed. Johns Hopkins University Press, Baltimore.

67. Meier, H., and MacPike, A. D. (1971): Three syndromes produced by two mutant genes in the mouse. *J. Hered.*, 62:297–302.

68. Meynert, E. W., Marczynski, T. J., and Browning, R. A. (1975): The role of the neurotransmitters in the epilepsies. *Adv. Neurol.*, 13:79–147.

69. Miller, C. A., and Benzer, S. (1983): Monoclonal antibody cross-reactions between *Drosophila* and human brain. *Proc. Natl. Acad. Sci.*, 80:7641–7645.

70. Milner, R. J., Bloom, F. E., Lai, C., Lerner, R. A., and Sutcliffe, J. G. (1984): Brain specific genes have identifier sequences in their introns. *Proc. Natl. Acad. Sci. USA*, 81:713–717.

71. Mody, I., Leung, P., and Miller, J. J. (1982): Role of norepinephrine in seizurelike activity of hippocampal pyramidal cells maintained in vitro: Alteration by 6-hydroxydopamine lesions of norepinephrine-containing systems. *Can. J. Physiol. Pharmacol.*, 61:841–846.

72. Moore, R. Y., and Bloom, F. E. (1979): Central catecholamine neuron systems: Anatomy and physiology of the norepinephrine and epinephrine systems. *Annu. Rev. Neurosci.*, 2:113–168.

73. Morrison, J. H., Molliver, M. E., Grzanna, R., and Coyle, J. T. (1981): The intracortical trajectory of the coeruleo-cortical projection in the rat: A tangentially organized cortical afferent. *Neuroscience*, 6:139–158.

74. Mueller, A. L., and Dunwiddie, T. V. (1983): Anticonvulsant and proconvulsant actions of alpha- and beta-noradrenergic agonists on epileptiform activity in rat hippocampus in vitro. *Epilepsia*, 24:57–64.

75. Mueller, A. L., Hoffer, B. J., and Dunwiddie, T. V. (1981): Noradrenergic responses in rat hippocampus: Evidence for mediation by a and b receptors in the in vitro slice. *Brain Res.*, 214:113–126.

76. Muramoto, O., Ando, K., and Kanazawa, I. (1982): Central noradrenaline metabolism in cerebellar ataxic mice. *Brain Res.*, 237:387–395.

77. Muramoto, O., Kanazawa, I., and Audo, K. (1981): Neurotransmitter abnormality in rolling mouse Nagoya, an ataxic mutant mouse. *Brain Res.*, 215:295–304.

78. Nadeau, J. H., and Taylor, B. A. (1984): The lengths of chromosomal segments conserved since divergence of man and mouse. *Proc. Natl. Acad. Sci. USA*, 81:814–818.

79. Nagatsu, I., Kondo, Y., Inagaki, S., Oda, S., and Nagatsu, T. (1980): Dopamine β-hydroxylase and tyrosine hydroxylase activities in brain

regions of rolling mouse nagoya. *Biomed. Res. (Jpn)*, 1:88–90.

80. Natali, J. P., McRae-Deguerce, A., Keane, P., Debilly, G., and Pujol, J. F. (1980): Genetic studies of daily variations of first step enzymes of monoamine metabolism in the brain of inbred mice and hybrids. II. Daily variations of tyrosine hydroxylase activity in the locus coeruleus. *Brain Res.*, 191:205–213.

81. Nelson, M. F. Zaczek, R., and Coyle, J. T. (1980): Effects of sustained seizures produced by intrahippocampal injection of kainic acid on noradrenergic neurons: Evidence for local control of norepinephrine release. *J. Pharm. Exp. Ther.*, 214:694–702.

82. Nishimura, Y. (1975): The cerebellum of rolling mouse Nagoya. *Adv. Neurol. Sci. (Jpn)* 19:670–672.

83. Noebels, J. L. (1979): Analysis of inherited epilepsy using single locus mutations in mice. *Fed. Proc.*, 38:2405–2410.

84. Noebels, J. L. (1982): Defined gene models of the inherited epilepsies. In: *Genetic Basis of the Epilepsies*, edited by V. E. Anderson, W. A. Hauser, and C. F. Sing. pp. 211–223. Raven Press, New York.

85. Noebels, J. L. (1984): A single gene error of noradrenergic axon growth synchronizes central neurons. *Nature*, 310:409–411.

86. Noebels, J. L. (1984): Isolating single genes of the inherited epilepsies. *Ann. Neurol.* (Suppl.), 16:18–21.

87. Noebels, J. L., and Sidman, R. L. (1979): Inherited epilepsy: Spike-wave and focal motor seizures in the mutant mouse tottering. *Science*, 204:1334–1336.

88. Noebels, J. L., and Sidman, R. L. (1982): Three mutations causing spike-wave seizures in the mouse. *Neuroscience*, (Suppl.), 7:159–160.

89. O'Brien, J. S. (1977): Neuraminidase deficiency in the cherry red spot–myoclonus syndrome. *Biochem. Biophys. Res. Commun.*, 79:1136–1141.

90. Oda, S. (1981): A new allele of the tottering locus, rolling mouse Nagoya, on chromosome no. 8 in the mouse. *Jpn. J. Genet.*, 56:295–299.

91. Olpe, H. R., Glatt, A., Laszlo, J., and Schellenberg, A. (1980): Some electrophysiological and pharmacological properties of the cortical noradrenergic projection of the locus coeruleus in the rat. *Brain Res.*, 186:9–19.

92. Palacios, J. M., and Wamsley, J. K. (1983): Microscopic localization of adrenoreceptors. In: *Adrenoreceptors and Catecholamine Action*, part B, edited by G. Kunos. pp. 295–313. John Wiley, New York.

93. Pauling, L., Itano, H. A., Singer, S. J., et al. (1949): Sickle cell anemia, a molecular disease. *Science*, 110:543–548.

94. Prince, D. A., and Conners, B. W. (1984): Mechanisms of epileptogenesis in cortical structures. *Ann. Neurol.*, 16(Suppl):59–64.

95. Reader, T. A., Ferron, A., Descarries, L., and Jasper, H. H. (1979): Modulatory role of biogenic amines in the cerebral cortex. Microiontophoretic studies. *Brain Res.*, 160:217–229.

96. Reis, D., Ross, R. A., Gilad, G., and Joh, T. H. (1978): Reaction of central catecholaminergic neurons to injury: Model systems for studying the neurobiology of central regeneration and sprouting. In: *Neuronal Plasticity*, edited by C. Cotman, pp. 197–226. Raven Press, New York.

97. Reisine, T. (1981): Adaptive changes in catecholamine receptors in the central nervous system. *Neuroscience*, 6:1471–1502.

98. Reuter, H. (1983): Calcium channel modulation by neurotransmitters, enzymes and drugs. *Nature*, 301:569–574.

99. Roach, A., Boylan, K., Horvath, S., Prusiner, S. B. and Hood, L. E. (1983): Characterization of cloned cDNA representing rat myelin basic protein: Absence of expression in brain of shiverer mutant mice. *Cell*, 34:799–806.

100. Roffler-Tarlov, S., and Zigmond, M. J. (1980): Effects of purkinje cell degeneration on the noradrenergic projection to mouse cerebellar cortex. *Soc. Neurosci. Abstr.* 6:600.

101. Rogawski, M. A., and Agajhanian, G. K. (1980): Activation of lateral geniculate neurons by norepinephrine: Mediation by an α-adrenergic receptor. *Brain Res.*, 182:345–359.

102. Russell, W. L., Kelly, E. M., Hunsicker, J. W., Bangham, J. W., Maddux, S. C., and Phipps, E. L. (1979): Specific-locus test shows ethylnitrosourea to be the most potent mutagen in the mouse. *Proc. Natl. Acad. Sci. USA*, 76:5818–5819.

103. Sachs, Ch., Pycock, C., and Jönsson, G. (1974): Altered development of central noradrenaline neurons during ontogeny by 6-hydroxydopamine. *Med. Biol.*, 52:55–65.

104. Sasa, M., and Takaori, S. (1973): Influence of the locus coeruleus on transmission in the spinal trigeminal nucleus neurons. *Brain Res.*, 55:203–208.

105. Sato, H., and Kayama, Y. (1983): Effects of noradrenaline applied iontophoretically on rat superior collicular neurons. *Brain Res. Bull.*, 10:453–457.

106. Segal, M. (1981): The action of norepinephrine in the rat hippocampus: Intracellular studies in the slice preparation. *Brain Res.*, 206:107–128.

107. Segal, M. (1982): Norepinephrine modulates reactivity of hippocampal cells to chemical stimulation in vitro. *Exp. Neurol.*, 77:86–93.

108. Seyfried, T. N., Itoh, T., Glaser, G. H., Miyazawa, N., and Yu, R. K. (1981): Cerebellar gangliosides and phospholipids in mutant mice with ataxia and epilepsy: The tottering leaner syndrome. *Brain Res.*, 216:429–436.

109. Sidman, R. L. (1983): Experimental neurogenetics. In: *Genetics of Neurological and Psychiatric Disorders*. edited by S. S. Kety, L. P. Roland, R. L. Sidman, and S. W. Matthysse, pp. 19–46. Raven Press, New York.

110. Sidman, R. L., Green, M. C., and Appel, S. H. (1965): *Catalog of the Neurological Mutants of the Mouse*. Harvard University Press, Cambridge, Massachusetts.

111. Siegelbaum, S., Camardo, J., and Kandel, E. R. (1982): Serotonin and cyclic AMP close single

K⁺ channels in aplysia sensory neurons. *Nature*, 299:413–417.

112. Sievers, H., Sievers, J., Baumgarten, H., Konig, N., and Schlossberger, H. G. (1983): Distribution of tritium label in the neonatal rat brain following intracisternal or subcutaneous administration of ³H 6-OHDA. An autoradiographic study. *Brain Res.*, 275:23–45.

113. Steindler, D. A. (1981): Locus coeruleus neurons have axons that branch to the forebrain and cerebellum. *Brain Res.*, 223:367–373.

114. Sutcliffe, J. G., Milner, R. J., and Bloom, F. E. (1983): Cellular localization and function of the proteins encoded by brain-specific mRNAs. *Cold Spring Harbor Laboratory Symposia on Quantitative Biology*, 48:477–484.

115. Sutin, J. and Minneman, K. P. (1984): Adrenergic receptor regulation in hyperinnervated neurons. *Soc. Neurosci. Abstr.* 10:236.

116. Szabadi, E. (1979): Adrenoceptors on central neurons: Microelectrophoretic studies. *Neuropharmacology*, 18:831–843.

117. Tillement, J. P., Debarl, M. C., Simon, P., and Boissier, J. R. (1971): Taux d'amines cerebrales d'une souche de souris "tremblentes." *Experientia*, 27:269.

118. Touret, M., Valatx, J. L., and Jouvet, M. (1982): The locus coeruleus: A quantitative and genetic study in mice. *Brain Res.*, 250:353–357.

119. Trimmer, P. A., Evans, T., Smith, M. M., Harden, T. K., and McCarthy, K. D. (1984): Combination of immunocytochemistry and radioligand receptor assay to identify beta adrenergic receptor subtypes on astroglia in vitro. *J. Neurosci.*, 4:1598.

120. Tsuji, S., and Meier, H. (1971): Evidence for allelism of leaner and tottering in the mouse. *Genet. Res.*, 17:83–88.

121. Unnerstall, J. R., Kopajtic, T. A., and Kuhar, M. J. (1984): Distribution of α_2 agonist binding sites in the rat and human central nervous system. *Brain Res. Rev.*, 7:69–101.

122. U'Prichard, D. C., Reisine, T. D., Mason, S. T., Fibiger, H. C., and Yamamura, H. I. (1980): Modulation of rat brain alpha- and beta-adrenergic receptor populations by lesion of the dorsal noradrenergic bundle. *Brain Res.*, 187:143–154.

123. VanderMaelen, C. P., and Agajhanian, G. K. (1980): Intracellular studies showing modulation of facial motoneurone excitability by serotonin. *Nature*, 287:346–347.

124. Van Dongen, P. (1981): The central noradrenergic transmission and the locus coeruleus: A review of the data, and their implications for neurotransmission and neuromodulation. *Prog. Neurobiol.*, 16:117–143.

125. Van Ness, J., Maxwell, I. H., and Hahn, W. E. (1979): Complex populations of nonpolyadenylated messenger RNA in mouse brain. *Cell*, 18:1341–1349.

126. Videen, T. O., Daw, N. W., and Rader, R. K. (1984): The effect of norepinephrine on visual cortical neurons in kittens and adult cats. *J. Neurosci.*, 4:1607–1617.

127. Waller, S. B., Ingram, D. K., Reynolds, M. A., and London, E. D. (1983): Age and strain comparisons of neurotransmitter synthetic enzyme activities in the mouse. *J. Neurochem.*, 41:1421–1428.

128. Waterhouse, B., Moises, H. C., and Woodward, D. (1980): Noradrenergic modulation of somatosensory cortical neuronal responses to iontophoretically applied putative neurotransmitters. *Exp. Neurol.*, 69:30–49.

129. Westfall, T. C. (1977): Local regulation of adrenergic neurotransmission. *Physiol. Rev.*, 57:659–729.

130. White, R. (1984): Looking for epilepsy genes. *Ann. Neurol. (Suppl.)*, 16:12–17.

131. White, S. R., and Neuman, R. S. (1980): Facilitation of spinal motoneurone excitability by 5-hydroxytryptamine and noradrenaline. *Brain Res.*, 188:119–127.

132. Wuenschell, C. W., Wandres, D. L., and Tobin, A. J. (1984): Localization of brain specific mRNAs in mouse cerebellum by in situ hybridization. *Soc. Neurosci. Abstr.*, 10:361.

133. Yeh, H. H., and Woodward, D. J. (1983): Beta-1 adrenergic receptors mediate noradrenergic facilitation of purkinje cell responses to gamma-aminobutyric acid in cerebellum of rat. *Neuropharmacology*, 22:629–639.

134. Yerkes, R. M. (1907): *The Dancing Mouse.* The Animal Behavior Series, No. 1. Macmillan Co., New York

Advances in Neurology, Vol. 44, edited by
A. V. Delgado-Escueta, A. A. Ward, Jr.,
D. M. Woodbury, and R. J. Porter.
Raven Press, New York © 1986.

5

Inherited Convulsive Disorders in Mice

*Thomas N. Seyfried, **Gilbert H. Glaser, **Robert K. Yu, and
**Sanjeewani T. Palayoor

*Department of Biology, Boston College, Chestnut Hill, Massachusetts 02617; and **Department of
Neurology, Yale University School of Medicine, New Haven, Connecticut 06510

SUMMARY   In this chapter, we review the major inherited convulsive disorders found in mice and discuss their possible relationship to specific clinical seizure disorders in humans. These disorders in mice include audiogenic seizures, the epilepsy (*El*) mouse, various spontaneous seizures, the tottering/leaner syndrome, seizures associated with cerebellar abnormalities, seizures associated with myelin disorders, and alcohol withdrawal seizures. We find that for most major types of epilepsy in humans, there exists a similar counterpart in the mouse. Because human and rodent nervous systems respond similarly to seizure-provoking stimuli, it is possible that biochemical and physiological mechanisms of naturally occurring convulsive disorders are also similar in these species. The use of recombinant inbred (RI) and congenic mouse strains for genetic and biochemical studies of audiogenic seizures is presented. Using these strains, we have identified a major gene, *Ias*, that inhibits the spread of seizure activity. This gene was found through its close linkage with the *Ah* locus on chromosome 17. We also found that juvenile-onset and adult-onset audiogenic seizures are controlled by different genetic systems. The problem of juvenile-onset audiogenic seizure susceptibility is especially interesting because these seizures are genetically associated with an ecto-Ca^{2+}-ATPase deficiency among the RI strains. This deficiency is the first neurochemical trait found to be inherited together with an idiopathic convulsive disorder, and may represent a potentially important basic mechanism of epilepsy. Because the brains of human epileptics are generally inaccessible for neurochemical research, the epileptic mouse mutants offer a convenient means of pursuing this type of research. The well-known genetic constitution of the mouse, together with the availability of numerous physiologically distinct convulsive disorders, makes the mouse ideally suited for molecular, genetic, and biochemical studies of convulsive behavior.

Convulsive disorders or the epilepsies represent a significant health problem in humans. With the exception of stroke, epilepsy is the most prevalent human neurological disorder. Anderson (2) estimates that the expectancy at birth of developing epilepsy by age 55 is 2%. All epilepsies can be classified into two broad etiological categories, i.e., acquired or symptomatic epilepsy and idiopathic or cryptogenic epilepsy. The acquired or symptomatic epilepsies can generally be attributable to some type of structural, metabolic, or organic brain lesion such as trauma, viral infection, tumor, or specific inherited disorder. The so-called idiopathic epilepsies, on the other hand, are not usually associated with an organic brain lesion. Although a number of "idiopathic" epilepsies are thought to be inherited, little is known about the genetic or biochemical mechanisms involved.

The inaccessibility of human epileptic brain tissue has hindered progress in understanding these mechanisms. Because human and rodent nervous systems respond similarly to seizure-provoking stimuli (57), it is possible that biochemical and physiological mechanisms of naturally occurring convulsive disorders are also similar in these species. Hence, the availability of several genetically and physiologically distinct forms of convulsive disorders in mice offers a convenient means of exploring these mechanisms. Our purpose is to review the major inherited convulsive disorders found in mice, and to discuss their possible relationship to specific clinical seizure disorders in humans. Because more is known about audiogenic seizures, we give more coverage of this convulsive disorder.

AUDIOGENIC SEIZURES

Audiogenic seizures (AGS) are clonic-tonic convulsions that occur in response to intense auditory stimulation. There are two types of AGS susceptibility in mice: (a) susceptibility that occurs spontaneously as an inherited trait; and (b) susceptibility that is acquired through a variety of physical and biochemical manipulations. The acquired types of AGS are discussed in a recent review (98). Spontaneous AGS can be classified as a form of inherited idiopathic epilepsy, since no organic brain disease is associated with these seizures. In the absence of sound stimulation, the behavior of mice with inherited AGS susceptibility is generally indistinguishable from the behavior of nonsusceptible mice.

The AGS consists of a progressive sequence of phases. There is usually a short latency period from the initiation of sound stimulation to the onset of an explosive burst of wild, frenzied running. The duration of this latency period is strain- and age-dependent. The wild running phase progresses into a clonic seizure as the mouse falls over on its side and displays violent kicking movements. The tonic seizure phase begins as the forelegs and then the hindlegs become rigidly extended to the rear (Fig. 1). During this phase, the pinnae are usually pressed down against the head. Respiratory arrest, signaled by a relaxation of the pinnae, can sometimes be a consequence of these seizures. If the mouse is not resuscitated, it will usually die. The AGS may not always progress through all of the phases. In some mice, the AGS may progress only as far as the wild running or clonic seizure phase. For statistical analyses, a mouse can be given a numerical score based on the severity of its response to the sound, e.g., no response = 0; wild running = 1; and clonic or

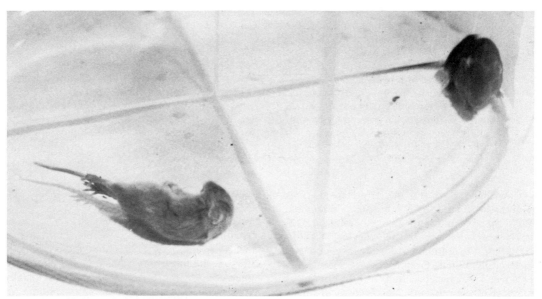

FIG. 1. Response to sound (120 db at 12.5 KHz) in 21-day-old B6 (*right*) and D2 (*left*) mice. The D2 mouse is experiencing a generalized tonic seizure.

tonic seizure = 2. In this way, the mean severity of seizure can be quantitated for a group of mice. The percentage of mice responding to each phase of the AGS can also be used as a means of quantitating seizure severity. Collins (14) and Schreiber et al. (96) present a detailed description of these and other phases of AGS in mice.

Developmental Profile

The ontogeny of inherited AGS susceptibility is strongly dependent on genetic background (14,94,98). In the prototype DBA/2 (D2) mice, AGS susceptibility is greatest at juvenile ages (16–30 days), and then gradually dissipates with age (Fig. 2). Mice of the C57BL/6 (B6) strain are mostly resistant to AGS at all ages, and the B6D2F1 hybrids are more susceptible at 30 days than at 21 days (Fig. 2). Several investigators found similar developmental profiles of susceptibility in the B6 and D2 mice (93,96,126). Other mouse strains, however, are more susceptible at older ages than at younger ages, and there are some strains that are susceptible at both young and adult ages (96,99,105).

Genetic Studies

Although the difference in AGS susceptibility between the B6 and D2 strains has been recognized since 1947 (39), the mode of inheritance of this susceptibility is still unclear. Genetic models supporting a single autosomal dominant gene with minor modifying factors (133), a single autosomal recessive gene, *asp*, loosely linked to the *b* locus on chromosome 4 (13,15), two unlinked autosomal loci with variable degrees of penetrance (32), and multiple genetic factors (27,28,92) have been proposed to explain the difference in AGS susceptibility between the C57 and DBA strains. Similar controversy exists for the inheritance of AGS susceptibility between sublines of mice selected for resistance or susceptibility to AGS. Lehman and Bosinger (59) suggested that the action of a dominant gene for resistance to AGS was responsible for the difference in AGS susceptibility between their selected lines, whereas Frings et al. (25) and Chen and Fuller (11) suggested that more than one gene was responsible for the difference between their selected lines.

The change in expression of AGS susceptibility with age has certainly contributed to the controversy surrounding the inheritance of these seizures. It is easy to see from Fig. 2 how the difference in AGS susceptibility between the B6 and D2 strains may simulate recessive inheritance at 21 days (since the AGS of the B6D2F1 hybrids is more similar to that of the B6 parent than that of D2 parent), but simulate dominant or multiple-factor inheritance around 30 days (since the AGS susceptibility of the B6D2F1 hy-

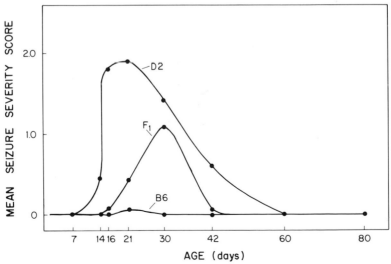

FIG. 2. Developmental profile of audiogenic seizure susceptibility in the B6 and D2 inbred strains and their F₁ hybrids. The mean seizure severity scores and number of mice tested at each age were determined as described previously in Seyfried, ref. 97, where this illustration appeared originally.

brids is somewhat intermediate or more similar to that of the D2 parent than that of the B6 parent). In addition to age, the phenomenon of acoustic priming may also complicate genetic studies of AGS susceptibility. This involves the transformation of a normally AGS-resistant mouse into an AGS-susceptible mouse by prior auditory stimulation (30,45,52,94). It is possible, therefore, that this phenomenon may have influenced the results from some of the earlier genetic studies in which susceptibility or resistance to AGS was determined after a mouse was tested daily over a period of days.

Genetic Analysis of Audiogenic Seizures in Recombinant Inbred Strains

We recently used recombinant inbred (RI) strains to understand the inheritance of AGS susceptibility better. Taylor (121) produced these strains by inbreeding the F2 generation derived from the B6 and D2 progenitor strains (Fig. 3). They are therefore designated BXD RI strains. RI strains are useful for studies of genetic determination, i.e., the number of genes controlling a trait, and for linkage analysis. If the difference in AGS susceptibility between the B6 and D2 strains is caused by the effects of a single pair of alleles, only two phenotypic classes, B6-like or D2-like, will be found among the RI strains. If more than one locus is responsible for the difference, however, the processes of reassortment and gene fixation through in-

breeding will generate new phenotypic classes among the RI stains. Moreover, since Taylor has already determined the inheritance of over 100 marker loci in the BXD RI strains (B. A. Taylor, *personal communication,* 1984), evidence of linkage or pleiotropy can be determined by observing an association between AGS susceptibility and a marker gene. Thus, the RI strains are a powerful analytical tool for studying the genetics of complex phenotypic traits (4).

The mean seizure severity scores of the B6 and D2 progenitor strains and the BXD RI strains are shown in Fig. 4. These scores were determined on 21-day-old mice as described previously (105,107). It is apparent that a dichotomy or bimodal distribution of seizure severity scores does not exist among the RI strains. Instead, a somewhat continuous distribution of scores is found. These findings indicate that the difference in AGS susceptibility between the B6 and D2 mice cannot be caused only by the action of alleles at a single locus. In addition to more than one gene, AGS susceptibility can also be influenced by intangible environmental factors. We previously discussed these concepts in detail (105).

Linkage Between the Ah Locus and a Major Gene That Inhibits Audiogenic Seizures

Although AGS susceptibility is not controlled by a single locus, an association was found between AGS and the *Ah* locus (105,107). The *Ah*

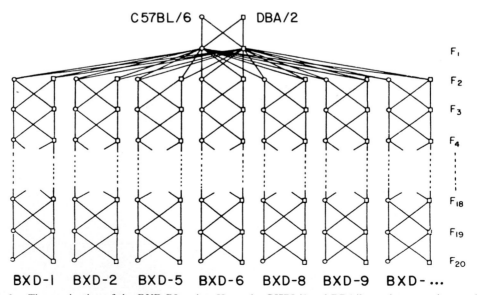

FIG. 3. The production of the BXD RI series. Here, the C57BL/6 and DBA/2 are the progenitor strains for the BXD series. Females (*circles*); males, (*squares*); genetic pathways (*line segments*). Modification of diagram from Bailey, ref. 4, with permission.

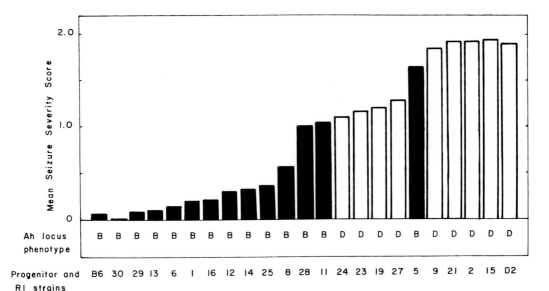

FIG. 4. Mean AGS severity scores and *Ah* locus phenotypes of the B6 and D2 progeniter strains and 21 BXD RI strains. The number of animals tested for each strain is given in Seyfried and Glaser, ref. 107, where this illustration appeared originally.

locus controls the induction of aryl hydrocarbon hydroxylase (AHH) activity by a number of aromatic hydrocarbons (73). B6 mice carry the Ah^b allele and have highly inducible AHH activity (designated as the B phenotype, Fig. 4); whereas D2 mice carry the Ah^d allele and have noninducible activity (designated as the D phenotype). The Ah^b allele is inherited as a Mendelian dominant in crosses between the B6 and D2 strains (73). The *Ah* locus was mapped recently to the distal portion of chromosome 17 (58a).

Most BXD RI strains with the B phenotype have lower seizure scores than do strains with the D phenotype (Fig. 4). The presence of one strain (BXD-5) that is clearly discordant for the association between the *Ah* locus and AGS susceptibility indicates that the association results from linkage rather than from a pleiotropic effect of the *Ah* locus on AGS susceptibility (4). In other words, the *Ah* locus is linked to a major gene influencing AGS susceptibility.

Further evidence of this linkage was obtained from the analysis of AGS susceptibility in B6 and D2 mice made congenic for the *Ah* locus. By backcrossing and selecting for the *Ah* locus, Nebert (73) transferred the Ah^b allele from the B6 strain to the D2 strain and transferred the Ah^d allele from the D2 strain to the B6 strain. Except for the *Ah* locus and a small amount of chromosomal material flanking this locus, the

genome of the D2.B6-Ah^b mice is similar to that of the D2 strain, and the genome of the B6.D2-Ah^b mice is similar to that of the B6 strain. If a gene influencing AGS susceptibility is closely linked to the *Ah* locus, it will "hitchhike" along with the *Ah* locus during each selective transfer.

The analysis of AGS susceptibility in the congenic strains is shown in Fig. 5. When the Ah^b allele was transferred from the B6 strain to the D2 strain, it caused a highly significant reduction in AGS susceptibility (D2N versus D2N-Ah^b, Fig. 5). An association between the Ah^b allele and reduced AGS susceptibility is also observed in the B6D2F1 × D2 backcross generation (Fig. 5) and in a survey of various inbred strains, for which information is available from the literature on both *Ah* locus phenotypes and AGS susceptibility (107). Thus, a gene closely linked to the *Ah* locus inhibits AGS susceptibility in 21-day-old mice. We have named this gene *Ias*, for inhibition of AGS. The alleles at this locus coming from the B6 and D2 stains are tentatively designated Ias^b and Ias^d, respectively. It is important to mention that *Ias* does not completely abolish AGS susceptibility, since many of the D2-Ah^b mice experience wild running (Fig. 5) (107). This wild running, however, rarely progresses into a clonic or tonic seizure. Thus, the Ias^b allele appears to inhibit the spread of seizure activity.

The transfer of the Ah^d allele into B6 genome,

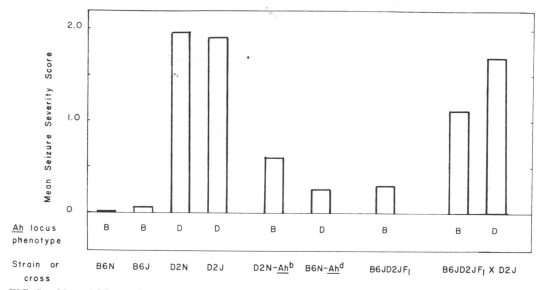

FIG. 5. Mean AGS severity scores and *Ah* locus phenotypes of inbred, congenic, hybrid, and backcross mice. The number of mice tested for each group is given in Seyfried and Glaser, ref. 107, where this illustration appeared originally.

or the removal of the *Ah*ᵇ allele, did not significantly enhance AGS susceptibility, since the B6N and B6N-*Ah*ᵈ mice had similar AGS susceptibilities (Fig. 5). This finding indicates that more than one gene inhibits AGS susceptibility in these mice and supports further the notion that the difference in AGS susceptibility between 21-day-old B6 and D2 mice cannot be under the control of a single locus.

Genetic Heterogeneity for the Development of Audiogenic Seizures

Genetic heterogeneity refers to a situation in which very similar clinical syndromes are produced by a number of distinctly different gene mutations (41). These gene defects may be either multiple alleles of a single locus or multiple loci. Alternatively, very different clinical syndromes can be produced from different mutant alleles at a single locus. The influence of genetic background and environment can be further causes of heterogeneity (41). The problem of heterogeneity has certainly hindered progress in understanding the genetic mechanisms responsible for idiopathic epilepsies in humans (2,19). Those idiopathic epilepsies with variable age of onset may be especially influenced by genetic heterogeneity. In this volume, V. E. Anderson addresses further aspects of heterogeneity in the epilepsies (see Chapter 2).

Although the B6 and D2 strains are not AGS-susceptible as adults, several of the BXD RI strains have a high incidence of AGS susceptibility as adults (105). Unlike AGS susceptibility at juvenile ages, no association is found between AGS susceptibility at adult ages and the expression of the *Ah* locus. Because the *Ias* and *Ah* loci are linked, it appears that *Ias* does not influence AGS susceptibility at adult ages. This situation is not unlike that found for the inheritance of diabetes mellitus in humans, in which an increased frequency of certain HLA antigens is associated only with the juvenile form, not the adult form of the disorder (87,110).

The developmental profile of AGS susceptibility in the BXD-15 RI strain is most interesting because these mice are susceptible at both young and adult ages (Fig. 6). It is difficult to imagine how a single genetic mechanism controlling seizure susceptibility might be turned on, turned off, and then turned on again at different ages. Rather, it is easier to envision two different genetic mechanisms, one controlling juvenile-onset AGS susceptibility, and the other controlling adult-onset susceptibility. Evidence for two genetic systems is supported by the results from breeding experiments.

Susceptibility to AGS is inherited as a recessive trait in the 21-day-old D2 and BXD-15 mice, since both the B6D2F1 and B6BXD-15F1 hybrids are mostly AGS-resistant at this age (Table

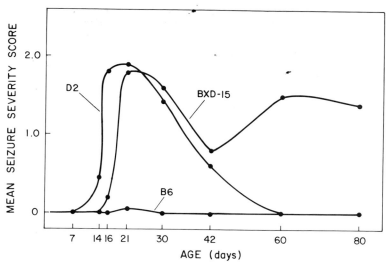

FIG. 6. Developmental profiles of audiogenic seizure susceptibility in the B6, D2, and BXD-15 inbred strains of mice. The mean seizure severity scores for the B6 and D2 strains were the same as described previously in Seyfried, ref. 97. The mean scores at each age for the BXD-15 mice were given in (99), where this illustration appeared originally.

1). This results in part from the dominantly expressed *Ias*[b] allele carried by the B6 mice. The high AGS susceptibility of the D2BXD-15F1 hybrids indicates that the genetic mechanism responsible for AGS susceptibility in the D2 and BXD-15 mice is similar at 21 days.

The inheritance of AGS susceptibility in these same crosses at adult ages is different from that at 21 days. As adults, the B6BXD-15F1 hybrids become partially susceptible, whereas the D2BXD-15F1 hybrids become completely resis-

TABLE 1. *Genetic analysis of audiogenic seizure susceptibility in juvenile (21 ± 1 days) and adult (60–80 days) mice*

Strain or cross	Percentage of seizures at 21 ± 1 days[a]		Percentage of seizures at 60–80 days	
	No. tested	Seizure (%)	No. tested	Seizure (%)
B6	55	1.8	18	0.0
D2	35	91.4	18	0.0
BXD-15	45	82.2	26	66.6
B6D2F₁	60	3.3	18	0.0
B6BXD-15F₁	18	0.0	25	24.0
D2BXD-15F₁	15	100.0	23	0.0

[a] Seizures include both clonic and tonic [from Seyfried, ref. 99, with permission].

tant to AGS (Table 1). D2 mice appear to carry a dominant gene, different from *Ias*[b], which inhibits AGS susceptibility at adult ages. The partial AGS susceptibility of the adult B6BXD-15F1 hybrids suggests that the B6 mice may share certain seizure genes with the BXD-15 mice or that an allele causing seizures in BXD-15 mice is partially dominant to the allele present in the B6 mice. When these findings are viewed together with the developmental profile of AGS susceptibility in the BXD-15 mice, they strongly suggest that juvenile-onset and adult-onset AGS susceptibility are controlled by different genetic mechanisms. Hence, the subtle differences between juvenile and adult BXD-15 mice for the latency period to seizure onset, for the type of seizures, and for the incidence of seizures in males and females (99), appear to be caused by the expression of different seizure-producing genes rather than by an age-related modification of a single genetic mechanism.

The extent of genetic heterogeneity for AGS susceptibility in mice is not known. The present findings indicate that genetic heterogeneity exists for the development of AGS susceptibility in the BXD-15 strain. Because this strain was derived from inbreeding the F2 generation of the B6 and D2 strains, it has obviously inherited a new gene combination, not present in either progenitor strain, affecting AGS susceptibility at adult ages. This suggests that both the B6 and

D2 strains contain genes that, when rearranged in a specific way, can enhance AGS susceptibility at adult ages. The partial AGS susceptibility of the B6BXD-15F1 hybrids supports this notion. Awareness of genetic heterogeneity for AGS susceptibility may facilitate an understanding of the biochemical defect underlying these seizures. It is likely that juvenile-onset and adult-onset AGS susceptibility in BXD-15 mice involve different physiological factors.

Although direct evidence of genetic heterogeneity for the development of a human idiopathic epilepsy has not yet been obtained, it is likely that such situations exist. In other words, phenotypically similar convulsive disorders may have different etiologies at young and adult ages. This situation may exist for the photoconvulsive reaction in humans. The photoconvulsive reaction involves the induction of electroencephalographic (EEG) abnormalities (with or without clinical manifestations) by stimulation with intermittent light (21). The developmental profile of photosensitivity appears biphasic, with girls more frequently affected than boys. Furthermore, the phenotype of the EEG abnormalities is noticeably different in children than in adolescents and adults (21). It is therefore possible that the childhood and adolescent-adult forms of the photoconvulsive response are caused by different genetic mechanisms.

Biochemical Studies

A necessary step for elucidating the biochemistry and physiology of AGS susceptibility is the establishment of correlations or associations between AGS and specific biochemical or physiological traits. Although numerous biochemical and physiological differences occur between 21-day-old AGS-resistant and AGS-susceptible mouse strains (98), it had not been determined whether these differences were genetically associated with AGS susceptibility or whether they were simply strain differences unrelated to AGS susceptibility. Although it may be possible to show that B6 and D2 mice differ significantly for a particular trait and that the experimental manipulation of the trait can reverse the AGS susceptibilities of these mice, this is not evidence that the trait is genetically associated with AGS susceptibility. A genetic association can be established between two traits by showing that both traits are inherited together. However, this may be difficult using mice from classical Mendelian crosses because AGS susceptibility is influenced by more than one gene and environ-

mental factors. Because the Ias^b allele can be studied in a homogenous D2 genetic background, any differences found between the D2 and the D2.B6-Ias^b mice should result from the effects of Ias^b or a closely linked gene. Consequently, the D2.B6-Ias^b congenic mice together with the BXD-RI strains offer a new and powerful system for testing associations between AGS susceptibility and specific biochemical or physiological traits.

Thyroid Hormone and Audiogenic Seizures

We found that serum T4 concentrations peak earlier and are significantly higher in D2 mice than in B6 mice during early postnatal life (103). Furthermore, the administration of 6-n-propylthiouracil (PTU) or radiothyroidectomy with ^{131}I suppressed AGS susceptibility in D2 mice, whereas treatment with excess T4 during early postnatal life (5–8 days) enhanced AGS susceptibility in 18 ± 1-day-old B6 mice (103). In a follow-up study, we found that T4 replacement from postnatal day 1 through day 17 could restore the AGS susceptibility of D2 mice made hypothyroid by PTU treatment from 3 days before birth until the time of AGS testing (19 days after birth) (106). These findings, together with those reported by Henry et al. (46), indicate that T4 can influence AGS susceptibility during early postnatal life, and that T4 is important for the development of AGS susceptibility in D2 mice.

In order to determine whether differences in neonatal thyroid hormone content were directly responsible for AGS susceptibility, we used the congenic and BXD RI strains. No significant correlations were found, however, between serum T4 content at 14 days of age and AGS susceptibility at 21 days of age (108). Although the experimental manipulation of thyroid hormone content can significantly influence AGS susceptibility in the B6 and D2 mice, it is unlikely that inherited differences in neonatal serum T4 content are directly responsible for differences in AGS susceptibility in 21-day-old mice. We (108) and Henry et al. (46) previously discussed the mechanisms by which thyroid hormone may influence AGS susceptibility. These studies illustrate the utility of the RI and congenic strains for testing possible mechanisms that may underlie AGS susceptibility.

Although more than one gene controls resistance to AGS in 21-day-old B6 mice, there are a variety of physical and biochemical factors that can enhance AGS susceptibility in B6 mice by overriding these inhibitory genes. In addition to the influence of T4, such factors include: the acoustic priming phenomenon (30,45,52); damage to the auditory system by a number of physical and chemical insults (12,76,78); withdrawal from drugs and alcohol (23,31); and the effects of single-locus mutations (98). It has not yet been determined whether each of these factors enhances AGS susceptibility through similar physiological mechanisms.

Mg^{2+} and Na^+,K^+-ATPase Activities and Audiogenic Seizures

Because abnormalities of cation transport in the brain have long been considered a potential cause of convulsive disorders (18,123), we used the RI and congenic strains to determine if AGS susceptibility was inherited together with changes in various cationic ATPase activities. Although the total and Mg^{2+}-ATPase activities of brainstem are significantly lower in 21-day-old D2 than B6 mice, these deficiencies are not genetically associated with differences in AGS (82). No significant associations were found between the strain-distribution patterns for these ATPase activities and AGS susceptibility among 13 BXD RI strains. Hence, differences in genetic background, rather than differences in AGS susceptibility, are probably responsible for the lower total and Mg^{2+}-ATPase activities in D2 mice.

We also found that the total Mg^{2+}, and Na^+,K^+-ATPase activities in the B6 brainstem did not change noticeably from 21 to 80 days of age (82). In the D2 brainstem, however, the Mg^{2+}-ATPase activity increased with age, and the Na^+,K^+-ATPase activity decreased from 30 to 80 days of age. Hence, the reduced total ATPase in 21-day-old D2 mice reflects a reduction in Mg^{2+}-ATPase activity, but the reduced total ATPase in 80-day-old D2 mice reflects a reduction in Na^+,K^+-ATPase activity (82).

The Na^+,K^+-ATPase activity in fresh brainstem homogenates is similar in 21-day-old B6 and D2 mice (82). These findings agree with those of Reichert (85) and Rosenblatt et al. (86), but disagree with those of Fromby (26), who reported lower activities in the D2 brain. The reason for this discrepancy is not clear. Nevertheless, the bulk of the evidence suggests that this enzyme is not involved with juvenile-onset AGS susceptibility.

Although little is known about the genetic control of Na^+,K^+-ATPase activity in brain, our findings indicate that more than one gene controls this activity. A significantly elevated activity in the B6D2F1 hybrids and the existence of BXD RI strains with Na^+,K^+-ATPase activities different from the B6 or D2 activities were found (82). Based on the "one gene—one enzyme" hypothesis (7,120), our findings support the evidence of two functional Na^+,K^+-ATPases in brain (91,116).

Genetic Association Between Ca^{2+}-ATPase Activity and Audiogenic Seizures

Calcium is known to play an important role in neuronal excitability and synaptic transmission (9,55,56,62). Because the influence of calcium on neuronal excitability is thought to be regulated in part by various Ca^{2+}-ATPase activities (9,38,61,112), a deficiency of Ca^{2+}-ATPase activity could cause defective synaptic transmission. Rosenblatt et al. (86) found a deficiency of Ca^{2+}-ATPase activity in the brains of D2 mice as compared with B6 and C3H mice. They did not, however, determine whether this deficiency was genetically associated with AGS susceptibility, or whether it was simply a strain difference unrelated to AGS susceptibility. Our findings with BXD RI strains show that a deficiency in brainstem Ca^{2+}-ATPase activity is genetically associated with AGS susceptibility.

We found a highly significant negative correlation ($r = -0.6624$) between Ca^{2+}-ATPase activity and seizure severity in the B6 and D2 progenitor strains and in 21 BXD RI strains ($p < 0.001$; $t = 4.05$ for 21 df) (83). In general, strains with mean Ca^{2+}-ATPase activities <2.40 are more AGS susceptible than strains with activities >2.40 (Fig. 7). Moreover, low Ca^{2+}-ATPase activity and high AGS susceptibility are inherited together in F1 hybrids produced from crosses between the D2, BXD-12, and BXD-28 strains (83). The BXD-12 and BXD-28 strains were used for these crosses because they have high Ca^{2+}-ATPase activities (Fig. 7), and prior breeding studies showed that neither strain carried the dominantly expressed Ias^b allele. Hence, the low AGS susceptibility in these mice may result largely from high Ca^{2+}-ATPase activity.

The Ca^{2+}-ATPase deficiency is the first neurochemical trait found to be inherited together with an idiopathic convulsive disorder. A deficiency in Ca^{2+}-ATPase activity may, therefore, be one of the underlying defects responsible for AGS susceptibility in mice.

The existence of a few discordant strains, e.g., BXD-1, BXD-14, and BXD-15 (Fig. 7) was not unexpected, because AGS susceptibility in

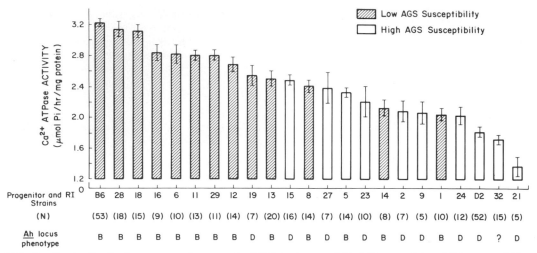

FIG. 7.   Strain distribution patterns for mean ($\pm$ SEM) brainstem Ca^{2+} ATPase activity, AGS susceptibility, and the *Ah* locus among the B6 and D2 progenitor strains and 21 BXD RI strains at 21 $\pm$ 2 days of age. The number of samples (N) analyzed for Ca^{2+}-ATPase activities is shown in parentheses below each strain. One brainstem was analyzed for each sample. The strains are arranged according to Ca^{2+}-ATPase activities. Strains with mean seizure severity scores >1.05 were classified as having high AGS susceptibility, whereas strains with mean seizure severity scores <1.05 were classified as having low AGS susceptibility. The mean seizure severity score for each strain was computed on a 0–2 scale (where 0 = no response, 1 = wild running; 2 = clonic or tonic seizure) from data presented previously by Seyfried et al., refs. 105 and 107. The *Ah* locus phenotypes were also determined previously by Wood and Taylor, ref. 134. Strains carrying the Ah^b allele are designated "B" and strains carrying the Ah^d allele are designated "D". From Palayoor and Seyfried, ref. 83, with permission.

21 day-old mice is influenced by more than one gene. Breeding studies showed that resistance to AGS in the BXD-1 strain was caused by the Ias^b allele; the Ias^b allele can inhibit AGS susceptibility even in the presence of low Ca^{2+}-ATPase activity. This notion is supported further from the finding of low Ca^{2+}-ATPase activities in the D2.B6-Ias^b congenic mice (Fig. 8). It appears that most of the difference in Ca^{2+}-ATPase activity between the B6 and D2 strains is not caused by the expression of Ias^b. If it were, the Ca^{2+}-ATPase activity in the D2.B6-Ias^b mice would be high, as is the activity in B6 mice. Although the difference in Ca^{2+}-ATPase activity between the D2 and D2.B6-Ias^b mice is slight, it is nevertheless significant (Fig. 8). Hence, Ias^b or a closely linked gene may exert a minor influence on Ca^{2+}-ATPase activity.

Our results also indicate that the difference in Ca^{2+}-ATPase activity between 21-day-old B6 and D2 mice cannot be under the control of a single locus, since we found a continuous, rather than biomodal, distribution of mean Ca^{2+}-ATPase activities among the BXD RI strains (Fig. 7). Nevertheless, an association was observed between Ca^{2+}-ATPase activity and the

Ah locus. In general, Ca^{2+}-ATPase activities were higher in strains with the *Ah* "B" phenotype than with the "D" phenotype (Fig. 7). The combined mean $\pm$ SEM Ca^{2+}-ATPase activity for the 12 BXD RI strains carrying the Ah^b allele (B phenotype, Fig. 7) was 2.63 $\pm$ 0.10, whereas the combined mean Ca^{2+}-ATPase activity for the 8 BXD RI strains carrying the Ah^d allele (D phenotype) was 2.14 $\pm$ 0.13. The difference between these means was significant ($p < 0.01$; as determined by the two-tailed t test).

The existence of two strains (BXD-1 and BXD-14) that were clearly discordant with the general association between Ca^{2+}-ATPase activity and *Ah* locus phenotype (Fig. 7) suggests that the association is not due to a direct pleiotropic effect of the *Ah* locus on Ca^{2+}-ATPase activity (4). It is possible that genetic information linked to the *Ah* locus or epistatic interactions between the *Ah* and another locus influences Ca^{2+}-ATPase activity in the brain. We propose as the simplest hypothesis a major gene that we designate *Caa*, for Ca^{2+}-ATPase activity. Because the *Ah* locus resides on the distal half of chromosome 17 (58a), it is possible that *Caa* also resides here.

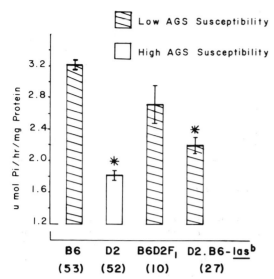

FIG. 8. Mean ($\pm$ SEM) brainstem Ca^{2+}-ATPase activities in 21-day-old B6, D2, B6D2F$_1$, and D2.B6-*Ias*[b] mice. Parameters are the same as shown in Fig. 7. Asterisks indicate that these means are significantly lower than the B6 means ($p < 0.001$). Number of independent brainstem samples analyzed is shown in parentheses.

Although *Ias* is closely linked to the *Ah* locus (105,107), it cannot be the same as *Caa*. If *Ias* and *Caa* were the same, the Ca^{2+}-ATPase activities in the D2.B6-*Ias*[b] and BXD-1 mice should be as high as in the B6 mice rather than lower as in the D2 mice. Further genetic studies are needed to determine the nature of the associations between *Caa* and the *Ias* and *Ah* loci. Neither do we rule out the possibility that these loci are part of a single genetic complex (73).

Our findings indicate that AGS susceptibility is influenced by two major genes, *Ias* and *Caa*, both associated with the *Ah* locus. In addition to these major genes, a number of minor genes, including the *asp* locus described previously by Collins, and Collins and Fuller (13,15), can also influence AGS susceptibility (107). *Ias* influences the spread of AGS activity by a yet unknown biochemical mechanism, whereas *Caa* may influence AGS by regulating Ca^{2+}-ATPase activity in brain tissue.

Although the Ca^{2+}-ATPase deficiency in D2 mice is expressed in brainstem and cerebral cortex, it is not expressed in cerebellum, where the activities in the B6 and D2 mice are similar. Moreover, Ca^{2+}-ATPase activity in cerebellum is significantly lower than the activities present in either brainstem or cerebral cortex (81). The Ca^{2+}-ATPase deficiency in D2 mice is also expressed in microsomes and intact synaptosomes prepared from fresh whole brains (81). This deficiency is not, however, present in mitochondria. Hence, the association between AGS and the Ca^{2+}-ATPase deficiency may occur at the plasma membrane.

Because the Ca^{2+}-ATPase activity is assayed in the absence of added magnesium and in the presence of high calcium concentration (83), it probably represents the ecto-ATPase described previously by Rosenblatt et al. (86). According to Trams (124) and Nagy et al. (72), this ecto-ATPase may modulate the action of ATP on the neuronal surface. A failure to modulate this action, as expressed in D2 mice, may lead to an uncontrolled cascading or avalanche of electrical impulses when the mice are exposed to intense auditory stimulation.

Audiogenic Seizures as a Genetic Animal Model of Epilepsy

There are a number of similarities between AGS in mice and certain inherited idiopathic convulsive disorders in humans. AGS are considered in the category of seizures of brainstem or centrencephalic origin (66,98), as are photosensitive and absence seizures in humans (1,21,70,127). Although seizures evoked by auditory stimuli (bells or music) also occur in humans, they are usually rare (22,84). Far more common, however, are seizures evoked by intermittent photic stimulation (8,21,74). Because the eye is the major sense organ in humans and the ear is the major sense organ in mice, the difference between mice and humans for sensory-induced seizures may be purely a species difference. Once the sensory impulses reach higher central nervous system (CNS) centers, the biochemical mechanism responsible for these convulsive disorders may be similar in mice and humans.

The photosensitive and "absence" seizures in humans, like AGS in mice, are thought to be influenced by more than one gene and are more prevalent at younger ages (21,42,70,74). The change in seizure incidence with age is an interesting similarity between the human and the mouse forms of epilepsy. Although Hertz et al. (48) suggested that AGS in D2 mice can serve as a valid animal model for febrile convulsions in humans, Maxson (65) was unable to substantiate this claim. On the other hand, AGS are remarkably sensitive to a number of anticonvulsant drugs, e.g., valproic acid, phenytoin, and phenobarbital (90,117). Anlezark et al. (3) recently showed that the order of anticonvulsant potency of dopamine agonist aporphines was the same in D2 mice and in photosensitive baboons. In view of these genetic, developmental, and pharmacological similarities, the audiogenic mouse can be considered an excellent animal model for the study of certain kinds of human epilepsy.

Perspectives

Although a deficiency of Ca^{2+}-ATPase activity is genetically associated with AGS susceptibility, little is known about the genetic control of this activity. According to Paigen (80), the realization of an enzyme activity can depend upon the expression of structural genes, processing genes, regulatory genes, and temporal genes. A structural gene can be thought of as the segment of DNA coding for a particular polypeptide sequence. On the other hand, genes that modify a primary protein sequence or determine the turnover or intracellular localization of an enzyme or protein are termed processing genes. The regulatory genes control the rate of synthesis of specific proteins. These regulatory genes can be systemic regulators, controllers of enzyme inducibility by effector molecules such as hormones or neuropeptides, or can control the level of a receptor molecule for hormones or neurotransmitters. Finally, the temporal genes control the developmental profile of the activity or concentration of a specific enzyme or protein. Because AGS susceptibility changes with age and is influenced by more than one gene, several actions and interactions among these gene categories are likely to be involved in this susceptibility.

The biochemical defects responsible for AGS susceptibility in 21-day-old mice may be different from the factors causing resistance to these seizures with age. Unlike AGS susceptibility, the Ca^{2+}-ATPase deficiency in D2 mice does not change significantly with age, but remains deficient through adult ages (83,86). The D2 mice may, therefore, have a developmental delay in a factor or structure that normally inhibits AGS susceptibility, that is, they may have a transient imbalance of excitatory and inhibitory factors in the brain (29). Further evidence for this notion comes from finding that these mice have accelerated myelinogenesis together with delayed cerebellar growth (101,102,104). It is also possible that an age-related hearing im-

pairment causes resistance to AGS susceptibility. Hence, it is not a necessary requirement for a particular biochemical or physiological trait to have the same developmental profile as AGS susceptibility in order to be involved with these seizures. Because more than one gene influences AGS, several biochemical mechanisms will probably be involved.

The sequence of events leading from the primary site of gene action at the DNA level to the AGS phenotype at the behavioral level will involve numerous biochemical and physiological processes. Some of the advances made in understanding the genetics and biochemistry of AGS are discussed above. With the exception of the studies of Willott et al. on the comparison of response properties of inferior collicular and cochlear nuclei neurons in the B6 and D2 strains (130,131), little information is available on the physiological properties of individual neurons in various brain regions of B6 and D2 mice. The mechanisms by which the *Ias* and *Caa* genes influence membrane physiology are largely unknown. Perhaps studies utilizing voltage clamps, patch clamps, or tissue slices, as outlined in this symposium, will shed light on these mechanisms. Only through a concerted approach involving genetics, biochemistry, and physiology can a clear picture emerge of the processes involved in AGS susceptibility.

El (EPILEPSY) MOUSE

The *El* mouse was discovered in 1954 (51), was registered internationally as a mutant mouse in 1964 (50), and was established electroencephalographically as an authentic epilepsy model in 1976 (113,114). The *El* gene is inherited as an autosomal dominant and causes a predisposition to tonic-clonic seizures (58). These seizures occur in response to vestibular stimulation (by repeated tosses into the air or by altering the equilibrium of the mouse). After experiencing 10–15 induced seizures, most *El* mice begin to experience spontaneous seizures during cage changing or when placed in an unfamiliar environment. These spontaneous seizures can sometimes occur, however, in older (>100 days) mice that never had induced vestibular stimulation. The seizures in *El* mice that receive weekly stimulations beginning at 30 days generally appear with the onset of sexual maturity (7–8 weeks of age), and then persist throughout life. It appears that the *El* mice inherit a predisposition to convulsions induced by various types of vestibular stimuli. These convulsions may represent an inherited type of "kindling" such as was produced in the rat (68).

The seizures in *El* mice appear to originate in the hippocampus or deep temporal lobe structures and then spread to other brain regions (113–115). The seizures are usually accompanied by excessive salivation and by head, limb, and chewing automatisms, i.e., resembling seizures produced by hippocampal stimulation. They are not enhanced by either photic or auditory stimulation, and our findings indicate that they are distinct, genetically and developmentally, from audiogenic seizures. They can be best classified as complex partial seizures with secondary generalization (temporal lobe epilepsy).

The seizures in *El* mice share a number of features with complex partial seizures in humans. In addition to the similarities in paroxysmal discharges and seizure focus (temporal lobe), the seizures are also similar in age of onset (generally occurring with sexual maturity) (19,20,33,34,95,122). The head, limb, and chewing automatisms expressed in the *El* mice also occur frequently in humans with complex partial seizures (33,122). *El* mice seizures can also be inhibited completely by phenytoin and phenobarbital (58,63), the anticonvulsant drugs of choice for treating complex partial seizures in humans (95). Although the inheritance of most partial epilepsies is not clear, dominant genes are thought to play a role (1). Because of these features, the *El* mouse can be considered an excellent animal model for complex partial seizures or temporal lobe epilepsy in humans.

SPONTANEOUS SEIZURE DISORDERS

Although there are a number of single-locus mutations that can produce spontaneous seizures in mice, such seizures are often found in association with organic brain lesions, inherited neuropathology, or other behavioral abnormalities, e.g., ataxia and tremor (98). There are relatively few examples of spontaneous seizures in mice that are unassociated with organic brain lesion. Maxson et al. (67) described a mutation (*sps*) in C57BL/10 Bg mice that caused repeated spontaneous seizures. These spontaneous seizures commence between 40 and 70 days of age and are often fatal. Abnormal cortical electroencephalographic patterns accompany these seizures (67). The *sps* mutation appears to be inherited as a Mendelian recessive and is not linked to the dilute, albino, or brown coat-color loci. No gross neural or myelin abnormalities were detected in the CNS of *sps* mice. The *sps*

mutation also enhances susceptibility to audiogenic seizures.

Spontaneous tonic-clonic seizures have also been described in mice carrying the autosomal recessive mutation epileptiform (*epf*) (40). These seizures are induced by subtle environmental changes, e.g., turning on room lights, moving the cage or lid, or handling the mice. About 98% of the *epf/epf* mice experience at least one seizure within 140 days after birth. Unlike the *sps* mice described above, the *epf* mice have a normal life span and rarely die from the seizures. The generalized seizure syndrome expressed in *epf* mice is indeed similar to certain types of idiopathic convulsive disorders in humans (40).

Violent generalized spontaneous seizures, similar to those described for *sps* and *epf* mice above, have also been observed in mice of the B6 × D2 RI strain 13 (T. N. S. *unpublished observations*, 1980). Adult mice of this strain are also highly susceptible to AGS (105). The spontaneous seizures experienced by these mice usually occur between 60 and 150 days of age and are often lethal. The seizures seldom occur before 60 days, i.e., a late-onset epilepsy. The factors that trigger these spontaneous seizures are not known, but the seizures seem to occur more frequently after a change of cage bedding. Males and females appear to be equally susceptible to these seizures. With the exception of audiogenic and spontaneous seizure susceptibility, BXD-13 mice show no other gross signs of behavioral abnormality. The biochemical–genetic relationship between the audiogenic and the spontaneous seizures is yet unknown.

TOTTERING/LEANER SYNDROME

The tottering (*tg/tg*) and leaner (*tg*^{la}/*tg*^{la}) mutants were initially classified as different disease entities because of their dramatically different clinical symptoms (125). The tottering mice are mildly ataxic and suffer from both simple partial seizures with motor symptoms (Jacksonian seizures) and "absence" seizures (37,44,54,77). Leaner mice, on the other hand, suffer from severe immobilizing ataxia and usually die by 25 days of age. Tsuji and Meier recognized that the *tg* and *tg*^{la} mutations were functional alleles, since mutant mice were found among progeny from crosses between *tg/tg* mice and known leaner heterozygotes (+/*tg*^{la}) (125). The *tg/tg*^{la} mutants are severely ataxic and suffer from a type of "epilepsia partialis continua" or status epilepticus (100). These *tg/tg*^{la} mice are noticeably ataxic at 16–17 days and begin to experience intermittent focal motor seizures by 21 days of age. Although the focal motor seizures in tg/tg^{la} mice are phenotypically similar to those seen in tg/tg mice, they are considerably more severe and of longer duration (125). We find that the tg/tg^{la} mice may have sustained motor seizures for >1 h. The seizures become completely manifest by 25 days and persist throughout life. The seizures are not apparent, however, during sleep. Noebels (77a) recently found that the tg/tg^{la} mice also express an abnormal electroencephalogram. To our knowledge, the tg/tg^{la} mutant mouse is the only natural animal model of status epilepticus.

Anatomical, histological, and biochemical abnormalities have been reported in the brains of mice with the tottering/leaner syndrome. Reduced weight and loss and shrinkage of neurons were found in the cerebellums of these mutants (47,100,118). Similar abnormalities were also found in the rolling (tg^{rol}) mutant mouse (71), which is another mutant allele at the tottering locus (79). We found highly significant reductions in total cerebellar ganglioside content in the tg/tg, tg/tg^{la}, and tg^{la}/tg^{la} (100). Because gangliosides are enriched in neuronal membranes, our findings agree with the anatomical and histological findings. On the other hand, tottering mice have a selective increase of locus ceruleus (LC) axons, together with elevated norepinephrine levels in hippocampus, cerebellum, dorsal lateral geniculate, and LC (60). The relationship between these anatomic and biochemical changes and convulsive behavior is not yet clear.

The tottering/leaner syndrome represents a classical example of genetic heterogeneity caused by multiple alleles (41). In other words, dramatically different clinical phenotypes are produced from alternate forms of alleles of a single gene. In the case of the tottering mutant, a single-gene defect is associated with two different types of seizures, i.e., "absence" and focal motor seizures. We feel that mice with this syndrome offer great potential for assessing the biochemical and physiological action of multiple alleles on convulsive behavior.

SEIZURES ASSOCIATED WITH CEREBELLAR ABNORMALITIES

A significant association has been found between epilepsy and cerebellar disorders in humans (43,75,88,89,111). Spontaneous convulsions also occur in certain mouse mutants with defective cerebellar development, e.g., weaver, staggerer (109), and tottering mice (discussed

above). Staggerer mice also experience severe tonic seizures when emerging from ether anesthesia (K. Herrup, *personal communication*, 1981). We have observed spontaneous generalized tonic seizures in lurcher mutant mice that lose both granule cell and Purkinje cells (128,129,132). These tonic seizures, which begin beyond 70 days of age, may last as long as 5 min and are accompanied by a continuous rolling-over of the body. Further studies of the cerebellar mutants, including mice with the tottering/leaner syndrome, may provide insight into the role played by the cerebellum in epileptogenesis.

SEIZURES ASSOCIATED WITH MYELIN DISORDERS

Seizures can be associated with myelin disorders in humans (34,69). Myelin abnormalities also occur in a number of childhood epilepsies of the West and Lennox-Gastaut syndromes (36). Little is known, however, about the role of myelin in epilepsy. Seizures associated with myelin defects are also found in several mouse mutants (5,49,98). In the hypomyelinating quaking mutant, for example, myoclonic seizures occur spontaneously or can be elicited through stress or arousal (10). These seizures start with facial twitches and gradually involve the flexor muscles of the neck, trunk, and forelimbs. Eventually, the whole body is involved in a brief, generalized clonic seizure. The entire myoclonic seizure, which is accompanied by EEG abnormalities, may last several minutes (10). Jimpy mice, on the other hand, experience severe tonic seizures in association with dysmyelination. Some jimpy mice may die during the ictal period (N. Herskowitz, *personal communication*, 1984). Ducky (du/du) mutant mice have a deficiency of myelin enriched glycolipids (cerebrosides) (Meier and McPike, 1970), and have seizures similar to those seen in tottering mice (77a). Because childhood convulsive disorders associated with myelin defects are notoriously difficult to control with anticonvulsant drugs (36), the myelin mutants of mice may be useful for evaluating such drugs. We also feel that the myelin mutants offer great potential for studying the role of myelin in convulsive behavior.

ALCOHOL WITHDRAWAL SEIZURES

Convulsions arising from drug or alcohol withdrawal is a frequent occurrence in man (35,64). Susceptibility to both audiogenic and spontaneous seizures in mice can also be significantly enhanced during withdrawal from barbiturate or alcohol (23,24,31,53,119). Through selective breeding, Crabb and co-workers (16,17) produced two lines of mice that differ markedly in susceptibility to alcohol withdrawal seizures. These lines will be especially useful for evaluating biochemical and physiological changes in the CNS that are associated with inherited differences in alcohol withdrawal convulsions.

CONCLUSION

Convulsive behavior, whether in humans or mice, is a complex phenomenon. The failure to make significant gains in our understanding of inherited convulsive behavior in humans has resulted in large part from the confounding nature of the epileptogenic phenotype (influenced by multiple genetic and environmental factors) and from the inaccessability of human epileptic brain tissue. Other problems in the assessment of epilepsy are discussed by Baumann (6).

It is difficult to determine whether age-related changes in convulsability result from developmental changes of single biochemical defects or from developmental changes in compensatory mechanisms. Consequently, naturally occurring animal models of convulsive behavior are extremely important for understanding abnormalities related to epileptogenesis. In this chapter, we discuss many of the inherited disorders in mice that influence convulsive behavior. We find that for most major types of epilepsy in humans, there exists a similar counterpart in mice. These disorders in humans and mice are summarized in Table 2. Because the genetic constitution of the mouse is better known and more easily manipulated than that of other mammalian species, the mouse may serve as an excellent animal model for genetic and biochemical studies of convulsive behavior.

ACKNOWLEDGMENTS

This work was supported by grants from the National Institutes of Health (NS 17704 and 21687), NSF (BNS 8305449) and by the Swebilius Fund. T. N. S. is a recipient of a Research Career Development Award (NS 00517) from the NINCDS, National Institutes of Health.

TABLE 2. *Seizure disorders of mice and their possible counterparts in humans*

Seizure disorder in mice	Seizure disorder in humans
Audiogenic seizures	Brainstem or centrencephalic epilepsies, e.g., photosensitive and "absence" seizures, musicogenic?
El (epilepsy)	Complex partial seizures with secondary generalization (temporal lobe-limbic epilepsy)
sps (spontaneous seizure)	Generalized seizures, adult onset
epf (epileptiform)	Generalized seizures, adult onset
BXD-13 (audiogenic and generalized spontaneous seizures)	Generalized seizures, adult onset
Tottering/leaner syndrome *tg/tg* (tottering)	Simple partial seizures (Jacksonian, focal motor), also "absence" seizures
*tg/tg*ˡᵃ	Partial status epilepticus (epilepsia partialis continua)
Cerebellar mutants *sg/sg* (staggerer), *wv/wv* (weaver) *Lc/+* (lurcher) *du/du* (ducky)	Tonic-clonic seizures associated with cerebellar pathology
Myelin mutants *qk/qk* (quaking), *jp* (jumpy)	West syndrome or Lennox-Gastaut syndrome
Alcohol withdrawal seizure susceptibility	Generalized tonic-clonic seizures of alcohol withdrawal

From Seyfried and Glaser (108a), with permission.

REFERENCES

1. Andermann, E. (1982): Multifactorial inheritance of generalized and focal epilepsy. In: *Genetic Basis of the Epilepsies*, edited by V. E. Anderson, W. A. Hauser, J. K. Penry, and C. F. Sing, pp. 355–374. Raven Press, New York.
2. Anderson, V. E. (1982): Family studies of epilepsy. In: *Genetic Basis of the Epilepsies*, edited by V. E. Anderson, W. A. Hauser, J. K. Penry, and C. F. Sing, pp. 103–112. Raven Press, New York.
3. Anlezark, G. M., Blackwood, D. H. R., Meldrum, B. S., Ram, V. J., and Neumeyer, J. L. (1983): Comparative assessment of dopamine agonist aporphines as anticonvulsants in two models of reflex epilepsy. *Psychopharmacology*, 81:135–139.
4. Bailey, D. W. (1981): Recombinant inbred strains and bilineal congenic strains. In: *The Mouse in Biomedical Research*, vol. I, edited by H. L. Foster, J. D. Small, and J. G. Fox, pp. 223–239. Academic Press, Orlando, Florida.
5. Baumann, N. (1980): *Neurological Mutations Affecting Myelination*, Elsevier, New York.
6. Baumann, R. J. (1982): Classification and population studies of epilepsy. In: *Genetic Basis of the Epilepsies*, edited by V. E. Anderson, W. A.

Hauser, J. K. Penry, and C. F. Sing, pp. 11–20. Raven Press, New York.

7. Beadle, G. W., and Tatum, E. L. (1941): Genetic control of biochemical reactions in *Neurospora. Proc. Natl. Acad. Sci. USA,* 27:499–506.

8. Bickford, R. G., and Klass, D. W. (1969): Sensory perception and reflex mechanisms. In: *Basic Mechanisms of the Epilepsies,* edited by H. H. Jasper, A. A. Ward, Jr. and A. Pope, pp. 543–564. Little, Brown and Co., Boston.

9. Blaustein, M. P., Retzlaff, R. W., and Schweitzer, E. S. (1980): Control of intracellular calcium in presynaptic nerve terminals. *Fed. Proc.,* 39:2790–2795.

10. Chauvel, P., Louvel, J., Kurcewicz, I., and Debono, M. (1980): Epileptic seizures of the quaking mouse: Electroclinical correlations. In: *Neurological Mutations Affecting Myelination,* edited by N. Baumann, pp. 513–516. Elsevier, New York.

11. Chen, C.-S., and Fuller, J. L. (1976): Selection for spontaneous or priming induced audiogenic seizure susceptibility in mice. *J. Comp. Physiol.,* 90:765–772.

12. Chen, C.-S., Gates, G. R., and Gregory, R. B. (1973): Effect of priming and tympanic membrane destruction on development of audiogenic seizure susceptibility in BALB/c mice. *Exp. Neurol.,* 39:277–284.

13. Collins, R. L. (1970): A new genetic locus mapped from behavioral variation in mice: Audiogenic seizure prone (*asp*). *Behav. Genet.,* 1:99–109.

14. Collins, R. L. (1972): Audiogenic seizures. In: *Experimental Models of Epilepsy—A Manual for the Laboratory Worker,* edited by D. P. Purpura, J. K. Penry, D. Tower, D. M. Woodbury, and R. Walter, pp. 347–372. Raven Press, New York.

15. Collins, R. L., and Fuller, J. L. (1968): Audiogenic seizure prone (*asp*): A gene affecting behavior in linkage group VIII of the mouse. *Science,* 162:1137–1139.

16. Crabbe, J. C., Kosobud, A., and Young, E. R. (1983): Peak ethanol withdrawal convulsions in genetically selected mice. *Proc. West. Pharmacol. Soc.,* 26:201–204.

17. Crabbe, J. C., Kosobud, A., and Young, E. R. (1983): Genetic selection for ethanol withdrawal severity: Differences in replicate mouse lines. *Life Sci.,* 33:955–962.

18. Delgado-Escueta, A. V., and Horan, M. P. (1980): Brain synaptosomes in epilepsy: Organization of ion channels and the Na$^+$-K$^+$ pump. In: *Antiepileptic Drugs: Mechanisms of Action,* edited by G. H. Glaser, J. K. Penry, and D. M. Woodbury, pp. 85–126. Raven Press, New York.

19. Delgado-Escueta, A. V., Treiman, D. M., and Enrile-Bascal, F. (1982): Phenotypic variations of seizures in adolescents and adults. In: *Genetic Basis of the Epilepsies,* edited by V. E. Anderson, W. A. Hauser, J. K. Penry, and C. F. Sing, pp. 49–81. Raven Press, New York.

20. Delgado-Escueta, A. V., Treiman, D. M., and Walsh, G. O. (1983): The treatable epilepsies. *N. Engl. J. Med.,* 308:1508–1514, 1576–1584.

21. Doose, H. (1982): Photosensitivity: Genetics and significance in the pathogenesis of epilepsy. In: *Genetic Basis of the Epilepsies,* edited by V. E. Anderson, W. A. Hauser, J. K. Penry, and C. F. Sing, pp. 113–121. Raven Press, New York.

22. Forster, F. M. (1977): Epilepsy evoked by auditory stimuli. In: *Reflex Epilepsy, Behavioral Therapy and Conditional Reflexes.* Charles C. Thomas, Springfield, Illinois, pp. 44–68.

23. Freund, G., and Walker, D. W. (1971): Sound induced seizures during ethanol withdrawal in mice. *Psychopharmacologia,* 22:45–49.

24. Freund, G. (1971): Prevention of ethanol withdrawal seizures in mice by local anesthetics and dextro-propranolol. *Adv. Exp. Biol. Med.,* 85B:1–13.

25. Frings, H., Frings, M., and Hamilton, M. (1956): Experiments with albino mice from stocks selected from predictable susceptibilities to audiogenic seizures. *Behavior,* 9:44–52.

26. Fromby, B. (1975): Age-dependent changes in (Na$^+$,K$^+$)-ATPase activity in brains of mice susceptible to audiogenic seizures. *Experientia,* 31:315–316.

27. Fuller, J. L., Easler, C., and Smith, M. E. (1950): Inheritance of audiogenic seizure susceptibility in the mouse. *Genetics,* 35:622–632.

28. Fuller, J. L., and Williams, E. (1951): Gene controlled time constants in convulsive behavior. *Proc. Natl. Acad. Sci. USA,* 37:349–456.

29. Fuller, J. L., and Smith, M. E. (1953): Kinetics of sound induced convulsions in some inbred mouse strains. *Am. J. Physiol.,* 172:661–670.

30. Fuller, J. L., and Collins, R. L. (1968): Temporal parameters of sensitization for audiogenic seizures in SJL/J mice. *Dev. Psychobiol.,* 1:185–188.

31. Gates, G. R., and Chen, C.-S. (1974): Effects of barbiturate withdrawal on audiogenic seizure susceptibility in BALB/c mice. *Nature,* 249:162–163.

32. Ginsburg, B. E., and Miller, D. S. (1963): Genetic factors in audiogenic seizures. In: *Psychophysiologie Neuropharmacologie et Biochimie de la Crise Audiogene,* edited by R. G. Busnel, pp. 217–228. CNRS, Paris.

33. Glaser, G. H. (1967): Limbic epilepsy in childhood. *J. Nerv. Ment. Dis.,* 144:391–397.

34. Glaser, G. H. (1982): The epilepsies. In: *Cecil, Textbook of Medicine,* 16th ed., edited by J. B. Wyngaarden and L. H. Smith, pp. 2114–2124. W.B. Saunders, Philadelphia.

35. Goldstein, G., Tarter, R. E., Shelly, C., Alterman, A. I., and Petrarulo, E. (1984): Withdrawal seizures in black and white alcoholic patients: Intellectual and neuropsychological sequelae. *Drug Alcohol Depend.,* 12:349–354.

36. Gomez, M. R., and Klass, D. W. (1982): Epilepsies of infancy and childhood. *Ann. Neurol.,* 13:113–124.

37. Green, M. C., and Sidman, R. L. (1962): Tot-

tering—A neuromuscular mutation in the mouse. *J. Hered.*, 53:233–237.

38. Hakim, G., Itano, T., Verma, A. K., and Penniston, J. T. (1982): Purification of the Ca^{2+} and Mg^{2+}-requiring ATPase from rat brain synaptic plasma membrane. *Biochem. J.*, 207:225–231.

39. Hall, C. S. (1947): Genetic differences in fatal audiogenic seizures. *J. Hered.*, 38:2–6.

40. Hare, J. E., and Hare, A. S. (1979): Epileptiform mice, a new neurological mutant. *J. Hered.*, 70:417–420.

41. Harris, H. (1974): Genetic heterogeneity in inherited disease. *J. Clin. Pathol.* (Suppl.), 27: (R. Coll. Pathol) 8:32–37.

42. Hauser, W. A. (1982): Genetics and the clinical characteristics of seizures. In: *Genetic Basis of the Epilepsies,* edited by V. E. Anderson, W. A. Hauser, J. K. Penry, and C. F. Sing, pp. 3–10. Raven Press, New York.

43. Heath, R. G., Franklin, D. E., and Shraberg, D. (1979): Gross pathology of the cerebellum in patients diagnosed and treated as functional psychiatric disorders. *J. Nerv. Ment. Dis.*, 167: 585–592.

44. Heller, A. H., Dichter, M. A., and Sidman, R. L. (1983): Anticonvulsant sensitivity of absence seizures in the tottering mutant mouse. *Epilepsia*, 24:25–34.

45. Henry, K. R. (1967): Audiogenic seizure susceptibility induced in C57BL/6J mice by prior auditory exposure. *Science*, 158:938–940.

46. Henry, K. R., McGinn, M. D., Berard, D. R., and Chole, R. A. (1981): Effects of neonatal thyroxine, genotype, and noise on the ear and audiogenic seizures. *J. Comp. Physiol. Psychol.*, 95:418–424

47. Herrup, K., and Wilczynski, S. L. (1982): Cerebellar cell degeneration in the leaner mutant mouse. *Neuroscience*, 7:2185–2196.

48. Hertz, L., Schousboe, A., Fromby, B., and Lennox-Buchthal, M. (1974): Some age-dependent biochemical changes in mice susceptible to seizures. *Epilepsia*, 15:619–631.

49. Hogan, E. (1977): Animal models of genetic disorders of myelin. In: *Myelin,* edited by P. Morell, pp. 489–531. Plenum Press, New York.

50. Imaizumi, K. (1964): *Mouse Newsletter*, 31:57.

51. Imaizumi, K., Ito, S., Kutsukake, G., Takizawa, T., Fujiwara, K., and Tutikawa, K. (1959): Epilepsy-like anomaly of mice. *Exp. Anim.* (Jpn.), 8:6–10.

52. Iturrian, W. B., and Fink, G. B. (1968): Effect of age and condition-test interval (days) on audio-conditioned convulsive response in CF #1 mice. *Dev. Psychobiol.*, 1:230–235.

53. Kakihana, R. (1979): Alcohol intoxication and withdrawal in inbred strains of mice: Behavioral and endocrine studies. *Behav. Neurol. Biol.*, 26:97–105.

54. Kaplan, B. J., Seyfried, T. N., and Glaser, G. H. (1979): Spontaneous polyspike discharges in an epileptic mutant mouse (tottering). *Exp. Neurol.*, 66:577–586.

55. Katz, B., and Miledi, R. (1972): Further study

of the role of calcium in synaptic transmission. *J. Physiol.* (Lond.), 207:789–801.

56. Kelly, R. B., Deutsch, J. W., Carlson, S. S., and Wagner, J. A. (1979): Biochemistry of neurotransmitter release. *Annu. Rev. Neurosci.*, 2:399–446.

57. Krall, R. L., Penry, J. K., Kupferberg, H. J., and Swinyard, E. A. (1978): Antiepileptic drug development: I. History and a program of progress. *Epilepsia*, 19:393–408.

58. Kurokawa, M., Naruse, H., and Kato, M. (1966): Metabolic studies on *ep* mouse, a special strain with convulsive predisposition. *Prog. Brain Res.*, 21A:112–130.

58a. Legraverend, C., et al. (1984): Aryl hydrocarbon hydroxylase induction by benzo[a]-anthracene: Regulatory gene localized to the distal portion of mouse chromosome 17. *Genetics*, 107:447–461.

59. Lehman, A., and Bosinger, E. (1964): Sur le determinisme genetique de l'epilepsie acoustique do *Mus Masculus* domestique, (Swiss, Rb). *C.R. Acad. Sci.* (Paris), 258:4858–4861.

60. Levitt, P., and Noebels, J. L. (1981): Mutant mouse tottering: Selective increase of locus ceruleus axons in a defined single-locus mutation. *Proc. Natl. Acad. Sci. USA*, 78:4630–4643.

61. Lin, S.-C., and Way, E. L. (1982): A high affinity Ca^{2+}-ATPase in enriched nerve-ending plasma membranes. *Brain Res.*, 235:387–392.

62. Llinas, R. R. (1982): Calcium in synaptic transmission. *Sci. Am.*, 247:56–65.

63. Matsumoto, Y., Hiramatsu, M., and Mori, A. (1983): Effects of phenytoin on convulsions and brain 5-hydroxytryptamine levels in El mice. *IRCS Med. Sci.*, 11:387.

64. Mattson, R. H. (1983): Seizures associated with alcohol use and alcohol withdrawal. In: *Epilepsy,* edited by T. R. Browne and R. G. Feldman, pp. 325–332. Little, Brown and Co. Boston.

65. Maxson, S. (1980): Febrile convulsions in inbred strains of mice susceptible and resistant to audiogenic seizures. *Epilepsia*, 21:637–645.

66. Maxson, S. C., and Cowen, J. S. (1976): Electroencephalographic correlates of the audiogenic response of inbred mice. *Physiol. Behav.*, 16:623–629.

67. Maxson, S. C., Fine, M. D., Ginsburg, B. E., and Koniecki, D. L. (1983): A mutant for spontaneous seizures in C57BL/10 Bg mice. *Epilepsia*, 24:15–24.

68. McNamara, J. D. (1980): Complex neuronal systems: Approach to development of new strategies in the treatment of epilepsy. In: *Antiepileptic Drugs: Mechanisms of Action,* edited by G. H. Glaser, J. K. Penry, and D. M. Woodbury, pp. 185–197. Raven Press, New York.

68a. Meier, H., and McPike, A. D. (1970): Ducky, a neurological mutation in mice characterized by deficiency of cerebrosides. *Exp. Med. Surg.*, 28:256–269.

69. Menkes, J. H. (1974): *Textbook of Child Neurology*. Lea & Febiger, Philadelphia.

70. Metrakos, J. D., and Metrakos, K. (1969): Ge-

netics in clinical epilepsy. In: *Basic Mecha-nisms of the Epilepsies*, edited by H. H. Jasper, A. A. Ward, Jr., and A. Pope, pp. 700–708. Little, Brown and Co., Boston.

71. Muramoto, O., Kanazawa, I., and Ando, K. (1981): Neurotransmitter abnormality in rolling mouse Nagoya, an ataxic mutant mouse. *Brain Res.*, 215:295–304.

72. Nagy, A., Shuster, T. A., and Rosenberg, M. D. (1983): Adenosine triphosphatase activity at the external surface of chicken brain synapto-somes. *J. Neurochem.*, 40:226–234.

73. Nebert, D. W. (1980): Pharmacogenetics: An approach to understanding chemical and biolog-ical aspects of cancer. *J. Natl. Cancer Inst.*, 64:1279–1290.

74. Newmark, M. E., and Penry, J. K. (1979): *Pho-tosensitivity and Epilepsy: A Review*. Raven Press, New York.

75. Newmark, M. E., and Penry, J. K. (1980): *Ge-netics of Epilepsy: A Review*. Raven Press, New York.

76. Niaussat, M. M. (1977): Experimentally in-duced otitis and audiogenic seizure in the mouse. *Experientia*, 33:473–474.

77. Noebels, J. L., and Sidman, R. L. (1979): In-herited epilepsy: Spike-wave and focal motor seizures in the mutant mouse tottering. *Science*, 204:1334–1336.

77a. Noebels, J. L. (1984): Isolating single genes of the inherited epilepsies. *Ann. Neurol.*, 16:s18–s21.

78. Norris, C. H., Cawthorn, T. H., and Carroll, R. C. (1977): Kanamycin priming for audiogenic seizures in mice. *Neuropharmacology*, 16:375–380.

79. Oda, S.-I. (1981): A new allele of the tottering locus, rolling mouse Nagoya, on chromosome No. 8 in the mouse. *Jpn. J. Genet.*, 56:295–299.

80. Paigen, K. (1979): Acid hydrolases as models of genetic control. *Ann. Rev. Genet.*, 13:417–466.

81. Palayoor, S. T., Seyfried, T. N., and Bernard, D. J. (1986): Calcium ATPase activities in syn-aptic plasma membranes of seizure prone mice. *J. Neurochem.* (*in press*).

82. Palayoor, S. T., and Seyfried, T. N. (1984): Ge-netic study of cationic ATPase activities and au-diogenic seizure susceptibility in recombinant inbred and congenic strains of mice. *J Neuro-chem.*, 42:529–533.

83. Palayoor, S. T., and Seyfried, T. N. (1984): Ge-netic association between Ca^{2+}-ATPase activity and audiogenic seizures in mice. *J. Neuro-chem.*, 42:1771–1774.

84. Poskanzer, D. C., Brown, A. E., and Miller, H. (1962): Musicogenic epilepsy caused by a dis-crete frequency band of church bells. *Brain*, 85:77–92.

85. Reichert, W. H. (1975): Cerebral magnesium and sodium-potassium ATPase following au-diogenic seizure in mce. *Exp. Neurol.*, 49:596–600.

86. Rosenblatt, D. E., Lauter, C. J., and Trans, E. G. (1976): Deficiency of a Ca^{2+}-ATPase in brains of seizure prone mice. *J. Neurochem.*, 27:1299–1304.

87. Rotter, J. I. (1981): The modes of inheritance of insulin-dependent diabetes mellitus. *Am. J. Hum. Genet.*, 33:835–851.

88. Salcman, M., Defendini, R., Correll., J., and Gilman, S. (1978): Neuropathological changes in cerebellar biopsies of epileptic patients. *Ann. Neurol.*, 3:10–19.

89. Sarnat, H. B., and Alcala, H. (1980): Human cerebellar hypoplasia: A syndrome of diverse causes. *Arch. Neurol.*, 37:300–305.

90. Schechter, P. J., Tranier, Y., and Grove, J. (1978): Effect of *n*-dipropylacetate on amino acid concentrations in mouse brain: Correla-tions with anti-convulsant activity. *J. Neuro-chem.*, 31:1325–1327.

91. Schellenberg, G. D., Pech, I. V., and Stahl, W. L. (1981): Immunoreactivity of subunits of the $(Na^+ + K^+)$-ATPase. *Biochem. Biophys. Acta.*, 649:691–700.

92. Schlesinger, K., Elston, R. C., and Boggan, W. (1966): The genetics of sound induced seizure in inbred mice. *Genetics*, 54:95–103.

93. Schlesinger, K., and Uphouse, L. L. (1972): Pyridoxine dependency and central nervous system excitability. *Adv. Biochem. Psycho-pharmacol.*, 4:105–140.

94. Schlesinger, K., and Sharpless, S. K. (1975): Audiogenic seizures and acoustic priming. In: *Psychopharmacogenetics*, edited by B. E. Eleftheriou, pp. 383–433. Plenum Press, New York.

95. Schomer, D. L. (1983): Current concepts in neurology: Partial epilepsy. *N. Engl. J. Med.*, 309:536–539.

96. Schreiber, R. A., Lehmann, A., Ginsburg, B. E., and Fuller, J. L. (1980): Development of susceptibility to audiogenic seizures in DBA/2J and Rb mice: Toward a systematic nomencla-ture of audiogenic seizure levels. *Behav. Genet.*, 10:537–544.

97. Seyfried, T. N. (1982): Developmental genetics of audiogenic seizures in mice. In: *Genetic Basis of the Epilepsies*, edited by V. E. An-derson, W. A. Hauser, J. K. Penry, and C. F. Sing, pp. 199–210. Raven Press, New York.

98. Seyfried, T. N. (1982): Convulsive disorders. In: *The Mouse in Biomedical Research*, edited by H. L. Foster, J. D. Small, and J. C. Fox, pp. 97–124. Academic Press, Orlando, Florida.

99. Seyfried, T. N. (1983): Genetic heterogeneity for the development of audiogenic seizures in mice. *Brain Res.*, 271:325–329.

100. Seyfried, T. N., Itoh, T., Glaser, G. H., Miya-zawa, N., and Yu, R. K. (1981): Cerebellar gan-gliosides and phospholipids in mutant mice with ataxia and epilepsy: The tottering/leaner syn-drome. *Brain Res.*, 216:429–436.

101. Seyfried, T. N., Glaser, G. H., and Yu, R. K. (1978): Cerebral, cerebellar, and brainstem gan-gliosides in mice susceptible to audiogenic sei-zures. *J. Neurochem.*, 31:21–27.

102. Seyfried, T. N., Glaser, G. H., and Yu, R. K. (1978): Developmental analysis of regional brain growth and audiogenic seizures in mice. *Ge-netics*, 88:s90.

103. Seyfried, T. N., Glaser, G. H. and Yu, R. K. (1979): Thyroid hormone influence on the sus-

ceptibility of mice to audiogenic seizures. *Science*, 205:598–600.

104. Seyfried, T. N., and Yu, R. K. (1980): Heterosis for brain myelin content in mice. *Biochem. Genet.*, 18:1229–1238.

105. Seyfried, T. N., Yu, R. K., and Glaser, G. H. (1980): Genetic analysis of audiogenic seizure susceptibility in C57BL/6J × DBA/2J recombinant inbred strains of mice. *Genetics*, 94:701–718.

106. Seyfried, T. N., Glaser, G. H. and Yu, R. K. (1981): Thyroid hormone can restore the audiogenic seizure susceptibility of hypothyroid DBA/2J mice. *Exp. Neurol.*, 71:220–225.

107. Seyfried, T. N., and Glaser, G. H. (1981): Genetic linkage between the *Ah* locus and a major gene that inhibits susceptibility to audiogenic seizures in mice. *Genetics*, 99:117–126.

108. Seyfried, T. N., Glaser, G. H., and Yu, R. K. (1984): Genetic analysis of serum thyroxine content and audiogenic seizures in recombinant inbred and congenic strains of mice. *Exp. Neurol.*, 83:423–428.

108a. Seyfried, T. N., and Glaser, G. H. (1985): A review of mouse mutants as genetic models of epilepsy. *Epilepsia*, 26(2):143–150.

109. Sidman, R. L., Green, M. C., and Appel, S. H. (1965): *Catalog of the Neurological Mutants of the Mouse.* Harvard University Press, Cambridge, Massachusetts.

110. Simpson, N. E. (1980): The genetics of diabetes mellitus in man. *Can. J. Genet. Cytol.*, 22:497–506.

111. Skre, H. (1975): A study of certain traits accompanying some inherited neurological disorders. *Clin. Genet.*, 8:117–135.

112. Sorensen, R. G., and Mahler, H. R. (1981): Calcium-stimulated adenosine triphosphatases in synaptic membranes. *J. Neurochem.*, 37:1407–1418.

113. Suzuki, J. (1976): Paroxysmal discharges in the electroencephalogram of the El mouse. *Experientia*, 32:336–337.

114. Suzuki, J., and Nakamoto, Y. (1977): Seizure patterns and electroencephalograms of El mouse. *Electroencephalogr. Clin. Neurophysiol.*, 43:299–311.

115. Suzuki, J., Nakamoto, Y., and Shinkawa, Y. (1983): Local cerebral glucose utilization in epileptic seizures of the mutant El mouse. *Brain Res.*, 226:359–363.

116. Sweadner, K. J. (1979): Two molecular forms of (Na⁺ + K⁺) stimulated ATPase in brain. *J. Biol. Chem.*, 254:6060–6067.

117. Swinyard, E. A. (1963): Some physiological properties of audiogenic seizures in mice and their alteration by drugs. In: *Psychophysiologie Neuropharmacologie et Biochemie de la Crise Audiogene*, edited by R. G. Basnel, pp. 405–428. CNRS, Paris.

118. Syapin, P. J. (1982): Effects of the tottering mutation in the mouse: Multiple neurological changes. *Exp. Neurol.*, 76:566–573.

119. Sze, P. Y., Yani, J., and Ginsburg, B. E. (1974): Adrenal glucocorticoids as a required factor in the development of ethanol withdrawal seizures in mice. *Brain Res.*, 80:155–159.

120. Tatum, E. L. (1959): A case history in biological research. *Science*, 129:1711–1715.

121. Taylor, B. A. (1978): Recombinant inbred strains: Use in gene mapping. In: *Origins of Inbred Mice*, edited by H. Morse, pp. 423–438. Academic Press, Orlando, Florida.

122. Theodore, W. H., Porter, R. J., and Penry, J. K. (1983): Complex partial seizures: Clinical characteristics and differential diagnosis. *Neurology*, 33:1115–1121.

123. Tower, D. (1969): Neurochemical mechanisms. In: *Basic Mechanisms of the Epilepsies*, edited by H. H. Jasper, A. A. Ward, Jr., and A. Pope, pp. 611–638. Little, Brown and Co., Boston.

124. Trams, E. G. (1974). Evidence for ATP action on the cell surface. *Nature*, 252:480–481.

125. Tsuji, S., and Meier, H. (1971): Evidence for allelism of leaner and tottering in the mouse. *Genet. Res.*, 17:83–88.

126. Vicari, E. M. (1951): Fatal convulsive seizures in the DBA mouse strain. *J. Psychol.*, 32:79–97.

127. Ward, A. A., Jr., Jasper, H. H. and Pope, A. (1969): Clinical and experimental challenges of the epilepsies. In: *Basic Mechanisms of the Epilepsies*, edited by H. H. Jasper, A. A. Ward, Jr., and A. Pope, pp. 1–12. Little, Brown and Co., Boston.

128. Wetts, R., and Herrup, K. (1982): Interaction of granule, Purkinje and inferior olivary neurons in lurcher chimaeric mice. I. qualitative studies. *J. Embryol. Exp. Morphol.*, 68:87–98.

129. Wetts, R., and Herrup, K. (1982): Interaction of granule, Purkinje, and inferior olivary neurons in lurcher chimaeric mice. II. granule cell death. *Brain Res.*, 250:358–362.

130. Willott, J. F. (1981): Comparison of response properties of inferior colliculus neurons of two inbred mouse strains during susceptibility to audiogenic seizures. *J. Neurophysiol.*, 45:35–46.

131. Willott, J. F., Demuth, R. M., and Lu, S.-M. (1984): Excitability of auditory neurons in the dorsal and ventral cochlear nuclei of DBA/2 and C57BL/6 mice. *Exp. Neurol.*, 83:495–506.

132. Wilson, D. B. (1976): Histological defects in the cerebellum of adult lurcher mice. *J. Neuropathol. Exp. Neurol.*, 35:40–45.

133. Witt, G., and Hall, C. S. (1949): The genetics of audiogenic seizures in the house mouse. *J. Comp. Physiol. Psychol.*, 90:373–381.

134. Wood, A. W., and Taylor, B. A. (1979): Genetic regulation of coumarin hydroxylase activity in mice: Evidence for single locus control on chromosome 7. *J. Biol. Chem.*, 254:5647–5651.

Section 3

EPILEPTOGENESIS I
Molecular Machinery of the Cell and Intracellular Communication

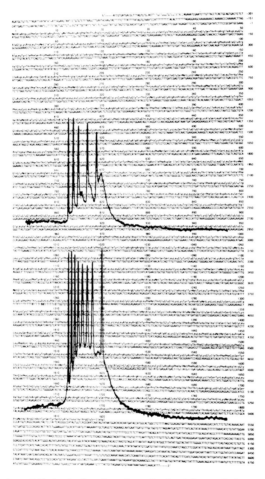

The paroxysmal depolarization shift is depicted against the backdrop of the nucleotide sequence of cloned cDNA encoding the EL electricus sodium channel protein. Exhibiting four repeated homology units, 1,820 amino acid residues are oriented in a pseudosymmetric fashion across the membrane. Each homology unit contains a unique segment with the clustered positively charged residues that may be involved in the gating structure. Nucleotide sequence from Noda, M., Shimuzu, S., Tanaba, T., et al. (1984) Primary structure of electrophorus electricus sodium channel deduced from cDNA sequence. *Nature*, 312:124. With permission from Macmillan Journals Limited.

Advances in Neurology, Vol. 44, edited by
A. V. Delgado-Escueta, A. A. Ward, Jr.,
D. M. Woodbury, and R. J. Porter.
Raven Press, New York © 1986.

6

Voltage-Dependent Currents of Vertebrate Neurons and Their Role in Membrane Excitability

Paul R. Adams and Martin Galvan

Department of Neurobiology and Behavior, SUNY at Stony Brook, Stony Brook, New York 11794; and Physiological Institute, University of Munich, D8000 Munich 2, F.R.G.

SUMMARY This chapter reviews what is known of the voltage-dependent conductances of three classes of vertebrate nerve cell, as assessed by somatic voltage clamping. These classes are: (1) bullfrog paravertebral sympathetic ganglion cells; (2) rodent superior cervical sympathetic ganglion cells; and (3) rodent hippocampal pyramidal cells. Of these, bullfrog neurons are the most thoroughly characterized. They possess at least seven distinct voltage-activated conductances. Two of these, called G_{Na} and G_{Ca}, carry inward, depolarizing current. They both activate rapidly, and can, under appropriate conditions, generate action potentials. The remaining five conductances are all potassium-mediated, and can thus in principle produce hyperpolarizations or repolarize the action potential. However, because each of these potassium conductances have different sizes, speeds, and voltage thresholds, they play a variety of hyperpolarizing, stabilizing, or braking roles. I_C is large, fast, and voltage dependent. Action potentials trigger calcium influx, which rapidly turns on I_C. This repolarizes the action potential and turns off I_C. However another Ca-dependent current, I_{AHP}, remains active even at negative potentials and leads to a prolonged hyperpolarization. If I_C is blocked, spike repolarization slows somewhat, allowing the Hodgkin-Huxley delayed rectifier current I_K to develop. This is also large enough to repolarize the spike rapidly, although it is normally preempted by I_C. I_A and I_M are other small potassium currents that activate at more negative potentials than do I_C, I_K, and I_{AHP}. I_A is a transient outward current that mainly influences voltage trajectories following hyperpolarizing current pulses. I_M activates progressively during prolonged depolarizing current pulses, and, together with I_{AHP}, explains most of the adaptation seen in these cells. The harmonious counterpoint of this septet of currents explains most of the electrical excitability properties of these cells. However, several of the currents are also synaptically regulated, as a result of transmitters acting on muscarinic or peptide receptors. These slow synaptic actions can lead to dramatic changes in the electrical behavior of the cells.

These currents all appear to be present in rat sympathetic ganglion cells also, although detailed analysis here has been hampered by the more complex geometry of these neurons. Furthermore, the roles of the various currents have not been completely defined. It seems possible that I_A can contribute to spike repolarization, and clean separation of I_C and I_{AHP} has not yet been achieved.

Hippocampal neurons have been even harder to study, because they are smaller, more fragile and inaccessible, and possess extensive dendrites. However, currents that are basically similar to those of bullfrogs are again present, plus several more. Rather little is known about the precise roles of many of these currents or about their anatomical distribution in the cells. Information about simpler cells such as bullfrog and rat sympathetic ganglia is thus particularly useful in devising experimental tests of central neuron behavior. In particular, it is reasonable to guess that the major properties of many of these currents are highly conserved between neuron types. This allows one to fill in gaps in direct biophysical characterizaton of central neurons.

In the illustrious predecessor to the present volume on basic mechanisms of the epilepsies, two chapters considered the voltage-dependent behavior of excitable membranes in relation to the spiking activity of normal and abnormal neurons. That by Woodbury described the rapid sodium and potassium currents discovered by Hodgkin and Huxley (91,92) that are responsible for the digital form of propagating electrical signals in the central nervous system (CNS). The intriguing preliminary report by Stevens discussed the frequency-modulating effects of a novel transient outward current subsequently named I_A by Connor and Stevens (52) and Neher (134). In the intervening years, work in this field has progressed rapidly. It is now clear that nerve cell bodies and processes are much more complicated than the squid axon studied by Hodgkin and Huxley, presumably because they must convert complex spatiotemporal arrays of voltages into varying instantaneous firing rates according to some functionally useful role. The work by Connor et al. was one of the first portents of this gathering complexity. Other heralds were the discovery of voltage-dependent calcium current (81,141) and of calcium-activated potassium current (129). A good example of the way in which the new currents can add to the possibilities inherent in the Hodgkin-Huxley equations is the study by Connor (53) of repetitive firing in crustacean axon, which documented the ability of the A-current to confer very low, minimum sustained firing rates, and to linearize the spike frequency–current relation. More recently, this approach has expanded further with the application of refined biophysical techniques to molluscan or dissociated cells on the one hand, and extensions into cells of the vertebrate nervous system, including the mammalian CNS, on the other (e.g., 8,9,66,82).

In this chapter, it would be quite impossible to survey all of these important developments. Instead, the focus will be on representative vertebrate neuron examples with which the authors have some first-hand experience—bullfrog sympathetic ganglion cells, rat superior cervical ganglion cells, and rodent hippocampal pyramidal cells.

The ultimate goal of the type of work to be discussed is the development of a complete empirical mathematical model of the electrical characteristics of these neurons. With this in hand, several exciting prospects would open up: (a) one could explore the emergent properties of interconnected arrays of such neurons (see Wong's chapter in this book); (b) one could explore the effect of pharmacological or pathological changes in the neuronal membrane; and (c) the model could be used as a tool in the refinement of techniques (such as impedance analysis) to be applied to other, more recalcitrant, neurons. It is not a primary goal of these studies to understand the molecular mechanisms underlying such electrical behavior, though of course any such insights that were achieved would be both welcome and useful.

VOLTAGE-DEPENDENT CURRENTS OF BULLFROG NEURONS

Bullfrog paravertebral sympathetic ganglia are among the most intensively investigated vertebrate nervous tissues. They contain two classes of neurons, "B" cells with diameters 35–60 μm, and "C" cells with diameters of 20–45 μm (60). Other than in size, they differ mainly in their synaptic responses (135,165).

The typical structure of a bullfrog ganglion cell, revealed by lucifer yellow injection for example, is very rudimentary. It consists of a compact cell body devoid of detectable dendrites, and a thin unbranched axon, which leaves the ganglion and is probably myelinated (160,165). Different subclasses of B cells probably differ in their extent of myelination, since they show different conduction velocities (60). A microelectrode voltage clamp in the soma, although only a point clamp, would thus be expected to reveal currents mostly arising in the soma itself, and thus amenable to quantitative analysis. Some contamination from axonal conductances is inevitable, but because of the high axial resistance, will be quite small. Furthermore, the nature of these nodal conductances is quite well understood (62,68,69,159).

The active currents that have been revealed by this approach are listed in Table 1. In the next sections, a summary of the principal characteristics of these various currents is presented. All the work discussed applies to B cells unless otherwise stated.

Sodium Current

Sodium current has not been studied in any detail, partly because of limitations of the microelectrode voltage-clamp technique. From the magnitudes of the rate of rise of the action potential in these cells and their total membrane capacity (about 100 V/sec and 200 pF), the peak amplitude of I_{Na} in these cells would probably be about 20 nA. Indeed, recent high-resolution two-electrode-clamp studies have revealed a rapidly peaking (1 msec) and rapidly and completely inactivating (3 msec) inward current in these cells when clamped to 0 mV from -40 mV (Fig. 1). Similar action potentials and currents can be seen in acutely dissociated ganglion cells which lack any visible axon stumps, and thus a large somatic Na current is real and not a result of nodal contamination. Space-clamp problems preclude accurate measurements of I_{Na} in intact bullfrog neurons, and for the moment we assume that the voltage dependence and kinetics of this current closely resemble that described for amphibian node of Ranvier (69,159). The major difference is likely to be that the somatic activation, and particularly inactivation, parameters are shifted to the right compared to node, since considerable Na current can be seen in bullfrog neurons held at

-40 mV or even -30 mV, which would inactivate I_{Na} in node of Ranvier (46).

Calcium Current

Figure 1 also shows that a small part of the early inward current in these cells is calcium-dependent. The existence of calcium current (I_{Ca}) in these cells has been suspected ever since Koketsu and Nishi demonstrated the occurrence of calcium-dependent action potentials in cells deprived of sodium and treated with tetraethylammonium (TEA) (109). The charge carried by calcium during normal spiking is probably itself insignificant, but it is important to understand the calcium current because it in turn triggers other conductance changes, primarily to potassium (see below). To this end, we have attempted to isolate the calcium current pharmacologically, and to measure its voltage sensitivity and kinetics (2,3,13,14). We decided to eliminate completely all other ionic currents which could coincide with I_{Ca} and distort it, and thus adopted the cesium-loading technique used by Eckert and Tillotson in *Aplysia* neurons (64), in combination with a suitable external medium [Na replaced by TEA, K by Cs, Ca raised to 10 mM with 5 mM 4-aminopyridine (4-AP) added]. The time course of the calcium current revealed under these conditions is shown in Fig. 2. The most striking features of I_{Ca} were: (a) the rapid, almost exponential rise time; and (b) the absence of any early inactivation. These points were explored in some detail; the activation time constant was slowest (about 4 msec) at -10 mV and became progressively faster at more positive potentials. The size of the current (about 5 nA at $+10$ mV) is adequate to account for the observed rate of rise of the calcium spike in these cells if allowance is made for the fact that the size of the current also (and unsurprisingly) depends on the external calcium concentration. It remains to be seen whether our measurements

TABLE 1. *Voltage-sensitive conductances of sympathetic neurons*

	Name		Size	Speed	Inactivation	Transmitter sensitivity
Inward currents		I_{NA}	Large	Very fast	Complete, fast	?
		I_{CA}	Small	Fast	Incomplete, very slow	Norepinephrine ↓
Outward currents		I_K	Large	Fast	Complete, very slow	?
		I_A	Medium	Fast	Complete, fast	?
		I_M	Small	Slow	None	ACh, Nucleotides, peptides ↓
	Ca Dependent	I_C	Large	Very fast	Incomplete, fast	?
		I_{AHP}	Small	Slow	None?	ACh ↓

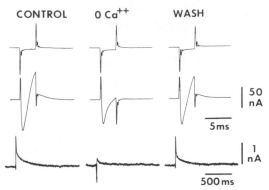

FIG. 1. Voltage-dependent currents in a bullfrog ganglion cell elicited by brief depolarizations. This cell was voltage clamped using two separate intracellular microelectrodes. The holding potential was -40 mV, and brief 40-mV pulses lasting 3 msec, either to -80 mV (top row) or to 0 mV (middle and bottom rows) were applied. The top row thus shows primarily leakage and capacity currents, whereas the bottom two rows show active currents in addition. The middle row shows fast sweep, low gain records of the currents elicited by brief depolarizations. In column one, row 2 an inward–outward sequence can be seen, followed by a rapid outward tail current; row 3 shows that the fast outward tail is followed by a slow, small, outward tail. The middle column shows the effect of omitting calcium ions from the Ringer's solution. Most of the inward current remains, and is thus probably sodium current. In other tests, it was shown that this rapid inward current is abolished by adding tetrodotoxin (TTX) or replacing Na by choline or TRIS. However, omitting Ca does abolish almost all the fast and slow outward currents; these correspond to I_C and I_{AHP} (from Pennefather et al., ref. 143).

of the voltage sensitivity of the size and time course of I_{Ca} (13,14) will permit a detailed accurate simulation of the calcium spike in these cells. One of the problems is that the calcium spike is much less stereotyped than is the normal Na-spike. In particular, the spike duration depends critically on the cell input resistance and on the past history of any previous calcium spiking. Spike repolarization seems to reflect the contribution of two processes that are not very well developed in these cesium-loaded cells $-I_{Ca}$ inactivation, and development of calcium-dependent outward current.

Both of these processes probably contribute to the slow droop of the calcium current seen in voltage-clamp experiments when the test depolarization is made hundreds of msec or even sec long, although when K-currents have been adequately eliminated, some net inward current always persists even after very long depolarizations (Fig. 3).

Evidence for genuine inactivation of I_{Ca} following 1-sec depolarizing commands was obtained by examining the "tail current" that follows the return of the membrane potential to the "resting" or "holding" value. Because the calcium conductance takes a finite time to return to its control, or zero, level, a brief inward kick of current is seen at pulse termination, which reflects the closing of those calcium channels that opened during the pulse. Recent detailed analyses of such tail currents in other cultured vertebrate cell preparations (66,82) have contributed greatly to our understanding of calcium current kinetics. However, for the present purpose, it is sufficient to realize that the amplitude of the tail current offers a precise measure of the extent to which the calcium conductance was activated, or became inactivated, during the test pulse. Figure 3 shows an example of such measurements, and reveals that significant, though not spectacular, inactivation does occur during 1-sec depolarizations.

Often the droop of the inward current itself *during* the pulse is much more impressive, raising the possibility that it is only partly caused by genuine inactivation and partly by development of a small residual outward current as a result of massive calcium influx. Some evidence for this was obtained by making large iontophoretic calcium injections into such cells and observing the development of an outward current. However, it is not known whether this outward current reflects outward movement of cesium or residual potassium or, conceivably, a reduction in a steady inward current (110).

A third procedure for assaying inactivation is to follow the long inactivating depolarizing command by a short test pulse, usually to a potential at which calcium current develops quickly and well. This is compared with the situation in which the test pulse is applied alone, evoking a standard amount of calcium current. Assayed in this way, several hundred msec conditioning pulses can produce quite dramatic inactivation, especially when they themselves elicit large inward currents (Fig. 4). This behavior was originally discovered by Brehm et al. (33) in *Paramecium* and by Eckert and Tillotson (64) in *Aplysia* neurons; they argued that this indicated that calcium conductance inactivation stems from the rise in intracellular calcium produced by the calcium current itself. Subsequent tail current experiments by Eckert and Ewald (65) have given strong support to this notion, although it is by no means universally accepted or indeed applicable (67,47).

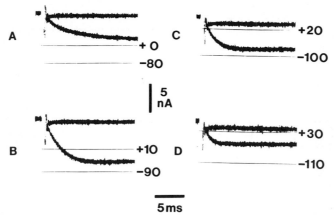

FIG. 2. Calcium current in bullfrog ganglion cells, loaded with cesium and voltage clamped with two CsCl microelectrodes. The holding potential was −40 mV, and pairs of traces with ±40-, 50-, 60-, and 70-mV clamp steps are shown. The speed of activation of the calcium current increases progressively as the membrane is depolarized more, whereas the size of the inward current first increases, then decreases, being largest at +10 mV (from ref. 3).

Both these processes—calcium-dependent inactivation and outward current development—progress during the plateau of the spike until the current–voltage relation no longer exhibits a negative conductance region, and repolarization rapidly occurs at a rate limited by the membrane capacity. Any intervention that reduces calcium current may thus have complex, unpredictable or even paradoxical effects on spike duration. A reduction in calcium current will simultaneously initially reduce the negative slope conductance and slow the rate at which further reductions in slope conductance (as a result of calcium accumulation) occurs. Conceivably, under certain conditions, the latter effect could predominate, so that partly blocking the calcium channels could prolong the calcium spike.

Frog ganglion cells, and probably even normal mammalian neurons, do not usually undergo the prolonged depolarizations that cause the phenomenon discussed above. However, under abnormal conditions, such as the administration of potent glutamate analogs such as kainic acid, prolonged depolarizations might occur, and may themselves include a certain regenerative element that will offset any tendency to desensitize the receptors (127). The sluggishness of inactivation of vertebrate neuron calcium currents, if it is a widespread phenomenon, could underlie the dramatic consequences of such depolarizations, particularly in cells or fine processes in which calcium current is unusually prominent or the internal volume is unusually small. This hypothesis is discussed in this volume by Meldrum (see Chapter 42).

Potassium Currents

The task of deciding just when, and with how many spikes, a nerve cell will fire in response to ongoing synaptic inputs is largely performed by the various outward current systems that are present, particularly potassium currents. Perhaps this is why nerve cells seem to have evolved a cornucopia of such K-currents, of all shapes, sizes, and speeds. The ganglion cell is a particularly striking example, for it exhibits five well-defined and distinct systems of this kind. One might suppose that one outward current was much like another, and that for practical purposes some rather sloppy average would be adequate for any but the nicest of analyses. However, the very dramatically different effects of various drugs, all "K-current blockers," indubitably result from their subtly different actions upon the various ionic currents. However, a nugget of truth remains, because it is experimentally very difficult to tease out the various strands that contribute to the amorphous outward current soup. Our original articles should be consulted for information on exactly how these distinctions were drawn (4,7,8,13,40,143). The following currents have been described.

I_A

The transient outward current reported by Stevens in this volume's predecessor, and subsequently termed I_A by Connor and Stevens (52) is found in essentially identical form in bullfrog

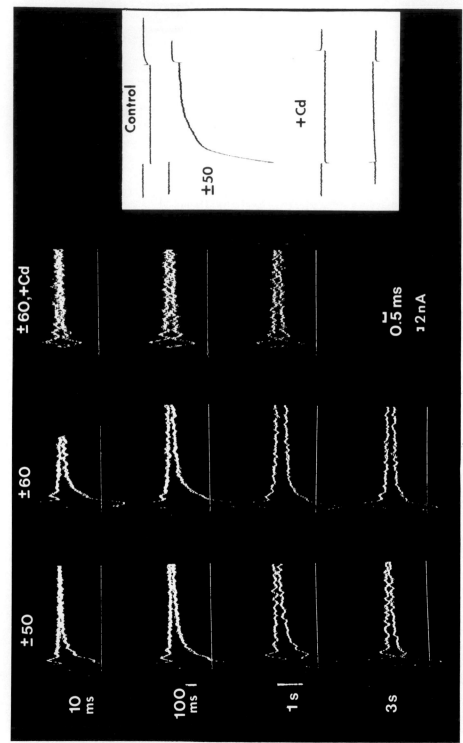

FIG. 3. Inactivation of calcium current in bullfrog neurons. *Right panel* Chart records of the time course of currents elicited by 4-sec long depolarizations or hyperpolarizations (50 mV in magnitude; holding potential −40 mV) before and after adding cadmium (100 μM). The oscilloscope pictures on the left show tail currents which follow the termination of the clamp steps (both negative and positive) at very fast sweep speeds. The positive-clamp step (which opens calcium channels) is followed by a brief cadmium-sensitive inward tail current, whereas the negative pulse is followed only by an under-damped capacity transient. The tail currents are shown for pulses lasting 10 msec, 100 msec, 1 sec, and 3 sec. The tail currents become smaller following 1-sec or especially 3-sec pulses, indicating the presence of genuine inactivation. Tail current is abolished by cadmium (P. R. Adams, *unpublished observations*).

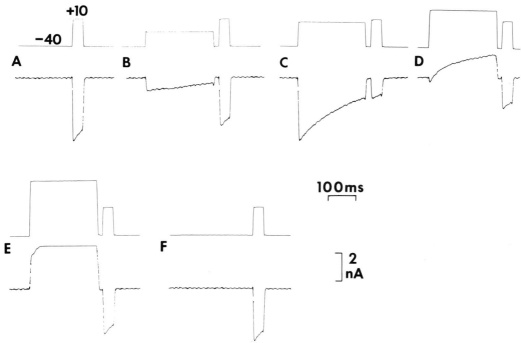

FIG. 4. Voltage dependence of I_{Ca} inactivation in bullfrog neurones. Top trace in each pair shows the membrane potential; bottom trace shows the clamp current (holding potential −40 mV). Traces A and F show the size of the calcium current elicited by a step to +10 mV at the beginning and at the end of the experiment, whereas traces A through E show the effects of a depolarizing prepulse of progressively increasing size. Inactivation of calcium current is maximal for depolarizing prepulses of intermediate size (C) (from Adams et al., ref. 8).

ganglion cells. A-current, by definition, shows two striking features: both its activation range and its inactivation range straddle rest potential, and activation is faster than inactivation. Thus, if the cell is held near rest potential and hyperpolarized, the steady ongoing inactivation is partly removed. When the cell is returned to rest potential, A-current first activates and then inactivates, resulting in a transient outward current (Fig. 5). The time course of activation is too fast to measure satisfactorily, but the current peaks in about 5 msec (Fig. 5). It then decays exponentially with a time constant of about 50 msec (Fig. 6).

Removal of inactivation also appears to occur exponentially, as shown by hyperpolarizing the cell for variable intervals, and measuring the size of the A-current that is subsequently attained during a fixed test depolarization (Fig. 5). The time constant of this process, about 150 msec (Fig. 6), does not obviously depend on membrane potential; however, if inactivation and removal of inactivation both represent a single kinetic step, it is possible that the under-

lying time constant does show some voltage dependence, obscured by measurement scatter (Fig. 6C).

A hyperpolarizing pulse of a half sec or more will result in some steady level of inactivation being reached, the magnitude of which depends on the size of the hyperpolarization (Fig. 7). In bullfrog neurons, this curve lies slightly more to the left than is the case in many other cells (27,52,75,134) with the result that fairly extreme hyperpolarization is needed to demonstrate the effects of this current on normal cell firing. These effects are two-fold. First, large hyperpolarizing electrotonic potentials do not decay back to baseline smoothly, but show a hyperpolarizing notch (51). Second, the development of this notch, and the underlying outward current, inhibit the development of anodal break action potentials. Thus, paradoxically, small hyperpolarizing stimuli are more effective in eliciting anodal break firing than are large stimuli.

If, starting from a hyperpolarized level, the cell is subjected to increasingly large depolarizations, the A-current elicited becomes larger

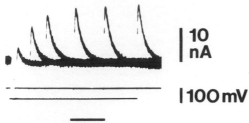

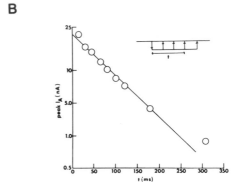

FIG. 5. A-current in a bullfrog ganglion cell; two-electrode voltage clamp. Muscarine (10 μM) was present to inhibit the M-current. The cell was held at −30 mV and stepped to −90 mV for various times. *Top trace:* membrane current; *bottom trace:* membrane potential. The A-current is seen as a rapidly rising but transient outward current that becomes larger as the repriming hyperpolarization is made longer. (D. A. Brown and P. R. Adams, *unpublished observations*.)

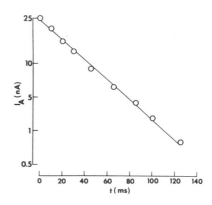

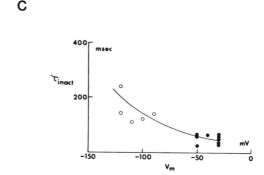

and larger (Fig. 7), partly because more and more A-conductance is being activated and partly because the driving force for K-currents is increasing. Presumably at some sufficiently positive potential, all of the A-channels transiently open, and any further increase in current magnitude with further depolarization would reflect only the ever-increasing driving force. If these effects could be separated, one could calculate the maximum attainable A-conductance. However, this experiment is impossible to perform, because other even larger K-currents intervene and distort the records. Unfortunately, 4-AP is not a selective blocker of I_A in bullfrog neurons as it is in many other systems; therefore, it has not yet been possible to dissect out the contribution of I_A to the total outward current seen at positive potentials. However, by assuming that the instantaneous I-V relation for A-channels is linear, that $E_K = -80mV$, and that G_A varies as a Boltzmann function of potential, it is possible to guess that the maximal A-conductance is about 100 nS and that the half-activation voltage is $\cong -40$ mV.

The contribution of I_A to normal cell firing is difficult to assess because the true resting potential of bullfrog neurons is uncertain (see below). If it is as negative as −70 mV, not all of the A-conductance will be inactive, and thus depolarizing excitatory postsynaptic potentials (EPSPs) might trigger enough I_A to slow or even to block spike discharge. Because the activation and inactivation ranges for I_A in bullfrog cells differ so widely, it is extremely unlikely that any

FIG. 6. Time course of inactivation and its removal of I_A in bullfrog ganglion cells. **A** shows a semilog plot of the time course of I_A following the initial peak elicited by a step depolarization from −100 mV to −40 mV. **B** shows a semilog plot of the peak apltude of A during depolarizations to −40 mV from an initial holding potential also of −40 mV with interposed hyperpolarizations of various durations. **C** collects time constants obtained from such plots for inactivation (●) and removal of inactivation (○) in several cells. The form of the line is quite speculative. (D. A. Brown and P. R. Adams, *unpublished observations*.)

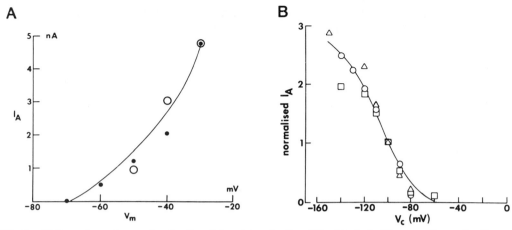

FIG. 7. Voltage dependence of activation (**A**) and inactivation (**B**) of I_A in bullfrog ganglion cells. The amplitude of the transient component of outward current (in the presence of muscarine) was measured for two different protocols. **A:** The cell was held at -110 mV for approximately 1 sec, and depolarized to the indicated potentials. **B:** The size of the 1-sec long conditioning hyperpolarizations varied. Different symbols represent different cells. From Adams et al., ref. 4.

"window current," i.e., steady state current resulting from the failure of I_A to inactivate completely, can contribute to the resting potential. If steady state activation and inactivation do show some overlap, yet inactivation is more voltage-dependent than activation, a maintained outward current that *decreases* with depolarization and that might confer a negative resistance characteristic could be observed (54).

I_K

In the Hodgkin-Huxley axon, as well as in real frog nodes of Ranvier [though not in rat nodes (48)], the delayed rectifier performs the vital role of swiftly repolarizing the membrane following the peak of the action potential. Although bullfrog neurons possess a large and quite respectable delayed rectifier system, we have recently concluded that in these cells it plays only a minor role in spike repolarization. The properties of the bullfrog system will first be reviewed; the reasons for exculpating it from a major role in spike repolarization will then be discussed.

The major similarities of the bullfrog cell body current I_K to the classical delayed rectifier of node of Ranvier are: (a) the sigmoidal turn-on of the current following step depolarizations; (b) the marked speeding of the turn on as the test potential is made more positive; and (c) clear sensitivity to TEA, the half-blocking concentration being about 1 mM in both cases (90). Indeed, the time course of activation could be described

by equations similar to those used by Frankenhauser (68), except that the absolute values of the rate constants are about 10 times less in ganglion cells.

Following depolarizing steps lasting several seconds, I_K was found to inactivate almost completely, with a time constant of about 5 sec. However, this inactivation can be largely removed by quite brief pulses to negative levels. This can lead to an awkward "swoop" phenomenon in voltage-clamp experiments on "M-current" (see below). In these experiments, the cell is often held at a relatively depolarized level— -30 mV or even -25 mV. When the membrane potential is set initially to -25 mV, a small degree of I_K activation occurs, followed by inactivation. This is seen as a transient overshoot in the outward current, which over several sec subsides to a constant level. This overshooting or "swoop" current will be evoked each time the membrane is briefly hyperpolarized and then returned to -25 mV.

Spike repolarization in bullfrog cells normally occurs at a velocity approaching 100 V/sec, and is followed by a distinct afterhyperpolarization (AHP). The magnitude of I_K (about 100 nA at $+50$ mV) is ample to provide the capacity current needed to repolarize the membrane at this rate; however, because the time constant of I_K's activation is larger than 10 msec at 0 mV, and still several msec even at $+50$ mV, it is unlikely that adequate outward current could be developed quickly enough by this system. This is supported by the finding that TEA is not much more effective than is cadmium in slowing spike repolarization (discussed in I_C below). Furthermore, virtually all of the outward current that develops during brief spike-like rectangular depolarizations to 0 mV is calcium-sensitive (Fig. 1), and thus, by definition, *not* I_K. However, until a specific blocker of the delayed rectifier becomes available, the possible role of I_K in the early part of the spike AHP, or in spike repolarization in situations in which I_C is not active, cannot be easily evaluated.

I_M

Both the potassium currents discussed so far show dramatic, and practically complete, inactivation. They are ubiquitous currents that were first well-described in molluscs, although they do not have major clearly defined roles in bullfrog neuron electrical behavior. The M-current, although it is another voltage-dependent potassium current, differs in that it shows no detectable inactivation, has not yet been clearly described in molluscs, and serves a pivotal role in influencing the excitability of bullfrog neurons. The latter feature has been relatively easy to document, because a wide range of specific blockers of M-current exist. The most significant feature of I_M is that many of these blockers are themselves neurotransmitters, and two of them are synaptically released onto the ganglion cells and thus physiologically modulate the firing pattern of the postsynaptic cells.

These unusual features have led to the paradoxical situation that this upstart among ionic currents is now the best characterized of all those present in bullfrog neurons. Hodgkin-Huxley equations describing its activation in the potential range − 100 mV to − 10 mV are available. Qualitatively, these can be summarized by saying that the average maximum conductance is 84 nS, the half-activation voltage is − 35 mV, the time constant at that voltage is 150 msec, and the effective "steepness factor" (corresponding to the valency of the gating particle) is 10 mV.

It is relatively easy to imagine how a theoretical neuron endowed with such a current, a membrane capacity, and some background voltage-independent leakage resistance would behave when subject to applied extrinsic current pulses. Suppose the leakage were such that the resting potential was about − 50 mV. At this potential, the M-conductance would take on a value of 15 nS, causing an outward current of

about 0.4 nA to flow. The inward leakage current would also be 0.4 nA or the membrane potential would change. If a small hyperpolarizing current (I_{hyp}) is suddenly applied to the "cell" from an extrinsic source (such as an intracellular microelectrode), the membrane potential will start to move negatively, and simultaneously the M-conductance will start to fall. If the cell time constant is much shorter than the time constant for I_M at − 50 mV, the first effect will occur faster than the second, and the result will be an initial hyperpolarization, followed by a "droop." However, the time course of the droop will not be exactly exponential, because the time constant for G_M deactivation is itself a function of membrane potential. The predicted membrane potential trajectory is obtained as the solution to the equation

$$I_{hyp} = C \frac{dV}{dt} + (V - E_K)\, G_M + (V - E_L) G_L$$

G_L, E_L are the leak conductance and battery, and G_M is the voltage and time-dependent value of the M-conductance. An example is given in Fig. 8. The overall effect is to stabilize the membrane potential near the resting value. A similar stabilization could also be achieved in principle by inserting a large parallel voltage-independent conductance with a "battery" equal to the resting potential. However, since this battery would represent the combined electromotive force (EMF) of several separate ionic species, it would be metabolically costly. Furthermore, it would not show the same time dependence as the M-current mechanism. Similar "droop" of the membrane potential back to rest can also be seen during the application of very small depolarizing current pulses; however, if the current pulse is made any larger, action potentials are generated, and their waveform obscures the underlying droop due to M-current activation. Nevertheless, such droop is probably still present in a latent form, and tends to raise the threshold for subsequent spikes if the current pulse is maintained. The result is striking adaptation of the initial discharge, such that a maximum of one to three spikes is normally seen. However, if the M-current is inhibited by applying muscarine, prolonged repetitive firing can be seen during quite weak current pulses.

In two common situations, the effects of M-current on membrane voltage trajectories are particularly obvious. The first is that the intracellularly recorded fast EPSP (FEPSP) in these cells often shows an AHP, which is abolished by muscarinic agonists (148,164). This is undoubt-

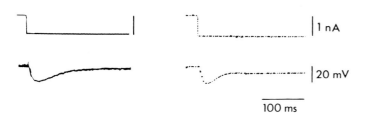

$|$ 1 nA

$|$ 20 mV

100 ms

FIG. 8. Observed (*left*) and predicted (*right*) "droop" during hyperpolarizing current injection. The top traces monitor the injected current waveform. The bottom traces show the intracellularly-recorded membrane potential of a ganglion cell (*left*), or the response of the analog current model of Adams et al. (*4*). (A. Constanti, D. A. Brown, and P. R. Adams, *unpublished observations.*)

edly caused by M-conductance, which is activated *during* the FEPSP but which outlasts it. We refer to this phenomenon as M-current bounce, since it can be mimicked by injection of a short depolarizing current pulse. FEPSPs recorded with external electrodes do not show this AHP component, perhaps because unimpaled cells have resting potentials sufficiently negative that negligible standing M-current is present (164). Certainly, very carefully impaled cells can have resting potentials up to -60 mV, and even here leakage shunting caused by microelectrode damage may still be present. This is also suggested by the observation that even higher leakage resistances are observed using whole-cell patch-clamp recording. An independent measurement of the true resting potential of bullfrog ganglion cells would be very useful.

The second situation occurs following an action potential. If the slow component of the AHP is absent (see below), the brief component can turn off sufficient resting M-conductance so that the membrane transiently depolarizes following the initially passive decay of the fast AHP, leading to a bouncy afterdepolarization. The slow component of the AHP, if prominent, will mask the M-generated afterdepolarization.

The primary effect of several neurotransmitters on the ganglion cell membrane is reduction of the size of the maximum available M-conductance G_M, without affecting the kinetics or voltage dependence of the remaining current. Because no convincing single-channel records of M-current have yet been obtained, it is not known whether this reduction of G_M is caused by a reduction in the effective number of channels or by a reduced single-channel conductance. The transmitters that exert this effect are acetylcholine (ACh), acting on muscarinic receptors, teleost leutinizing hormone-releasing hormone (T-LHRH), and substance P acting on their appropriate peptide receptors, and uridine triphosphate (UTP) and ATP, acting on a rather poorly defined nucleotide receptor (1,5,11,104). Dose–response curves for some of these agents,

or for closely related molecules, are now available (5,104,105). The EC_{50}s for T-LHRH and muscarine are 0.3 and 1 μM, respectively, with the curves exhibiting Hill coefficients of ≤ 1.0. EC_{50}s for substance P are extremely variable, but range down to 2 nM, a concentration at which many neuropeptides are active in isolated systems.

Synaptic Responses in Bullfrog Neurons

M-current is also intimately involved in the generation of some of the synaptic responses in these cells. These are generated by preganglionic axons (usually one per cell) that form many *en passant* boutons over the cell body and initial segment (169). The synaptic circuitry of the ganglion is shown in Fig. 9. Both B and C cells exhibit fast EPSPs generated by ACh acting on nicotinic receptors that are probably located under the presynaptic boutons (124). In both B and C cells, some of this ACh can also reach muscarinic receptors (of unknown location). In B cells, the activation of muscarinic receptors leads, after a latency of about 100 msec, to the generation of a slow low-amplitude depolarization, the slow EPSP (SEPSP) which peaks in 1–2 sec, and lasts half a min. During the SEPSP, the excitability of the cell is enhanced, so that, for example, test depolarizing current pulses that normally evoke only one or two spikes can now trigger trains of spikes (Fig. 10). This enhanced excitability is *not* caused by the slow depolarization, since it is not mimicked by depolarizing the cell with extrinsic steady current (Fig. 10). Neither is it caused by a simple change in cell resistance, since the effect cannot be obtained by increasing the size of the testing current pulse. It has been shown that during the SEPSP M-current is, as expected, depressed (6), and this is probably responsible for the increased excitability. Depolarization during the SEPSP also partly reflects M-current suppression, but is also caused by some increase in membrane conductance to ions with a net positive reversal

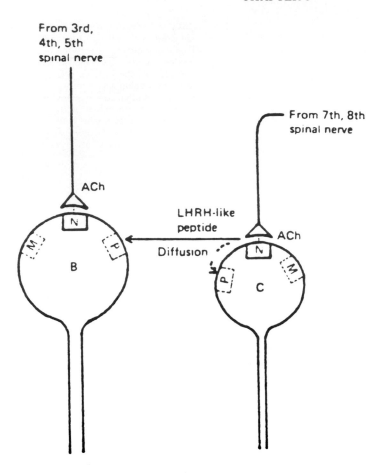

From 3rd,
4th, 5th
spinal nerve

From 7th, 8th
spinal nerve

ACh

LHRH-like
peptide

Diffusion

ACh

B

C

FIG. 9. A diagram of the probable synaptic circuitry in the bullfrog sympathetic ganglion. (From ref. 101, with permission.)

potential, especially in cells in which impalement damage is minimal or absent (22,105,114).

In C cells, muscarinic receptor activation following nerve stimulation results mainly in a potassium conductance *increase* (61). Although C cells show normal M-current, it is much less sensitive to muscarinic receptor activation than in B cells (106). The effect of the K-conductance increase is to hyperpolarize the cell (i.e., generate a SIPSP) as well as to inhibit it.

Preganglionic axons innervating C cells contain and release a peptide resembling LHRH in addition to ACh (100). Peptide release is particularly marked following short trains of stimuli at about 10 Hz. The peptide is now thought to be similar or identical to the LHRH of teleost fish, T-LHRH. Following release it acts to reduce M-current in C cells and, particularly, in neighboring B cells (105,106). This effect again leads to enhanced excitability and depolarization, this time reaching a peak in about 1 min and lasting nearly 10 min. For this reason, the depolarization is called the late slow EPSP.

Although the depolarizing slow synaptic events in these ganglion cells are commonly referred to as the SEPSP and late SEPSP, it should be remembered that the depolarizations themselves are rather weak, and that the most important feature of the synaptic *responses* is instead the enhanced excitability. For this reason, it might in some ways be better to refer to slow and late excitatory postsynaptic responses (SEPSR and LEPSR).

The ability of transmitters to regulate properties of voltage-dependent conductances represents an important new class of synaptic action, which was first clearly described for the heart (146). Previously, transmitters had been simply regarded as either excitatory or inhibitory, based largely on whether their reversal potentials were above or below spike threshold. However, transmitter actions of the "modulatory" type cannot be so simply classified. In general, inhibition of M-current will be excitatory in overall effect, yet because the resulting depolarization is small or negligible, no direct or

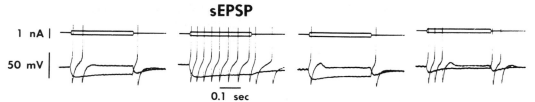

FIG. 10. Excitability changes during the slow excitatory postsynaptic potential SEPSP in bullfrog neurons. The records on the left was obtained by injecting small current pulses into the cell (monitored in top traces). The second pair of records was obtained during similar current injections, but at the peak of a SEPSP elicited by repetitive preganglionic nerve stimulation (10 stimuli at 10 Hz). The third pair of records shows recovery after the end of the SEPSP, whereas the fourth pair (*right*) shows the effect of depolarizing the cell to the level obtained during the SEPSP (from S. W. Jones, *unpublished observations*).

subliminal tendency to fire action potentials may be seen. However, the excitatory effect of a classical synaptic input may be enhanced by concurrent activation of the M-current inhibiting input providing a form of "enabling" device (Fig. 11). One can easily imagine other nonclassical synaptic actions that would change *statistical* features of neuronal discharge (e.g., random vs burst firing rate). It would be difficult to call such an input "excitatory." Another example is a persistent nonregenerative inward current triggered by depolarization and operating near the resting potential region. Because such a system operates as a negative conductance, it can cancel out cable attenuation produced by low membrane resistance. It can thus make an extended neuronal structure look smaller electrically, thereby boosting remote dendritic EPSPs (117). A transmitter that regulated the size of such a conductance would thus control the "listening area" or "field of view" accessible to the somatic readout mechanisms.

Fast Ca-activated K-current: I_C

Patch recording reveals that the ganglion cell membrane contains high-conductance, voltage-dependent K channels closely resembling those seen in a variety of other vertebrate membranes (125,142). These channels require both membrane depolarization and physiological levels of intracellular calcium (0.1–10 μM) to open. At a fixed level of Ca, both the opening frequency and the mean open time increase with depolarization. These channels are blocked by low concentrations of external TEA and by internal barium (32,115,173). They are often referred to as *the* Ca-activated K channel, but since other quite different potassium channels can also be activated by internal Ca, this term is unsatisfactory. They have also been called the Big-K or

maxi-K channel. Here they will be referred to as the I_C channel. A typical patch, with an area of perhaps 5 μm^2, exhibits one to two such channels, so that a cell with a diameter of 50 μm could, if all these channels were open, generate an outward current of 50 nA at about +20 mV membrane potential. There is much evidence that such a large C-current can be generated, as, for example, by depolarizing voltage-clamp commands or by intracellular Ca injections. Results of such experiments are shown in Fig. 12. The upper section shows that the peak outward current generated by depolarizing step commands of 50-msec duration is greatly reduced by adding the Ca-antagonist manganese to the external solution. Furthermore, the dip in the current-voltage relation that occurs near +80 mV and that causes a characteristic N-shape is nearly eliminated in these conditions. The N-shape has been traditionally ascribed to a decrease in Ca-activated K-current concomitant with diminished Ca entry at very positive potentials (130). Threshold activation for the Ca-dependent outward current occurs at about −20 mV, corresponding to the threshold for I_{Ca} in this preparation.

Iontophoretic Ca injection elicits a large outward current that is both voltage dependent and TEA sensitive. Furthermore, the same amount of Ca entry, whether by iontophoresis or by voltage-dependent influx through the surface membrane, results in about the same size of outward current (14). If I_C conductance is activated by a combination of prolonged Ca-injection and maintained depolarization, a subsequent hyperpolarization will rapidly close the I_C channels. Although the detailed time course of such relaxations has not yet been analyzed, it is clear that the shut-down of these channels takes 5–20 msec, the shorter values being seen at more negative potentials. When the depolarization is re-

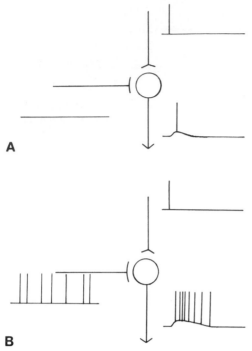

FIG. 11. Heterosynaptic facilitation by M-channel inhibition. An idealized nerve cell is shown receiving both a classical input (from the top) and a nonclassical M-current inhibiting input (from the side). Two cases are illustrated. **A:** the nonclassical input is silent, while a single spike in the classical input generates an excitatory postsynaptic potential EPSP and a spike in the postsynaptic cell. **B:** tonic input via the nonclassical pathway inhibits voltage dependent currents such as the M-current, such that the classical EPSP is enhanced and excitability is increased. The result of this form of heterosynaptic action is a change in the input–output relation of the cell.

stored, I_C channels reopen along a roughly exponential time course.

The response to Ca injection is on the whole very robust, although rather variable from cell to cell. For example, it can still be seen in cells that have virtually no membrane potential and are probably "dead." However, if large injections are repeatedly made, the response eventually gets slower, smaller, and rides an increasingly outward baseline. Our interpretation of these observations is that all the Ca injected can initially be rapidly taken up into an intracellular storage compartment (30,31,88), perhaps lying close to the plasma membrane (161). As this store fills up, the calcium loads presented to the cell are less and less efficiently disposed of, until stores are completely full and the last injection provokes an irreversible increase in outward current. This irreversible outward current still has all the hallmarks of I_C: it can be turned off by hyperpolarization or by TEA, and is accompanied by membrane noise characteristic of these highly conducting channels. Such a Ca-loaded state may also occur when cells are depolarized in isotonic potassium. These cells appear to be very leaky, but can be restored to a high resistance state by hyperpolarization. If such calcium loading were to occur under physiological conditions, presumably the cell would hyperpolarize until I_C became small enough to match depolarizing influences exactly. The calcium load would then be sequestered or pumped out.

The kinetics of I_C produced by voltage steps and normal Ca entry are quite complicated and variable. Typically, the current rises within a few msec without any initial sigmoidicity, reaches a peak at about 5 msec, and then quickly droops to a lower level. It then decays very slowly if the step is maintained for sec or min. It is the droop that is the most variable. In a study by MacDermott and Weight, (121; see also 36) the droop was very prominent, which led them to speak of a Ca-dependent transient outward current; in our own records, the droop is often partly concealed by the concomitantly developing delayed rectifier current. The droop likely is real and not just a result of massive K-accumulation in the space between the neuron surface and surrounding glia because it is still seen in raised potassium (Brown and Adams, *unpublished observations*) and in cultured "naked" ganglion cells. Furthermore, the corresponding tail current seen if repolarization is made at the peak of the outward current or into the droop shows parallel decreases in magnitude.

The time course of these tail currents has also been explored, either by making small probing jumps during the 30-sec to 1-min maintained phase of the current, or by quick repolarization early in the current (1–10 msec). The former experiment revealed turn-off kinetics in the 4- to 20-msec range, depending on test potential. At least near -10mV, similar kinetics were also obtained by steps during iontophoresis (see above) or by noise analysis during prolonged depolarizations (7). The latter method gave a faster result, around 2 msec at -40 mV (Fig. 1). The simplest explanation of this discrepancy is different weighting of the amplitudes of components of a multiexponential relaxation in different types of experiments. Nevertheless, the transient early and maintained late components of "I_C" may in fact be contributed by channels with different properties.

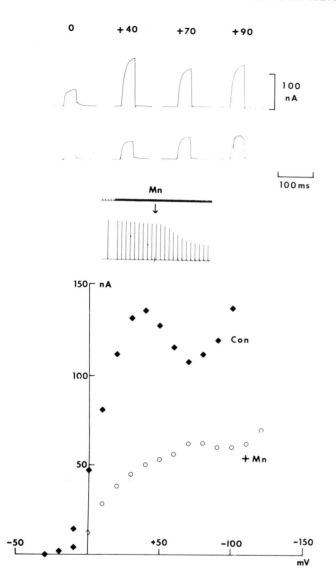

FIG. 12. Calcium-dependence of large outward currents in bullfrog ganglion cells. The holding potential was −40 mV and the cell was stepped to various depolarized levels for 50 msec, using a two-electrode voltage clamp. The records in the upper panel show specimens of the outward currents before (*top row*) and after (*bottom row*) adding 4 mM manganese chloride to the external Ringer's solution. The middle panel shows a slow time base chart recording of the large outward currents elicited by 50 msec depolarizations to +50 mV every 10 sec. The graph shows the current-voltage relation for the peak outward current before and after adding 4 mM manganese (A. Constanti, D. A. Brown, and P. R. Adams, *unpublished observations*.)

If this is *not* the case, a puzzle arises. I_{Ca} in bullfrog cells shows no sign of early rapid inactivation (cf. 46). A transient component of I_{Ca} could of course be missed if the rigorous conditions used to block outward currents also eliminate a component of I_{Ca} (cf. 14,16). Neither does I_C elicited by Ca iontophoresis ever show an early rapid inactivation. The temporal resolution of the iontophoretic method may be inadequate to reveal this, if it is present, but no sign of transience is seen when I_C is activated by depolarizing steps applied in the presence of steady internal Ca. Therefore, why is I_C itself partly transient, often showing a prominent early droop? At first, we felt that this could occur if internal Ca buffering mechanisms acted with a delay (corresponding to a finite, and realistic, forward binding rate constant). However, such a buffering delay would probably only act to enhance the rate of rise of the internal Ca concentration following a step increase in surface Ca permeability. The rise would still be monotonic. Transience could arise simply from some geometrical relationship of I_{Ca} and I_C channels. The only obvious solution to this puzzle is to postulate that initial Ca entry can produce a sudden release of Ca from an internal store very near the inner surface of the plasma membrane (88,138). This store would have to be very readily depleted. Such a component of release has been described in cardiac cells (97), although there it seems to be rather slow.

There is other evidence for activation of I_C by Ca-release from internal stores. For example, spontaneous miniature outward currents (SMOCs) seen in some cultured cells have been postulated to result from random opening of Ca-channels in such stores (10,13,40,147). This release appears to be triggered by surface membrane potential, however. Much longer-lasting spontaneous hyperpolarizations in xanthine-treated or internal citrate-treated preparations seem to be potassium conductances triggered by synchronized internal calcium release (112,155). Voltage-clamp analysis has revealed two components of outward current underlying these slow spontaneous events (108), the earlier one of which is TEA sensitive and may thus correspond to I_C.

A transient Ca-dependent outward current that is probably related to I_C can be seen with a slightly different protocol, one that is similar to that used to study A-current. The cell is hyperpolarized to -100 mV for about 100 msec and then stepped to various potentials in the -50 mV to -10 mV range. This procedure elicits a transient outward current. Steps to -50 to -30 mV elicit a conventional A-current, but steps to -20 or -10 mV elicit an additional rapidly decaying outward component that, unlike A-current, is readily blocked by TEA or by omitting extracellular Ca from the Ringer's solution (Fig. 13). These latter two features suggest that it is related to, or identical with, C-current. It is clearly quite distinct from A-current in terms of pharmacology, voltage sensitivity, and kinetics.

The main role of I_C seems to be to produce rapid spike repolarization (7,121). It is ideally suited to this task since it activates very rapidly at positive potentials and rapidly turns off at the

potential achieved at the peak of the AHP. Although TEA does block the delayed rectifier, the observed broadening of the action potential in this drug (34) is almost certainly mainly caused by the equally potent action of this drug on I_C. In many cells, especially those damaged by electrode impalement, the spike AHP then decays essentially passively back to rest, perhaps with an M-current "bounce." Nevertheless, the I_C system has not been reset to zero following such a spike, because internal Ca is still elevated. It is thus theoretically possible that I_C would activate even more rapidly in the wake of such a "priming" spike were another spike to follow within a short interval.

In other cells, particularly those that have suffered little impalement damage, the spike AHP does not decay passively, and can last as long as 1 sec. This slow AHP component also reflects Ca-activated K current (45,113,163), but the current involved is quite different from I_C.

Slow Ca-activated K-current: I_{AHP}

It has been recently shown that the slow component of the AHP is generated by an outward current that, like I_C, is a calcium-dependent potassium current (38, 63, 143; see also 131–133). This current, which we call I_{AHP}, differs from I_C so radically that it is likely to be generated by a separate set of ionic channels, although the individual channels have not yet been resolved. The two currents differ in size, kinetics, voltage-dependence, and pharmacology. Thus, I_{AHP} is small (typically 1 nA at -50 mV) and slow (deactivating with a time constant of about 250 msec). The underlying conductance change, G_{AHP}, does not appear to be directly voltage sen-

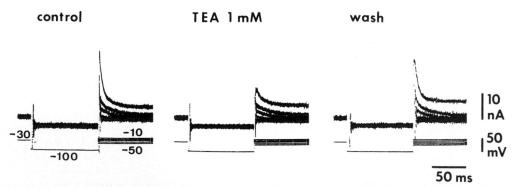

FIG. 13. Components of transient outward current in bullfrog ganglion cells clamped with two microelectrodes. Muscarine (10 μM) was present to inhibit M-current, and the cell was held at -30 mV and stepped for 100 msec to -100 mV. Superimposed traces were obtained with this protocol before, during, and after washing out 1 mM TEA. (D. A. Brown and P. R. Adams, *unpublished observations.*)

sitive in the range -40 to -130 mV, apart from a small effect in the direction expected for constant field rectification. Of course G_{AHP} is indirectly voltage sensitive because of the requirement for calcium influx. It appears that G_{AHP} can be fully activated by very short depolarizations (3 to 5 msec). These depolarizations must be in the range -10 to $+70$ mV, which is also the range for activation of I_{Ca}. However, there does not seem to be perfect parallelism between the size of I_{Ca} and of the subsequent G_{AHP} increase, probably because G_{AHP} can be fully activated by very small rises in internal Ca. In Fig. 1, I_{AHP} shows as a very small, slow, Ca-dependent component of the tail current that follows brief depolarizations.

The pharmacological differences between I_C and I_{AHP} are even more striking. Only one blocker, TEA, has been found to prefer I_C to I_{AHP}. A range of other drugs, such as apamin, curare, pancuronium, and barium, select for I_{AHP} over I_C (40,97,143; Pennefather and Adams, *unpublished observations*). Several neurotransmitter-like drugs, such as muscarine, oxotremorine, and ATP also have appreciable activity against I_{AHP} (143,162). Nevertheless, the effects of these agents on I_M is more dramatic, and it is not yet known whether the same receptors or internal messengers are involved in regulation of I_M and I_{AHP}.

The shapes of the AHPs of bullfrog ganglion cells show great variability, being very sensitive to damage by microelectrode impalement. Injured cells often show a rapid passively decaying AHP, which may exhibit a small, slow tail. In healthier cells, the slower component becomes more prominent, reaching a point where the fast initial decay may be almost absent. Finally, in minimally damaged cells, the slow component is actually larger than the fast component, so that the slow AHP shows a rising phase. Although the AHP current itself may be absent in severely damaged cells, both I_C and I_{AHP} may be essentially constant as a cell evolves through all these various shapes, as shown in Fig. 14. The spike AHP is considered to be generated by the injection of an outward current, comprised of a delta (Δ) function plus a slow exponentially decaying function, into a passive RC circuit. The Δ function represents I_C (actually a very rapidly decaying outward current) and the exponential term I_{AHP}. As the "cell" input resistance is varied from 25 to 50 and 100 MΩ, the predicted AHP shape varies much as is seen in real neurons as the microelectrode seals in and the impalement leak diminishes. The two main defects

of this model are: (1) current saturation as V approaches E_K is not included; and (2) the role of I_M in sculpting AHPs when the initial membrane potential is worse than -60 mV is neglected.

Because I_{AHP} is a small slow potassium current like I_M, one might expect it to play a similar role. Selective blockers of I_{AHP} can enhance repetitive firing in much the same way as already described for I_M. The relative contribution of these two currents to spike frequency adaptation and its modulation by transmitters must be evaluated. In principle, I_{AHP} should act only as a temporary brake, because following cessation of spike firing internal calcium will eventually decay back to its resting level, whereas I_M will remain elevated throughout a depolarizing stimulus.

RAT SYMPATHETIC GANGLION CELLS

There are now about 11 published voltage-clamp studies of rat superior cervical sympathetic ganglion cells, utilizing both one and two microelectrodes, and both intact *in vitro* and tissue-cultured preparations (27,28,39,41,56,70, 72–75,152). These neurons represent an interesting half-way house between the adendritic frog cells and the elaborately arborized hippocampal pyramidal cells. They also represent an intermediate cell type in terms of fragility and richness of synaptic inputs. However, no major new general insight has been yet obtained with these cells.

Two studies have been made of cable properties, utilizing the equivalent cylinder approximation (27,89). McAfee and colleagues reported that ρ and L (see section below) were about 2 and 0.7, meaning that the cells were electrically compact, but not isopotential. Belluzzi et al. found that most of their cells were strictly isopotential, judging by the excellence of fits of charging curves to single exponentials. A few cells showed a fast component in the charging curve, which on analysis gave $L \cong 1.7$ and $\rho \cong 1.6$. However, the cells studied by this group had much lower input resistances and shorter time constants than those of Henon et al., suggesting either a temperature difference or impalement damage. Therefore, the possibility certainly exists that space-clamp problems may distort the time course of rapid clamp currents in rat neurons.

Inward Currents

Figure 15 illustrates typical currents observed with a two-electrode voltage clamp. Part A

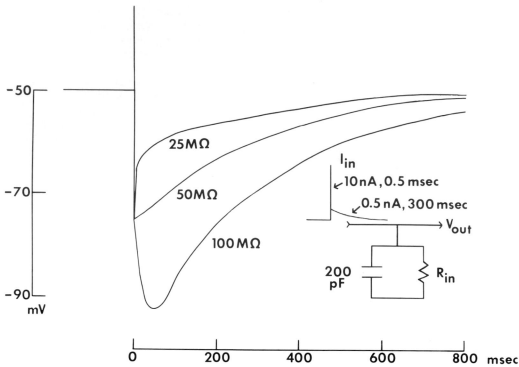

FIG. 14. A passive circuit model of afterhyperpolarizations in bullfrog ganglion cells. The ganglion cell was modelled as a fixed leakage resistor in parallel with a membrane capacity. An outward current waveform was injected into this circuit consisting of the sum of a Δ function (representing I_c) and an exponentially decaying component (representing I_{AHP}). Calculations were done for three different values of the leakage resistor R_L. For $R_L = 25$ MΩ, the predicted AHP shows a rapidly rising phase which merges into a small slowly decaying component. For $R_L = 50$ MΩ only a slowly decaying phase is seen. For $R_L = 100$ MΩ the AHP rises very rapidly, shows a further rapid rise, and then decays slowly.

shows that starting from a relatively depolarized holding potential a step to -25 mV evokes a very brief inward current which is blocked by TTX (28,74). This is thought to be a Hodgkin-Huxley sodium current. After blockage of I_{Na} and suppression of some of the outward K-currents by external TEA (28) preferably combined with cesium loading (74) a smaller, better sustained inward current can be recorded, with a slightly more positive threshold (74) (Fig.16). This can be blocked by removing Ca from the external medium or by adding cadmium, and thus is probably a calcium current. It reaches its peak within a few msec, and thereafter slowly declines. In normal external Ca, the peak current is about 2 nA, and it is as large as 10 nA in 10 mM external Ca (74). It has been suggested that the activation of I_{Ca} is highly sigmoidal (28) or approximately exponential (74); however, in view of space-clamp problems, this discrepancy may be more apparent than real. It is at least clear that both activation and deactivation are

very fast (28,74) (Fig. 17), and this hampers determination of the activation curve. The time for the current to decay back to zero during maintained depolarizations is rather variable, probably partly because of variable contamination by outward current, but is usually several hundred msec (Fig. 18). After repolarizing to the holding potential, the inactivation wears off, with a time constant of several sec (Fig. 18). The extent of inactivation, assayed by a prepulse/test pulse sequence, is maximal for depolarizations yielding maximum inward current (Fig. 19), suggesting that it largely reflects Ca-mediated inactivation.

One of the most interesting features of I_{Ca} in this preparation is that it is inhibited by low concentrations of norepinephrine (74) (Fig. 20). This in turn affects several calcium-dependent potentials that can be recorded in these ganglion cells (93).

Last, large, long-lasting hyperpolarizations can evoke a slowly developing inward current (70) (Fig. 21). It now appears that this may re-

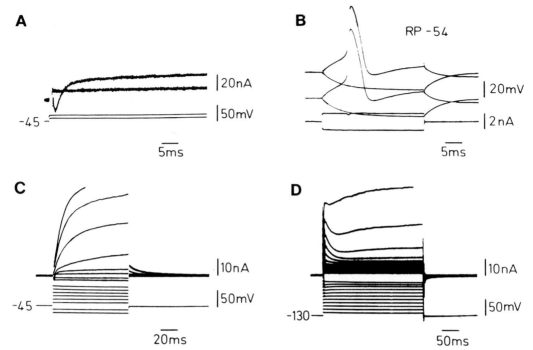

FIG. 15. Current and voltage responses in a rat sympathetic neuron recorded with two intracellular KCl microelectrodes at room temperature. Normal Krebs' solution was used; other conditions are as in ref. 74. **A** shows currents elicited in dual microelectrode voltage clamp by step depolarizations from a holding potential of −45 mV. **B** shows the current clamp responses at the resting potential recorded by both microelectrodes. **C** shows the large outward currents elicited by steps from −45 mV. **D** shows currents for various depolarizations from a holding potential of −130 mV. Note that the threshold for A-current is 30 mV negative to that for the sustained outward currents (M. Galvan and P. R. Adams, *unpublished observations.*)

flect a cadmium-sensitive voltage-dependent chloride current (152).

Outward Currents

Under normal conditions, the various outward currents elicited by depolarizing steps tend to dwarf the inward current (Fig. 15). Furthermore, the shape of the outward currents depends critically on the holding potential. Starting from rest potential or slightly depolarized to rest, the outward currents rise monotonically, whereas if the holding potential is very negative to rest, an early transient component becomes prominent (Fig. 15). As one might anticipate, this transient current behaves as an A-current, though there is some disagreement as to whether it is Ca-dependent (27,75). Both groups report similar activation threshold ($\cong$ −60 mV), although the current is larger in the study by Galvan and Sedlmeir (ref. 75, 40 nA at −30 mV) than in the study by Belluzzi et al. (ref. 27, 10 nA at −30 mV). In both studies, the time to peak is very rapid

(1–3 msec), and thus the time course of activation is difficult to analyze. In cultured cells, the activation seems to be somewhat slower (70).

Steady state removal of inactivation starts at about −60 mV, and is complete by −110 to −130 mV (27,75). Removal of inactivation procedes exponentially with a voltage-dependent time constant in the 10–40 msec range. Onset of inactivation has a time constant around 10 msec, although again it shows voltage dependence. In summary, the A-current of rat sympathetic neurons resembles that of bullfrog neurons, except that it is rather larger, faster, and steady state curves lie about 10 mV more positive. Belluzzi et al. suggest that in rat, I_A may be an important contributor to spike repolarization, although a major contribution from other large outward currents was not ruled out.

The outward currents that survive holding at $\cong$ −50 mV (Fig. 15) have been separated into Ca-dependent and -independent components by both Galvan and Sedlmeier (75) and Belluzzi et

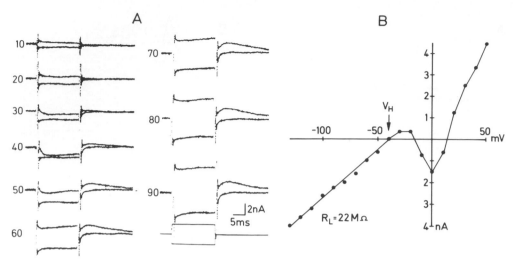

FIG. 16. Two-electrode voltage clamp in Cs-loaded cells (74). **A:** The holding potential was −40 mV, and in each pair of traces equal and opposite voltage steps of the indicated size applied. Note that hyperpolarizing steps are followed by an A-current, whereas depolarizing steps are followed by inward tail currents. **B:** a plot of the peak inward currents during the steps (M. Galvan and P. R. Adams, *unpublished observations*).

al. (27). Both groups assume that the Ca-resistant component of large outward current is delayed rectifier. This identification is supported by TEA sensitivity and slow inactivation, as well as by potassium dependence (70). However, its activation does not appear to be sigmoidal, which is normally part of the definition of "delayed rectification."

Two separate Ca-dependent K-currents analogous to I_C and I_{AHP} of bullfrog have not yet been clearly identified, but it seems probable that the complexity of the time course of the Ca-dependent outward currents reflects such a distinction. The tail currents shown by Belluzzi et al. (28) are very fast, whereas those illustrated by Brown et al. (39) are small and slow. Freschi (70) has separated a fast, large tail from a slow, small one, and comments that the slow tail is less susceptible to TEA than part of the fast one. The late part of the spike AHP in these cells is TEA resistant (128). The I_C-like component is presumably responsible for the N-shaped I-V relation in these cells (73) and may contribute to spike repolarization.

The remaining outward current is M-like, and clearly responsive to muscarinic agonists (56) (Fig. 21). Its properties are very similar to those of the bullfrog homologue. Some of the differences, such as the somewhat more negative activation range, accord with the different resting potentials of these cells. Belluzzi et al. (28) claim that I_M may be identical to a component of cal-

cium-activated K-current, but this is difficult to reconcile with observation of I_M in the presence of cadmium (41). These conflicting data may reflect the presence of an I_{AHP}-like current. It has been shown recently that muscarinic agonists reduce a resting chloride conductance as well as G_M in these cells, especially when artificially chloride-loaded (41). Inhibition of both these systems seems to occur during the SEPSP (151).

Rat ganglion cells show even more dramatic adaptation than bullfrog neurons, usually showing only one spike in response to prolonged depolarizing current pulses. However, after muscarinic stimulation, the cells fire repetitively in response to current pulses, presumably because of inhibition of I_M. Possible contributions of I_{AHP} remain to be evaluated.

HIPPOCAMPAL PYRAMIDAL CELLS

CA1 and CA3 pyramidal cells are the vertebrate central neurons that have been most intensively studied using voltage-clamp techniques. Three types of preparation have been used: slices (15,37,38,42,76,85,86,101,102,116,176), freshly isolated adult neurons (140,170) and long-term dissociated or organotypic cultures from young animals or embryos (71,153,154). In addition, several different clamp techniques were used, ranging from two-microelectrode clamping, single-electrode switch clamping,

A

B

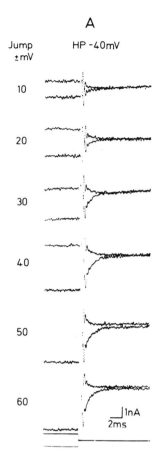

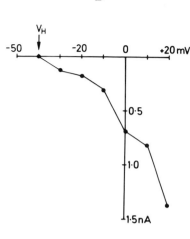

FIG. 17. Calcium tail currents in rat SCG cells; two-electrode clamp. Tail currents following steps to various potentials are shown. Note that the tails for depolarizing and hyperpolarizing steps are asymmetrical. The inward tail following depolarizing steps minus the reverse of the hyperpolarizing tail (capacity current) is assumed to reflect I_{Ca}, and is plotted in part **B**. (M. Galvan and P. R. Adams, *unpublished observations.*)

whole-cell patch recording, and on-cell single-channel recording. Because of this range of techniques and preparations, and because of intrinsic limitations of pyramidal cells themselves, the situation is much less clear-cut for these cells than for sympathetic ganglion cells. Nevertheless, these cells seem to display a richer palette of ionic conductances than do peripheral neurons, and a fair case can be made for the separate identity of the 10 listed in Table 2.

Before considering these currents one by one, the primary technical limitations of such studies should be emphasized. All the cells studied have dendrites, which are truncated in the acutely isolated cells and very extensive in slices. It is thus inevitable that perfect space-clamp conditions do not exist throughout these neurons when they are point-clamped at the soma. This problem is avoided by on-cell single-channel recordings, but such studies have other drawbacks, such as identification and quantitation of the channel types present. It is rather as though

objects were observed through a fish-eye lens, which affords a distorted but global view, or through a microscope, which gives an accurate but too detailed image.

The extent to which lack of space-clamp vitiates voltage-clamp measurement depends on numerous factors, such as the detailed cable properties of the cell, the characteristics of the conductance under study (kinetics, ionic selectivity, size, and spatial location), and the optimism of the experimenter. Two extreme views are: (a) unless space clamp is perfect wherever the conductance under study is present any data will be worse than misleading; and (b) any degree of voltage control, however bad, still represents an improvement on current clamp for the measurement of voltage-dependent conductances. Our own view lies somewhere between these, and can be summarized by the following statement. If the currents observed with an imperfect voltage clamp resemble in certain aspects those that would be observed in a perfectly

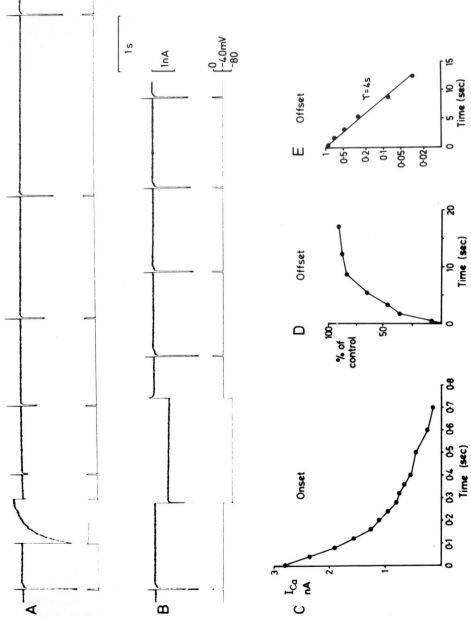

FIG. 18. Time course of inactivation of I_{Ca} in rat ganglion cell. Single-electrode voltage clamp (74). A: The recovery of the inward current assayed by a brief test pulse following a 700-msec conditioning pulse. Both test and conditioning pulses are to 0 mV. B: shows the lack of effect of a prolonged conditioning hyperpolarization. C: plots the size of the I_{Ca} during the conditioning pulse as a function of the peak current, using linear leak substraction. Parts D and E shows linear and semilog plots of the recovery time course. (M. Galvan and P. R. Adams, *unpublished observations*.)

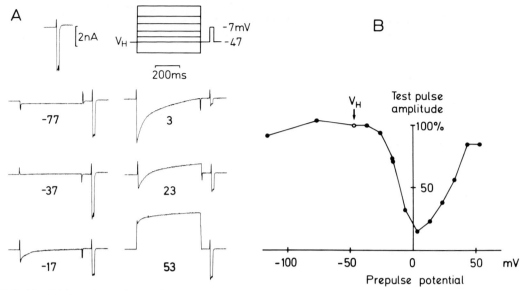

FIG. 19. Voltage dependence of I_{Ca} inactivation in rat ganglion cells. Single electrode clamp (see ref. 75). **A** shows the voltage protocol and the recorded membrane currents. **B** shows the test pulse current amplitude as a function of the conditioning potential. (M. Galvan and P. R. Adams, *unpublished observations.*)

clamped neuron, the clamp is useful. However, implementation of this criterion is not easy, since it requires simulation of voltage-clamp data from an active cable endowed with an appropriate collage of ionic channels.

Several authors have attempted to determine the cable structure of pyramidal cells, using an equivalent cylinder approximation (44,103,167). This model, originated by Rall (145), is also very useful for gaining insight into the limitations of

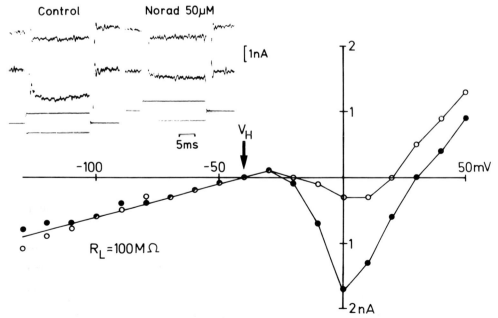

FIG. 20. Inhibition of I_{Ca} by 50 μM norepinephrine. Two-electrode clamp (74). Note that norepinephrine decreases inward current without changing the shape of the $I-V$ relation or affecting leakage resistance. (M. Galvan and P. R. Adams, *unpublished observations.*)

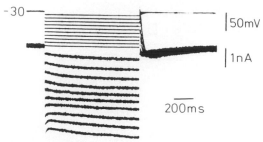

FIG. 21. M, A, and creep currents in a rat ganglion cell. Single-electrode voltage clamp. The cell was held at − 30 mV and subjected to long hyperpolarizations of various magnitudes. The smaller steps evoke a slowly relaxing M-current that becomes faster and reverses at about − 90 mV. The largest hyperpolarizations evoke an inward creep current. Returns to − 30 mV evoke a transient outward current, followed by reactivation of M-current. (M. Galvan and P. R. Adams, *unpublished observations.*)

the somatic point-clamp technique. The total clamp current supplied by the somatic electrode following a step command will, for a linear system, be given by the superimposition of the somatic current (ideally a Δ function plus a constant) and the current injected into the processes. The latter is given by simple cable theory (98). For a finite cable of length *l* and length constant λ (L = *l*/τ) the major transient component of the current is exponential with time constant $\tau_1 = \tau_m/ (\pi^2/4L^2 + 1)$ where τ_m is the dendritic membrane time constant and ρ is the dendritic/somatic input conductance ratio. τ_m can easily be obtained from the charging of the soma following a *current* step, and thus L can be evaluated. The reported values are about 1. This allows immediate evaluation of *steady state*-clamp nonuniformities from the classic short cable equation $V_x = V_o \cosh (L - X)/\cosh L$ where V_x is the steady state voltage achieved at distance X = x/λ from the soma. For example, with L = X = 1, the voltage at the tips of the dendrites is about 70% of that applied to the soma. In the worst case, the apparent steady state voltage sensitivity and reversal potential for a *small* (compared to passive) voltage-dependent conductance would be underestimated by about this amount. Furthermore, if the kinetics of the channel were slow as compared with τ_m, the observed kinetics would be roughly right. In a more favorable situation, with the conductance uniformly distributed along soma and dendrites, the clamp fidelity is quite good. However, if the conductance is not small, and particularly if the conductance can become neg-

ative, extreme steady state nonuniformities could develop in such a cable. A good introductory discussion of this problem can be found in Jack et al.(98) (see Chapter 7). Fortunately there is a simple test for this unhappy but likely condition, and that is to investigate the way in which diminishing the current size affects the apparent voltage dependence of the current. It is usually possible to do this with appropriate drugs or ionic manipulations. The current should be reduced in size until it can be shown that further reductions in current size have no residual effect on the voltage sensitivity of the current.

If the kinetics of the current being studied are comparable to or faster than τ_m, severe distortions must be expected. In our own work, we wait about 20 msec before making "instantaneous" current measurements, at which time the capacity transient has completely decayed, and even remote membrane is quite close to its final (but deviated) potential. It is tempting of course to subtract the capacity transient from experimental records to "improve" the resolution, but unless it is known that the conductance under study is mainly somatic or else very proximal, this procedure is, at best, a last resort. In particular, any kinetic "information" obtained by such a procedure should be regarded with extreme skepticism. It is usually best to display the unvarnished experimental records. These points have been labored at some length in connection with synaptic inputs to dendrites by Johnston and Brown (102). They have argued that mossy fiber synapses on CA3 apical dendrites are sufficiently close to the soma to allow adequate voltage clamping, even though the observed currents have time courses comparable to or faster than the capacity transients. However, in the absence of direct measurements of the time course of the synaptic current itself, it is not possible to be certain that considerable distortion does not occur.

It has been recently shown that pyramidal cells do *not* anatomically conform to the requirements of the equivalent cylinder approximation (168). Nevertheless, the transients exhibited by a realistic electrical model of the non-ideal anatomy could be successfully analyzed as though they had originated in an ideal cable model and gave length constants identical to those deduced by purely electrical measurements on the original cell itself. For practical purposes then, the equivalent cylinder model is valid, provided that the "somatic" isopotential compartment is allowed to include some proximal dendrite.

TABLE 2. *Voltage-dependent conductances of hippocampal pyramidal cells*

		Activation	Inactivation	Blockers
Inward	$I_{Na,t}$	Very fast	Fast	TTX
	$I_{Na,s}$	Very fast	Absent	TTX
	$I_{Ca,s}$	Fast	Very slow	Cd
	$I_{Ca,t}$	Fast	Fast	Cd
	I_Q	Slow	Absent	Cs
Outward	I_K	Slow	Slow	TEA
	I_A	Fast	Fast	4-AP
	I_C	Complex	Absent?	
	I_M	Slow	Absent	TEA
	I_{AHP}	Slow	Absent?	Carbachol Norepinephrine, cAMP, ACh, histamine

Inward Currents

It appears likely that hippocampal pyramidal cells exhibit separate sodium and calcium currents, and that these both exist in sustained and transient forms. The transient Na current, $I_{Na,t}$, is responsible for the upswing of the neuronal action potential in these cells. It can be blocked by TTX or intracellularly applied QX-314 (54). Intradendritic recordings (29,172; see also 118) often reveal only small passively conducted remnants of the intrasomatically recorded Na spike, presumably because dendritic membrane is largely devoid of $I_{Na,t}$. It is not clear how well developed the $I_{Na,t}$ mechanism is in the soma as compared with the initial segment of the axon, nor to what extent inward currents that could be recorded by a somatic point clamp of high temporal resolution would represent the true channel kinetics. Single-channel recording offers the best hope of reconstructing $I_{Na,t}$ in mammalian central neurons.

A noninactivating voltage-dependent sodium current that is also sensitive to TTX and intracellular QX-314 has been clearly described in cerebellum, thalamus, and cortex (99,117,157), and seems to be present in CA1 cells (95). It remains to be seen whether $I_{Na',t}$ and $I_{Na',s}$ flow through separate channels or represent incomplete inactivation of a single channel type.

Calcium currents have been recorded from pyramidal cells after partial suppression of outward current, either by external TEA application (42) or use of CsCl recording electrodes (86,101). The responses seem to fall into two classes. If the holding potential is rather positive (-50 to -30 mV) depolarizing steps to about -40 mV or beyond elicit slowly rising, sometimes slightly bumpy inward currents, that can remain inward for depolarizations lasting several sec. If the initial holding potential is closer to the normal resting potential (-70mV), depolarization to about -55mV elicits a rapidly activating but transient inward current. Both these inward currents are blocked by cadmium and reduced in low calcium solutions, and are thus probably calcium mediated. Similar sustained and transient calcium-currents are seen in sensory ganglion cells (47,139). These currents also seem to be present in many other central neurons, where they can generate low- and high-threshold Ca-spikes (99).

To what extent do the time courses of the observed currents reflect the kinetics of the underlying channels rather than space-clamp problems? The sustained current at least is probably partly or even totally dendritic (29,117,172). The existence of a large negative resistance and apparent kinetics similar to the membrane time constant are unfavorable. In general, the existence of poor voltage control will not necessarily be evinced by notches or spike-like somatic currents, but will show up in the form of a distorted I-V relation. The overall effect resembles that produced by uncompensated series resistance: the voltage for peak current will be shifted to the left, and the negative slope will be steepened (see Fig. 12.13 in Jack et al., ref. 98). The peak of the I-V would shift to the right as the magnitude of I_{Ca} were reduced by lowering external Ca or adding blockers. Although the published data are not completely clear-cut, there does not appear to be any such rightward shift (38,42), suggesting that adequate space clamp exists at least in the steady state. However, in other unpublished experiments, such rightward shifts on lowering external calcium have been seen (B. Lancaster, H. V. Wheal, and P. R. Adams, *unpublished observations*).

What might be the function of persistent inward currents in these cells? One obvious possibility is that calcium influx provides a way of coupling membrane potential to other processes, such as potassium channel activation or metabolic events. A more tantalizing possibility is that they act to cancel out leakage conductances in relation to "passive" cable properties such as τ and ρ. This is again well illustrated in Fig. 12.13. in Jack et al. (98). This shows that whereas a small depolarization applied to an active cable will show normal spatial decrement, a slightly larger depolarization will spread without decrement. That this can actually be the case in cerebellar Purkinje cells has been recently directly demonstrated by Llinas and Sugimori (117). Recent work exploiting cuts between the cell body region and the main apical dendrites suggests that the persistent Na and Ca currents contributing to "anomalous rectificaton" may have different dendritic/somatic locations (29).

There is another important way in which neutralization of leak conductance by negative conductance can influence simple cable properties, and that is in charging behavior. If the overall steady state I-V relation is completely flat over a certain range, and the active conductances have kinetics that are fast as compared with the intrinsic membrane time constant, the membrane will charge up infinitely slowly following a current injection. In fact, because the input resistance is also infinite, the membrane will spontaneously ramp. The situation is rather like that described by Connor (ref. 54, p. 191). Thus, what one can gain in terms of spatial uniformity, one can lose in terms of cable frequency response.

The remaining inward current, I_Q, is even more unconventional, for it is activated by *hyperpolarization* from rest (85). Activation starts at about -80 mV, and maximum activation time constant (at 25°C) ranged from 100 msec at -120 mV to 600 msec at -80 mV. No inactivation is seen. The reversal potential for I_Q is $\cong -55$ mV, and seems to reflect a mixed Na-K conductance. I_Q is insensitive to Ba but quite sensitive to millimolar cesium concentrations (Fig. 22). Because it is not a pure K-current, nor is it sensitive to barium, it does not appear to be an anomalous rectifier, at least in the strict sense of the term (83,84,158). It is very reminiscent of an inward current activated by hyperpolarization that is found in various cardiac cells (43,175). The cardiac current activates in a somewhat more positive voltage range and can thus give rise to

slow spontaneous depolarizatons. In hippocampal cells, its influence is seen most clearly as a sag in long-duration hyperpolarizing electrotonic potentials (85). An almost identical current is found in photoreceptors (26), in cultured dorsal root ganglion cells (126), and in neocortical pyramidal cells (156). On the other hand, a somewhat similar current seen in olfactory cortex cells seems more akin to a true anomalous rectifier (59).

Outward Currents

All the outward currents that are found in bullfrog ganglion cells seem to be present also in hippocampal pyramidal cells: I_M (85), I_K (153), I_A (76), I_C (15,37,176) and I_{AHP} (15,116,122,123). However, in each case there are some differences, varying from rather minor (e.g., I_M) to impressive (e.g., I_{AHP}). These differences could conceivably reflect space-clamp distortions or temperature effects rather than intrinsic channel properties.

I_M

The activation range for this current has not been properly determined and may not be determinable by single-electrode voltage-clamp techniques (57,87). Added to the usual space-clamp difficulties are other overlapping currents at both extremes of the activation range, smallness of the current, and sensitivity of currents other than I_M to muscarine. Nevertheless, it seems likely that most of the activation range lies between -70 mV and -30 mV, thus lying some 10 mV hyperpolarized with respect to bullfrog ganglion. The activation time constant at -50 mV (23°C) was about 280 msec, and clearly became smaller at more negative potentials. I_M could be blocked by muscarinic agonists or by barium. It seems to be responsible for an early component of spike frequency adaptation (123). Halliwell and Adams (85) predicted that activation of septal cholinergic afferents to hippocampal cells would inhibit M-current in pyramidal cells and produce a heterosynaptic facilitation of homosynaptic excitation much as sketched in Fig. 11. It is known that selective septal stimulation will indeed produce a cholinergic facilitation (25,111), but it is not yet clear whether the mechanism is M-current inhibition. Other possibilities are disinhibition (111) or reduction of AHP current (49,50). In recent work, two groups have tested some of these hy-

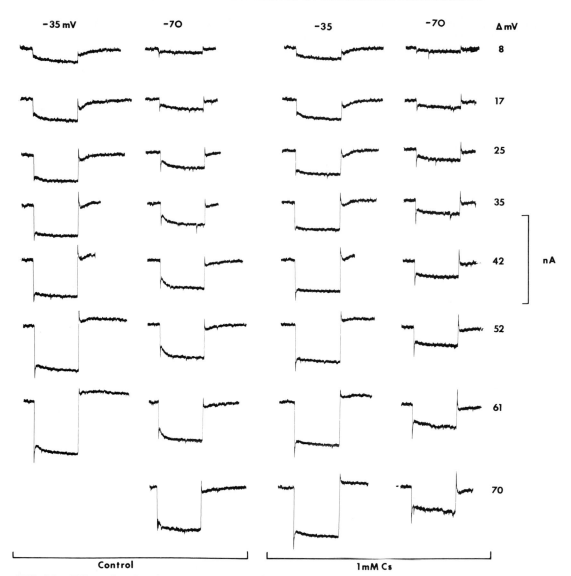

FIG. 22. Effect of cesium ions on M-current and Q-current in guinea-pig hippocampal pyramidal cell (85). The cell was held at either -35 mV or -70 mV, and subjected to various hyperpolarizing clamp commands (*right*). Small hyperpolarizations from -35 mV elicit relaxing M-current, whereas hyperpolarizations from -70 elicit Q-current. Application of Cs selectively inhibits I_Q. (J. V. Halliwell and P. R. Adams, *unpublished observations.*)

potheses in voltage-clamp experiments. Gahwiler and Brown (*personal communication*) using a hippocampal slice–septal explant culture system, indeed found synaptic suppression of I_M. On the other hand, Madison, Lancaster, and Nicoll, using selective activation of cholinergic afferents coursing through slices (*personal communication*), found that I_{AHP} rather than I_M was suppressed.

I_K

This is quite a large current and requires the dual microelectrode method (153). Its threshold was about -45 mV, but the maximum conductance could not be determined. The current then inactivated; steady inactivation was nearly complete at -50 mV and almost completely removed at -90 mV. The activation and inactivation time constants (at room temperature) were around 180 msec and 4 sec, respectively.

I_A

The A-current in these cells exhibits a conventional pharmacological profile: sensitivity to 4AP in the millimolar range, and relative insensitivity to TEA and calcium blockers. Inactivation is almost complete at -45 mV, and essentially removed at -70 mV, whereas activation has a threshold near -50 mV. The kinetics of activation are too fast to resolve, while inactivation onsets with a time constant around 400 msec. However, in whole-cell patch-clamp experiments, a much more rapidly inactivating A-current has been detected (170). Two roles for the A current can be suggested: (1) it may raise the threshold for spikes, especially early in the stimulus pulse; and (2) it may account for the early transient dip in the spike amplitude during repetitive firing induced by a current pulse (e.g., 122,123).

I_C

A rapidly activating outward current that is blocked by calcium removal or addition of calcium blockers has been described by two groups of workers (37,176). As expected, this current is quite sensitive to TEA. In the Brown and Griffith experiments (37), I_C was found to be sustained, whereas in the Zbicz and Weight study (176), it was found to inactivate rapidly (within 20 msec). These differences could reflect holding potential differences, space-clamp problems in one or both studies, or the coexistence of two distinct currents. Until one understands the rather similar results found in bullfrog cells, it is probably premature to proceed much further with the hippocampal analysis. Whole-cell patch-clamp recording has also revealed the existence of an I_C-like current (170). Single-channel recording has given a preliminary single-channel conductance of 100 picosiemens (pS), similar to that seen in other systems.

It has been suggested that one role of I_C in hippocampal neurons may be the generation of postburst hyperpolarizations (37). However, there are a number of objections to this conclusion: (1) the kinetics of I_C seem too fast at negative potentials to account for the long-lasting postspike hyperpolarizatons; (2) whereas both norepinephrine and acetylcholine readily abolish spike AHPs, they seem to have little effect on I_C; and (3) TEA, which blocks I_C, seems to enhance AHPs. Instead it seems likely that a current similar to the bullfrog I_{AHP} is responsible for slow AHPs in hippocampal neurons (see below).

I_{AHP}

Recently voltage-clamp and hybrid-clamp experiments have revealed a slowly activating, slowly deactivating (3-sec) calcium-dependent K-current in rat CA1 pyramidal cells (15,116). This current is TEA resistant and norepinephrine sensitive, and therefore fits the bill for the AHP conductance suggested by the current clamp data of Madison and Nicoll (122,123; see also 94). It seems that this current was overlooked in the study by Brown and Griffith, partly because they used rather positive holding potentials, where it may be constantly activated, and partly because it is small and very slow. It seems to be very important in controlling the dramatic slow firing adaptation shown by these neurons (123). It is attractive to suppose that activation of ascending noradrenergic fibers during behavioral arousal could, by inhibition of I_{AHP}, heterosynaptically facilitate pyramidal cell discharge.

Hippocampal Excitability and Epilepsy

Exploration of the voltage-dependent conductances of hippocampal neurons is in its infancy, and one can expect that over the next few years many of the apparent contradictions and uncertainties will disappear as work progresses. It is very likely that almost all the reported currents can be brought into play by appropriate current stimulation protocols. However, it is unknown whether any of these currents are important in controlling normal physiological activation of these cells, or whether the remarkable modulation by various transmitters is made use of in the intact brain. Presumably, all these mechanisms can be brought into play and are not present merely for the delectation of the electrophysiologist. If this is so, in epileptic tissue some of these currents may be modified, either as a result of abnormal discharging, or even as a cause. Also, even if these mechanisms are largely intact, they will participate in the abnormal activity, and help to abate or intensify it. An excellent example of this is the work of Traub and Wong (166) on epileptiform activity in interconnected arrays of realistically modelled excitable neurons. Clearly, such models are only as good as the equations used to describe the neurons' membrane, and it is imperative to make as many direct measurements as possible, so as to restrict arbitrariness in such calculations.

A more restricted but perhaps more attainable goal is to ask whether any of the chemical treatments that precipitate paroxysomal activity in slices might do so in part by inhibition of outward currents that normally stabilize repetitive characteristics. Two examples are 4-AP, which affects A-current, and tubocurare, which blocks I_{AHP}. Of course these agents also have other actions, such as enhancing transmitter release or blocking γ-aminobutyric acid (GABA). However, other agents which have these actions do not mimic all aspects of the convulsant effect of these drugs. There are many other drugs as well, such as bemigride, pentylenetetrazol (PTZ), and convulsant barbiturates, whose mechanism of action has not yet been explained. Clearly, the neuropharmacology of central voltage-dependent conductances will become a very active field.

ACKNOWLEDGMENT

Work in P.R.A.'s laboratory is supported by NINCDS grant no. NS18579. We thank D. A. Brown, A. Constanti, M. Galvan, J. V. Halliwell, P. Pennefather, S. W. Jones, and B. Lancaster for their participation in many of the experiments discussed above, as well as for ideas and criticisms. We thank Linda Cerracchio, Peter Pennefather, Steve Jones, and Claire Adams for help with the manuscript.

REFERENCES

1. Adams, P. R., and Brown, D. A. (1980): LHRF and muscarinic agonists act on the same voltage-sensitive K^+-current in bullfrog sympathetic neurones. *Br. J. Pharmacol.*, 68:353–355.

2. Adams, P. R. (1980): The calcium current of a vertebrate neurone. *Fed. Proc.*, 39:282.

3. Adams, P. R. (1980): The calcium current of a vertebrate neurone. *Advances in Physiological Science*, 4, *Physiology of Excitable Membranes*, edited by J. Salanki. Akademiai Kiado, Budapest.

4. Adams, P. R., Brown, D. A., and Constanti, A. (1982): M-currents and other potassium currents in bullfrog sympathetic neurons. *J. Physiol.*, 30:537–572.

5. Adams, P. R., Brown, D. A., and Constanti, A. (1982): Pharmacological inhibition of the M-current. *J. Physiol.*, 332:223–262.

6. Adams, P. R., and Brown, D. A. (1982): Synaptic inhibition of the M-current: Slow excitatory postsynaptic potential mechanism in bull-

frog sympathetic neurones. *J. Physiol.*, 332:263–272.

7. Adams, P. R., Constanti, A., Brown, D. A., and Clark, R. B. (1982): Intracellular Ca^{2+} activates a fast voltage sensitive K^+ current in vertebrate sympathetic neurones. *Nature*, 296:746–749.

8. Adams, P. R., Brown, D. A., and Constanti, A. (1982): Voltage clamp analysis of membrane currents underlying repetitive firing of bullfrog sympathetic neurons. In: *Physiology and Pharmacology of Epileptognic Phenomenon*, edited by M. R. Klee, H. D. Lux, and E. J. Speckman. Raven Press, New York.

9. Adams, P. R. (1982): Voltage-dependent conductances of vertebrate neurones. *Trends Neurosci.*, 5:116–119.

10. Adams, P. R., Brown, D. A., Constanti, A., and Adams, C. E. Y. (1982): Spontaneous hyperpolarizations in cultured bullfrog ganglion cells reflect K-channels opened by internal calcium packets. *Biophys. J.*, 37:308a.

11. Adams, P. R., Brown, D. A., and Jones, S. W. (1983): Substance P inhibits the M-current in bullfrog sympathetic neurones. *Br. J. Pharmacol.*, 79:330–333.

12. Adams, P. R., Brown, D. A., Constanti, A., Clark, R. B., and Satin, L. (1984): Calcium-activated potassium channels in bullfrog sympathetic ganglion cells. In: *Calcium in Biological Systems*, edited by R. Rubin, pp. 181–191. Plenum, New York.

13. Adams, P. R. (1985): Activation of calcium current in bullfrog ganglion cells. *J. Physiol.* (in press).

14. Adams, P. R. (1985): Inactivation of calcium current in bullfrog ganglion cells. *J. Physiol.* (in press).

15. Adams, P. R., and Lancaster, B. (1985): Components of Ca-activated K current in rat hippocampal neurones. *J. Neurophys.*, (in press).

16. Akasu, T., and Koketsu, K. (1981): Voltage-clamp studies of a slow inward current in bullfrog sympathetic ganglion cells. *Neurosci. Lett.*, 26:259–262.

17. Akasu, T., and Koketsu, K. (1982): Modulation of voltage-dependent currents by muscarinic receptor in sympathetic neurones of bullfrog. *Neurosci. Lett.*, 29:41–45.

18. Akasu, T., Kojima, M., and Koketsu, K. (1983): Substance P modulates the sensitivity of the nicotinic receptor in amphibian cholinergic transmission. *Br. J. Pharmacol.*, 80:123–131.

19. Akasu, T., Nishimura, T., and Koketsu, K. (1983): Substance P inhibits the action potentials in bullfrog sympathetic ganglion cells. *Neurosci. Lett.*, 41:161–166.

20. Akasu, T., Kojima, M., and Koketsu, K. (1983): Luteinizing hormone-releasing hormone modulates nicotinic ACh-receptor sensitivity in amphibian cholinergic transmission. *Brain Res.*, 279:347–351.

21. Akasu, T., Nishimura, T., and Koketsu, K. (1983): Modulation of action potential during the late slow excitatory postsynaptic potential

in bullfrog sympathetic ganglia. *Brain Res.*, 280:349–354.

22. Akasu, T., Gallagher, J. P., Koketsu, K., and Shinnick-Gallagher, P. (1984): Slow excitatory post-synaptic currents in sympathetic neurones of *Rana catesbiana. J. Physiol.*, 351:583–593.

23. Akasu, T., Hirai, K., and Koketsu, K. (1983): Modulatory actions of ATP on membrane potentials of bullfrog sympathetic ganglion cells. *Brain Res.*, 258:313–317.

24. Alger, B. E., and Nicoll, R. A. (1981): Epileptiform burst after hyperpolarization: Calcium dependent potassium potential in hippocampal CA1 pyramidal cells. *Science,* 210:1122–1124.

25. Alvarez-Leefmans, F. J., and Gardner-Medwin, A. R. (1975): Influences of septum on the hippocampal dentate area which are unaccompanied by field potentials. *J. Physiol. (Lond.),* 249:14–16P.

26. Attwell, D., and Wilson, M. (1980): Behavior of the rod network in the tiger salamander retina mediated by membrane properties of individual rods. *J. Physiol. (Lond.),* 309:287–315.

27. Belluzzi, O., Sacchi, O., and Wanke, E. (1985): A fast transient outward current in the rat sympathetic neurone studied under voltage-clamp conditons. *J. Physiol.*, 358:91–108.

28. Belluzzi, O., Sacchi, O., and Wanke, E. (1985): Identification of delayed potassium and calcium currents in the rat sympathetic neurone under voltage clamp. *J. Physiol.*, 358:109–130.

29. Benardo, L. S., Masukawa, L. M., and Prince, D. A. (1982): Electrophysiology of isolated hippocampal pyramidal dendrites. *J. Neurosci.*, 2:1614–1622.

30. Blaustein, M. P., Ratzkaff, R. W., Kendrick, N. C., and Schweitzer, E. S. (1978): Calcium buffering in presynaptic nerve terminals. I. Evidence for involvement of a nonmitochondrial ATP-dependent sequestration mechanism. *J. Gen. Physiol.*, 72:15–41.

31. Blaustein, M. P., Ratzkaff, R. W., and Schweitzer, E. S. (1980): Control of intracellular calcium in presynaptic nerve terminals. *Fed. Proc.*, 39:2790–2795.

32. Blatz, A., and Magleby, K. L. (1984): Ion conductance and selectivity of single calcium-activated potassium channels in cultured rat muscle. *J. Gen. Physiol.*, 84:1–23.

33. Brehm, P., Eckert, R., and Tillotson, D. O. (1980): Calcium mediated inactivation of calcium current in *Paramecium. J. Physiol.*, 306:193–203.

34. Brown, D. A., and Adams, P. R. (1980): Muscarinic suppression of a novel voltage-sensitive K⁺-current in a vertebrate neurone. *Nature (Lond.),* 283:673–676.

35. Brown, D. A., Constanti, A., and Marsh, S. (1980a): Angiotensin mimics the action of muscarinic agonists on rat sympathetic neurones. *Brain Res.*, 193:673–676.

36. Brown, D. A., Constanti, A., and Adams, P. R. (1982): Calcium-dependence of a component of transient outward current in bullfrog ganglion cells. *Soc. Neurosci., Abstr.*, 8:252.

37. Brown, D. A., and Griffith, W. H. (1983): Cal-

38. Brown, D. A., Halliwell, J. V., Constanti, A., Docherty, R. J., and Galvan, M. (1985): Pharmacology of neuronal calcium currents. 9th International Congress of Pharmacology Abstracts, S19-8.

39. Brown, D. A., Adams, P. R., and Constanti, A. (1982): Voltage-sensitive K currents in sympathetic neurones and their modulation by neurotransmitters. *J. Auton. Nerv. Syst.*, 6:23–35.

40. Brown, D. A., Constanti, A., and Adams, P. R. (1983): Ca-activated potassium current in vertebrate sympathetic neurones. *Cell Calcium*, 4:407–420.

41. Brown, D. A., and Selyanko, A. A. (1985): Two components of muscarine-sensitive membrane current in rat sympathetic neurones. *J. Physiol.*, 358:335–364.

42. Brown, D. A., and Griffith, W. H. (1983): Persistent slow inward calcium current in voltage-clamped hippocampal neurones of the guinea-pig. *J. Physiol.*, 337:303–320.

43. Brown, H., and DiFrancesco, D. (1980): Voltage-clamp investigations of membrane currents underlying pace-maker activity in rabbit sino-atrial node. *J. Physiol. (Lond.),* 308:331–351.

44. Brown, T. H., Fricke, R. A., and Perkel, D. H. (1980): Passive electrical constants in three classes of hippocampal neurons. *J. Neurophysiol.*, 358:335–364.

45. Busis, N. A., and Weight, F. F. (1976): Spike after-hyperpolarization of a sympathetic neurone is calcium sensitive and is potentiated by theophylline. *Nature (Lond.),* 263:434–436.

46. Campbell, D. T., and Hille, B. (1976): Kinetic and pharmacological properties of the sodium channel of frog skeletal muscle. *J. Gen. Physiol.*, 67:309–323.

47. Carbone, E., and Lux, H. D. (1984): A low voltage-activated, fully inactivating Ca channel in vertebrate sensory neurones. *Nature,* 310:501–502.

48. Chiu, S. Y., and Ritchie, J. M. (1980): Evidence for the presence of potassium channels in the paranodal region of acutely demyelinated mammalian single nerve fibres. *J. Physiol.*, 313:415–438.

49. Cole, A. E., and Nicoll, R. A. (1983): Acetylcholine mediates a slow synaptic potential in hippocampal cells. *Science,* 221:1299–1301.

50. Cole, A. E., and Nicoll, R. A. (1984): Characterization of a slow cholinergic postsynaptic potential recorded *in vitro* from rat hippocampal pyramidal cells. *J. Physiol.*, 352:173–188.

51. Connor, J. A., and Stevens, C. F. (1971): Prediction of repetitive firing behavior from voltage clamp data on an isolated neurone soma. *J. Physiol.*, 213:31–53.

52. Connor, J. A., and Stevens, J. A. (1971): Voltage clamp studies of a transient outward membrane current in gastropod neural somata. *J. Physiol. (Lond.),* 213:21–30.

53. Connor, J. A. (1978): Slow repetitive activity

from fast conductance changes in neurones. *Fed. Proc.*, 37:2139–2145.

54. Connor, J. A. (1982): Mechanisms of pacemaker-discharge in invertebrate neurons. In: *Cellular Pacemakers*, vol. 1, edited by D. O. Carpenter. John Wiley, New York.

55. Connors, B. W., and Prince, D. A. (1982): Effects of local anesthetic QX-314 on the membrane properties of hippocampal pyramidal neurons. *J. Pharmacol. Exp. Ther.*, 200:476–481.

56. Constanti, A., and Brown, D. A. (1981): M-currents in voltage-clamped mammalian sympathetic neurones. *Neurosci. Lett.*, 24:289–294.

57. Constanti, A., and Galvan, M. (1983): M-current in voltage-clamped olfactory cortex neurones. *Neurosci. Lett.*, 39:65–70.

58. Constanti, A., Adams, P. R., and Brown, D. A. (1981): Why do barium ions imitate acetylcholine? *Brain Res.*, 206:244–250.

59. Constanti, A., and Galvan, M. (1983): Fast inward-rectifying current accounts for anomalous rectification in olfactory cortex neurones. *J. Physiol.*, 385:153–178.

60. Dodd, J., and Horn, J. P. (1983): A reclassification of B and C neurones in the 9th and 10th paravertebral sympathetic ganglia of the bullfrog. *J. Physiol.*, 344:255–269.

61. Dodd, J., and Horn, J. P. (1983): Muscarinic inhibition of sympathetic C neurons in the bullfrog. *J. Physiol.*, 334:271–291.

62. Dubois, J. M. (1981): Evidence for the existence of three types of potassium channels in the frog Ranvier node membrane. *J. Physiol.*, 318:297–316.

63. Dunlap, K., and Fischbach, G. D. (1981): Neurotransmitters decrease the calcium conductance activated by depolarization of embryonic chick sensory neurones. *J. Physiol.*, 317:519–535.

64. Eckert, R., and Tillotson, D. L. (1981): Calcium-mediated inactivation of the calcium conductance in cesium-loaded giant neurones of *Aplysia california*. *J. Physiol.*, 314:265–280.

65. Eckert, R., and Ewald, D. (1983): Calcium tail currents in voltage clamped intact nerve cell bodies of *Aplysia california*. *J. Physiol.*, 345:533–548.

66. Fenwick, E. M., Marty, A., and Neher, E. (1982): Sodium and calcium channels in bovine chromaffin cells. *J. Physiol.*, 331:599–635.

67. Fox, A. (1981): Voltage-dependent inactivation of a calcium-channel. *Proc. Natl. Acad. Sci. USA*, 78:953–956.

68. Frankenhauser, B. (1963): A quantitative description of potassium currents in myelinated nerve fibres of *Xenopus laevis*. *J. Physiol.*, 169:424–430.

69. Frankenhauser, B., and Huxley, A. F. (1964): The action potential in the myelinated nerve fiber of *Xenopus laevis* as computed on the basis of voltage clamp data. *J. Physiol.*, 171:302–315.

70. Freschi, J. E. (1983): Membrane currents of cultured rat sympathetic neurons under voltage clamp. *J. Neurophysiol.*, 50:1460–1478.

71. Gahwiler, B. H., and Brown, D. A. (1984): GABA-receptor activated K^+ current in voltage-clamped CA_3 pyramidal cells in hippocampal cultures. *Proc. Natl. Acad. Sci.*, 82:1558–1562.

72. Galvan, M. (1982): A transient outward current in rat sympathetic neurones. *Neurosci. Lett.*, 31:295–300.

73. Galvan, M., Sedlmeir, C. (1982): An N-shaped current-voltage relationship in rat sympathetic neurones. *Pflugers Arch.*, 398:78–80.

74. Galvan, M., and Adams, P. R. (1982): Control of calcium current in rat sympathetic neurones by norepinephrine. *Brain Res.*, 244:135–144.

75. Galvan, M., and Sedlmeir, C. (1984): Outward currents in voltage clamped rat sympathetic neurones. *J. Physiol.*, 356:115–133.

76. Gustafsson, B., Galvan, M., Grafe, P., and Wigstrom, H. (1982): A transient outward current in a mammalian central neurone blocked by 4-aminopyridine. *Nature (Lond.)*, 299:252–254.

77. Gustafsson, B., and Wigstrom, H. (1981): Evidence for two types of afterhyperpolarization in CA 1 pyramidal cells in the hippocampus. *Brain Res.*, 206:462–468.

78. Haas, H. L., and Konnerth, A. (1983): Histamine and noradrenaline decrease calcium-activated potassium conductance in hippocampal pyramidal cells. *Nature*, 302:432–434.

79. Hablitz, J. J. (1981a): Altered burst responses in hippocampal CA_3 neurones injected with EGTA. *Exp. Brain Res.*, 42:483–485.

80. Hablitz, J. J. (1981b): Effects of intracellular injections of chloride and EGTA on postepileptiform burst-hyperpolarizations in hippocampal neurones. *Neurosci. Lett.*, 22:159–163.

81. Hagiwara, S., and Byerly, L. (1981): Calcium channel. *Annu. Rev. Neurosci.*, 4:69–125.

82. Hagiwara, S., and Ohmari, H. (1982): Studies of calcium channels in rat cloned pituitary cells with patch electrode voltage clamp. *J. Physiol.*, 331:231–252.

83. Hagiwara, S., Miyazaki, S., Moody, W., and Patlak, J. (1978): Blocking effects of barium and hydrogen ions on potassium current during anomalous rectification in the starfish egg. *J. Physiol. (Lond.)*, 279:167–185.

84. Hagiwara, S., Miyazaki, S., and Rosenthal, N. P. (1976): Potassium current and the effect of cesium on this current during anomalous rectification of the egg cell membranes of a starfish. *J. Gen. Physiol.*, 67:621–638.

85. Halliwell, J. V., and Adams, P. R. (1982): Voltage-clamp analysis of muscarinic excitation in hippocampal neurons. *Brain Res.*, 250:71–92.

86. Halliwell, J. V. (1983): Calcium-loading reveals two distinct Ca-currents in voltage-clamped guinea-pig hippocampal neurones *in vitro*. *J. Physiol.*, 341:10–11.

87. Hashiguchi, T., Kobayashi, H., Tosaka, T., and Libet, B. (1982): Two muscarinic depolarizing mechanisms in mammalian sympathetic neurons. *Brain Res.*, 242:378–382.

88. Henkart, M. (1980): Identification and function

of intracellular calcium stores in axons and cell bodies of neurons. *Fed. Proc.*, 39:2783–2798.

89. Henon, B. K., Brown, T. H., and McAfee, D. A. (1981): Electrotonic structure of the rat sympathetic postganglionic neurons. *Soc. Neurosci. Abstr.*, 7:518.

90. Hille, B. (1967): The selective inhibition of delayed potassium currents in nerve by tetraethylammonium ion. *J. Gen. Physiol.*, 50:1287–1302.

91. Hodgkin, A. L., and Huxley, A. F. (1985): A quantitative description of membrane current and its application to conduction and excitation in nerve. *J. Physiol.*, 117:500–544.

92. Hodgkin, A. L., and Huxley, A. F. (1952): The dual effect of membrane potential on sodium conductance in the giant axon of *Loligo*. *J. Physiol. (Lond.)*, 116:497–506.

93. Horn, J. P., and McAffee, D. A. (1980): Alpha-adrenergic inhibition of calcium-dependent potentials in rat sympathetic neurones. *J. Physiol.*, 301:191–204.

94. Hotson, J. R., and Prince, D. A. (1980): A calcium-activated hyperpolarization follows repetitive firing in hippocampal neurons. *J. Neurophysiol.*, 43:409–419.

95. Hotson, J. R., Prince, D. A., and Schwartzkroin, P. A. (1979): Anomalous inward rectification in hippocampal neurons. *J. Neurophysiol.*, 42:889–895.

96. Hugues, M., Romey, G., Duval, D., Vincent, J. P., and Lazdunski, M. (1982): Apamin as a selective blocker of the calcium-dependent potassium channel in neuroblastoma cells: Voltage-clamp and biochemical characterization of the toxin receptor. *Proc. Natl. Acad. Sci. USA*, 79:1308–1312.

97. Isenberg, G., and Kloeckner, V. (1982): Calcium currents of isolated bovine ventricular myocytes are fast and of large amplitude. *Plugers Arch.*, 395:30–41.

98. Jack, J. J. B., Noble, D., and Tsien, R. W. (1975): *Electric Current Flow in Excitable Cells*. Clarendon Press, Oxford.

99. Jahnsen, H., and Llinas, R. (1984): Electrophysiological properties of guinea-pig thalamic neurones: An *in vitro* study. *J. Physiol.*, 349:205–226.

100. Jan, L. Y., and Jan, Y. N. (1982): Peptidergic transmission in symapathetic ganglia of the frog. *J. Physiol.*, 327:219–246.

101. Johnston, D., Hablitz, J. J., and Wilson, W. A. (1980): Voltage clamp discloses slow inward currents in hippocampal burst firing neurones. *Nature*, 286:391–393.

102. Johnston, D., and Brown, T. H. (1983): Interpretation of voltage-clamp measurements in hippocampal neurons. *J. Neurophysiol.*, 50:464–486.

103. Johnston, D. (1981): Passive cable properties of hippocampal CA3 pyramidal neurons. *Cell Molec. Neurobiol.*, 1:100–110.

104. Jones, S. W., Adams, P. R., Brownstein, M. J., and Rivier, J. E. (1984): Teleost leutinizing hormone-releasing hormone: Action on bullfrog

sympathetic ganglia is consistent with role as neurotransmitter. *J. Neurosci.*, 4:420–429.

105. Jones, S. W. (1985): Muscarinic and peptidergic excitation of bullfrog sympathetic neurons. *J. Physiol.*, 366:63–87.

106. Jones, S. W. (1984): Muscarinic and peptidergic actions on C cells of bullfrog sympathetic ganglia. *Soc. Neurosci. Abstr.*, 10:207.

107. Katayama, Y., and Nishi, S. (1982): Voltage-clamp analysis of peptidergic slow depolarizations in bullfrog sympathetic ganglion cells. *J. Physiol.*, 333:305–313.

108. Koketsu, K., Akasu, T., and Miyagawa, M. (1982): Identification of K systems activated by $[CA^{2+}]$. *Brain Res.*, 243:369–372.

109. Koketsu, K., and Nishi, S. (1969): Calcium and action potentials of bullfrog sympathetic ganglion cells. *J. Gen. Physiol.*, 53:608–623.

110. Kramer, R. H., and Zucker, R. S. (1985): Calcium dependent inactivation of persistent calcium underlies the interburst hyperpolarization of *Aplysia* bursting pacemaker neurones. *J. Physiol.* (in press).

111. Krnjevic, K., and Ropert, N. (1981): Septo-hippocampal pathway modulates hippocampal activity by a cholinergic mechanism. *Can. J. Physiol., Pharmacol.*, 59:911–914.

112. Kuba, K. (1980): Release of calcium ions linked to the activation of potassium conductance in a caffeine-treated sympathetic neurone. *J. Physiol. (Lond.)*, 298:251–269.

113. Kuba, K., Morita, K., and Nohmi, M. (1983): Origin of calcium ions involved in the generation of a slow after-hyperpolarization in bullfrog sympathetic neurones. *Pflugers Arch.*, 399:194–202.

114. Kuffler, S. W., and Sejnowski, T. J. (1983): Peptidergic and muscarinic excitation at amphibian sympathetic synapses. *J. Physiol.*, 341:257–278.

115. Latorre, R., Vergara, C., and Hidalgo, C. (1982): Reconstitution in planar lipid bilayers of a Ca^{2+}-dependent K^+ channel from transverse tubule membranes isolated from rabbit skeletal muscle. *Proc. Natl. Acad. Sci. USA*, 79:805–809.

116. Lancaster, B., and Adams, P. R. (1984): Single electrode voltage clamp of the slow AHP current in rat hippocampal pyramidal cells. *Soc. Neurosci. Abstr.*, 10:872.

117. Llinas, R., and Sugimori, M. (1984): Simultaneous intracellular somatic and dendritic recording from Purkinje cells *in vitro* dynamic somadendritic coupling. *Soc. Neurosci. Abstr.*, 10:659.

118. Llinas, R., and Sugimori, M. (1980): Electrophysiological properties of *in vitro* Purkinje cell dendrites in mammalian cerebellar slices. *J. Physiol. (Lond.)*, 305:197–213.

119. Llinas, R., and Sugimori, M. (1980): Electrophysiological properties of *in vitro* Purkinje cell somata in mammalian cerebellar slices. *J. Physiol. (Lond.)*, 305:171–195.

120. Llinas, R., and Yarom, Y. (1981): Electrophysiology of mammalian inferior olivery neurones

in vitro. Different types of voltage-dependent ionic conductances. *J. Physiol.,* 315:549–567.

121. MacDermott, A. B., and Weight, F. F. (1982): Action potential repolarization may involve a transient Ca^{2+}-sensitive outward current in a vertebrate neurone. *Nature (Lond.),* 300:185–188.

122. Madison, D. V., and Nicoll, R. A. (1982): Noradrenaline blocks accommodation of pyramidal cell discharge in the hippocampus. *Nature,* 299:636–638.

123. Madison, D. V., and Nicoll, R. A. (1984): Control of the repetitive discharge of rat (CA1) pyramidal neurones *in vitro. J. Physiol.,* 354:319–331.

124. Marshall, L. M. (1981): Synaptic localization of alpha-bungarotoxin binding which blocks nicotinic transmission at frog sympathetic neurons. *Proc. Natl. Acad. Sci. USA,* 78:1948–1952.

125. Marty, A. (1981): Ca-dependent K channels with large unitary conductance in chromaffin cell membranes. *Nature (Lond.),* 291:497–500.

126. Mayer, M. L., and Westbrook, G. L. (1983): A voltage-clamp analysis of inward (anomalous) rectification in mouse spinal sensory ganglion neurones. *J. Physiol.,* 340:19–45.

127. Mayer, M. L., Westbrook, G. L., and Guthrie, P. B. (1984): Voltage dependent block by Mg^{2+} of NMDA responses in spinal cord neurones. *Nature,* 309:261–263.

128. McAfee, D. A., and Yarowsky, P. J. (1979): Calcium-dependent potentials in the mammalian sympathetic neurone. *J. Physiol. (Lond.),* 290:507–523.

129. Meech, R. W. (1972): Intracellular calcium injection causes increased potassium conductance in *Aplysia* nerve cells. *Comp. Biochem. Physiol.,* 42A:493–499.

130. Meech, R. W., and Standen, N. B. (1975): Potassium activation in Helix asperase neurones under voltage clamp: A component mediated by calcium influx., *J. Physiol. (Lond.)* 249:211–239.

131. Minota, S. (1974): Calcium ions and the posttetanic hyperpolarization of bullfrog sympathetic ganglion cells. *Jpn. J. Physiol.,* 24:501–512.

132. Morita, K., North, R. A., and Tokimasa, T. (1982): Muscarinic agonists inactivate potassium conductance of guinea-pig myenteric neurons. *J. Physiol.,* 333:124–139.

133. Morita, K., North, R. A., and Tokimasa, T. (1982): The calcium-activated potassium conductance in guinea-pig myenteric neurones. *J. Physiol. (Lond.),* 329:341–354.

134. Neher, E. (1971): Two fast transient current components during voltage clamp on snail neurones. *J. Gen. Physiol.,* 58:36–53.

135. Nishi, S., Soeda, H., and Koketsu, K. (1965): Studies on sympathetic B and C neurons and patterns of preganglionic innervation. *J. Cell Comp. Physiol.,* 66:19–32.

136. Nishi, S., and Koketsu, K. (1960): Electrical properties and activities of single sympathetic neurones of frogs. *J. Cell Comp. Physiol.,* 55:15–30.

137. Noble, D., and Tsien, R. W. (1968): The kinetics and rectifier properties of the slow potassium current in cardiac purkinje fibres. *J. Physiol. (Lond.),* 195:185–214.

138. Nohmi, M., Kuba, K., and Morita, K. (1983): Does intracellular release of Ca^{2+} participate in afterhyperpolarization of a sympathetic neurone? *Brain Res.,* 268:158–161.

139. Nowycky, M. C., Fox, A. P., and Tsien, R. W. (1984): Multiple types of calcium channel in dorsal root ganglion cells distinguished by sensitivity to cadmium and single channel properties. *Soc. Neurosci. Abstr.,* 10:526.

140. Numann, R., Wong, R. K. S., and Clark, R. (1982): Electrophysiology of single dissociated cortical neurones. *Soc. Neurosci. Abstr.,* 8:413.

141. Oomura, Y., Ozeki, S., and Maena, T. (1961): Electrical activity of a giant nerve cell under abnormal conditions. *Nature,* 191:1265–1267.

142. Pallotta, B. S., Magleby, K. L., and Barrett, J. N. (1981): Single channel recordings of Ca^{2+}-activated K^+ currents in rat muscle cell culture. *Nature (Lond.),* 292:471–474.

143. Pennefather, P., Lancaster, B., Adams, P. R., and Nicoll, R. A. (1985): Two distinct Ca-dependent K currents on bullfrog sympathetic ganglion cells. *Proc. Natl. Acad. Sci. USA,* 82:3040–3044.

144. Pick, J. (1963): The submicroscopic organization of the sympathetic ganglion in the frog (*Rana pipiens*). *J. Comp. Neurol.,* 120:409–462.

145. Rall, W. (1977): Core conductor theory and cable properties of neurons. In *Handbook of Physiology, Section 1—The Nervous System,* edited by E. Kandel, pp. 39–97. Williams & Wilkins, Baltimore.

146. Reuter, H. (1983): Calcium channel modulation by neurotransmitters, enzymes and drugs. *Nature,* 301:569–574.

147. Satin, L., and Adams, P. R. (1984): Miniature outward currents in autonomic neurons. *Soc. Neurosci. Abstr.,* 10:146.

148. Shulman, J., and Weight, F. (1976): Synaptic transmission: Long-term potentiation by a postsynaptic mechanism. *Science (NY),* 194:1437–1439.

149. Schwartzkroin, P. A., and Prince, D. A. (1980): Effects of TEA on hippocampal neurons. *Brain Res.,* 185:169–181.

150. Schwartzkroin, P. A., and Stafstrom, C. E. (1980): Effects of EGTA on the calcium-activated afterhyperpolarization in hippocampal CA3 pyramidal cells. *Science,* 210:1125–1126.

151. Selyanko, A. A., and Brown, D. A. (1985): Cholinergic synaptic inhibition of potassium and chloride currents in a mammalian sympathetic neurone. *Neurosci. Lett.* (in press).

152. Selyanko, A. A. (1984): Cd^{2+} suppresses a time-dependent Cl-current in rat sympathetic neurone. *J. Physiol.,* 350:49P.

153. Segal, M., and Barker, J. L. (1984): Rat hippocampal neurons in culture: Potassium conductances. *J. Neurophysiol.,* 51:1409–1433.

154. Segal, M., Rogawski, M. A., and Barker, J. L.

(1984): A transient potassium conductance depresses the excitability of cultured hippocampal and spinal neurons. *J. Neurosci.*, 4:604–609.

155. Smith, S. J., MacDermott, A. B., and Weight, F. F. (1983): Detection of intracellular Ca^{2+} transients in sympathetic neurones using arsenazo III. *Nature (Lond.)*, 304:350–352.

156. Spain, W. J., Schwindt, P. C., Stafstrom, C. E., and Crill, W. E. (1984): Voltage clamp analysis of an inwardly rectifying ionic current in neurons from cat sensorimotor cortex. *Soc. Neurosci. Abstr.*, 10:871.

157. Stafstrom, C. E., Schwindt, P. C., and Crill, W. E. (1982): Negative slope conductance due to a persistent subthreshold sodium current in cat neocortical neurons *in vitro*. *Brain Res.*, 236:221–226.

158. Standen, N. B., and Stanfield, P. R. (1978): A potential—and time-dependent—blockade of inward rectification in frog skeletal muscle by barium and strontium ions. *J. Physiol. (Lond.)*, 280:169–191.

159. Stampfli, R., and Hille, B. (1976): Electrophysiology of the peripheral myelinated nerve. In: *Frog Neurobiology*, edited by R. Llinas and W. Precht, pp. 3–32. Springer Verlag, Berlin.

160. Taxi, J. (1976): Morphology of the autonomic nervous system. In: *Frog Neurobiology*, edited by R. Llinas and W. Precht, pp. 93–150. Springer Verlag, Berlin.

161. Tillotson, D., and Gorman, A. L. F. (1980): Non-uniform Ca^{2+} buffer distribution in a nerve cell body. *Nature*, 286:816–817.

162. Tokimasa, T. (1984): Muscarinic agonists depress calcium dependent K in bullfrog sympathetic neurons. *J. Auton. Nerv. Syst.*, 10:107–116.

163. Tokimasa, T. (1984): Calcium-dependent hyperpolarizations in bullfrog sympathetic neurons. *Neuroscience*, 12:919–937.

164. Tosaka, T., Takasa, J., Miyazaki, T., and Libet, B. (1983): Hyperpolarization following activation of K^+ channels by excitatory postsynaptic potentials. *Nature (Lond.)*, 308:143–150.

165. Tosaka, T., Chichibu, S., and Libet, B. (1968): Intracellular analysis of slow inhibitory and excitatory postsynaptic potentials in sympathetic ganglia of the frog. *J. Neurophysiol.*, 31:396–409.

166. Traub, R. D., and Wong, R. K. S. (1983): Synchronized burst discharge in disinhibited hippocampal slice II. Model of cellular mechanism., *J. Neurophysiol.*, 49:459–471.

167. Turner, D. A., and Schwartzkroin, P. A. (1980): Steady state electronic analysis of intracellularly stained hippocampal neurons. *J. Neurophysiol.*, 44:184–199.

168. Turner, D. (1984): Segmental cable evaluation of somatic transients in hippocampal neurons (CA1, CA3 and dentate). *Biophys. J.*, 46:73–84.

169. Weitsen, H. A., and Weight, F. F. (1977): Synaptic innervations of sympathetic ganglion cells in the bullfrog. *Brain Res.*, 128:197–211.

170. Wong, R. K. S., and Clark, R. B. (1983): Single K^+ channel currents from hippocampal pyramidal cells of adult guinea-pig. *Soc. Neurosci. Abstr.*, 9:602.

171. Wong, R. K. S., and Prince, D. A. (1981): Afterpotential generation in hippocampal pyramidal cells. *J. Neurophysiol.*, 45:86–97.

172. Wong, R. K. S., Prince, D. A., and Basbaum, A. I. (1979): Intradendritic recording from hippocampal neurons. *Proc. Natl. Acad. Sci. USA*, 76:986–990.

173. Wong, B. S., Lecar, H., and Adler, M. (1982): Single calcium-dependent potassium channels in clonal anterior pituitary cells. *Biophys. J.*, 39:313–317.

174. Yamamoto, T. (1963): Some observations on the fine structure of the sympathetic ganglion of bullfrog. *J. Cell Biol.*, 16:159–170.

175. Yanigahara, K., and Irisawa, H. (1980): Inward current activated during hyperpolarization in the rabbit sino atrial node cell. *Pflugers Arch. Ges. Physiol.*, 385:11–19.

176. Zbicz, K. L., and Weight, F. F. (1984): Voltage-clamp analysis reveals two transient outward currents in hippocampal CA3 pyramidal neurons. *Soc. Neurosci. Abstr.*, 10:657.

Advances in Neurology, Vol. 44, edited by
A. V. Delgado-Escueta, A. A. Ward, Jr.,
D. M. Woodbury, and R. J. Porter.
Raven Press, New York © 1986.

7

Toward a Mechanism of Gating of Chemically Activated Channels

Meyer B. Jackson

Department of Biology, University of California, Los Angeles 90024

SUMMARY   Chemically activated channels are membrane proteins that have various functions, including the generation of postsynaptic responses. Receptor activation of channels produces excitation, inhibition, or modulation of the responsiveness of a neuron. Synaptic transmission can be altered by many drugs that act on receptors or channels, and many such drugs are important to epilepsy research and treatment.

The analysis of channel-gating mechanisms proceeds by the identification of conformations of the receptor channel complex with high or low conductance. These "open" and "closed" states are correlated with the state of occupancy of the receptor binding sites. The patch-clamp technique is ideally suited for the study of channel gating, since it permits the detection of different conductance states of a single channel. Analysis of single-channel current data yields information about the number of such conformations available to channels.

Single-channel current analysis of the nicotinic acetylcholine (Ach) receptor of skeletal muscle has shown that there are several different open and closed states. Two of the closed states open very rapidly and are probably activated closed states with bound agonists. The ACh receptor channel can open spontaneously at a very low rate in the absence of bound agonist.

Work with other chemically activated channels offers hope that channels activated by neurotransmitters in the mammalian central nervous system can be understood. Glutamate-activated channels can be studied in arthropod muscle and GABA-activated channels can be studied in mammalian spinal cord and hippocampus. In addition, the action of serotonin can be studied in molluscan neurons.

One goal of such studies is to understand the mechanisms of responses to neurotransmitters well enough to test for the normal and defective activity of receptor channels as hypotheses for epilepsy. Another goal is to understand the molecular mechanism of action of drugs that are relevant to epilepsy.

The union of a stereospecific receptor with an ion-selective transmembrane pore forms a chemically activated channel. This membrane-bound complex transduces a change in the local concentration of a specific neurotransmitter into a change in the cell membrane's ionic conductance.

The receptor and channel represent two distinct functions that are coupled within the receptor–channel complex. A channel modifies the electrical properties of its hosting cell membrane by giving it at least two discrete states of high and low conductance corresponding to "open" and "closed" states respectively. Depending on the type of ions that permeate an open channel, and depending on the gradients of these ions across the membrane, the gating of these channels can excite or inhibit the postsynaptic cell or modulate its responsiveness to other synaptic inputs. Receptors bind specific molecules from a solution. Depending on the stereospecificity of the receptor binding site, homologous drugs can be strong or weak agonists or strong or weak antagonists of a synaptic response.

The molecular identity of receptor–channel complexes has been established by biochemical and molecular biological techniques. Receptor–channel complexes can be labeled by various specific agents (56,62), and they can be purified (56) and functionally reconstituted (33,84,101). They can be used as immunogens to raise highly specific antibodies (91,109). Finally, a receptor channel gene has been cloned and sequenced (86,111). Receptor–channel complexes are among the molecular building blocks that form a functional chemical synapse; an understanding of their activation and inactivation is a necessary part of a complete description of the postsynaptic response.

The striking electrophysiological correlates of epilepsy may have an explanation in terms of basic synaptic mechanisms. One interesting hypothesis suggests that seizures arise from a failure of inhibitory synaptic transmission. The paroxysmal depolarization shift (PDS)—an experimentally induced prolonged bursting depolarization that has a striking correlation with interictal epileptic behavior—can be induced in experimental animals by a number of compounds that block the action of the inhibitory transmitter γ-aminobutyric acid (GABA), at its receptor or channel (73,74,92).

GABA-activated channels are known to be a site of action of important antiepileptic drugs including barbituates and benzodiazepines (64, 65,71,108), and may be the site of action of other antiepileptic drugs as well. Many of these drugs facilitate the response to GABA, suggesting a possible role of GABA in controlling or preventing seizure activity.

Seizures may also involve an excess of synaptic excitation. Some antiepileptic drugs also antagonize excitatory synaptic transmission (65). Model studies of neuronal circuits with re-

current excitation show synchronized bursting behavior (115). The PDS shares many of the characteristics of a very large excitatory synaptic potential (55).

At a basic level, studies of mechanisms of channel gating may contribute to a better understanding of how synaptic transmission participates in epileptogenesis. At a more practical level, studies of gating mechanisms are often easily extended to mechanisms by which drugs act on a receptor. A better understanding of how neurotransmitters affect channel gating could help in finding the precise site at which a drug binds and the specific process that the drug modifies.

In this chapter, a conceptual framework is developed for the understanding of chemically activated channels. Channel-gating mechanisms are then discussed in detail, emphasizing experiments with patch-clamp techniques to illustrate interesting features of channel behavior. A great variety of membrane channels have been investigated intensively with many different methods. For a broader view of channels, the reader is referred to Jackson et al., Parsegian, and Sakmann and Neher (53,89,98).

PRINCIPLES OF CHANNEL GATING

A conceptual leap in understanding the electrical properties of a membrane is taken when one localizes a selective ionic conductance to a molecular-sized membrane protein and ascribes to it a few relatively stable conformations. Considering only an open (O) and closed (C) conformation in equilibrium, we have

$$C \leftrightharpoons O$$

This simple two-state model is a starting point in developing ideas about channel gating.

Depending on the specific nature of the channel, this equilibrium might be coupled to some other property of the environment. Among the more important variables might be membrane potential or the concentration of some soluble molecule. The influence of these different variables on the open-closed equilibrium can be put into similar forms. If the equilibrium depends on voltage (V), then this dependence can be described by the relation

$$\frac{d \ln K}{dV} = \frac{-qx}{kT} \qquad \text{(Eq. 1)}$$

where $K = [O]/[C]$, k is Boltzmann's constant, T is the temperature, q is the charge that moves during gating, and x is the fraction of the field traversed by the charge during gating. If more than one charge moves, then qx is replaced by a sum over all products of q and x for each charge. Behavior qualitatively similar to this is responsible for the propagation of an action potential along an axon. This simple dependence of a gating equilibrium on voltage has been studied in detail in artificial membranes and has been used to explain negative resistance or N-shaped current-voltage curves that are the essence of voltage excitation of membranes (31).

Gating can be coupled to the binding of n ligands A to a receptor. The gating equilibrium can then assume the form

$$C + nA \rightleftharpoons OA_n \qquad \text{(Eq. 2)}$$

where it is assumed that the fully bound complex is always open, and only the fully bound complex can open. The ligand concentration dependence of the open-closed equilibrium is described by

$$\frac{d \ln K}{d \ln [A]} = n \qquad \text{(Eq. 3)}$$

where [A] is the concentration of free A. Thus, the relative effectiveness with which voltage or ligand can influence the channel gating equilibrium in the above simple examples depends on $-qx/kT$ or n, respectively.

Equation 3 is the natural starting point in an analysis of chemically activated channels. Because K can be estimated from measurements of membrane current, plots of $\ln K$ verses $\ln [A]$ can be used to determine n.

Because channel gating is a dynamic process, it is natural to apply kinetic techniques to the study of gating mechanisms. A two-state equilibrium exhibits a characteristic dynamic response. When the variable to which the equilibrium is coupled (membrane potential or ligand concentration) undergoes a sudden change, the equilibrium is altered. The concentrations of the two states relax exponentially with time to a new equilibrium. The time for e-fold decay is the reciprocal of the sum of the forward and reverse rate constants.

Using photolytic techniques, the concentration of agonist near the postsynaptic muscle membrane can be subjected to a virtually instantaneous increase (63). The fact that the membrane current then increases with a rate comparable to the rate following a sudden change in voltage suggests that agonist binding is not rate-limiting under these conditions. The exponential decay of an endplate current is consistent with a virtually instantaneous removal of transmitter (67,68). A change in the endplate current following a voltage jump indicates that, although a chemically activated channel does not have a primary functional requirement for voltage dependence, the gating of the ACh receptor channel is accompanied by some charge movement (2,24,68,96,102).

The kinetic response following a perturbation has an equilibrium or steady state counterpart in the autocorrelation function and power spectrum of fluctuations in the membrane current. Measurable fluctuations result from the random opening and closing of many channels. Analysis of channel noise in membrane currents in many different systems has been made in terms of an open–closed channel equilibrium (4,31,57,58,71, 95). In these experiments, noise power is measured as a function of frequency and compared with the theoretical predictions of simple models to infer some of the unitary channel properties.

Most of the methods used to study channel-gating mechanisms have on at least some occasions shown deviations from the predictions of the two-state model. For example, receptor desensitization implies the existence of receptor states in which ligand is bound but in which the channel remains closed (60,112). Desensitization is often manifest in dynamic studies as the current increases at the onset of application of a drug and then decreases to a lower steady state with continued drug application.

In an initial period during which various kinetic methods were being developed, most observed kinetic relaxations were simply exponential, supporting a two-state model for synaptic channels. As the various methods were improved and refined, some of them revealed more complex responses. Voltage relaxation and noise studies (21,93) have resolved more than one exponential component, indicating additional steps in the underlying kinetic process. These and other findings point towards mechanisms of channel gating that are more complex than the two-state model. In light of these observations investigators have retained the concept of stable interconverting states, but have augmented the two-state model by adding more states. Currently, much work on gating mechanisms is centered on the task of identifying and characterizing kinetic intermediates and determining their relative stabilities and the rates with which they interconvert.

PATCH CLAMP

Among the many techniques used to study channels, the patch clamp is particularly well suited for the elucidation of channel-gating mechanisms. The stepwise changes in membrane current seen with the patch clamp as single channels open and close are some of the more compelling evidence for the existence of channels in biological membranes. In a patch-clamp experiment (Fig. 1), a small area of cell membrane is covered with the tip of a smooth-edged saline-filled glass micropipet with an inner diameter of roughly 1 μm. Gentle suction pulls the membrane into the electrode, and a tight, high-resistance seal forms between the edges of the electrode tip and the cell membrane. Under these conditions, the intrinsic current noise of the circuit falls below 1 pA (10^{-12} A), and an amplifier with very low noise can resolve single-channel currents, which are typically of the order of 1 pA.

Obtaining a high-resistance seal is a critical requirement for good single-channel recordings, since part of the current noise power of the circuit is inversely proportional to the square root of this resistance. In the first successful experiments, seals ranged from 20 to 50 MΩ (80–83). Using suction and extremely clean patch elec-trodes, Neher, Sakmann, and their colleagues obtained "gigaseals," where the seal resistance surpassed the 10^9Ω (1 GΩ) landmark (44,105), occassionally reaching 100 GΩ or more. The tight electrode is pulled away from the cell, giving rise to excised membrane patches, providing a cell-free system for single-channel current recording (44,48). Extensive reviews of patch-clamp methodology are available (44, 53,98).

MOLECULAR ACTIVITY OF CHANNELS

Carrying the two-state model to the single-channel level requires a replacement of concentrations of open and closed channels with the probabilities that channels are open and closed. In single-channel current records (Fig. 2), we see that the current changes abruptly between well-defined levels, but that the time at which transitions occur is random. The randomness in time of transition reflects the intrinsic randomness of molecular processes. We must then ask what is the probability that a state will endure for a certain time. This analysis has been carried out for the two-state model to show that the probabilities of open-state and closed-state lifetimes are exponentially decreasing functions with rates of decay equal to the closing rate and opening rate, respectively (32). Thus, an analysis of the distributions of lifetimes of these states allows the determination of rate constants

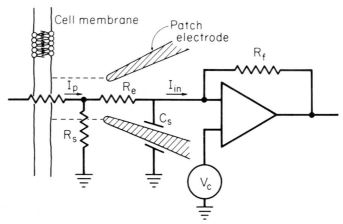

FIG. 1. A patch electrode is pushed up against the cell membrane (not drawn to scale). The current through the patch of membrane, I_p, is divided by two resistances, the seal resistance, R_s, and the electrode resistance, R_e. As the seal resistance increases, a larger portion of the membrane current is captured by the electrode and the input noise goes down. The membrane current is converted to a voltage by the operational amplifier and the feedback resistor, R_f. C_s, the source capacitance, is an important source of noise. C_s is reduced by coating the electrode with a low dielectric material. A command voltage, V_c, to the noninverting input of the amplifier controls the potential at the tip of the electrode when the seal resistance is sufficiently high.

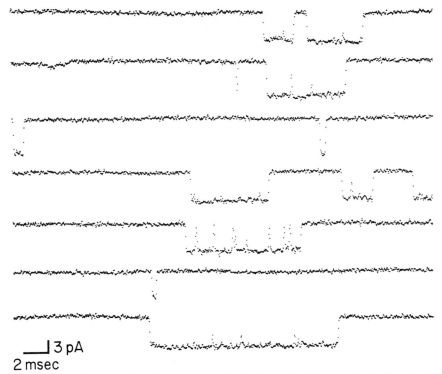

FIG. 2. Single-channel currents in cultured mouse skeletal muscle. Cells were bathed in physiological saline at room temperature (23°C). The patch electrode contained 40 nM suberyldicholine in the same saline used to bathe the cells. The signal was filtered at 5 kHz with a low-pass 8-pole Bessel filter. The command voltage (see Fig. 1), V_c, was held at $+50$ mV. Because the membrane potential was about -60 mV, a net driving force of about -110 mV produced inward current flow. Thus, the opening of a channel produces a step in the negative direction.

for each process independently. By comparison, measurements of rate processes at a macroscopic level yield the sum of the forward and reverse rates, and knowledge of additional quantities is necessary to separate these two numbers.

The patch clamp has proven extraordinarily useful in revealing new channel states relevant to the gating process. Direct analysis of single-channel current amplitudes has in many cases revealed multiple conductance states. The current is seen to flicker between different conducting states, suggesting that some channels have multiple open structures (7,8,43,45,116). Different states with the same conductance are not apparent from an analysis of current amplitudes. But, just as for macroscopic rate processes, the distribution of state lifetimes will have more exponential components. A mathematical analysis of the stochastic behavior of multistate models provides a number of examples of distributions that are sums of two or more exponential components (13,46). The number of exponential components in a lifetime

distribution of a particular conductance level is formally a lower bound to the number of stable states with the same conductance.

The information content of a single-channel current record is still not known. Lifetime distributions are only one way of analyzing the stochastic behavior of channels. It is also possible to analyze channel state lifetimes subject to a condition of prior behavior (49), or to look for correlations in the lifetimes of different channel states (54,76). This approach can be made more systematic by deriving two-dimensional or joint probability distributions for different models and comparing them with observed joint distributions (36). Perhaps the most general method of analysis is to calculate the likelihood of a long sequence of channel currents given a specific model. For data with many channel events, the likelihood can have a very sharp maximum with respect to variation of the parameters of this model. Using the method of likelihood maximization, different models can be evaluated, and the rate constants of the kinetic processes can be estimated (47).

CHEMICALLY ACTIVATED CHANNELS

By far the most thoroughly studied chemically activated channel is the nicotinic ACh receptor channel of skeletal muscle. It was the first membrane channel studied *in situ* with noise analysis (4,57,58,95) and with the patch clamp (80). The techniques of noise analysis and patch clamp, pioneered with the nicotinic receptor channel, have been applied to many other chemically activated channels. We now know the unitary properties of channels activated by ACh at excitatory (6) and inhibitory (5) receptors in neurons of *Aplysia,* at nicotinic receptors in bovine chromaffin cells (35), and at muscarinic receptors of heart muscle (99). The channels activated by glutamate in locust muscle (3,90) and crayfish muscle (17); by GABA in crayfish muscle (29), locust muscle (18), and mouse spinal cord (43,52,75,97); and by glycine in brainstem of lamprey (37), spinal cord of goldfish (34), and mouse (9,43,97) have all been described. In addition, channels modulated by second messengers by serotonin in *Aplysia* (103) and by cholecystokinin (CCK) and ACh in pancreatic cells (69,70) have been studied.

Most of these studies have not gone beyond a determination of single-channel conductance and mean open time or mean duration of a burst of openings. The higher resolution afforded by current techniques shows that a single channel can have multiple conductance states and multiple rate processes that control gating. These more complex features have been revealed in the GABA-activated (43,52,97) and glycine-activated (43,97) channels in cultured spinal cord; the glutamate-activated channel of locust muscle (20,38,39,90); and the nicotinic ACh receptor channel of vertebrate skeletal muscle (7,8, 15,16,21,22,45,51,54,76,78,83,100,106,116). Because these observations offer some of the newest insights into gating mechanisms, they will be reviewed in detail.

The work on the nicotinic receptor is the most extensive, although even for this channel we do not have a complete mechanism. Reviewing this work helps in presenting the current scope of channel-gating mechanisms, and suggests the direction in which work on CNS channels may be heading.

NICOTINIC RECEPTOR CHANNEL

ACh opens a cation-selective channel at the vertebrate neuromuscular junction. The response exhibits strong desensitization, but even early studies of the dose-response behavior suggested that the binding of two agonists to the receptor was necessary for channel opening (60). More quantitative studies supported this view (1,23,27), although one study raised the possibility that singly liganded receptors have a small but finite probability of opening (23).

Binding of ligands to purified receptors suggests that each receptor has two ligand binding sites (56,94). There are also two binding sites for α-bungarotoxin (56,94), a toxin derived from snake venom that blocks neuromuscular transmission (62). The binding between toxin and cholinergic ligand is competitive, indicating that they bind to overlapping domains of the receptor (56). The two sites that bind toxin and ligand are not identical in their pharmacological selectivity (107). A high-affinity receptor state that forms slowly in the presence of agonist may correspond to a densensitized state of the receptor (10,85,110).

Many of the features of channel activation by ACh compare well with the properties of the endplate current. The rate of decay of the endplate current is similar to the apparent mean channel open time obtained from analysis of ACh-induced noise (4,58). This suggests that the time course of the endplate current is determined by the lifetime of the open state, with channels opening only once, and with diffusion and hydrolysis preventing the rebinding reaction. Other agonists produce channel currents with the same conductance, but with different mean open times (12,51,58,79). As the membrane potential is hyperpolarized, both the endplate current and the channel mean open time are prolonged (4,24,68). The ACh in motor terminals can be replaced with an artificial transmitter, acetylmonoethylcholine (14), since monoethylcholine is transported by the choline uptake system and esterified with acetate by the enzyme, choline acetyltransferase. Following this replacement, the endplate current assumed a decay time similar to the channel mean open time for acetylmonoethylcholine (14).

The inclusion of a binding step in the gating process raises the possibility that binding and gating are not necessarily concomitant, as in Eq. 2, but occur separately. The rate of agonist binding appeared to be faster than the rate of the gating step (63). However, with cooled preparations, the noise relaxation time for a weaker agonist, carbamylcholine, saturates, such that at sufficiently high concentrations the binding rate is greater than the rate of the channel opening conformational change (96). This suggests that a small but detectable time elapses between binding and gating. Voltage relaxation experiments showing two exponential components have also been interpreted in terms of a model with separate binding and channel opening steps (21).

Patch-clamp studies have opend a Pandora's box of multiple states of the ACh receptor-channel. Nelson and Sachs (83) reported the first direct observation of short-duration closed states. These closures broke a long-duration event into a burst of repeated openings. With desensitizing concentrations, even more complex behavior was observed (100). The closed times could have been the closed-liganded complexes inferred by others (21,96), but Nelson and Sachs (83) were also compelled to consider the possibility that the agonist they used, suberyldicholine, blocked the channel. This possibility carried considerable weight at the time because of an important study by Neher and Steinbach (82), showing similar short-duration closed times to be periods of channel blockade by local anesthetic. Colquhoun and Sakmann (15) resolved this issue by showing that the frequency of short-duration closures in agonist-induced openings were independent of agonist concentration, ruling out the possibility of agonist blockade of an open channel.

This observation required a reinterpretation of earlier noise studies and of comparisons of mean channel open time with endplate current decay time. Noise studies were not capable of resolving the relaxation time associated with the very rapid channel closures. The observed relaxation time of the noise corresponded to the duration of a burst of repeated openings of a liganded receptor channel. With these reopenings, the endplate current decay time is also governed by the duration of such a burst. The relaxation times in noise experiments are comparable to the endplate current decay times, and both measurements are of times that are essentially bounded by the lifetime of the receptor ligand complex.

Colquhoun and Sakmann (15) performed a quantitative analysis, demonstrating without ambiguity a second exponential component in their closed-time distributions and determining separate rate constants for agonist dissociation and channel opening. Dionne and Liebowitz (22) analyzed a similar fast component of closed times in nicotinic receptor channels of snake muscle. The observation of brief channel closures, and their interpretation as times during

which the channel is closed while the binding site is occupied, suggests that there is an equilibrium between the liganded open and liganded closed channel, with the open state favored. Others have since found that there are as many as five kinetic components in closed-time distributions, suggesting that there are additional closed states that may or may not be in rapid equilibrium with an open state (16,106).

Colquhoun and Sakmann (15), and others (51,106) also found two exponential components in the open-time distribution. Previous noise analysis had not revealed this process because of poorer time resolution and because of an inherent weighting by noise analysis of slower processes (51,52). In a tentative interpretation of the population of brief duration openings, Colquhoun and Sakmann (15) suggested that it results from openings in which only one of the receptor binding sites was occupied. This interpretation was consistent with some earlier dose–response studies (23). The same phenomenon was observed in cultured human muscle (51), in which an interpretation of two separate channel populations was suggested based on the variability in the proportion of long- and short-duration channel openings. Subsequent studies in numerous skeletal muscle preparations confirmed the complexity of open-time and closed-time distributions (7,8,16,54,76,78,106) (Fig. 3), but failed to provide a clear interpretation.

In a companion study to that of Colquhoun and Sakmann (15), Hamill and Sakmann (45) reported three open states of the ACh receptor channel in cultured rat muscle with different conductances. Two larger conductance levels, one of 23 pS and one of 33 pS, did not interconvert. These levels were similar to the two different conductance levels previously found in skeletal muscle, in which the larger conductance channel was localized to the endplate region. The smaller conductance level appeared over the entire muscle fiber following denervation and had openings of longer duration (26,28,79). It was striking to find both conductance levels coexisting in cultured muscle (45), but it was also common to find muscle cultures with mostly one conductance level or the other (54). With either one of the two conducting species in the majority, two exponential components in the open-time distributions were still found, and the average current amplitude of the short-duration openings was found to be equal to the average current amplitude of the long-duration openings (54). Thus, there are two different ACh-receptor-channel populations with dif-

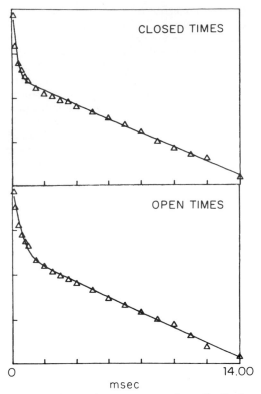

FIG. 3. Closed-time and open-time distributions were prepared from records such as those in Fig. 2 by counting the number of closed times and open times of duration t or longer. The solid curves are best-fitting sums of two exponentials.

ferent conductances, but each has two open states. The factors that determine which receptor-channel type will appear in a muscle cell culture are not known at the present time.

Hamill and Sakmann (45) found that either major conductance level can undergo a "partial closure" to the third conductance state of only 8 pS. Trautmann (116) and Auerbach and Sachs (7,8) observed a similar process. These partial closures remain a mysterious aspect of channel behavior.

The observation of multiple conductance levels by Trautmann (116) was an offshoot of his surprising find that curare, a classical ACh antagonist, could activate ACh receptor channels. Morris et al. (77) also reported single-channel currents activated by curare. These results were consistent with a previous report of curare-induced depolarization of embryonic skeletal muscle (117). Curare only activates in embryonic and cultured muscle, including cultured muscle derived from adult humans (51). The ca-

pacity of the receptor to be activated by curare is an interesting and yet unexplained feature, apparently subject to developmental control.

Trautmann noted that the mean open time of curare-activated channels was shorter when higher concentrations of curare were used (116). His interpretation was that curare blocked the open channel. A conclusion of channel blockade could be further supported by an appropriate analysis of close times, similar to that used for local anesthetics (82).

In the original report of curare-induced depolarization it was noted that the muscle had to be hyperpolarized to see an effect, and that the depolarization never went beyond -50 mV (117), as though the reversal potential were different from that of the depolarization elicited by agonists. A response was never seen from a holding potential above -50 mV. The conclusion that curare caused this depolarization by opening the ACh receptor channel was based primarily on the fact that the response was blocked by α-bungarotoxin (117), but the failure to depolarize past -50 mV represented a serious discrepancy with the normal agonist response.

Morris et al. (78) analyzed curare-activated single-channel currents to show that the rate of channel opening had a strong voltage dependence that could explain a failure to depolarize beyond -50 mV. The single-channel current–voltage curve was linear and extrapolated to 0 mV, as it should for the ACh receptor channel. At membrane potentials above -50 mV, the rate of curare-induced channel opening was insignificant. This effect is not unique to channel activation by curare, but bears a strong resemblance to the response of the desensitized endplate, in which an extrapolated reversal potential can differ from the true reversal potential, possibly because of strongly voltage-dependent channel gating (59).

In some respects, curare activation of the ACh receptor is similar to agonist activation of the receptor: two main conductance levels are seen as are partial closures (116), and open-time distributions have two exponential components (78).

In the absence of an agonist, the equilibrium between the open and closed states should favor the closed state. The unfavored open state is still present, but occurs rarely. Upper boundaries to the frequency of spontaneous openings of the nicotinic receptor channel have been estimated previously (23,85).

With the patch clamp, one can observe

channel currents in cultured muscle in the absence of ligand (Fig. 4) (50). These currents are of the same amplitude as currents activated by agonist, and are blocked by α-bungarotoxin (50). Agonist-activated channel currents and spontaneously occurring channel currents have similar ion selectivity (50). Chemical modification of the binding site prevented agonist binding and activation, but spontaneous openings occurred more frequently (50). Although these spontaneous openings reflect an unliganded open–closed equilibrium, it is not possible to estimate the equilibrium constant quantitatively because the number of receptors in a patch of membrane is not known.

An analysis of the open-time distribution of spontaneous openings reveals two exponential components (Fig. 5). Thus, even a receptor that has not been activated by ligand has access to two different open states. This adds a new element of complexity to the two exponential components in the open-time distributions of agonist-activated channels, since one interpretation considered previously was that they were singly and doubly liganded gatings (15).

In order to explain the double exponential open-time distributions seen with agonist activation, investigators have examined single-channel records more closely, trying to extract more information. This led to questions concerning the relationships between open times of different channel currents. One can see in Fig. 2 that long- and short-duration openings are not intermingled randomly. Instead, channels of similar duration are often grouped in clusters. A statistical analysis of pairs of channel currents separated by closed times of less than 5 msec showed a striking correlation in open times (54). The majority of closely spaced pairs were either both relatively long or both relatively short, with few mixed pairs of long and short openings together. This indicates that there are two distinct activated closed states that can open, with one closed state opening for relatively long times, and the other closed state opening for relatively short times. Considering the five closed states inferred from analysis of closed-time distributions (16,106), the analysis of correlations in open times suggests that two closed states are activated and open rapidly.

Figure 6A shows the results of a quantitative analysis of open-state closed-state correlations. Short-duration closed times are associated with a higher proportion of long-duration openings, and intermediate-duration closed times are associated with a higher proportion of short-duration openings. Thus, one open state not only closes more rapidly, but its associated activated closed state also opens more slowly than the other activated closed state.

An approach described by Montal et al. (76) to the analysis of correlations involves a deter-

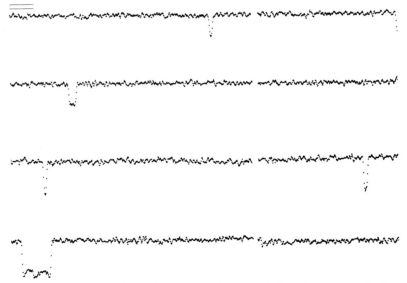

FIG. 4. Channel currents recorded as in Fig. 2, but without a cholinergic substance in the patch-electrode filling solution. These spontaneous openings of the acetylcholine receptor-channel occur infrequently and have the same amplitude as channel currents seen when suberyldicholine or some other agonist is in the patch electrode. Calibration bar 1 pA × 2 msec.

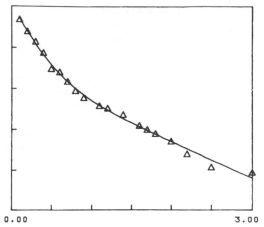

0.00   3.00

FIG. 5. The open-time distribution for spontaneous openings of the acetylcholine receptor channel. The solid curve is a best-fitting sum of two exponentials.

mination of the frequency of short-duration openings in a record subject to the condition of having a given number of long-duration openings. The probability of observing a long opening was dependent upon the probability of observing a short opening, suggesting that the two activated closed states could interconvert.

If the two identified open states were distinguished by having one or two binding sites occupied, the ratio in number of long-duration openings to short-duration openings should depend on agonist concentration. Sine and Steinbach (106) found only a very weak concentration dependence; however, on closer analysis, they found that at high agonist concentrations short-duration openings were more likely to occur within bursts of openings that also included long-duration openings. At low concentrations, there were many isolated short- and long-duration openings. This may mean that doubly liganded receptors produce bursts comprising openings of both the rapidly and slowly closing components.

A more detailed analysis of correlations in open times of pairs of very closely spaced openings bears out the suggestion by Sine and Steinbach (106) that a burst produced by one channel can include channel openings of both the long- and short-duration components. When the lifetimes of channel openings associated with short-duration closures are analyzed, the fraction of slowly closing channels is lower if the closed time is longer (Fig. 6A). The slowly closing channels outnumber the rapidly closing channels by about four to one for very short intervening closed times (0.075–0.125 msec), but the fraction of rapidly closing channels in this group is significantly higher than expected. This supports the notion that the rapidly opening closed state can produce both long- and short-duration openings.

A statistical analysis of pairs of openings separated by closed times of between 0.075 and 0.125 msec shows that within these bursts of long and short openings, there is relatively little correlation (Fig. 6B), indicating that these long- and short-duration openings can arise from the same activated closed state. For pairs separated by intermediate closed times, there is a high correlation, since both activated states produce closed-time intervals in this range and, on the average, the open times produced by the two activated states are different. For long closed-time intervals, there is no significant correlation, as expected for randomly composed pairs (54).

The goal of such studies of channel gating is a picture of how many open and closed states there are, how they interconvert, and how the interconversion rates are influenced by the occupation of the different binding sites by different drugs. To summarize the above discussion, there may be as many as 5 closed states, at least 1 of which is unliganded, 2 of which can open rapidly, and 2 of which are probably desensitized. The unliganded and the most rapidly opening activated closed states can each open into two different open states.

GLUTAMATE RECEPTOR CHANNEL

In the arthropod neuromuscular junction, glutamate is a transmitter. Noise analysis suggested that in insect (locust) muscle, the glutamate receptor channel has a very high conductance (3), in contrast to crustaceans (17). In crayfish muscle, an important comparison was made between endplate current decay time, and noise relaxation time for different agonists. The similarity between the glutamate-induced mean burst duration and the endplate current decay time offers convincing support for the role of glutamate as a neurotransmitter (17).

Before the development of high-resistance GΩ seals, the large channel conductance of locust muscle was especially appealing since it offered a high signal when low noise could not be obtained. Patlak et al. (90) confirmed the report of a high conductance and also showed that the

FIG. 6. Data such as that shown in Fig. 2 was analyzed for correlations in the durations of successive dwell times. Pairs of channel openings separated by various closed-time intervals (abscissa) were tabulated. The probability that a particular opening was a member of the rapidly decaying as opposed to the slowly decaying exponential component was determined from the best fitting open-time density (the derivative of a curve such as that in Fig. 3B). This probability is denoted by P_f and is plotted in **A** versus the closed time between the pair of openings. Openings adjacent to long closed times have higher values of P_f and are thus more likely to be brief in duration. Openings adjacent to brief closed times have lower values of P_f and are thus more likely to be long in duration. This indicates that there is an inverse correlation between open times and their neighboring closed times. **B:** Correlation between successive open times was tested by using a two by two contingency test. χ^2 reflects the deviation from randomness. A high χ^2 means that pairs

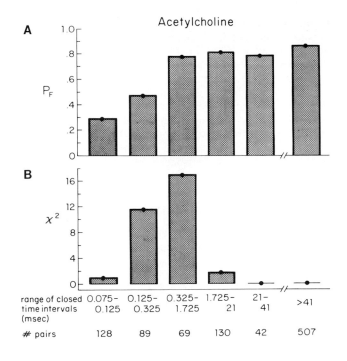

of openings are more often similar in open time; members of the same exponential component are segregated. A low χ^2 suggests that members of the two exponential components mix randomly. Pairs of openings separated by intermediate closed times are highly correlated in open time. The second opening of such a pair has a high probability of being a reopening of the same channel that produced the first opening. This defines one specific pathway between an open channel configuration with a characteristic closing rate and a closed channel configuration with a characteristic opening rate. Pairs of openings separated by long closed times are uncorrelated in open time, suggesting that the gating of different channels is independent. Pairs of openings separated by very short closed times are essentially uncorrelated in open time, suggesting that there is an additional pathway between another pair of open and closed states. This pathway is different from the pathway represented by the intermediate closed times.

channel undergoes a transition in its kinetic behavior. The channel spends relatively long times in either a state in which openings are brief and infrequent or in a state in which openings are long and frequent.

Because the receptor density is low in some regions of the muscle fiber, and because receptor desensitization can be removed by prior treatment with concanavalin A (ConA) (72), very high agonist concentrations can be used. Two different laboratories working on this preparation have undertaken dose–response studies with patch-clamp techniques, finding values for the number of bound ligands needed to activate a channel of 1 (40) and 2 (19). Cull-Candy et al. (19) made many measurements from a single patch of membrane using a perfused patch electrode. Gration et al. (39) found a change in

channel open time at very high agonist concentration.

The number of channel openings in a record is not well described by a Poisson distribution (39), indicating the existence of more than one channel closed state. An activated closed state has been suggested by the observation of a fast second exponential component in the distribution of closed times (20,35,38). This fast component is more pronounced with the strong agonist, quisqualate, than with the weak agonist, fluoroglutamate (40). This can be explained by a lower rate of dissociation or a higher rate of opening of the quisqualate-liganded complex.

Cull-Candy and Parker (20) showed that there are two exponential components in the open-time distribution, providing an appealing similarity with the ACh receptor channel. Because in one of their experiments only one channel was present in the patch of membrane and two exponentials were still seen, the hypothesis that there are two separate populations of channels that close with different rates can be eliminated.

In sharp contrast to Cull-Candy and Parker (20), Gration et al. (38) see a dearth of fast openings and suggest a cyclical scheme of binding, opening, unbinding, and closing. Until the discrepancies in the literature are resolved, it will be difficult to discuss the specific gating mechanism.

INHIBITORY CHLORIDE CHANNELS

The gating of a chloride selective channel is an important inhibitory mechanism in nerve and muscle. The inhibitory amino acids GABA and glycine operate by this mechanism. Studies of arthropod muscle characterized the basic nature of inhibitory transmission. These studies showed relatively little desensitization (113), and suggested that the binding of two GABA molecules to the receptor was necessary for channel opening (114). In addition, a slower time course of decay of responses to GABA in crayfish muscle as compared to ACh responses in vertebrate muscle (112) was eventually explained in terms of a longer channel mean open time (29). In lamprey brainstem, a favorable comparison between channel noise relaxation time and synaptic current decay time supports the status of glycine as a neurotransmitter (37).

Because the mouse spinal cord cell culture is derived from a mammalian central nervous system (CNS), it is a very promising preparation for the study of various questions relevant to epilepsy. These include basic mechanisms of gating of the GABA receptor channel and the mechanisms by which antiepileptic and epileptogenic drugs interact with this receptor. There is a considerable body of molecular pharmacology of convulsants and anticonvulsants that has been obtained through iontophoretic studies and noise analysis in this preparation (64, 65,108).

The first patch-clamp studies of the GABA receptor channel in spinal neurons were done with low-resistance seals. Simultaneous intracellular impalement with a microelectrode filled with 3 M KCl filled the cell with chloride, reversing the chloride driving force. When the cell was hyperpolarized to −80 mV and the signal was filtered to 100 Hz, inward single-channel currents of nearly 2 pA could be seen as chloride left the cell and entered the patch electrode (52).

Channel currents produced by three agonists— GABA, muscimol, and (−)-pentobarbital— were similar in amplitude (52). When GΩ seals were formed, the electrode could be depolarized, producing outward channel currents as chloride entered the cell from the electrode (Fig. 7).

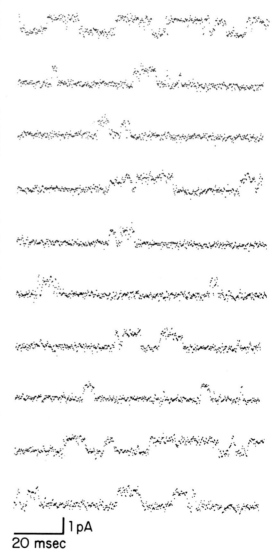

1 pA

20 msec

FIG. 7.   Channel currents activated by GABA in cultured mouse spinal cord. The cells were bathed in a solution of 140 mM Tris Cl buffered with Hepes to pH 7.4; 2 mM MgCl₂ and 1 mM CaCl₂ were also present. The patch electrode contained the bathing solution with 0.3 μM GABA added. The signal was filtered at 500 Hz with a low-pass 8-pole Bessel filter. The patch-electrode potential was held at −80 mV. Outward channel currents were produced as chloride entered the cell from the patch electrode.

Kinetic analysis of single-channel current records revealed two open states with open-time distributions being well fit by a sum of two exponentials (52,97) (Fig. 8A). Two exponentials are found in the closed-time distribution as well (97) (Fig. 8B). When the cell body of a cultured spinal neuron was clamped, dose–response studies indicated that the binding of two GABA molecules opened a channel (97). This revealed an interesting similarity with arthropod muscle (114). GABA-receptor binding studies suggest that there are two distinct binding sites for GABA in the mammalian brain (88).

With at least two closed states and two open states, it should be possible to ask questions about correlations of state lifetimes similar to those asked about the ACh receptor channel and in this way to probe the gating mechanism in greater detail. Analyzing pairs of openings, as was done above for the ACh receptor, and dividing open times into the fast or slow variety, we find very little correlation in the open times of closely spaced openings (Fig. 9B). The χ^2 for pairs of openings separated by 2–5 msec is so low that as an isolated observation, it would not be significant. However, by comparison with the suitable control distribution of pairs separated by longer times, the χ^2 of this group can be taken as a sign of weak correlation.

The proportion of short open-time to long open-time events seems to be independent of the intervening closed time (Fig. 9A). In the case of the GABA receptor channel, this method of analysis does not offer a clear interpretation. The nature of the interconversion between the various open and closed states remains unknown.

Studies of the open channel in hippocampal pyramidal cells suggest that it rectifies, i.e., it has a different conductance when the potential is positive than when the potential is negative (41).

Fluctuations between different conducting states have been resolved for both glycine- and GABA-activated channels in mouse spinal cord (43). The major conducting state of the glycine receptor channel has a higher conductance than that of the major conductance state of the

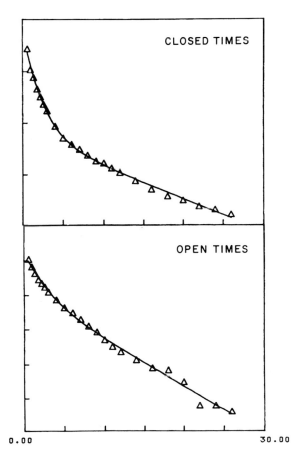

CLOSED TIMES

OPEN TIMES

1.00

0.00   30.00

FIG. 8. Closed-time and open-time distributions for GABA-activated channel currents, including those shown in Fig. 7. The solid curves are best-fitting sums of two exponentials.

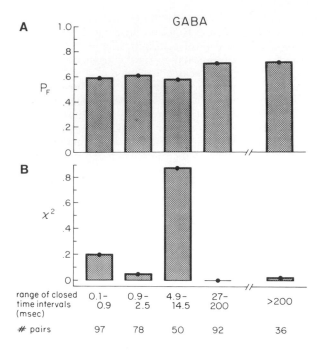

FIG. 9. An analysis of pairs of open times for GABA-activated channel currents. The analysis was identical to that described for the acetylcholine receptor in Fig. 6. **A:** The plot of P_f, the probability that a channel current is of the rapidly decaying exponential component of open times, versus the intervening closed times shows no significant correlation between neighboring open times and closed times. **B:** The χ^2 are much lower than those for the acetylcholine receptor channel. The value of χ^2 for intermediate closed times is small, but by comparison with χ^2 for longer and shorter duration closed times, a weak correlation in open times of successive openings can be inferred.

GABA receptor channel, consistent with previous noise analysis (9). The second highest conducting state for glycine has the same conductance as the major conducting state for GABA. A third conducting state for glycine and a second conducting state for GABA also have identical conductances. These open states have different conductances when different permeant anions are used, but the conductances change in exactly the same way for both the glycine and GABA receptor channels. These observations raise the intriguing possibility that the same basic channel structure can be coupled to either the glycine receptor or the GABA receptor (43).

NEUROTRANSMITTERS AS CHANNEL MODULATORS

The classical mechanism that dominates the above discussion involves a direct interaction between the receptor and channel with the binding of ligand causing the opening of the channel. This mechanism is by no means universal. Some transmitters, rather than open a channel, affect membrane conductance by closing or modifying the behavior of a membrane channel that gates freely in the absence of ligand. Many responses involve second messengers; the receptor and channel are not coupled by a direct interaction

within the membrane, but by additional components within the cytoplasm. These responses add an important dimension of diversity to synaptic responses, and could easily become the subject of an entire chapter (61,104). The following discussion will highlight some of the more interesting developments in this exciting and rapidly advancing field.

An important form of excitation occurs through a mechanism involving a decrease in the potassium conductance of a membrane. Because different classes of potassium channels maintain the negative resting potential of a cell and repolarize the membrane after an action potential, the closure of the appropriate group of potassium channels can initiate a depolarization or retard the termination of a depolarization. Muscarinic ACh receptors in central and peripheral mammalian neurons (61,25,11), substance P in mammalian spinal neurons (87), and serotonin in *Aplysia* neurons (103) involve the receptor-mediated closure of potassium channel. In many of these responses, a delay between application of the chemical stimulus and the onset of the potassium conductance decrease is caused by the time it takes for a receptor-activated adenylate cyclase to produce enough cyclic adenosine monophosphate (cAMP) to activate a protein kinase and bring about the phosphorylation of a potassium channel.

The excitatory response of *Aplysia* neurons to serotonin has been the subject of a patch-clamp study (103). Patch-clamp recordings from serotonin-sensitive cells show the simultaneous gating activity of several identical potassium channels that are unique in their conductance and gating behavior. Following serotonin application to the membrane outside the area of contact of the patch electrode, the potassium channels close. Leak of serotonin through the very tight GΩ seal is very unlikely. Thus, a response was generated without direct interactions between the receptor outside the patch and the channel inside the patch. The same potassium channels are closed by injection of cAMP. These experiments are exceptionally strong evidence for the ionic mechanism and second messenger aspect of this response.

Experiments with excised patches (44,48), in which the inner face of the membrane is accessible to manipulations, will be very valuable in determining how cytoplasmic components modify these potassium channels in *Aplysia* neuronal membranes. Recording channel currents from patches exposed to enzymes that phosphorylate and dephosphorylate the channel will provide some important insights into how the channel activity is regulated by the cytoplasm. This will probably become a very powerful and widely used approach in the study of slow synaptic potentials and responses modulated by transmitters through second messengers.

ACh has a more subtle effect on a potassium channel in bullfrog sympathetic ganglion. A potassium current is normally activated by depolarization. This current, called the M-current, is suppressed by ACh acting at a muscarinic receptor (11). An important feature of this synaptic mechanism is that muscarinic agonists have little influence on a cell at rest. The effect is only seen if the cell is suddenly depolarized; if the M-current is suppressed, the cell becomes more excitable. This is an example of a transmitter that has little action by itself but which can alter or modulate the response of a cell to other stimuli.

The action of norepinephrine (NE) and histamine on hippocampal pyramidal cells has some features in common with the muscarinic response in sympathetic ganglia. These two amines, in a cAMP mediated response, suppress the activation of the calcium-activated potassium channel (66,42). Because this channel is normally closed when a cell is at rest, NE or histamine produces no response. However, the calcium-activated potassium channel plays a key role in terminating a train of action potentials evoked by depolarizing current. In the presence of NE or histamine, an evoked train of action potentials lasts much longer (66,42).

Calcium channels can also be modulated by transmitters. In chick sensory neurons, compound action potentials could be recorded in which a fast sodium action current was followed by a long-lasting calcium action current. 5-HT, GABA, and NE all reduce the duration of the calcium component (30). Thus, they inhibit the opening or accelerate the inactivation of a voltage-activated calcium channel. Again, a quiescent cell gives little if any response. Although the effect was seen in the cell soma, the same mechanism would be very effective at the presynaptic level in reducing transmitter release.

CONCLUSION

Patch-clamp techniques have contributed very detailed insight into the gating mechanism of the nicotinic receptor channel, paving the way for similar studies in nervous systems. This reductionist approach of determining molecular conformations and rate processes of channel proteins that underlie synaptic responses has important applications to epilepsy.

The pharmacological significance is straightforward. With detailed knowledge of channel-gating mechanisms, studies of drug-induced changes in channel gating will indicate what are the molecular sites of drug action. Such studies will complement receptor binding studies (88) (see Chapter 17) and add information about the functional consequences of drug treatment. Such information should be very useful in making decisions about drug therapy.

Studies of chemically activated channel-gating mechanisms may also contribute more fundamental insights into the mechanisms of generation of epileptic activity. Essentially, every experimental model of epilepsy has some associated abnormality in an important neurotransmitter system, although it is often unclear whether an abnormality is a cause or consequence of bursting activity. The GABA antagonist models of epilepsy suggest that a defective GABA receptor can cause bursting behavior. An animal with a completely dysfunctional receptor would not be viable; however, if the channel has many different closed states, open states, and transition rates, there are a number of possibilities for nonlethal defects and interventions. Thus, as the GABA receptor integrates the effects of GABA and other pharmacological and endogenous ligands (64,68), and the channel pursues a stochastic trajectory through various closed states to different open states, a modification of one or a few of the rate processes or conductance states could, under special circumstances, alter the inhibitory efficacy of the channel. This could indeed be a basis for epileptic activity.

On the other hand, voltage, second messenger, and calcium-gated potassium currents that control excitability and are turned off by neurotransmitters (11,25,42,66,103) are intricately regulated. The molecular complexity of these responses provides a plethora of sites where function can be subtly altered to facilitate the development of bursts. The various transmitter hypotheses of epilepsy all become more testable as our understanding of the synaptic mechanisms improves.

REFERENCES

1. Adams, P. R. (1975): An analysis of the dose-response curve at voltage-clamped frog endplates. *Pflugers Arch.*, 360:145–153.
2. Adams, P. R. (1975): Kinetics of agonist-induced conductance changes during hyperpolarization at frog endplates. *Br. J. Pharmacol.*, 53:308–310.
3. Anderson, C. R., Cull-Candy, S. G., and Miledi, R. (1976): Glutamate and quisqualate noise in voltage clamped locust muscle fibers. *Nature*, 261:151–153.
4. Anderson, C. R., and Stevens, C. F. (1973): Voltage clamp analysis of acetylcholine produced end plate current fluctuations at frog neuromuscular junction. *J. Physiol.*, 235:655–691.
5. Ascher, P., and Erulkar, S. (1983): Cholinergic chloride channels in snail neurons. In: *Single Channel Recording*, edited by B. Sakmann and E. Neher, pp. 401–407. Plenum, New York.
6. Ascher, P., Marty, A., and Neild, T. O. (1978): Life time and elementary conductance of the channels mediating the excitatory effects of acetylcholine in *Aplysia* neurones. *J. Physiol.*, 278:177–206.
7. Auerbach, A., and Sachs, F. (1983): Flickering of a nicotinic ion channel to a subconductance state. *Biophys. J.*, 42:1–10.
8. Auerbach, A., and Sachs, F. (1984): Single channel currents from acetylcholine receptors in embryonic chick muscle: Kinetic and conductance properties of gaps within bursts. *Biophys. J.*, 45:157–164.
9. Barker, J. L., and McBurney, R. N. (1979): GABA and glycine may share the same conductance channel on cultured mammalian neurones. *Nature*, 277:234–236.
10. Barrantes, F. J. (1978): Agonist mediated changes in the acetylcholine receptor in its membrane environment. *J. Mol. Biol.*, 124:1–26.
11. Brown, D. A., and Adams, P. R. (1980): Mus-carinic suppression of a novel voltage-sensitive K^+ current in a vertebrate neurone. *Nature*, 283:673–676.
12. Colquhoun, D., Dionne, V. E., Steinbach, J. H., and Stevens, C. F. (1975): Conductance of channels opened by acetylcholine-like drugs in muscle-endplate. *Nature*, 253:204–206.
13. Colquhoun, D., and Hawkes, A. G. (1981): On the stochastic properties of single ion channels. *Proc. R. Soc. Lond. [Biol.] B*, 211:205–235.
14. Colquhoun, D., Large, W. A., and Rang, H. P. (1977): An analysis of the action of a false transmitter at the neuromuscular junction. *J. Physiol.*, 266:361–395.
15. Colquhoun, D., and Sakmann, B. (1981): Fluctuations in the microsecond time range of the current through single acetylcholine receptor ion channels. *Nature*, 294:464–466.
16. Colquhoun, D., and Sakmann, B. (1983): Bursts of openings in transmitter-activated ion channels. In: *Single Channel Recording*, edited by B. Sakmann and E. Neher, p. 345–364. Plenum, New York.
17. Crawford, A. C., and McBurney, R. N. (1976): The post-synaptic action of some putative excitatory transmitter substances. *Proc. R. Soc. Lond. B*, 192:481–489.
18. Cull-Candy, S. G., and Miledi, R. (1981): Junctional and extrajunctional membrane channels activated by GABA in locust muscle fibers. *Proc. R. Soc. Lond. [Biol.] B*, 211:527–535.
19. Cull-Candy, S. G., Miledi, R., and Parker, I. (1981): Single glutamate-activated channels recorded from locust muscle fibers with perfused patch clamp electrodes. *J. Physiol.*, 321:195–210.
20. Cull-Candy, S. G., and Parker, I. (1982): Rapid kinetics of single glutamate receptor channels. *Nature*, 295:410–412.
21. Dionne, V. E., and Parsons, R. L. (1981): Characteristics of the acetylcholine operated channels at twitch and slow fibre neuromuscular junctions of the garter snake. *J. Physiol.*, 310:145–158.
22. Dionne, V. E., and Liebowitz, M. D. (1982): Acetylcholine receptor kinetics. A description from single-channel currents at snake neuromuscular junctions. *Biophys. J.*, 39:253–261.
23. Dionne, V. E., Steinbach, J. H., and Stevens, C. F. (1978): An analysis of the dose-response relationship at voltage-clamped frog neuromuscular junctions. *J. Physiol.*, 281:421–444.
24. Dionne, V. E., and Stevens, C. F. (1975): Voltage dependence of agonist effectiveness at the frog neuromuscular junction: The resolution of a paradox. *J. Physiol.*, 251:245–270.
25. Dodd, J. E., Dingledine, R., and Kelly, J. S. (1981): The excitatory action of acetylcholine on hippocampal neurones of the guinea pig and rat maintained *in vitro*. *Brain Res.*, 207:109–127.
26. Dreyer, F., Muller, K. D., Peper, K., and Sterz, R. (1976): The *m. omohyoideus* of mouse as a convenient mammalian muscle preparation. A study of junctional and extrajunctional acetyl-

choline receptors by noise analysis and cooperativity. *Pflugers Arch.*, 367:115–122.

27. Dreyer, F., Peper, R., and Stertz, R. (1978): Determination of dose-response curves by quantitative iontophoresis at the frog neuromuscular junction. *J. Physiol.*, 281:395–419.

28. Dreyer, F., Walther, F., and Peper, K. (1976): Junctional and extrajunctional acetylcholine receptors in normal and denervated frog muscle fibers. Noise analysis with different agonists. *Pflugers Arch.*, 366:1–9.

29. Dudel, J., Finger, W., and Stettmeier, H. (1980): Inhibitory synaptic channels activated by γ-aminobutyric acid (GABA) in crayfish muscle. *Pflugers Arch.*, 387:143–151.

30. Dunlap, K., and Fischbach, G. D. (1978): Neurotransmitters decrease the calcium component of sensory neurone action potentials. *Nature*, 276:837–839.

31. Ehrenstein, G., Lecar, H., and Nossal, R. (1970): The nature of the negative resistance in bimolecular lipid membranes containing excitability-inducing-material. *J. Gen. Physiol.*, 55:119–133.

32. Ehrenstein, G., Blumenthal, R., Latorre, R., and Lecar, H. (1974): Kinetics of opening and closing of individual excitability-inducing-material channels in a lipid bilayer. *J. Gen. Physiol.*, 63:707–721.

33. Epstein, M., and Racker, E. (1978): Reconstitution of carbamylcholine-dependent sodium ion flux and desensitation of the acetylcholine receptor from *Torpedo california*. *J. Biol. Chem.*, 253:6660–6662.

34. Faber, D. S., and Korn, H. (1982): Transmission at a central inhibitory synapse I. Magnitude of unitary postsynaptic conductance change and kinetics of channel activation. *J. Neurophysiol.*, 48:654–678.

35. Fenwick, E. M., Marty, A., and Neher, E. (1982): A patch clamp study of bovine chromaffin cells and of their sensitivity to acetylcholine. *J. Physiol.*, 331:577–597.

36. Fredkin, D. R., Montal, M., Rice, J. A. (1983): Identification of aggregated Markovian models: Applications to the nicotinic acetylcholine receptor. *Proceedings of the Neyman-Kiefer Memorial Symposium*, edited by L. Le Cam.

37. Gold, M. R., and Martin, A. R. (1983): Analysis of glycine-activated inhibitory post-synaptic channels in brain-stem neurones of the lamprey. *J. Physiol.*, 342:99–117.

38. Gration, K. A. F., Lambert, J. J., Ramsey, R. L., Rand, R. P., and Usherwood, P. N. R. (1982): Closure of membrane channels gated by glutamate receptors may be a two step process. *Nature*, 295:599–601.

39. Gration, K. A. F., Lambert, J. J., Ramsey, R. L., and Usherwood, P. N. R. (1981): Nonrandom openings and concentration-dependent lifetimes of glutamate gated channels in muscle membranes. *Nature*, 291:423–425.

40. Gration, K. A. F., Ramsey, R. L., and Usherwood, P. N. R. (1983): Analysis of single-channel currents from glutamate receptor-channel complexes on locust muscle. In: *Single Channel Recording*, edited by B. Sakmann and E. Neher, pp. 377–388. Plenum, New York.

41. Gray, R., Kellaway, J., and Johnston, D. (1983): Recordings of single GABA-activated channels from acutely-isolated hippocampal neurons. *Soc. Neurosci. Abstracts*, 9:345.7.

42. Haas, H. L., and Konnerth, A. (1983): Histamine and norepinephrine decrease calcium-activated potassium conductance in hippocampal pyramidal cells. *Nature*, 302:432–434.

43. Hamill, O. P., Bormann, J., and Sakmann, B. (1983): Activation of multiple conductance state chloride channels in spinal neurones by glycine and GABA. *Nature*, 305:805–808.

44. Hamill, O. P., Marty, A., Neher, E., Sakmann, B. and Sigworth, F. J. (1981): Improved patch-clamp techniques for high-resolution current recording from cells and cell-free membrane patches. *Pflugers Arch.*, 391:85–100.

45. Hamill, O. P., and Sakmann, B. (1981): Multiple conductance states of single acetylcholine receptor channels in embryonic muscle cells. *Nature*, 291:426–427.

46. Horn, R. (1984): Gating of channels in nerve and muscle: A stochastic approach. In: *Ion channels: Molecular and physiological aspects*, edited by W. D. Stein, pp. 53–97. Academic Press, Orlando, Fla.

47. Horn, R., and Lange, K. (1983): Estimating kinetic constants from single channel data. *Biophys. J.*, 43:207–223.

48. Horn, R., and Patlak, J. B. (1980): Single channel currents from excised patches of muscle membrane. *Proc. Natl. Acad. Sci. USA*, 77:6930–6934.

49. Horn, R., Patlak, J., and Stevens, C. F. (1981): Sodium channels need not open before they inactivate. *Nature*, 291:426–427.

50. Jackson, M. B. (1984): Spontaneous openings of the acetylcholine receptor channel. *Proc. Natl. Acad. Sci. USA*, 81:3901–3904.

51. Jackson, M. B., Lecar, H., Askanas, V., and Engel, W. K. (1982): Single cholinergic channel currents in cultured human muscle. *J. Neurosci.*, 2:1465–1473.

52. Jackson, M. B., Lecar, H., Mathers, D. A., Barker, J. L. (1982): Single channel currents activated by GABA, muscimol, and (−) pentobarbital in cultured mouse spinal neurons. *J. Neurosci.*, 2:889–894.

53. Jackson, M. B., Lecar, H., Morris, C. E., and Wong, B. S. (1983): Single-channel current recording in excitable cells. In: *Current Methods in Cellular Neurobiology*, edited by J. L. Barker and J. F. McKelvy, pp. 61–99. Wiley, New York.

54. Jackson, M. B., Wong, B. S., Morris, C. E., Lecar, H., and Christian, C. N. (1983): Successive openings of the same acetylcholine receptor channel are correlated in open-time. *Biophys. J.*, 42:109–114.

55. Johnston, D., and Brown, T. H. (1981): Giant synaptic potential hypothesis for epileptiform activity. *Science*, 211:294–297.

56. Karlin, A. (1980): Molecular properties of nicotinic acetylcholine receptors. In: *The Cell Surface and Neuronal Function*, edited by C. W. Cotman, G. Poste, and G. L. Nicolson, pp. 192–260. Elsevier/North-Holland, Karlin, The Netherlands.

57. Katz, B., and Miledi, R. (1970): Membrane noise produced by acetylcholine. *Nature*, 226:962–963.

58. Katz, B., and Miledi, R. (1972): The statistical nature of the acetylcholine potential and its molecular components. *J. Physiol.*, 224:665–699.

59. Katz, B., and Miledi, R. (1977): The reversal potential of the desensitized endplate. *Proc. R. Soc. Lond. [Biol.] B*, 199:329–334.

60. Katz, B., and Thesleff, S. (1957): A study of desensitization produced by acetylcholine at the motor endplate. *J. Physiol.*, 138:63–80.

61. Kehoe, J. S., and Marty, A. (1980): Certain slow synaptic processes: Their properties and possible underlying mechanisms. *Annu. Rev. Biophys. Bioeng.*, 9:437–465.

62. Lee, C. Y. (1979): Recent advances in chemistry and pharmacology of snake toxins. In: *Neurotoxins: Tools in Neurobiology*, edited by B. Ceccarelli and F. Clementi, pp. 1–16. Raven Press, New York.

63. Lester, H. A., and Chang, H. W. (1977): Response of acetylcholine receptors to rapid photochemically produced increases in agonist concentration. *Nature*, 266:373–374.

64. Macdonald, R. L., and McLean, M. J. (1986): Anticonvulsant drug mechanisms of action. In: *Basic Mechanisms of the Epilepsies*, Chapter 36, edited by A. V. Delgado-Escueta, A. A. Ward, Jr., and R. I. Porter. Raven Press, New York.

65. Macdonald, R. L., and Barker, J. L. (1979): ticonvulsant and anesthetic barbiturates: Different postsynaptic actions in cultured mammalian neurons. *Neurology*, 29:432–447.

66. Madison, D. V., and Nicoll, R. A. (1982): Noradrenaline blocks accommodation of pyramidal cell discharge in the hippocampus. *Nature*, 299:636–638.

67. Magleby, K. L., and Stevens, C. F. (1972): A quantitative description of endplate currents. *J. Physiol.*, 223:173–197.

68. Magleby, K. L., and Stevens, C. F. (1972): The effect of voltage on the timecourse of endplate currents. *J. Physiol.*, 223:151–171.

69. Maruyama, Y., and Petersen, O. H. (1982): Single channel currents in isolated patches of plasma membrane from basal surface of pancreatic acini. *Nature*, 299:159–161.

70. Maruyama, Y., and Petersen, O. H. (1982): Activation of single channel currents by cholecystokinin is mediated by internal messenger in pancreatic acinar cells. *Nature*, 300:61–63.

71. Mathers, D. A. (1983): Electrical noise in biological membranes: In: *Current Methods in Cellular Neurobiology*, edited by J. L. Barker and J. F. McKelvy, pp. 101–127. Wiley, New York.

72. Mathers, D. A., and Usherwood, P. N. R. (1976); Concanavalin A blocks desensitization

73. Matsumoto, H., and Ajmone-Marsan, C. (1964): Cortical cellular phenomena in experimental epilepsy: Ictal manifestations. *Exp. Neurol*, 9:305–326.

74. Matsumoto, H., and Ajmone-Marsan, C. (1964): Cortical cellular phenomena in experimental epilepsy: Interictal manifestations. *Exp. Neurol.*, 9:286–304.

75. McBurney, R. N., and Barker, J. L. (1978): GABA-induced conductance fluctuations in cultured spinal neurons. *Nature*, 274:596–597.

76. Montal, M., Labarca, P., Fredkin, D. R., Suarez-Isla, B. A., and Lindstrom, J. (1984): Channel properties of the purified acetylcholine receptor from *Torpedo californica* reconstituted in planar lipid bilayer. *Biophys. J.*, 45:141–148.

77. Morris, C. E., Jackson, M. B., Lecar, H., Wong, B. S., and Christian, C. N. (1982): Activation of individual acetylcholine channels by curare in embryonic rat muscle. *Biophys. J.*, 37:19a.

78. Morris, C. E., Wong, B. S., Jackson, M. B., and Lecar, H. (1983): Single-channel currents activated by curare in cultured embryonic rat muscle. *J. Neurosci.*, 3:2525–2531.

79. Neher, E., and Sakmann, B. (1976): Noise analysis of drug induced voltage clamp current in denervated frog muscle fibers. *J. Physiol.*, 258:705–730.

80. Neher, E., and Sakmann, B. (1976): Single channel currents recorded from membrane of denervated frog muscle fibers. *Nature*, 260:799–801.

81. Neher, E., Sakmann, B., and Steinbach, J. H. (1978); The extracellular patch clamp: A method for resolving current through individual open channels in biological membranes. *Pflugers Arch.*, 375:219–228.

82. Neher, E., and Steinbach, J. H. (1978): Local anaesthetics transiently block currents through single acetylcholine-receptor channels. *J. Physiol.*, 277:153–176.

83. Nelson, D. J., and Sachs, F. (1979): Single ionic channels observed in tissue cultured muscle. *Nature*, 282:861–863.

84. Nelson, N., Anholt, R., Lindstrom, J., and Montal, M. (1980): Reconstitution of purified acetylcholine receptors with functional ion channels in planar lipid bilayers. *Proc. Natl. Acad. Sci. USA*, 77:3057–3061.

85. Neubig, R. R., Boyd, N. D., and Cohen, J. B. (1982): Conformations of *Torpedo* acetylcholine receptor associated with ion transport and desensitization. *Biochemistry*, 21:3460–3467.

86. Noda, M., Takahashi, H., Tanabe, T., Toyosato, M., Kikyotani, S., Furutani, Y., Hirose, T., Takashima, H., Inayama, S., Miyata, T., and Numa, S. (1983): Structural homology of *Torpedo californica* acetylcholine receptor subunits. *Nature*, 302:528–532.

87. Nowak, L. M., and McDonald, R. L. (1982): Substance P: Ionic basis for depolarizing re-

sponses of mouse spinal cord neurons in cell culture. *J. Neurosci.*, 2:1119–1128.

88. Olsen, R. W., Bergman, M. O., Van Ness, P. C., Lummis, S. C., Watkins, A. E., Napias, C., and Greenlee, D. V. (1981): γ-Aminobutyric acid receptor binding sites in mammalian brain: Heterogeneity of binding sites. *Mol. Pharmacol.*, 19:217–227.

89. Parsegian, V. A. (1984): Fourth biophysical discussion. Ionic channels in membranes. *Biophys. J.*, 45.

90. Patlak, J., Gration, K. A. F., Usherwood, P. N. R. (1979): Single glutamate-activated channels in locust muscle. *Nature*, 278:643–644.

91. Patrick, J., Lindstrom, J., Culp, B., and McMillan, J. (1973): Studies on purified eel acetylcholine receptor and anti-acetylcholine receptor antibody. *Proc. Natl. Acad. Sci. USA*, 70:3334–3338.

92. Prince, D. A. (1978): Neurophysiology of epilepsy. *Annu. Rev. Neurosci.*, 1:395–416.

93. Rang, H. P. (1981): The characteristics of synaptic currents and responses to acetylcholine of rat submandibular ganglion cells. *J. Physiol.*, 311:23–55.

94. Reynolds, J., and Karlin, A. (1978): Molecular weight in detergent solution of acetylcholine receptor from *Torpedo californica*. *Biochemistry*, 17:2035–2038.

95. Sachs, F., and Lecar, H. (1973): Acetylcholine noise in tissue cultured muscle cells. *Nature New Biol.*, 246:214–216.

96. Sakmann, B., and Adams, P. R. (1978): Biophysical aspects of agonist action at the frog end-plate, In: *Advances in Pharmacology and Therapeutics 1*, edited by J. Jacobs, pp. 81–90. Pergammon Press, Oxford.

97. Sakmann, B., Hamill, O. P., and Bormann, J. (1983): Patch-clamp measurements of elementary chloride currents activated by the putative inhibitory transmitters GABA and glycine in mammalian spinal cord. *J. Neural. Transm.* (Suppl.), 18:83–95.

98. Sakmann, B., and Neher, E. (1983): *Single-Channel Recording*, Plenum Press, New York.

99. Sakmann, B., Noma, A., and Trautwein, W. (1983): Acetylcholine activation of single muscarinic K^+ channels in isolated pacemaker cells of the mammalian heart. *Nature*, 303:250–253.

100. Sakmann, B., Patlak, J., and Neher, E. (1980): Single acetylcholine-activated channels show burst-kinetics in presence of desensitizing concentrations of agonist. *Nature*, 286:71–73.

101. Schindler, H., and Quast, U. (1980): Functional acetylcholine receptor from *Torpedo marmorata* in planar membranes. *Proc. Natl. Acad. Sci. USA*, 77:2052–2056.

102. Sheridan, R. E., and Lestner, H. A. (1975): Relaxation measurements on the acetylcholine receptor. *Proc. Natl. Acad. Sci. USA*, 72:3496–3500.

103. Siegelbaum, S. A., Camardo, J. S., and Kandel, E. R. (1982): Serotonin and cyclic AMP close single K^+ channels in *Aplysia* sensory neurones. *Nature*, 299:413–417.

104. Siegelbaum, S. A., and Tsien, R. W. (1983): Modulation of channel gating as a mode of transmitter action. *Trends Neurosci.*, 6:307–312.

105. Sigworth, F. J., and Neher, E. (1980): Single Na channel currents observed in cultured rat muscle cells. *Nature*, 287:447–449.

106. Sine, S. M., and Steinbach, J. H. (1984): Activation of a nicotinic acetylcholine receptor. *Biophys. J.*, 45:149–156.

107. Sine, S. M., and Tayler, P. (1981): Relationship between reversible antagonist occupancy and the functional capacity of the acetylcholine receptor. *J. Biol. Chem.*, 256:6692–6699.

108. Study, R. E., and Barker, J. L. (1981): Diazepam and ($-$)-pentobarbitol. Fluctuation analysis reveals different mechanisms of potentiation of GABA responses in cultured neurons. *Proc. Nat. Acad. Sci. USA*, 78:7180–7184.

109. Sugiyama, H., Benda, P., Meunier, J.-C., Changeux, J.-P. (1973): Immunological characterization of the cholinergic receptor protein from *Electrophorus electricus.*, *FEBS Lett.*, 35:124–128.

110. Sugiyama, H., Popot, J. L., and Changieux, J. P. (1976): Studies on the electrogenic action of acetylcholine with *Torpedo marmorata* electric organ. III. Pharmacological densensitization *in vitro* of the receptor-rich membrane fragments by cholinergic agonists. *J. Mol. Biol.*, 106:485–496.

111. Sumikawa, K., Houghton, M., Smith, J. C., Bell, L., Richards, B. M., and Barnard, E. A. (1982): The molecular cloning and characterization of cDNA coding for the δ subunit of the acetylcholine receptor. *Nucleic Acid Res.*, 10:5809–5822.

112. Takeuchi, A. (1977): Junctional transmission I. Postsynaptic mechanisms. In: *Handbook of Physiology*, section I, volume I, edited by E. R. Kandel. American Physiological Society, Bethesda, Md.

113. Takeuchi, A., and Takeuchi, N. (1966): A study of the inhibitory action of γ-aminobutyric acid on neuromuscular transmission in the crayfish. *J. Physiol.*, 183:418–432.

114. Takeuchi, A., and Takeuchi, N. (1969): A study of the action of picrotoxin on the inhibitory neuromuscular junction of crayfish. *J. Physiol.*, 205:377–391.

115. Traub, R. D., and Wong, R. K. S. (1982): Cellular mechanism of neuronal synchronization in epilepsy. *Science*, 216:745–747.

116. Trautmann, A. (1982): Curare can open and block ionic channels associated with cholinergic receptors. *Nature*, 298:272–275.

117. Ziskind, L., and Denis, M. J. (1978): Depolarizing effect of curare on embryonic rat muscles. *Nature*, 276:622–623.

Advances in Neurology, Vol. 44, edited by
A. V. Delgado-Escueta, A. A. Ward, Jr.,
D. M. Woodbury, and R. J. Porter.
Raven Press, New York © 1986.

8

Conducting Sites in Excitable Membranes

E. Schoffeniels

Laboratory of General and Comparative Biochemistry, University of Liege, Liege, Belgium

SUMMARY   Electrical activity of conducting membranes is produced by transient changes in membrane conductance to Na and K ions (66). These time- and voltage-dependent conductance changes are controlled by intrinsic proteins that span the membrane and provide a pathway for ion movement. Several lines of evidence indicate that the membrane conducting sites are indeed largely or entirely protein structures. Proteolytic enzymes, when applied on unmyelinated axonal membrane such as the gar olfactory nerve (19) or on eel electroplax (119), completely destroyed tetrodotoxin (TTX) binding. Treatment of the internal face of the giant axon of the squid with proteases resulted in the loss of the inactivation mechanism of the increased sodium conductance (9,124,125). The binding site of the TTX component in membrane isolated from eel electroplax, estimated by the method of irradiation inactivation, revealed MWs in the range of 230–240 kd (94). Moreover, this membrane component undergoes a cycle of phosphorylation–dephosphorylation that is affected by electrical activity and various neurotropic compounds and has also been shown to be a protein by the use of proteolytic enzymes (129,131–133,137).

The membrane conducting sites through which ions are flowing are generally called "channels," and the activated "channels" are thought to form "pores" through which ions diffuse according to their electrochemical potential. The channel behaves as though it exists in open or closed permeability or "gating" states. The gating is generally assumed to be solely controlled by the voltage gradient across the membrane.

Hence, the denominations of "gating proteins" are often attributed to the specific protein forming the membrane conducting sites. These proteins are intrinsic membrane proteins whose conformational changes, driven by the electric field in the membrane, are responsible for the ion fluxes generating the electrical activity in excitable cells. Electrical excitation of conducting cells involves transient permeability increases to Na^+, K^+, and Ca^+ ions. In some specific cases, Cl^- ions may also be involved. These ionic permeabilities are voltage-dependent and can be modified selectively and *independently* by a variety of compounds, thus leading to the idea that specific entities are spatially separated in the membrane and are acting independently. However, some data of patch-clamp analysis are best interpreted if one assumes that the activation of a specific entity may control the activation of another entity, thereby suggesting a kind of cooperation among some specific ionic sites. The idea of separate sites for Na^+ and K^+ ions in axonal membranes was already contained in Hodgkin-Huxley formulation of the ionic theory of action potential, since in voltage-clamp conditions, the evolution of the conductance change for Na^+ ions is quite different from that for K^+ ions. The discovery of toxins or compounds blocking specifically the conductance change of single ionic species offers further evidence of the specific identity of the various conducting sites (or ionic translocator) in an excitable membrane. The goal is to elucidate the molecular mechanisms of operation of these sites. My purpose therefore is to review the major problems posed in studies of ionic movements in conducting membranes, thus presenting the most coherent picture that emerges from present-day investigation, together with an outline of the most promising approaches for the near future.

Because an "epileptic" neuron is characterized by an enhanced electrical activity, it may also be worthwhile to investigate the properties of the various conducting sites in pathological cases. Preliminary results that we have obtained on the photosensitive baboon indicate differences in the content of thiamine-phosphorylated derivatives in the frontal lobe with respect to the values found in slightly photosensitive animals. Because thiamine-phosphorylated derivatives are involved in bioelectrogenesis, this observation may open new vistas with regard to our interpretation of the epileptic process.

The study of conducting sites in excitable membrane has greatly benefited from the application of biophysical techniques such as the voltage clamp (35,66,67), fluctuation analysis (8,88), and recording of single-channel activity (108). In addition, the use of biochemical methods aiming at disassembling the membrane by mild disruption of noncovalent lipid–protein and lipid–lipid interactions, together with the use of toxins binding specifically to the proteins involved in the conductance change, have led to the solubilization of the protein(s) forming the Na translocator, which is, together with the acetylcholine (ACh) receptor, the best conducting site yet studied at the molecular dimension.

GATED ION CHANNELS, GATING PROTEINS, AND CONDUCTINS

First, it seems appropriate to question the validity of the name "channel" as applied to the protein controlling the ion flux. It is not just a matter of semantics, since it is obvious that the word conceals a conceptual and logical framework that may well bias our interpretation of the biological reality. It is clear that physiologists or electrophysiologists, who are thinking essentially in terms of analogy, are prone to use a picturesque and imaginative vocabulary to describe their observations. Thus, when dealing with ion movements across biological membrane, they refer to ion "channel," "rectifier," "gating" charges, selectivity "filter," etc.

These words are taken from our daily vocabulary or from other fields of investigation, therefore producing different images in the brain, depending on the type of education of the reader. A word such as "channel" generally evokes for most of us a rigid structure filled with water, through which ions are diffusing freely. The fact that some ionic species move through sites having electrical conductance close to 1–10 pS corresponds to a rather high permeability. This is interpreted by many research workers as indicating that "because of this prodigious throughput rate, Na and K channels are now accepted to be pores. The open pore provides an aqueous pathway for ions to cross the membrane" (65).

However, this view, in terms of a precise description at the molecular scale of dimension, is challenged by many (e.g., ref. 55). It seems profitable and appropriate to select for a given level of description a rather precise terminology. Because the word "channel" is now so widely used, it will certainly be difficult to reverse the trend. The word "channel" should, however, be replaced by a word describing solely the phenomenology used in electrophysiology and devoid of mechanistic connotation. I propose the use of the term "conducting site," which is a rather concise way of describing either at a macroscopic or even at a microscopic level the behavior of a membrane toward a given ionic species. We are referring to the various K^+ conducting sites existing in a given membrane, thus meaning that the membrane has different sites through which K^+ ions are moving, a given category of sites having properties that distinguishes it from another category of sites.

What we know about the conducting sites in membrane is certainly far from the image carried by the word "channel" and more close to a dynamic entity that bears no resemblance whatsoever to the picture we have of a channel.

We may also phrase the question as follows: Are these intrinsic proteins "porous" in the common sense of the term? It is not easy to answer this question because the proteins forming the ACh receptor are the only ones to have been purified so far; despite the remarkable progress achieved, we do not have a precise picture of how ions cross the postsynaptic membrane.

Because we know today that a category of sites is made of specific proteins, we may refer to these proteins by naming the class to which they belong under the general name of *conductins,* since they control the conductance of permanent ions.

This name is less restrictive and simply describes what we already knew, i.e., a given protein, such as an oligomeric structure, controls specifically the conductance of one ionic species: thus, Na^+-conductin, K^+-conductin, Ca^{2+}-conductin, etc. They are also named "gating proteins," since in most instances they "gate" the movement of permanent ions. For the very same reasons that force me to reject the word "channel," this last term appeals less to me because it is already too suggestive of a possible mechanism of action. As Hille (65) points out, "they gate the movement of permanent ions by opening and closing the pore." This gives rise to the model shown in Fig. 1. I suggest that only two names be used, according to the level of description: conducting site or ionic translocator for the phenomenological approach; and *conductin* when referring to the molecular dimen-

sion and, more specifically, to the specific protein controlling the site activity.

The "gating process" resulting from conformation charges of *conductin* should preferably be referred to as a "transition" from a low-conductance state (LCS) to a high-conductance state (HCS) rather than to a closed or open configuration respectively.

We may now ask ourselves what are the minimal structural characteristics of an intrinsic protein controlling the ionic conductance of a membrane. It should have some kind of transmembrane symmetry axis, be stable in a lipid environment, and should include a strong polar component. If the intrinsic protein were an oligomeric structure, these polar components could be located in the intersubunit links. Next we ask if it is reasonable to assume that the transmembrane symmetry axis provides a plausible location for the translocation of ions and if this must be seen as a polar site. From the consideration of the vectorial activities of transport proteins, such as the Na^+,K^+-ATPase or Ca^{2+}-ATPase, an absence of symmetry axis from the plane of the membrane is generally implied. A tetrameric structure in this case is therefore unlikely to be found among the proteins of membrane transport that must then possess a cyclic symmetry and, of course, a transmembrane symmetry axis. The Na^+-conductin isolated from rat brain (62) or rat muscle (15) is a trimeric structure ($\alpha = 270$ kd; $\beta_1 = 39$ kd; $\beta_2 = 37$ kd), whereas the Na^+ conductin isolated from the electric organ of electric eel (5,6) seems to be made of the sole α subunit; attempts to identify the β subunits have failed so far.

BIOCHEMICAL INTRODUCTION TO ELECTROPHYSIOLOGY

Before attempting to explain at the molecular dimension conductance changes occurring in a membrane, it seems relevant to consider possible theoretical mechanisms that could explain the conformation changes of the conductins from a LCS to a HCS.

Although it is generally believed that permeability changes leading to action currents arise from conformation changes of a specific protein, a process that is dissipative and entropy-producing (65), researchers differ greatly on the source of energy needed to power the process. Are we dealing with an electric-field–dependent process—i.e., a unimolecular reaction system, or must we postulate that a substrate has to be

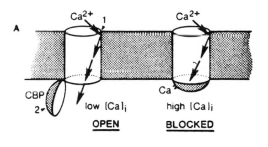

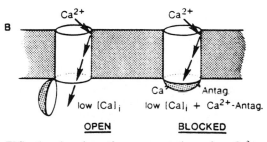

FIG. 1. A schematic representation of a Ca^{2+}-channel. From Johnson, ref. 84, with permission.

used in order to explain the energetics of the conductance change in axonal membranes?

The main lines of argument developed by the two school of thoughts will not be reviewed here. This has been done elsewhere (135,136). The bases for chemical energy input are drawn from theoretical as well as from experimental evidence. Unimolecular models fail to simulate experimental observations (46–48,82,109). However, membrane capacitance measurements (10), conformational transitions (34,39), and heat production analysis (100,140) point to the existence of endogenous energy input to the axonal membrane.

The only alternative to intramolecular representations is the reaction model that allows for bimolecular reaction steps. As already shown by Dubois and Schoffeniels (49), it is possible to reproduce accurately g_{Na}, g_K, and the membrane potential (E_m) on the basis of kinetic equations corresponding to a biomolecular model in which a chemical is used.

DESCRIPTION OF MAIN CONDUCTING SITES

Sodium Translocator

Description

Under voltage-clamp conditions, sodium conducting sites of axonal membranes undergo a cycle of conductance change. Thus, although the electric field across the membrane is kept constant, the sites go back to a LCS. Na^+-conducting sites in different tissues have similar properties, suggesting that protein(s) are homologous (122).

Models describing the Na^+ translocator generally assume the presence of two conducting states, in agreement with the phenomenological approach developed by Hodgkin and Huxley (66). At the resting potential, center m is in LCS, and center h is in HCS. Ion flow is only possible if both centers are in HCS. Depolarization induces the m center to undergo a conformation change leading to HCS, thus permitting the ion flow. Depolarization also induces a transition of the h center from HCS to LCS with slower kinetics, thereby stopping ion flow. To reactivate the conducting site, the h center must first go back to HCS. Analysis of single-site activity shows that the conductance is on the order of 5–20 pS (144).

To be inactivated, the sites do not have to pass through the HCS configuration (69), suggesting that the m and h centers function independently.

The basic pharmacological observations concerning the Na current are as follows. Two toxins, tetrodotoxin (TTX) and saxitoxin (STX), completely block I_{Na} in both myelinated and unmyelinated fibers at low concentrations (0.1 μM) when applied *outside*. The other ionic currents, I_K and I_L (leakage current) are not affected even by 100-fold greater concentrations. The specificity of the Na^+ conducting sites is far from being absolute, and the relative permeability of a site to other ionic species has been estimated (64,103,152). Thus, neurotoxins that increase the rate of Na^+ influx through the specific sites also give rise to an extra efflux of K^+ ions through the same sites (81).

Other compounds, such as batrachotoxin (BTX) and veratridine, bind the Na translocator at a different site in the lipophilic domain. Occupancy of this category of site persistently induces the HCS transition (7).

A third class of ligands are toxins from scorpion or sea anemones. These peptides exhibit a voltage-sensitive binding to the Na^+-conducting site and act at the cell exterior (28). As a result of their binding, return to LCS—the so-called inactivation—is inhibited. Moreover, they enhance the activation, i.e., the HCS observed when alkaloid ligands are applied.

The fact that binding by peptide ligands is voltage-sensitive indicates that the Na^+-conducting site proteins must be in the configuration imposed by the electric field existing normally across the membrane. Although these toxins may be radiolabeled, they are of little use for purification of the specific proteins.

However, by using *Arylazido* (^{125}I)-scorpion toxin, Beneski and Catterall (18) labeled two subunits of Na^+-conducting sites in rat brain synaptosomes (subunits α and β). Thus, two polypeptides with apparent MWs of 250 kd and 32 kd were identified.

The Na^+-conducting site isolated from the electroplax of *E. electricus* L. appears to be formed by a single polypeptide chain of 270 kd since it copurifies with the fraction containing the STX-binding activity (6).

This polypeptide contains 30% carbohydrates and behaves anomalously during electrophoresis (105). It is likely that the estimate of 270 kd is only an approximation of the MW. Besides the subunit of 270 kd (α-subunit), the conducting sites isolated from mammalian brain seem to be formed by two other subunits, $β_1$ with an apparent MW of 39 kd, and $β_2$, with an apparent MW weight of 37 kd (62,63). $β_1$ is linked to the α subunit by disulphide bonds.

It has also been possible to isolate from rat muscle the proteins of the Na$^+$-conducting site: a glycoprotein behaving anomalously on polyacrylamide gel and two subunits closely related to β_1 and β_2 found in rat brain. But here a protein of 45 kd is also isolated (13), the significance of which will be discussed later. Na$^+$-conducting sites have been found in some dendrites (156). The initiation sites for action potentials in neurons have a high density of Na$^+$-conducting sites, an observation that may explain the lower threshold of excitation at this part of the neuron (29).

In the nodes of Ranvier, the sites density is several hundred-fold higher than in internodal segments: thus, 3,000–5,000 sites per μm^2 are found (122,123) indicating that the Na$^+$ conducting must be a predominant membrane protein in that part of the axon (53). In the case of unmyelinated axons, the density of the sites is far less, some 30-fold lower, but the distribution is more uniform (77,123).

Phosphorylation of Na$^+$-Conducting Sites

The first observations on the phosphorylation of the Na$^+$-conducting sites were reported in 1976 by Schoffeniels (131–133) working on isolated nerves submitted to electrical stimulation or to the action of neurotropic compounds. Later, these observations were extended to axonal membranes prepared from crustacean nerve or to membranes obtained from the electric organ of *E. electricus* L. or from rat and mouse brain (for review, see ref. 133).

Partially purified proteins isolated from walking nerves of crabs, electric organ, or brain have also been studied. It was concluded that a protein of roughly 250 kd is phosphorylated, and that its level of phosphorylation is influenced by neurotropic compounds such as TTX, veratridine, local anesthetics, diphenylhydantoin, etc. (21,133). A lower MW protein, i.e., 40–50 kd, seems to be involved in the phosphorylation activity in nerves.

Experiments using low concentration of ATP (5.10^{-8}M) indicated an incorporation of 10 picomoles of ^{32}P per mg protein, after 10 min of incubation, a value five times higher than the one reported when membrane fragments were used in the same experimental conditions. In addition, even in the absence of added ATP (exogenous ATP), a net phosphorylation of the proteins was observed, suggesting the existence of an endogenous phosphate donor copurifying with the proteins.

We were thus able to show that the protein that binds specifically TTX, i.e., the principal component of the Na$^+$-conducting site, is associated with different phospholipids (45), adenine nucleotides (22), and phosphate derivatives of thiamine (Table 1) (135,136,138). Because the presence of thiamine-phosphorylated derivatives in the nervous system, central or peripheral, is a well-documented fact (12,23,42, 59,78,79,106,115,116,153,154), we believe that thiamine triphosphate is the phosphate donor involved in the phosphorylation cycle of the Na$^+$-conducting site. This would explain on a molecular basis such pathological conditions as beriberi, as well as the symptomatology associated with a vitamin B$_1$-deficient diet. Moreover, the fact that electrical activity of nerves or the application of neurotropic compounds—such as TTX, local anesthetics, ACh, diisopropylfluorophosphonate (DPF), and 5-hydroxytryptamine

TABLE 1. *Thiamine Derivatives (pM/mgr protein) Associated With the Na$^+$-conductin Isolated From the Main Electric Organ of* Electrophorus electricus *L.*

Fraction	TTP	TDP	TMP	T
DEAE wash				
Control	—	2.6–4.6	—	—
TTX	—	1.1–6.6	14.0–15.1	0.92–4.3
Veratridine	0.3–0.9	2.6	0.3–1.1	—
Na$^+$-conductin				
Control	7.4–11.6	10.6–15.7	33.3–98	—
TTX	0.7–2.2	2.2–3.7	5.1	1.5
Veratridine	7.4–17.2	12.3–38	34.0–67.5	—

TTP, thiamine triphosphate; TDP, thiamine diphosphate, TMP, thiamine monophosphate; T, thiamine; TTX, tetrodotoxin.

TTX (3×10^{-7}M) and veratridine (10^{-4}) are added during the purification procedure before the DEAE step. Thiamine derivatives are determined as fluorescent compounds in HPLC. The figures quoted are extreme values obtained by measuring several aliquots of the same sample.

From Schoffeniels et al., ref. 138, with permission.

(5-HT)—are accompanied by a contemporary release of thiamine into the extracellular fluid (42,59,106,153,154) gives even more weight to our interpretation. As shown in Table 1, the addition of TTX during the purification procedure of the Na^+-conductin displaces the thiamine derivatives and shifts the equilibrium toward the less phosphorylated derivatives. The fact that thiamine monophosphate (TMP) is the main compound that appears to copurify with the Na^+-conductin may indicate that this thiamine ester is the end product of a Na^+-conducting site phosphorylation occurring during the purification procedure. Lack of effect of veratridine on thiamine-phosphorylated compounds bound to the Na^+-conductin is in accord with previous results showing that the Na^+-conducting site has at least four different binding sites in addition to the Na^+-binding sites (134) and that veratridine together with BTX and dihydrograyanotoxin II binds to a site category different from that of TTX (27). Because TTX and veratridine have different effects on the configuration of the Na^+-conductin, our results suggest strongly that the conductance state of the Na^+-conducting sites could well be controlled by their net state of phosphorylation (136). The phosphorylation of the Na^+-conductin has also been reported by Costa et al. (43).

Reconstitution in Phospholipid Vesicles

Early attempts to reconstitute ion-conducting sites into lipid bilayers (139) have been followed by experiments using crude preparations of Na^+-conducting site proteins obtained from rat brain and rat muscle and reconstituted into liposomes. In one type of experiment, the reconstituted liposomes were preloaded with Cs^+ and subjected to the action of veratridine. As a consequence, the liposomes having functional proteins would lose Cs^+, thus diminishing their density. Therefore a 50-fold purification of the vesicles containing the specific proteins could be achieved (57).

In other experiments in which a Na^+ gradient was established across the membrane of the vesicles, veratridine was applied, thus generating a diffusion potential that was assayed by the voltage-dependent binding of scorpion toxin (149). Other experiments have also shown an induction of Na^+ uptake by veratridine that is sensitive to TTX and STX (148,155).

By means of quenched-flow kinetic technique (150), it was shown that the selectivity to cations of the purified proteins is very close to that found with the intact cell, indicating that no major alteration resulted from the purification procedure. Barchi (1983) has attempted to patch clamp reconstituted vesicles. Although the results indicate that it is certainly feasible, there are still some ambiguities as to the interpretation. The reconstitution experiments have not been able to reproduce convincingly either the behavior of the Na^+-conducting sites as found in the cell membrane, or, more specifically, the relation between the conformation states and the free energy source or the response to transmembrane potential changes.

Moreover, the conductance and the opening time gave values higher than the ones determined on intact membrane. It seems that the activation of the Na^+-conducting sites as obtained with BTX is not comparable to the physiological process. More recently Rosenberg et al. (127) have considerably improved the technique. They were able to demonstrate the voltage-dependent activation using a single depolarization pulse. Sixty percent of the observed transitions to the HCS occurred within the first 2 msec of the depolarization step. Moreover, the conductance found for a single site is 11.2 picosiemens (pS), a value in close agreement with that recorded from patch of native membranes (15–18 pS) (70,71,144).

By comparing the characteristics of the Na^+-conducting site in the presence of BTX, a discrepancy between the conductance of BTX-associated sites in reconstituted membranes compared with native membranes was shown. Values of 20–25 pS were found. The duration of the HCS was also some 20-fold longer, and the transition LCS–HCS occurred much later after the onset of depolarization. As mentioned (138), it seems therefore that the properties of the Na^+-conducting site as revealed by BTX are significantly different from that found *in vivo*. It is unfortunate that Rosenberg et al. (127) did not assay thiamine triphosphate or thiamine pyrophosphate on their preparation since their results are certainly compatible with our model shown in Fig. 2 (see p. 209). They found a threshold behavior, a limited number of transition LCS–HCS shortly after (2 msec) the onset of depolarization, and a conductance close to that found in the native membrane (11 pS). However, their data collected through a filter at 1,000 Hz may still be subject to some revisions since we do not know the precise conditions of use of this filter. Therefore, the 2-msec delay could be shorter, the activation faster, and the lifetime of the HCS could be longer.

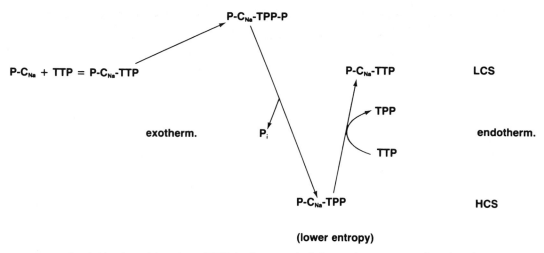

FIG. 2. Role of thiamine triphosphate (TTP) in the control of the conductance to sodium ions in crustacean nerve.

Homology

The α subunits identified in brain, muscle, nerve, and electric organ seem to be homologous, having the same size, carbohydrate and lipid content, phosphorylation cycle, toxin affinity, etc. However, definite confirmation will require sequence analysis. One result, that should be investigated in more detail, concerning the amino acid composition of four specific membrane proteins isolated from the electroplax of *E. electricus* L. (Table 2), has been demonstrated by Miller et al. (105).

Although it is certainly impossible to look for homology without having the sequence, the amino acid composition of the α-subunit of the Na^+-conducting site, the ACh receptor, the α-subunit of the Na^+,K^+-ATPase and the acetylcholinesterase is sufficiently similar to permit us to think that these four molecules that play an important role in controlling the permeability of cell membrane to inorganic ions are homologous, particularly since the α-subunit of the ATPase as well as the ACh receptor are also phosphorylated. The α-subunit of the ATPase is dephosphorylated by diphenylhydantoine exactly as is the Na^+-conductin. The phosphorylation of the α-subunit of the ATPase is favored by Na^+ ions, whereas the reverse is true with Na^+-conductin. It would be worthwhile to compare the properties of these proteins further in the light of the concept of homology. If, as we have already proposed, the transconformation LCS–HCS–LCS is associated with a phosphorylation cycle of the Na^+-conductin, the process

may well be similar to the one involved in the translocation of Na^+ ions upon hydrolysis of ATP by the Na^+,K^+-ATPase. This problem will be discussed below in the description of the model of nerve excitation.

Electron Microscopy

The TTX-binding protein isolated from *E. electricus* L. has been visualized by negative staining as clusters of 40 A × 170 A rods (52). The rod-like image is a cylindrical structure as shown by stereoscopic imaging. Assuming that the rod-like structure is only the protein moiety of the Na^+ conductin, it is easy to calculate that the MW of the cylinder is ~180 kd. Because 30% of the Na^+ conductin is carbohydrates, this estimate implies that the actual MW of the Na^+ conductin is about 257 kd, a value close to those estimated by irradiation inactivation (94) and by sedimentation studies (16,62).

Various K^+-Conducting Sites

K^+ Sites in HCS at Rest

Patch-clamp studies of rat muscle cells (112) have demonstrated the existence of K^+-conducting sites present at low density, 1 μm^{-2}, having in resting conditions a rather high conductance (around 10 pS), whose kinetics are not different from those of other ionic translocators. They have also been found in molluscan neurons (1) and tunicate egg cells (111).

TABLE 2. *Amino Acid Composition and Hydrophobicity Parameters of TTX-Binding Protein and of Related Membrane and Peripheral Proteins of Electroplax of* Electrophorus.

	TTX-binding component	Eel ACHR	Eel ATPase (large subunit)	Eel ACHease
Asx	10.1	11.4	10.6	9.7
Thr	5.0	5.6	6.0	4.4
Ser	7.1	6.2	7.6	6.9
Glx	10.8	10.2	9.8	9.5
Pro	4.7	5.7	5.2	8.4
Gly	6.5	5.9	8.3	8.0
Ala	6.0	5.8	7.6	5.7
Cys	2.0	2.0	ND	1.1
Val	5.3	8.6	7.2	7.2
Met	3.4	2.0	2.6	2.9
Ile	5.5	6.4	6.4	3.8
Leu	9.3	10.5	10.7	9.1
Tyr	2.8	4.0	2.0	3.8
Phe	5.9	5.7	4.5	5.3
His	2.8	2.2	1.6	2.3
Trp	3.5	ND	ND	2.1
Lys	5.0	4.6	5.7	4.4
Arg	4.3	6.2	5.0	5.5
$H\phi_{av}$	1073	1177	(1248)**	957
z^*	0.29	0.40	(0.42)**	0.24

ACHR, acetylcholine receptor; ACHease, acetylcholinesterase; TTX, tetrodotoxin; ND, not determined.

The $H\phi_{av}$ parameter indicates that the TTX binding protein is in the more polar range of membrane proteins and in the more hydrophobic range of soluble proteins. The z parameters indicates even more clearly that the peptide is clearly intermediate between the z classes.

* Hydrophobicity parameters.

** Values given are for native eel ATPase (large and small subunits).

Modified from data in Miller, ref. 105, with permission.

Neurotransmitter release, mediated by cyclicAMP, further increases the conductance of this category of K$^+$ sites, affording a means to modulate the neuronal response (4). In tunicate egg cells, the unit conductance (γ) at a site is related to external K$^+$ concentration, which is without effect on the number (n) of sites activated. However (n) is related to the calcium concentration. Mg^{2+} decreases the conductance of the site.

K$^+$ Sites Responsible for A-Current

Another class of K$^+$ sites involves translocators activated at membrane potential more positive than -60 mV, the characteristic of which is rapid inactivation. The transient current thus produced is the A-current (3,36,37). Translocators of this category play a fundamental role in neuronal excitability since they control the rate of depolarization, therefore regulating the rate of action potential production. This is best illustrated through the study of *Drosophila* mutants. *Drosophila shaker* mutants are characterized by a rather prolonged transmitter release and an alteration in A-current produced in a muscle and

nerve (128). The voltage dependency of the conducting sites inducing the A-current is also affected by the mutations. Thus, this class of translocator controls the transmitter release by modulating the repolarization of nerve terminals (83).

Voltage-Sensitive K$^+$ Translocators in Axonal Membranes

In the formulation of the ionic theory of action potential by Hodgkin and Huxley, the late current is a K$^+$-current resulting from the activation of K$^+$ conducting sites. These sites are further characterized by their delayed inactivation and the fact that when TEA (tetraethylammonium ions) is applied from inside the cell, there is a blockade of the transconformation in the LCS. This translocator is widely distributed in conducting membranes. When analyzed by patch-clamping method, it has a conductance (γ) of about 10 pS and a mean opening time (τ) of 12 msec, although short interruptions of conductance are sometimes noticed during the HCS. The probability of observing a transition to HCS is voltage-dependent, though γ and τ are not affected (40).

In muscle, the density of the K^+ sites is lower than that for Na^+ sites by a factor of five (146). This category of sites has not been isolated and purified because a specific toxin is lacking. However, a recent observation that a scorpion toxin binds specifically to this translocator opens interesting perspectives in that direction (26).

Ca^{2+}-Activated K^+-Conducting Sites

The Ca^{2+}-activated K^+-conducting sites are widely distributed. They exist not only in conducting cells such as neurons (3,102) chromaffin cells (101), and muscle (113), but also in red blood cells and hepatocytes (59,95).

The conductance is some 10 times higher than that of the voltage-sensitive K^+ sites, indicating that their density must be much lower since they carry currents comparable in magnitude to the late K^+ current. The translocator requires the presence of Ca^{2+} ions for activation, but is also sensitive to the membrane electric field, particularly at suboptimal calcium concentration (3,101,113).

The transition LCS–HCS seems to be controlled by the intracellular calcium concentration: an increase in $(Ca^{2+})_i$ that increases the number of translocators seems to be insensitive to calmodulin (e.g., red cells); (56) in dog heart, it is blocked by trifluoperazine, a potent inhibitor of calmodulin action.

Apamin, a neurotoxin extracted from bee venom (60) is a polypeptide of 18 amino acids with two disulfide bridges. By K^+ flux studies, it was demonstrated that apamin prevented the rise in potassium permeability in guinea pig hepatocytes and taenia coli (11,98), suggesting that it may act as a specific blocker of the Ca^{2+}-activated K^+-conducting sites. A direct demonstration of this action was obtained on neuroblastoma cells and rat muscle cells, using the voltage-clamp technique (74,76). ^{125}I-Apamine has now been used to identify the specific K^+ translocators in various cell types such as neuroblastoma cells (74), skeletal muscle cells in culture (76), guinea pig colon (73), and hepatocytes (41). A high affinity for the translocator together with a low number of binding sites have consistently been found in all systems. In neuroblastoma or muscle cells, their density is five to seven times lower than that of the Na^+-conducting sites (74,76). The toxin has a high affinity and dissociates very slowly from its receptor sites, thus offering a tool to purify the Ca^{2+}-activated K^+ translocator. However, the low density of this translocator at the cell surface caused some difficulties in visualizing this purification. In brain synaptosomes (72), the best source of apamin receptors, the Na^+ translocators, are 150–300 times more numerous than the apamin-sensitive Ca^{2+}-dependent K^+-conducting sites. Thus, available data concerning the structure of identical subunits (8 to 10) with MW of 30 kd or results from the association of other polypeptide chains not labeled by apamin is not known at the present time.

Clearly, the K^+-conducting sites sensitive to apamin are only one of several types of Ca^{2+}-dependent K^+ translocators. Thus, in rat skeletal muscle cells in culture, Ca^{2+}-dependent K^+-conducting sites identified by patch-clamp techniques are blocked by TEA whereas they are insensitive to apamin. Conversely, Ca^{2+}-dependent K^+-conducting sites responsible for the positive afterpotential and identified by voltage-clamping are very sensitive to apamin but not at all affected by TEA. The same results are obtained with neuroblastoma cells. The properties of these sites indicate that the apamin-sensitive sites are involved in the production of positive afterpotentials, whereas the other Ca^{2+}-dependent K^+ translocators are involved in the control of the membrane potential by preventing too long a depolarization.

Neurotransmitter-Activated K^+ Sites

Some neurotransmitters are specific ligands for selective K^+ conducting sites: they induce either the transconformation LCS or HCS. Among the K^+ sites sensitive to transmitters in sympathetic neurons, the so-called M translocator selective for K^+ ions, is in HCS at subthreshold membrane potential and does not inactivate with time. As a consequence, there is a stabilization of the membrane of the cells that are depolarized by other actions. ACh, together with muscarinic agonists, abolishes this current, thus increasing the excitability of sympathetic neurons (2). The LCS transition of these sites is induced by Ba^{2+} (38). In *Aplysia* sensory neurons, the S translocator is in HCS at rest, insensitive to membrane field and Ca^{2+} (89,117). Application of serotonin induces the transition LCS, and the response is mediated by cyclic-AMP (87,143). The M and S translocators are specific entities that are different from the other K^+-conducting sites that we have examined. Different K^+ translocators do coexist in the same cell membrane, and their activity is often regulated by transmitters of peptidic nature (44).

Distribution of K$^+$-Conducting Sites

There is a large variety of K$^+$-conducting sites whose properties control the overall activity of a neuron. The very fact that the given neuron has many different K$^+$ translocators offers an explanation for the diversity of the electrophysiological response seen in different neurons. The efficiency of synaptic transmission is also under the control of these K$^+$ sites. Moreover, agents affecting behavior and memory are often effective on the K$^+$ sites (87).

It is also clear that the specific distribution of the various K$^+$ conducting sites among a population of neurons introduces the selectivity of the response of particular neuronal aggregates in response to an identical second messenger.

The only specific ligand that has been found is apamin. Thus, it is difficult to offer a precise distribution of the different species of K$^+$-conducting sites among the various types of cellular differentiation, although it should be realized that we need this information to understand better not only the properties of specific neurons but also the complexity of the neuronal circuitry.

Electrophysiological studies have so far shown the unequal distribution of K$^+$ conducting sites even along the same cell membrane. Thus, in mammalian myelinated fibers, the K$^+$-conducting sites are not found in the Ranvier node (33) although they are present in the paranodal axolemma (31), in contradistinction to frog myelinated axons, where they exist in nodal, paranodal, and internodal regions (32).

Phosphorylation of Ca^{2+}-Dependent K$^+$-Conducting Sites

In neurons of the snail *Helix* or in *Aplysia* bag cells, as well as in mammalian pyramidal cells, there is evidence that a covalent modification by phosphorylation is involved in controlling the activity of the Ca^{2+}-dependent K$^+$-conducting sites.

For instance, the catalytic subunit of the cyclicAMP-dependent protein kinase reduces the conductance of the Ca^{2+}-activated K$^+$ translocator. Thus, application of cyclicAMP or the intracellular injection of the catalytic subunit of the cyclicAMP-dependent protein kinase into *Aplysia* bag cells (85) reduces the late K$^+$-current. Because the activity of the translocator is abolished by Co^{2+} or Ni$^+$, it is argued that it is in fact a Ca^{2+}-activated site (86). An elevation of cyclicAMP in the cell interior induces a prolonged period of spontaneous activity in response to a train of stimulus. Internally perfused neurons of *Helix* with the catalytic subunit of the cyclicAMP-dependent protein kinase show an increased Ca^{2+}-dependent K$^+$ conductance, and Ca^{2+} is still necessary to induce the conformation state of HCS. In mammalian pyramidal cells, catecholamines promote the transition HCS of the Ca^{2+}-activated K$^+$ sites, suggesting that a cyclicAMP-dependent phosphorylation is also present here (20,99). We shall discuss in a more synthetic way the importance of phosphorylation cycle in the activity of the translocators below.

Voltage-Sensitive Calcium Translocator

Description

The patch-clamp technique has permitted identification in heart cells, chromaffin cells and snail neurons of Ca^{2+}-conducting sites that are voltage-dependent. The duration τ of HCS is 1–2 msec with a current of 0.5–2 pA; clusters are observed at high depolarization. Flickering is also noticed (121).

In heart cells, the Ca^{2+} translocator has a conductance γ of about 25 pS and inactivates if depolarization is sustained (121). In nerve terminals of squid stellate ganglion, the transition to HCS is delayed after voltage pulse is applied, i.e., the transconformation takes place during the falling phase of the action potential (96) and the current is approximately five times lower than the sodium current.

Arsenazo III has been used to probe the entry of Ca^{2+}, since the complex Ca^{2+}–Arsenazo III absorbs light. Light absorption is maximum at the peak of transmitter release and absorption increases with the number of stimuli (30,104).

The density of the Ca^{2+} translocators is higher at the nerve terminals than in the preterminal part of the axon, and the use of Ca^{2+}–Arsenazo III complex permits estimation at 2.10^8 the number of Ca^{2+} ions entering the nerve terminal during a single action potential. If one assumes that the clusters of large particles that are seen at the nerve terminal are made of Ca^{2+} translocators, one can estimate at 150 the number of Ca^{2+} ions entering the cell per conducting site, thus giving a conductance of 0.14–0.21 pS per translocator (118).

This is in close agreement with values obtained by noise analysis in *Helix* neurons (92), but much lower than that obtained by the patch-clamp technique (24). Ca^{2+}-conducting sites rapidly lose their properties in perfused cells (25). This observation is not explained and adds to the already difficult problem of isolation and purification of the Ca^{2+} translocator, since we have not yet found a specific toxin. We know that BTX, thought to be specific only to the Na^+ conduction, also inhibits Ca^{2+} conducting sites in a neuroblastoma cell line (126). However, the lipophilic nature of this toxin will limit its usefulness.

Maitotoxin increases Ca^{2+} influx in pheochromocytome cells (147), and its action is prevented by verapamil, tetracain, and dihydropyridine derivatives, thus inhibiting the Ca^{2+} translocators. [3H]Nitrendipine seems to bind to the same sites, provided that Ca^{2+} or Sr^{2+} ions are present. La^{3+} or Co^{3+} ions prevent the binding. Because verapamil and D-600 do not interfere with the binding of [3H]nitrendipine, it is accepted that these inhibitors bind to different sites on the Ca^{2+} translocator (58).

Regulation of Ca^{2+}-Conducting Sites

Regulation of Ca^{2+}-conducting sites is controlled by Ca^{2+}, neurotransmitters, and hormones. These mechanisms are particularly important at synapses, since it is now well-established that synaptic facilitation, i.e., the increase in transmitter release, is caused by accumulation of Ca^{2+} in the nerve terminal (91). Therefore, the short-time plasticity of a synaptic junction is narrowly dependent on the balance between influx and efflux of Ca^{2+}. Efflux of Ca^{2+} is an enzyme-controlled process involving the hydrolysis of ATP, whereas influx is associated with the activation of Ca^{2+}-conducting sites and steady state Ca^{2+}-currents (141). Alteration of steady state currents per se is not the direct cause of synaptic facilitation, as shown by the results of Charlton et al. (30) obtained on the stellate ganglion of squid. Although the importance of the Ca^{2+} concentration at the nerve terminal is easily demonstrated, for instance on neuron L10 of *Aplysia* (91), it is shown here that the intracellular concentration of Ca^{2+} in turn controls the activity of Ca^{2+}-activated K^+-conducting sites. Therefore, Ca^{2+} removal by cellular sequestration determines the kinetics of facilitation disappearance (114) by inactivation of Ca^{2+}-dependent K^+-conducting sites. The work on neuron L10 of *Aplysia* has also shown that internal Ca^{2+} is somehow membrane-field dependent in the following way. Depolarization enhances the steady state inward Ca^{2+}-current and inactivates voltage-sensitive K^+ translocators. As a result, there is an increase in the duration of the action potential (142). Increase in the internal Ca^{2+} concentration slowly inactivates

Ca^{2+}-conducting sites (145,151). Half-times of inactivation range from 5 to 1,000 msec (61). Because Ca^{2+} ions in the cell interior control inactivation, one should take into account the surface-volume ratio in order to explain the differences in observed inactivation rates (120).

Noradrenaline, GABA, enkephalin, and somatostatin induce a decrease in the duration and amplitude of Ca^{2+}-dependent potentials in the rat superior cervical ganglion (68) and in cell bodies of the chick dorsal root ganglia (50,107). As demonstrated by voltage clamping of the membrane, this results from a decreased activity of the Ca^{2+}-conducting sites, leading to a reduced Ca^{2+}-current (51). This seems to be solely dependent on a direct action of the neurotransmitter on the Ca^{2+} translocator without involvement of a second messenger: neither dibutyryl cyclicAMP nor Ca^{2+} has an effect on the Ca^{2+} current (142). Patch-clamp analysis of heart muscle reveals that τ, the duration of HCS, is increased under the influence of epinephrine (121). Therefore, unlike sensory or sympathetic neurons, epinephrine increases Ca^{2+}-current. In cardiac muscle cells, a cycle of phosphorylation–dephosphorylation of some specific protein(s) seems to be involved in the production of the Ca^{2+} action potential, as revealed by the following observations: (a) by injecting the catalytic subunit, a prolongation and enhancement of the Ca^{2+} action potential is seen. Influx of Ca^{2+} is increased by a factor of 3, and epinephrine has no further effect; and (b) by injecting regulatory subunit the opposite effect is seen, i.e., a decrease in duration and amplitude of the Ca^{2+} current.

A cyclicAMP-dependent phosphorylation can therefore be reasonably presumed to explain the effect of epinephrine. Whether or not the protein phosphorylated is the Ca^{2+} translocator or a protein regulating its activity is still a matter of conjecture. Membranes prepared from cardiac cells retain their ability to exhibit a voltage-sensitive Ca^{2+} uptake (17). If one adds ATP and the catalytic subunit of protein kinase, it can be shown that a protein of 23 kd is phosphorylated. This is the so-called regulatory subunit, assumed because of its low MW to be a kind of regulatory subunit rather than the Ca^{2+} translocator itself. This suggestion is also made by analogy with the heart-specific protein phospholamban associated to the enzyme catalyzing the ATP-dependent sequestration of Ca^{2+} in the endoplasmic reticulum. Although not the enzyme, the phosphorylation of phospholamban results in an enhanced sequestration of Ca^{2+} ions (90,97).

ATP is released together with some neurotransmitters. It is therefore of interest to notice that in the nanomolar range, ATP applied extracellularly increases the Ca^{2+}-current (157). This does not involve a hydrolysis of ATP. In view of marked differences in the kinetics of the transition LCS–HCS–LCS observed when considering Ca^{2+}-conducting sites in various types of cell differentiation, it has been assumed that there is more than one type of Ca^{2+} translocator. However, the observations made using the patch-clamp technique when applied to different cells (54,121) seen more in favor of a single type of translocator, since the kinetics of the transconformation is remarkably similar. This problem is still much debated, however, and requires more investigation before a definite answer can be given.

EVOLUTIONARY SIGNIFICANCE OF PHOSPHORYLATION OF THE VARIOUS IONIC TRANSLOCATORS

Na^+ Translocator

As shown above, the α-subunit of the Na^+ translocator is phosphorylated in a way that is controlled by the electrical stimulation and compounds known to affect the electrical activity, such as TTX, veratridine, diphenylhydantoin, local anesthetics, etc. Therefore, I have suggested that the net state of phosphorylation directly controls the conductance of the Na^+ translocator (132,133). We have already mentioned the importance of thiamine-phosphorylated derivatives in the process.

Therefore, our data can be integrated to fit in a biochemical cycle involving phosphorylation–dephosphorylation processes explaining the impedance variation cycle.

Figure 2 shows (*right*), the conducting state of the sodium conductin. In this model, the sodium-conductin, C_{Na}, can assume two configurations: LCS and HCS.

In resting conditions, the LCS consists of a population of P-C_{Na} that is partially associated with thiamine triphosphate (P-C_{Na}–TTP). On electrical stimulation, i.e., an adequate change in the electric field across the membrane, the terminal phosphate is liberated *cooperatively* in a large population of P-C_{Na}–TTP, but remains fixed on the protein. This is the activated complex P-C_{Na}–TDP-P that undergoes a dephosphorylation leading to the HCS configuration of the sodium-conductin: P-C_{Na}–TDP, giving rise to the ascending phase of the action potential. It is an exothermic process characterized by a

decrease in entropy (39,100). The change in electric field that follows favors the displacement of TDP (which is replaced by TTP), an endothermic process corresponding to the descending phase of the action potential because it brings back the sodium conductin to its resting state (LCS). Notice that C_{Na}, as shown in patch-clamp studies of reconstituted liposomes (14) can exist in the two configurations, LCS and HCS, in an electric field, but does not exhibit the cooperativity or the threshold behavior. However, a synchronization of the transition of many Na conductin molecules under the influence of a threshold depolarization causes an action potential. In our model, this cooperativity can only be obtained if C_{Na} is phosphorylated and associated to TTP. The form P-C_{Na}–TTP does not change configuration in the electric field as is the case with C_{Na} and should be electrically silent in reconstituted liposomes. To activate the complex P-C_{Na}–TTP, a *threshold* depolarization must be applied. The effect of cyclicAMP deserves further comment. As shown by our data as well as those of Costa et al. (43), the phosphorylation of C_{Na} is controlled by cyclicAMP. Species differences are observed: in extracts from crustacean nerves or electroplax of electric eel, cyclicAMP displaces the equilibrium $C_{Na} = C_{Na} - P$ in favor of C_{Na}, whereas the converse is true when the protein is extracted from rat brain.

Because thiamine-phosphorylated derivatives are copurified with C_{Na} from different species (crustacean, electric eel, mammalian brain) one may ask if the cyclicAMP-controlled process is not related to the regulation of the density of the Na^+ translocators available for conductin. According to our data regarding the volume regulation of crustacean nerve during an osmotic stress, there seems to be a temporary increase in cAMP when fresh water is replaced by sea water (130). Because the speed of conduction in peripheral nerve is unchanged although the ionic concentration of the extracellular fluid is doubled, this could well result in a decrease in the density of the Na^+-conducting sites in sea water. This would accord with the belief that the affinity of C_{Na} for TTP would be much lower than that of C_{Na}-P, and would imply two levels of phosphorylation: (a) one process, cAMP-dependent, controlling the density of the sites available for the production of action potential; and (b) one process, TTP-dependent, controlling the transition LCS–HCS.

According to available data, process a would be species-specific in that in mammalian brain,

C_{Na} would have higher affinity for TTP, whereas in lower vertebrates or invertebrates, C_{Na}-P would have higher affinity. In all cases, not only TTP but also ATP would be endogenous phosphate donors, TTP for the fast transition LCS–HCS leading to the production of an action potential; and ATP for the control of the equilibrium C_{Na}-C_{Na}-P, i.e., the regulation of the density of the Na^+ translocator available for electrical activity. In the case of mammalian brain, the model shown in Fig. 2 still applies, provided that P-C_{Na} is replaced by C_{Na}.

Ca^{2+}-Dependent K^+-Conducting Site

As discussed above, the phosphorylation of the Ca^{2+}-activated K^+ translocator leads to the transition LCS, but also seems to increase the density of the sites easily available to Ca^{2+} activation, as though the K^+ translocator had to be in a phosphorylated state in order to undergo the transition HCS. Because we have so little information regarding the influence of compounds affecting the transition of this conducting site in relation to its phosphorylated state, more definite conclusions should not be drawn.

Ca^{2+}-Conducting Site

Available evidence favors the existence of a regulatory subunit, the phosphorylation of which controls in turn the activity of the Ca^{2+} translocator.

From available data, it is clear that neuronal excitability is controlled by the phosphorylation of the specific proteins involved in the process. This is not at all surprising if one considers how important this mechanism is in cellular regulation in general. Therefore, such subtle processes as synaptic plasticity and neuronal excitability are no exception to what seems a rather general rule.

We now must face the problem of the fast conductance changes leading to the early and late Na^+- and K^+-currents, respectively. Much of the evidence points to a bimolecular model involving a substrate that is consumed, as occurs in any biochemical cycle requiring the input of energy. Neither electrophysiologists nor biophysicists take such a model seriously: they prefer to think in terms of a protein changing its configuration back and forth—from LCS to HCS, and returning to LCS in a constant electric field. Although all patch-clamp experiments indicate that all conducting sites studied, either *in situ* or in reconstituted liposomes or bilayers, exhibit conductance changes that are membrane-field–dependent, it must be made clear that the transition still requires an input of external energy, which in this case is the thermal agitation. Even transmitter-activated conducting sites such as the ACh receptor exhibit this behavior *in the absence of an agonist* (80). This question is raised to give a meaning to these observations and to illustrate how they relate to the in vivo situation, and is even more pertinent when considering the data of Conti (39) who showed [in agreement with my previous analysis (100)] that the HCS of the Na^+ conductin has a lower entropy than that of the LCS, the transition involving some 20 entropy units—a value much too high to be accommodated by thermal energy when the membrane voltage is clamped. Therefore, it is obvious that thiamine triphosphate is the energy source and thus the specific operating substance responsible for the impedance variation cycle.

This model gives an interpretation at the molecular scale of the dimension of beri-beri and also explains the symptomatology observed in patients with a vitamin B_1-deficient diet.

PERSPECTIVES

A brief survey of the ionic translocators in conducting membranes would be incomplete without presenting perspectives for the future as they are opened by the recent introduction of new approaches such as the patch-clamp technique and the use of such powerful tools as the various toxins available. Although specific conducting sites for water and for anions have been described in red blood cells and various epithelial cells, they have not been thoroughly investigated in neurons and other conducting membranes. The same is true with regard to amino acid transporting sites, although the ways in which amino acids are important in cerebral metabolism are now well established. Cell volume regulation requires special mention since it involves not only the enzyme-controlled ionic flux but also the various ionic conducting sites, water conducting sites, and control of amino acids metabolism (130). More specifically, in disease such as epileptic status, all that remains is to define the biochemical lesion responsible for the anomalous electrical discharges in the neuron aggregates involved. It is clear that the coherent model we now have regarding the ionic basis of bioelectrogenesis in normal neurons induces us to look for possible defect(s) in the properties of the ionic translocators in ''epileptic'' neurons.

TABLE 3. *Effect of photostimulation on the content in thiamin (Th) and its phosphorylated derivatives in three cortical areas of the brain of the baboon Papio papio*

| | Photosensitive (Ps) | | | | | | Nonphotosensitive (NPS) | | | | | |
| | Occ | | PM | | M | | Occ | | PM | | M | |
	NSt	St	NSt	St	NSt	St	NSt	St	NSt	St	NSt	St
ThTP	2.3 ± 1.0	1.3 ± 0.3*	3.9 ± 0.8	3.0 ± 0.9*	3.6 ± 1.6	1.9 ± 0.4*	2.6 ± 0.8	1.8 ± 0.5**	5.0 ± 0.9	2.8 ± 0.6*	3.4 ± 0.8	2.3 ± 0.7*
ThDP	80 ± 11	76 ± 5	80 ± 8	77 ± 5	82 ± 9	77.3 ± 2.6**	76.5 ± 4.0	80 ± 2**	79.5 ± 2	82 ± 2*	74 ± 7	82 ± 6*
ThMP	3.1 ± 0.8	7.9 ± 3.5*	3.4 ± 0.9	5.6 ± 3.2**	3.3 ± 0.7	4.9 ± 3.1*	4.5 ± 2.0	3.7 ± 1.1	3.1 ± 1.0	3.2 ± 1.0	7.4 ± 5	2.9 ± 1.3*
Th	14.3 ± 10.5	15.1 ± 3.0	12.1 ± 8.0	13.5 ± 2.9	11.8 ± 7.1	15.9 ± 2.9**	16.5 ± 3.8	14.3 ± 1.3*	12.5 ± 3.3	12.0 ± 1.4	15.0 ± 4.8	13 ± 4

Occ = occipital; PM = pre-motor; M = motor. Two sets of four animals were used: photosensitive individuals (PS), little or no photosensitive animals (NPS). NSt = no photostimulation; St = photostimulation.

Results are expressed as percent of the total sum of thiamin and its phosphorylated derivative ± SD. Four monkeys were studied in each group. Three pieces of the same brain area were analyzed. The results obtained with both hemispheres separately were pooled; each value is thus the average of 12 determinations. Probability to the equivalence of the means (Student's t-test): *very significant (P < 0.01, **significant (P < 0.05); otherwise, not significant. (*Unpublished results.*)

More specifically, the idea that thiamine-phosphorylated derivatives are directly involved in the impedance variation cycle (IVC), prompts us to investigate more specifically the properties of the Na^+-conducting sites protein in epileptic brain areas isolated from various species including humans. The following steps may be envisioned:

1. Purification of the Na^+ conductin and partial determination of the amino acid sequence.
2. Concentration of thiamine compounds in various areas of the brain.
3. Elucidation of the binding capacity and affinity for thiamine-phosphorylated compounds and TTX.
4. Regulation of the net state of phosphorylation with or without phosphate donors (ATP, thiamine triphosphate, etc.) in various experimental conditions (antiepileptic drugs, neurotropic compounds).
5. Cloning of the specific cDNA(s) and gene(s).
6. Search for mutations in epileptic versus normal brains.
7. Examination of regulation of gene expression in epileptic versus normal neurons.
8. Investigation in more details of postranslational modification of Na^+ conductin.
9. Investigation in detail of properties of the various K^+ translocators and of the voltage-sensitive Ca^{2+}-conducting site in epileptic neurons, since they appear to control the overall electrical activity of the neuron together with its electrical plasticity.

With respect to 2 above, available data, indicates that in the frontal area of the photosensitive baboon, *Papio papio,* there is a marked decrease of thiamine triphosphate and an increase in thiamine monophosphate concentrations with respect to the situation found in the "normal" animal, i.e., the one with very little sensitivity to light (Table 3). As shown in Fig. 2, one should expect in very active neurons a higher turnover rate of thiamine-phosphorylated derivatives as well as an increase in thiamine monophosphate concentration. This could be achieved at the expense of thiamine triphosphate concentration or of thiamine diphosphate. However, the exact significance of the increase in thiamine monophosphate will be better grasped when we know more about the metabolic interrelationships between the various thiamine derivatives.

Finally, a more extensive use of *Drosophila* genetic mutants or the discovery of other species that may lend themselves to genetic studies will certainly be of great help in our understanding of bioelectrogenesis at the molecular scale.

ACKNOWLEDGMENT

This work was aided by a grant No. 2.4518.80 from the Fonds de la Recherche Fondamentale Collective.

REFERENCES

1. Adams, D. J., Smith, S. J., and Thompson, S. H. (1980): Ionic currents in molluscan soma. *Annu. Rev. Neurosci.,* 3:141–167.
2. Adams, P. R., Brown, D. A., and Constanti, A. (1982b): M-currents and other potassium currents in bullfrog sympathetic neurones. *J. Physiol.,* 330:537–572.
3. Adams, P. R., Constanti, A., Brown, D. A., and Clark, R. B. (1982a): Intracellular Ca^{2+} activates a fast voltage-sensitive K^+ current in vertebrate sympathetic neurones. *Nature,* 296:746–749.
4. Adams, W. B., and Levitan, I. B. (1982): Intracellular injection of protein kinase inhibitor blocks the serotonin-induced increase in K^+ conductance in *Aplysia* neuron R15. *Proc. Natl. Acad. Sci. USA,* 79:3877–3880.
5. Agnew, W. S., Levinson, S. R., Brabson, J. S., and Raftery, M. A. (1978): Purification of the tetrodotoxin-binding component associated with the voltage-sensitive sodium channel from *Electrophorus electricus* electroplax membranes. *Proc. Natl. Acad. Sci. USA,* 75:2606–2610.
6. Agnew, W. S., Moore, A. C., Levinson, S. R., and Raftery, M. A. (1980): Identification of a large molecular weight peptide associated with a tetrodotoxin binding protein from the electroplax of *Electrophorus electricus. Biochem. Biophys. Res. Commun.,* 92:860–866.
7. Albuquerque, E. X., and Daly, J. W. (1976): The specificity of animal and plant toxins. In: *Receptors and Recognition,* edited by P. Cuatracasas, pp. 297–338. Chapman and Hall, London.
8. Anderson, C. R., and Stevens, C. F. (1973): Voltage clamp analysis of acetylcholine produced end-plate current fluctuations at frog neuromuscular junction. *J. Physiol.,* 235:655–691.
9. Armstrong, C. M., Benzanilla, F., and Rojas, E. (1973): Destruction of sodium conductance inactivation in squid axons perfused with pronase. *J. Gen. Physiol.,* 62:375–391.
10. Armstrong, C. M., and Gilly, W. F. (1979): Fast and slow steps in the activation of sodium channels. *J. Gen. Physiol.,* 74:691–711.
11. Banks, B. E. C., Brown, C., Burgess, G. M., Burnstock, G., Claret, M., Cocks, T. M., and Jenkinson, D. H. (1979): Apamin blocks certain neurotransmitter-induced increases in potassium permeability. *Nature,* 282:415–417.
12. Barchi, R. L. (1976): The non-metabolic role of thiamine in excitable membrane function. In: *Thiamine,* edited by C. J. Gubler, M. Fujiwara, and P. M. Dreyfus. Wiley, New York.
13. Barchi, R. L. (1983a): Protein components of the purified sodium channel from rat skeletal muscle sarcolemma. *J. Neurochem.,* 40:1377–1385.
14. Barchi, R. L. (1983b): Properties of Na channel

reconstituted in liposomes. 9th Meeting of International Society of Neurochemistry, Vancouver, B.C., July 10–15.

15. Barchi, R. L., Cohen, S. A., and Murphy, L. E. (1980): Purification from rat sarcolemma of the saxitoxin-binding componed of the excitable membrane sodium channel. *Proc. Natl. Acad. Sci. USA*, 77:1306–1310.

16. Barchi, R. L., and Murphy, L. E. (1981): Estimate of the molecular weight of the sarcolemmal sodium channel using H_2O-D_2O centrifugation. *J. Neurochem.*, 36:2097–2100.

17. Bartschat, D. K., Cyr, D. L., and Lindenmayer, G. E. (1980): Depolarization-induced calcium uptake by vesicles in a highly enriched sarcolemma preparation from canine ventricle. *J. Biol. Chem.*, 225:10044–10047.

18. Beneski, D. A. and Catterall, W. A. (1980): Covalent labeling of protein components of the sodium channel with a photoactivable derivation of scorpion toxin. *Proc. Natl. Acad. Sci. USA*, 77:639–643.

19. Benzer, T. I., and Raftery, M. A. (1972): Partial characterization of a tetrodotoxin-binding component from nerve membrane. *Proc. Natl. Acad. Sci. USA*, 69:3634–3637.

20. Bernardo, L. S., and Prince, D. A. (1982): Dopamine modulates as Ca^{2+} activated potassium conductance in mammalian hippocampal pyramidal cells. *Nature*, 297:76–79.

21. Bontemps, J., Dandrifosse, G., and Schoffeniels, E. (1980): Protein phosphorylation in nerve and electric organ: Isolation and partial characterization of a high affinity system for ATP. *Neurochem. Int.*, 2:101–110.

22. Bontemps, J., Dandrifosse, G., and Schoffeniels, E. (1981): Extraction of a nerve protein complex containing a self phosphorylating system influenced by tetrodotoxin and carbamylcholine. *IRCS Med. Sci.*, 9:70.

23. Breslow, R. (1958): On the mechanism of thiamine action. Evidence from studies on model systems. *J. Am. Chem. Soc.*, 80:3719–3726.

24. Brown, A. M., Camerer, H., Kunze, D. L., and Lux, H. D. (1982): Similarity of unitary Ca^{2+} currents in three different species. *Nature*, 299:156–158.

25. Byerli, L., and Hagiwara, S. (1982): Calcium currents in internally perfused nerve cell bodies of *Limnea stagnalis*. *J. Physiol.*, 322:503–528.

26. Carbone, E., Wanke, E., Prestipino, G., Possani, L. D., and Maelicke, A. (1982): Selective blockage of voltage-dependent K^+ channels by a novel scorpion toxin. *Nature*, 296:90–91

27. Catterall, W. A. (1975): Cooperative activation of action potential Na^+ ionophore by neurotoxins. *Proc. Natl. Acad. Sci. USA*, 72:1782–1786.

28. Catterall, W. A. (1977): Activation of the action potential C_{Na} ionophore by neurotoxins in allosteric model. *J. Biol. Chem.*, 252:8669–8676.

29. Catterall, W. A. (1981): Localization of sodium channels in cultured neural cells. *J. Neurosci.*, 1:777–783.

30. Charlton, M. P., Smith, S. J., and Zucker, R. S. (1982): Role of presynaptic calcium ions and channels in synaptic facilitation and depression

at the squid giant synapse. *J. Physiol.*, 323:173–193.

31. Chiu, S. Y., and Ritchie, J. M. (1981): Evidence for the presence of potassium channels in the paranodal region of acutely demyelinated mammalian single nerve fibres. *J. Physiol.*, 313:415–437.

32. Chiu, S. Y., and Ritchie, J. M. (1982): Evidence for the presence of potassium channels in the internode of frog myelinated nerve fibres. *J. Physiol.*, 322:485–501.

33. Chiu, S. Y., Ritchie, J. M., Rogart, R. B., and Stagg, D. (1979): A quantitative description of membrane currents in rabbit myelinated nerve. *J. Physiol.*, 292:149–166.

34. Cohen, L. B. (1973): Changes in neuron structure during action potential propagation and synaptic transmission. *Physiol. Rev.*, 53:373–418.

35. Cole, K. S. (1949): Dynamic electrical characteristics of the squid axon membrane. *Arch. Sci. Physiol.*, 3:253–258.

36. Connor, J. A., and Stevens, C. F. (1971a): Voltage clamp studies of a transient outward membrane current in gastropod neural somata. *J. Physiol.*, 213:21–30.

37. Connor, J. A., and Stevens, C. F. (1971b): Prediction of repetitive firing behaviour from voltage clanip data on an isolated neurone soma. *J. Physiol.*, 213:31–53.

38. Constanti, A., Adams, P. R., and Brown, D. A. (1981): Why does barium imitate acetylcholine? *Brain Res.*, 206:244–250.

39. Conti, F. (1983): Volume and entropy changes accompanying the isomerization of Na channels in nerves. Ninth Meeting of International Society of Neurochemistry, Vancouver, B.C., July 10–15.

40. Conti, F., and Neher, E. (1980): Single channel recordings of K^+ currents in squid axons. *Nature*, 285:140–143.

41. Cook, N. S., Haylett, D. G., and Strong, P. N. (1983): High affinity binding of (^{125}I) monoiodoapamin to isolated guinea-pig hepatocytes. *FEBS Lett.*, 152:265–269.

42. Cooper, J. R., Roth, R. H., and Kini, M. M. (1963): Biochemical and physiological function of thiamine in nervous tissue. *Nature*, 199:609–610.

43. Costa, M. R. C., Casnellie, J. E., and Catterall, W. A. (1982): Selective phosphorylation of the alpha subunit of the sodium channel by cAMP-dependent protein kinase. *J. Biol. Chem.*, 257:7918–7921.

44. Cottrell, G. A. (1982): FMR famide neuropeptides simultaneously increase and decrease K^+ currents in a identified neurone. *Nature*, 296:87–89.

45. Dandrifosse, G., Chapelle, S., Zwingelstein, G., and Schoffeniels, E. (1982): Fatty acid and phospholipid composition of excitable membranes and of a preparation enriched in sodium channel extracted from these organites. *Physiologist*, 25:220.

46. Dorogi, P. L., and Neumann, E. (1978): Asymmetric displacement currents in giant axons and

macromolecular gating processes. *Proc. Natl. Acad. Sci. USA*, 75:4911–4915.

47. Dorogi, P. L., and Neumann, E. (1980a): Theoretical implication of liganding reactions in axonal sodium channel gating. *Neurochem. Int.*, 2:45–51.

48. Dorogi, P. L., and Neumann, E. (1980b): Kinetic models suggest bimolecular reaction steps in axonal Na⁺-channel gating. *Proc. Natl. Acad. Sci. USA*, 77:6582–6586.

49. Dubois, D., and Schoffeniels, E. (1974): A molecular model of action potentials. *Proc. Natl. Acad. Sci. USA*, 71:2858–2862.

50. Dunlap, K., and Fischbach, G. D. (1978): Neurotransmitters decrease the calcium component of sensory neurone potentials. *Nature*, 276: 837–839.

51. Dunlap, K., and Fischbach, G. D. (1981): Neurotransmitters decrease the calcium conductance activated by depolarization of embryonic chick sensory neurones. *J. Physiol.*, 317:519–535.

52. Ellisman, M. H., Agnew, W. S., Miller, J. A., and Levinson, S. R. (1982): Electron microscopic visualization of the tetrodotoxin-binding protein from *Electrophorus electricus*. *Proc. Natl. Acad. Sci. USA*, 79:4461–4465.

53. Ellisman, M. H., and Levinson, S. R. (1982): Immunocytochemical localization of sodium channel distributions in the excitable membranes of *Electrophorus electricus*. *Proc. Natl. Acad. Sci. USA*, 79:6707–6711.

54. Fenwick, E. M., Marty, A., and Neher, E. (1981): Voltage clamp and single-channel recording from bovine chromaffin cells. *J. Physiol.*, 319:100–101P.

55. Fröhlich, O. (1984): How channel-like is a biological carrier? Biophysical discussion, Oct. 2–5, 1983. In: *Biophys. J.*, 45:93–94.

56. Garcia-Sancho, J., Sanchez, A., and Herreros, B. (1982): All-or-none response of the Ca²⁺-dependent K⁺ channel in inside-out vesicles. *Nature*, 296:744–746.

57. Goldin, S. M., Rhoden, V., and Hess, E. J. (1980): Molecular characterization, reconstitution, and "transport-specific fractionation" of the saxitoxin binding protein/Na⁺ gate of mammalian brain. *Proc. Natl. Acad. Sci. USA*, 77:6884–6888.

58. Gould, R. J., Murphy, K. M. M., and Snyder, S. H. (1982): (³H)Nitrendipine-labeled calcium channels discriminate inorganic calcium agonists and antagonists. *Proc. Natl. Acad. Sci. USA*, 79:3656–3660.

59. Gurtner, H. P. (1961): Aneurin and nervenerregung. Versuche mit ³⁵S-markiertem Aneurin and Aneurinantimetaboliten. *Helv. Physiol. Pharm. Acta*, XI (Suppl.): 1–47.

60. Habermann, E. (1972): Bee and wasp venoms. *Science*, 177:314–322.

61. Hagiwara, S., and Byerly, L. (1981): Calcium channel. *Annu. Rev. Neurosci.*, 4:69–125.

62. Hartshorne, R. P., and Catterall, W. A. (1981): Purification of the saxitoxin receptor of the sodium channel from rat brain. *Proc. Natl. Acad. Sci. USA*, 78:4620–4624.

63. Hartshorne, R. P., Messner, D. J., Copper-

smith, J. C., and Catterall, W. A. (1982): The saxitoxin receptor of the sodium channel from rat brain. *J. Biol. Chem.*, 257:13888–13891.

64. Hille, B. (1975): Ionic selectivity of Na and K channels of nerve membranes. *Membranes*, 3:255–324.

65. Hille, B. (1978): Ionic channels in excitable membranes. Current problems and biophysical approaches. *Biophys. J.*, 22:283–294.

66. Hodgkin, A. L., and Huxley, A. F. (1952a): Currents carried by sodium and potassium ions through the membrane of the giant axon of *loligo*. *J. Physiol.*, 116:449–472.

67. Hodgkin, A. L., and Huxley, A. F. (1952b): A quantitative description of membrane current and its application to conduction and excitation in nerve. *J. Physiol.*, 117:500–544.

68. Horn, J. P., and McAfee, D. A. (1980): Alpha-adrenergic inhibition of calcium-dependent potentials in rat sympathetic neurones. *J. Physiol.*, 301:191–204.

69. Horn, R., Patlak, J., and Stevens, C. R. (1981a): Sodium channels need not open before they inactivate. *Nature*, 291:426–427.

70. Horn, R., Patlak, J., and Stevens, C. F. (1981b): The effect of tetramethylammonium on single sodium channel currents. *Biophys. J.*, 36:321–327.

71. Horn, R., Vandenberg, C. A., and Lange, K. (1984): Statistical analysis of single sodium channels: Effects of *N*-bromoacetamide. *Biophys. J.*, 45:323–335.

72. Hugues, M., Duval, D., Kitabgi, P., Lazdunski, M., and Vincent, J. P. (1982d): Preparation of a pure monoiodo derivative of the bee venom neurotoxin apamin and its binding properties to rat brain synaptosomes. *J. Biol. Chem.*, 257: 2762–2769.

73. Hugues, M., Duval, D., Schmid, H., Kitabgi, P., Lazdunski, M., and Vincent, J. P. (1982c): Specific binding and pharamacological interactions of apamin, the neurotoxin from bee venom, with guinea pig colon. *Life Sci.*, 31:437–443.

74. Hugues, M., Romey, G., Duval, D., Vincent, J. P., and Lazdunski, M. (1982a): Apamin as a selective blocker of the calcium-dependent potassium channel in neuroblastoma cells: Voltage-clamp and biochemical characterization of the toxin receptor. *Proc. Natl. Acad. Sci. USA*, 79:1308–1312.

75. Hugues, M., Schmid, H., and Lazdunski, M. (1982e): Identification of a protein component of the Ca²⁺-dependent K⁺ channel by affinity labelling with apamin. *Biochem. Biophys. Res. Commun.*, 107:1577–1582.

76. Hugues, M., Schmid, H., Romey, G., Duval, D., Frelin, C., and Lazdunski, M. (1982b): The Ca²⁺-dependent slow K⁺ conductance in cultured rat muscle cells: Characterization with apamin. *EMBO J.*, 1:1039–1042.

77. Huxley, A. F., and Stampfli, R. (1949): Evidence for saltatory conduction in peripheral myelinated nerve fibres. *J. Physiol.*, 108:315–339.

78. Itokawa, Y., and Cooper, J. R. (1970): Ion movements and thiamine in nervous tissue. I.

Intact nerve preparations. *Biochem. Pharmacol.*, 19:985–992.

79. Itokawa, Y., Schulz, R. A., and Cooper, J. R. (1972): Thiamine in nerve membranes. *Biochim. Biophys. Acta*, 266:293–299.

80. Jackson, M. B. (1984): Spontaneous openings of the acetylcholine-receptor channel. *Proc. Natl. Acad. Sci. USA*, 81:3901–3904.

81. Jacques, Y., Romey, G., Fosset, M., and Lazdunski, M. (1980): Properties of the interaction of the sodium channel with permeant monovalent cations. *Eur. J. Biochem.*, 106:71–83.

82. Jakobsson, E. (1978): A fully coupled transient excited state model for the sodium channel. *J. Math. Biol.*, 5:121–142.

83. Jan, Y. N., Jan, L. Y., and Dennis, M. J. (1977): Two mutations of synaptic transmission in *Drosophila*. *Proc. R. Soc. Lond. B*, 198:87–108.

84. Johnson, J. D. (1984): A calmodulin-like Ca^{2+} receptor in the Ca^{2+} channel. Biophysical discussion, Oct. 2–5, 1983. *Biophys. J.*, 45:134–136.

85. Kaczmarek, L. K., Jennings, K. R., Strumwasser, F., Nairn, A. C., Wilson, F. D., and Greengard, P. (1980): Microinjection of catalytic subunit of cyclic AMP-dependent protein kinase enhances calcium action potentials of bag cell neurons in cell culture. *Proc. Natl. Acad. Sci. USA*, 77:7487–7491.

86. Kaczmarek, L. K., and Strumwasser, F. (1981): Net outward currents of bag cell neurons are diminished by a cAMP analogue. *Soc. Neurosci. Abstr.*, 7:932.

87. Kandel, E. R., and Schwartz, J. H. (1982): Molecular biology of learning: Modulation of transmitter release. *Science*, 218:433–442.

88. Katz, B., and Miledi, R. (1972): The statistical nature of the acetylcholine potential and its molecular components. *J. Physiol.*, 244:665–699.

89. Klein, M., Camardo, J., and Kandel, E. R. (1982): Serotonin modulates a specific potassium current in the sensory neurons that show presynaptic facilitation in *Aplysia*. *Proc. Natl. Acad. Sci. USA*, 79:5713–5717.

90. Kranias, E. G., and Solaro, R. J. (1982): Phosphorylation of troponin I and phospholamban during catecholamine stimulation of rabbit heart. *Nature*, 298:182–184.

91. Kretz, R., Shapiro, E., and Kandel, E. R. (1982): Post-tetanic potentiation at an identified synapse in *Aplysia* is correlated with a Ca^{2+}-activated K^+ current in the presynaptic neuron: Evidence for Ca^{2+} accumulation. *Proc. Natl. Acad. Sci. USA*, 79:5430–5434.

92. Krishtal, O. A., Pidoplichko, V. I. and Shakhovalov, Y. A. (1981): Conductance of the calcium channel in the membrane of snail neurones. *J. Physiol.*, 310:423–434.

93. Lazdunski, M. (1983): Apamin, a neurotoxin specific for one class of Ca^{2+}-dependent K^+ channels. *Cell Calcium* 4:421–428.

94. Levinson, S. R., and Ellory, J. C. (1973): Molecular size of the tetrodotoxin binding site estimated by irradiation inactivation. *Nature New Biol.*, 245:122–123.

95. Lew, V. L., Muallem, S., and Seymour, C. A. (1982): Properties of the Ca^{2+} activated K^+

channel in one-step inside-out vesicles from human red cell membranes. *Nature*, 296:742–744.

96. Llinas, R., Sugimori, M., and Simon, S. M. (1982): Transmission by presynaptic spike-like depolarization in the squid giant synapse. *Proc. Natl. Acad. Sci. USA*, 79:2415–2419.

97. Louis, C. F., Maffitt, M., and Jarvis, B. (1982): Factors that modify the molecular size of phospholamban, the 23.000 dalton cardiac sarcoplasmic reticulum phosphoprotein. *J. Biol. Chem.*, 257:15182–15186.

98. Maas, A. J. J., Den Hertog, A., Ras, R., and Van Den Akker, J. (1980): The action of apamin on guinea-pig *Taenia coli*. *Eur. J. Pharmacol.*, 67:265–274.

99. Madison, D. V., and Nicoll, R. A. (1982): Dual action of norepinephrine in hippocampus. *Soc. Neurosci. Abstr.*, 8:922.

100. Margineanu, D. G., and Schoffeniels, E. (1977): Molecular events and energy changes during the action potential. *Proc. Natl. Acad. Sci. USA*, 74:3810–3813.

101. Marty, A. (1981): Ca-dependent K channels with large unitary conductance in chromaffin cell membranes. *Nature*, 291:497–500.

102. Meech, R. W. (1978): Calcium dependent potassium activation in nervous tissues. *Annu. Rev. Biophys. Bioeng.*, 7:1–18.

103. Meves, H. (1975): Calcium currents in squid giant axon. *Philos. Trans. R. Soc. B*, 270:377–387.

104. Miledi, R., and Parker, I. (1981): Calcium transients recorded with arsenazo III in the presynaptic terminal of the squid giant synapse. *Proc. R. Soc. Lond. B*, 212:197–211.

105. Miller, J. A., Agnew, W. S., and Levinson, S. R. (1983): Principal glycopeptide of the tetrodotoxin/saxitoxin binding protein from *Electrophorus electricus:* Isolation and partial chemical and physical characterization. *Biochemistry*, 22:462–470.

106. Minz, B. (1938): Sur la libération de la vitamine B1 par le tronc isolé du nerf pneumogastrique soumis à l'excitation électrique. *C.R. Soc. Biol. (Paris)*, 127:1251–1253.

107. Mudge, A. W., Leeman, S. E., and Fischbach, G. D. (1979): Enkephalin inhibits release of substance P from sensory neurons in culture and decreases action potential duration. *Proc. Natl. Acad. Sci. USA*, 76:526–530.

108. Neher, E., and Sackman, B. (1976): Single channel currents recorded from membrane of denervated frog muscle fibres. *Nature*, 206:799–801.

109. Neumann, E. (1980): Chemical representation of ion flux gating in excitable biomembranes. *Neurochem. Intl.*, 2:27–43.

110. Norman, R. I., Borsotto, M., Fosset, M., Lazdunski, M., and Ellory, J. C. (1983): Determination of the molecular size of the nitrendipine-sensitive Ca^{2+} channel by radiation inactivation. *Biochem. Biophys. Res. Commun.*, 111:878–883.

111. Ohmori, H. (1978): Inactivation kinetics and steady-state current noise in the anomalous rec-

tifier of tunicate egg cell membranes. *J. Physiol.*, 281:77–99.

112. Ohmori, H., Yoshida, S., and Hagiwara, S. (1981): Single K^+ channel currents of anomalous rectification in cultured rat myotubes. *Proc. Natl. Acad. Sci. USA*, 78:4960–4964.

113. Pallotta, B. S., Magleby, K. L., and Barrett, J. N. (1981): Single channel recordings of Ca^{2+}-activated K^+ currents in rat muscle cell culture. *Nature*, 293:471–475.

114. Parnas, I., Parnas, H., and Dudel, J. (1982): Neurotransmitter release and its facilitation in crayfish. II. Duration of facilitation and removal processes of calcium from the terminal. *Pflugers Arch.*, 393:232–236.

115. Peters, R. A. (1936): The biochemical lesion in vitamin B1 deficiency. *Lancet*, 1:1161–1164.

116. Peters, R. A. (1963): *Biochemical Lesions and Lethal Synthesis*. Pergamon Press, Oxford.

117. Pollock, J. D., Camardo, J. S., Bernier, L., Schwartz, J. H., and Kandel, E. R. (1982): Pleural sensory neurons of *Aplysia*: A new preparation for studying the biochemistry and biophysics of serotonin modulation of K^+ currents. *Soc. Neurosci. Abstr.*, 8:523.

118. Pumplin, D. W., Reese, T. S., and Llinas, R. (1981): Are the presynaptic membrane particles the calcium channels? *Proc. Natl. Acad. Sci. USA*, 78:7210–7213.

119. Reed, J. K., and Raftery, M. A. (1976): Properties of the tetrodotoxin binding component in plasma membranes isolated from *Electrophorus electricus*. *Biochemistry*, 15:944–953.

120. Reichardt, L. F., and Kelly, R. B. (1983): A molecular description of nerve terminal function. *Annu. Rev. Biochem.*, 52:871–926.

121. Reuter, H., Stevens, C. F., Tsien, R. W., and Yellen, G. (1982): Properties of single calcium channels in cardiac cell culture. *Nature*, 297:501–504.

122. Ritchie, J. M. (1979): A pharmacological approach to the structure of sodium channels in myelinated axons. *Annu. Rev. Neurosci.*, 2:341–362.

123. Ritchie, J. M., and Rogart, R. B. (1977): Density of sodium channels in mammalian myelinated nerve fibers and nature of the axonal membrane under the myelin sheath. *Proc. Natl. Acad. Sci. USA*, 74:211–215.

124. Rojas, E., and Armstrong, C. (1971): Sodium conductance activation without inactivation in pronase-perfused axons. *Nature New Biol.*, 229:177–178.

125. Rojas, E., and Rudy, E. (1976): Destruction of the sodium conductance inactivation by a specific protease in perfused nerve fibres from *Loligo*. *J. Physiol.*, 262:502–531.

126. Romey, G., and Lazdunski, M. (1982): Lipid-soluble toxins thought to be specific for Na^+ channels block Ca^{2+} channels in neuronal cells. *Nature*, 297:79–80.

127. Rosenberg, R. L., Tomiko, S. A., and Agnew, W. S. (1984): Single-channel properties of the reconstituted voltage-regulated Na channel isolated from the electroplax of *Electrophorus electricus*. *Proc. Natl. Acad. Sci. USA*, 81:5594–5598.

128. Salkoff, L., and Wyman, R. (1981): Genetic modification of potassium channels in *Drosophila shaker* mutants. *Nature*, 293:228–230.

129. Schoffeniels, E. (1976a): Protein phosphorylation and bioelectrogenesis. 2nd International Meeting on *Torpedo*, Arcachon, France.

130. Schoffeniels, E. (1976b): Biochemical aspects of adaptation: Adaptation to salinity. *Biochem. Soc. Symp.*, 41:179–204.

131. Schoffeniels, E. (1979): Protein phosphorylation and nerve conduction. In: *Epithelial Transport in Lower Vertebrates*, edited by B. Lahlou, pp. 285–297. Cambridge University Press, Cambridge.

132. Schoffeniels, E. (1980a): Protein phosphorylation and bioelectrogenesis. *Adv. Chem. Series Am. Chem. Soc.*, 188:285–297.

133. Schoffeniels, E. (1980b): The biochemical cycle of impedance variation in axonal membranes. *Neurochem. Int.*, 2:81–93.

134. Schoffeniels, E. (1981): Identification of Na gating proteins in conducting membranes. In: *Membranes and Transport*, edited by A. N. Martonosi, pp. 379–383. Wiley, New York.

135. Schoffeniels, E. (1983a): Workshop on characterization and isolation of Na^+-gating proteins. Ninth Meeting of International Society of Neurochemistry, Vancouver, B.C., July 10–15.

136. Schoffeniels, E. (1983b): Thiamine phosphorylated derivatives and bioelectrogenesis. *Arch. Int. Physiol. Biochim.*, 91:233–242.

137. Schoffeniels, E., and Dandrifosse, G. (1980): Protein phosphorylation and sodium conductance in nerve membrane. *Proc. Natl. Acad. Sci. USA*, 77:812–816.

138. Schoffeniels, E., Dandrifosse, G., and Bettendorff, L. (1984): Phosphate derivatives of thiamine and Na^+ channel in conducting membranes. *J. Neurochem.*, 43:269–271.

139. Schoffeniels, E., and Dubois, D. M. (1974): Un modèle moléculaire de la bioélectrogenèse. *Bull. Acad. R. Med. Belg.*, 129:509–525.

140. Schoffeniels, E., and Margineanu, D. G. (1981): Intramembrane events during the nerve impulse. *J. Theor. Biol.*, 92:1–13.

141. Shapiro, E., Castellucci, V. F., and Kandel, E. R. (1980a): Presynaptic membrane potential affects transmitter release in an identified neuron in *Aplysia* by modulating the Ca^{2+} and K^+ currents. *Proc. Natl. Acad. Sci. USA*, 77:629–633.

142. Shapiro, E., Castellucci, V. F., and Kandel, E. R. (1980b): Presynaptic inhibition in *Aplysia* involves a decrease in the Ca^{2+} current of the presynaptic neuron. *Proc. Natl. Acad. Sci. USA*, 77:1185–1189.

143. Siegelbaum, S. A., Camardo, J. S., and Kandel, E. R. (1982): Serotonin and cyclic AMP close single K^+ channels in *Aplysia* sensory neurones. *Nature*, 299:413–417.

144. Sigworth, F. J., and Neher, E. (1980): Single Na^+ channel currents observed in cultured rat muscle cells. *Nature*, 287:447–449.

145. Standen, N. B. (1981): Ca channel inactivation by intracellular Ca injection into *Helix* neurones. *Nature*, 293:158–159.

146. Stefani, E., and Chiarandini, D. J. (1982): Ionic

channels in skeletal muscle. *Annu. Rev. Physiol.*, 44:357–372.

147. Takahashi, M., Ohizumi, Y., and Yasumoto, T. (1982): Maitotoxin, a Ca^{2+} channel activator candidate. *J. Biol. Chem.*, 257:7287–7289.

148. Talvenheimo, J. A., Tamkun, M. M., and Catterall, W. A. (1982): Reconstitution of neurotoxin stimulated sodium transport by the voltage-sensitive sodium channel purified from rat brain. *J. Biol. Chem.*, 257:11868–11871.

149. Tamkun, M. M., and Catterall, W. A. (1981): Reconstitution of the voltage-sensitive sodium channel of rat brain from solubilized components. *J. Biol. Chem.*, 256:11457–11463.

150. Tanaka, J. C., Eccleston, J. F., and Barchi, R. L. (1983): Cation selectivity characteristics of the reconstituted voltage-dependent sodium channel purified from rat skeletal muscle sarcolemma. *Biophys. J.*, 41:50(abstr.). *J. Biol. Chem.*, 258:7519–7526.

151. Tillotson, D. (1979): Inactivation of Ca conductance dependent on entry of Ca ions in mol-luscan neurons. *Proc. Natl. Acad. Sci. USA*, 76:1497–1500.

152. Ulbricht, W. (1974): Drugs to explore the ionic channels in the axon membrane. In: *Biochemistry of Sensory Functions*, edited by L. Jaenicke, pp. 351–366. Springer Verlag, Berlin.

153. Von Muralt, A. (1947): Thiamine and peripheral neurophysiology. *Vitam. Horm.* 5:93–118.

154. Von Muralt, A. (1958): The role of thiamine (vitamin B1) in nervous excitation. *Exp. Cell Res.*, 5:72–79.

155. Weigele, J. B., and Barchi, R. L. (1982): Functional reconstitution of the purified sodium channel protein from rat sarcolemma. *Proc. Natl. Acad. Sci. USA*, 79:3651–3655.

156. Wong, R. K. S., Prince, D. A., and Basbaum, A. I. (1979): Intradendritic recordings from hippocampal neurons. *Proc. Natl. Acad. Sci. USA*, 76:986–990.

157. Yatani, A., Tsuda, Y., Akaike, N., and Brown, A. M. (1982): Nanomolar concentrations of extracellular ATP activate membrane Ca channels in snail neurones. *Nature*, 296:169–171.

Advances in Neurology, Vol. 44, edited by
A. V. Delgado-Escueta, A. A. Ward, Jr.,
D. M. Woodbury, and R. J. Porter.
Raven Press, New York © 1986.

9

Modulators Acting on Sodium and Calcium Channels: Patch-Clamp Analysis

Toshio Narahashi

Department of Pharmacology, Northwestern University Medical School, Chicago, Illinois 60611

SUMMARY   Certain antiepileptic drugs are known to block sodium and calcium channels of excitable membranes. These channels are responsible for generation of action potentials. Various natural toxins, chemicals, and therapeutic drugs have been found to modify the gating kinetics of the sodium and/or calcium channels, thereby altering the excitation. Studies of such chemical modulations of the sodium and calcium channel gating provide the basis for understanding the mechanisms underlying epilepsies and the actions of antiepileptic drugs. Tetrodotoxin blocks the sodium channels, whereas batrachotoxin (BTX), grayanotoxin (GTX), and pyrethroids modify a population of the sodium channels to give rise to an extremely slow opening and/or closing. Patch-clamp techniques developed during the past few years permit measurements of opening and closing of individual ionic channels. When a membrane patch isolated from a neuroblastoma cell is depolarized, square inward currents of about 1 pA in amplitude and 2 msec in duration are observed at 10°C. After exposure of the membrane to BTX, the open time is prolonged, the single-current amplitude is reduced, and channel opening is observed at large negative potentials at which no opening is expected to occur in normal preparations. In the BTX-poisoned membrane, there are two separate groups of the sodium channels, one exhibiting the normal characteristics and the other exhibiting a prolonged opening and reduced amplitude. Tetramethrin also modifies the single sodium channel in a similar manner to BTX, but fails to affect the amplitude of single-channel current. Neuroblastoma cells are also endowed with calcium channels, which undergo inactivation in a manner dependent upon membrane potential.

Antiepileptic drugs have been shown to exert potent actions on excitable cells, and an exhaustive literature has accumulated to account for their mechanisms of action. These actions of antiepileptic drugs include stimulation of Na–K ion pump, inhibition of voltage-dependent sodium influx during excitation, reduction of passive calcium influx, reduction of posttetanic potentiation, and enhancement of postsynaptic inhibition primarily at GABAergic synapses (117).

Particularly important is the block of sodium and calcium channels of various excitable cells. For example, phenytoin has been shown to block sodium channels in squid giant axons (54,86,122), in myelinated nerve fibers (96), and in neuroblastoma cells (62,87,115). It also inhibits the calcium-dependent component of the action potential in neuroblastoma cells (112). Bursting activity associated with the negative slope resistance in the current–voltage relation is inhibited by phenytoin (47), and calcium currents have been implicated in the generation of burst firing (46,116). It has been demonstrated recently that phenytoin decreases calcium current in cardiac fibers (96).

These studies clearly indicate that sodium and calcium channels are important target sites of phenytoin and are possibly target sites of some other antiepileptic drugs. Voltage-clamp methods provide us with the most straightforward and powerful approach to the study of these channels, because the activity and kinetics of sodium and calcium channels can be measured separately. More recently, patch-clamp single-channel recording techniques have been developed, enabling us to analyze the kinetics of opening and closing of individual ionic channels. The voltage-clamp and patch-clamp techniques have been used extensively for the study of the mechanisms of action of various drugs. This chapter gives a brief account of recent developments in our laboratory, with special reference to the actions of agents that modify the kinetics of sodium and calcium channels. Before explaining the actions of these agents, the mechanism of action potential generation and the principle of voltage clamp and patch clamp will be described briefly.

MECHANISM OF ACTION POTENTIAL GENERATION

Action potentials are generated as a result of increases in membrane conductance to certain cations (Fig. 1). In the case of squid giant axons, the membrane undergoes a conductance increase to sodium upon depolarizing stimulation, generating the rising phase of an action potential. The increased sodium conductance begins decreasing quickly, and the potassium conductance begins increasing with some delay. These changes in sodium and potassium conductances bring the membrane potential back to the resting level. However, in certain excitable cells, including some of the central neurons, calcium conductance changes take the place of sodium conductance. In any case, ions flow in or out of the cell according to their electrochemical gradient across the membrane while the membrane conductance is increased. It should be noted that these ionic conductance changes occur as a result of opening and closing of ionic channels in the membrane. The channel-gating mechanisms are totally independent of the metabolic energy. These ionic channels are indeed the sites of action of a variety of neuroactive agents.

In summary, there are at least three or four ionic permeability components: (a) increase in sodium and/or calcium permeability, responsible for the rising phase of action potential; (b) decrease in sodium and/or calcium permeability (inactivation); and (c) increase in potassium permeability ((b) and (c) are responsible for the falling phase of the action potential).

VOLTAGE CLAMP

Activity of ionic channels can be measured as electric conductance of the membrane. Conductance is given by current and potential. Therefore, if we can measure the membrane current carried by any particular ion species (e.g., Na) and the membrane potential at the same time, the membrane conductance to that ion can easily be calculated. This method is called voltage clamp, and was originally developed by Cole (15) and further improved and extensively utilized in the study of ionic mechanism of excitation in squid giant axons (37–41). According to Ohm's law, membrane sodium conductance (g_{Na}), potassium conductance (g_K), and calcium conductance (g_{Ca}) are given by

$$g_{Na} = I_{Na}/(E_m - E_{Na}),   \text{(Eq. 1)}$$

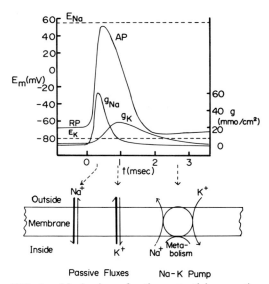

FIG. 1.   Mechanism of action potential generation. **Top:** changes in membrane sodium conductance (g_{Na}) and potassium conductance (g_K) during an action potential (AP). Resting potential (RP) is close to the potassium equilibrium potential (E_K), and the peak of the action potential approaches the sodium equilibrium potential (E_{Na}). **Bottom:** ionic fluxes during the action potential and recovery (67a).

$$g_K = I_K/(E_m - E_K), \text{ and} \qquad \text{(Eq. 2)}$$

$$g_{Ca} = I_{Ca}/(E_m - E_{Ca}), \qquad \text{(Eq. 3)}$$

where I_{Na}, I_K, and I_{Ca} represent sodium, potassium, and calcium currents, respectively; E_m represents the membrane potential; and E_{Na}, E_K, and E_{Ca} represent the sodium, potassium, and calcium equilibrium potentials, respectively. Therefore, if we can measure I_{Na}, E_m, and E_{Na}, we will be able to calculate g_{Na}. Likewise, we can calculate g_K and g_{Ca}.

However, in order to measure membrane ionic current density, both ionic current and membrane potential must be uniform over an area of the membrane where the measurement is made. This can be accomplished by short-circuiting external and internal resistances of the cell. Depending on the shape of the cell and the area of the membrane in question, a variety of methods can be used for the short-circuiting. In the squid giant axon, for instance, an axial wire can be inserted longitudinally, and large electrodes can be placed externally for current delivery. For a smaller axon such as the crayfish giant axon, the sucrose-gap method can be applied. For a nerve cell, an intracellular microelectrode for current delivery will be satisfactory for establishing the space-clamp condition unless the cell is very large or has branches.

By means of a feedback circuit, the membrane potential can be changed and maintained at any level. The membrane current thus recorded is the current necessary to change or hold the membrane potential. However, since the membrane has an electric capacity, the current across the membrane capacity must be eliminated in order to measure membrane ionic currents. This can be accomplished by changing the membrane potential quickly and maintaining it at a new level. Thus, in the conventional voltage-clamp experiments, step depolarizing or hyperpolarizing pulses are applied to the membrane, and the membrane currents associated with them are recorded.

Records under voltage-clamp conditions are compared with those under current-clamp conditions in Fig. 2. If a step depolarizing (outward) current is applied to the nerve membrane, the membrane will be depolarized and will generate an action potential if the depolarization reaches the threshold membrane potential (current clamp). Under voltage-clamp conditions, however, the membrane is step-depolarized and the membrane current necessary for the membrane potential change will be recorded. The membrane current is composed of three elements: (a) capacitative currents associated with a step depolarization and a step repolarization are brief in duration; (b) a transient current, either inward or outward depending on the membrane potential, is carried mostly by sodium ions and represents kinetics of sodium channels; and (c) a late steady state outward current, carried mostly by potassium ions, represents kinetics of potassium channels.

Internal perfusion techniques add a great degree of flexibility to measurements of ionic channel activity. In 1961, Baker et al. (9) and Oikawa et al. (82) independently developed internal perfusion methods for squid giant axons. In short, the axoplasm is removed by squeezing the axon with a small roller or by sucking it through glass capillaries inserted longitudinally to the axon. The axon can then be continuously perfused intracellularly as well as extracellularly and maintained excitable over a much longer period of time than that for the intact axon because the internal ionic composition can be maintained constant without help from Na-K pump. With

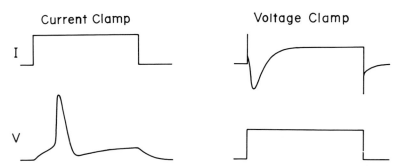

FIG. 2. Comparison of current clamp and voltage clamp. Application of a step-depolarizing current causes membrane depolarization, which in turn triggers an action potential (current clamp). Under voltage-clamp condition, a step depolarization causes a transient inward (Na) current, which is followed by a late steady state (K) current. I, current record; V, voltage record.

the internal perfusion techniques, the ionic compositions and pH, both inside and outside, can be changed at will and maintained, providing a great degree of flexibility of measurements. For example, for measurements of sodium channel activity, potassium ions can be removed from both outside and inside, and cesium ions can substitute for internal potassium ions to block the potassium channels. Internal perfusion techniques have recently been applied to nerve cells such as *Aplysia* neurons (53) and neuroblastoma cells (87,91).

DRUG–CHANNEL INTERACTIONS AS STUDIED BY CONVENTIONAL VOLTAGE CLAMP

The modern era of the study of drug–channel interactions began when voltage-clamp techniques were used to demonstrate the block of sodium and potassium channels of squid axons caused by procaine and cocaine (101,109). The discovery of the highly selective and potent sodium channel blocking action of tetrodotoxin (TTX) (Fig. 3) (74,76) ignited a widespread interest in using specific chemicals as probes for the study of ionic channels. A large number of articles have since been published, dealing with the mechanisms whereby various chemicals block sodium and potassium channels [see reviews by Hille (34), Narahashi (66), Ritchie (93), and Yeh (126)].

Voltage-clamp techniques have been used for the study of other types of drug action also. One of the first such studies is the demonstration that the insecticide DDT inhibits the sodium inactivation, thereby elevating the depolarizing afterpotential, which in turn causes repetitive afterdischarges (33,69,70). Polypeptide neurotoxins, another important group of chemicals isolated

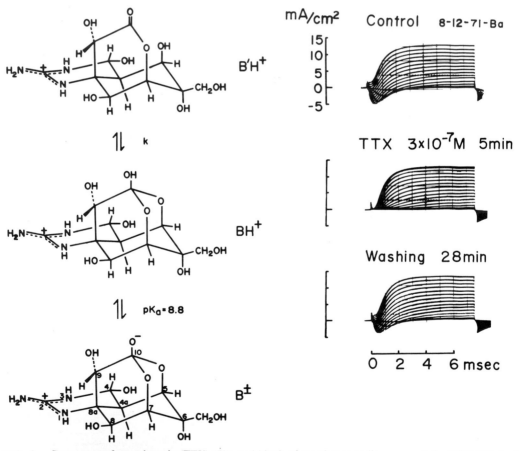

FIG. 3. Structures of tetrodotoxin (TTX) (73), and block of membrane sodium currents by TTX (67). In the control, the membrane current associated with a step depolarization to various levels is composed of a transient inward or outward (Na) current and a late steady state (K) current. TTX (3×10^{-7}M) blocks the sodium currents with no effect on the potassium currents.

from the sea anemone [*Condylactis* (75), *Anemonia sulcata* (94), and *Anthopleura xanthogrammica* (55)] also inhibit the sodium inactivation. These polypeptide neurotoxins provide important tools for the study of sodium channels, since they can be tagged with isotopes such as [125]I (29).

Ionic channel modulators are another important group of chemicals. They modify the kinetics of channels, causing, in most cases, a prolonged opening (13,66). The sodium channel modulators include batrachotoxin (BTX) isolated from the skin secretion of the Colombian arrow poison frog, *Phyllobates aurotaenia;* grayanotoxins (GTXs) isolated from the leaves of various plants (*Leucothoe, Rhododendron, Andromeda, Kalmia*) that belong to the family Ericaceae; and pyrethroids, synthetic derivatives of pyrethrins contained in the flowers of *Chrysanthemum cinerariaefolium.* Pyrethrins and pyrethroids have been used as insecticides extensively.

Batrachotoxin exerts a potent depolarizing action on squid axon membranes (72). This effect was found to be caused primarily by opening of sodium channels at the resting potential level. Khodorov and his associates later discovered drastic changes in sodium channel kinetics by BTX in frog nodes of Ranvier (48–50). The amplitude of peak sodium current decreased, a noninactivating slow sodium current appeared, and the slow current occurred at large negative potentials at which no sodium current was observed under normal conditions. Recently, we have also found similar changes in sodium channel kinetics in squid giant axons poisoned by BTX (107). It was found that BTX blocked the receptor site of the sodium inactivation located near the inner mouth of the channel rather than blocking the inactivation gate per se.

GTXs also have a depolarizing action on squid axons (36,71,99), and a sodium channel modulating action (Fig. 4) (100). An extensive kinetic analysis had led to the following scheme for the action of GTXs:

$$C \rightleftharpoons O \rightleftharpoons I$$
$$\Updownarrow \quad \Updownarrow \qquad \qquad \text{(Scheme 1)}$$
$$C^* \rightleftharpoons O^* \rightleftharpoons I^*$$

where C, O, and I refer to the closed, open, and inactivated states of normal sodium channel, respectively, and C^*, O^*, and I^* are the corresponding states of the GTX-modified sodium channel. The reaction from O^* to I^* may be extremely slow or absent. Kinetic scheme 1 can also be applied to BTX. Thus, two separate populations of sodium channels are predicted in the presence of the toxins. This has proved true by single-channel recording experiments (described below).

Pyrethroids are highly potent sodium channel toxins. Various pyrethroids have been studied for their effects on the sodium channels. Tetramethrin and allethrin cause repetitive afterdischarges to be induced by a single stimulus as a result of an elevation of the depolarizing afterpotential (64,65,68), which in turn results from a prolongation of sodium current (Fig. 5) (56,57,68,114).

PATCH-CLAMP TECHNIQUES

The conventional voltage-clamp methods described in the foregoing sections permit measurements of membrane ionic currents from a large membrane area. The currents recorded are derived from a large number of ionic channels contained in the membrane area and therefore represent an algebraic sum of the activities of individual ionic channels.

A quantum jump in technological developments was made for the study of ionic channels when Neher and Sakmann (78) successfully recorded opening and closing of individual ionic channels associated with extrajunctional acetylcholine (ACh) receptors from the denervated skeletal muscle, using a glass capillary applied onto the membrane surface. More recently, a gigaohm (GΩ) seal patch-clamp technique was developed whereby the activity of a limited number of ionic channels confined in a very small area of the membrane could be clearly observed (32,77,103). During the past few years, these techniques have been applied to a variety of ionic channels, including those associated with: the ACh receptor (16,32,80,95,108); those associated with the glutamate receptor (20,28, 85); sodium channels (27,42–45,63,84,89,103, 120,121); potassium channels (26,59,60,81,83); and calcium channels (11,14,24,30,58). Unlike the conventional "macroscopic" current recording techniques, the patch-clamp techniques permit observation and analysis of single-channel behavior at a level very close to the molecular events.

Single-channel analysis has proved extremely powerful in elucidating the mechanisms whereby a chemical or ion blocks the channel. This is not only because the opening and closing of individual channels can be measured directly in the absence and in the presence of a test chemical, but also because the step from the

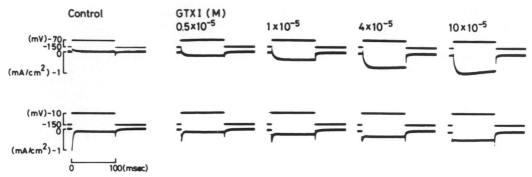

FIG. 4. Membrane sodium currents associated with step depolarizations from the holding potential of -150 mV to -70 mV (*upper set*) and to -10 mV (*lower set*) before and during internal perfusion of various concentrations of grayanotoxin I (GTX I) in a squid giant axon in the presence of 20 mM tetraethylammonium inside to block the potassium channels. Note that at -70 mV only slow sodium currents are generated in the presence of GTX I, and that at -10 mV the peak transient sodium currents are followed by slow sodium currents in GTX I (100).

open channel to the drug-bound blocked channel can be directly measured (for open channel blockers) without complication caused by the channel-gating mechanism.

We have adapted the $G\Omega$ seal patch-clamp technique to cultured neuroblastoma N1E-115 cells (88–90,92,119–121). A patch pipette with a tip opening diameter of <1 μm and a resistance of 2–10 megohms will be applied to the surface of the cell. The pipette-membrane seal resistance can be increased to as high as 10 $G\Omega$. However, since it is difficult to change the solution inside the patch pipette, an isolated patch of the membrane is more convenient and pro-

vides us with a great degree of flexibility in carrying out the experiments. This method permits obtaining either an "outside-out" or "inside-out" patch at the pipette tip (32). Thus, either external or internal surface of the cell membrane can be easily exposed to test solutions.

BLOCK OF IONIC CHANNELS

Block of ionic channels may be classified into two large groups, closed-channel block and open-channel block. In the closed-channel block, a blocking agent binds to a channel site while the channel is closed. The drug-bound

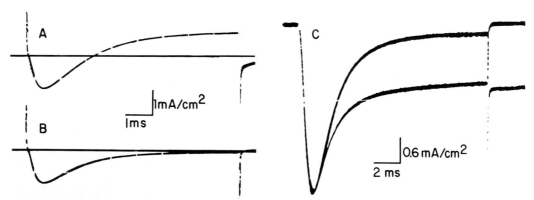

FIG. 5. Membrane currents associated with step depolarizations in a squid giant axon before and during internal perfusion of 1 μM (+)-*trans* allethrin **A:** Peak inward sodium current followed by a steady state outward potassium current when the membrane is step-depolarized from -80 mV to 0 mV. **B:** Sodium current after cesium was substituted for potassium in the internal perfusate and tetramethylammonium was substituted for potassium in the external perfusate to eliminate the potassium current. **C:** Sodium current associated with a step depolarization from -100 mV to -20 mV in the K-free media before (current with a small residual component) and during (with a large residual component) internal perfusion of allethrin (67a).

channel may undergo opening and inactivation as does the normal channel, but remains non-conducting even when it is open. An example of a closed-channel block that can still lead to opening and inactivation is given by TTX. In the presence of TTX, the sodium channel is not conducting (74), yet gating current remains unaffected (4,7). Polyarginine, which blocks both sodium current and gating current of squid axon membranes (118), causes the situation in which the closed sodium channel is bound by the blocking agent and cannot open.

Open-channel block has been demonstrated for various agents and channels. Examples include: the potassium channel block caused by tetraethylmammonium derivatives (5,6); the sodium channel block by pancuronium (127), local anesthetics (17–19,35,51,106,122,125), 9-aminoacridine (124), N-alkylguanidines (52), strychnine (102), and N-methylstrychnine (12); and the ACh-activated channel block by local anesthetics (1,79,104,105), amantadine (111), histrionicotoxin (61), tetraethylammonium (3), decamethonium (2), and N-alkylguanidines (23,113).

Depending on the rate of drug binding to the open channel relative to the channel-opening kinetics, the time course of membrane ionic current could undergo a drastic change. For example, pancuronium accelerated the falling phase of sodium current. This was interpreted as resulting from an open-channel block and not from a change in inactivation, because a similar acceleration by pancuronium was observed in the axon treated with pronase, which destroyed the inactivation mechanism. The block of sodium channel at its open state also results in a frequency- or use-dependent block by local anesthetics (17,98,106).

SINGLE SODIUM CHANNELS

Responses of individual sodium channels of neuroblastoma cell to a step depolarization from a holding potential of -90 mV to -50 mV are illustrated in Fig. 6A. Opening of individual channels is seen as a square downward deflection (inward current). The amplitude histogram shown in Fig. 6B gives a mean value of 1.12 pA at 11°C. These currents were completely abolished by external application of 500 nM TTX, indicating that the currents flowed through the sodium channels. The open time followed a Poisson distribution. In Fig. 6C, the number of channel openings that have durations greater than the times on the abscissa is plotted. The

measurements are fitted by a single exponential curve with the mean open time of 2.2 msec. The probability of channel openings as a function of time during a step depolarization is expected to follow the same time course as the "macroscopic" sodium current recorded from the whole cell. This is actually the case, as shown in Fig. 6D.

TTX BLOCK OF SINGLE SODIUM CHANNELS

External application of 3 nM TTX decreased the number of conducting channels observed for a given number of step depolarizations by about 50%, but the channel open time and current amplitude remained unchanged (92). Analyses of the dose–response curve indicated that TTX blocked the individual sodium channel on the one-to-one stoichiometric basis with the apparent dissociation constant of 2 nM. These results lend support to the notion that TTX blocks the sodium channel regardless of its gating state.

BTX MODULATION OF SINGLE SODIUM CHANNELS

As expected from the macroscopic effects of BTX on sodium channels described in a preceding section, BTX has been found to cause drastic effects on single sodium channels of neuroblastoma cells (Fig. 7) (89). The open time was greatly prolonged from the control value of 2–3 msec to more than 100 msec, the current amplitude was reduced drastically by about 50%, the probability of openings during a prolonged step depolarization remained constant indicating the lack of inactivation, and the channels opened at large negative membrane potentials (e.g., -80 mV) at which normal channels did not open. These prolonged currents were blocked by TTX, indicating that they passed through the sodium channels. When the amplitude of individual sodium channel current is plotted against the open time, the entire channel population in the presence of BTX can be divided into two distinct groups, one having normal characteristics, and the other having a reduced amplitude and a prolonged open time (Fig. 8). This strongly suggests that BTX modifies individual sodium channels in an all-or-none manner, and that in the presence of BTX both normal and modified channels open upon depolarization generating two distinct types of currents. In terms of Scheme 1, the normal and modified channels are repre-

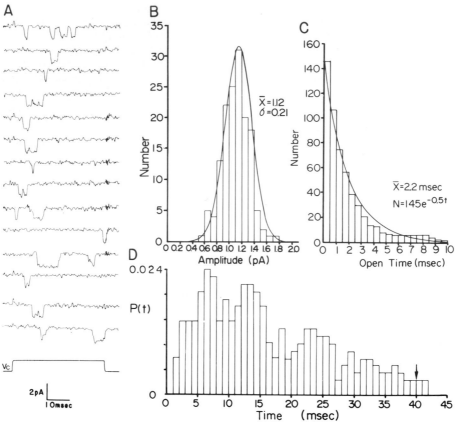

FIG. 6. Single sodium channel activity in a normal neuroblastoma cell N1E-115 as recorded by the patch clamp method. **A:** Sample records of sodium channel currents (*downward deflections*) during step depolarizations from a holding potential of -90 mV to -50 mV (V_c). **B:** Amplitude histogram of sodium channel currents. **C:** Poisson distribution of channel open time. **D:** Probability of channel openings during the step depolarization. Arrow indicates the point of step repolarization. The probability curve resembles the time course of macroscopic sodium current (89).

sented by C, O, and I and C*, O*, and I*, respectively.

TETRAMETHRIN MODULATION OF SINGLE SODIUM CHANNELS

Single sodium channel behavior in response to exposure to tetramethrin also reflects its behavior at the whole cell level. Patch-clamp single-channel recording experiments with neuroblastoma cells have revealed a drastic prolongation of the open time of sodium channels (Fig. 9). Unlike BTX, tetramethrin had no effect on single-channel current amplitude and did not significantly shift the conductance curve in the direction of hyperpolarization (119,120).

CALCIUM CHANNELS

Neuroblastoma cells (N1E-115 line) are also endowed with potassium channels (90) and calcium channels (91). Calcium channel currents were measured after replacement of internal and external K^+ with Cs^+ in order to eliminate currents through potassium channels, and with 0.5 μM TTX added to the external solution to block sodium channels. The calcium channel current thus recorded mimicked the sodium channel current except for a smaller amplitude and a slower time course. The time constants for activation and inactivation were in the range of 1–4 msec and 4–6 msec, respectively, at the membrane potentials of $+60$ mV to 0 mV (28°C).

One interesting property of calcium channel inactivation in many preparations is its depen-

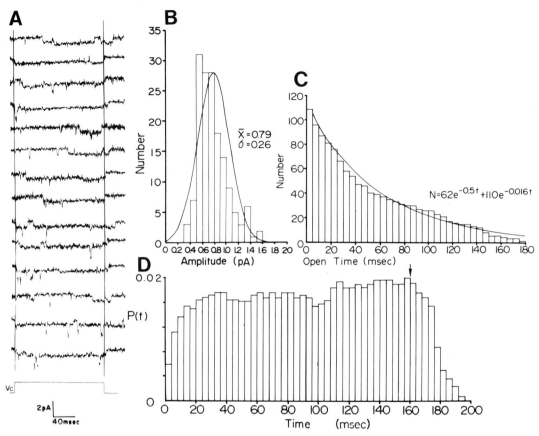

FIG. 7   Same as Fig. 6, but in the presence of 10 μM batrachotoxin (89).

dence of Ca^{2+} influx rather than on membrane potential. The calcium channels of gastropod neurons have been shown to inactivate as a result of an increase in internal calcium concentration (22,110). This was also the case in some other preparations (8,10,21). However, voltage-dependent inactivation of calcium channels was also found (25). We have not performed experiments specifically designed to determine the proportion of calcium versus voltage dependency of inactivation in the neuroblastoma cell calcium channel. However, the following two types of experiments suggest the existence of voltage-dependent inactivation of calcium channels. Calcium channel currents were measured either in the presence or in the absence of EGTA, a calcium chelator, in the internal perfusate. No quantitative difference was found in calcium current under these two conditions.

In another experiment, a two-pulse protocol was used. A conditioning pulse was applied to inactivate calcium channels, and the proportion

of channels not inactivated was determined by measuring the peak calcium current in response to a test depolarization, which followed the conditioning pulse after a short interval. If inactivation were dependent on calcium influx, it would decrease with an increase in conditioning pulse depolarizations approaching the null potential for calcium current. However, the peak calcium current was reduced and maintained at a low level, with an increase in depolarizing conditioning pulse even when it reached the value that should cause calcium influx during this pulse to be reduced. These results support the conclusion that inactivation recorded under the conditions described here is primarily a process that is gated by membrane potential alone. However, we cannot exclude a Ca-dependent inactivation in the intact cell.

Our most recent experiments with the neuroblastoma cell line N1E-115 have revealed two types of calcium channels currents, one with inactivation as described above and the other

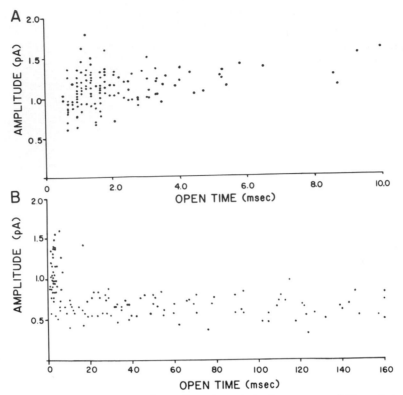

FIG. 8. Two populations of open states for sodium channels in the presence of 10 μM batrachotoxin in a neuroblastoma cell. **A:** Control data before application of batrachotoxin. **B:** After application of the toxin. Note that in the presence of toxin there are modified channels that show lower current amplitudes and prolonged open times (89).

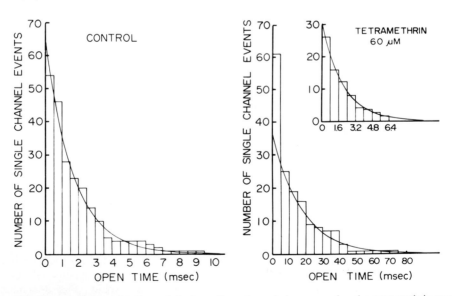

FIG. 9. Distribution of the open time of single sodium channels in a normal and a tetramethrin-treated neuroblastoma cell (N1E-115). The number of events having an open time longer than that indicated on the abscissa is plotted. In the control preparation, the distribution can be fitted by a single exponential function with a decay rate constant of 0.59 msec^{-1}. In the tetramethrin-treated preparation, the distribution of the open time >5 msec is fitted by a single exponential function with a decay rate constant of 0.06 msec^{-1}. The distribution of the open time <5 msec can be divided ino two components: the component obtained by subtraction of the long time constant component from the total population is plotted in the inset, using an expanded time scale, and can be fitted by a single exponential function with a decay rate constant of 0.53 msec^{-1}. This value is very close to the rate constant obtained before application of tetramethrin, and this component likely represents the unmodified population of sodium channels in the presence of tetramethrin (120).

without inactivation (128). The latter was observed only with large depolarizations of the membrane. It appears that these two types of calcium currents represent the activities of two types of calcium channels.

ACKNOWLEDGMENTS

This work was supported by Nos. NS14143 and NS14144 from the National Institutes of Health. I thank Janet Henderson for secretarial assistance.

REFERENCES

1. Adams, P. R. (1977): Voltage jump analysis of procaine action on frog end-plate. *J. Physiol. (Lond.)*, 268:291–318.
2. Adams, P. R., and Sakmann, B. (1978): Decamethonium both opens and blocks endplate channels. *Proc. Natl. Acad. Sci. USA*, 75: 2994–2998.
3. Adler, M., Oliveira, A. C., Albuquerque, E. X., Mansour, N. A, and Eldefrawi, A. T. (1979): Reaction of tetraethylammonium with the open and closed conformations of the acetylcholine receptor ionic channel compex. *J. Gen. Physiol.*, 74:129–152.
4. Almers, W. (1978): Gating currents and charge movements in excitable membranes. *Rev. Physiol. Biochem. Pharmacol.*, 82:96–190.
5. Armstrong, C. M. (1969): Inactivation of the potassium conductance and related phenomena caused by quaternary ammonium ion injection in squid axons. *J. Gen. Physiol.*, 54:553–575.
6. Armstrong, C. M. (1971): Interaction of tetraethylammonium ion derivatives with the potassium channels of giant axons. *J. Gen. Physiol.*, 58:413–437.
7. Armstrong, C. M. (1975): Ionic pores, gates and gating currents. *Q. Rev. Biophys.*, 7:179–210.
8. Aschroft, F. M., and Stanfield, P. R. (1980): Calcium dependence of the inactivation of calcium currents in the skeletal muscle fibres of an insect. *Science*, 213:224–226.
9. Baker, P. R., Hodgkin, A. L., and Shaw, T. I. (1961): Replacement of the protoplasm of a giant nerve fibre with artificial solutions. *Nature*, 190:885–887.
10. Brehm, P., and Eckert, R. (1978): Calcium entry leads to inactivation of calcium channel in *Paramecium*. *Science*, 202:1203–1206.
11. Cachelin, A. B., de Peyer, J. E., Kokubun, S., and Reuter, H. (1983): Ca^{2+} channel modulation by 8-bromocyclic AMP in cultured heart cells. *Nature*, 304:462–464.
12. Cahalan, M. D., and Almers, W. (1979): Interactions between quaternary lidocaine, the sodium gates and tetrodotoxin. *Biophys. J.*, 27:39–56.
13. Catterall, W. A. (1980): Neurotoxins that act on voltage-sensitive sodium channels in excitable membranes. *Annu. Rev. Pharmacol. Toxicol.*, 20:15–43.
14. Cavalie, A., Ochi, R., Pelzer, D., and Trautwein, W. (1983): Elementary currents through Ca^{2+} channels in guinea pig myocytes. *Pflugers Arch.*, 398:284–297.
15. Cole, K. S. (1949): Dynamic electrical characteristics of the squid axon membrane. *Arch. Sci. Physiol.*, 3:253–258.
16. Colquhoun, D., and Sakmann, B. (1981): Fluctuations in the microsecond time range of the current through single acetylcholine receptor ion channels. *Nature*, 294:464–466.
17. Courtney, K. R. (1975): Mechanism of frequency-dependent inhibition of sodium currents in frog myelinated nerve by the lidocaine derivative GEA 968. *J. Pharmacol. Exp. Ther.*, 195:225–236.
18. Courtney, K. R. (1980): Structure-activity relations for frequency-dependent sodium channel block in nerve by local anesthetics. *J. Pharmacol. Exp. Ther.*, 213:114–119.
19. Courtney, K. R., Kendig, J. J., and Cohen, E. N. (1978): The rates of interaction of local anesthetics with sodium channels in nerve. *J. Pharmacol. Exp. Ther.*, 207:594–604.
20. Cull-Candy, S. G., Miledi, R., and Parker, I. (1980): Single glutamate-activated channels recorded from locust muscle fibers with perfused patch-clamp electrodes. *J. Physiol. (Lond.)*, 321:195–210.
21. Dunlap, K., and Fischbach, G. D. (1981): Neurotransmitters decrease the calcium conductance activated by depolarization of embryonic chick sensory neurones. *J. Physiol. (Lond.)*, 317:519–535.
22. Eckert, R., and Ewald, D. (1982): Residual calcium ions depress activation of calcium-dependent current. *Science*, 216:730–733.
23. Farley, J. M., Watanabe, S., Yeh, J. Z., and Narahashi, T. (1981): Endplate channel block by guanidine derivatives. *J. Gen. Physiol.*, 77:273–293.
24. Fenwick, E. M., Marty, A., and Neher, E. (1982): Sodium and calcium channels in bovine chromaffin cells. *J. Physiol. (Lond.)*, 331:599–635.
25. Fox, A. P. (1981): Voltage-dependent inactivation of a calcium channel. *Proc. Natl. Acad. Sci. USA*, 78:953–956.
26. Fukushima, Y. (1981): Single channel potassium currents of the anomalous rectifier. *Nature*, 294:368–371.
27. Fukushima, Y. (1981): Identification and kinetic properties of the current through a single Na^+ channel. *Proc. Natl. Acad. Sci. USA*, 78:1274–1277.
28. Gration, K. A. F., Lambert, J. J., Ramsey, R., and Usherwood, P. N. R. (1981): Non-random openings and concentration-dependent lifetimes of glutamate-gated channels in muscle membrane. *Nature*, 291:423–425.
29. Habermann, E., and Beress, L. (1979): Iodine labelling of sea anemone toxin II, and binding to normal and denervated diaphragm. *Naunyn*

Schmiedeberg's Arch. Pharmacol., 309:165–170.

30. Hagiwara, S., and Ohmori, H. (1983): Studies of single calcium channel currents in rat clonal pituitary cells. *J. Physiol. (Lond.)*, 336:649–661.

31. Hamill, O. P., and Sakmann, B. (1981): Multiple conductance states of single acetylcholine receptor channels in embryonic muscle cells. *Nature*, 294:462–464.

32. Hamill, O. P., Marty, A., Neher, E., Sakmann, B., and Sigworth, F. J. (1981): Improved patch-clamp techniques for high-resolution current recording from cells and cell-free membrane patches. *Pflugers Arch.*, 391:85–100.

33. Hille, B. (1968): Pharmacological modifications of the sodium channels of frog nerve. *J. Gen. Physiol.*, 51:199–219.

34. Hille, B. (1976): Gating in sodium channels of nerve. *Annu. Rev. Physiol.*, 38:139–152.

35. Hille, B. (1977): Local anesthetics: Hydrophilic and hydrophobic pathways for the drug-receptor reaction. *J. Gen. Physiol.*, 69:497–515.

36. Hironaka, T., and Narahashi, T. (1977): Cation permeability ratios of sodium channels in normal and grayanotoxin-treated squid axon membranes. *J. Membrane Biol.*, 31:359–381.

37. Hodgkin, A. L., and Huxley, A. F. (1952): Currents carried by sodium and potassium ions through the membrane of the giant axon of *Loligo*. *J. Physiol. (Lond.)*, 116:449–472.

38. Hodgkin, A. L., and Huxley, A. F. (1952): The components of membrane conductance in the giant axon of *Loligo*. *J. Physiol. (Lond.)*, 116:473–496.

39. Hodgkin, A. L., and Huxley, A. F. (1952): The dual effect of membrane potential on sodium conductance in the giant axon of *Loligo*. *J. Physiol. (Lond.)*, 116:497–506.

40. Hodgkin, A. L., and Huxley, A. F. (1952): A quantitative description of membrane current and its application to conduction and excitation in nerve. *J. Physiol. (Lond.)*, 117:500–544.

41. Hodgkin, A. L., Huxley, A. F., and Katz, B. (1952): Measurements of current-voltage relations in the membrane of the giant axon of *Loligo*. *J. Physiol. (Lond.)*, 116:424–448.

42. Horn, R., and Patlak, J. (1980): Single channel currents from excised patches of muscle membrane. *Proc. Natl. Acad. Sci. USA*, 77:6930–6934.

43. Horn, R., Patlak, J., and Stevens, C. (1981): Single sodium channel currents in excised membrane patches. *Biophys. J.*, 33:210a.

44. Horn, R., Patlak, J., and Stevens, C. (1981): Sodium channels need not open before they inactivate. *Nature*, 291:426–427.

45. Horn, R., Patlak, J., and Stevens, C. (1981): The effect of tetramethylammonium on single sodium channel currents. *Biophys. J.*, 36:321–327.

46. Johnston, D. (1976): Voltage clamp reveals basis for calcium regulation of bursting pacemaker potentials in *Aplysia* neurons. *Brain Res.*, 107:418–423.

47. Johnston, D., and Ayala, G. F. (1975): Diphe-nylhydantoin: Action of a common anticonvulsant on bursting pacemaker potentials in *Aplysia*. *Science*, 189:1009–1011.

48. Khodorov, B. I. (1978): Chemicals as tools to study nerve fiber sodium channels; effects of batrachotoxin and some local anesthetics. In: *Membrane Transport Processes*, vol. 2, edited by D. C. Tosteson, A. O. Yu, and R. Latorre, pp. 153–174. Raven Press, New York.

49. Khodorov, B. I., and Revenko, S. V. (1979): Further analysis of the mechanisms of action of batrachotoxin on the membrane of myelinated nerve. *Neuroscience*, 4:1315–1330.

50. Khodorov, B. I., Peganov, E. M., Revenko, S. V., and Shishkova, L. D. (1975): Sodium currents in voltage clamped nerve fiber of frog under the combined action of batrachotoxin and procaine. *Brain Res.*, 84:541–546.

51. Khodorov, B., Shishkova, L., Peganov, E., and Revenko, S. (1976): Inhibition of sodium currents in frog Ranvier node treated with local anesthetics. Role of slow sodium inactivation. *Biochim. Biophys. Acta*, 433:409–435.

52. Kirsch, G. E., Yeh, J. Z., Farley, J. M., and Narahashi, T. (1980): Interaction of *n*-alkyl-guanidines with the sodium channels of squid axon membrane. *J. Gen. Physiol.*, 76:315–335.

53. Lee, K. S., Akaike, N., and Brown, A. M. (1978): Properties of internally perfused, voltage-clamped, isolated nerve cell bodies. *J. Gen. Physiol.*, 71:489–507.

54. Lipicky, R. J., Gilbert, D. L., and Stillman, I. M. (1972): Diphenylhydantoin inhibition of sodium conductance in squid giant axon. *Proc. Natl. Acad. Sci. USA*, 69:1758–1760.

55. Low, P. A., Wu, C. H., and Narahashi, T. (1979): The effect of anthopleurin-A on crayfish giant axon. *J. Pharmacol. Exp. Ther.*, 210:417–421.

56. Lund, A. E., and Narahashi, T. (1981): Modification of sodium channel kinetics by the insecticide tetramethrin in crayfish giant axons. *Neurotoxicology*, 2:213–229.

57. Lund, A. E., and Narahashi, T. (1981): Kinetics of sodium channel modification by the insecticide tetramethrin in squid axon membranes. *J. Pharmacol. Exp. Ther.*, 219:464–473.

58. Lux, H. D., and Nagy, K. (1981): Single channel Ca^{2+} currents in *Helix pomatia* neurons. *Pflugers Arch.*, 391:252–254.

59. Lux, H. D., Neher, E., and Marty, A. (1981): Single channel activity associated with the calcium dependent outward current in *Helix pomatia*. *Pflugers Arch.*, 389:293–295.

60. Marty, A. (1981): Ca-dependent K channels with large unitary conductance in chromaffin cell membranes. *Nature*, 291:497–500.

61. Masukawa, L. M., and Albuquerque, E. X. (1978): Voltage- and time-dependent action of histrionicotoxin on the endplate current of the frog muscle. *J. Gen. Physiol.*, 72:351–367.

62. Matsuki, N., Quandt, F. N., Ten Eick, R. E., and Yeh, J. Z. (1984): Characterization of the block of sodium channels by phenytoin in mouse neuroblastoma cells. *J. Pharmacol. Exp. Ther.*, 228:523–530.

63. Nagy, K., Kiss, T., and Hof, D. (1983): Single Na channels in mouse neuroblastoma cell membrane. Indications for two open states. *Pflugers Arch.*, 299:302–308.

64. Narahashi, T. (1962): Effect of the insecticide allerthrin on membrane potentials of cockroach giant axons. *J. Cell. Comp. Physiol.*, 59:61–65.

65. Narahashi, T. (1962): Nature of the negative after-potential increased by the insecticide allethrin in cockroach giant axons. *J. Cell. Comp. Physiol.*, 59:67–76.

66. Narahashi, T. (1974): Chemicals as tools in the study of excitable membranes. *Physiol. Rev.*, 54:813–889.

67. Narahashi, T. (1975): Mode of action of dinoflagellate toxins on nerve membranes. In: *Proceedings of the First International Conference on Toxic Dinoflagellate Blooms*, edited by V. R. LoCicero, pp. 395–402.

67a. Narahashi, T. (1984): Drug-ionic channel interactions: Single-channel measurements. *Ann. Neurol.*, 16:539–551.

68. Narahashi, T., and Anderson, N. C. (1967): Mechanism of excitation block by the insecticide allethrin applied externally and internally to squid giant axons. *Toxicol. Appl. Pharmacol.*, 10:529–547.

69. Narahashi, T., and Haas, H. G. (1967): DDT: Interaction with nerve membrane conductance changes. *Science*, 157:1438–1440.

70. Narahashi, T., and Haas, H. G. (1968): Interaction of DDT with the components of lobster nerve membrane conductance. *J. Gen. Physiol.*, 51:177–198.

71. Narahashi, T., and Seyama, I. (1974): Mechanism of nerve membrane depolarization caused by grayanotoxin I. *J. Physiol. (Lond.)*, 242:471–487.

72. Narahashi, T., Albuquerque, E. X., and Deguchi, T. (1971): Effects of batrachotoxin on membrane potential and conductance of squid giant axons. *J. Gen. Physiol.*, 58:54–70.

73. Narahashi, T., Moore, J. W., and Frazier, D. T. (1969): Dependence of tetrodotoxin blockage of nerve membrane conductance on external pH. *J. Pharmacol. Exp. Ther.*, 169:224–228.

74. Narahashi, T., Moore, J. W., and Scott, W. R. (1964): Tetrodotoxin blockage of sodium conductance increase in lobster giant axons. *J. Gen. Physiol.*, 47:965–974.

75. Narahashi, T., Moore, J. W., and Shapiro, B. I. (1969): Condylactis toxin: Interaction with nerve membrane ionic conductances. *Science*, 163:680–681.

76. Narahashi, T., Deguchi, T., Urakawa, N., and Ohkubo, Y. (1960): Stabilization and rectification of muscle fiber membrane by tetrodotoxin. *Am. J. Physiol.*, 198:934–938.

77. Neher, E. (1982): Unit conductance studies in biological membranes. In: *Techniques in Cellular Physiology*, Vol. Pl/II, edited by P. F. Baker, pp. 1–16. Elsevier/North-Holland, County Clare, Ireland.

78. Neher, E., and Sakmann, B. (1976): Single-channel currents recorded from membrane of denervated frog muscle fibres. *Nature*, 260:779–802.

79. Neher, E., and Steinbach, J. H. (1978): Local anaesthetics transiently block currents through single acetylcholine-receptor channels. *J. Physiol. (Lond.)*, 277:153–176.

80. Ogden, D. C., Siegelbaum, S. A., and Colquhoun, D. (1981): Block of acetylcholine-activated ion channels by an uncharged local anaesthetic. *Nature*, 289:596–598.

81. Ohmori, H., Yoshida, S., and Hagiwara, S. (1981): Single K^+ channel currents of anomalous rectification in cultured rat myotubes. *Proc. Natl. Acad. Sci. USA*, 78:4960–4964.

82. Oikawa, T., Spyropoulos, C. S., Tasaki, I., and Teorell, T. (1961): Methods for perfusing the giant axon of *Loligo paelii*. *Acta Physiol. Scand.*, 52:195–196.

83. Pallotta, B. S., Magleby, K. L., and Barrett, J. N. (1981): Single channel recordings of Ca^{2+}-activated K^+ currents in rat muscle cell culture. *Nature*, 293:471–474.

84. Patlak, J., and Horn, R. (1982): Effect of N-bromoacetamide on single sodium channel currents in excised membrane patches. *J. Gen. Physiol.*, 79:333–351.

85. Patlak, J. B., Gration, K. A. F., and Usherwood, P. N. R. (1979): Single glutamate-activated channels in locust muscle. *Nature*, 278:643–645.

86. Perry, J. G., McKinney, L., and DeWeer, P. (1978): The cellular mode of action of the antiepileptic drug 5,5-diphenylhydantoin. *Nature*, 272:271–273.

87. Quandt, F. N., and Narahashi, T. (1980): Internal perfusion of neuroblastoma cells and the effects of diphenylhydantoin on voltage-dependent currents. *Soc. Neurosci. Abstr.*, 6:97.

88. Quandt, F. N., and Narahashi, T. (1981): Characteristics of single sodium channel currents and their modification by batrachotoxin in neuroblastoma cells. *Soc. Neurosci. Abstr.*, 7:902.

89. Quandt, F. N., and Narahashi, T. (1982): Modification of single Na^+ channels by batrachotoxin. *Proc. Natl. Acad. Sci. USA*, 79:6732–6736.

90. Quandt, F. N., and Narahashi, T. (1982): Properties of delayed rectified K channels in neuroblastoma cells. *Soc. Neurosci. Abstr.*, 8:124.

91. Quandt, F. N., and Narahashi, T. (1984): Isolation and kinetic analysis of inward currents in neuroblastoma cells. *Neuroscience*, 13:249–262.

92. Quandt, F. N., Yeh, J. Z., and Narahashi, T. (1982): Contrast between open and closed block of single Na channel currents. *Biophys. J.*, 37 (2):319a.

93. Ritchie, J. M. (1979): A pharmacological approach to the structure of sodium channels in myelinated axons. *Annu. Rev. Neurosci.*, 2:341–362.

94. Romey, G., Abita, J. P., Schweitz, H., Wunderer, G., and Lazdunski, M. (1976): Sea anemone toxin: A tool to study molecular mechanisms of nerve conduction and excitation-secre-

tion coupling. *Proc. Natl. Acad. Sci. USA*, 73:4055–4059.

95. Sakmann, B., Patlak, J., and Neher, E. (1980): Single acetylcholine-activated channels show burst-kinetics in presence of desensitizing concentrations of agonist. *Nature*, 286:71–73.

96. Scheuer, T., and Kass, R. S. (1983): Phenytoin reduces calcium current in the cardiac Purkinje fiber. *Circulation Res.*, 53:16–23.

97. Schwarz, J. R., and Vogel, W. (1977): Diphenylhydantoin: Excitability reducing action in single myelinated nerve fibres. *Eur. J. Pharmacol.*, 44:241–249.

98. Schwarz, W., Palade, P. T., and Hille, B. (1977): Local anesthetics. Effect of pH on use-dependent block of sodium channels in frog muscle. *Biophys. J.*, 20:343–368.

99. Seyama, I., and Narahashi, T. (1973): Increase in sodium permeability of squid axon membranes by α-dihydrograyanotoxin II. *J. Pharmacol. Exp. Ther.*, 184:299–307.

100. Seyama, I., and Narahashi, T. (1981): Modulation of sodium channels of squid nerve membranes by grayanotoxin I. *J. Pharmacol. Exp. Ther.*, 219:614–624.

101. Shanes, A. M., Freygang, W. H., Grundfest, H., and Amatniek, E. (1959): Anesthetic and calcium action in the voltage clamped squid giant axon. *J. Gen. Physiol.*, 42:793–802.

102. Shapiro, B. I. (1977): Effects of strychnine on the sodium conductance of the frog node of Ranvier. *J. Gen. Physiol.*, 69:915–926.

103. Sigworth, F. J., and Neher, E. (1980): Single Na$^+$ channel currents observed in cultured rat muscle cells. *Nature*, 287:447–449.

104. Steinbach, A. B. (1968): Alteration by Xylocaine (lidocaine) and its derivatives of the time course of the endplate potential. *J. Gen. Physiol.*, 52:144–161.

105. Steinbach, A. B. (1968): A kinetic model for the action of Xylocaine on receptors for acetylcholine. *J. Gen. Physiol.*, 52:162–180.

106. Strichartz, G. (1973): The inhibition of sodium currents in myelinated nerve by quaternary derivatives of lidocaine. *J. Gen. Physiol.*, 62:37–57.

107. Tanguy, J., Yeh, J. Z., and Narahashi, T. (1984): Interaction of batrachotoxin with sodium channels in squid axons. *Biophys. J.*, 45:184a.

108. Tank, D. W., Huganir, R. L., Greengard, P., and Webb, W. W. (1983): Patch-recorded single-channel currents of the purified and reconstituted *Torpedo* acetylcholine receptor. *Proc. Natl. Acad. Sci. USA*, 80:5129–5133.

109. Taylor, R. E. (1959): Effect of procaine on electrical properties of squid axon membranes. *Am. J. Physiol.*, 196:1071–1078.

110. Tillotson, D. (1979): Inactivation of Ca conductance dependent on entry of Ca ions in molluscan neurons. *Proc. Natl. Acad. Sci. USA*, 76:1497–1500.

111. Tsai, M-C., Mansour, N A., Eldefrawi, A. T., Eldefrawi, M. E., and Albuquerque, E. X. (1978): Mechanism of action of amantadine on neuromuscular transmission. *Mol. Pharmacol.*, 14:787–803.

112. Tuttle, J. B., and Richelson, E. (1979): Phenytoin action on the excitable membrane of mouse neuroblastoma. *J. Pharmacol. Exp. Ther.*, 211:632–637.

113. Vogel, S. M., Watanabe, S., Yeh, J. Z., Farley, J. M., and Narahashi, T. (1984): Current-dependent block of endplate channels by guanidine derivatives. *J. Gen. Physiol.*, 83:901–918.

114. Wang, C. M., Narahashi, T., and Scuka, M. (1972): Mechanism of negative temperature coefficient of nerve blocking action of allethrin. *J. Pharmacol. Exp. Ther.*, 182:442–453.

115. Williow, M., and Catterall, W. A. (1982): Inhibition of binding of [^{3}H]batrachotoxin A 20-α-benzoate to sodium channels by the anticonvulsant drugs diphenylhydantoin and carbamazepine. *Mol. Pharmacol.*, 22:627–635.

116. Wilson, W. A., and Wachtel, H. (1974): Negative resistance characteristic essential for the maintenance of slow oscillations in bursting neurons. *Science*, 186:932–934.

117. Woodbury, D. M. (1980): Phenytoin: Proposed mechanisms of anticonvulsant action. *Adv. Neurol.*, 27:447–472.

118. Wu, C. H., and Yeh, J. Z. (1982): Effects of polyarginine on gating current of squid sodium channels. *Biophys. J.*, 37(2):314a.

119. Yamamoto, D., Quandt, F. N., and Narahashi, T. (1982): Modification of single sodium channels by the insecticide tetramethrin. *Soc. Neurosci. Abstr.*, 8:251.

120. Yamamoto, D., Quandt, F. N., and Narahashi, T. (1983): Modification of single sodium channels by the insecticide tetramethrin. *Brain Res.*, 274:344–349.

121. Yamamoto, D., Yeh, J. Z., and Narahashi, T. (1984): Voltage-dependent calcium block of normal and tetramethrin-modified single sodium channels. *Biophys. J.*, 45:337–344.

122. Yeh, J. Z. (1978): Sodium inactivation mechanism modulates QX-314 block of sodium channels in squid axons. *Biophys. J.*, 24:569–574.

123. Yeh, J. Z. (1979): Frequency- and voltage-dependent block of Na channels in squid axon membranes by antiarrhythmic drugs. *Fed. Proc.*, 38:589.

124. Yeh, J. Z. (1979): Dynamics of 9-aminoacridine block of sodium channels in squid axons. *J. Gen. Physiol.*, 73:1–21.

125. Yeh, J. Z. (1980): Blockage of sodium channels by stereoisomers of local anesthetics. In: *Molecular Mechanisms of Anesthesia*, edited by B. R. Fink, pp. 35–44. Raven Press, New York.

126. Yeh, J. Z. (1982): A pharmacological approach to the structure of the Na channel in squid axon. In: *Proteins in the Nervous System: Structure and Function*, edited by B. Haber, J. Preg-Polo, and J. Coulter, pp. 17–49. Alan R. Liss, New York.

127. Yeh, J. Z., and Narahashi, T. (1977): Kinetic analysis of pancuronium interaction with sodium channels in squid axon membranes. *J. Gen. Physiol.*, 69:293–323.

128. Yoshii, M., Tsunoo, A., and Narahashi, T. (1985): Different properties in two types of calcium channels in neuroblastoma cells. *Biophys. J.*, 47:433a.

Advances in Neurology, Vol. 44, edited by
A. V. Delgado-Escueta, A. A. Ward, Jr.,
D. M. Woodbury, and R. J. Porter.
Raven Press, New York © 1986.

10

Role of Persistent Inward and Outward Membrane Currents in Epileptiform Bursting in Mammalian Neurons

Wayne E. Crill and Peter C. Schwindt

Departments of Physiology and Biophysics and Medicine (Neurology), University of Washington, Seattle, Washington 98195

SUMMARY During the last five years, work in many laboratories has extended our knowledge of the ionic mechanisms of action potential generation in normal cells of the mammalian central nervous system (CNS). Here we review some of the important voltage-dependent currents present in mammalian CNS neurons. We discuss their possible role in epileptogenesis and normal behavior. We also emphasize the importance of these recent findings in relation to general models of neuronal behavior.

Fifteen years ago at the Colorado Springs Conference on the Basic Mechanisms of The Epilepsies, we had only a minimal understanding of the normal synaptic and excitable properties of neurons. Nevertheless, the mechanism of the recently described paroxysmal depolarization shift (PDS) was being discussed in and out of the literature (2,25,26,28). At that time, the primary conceptual framework for any proposed model of central epileptic cellular mechanisms was the elegant work of Hodgkin and Huxley on the squid axon (14) and of Eccles on the motoneuron (11). The initial studies on cell bodies of invertebrate neurons were just beginning to reveal the complex ionic conductances present in cell bodies (1). Experimentalists studying epileptic processes were severely limited because of the lack of fundamental information about the properties of central mammalian neurons. In the latter part of the past decade, however, we have made significant progress in our understanding of excitable

and synaptic mechanisms in these neurons (3,4,7,9,13,16,20,21,27,29,31,35). Although we do not understand any central neuron in detail, we at least have qualitative information about the properties of a number of neuron types. There is no shortage of hypothetical mechanisms to explain many aspects of epileptic behavior at the cellular level (3,15). In this brief review, we will extend Paul Adams' discussion (see Chapter 6) of vertebrate neuron membrane properties to mammalian central neurons. The emphasis will be on the excitable properties of cat spinal motoneurons and Betz cells of cat motor cortex and their relationship to epileptic behavior. We will also present briefly some findings in experimental spinal seizures.

METHODS

In the experiments discussed below, cat lumbar spinal motoneurons were impaled with two separate microelectrodes for either passing constant current or voltage clamp (3,4,30,31). Large Betz cells were impaled with single electrodes using the tissue slice preparation (38) and the single-electrode voltage clamp (39). For accurate voltage-clamp measurements of ionic currents, the membrane potential must be controlled over the spatial regions of the cell that generates active currents. Neurons of the mammalian central nervous system (CNS), however, have complex geometry. During voltage clamp, the membrane potential is controlled only over the soma and proximal dendrites, and active voltage-dependent currents from the dendrites can give a distorted view of ionic channel properties. In addition, the microelectrode properties and the capacitive properties of the neurons themselves often obscure the fastest ionic currents. The ionic currents of mammalian central neurons cannot be described with the precision of experiments on neurons with simpler geometry. Nevertheless, the voltage-clamp experiments of central neurons have given us an insight into the active properties of central neurons that has not been obtained with other methods.

IONIC MECHANISMS OF THE ACTION POTENTIAL

All of the experimental studies on the excitable properties of mammalian CNS neurons in the spinal cord, brainstem, and cerebral hemispheres reveal a Hodgkin-Huxley-like mechanism for generation of the action potential (4,8,9,20,21). The normally recorded spike is blocked by tetrodotoxin (TTX) in every cell type studied so far. Sodium currents, however, have only been measured in spinal motoneurons (4) (Fig. 1). The initial segment has the lowest threshold for sodium spike generation. The soma sodium current is not activated until the cell is depolarized by 25–40 mV. Figure 1C shows the steady state inactivation of sodium conductance for another motoneuron. Note that appreciable inactivation does not occur until the neuron is depolarized by 10–20 mV. In motoneurons, the initial segment region accommodates during repetitive firing in response to steady depolarizing currents (34). This accommodation and the absence of somatic sodium conductance inactivation allows the summation of synaptic potentials over a membrane potential range of 20–25 mV. It is the regenerative relationship between sodium conductance and membrane potential that causes the all-or-nothing upstroke of the action potential. Repo-

larization is caused by the voltage-dependent activation of a potassium conductance system with relatively fast kinetic properties (3,33), inactivation of the transient inward sodium conductance, and the passive properties of the soma and dendrites. Time constants for activation of the fast potassium current, I_{Kf}, vary from 2 to 4 msec, and I_{Kf} is not activated until the motoneuron soma is depolarized 20–25 mV above resting potential. As shown in Fig. 2, I_{Kf} is selectively blocked by extracellular tetraethylammonium (TEA) ions (33).

SUBTHRESHOLD CURRENTS

In all central neuron types examined, active or voltage-dependent currents have been described in the membrane potential region between rest and spike threshold (8,16,20,21,31,35,36,38). Both the ionic characteristics and the kinetic properties of these subthreshold currents vary, to some extent, in different neuron types. The significance of this variation is not known. It is likely that most neurons have similar ionic channels, but that specific channels dominate in different neuron types.

Two subthreshold currents in motoneurons have been identified: an inward current, I_i, primarily carried by calcium ions (31), and a much slower potassium current, I_{Ks}, that underlies the long afterhyperpolarization of spinal motoneurons (3,33). Figure 3 shows the effect of the persistent inward current on the near-steady state current–voltage (I/V) curve. The presence of the persistent inward current gives the steady I/V curve a region of negative slope conductance just positive to resting potential; in most normal motoneurons, however, the ionic current is not net inward in the negative conductance region. I_i is not blocked by intracellular QX314, a lidocaine derivative that blocks sodium currents, and is markedly potentiated in the presence of extracellular barium ions (32). I_i is, therefore, carried primarily by calcium ions although sodium ions may contribute to the current.

In many motoneurons I_{Ks} can be detected only a few millivolts above resting potential. Both the slow potassium current and the persistent I_i have slow time constants in the subthreshold voltage range, varying from 20–40 msec (3,31). Each current is activated with faster time constants at larger depolarizations. It is clear from these observations that tonic depolarization occurring in the interspike interval during repetitive firing (Fig. 4) will activate the slow

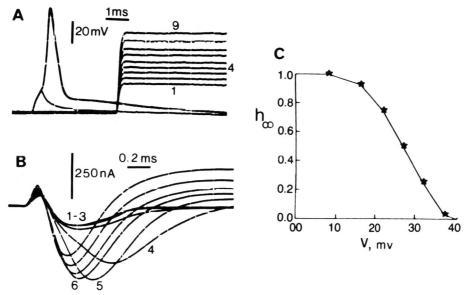

FIG. 1. The fast transient inward current recorded from a cat spinal motoneuron impaled with two micro-electrodes. **A:** Superimposed traces of intracellularly recorded action potential evoked by an intracellularly applied current pulse and a series of numbered voltage-clamp steps. **B:** Voltage-clamp currents recorded during voltage-clamp steps shown in **A. C:** Steady state inactivation of the rapid transient inward current from a different motoneuron plotted as a function of membrane potential (mV) positive to resting potential. From Crill and Schwindt, ref. 9, with permission.

persistent currents (34). Only a small amount of the persistent currents will be activated during the spikes because of their brief duration.

Figure 4C shows a typical relationship between steady injected current and firing frequency recorded from cat spinal motoneurons. The minimal repetitive firing rate is highly correlated with the duration of the long afterhyperpolarization present in spinal motoneurons (19).

The lower slope at small injected currents is called the primary range of repetitive firing. At larger steady injected currents, the slope of the frequency–current curve dramatically increases, producing the so-called secondary range of repetitive firing. As the steady stimulating current is increased, I_{Ks} is activated both by the tonic depolarization and the individual spikes themselves. The activation of I_{Ks} coun-

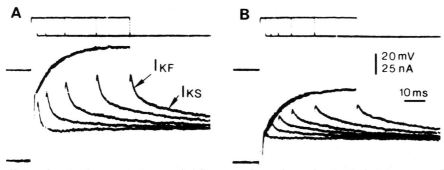

FIG. 2. Outward potassium currents recorded from a voltage-clamped cat spinal motoneuron. **A** and **B:** Superimposed voltage traces (*top*) and superimposed current traces (*bottom*) **A:** Records from a normal spinal motoneuron. **B:** Voltage and current traces from the same neuron as in **A** after the extracellular iontophoresis of tetraethylammonium ions (TEA). Note that in the presence of TEA the steady outward current is decreased, with a selective decrease in the fast decaying portion of the tail currents. From Schwindt and Crill, ref. 33, with permission.

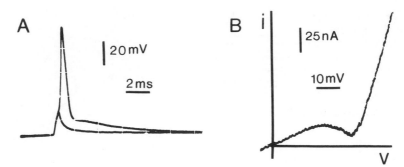

FIG. 3.   **A:** Subthreshold response and action potential recorded from a cat spinal motoneuron impaled with two microelectrodes. **B:** Steady state current-voltage relationship for the same neuron obtained by using a slowly rising ramp voltage-clamp command. The origin is the resting potential. From Schwindt and Crill, ref. 30, with permission.

teracts the effect of the applied current and inhibits repetitive firing. Another important characteristic of spinal motor neurons is the progressive increase in spike firing level caused by accommodation of the initial segment region. The increase in firing level (Fig. 4A) allows tonic activation of I_i. Mathematical reconstruction of motoneuron repetitive firing using measured

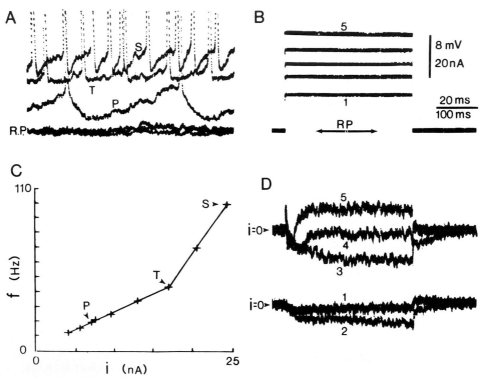

FIG. 4.   Repetitive firing properties and ionic currents recorded from a single cat spinal motoneuron. **A:** Superimposed repetitive firing in response to constant current stimulation of progressively larger amplitude. P shows the interspike trajectory during primary range firing; T labels trajectory during the transition to secondary range (S). Top of the spikes are clipped. **B:** Series of depolarizing voltage change steps in the same neuron. Membrane potential values in B correspond to those in A. **C:** Plot of steady state firing frequency as function of constant stimulating current. P, T, and S mark frequencies from which records in A were obtained. **D:** Voltage-clamp current traces recorded during like-numbered step voltage-clamp records in B. From Schwindt and Crill, ref. 34, with permission.

characteristics of the transient sodium conductance, the fast and slow potassium currents shows only repetitive firing in the primary range (3). Motoneurons studied with somatic voltage clamp that have lost I_i as a result of impalement injury also fire only repetitively in the primary range. These observations are compatible with the hypothesis that the tonic activation of the persistent inward calcium current maintains a linear frequency–current relationship and, in many cells, allows the cell to fire at faster rates in the secondary range if a relatively large amount of I_i is activated. Thus, it appears that the spike output of motoneurons in response to synaptic depolarization is determined by the balance of the subthreshold inward and outward ionic currents. The hypothesis that persistent inward currents activated in the subthreshold region are responsible for tonic firing at faster rates cannot be directly tested, since I_i cannot be manipulated independently of the other ionic currents. Nevertheless, our findings of subthreshold currents in cat neocortical neurons support the above hypothesis.

PROPERTIES OF NEOCORTICAL NEURONS

Stafstrom et al. have been studying in our laboratory the properties of Betz cells from cats using the tissue-slice preparation and the single-electrode voltage clamp (38). Betz cells also have a slow potassium conductance system with time constants similar to those measured in cat spinal motoneurons, yet these neurons have frequency–current curves with a slope 10 to 20 times greater than motoneurons. This difference is best explained by the presence of a subthreshold persistent inward current that is relatively larger (35,37). Figure 5 shows the steady state I/V curve from a Betz cell measured by using both a slowly rising voltage-clamp ramp command and step voltage commands. The presence of extracellular calcium channel blockers such as cobalt or manganese have no effect on the subthreshold inward current in Betz cells. TTX, however, completely blocks the persistent inward current (Fig. 5B). The persistent inward current is therefore assumed to be carried by sodium ions. In contrast to I_i of spinal motoneurons, the persistent inward subthreshold sodium current, I_{Nap}, in neocortical neurons is rapidly activated. In our experiments, I_{Nap} is turned on within the time resolution of the single-electrode voltage clamp (2–4 msec). Whether I_{Nap} is carried through the transient sodium channels or a

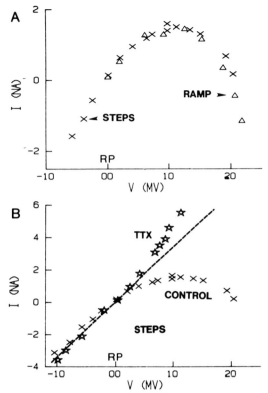

FIG. 5. Plots of current–voltage relationship from a Betz cell in cat *in vitro* neocortex slice recorded using the single-electrode voltage clamp. **A:** Current–voltage relationship obtained using both a step-clamp command and a slowly rising voltage-clamp ramp command. **B:** Current–voltage relationship from another neuron before and after the application of tetrodotoxin to identify the persistent inward sodium current. RP is the resting potential. From Stafstrom et al., ref. 35, with permission.

separate sodium channel remains to be determined. If the activation and inactivation curves for the transient sodium conductance had a significant overlap, a persistent inward sodium current would result. The experiments of Stafstrom et al. (35,36) show evidence for the existence of a cobalt-resistant, TTX-sensitive persistent inward current at depolarizations as large as 52 mV positive to resting potential. If I_{Nap} is caused by an overlap of activation and inactivation curves for sodium conductance, the overlap must be extensive. Regardless of the channel mechanism, I_{Nap} is activated in the subthreshold region and likely plays an important role in repetitive firing mechanisms. Figure 6 shows the tonic activation of I_{Nap} in the voltage range covered by the interspike trajectory during repeti-

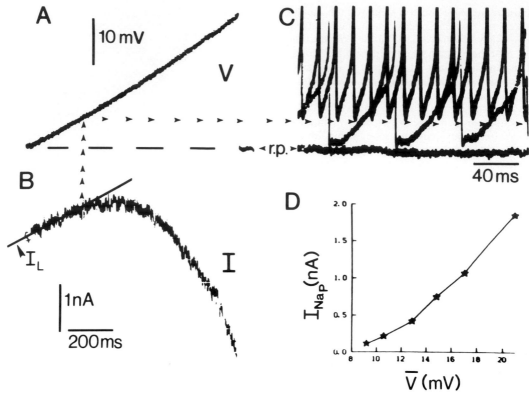

FIG. 6. Relationship of the interspike trajectory to the persistent inward sodium current in neocortical Betz cell from cat using the *in vitro* slice preparation. **A:** Membrane potential during a ramp voltage-clamp command; **B,** the associated membrane current. I_L is linear leakage current. **C:** Repetitive firing response to injected constant current. Arrows show corresponding voltage from **A** where persistent inward current first appears, and the relationship to the interspike trajectory (**C**) during repetitive firing. **D:** Plot of persistent inward sodium current as a function of mean membrane depolarization during interspike intervals obtained during adapted repetitive steady state firing. From Schwindt and Crill, ref. 33, with permission.

tive firing. Because I_{Nap} is activated so rapidly and is persistent, it can have an effect even upon single excitatory postsynaptic spike potentials (EPSPs) as shown in Fig. 7. A similar current probably underlies the subthreshold TTX-sensitive responses measured in Purkinje cells by Llinas and Sugamori (20), in guinea pig neocortex by Conners et al. (8), and recently, by Wong in isolated hippocampal pyramidal neurons (*personal communication*). The important point, with regard to epileptic behavior, is that minor changes in the relative dominance of subthreshold voltage-dependent currents can cause major alterations in a neuron's firing properties. This principle is illustrated by the effects of penicillin on spinal motoneurons.

PENICILLIN-INDUCED SPINAL SEIZURES

Several laboratories have reported that the direct application of penicillin (PCN) to the spinal cord causes episodic bursting of spinal motoneurons (17,18,23) within a few minutes. Our experiments (30) indicate that this behavior involves more than just motoneuron repetitive firing superimposed upon prolonged postsynaptic potentials: the episodic bursts in motoneurons far outlast the synaptic currents measured by holding the neuron voltage clamped at resting potential. When penicillin is applied directly to the spinal cord we could identify no specific effects on the ionic currents of spinal moto-

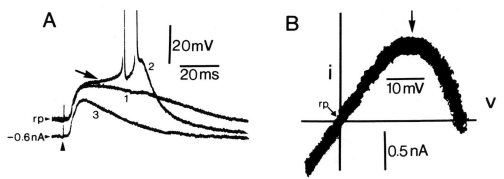

FIG. 7. Effect of persistent inward current upon the shape of excitatory postsynaptic spike potentials (EPSPs) evoked in cat Betz cell recorded in the *in vitro* slice preparation. **A:** Superimposed EPSPs evoked by subcortical white matter stimulation with the neuron at resting potential and hyperpolarized by a 0.6 nA current. **B:** Current–voltage relationship from the same neuron as **A**. Arrows mark identical membrane potential where in **A** the self-sustained depolarization appears, and where in **B** the persistent inward current causes zero slope conductance. From Stafstrom et al., ref. 35, with permission.

neurons. More interesting was the consistent observation of fluctuating I/V responses of a given motoneuron as shown in Fig. 8. When the neuron was not showing prolonged bursts, no inward current was detected in the I/V curve. However, a few seconds later, during the bursting, a decrease in outward and an increase in steady inward currents were detected. Nonstationary behavior of the I/V curves of motoneurons never occurred in normal cells, but was always present during the intense PCN bursting. Figure 8B shows the response of the cell to a ramp-and-hold voltage clamp potential. When bursts were not present, the holding potential was associated with a steady outward current; termination of the clamp led to repolarization of the neuron. A few seconds later, the holding I/V was associated with a net inward current. When the clamp was turned off, persistent self-sustained firing occurred. The lack of change in the I/V curve near resting potential indicates that the observed fluctuations are not caused by fluctuations in nonvoltage-dependent synaptic currents. The transient dominance of the inward current could be explained by the decrease in outward potassium currents or an increase in the inward calcium currents. The simplest explanation for the fluctuation of ionic currents is a relative increase of inward currents caused by a decrease in outward potassium currents (30). The fluctuation in outward current is caused by a transient increase in extracellular potassium

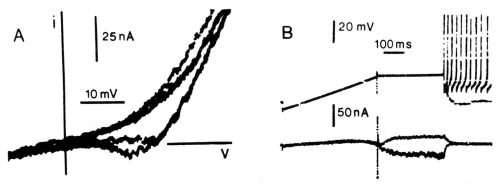

FIG. 8. Fluctuation of the current–voltage relationship in cat spinal motoneuron during penicillin-induced spinal seizures. **A:** Superimposed traces of current–voltage curves obtained at about 1-sec intervals during the onset of intense penicillin-induced bursting. The current–voltage curve shows that a persistent inward current and negative slope conductance occurred during synchronized bursting. **B:** Ramp-hold voltage clamp recorded between bursts shows net outward current during the holding potential and a net inward current during intense bursting. From Schwindt and Crill, ref. 30, with permission.

concentration associated with the bursting behavior (22). We emphasize that this is not the sole mechanism underlying epileptic behavior in the PCN spinal model. However, it is one mechanism whereby normal neurons can be recruited into the epileptic process.

Other mechanisms can alter the balance of currents in the subthreshold region. Paul Adams and colleagues have described the effect of muscarinic agents upon outward potassium currents in sympathetic ganglion neurons and upon similar currents in hippocampal neurons (5,6,13). This effect of putative neurotransmitters upon active membrane currents has major importance for our understanding of normal integrative mechanisms in neurons and could be a significant factor in epileptic behavior.

Some excitatory amino acids activate voltage-dependent currents in mammalian neurons (10,24). Flatman et al., working in our laboratory, has examined the effects of N-methyl-D-aspartic acid (NMDA) on Betz cells (12). NMDA activates one type of receptor for excitatory amino acids. When NMDA is iontophoresed on cat Betz cells in the slice preparation, self-sustained, prolonged bursting occurs. Voltage-clamp studies reveal that NMDA induces an inward current with marked voltage dependence. Single-channel studies (27) indicate that the voltage-dependence of the NMDA current is caused by a voltage-dependent block of the channel by magnesium ions.

In conclusion, we emphasize the following principles that have important implications in both normal and epileptic behavior. First, the concept of a subthreshold region of membrane potential lacking active, voltage-dependent currents is not supported by the experimental data. One can question whether or not there is any range of membrane potential in which voltage-dependent conductances are not active. The concept of algebraic addition of synaptic currents by a soma with passive properties appears to be an oversimplification.

Second, the voltage- and time-dependent conductances activated in the subthreshold region have a major influence upon the transduction of synaptic currents into spike trains. It is these currents that largely determine the firing frequency of a neuron and whether or not the cell fires in a steady or burst pattern in response to synaptic depolarization.

Third, several examples have now shown that transmitter–receptor activation can markedly affect voltage- and time-dependent ionic currents. Brown and colleagues have shown that activation of muscarinic receptors decreases a voltage-dependent outward current (5,6,13). Workers in several other laboratories (10,12,24) have also shown that activation of certain receptors by excitatory amino acids induces highly voltage-dependent currents. Furthermore, changes in extracellular ion concentrations can affect the magnitude of ionic currents flowing through voltage-dependent ion channels. The functional implication of these observations is that the excitable properties of neurons are dynamic and not stationary. Thus, the concept that synaptic currents sum together and excite a neuron with a fixed set of excitable properties is also an oversimplification.

Finally, with regard to epileptic behavior, it is now clear that modest changes in the dynamic effects discussed above can markedly alter the pattern of information transfer through circuits of neurons. More drastic changes can even cause such behavior as self-sustained neuronal firing. At present, we cannot determine which of the properties are responsible for the generation of epileptic behavior in patients, but is likely that the mechanisms discussed here play a role; this may be particularly prominent in the process whereby normal neurons and neural circuits are recruited into synchronized epileptic behavior and large synaptic depolarizations (15).

ACKNOWLEDGMENT

This work was supported by grant No. NS16792 from the National Institutes of Health.

REFERENCES

1. Adams, D. J., Smith, S. J., and Thompson, S. H. (1980): Ionic currents in molluscan soma. *Annu. Rev. Neurosci.*, 3:141–168.
2. Ayala, G. F., Dichter, M., Gumnit, R., Matsumoto, H., and Spencer, W. A. (1973): Genesis of epileptic interictal spikes. New knowledge of cortical feedback systems suggests a neurophysiological explanation of brief paroxysms. *Brain Res.*, 52:1–17.
3. Barrett, E. F., Barrett, J. N., and Crill, W. E. (1980): Voltage-sensitive outward currents in cat motoneurones. *J. Physiol. (Lond.)*, 304:251–276.
4. Barrett, J. N., and Crill, W. E. (1980): Voltage clamp of cat motoneurone somata: Properties of a fast inward current. *J. Physiol. (Lond.)*, 304:231–249.
5. Brown, D. A. (1983): Slow cholinergic excitation—A mechanism for increasing neuronal excitability. *Trends Neurosci.*, 6:302–306.
6. Brown, D. A., and Adams, P. R. (1980): Muscarinic suppression of a novel voltage-sensitive K^+ current in a vertebrate neurone. *Nature*, 283:673–676.

7. Brown, D. A., and Griffith, W. H. (1983): Persistent slow inward calcium current in voltage-clamped hippocampal neurones of guinea-pig. *J. Physiol. (Lond.)*, 337:303–320.

8. Conners, B. W., Gutnick, M. J., and Prince, D. A. (1982): Electrophysiological properties of neocortical neurons in vitro. *J. Neurophysiol.*, 48:1302–1320.

9. Crill, W. E., and Schwindt, P. C. (1983): Active currents in mammalian central neurons. *Trends Neurosci.*, 6:236–240.

10. Dingledine, R. (1983): *N*-Methyl aspartate activates voltage-dependent calcium conductance in rat hippocampal pyramidal cells. *J. Physiol. (Lond.)*, 343:385–405.

11. Eccles, J. C. (1957): *The Physiology of Nerve Cells.* Johns Hopkins Press, Baltimore.

12. Flatman, J., Schwindt, P. C., Crill, W. E., and Stafstrom, C. E. (1983): Multiple actions of *N*-methyl-D-aspartate on cat neocortical neurons in vitro. *Brain Res.*, 266:169–173.

13. Halliwell, J. V., and Adams, P. R. (1982): Voltage-clamp analysis of muscarinic excitation in hippocampal neurons. *Brain Res.*, 250:71–92.

14. Hodgkin, A. L., and Huxley, A. F. (1952): Currents carried by sodium and potassium ions through the membrane of giant axon of Loligo. *J. Physiol. (Lond.)*, 116:449–472.

15. Johnston, D., and Brown, T. H. (1981): Giant synaptic hypothesis for epileptiform activity. *Science*, 211:274–277.

16. Johnston, D., Hablitz, J. J., and Wilson, W. A. (1980): Voltage clamp discloses slow inward current in hippocampal burst-firing neurons. *Nature*, 286:391–393.

17. Kao, L. I., and Crill, W. E. (1972): Penicillin induced segmental myoclonus. Motor responses and intracellular recording from motoneurons. *Arch. Neurol.*, 26:156–161.

18. Kao, L. I., and Crill, W. E. (1972): Penicillin induced segmental myoclonus. Membrane properties of cat spinal motoneurons. *Arch. Neurol.*, 26:162–168.

19. Kernell, D. (1965): The limits of firing frequency in cat lumbosacral motoneurones possessing different time course of afterhyperpolarization. *Acta Physiol. Scand.*, 65:87–100.

20. Llinas, R., and Sugamori, M. (1980): Electrophysiologic properties of in vitro purkinje cell somata in mammalian cerebellar slices. *J. Physiol. (Lond.)*, 305:171–195.

21. Llinas, R., and Yarom, Y. (1981): Electrophysiology of mammalian inferior olivary neurones in vitro. Different types of voltage-dependent ionic conductances. *J. Physiol. (Lond.)*, 315:549–567.

22. Lothman, E. W., and Somjen, G. G. (1975): Extracellular potassium activity, intracellular and extracellular potential responses in the spinal cord. *J. Physiol. (Lond.)*, 252:115–136.

23. Lothman, E. W., and Somjen, G. G. (1976): Motor and electrical signs of epileptic activity induced by penicillin in the spinal cords of decapitate cats. *Electroencephalogr. Clin. Neurophysiol.*, 41:237–252.

24. MacDonald, J. F., Porietis, A. V., and Wojtowicz, J. M. (1982): Aspartic acid induces a region of negative slope conductance in the current-voltage relationship of cultured spinal cord neurons. *Brain Res.*, 237:248–253.

25. Matsumoto, H., and Ajmone Marsan, C. (1964): Cortical cellular phenomena in experimental epilepsy: Interictal manifestations. *Exp. Neurol.*, 9:286–304.

26. Matsumoto, H., and Ajmone Marsan, C. (1964): Cortical cellular phenomena in experimental epilepsy: Ictal manifestations. *Exp. Neurol.*, 9:305–326.

27. Nowak, L., Bregestovski, P., Ascher, P., Herbet, A., and Prochlantz, A. (1984): Magnesium gates glutamate-activated channels in mouse central neurones. *Nature*, 307:462–465.

28. Prince D. A. (1968): The depolarization shift in epileptogenic neurones. *Exp. Neurol.*, 21:467–485.

29. Schwartzkroin, P. A., and Slawsky, M. (1977): Probable calcium spikes in hippocampal neurons. *Brain Res.*, 135:157–161.

30. Schwindt, P. C., and Crill, W. E. (1980): Role of a persistent inward current in motoneuron bursting during spinal seizures. *J. Neurophysiol.*, 43:1296–1318.

31. Schwindt, P. C., and Crill, W. E. (1980): Properties of a persistent inward current normal and TEA-injected motoneurons. *J. Neurophysiol.*, 43:1700–1724.

32. Schwindt, P. C., and Crill, W. E. (1980): Effects of barium on cat spinal motoneurons studied by voltage clamp. *J. Neurophysiol.*, 44:827–846.

33. Schwindt, P. C., and Crill, W. E. (1981): Differential effects of TEA and cations on the outward ionic currents of cat motoneurons. *J. Neurophysiol.* 46:1–16.

34. Schwindt, P. C., and Crill, W. E. (1982): Factors influencing motoneuron rhythmic firing: Results from a voltage clamp study. *J. Neurophysiol.*, 48:875–890.

35. Stafstrom, C. E., Schwindt, P. C., Chubb, M. C., and Crill, W. E. (1985): Properties of the persistent sodium conductance and the calcium conductance of layer V neurons from cat sensorimotor cortex in vitro. *J. Neurophysiol.*, 53:153–170.

36. Stafstrom, C. E., Schwindt, P. C., and Crill, W. E. (1982): Negative slope conductance due to a persistent subthreshold sodium current in cat neocortical neurons in vitro. *Brain Res.*, 236:221–226.

37. Stafstrom, C. E., Schwindt, P. C., and Crill, W. E. (1984): Repetitive firing in layer V neurons of cat neocortex in vitro. *J. Neurophysiol.*, 52:264–277.

38. Stafstrom, C. E., Schwindt, P. C., Flatman, J. A., and Crill, W. E. (1984): Properties of subthreshold response and action potential recorded in layer V neurons from cat sensorimotor cortex in vitro. *J. Neurophysiol.*, 52:244–263.

39. Wilson, W. A., and Goldner, M. M. (1975): Voltage clamping with a single microelectrode. *J. Neurobiol.*, 6:411–422.

Advances in Neurology, Vol. 44, edited by
A. V. Delgado-Escueta, A. A. Ward, Jr.,
D. M. Woodbury, and R. J. Porter.
Raven Press, New York © 1986.

11

Membrane Currents Underlying Bursting Pacemaker Activity and Spike Frequency Adaptation in Invertebrates

*Darrell V. Lewis, **John R. Huguenard, †William W. Anderson, and †Wilkie A. Wilson

*Departments of *Pediatrics, Medicine, and †Pharmacology, Duke University, Durham, North Carolina, and Department of **Neurology, Stanford University Medical Center, Stanford, California 94305*

SUMMARY   Invertebrate systems have proved to be quite useful for the development of an understanding of some processes in the central nervous system (CNS). An understanding of the basic mechanisms of epilepsy will result from understanding not only how populations of neurons interact but also how the physiological processes in individual neurons are altered in epileptogenesis. Because invertebrate neurons have been so accessible to experimentation, it has been possible to explore in detail the basic mechanisms controlling neuronal excitability using these cells and to make some useful predictions about electrophysiological mechanisms that may be present in central neurons.

This chapter deals with two electrophysiological processes that have been observed in invertebrate neurons and that may have some relevance to understanding the basic mechanisms of epilepsy. We review first the past and current studies of invertebrate burst firing neurons. It appears that the electrophysiological mechanisms producing burst firing may be present in CNS neurons participating in epileptogenesis. With caution, the information gleaned from invertebrate studies may be applicable to higher systems.

The second process we consider is the phenomenon of spike frequency adaptation seen in invertebrates. Spike frequency adaptation is the process by which the firing rate of the neuron declines despite the maintenance of a constant stimulus. This process is not so thoroughly studied as burst firing, but it appears to represent a cellular mechanism designed to suppress prolonged periods of repetitive firing. Clearly, the suppression of such a process would produce excessive neuronal excitability, while its enhancement might have some anticonvulsant effects. The extreme sensitivity of spike frequency adaptation to barbiturates suggests such a possibility.

These two electrophysiological processes are interesting in themselves and also because they may underlie the genesis or control of seizures. However, the greater significance is that, to understand the basic mechanisms of epilepsy, we may be well advised to examine neuronal processes in systems not considered to have seizure susceptibility.

The rhythmic, repetitive bursts of action potentials generated by certain autoactive invertebrate neurons have fascinated many neurobiologists. These bursting pacemaker neurons (BPNs) are large, identifiable cells which generate, independent of any synaptic input, rhythmically recurring bursts of action potentials. After each burst, the BPN abruptly hyperpolarizes. Subsequently, the cell slowly depolarizes until spike threshold is reached many seconds later and the next burst begins and the cycle is repeated. Numerous experiments have confirmed that the slow membrane currents underlying the bursting rhythm are not synaptic but are endogenous to the BPN membrane (6,24,92). The marked influx of calcium with each burst is a crucial modulator of these slow currents (Fig. 1). In addition, neurotransmitters and peptides can modulate bursting pacemaker activity (BPA) by altering these endogenous conductances.

The BPA of invertebrate neurons resembles the bursting activity encountered in neurons in experimental vertebrate models of epilepsy. This resemblance has suggested that understanding the basic mechanisms of invertebrate BPA might give some insight into mechanisms of bursting in epilepsy. Indeed, several ionic conductances underlying BPA initially described in studies of invertebrates have been paralleled by later discoveries of similar currents involved in bursting in hippocampal pyramidal cells. Nevertheless, the superficial similarity between BPA and epileptiform bursting should not be assumed to imply identical underlying mechanisms.

This review will concentrate on the evolution of our concepts of BPA, which, as will become apparent, are still developing. In spite of the relative ease of experimenting with these large, hardy, easily identifiable neurons and the intensive efforts expended upon them in the last 10 to 15 years, new insights into the nature and control of the slow currents governing bursting are still occurring. Direct comparisons with the literature of epilepsy will not be attempted, but it is hoped that reading this account of the efforts to understand bursting will be of some indirect, philosophical, and perhaps scientific, value to the epileptologist who is grappling with the even more complex problem of epileptiform bursting.

OVERVIEW OF BURSTING PACEMAKER ACTIVITY

A brief description of the currents regulating BPA will be helpful in understanding the detailed review of their mechanisms to follow. Present models of bursting (12,20,21,40,47,75,83,92) attribute to slow potential oscillations to two slow current systems. These currents are smaller and slower in their activation and inactivation kinetics than the classical action potential currents. The slow inward current (SIC) is a calcium and/or sodium current, activated by depolarization. It has very gradual and incomplete inactivation; thus, it is frequently referred to as a persistent inward current or steady state inward current. The slow outward current (SOC) is a hyperpolarizing current that is activated by increased intracellular calcium activity, [Ca]$_i$, and has a very slow time course (many seconds) often appearing to reflect the time course of changes in [Ca]$_i$. As will be discussed, the exact

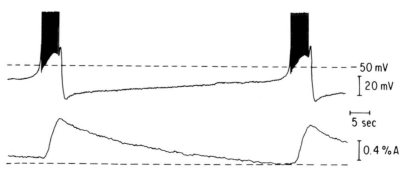

FIG. 1. Bursting pacemaker activity and the corresponding changes of intracellular calcium. **Upper trace:** voltage-measured at soma during spontaneous bursting. In this example, each burst contains about 50 spikes. **Lower trace:** absorbance of intracellular Arsenazo III measured at the soma (660–700 nM). As intracellular calcium activity, [Ca]$_i$, increases, the absorbance increases. Thus, during the burst, there is a rise of [Ca]$_i$ indicated by the upswing of the absorbance trace. During the interburst interval [Ca]$_i$ slowly declines. (D. V. Lewis, unpublished data, July 1981.)

ionic basis of the SOC and SIC are at present debated.

The SIC and SOC can be demonstrated using voltage clamp commands in a BPN. In Fig. 2A, the cell is held at -50 mV, and then is given depolarizing commands to several membrane voltages at which the SIC is activated. The commands are 10 sec in duration because of the slow kinetics of the currents being measured. When the current values 1.5 sec after the beginning of the commands are plotted, the current–voltage (I/V) curve shows a prominent region of negative slope (Fig. 2B), in this instance above -50 mV. This negative slope resistance (NSR) region of the I/V curve is caused by the voltage-dependent activation of the SIC. The NSR region clearly implies an unstable situation. If the cell were to come to rest at any voltage in this region, the inward membrane current would depolarize the cell further, activating more SIC, causing more depolarization, etc.

The SOC also can be seen in Fig. 2A. Note the outward tail current following the 10-sec depolarizations. This tail, the SOC, becomes larger with the larger depolarizations and decays with a slow, many seconds long, time course (57). The partial relaxation of the SIC seen during the commands, which also is more prominent with the greater depolarizations, may represent the same process that gives rise to the SOC tails. Evidence yet to be discussed in detail indicates that the SOC is caused by calcium that enters the cell during depolarization (Fig. 2C).

These illustrations reflect current concepts of the roles of the SIC and SOC in bursting. Beginning at the most hyperpolarized point in the bursting cycle, the SOC is maximum as a result of the massive increase of [Ca]$_i$ during the spikes of the preceding burst (Fig. 1). As the [Ca]$_i$ gradually declines as a result of sequestration and extrusion, the SOC also decreases, allowing the cell to begin to depolarize slightly. The depolarization ultimately begins to activate the regenerative SIC, which drives the depolarization more rapidly. Soon spike threshold is reached and the burst begins. The repetitive firing during the burst is maintained by the regenerative SIC and by the summation of transient depolarizing afterpotentials or DAPs following each spike. As the burst continues, the [Ca]$_i$ level climbs rapidly because calcium enters with each spike, and the SOC builds up, ultimately terminating the burst. At this point, the cycle begins again.

This model of bursting is not necessarily complete. In the sections to follow, we will discuss possible additions to and changes in this scheme. Very likely, the alterations we suggest will, in time, themselves be altered as new insights to this complex neuronal activity occur.

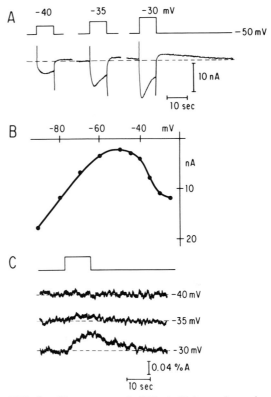

FIG. 2. Slow currents in R15. **A:** Voltage clamp depolarizations disclose slow inward current (SIC) and slow outward current (SOC). **Top traces:** voltage of cell during steps for 10 sec to -40, -35, and -30 mV from holding potential of -50 mV. **Bottom traces:** current (whole cell) during these steps, downward deflection is inward current. Note SIC peaks within 1–5 sec and then begins to relax, more prominently with the larger depolarizations. At these voltages, relaxation is incomplete and longer steps show sustained inward current. After the command, a SOC is seen as a tail current following the steps. The SOC is larger after the greater depolarizations. **B:** The I/V curve of this cell obtained by plotting the peak inward current value versus voltage (holding potential -50 mV). **C: Top trace:** duration and timing of the depolarizing commands given to elicit the SIC. Below it are three traces of the Arsenazo III absorbance at the soma (655–700 nM) during 10-sec depolarizations to -40, -35 and -30 mV. Each absorbance trace is the average of 10 traces (10 depolarizations) to the indicated voltage. The rise of the absorbance signal during the steps to -35 and -30 mV indicate calcium influx produced a detectable rise in [Ca]$_i$ during these commands, whereas at -40 mV no rise in [Ca]$_i$ was detectable. (D. V. Lewis, unpublished data, September 1981.)

IONIC BASIS OF SLOW
INWARD CURRENT

In spite of its crucial role in depolarizing the BPN preparatory to the next burst, there is still disagreement about the ionic basis of the SIC. Early experiments demonstrated that elimination or reduction of extracellular sodium reduced or stopped BPA in certain neurons (23, 36,89). This blockage of the slow depolarizing and hyperpolarizing waves of BPA was not simply a result of the blockade of sodium spikes. Cell 11 of *Otala* continued to generate calcium spikes in the absence of sodium (36), and R15 of *Aplysia* generated slow rhythmic depolarizing waves when its spikes were blocked by tetrodotoxin (TTX) and low calcium (89). The sensitivity of BPA to sodium suggested to these investigators that a high resting sodium conductance was responsible for the depolarizing phase of BPA. This sodium conductance was different from that of the spike by being resistant to TTX, and not inactivated by depolarization.

The application of voltage-clamp analysis to BPNs in *Aplysia* and *Otala* added a new dimension to the bursting mechanism, a voltage-sensitive regenerative SIC (20,38,87,93). BPNs seemed to have both a high resting, voltage-insensitive, sodium conductance and a sodium-mediated SIC that was activated by depolarization. The SIC was reduced progressively as the extracellular sodium was reduced and replaced by Tris, lithium, or sucrose (20,87,94). With the elimination of the SIC, the NSR region of the I/V curve was also eliminated, and the I/V curve was identical to that of a nonbursting neuron. The dependence of the SIC on calcium was also tested. Lowering extracellular calcium had not previously blocked BPA (23,36). In voltage-clamp studies, the amplitude of the SIC seemed to vary inversely with the concentration of extracellular calcium. High calcium suppressed the NSR and SIC, whereas low calcium enhanced them (12).

Most of these experiments were performed on BPNs of the molluscan species *Aplysia* and *Otala*. Using *Helix,* a different species of snail, Eckert and Lux (31) suggested that the SIC was carried by calcium ions, not sodium. In *Helix,* elimination of extracellular sodium had little effect on the SIC. Furthermore, the SIC was blocked by calcium blockers such as lanthanum, cobalt, and D-600. Barium, which readily passes through calcium channels (48), enhanced the SIC. Attempts to eliminate extracellular calcium with EGTA were inconclusive because of a marked increase in membrane conductance. It is worth noting that Eckert and Lux (31) utilized a novel voltage-clamp technique. They recorded currents from a small patch of soma membrane by placing a current measuring pipette directly onto the soma. It is uncertain how much differing voltage-clamp techniques contributed to the apparent difference in effects of low sodium on the SIC of *Helix* versus *Aplysia* and *Otala* BPNs.

With the demonstration of a calcium-mediated SIC in *Helix* BPNs, data began to appear suggesting that *Aplysia* BPNs might not have purely sodium-mediated SICs. Addition of calcium channel blockers, manganese, and cobalt to the bathing medium reduced the SIC (and the SOC), and it was suggested that both calcium and sodium carried the SIC in *Aplysia* BPNs (56). A series of elegant studies appeared, using Arsenazo III as an intracellular calcium indicator to monitor calcium influx into invertebrate neurons. Gorman and Thomas (41) clearly demonstrated increases of intracellular calcium in the soma during small prolonged depolarizations that elicited the SIC in R15 of *Aplysia*. The NSR region usually begins between -65 and -55 mV in R15, and Arsenazo III spectrophotometry detected $[Ca]_i$ increments with depolarizations to between -45 and -40 mV or above (41) (Fig. 2C). Smaller calcium influx at more hyperpolarized voltages may occur but could be below the detection limit of the Arsenazo III technique as a result of effective intracellular calcium buffering (42).

Therefore, calcium enters the soma during depolarizations eliciting the SIC, and the SIC is blocked by agents that can block calcium channels; nevertheless, removal of extracellular sodium seems to eliminate the SIC in some BPNs. In a recent paper, Gorman et al. (40) have attempted to resolve this apparent paradox. In experiments using R15 of *Aplysia* exclusively, these investigators placed the neuron in potassium current blockers tetraethylammonium (TEA) and 4-aminopyridine (4-AP) and injected the calcium buffer EGTA intracellularly. Under these conditions, removal of extracellular sodium had minimal effect on the I/V curve of the cell, whereas removal of calcium eliminated the NSR region of the I/V curve. Gorman et al. (40) suggest that removal of extracellular sodium under conditions in which potassium currents are not blocked somehow produces large outward currents that mask the SIC. Thus, the apparent sodium sensitivity of the SIC may actually not be caused by blockade of the SIC, but rather may represent summation of the SIC with larger outward currents. These authors were also able to demonstrate that SIC varied directly with the extracellular calcium level as the latter was raised or lowered when outward currents were suppressed (TEA and 4-AP) and intracellular calcium accumulation was prevented (intracellular EGTA injection). With this treatment, reduction of extracellular calcium reduced the slope of the NSR region. Again they attribute the previous opposite observations (12) to complex effects of altered extracellular calcium. For example, high extracellular calcium might cause intracellular calcium accumulation and activate calcium-dependent outward potassium currents which would summate with the SIC, eliminating the NSR region of the I/V curve. In addition, high extracellular calcium may alter the surface potential of the outer membrane, shifting the I/V curve such that the SIC is activated at higher apparent depolarizations (52). It appears that much of the difficulty in determining the ionic basis of the SIC could result from the variable amplitude of simultaneous outward potassium currents that occur during the SIC. These currents could change magnitude unbeknownst to the experimenter who is attempting to change only the SIC. This complication has been discussed at length by Lux and Heyer (69) also.

In our view, several questions must be answered before it can be concluded that SICs of BPNs are exclusively calcium mediated. The influx of calcium as measured by Arsenazo III spectrophotometry is first detectable at membrane potentials significantly more depolarized than those at which the SIC first appears (40) (Fig. 2). Does this indicate that a sodium component of the SIC is activated at more hyperpolarized potentials than the calcium component, or that the threshold of the Arsenazo III technique is too high to detect the earliest physiological calcium influx? There also appear to be species differences in the response of BPNs to reduced extracellular sodium (31) and even differences between different BPNs within the same animal (23). Do certain neurons, e.g., R15 of *Aplysia* which is very sensitive to removal of extracellular sodium (12,23,94), have a greater sodium component of the SIC than others, e.g., *Helix* BPNs, which seem insensitive to low sodium? Finally, what is the ionic mechanism and the cause of the hypothetical outward current induced by low extracellular sodium which is proposed (40) to mask the calcium-mediated SIC in *Aplysia* BPNs? It is possible that low sodium causes calcium-activated potassium current by reducing sodium–calcium exchange and causing accumulation of intracellular calcium (30). However, Arsenazo III spectrophotometry has not shown increases of baseline intracellular calcium when R15 is bathed in zero sodium (D. V. Lewis, unpublished observations, June 1982). Neither does low sodium appear to reduce depolarization-induced calcium influx (D. V. Lewis, unpublished observations; 40), whereas, if [Ca]$_i$ were rising in low sodium solutions, one might expect to see reduced calcium influx (33). Until these issues are resolved, it is reasonable to assume that both calcium and sodium may contribute to the SIC.

IONIC BASIS OF SOC

The SOC or slow outward current is found in all BPNs and causes the postburst hyperpolarization. Following either depolarizing voltage-clamp commands or single or multiple spikes, the SOC appears as a slowly peaking (seconds) and very slowly decaying (many seconds) outward current. During the burst of spikes, there is a progressive increase of the SOC that ultimately exceeds the inward current generated during the burst and repolarizes the cell (12, 21,40,75). Activation of the SOC requires an increase in [Ca]$_i$ such as occurs during action potentials or voltage-clamp depolarization (41, 56,66,67,73). The most reasonable explanation of the SOC has been that it represents a calcium-activated potassium conductance. However, recent investigations of this current have suggested that even this accepted explanation may need to be revised.

Early studies of BPNs implicated increased potassium conductance in the termination of the typical bursts of spikes. Junge and Stevens (58) and Gainer (36) suggested that during the postburst hyperpolarization there was a conductance increase that slowly declined as the cell gradually depolarized in advance of the succeeding burst. Periodic injection of identical hyperpolarizing current pulses during the interburst interval was the means used to illustrate the conductance change. However, because of the nonlinear I/V curve of BPNs, this method may give misleading results (47). The voltage change during hyperpolarizing current pulses can be used as an index of voltage-insensitive conductance. However, this deflection can also vary as different voltage sensitive conductances, e.g., the SIC are activated or inactivated during the test pulse itself. For example, as the BPN gradually depolarizes during the interburst interval, more SIC is turned on as the membrane potential enters the region of decreasing positive slope, just preceding the NSR region of the I/V curve. A brief hyperpolarizing current pulse at this potential will inactivate some SIC, resulting in an augmented voltage deflection during the pulse. This phenomenon would cause increasing deflections with successive current pulses during the interburst interval, resembling what could also be seen during the gradual decay of a voltage-insensitive potassium conductance. Still using current clamp methods, Junge and Stevens (58) seemed to be able to reverse the postburst hyperpolarization to a depolarization with the constant injection of a large hyperpolarizing current. In addition, the reversal potential was sensitive to changes in extracellular potassium as expected of a potassium conductance. Carnevale (20), Gola (38) and Smith et al. (87) used voltage clamp to study the SOC following spikes or voltage-clamp depolarizations. All found the current to decrease in amplitude with hyperpolarization and to be sensitive to changes in extracellular potassium. Some demonstrated inversion of the SOC near the potassium equilibrium potential (12), whereas in other studies inversion was not attained (20,57). It should be mentioned that activation of an electrogenic sodium pump had also been considered as a possible mechanism of the SOC or postburst hyperpolarization (89). However, this hypothesis was abandoned when pump blockers and metabolic poisons failed to eliminate the postburst hyperpolarization (20,22,58).

While the SOC was being characterized as a potassium current, other investigators were demonstrating that calcium injection into molluscan and vertebrate neurons also elicited potassium current (63,72). Stinnakre and Tauc (88), using the calcium indicator aequorin, showed marked rises in [Ca]$_i$ during spikes in R15 of *Aplysia*. It was logical to suggest that the SOC was a calcium-activated potassium conductance (58) such as that described by Meech (72) in *Aplysia* neurons. Subsequent voltage-clamp studies clearly demonstrated that depolarization sufficient to produce large calcium influx activated outward potassium currents (28,33,51, 57,76). The potassium current was clearly dependent upon calcium influx because calcium channel blockers and depolarizing commands exceeding the calcium equilibrium potential eliminated it. In addition, buffering the increases in [Ca]$_i$ by intracellular injection of EGTA appeared to eliminate the component of potassium current attributed to calcium influx (28,64,75).

Using intracellular calcium indicators, the increase in potassium conductance was found to correlate with the increase in [Ca]$_i$ during and after voltage-clamp commands (4,32,43).

These investigations produced general agreement that calcium activates potassium currents, although some disagreement remains on the details of this system. Most investigators think that the rise of [Ca]$_i$ at the inner membrane surface increases the potassium conductance, resulting in the delayed potassium current seen during depolarizing commands and causing the slowly decaying outward currents after a train of spikes (4,28,32,43,56,64,68,75). However, Lux and Heyer (69) have presented a significantly different interpretation. Using an extracellular potassium-sensitive microelectrode to monitor potassium efflux, these investigators have concluded that it is the actual passage of calcium through the membrane that activates the delayed potassium current seen during depolarizing commands. Thus, the passage of calcium through the membrane rather than the resultant rise in [Ca]$_i$ activates a potassium conductance. Lux and Heyer (69) suggest that the current activated by increased [Ca]$_i$ is a different potassium current, a potassium leakage (not time-dependent) current. Although this issue may not yet be entirely resolved, we make the simplifying assumption that there is one calcium-activated potassium conductance, and that it is activated by increased [Ca]$_i$ rather than by transmembrane calcium flux.

Returning to the role of calcium-activated potassium currents in BPA, Gorman and Thomas (41) used Arsenazo III spectrophotometry to follow changes in [Ca]$_i$ in R15 during the bursting cycle (Fig. 1). They illustrated marked rises in [Ca]$_i$ during the burst and slow decline of [Ca]$_i$ during the interburst interval (Fig. 1). Thus, there existed abundant evidence that increased [Ca]$_i$ activated a potassium conductance in BPNs, and that [Ca]$_i$ increased during a burst. However, there was little direct and conclusive evidence that the postburst hyperpolarization resulted entirely from the calcium-activated potassium current. In fact, the demonstration that intracellular calcium accumulation might inactivate inward calcium currents (33) prompted speculation that a component of the postburst hyperpolarization might be caused by a calcium-mediated inactivation of the SIC (92).

Within the last several years, evidence suggesting that inactivation of inward current, most probably the SIC, may account for the SOC and the postburst hyperpolarization has been independently presented by several investigators (1,61,62,67). These experiments, using *Aplysia* BPNs, have shown no inversion of the SOC at hyperpolarized holding potentials well below the presumed potassium equilibrium potential, nor sensitivity of the SOC to altered extracellular potassium concentration. Another source of evidence that the SOC may not be a calcium-activated potassium current is its insensitivity to TEA. Although there has been some disagreement (90), several investigators have shown that extracellular TEA will block the potassium currents elicited by either intracellular calcium injection or calcium influx during large depolarizing commands (1,50,61,62,76) in *Aplysia* and *Helix* neurons. However, at least in *Aplysia* neurons, TEA does not block the prolonged outward tail currents or SOC following calcium influx during depolarization (1,61,62).

Therefore, although the SOC followed depolarization-induced calcium influx, it did not have the properties expected of a potassium current. There was no question, however, that the SOC was dependent upon an increase in $[Ca]_i$. It was eliminated by intracellular EGTA, depolarization to voltages exceeding the calcium equilibrium potential did not elicit an SOC, and the SOC was blocked by calcium channel blockers or by elimination of extracellular calcium. The interpretation of these data was the same by several groups (1,61,62,67); the SOC represented, in BPNs, a calcium-mediated inactivation of a persistent inward current. The inward current being inactivated appeared to be identical to the SIC. The voltage sensitivity of the SOC agrees with the voltage activation characteristics of the SIC. At hyperpolarized potentials at which the SOC is small, very little SIC is tonically activated; thus, there is very little to inactivate. At depolarized potentials at which most SIC is tonically activated, the SOC is larger, there being more SIC to be inactivated by calcium influx.

Given the clear presence of calcium-activated potassium channels and the marked increase in intracellular calcium during a burst, it seems premature to conclude that the SOC underlying the postburst hyperpolarization has no component of potassium conductance. We have discussed evidence that under some circumstances the SOC seemed sensitive to altered extracellular potassium. The explanation for conflicting data is not clear. The outstanding conflicting observations seem to involve the response of the SOC to altered extracellular potassium and whether or not the SOC reverses at hyperpolarized potentials. Very likely, the slow outward tail currents following depolarization of BPNs, collectively referred to as the SOC, can be composed of varying proportions of SIC inactivation and calcium-activated potassium current, with the relative proportions determined by differing experimental techniques and biological factors. Obviously, these concepts are still evolving, and it may be some time before the final answer will be known.

CALCIUM-ACTIVATED INWARD CURRENTS IN BPNs

As discussed above, numerous studies have shown that pressure injection or iontophoresis of calcium intracellularly in BPNs and other neurons produces outward potassium currents (17,39,63,72,74). Occasionally, there has been mention of calcium injection producing transient inward currents as well. Meech (74) pressure-injected calcium salts into *Helix* neurons and observed occasional biphasic responses consisting of an early transient depolarization followed by a prolonged hyperpolarization. With smaller injections, only hyperpolarizing potassium-mediated responses were observed. While pressure-injecting calcium into the nonbursting neuron R2 of *Aplysia*, Brown and Brown (17) noted that very large injections occasionally caused initial depolarization followed by prolonged hyperpolarization. Hofmeier and Lux (53) extensively studied the inward current associated with calcium injection and proposed that it was not an artifact of excessive calcium injection but reflected a physiological effect of normal calcium influx. By pressure-injection of calcium in *Helix* BPNs, they could consistently elicit a transient inward current peaking in several seconds, followed by a more prolonged outward current peaking many seconds later. The inward current was increased by hyperpolarization, was associated with a simultaneous conductance increase, and had an extrapolated reversal potential between -20 and $+20$ mV. Nickel, an effective calcium channel blocker, did not eliminate the inward current, nor did replacement of extracellular sodium with sucrose; therefore, the ionic basis of the current was unclear. The authors speculated that previous studies elicited primarily outward currents because calcium was injected or iontophoresed intracellularly in smaller amounts and relatively slowly. They surmised that rapid, large injections were required to raise $[Ca]_i$ sufficiently at the inner membrane surface to activate the inward current. By reducing the size of their calcium injections, Hofmeier and Lux (53) could elicit pure outward current responses.

The physiological role of calcium activated inward currents in BPNs is also being clarified. Following spikes in BPNs are prominent depolarizing afterpotentials or DAPs (91) which precede the later-occurring, previously discussed, SOC or hyperpolarizing aftercurrent (Fig. 3). Lewis (66) presented evidence that DAPs in R15 of *Aplysia* might be activated by increased $[Ca]_i$. DAP current was very sensitive to reduced extracellular calcium, calcium channel blockers, and intracellular injection of calcium buffers EGTA or EDTA. The ionic conductance underlying DAPs had many similarities to the SIC, and Lewis (66) suggested that DAPs might arise from a calcium-mediated activation of the SIC.

A calcium-activated inward current has also been studied by Kramer (61) in left upper quadrant BPNs in *Aplysia*, which, like R15, are in the abdominal ganglion. This current causes DAPs in these neurons and shows the same dependence upon increased $[Ca]_i$ as the DAP current described by Lewis (66). In addition, Kramer (61) was able to show that the current was not activated by depolarizing commands that exceeded the calcium equilibrium potential, thus further excluding any role of depolarization per se in activating it. Kramer (61) also demonstrated that calcium iontophoresis intracellu-

larly in these BPNs activated a voltage-independent inward current that could be seen when the superimposed larger outward potassium current (39) was blocked by extracellular TEA. This observation has been repeated in R15 by Lewis (unpublished observations, December 1983). Kramer suggests that both the DAP current and the inward current activated by calcium injection are identical and are examples of the nonselective calcium-activated cation channels found in neuroblastoma, cardiac cells, and pancreatic acinar cells (27,70,96).

An alternative interpretation of the DAP current has been offered by Adams and Levitan (2) working with R15. These investigators suggest that DAPs result from electronic spread of action potential currents from the axon. They note that axotomy of R15 eliminates DAPs, and that, like the action potentials of R15, the DAPs are dependent upon both extracellular sodium and calcium.

We suggest that the increasing evidence for calcium-activated inward currents in BPNs justifies adding this mechanism to the model of BPA. Previous concepts of the DAP were that it is simply a manifestation of the SIC, and therefore its role in producing bursting activity was lumped with the role of the SIC (47). However, if the DAP current is a calcium-activated inward current, it is therefore removed from the cate-

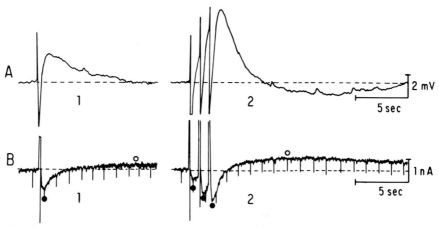

FIG. 3. Depolarizing after potentials in R15. **A1:** R15 in current clamp at -59 mV showing the DAP after one spike triggered by a 5-msec pulse of depolarizing current. The initial positive (*upward*) deflection is the spike (overshoot is clipped by the pen recorder), the following negative (*downward*) deflection is the spike undershoot and the final prolonged positive deflection is the DAP. **A2:** By triggering three consecutive spikes, summation of DAPs can be observed; following the DAPs, a prolonged hyperpolarization reflecting the SOC can be seen. **B1:** By placing the cell in voltage clamp, except for a brief 50-msec interval when the spike is triggered, the currents underlying the DAP (●) and the succeeding hyperpolarization (○) can be measured after one (**B1**) or several (**B2**) spikes. The prolonged outward current (○) following the DAP current is the SOC. Monophasic downward deflections in **B** are excitatory postsynaptic currents. From Lewis, ref. 66, with permission.

gory of simply a manifestation of the voltage-activated SIC and there is a need for further consideration of its role in BPA.

EXPANDED MODEL OF BPA

Here we will attempt to incorporate several additional mechanisms into the previously described model of bursting based on the SIC and SOC. The additional features will be the role of DAPs in initiating and maintaining the burst (91), the activation of inward DAP current by increased [Ca]$_i$ (61,66) and the inactivation of inward current by increased [Ca]$_i$ (1,61,62,67). We stress that any model of bursting must be considered tentative, awaiting new research in this area. Furthermore, the suggested role of [Ca]$_i$ in activation and inactivation of inward currents during BPA has yet to be observed in species other than *Aplysia* and *Helix*. Therefore, this is not intended to be a generalized model of BPA; there are undoubtedly many other existing mechanisms of BPA just as there are other neurons exhibiting bursting behavior.

The importance of DAPs in BPA was stressed by Thompson and Smith (91) in a study of BPNs from *Archidoris, Anisodoris, Aplysia, Helix,* and *Tritonia*. Spikes in these cells were followed by DAPs that were seconds in duration. Thompson and Smith showed that DAPs from successive spikes underwent temporal summation (Fig. 3) creating a significant depolarizing current that very likely had a role in maintaining the burst of spikes and causing the acceleration of firing rate typically seen in the initial half of a burst. We agree that DAP currents have a significant role in many BPNs and suggest that reconsideration of DAP function is warranted by recent suggestions that DAPs may represent calcium-activated inward currents.

The sequence of inward and then outward aftercurrents activated by the calcium influx during spikes in BPNs seems ideally suited to support BPA. As seen in Fig. 3, the DAP current is larger and briefer than the following SOC, and both aftercurrents show temporal summation (66,91). A very rough approximation of the way in which these aftercurrents might summate during a burst to produce the initial acceleration of spiking, then deceleration and cessation of the burst, can be illustrated by attempting to imitate a burst with voltage-clamp commands (Fig. 4). A spike-like depolarization of the cell, e.g., a command to +40 msec for 15 msec, will elicit a DAP current and subsequent SOC similar to those following a spike. By delivering a train of

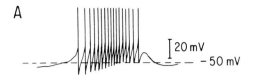

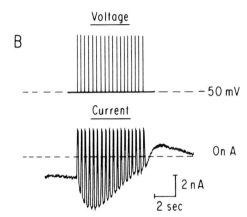

FIG. 4. Burst structure and summation of spike aftercurrents. **A:** R15 was allowed to burst spontaneously. The typical burst illustrated here contained 18 spikes and demonstrates the increasing and then the decreasing spike firing rate followed by the interburst hyperpolarization. **B:** A simulation of a burst was attempted with the cell in voltage clamp. **Upper trace:** (voltage) shows the train of 17 depolarizing steps to +40 mV for 15 msec, each from a holding potential of −50 mV. **Lower trace:** (current) shows the current trace during the train of depolarizing commands (the large brief outward currents during the commands are clipped by limited pen recorder motion). Note that the baseline net membrane current initially becomes more inward and then shifts in an outward direction, becoming briefly net outward at the end of the train. (D. V. Lewis, unpublished data, June 1984.)

such depolarizations, one can observe an initial increase of net inward current followed by a gradual decrease of net inward current and, ultimately, a net outward current. This same sequence probably occurs during a spontaneous burst, causing the initial acceleration, then deceleration, and cessation of spiking typical of a burst.

In summary, we think an expanded model of BPA is appropriate at this time (Fig. 5). Beginning at the nadir of hyperpolarization following a burst, [Ca]$_i$ has been elevated by the burst and has inactivated a significant proportion of the SIC and activated an unknown amount of calcium-dependent potassium current. As the [Ca]$_i$ declines during the interburst interval, the SIC is reactivated and the potassium conductance

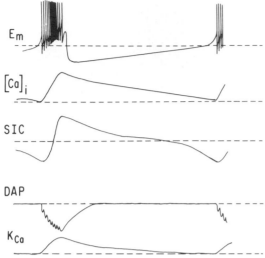

FIG. 5. Illustration of hypothetical model of bursting pacemaker activity. Em, membrane voltage; [Ca]$_i$, intracellular calcium activity measured at the soma. This represents average [Ca]$_i$ as seen with Arsenazo III; here the rise in [Ca]$_i$ is depicted as a smooth rise, but with optimal records it can be seen to increment in a pulsatile manner with each spike, e.g., Gorman and Thomas (41). SIC, slow inward current (a decrease in SIC is depicted as an upward deflection); DAP, summating DAP currents which are inward, hence downward deflection; K$_{Ca}$, calcium activated potassium current. The time courses of inactivation of the SIC, decay of the DAP currents, and increase and decline of K$_{Ca}$ are at this point uncertain. The traces are illustrative only and should not be taken to represent actual current magnitudes. Baselines are also relative and in the case of the SIC do not represent zero current level.

decreases. This causes depolarization, which in turn activates more SIC, driving the depolarization incessantly toward spike threshold. During the first spike, there is a marked increase in [Ca]$_i$ at the inner membrane surface, and the DAP is activated, bringing the cell out of the spike undershoot and to threshold for the next spike. The DAPs summate and accelerate the spiking. With a slight delay, the increased [Ca]$_i$ begins to inactivate the SIC and perhaps to activate a potassium conductance. These combined features decelerate spiking and terminate the burst, and the cycle begins again.

MODULATION OF BURSTING PACEMAKER ACTIVITY BY NEUROTRANSMITTERS

The currents generating BPA are, in the neurons discussed above, nonsynaptic and endogenous to the BPN membrane. However, neuro-

transmitters and other neuroregulators can alter BPA either by controlling the voltage-sensitive SIC or by superimposing discrete postsynaptic currents which transiently accelerate or retard a burst. A large number of interesting studies exist concerning modulation of BPA by exogenous peptides and steroids (11), endogenous peptides (71), and spontaneous synaptic input (79,82). Synaptic input can either inhibit or enhance BPA. Inhibition of long duration will stop BPA in R15 for many minutes (3,79). Stimulation of the right pleurovisceral connective can enhance BPA for hours in R15 (79). Synaptic input can also induce BPA in silent neurons, as in the lobster stomatogastric ganglion in which neurons will generate BPA only when afferent input is intact even though the BPA is not caused by discrete postsynaptic currents (7,77). As with nonbursting neurons, cyclic nucleotides may often be the intracellular messengers mediating the effects of the neurotransmitters on BPA (65).

This brief review cannot adequately encompass the literature on neuroregulators and BPA. Therefore, we will focus on one example of such modulation, the inhibition of BPA in R15 by dopamine. Dopamine is found in high concentrations in molluscan nervous tissue, including that of *Aplysia* (44). Ascher (9) characterized the dopamine responses of multiple neurons of *Aplysia*. Dopamine application was effective on the axons rather than the somata and had both inhibitory and excitatory effects. The response of the BPN R15 was purely hyperpolarizing and, unlike most of the other hyperpolarizing responses, was not inverted by hyperpolarization to below the presumed potassium equilibrium potential, nor was it sensitive to alterations in extracellular potassium. However, with the application of sodium pump inhibitors and with cooling, the response appeared to invert near -90 mV, and the inversion became sensitive to extracellular potassium. These and other considerations led Ascher (9) to propose that dopamine was increasing potassium conductance in R15, thus hyperpolarizing the cell and stopping bursting. To explain the failure of the dopamine response to invert under normal conditions, Ascher (9) speculated that the site of dopamine action was electrically distant from the soma and therefore difficult to invert with hyperpolarization at the soma. He further speculated that the extracellular surface of R15 was protected from changes in extracellular potassium by an unspecified diffusion barrier, explaining the insensitivity of the dopamine response to altered extracellular potassium.

Wilson and Wachtel (94) proposed the alternative interpretation that dopamine was blocking the regenerative SIC. They iontophoresed dopamine onto the axodendritic region of the cell and eliminated the NSR region of the I/V curve without increasing conductance in the hyperpolarized voltage range. Transient outward shifts of membrane current elicited by dopamine iontophoresis were not affected by increasing extracellular potassium, but were eliminated by removing extracellular sodium which also eliminated the SIC and NSR region of the I/V curve. These observations suggested that dopamine was blocking the voltage-sensitive SIC. Furthermore, when BPA was blocked by bath-applied dopamine, injection of depolarizing current could not restore bursting, arguing that dopamine was not simply superimposing a constant hyperpolarizing current (45). Gospe and Wilson (45) established a dose–response curve for the effect of bath applied dopamine on the I/V curve of R15 showing maximum effect at 500 μM. The dopamine effect was antagonized by dihydroergotamine and lysergic acid diethylamide, but not by neuroleptics or certain adrenergic antagonists. Therefore, Gospe and Wilson (46) concluded that the receptor mediating BPA inhibition in R15 was different from previously described dopamine receptors.

Adams et al. (3) compared the effects of branchial nerve stimulation to those of dopamine application. In R15, branchial nerve stimulation produced an outward current that had two components. The early component was associated with a slope conductance increase resembling a potassium conductance. The late component was a reduction in the NSR without a conductance increase in the hyperpolarized limb of the I/V curve. Dopamine application eliminated the late but not the early component. Adams et al. interpreted these results as indicating that both the dopamine effect and the late component of branchial nerve stimulation resulted from elimination of the SIC and that they therefore occluded one another.

Understanding the action of dopamine, as with the SIC and SOC, seemed to hinge upon the differentiation of increased outward current from decreased inward current. Lewis et al. (67) attempted to overcome this dilemma, at least insofar as calcium influx was concerned, by using Arsenazo III spectrophotometry. During small, subthreshold depolarizations, in the range of the SIC, a rise in $[Ca]_i$ was seen in the soma of R15. A maximum dopamine concentration of 500 μM did not reduce the rise in $[Ca]_i$ at the soma.

Next, axodendritic absorbance changes were monitored, and rises in $[Ca]_i$ in the axon region could also be seen during the activation of the SIC. In the axodendritic region, dopamine markedly attenuated the $[Ca]_i$ rise. It appeared that, just as dopamine application is only effective in the axodendritic region in producing current responses, so is it effective in reducing axodendritic, but not somatic, calcium influx. During voltage clamp, simultaneous voltage measurements in the soma and axon showed that dopamine application had little effect on voltage control in the axon, suggesting that the decreased calcium influx resulted from a decrease in calcium conductance rather than from altered space clamp properties.

Recently, dopamine has been shown to affect not only the SIC, but the DAP current (66) and the SOC (67) as well (Fig. 6). DAP currents following single spikes and voltage-clamp commands are reduced and ultimately eliminated by dopamine in a dose-dependent manner (66). The effect of dopamine on the DAP current is equally effective whether the dopamine is bath-applied or applied locally to the axodendritic region, but is not seen when dopamine is applied locally to the soma. One could speculate therefore, that dopamine may reduce the DAP by reducing axodendritic calcium influx during a spike.

Dopamine effects on the SOC are more complex. Low concentrations of dopamine will increase the magnitude of the outward current following a train of action potentials in R15 (8) (Fig. 7A). However, after single or very few spikes or after a brief depolarizing command, dopamine reduces the SOC (Fig. 6). The explanation of these apparently contradictory observations is not yet known. Possibly the currents contributing to the SOC after a burst of spikes are different from those comprising the SOC after one spike. Furthermore, since the net posttetanic current after a burst of spikes may reflect algebraic summation of several different currents including DAP currents, inactivation of SIC, and calcium-activated potassium current, the exact cause of a change in the net current will be difficult to ascertain.

It would be ideal to account for all of the effects of dopamine with one unifying hypothesis. An attractive hypothesis would be that dopamine reduces voltage-sensitive axodendritic calcium influx. This would explain the reduction of the SIC, the reduced calcium dependent DAPs, and decreased SOC. However, it will not explain the increased posttetanic current following a long burst of spikes. Clearly, more effort is re-

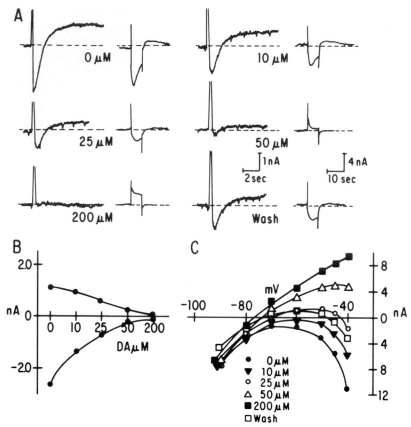

FIG. 6. Dopamine effects on membrane currents in R15. **A:** These current traces show the concentration-dependent effects of dopamine on the DAP current, and the slow outward and slow inward currents (SOC and SIC). Six pairs of traces are illustrated, each consisting of one trace (*left*) of the inward DAP current and SOC following one spike (cell placed in voltage clamp at −50 mV after the spike) and one trace (*right*) of the SIC and following SOC activated by a depolarization from −50 to −40 mV for 8 sec. Before dopamine exposure (0 μM), the usual currents are present. With progressively higher dopamine concentration in the bath, the DAP current, SOC following the DAP current, the SIC, and the SOC following the SIC are all eliminated. Partial recovery follows the wash. Often, after prolonged exposure to high concentrations (as in this example) of dopamine recovery is incomplete or takes several hours. **B:** Graph of the amplitude of the DAP current (*lower curve*) and of the SOC (after one spike) (*upper curve*) versus dopamine concentration in the bath. **C:** I/V curves of the cell in the various concentrations of dopamine (holding potential −50 mV, current at 1.5 sec after beginning of command). From Lewis, ref. 66, with permission.

quired to explain all these phenomena. It is of interest in this regard that dopamine application to hippocampal pyramidal cells increases the hyperpolarization following a train of spikes (16). Even lacking a full understanding of the mechanisms, knowing the diversity of the dopamine effects helps to clarify the ways in which this neurotransmitter could modulate BPA. Reducing the SIC would tend to prevent regenerative depolarization of the cell. Reducing the DAP current would tend to reduce the depolarizing drive during a burst, hence reducing spike frequency during the burst; enhancing the SOC generated during a burst would also tend to

shorten the burst. Indeed, the most clear-cut effect of low concentrations of dopamine is to reduce the number of spikes per burst and increase the interspike intervals (Fig. 7B), whereas higher concentrations halt BPA entirely.

CONCLUSION

From this synthesis of the studies of burst-firing neurons, it is clear that what seemed initially to be a quite simple process is actually much more complicated. The regulation of burst firing by neurotransmitters, such as dopamine regulation of bursting in R15, has proven much

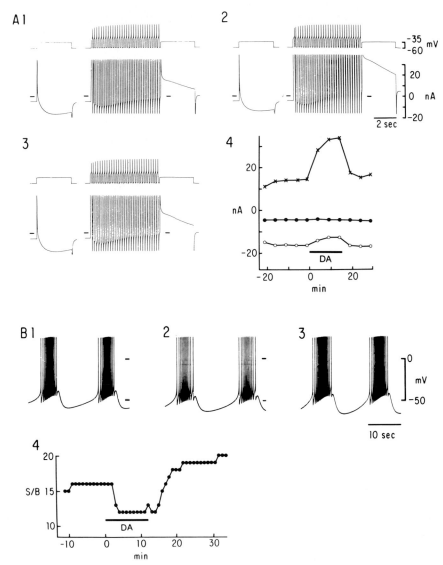

FIG. 7. **A:** Enhancement of spike-evoked slow outward current (SOC) in neuron R15 by a low concentration of dopamine. Every 30 sec, the cell was depolarized from a holding potential of -60 mV to a pulse voltage of -35 mV for 3 sec, which produced a persistent slow inward current (SIC). Every 5 min (i.e., every 10th pulse), a 5.8-sec, 5.0-Hz train of action potentials (in current clamp) preceded the depolarizing clamp pulse, which now produced a SOC. **A1:** Normal saline control. The SIC during a depolarizing clamp pulse (*left*) was converted to a SOC following a train of spikes (right). **A2:** In 5 μM dopamine, the inward current was reduced slightly (*left*) as compared with control values, but the SOC following the spike train (*right*) was doubled. The increase in SOC was five times the decrease in SIC. **A3:** Recovery in normal saline. **A4:** Plot of the experiment in A1–A3. Solid circles, holding current; open circles, peak SIC; Xs, SOC. **B:** The effect of a low concentration of dopamine on spontaneous bursting in R15. **B1:** Normal saline control; **B2:** 5 μM dopamine. There was a 25% decrease in spikes/burst, and a 43% increase in mean interspike interval. **B3:** Recovery in normal saline. **B4:** Plot of spikes/burst (S/B) from the experiment in **B1–B3**. **A** and **B** are from different preparations. (W. W. Anderson, unpublished observations, April 1984.)

more difficult to analyze than are more conventional synaptic processes.

Because analogies are often drawn between invertebrate burst-firing neurons and neurons

participating in epileptogenic activity, it is appropriate to recognize the complexity of these neuronal burst-firing processes. Even in cells as amenable to study as the *Aplysia* neurons, the data can be complex and, at times, confusing. The situation is much more difficult in the mammalian central nervous system (CNS), and extreme caution would be appropriate in the interpretation of experiments to study bursting in these cells.

SPIKE FREQUENCY ADAPTATION

Spike frequency adaptation (SFA), or accommodation, is the process in which a neuron responds to a constant stimulus with a decreasing rate of firing of action potentials. The result of this process is that the firing rate of a neuron is more closely related to the rate of change of the stimulus than to the steady state level of the stimulus. It seems plausible to postulate that the process of SFA may be an endogenous "anticonvulsant" mechanism in certain neurons, and that the suppression of SFA might promote epileptiform activity. This hypothesis is based on the assumption that seizures are related to the supranormal activity of certain foci in the CNS, and that a decrease in the ability of individual neurons to sustain a high level of activity may help to prevent either the initiation of a seizure focus or the spread of activity from the seizure focus to other areas of the CNS.

Adaptation is a somewhat universal phenomenon in neurophysiology. Not only has it been extensively studied in invertebrates (25,80,81), but it has also been demonstrated in the mammalian CNS, with adaptation responses having been shown in the spinal cord (10,55,59,60).

Several mechanisms that contribute to the process of adaptation have been elucidated. In general, these mechanisms have a slow hyperpolarizing effect on the membrane during a train of action potentials that leads to increasing interspike intervals. Baylor and Nichols (15) demonstrated a prolonged hyperpolarization after a train of spike in leech sensory neurons. The hyperpolarization was blocked by cooling and the cardiac glycosides, ouabain and strophanthidin, and therefore was attributed to the action of an electrogenic pump. Brodwick and Junge (19) studied a posttetanic hyperpolarization in *Aplysia* giant neuron R2. They showed that the hyperpolarization was not blocked by inhibitors of electrogenic pumping (cooling, ouabain, cyanide, and removal of extracellular Na^+ or K^+), but instead was caused by an increase in potassium conductance. Furthermore, since the hyperpolarization persisted in the absence of action potentials (blocked by TTX), it could not be accounted for by the summation of spike afterhyperpolarizations. Partridge and Stevens (81) were able to show that a SOC of this type could account for adaptation in the marine molluscs *Archidoris* and *Anisodoris*. In response to a constant current step, these neurons showed an adapting response. However, when Partridge and Stevens superimposed an exponentially rising current onto the constant current step, they were able to "frequency clamp" the cell. That is, they blocked adaptation by negating the effects of a SOC. Using this method, they were able to explain adaptation in these cells.

Colmers et al. (26) showed that in the presence of Cs^+ (a blocker of K^+ currents), there is a net inward current in response to subthreshold depolarizations in *Aplysia* giant neurons. The activation of this inward current would result in an increase in firing rate of a neuron. The inward current inactivates somewhat during the first 5–10 sec of depolarization of the membrane. Therefore, this process may also contribute to adaptation.

Lewis and Wilson (68) have demonstrated another mechanism that is important in early adaptation. Using the calcium-sensitive dye, Arsenazo III, in conjunction with differential absorbance spectrophotometry, they were able to measure changes in the intracellular levels of Ca^{2+} in *Aplysia* giant neurons. They showed that during the first 5–10 sec of an adaptation response, there is a rapid increase in intracellular Ca^{2+}, and that this portion of adaptation could be accounted for by the onset of a Ca^{2+}-activated K^+ conductance.

Cote et al. (29) used a voltage-clamp analysis to study a SOC in *Aplysia* giant neurons. They showed that the SOC was a potassium current that was activated by subthreshold depolarizations, that the current could account for adaptation, and that the current was enhanced by submillimolar concentrations of barbiturates (pentobarbital and phenobarbital). It has been further proposed that enhancement of SOC by barbiturates is an anticonvulsant effect (97).

The phenomenon of spike frequency adaptation and the effect of an anticonvulsant barbiturate on it is shown in Fig. 8. In this case, diphenylbarbituric acid (DPB) (54,85) was used to enhance SFA. Adaptation in these cells occurs in two phases. In response to a constant depolarizing stimulus current (indicated by the arrows in Fig. 8) the firing of the cell declines rapidly at first, and then slowly. This is best seen in part B of the figure in which the interspike interval is plotted versus time. In control artificial seawater (ASW), the interspike interval in-

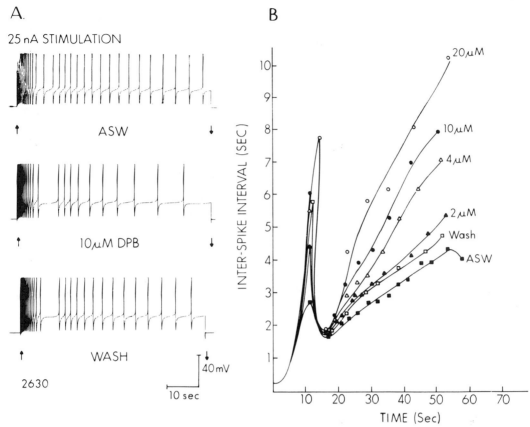

FIG. 8. Typical repetitive firing pattern of giant cell R2, and changes produced by DPB. **A:** Adaptation in response to a 60-sec, 25-nA constant current depolarization obtained in control, with 10 μM DPB, and with wash. Arrows mark the beginning and end of the stimulus. **B:** To elucidate the relationship between DPB concentration and adaptation, data from the experiment in part **A** are plotted as the interspike interval (ISI) versus time of depolarization. DPB causes a dose-related, reversible increase in adaptation as evidenced by an increased rate of development of ISI. Adaptation within the first 5 sec was unchanged by DPB. From Huguenard and Wilson, ref. 54, with permission.

creases rapidly during the first few seconds of stimulation, and then increases more slowly as the stimulus is maintained. DPB enhances the slow adaptation process, without altering the firing rate during the first few seconds, as is best seen in Fig. 8A.

The fast phase of adaptation appears to be the direct result of a calcium-activated potassium current (68), and is not sensitive to barbiturates (97). Therefore, we have concentrated our efforts on understanding the slow phase of adaptation, which is barbiturate enhanced. In this review, we explain how we have studied this process and the membrane current underlying it. We present some additional data implicating potassium as the primary current carrier for the SOC producing the slow phase of SFA, discuss the unusual sensitivity of the process to calcium,

and then present an admittedly speculative model describing the process.

Our previous studies linked a SOC (as shown in Fig. 9) to the slow phase of SFA (97) and provided a qualitative description of the effects of barbiturates on this current. However, to study this SOC and the effects of drugs on it thoroughly, an accurate means of quantitating the current is necessary. Unfortunately, there are a number of problems involved in directly measuring the onset of SOC. First, the study by Colmers et al. (26) showed that during the initial 5 sec of a subthreshold depolarization, there is an activation and a partial inactivation of an inward current. These changes in the inward current are occurring at a time course similar to the initial changes in SOC. Therefore, one cannot use the change in whole cell current during a

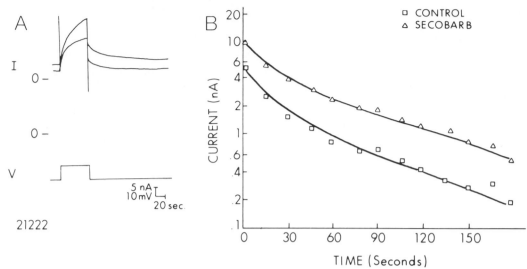

21222

FIG. 9. Example of the change in tail current produced by barbiturates: **A**: Slow outward currents obtained in control and with 100 μM secobarbital. *Upper trace;* current (up, outward); *lower trace;* voltage. **B**: Semilog plots of tail currents from part **A**. Stimulus, 60-sec depolarization to −34 mV from a holding potential of −50 mV.

depolarizing pulse as a measure of the change in outward current. Second, the rise in SOC is an extremely slow process; depolarizations of up to 30–40 min are required even to approach a maximum effect. The slope of SOC during the first 60 sec of depolarization represents less than 5% of the total SOC activation curve. With this limited sample of the time course of activation, it is difficult to determine accurately the parameters describing the process.

Considering the difficulties involved in analyzing the onset of SOC, alternatives must be considered. A good option is the analysis of "tail currents," the decay of a stimulus-induced current; in this case, the stimulus was SOC. Upon repolarization to the holding potential after SOC activation, there was a very slow return of the current to baseline levels. After some initial studies, which showed that tail currents could easily be represented by the sum of exponential decay processes, it was decided that tail current analysis was suitable for the quantitation of SOC.

Analysis of tail currents has several advantages over analysis of the SOC itself. First, with a stable holding current, the endpoint of decay is known. This greatly simplifies the analysis of an exponential decay process. Second, since the tails could be represented as the sum of exponential decay processes, we could use simple, readily available analysis routines to determine

the parameters of decay. Last, it was found quite early in this study that barbiturate-induced changes in SOC correlated very well with changes in the parameters describing tail currents. Therefore, tail current analysis provided a means to measure accurately and reproducibly (albeit indirectly) barbiturate-induced changes in SOC.

EXPERIMENTAL DESIGN

Preparation

The giant cells of *Aplysia* were chosen for this study for several reasons. Homologous cells LP1 and R2 are extremely easy to identify, and the membrane properties in these neurons are very constant from preparation to preparation. The somata are large (up to 1 mm in diameter) and are physically very accessible for complex neurophysiological manipulations. Several microelectrodes can be positioned in or around the soma or initial axon segment, and fiberoptic light pipes can even be positioned in order to monitor optical changes within the neuron.

Aplysia giant neurons have been the subject of many neurophysiological studies (19,26,37, 68,97); therefore, background data are available concerning the known Ca^{2+}, Na^+, and K^+ conductances of these cells. A very important reason for the use of this preparation in the study of slow currents is that the giant cells are very stable *in vivo* and can remain viable for greater than 12 hr. Long-term stability and viability was crucial for this type of study because of the extended periods of time necessary to obtain SOC tail data with drugs. Often, 2 hr are required for each concentration of drug and to obtain responses across a wide concentration range requires that an experiment continue for up to 10–16 hr. In most cases, the giant cell preparations are able to sustain this long-term viability.

Tail Analysis

Plotting the tail currents on semilogarithmic graph paper revealed that SOC tail currents appeared to be made up of at least two exponential decay processes. A more rigorous method of analysis was developed in order to determine the kinetics and amplitudes of tail currents more accurately. A compartmental analysis program was modified to perform an automatic curve peel (98) on tail current data. Figure 3 shows an example of SOC and tail current obtained in control solutions and with added barbiturate, in this case 100 μM secobarbital. The raw data are shown in panel A, whereas panel B shows semilogarithmic plots of the tail currents and the best-fit curves obtained from the analysis program (solid lines).

The analysis program relies on the following assumptions: (a) the process under study is made up of multiple exponential decay components; and (b) the individual decay components are of reasonably different kinetics. A subtle requirement of the program is that data must be collected in such a fashion that there are enough points to represent each component of decay adequately, i.e., relatively more points are needed during the early portions of tail than the late portions of tail. This was usually accomplished by collecting the first points in a tail at twice the rate (0.5 Hz) of the second half (0.25 Hz).

The method of the tail analysis was similar to a manual "peel": (a) the slowest component of decay was determined; (b) the contribution of the slow component was removed from fast components by subtraction; and (c) the next slower component of decay was determined. The process was repeated until there were no more points.

More sophisticated methods than peeling are available for the determination of the parameters describing a multicomponent exponential decay process, such as nonlinear least-squares fitting routines. However, when these methods were applied to the analysis of tail currents, it was found that the results were not appreciably different from those obtained with the peeling routine. Therefore, the advantages of ease and rapidity of peeling were chosen at the expense of a small decrement in the accuracy of the estimates for the parameters, as compared with least-squares fitting routines.

The results of tail analysis most often yielded two components with half-lives of ~10 and ~60 sec. However, in some cases, three components were described. In these cases, it was found that the tails could be reasonably well fit with a two-component tail. In all cases in which an equally good fit would be obtained with models of differing complexity, the least complex model (that with fewest components) was assumed.

K⁺ Sensitivity

The rate of rise of SOC and the reversal potential for SOC tails have previously been shown to depend on the level of extracellular K^+ (29). Using tail-current analysis, we tested the sensitivity of both of the components of tail current and found that each component was approximately equally affected by changes in $[K^+]_o$. Figure 10 shows tail currents obtained by depolarizing from a holding potential of -50 mV to -35 mV for 60 sec in artificial seawater (ASW) with three different levels of $[K^+]_o$. Panel A is a linear plot of the tail currents; panel B shows the tail currents on a semilog plot. In the semilog plot, the currents are paralleled over the entire time course of the tail. This indicates that the major difference between the currents is one of *magnitude,* as one would expect with the change in driving force produced by altering the potassium equilibrium potential.

The tail currents can be converted to conductance measurements based on these assumptions:

1. Tail currents are the result of K^+ conductance changes according to the following rearrangement of Ohm's law:

$$I_K = g_K(E_K - E_m), \qquad \text{(Eq. 1)}$$

where I_K is the potassium current, g_K is the potassium conductance, E_K is the potassium equilibrium potential, and E_m is the membrane potential.

2. E_K was calculated based on the Nernst equation:

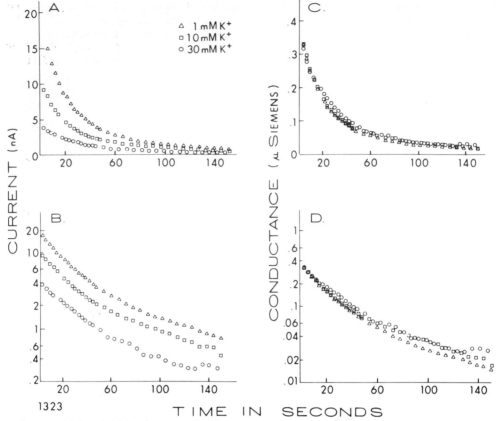

FIG. 10. Sensitivity of SOC tail currents to extracellular potassium levels. **A:** Linear plots of tail currents obtained with different levels of extracellular potassium. **B:** Semilog plots of the data in **A**. **C:** Tail currents from **A** converted to tail conductances based on the assumptions stated in test, linear plot. **D:** Semilog plots of the data in **C**. Stimulus was a 60-sec depolarization to −30 mV from a holding potential of −50 mV. From Huguenard et al., ref. 54a, with permission.

$$E_K = \frac{RT}{Fz} \times Ln\left(\frac{[K^+]_o}{[K^+]_i}\right) \qquad \text{(Eq. 2)}$$

where R is the universal gas constant, T is the temperature in °K, F is the Faraday constant, and z is the valence of the ion, in this case, 1.

3. Intracellular $[K^+]$ was assumed to be 158 mM (measured as described in the following section).

These conductance curves are plotted in panel C on a linear scale and again in panel D on a semilog scale. The curves largely overlap each other, verifying the assumption that tail currents are primarily caused by changes in K^+ conductance.

Tail reversal experiments were performed in order to verify that SOC tails were strictly dependent on the potassium equilibrium potential. These experiments proved fairly difficult to per-

form as a result of slow changes in other currents which occurred at very hyperpolarized potentials. However, in some cases we were able to reverse the tail currents, and as previously shown (29), the reversal potential was found to depend on the extracellular level of potassium.

Extracellular Potassium Accumulation

In two experiments, a K^+-sensitive microelectrode was positioned near the soma of the giant neuron R2 to examine changes in extracellular K^+-induced during SOC. Figure 11 shows that the results of one of these experiments. In this case, the K^+-sensitive electrode was placed so that it was actually touching the membrane of neuron R2. The extracellular K^+ levels follow the kinetics of SOC activation and tail inactivation reasonably well.

At the end of the experiment, the K^+-sensi-

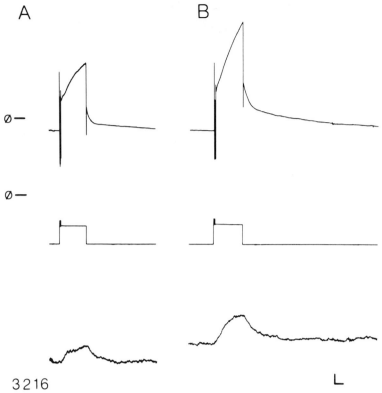

3 2 16   L

FIG. 11. Extracellular potassium accumulation during slow outward current (SOC) and tail currents; effects of pentobarbital. *Upper traces:* voltage clamp currents; *middle traces:* voltage levels; *lower traces:* potential measured at the potassium sensitive electrode. A: Control. B: Pentobarbital, 100 μM. Calibration: vertical 5 nA, 10 mV, and 5 mM K^+; horizontal 20 sec.

tive electrode was put into the neuron in order to obtain an estimate of $[K^+]_i$. According to the calibration obtained with different levels of K^+ in ASW, $[K^+]_i$ was 158 mM.

Sensitivity of Tail Currents to Alterations of Other Ions

The results of sodium substitution experiments were somewhat variable. In general, replacement of $[Na^+]_o$ by equiosmolar concentrations of sucrose or *bis*-tris-propane markedly reduced the SOC and tail currents. The tail currents were usually reduced to such levels that analysis became impractical because of the decreased signal to noise ratio. However, in every case, the addition of pentobarbital to the perfusate was able to reverse the inhibition. Although the sensitivity of SOC or Cl^- was not specifically studied, the sucrose substitution experiments resulted in removal of most of the extracellular Cl^-, and as mentioned above, SOC

persisted in these experiments, especially with barbiturate added.

Removal of Ca^{2+} from the ASW resulted in depression of SOC and tail current. To reduce further the extracellular Ca^{2+} to very low levels, the specific calcium chelator EGTA (2 mM) was added to 0 Ca^{2+} ASW. Surprisingly, in the presence of EGTA, the SOC and tail current were restored to near control levels. This may be caused by the removal of membrane screening charges (35), which would result in a stronger net depolarization of the membrane. Moderate doses of pentobarbital were also able to restore, and usually exceed, control SOC and tail current levels.

Figure 12 shows the tail currents from a Ca^{2+} experiment. As can be seen, removal of extracellular Ca^{2+} caused a marked decrease in the amplitude of the tail current, with any slow component becoming indistinguishable from noise. The addition of 2 mM EGTA restored the tail currents towards control levels, and the addition

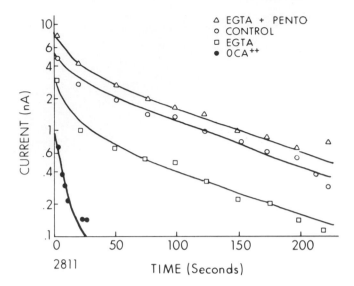

FIG. 12. Effect of removal of extracellular calcium on tail currents; effects of pentobarbital. Stimulus, 60-sec depolarization to -32 from a holding potential of -50 mV. EGTA, 2 mM; pentobarbital, 100 μM.

of 100 μM pentobarbital further increased the amplitude of tail current.

Lewis and Wilson (68) have shown that the initial portion of adaptation (5 sec) in *Aplysia* giant cells is caused by Ca^{2+} entry which leads to activation of a potassium current. As shown in Fig. 12, removal of extracellular Ca^{2+} does not block tail currents (nor does it block SOC). Adaptation responses were obtained in this situation to verify that late adaptation does occur

in the absence of Ca^{2+}. As shown in Fig. 13, slow adaptation does persist (although at a different level) in the absence of extracellular Ca^{2+}, and pentobarbital does enhance the slow adaptation.

It should be pointed out here that the tail currents obtained in these neurons after a brief (2 sec) burst of action potentials are qualitatively quite similar to SOC tail currents. Both types of tail currents can be represented by multicom-

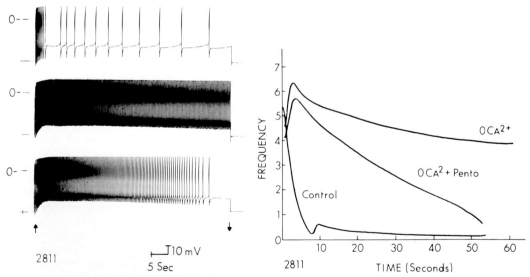

FIG. 13. Effect of removal of extracellular calcium on adaptation; effects of added pentobarbital. **A:** Adaptation responses in control, *upper trace;* OCa^{2+}, *middle trace;* and OCa^{2+} with pentobarbital, *lower trace.* **B:** Spike frequency plots of the data in part **A.** Stimulus, 60-sec constant current depolarization of 25 nA from a holding potential of -50 mV; pentobarbital, 100 μM.

ponent exponential decay processes with similar kinetics. However, there are differences between the two currents. The tail current after a brief burst of spikes (postspike current, PSC) is not affected by concentrations of barbiturates that cause a marked enhancement of SOC tail currents (34). The PSC is totally eliminated by the removal of extracellular Ca^{2+}, but the SOC tail current does not require extracellular Ca^{2+} (see Fig. 12). Intracellular injection of the Ca^{2+} chelator, EGTA, resulted in blockade of PSC at concentrations that did not affect SOC or tail current. However, much higher concentrations of EGTA did diminish both SOC and tail current. Both the Ca^{2+}-dependent light response (14) and the response to iontophoretic injection of Ca^{2+} were unaffected by 100 μM pentobarbital. Therefore, although SOC is somewhat sensitive to Ca^{2+}, it does not seem to be dependent on Ca^{2+} entry. In addition, it appears that barbiturates are *not* exerting their effect by producing an increased sensitivity to the intracellular level of Ca^{2+}.

Kinetic Model of Slow Outward Current

The existence of *two* components of outward tail current along with the selective enhancement of one of the components by barbiturates led us to develop several models that might explain these phenomena.

We originally hypothesized that SOC may result from the activation of two different types of potassium channels. However, there was much evidence to indicate that the two components of tail current were not independent. Any manipulation that resulted in a diminution of SOC and tail current could be reversed by the addition of barbiturate, and the barbiturate-induced restoration normally affected *both* components of tail. For example, although removal of extracellular Ca^{2+} or the addition of Ca^{2+} channel blockers La^{3+} or Co^{2+} resulted in a marked decrease in SOC and the amplitude of both tail components, barbiturate restored all of these parameters to at least control levels. We were unable to find any one agent that would selectively block one of the components. Therefore, it appeared that SOC could not be easily explained by the existence of two conductance mechanisms, one of which is enhanced by barbiturates. A more reasonable mechanism seemed to be that there were several regulatory factors affecting one conductance mechanism.

Several sequential models were developed to explain how alterations in one type of channel

could result in tail current kinetics that resembled two types of channel. These sequential models involved such events as the activation of a channel by depolarization of the membrane, followed by binding of the channel by Ca^{2+}, which would further activate the channel. Another possibility was that Ca^{2+} was an enabling agent for the ionic channels underlying SOC. The enabling action of Ca^{2+} allowed membrane depolarization to activate the channels. Some of these models were quite complex; however, none of them could easily explain SOC and the enhancement produced by barbiturates. In each case, complex alterations by barbiturates of more than one parameter of the model were necessary to obtain predicted curves similar to those obtained in actual experiments.

Two factors led us to develop a different type of model. First, an early study by Pallotta et al. (78) of Ca^{2+}-activated K^+ channels in cultured rat myotubules demonstrated that these channels were regulated by two factors: intracellular level of Ca^{2+}, and membrane potential. Because SOC is caused by a K^+ conductance and is somewhat dependent on Ca^{2+}, we hypothesized that a Ca^{2+} activated K^+ mechanism such as that elucidated by Pallotta might underlie SOC. Second, we found evidence in the literature (5,49,84) that there may be a voltage-sensitive intracellular release of Ca^{2+} in neurons and other cells, similar to the release of Ca^{2+} from sarcoplasmic reticulum in muscle (95). We hypothesized that the combination of these two mechanisms (Ca^{2+}-activated K^+ conductance and depolarization-activated Ca^{2+} release) would explain SOC, and that barbiturate alteration of one of these mechanisms would explain the changes in SOC produced by barbiturates.

To test the model, we developed a mathematical relationship describing all of the parameters of the model. The simplest basis of the model is the potassium channel itself;

$$CH_{closed} \underset{KC}{\overset{KO}{\rightleftharpoons}} CH_{open} \qquad \text{(Eq. 3)}$$

In this simple model, KC, the channel-closing rate, is constant. KO, the channel-opening rate, is a function of membrane potential and intracellular Ca^{2+}. Ca^{2+} is an agonist which increases KO according to the Michaelis-Menton relationship:

$$KO = \frac{KO_{max}}{(Km/[Ca]) + 1} \qquad \text{(Eq. 4)}$$

However, membrane potential also affects this

relationship such that hyperpolarization is antagonistic to the effects of Ca^{2+}. A competitive antagonist effectively increases the Km for a reaction. With this in mind, we developed the following relationship for the value of Km in equation 4:

$$Km = Km_{min} (1 + e^{((Kv - V)/SF)}) \qquad \text{(Eq. 5)}$$

Km is the apparent Km, Km_{min} is the minimum Km, V is the membrane potential, Kv is the membrane potential at which Km is $2 \times Km_{min}$, and SF is a factor that determines the steepness of the relationship between voltage and apparent Km. As V becomes hyperpolarized, the apparent Km becomes larger, so that a higher concentration of Ca^{2+} is necessary to attain the same channel-opening rate. A three-dimensional representation of this relationship at equilibrium can be seen in Fig. 14. The parameters that were used to generate Fig. 14 are as follows: KO_{max} = 10/sec; KC = .05/sec; Km_{min} = 50 μM, SF (slope factor) = 13; and Kv = 0 mV. As can be seen, Ca^{2+} becomes less effective at opening channels with more negative (hyperpolarized) potentials. In fact, there is further evidence that this is exactly the character of these channels. Compare this figure with Fig. 8D in Barrett et al. (13). Although the vertical axis in that figure indicates percentage of time open, this could be easily converted to percentage of channels open by multiplying this value by the total number of channels. Thus, the description of the channels in this model closely resembles the actual voltage and calcium sensitivity of the channels studied in isolation.

Thus far, we have described the channels that may underlie slow outward current. To understand how this might work, we must discuss part 2 of the model, which states that there is a voltage-dependent release of Ca^{2+} inside the neuron. The control of Ca^{2+} within this system can be described by the following equation:

$$Ca_{bound} \underset{KU}{\overset{KR}{\rightleftharpoons}} Ca_{free} \qquad \text{(Eq. 6)}$$

Ca_{bound} is the releasable Ca^{2+} which is available to interact with the K^+ channels, KU is the rate of Ca^{2+} uptake, a constant, and KR is the rate of Ca^{2+} release, which is a sigmoidal function of membrane potential according to the following relationship:

$$KR = \frac{KR_{max}}{1 + e^{(Kvr - V/SF2)}} \qquad \text{(Eq. 7)}$$

KR_{max} is the maximum rate of Ca^{2+} release, Kvr is the membrane potential at which the Ca^{2+} release is half maximal, V is the membrane potential, and SF2 is the scaling factor that determines the steepness of the relationship between voltage and the rate of Ca^{2+} release.

Based on these mathematical relationships,

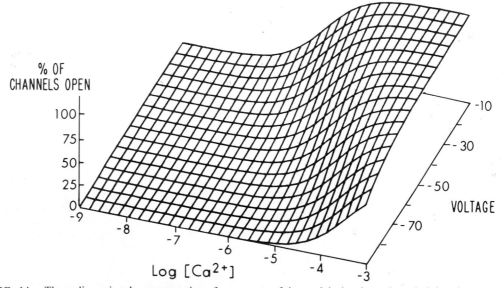

FIG. 14. Three-dimensional representation of one aspect of the model, the channels underlying slow outward current. The dependence on calcium levels and membrane potential is indicated. Either increased free intracellular calcium or depolarization of the membrane results in a greater percentage of open channels.

we were able to describe an equilibrium level of Ca^{2+} and the equilibrium number of channels open at any one membrane potential and to study the time-dependent changes in the current (number of channels open). The effects of perturbation of the system from equilibrium were predicted using standard kinetic procedures. An iterative procedure was used in which the voltage-induced change in Ca^{2+} was calculated for a short time interval; the resultant change in the channel opening rate and the number of channels opened during that interval could then be determined. This iteration was repeated for the duration of the stimulated depolarization. In this way, we could predict the time course of both the change in intracellular Ca^{2+} and the change in number of channels open. Finally, we predicted that barbiturates altered the voltage sensitive calcium release, so that depolarization became more effective at releasing calcium. To test this theory, we studied the effects of changes in Kvr (in equation 7) on the voltage- and time-dependent kinetics of intracellular Ca^{2+} and the number of channels open.

Figure 15 is a three-dimensional representation of what the time-dependent onset of SOC might look like with various concentrations of barbiturate. The time axis represents the time of

depolarization to -30 mV from a holding potential of -50 mV. The number of channels open at time = 0 is equivalent to the number of channels that are open at the holding potential. With increasing duration of depolarization, there is a slow increase in the number of channels open. The effect of increased barbiturate concentration are twofold: first, there is an increase in the rate of development of open channels with depolarization; second, with high concentrations of barbiturate, there is an increase in the number of channels open at the holding potential. Both of these effects predicted by the model are quite evident in barbiturate experiments. Increasing concentrations of barbiturates do result in an increased rate of SOC (channel opening), and at higher doses there is a large increase in outward current at the holding potential.

We also looked at the predictions that the model makes for tail currents and the changes produced by barbiturates. Figure 16A shows the tail currents that are predicted from the model with changes in Kvr (the voltage at which the half-maximal rate of Ca^{2+} release occurs). Curves 1 through 4 are the predicted tail currents after a 60-sec depolarization to -30 mV from a holding potential of -50 mV. Curve 4 corresponds to a Kvr of 0 mV; curve 3 to -5

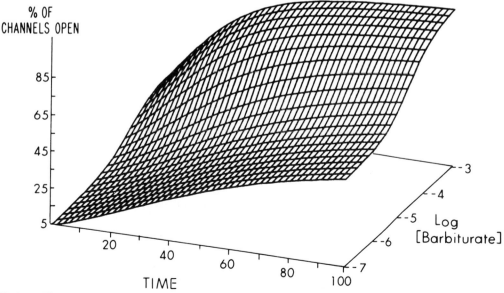

FIG. 15. Illustration of the time dependence of channel opening and alterations produced by the addition of barbiturate. Time in this figure indicates the duration of depolarization to -30 mV from a holding potential of -50 mV. With depolarization, intracellular free calcium slowly increases toward a new steady state; this underlies the slow time course of the slow outward current. In this model, barbiturates are thought to enhance the voltage-dependent increase in intracellular calcium and the resultant activation of potassium channels.

mV; curve 2 to −10 mV; and curve 1 corresponds to −15 mV. The result of making depolarization more effective in releasing Ca^{2+} is an increase in tail amplitude, with a somewhat selective enhancement of the amplitude of the slow component of tail. Part B of Fig. 16 shows the results of an actual barbiturate experiment (in this case, secobarbital) for comparison purposes. Although the actual currents in Fig. 16C are somewhat more noisy than the predicted currents (as a result of small spontaneous synaptic events), the model is quite capable of describing the effects of barbiturates qualitatively.

Therefore, we have a model that can explain not only the two components of tail current, but the alterations in SOC and tail current produced by barbiturate as well. Obviously, this is only one of several models or derivations of this model that can explain the data. In general, this type of current can be explained by the voltage-dependent levels of some factor; this factor affects the voltage sensitivity of the ionic channels underlying the current.

ACKNOWLEDGMENTS

We would like to thank Drs. Robert Zucker, Richard Kramer, William Adams, and Irwin Levitan for their valuable advice and assistance and for allowing us to refer to their most recent work in this review.

REFERENCES

1. Adams, W. B., and Levitan, I. B. (1981): Ionic dependence and charge carriers of the currents underlying bursting in *Aplysia* neuron R15. *Soc. Neurosci. Abstr.*, 7:863.
2. Adams, W. B., and Levitan, I. B. (1982): Origin of the depolarizing after-potential in *Aplysia* cell R15. *Soc. Neurosci. Abstr.*, 8:126.
3. Adams, W. B., Parnas, I., and Levitan, I. B. (1980): Mechanism of long lasting inhibition in *Aplysia* neuron R15. *J. Neurophysiol.*, 44:1148–1160, 1980.
4. Ahmed, Z., and Connor, J. A. (1979): Measurement of calcium influx under voltage clamp in molluscan neurones using the metallochronic dye Arsenazo III. *J. Physiol (Lond.)*, 286:61–82.
5. Akaike, A. M., Brown, A. M., Dahl, G., Highashi, H., Isenberg, G., Tsuda, Y., and Yatani, A. (1983): Voltage-dependent activation of potassium current in *Helix* neurones by endogenous cellular calcium. *J. Physiol.*, 334:309–324.
6. Alving, B. O. (1968): Spontaneous activity in isolated somata of *Aplysia* pacemaker neurons. *J. Gen. Physiol.*, 51:29–45.
7. Anderson, W. W., and Barker, D. L. (1981): Synaptic mechanisms that generate network oscillations in the absence of discrete postsynaptic potentials. *J. Exp. Zool.*, 216:187–191.
8. Anderson, W. W., Wilson, W. A., and Lewis, D. V. (1984): Dopamine enhancement of a spike-evoked current in the *Aplysia* bursting neuron R15. *Neurosci. Abstr.* 10:204.
9. Ascher, P. (1972): Inhibitory and excitatory effects of dopamine on *Aplysia* neurons. *J. Physiol. (Lond.)*, 225:173–209.
10. Baldissera, F., and Gustafsson, B. (1971): Regulation of repetitive firing in motoneurones by the afterhyperpolarization conductance. *Brain Res.*, 30:431–434.
11. Barker, J. L., Ifshin, M. S., and Gainer, H. (1975): Studies on bursting pacemaker potential

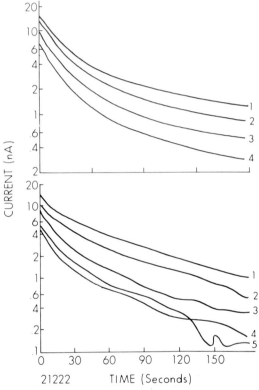

FIG. 16. Tail currents predicted by the model compared with results of an actual secobarbital concentration-response experiment. **A:** Tail currents predicted as a result of changing the voltage sensitivity of calcium release. Curves 1–4 represent the effects of decreasing the voltage-sensitive calcium release (i.e., depolarization becomes less effective in releasing calcium). **B:** Tail currents from a secobarbital concentration-response experiment: 4, control; 3, 25 μM secobarbital; 2, 50 μM secobarbital; 1, 100 μM secobarbital; 5, wash. Thus, the effects of increasing concentrations of barbiturates can be paralleled in the model by shifts in the voltage sensitivity of calcium release. Stimulus, 60-sec depolarization to −34 from a holding potential of −50 mV.

activity in molluscan neurons. III. Effects of hormones. *Brain Res.*, 84:501–515.

12. Barker, J. L., and Smith, T. G., Jr. (1978): Electrophysiological studies of molluscan neurons generating bursting pacemaker potential activity. In: *Abnormal Neuronal Discharges*, edited by N. Chalazonitis and M. Buisson, pp. 359–387. Raven Press, New York.

13. Barrett, J. N., Magleby, K. L., and Pallotta, B. S. (1982): Properties of single calcium-activated potassium channels in cultured rat muscle. *J. Physiol.*, 331:211–230.

14. Baur, P. S., Jr., Brown, A. M., Rogers, T. D., and Brower, M. E. (1977): Lipochondria and the light response of *Aplysia* giant neurons. *J. Neurobiol.*, 8:19–42.

15. Baylor, D. A., and Nichols, J. G. (1969): After-effects of nerve impulses on signalling in the central nervous system of the leech. *J. Physiol.*, 203:571–589.

16. Benardo, L. S., and Prince, D. A. (1982): Dopamine action on hippocampal pyramidal cells. *J. Neurosci.*, 2:415–423.

17. Brown, A. M., and Brown, H. M. (1973): Light response of a giant *Aplysia* neuron. *J. Gen. Physiol.*, 62:239–254.

18. Bragdon, A. C., and Wilson, W. A. (1982): CA1 pyramidal cells exhibit spike frequency adaptation and a slow outward current. *Soc. Neurosci, Abstr.*, 287.16.

19. Brodwick, M. S., and Junge, D. (1972): Post-stimulus hyperpolarization and slow potassium conductance increase in *Aplysia* giant neurons. *J. Physiol.*, 223:549–570.

20. Carnevale, N. T. (1973): Voltage clamp analysis of the slow oscillations in bursting neurons reveals two underlying current components. PhD Dissertation, Duke University, Durham, N.C.

21. Carnevale, N. T., and Wachtel, H. (1980): Two reciprocating current components underlying slow oscillations in *Aplysia* bursting neurons. *Brain Res. Rev.*, 2:45–68.

22. Carpenter, D. O., and Alving, B. O. (1968): A contribution of an electrogenic Na$^+$ pump to membrane potential in *Aplysia* neurons. *J. Gen. Physiol.*, 52:1–21.

23. Carpenter, D., and Gunn, R. (1970): The dependence of pacemaker discharge of *Aplysia* neurons on Na$^+$ and Ca^{++}. *J. Cell. Physiol.*, 75:121–128.

24. Chen, C. F., von Baumgarten, R., and Takeda, R. (1971): Pacemaker properties of completely isolated neurons in *Aplysia californica*. *Nature New Biol.*, 233:27–29.

25. Colding-Jorgensen, M. (1977): Impulse dependent adaptation in *Helix Pomatia* neurones: Effect of the impulse on the firing pattern. *Acta. Physiol. Scand.*, 101:369–381.

26. Colmers, W. F., Lewis, D. V., Jr., and Wilson, W. A. (1982): Cs$^+$ loading reveals Na$^+$-dependent persistent inward current and negative slope resistance region in *Aplysia* giant neurons. *J. Neurophys.*, 48:1191–1200.

27. Colquhoun, D., Neher, E., Reuter, H., and Stevens, C. F. (1981): Inward current channels activated by intracellular Ca in cardiac cells. *Nature*, 294:752–754.

28. Connor, J. A. (1979): Calcium current in molluscan neurones: Measurement under conditions which maximize its visibility. *J. Physiol. (Lond.)*, 286:41–60.

29. Cote, I. L., Zbicz, K. L., and Wilson, W. A. (1978): Barbiturate-induced slow outward currents in *Aplysia* neurones. *Nature*, 274:594–596.

30. Dipolo, R., Requena, J., Brinley, F. J., Jr., Mullins, L. J., Scarpa, A., and Tiffert, T. (1976): Ionized calcium concentrations in squid axons. *J. Gen. Physiol.*, 67:433–467.

31. Eckert, R., and Lux, H. D. (1976): A voltage-sensitive persistent calcium conductance in neuronal somata of *Helix*. *J. Physiol.*, 254:129–151.

32. Eckert, R., and Tillotson, D. (1978): Potassium activation associated with intraneuronal free calcium. *Science*, 200:437–439.

33. Eckert, R., and Tillotson, D. L. (1981): Calcium-mediated inactivation of the calcium conductance in caesium loaded giant neurones of *Aplysia californica*. *J. Physiol. (Lond.)*, 314:265–280.

34. Evans, G. J., Huguenard, J. R., Wilson, W. A., and Lewis, D. V. (1982): Enhancement of slow outward current by pentobarbital is independent of Ca^{++} entry. *Soc. Neurosci. Abstr.*, 194.3.

35. Frankenhaeuser, B., and Hodgkin, A. L. (1957): The action of calcium on the electrical properties of squid axons. *J. Physiol.*, 137:218.

36. Gainer, H. (1972): Electrophysiological behavior of an endogenously active neurosecretory cell. *Brain. Res.*, 39:403–418.

37. Geduldig, D., and Junge, D. (1968): Sodium and calcium components of action potentials in the *Aplysia* giant neurones. *J. Physiol.*, 199:347–365.

38. Gola, M. (1974): Neurones a ondes-salves des mollusques. Variations cycliques lentes des conductances ioniques. *Eur. J. Physiol.*, 352:17–36, 1974.

39. Gorman, A. L. F., and Hermann, A. (1979): Internal effects of divalent cations on potassium permeability in molluscan neurons. *J. Physiol. (Lond.)*, 296:393–410.

40. Gorman, A. L. F., Hermann, A., and Thomas, A. V. (1982): Ionic requirements for membrane oscillations and their dependence on calcium concentration in a molluscan pace-maker neurone. *J. Physiol. (Lond.)*, 327:185–217.

41. Gorman, A. L. F., and Thomas, M. V. (1978): Changes in the intracellular concentration of free calcium ions in a pace-maker neurone measured with the metallochromic indicator dye Arsenazo III. *J. Physiol. (Lond.)*, 275:357–376.

42. Gorman, A. L. F., and Thomas, M. V. (1980a): Intracellular calcium accumulation during depolarization in a molluscan neurone. *J. Physiol. (Lond.)*, 308:259–285.

43. Gorman, A. L. F., and Thomas, M. V. (1980b): Potassium conductance and internal calcium accumulation in a molluscan neurone. *J. Physiol. (Lond.)*, 308:287–313.

44. Gospe, S. M., Jr. (1983): Minireview: Studies of

dopamine pharmacology in molluscs. *Life Sci.*, 33:1945–1957.

45. Gospe, S. M., Jr., and Wilson, W. A., Jr. (1980): Dopamine inhibits burst-firing of neurosecretory cell R15 in *Aplysia californica:* Establishment of a dose response relationship. *J. Pharmacol. Exp. Ther.*, 214:112–118.

46. Gospe, S. M., Jr., and Wilson, W. A., Jr. (1981): Pharmacological studies of a novel dopamine-sensitive receptor mediating burst-firing inhibition of neurosecretory cell R15 in *Aplysia californica. J. Pharmacol. Exp. Ther.*, 216:368–377.

47. Gulrajani, R. M., and Roberge, F. A. (1978): Possible mechanisms underlying bursting pacemaker discharges in invertebrate neurons. *Fed. Proc.*, 37:2146–2152.

48. Hagawara, S., and Byerly, L. (1981): Calcium channel. *Annu. Rev. Neurosci.*, 4:69–125.

49. Henkart, M. P., and Nelson, P. G. (1979): Evidence for an intracellular calcium store releasable by surface stimuli in fibroblasts (L cells). *J. Gen. Phys.*, 73:655–673.

50. Hermann, A., and Gorman, A. L. F. (1979): External and internal effects of tetraethylammonium on voltage-dependent and Ca-dependent K^+ currents components in molluscan pacemaker neurons. *Neurosci. Lett.*, 12:87–92.

51. Heyer, C. B., and Lux, H. D. (1976): Control of the delayed outward potassium currents in the bursting pacemaker neurons of the snail, *Helix pomatia. J. Physiol. (Lond.)*, 262:349–382.

52. Hille, B., Woodhull, A. M., and Shapiro, E. I. (1975): Negative surface charge near sodium channels of nerve: Divalent ions, monovalent ions and pH. *Philos. Trans. R. Soc. (Lond.) B* 270:301–318.

53. Hofmeier, G., and Lux, H. D. (1981): The time courses of intracellular free calcium and related electrical effects after injection of $CaCl_2$ into neurons of the snail, *Helix pomatia. Pflugers Arch.*, 391:242–251.

54. Huguenard, J. R., and Wilson, W. A. (1985): Suppression of repetitive firing of neurons by diphenylbarbituric acid. *J. Pharmacol. Exp. Ther.*, 232:228–231.

54a. Huguenard, J. R., Zbicz, K. L., Lewis, D. V., Evans, G. J., and Wilson, W. A. (1985): The ionic mechanism of the slow outward current in *Aplysia* neurons. *J. Neurophysiol.*, 54:449–461.

55. Ito, M., and Oshima, T. (1962): Temporal summation of after-hyperpolarisation following a motoneurone spike. *Nature*, 195:910–911.

56. Johnston, D. (1976): Voltage clamp reveals basis for calcium regulation of bursting pacemaker potentials in *Aplysia* neurons. *Brain Res.*, 107:418–423.

57. Johnston, D. (1980): Voltage, temperature and ionic dependence of the slow outward current in *Aplysia* burst-firing neurones. *J. Physiol. (Lond.)*, 289:145–157.

58. Junge, D., and Stephens, C. L. (1973): Cyclic variation of potassium conductance in a burst-generating neurone in *Aplysia. J. Physiol. (Lond.)*, 235:155–181.

59. Kernell, D. (1965): The adaptation and the relation between discharge frequency and current strength of cat lumbosacral motoneurones stim-

ulated by long-lasting injected currents. *Acta Physiol. Scand.*, 65:65–73.

60. Kernell, D., and Monster, A. W. (1982): Time course and properties of late adaptation in spinal motoneurons of the cat. *Exp. Brain Res.*, 46:191–196.

61. Kramer, R. H. (1984): The ionic mechanism of bursting pacemaker activity in *Aplysia* neurons. Ph.D. Dissertation. University of California at Berkeley.

62. Kramer, R. H., and Zucker, R. S. (1983): Inactivation of persistent inward current mediates post-burst hyperpolarization in *Aplysia* bursting pacemaker cells. *Soc. Neurosci. Abstr.*, 9:510.

63. Krnjevic, K., and Lisiewicz, A. (1972): Injections of calcium ions into spinal motoneurons. *J. Physiol. (Lond.)*, 225:363–390.

64. Krnjevic, K., Puil, E., and Werman, R. (1978): EGTA and motoneuron afterpotentials. *J. Physiol. (Lond.)*, 275:199–223.

65. Levitan, I. B., Harmon, A. J., and Adams, W. B. (1979): Synaptic and hormonal modulation of a neuronal oscillator: A search for molecular mechanisms. *J. Exp. Biol.*, 81:131–151.

66. Lewis, D. V. (1984): Spike aftercurrents in R15 of *Aplysia*. Their relationship to slow inward current and calcium influx. *J. Neurophysiol.*, 51:403–419.

67. Lewis, D. V., Evans, G. B., and Wilson, W. A. (1984): Dopamine reduces slow outward current and calcium influx in burst firing neuron R15 of *Aplysia. J. Neurosci.*, 4:3014–3020.

68. Lewis, D. V., and Wilson, W. A. (1982): Calcium influx and poststimulus current during early adaptation in *Aplysia* giant neurons. *J. Neurophysiol.*, 48:202–216.

69. Lux, H. D., and Heyer, C. B. (1979): A new electrogenic calcium-potassium system. In: *The Neurosciences Fourth Study Program*, edited by F. O. Schmitt and F. G. Worden, pp. 601–615. M.I.T. Press, Cambridge, Mass.

70. Maruyama, Y., and Peterson, O. H. (1982): Single channel currents in isolated patches of plasma membrane from basal surface of pancreatic acini. *Nature*, 299:159–161.

71. Mayeri, E., Brownell, P., Branton, W. D., and Simon, S. B. (1979): Multiple, prolonged actions of neuroendocrine bag cells on neurons in *Aplysia*. I. Effects on bursting pacemaker neurons. *J. Neurophysiol.*, 42:1165–1184.

72. Meech, R. W. (1972): Intracellular calcium injection causes increased potassium conductance in *Aplysia* nerve cells. *Comp. Biochem. Physiol.*, 42A:493–499.

73. Meech, R. W. (1974): Calcium influx induces a post tetanic hyperpolarization in *Aplysia* neurones. *Comp. Biochem. Physiol.*, A48:387–395.

74. Meech, R. W. (1974): The sensitivity of *Helix aspersa* neurones to injected calcium ions. *J. Physiol. (Lond.)*, 237:259–277.

75. Meech, R. W. (1979): Membrane potential oscillations in molluscan "burster" neurones. *J. Exp. Biol.*, 81:93–112.

76. Meech, R. W., and Standen, N. B. (1975): Potassium activation in *Helix Aspersa* neurones under voltage clamp. A component mediated by calcium influx. *J. Physiol. (Lond.)*, 249:211–239.

77. Moulins, M., and Cournil, I. (1982): All-or-none control of the bursting properties of the pacemaker neurons of the lobster pyloric pattern generator. *J. Neurobiol.*, 13:447–458.

78. Pallotta, B. S., Magleby, K. L., and Barrett, J. N. (1981): Single channel recordings of Ca^{2+} activated K^+ currents in rat muscle cell culture. *Nature*, 293:471–474.

79. Parnas, I., Armstrong, D., and Strumwasser, F. (1974): Prolonged excitatory and inhibitory synaptic modulation of a bursting pacemaker neuron. *J. Neurophysiol.*, 37:594–609.

80. Partridge, L. D. (1980): Calcium independence of slow currents underlying spike frequency adaptation. *J. Neurobiol.*, 11:613–622.

81. Partridge, L. D., and Stevens, C. F. (1976): A mechanism for spike frequency adaptation. *J. Physiol.*, 256:315–332.

82. Pinsker, H. M. (1977): *Aplysia* bursting neurons as endogenous oscillators. I Phase response curves for pulsed inhibitory synaptic input. *J. Neurophysiol.*, 40:527–543.

83. Plant, R. E. (1978): The effects of calcium on bursting neurons: A modeling study. *Biophys. J.*, 21:217–237.

84. Poggioli, J. and Putney, J. W., Jr. (1982): Net calcium fluxes in rat parotid acinar cells: Evidence for a hormone-sensitive calcium pool in or near the plasma membrane. *Pflugers Arch.*, 392:239–243.

85. Raines, A., Niner, J. M., and Pace, D. G. (1973): A comparison of the anticonvulsant, neurotoxic and lethal effects of diphenylbarbituric acid, phenobarbital and diphenylhydantoin in the mouse. *J. Pharmacol. Exp. Ther.*, 186:315–322.

86. Schwartzkroin, P. A. (1978): Secondary range rhythmic spiking in hippocampal neurons. *Brain Res.*, 149:247–250.

87. Smith, T. G., Jr., Barker, J. L., and Gainer, H. (1975): Requirements for bursting pacemaker potential activity in molluscan neurones. *Nature*, 253:450–452.

88. Stinnakre, J., and Tauc, L. (1973): Calcium influx in active *Aplysia* neurones detected by injected aequorin. *Nature New Biol.*, 242:113–115.

89. Strumwasser, F. (1973): Neural and humoral factors in the temporal organization of behavior (Seventeenth Bowditch Lecture). *Physiologist*, 16:9–42.

90. Thompson, S. H. (1977): Three pharmacologically distinct potassium channels in molluscan neurones. *J. Physiol. (Lond.)*, 265:465–488.

91. Thompson, S. H., and Smith, S. J. (1976): Depolarizing afterpotentials and burst production in molluscan pacemaker neurons. *J. Neurophysiol.*, 39:153.

92. Wilson, W. A. (1982): Patterned bursting discharge of invertebrate neurons. In: *Cellular Pacemakers*, vol. I., edited by D. Carpenter, pp. 219–235. Wiley, New York.

93. Wilson, W. A., and Wachtel, H. (1974): Negative resistance characteristic essential for the maintenance of slow oscillations in bursting neurons. *Science*, 186:932–934.

94. Wilson, W. A., and Wachtel, H. (1978): Prolonged inhibition in burst firing neurons: Synaptic inactivation of the slow regenerative inward current. *Science*, 202:772–775.

95. Winegard, S. (1982): Calcium release from cardiac sarcoplasmic reticulum. *Annu. Rev. Physiol.*, 44:451–462.

96. Yellen, G. (1982): Single Ca^{+2} activated non-selective cation channels in neuroblastoma. *Nature*, 296:357–359.

97. Zbicz, K. L., and Wilson, W. A. (1981): Barbiturate enhancement of spike frequency adaptation in *Aplysia* giant neurons. *J. Pet.*, 217:222–227.

98. Zierler, K. (1981): A critique of compartmental analysis. *Annu. Rev. Biophys. Bioeng.*, 10:531–562.

Advances in Neurology, Vol. 44, edited by
A. V. Delgado-Escueta, A. A. Ward, Jr.,
D. M. Woodbury, and R. J. Porter.
Raven Press, New York © 1986.

12

Control Theory Applied to Neural Networks Illuminates Synaptic Basis of Interictal Epileptiform Activity

*Daniel Johnston and **Thomas H. Brown

*Program in Neuroscience, Section of Neurophysiology, Department of Neurology, Baylor College of
Medicine, Houston, Texas 77030 and **Department of Cellular Neurophysiology, Division of Neurosciences,
Beckman Research Institute of the City of Hope, Duarte, California 91010*

SUMMARY   A brief historical account is presented of the formulation of two
hypotheses that have been proposed to explain the mechanisms underlying the
paroxysmal depolarizing shift (PDS) in experimental epilepsy. The two hypotheses are called the *giant EPSP hypothesis* and the *endogenous burst hypothesis*. The giant EPSP hypothesis states that the PDS (the intracellular correlate of the interictal discharge) is comprised of a larger-than-normal-strength
excitatory synaptic input, whereas the endogenous burst hypothesis states that
the PDS is an endogenous burst triggered by an excitatory postsynaptic potential
of normal strength.

Two sets of four experimentally testable predictions, which were derived from
these two hypotheses for the PDS, are presented. These predictions describe the
expected behavior of the PDS in response to changes in membrane potential and
under conditions of voltage clamping. With the advent of single-electrode current-
and voltage-clamp techniques and improved intracellular recording conditions,
the testing of these predictions has become possible.

Experiments are described in which each of the predictions from the two hypotheses were tested. The results strongly support the giant EPSP hypothesis
and are not easily reconciled with the endogenous burst hypothesis.

Because the PDS is a network-driven event, it is important to understand the
properties of the neuronal network responsible for the genesis of the PDS. Others
have proposed that there are three necessary conditions for epileptiform activity
in any neuronal network: endogenous bursting, disinhibition, and recurrent excitatory synapses. Using control theory as a frame of reference, we argue that it
is premature to raise these three phenomena to the level of general theoretical
requirements for interictal activity. Insufficient quantitative information exists
about the properties of neurons, synapses, and connectivity patterns in any cortical neuronal network to conclude that the three preposed requirements are
necessary and sufficient general conditions for epileptiform activity.

Because all of the key predictions of the giant EPSP hypothesis have now been
experimentally verified, we conclude that the PDS is a large, network-driven
EPSP. The current challenge to neurophysiologists is to describe in detail the
properties of neurons and synapses in a cortical neuronal network and then to
evaluate the relative contributions of network and individual neuronal properties
to the expression of interictal epileptiform activity.

The paroxysmal depolarizing shift (PDS), which is defined below, is a particular intracellular consequence in one neuron of a series of complicated processes in a synaptically connected network of neural tissue. The neuronal mechanisms responsible for the PDS have been studied extensively during the past 20 years. What has emerged from these studies is not only a clarification of the mechanisms, but also better insight into the important questions for further investigation. There is general consensus that further knowledge of the mechanisms underlying the genesis of the PDS could provide insights into the causes and treatment of epilepsy.

In this review, we first present a brief historical account of some key investigations that led to our recent experimental and theoretical studies of the cellular and network events responsible for the PDS. We then summarize some of these recent studies and show how they furnished the basis of our present understanding of the neurophysiology of the PDS. We reject a strict reductionistic perspective and suggest that epileptiform activity can be understood only in terms of interactions between cellular and network properties—a viewpoint that is generally compatible with the emergent determinism of Sperry (67) or the hierarchical control systems of Evarts (23).

HISTORICAL PERSPECTIVE ON THE PDS

To review some of the previous research and hypotheses about the mechanisms responsible for interictal epileptiform discharges, we must define some terms. The four-way classification scheme (Table 1), proposed elsewhere (33), is a conceptually useful starting point. However, we hasten to point out that this classification scheme is perhaps overly rigid because it is based on dichotomies and therefore does not explicitly address transitions or intermediate states (see Chapter 27). Although we recognize the obvious linguistic or conceptual limitations of this simple classification scheme, we continue to use this language here, dividing bursts into those that are spontaneous versus those that are triggered and those that are network-driven versus those that are endogenous or intrinsic.

Studies of the cellular basis of epileptiform activity have led to two hypotheses for the generation of the PDS. Early formulations of the *first hypothesis* suggested that the PDS is an intrinsic membrane response, such as an abnormally prolonged action potential, whereas more recent versions of this same hypothesis emphasize endogenous bursting. For the purposes of this discussion, we will call this viewpoint the *endogenous burst hypothesis*. The *second hypothesis* proposes that the PDS results from an excitatory postsynaptic potential (EPSP) that is much larger than normal, possibly mediated through recurrent excitatory circuitry. We call this viewpoint the *giant EPSP hypothesis*. Both of these seemingly different viewpoints have permeated the literature for over 20 years.

High-quality intracellular recordings that contributed to our understanding of the PDS (and seizure activity) were made 25 years ago *in vivo* by Kandel and Spencer (38) in the feline hippocampus. The seizures were electrically induced. Kandel and Spencer observed that tetanic stimulation of the fornix caused oscillations superimposed upon prolonged depolarizing shifts of the membrane potential of hippocampal pyramidal neurons. They proposed that the oscillations were either large EPSPs or some type of graded response. They further proposed that the steady depolarization was produced by the smooth summation of EPSPs. The seizures that resulted from fornix tetanization were postulated to result from synaptic bombardment and not from a change in the intrinsic properties of the cells. This interpretation thus set the stage for the giant EPSP hypothesis.

A contrary interpretation was provided by Matsumoto and Ajmone Marsan (49) based on a series of *in vivo* experiments in which epileptiform activity was induced by the topical application of penicillin to the feline cortex (49,50). Intracellular recordings were made from neocortical neurons during interictal and ictal events. In these studies, they coined the phrase "paroxysmal depolarizing shift (PDS)" to describe the sudden depolarization of the membrane potential (which can last 90–150 msec) that occurred during the surface EEG spike. Al-

TABLE 1. *Classification of bursts in hippocampal neurons*

Origin of burst-sustaining currents	Cause of onset	
	Spontaneously occurring	Experimentally triggered
Endogenous or intrinsic	Spontaneous endogenous burst	Triggered endogenous burst
Network-driven	Spontaneous network burst (spontaneous PDS)	Triggered network burst (triggered PDS)

though conclusive data could not be presented at the time, Matsumoto and Ajmone Marsan speculated that " . . . excessive, oversustained response to relatively unaltered synaptic influences should be mainly determined by intrinsic alterations within the cell itself" (49).

From 1966 through 1971, a consistent view of the PDS began to emerge from the work of Prince (56,57), Ayala et al. (7), Matsumoto et al. (51), and Dichter and Spencer (20,21). The penicillin model for focal epilepsy became an established preparation in these investigations, which involved both neocortex (7,51,56,57) and hippocampus (20,21). In 1966, two explicit hypotheses were put forth by Prince (56) to explain the origin of the PDS: (a) the PDS could be a graded response to synaptic input, or (b) the PDS could be a regenerative electrical response in individual neurons whose membrane properties had been altered by the convulsant agent. Because the amplitude of the PDS varied with the membrane potential and because there appeared to be no constant "firing level" for the PDS, Prince favored the first hypothesis.

In 1968, Prince (57) provided further evidence that he interpreted as supporting a synaptic hypothesis for the PDS. The amplitude of the PDS was observed to vary over a wide range of membrane potentials, and even a possible reversal of the PDS was reported to occur at extreme depolarizations. The graded nature of the PDS observed in some cells also supported the view that the envelope of depolarization during the PDS reflects " . . . a series of high amplitude EPSPs summated temporally" (57).

A similar line of reasoning was used by Ayala et al. (6,7,51), Matsumoto et al. (57), and Dichter and Spencer (20,21) in their description of the PDS. The giant EPSP hypothesis was stated more explicitly by these authors. They concluded that the PDS was a large, compound EPSP produced by recurrent excitatory feedback synapses in the area of the focus. The basis for this conclusion was that: (a) the PDS was graded in amplitude when repeatedly elicited, (b) the PDS was associated with a conductance increase, and (c) the PDS could be reversed in polarity with strong depolarization. Although the large or "giant" EPSP hypothesis for the PDS was now clearly established in the literature, most of the evidence marshaled in favor of this hypothesis was still indirect. Even the possible reversal of the PDS reported by Prince (57) and Matsumoto et al. (51) might be considered suspect because the health of the neurons was questionable, and the data may have been corrupted by the presence of inhibitory synaptic potentials or field effects.

By the mid-1970s, the use of *in vitro* brain slices (particularly hippocampal slices) was beginning to prove useful for cellular studies of epilepsy. The brain-slice preparation provided sufficient mechanical stability to permit high-quality intracellular recordings to be made, and allowed the experimenter to control more accurately and conveniently the extracellular environment. In addition, the properties of the neurons and synapses in the slices appeared similar to those found *in vivo* (61,62). Application of penicillin or other convulsant agents, such as picrotoxin or bicuculline, to the bath caused large areas of a slice to display synchronous burst discharges (63,64). Intracellular recordings during these synchronous discharges revealed an intracellular PDS that was similar to that found in the *in vivo* penicillin model (63,64). The hippocampal slice quickly became a popular model system for investigating the PDS.

In addition to its utility for studying epileptiform activity, the brain-slice preparation also provided greatly needed information about the basic physiology of hippocampal neurons. Schwartzkroin and Slawsky (65) showed that hippocampal neurons could display what appeared to be calcium-dependent regenerative membrane responses, which were termed calcium spikes. Wong et al. (77) provided evidence suggesting that hippocampal dendrites themselves are capable of generating calcium-dependent regenerative responses. The original *in vivo* findings of Kandel and Spencer (37), showing that hippocampal CA3 neurons can display burst responses under normal conditions, were found to be true *in vitro* as well (27,74). In the slice, these bursts appeared to be generated largely by intrinsic properties of the neurons (27,33,76,78). Given the evidence for calcium spikes in hippocampal neurons, the later demonstration that a single action potential was followed by a calcium-dependent afterhyperpolarization (29) came as no surprise. The afterhyperpolarization is thought to be a calcium-gated potassium conductance (see Fig. 5 of ref. 33), similar to that found in many other cell types (52).

With the new evidence that hippocampal neurons are apparently capable of generating calcium spikes, endogenous burst responses, and other interesting voltage-dependent responses, attention shifted away from the giant EPSP hypothesis and toward the hypothesis that the PDS was an intrinsic membrane response. Between 1977 and 1984, several investigators (1,58,64,66) concluded that the PDS was not a "giant" synaptic potential but instead was an intrinsic depolarization produced by calcium-mediated burst mechanisms in the dendrites. The endogenous burst hypothesis was then further defined to state specifically that normal-amplitude EPSPs trigger these endogenous burst mechanisms whenever the usual concomitant synaptic inhibition is reduced (75).

In 1978, a new technique was being developed for use on brain slices—a technique that permitted quantitative investigation of the biophysical properties of hippocampal neurons and their synapses (35). Using a time-share, single-electrode recording technique (SEC), it became possible to provide a point voltage clamp to the soma of hippocampal neurons and to measure voltage-dependent and synaptic currents. Moreover, in the current-clamp mode, the SEC permitted injection of larger currents than those possible with traditional bridge-balance techniques, while maintaining a more accurate monitor of membrane potential. This experimental approach was first described by Wilson and Goldner (72) for studies of large *Aplysia* neurons, and was then further refined and developed by Johnston et al. (36) for use on hippocampal neurons in the slice. Using this technique, a voltage-dependent calcium current and a calcium-dependent potassium current were described in CA3 neurons (33,36).

Because much of the evidence in favor of either the giant EPSP hypothesis or the endogenous burst hypothesis was indirect, Johnston and Brown (30) decided to apply the newly developed SEC technology to the PDS in hippocampal slices exposed to penicillin and several other convulsants (33,34,42,43,60). The SEC permitted the testing of quantitative predictions derived from the two hypotheses—predictions that could not be tested properly by using conventional intracellular recording techniques.

DIFFERENTIAL PREDICTIONS DERIVED FROM THE TWO HYPOTHESIZED MECHANISMS FOR PDS

The fundamental characteristics of endogenous bursts have been well described (33). One well-known feature of endogenous bursts is their voltage dependence (see ref. 33 for details). Both the frequency of spontaneously occurring endogenous bursts and the probability of triggering an endogenous burst are strongly dependent on the membrane potential. This dependency can be easily demonstrated by observing the frequency of spontaneous or triggered bursting as a function of the membrane potential. Endogenous bursts have several other defining features (33).

Based on knowledge of the well-known properties of endogenous bursts, Johnston and Brown (30) tested four key quantitative predictions, derived from the two hypotheses, concerning the behavior of the PDS in response to changes in membrane potential. The giant EPSP hypothesis and the endogenous burst hypothesis were shown to make different quantitative or qualitative predictions about the behavior of the PDS in response to the same manipulations of the membrane potential:

1. The first prediction of the giant EPSP hypothesis was that the frequency or probability of occurrence of PDSs should be independent of the membrane potential. In contrast, the endogenous burst hypothesis predicted that the frequency or probability of occurrence of PDSs should be highly dependent on the membrane potential.

2. The second prediction of the giant EPSP hypothesis was that the amplitude of the PDS should be a monotonically decreasing function of the membrane potential, consistent with the decrease in synaptic driving force. In contrast, the endogenous burst hypothesis predicted that the amplitude of the underlying depolarization responsible for the PDS should be a discontinuous and highly nonlinear function of the membrane potential. According to the latter hypothesis, the PDS amplitude should change from zero to some positive value and then back to zero as the membrane potential was depolarized from very negative to positive values.

3. The third prediction of the giant EPSP hypothesis was that the polarity of the PDS should reverse when the membrane was depolarized beyond the synaptic equilibrium potential, which was found to be about -5 mV (14,32). In contrast, the prediction of the endogenous burst hypothesis was that the polarity of the PDS should not reverse at the synaptic equilibrium potential. Instead, the PDS amplitude should asymptotically approach zero as the membrane potential approaches the calcium equilibrium potential, which has not been accurately measured in hippocampal neurons but is presumably much more positive than -5 mV (24,36). Furthermore, unless one wished to make additional ad hoc and untested assumptions, the PDS should *never* reverse polarity if it were simply a calcium spike—even at extremely positive membrane potentials.

4. The fourth prediction of the giant EPSP hypothesis was that the synaptic conductance underlying the PDS should be large in comparison to that accompanying normal EPSPs. The endogenous burst hypothesis specifically stated that the strength of the synaptic input that triggered the endogenous burst was normal. According to the endogenous burst hypothesis, a larger-than-normal-strength synaptic input was not present in neurons from convulsant-treated slices. The test of this fourth prediction hinged on the *relative conductances of normal and PDS-associated synaptic inputs.*

The experimental test of the first three predictions required accurate measurement of the membrane potential during the passage of large transmembrane currents. The experimental test of the fourth prediction required voltage-clamp techniques. These types of experiments were now feasible with the newly developed SEC technology.

RESULTS SUPPORT THE GIANT EPSP HYPOTHESIS

The results from experiments in which the four key predictions were tested have been described in detail elsewhere (30,33,34,42,43) but will be summarized briefly here. To test the first prediction, the membrane potentials of both CA1 and CA3 neurons were varied between about -150 and $+65$ mV (an extreme range that could not have been achieved without the SEC and more optimal recording conditions, including improved microelectrode characteristics). The frequency of spontaneous PDSs and the probability of triggering a PDS with orthodromic stimulation were measured as a function of the membrane potential. Both the frequency and the probability of occurrence of PDSs were found to be independent of the membrane potential (see Fig. 1 of ref. 30 and Fig. 6 of ref. 33). No significant relationship between membrane potential and the occurrence of a PDS could be detected. The results from these experiments therefore supported the giant EPSP hypothesis.

The test of the second prediction also required measurement of the amplitude of the PDS as a function of membrane potential (the use of the SEC and improved recording conditions were also necessary for these experiments). Again, in both CA1 and CA3 neurons, the membrane potentials were varied over extreme ranges, sometimes from -100 to $+50$ mV (30,33,34,42,43).

In all of these experiments, there was a monotonic relationship between the amplitude of the PDS and the membrane potential (see Fig. 2 of ref. 30 and Fig. 8 of ref. 33). Usually the relationships were not only monotonic but linear. The linearity was easily explained, but not required, by the giant EPSP hypothesis. (It results from the fact that *the synaptic conductance was large relative to the sum of all other membrane conductances that were activated.*) The results from these experiments supported the giant EPSP hypothesis.

The test of the third prediction again required depolarization of the membrane potential to extremely positive and known values (again requiring the SEC and improved recording conditions). In both CA1 and CA3 neurons, the polarity of the PDS was reversed at potentials more positive than the synaptic reversal potential (see Fig. 2 of ref. 30, Fig. 9 of ref. 33, and Fig. 2 of ref. 34). The polarity of a PDS was always reversed when the membrane was depolarized beyond 0 mV. The results from these experiments furnished the third line of evidence in favor of the giant EPSP hypothesis.

Testing the fourth prediction required the use of voltage-clamp techniques (and therefore the SEC and improved recording conditions). Both CA1 and CA3 neurons were voltage-clamped, and the currents underlying spontaneous EPSPs, evoked EPSPs, spontaneous PDSs, and orthodromically evoked (triggered) PDSs were measured. The peak synaptic conductance increase associated with the PDS was compared to the peak conductance increase responsible for normally occurring EPSPs. The synaptic conductance increase underlying the spontaneous PDS was about 5–10 times larger than the conductance increase responsible for the normal spontaneous EPSP (30). Similarly, the synaptic conductance increase underlying the evoked PDS was 5–10 times larger than the conductance increase responsible for the normally occurring evoked EPSP (Fig. 1). These results, when combined with the preceding evidence, offer a fourth and compelling argument in favor of the giant EPSP hypothesis.

Prior to the preceding four types of experiments, the existence of giant (unusually large) synaptic responses in hippocampal neurons had been discounted by a number of investigators (1,58,64,66). However, the use of the SEC-based techniques and improved recording conditions (32) demonstrated beyond reasonable doubt the existence of such large synaptic responses. Until an alternative viable hypothesis that can account

A

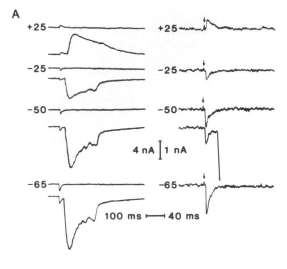

B

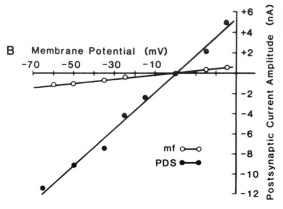

FIG. 1. Triggered mossy fiber and PDS currents as a function of membrane potential. A hippocampal neuron from a slice bathed in 10 μM picrotoxin was voltage-clamped using a Cs_2SO_4-filled micropipette and a single-electrode clamp system (SEC). **A:** Mossy fiber and PDS currents at four different holding potentials. Traces on the left were filmed at a lower gain and slower time base than the corresponding traces on the right. Stimulus artifact is indicated by the arrow. Occasionally, mossy fiber stimulation triggered an interictal discharge. The PDS currents occurred during the decay phase of the mossy fiber currents and were about nine times larger than the latter. Both the PDS and mossy fiber currents reversed at about the same potential. **B:** Current–voltage relationship for the early mossy fiber currents and the delayed PDS currents. Each data point represents the mean of 3–6 trials (for the PDS currents) or 5–15 trials (for the mossy fiber currents). The conductance increase associated with the PDS was 180 nS, compared with 21 nS for the mossy fiber input. The reversal potentials were close to 0 mV for both the mossy fiber and PDS currents. From Johnston and Brown, ref. 34, with permission.

for the preceding facts is put forth, we shall conclude that giant EPSPs do indeed exist and play a causal role in the genesis of the PDS in hippocampal slices made epileptic by the application of convulsant agents.

THEORETICAL ASPECTS OF NEURONAL NETWORK INTERACTIONS

It is generally recognized that there are two types of burst discharges in neuronal systems (33). They are called endogenous and network bursts. Because the interictal discharge is *defined* as the synchronous activity of a group of neurons, this activity is of necessity a network phenomenon. The PDS is a burst discharge that is recorded intracellularly during the network synchronization that is termed the interictal event. The genesis of the PDS is obviously dependent on the properties and interactions of a group of neurons. As the experiments just described show, the PDS is accompanied by a large synaptic input from elements of the synchronized neuronal network. This is hardly surprising, because the network is known to be rich in excitatory synaptic interconnections and, by definition, activity in the network must become synchronized during the PDS.

Now that this issue appears to have been settled, it is time to proceed to the next challenge to neurophysiologists, which is to define the necessary and sufficient conditions for producing epileptiform activity in a neuronal network. Others have proposed that there are three requirements, perhaps even ''absolute requirements'' (1), for the development of paroxysmal discharges in neuronal systems (1,59,69–71,73). A priori, we see no logical basis for these claimed theoretical requirements, which are listed and then discussed below:

1. Endogenous bursting: For paroxysmal discharges to occur, neurons within a network must be capable of generating endogenous burst discharges (that is, they must be endogenous oscillators) in order for the neuronal network to be capable of generating spontaneous or triggered paroxysmal discharges. According to this view, networks that do not contain such endogenous oscillators cannot synchronize their activity in an epileptiform manner.

2. Disinhibition: For such synchronization to occur, there must be a reduction in inhibition within the network. In a network of interconnected neurons, inhibition would take the form

of negative feedback. According to this view, there must be a reduction in negative feedback in order for the network to display oscillations.

3. Recurrent excitation: Recurrent excitatory synaptic pathways must be present. In a system of interconnected neurons, recurrent excitation would take the form of positive feedback among the neuronal elements. The explicit interpretation of this requirement is that positive feedback among elements must be present and be synaptic in nature. A more general interpretation would simply be that some form of positive feedback must be present.

The theoretical basis for the behavior of a network of interconnected neurons with realistic membrane properties is complicated. However, if the problem is viewed from the perspective of control theory, perhaps a better intuitive feel for the issues involved can be obtained. In a simple feedback system, the *individual neurons* would be in the *open loop,* and the *excitatory and inhibitory synaptic interconnections* would be in the *feedback loop* (Fig. 2).

The general features of such a control system are well known. There are two general requirements for the output of a closed-loop system to be unstable (that is, to undergo spontaneous oscillations or to saturate). If the net feedback is negative, 180° out of phase with the output, and has an overall gain greater than unity, or if the net feedback is positive and has an overall gain greater than unity, the system will always oscillate. *There are no general requirements for sta-bility of the system in the open loop (that is, the neuronal elements need not be spontaneous oscillators) in order for instabilities to be present in the closed loop.* The closed-loop system can be unstable even if the open-loop system is stable (that is, the neuronal elements in the open loop are not spontaneous oscillators). Also, there is no specific requirement regarding the nature of the feedback. The latter can be any combination of positive (excitatory) or negative (inhibitory) feedback as long as the sum satisfies either of the two criteria given above.

We are not suggesting that the three proposed requirements given above are unimportant factors in the genesis of epileptiform activity in the hippocampus. Rather, for two reasons, we believe that it is premature to elevate these three particular experimental observations in selected cortical tissues to the level of general theoretical requirements. First, no such theoretical network requirements apparently exist. Second, there are insufficient quantitative data pertinent to understanding the true causes of epileptiform activity, even in the particular case of the hippocampal brain slice.

There are numerous examples in the literature in which network oscillations can be obtained even though the individual neurons of the network are not endogenous oscillators (3,16–19,22,40,44,45,48,54,55). In general, oscillations can occur regardless of whether the feedback among the elements is inhibitory (negative feedback) or excitatory (positive feedback). Obviously, what is important about the nature of the feedback is that, by virtue of its sign or phase, it results in an unstable system. Therefore, there is *no theoretical requirement* for there to be a population of endogenously bursting cells, a decrease in inhibition, or the presence of excitation to produce system oscillations.

Thus, the specific question that must be addressed concerning the requirements for PDSs in hippocampal neurons is not "How *can* the system work?", because there seem to be a large number of possible mechanisms, but rather "How *does* the system work?" The answers to this question require the knowledge of specific details within each of the boxes depicted in Fig. 2, including quantitative information about the membrane and synaptic properties of the neurons involved as well as the connectivity patterns among them. Because such information is not yet available, any general conclusions regarding the specific requirements for oscillations

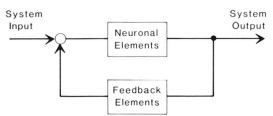

FIG. 2. Block diagram of hypothetical control system. The control system represents the neuronal network responsible for epileptiform activity. The output of the system could be spontaneous or evoked interictal discharges or seizure activity. The input to the system could either be experimentally triggered or naturally occurring. All the neuronal elements of the network are represented by a single box, and all forms of feedback (for example, excitatory and inhibitory synaptic pathways, ephaptic or electrotonic interactions, extracellular ions) are represented by another box. As conceptualized, in this control system a neuronal element in the open loop has no causal influence on any other neuronal elements of the network.

of neuronal networks in general is presently unwarranted.

PROPERTIES OF SYNAPSES RESPONSIBLE FOR THE PDS

Because the PDS is a network-driven burst that is sustained by a strong synaptic input, we concluded that additional knowledge about the properties of the synapses in this network would be valuable. In both the neocortex and the CA3 region of the hippocampus, a reasonable working hypothesis is that synapses responsible for the PDS arise from excitatory recurrent collaterals, either through monosynaptic connections or excitatory interneurons. In the CA1 region of the hippocampus, however, there is little direct evidence for recurrent excitatory connections (41). The synapses responsible for the PDS in region CA1 may simply be the Schaffer collateral fibers from the CA3 region. Nevertheless, the possibility still remains that previously undiscovered recurrent excitatory synapses may contribute to the PDS in region CA1. Slow and irregular spontaneous network discharges can, in fact, be generated in isolated pieces of tissue from the CA1 region following exposure to solutions containing picrotoxin (26). Whether recurrent excitatory connections might contribute to network synchronization in region CA1 is still an open question. If such synaptic connections do not in fact exist, further emphasis must be placed on the role of nonsynaptic forms of feedback in region CA1 (see Chapter 30).

The only synapses in the mammalian brain about which quantitative biophysical and physiological information is available are the mossy fiber synapses that project from dentate granule cells onto pyramidal neurons of the CA3 region (Fig. 3). The peak conductance increase, reversal potential, and kinetics of the conductance change associated with activation of this pathway have been described (9,14,31,32). Because the mossy fiber endings are located electrotonically near the somata of CA3 neurons (31), this input has been particularly amenable to voltage-clamp analysis. Whether the Schaffer collateral input to CA1 and the recurrent excitatory pathways in the CA3 region can be voltage-clamped with reasonable accuracy is not yet known, but this is obviously an extremely important question for future study.

Although the voltage-clamp experiments have shown the existence of a large synaptic conductance associated with the PDS, it is not known whether that conductance reflects an abnormally large number of synapses that are simultaneously active or whether the efficacy of individual synapses is abnormally large. The summation of individual EPSPs can often be seen on the rising phase of the PDS. In particular, under voltage-clamp conditions, the synaptic currents appear to summate on the leading edge of the waveform. These results suggest that there is some asynchrony in the activation of the synapses that are responsible for the PDS. However, it is not known whether the individual synapses are potentiated over their baseline levels. Long-term potentiation (LTP) is a prominent feature of excitatory synapses in the hippocampus and dentate gyrus. It is reasonable to wonder whether LTP of recurrent excitatory synapses or of Schaffer collateral synapses plays a role in the development and/or maintenance of the large synaptic drive that sustains the PDS.

LTP is defined as a long-lasting increase in the efficacy of a synaptic input following a brief high-frequency stimulation of the synaptic pathway (10–13,68). Because posttetanic potentiation generally decays within a few minutes, LTP is defined as an increase in synaptic efficacy lasting 15 min or longer (8,9,15,25,28). The definition is operational in nature in that it does not necessarily imply a single phenomenon or mechanism. Any use-dependent mechanism that produces an enhanced synaptic efficacy lasting more than 15 min following brief repetitive stimulation of the synaptic input would currently be defined as LTP. The recent successful application of voltage-clamp techniques to the study of LTP (9,25) promises further insights into the cellular neurophysiology of this interesting phenomenon. Experiments in progress should soon provide needed biophysical, biochemical, and pharmacological information about the induction and maintenance of LTP and its role in epileptiform activity.

SUMMARY AND CONCLUSIONS

The interictal discharge is a brief, synchronous activation of a group of neurons. The synchronization begins and ends abruptly. During the interictal discharge, individual neurons within the group sustain a brief and apparently simultaneous depolarization called the PDS, which normally triggers a burst of action potentials. The PDS is graded in amplitude when repeatedly elicited; its amplitude varies with the membrane potential; it can be reversed in polarity with depolarization; its frequency and probability of occurrence are independent of the membrane po-

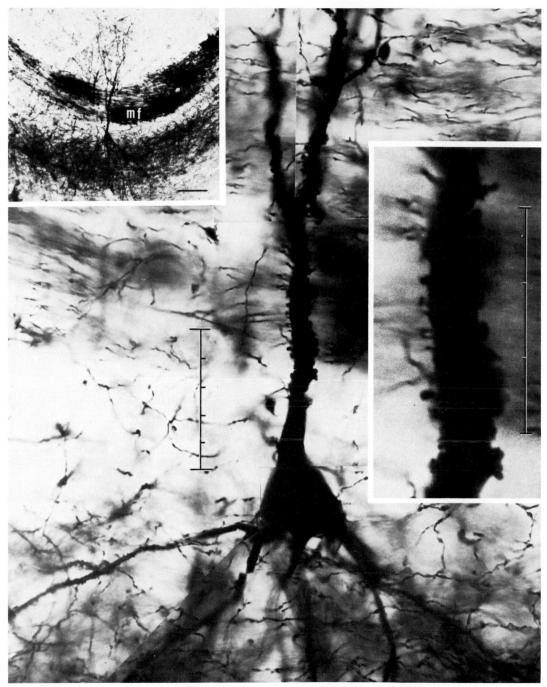

FIG. 3. Photomicrograph of a transverse section through the hippocampus that was stained by the use of the rapid Golgi method. *Upper left:* Low-power view of a CA3 neuron, indicating its location within the regio inferior. The dark band passing through the apical region (stratum lucidum) represents numerous Golgi-stained mossy fiber synaptic expansions (scale, 100 μm). *Center:* A higher-power view of the same CA3 pyramidal neuron. Several large mossy fiber synaptic expansions can be seen within the plane of focus. The dendritic thorny excrescences (the characteristic large postsynaptic spines on which the mossy fiber synapses are located) are also apparent (scale, 50 μm). *Lower right:* Higher magnification of a portion of the apical dendrite of the same neuron, illustrating the thorny excrescences more clearly (scale, 30 μm). From Johnston and Brown, ref. 31, with permission.

tential; and it is associated with a larger-than-normal excitatory synaptic conductance increase. The giant EPSP hypothesis for the PDS has been extremely useful in guiding experimental investigations of epileptiform activity, and all four key predictions of this hypothesis have now been experimentally verified.

The properties or size of the network of neurons capable of generating a PDS are not known. The network can be viewed as a complex control system consisting of neuronal elements among which are various forms of feedback. The interictal discharge represents the output of the control system, and the PDS represents the event taking place within the individual neuronal elements. In the hippocampus, the required size of an adequate network need be no greater than the CA3 subfield, because Miles et al. (53) recently showed that pieces of a hippocampal slice consisting primarily of the CA3 region are capable of generating spontaneous interictal discharges.

Pyramidal neurons of the CA3 region possess many types of voltage-dependent conductances, although the quantitative details of those conductances are not known. In the CA3 region, there is substantial evidence for recurrent excitatory synaptic connections (46,47) as well as for recurrent and feed-forward inhibition (2,4,5,39). There is also evidence for some electrotonic junctions and for ephaptic interactions among the neurons (see Chapter 30). Each of these neurophysiological properties possibly plays some role in the generation of spontaneous epileptiform activity in the CA3 region. However, what that role is and whether each is required in some way for the PDS are not known. Even less is known about the CA1 region. We believe that an increased knowledge of the quantitative details of the neuronal and synaptic properties and connectivity patterns will give us more insight into the network mechanisms responsible for the PDS. The biophysical studies currently underway should provide some of this information. When this essential information becomes available, it will be possible, by combining quantitative experiments with realistic computer simulations of the neuronal networks, to generate and then critically examine competing hypotheses about epileptiform activity in cortical neuronal networks.

ACKNOWLEDGMENTS

This work was supported by Grant Nos. NS11535, NS15772, and NS18295 from the National Institutes of Health; by McKnight Foundation Scholar's and Development Awards; and by AFOSR contract F49620.

REFERENCES

1. Alger, B. E. (1984): Hippocampus: Electrophysiological studies of epileptiform activity *in vitro*. In: *Brain Slices*, edited by R. Dingledine, pp. 155–193. Plenum Press, New York.
2. Alger, B. E., and Nicoll, R. A. (1982): Feed-forward dendritic inhibition in rat hippocampal pyramidal cells studied *in vitro*. *J. Physiol. (Lond.)*, 328:105–123.
3. Amari, S. (1971): Characteristics of randomly connected threshold-element networks and network systems. *Proc. IEEE*, 59:35–47.
4. Andersen, P., Eccles, J. C., and Løyning, Y. (1964): Location of postsynaptic inhibitory synapses on hippocampal pyramids. *J. Neurophysiol.*, 27:592–607.
5. Andersen, P., Eccles, J. C., and Løyning, Y. (1964): Pathway of postsynaptic inhibition in the hippocampus. *J. Neurophysiol.*, 27:608–619.
6. Ayala, G. F., Dichter, M., Gumnit, R. J., Matsumoto, H., and Spencer, W. A. (1973): Genesis of epileptic interictal spikes. New knowledge of cortical feedback systems suggests a neurophysiological explanation of brief paroxysms. *Brain Res.*, 52:1–18.
7. Ayala, G. F., Matsumoto, H., and Gumnit, R. J. (1970): Excitability changes and inhibitory mechanism in neocortical neurons during seizures. *J. Neurophysiol.*, 33:73–85.
8. Barrionuevo, G., and Brown, T. H. (1983): Associative long-term potentiation in hippocampal slices. *Proc. Natl. Acad. Sci. USA*, 80:7347–7351.
9. Barrionuevo, G., Kelso, S. R., Johnston, D., and Brown, T. H. (1985): Voltage-clamp analysis of long-term potentiation in monosynaptic and isolated excitatory inputs to hippocampus. *J. Neurophysiol.* (in press).
10. Bliss, T. V. P. (1979): Synaptic plasticity in the hippocampus. *Trends Neurosci.*, 2:42–45.
11. Bliss, T. V. P., and Dolphin, A. C. (1982): What is the mechanism of long-term potentiation in the hippocampus? *Trends Neurosci.*, 5:289–290.
12. Bliss, T. V. P., and Gardner-Medwin, A. R. (1973): Long-lasting potentiation of synaptic transmission in the dentate area of the unanaesthetized rabbit following stimulation of the perforant path. *J. Physiol. (Lond.)*, 232:357–374.
13. Bliss, T. V. P., and Lømo, T. (1973): Long-lasting potentiation of synaptic transmission in the dentate area of the anaesthetized rabbit following stimulation of the perforant path. *J. Physiol. (Lond.)*, 232:331–356.
14. Brown, T. H., and Johnston, D. (1983): Voltage-clamp analysis of mossy fiber synaptic input to hippocampal neurons. *J. Neurophysiol.*, 50:487–507.
15. Brown, T. H., and McAfee, D. (1982): Long-term synaptic potentiation in the superior cervical ganglion. *Science*, 215:1411–1413.

16. Carpenter, G. A., and Grossberg, S. (1983): A neural theory of circadian rhythms: The gated pacemaker. *Biol. Cybern.*, 48:35–59.

17. Carpenter, G. A., and Grossberg, S. (1985): A neural theory of circadian rhythms: Aschoff's rule in diurnal and nocturnal mammals. *Am. J. Physiol.* (in press).

18. Carpenter, G. A., and Grossberg, S. 1985: A neural theory of circadian rhythms: Split rhythms, after-effects, and motivational interactions. *J. Theor. Biol.* (in press).

19. Cohen, M. A., and Grossberg, S. (1983): Absolute stability of global pattern formation and parallel memory storage by competitive neural networks. *IEEE Trans. Syst. Man Cybern.*, 13:815–826.

20. Dichter, M., and Spencer, W. A. (1969): Penicillin-induced interictal discharges from the cat hippocampus. I. Characteristics and topographical features. *J Neurophysiol.*, 32:649–662.

21. Dichter, M., and Spencer, W. A. (1969): Penicillin-induced interictal discharges from the cat hippocampus. II. Mechanisms underlying origin and restriction. *J. Neurophysiol.*, 32:663–687.

22. Ellias, S. A., and Grossberg, S. (1975): Pattern formation, contrast control, and oscillations in the short term memory of shunting on-center off-surround networks. *Biol. Cybern.*, 20:69–98.

23. Evarts, E. V. (1984): Hierarchies and emergent features in motor control. In: *Dynamic Aspects of Neocortical Function*, edited by G. Edelman, W. E. Gall, and W. M. Cowan, pp. 557–579. John Wiley, New York.

24. Gray, R., and Johnston, D. (1985): Macroscopic calcium currents in acutely-exposed neurons from adult hippocampal slices. *Biophys. J.* 47:66a.

25. Griffith, W. H., Brown, T. H., and Johnston, D. (1985): Voltage-clamp analysis of synaptic inhibition during long-term potentiation in hippocampus. *J. Neurophysiol.* (in press).

26. Hablitz, J. J. (1984): Picrotoxin-induced epileptiform activity in the hippocampi: Role of endogenous versus synaptic factors. *J. Neurophysiol.*, 51:1011–1027.

27. Hablitz, J. J., and Johnston, D. (1981): The endogenous nature of spontaneous bursts in hippocampal pyramidal neurons. *Cell Mol. Neurobiol.*, 1:325–334.

28. Hopkins, W. F., and Johnston, D. (1984): Frequency-dependent noradrenergic modulation of long-term potentiation in the hippocampus. *Science*, 226:350–352.

29. Hotson, J. R., and Prince, D. A. (1980): A calcium-activated hyperpolarization follows repetitive firing in hippocampal neurons. *J. Neurophysiol.*, 43:409–419.

30. Johnston, D., and Brown, T. H. (1981): Giant synaptic potential hypothesis for epileptiform activity. *Science*, 211:294–297.

31. Johnston, D., and Brown, T. H. (1983): Interpretation of voltage clamp measurements in hippocampal neurons. *J. Neurophysiol.*, 50:464–486.

32. Johnston, D., and Brown, T. H. (1984): Bio-

physics and microphysiology of synaptic transmission in hippocampus. In: *Brain Slices*, edited by R. Dingledine, pp. 51–86. Plenum Press, New York.

33. Johnston, D., and Brown, T. H. (1984): Mechanisms of neuronal burst generation. In: *Electrophysiology of Epilepsy*, edited by P. A. Schwartzkroin and H. Wheal, pp. 277–301. Academic Press, New York.

34. Johnston, D., and Brown, T. H. (1984): The synaptic nature of the paroxysmal depolarizing shift in hippocampal neurons. *Ann Neurol.*, 16:S65–S71.

35. Johnston, D., and Hablitz, J. J. (1979): Voltage clamp analysis of CA3 neurons in hippocampal slices. *Soc. Neurosci. Abstr.*, 5:292.

36. Johnston, D., Hablitz, J. J., and Wilson, W. A. (1980): Voltage clamp discloses slow inward current in hippocampal burst-firing neurones. *Nature*, 286:391–393.

37. Kandel, E. R., and Spencer, W. A. (1961): Electrophysiology of hippocampal neurons. II. Afterpotentials and repetitive firing. *J. Neurophysiol.*, 24:243–259.

38. Kandel, E. R., and Spencer, W. A. (1961): Excitation and inhibition of single pyramidal cells during hippocampal seizure. *Exp. Neurol.*, 4:162–179.

39. Kandel, E. R., Spencer, W. A., and Brinley, F. J. (1961): Electrophysiology of hippocampal neurons. I. Sequential invasion and synaptic organization. *J. Neurophysiol.*, 24:225–242.

40. Kitatsuji, Y., and Kuroda, T. (1983): Statistical study on reverberation between two mutually excitatory neuron groups. *J. Theor. Biol.*, 100:25–55.

41. Knowles, W. D., and Schwartzkroin, P. A. (1981): Local circuit synaptic interactions in hippocampal brain slices. *J. Neurosci.*, 1:318–322.

42. Lebeda, F. J., Rutecki, P. A., Brown, T. H., and Johnston, D. (1985): Large synaptic currents during epileptiform activity in the hippocampus (in preparation).

43. Lebeda, F. J., Hablitz, J. J., and Johnston, D. (1982): Antagonism of GABA-mediated responses by *d*-tubocurarine in hippocampal neurons. *J. Neurophysiol.*, 48:622–632.

44. Lebeda, F. J., Rutecki, P. A., and Johnston, D. (1983): Synaptic mechanisms of action of convulsion-producing anticholinesterases: Characterization of di-isopropyl phosphorofluoridate-induced epileptiform activity in the mammalian hippocampus. U.S. Army Medical Research and Development Command. Report No. 1.

45. Lebeda, F. J., Rutecki, P. A., and Johnston, D. (1984): Synaptic mechanisms of action of convulsion-producing anticholinesterases: Further characterization of organophosphate-induced epileptiform activity in the mammalian hippocampus. U.S. Army Medical Research and Development Command. Report No. 2.

46. Lebovitz, R. M., Dichter, M., and Spencer, W. A. (1971): Recurrent excitation in the CA3 region of cat hippocampus. *Int. J. Neurosci.*, 2:99–108.

47. MacVicar, B. A., and Dudek, F. E. (1980): Local synaptic circuits in rat hippocampus: Interactions between pyramidal cells. *Brain Res.,* 184:220–223.

48. Martin, T. P., and Taylor, J. G. (1973): Solutions of probabilistic equations for neural networks. *Int. J. Neurosci.,* 6:7–16.

49. Matsumoto, H., and Ajmone Marsan, C. (1964): Cortical cellular phenomena in experimental epilepsy: Interictal manifestations. *Exp. Neurol.,* 9:286–304.

50. Matsumoto, H., and Ajmone Marsan, C. (1964): Cortical cellular phenomena in experimental epilepsy: Ictal manifestations. *Exp. Neurol.,* 9:305–326.

51. Matsumoto, H., Ayala, G. F., and Gumnit, R. J. (1969): Neuronal behavior and triggering mechanism in cortical epileptic focus. *J. Neurophysiol.,* 32:688–703.

52. Meech, R. W. (1978): Calcium-dependent potassium activation in nervous tissue. *Annu. Rev. Biophys. Bioeng.,* 7:1–18.

53. Miles, R., Wong, R. K. S., and Traub, R. D. (1985): Synchronized afterdischarges in the hippocampus: contribution of local synaptic interactions. *Neuroscience* (in press).

54. Palmay, F. V., Davison, E. J., and Duffin, J. (1974): The simulation of multi-neurone networks: Modelling of the lateral inhibition of the eye and the generation of respiratory rhythm. *Bull. Math. Biol.,* 36:77–89.

55. Perkel, D. H., and Mulloney, B. (1974): Motor pattern production in reciprocally inhibitory neurons exhibiting postinhibitory rebound. *Science,* 185:181–182.

56. Prince, D. A. (1966): Modification of focal cortical epileptogenic discharge by afferent influences. *Epilepsia,* 7:181–201.

57. Prince, D. A. (1968): The depolarization shift in "epileptic" neurons. *Exp. Neurol.,* 21:467–485.

58. Prince, D. A. (1978): Neurophysiology of epilepsy. *Annu. Rev. Neurosci.,* 1:395–415.

59. Prince, D. A., and Connors, B. W. (1984): Mechanisms of epileptogenesis in cortical structures. *Ann. Neurol.,* 16:S59–S64.

60. Rutecki, P. A., Lebeda, F. J., and Johnston, D. (1985): Epileptiform activity induced by changes in extracellular potassium in hippocampus. *J. Neurophysiol.,* 54:1363–1374.

61. Schwartzkroin, P. A. (1975): Characteristics of CA1 neurons recorded intracellularly in the hippocampal *in vitro* slice preparation. *Brain Res.,* 85:423–436. ·

62. Schwartzkroin, P. A. (1977): Further characteristics of hippocampal CA1 cells *in vitro.* *Brain Res.,* 128:53–68.

63. Schwartzkroin, P. A., and Prince, D. A. (1978): Cellular and field potential properties of epileptic hippocampal slices. *Brain Res.,* 147:117–130.

64. Schwartzkroin, P. A., and Prince, D. A. (1980): Changes in excitatory and inhibitory synaptic potentials leading to epileptogenic activity. *Brain Res.,* 183:61–76.

65. Schwartzkroin, P. A., and Slawsky, M. (1977): Probable calcium spikes in hippocampal neurons. *Brain Res.,* 135:157–161.

66. Schwartzkroin, P. A., and Wyler, A. R. (1980): Mechanisms underlying epileptiform burst discharge. *Ann Neurol.,* 7:95–107.

67. Sperry, R. W. (1980): Mind-brain interaction: Mentalism, yes; dualism, no. *Neuroscience,* 5:195–206.

68. Swanson, L. W., Tyler, T. J., and Thompson, R. F. (1982): Hippocampal long-term potentiation: Mechanisms and implications for memory. *Neurosci. Res. Program Bull.,* 20:613–769.

69. Traub, R. D., Knowles, W. D., Miles, R., and Wong, R. K. S. (1985): Synchronized afterdischarges in the hippocampus: Simulation studies of the cellular mechanism. *Neuroscience* (in press).

70. Traub, R. D., and Wong, R. K. S. (1982): Cellular mechanism of neuronal synchronization in epilepsy. *Science,* 216:745–747.

71. Traub, R. D., and Wong, R. K. S. (1983): Synchronized burst discharge in disinhibited hippocampal slice. II. Model of cellular mechanism. *J. Neurophysiol.,* 49:442–458.

72. Wilson, W. A., and Goldner, M. M. (1975): Voltage clamping with a single microelectrode. *J. Neurobiol.,* 6:411–422.

73. Wong, R. K. S., Miles, R., and Traub, R. D. (1984): Local circuit interactions in synchronization of cortical neurons. *J. Exp. Biol.,* 112:169–178.

74. Wong, R. K. S., and Prince, D. A. (1978): Participation of calcium spikes during intrinsic burst firing in hippocampal neurons. *Brain Res.,* 159:385–390.

75. Wong, R. K. S., and Prince, D. A. (1979): Dendritic mechanisms underlying penicillin-induced epileptiform activity. *Science,* 204:1228–1230.

76. Wong, R. K. S., and Prince, D. A. (1981): Afterpotential generation in hippocampal pyramidal cells. *J. Neurophysiol.,* 45:86–97.

77. Wong, R. K. S., Prince, D. A., and Basbaum, A. I. (1974): Intradendritic recordings from hippocampal neurons. *Proc. Natl. Acad. Sci. USA,* 76:986–990.

78. Wong, R. K. S., and Schwartzkroin, P. A. (1982): Pacemaker neurons in the mammalian brain: Mechanisms and function. In: *Cellular Pacemakers,* vol. 1, edited by D. O. Carpenter, pp. 237–254. John Wiley, New York.

Advances in Neurology, Vol. 44, edited by
A. V. Delgado-Escueta, A. A. Ward, Jr.,
D. M. Woodbury, and R. J. Porter.
Raven Press, New York © 1986.

13

Mechanisms of Interictal Epileptogenesis

David A. Prince and Barry W. Connors

From the Department of Neurology, Stanford University School of Medicine, Stanford, California 94305

SUMMARY The interictal discharge is a brief epileptiform event that provides the simplest experimental system available for investigating some of the basic mechanisms of epilepsy. Interictal discharges are characterized by two major abnormal properties: each involved neuron exhibits a transient large amplitude depolarization (the "depolarization shift") associated with repetitive spike generation, and this excitation arises with virtual synchrony in the majority of cells in a local population. Recent studies have attempted to define the cellular properties that predispose a cortical circuit to this pathological behavior. There appear to be three general factors that interactively determine cortical susceptibility to epilepsy:

1. Intrinsic membrane properties of neurons. The intrinsic excitability of individual cells may vary greatly within a cortical area; the initiation of a synchronous discharge usually occurs in the subpopulation of cells that has the endogenous ability to generate bursts of action potentials.
2. Efficacy of local inhibitory synaptic mechanisms. Normal integrative functions of the cortex require robust inhibition; depression of inhibition is one of the most reliable ways to trigger a seizure.
3. Effectiveness of excitatory synaptic connections and other synchronizing mechanisms. Highly synchronized discharge among a large number of neurons requires widely divergent excitatory interactions.

Differences in these factors for different cortical areas can confer relative susceptibility or resistance to development of epileptiform discharge. Pharmacologic, pathologic, developmental, and genetic processes can presumably mitigate or aggravate focal cortical epileptogenesis by affecting any of these three general factors.

Since the meeting in Colorado Springs in 1968 that led to the first volume on basic mechanisms of the epilepsies (56), we have learned much more about the cellular mechanisms that normally regulate the excitability of groups of neurons in the cortex, and the disorders of function that occur during epileptogenesis. Various aspects of this problem are considered in recent

reviews and symposia (4,5,19,98–103,105,106, 119,126).

In this chapter, we review the cellular mechanisms of interictal epileptogenesis. To put the experimental studies in proper perspective, it is important to consider some definitions and common clinical phenomenology of epilepsy. It will also be useful to discuss normal cortical organization, patterns of connectivity, and the modulation of neuronal electrophysiological properties as a background for examining changes that render cortices epileptogenic. Finally, we will describe the types of abnormality that give rise to synchronous interictal discharges in experimental systems and speculate about the pathophysiological alterations that might lead to epileptogenesis following naturally occurring injuries or other events.

CLINICAL DEFINITIONS AND ISSUES

Ordinarily the neurologist distinguishes between focal *interictal* and *ictal* seizure activity. During the interictal period, the electroencephalogram (EEG) shows brief single paroxysmal waves, termed interictal spikes, that are not accompanied by obvious behavioral manifestations of the seizure. Each interictal epileptiform discharge has widespread consequences, even for aggregates of neurons at sites distant from the area of focal abnormality (16,41,96,97). This may explain why closely spaced interictal events can produce a subtle behavioral disturbance (90,129). From time to time an electrographic ictal episode may occur, characterized by a more continuous EEG epileptiform abnormality and associated with a stereotyped behavioral disturbance followed by a postictal period of disturbed function. In this chapter, we will focus on the mechanisms underlying interictal discharges. It is important to note, however, that the factors leading to the transition from interictal to ictal activity or to sustained ictal discharge may be somewhat different from those that initiate the interictal discharge in the first place (103).

Epilepsy is a symptom of disordered brain function, rather than a disease itself. This implies that multiple etiologies can give rise to clinical epilepsy. However, it is not known whether all forms of epilepsy in humans have the same common mechanism at the cellular level. Such a generalization appears unlikely, since seizures follow a wide variety of pathological processes, including trauma, genetic defects, tumors, metabolic derangements and toxicological events, which presumably have widely different effects on the anatomy, chemistry, and excitability of neurons and their connections.

Despite the remarkable advances in neuroscience over the past decade, the answers to many of the critical problems in epilepsy are still very incomplete. For example, the mechanisms for development of posttraumatic epilepsy, and the reasons for the long latency that often intervenes between the time of injury and the time of development of seizures, remain unclear. At present, we cannot predict which brain injuries will lead to focal epileptogenesis and which will not. There is a well-known differential susceptibility to epileptogenesis in different brain regions; some recent data allow speculations about the reasons for these differences. We know that there is a strong hereditary component in certain forms of epilepsy; however, the techniques for studying genetic regulation of neuronal excitability have not yet been applied to the problem of inherited epilepsies in animals and in humans. Another critical relationship is that of epilepsy and brain development. The effects of epileptogenesis on anatomic, physiologic, and metabolic development of immature neuronal systems are largely unknown. Although it seems likely that mechanisms of epileptogenesis will vary between immature and mature brain, incomplete information is available in this area as well. Other problems of great interest are the mechanisms for transition between interictal and ictal discharge and the ways in which epileptic discharge influences normal brain function or gives rise to nerve cell death.

PRINCIPLES OF NORMAL CORTICAL STRUCTURE AND FUNCTION

Clinical epilepsy is largely a condition of telencephalic cortical structures. Epileptogenesis may thus be one of the risks that higher vertebrates have had to balance against the advantages conferred by the cortical circuit. Although subcortical or humoral influences may trigger or modulate seizure discharges, local cortical circuitry is both necessary and sufficient to support synchronized paroxysms. For example, even when surgically separated from surrounding neural tissue, islands of neocortex can display rhythmic seizures when chemically or electrically stimulated (65). When reduced even further, to thin slices maintained *in vitro*, tissues from hippocampus (152), neocortex (21,40), and olfactory cortex (37) still generate convulsant-induced synchronized bursts. These autonomous behaviors are basically similar in each cortical area. We may infer, then, that: (a) cortical structures per se have all of the properties necessary to initiate and propagate epileptiform activity; and (b) these properties are likely to be similar in different cortical structures. An examination of the specific and general characteristics of cortical neurons and their local connections will be necessary in defining the mechanisms of cortical epileptogenesis.

As an initial characterization, we may describe a cortical circuit in terms of the types of neurons, defined by their shapes and membrane properties, and the synaptic connections, defined by their physiological consequence and cellular location. At this admittedly myopic level of analysis, certain general principles of cortical structure nevertheless reveal themselves.

Morphology and Circuitry of Cortical Neurons

Traditionally, cortical neurons have been grouped into two general classes, pyramidal cells and nonpyramidal, or stellate, cells. Pyramidal cells are the principal cortical neurons; that is, they constitute the majority of cells, they are generally the largest, and their axons project out of the cortex as well as ramify locally. Nonpyramidal cells are a diverse group, with axons largely restricted to a local cortical region. These simple designations belie a wide array of neuronal subtypes within each group, each cortex, and across species. The labels "pyramidal" and "stellate" are not meant to imply evolutionary homologies or similarities of function (130). As we shall see, cells within a group can behave very differently. Nevertheless, for the sake of comparison, there is heuristic value in these distinctions.

Cortical pyramidal cells usually have a distinctive morphology, which includes a prominent apical dendrite extending toward the pia, a high density of spinous dendritic processes and a long projection axon (109). Thus, superficial and deep pyramidal cells of olfactory cortex, pyramidal cells and dentate granule cells of hippocampus, and pyramidal cells of all neocortical areas meet these criteria. There are exceptions to these rules; for example, some superficial neocortical pyramidal cells lack a prominent apical dendrite. Of paramount importance, however, is the observation that all cortical pyramidal cells possess axons with excitatory synaptic endings. This implies that pyramidal cell activity yields projected excitation as well as direct local excitation, within the sphere of influence defined by local axon ramifications. The relevance of this to epilepsy is profound.

Nonpyramidal cells of cortex have been variously subdivided based on overall shape, ultrastructure, and immunohistochemical character (91). The best defined of these is the group of cells that stains positively for glutamic acid decarboxylase (GAD) immunoreactivity, a trait that is very probably linked with the synthesis and utilization of the inhibitory transmitter γ-aminobutyric acid (GABA) (114). GAD-staining neurons are common in all cortical areas, and have aspinous, or poorly spinous, dendrites of various configurations (110). Their importance in epileptogenesis cannot be overemphasized. Suppression of their efficacy, by any of a variety of means, is one of the simplest methods of inducing seizures.

A variety of nonpyramidal cells in cortical structures may subserve an excitatory function. These include the spiny multipolar cells of neocortical layer IV (143) and some of the nonspiny bipolar cells, which are immunoreactive for vasoactive intestinal polypeptide (VIP) or cholecystokinin (CCK) (33). The latter two peptides are potent neuronal excitants. The evidence for excitatory interneurons in all cortical areas is entirely morphological, and their relevance to normal function and epileptogenesis is obscure. As more data become available, however, it will be of great interest to examine the role of excitatory interneurons in paroxysmal activity. For example, the terminals of both CCK- and VIP-immunoreactive neurons associate intimately with cerebral blood vessels (31,47), raising the possibility that they mediate between neuronal function and local blood flow.

Figure 1A illustrates simplified and qualitative aspects of synaptic connectivity in olfactory cortex, hippocampus, and neocortex. The general cell types are schematized, with the exception of the enigmatic excitatory interneurons. The flow of neural activity begins with a set, or sets, of afferent axons that arise in extracortical or association areas. In olfactory cortex, these may be lateral olfactory tract axons; in neocortex, they may be thalamocortical afferents. In the latter case, most fibers do not enter via the superficial layers (as illustrated in Fig. 1), but penetrate radially from the subcortical white matter. In all cases, however, monosynaptic excitatory connections are formed with the dendrites of pyramidal cells, which in turn send their axons out of the local cortical region. Imposed upon this simple relay scheme is a set of local synaptic interactions that largely define the uniqueness of each cortical circuit.

A very common, if not universal, feature of cortices is reciprocal excitation between pyramidal cells. It has been proposed for opossum pyriform cortex (43) and demonstrated directly in the CA3–CA4 region of rat hippocampus (77), but not in the CA1 hippocampal area of guinea pigs (61). The evidence for direct excitatory interactions between pyramidal cells in neocortex is compelling. Lorente de No (76) commented on the widespread occurrence of recurrent axon collaterals from pyramidal cells, and physiolog-

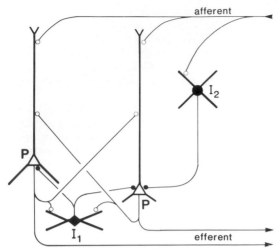

FIG. 1. Simplified schematic diagram of local cortical circuitry. Telencephalic cortical structures are primarily composed of pyramidal cells (P) and stellate-shaped interneurons (I). Afferent axons make excitatory synaptic contacts (open circles) with the dendrites of both types of cells. The axons of pyramidal cells project out of the cortex (efferents) as well as locally. *Recurrent excitation* of pyramidal cells can be mediated by these local contacts. *Recurrent inhibition* is generated by inhibitory interneurons, such as I_1, that are excited by pyramidal cells and, in turn, make inhibitory contacts (closed circles) with pyramidal cells. Interneurons such as I_2 may be directly excited by afferent input, and induce a *feed-forward inhibition* of pyramids.

ical experiments in pyramidal tract cells (94,137) suggest that these collaterals make direct contact with adjacent pyramidal cells. Direct electrical synapses between pyramidal cell dendrites have also been hypothesized (42), based upon the cell–cell movement of intracellularly injected dyes. These chemical and electrical interactions may serve to spread and synchronize excitation locally.

Two general forms of inhibition have been repeatedly hypothesized for mammalian cortices. In the first, afferent axons directly excite both principle cells and a class of inhibitory interneurons (I_2 in Fig. 1); the interneurons then feed-forward onto the principal cells, thus rapidly terminating the initial excitation induced by an afferent volley. Physiological evidence for this mechanism has been reported for pyriform cortex (43) and the CA1 area of hippocampus (2,108). The data for neocortex are indirect, but very suggestive of the feed-forward scheme. The requisite anatomic circuitry appears to be present, in that thalamocortical axons terminate on the dendrites of presumed inhibitory inter-

neurons (38), and the interneurons then form direct connections with pyramidal cells (25,92). When afferents are electrically stimulated, the timing of excitation to identified interneurons (78) and the inhibitory postsynaptic potential (IPSP) latency in pyramidal cells (139) are also compatible. The significance and generality of feed-forward inhibitory circuitry are unknown. A better-documented form of inhibition is that mediated by feedback, or recurrent circuits. Collaterals from principal cells may directly excite a set of interneurons (I_1 in Fig. 1), which in turn inhibit the same or other principal cells. In olfactory cortex, recurrent IPSPs appear to be the dominant form of inhibition evoked by afferent excitation (12,44,116). Recurrent inhibition is also very prominent in hippocampus (3) and neocortex (94,134). The soma-dendritic morphology of the cells mediating cortical inhibition is diverse but well described (52,59,93,112,113). Unfortunately, the details of their synaptic connections with pyramidal cells, and among themselves, is very poorly understood. New anatomical methodologies are just beginning to address this important set of questions (cf. ref. 132).

Cortical structures are influenced by several other extrinsic and intrinsic neurotransmitter systems, including adrenergic, serotonergic, cholinergic, and several peptidergic innervations (33). Their relative densities in each cortical area may vary greatly. Most of these appear to have a relatively slowly acting modulatory role on cortical activity. Little is known about their potential role in epileptogenesis; however, their relatively widespread and long-term actions lead to speculations regarding possible roles in the initiation, spread, or termination of seizure activity.

Electrophysiology of Cortical Neurons

Although the synaptic circuitry of a cortical area is critical to its function, the intrinsic properties of its neurons are equally important. The modern view of nerve membrane excitability was inspired by the seminal analysis of the squid axon by Hodgkin and Huxley (48). However, subsequent work has shown that axons, whose membranes are dominated by one type of sodium channel and one type of potassium channel, are much simpler physiologically than central neurons. A large variety of voltage- and chemical-sensitive membrane channels, complex dendritic geometries, and diverse intercellular relationships yield a vast and flexible repertoire of central neuronal function in mammals (see refs. 23 and 73 for reviews). The electro-physiological behavior of neurons in different brain areas may vary greatly; within a particular brain area, neurons with dissimilar morphological features may also exhibit very different membrane properties. It is even possible for two neurons of apparently identical morphology to have disparate membrane properties. In any case, a knowledge of the intrinsic physiological characteristics of cortical neurons plays a central role in our understanding of the genesis of epileptiform discharge.

Figure 2 illustrates some of the diversity of cortical neuronal properties. Within the hippocampus, the various principal cell types have consistently different action potential characteristics. Dentate granule cells (Fig. 2) are rather conventional, with sodium-dependent spikes, a monotonic relationship between action potential frequency and intracellularly injected current, and very little calcium current (35). Pyramidal cells of the CA3a area are strikingly different; at a critical voltage threshold, most cells display an all-or-none burst of several action potentials

(Fig. 2) (60,145,148). This intrinsically generated spike burst consists of both sodium-dependent fast spikes and more slowly rising calcium-dependent electrogenesis (58,145). Thus, the output frequency of a CA3 pyramid can be an abruptly discontinuous function of the input current. CA1 pyramidal cells are intermediate in their membrane properties. Some of them can burst, whereas most generate only fast sodium spikes with prominent depolarizing afterpotentials (79,118). Some hippocampal stellate cells possess yet another mode of spiking—their action potentials are uniquely fast, they can fire repetitively at exceptionally high rates, and they do not burst in an all-or-none fashion (Fig. 2) (121). There may also be electrophysiologically distinctive subtypes of hippocampal interneurons (84).

Within neocortex, a similar spectrum of neuronal properties has been found. Most pyramidal cell recordings are reminiscent of hippocampal CA1 or dentate granule cells (Fig. 2) (22,136). Intrinsic bursts of action potentials similar to those of hippocampal CA3a cells occur in a

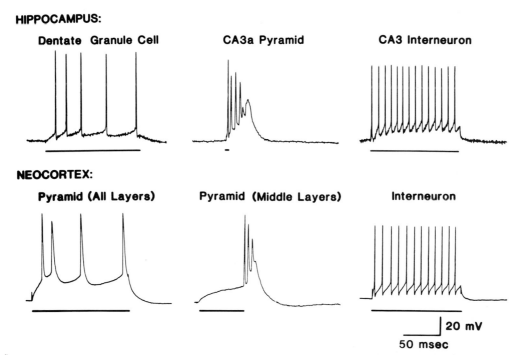

FIG. 2. Comparative electrophysiology of mammalian cortical neurons. Membrane potentials were recorded intracellularly and suprathreshold current pulses were delivered during the times represented by the horizontal lines. Three basic types of behavior are observed in both hippocampus and neocortex. Many of the principle cells (e.g., dentate granule and most neocortical pyramidal cells) generate trains of simple action potentials; the frequency of firing adapts, or slows down, when stimulating current is maintained. Some principal cells (e.g., CA3a pyramidal cells and some neocortical pyramids of the middle layers) generate an intrinsic burst of action potentials that can outlast the duration of the stimulus. In both cortices, inhibitory interneurons have uniquely fast action potentials and the ability to fire at high frequency without adaptation.

small subpopulation of cells located only in middle layers (Fig. 2) (18). Intracellular dye injections have revealed that the bursting neurons can be either pyramidal cells (77a) or spiny stellate neurons (M. J. Gutnick and E. L. White, *personal communication*). A third distinct type of recording closely resembles that obtained from the interneurons of hippocampus (Fig. 2); such cells occur in all layers, and labeling studies show that they correspond to sparsely spiny stellates (77a). In general, the array of neocortical cell membrane properties resembles that of hippocampus, although the prevalence of bursting neurons appears to be much lower in neocortex.

Intracellular recordings from pyramidal neurons of olfactory cortex have not revealed intrinsic bursting tendencies (12,20,117). Pyramidal cell properties closely resemble those of typical nonbursting neocortical pyramidal cells (cf. ref. 18). It is unfortunate that there are few biophysical studies of olfactory cortical neurons; further experiments may reveal membrane heterogeneity. Stellate interneurons that presumably mediate GABAergic inhibition have been recorded from, and their characteristics are consistent with, identified interneurons of other cortical areas (116).

The neuronal membrane properties of a cortical region correlate closely with its general susceptibility toward seizures (discussed below). Pharmacologic and ionic manipulations of these properties may bias the epileptogenicity of a network of neurons. We can therefore expect that further information about the genetic, pathologic, and pharmacologic control of intrinsic excitability will be invaluable to our understanding of the genesis, prevention, and treatment of epilepsy.

MECHANISMS OF CORTICAL EPILEPTOGENESIS

A variety of experimental studies indicate that the electrographic hallmark of focal epilepsy, the interictal spike of the electroencephalographer, is associated with long-duration, large-amplitude depolarizations that elicit bursts of action potentials in a large number of neurons within the focus (see refs. 1,98,101,102 for reviews). These events, termed paroxysmal depolarization shifts by Matsumoto and Ajmone Marsan (81), occur in all acute foci such as those produced by strychnine (71) and penicillin (81); in acute freeze foci (39); and in chronic epileptogenic foci of monkey (104) and humans (107). It is there-

fore important to consider several different issues regarding the generation of these potentials. First, what is the nature of the membrane events underlying the depolarization shift (DS)? What sorts of neuronal dysfunction might give rise to such synchronous behavior in a large aggregate of neurons? Also, where are the sites of origin of focal epileptiform discharge within the cortex, what factors determine them, and why are some cortical sites more susceptible to epileptogenesis than others?

The advantages of the *in vitro* cortical slice preparation and its application to studies of epileptogenesis (122,152), have led to a more detailed understanding of the basic mechanisms underlying epileptogenic discharge. There are, however, some limitations in the use of this preparation, including loss of modulatory synaptic connectivity and influences from distant and surrounding structures (e.g., most cholinergic and all of the dopaminergic, noradrenergic, and serotonergic inputs to cortex are derived from subcortical nuclei), and absence of humoral influences. Fortunately, most of the phenomenology of epileptogenesis *in vivo* can be recapitulated *in vitro,* including spontaneous interictal events (122), interictal–ictal transitions (37), associated changes in extracellular ionic environment (11; see Chapter 32) and persistence *in vitro* of abnormalities associated with chronic epileptogenesis (72,107).

Studies of hippocampal and neocortical slice preparations have furnished a detailed view of neuronal function during epileptogenesis (4,5,17,37,40,50,57,107,122,124,125,140, 141,146, 149). The most specific hypotheses have arisen from studies of a particular model of focal epileptogenesis: interictal discharges induced by GABA antagonists in mammalian cortices. Although this model is somewhat restricted in scope, it has yielded very important general principles that we will discuss in detail. The data suggest that several interacting factors determine whether a given population of neurons will become involved in epileptogenesis. These factors include: (a) the intrinsic membrane properties of individual neurons and neuronal capacities to generate pacemaker-like slow depolarizations; (b) the loss of inhibitory control mechanisms within the neuronal aggregate (disinhibition); and (c) the intensity of excitatory coupling among members of the neuronal population. A consideration of these variables serves as a framework for understanding differences in the susceptibility to epileptogenesis in different brain areas, and leads to predictions about the kinds of underlying abnormality by which a given pathological process in the brain might give rise to epilepsy.

Intrinsic Membrane Properties in Epileptogenesis

As Hughlings Jackson predicted in 1870 (54), focal epileptogenesis is characterized by intense and synchronous activity in large groups of neurons within the cortex. The mechanisms by which amplified and synchronized activities occur involve a complex interaction between the intrinsic membrane properties of individual neurons and the network properties of the population of neurons. Data indicate that the membranes of central nervous system (CNS) neurons possess a variety of voltage-dependent conductances that will modify their responses and, under some circumstances, serve to amplify the synaptic signals and increase neuronal output. For example, in some cells, subthreshold slow conductances for Na^+, Ca^{2+}, and K^+ are activated as the membrane is depolarized toward firing level; these conductances may influence the amplitude of synaptic potentials. Figure 3A illustrates a current–voltage (I/V) plot for a neuron

from a human cortical slice. As the neuron is depolarized (right upper quadrant), a nonlinearity develops in the I/V relationship. This is presumably a consequence of the activation of voltage-dependent ion channels. As can be seen in the inset of Fig. 3 (upper left quadrant), depolarizing current pulses tend to produce a larger change in membrane potential than do hyperpolarizing ones of similar amplitude, because of the addition of an active slow depolarizing component to the passive membrane response. In guinea pig and cat cortical neurons, this depolarizing anomalous rectification is caused by activation of a subthreshold slow Na^+ conductance (18,133). In hippocampal neurons, in which depolarizing rectification has been compared in dendrites and somata (7,49), it appears that the slow voltage-dependent depolarization is predominantly caused by a Ca^{2+} conductance in dendrites and a Na^+ conductance in the cell body. The data of Fig. 3B show that blockade of voltage-dependent Na^+ channels in hippocampal neurons by intracellular injection of QX-314, a local anesthetic, eliminates depolarizing anomalous rectification in the cell body, but not in dendrites (cf. depolarizing versus hy-

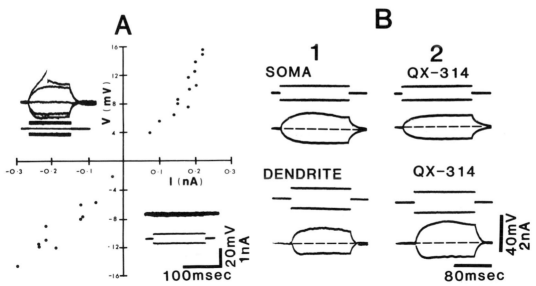

FIG. 3. Subthreshold voltage-dependent conductances in cortical **(A)** and hippocampal **(B)** neurons. A: I/V plot from neuron of human neocortical slice. Membrane shows apparent increase in resistance in the depolarizing quadrant due to development of inward rectification. *Upper inset:* representative traces show that responses to depolarizing current pulses are larger than those to equal hyperpolarizing current pulses. *Lower inset:* Responses to similar current pulses outside the neuron. **B:** Representative responses of soma and dendrite of hippocampal CA1 pyramidal cells to equal and opposite current pulses under normal conditions (1) and in elements impaled with electrodes containing QX-314 (2). Responses to depolarizing current are larger in somata and dendrites (1). The inward depolarizing rectification is blocked in somata but not dendrites by QX-314 **(B2).** Each frame is from a different neuron. A from Prince and Wong, unpublished observations; B from Benardo et al. (7) with permission.

perpolarizing responses to current in B1 and B2).

The potential importance of subthreshold activation of slow Na^+ or Ca^{2+} conductances is shown in Fig. 4. The recording of Fig. 4A is from a neuron in the area of chronic cortical epileptogenesis produced by a local freeze lesion and subsequently studied *in vitro* (72). The excitatory postsynaptic potential (EPSP) evoked at resting potential has a slower falling phase than the EPSP elicited by the same stimulus when the membrane is hyperpolarized (cf. traces 1 and 2). At times, the EPSP evoked at rest is larger in amplitude and markedly prolonged (trace 4), resulting in spike generation (trace 3). Figure 4 (A2 − 1 and A4 − 1), derived by subtracting trace 1 from trace 2, and trace 1 from trace 4, respectively, show that the EPSP has evoked a slow membrane depolarization which, in this instance, lasted longer than 50 msec and reached an amplitude of about 20 mV (A4 − 1). Similar EPSPs containing active components have also been recorded from isolated hippocampal dendrites (80). In the dendrite of Fig. 4B, depolarization allowed the EPSP to evoke a slow voltage-dependent component (Fig. 4B, cf. traces 1 and 2) that is seen in isolation in the subtracted trace of Fig. 4B, 1 − 2. From these observations, it appears that synaptically evoked membrane depolarizations may activate intrinsic membrane currents in the subthreshold voltage region, and that the intrinsic currents may increase the probability that a cell will fire to a given input. Similar findings have been reported in Purkinje cells (74). The effect of these inward currents may be modified by the simultaneous activation of synaptic inhibition, or when the cell membrane possesses significant voltage-dependent K^+ conductances that are activated by depolarization in the subthreshold range. Under conditions in which inhibition or K^+ conductances are depressed, the synaptically evoked, intrinsic "booster" currents would become much more effective in bringing the neuron to its firing threshold.

Application of convulsant agents such as penicillin, bicuculline, or picrotoxin (all of which are GABA antagonists) to the *in vitro* hippocampal or neocortical slice produces a significant change in spontaneous and evoked activities. As

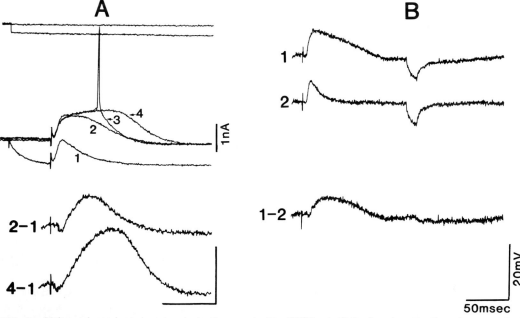

FIG. 4. Voltage-dependent slow depolarizations evoked by EPSPs. **A:** Orthodromic activation of a neocortical neuron in the area of a freeze lesion elicits an EPSP at hyperpolarized membrane potentials (trace 1) and EPSPs with variable duration slow falling phase at resting membrane potential (traces 2 and 4). Evoked slow depolarizations sometimes reaches threshold for spike generation (trace 3). Results of subtraction of trace 1 from trace 2 and trace 4, respectively (2 − 1 and 4 − 1). From Lighthall and Prince, unpublished observations **B:** Orthodromic responses from a dendrite at resting V_m (B2) and following DC depolarization of V_m by about 15 mV (B1). Subtraction of trace 2 from trace 1 (1 − 2). Orthodromic stimuli in traces 1 and 2 are identical. Evoked responses are followed by electrotonic responses to hyperpolarizing current pulses in 1 and 2. Calibrations in **A** are 50 msec and 20 mV; **B** from Masukawa and Prince, (80), with permission.

shown in Fig. 5A, the single peak field potential recorded in the pyramidal cell layer of the hippocampus following stimulation of afferents (A1) becomes multipeaked (A2) after the addition of penicillin. Intracellular recordings show that most neurons generate large-amplitude DSs and spike bursts coincident with the spontaneous or evoked epileptiform field potentials (Fig. 5C). These characteristics are similar to those of penicillin foci within the hippocampus *in vivo*. The potential for initiating interictal activity is not the same for all hippocampal areas. As shown in Fig. 5B1, spontaneous epileptiform events always begin in the CA2–CA3 pyramidal region and propagate into the CA1 area (123,149). Recordings from pairs of neurons in these two areas confirm that the onset of DS generation in CA2–CA3 pyramidal neurons leads that in CA1 cells (Fig. 5C). When connec-

tions between CA3 and CA1 pyramidal regions are cut, the CA2–CA3 region continues to generate spontaneous interictal discharges, whereas the CA1 region becomes silent (Fig. 5B2). Electrical stimulation of the synaptic pathway onto CA1 cells distal to the cut may, however, elicit epileptiform DSs in the CA1 neuron population (123). In a study of picrotoxin-treated hippocampal slices, the isolated CA1 area discharged spontaneously (as it may *in situ*; cf. ref. 26), but was still paced by CA3 when the slice was left intact (45). These observations suggest two conclusions: (a) that both areas of hippocampus are capable of generating interictal discharge, but that the CA2–CA3 area is intrinsically more excitable than CA1; and (b) that discharge in the CA2–CA3 region is capable of initiating a synchronized interictal discharge in CA1, presumably through a collateral system of excitatory connections.

What are the properties of the CA3 area that render it the pacemaker for epileptogenic activity in hippocampus? The most important factor may be the intrinsic characteristics of its neuronal membranes. The behavior of typical region CA3a pyramidal neurons is shown in Fig. 6. At resting membrane potential, such cells generate intrinsic rhythmic burst activity (6A) that is dependent on the membrane potential and can be blocked either by membrane depolarization (Fig. 6B) or hyperpolarization (not shown). Brief depolarizing pulses (Fig. 6C1), can elicit a slow depolarization and spike burst in these cells (see also Fig. 2B), but stimulation of synaptic inputs is ordinarily not effective (146,148). As is shown in Fig. 6C2, following a directly evoked spike, there may occur a prolonged depolarizing afterpotential (DAP). The latter may serve as a generator for the the next spike in the burst. The DAP, the slow, high-threshold spikes associated with the burst, and the underlying slow depolarization are thought to be mediated largely by Ca^{2+} (58,145,147). Slowly activating Na^+ currents also probably contribute to intrinsic slow depolarizations (49), but their importance is not well established. Both cell bodies and dendrites of CA3a pacemaker neurons appear to have burst-generating properties (148). The termination of the slow depolarization and burst discharge is accompanied by a large afterhyperpolarization (Fig. 6A) that is probably owing to some combination of Ca^{2+} mediated K^+ conductance, voltage-dependent K^+ conductances, or perhaps even inactivation of inward Ca^{2+} currents by accumulation of Ca^{2+} within the neuron (32).

The coincident location of uniquely strong in-

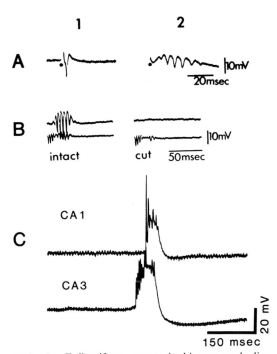

FIG. 5. Epileptiform events in hippocampal slice treated with penicillin. A: Extracellular response in normal solution (1) and following development of epileptiform field potential (2). **Dots:** Single stimuli to stratum radiatum. B: Spontaneous multipeaked field potentials in CA1 (upper trace) and CA3 (lower trace) regions. In intact slice (**B1**) epileptiform discharge in CA3 always leads that in CA1. **B2:** Recordings of field potentials after cut between CA3 and CA1. C: Simultaneous recordings from a pair of CA1 and CA3 pyramidal neurons. **A** from Schwartzkroin and Prince, (122); **B** from Schwartzkroin and Prince, (123); and **C** from P. A. Schwartzkroin and D. A. Prince, unpublished observations, with permission.

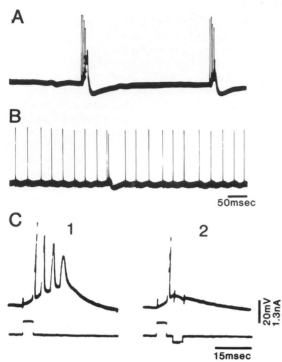

FIG. 6. Recordings from CA3 hippocampal pyramidal cells. **A** and **B**: Change in pattern of firing in bursting hippocampal pyramidal cells at resting potential (A) and during DC depolarization (B). Intracellular records are AC coupled. **C1**: Burst response evoked by brief depolarizing current pulse. **C2**: When a hyperpolarizing current pulse was applied immediately following the depolarizing pulse, the burst was blocked and a prominent depolarizing afterpotential was uncovered. From Wong and Prince, (147); with permission.

trinsic burst capabilities and epileptogenic pacemaker activity in the CA2–CA3 region of the hippocampus suggests that these phenomena are related. A similar coincidence has recently been found in neocortical slices. Experiments in normal guinea pig sensorimotor neocortex have shown that there is a population of neurons located in middle cortical layers that possesses intrinsic burst-generating capacities (Fig. 7A) (18). These neurons do not generate spontaneous bursts in the slice as do CA2–CA3 pyramidal neurons in hippocampus; however, intrinsic prolonged depolarizations may be evoked by current pulses and, occasionally, by synaptic inputs. Several lines of evidence suggest that focal epileptiform discharge develops at lowest threshold within this same area of the neocortex (14,75). Figure 7A,B shows data from one such experiment. Focal application of the excitatory amino acid L-glutamate was used to map the threshold of synchronized discharge in bicucul-

line-treated neocortex. The minimum threshold was consistently located in the middle layers. Other data, including current source density analysis and focal bicuculline application, confirm the unique role of the same middle layers and suggest that epileptiform events in the neocortex, as in the hippocampus, are initiated at sites where intrinsic burst-generating pacemaker neurons exist (17).

Thus, one prerequisite for the development of epileptogenic discharge may be the presence of a population of neurons that have burst-generating capacities. Pathological processes that induce pacemaker activity in neurons might facilitate the occurrence of epileptiform events in a neuronal population that otherwise would not support them. The membranes of many non-bursting neurons possess voltage-dependent Ca^{2+}, Na^+, and K^+ conductances that are in delicate balance during depolarization. Events that decrease outward (K^+-mediated) currents and/or facilitate inward (Na^+, Ca^{2+}-mediated) currents may convert such cells to intrinsic bursting pacemakers. The potential for producing this change in neuronal behavior in the hippocampal CA1 region is shown in Fig. 8. Tetraethylammonium (TEA) ions, which block several K^+ conductances, cause the development of rhythmic slow spontaneous depolarizations and burst discharges that can be directly evoked by depolarizing pulses (Fig. 8A1 and 8A2). When Ba^{2+}, a cation that readily passes through Ca^{2+} channels and in addition blocks K^+ channels, is added to the bathing solution, spontaneous depolarizations and spikes occur; these are resistant to tetrodotoxin (TTX) and presumably mediated by divalent cations (49). Although TEA and Ba^{2+} are not present in the brain, their actions may mimic those of endogenous substances. Acetylcholine (ACh), a transmitter that is known to block both voltage-dependent (8,9,46) and Ca^{2+}-activated K^+ conductances (8–10,15) in these neurons, can also convert CA1 cells to burst generators (Fig. 8B). Other experiments have shown that transmitters or modulators such as ACh (64) and dopamine (135) can significantly alter ongoing epileptiform activity within the hippocampal slice. As is shown in Fig. 8C, increases in $[K^+]_0$ that are well within the range of those seen during intense excitation of normal neuronal aggregates (34,85) can result in development of synchronous burst generation, perhaps by shifting the K^+ equilibrium potential and reducing the inhibitory efficacy of K^+-mediated conductances (98,103,106,127). Under some circumstances, increased $[K^+]_0$ may contribute to

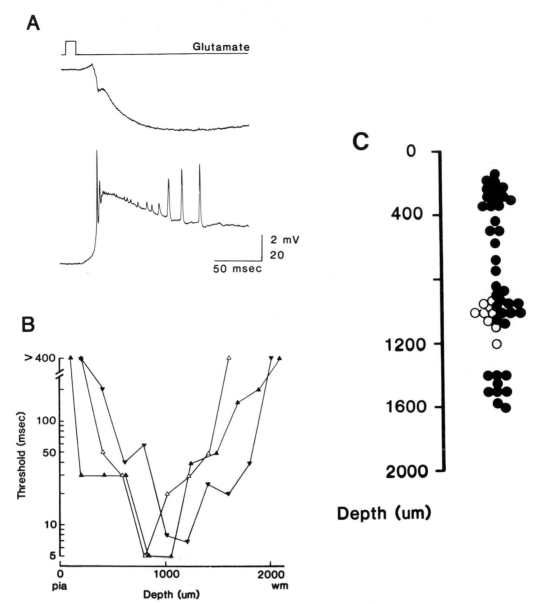

FIG. 7. **A:** Extracellular pressure pulse of glutamate evokes an epileptiform field potential (upper trace) and intracellular depolarization shift (lower trace) in a neocortical slice treated with bicuculline. **B:** Plot of threshold glutamate pulse duration to evoke epileptiform event as in A against cortical depth. Lowest threshold occurred in the middle of the cortex. **C:** Plot of cortical depth (*left,* pia surface corresponds to 0 μ*M*) for 48 neurons recorded under control conditions in neocortical slices. Intrinsically bursting cells, ○; nonbursting cells, ●. (see Fig. 2). **A−B** from Connors, (17); **C** from Connors et al., (18) with permission.

propagation and synchronization of epileptiform discharge even when synaptic transmission is blocked (63) (see Chapter 32).

The significance of an intrinsic burst-generating capability lies in its potential effects as a high-gain amplifier of stimuli. A somatic burst generator coupled to a widely diverging axon with excitatory terminals would also be particularly important in synchronizing discharges. Burst discharges arising from synaptic terminals themselves would effect transmitter release and therefore would be particularly important in amplifying synaptic events. An example of such a phenomenon is found in the neuromuscular

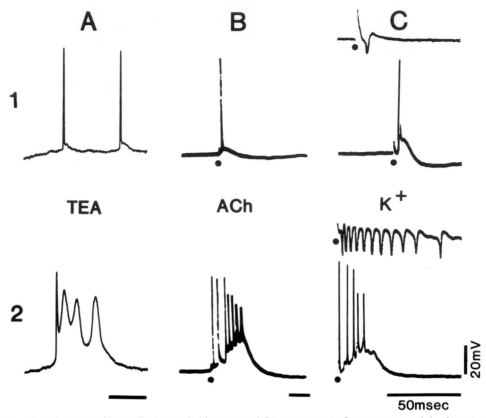

FIG. 8. Development of burst discharges in hippocampal CA1 neurons. **A:** Spontaneous activity from 1 neuron immediately after (1), and 10 min after (2) impalement with microelectrode containing tetraethylammonium. **B:** Orthodromic response of one neuron before **(B1)** and 90 sec after **(B2)** focal application of acetylcholine. **C:** Extracellular field potential (upper trace) and intracellular recording (lower trace) in slices when $[K^+]_0 = 5$ mM **(C1)** and 10 mM **(C2). Dots, B** and **C:** Stimuli in stratum radiatum. Field potentials and intracellular events in **C** were not recorded simultaneously. **A** and **C** from P. A. Schwartzkroin and D. A. Prince, unpublished observations; **B** from Benardo and Prince (8), with permission.

system of *Drosophila*. In some mutant flies, absence of particular K^+ channels in the axonal membrane can cause relatively long-duration and large-amplitude excitatory junctional potentials in the postsynaptic (muscle) cell (cf. Fig. 9A1–A2) as well as spontaneous firing in the presynaptic terminals (Fig. 9A3–A4) (151). Synaptic events may be an order of magnitude longer in duration than those in wild-type flies, presumably because of large inward Ca^{2+} currents at terminals that release excessive amounts of transmitter (Fig. 9A4). Similar genetic defects in the types, distribution, or regulation of channel proteins within the mammalian cortex have not yet been described, however such effects could certainly give rise to a brain prone to epilepsy.

Other processes are known to affect intrinsic membrane properties, and are of potential importance in epileptogenesis. For example, injury

to neurons may produce a fundamental reorganization of membrane ionic channels. Such alterations have been demonstrated in a variety of subcortical neurons from a wide range of vertebrate and invertebrate species during retrograde changes following axotomy (Fig. 9B) (30,67,68). At this time, it is not known whether mammalian cortical neurons develop new mechanisms of spike generation, burst firing patterns, and changes in behavior similar to those that occur in other preparations following injury.

Disinhibition

If cortical structures possess populations of neurons capable of generating intrinsic burst discharges, and these neurons can excite other cortical neurons (see below), why are seizures relatively unusual in the mammalian brain? The infrequency of epileptiform activity is probably a

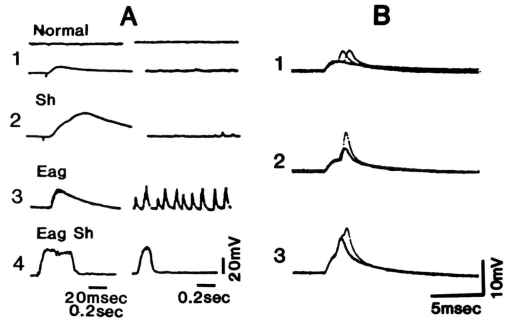

FIG. 9. Alterations in intrinsic membrane properties produced by pathological processes. **A:** Excitatory junctional potentials (EJPs) from larval neuromuscular junctions in normal (1); Shaker mutant (2); Eag mutant (3); and double Eag Shaker mutant (4) *Drosophila*. *Right column:* Spontaneous activities; *left column:* Evoked activities. Calcium concentrations of bathing media are .1 mM in upper traces of 1 and in 2 and 4. $[Ca^{2+}]$ is 0.2 mM in lower traces of 1 and in 3. Time calibrations for traces of left column are 20 msec. except that A4 is 0.2 sec. Time calibrations in right column are all 0.2 sec. as in A4. From Wu et al., (151), with permission. **B:** Responses of a chromatolyzed motoneuron to muscle afferent volleys from triceps surae, 18 days after axotomy. Afferent stimulation was gradually increased in intensity from B1–B3. Spike-like partial responses are superimposed upon monosynaptic EPSPs. Partial spikes have multiple threshold levels. From Kuno and Llinas, (67), with permission.

consequence of the powerful postsynaptic inhibition that is present at all levels of the CNS. The ways in which synaptic inhibition limits the development of epileptogenic discharge have been most completely studied in hippocampal pyramidal cells. As noted above, CA3 pyramidal neurons have the capacity to generate intrinsic burst discharges when direct depolarizing current is passed through an intrasomatic microelectrode. Both CA3 and CA1 pyramidal cell dendrites also have intrinsic burst-generating properties when directly polarized (7,80,146,148). However, when excitatory orthodromic pathways that terminate on these dendrites are electrically stimulated, burst discharges do not occur. The apparent reasons for this discrepancy are illustrated in Fig. 10. In the dendrite of Fig. 10A–10B, orthodromic stimuli evoke a single spike and an EPSP–IPSP sequence (A); however, direct depolarization elicits a burst discharge (B). When the orthodromic stimulus is timed so that the IPSP coincides with the direct depolarization, the burst-generating capacity is blocked because the membrane is hyperpolar-

ized and shunted by the IPSP conductance increase (superimposed sweep of Fig. 10B). However, after exposure of slices to penicillin, orthodromic stimuli that had previously only elicited EPSP–IPSP sequences (Fig. 10C) evoke large depolarizations and burst discharges in dendrites (Fig. 10D). Hyperpolarization of the membrane with a current pulse (superimposed sweep in D) blocks the burst discharge and uncovers the small prolonged EPSP that has triggered the intrinsic burst. Thus, any event that decreases postsynaptic inhibition may allow certain subsets of neurons to express their own intrinsic burst-generating capacities when stimulated orthodromically. If disinhibition occurs in a group of neurons that have excitatory interconnections via recurrent EPSPs, or a common excitatory input, a synchronized ringing field potential and DS generation is seen (123,124,146). These relationships between disinhibition, intrinsic burst generation and recurrent excitatory interconnections within a population of neurons have been modeled by Traub and Wong (141) and are described in more detail in Chapter 29.

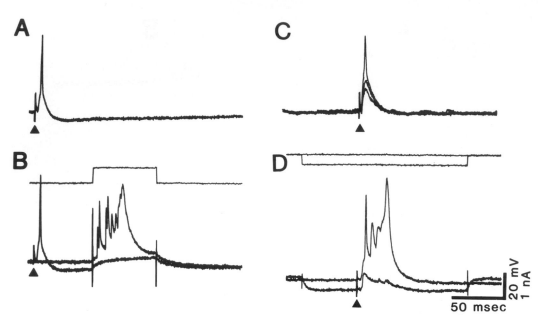

FIG. 10. Disinhibition in hippocampal CA1 pyramidal dendrites. **A** and **C:** Orthodromic stimuli (arrowheads) elicit excitatory postsynaptic spike potentials–inhibitory postsynaptic spike potentials (EPSP–IPSP) sequences in two dendrites. **B:** Direct depolarization of the dendrite of **A** elicits a complex burst with fast and slow spikes. When the direct burst response falls during the orthodromically evoked IPSP (lower superimposed trace), the burst response is blocked. **D:** Following perfusion with penicillin solution, orthromic stimulation elicits burst discharge in another dendrite. When the stimulus falls during the hyperpolarizing current pulse (lower superimposed sweep), a prolonged EPSP is uncovered which serves to trigger the intrinsic burst discharge at resting potential. From R. K. S. Wong and D. A. Prince, unpublished observations, with permission.

The results of intradendritic recordings from hippocampal pyramidal neurons suggest that somatic IPSPs are not the only inhibitory influence that controls neuronal burst generation. Isolated hippocampal pyramidal cell dendrites that have been surgically separated from most of the inhibitory circuitry within the hippocampus do not generate phasic hyperpolarizing IPSPs when orthodromically stimulated (cf. Figs. 11A1–A2 and B1–B2) (80). In spite of this, burst discharges of the sort that are seen following chemical disinhibition are not evoked (Fig. 11B). However, such dendrites do generate orthodromic burst discharges after exposure to bicuculline, as do intact dendrites (Fig. 11C2–113). These findings suggest that there may be a tonic inhibitory control in hippocampal dendrites that is effective in blocking intrinsic burst capabilities of the membrane, independent of somatically generated IPSPs.

Disinhibition alone may be insufficient to allow the development of epileptogenic discharge unless the proper intrinsic membrane properties and connectivity are present. For example, in contrast to the results in neocortex or the pyramidal cell layer of the hippocampus, dentate gyrus granule cells exposed to low concentrations of convulsant agents such as penicillin or bicuculline do not generate DSs, even though IPSPs are blocked (35). One reason for this may be the absence of recurrent excitatory connections between granule cells in normal hippocampus (69). The membrane properties of dentate granule cells may also play a role. Presumed intradendritic recordings show that depolarizing current can elicit trains of small spikes; however, intrinsic burst discharges similar to those seen in hippocampal dendrites have not been seen in a limited number of penetrations. I/V plots from such neurons also show that their membranes are different from those of hippocampal pyramidal cells in that inward rectification is not prominent (35). This may reflect a different distribution of voltage-dependent ion channels in their membranes.

Temporary disinhibition might predispose an otherwise normal cortical area to epileptiform activity. This could occur in several ways. One possible mechanism is desensitization of the postsynaptic GABA receptors. Results of electrophysiological studies (66,89,150) suggest that repeated applications of GABA may reduce its effectiveness; this might also occur during repetitive activation of cortical circuits. Inhibition

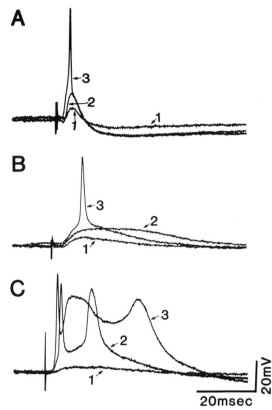

FIG. 11. Recordings from intact (**A**) and isolated (**B,C**) hippocampal CA1 dendrites. **A:** Three super-imposed sweeps of responses to stimuli of increasing intensity. Stimulus 1 elicits an excitatory postsynaptic spike potential–inhibitory postsynaptic spike potential (EPSP–IPSP) sequence. Increasing stimulus intensity evokes a larger EPSP and IPSP (trace 2). A further increase in intensity elicits an EPSP which triggers an orthodromic spike followed by an IPSP (trace 3). **B:** Postsynaptic responses from an isolated dendrite to stimuli of increasing intensity. Low-intensity stimulus evokes a simple EPSP (trace 1). More intense stimulation evokes an EPSP which has a prolonged time course (trace 2). Further increase in stimulus intensity evokes a faster rising EPSP which triggers a spike (trace 3). Note that no hyperpolarizing IPSPs are evoked. **C:** Responses from an isolated dendrite to increasing intensity orthodromic stimuli following exposure to bicuculline (5 μM). Subthreshold stimulus evokes a slow EPSP (trace 1). Small increases in stimulus intensity evoke slow depolarizations with fast and slow spike components (traces 2 and 3). From Matsukawa and Prince, ref. 80, with permission.

could also be depressed if neurons failed to maintain the necessary ionic gradients, e.g., if there were accumulation of intracellular Cl⁻ (53). Alternatively, the release of GABA from terminals may be depressed by presynaptic actions of neuromodulators such as ACh (6). This effect of ACh might act synergistically with its direct excitatory influences on intrinsic membrane properties noted above.

Recent anatomic studies in juvenile monkeys subjected to hypoxia (131), and in monkeys with alumina cream epileptic foci (111,112), suggest that inhibitory interneurons may be especially vulnerable to cortical insult (see Chapter 37). A similar sensitivity has been shown by glycinergic inhibitory interneurons in spinal cord following ischemia (24). Although loss of inhibition alone might account for focal epileptogenesis following cortical injury, it must be pointed out that a variety of other pathologic changes also occur, including gliosis, disturbances in the blood–brain barrier, presumed injury and distortion of portions of nerve cells and dendrites, possible reorganization of intrinsic excitatory circuitry or cortical afferents, etc. As pointed out by Jasper (55), adequate anatomic and physiologic controls have not yet been obtained from injured but nonepileptic cortex to determine which, if any, of these pathological substrates is important for epileptogenesis. Also, the co-occurrence of anatomic disinhibition (e.g., loss of symmetrical axo-somatic synapses), physiologic disinhibition (loss of IPSPs), and the development of abnormal orthodromically evoked burst discharges have not been demonstrated in the same neuron. Nonetheless, recent studies of chronic epileptogenic foci produced by freeze lesions (Lighthall and Prince, *manuscript in preparation*) do suggest that postsynaptic IPSPs may be depressed in neurons of injured cortex that generate prolonged DSs following orthodromic stimuli. Figure 12 shows recordings from three neurons in the region of an epileptogenic freeze focus. Prolonged DSs with repetitive spike activity are occasionally elicited (A2,B1), whereas other stimuli evoke only EPSPs (B1). DSs can have long and variable latencies and behavior similar to those of slice neurons exposed to convulsants. The analysis of these potentials is incomplete, however both voltage-dependent and synaptic components appear to be present (72). Neurons with varying degrees of burst generation evoked by slow PSPs are present (cf. Fig. 12A1 and B1). Rare spontaneous bursts have also been recorded (B2). Such events are not seen in neurons in normal neocortical slices.

Genetic abnormalities may also decrease the effectiveness of inhibitory control mechanisms in the brain. One example may be the occurrence of pyridoxine-dependent seizures in newborn infants (see ref. 138 for review). It seems likely that a variety of genetic abnormalities affecting transmitter systems in the CNS will be

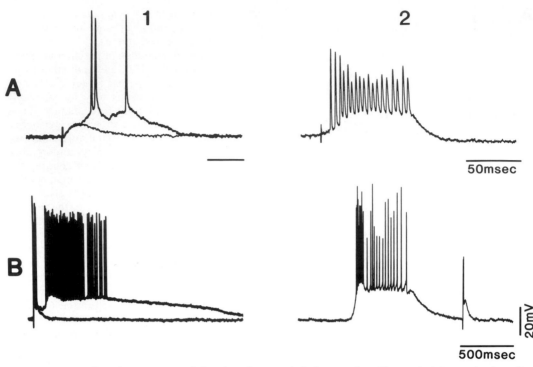

FIG. 12. Recordings from neurons of chronic epileptogenic lesions produced by cortical freeze; *in vitro* slice preparations. **A1:** Orthodromic stimuli evoke slow excitatory postsynaptic spike potentials (EPSPs) alternating with prolonged multiphasic depolarizing responses which trigger multiple spikes. **A2:** More prolonged spike burst response in another neuron. **B:** In another cell, consecutive stimuli of the same intensity evoke EPSP and brief burst of three spikes and a similar short latency response followed by a prolonged depolarization and spike burst. **B2:** Spontaneous burst followed by orthodromic EPSP and spike in the cell of **B1.** Time calibration marks in **A:** 50 msec. Time calibration in **B2** for traces of **B:** Spike amplitudes attenuated in portions of B because of slow digitization rate.

found in future experiments. The defects in spinal inhibitory receptors for glycine in the "spastic" mouse (144), and the anatomic abnormalities of the ascending noradrenergic system in the seizure-prone totterer mouse (70) provide prototypes.

Excitatory Interactions

Excitatory synaptic potentials generated as a consequence of propagation of impulses through the intracortical and extracortical connections shown in Fig. 1 have three general roles in the development of focal epileptogenesis: (a) they provide a mechanism for synchronization of epileptiform discharges; (b) they contribute significantly to the generation of DSs in individual neurons during interictal discharge; and (c) they may trigger intrinsic slow depolarizations and burst discharges in subpopulations of neurons with particular membrane properties. The latter role is discussed above and illustrated in Fig. 10.

EPSPs and Synchronization of Interictal Discharges

Although nonsynaptic synchronizing mechanisms may be present (see Chapter 30), the predominant mechanism for synchronization of epileptiform activities in all cortical structures appears to be synaptic excitation. The reciprocal excitatory connections between principal cells provide one anatomic substrate for synchronization (see Fig. 1). Axons of pyramidal neurons possess large numbers of collaterals through which recurrent excitation of surrounding neurons takes place. These anatomic arrangements assure that discharge in a small group of cells result in divergent excitation of a population of neurons. The divergent excitatory afferents arising from more remote structures form a second substrate for synchronization. For example, activation of a few thalamocortical relay cells and their extensive axonal arborizations may excite thousands of cortical neurons synchronously. Electrophysiological studies in very small epileptiform foci made in visual cortex (29,36), and functional mapping in and around cortical foci using 2-deoxyglucose techniques (16) show that focal epileptiform discharges utilize normal cortical circuitry, with strong columnar and specific lateral connections. It seems likely that the type or intensity of excitatory interaction mediated by chemical EPSPs will vary according to the local circuitry present in the structure being studied. An example of low susceptibility to epileptogenesis is provided by the cerebellar cortex. Here Purkinje cells have GABA-mediated inhibition which may be blocked by convulsant agents, and intrinsic burst-generating capabilities on dendrites are prominent (74). There is, however, no recurrent excitatory connectivity between these neurons, perhaps accounting for the fact that the cerebellar cortex is not prone to epileptogenesis either experimentally or clinically.

Another mechanism by which intense ampli-fication, synchronization, and spread of excitatory synaptic inputs to the cortex may occur is through alterations at the level of the presynaptic terminals. These elements presumably possess membrane properties similar to those in cortical dendrites where prominent Ca^{2+} conductances are present. Disorders in membrane excitability that induce repetitive spike firing or prolonged slow depolarizations in terminals may be translated directly into increased release of transmitter. Experiments in mammalian cortex indicate that such disruptions in function may occur. Thalamocortical and transcallosal axonal terminals in the area of a chemical epileptogenic focus can generate bursts of spikes that antidromically invade the cell body (Fig. 13A) (41,86,120,128). Similar bursts can be elicited in neuromuscular terminals in the rat phrenic nerve-diaphragm preparation following exposure to the convulsant penicillin (87). Of more significance is the finding that similar bursts in

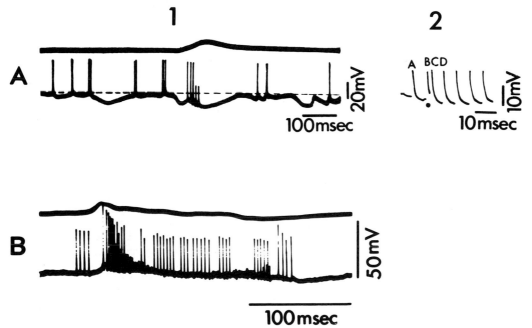

FIG. 13. Spikes initiated in axonal terminal regions during focal epileptogenesis. **A1:** Intracellular recording from a thalamocortical relay neuron in the ventral posterolateral nucleus of the cat. During this segment of spontaneous activity, the neuron generates a train of spikes coincident with the interictal epileptiform event shown in the EEG (upper trace). Spikes during the burst associated with the EEG event arise from below the firing level for spontaneous spikes (dashed line). **A2:** Stimulation of the ipsilateral cortex during the course of an epilepsy-related burst evokes an antidromic spike **(C)** and resets the intervals between the spikes of the burst without colliding with spike B. The interval between spikes B and C is less than twice the antidromic latency plus spike refractory period, proving that both B and C originate in the cortex. From Gutnick and Prince, (41), with permission. **B:** Intracellular recording from an identified thalamocortical relay neuron during cortical afterdischarges initiated by repetitive electrical stimulation. Constant-amplitude, regular-interval (3.5–4.5 msec.) action potentials appear prior to and during the prolonged plateau depolarization. Regular-interval spike burst is present during period when dendritic and somatic spike-generating zones are inactivated. From Noebels and Prince, (88), with permission.

axonal terminals, independent of depolarization of the cell body, can occur during electrically induced afterdischarges in the cortex (Fig. 13B) (88). This suggests that similar activities may be present in presynaptic terminals in all forms of epileptogenesis, and that these events may be important in the spread of epileptiform activity into normal cortical areas, as is the case during propagation of electrically induced afterdischarge. The mechanisms by which these bursts occur are not understood. Because thalamocortical or callosal terminals do not appear to be sites for axo-axonal presynaptic synapses, some nonsynaptic excitatory process must produce significant alterations in terminal excitability. For example, it may be that nonjunctional presynaptic receptors are normally present for agents such as GABA (13), ACh (51), or other modulatory agents. Interruption of tonic inhibitory influences by convulsant agents such as penicillin, at times when excitatory substances such as ACh and K^+ are being released, may be sufficient to produce depolarization and repetitive firing in terminals. Whatever the underlying mechanism, this phenomenon would produce significant amplification and synchronization of responses in postsynaptic neurons. This is clearly a problem that deserves further study in models of focal epileptogenesis, especially since anatomic experiments show a significant pathological alteration in axons within the area of cortical injury (142), and studies in peripheral axons show that significant changes in axonal membrane properties may follow local injury (62). It even seems possible that some focal epileptiform discharges may be initiated in areas of axonal damage where spontaneous bursts are initiated by normal impulse traffic. Tonic seizures possibly originating from axons in areas of subcortical demyelination are known to occur in patients with multiple sclerosis (28).

Once EPSPs are evoked on postsynaptic neurons, various factors will influence the "strength" of the synaptic input and determine whether it will be effective in bringing the membrane to the firing level for a single spike or burst. Stimulus-evoked EPSPs are normally quite brief in cortical neurons in part because of the concurrent activation of feed-forward or recurrent IPSPs (Fig. 1). When the latter potentials are no longer present owing to disinhibition, the falling phase of the EPSP becomes prolonged (27,146), and the EPSP becomes more effective in depolarizing the postsynaptic cell to the activation level for various voltage-dependent conductances, including those that underlie burst generation. The location of the synaptic event in relation to the voltage-dependent channels in the dendritic membrane (Fig. 4B) is also an important factor in determining EPSP efficacy. Some of the pathological changes that occur following injury, such as loss of dendritic branches and spines and changes in dendritic diameter (142), could make dendritic excitatory events more effective in evoking somatic spikes.

EPSPs and DS Generation

Recent studies of disinhibited cortical models have demonstrated unequivocally that uniquely large and prolonged EPSPs contribute significantly to DSs that occur in single neurons during interictal discharges (19,40). In neocortical (40) and hippocampal pyramidal (57) neurons, the DS can be inverted when the membrane is depolarized to ~0 mV, showing that there are significant excitatory synaptic currents contributing to this potential. The results of one experiment in a neocortical neuron from a biculline-treated slice are shown in Fig. 14. Stimuli elicit EPSPs alternating with complexes containing EPSPs and DSs (Fig. 14A2,B2). As the membrane is depolarized, the EPSP and DS appear to invert to negative-going potentials (Fig. 14A1,B1). The results of such experiments confirm earlier reports (82,95) on inversion of DSs in neocortical neurons studies in vivo. These results cannot, however, be used to estimate the contributions of voltage-dependent events to generation of DSs at the resting potential, since Na^+ and Ca^{2+} currents would be inactivated at depolarized membrane potentials. The relative contributions of intrinsic and synaptic currents to slow depolarizations should vary from structure to structure and neuron to neuron depending upon the intrinsic properties of a given cell and its synaptic connections. For example, in neurons with prominent voltage-dependent conductances for Na^+ and/or Ca^{2+} (Figs. 3, 4, and 10), there is no way to achieve significant synaptic depolarization without activating these intrinsic membrane currents which will contribute to the total postsynaptic depolarization. Burst-generating pacemaker neurons that are recurrently excited will also generate DSs that are dependent both on synaptic and intrinsic currents (140).

A recapitulation of the factors influencing epileptogenesis in different populations of cells is provided in Table 1. The pacemaker hippocampal CA3 pyramidal neurons possess low-threshold, intrinsic burst-generating capabilities on both their somata and dendrites, and have recurrent excitatory interconnections. When

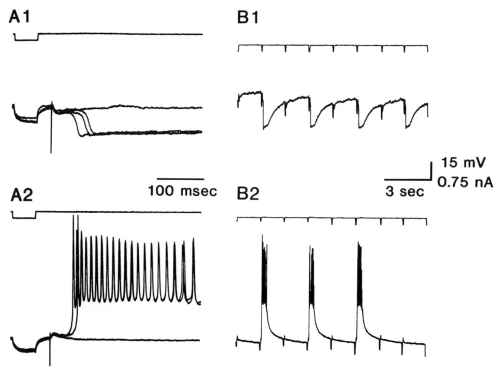

FIG. 14. Reversal of depolarizing shift (DS)-associated synaptic potentials. Recordings were obtained from a neocortical pyramidal cell that was injected with Cs^+, to reduce K^+ conductances, and bathed in 50 μM bicuculline. *Upper traces:* monitoring injected current pulses. *Lower traces:* transmembrane voltage. **A:** At resting potential (-60 mV, **A2**) excitatory postsynaptic spike potent repetitive stimuli to the white matter evoked alternating EPSPs and EPSP–DS complexes (three superimposed traces). When steady depolarizing current was applied to shift the membrane potential to about $+35$ mV (**A1**) similar stimuli evoked only negative-going, small, short-latency potentials (the early EPSP) alternating with reversed EPSPs plus much larger potentials of long and shifting latency. Small intracellular current pulses preceding stimuli were used to monitor input resistance. **B:** Slower sweep speeds of data from which traces in *A* were derived. Note the prolonged time course of both DSs (**B2**) and inverted paroxysmal potentials (**B1**). From Connors and Gutnick, (19), with permission.

this group of cells is disinhibited, it becomes a pacemaker for epileptiform discharges in the hippocampus. Recent work (83) shows clearly that even stimulation of single CA3 pyramidal neurons after exposure to a convulsant agent may, under proper experimental circumstances, influence discharges in the aggregate. The CA1 pyramidal neurons possess burst-generating capacities on their dendrites. However, recurrent excitatory interconnections have not yet been

TABLE 1. *Properties of neuronal aggregates in relationship to epileptogenic capacities*

	Burst generation	Recurrent excitation	Epileptogenesis following disinhibition
Hippocampus			
CA1b pyramidal cells	+ Dendrites only	0	Followers
CA3 pyramidal cells	+ Dendrites and probably somata	+	Pacemakers
Dentate granule cells	0	0	0
Neocortex			
Nonbursting pyramidal cells	0	+	Followers
Bursting pyramidal cells layer IV–V	+ Site unknown	+	Pacemakers
Purkinje cells	+ Dendrites	0	0

demonstrated; following disinhibition, this area acts as a follower region but usually cannot spontaneously initiate interictal discharges. Granule cells of the dentate gyrus possess neither recurrent excitatory connections nor intrinsic membrane properties that promote burst generation, and are relatively nonsusceptible to participation in epileptogenesis *in vivo* or *in vitro* following disinhibition. It is important to note that this incapacity of dentate and CA1 neurons to generate epileptic events spontaneously may be altered significantly depending on the experimental paradigm. For example, nonsynaptic, or as yet undescribed synaptic interconnections in CA1 might, under some circumstances, allow this structure to become spontaneously epileptogenic. It is known that some subclasses of CA1 pyramidal cells have intrinsic burst-generating capacities following somatic depolarization (79).

CONCLUSIONS

There are several important factors that determine whether a given population of neurons will develop epileptogenesis. The first factor is the capacity of subpopulations of cells to generate intrinsic burst discharges and pacemaker potentials. Such capacities are normally present in some groups of neurons and might be induced in others by genetic disorders affecting voltage-dependent channels, release of substances in the brain that alter the balance between inward Na^+-Ca^{2+} currents and outward K^+ currents, or even changes in the structure of the cell membrane that occur following trauma. Second, disinhibition may develop. Inhibitory postsynaptic events that ordinarily control intrinsic membrane excitability and burst-generating capacity may be depressed during repetitive activation, as the result of selective vulnerability of inhibitory interneurons and synapses following various cortical traumata, or secondary to specific defects in receptors or transmitter metabolism that might result from genetic disorders or other disturbances that affect ionic gradients across the cell membrane. Third, excitatory interconnections may be present. The consequence of these will vary depending on the specific synaptic circuitry. EPSPs may contribute to the slow envelope of the DS, serve as trigger potentials for intrinsic depolarizations, and as synchronizing potentials within the epileptic neuronal aggregate. It seems likely that different pathological processes may produce epileptogenesis by influencing each of these mechanisms to a different degree, and that cellular mechanisms underlying interictal discharge may vary at different sites in the brain.

ACKNOWLEDGMENTS

We thank Cheryl Joo and Terry Alter for assistance in manuscript preparation. Portions of this work were supported by National Institutes of Health grant Nos. NS 06477, NS 12151, and NS 19510 from the National Institute of Neurological and Communicative Disorders and Stroke (NINCDS), and the Morris Research Fund.

REFERENCES

1. Ajmone Marsan, C. (1969): Acute effects of topical epileptogenic agents. In: *Basic Mechanisms of the Epilepsies*, edited by H. H. Jasper, A. A. Ward, Jr., and A. Pope, pp. 299–319, Little, Brown, and Co., Boston.
2. Alger, B. E., and Nicoll, R. A. (1980): Feedforward dendritic inhibition in rat hippocampal pyramidal cells studied *in vitro*. *J. Physiol. (Lond.)*, 328:105–123.
3. Andersen, P., Eccles, J. C. and Loyning, Y. (1964): Location of postsynaptic synapses on hippocampal pyramids. *J. Neurophysiol.*, 27:592–607.
4. Andersen, P., Gjerstad, L., Hablitz, J. J. and Langmoen, I. A. (1982): Two types of burst discharges in penicillin-treated brain slices. In: *Physiology and Pharmacology of Epileptogenic Phenomena*, edited by M. R. Klee, H. D. Lux, and E. J. Speckman, pp. 93–95, Raven Press, New York.
5. Andersen, P., Gjerstad, L., and Langmoen, I. A. (1978): A cortical epilepsy model *in vitro*. In: *Abnormal Neuronal Discharges*, edited by N. Chalazonitis and M. Boisson, pp. 29–36, Raven Press, New York.
6. Ben-Ari, Y., Krnjevic, K., Reinhardt, W., and Ropert, N. (1981): Intracellular observations on the disinhibitory action of acetylcholine in the hippocampus. *Neuroscience*, 6:2475–2484.
7. Benardo, L. S., Masukawa, L. M., and Prince, D. A. (1982): Electrophysiology of isolated hippocampal dendrites. *J. Neurosci.*, 2:1614–1622.
8. Benardo, L. S., and Prince, D. A. (1982): Cholinergic excitation of mammalian hippocampal pyramidal cells. *Brain Res.*, 249:315–331.
9. Benardo, L. S., and Prince, D. A. (1982): Ionic mechanisms of cholinergic excitation in mammalian hippocampal pyramidal cells. *Brain Res.*, 249:333–344.
10. Benardo, L. S., and Prince, D. A. (1982): Cholinergic pharmacology of mammalian hippocampal pyramidal cells. *Neuroscience*, 7:1703–1712.
11. Benninger, C., Kadis, J., and Prince, D. A. (1980): Extracellular calcium and potassium changes in hippocampal slices. *Brain Res.*, 180:165–182.
12. Biedenbach, M. A., and Stevens, C. F. (1969): Synaptic organization of cat olfactory cortex

as revealed by intracellular recording. *J. Neurophysiol.*, 32:204–214.

13. Brown, D. A., Adams, P. R., Higgins, A. J., and Marsh, S. (1979): Distribution of GABA-receptors and GABA-carriers in the mammalian nervous system. *J Physiol. (Paris)*, 75:667–671.

14. Chatt, A. B., and Ebersole, J. S. (1982): The laminar sensitivity of cat striate cortex to penicillin-induced epileptogenesis. *Brain Res.*, 241:382–387.

15. Cole, A. E., and Nicoll, R. A. (1984): The pharmacology of cholinergic excitatory responses in hippocampal pyramidal cells. *Brain Res.*, 305:283–290.

16. Collins, R. C. (1978): Use of cortical circuits during focal penicillin seizures: An autoradiographic study with [^{14}C]-deoxyglucose. *Brain Res.*, 150:487–501.

17. Connors, B. W. (1984): Initiation of synchronized neuronal bursting in neocortex. *Nature*, 310:685–687.

18. Connors, B. W., Gutnick, M. J., and Prince, D. A. (1982): Electrophysiological properties of neocortical neurons *in vitro*. *J. Neurophysiol.*, 48:1302–1320.

19. Connors, B. W., and Gutnick, M. J. (1984): Cellular mechanisms of neocortical epileptogenesis in an acute experimental model. In: *Electrophysiology of Epilepsy*, edited by P. Schwartzkroin, and H. Wheal, pp. 79–105. Academic Press, London.

20. Constanti, A., and Galvan, M. (1983): Fast inward-rectifying current accounts for anomalous rectification of olfactory cortex neurons. *J. Physiol.*, 335:153–178.

21. Courtney, K. R., and Prince, D. A. (1977): Epileptogenesis in neocortical slices. *Brain Res.*, 127:191–196.

22. Creutzfeldt, O. D., Lux, H. D., and Watanabe, S. (1966): Electrophysiology of cortical nerve cells. In: *The Thalamus*, edited by D. P. Purpura, and M. Yahr, pp. 209–235. Columbia University Press, New York.

23. Crill, W. E., and Schwindt, P. C. (1983): Active currents in mammalian central neurons. *Trends Neurosci.*, 6:236–240.

24. Davidoff, R. A., Graham, L. T., Jr., Shank, R. P., Werman, R., and Aprison, M. J. (1967): Changes in amino acid concentrations associated with loss of spinal interneurons. *J. Neurochem.*, 14:1025–1031.

25. DeFelipe, J., and Fairen, A. (1982): A type of basket cell in superficial layers of the cat visual cortex. A golgi-electron microscope study. *Brain Res.*, 244:9–16.

26. Dichter, M., Hermann, C., and Selzer, M. (1973): Penicillin epilepsy in isolated islands of hippocampus. *Electroenceph. Clin. Neurophysiol.*, 34:631–638.

27. Dingledine, R., and Gjerstad, L. (1980): Reduced inhibition during epileptiform activity in the *in vitro* hippocampal slice. *J. Physiol.*, 305:297–313.

28. Drake, W. E., and MacRae, D. (1961): Epilepsy in multiple sclerosis. *Neurology*, 11:810–816.

29. Ebersole, J. S. (1977): Initial abnormalities of neuronal response during epileptogenesis in visual cortex. *J. Neurophysiol.*, 40:514–526.

30. Eccles, J. C., Libet, B., and Young, R. R. (1958): The behaviour of chromatolysed motoneurones studied by intracellular recording. *J. Physiol. (Lond.)*, 143:11–40.

31. Eckenstein, F., and Baughman R. W. (1984): Two types of cholinergic innervation in cortex, one co-localized with vasoactive intestinal polypeptide. *Nature*, 309:153–155.

32. Eckert, R., and Tillotson, D. L. (1981): Calcium-mediated inactivation of the calcium conductance in cesium-leaded giant neurons of *Aplysia californica*. *J. Physiol.*, 314:265–280.

33. Emson, P. C., and Hunt, S. P. (1981): Anatomical chemistry of the cerebral cortex. In: *The Organization of the Cerebral Cortex*, edited by F. O. Schmitt, F. G. Worden, G. A. Adelman, and S. G. Dennis, pp. 325–346. MIT Press, Cambridge, Massachusetts.

34. Fisher, R. F., Pedley, T. A., Moody, W. J., Jr., and Prince, D. A. (1976): The role of extracellular potassium in hippocampal epilepsy. *Arch. Neurol.*, 33:76–83.

35. Fricke, R. A., and Prince, D. A. (1984): Electrophysiology of dentate gyrus granule cells. *J. Neurophysiol.*, 51:195–209.

36. Gabor, A. J., Scobey, R. P., and Wehrli, C. J. (1979): Relationship of epileptogenicity to cortical organization. *J. Neurophysiol.*, 42:1609–1625.

37. Galvan, M., Grafe, P., and ten Bruggencate, G. (1982): Convulsant actions of 4-aminopyridine on the guinea pig olfactory cortex slice. *Brain Res.*, 241:75–86.

38. Globus, A., and Scheibel, A. B. (1967): Synaptic loci on visual cortical neurones of the rabbit. The specific afferent radiation. *Exp. Neurol.*, 18:116–131.

39. Goldensohn, E. S., and Purpura, D. P. (1963): Intracellular potentials of cortical neurons during focal epileptogenic discharges. *Science*, 139:840–842.

40. Gutnick, M. J., Connors, B. W., and Prince, D. A. (1982): Mechanisms of neocortical epileptogenesis *in vitro*. *J. Neurophysiol.*, 48:1321–1335.

41. Gutnick, M. J., and Prince, D. A. (1972): Cortical relay neurons: Antidromic invasion of spikes from a cortical epileptogenic focus. *Science*, 176:424–426.

42. Gutnick, M. J., and Prince, D. A. (1981): Dye-coupling and possible electrotonic coupling in the guinea pig neocortical slice. *Science*, 211:67–70.

43. Haberly, L. B., and Bower, J. M. (1984): Analysis of association fiber systems in piriform cortex with intracellular recording and staining techniques. *J. Neurophysiol.*, 51:90–112.

44. Haberly, L. B., and Shepherd, G. M. (1973): Current-density analysis of summed evoked potentials in opossum prepyriform cortex. *J. Neurophysiol.*, 36:789–802.

45. Hablitz J. J. (1984): Picrotoxin-induced epileptiform activity in hippocampus: Role of endogenous versus synaptic factors. *J. Neurophysiol.*, 51:1011–1027.

46. Halliwell, J. V., and Adams, P. R. (1982): Voltage-clamp analysis of muscarinic excitation in hippocampal neurons. *Brain Res., 250:*71–92.

47. Hendry, S. H. C., Jones, E. G., and Beinfeld, M. C. (1983): Cholecystokinin-immunoreactive neurons in rat and monkey cerebral cortex make symmetric synapses and have intimate associations with blood vessels. *Proc. Natl. Acad. Sci. USA,* 80:2400–2404.

48. Hodgkin, A. C., and Huxley, A. F. (1952): A quantitative description of membrane current and its application to conduction and excitation in nerve. *J. Physiol. (Lond.),* 117:500–544.

49. Hotson, J. R., Prince, D. A., and Schwartzkroin, P. A. (1979): Anomalous rectification in hippocampal neurons. *J. Neurophysiol.,* 42:889–895.

50. Hotson, J. R., and Prince, D. A., (1981): Penicillin- and barium-induced epileptiform bursting in hippocampal neurons: Actions on Ca^{++} and K^+ potentials. *Ann. Neurol.,* 10:11–17.

51. Hounsgaard, J. (1978): Pre-synaptic inhibitory action of acetylcholine in area CA1 of the hippocampus. *Exp. Neurol.,* 62:787–797.

52. Houser, C. R., Hendry, S. H. C., and Vaughn, J. E. (1983): Morphological diversity of immunocytochemically identified GABA neurons in the monkey sensory-motor cortex. *J. Neurocytol.,* 12:617–638.

53. Huguenard, J. R., and Alger, B. E. (1984): Repetitive GABA activation leads to shifts in GABA reversal potential: A voltage clamp study in acutely isolated hippocampal cells. *Soc. Neurosci. Abstr.,* 10:204.

54. Jackson, J. H. (1870): A study of convulsions. *Trans. St. Andrews Med. Grad. Assn.,* 3:1–45.

55. Jasper, H. H. (1970): Physiopathological mechanisms of post-traumatic epilepsy. *Epilepsia,* 11:73–80.

56. Jasper, H. H., Ward, A. A., Jr., and Pope, A., (editors) (1969): *Basic Mechanisms of the Epilepsies.* Little, Brown, and Co., Boston.

57. Johnston, D., and Brown, T. H. (1981): Giant synaptic potential hypothesis for epileptiform activity. *Science,* 211:294–297.

58. Johnston, D., Hablitz, J. J., and Wilson, W. A. (1980): Voltage clamp discloses slow inward current in hippocampal burst-firing neurones. *Nature,* 285:391–393.

59. Jones, E. G. (1975): Varieties and distribution of nonpyramidal cells in the somatic sensory cortex of the squirrel monkey. *J. Comp. Neurol.,* 160:167.

60. Kandel, E. R., and Spencer, W. A. (1961): Electrophysiology of hippocampal neurons. II. Afterpotentials and repetitive firing. *J. Neurophysiol.,* 24:243–259.

61. Knowles, W. D., and Schwartzkroin, P. A. (1981): Local circuit synaptic interactions in hippocampal brain slices. *J. Neurosci.,* 1:318–322.

62. Kocsis, J. D., and Waxman, S. G. (1983): Long term regenerating nerve fibres retain sensitivity to potassium channel blocking agents. *Nature,* 304:640–642.

63. Konnerth, A., Heinemann, U., and Yaari, Y. (1984): Slow transmission of neural activity in hippocampal area CA1 in absence of active chemical synapses. *Nature,* 307:69–71.

64. Kriegstein, A. R., Suppes, T. A., and Prince, D. A. (1983): Cholinergic enhancement of penicillin-induced epileptiform discharges in pyramidal neurons of the guinea pig hippocampus. *Brain Res.,* 266:137–142.

65. Kristiansen, R., and Courtois, G. (1949): Rhythmic electrical activity from isolated cerebral cortex. *EEG Clin. Neurophysiol.,* 1:265–277.

66. Krnjevic, K. (1981): Desensitization of GABA receptors. *Adv. Biochem. Psychopharmacol.,* 26:111–120.

67. Kuno, M., and Llinas, R. (1970): Enhancement of synaptic transmission by dendritic potentials in chromatolysed motoneurones of the cat. *J. Physiol. (Lond.),* 210:807–821.

68. Kuwada, J. Y., and Wine, J. J. (1981): Transient, axotomy-induced changes in the membrane properties of crayfish central neurones. *J. Physiol. (Lond.),* 317:435–461.

69. Laurberg, S., and Zimmer, J. (1981): Lesion induced sprouting of hippocampal mossy fiber collaterals to the fascia dentata in developing and adult rats. *J. Comp. Neurol.,* 200:433–459.

70. Levitt, P., and Noebels, J. L. (1981): Mutant mouse tottering: Selective increase of locus ceruleus axons in a defined single-locus mutation. *Proc. Natl. Acad. Sci. USA,* 78:4630–4636.

71. Li, C.-L., (1959): Cortical intracellular potentials and their responses to strychnine. *J. Neurophysiol.,* 22:436–450.

72. Lighthall, J. W., and Prince, D. A. (1984): Further observations on neuronal activity in areas of chronic cortical epileptiform foci. *Soc. Neurosci. Abstr.,* 10:551.

73. Llinas, R. R. (1984): Comparative electrobiology of mammalian central neurons. In: *Brain Slices,* edited by R. Dingledine, pp. 7–24. Plenum Press, New York.

74. Llinas, R., and Sugimori, M. (1980): Electrophysiological properties of *in vitro* Purkinje cell dendrites in mammalian cerebellar slices. *J. Physiol. (Lond.),* 305:197–213.

75. Lockton, J. W., and Holmes, O. (1983): Penicillin epilepsy in the rat: The responses of different layers of the cortex cerebri. *Brain Res.,* 258:79–90.

76. Lorente de No, R. (1938): The cerebral cortex: Architecture, intracortical connections and motor projections. In: *Physiology of the Nervous System,* edited by J. F. Fulton, pp. 291–339. Oxford University Press, Oxford.

77. MacVicar, B. A., and Dudek, F. E. (1980): Local synaptic circuits in rat hippocampus: Interactions between pyramidal cells. *Brain Res.,* 184:220–223.

77a. McCormick, D. A., Connors, B. W., Lighthall, J. W., and Prince, D. A. (1985): Comparative electrophysiology of pyramidal and sparsely spiny stellate neurons of the neocortex. *J. Neurophysiol.,* 54:782–806.

78. Martin, K. A. C., Somogyi, P., and Whitteridge, D. (1983): Physiological and morpholog-

ical properties of identified basket cells in cat's visual cortex. *Exp. Brain Res.*, 50:193–220.

79. Masukawa, L. M., Benardo, L. S., and Prince, D. A. (1982): Variations in electrophysiological properties of hippocampal pyramidal neurons in different subfields. *Brain Res.*, 242:341–344.

80. Masukawa, L. M., and Prince, D. A. (1984): Synaptic control of excitability in isolated dendrites in hippocampal neurons. *J. Neuroscience*, 4:217–227.

81. Matsumoto, H., and Ajmone Marsan, C. (1964): Cortical cellular phenomena in experimental epilepsy: Interictal manifestations. *Exp. Neurol.*, 9:286–304.

82. Matsumoto, H., Ayala, G. F., and Gumnit, R. J. (1969): Neuronal behavior and triggering mechanisms in cortical epileptic focus. *J. Neurophysiol.*, 32:688–703.

83. Miles, R., and Wong, R. K. S. (1983): Single neurones can initiate synchronized population discharge in the hippocampus. *Nature*, 306:371–373.

84. Miles, R., and Wong, R. K. S. (1984): Unitary inhibitory synaptic potentials in the guinea pig hippocampus *in vitro*. *J. Physiol.* 356:97–113.

85. Moody, W. J., Jr., Futamachi, K. J., and Prince, D. A. (1974): Extracellular potassium activity during epileptogenesis, *Exp. Neurol.*, 42:248–263.

86. Noebels, J. L., and Prince, D. A. (1978): Development of focal seizures in cerebral cortex: Role of axon terminal bursting. *J. Neurophysiol.*, 41:1267–1281.

87. Noebels, J. L., and Prince, D. A. (1978): Presynaptic origin of penicillin afterdischarges at mammalian nerve terminals. *Brain Res.*, 138:59–74.

88. Noebels, J. L., and Prince, D. A. (1978): Excitability changes in thalamocortical relay neurons during synchronous discharges in cat neocortex. *J. Neurophysiol.*, 41:1282–1296.

89. Numann, R., and Wong, R. K. S. (1983): Desensitization of the GABA receptor in hippocampal neurons isolated from the adult guinea pig. *Soc. Neurosci. Abstr.*, 9:738.

90. Penfield, W. (1952): Ablation of abnormal cortex in cerebral palsy. *J. Neurol. Neurosurg. Psychiatry*, 15:73–78.

91. Peters, A., and Jones, E. G. (1984): *Cerebral Cortex, Cellular Components of the Cerebral Cortex*, Vol. 1, pp. 565. Plenum Press, New York.

92. Peters, A., and Proskauer, C. C. (1980): Synaptic relations between a multipolar stellate cell and a pyramidal neuron in the rat visual cortex. A combined Golgi-electron microscope study. *J. Neurocytol.*, 9:163–183.

93. Peters, A., and Regidor, J. (1981): A reassessment of the forms of nonpyramidal neurons in area 17 of cat visual cortex. *J. Comp. Neurol.*, 203:685-716.

94. Phillips, C. G. (1959): Actions of antidromic pyramidal volleys on single Betz cells in the cat. *J. Exp. Physiol.*, 44:1–25.

95. Prince, D. A. (1968): The depolarization shift in "epileptic" neurons. *Exp. Neurol.*, 21:467–485.

96. Prince, D. A. (1969): Microelectrode studies of penicillin foci. In: *Basic Mechanisms of the Epilepsies*, edited by H. H. Jasper, A. A. Ward, Jr., and A. Pope, pp. 320–328. Little, Brown and Co., Boston.

97. Prince, D. A. (1976): Cellular activities in focal epilepsy. In: *Brain Dysfunction in Infantile Febrile Convulsions*, edited by M. A. B. Brazier and F. Coceani, pp. 187–212. Raven Press, New York.

98. Prince, D. A. (1978): Neurophysiology of epilepsy. *Annu. Rev. Neurosci.*, 1:395–415.

99. Prince, D. A. (1982): Neuronal events underlying epileptogeneis. In: *Topics in Child Neurology*, Vol. 2, edited by R. R. Ouvrier, and P. G. Procopis, pp. 35–53. Spectrum, New York.

100. Prince, D. A. (1982): Epileptogenesis in hippocampal and neocortical neurons. In: *Physiology and Pharmacology of Epileptogenic Phenomena*, edited by M. R. Klee, H. D. Lux, and E. J. Speckmann, pp. 151–162. Raven Press, New York.

101. Prince, D. A. (1983): Mechanisms of epileptogenesis in brain slice model systems. In: *Epilepsy*, edited by A. A. Ward, Jr., J. K. Penry, and D. Purpura, pp. 29–52. Raven Press, New York.

102. Prince, D. A. (1983): Ionic mechanisms in cortical and hippocampal epileptogenesis. In: *Basic Mechanisms of Neuronal Hyperexcitability*, edited by H. H. Jasper and N. M. van Gelder, pp. 217–243. Alan R. Liss, New York.

103. Prince, D. A., Connors, B. W., and Benardo, L. S. (1982): Mechanisms underlying interictal–ictal transitions. In: *Advances in Neurology: Status Epilepticus*, vol. 34: edited by A. V. Delgado-Escueta, C. Wasterlain, D. M. Treiman, and R. J. Porter, pp. 179–189. Raven Press, New York.

104. Prince, D. A., and Futamachi, K. J. (1968): Intracellular recording in chronic focal epilepsy. *Brain Res.*, 11:681–684.

105. Prince, D. A., Pedley, T. A., and Ransom, B. R. (1978): Fluctuations in ion concentrations during excitation and seizures. In: *Dynamic Properties of Glia Cells*, edited by G. Frank, L. Hertz, E. Schoffeniels, and D. B. Tower, pp. 281–303. Pergamon Press, New York.

106. Prince, D. A., and Schwartzkroin, P. A. (1978): Nonsynaptic mechanisms in epileptogenesis. In: *Abnormal Neuronal Discharges*, edited by N. Chalazonitis, and M. Boisson, pp. 1–12. Raven Press, New York.

107. Prince, D. A., and Wong, R. K. S. (1981). Human epileptic neurons studied *in vitro*. *Brain Res.*, 210:323–333.

108. Purpura, D. P., Prelevic, S., and Santini, M. (1968): Postsynaptic potentials and spike variations in feline hippocampus during postnatal ontogenesis. *Exp. Neurol.*, 22:408–417.

109. Ramon y Cajal, S. (1911): *Histologie du Systeme Nerveux de l'Homme et des Vertebres* (translated by L. Azoulay), vol. II, Instituto Ramon y Cajal, Madrid.

110. Ribak, C. E. (1978): Aspinous and sparsely-spinous stellate neurons in the visual cortex of rats

contain glutamic acid decarboxylase. *J. Neurocytol.*, 7:461–478.

111. Ribak, C. E., Bradburne, R. M., and Harris, A. B. (1982): A preferential loss of GABAergic symmetric synapses in epileptic foci: A quantitative ultrastructural analysis of monkey neocortex. *J. Neurosci.*, 2:1725–1735.

112. Ribak, C. E., Harris, A. B., Vaughn, J. E., and Roberts, E. (1979): Inhibitory, GABAergic nerve terminals decrease at sites of focal epilepsy. *Science*, 205:211–214.

113. Ribak, C. E., and Seress, L., (1983): Five types of basket cell in the hippocampal dentate gyrus: A combined Golgi and electron microscopic study. *J. Neurocytol.*, 12:577–597.

114. Roberts, E., Chase, T. N. and Tower, D. B. (1976): *GABA in Nervous System Function*, Raven Press, New York.

115. Satou, M., Mori, K., Tazawa, Y., and Takagi, S. F. (1982): Two types of postsynaptic inhibition in pyriform cortex of the rabbit: Fast and slow inhibitory postsynaptic potentials. *J. Neurophysiol.*, 48:1142–1156.

116. Satou, M., Mori, K., Tazawa, Y., and Takagi, S. F. (1983): Interneurons mediating fast postsynaptic inhibition in pyriform cortex of the rabbit. *J. Neurophysiol.*, 50:89–101.

117. Scholfield, C. N. (1978): Electrical properties of neurones in the olfactory cortex slice *in vitro*. *J. Physiol. (Lond.)*, 275:535–546.

118. Schwartzkroin, P. A. (1975): Characteristics of CA1 neurons recorded intracellularly in the hippocampal *in vitro* slice preparation. *Brain Res.*, 85:423–436.

119. Schwartzkroin, P. A. (1983): Local circuit considerations and intrinsic neuronal properties involved in hyper-excitability and cell synchronization. In: *Basic Mechanisms of Neuronal Hyperexcitability*, edited by H. H. Jasper and N. M. van Gelder, pp. 75–108. Alan R. Liss, New York.

120. Schwartzkroin, P. A., Futamachi, K. J., Noebels, J. L., and Prince, D. A. (1975): Transcallosal effects of a cortical epileptiform focus. *Brain Res.*, 99:59–68.

121. Schwartzkroin, P. A., and Mathers, L. H. (1978): Physiological and morphological identification of a nonpyramidal hippocampal cell type. *Brain Res.*, 157:1–10.

122. Schwartzkroin, P. A., and Prince, D. A. (1977): Penicillin-induced epileptiform activity in the hippocampal *in vitro* preparation. *Ann. Neurol.*, 1:463–469.

123. Schwartzkroin, P. A., and Prince, D. A. (1978): Cellular and field potential properties of epileptogenic hippocampal slices. *Brain Res.*, 147:117–130.

124. Schwartzkroin, P. A., and Prince, D. A. (1980): Changes in excitatory and inhibitory synaptic potentials leading to epileptogenic activity. *Brain Res.*, 183:61–73.

125. Schwartzkroin, P. A., and Prince, D. A. (1980): Effects of TEA on hippocampal neurons. *Brain Res.*, 185:169–181.

126. Schwartzkroin, P. A., and Wyler, A. R. (1980): Mechanisms underlying epileptiform burst discharge. *Ann. Neurol.*, 7:95–107.

127. Schwindt, P., and Crill, W. (1980): Role of a persistant inward current in motoneuron bursting during spinal seizures. *J. Neurophysiol.*, 43:1296–1318.

128. Scobey, R. P., and Gabor, A. J. (1975): Ectopic action potential generation in epileptogenic cortex. *J. Neurophysiol.*, 38:383–394.

129. Seino, M., and Wada, J. A. (1964): Chronic focal cortical epileptogenesis lesion and behavior: Comparison of behavioral performance in monkeys with either epileptogenic or ablative unilateral lesion. *Epilepsia*, 5:321–333.

130. Shepherd, G. M. (1979): *The Synaptic Organization of the Brain*. Oxford University Press, New York.

131. Sloper, J. J., Johnston, P., and Powell, T. T. S. (1980): Selective degeneration of interneurons in the motor cortex of infant monkeys following controlled hypoxia: A possible cause of epilepsy. *Brain Res.*, 198:204–209.

132. Somogyi, P., Freund, T. F., Halasz, N., and Kisvarday, Z. F. (1981): Selectivity of neuronal [^{3}H]-GABA accumulation in the visual cortex as revealed by Golgi staining of the labeled neurons. *Brain Res.*, 225:431–436.

133. Stafstrom, C. E., Schwindt, P. C., and Crill, W. E. (1982): Negative slope conductance due to a persistant subthreshold sodium current in cat neocortical neurons *in vitro*. *Brain Res.*, 236:221–226, 1982.

134. Stefanis, C., and Jasper, H. (1964): Intracellular microelectrode studies of antidromic responses in cortical pyramidal tract neurons. *J. Neurophysiol.*, 27:828–954.

135. Suppes, T. A., Kriegstein, A. R., and Prince, D. A. (1985): The influence of dopamine on epileptiform burst activity in hippocampal pyramidal cells. *Brain Res.*, 326:273–280.

136. Takahashi, K. (1965): Slow and fast groups of pyramidal tract cells and their respective membrane properties. *J. Neurophysiol.*, 28:908–924.

137. Takahashi, K., Kubota, K., and Uno, M. (1967): Recurrent facilitation in cat pyramidal tract cells. *J. Neurophysiol.*, 30:22–34.

138. Tower, D. B. (1969): Neurochemical mechanisms. In: *Basic Mechanisms of the Epilepsies*, edited by H. H. Jasper, A. A. Ward, Jr., and A. Pope, pp. 611–638. Little, Brown and Co., Boston.

139. Toyama, K., Matsunami, K., Ohno, T., and Tokashiki, S. (1974): An intracellular study of neuronal organization in the visual cortex. *Exp. Brain Res.*, 21:45–66.

140. Traub, R. D., and Wong, R. K. S. (1982): Cellular mechanism of neuronal synchronization in epilepsy. *Science*, 216:745–747.

141. Traub, R. D., and Wong, R. K. S. (1983): Synchronized burst discharge in the disinhibited hippocampal slice. II. Model of the cellular mechanism. *J. Neurophysiol.*, 49:459–471.

142. Westrum, L. E., White, L. E., Jr., and Ward, A. A., Jr. (1964): Morphology of the experimental epileptic focus. *J. Neurosurg.*, 21:1033–1046.

143. White, E. L., and Rock, M. P. (1980): Three-dimensional aspects and synaptic relationships

of a Golgi-impregnated spiny stellate cell reconstructed from serial thin sections. *J. Neurocytol.*, 9:615–636.

144. White, W. F., and Heller, A. H. (1982): Glycine receptor alteration in the mutant mouse spastic. *Nature*, 298:655–657.

145. Wong, R. K. S., and Prince, D. A. (1978): Participation of calcium spikes during intrinsic burst firing in hippocampal neurons. *Brain Res.*, 159:385–390.

146. Wong, R. K. S., and Prince, D. A. (1979): Dendritic mechanisms underlying penicillin-induced epileptiform activity. *Science*, 204:1228–1231.

147. Wong, R. K. S., and Prince, D. A. (1981): Afterpotential generation in hippocampal pyramidal cells. *J. Neurophysiol.*, 45:86–97.

148. Wong, R. K. S., Prince, D. A., and Basbaum, A. I. (1979): Intradendritic recordings from hippocampal neurons. *Proc. Nat. Acad. Sci. USA*, 76:986–990.

149. Wong, R. K. S., and Traub, R. D. (1983): Synchronized burst discharge in disinhibited hippocampal slice. I. Initiation in CA2-CA3 region. *J. Neurophysiol.*, 49:442–458.

150. Wong, R. K. S., and Watkins, D. J. (1982): Cellular factors influencing the GABA response in hippocampal pyramidal cells. *J. Neurophysiol.*, 48:938–951.

151. Wu, C. F., Ganetzky, B., Haugland, F. N., and Liu, A.-X. (1983): Potassium currents in *Drosophilia:* Different components affected by mutations of two genes. *Science*, 220:1076–1078.

152. Yamamoto, C. (1972): Intracellular study of seizure-like afterdischarge elicited in thin hippocampal sections *in vitro. Exp. Neurol.*, 35:154–164.

EPILEPTOGENESIS II
Cell-to-Cell Communication: Neurotransmitters, Neuromodulators, and Receptors

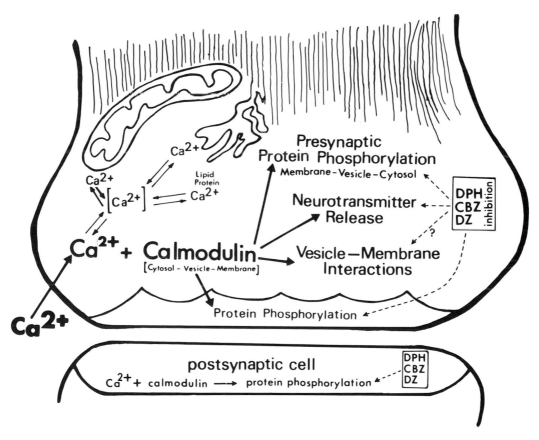

DeLorenzo's schematic model showing the roles of calcium and calmodulin in regulating synaptic protein phosphorylation, neurotransmitter release and turnover, and vesicle membrane interactions. The inhibitory effects of phenytoin (DPH), carbamezapine (CBZ), and diazepam (DZ) on these calcium calmodulin-stimulated processes are also shown. From Chapter 22 in this volume by R. J. DeLorenzo.

Advances in Neurology, Vol. 44, edited by
A. V. Delgado-Escueta, A. A. Ward, Jr.,
D. M. Woodbury, and R. J. Porter.
Raven Press, New York © 1986.

14

Kindling Model of Epilepsy

James O. McNamara

Departments of Medicine (Neurology) and Pharmacology, Duke University Medical Center, and Veterans Administration Hospital, Durham, North Carolina 27705

SUMMARY Kindling is an animal model of epilepsy produced by focal electrical stimulation of the brain. This chapter: (a) describes the kindling phenomenon; (b) considers the validity of kindling as an animal model and proposes a hypothesis as to how kindling might contribute to human epileptogenesis; (c) presents a critical review of current insights into the underlying mechanisms; and (d) emphasizes that, if progress is to be made in understanding the mechanisms, the *network* of brain structures underlying kindling must be elucidated.

Recent investigations directly related to the network issue are considered, namely studies demonstrating that a brainstem structure, the substantia nigra (SN), can regulate the kindled seizure threshold. Thus, either microinjection of a GABA receptor agonist or a GABA transaminase inhibitor into SN, but not into nearby sites, elevates kindled-seizure threshold. Likewise, destruction of SN, but not of adjacent structures, is associated with an increase of kindled-seizure threshold. These treatments suppress not only clonic motor seizures, but also complex partial seizures and afterdischarge at the site of stimulation. These findings demonstrate that the SN can regulate the intrinsic neuronal excitability of forebrain structures.

A hypothesis is advanced that generation of a complex partial seizure requires activation of neurons in the SN which in turn feed back through polysynaptic connections to influence neurons at the site of seizure origin. This nigral influence on neurons at the site of seizure origin is either a direct excitation or a disinhibition. Thus, the seizure represents reverberatory activity within a network of brain structures which includes the SN. Other investigators have proposed that the centrencephalic system subserved seizure propagation; the relationship of the hypothesis proposed here to these earlier ideas is discussed.

The kindling phenomenon represents a model of epilepsy and neuronal plasticity. This intriguing phenomenon has attracted the interest of many investigators with widely differing scientific backgrounds. The goals of this review are several: (a) to describe the kindling phenomenon; (b) to consider its validity as a model of human epilepsy; (c) to present hypotheses as to how kindling might participate in human epileptogenesis; (d) to review critically current insights into basic mechanisms of kindling; and (e) to summarize recent work from the author's laboratory pertaining to the role of the substantia nigra (SN) in kindling.

HISTORICAL PERSPECTIVE

The seizure-inducing potential of focal electrical stimulation of the brain was recognized by numerous investigators in the 1950s and 1960s.

Delgado and Sevillano (9) demonstrated in 1961 that repeated administration of low levels of electrical current to the hippocampus induced progressive intensification of stimulus-induced seizure activity. The potential importance of this observation was recognized by Goddard et al. in the late 1960s (16,17).

"The progressive changes that result from repeated electrical stimulation will be referred to as the 'kindling effect'." This statement by Goddard in 1969 reflected his perception of this phenomenon (17). He coined the term kindling because of the analogy to lighting a fire. He carefully characterized the kindling effect and demonstrated its permanence; he recognized its potential as a model of human epileptogenesis, learning, and memory. His landmark paper on the subject ushered in a new era for investigation of this intriguing phenomenon (17). This growth is attested to by the hundreds of articles published on this subject in the past decade.

KINDLING PHENOMENON

The term kindling refers to a phenomenon whereby repeated administration of an initially subconvulsive electrical stimulus results in progressive intensification of seizure activity culminating in a generalized seizure. In rats stimulated in the amygdala, the initial stimulus often elicits focal electrical seizure activity (after discharge recorded on electroencephalogram [EEG]) without overt clinical seizure activity. Subsequent stimulations induce the development of seizures, generally evolving through the following classes: class 1, facial clonus; class 2, head nodding; class 3, forelimb clonus; class 4, rearing; and class 5, rearing and falling (46). The behavior observed in classes 1 and 2 mimics that found in human complex partial or limbic seizures; the behavior in later classes is consistent with limbic seizures evolving into secondarily generalized clonic motor seizures. Henceforth, the term limbic seizure will be used to refer to behavior in which the rat is immobilized with or without associated facial clonus or head nodding; these behaviors are defined as limbic seizures when correlated with focal afterdischarge recorded between the tips of the bipolar electrode. The term motor seizure will be used to refer to the clonic or tonic activity of the extremities during a class 4 or 5 seizure.

Once the enhanced sensitivity (as evidenced by a class 5 seizure) has developed, the animal is said to be "kindled." This effect is long-lasting, and use of the term "kindling" implies that the change is permanent. Animals left un-

stimulated for as long as 12 months will respond to one of the first two electrical stimuli with a class 5 seizure. No widely accepted method exists whereby the kindling effect can be reversed.

Kindling can be induced by electrical stimulation of many, but not all, sites in the brain. The amygdala is the structure most commonly used, mainly because relatively few stimulations are required to induce kindling. The hierarchy of sensitivity (progressing from most to least sensitive) with the various sites was characterized by Goddard as follows: amygdala, globus pallidus, pyriform cortex, olfactory area, anterior neocortex, entorhinal cortex (EC), olfactory bulb, septal area, preoptic area, caudate-putamen, and hippocampus (17). These experiments were performed before the importance of local afterdischarge in the development of kindling was appreciated; sensitivities have not been systematically studied recently. Kindled seizures have not been elicited with electrodes in superior colliculus, reticular formation, or cerebellum. The pattern of development of kindled seizures elicited by stimulation of many sites in the limbic system is similar to those from the amygdala. Kindling induced by anterior neocortical stimulation differs in that motor seizures, although mild, accompany the initial stimulation (48). These seizures intensify with subsequent stimulations and assume more tonic components than do limbic kindled seizures. If neocortical stimulations are continued, seizures typical of limbic-kindled seizures follow or occur simultaneously with the neocortical-kindled seizures.

Kindling can be established in numerous species, including: frog (34); reptile (50); mouse (26); rat (17); rabbit (54); dog (65); cat (60); rhesus monkey (17); and baboon (61). Although some differences exist, the behavioral patterns of amygdaloid-kindled seizures are remarkably similar in many of these species. Differences exist in the sensitivity to kindling among strains within a species as well as among species.

The nature of the electrical stimulus is an important determinant of the development of kindling. The standard paradigm consists of the periodic administration of a 1-sec train of 1 msec biphasic square wave pulses at a frequency of 60 Hz. Stimulations with pulse frequencies of 25, 60, or 150 Hz are equally effective in inducing the development of kindling (17). Early studies indicated that low-frequency (i.e., pulses less than 10 Hz) stimuli were ineffective in eliciting kindling. Recent investigations indicate that long trains (60 sec) of high-intensity, low-frequency (down to 0.875 Hz) stimuli can elicit the kindling phenomenon with relatively few stimulations (4); whether this method proves to be as reliable as the standard paradigm remains to be determined. Kindling develops at comparable rates regardless of whether sine wave or rectangular pulses are used, and regardless of whether train durations of 2 sec or 60 sec are used (17).

The interval between stimulations represents a key variable in establishment of kindling. Stimulations (1-msec pulses at 60 Hz for 1 sec) administered at intervals ranging from 15 min to 7 days can induce kindling. Greater numbers of stimulations are required when intervals of 15 or 30 min are used (47). Administration of 1 msec pulses at 60 Hz continuously for several hours does not induce kindling (17).

The electrical stimulus must induce local afterdischarge in order for kindling to develop. However, subthreshold stimulation causes a lowering of the afterdischarge threshold (45). If the current intensity is set slightly below the afterdischarge threshold, repeated stimulation will lower the threshold and can lead to afterdischarge production and subsequent kindling.

A necessary criterion for an animal model of epilepsy is that seizures occur spontaneously, since epilepsy by definition implies the presence of spontaneous seizures (as opposed to seizures elicited by an electrical stimulus). Most kindling experiments are terminated after elicitation of a single or several class 5 motor seizures. Spontaneous generalized motor seizures are infrequently observed in rats stimulated to this extent. However, Pinel and Rovner found that continued periodic stimulation of amygdala, hippocampus, or EC of the rat leads to spontaneous motor seizures (42). In contrast to the 15–30 stimulations required to elicit a class 5 seizure, additional stimulations (a mean of 348) result in spontaneous motor seizures in all subjects. Among subjects manifesting at least three spontaneous class 5 seizures, spontaneous seizures persist for as long as 7 months following termination of the stimulation, suggesting that the epilepsy is permanent. Because limbic seizure with subtle or absent motor features are difficult to detect in the rat, the large numbers of seizures during the relatively brief observation sessions in this study indicate that kindling is a potent means of inducing epilepsy. Spontaneous seizures have been identified in additional species, including baboons, cats, and dogs.

If the term kindling is expanded to imply the evolution of progressively more severe seizures in response to the periodic administration of a constant stimulus, kindling can be induced by a variety of pharmacologic agents and even electroconvulsive shock. Drugs administered by local brain injection (carbamyl choline or penicillin) or systemically (e.g., cocaine, lidocaine, or pentylenetetrazol) can induce kindling-like effects (6,23,43,44,58).

VALIDITY OF KINDLING AS A MODEL OF HUMAN COMPLEX PARTIAL SEIZURES AND EPILEPSY

Whether similar mechanisms are operative in kindling and human complex partial seizures and epilepsy is unknown. Several features of kindled seizures support the validity as a model of human seizures. First, the behavioral patterns of kindled seizures mimic human complex partial seizures with secondarily generalized tonic-clonic seizures. Second, the EEG abnormalities during kindled seizures are similar to those recorded from electrodes in the amygdala and hippocampal formation during human complex partial seizures. Third, interictal spikes are present in the EEG of both kindled animals and human epileptic subjects. Fourth, there is a close correspondence between the anticonvulsants which are effective against kindled and human seizures. One exception to the pharmacology is the ineffectiveness of phenytoin against amygdaloid-kindled seizures; whether this is owing to pharmacokinetic factors is presently unclear (62).

Whether similar mechanisms are operative in the development of epilepsy in kindling and the human condition is also unknown. Three clinical observations suggest that kindling-like phenomena may contribute to human epileptogenesis. One observation is that of the mirror focus. Adults with complex partial epilepsy arising from one temporal lobe may progress so that both temporal lobes eventually trigger complex partial seizures. The common occurrence of interictal epileptiform activity independently in each temporal lobe supports this notion. This notion was strengthened by identifying patients with brain tumors, apparently confined to one temporal lobe, in whom distinct clinical seizures were initiated independently by each temporal area (35). Although multiple interpretations of this observation exist, one possibility is that repeated seizure activity from an abnormal temporal lobe could itself induce epilepsy in an originally normal temporal lobe.

A second observation arises from a single case which suggests that kindling can occur in humans (52). In this instance, repeated periodic electrical stimulation was being administered through depth electrodes implanted in the left thalamus of the patient. The goal was to ameliorate intractable pain which had developed as a consequence of traumatic amputation of the fingers of the patient's right hand. Unfortunately, during this treatment course, the patient developed partial motor seizures of the right upper extremity that proceeded to generalized tonic-clonic seizures. The absence of other complications (e.g., abscess, hemorrhage, etc.) strongly suggested that repeated periodic electrical stimulation caused the epilepsy.

A third observation, namely the latency between head trauma and the onset of posttraumatic epilepsy, raises the possibility of a kindling-like process. The silent period between head trauma and onset of spontaneous seizures ranges from weeks to years. One hypothesis is that the brain injury leads to formation of new neural connections (e.g., sprouting) which in turn lead to abnormal neuronal excitability, repetitive neuronal firing, and a kindling-like process culminating in epilepsy.

INITIATION OF KINDLED EPILEPTOGENESIS IN HUMANS: A HYPOTHESIS

These clinical observations notwithstanding, one striking difference exists between kindling and human epilepsy, namely the absence of a histologically detectable lesion in the brains of kindled animals (in comparison to electrode-implanted unstimulated controls). Indeed a lesion, often including Ammon's horn sclerosis, is readily detectable with standard histologic techniques in most temporal lobes resected from patients with medically intractable complex partial epilepsy (12). Epileptologists have long speculated that these lesions may somehow increase local neuronal excitability, which in turn contributes to human epileptogenesis. Studies of Ammon's horn sclerosis induced by the excitatoxin, kainic acid, lends support to this idea. The principal target of the axons of the dentate granule cells of hippocampal formation are the CA3 pyramidal cells. These axons exert a powerful excitatory influence on the CA3 cells. Destruction of some of these CA3 pyramidal cells deprives the granule cells of their normal targets. One consequence is that the axons of the granule cells appear to innervate themselves, apparently forming synapses on their soma and proximal dendrites, thereby potentially forming a recurrent excitatory synapse (37). Studying hippocampal slices removed from animals with Ammon's horn sclerosis, Nadler and his col-

leagues (38) have demonstrated the presence of repetitive firing of granule cells in response to a single orthodromic excitatory pulse. Such repetitive firing was not observed in slices from control animals. Thus, repetitive firing might develop in response to a physiologic afferent input. We speculate that such repetitive firing could "kindle" target structures in a pattern similar to that observed in the kindling model. The presence of spontaneous seizures months after a single treatment with kainic acid supports this idea (5,55).

If correct, this hypothesis would predict that the presence of Ammon's horn sclerosis—induced by hypoxic damage in infancy or adulthood—would increase the risk of developing epilepsy. Moreover, since repeated seizures can induce Ammon's horn sclerosis in experimental animals, this might account for the apparent progression of the epileptic condition observed in some patients after frequent seizures.

APPROACHES TO BASIC MECHANISMS

Electrophysiologic

The leading hypothesis for the cellular mechanism underlying kindling is that excitatory synapses undergo long-term potentiation (LTP) (10). Studies by four different groups have produced different experimental findings and some differences in conclusions. Sutula and Steward (53) kindled animals by stimulation of the angular bundle (which carries the principal extrinsic excitatory afferents to hippocampal formation), and examined the field excitatory postsynaptic spike potential (EPSP) and population spike of the granule cells elicited by single shocks of the angular bundle. They found long-lasting increases of the slope of the EPSPs, increases of the amplitude of the population spike, and more efficient coupling of the EPSP-population spike in the kindled animals. By contrast, Maru et al. (29) and Tuff et al. (56) found no consistent evidence of LTP in kindled animals. Likewise, Giacchino et al. (15) found no LTP of the monosynaptic EPSPs of granule cells following stimulation of lateral entorhinal cortex (LEC) in animals kindled by LEC stimulation.

A number of considerations arise in regard to these paradoxical findings. First, technical difficulties of these long-term recordings are considerable. These include damage induced by the electrodes and movement of either the stimulating and/or recording electrodes from the site of initial placement. Meaningful interpretation of positive or negative findings requires demonstration of stable responses in electrode-implanted but unkindled control animals paired to the kindled animal for the entire duration of the experiment. Second, neither the absence nor presence of LTP in identified synaptic connections alone is a sufficient test of the hypothesis. Correlative experiments (with lesions, microinjections, etc.) will be necessary to assess the importance of the identified neuronal populations in the kindling phenomenon. The possibility exists that destruction of only potentiated neuronal populations will retard kindling development or reverse kindling, whereas destruction of unpotentiated populations will have no effect. Careful attention to these considerations will be necessary to confirm or exclude the hypothetical role of LTP in the kindling phenomenon.

Biochemical

Numerous biochemical studies have been conducted to elucidate the molecular basis of kindling. These biochemical studies can be divided into two general categories: first, molecules immediately related to neurotransmission, e.g., synthesis or degradation of a putative neurotransmitter, steady state levels of the neurotransmitter, neurotransmitter membrane receptors, etc.; and second, molecules that might participate in the chain of events triggered by interaction of a neurotransmitter with its receptor.

Most of the studies have focused on molecules immediately related to neurotransmission. Putative neurotransmitters examined include GABA and benzodiazepines, glutamate, norepinephrine (NE), dopamine, serotonin, acetylcholine (ACh), and Leu- and Met-encephalin. Reviews of these studies have been published recently (22,31) and will not be repeated here. These studies have not provided a coherent explanation of the kindling phenomenon. Discovery of some transient molecular changes following kindling has provided insight into some aspects of the brain's response to seizures. If the working hypotheses are correct, these represent the molecular basis of endogenous mechanisms attempting to stabilize neuronal excitability.

Whether a modification of neurotransmitter mechanisms per se is responsible for the kindling phenomenon is unclear. There are numerous ways of regulating neuronal excitability without directly affecting neurotransmitter mechanisms (e.g., regulating the voltage sensitivity of ionic conductances; e.g., modifying in-

ternal resistance to current flow by regulating diameter of dendritic spines). Study of molecules participating in the chain of events triggered by the interaction of a transmitter with its receptor may be one way of approaching this issue. Three such lines of investigation with respect to kindling have focused on the role of cyclic nucleotides, calcium binding protein and calmodulin, and protein phosphorylation.

The cyclic nucleotides have been implicated in control of neuronal excitability (25). Measurement of steady state concentrations of cyclic AMP and cyclic GMP in amygdala and cerebral cortex disclosed no significant differences between kindled and control animals (64).

Decreased amounts of immunoreactivity of calcium-binding protein have been detected in the hippocampus (but not in the cerebellum, caudate, or cerebral cortex) 24 hr and 10 days after completion of kindling of the hippocampal commissure (33). No alterations in total soluble protein or calmodulin immunoreactivity were found. Immunocytochemical studies disclosed the most marked reductions of calcium-binding protein to be in the areas overlying the dendrites, cell bodies, and axons of the granule cells; thus, the reduced immunoreactivity almost certainly resides in the granule cells. This interesting observation raises a number of questions: Does this reduction of calcium binding protein immunoreactivity modify granule cell excitability, and if so how? Is this reduction a cause or a consequence of kindling? Do the granule cells play a pivotal role in kindling induced by commissural stimulation?

Similar questions have been raised by previous observations that demonstrated altered numbers of receptors (decreased numbers of muscarinic cholinergic and increased numbers of benzodiazepine receptors) in the granule cells following amygdaloid kindling (51,57). The data indicate that these receptor changes likely represent a consequence of kindled seizures and not the cause of kindling. The receptor changes appear to contribute to a net increase of inhibition of the granule cells that has been found in electrophysiologic investigations of kindled animals both *in vivo* (56) and *in vitro* (24). Removal of the granule cells prior to kindling (with the neurotoxin colchicine) suppresses the rate of development of amygdaloid kindling (8). Together, these data point to the hippocampal formation in general and the granule cells in particular as mediating a facilitating role in the development of kindling. The mechanisms by which the granule cells fulfill this role, and how changes in calcium-binding protein immunoreactivity or these receptors might contribute to these mechanisms, remains to be elucidated.

Other investigators have found reductions in radioactive phosphorus incorporation into multiple proteins in hippocampal synaptic membranes after septal kindling (see Chapter 21) (66). This finding is particularly interesting because the reductions persist as long as 2 months following completion of kindling. Understanding the functional implications of these alterations will require determination of the cellular location of these proteins, and the cell functions mediated by phosphate turnover on these proteins.

Morphological

Morphological studies have not detected clear differences between kindled animals and electrode-implanted, unstimulated controls (7,17, 49). These studies have utilized Nissl stains, Golgi studies, and some ultrastructural analyses. Possible explanations for these negative findings are: (a) the available methods are not adequate to identify subtle differences; (b) the differences exist but not in the areas studied; and (c) technical shortcomings in implementing these experiments obscured the positive findings. Because ultrastructural differences have been found after repeated electrical stimulation in acute experiments *in vivo,* we suspect that similar differences exist between kindled and control animals. If so, the contribution of such morphologic changes to the kindling phenomenon would require elucidation.

Network of Kindling

Consideration of these different approaches to elucidating the mechanisms of kindling underscores the key limiting factor, namely our ignorance of the spatial distribution of the network of brain structures containing the alterations responsible for kindling. Knowing where the alterations reside is necessary to delineating the nature of the alterations at a cellular and molecular level.

Two major hypotheses have been advanced to address this network issue. One hypothesis states that the neural reorganization responsible for kindling involves neurons restricted to the area of the kindling electrode. An alternate hypothesis claims that alterations residing in targets (i.e., neurons remote from the kindled area and related to the kindled area by monosynaptic or polysynaptic connections) of the kindled structure contribute to the kindling effect.

Evidence supporting the first hypothesis has

been obtained from 2-deoxyglucose autoradiographic study of "penicillin kindling" of the neocortex (6). Injection of large amounts (100 U) of penicillin caused an intense motor convulsion on the first injection; subsequent injections caused *milder* convulsions. By contrast, injection of smaller amounts (25 U) of penicillin caused a relatively minor focal motor seizure initially; repeated injections at 4-day intervals caused a progressive intensification of the focal motor seizure and frequently bilateral clonic jerks of the upper extremities. In this paradigm, 2-deoxyglucose autoradiography was used to measure neuronal metabolic activity. The animals "kindled" with 25 U of penicillin disclosed an increase in size and metabolic activity of the seizure focus, together with an increase in size and intensity of most transsynaptic sites. Comparison of these findings with the autoradiographic results of animals receiving 100 U of penicillin for the first time suggested that the major change during kindling takes place in the focus itself. Although alterations inherent in the transsynaptic targets of the kindled focus could not be excluded, the magnitude of the increase in the targets could be accounted for by enhanced intensity of the primary focus itself. Therefore, it seems possible that the principle alteration in "penicillin kindling" involves alterations mainly at the primary seizure focus.

The second hypothesis is supported by two experimental results. Establishment of kindling by electrical stimulation in one brain region (e.g., amygdala) results in fewer stimulations required to establish kindling in a second region (e.g., opposite amygdala) (17). This phenomenon has been termed transfer. The transfer phenomenon suggests that key alterations occur in brain regions anatomically remote from the kindled structure. This suggestion was strengthened when transfer persisted despite destruction of the primary kindled structure (44).

Additional support for the second hypothesis was obtained in a series of experiments utilizing kindling of the EC (32). Each EC projects heavily to the ipsilateral dentate gyrus of the hippocampal formation, but only sparsely to the contralateral dentate gyrus (DG). Unilateral EC lesions massively deafferent the ipsilateral DG; this is followed within 2 weeks by a partial reinnervation of the DG owing to sprouting of surviving afferent systems. Among these sprouting afferent fibers is a sparse projection from contralateral EC, which reinnervates some of the dendritic territory in the DG that was previously occupied by the ipsilateral EC projection. These authors reasoned that if kindling via EC stimulation induced transynaptic alterations in either the DG or further "downstream," the neural reorganization underlying kindling should survive destruction of the primary site of kindling. The presynaptic structures that were directly activated by the kindling stimulations (the projection from the "kindled" EC) would be replaced by a system (the sprouted connections from the contralateral side) not subjected to the direct application of the kindling stimulus. If the sprouting projections from the contralateral EC gain access to circuitry that had been transsynaptically modified during primary kindling, activation of the lesion-induced crossed EC projections might precipitate a kindled convulsion. The experimental results were consistent with this possibility.

In normal rats, a mean of 23 daily stimulations were required to establish kindling (five class 5 motor seizures). When the primary kindled EC site was destroyed and 2 weeks were allowed for the contralateral EC to sprout in response to the lesion, kindling stimulation of the surviving EC evoked class 5 seizures on the first or second stimulation. If the primary site was not destroyed, kindling via a contralateral EC required an average of more than five stimulations (transfer phenomenon). If sprouting was induced by unilateral EC lesion prior to any kindling stimulations, kindling by the surviving "sprouted" EC contralateral to the lesion occurred at a rate similar to normal. If kindling via the secondary site was initiated 1 day after a primary site lesion, at a time prior to completion of sprouting, the relatively immediate expression of generalized seizures via secondary site stimulation was not observed. These results were consistent with the hypothesis that EC kindling results in transsynaptic alterations either in the immediate targets of the EC (e.g., DG) or further "downstream" synaptically.

None of these three experimental approaches provides an unequivocal answer to the question. First, the relevance of penicillin kindling to electrical kindling is unclear; likewise different circuits may be operative in limbic and neocortical kindling. Second, although the transfer phenomenon implies the presence of alterations in anatomically remote brain regions, whether these alterations are essential to primary site kindling is unclear. Finally, EC kindling of the primary site may induce direct alterations in the contralateral unstimulated EC, either transsynaptically or by backfiring EC-EC projections; increase of the synaptic targets of the contralateral EC through lesion-induced sprouting could account for the more rapid "transfer" observed. This in-

terpretation of the results would not require alterations inherent in targets of the kindled structures.

These various limitations notwithstanding, it appears likely that the neural reorganization underlying electrically induced kindling in the limbic system involves both the kindled structure and its synaptically related targets. Defining the precise spatial extent of these circuits is essential to understanding the mechanisms of the kindling phenomenon.

Network of Kindled Seizures

One approach to determining the structures responsible for kindling is to delineate the structures responsible for generation of kindled seizures. It seems likely that at least some of the alterations involved in generating the seizures may be sites of the alterations subserving kindling itself.

To delineate these structures, several investigators have examined the distribution of afterdischarge from electrodes implanted in multiple brain structures during kindled seizures (28, 59,63). The results obtained by different investigators are not easy to compare since different species and different recording sites have been studied. All have found afterdischarge in electrodes placed in cortical, limbic, and brainstem sites in class 4 or 5 seizures induced by amygdaloid stimulation. Although some useful information has been obtained with this approach, several shortcomings exist: (a) the number of possible structures is vast and the number which can be sampled in a single experiment is limited; (b) the response time of the paper-based EEG recordings is often too slow to record the temporal sequence of afterdischarge appearance in the various structures; (c) the EEG is recording slow waves (mainly synaptic potentials) and does not permit inferences as to alterations in firing patterns of neuronal populations; and (d) the studies to date have not addressed the issue of the spatial extent of the neuronal populations which generate the afterdischarge recorded in the various electrodes.

More recently, the 2-deoxyglucose autoradiographic method has been utilized to address this issue in kindled rats. Engel et al. (11) found increased glucose uptake in the stimulated amygdala and related limbic sites (medial septum, EC, and pyriform cortex) during class 1 and 2 seizures. During class 4 and 5 seizures, the most prominent increases were found in the SN, globus pallidus, thalamic nuclei, and neocortex. The method used in this study departed from the standard 2-deoxyglucose approach (isotope infusion followed by relatively stable behavioral events for 45 min and then killing of the animals) in that a seizure (lasting approximately 80 sec) was induced 3 sec after the infusion followed by killing 5 min later. Thus, the altered 2-deoxyglucose uptake may reflect a mixture of altered patterns of metabolism as well as altered blood flow. It is also unclear whether the altered 2-deoxyglucose uptake is caused by events underlying seizure generation, seizure termination, or behavioral events that represent a consequence of either seizure generation or termination. Increased 2-deoxyglucose uptake does not necessarily imply increased neuronal firing (1). The extent to which this method will contribute to understanding which brain structures subserve kindled seizure generation remains to be determined.

ROLE OF SUBSTANTIA NIGRA IN REGULATION OF KINDLED-SEIZURE THRESHOLD

The preceding section indicates that current insights into the brain structures subserving generation of kindled seizures are limited. We reasoned that identification of a synaptically downstream structure that was pivotal to the expression of a kindled seizure would be an important step in resolving this problem. Knowing the site of origin (site of stimulating electrode) and a downstream target, together with knowledge of the anatomic connections, would provide a model testable with currently available techniques. Such information could reduce the number of candidate structures so that the hypotheses could be tested with electrophysiologic, lesion, and pharmacologic techniques.

Observations by other investigators led us to postulate that the SN may be a synaptically downstream structure playing a key role in the expression of kindled seizures. Myslobodsky et al. (36) found that systemic administration of γ-vinyl GABA (GVG), a GABA transaminase inhibitor, blocked the motor component of kindled seizures. Iadarola and Gale (21) found that the SN appears to be a key site of GABA-mediated anticonvulsant action, since microinjection of muscimol, an agonist of the inhibitory neurotransmitter GABA, into SN decreased susceptibility to seizures induced by electroshock and chemoconvulsants. Therefore, we hypothesized that SN may also regulate the expression of motor seizures in the kindling model.

Methods and Results

To test this hypothesis, we studied the effects of microinjected drugs and brainstem lesions on motor and limbic seizures in kindled rats. These animals were stimulated through stereotactically implanted bipolar electrodes until kindling was established. Daily stimulations were then initiated and continued until a stable generalized seizure threshold (GST) was obtained by determining responses to a specified current intensity on 4 consecutive days. A stable GST refers to a current intensity at which stimulations 20 μA above this value resulted in motor seizures, whereas stimulations 20 μA below this value did not. The duration of motor seizures was determined by timing the clinic and tonic movements of the extremities. The duration of limbic seizures was determined by measuring afterdischarge recorded on the EEG (Fig. 1). Drugs were microinjected via injection cannulas inserted through guide cannulas in awake, gently restrained rats; all injections were made bilaterally. Electrode and cannula placements were histologically verified with a Nissl stain of coronal sections in all animals.

Bilateral microinjections of muscimol (a GABA agonist) (50 ng per side) into or adjacent to SN markedly suppressed motor seizures (Fig. 2, top; Table 1). The 91% suppression was highly significant ($p < 0.001$) in comparison to either the day preceding or the day following the injection. Motor seizures were abolished in seven of the eight animals. Microinjection of saline into equivalent areas did not suppress motor seizures (Fig. 2, middle; Table 1).

Muscimol microinjections into the region of SN also suppressed limbic seizures. This was evident from both behavioral and EEG observations. The 85% suppression of afterdischarge duration in these animals was statistically significant (Fig. 2, top; Table 1). Data on afterdischarge duration are presented in Table 1 in only four of the eight animals receiving muscimol in the region of SN; the reason for excluding four of the animals was that the data on afterdischarge were not available on either pretreatment or posttreatment day because recording electrodes were dislodged during intense motor seizures. The data were available for all eight of these animals on the day of muscimol treatment because motor seizures were suppressed. The afterdischarge duration (mean $\pm$ SEM) was 17 $\pm$ 8 sec, which is not significantly different from the value of 10 $\pm$ 8 sec reported for the four animals in Table 1. Four of these eight animals

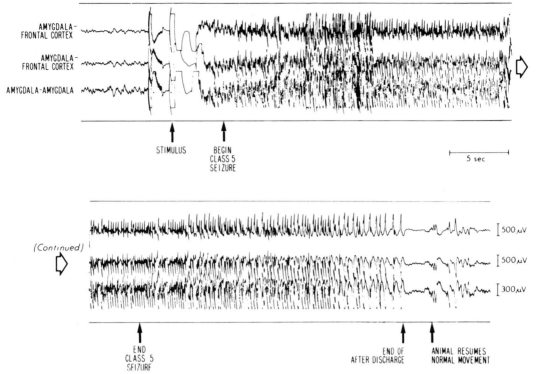

FIG. 1. Typical EEG patterns observed during a class 5 seizure. Behaviorally, the animal was immobilized with mild facial clonus for several seconds after cessation of the stimulus prior to exhibiting the class 5 seizure consisting of rearing, loss of postural tone, and clonic and tonic movements of the extremities. After completion of the clonic and tonic components of the seizure, the animal regained his normal posture, but remained immobilized with facial clonus and head nodding. This persisted for approximately 35 sec and was followed by resumption of normal movement about the cage and frequent "wet-dog shakes." The afterdischarge terminated a few seconds prior to resumption of normal movement.

exhibited no afterdischarge at all. In contrast to these results, no statistically significant depression of afterdischarge duration was observed after saline injection into the area of SN or after muscimol injection into brainstem sites dorsal to the area of SN (Fig. 2, middle and bottom; Table 1). Further evidence for spatial specificity was obtained when bilateral microinjections of muscimol into areas of neocortex of eight rats (50 ng per side in seven rats and 100 ng per side in one rat) did not significantly attenuate motor seizure duration (Table 1).

To determine whether the seizure suppressant action of muscimol was unique to kindled seizures elicited from amygdala, we examined the effects of muscimol in animals kindled from lateral entorhinal cortex or olfactory structures. Intranigral muscimol was highly effective in suppressing both motor and limbic seizures triggered from these sites (30).

In additional experiments, we found that the suppressive effect of muscimol dissipated after several hours and was dependent upon dose. We also found that this effect was caused by an elevation of the seizure threshold, since typical seizures could be elicited with electrical current far exceeding the threshold.

The actions of muscimol were likely mediated by its GABA agonist properties, since microinjection of an irreversible inhibitor of GVG into the area of SN also suppressed kindled seizures (30).

We postulated that the seizure-suppressant action of muscimol was mediated by reducing neuronal activity in the SN. This hypothesis was based on two observations: (a) the spatial selectivity of seizure-suppressing effects of muscimol suggested that SN was the site of action; and (b) iontophoretic application of muscimol inhibited unit activity in SN (67). This hypothesis predicts

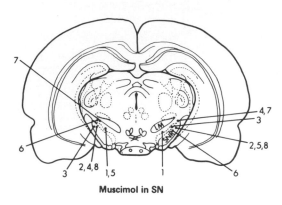

Muscimol in SN

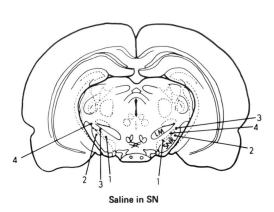

Saline in SN

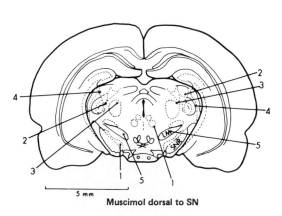

Muscimol dorsal to SN

that destruction of SN would suppress kindled seizures.

To test this postulate, we studied the effects of neurotoxin lesions produced with N-methyl-D,L-aspartate on kindled seizures. Following establishment of a stable GST, 20 μg of N-methyl-D,L-aspartate in 0.5 μl of saline were injected into various sites of the brainstem. Three days later, the animals received a test stimulation at a current intensity 10% above the GST. Following completion of the experiment, the animals were killed, and the extent of the lesion was reconstructed from Nissl stains of serial coronal sections. The reconstructions were done without prior knowledge of the seizure responses after lesions.

We divided the animals into three groups: animals with no SN destruction (group 1); animals with unilateral SN destruction (group 2); and animals with bilateral SN destruction (group 3) (Table 2). Reconstructions of the lesions in representative animals from these groups are depicted in Fig. 3. Motor seizures and afterdischarges after the lesion were suppressed by 81 and 71%, respectively, in animals with bilateral SN destruction as compared with prelesion seizure durations. Animals with unilateral SN destruction exhibited suppression of motor seizures (30%) and afterdischarges (32%), which was less than that with bilateral destruction but which exceeded that in which SN was spared (21% suppression of motor seizures and 7% reduction of afterdischarges). The reductions after bilateral lesions were statistically significant ($p < 0.001$), whereas reductions in neither of the other groups were significant ($p > 0.05$).

The destruction of structures other than SN

FIG. 2. Locations of injection cannula tips plotted on the drawings of coronal sections through the brainstem according to the stereotaxic atlas of Konig and Klippel (25a). The right side of the brain corresponds to the right side of the figure. The numbers refer to the sites of injection cannula tips in each side of a single animal determined by examination of Nissl stains of serial frozen sections. **Top:** Location of the cannulas of animals receiving muscimol in the region of substantia nigra (SN). **Middle:** Location of the cannulas of animals receiving saline in the area of SN. **Bottom:** Location of the cannulas in animals receiving muscimol dorsal to the area of SN. The rostral and caudal extent of locations of cannula tips ranged approximately 500 μm on either side of this level with the exception of animal 1 in Fig. 2 **(bottom):** the cannula on the right side of this animal was situated 1.2 mm rostral to this level. The data from these animals are presented in Table 1. SNR, pars reticulata of SN; LM, medial lemniscus.

TABLE 1. *Effects of microinjections of muscimol or saline on the duration of amygdaloid-kindled seizures*

Drug	Injection site	Pretreatment day	Treatment day	Posttreatment day
Muscimol	SN			
(50 ng)				
Motor seizure (N = 8)		34 ± 3	3 ± 3[b]	31 ± 4
Afterdischarge (N = 4)[a]		70 ± 7	10 ± 8[b]	66 ± 10
Saline	SN			
Motor seizure (N = 4)		39 ± 5	39 ± 8	36 ± 4
Afterdischarge (N = 2)[a]		69 ± 0	64 ± 2	55 ± 0
Muscimol	Dorsal to SN			
(50 or 100 ng)				
Motor seizure (N = 5)		38 ± 4	27 ± 3	35 ± 4
Afterdischarge (N = 4)[a]		65 ± 11	55 ± 15	62 ± 6
Muscimol	Neocortex			
(50 ng)				
Motor seizure (N = 8)		36 ± 3	28 ± 7	36 ± 4

SN, substantia nigra.

Values represent mean ± SEM of seizure duration in seconds; N refers to number of individual animals from which these data were taken.

[a] Discrepancy in N between motor seizure and afterdischarge occurs because data on afterdischarge were not available in all animals as a result of dislodging of recording electrodes during intense motor seizures.

[b] Data from muscimol injections into the region of SN are significantly different (Student's t-test, two-tailed, $p < 0.001$) from pretreatment days.

in these cases warranted careful consideration of the potential role of these structures in seizure suppression. We examined the correlation between bilateral destruction of each structure listed in the legend of Fig. 3 and total suppression of motor seizures. Motor seizure suppression correlated best with bilateral destruction of SN. An effect caused by destruction of the reticular formation situated between pars compacta of SN and the medial lemniscus could not be excluded, since the destruction of this area in the lesion paralleled that of SN. By contrast, the mamillary body and interpeduncular nucleus could be readily excluded since these structures

were spared in all animals with seizure suppression. Destruction of the ventral tegmental area correlated less well with seizure suppression than with destruction of SN. Among animals in which motor seizures were abolished, SN was destroyed bilaterally in seven of eight animals, whereas the ventral tegmental area was destroyed bilaterally in five of eight. The results of these analyses were consistent with the idea that destruction of SN was the factor responsible for seizure suppression.

The effect of SN destruction represented an increase in seizure threshold rather than an elimination of the ability to generate seizures. Ad-

TABLE 2. *Effects of lesions on the duration of amygdaloid-kindled seizures*

	Group 1		Group 2		Group 3	
	Prelesion	Postlesion	Prelesion	Postlesion	Prelesion	Postlesion
Motor seizure	34 ± 4	27 ± 1	37 ± 3	26 ± 11	32 ± 2	6 ± 3[a]
	(5)	(5)	(4)	(4)	(10)	(10)
Afterdischarge	96 ± 8	89 ± 12	107 ± 14	73 ± 23	89 ± 5	26 ± 10[a]
	(4)	(4)	(4)	(4)	(10)	(10)

Values represent the mean ± SEM of seizure duration in seconds. Number in parentheses refers to number of animals. Substantia nigra was spared in animals in group 1, but was at least partially destroyed unilaterally among animals in group 2, and at least partially destroyed bilaterally among animals in group 3. Data on afterdischarge were available in fewer animals than were data on motor seizure duration (group 1) because one animal dislodged a recording electrode during the seizure. Differences between prelesion and postlesion values were not significant ($p > 0.05$) unless denoted by asterisk.

[a] $p < 0.001$, Student's t-test, two-tailed.

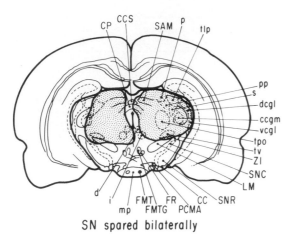

SN spared bilaterally

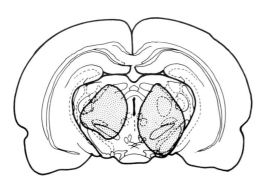

SN destroyed unilaterally

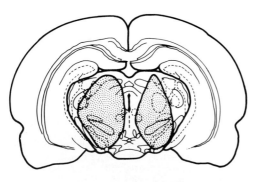

SN destroyed bilaterally

5 mm

ditional stimuli equivalent to the test stimulus were administered at intervals of at least 1 hr to three animals in which motor seizures were abolished and brief or no afterdischarges were obtained. None of these subsequent stimuli elicited motor seizures, and the duration of afterdischarge elicited was 20 sec or less. However, administration of an additional stimulus in which both current intensity and train duration were doubled resulted in long afterdischarges in all three animals (98, 70, and 42 sec, respectively) accompanied by class 4 seizures in two of the three animals. Extensive destruction of SN bilaterally was found in all three animals.

Discussion

Two lines of evidence from these studies point to SN as a crucial site responsible for seizure suppression: first, the spatial delectivity of microinjections of the GABA agonist, muscimol, together with the fact that SN is the principal site of GABA receptors in ventral midbrain; and second, the correlation between seizure suppression and neurotoxin-mediated destruction of SN.

Precisely which neuronal constituents within SN are responsible for the seizure suppressant effect is unclear. The dopaminergic neurons of pars compacta are not likely to be involved, since neither dopamine receptor agonists nor antagonists suppress kindled seizures (2). The much greater sensitivity to muscimol of neurons

FIG. 3. The darkened areas reflect the extent of lesions produced by the neurotoxin, *N*-methyl-D,L-aspartate, in animals shown in Table 1. Nissl-stained serial coronal frozen sections were analyzed to determine the extent of the lesions. Only a representative section from each group is presented. **Top:** Lesion spared substantia nigra (SN) bilaterally (Table 1, group 1). **Middle:** Lesion destroyed SN only unilaterally (Table 2, group 2). **Bottom:** Lesion destroyed SN bilaterally (Table 3, group 3). CC, cerebral peduncle; CP, posterior commissure; CCS, commissure of superior colliculus; ccgm, central nucleus of medial geniculate; d, nucleus Darkschewitsch; dcgl, dorsal nucleus of lateral geniculate; FMT, mamillothalamic tract; FMTG, mamillotegmental tract; FR, fasciculus retroflexus; i, intersitial nucleus of Cajal; LM, medial lemniscus; mp, posterior mamillary nucleus; p, pretectal nucleus; PCMA, peduncle of mamillary body; pp, pretectal nucleus, pars profundus; s, suprageniculate nucleus; SAM, stratum album of superior colliculus; SNC, substantia nigra, pars compacta; SNR, substantia nigra, pars reticulata; tlp, lateral thalamic nucleus, pars posterior; tpo, posterior thalamic nucleus; tv, ventral thalamic nucleus; vcgl, ventral nucleus of lateral geniculate; and ZI, zona incerta.

in reticulata than in compacta (67) supports reticulata as the key site. The pars reticulata also seems more likely in view of its extensive, often bilateral, and often collateralized projections to numerous thalamic and brainstem nuclei (14,39); these connections render it capable of modulating neuronal activity diffusely throughout the brain.

Speculation Regarding Role of SN in Kindled Seizures

Our results suggest that reduction of neuronal activity within SN underlies the seizure suppressant effect. Injection of muscimol, which inhibits SN unit activity (67), suppresses seizures. Destruction of SN also suppresses seizures. Indeed, the presence of afterdischarge recorded from electrodes in SN during limbic seizures (59,63) raises the possibility that SN must exhibit increased and/or synchronized neuronal firing in order for seizures to occur.

The suppression of motor seizures is consistent with the idea that SN transmits seizure information directly from rostral sites of origin to caudal motor targets. Alternatively, SN could regulate other neuronal structures that propagate the seizure information. The present findings extend previous observations that application of muscimol in the area of SN suppresses motor seizures induced by electroshock and pentylenetetrazol (21).

The most striking finding of the present work is that focal application of muscimol and GVG to SN can suppress limbic seizure activity, including electrical afterdischarge at the site of stimulation. If SN is actively involved in limbic seizure generation, it is not simply transmitting or regulating transmission of seizure information from rostral sites of origin to caudal targets. Rather, this nucleus in the midbrain is regulating the intrinsic neuronal excitability of multiple sites in the cerebral hemispheres, including lateral EC, amygdala, and olfactory structures.

This regulatory influence is almost certainly mediated through polysynaptic pathways, since no direct connections either to or from SN on the one hand, and olfactory structures and lateral EC on the other have been identified (14). Whether the interactions between amygdala and SN are mediated through polysynaptic connections is less clear, since reciprocal connections do exist between the central nucleus of the amygdala and pars lateralis of SN (3,27).

These findings lead us to propose the following hypothesis to explain how these structures interact to generate a limbic seizure in the kindling model. The train of stimuli activates neurons in the immediate vicinity (e.g., lateral EC) of the electrode. The repetitive firing of these neurons activates targets (e.g., in hippocampal formation and subsequently in ventral striatum), which in turn activate neurons in pars reticulata of SN. Working through polysynaptic connections, the output from SN mediates net excitation (either through disinhibition or a direct excitation) of neurons at the site of the stimulating electrode and increases the likelihood of neuronal firing lasting beyond cessation of the stimulation train. Thus, reduction of neuronal excitability in SN would reduce the likelihood of reverberatory activity in the network and thereby raise the seizure threshold.

SN in Epilepsy and Parkinsonism

The present findings may shed light on a long-standing clinical observation relating epilepsy to Parkinson's syndrome. Yakovlev (68) reported that development of Parkinson's syndrome in patients with epilepsy was temporally associated with a dramatic reduction in seizure frequency. A number of hypotheses have been advanced to explain this phenomenon (13). A central feature of the pathology underlying Parkinson's syndrome is degeneration of SN (18). Based upon the present data, it seems plausible that destruction of SN is one factor responsible for the observed reduction in seizure frequency.

Relationship to Previous Hypotheses of Seizure Generation

Previous investigators have proposed the involvement of subcortical and brainstem structures in the propagation of seizure activity from cortical sites and in the synchronization of hemispheres in seizure activity. Hayashi (19,20) suggested that the SN was one component of an efferent pathway mediating propagation of seizures from motor cortex. He based this suggestion on the observation that lesions in rostral midbrain suppress seizures induced by application of nicotine at cortical sites.

Drawing from his neurosurgical experience in epileptic patients, Penfield (40) proposed a concept of a centrencephalic coordinating and integrating system that is symmetrically related to both hemispheres. The anatomic substrate of this system was proposed to be two areas of gray matter symmetrically placed in the higher brainstem. He suggested that cortical discharges can lead to generalized convulsions by activation of this centrencephalic system. He further subdivided this system, one part having to do with motor control, which became affected during generalized motor seizures. The other part was involved in consciousness or perception and became involved during epileptic automatisms equivalent to limbic seizures (41).

The present work demonstrates that a specific anatomic structure, SN, may mediate the functions ascribed to the centrencephalic system. The work further suggests that SN may be operative not only in the propagation of motor seizure information but also in the generation of limbic seizures at the site of origin. Identification of the nuclei mediating the interactions between limbic structures and SN will be necessary to determine whether and how these structures interact to generate seizures.

CONCLUSIONS

The fundamental mechanisms of kindling remain obscure. The complexity of mammalian brain stands as a massive barrier to our feeble attempts to unlock its secrets. Progress in elucidating these mechanisms is slow yet proceeding. This is perhaps best exemplified in the studies testing LTP as the underlying cellular mechanism. If LTP proves to be the key, the extensive studies searching for the mechanism of LTP will guide the search for the mechanism of kindling. Alternatively, the absence of LTP could focus efforts on the possible contribution of nonsynaptic mechanisms of synchronizing firing of neuronal populations to the kindling phenomenon. Elucidating the network of brain structures subserving kindling would likely accelerate insights into the basic mechanisms.

Studies of kindling may provide insight into human epileptogenesis. Even if kindling-like processes do not contribute to human epileptogenesis, understanding of the network of structures generating limbic seizures would provide a framework for devising pharmacologic (i.e., key neurotransmitters in network) and surgical (i.e., destruction of pivotal sites in the network) strategies aimed at eliminating the seizures. Finally, regardless of its potential implications for understanding human seizures or epilepsy, insights into kindling will teach us many valuable lessons regarding normal brain function.

ACKNOWLEDGMENTS

This work was supported by grant No. NS17771 from the National Institutes of Health and by a grant from the Veterans Administration.

The secretarial assistance of Mrs. Eloise Pittman and Mrs. Rena Wethington is gratefully acknowledged.

REFERENCES

1. Aiker, C. R., Messler, R. M., and Carpenter, D. O. (1983): Apparent discrepancy between single-unit activity and [^{14}C] deoxyglucose labeling in optic tectum of the rattlesnake. *J. Neurophysiol.*, 49:1504–1516.
2. Babington, R. G., and Wedeking, P. W. (1973): The pharmacology of seizures induced by sensitization with low intensity brain stimulation. *Pharmacol. Biochem. Behav.*, 1:461–467.
3. Bunney, B. S., and Aghajanian, G. K. (1976): The precise localization of nigral afferents in the rat as determined by a retrograde tracing technique. *Brain Res.*, 117:423–435.
4. Cain, D. P., and Corcoran, M. E. (1981): Kindling with low-frequency stimulation: Generality, transfer, and recruiting effects. *Exp. Neurol.*, 73:219–232.
5. Cavalheiro, E. A., Riche, D. A., and Le Gal La Salle, G. (1982): Long-term effects of intrahippocampal kainic acid injection in rats: A method for inducing spontaneous recurrent seizures. *Electroencephalogr. Clin. Neurophysiol.*, 53: 581–589.
6. Collins, R. C. (1978): Kindling of neuroanatomic pathways during recurrent focal penicillin seizures. *Brain Res.*, 150:503–517.
7. Crandall, J. E., Bernstein, J. J., Boast, C. A., and Zornetzer, S. F. (1979): Kindling in the rat hippocampus: Absence of dendritic alterations. *Behav. Neurol. Biol.*, 27:516–522.
8. Dasheiff, R. M., and McNamara, J. O. (1983): Intradentate colchicine retards the development of amygdala kindling. *Ann. Neurol.*, 11:347–352.
9. Delgado, J. M. R., and Sevillano, M. (1961): Evolution of repeated hippocampal seizures in the cat. *Electroencephalogr. Clin. Neurophysiol.*, 13:722–733.
10. Douglas, R. M., and Goddard, G. V. (1975): Long-term potentiation of the perforant path-granule cell synapse in the rat hippocampus. *Brain Res.*, 86:205–215.
11. Engel, J., Wolfson, L., and Brown, L. (1978): Anatomical correlates of electrical and behavioral events related to amygdaloid kindling. *Ann. Neurol.*, 3:538–544.
12. Falconer, M. A. (1971): Genetic and retarded aetiological factors in temporal lobe epilepsy. A review. *Epilepsia*, 12:13–31.
13. Frigyesi, T. L. (1976): Parkinson and epilepsy. In: *Advances in Experimental Medicine and Biology*, Vol. 90, edited by F. S. Messiha, and A. D. Kenny, pp. 63–107. Plenum Press, New York.
14. Gerfen, C. R., Staines, W. A., Arbuthnott, G. W., and Fibiger, H. C. (1982): Crossed connections of the substantia nigra in the rat. *J. Comp. Neurol.*, 207:283–303.
15. Giacchino, J. L., Somjen, G. G., Frush, D. P., and McNamara, J. (1984): Lateral entorhinal cortical kindling can be established without poten-

tiation of the entorhinal-granule cell synapse. *Exp. Neurol.*, 86:483–492.

16. Goddard, G. V. (1967): Development of epileptic seizures through brain stimulation at low intensity. *Nature*, 214:1020–1021.

17. Goddard, G. V., McIntyre, D. C., and Leech, C. K. (1969): A permanent change in brain function resulting from daily electrical stimulation. *Exp. Neurol.*, 25:295–330.

18. Greenfield, J. G. (1955): The pathology of Parkinson's disease. In: *James Parkinson (1755–1824)*, edited by M. Critchley, pp. 219–243, Macmillan, London.

19. Hayashi, T. (1953a): A physiological study of epileptic seizures following cortical stimulation in animals and its application to human clinics. *Jpn. J. Physiol.*, 3:46–54.

20. Hayashi, T. (1953b): The efferent pathway of epileptic seizures for the face following cortical stimulation differs from that for limbs. *Jpn. J. Physiol.*, 3:306–321.

21. Iadarola, M. J., and Gale, K. (1982): Substantia nigra: Site of anticonvulsant activity mediated by γ-aminobutyric acid. *Science*, 218:1237–1240.

22. Kalichman, M. W. (1982): Neurochemical correlates of the kindling model of epilepsy. *Neuroscience Biobehav. Rev.*, 6:165–181.

23. Kilbey, M. M., Ellinwood, E. H., and Easler, M. E. (1979): The effects of chronic cocaine pretreatment on kindled seizures and behavioral stereotypes. *Exp. Neurol.*, 64:306–314.

24. King, G. L., Dingledine, R., Giacchino, J., and McNamara, J. O. (1985): Enhanced inhibition and epileptiform bursting in hippocampal slices from kindled rats. *J. Neurophysiol.*, 54:1295–1304.

25. Klein, M., and Kandel, E. R. (1978): Presynaptic modulation of voltage-dependent CA^{2+} current: Mechanism for behavioral sensitization in *Aplysia californica. Proc. Natl. Acad. Sci. USA*, 75:3512–3516.

25a. Konig, J. F. R., and Klippel, R. A. (1963): *The Rat Brain. A Stereotoxic Atlas*. R. A. Krieger Publishing Co., Inc., Huntington, New York.

26. Leech, C. K., and McIntyre, D. C. (1976): Kindling rates in inbred mice: An analog to learning? *Behav. Biol.*, 16:439–452.

27. Loughlin, S. E., and Fallon, J. H. (1983): Dopaminergic and non-dopaminergic projections to amygdala from substantia nigra and ventral tegmental area. *Brain Res.*, 262:334–338.

28. Mars, N. J. I, and Lopes Da Silva, F. H. (1983): Propagation of seizure activity in kindled dogs. *Electroencephalogr. Clin. Neurophysiol.*, 56:194–209.

29. Maru, E., Tatsuno, J., Okamoto, J., and Ashida, H. (1982): Development and reduction of synaptic potentiation induced by perforant path kindling. *Exp. Neurol.* 78:409–424.

30. McNamara, J. O., Rigsbee, L. C., and Galloway, M. T. (1983): Evidence substantia nigra is crucial to neural network of kindled seizures. *Eur. J. Pharmacol.*, 86:485–486.

31. McNamara, James O. (1984): The role of neurotransmitters in seizure mechanisms in the kindling model of epilepsy. *Fed. Proc.*, 43:2516–2520.

32. Messenheimer, J. A., Harris, E. W., and Stew-
ard, O. (1979): Sprouting fibers gain access to circuitry transynaptically altered by kindling. *Exp. Neurol.*, 64:469–481.

33. Miller, J. J., and Baimbridge, K. G. (1983): Biochemical and immunohistochemical correlates of kindling-induced epilepsy: Role of calcium binding protein. *Brain Res.*, 278:322–326.

34. Morrell, F., and Tsura, N. (1976): Kindling in the frog: Development of spontaneous epileptiform activity. *Electroencephalogr. Clin. Neurophysiol.*, 40:1–11.

35. Morrell, F. (1979): Human secondary epileptogenic lesions. *Neurology*, 29:558.

36. Myslobodsky, M. S., Ackerman, R. F., and Engel, J. (1979): Effects of γ-acetylenic GABA and γ-vinyl GABA on metrazol-activated, and kindled seizures. *Pharmacol. Biochem. Behav.*, 11:265–271.

37. Nadler, J. V., Perry, B. W., Gentry, C., and Cotman, C. W. (1981): Fate of the hippocampal mossy fiber projection after destruction of postsynaptic targets with intraventricular kainic acid. *J. Comp. Neurol.*, 196:549–569.

38. Nadler, J. V., Tauck, D. L., Evenson, D. A., and Davis, J. N. (1983): Synaptic rearrangements in the kainic acid model of Ammon's horn sclerosis. In: *Excitatoxins, Wenner-Gren International Symposium 39,* edited by K. Fuxe, P. J. Roberts, and R. Schwarcz, pp. 256–270. Macmillan, Houndmills.

39. Parent, A., Mackey, A., Smith, Y., and Boucher, R. (1983): The output organization of the substantia nigra in primate as revealed by a retrograde double labeling method. *Brain Res. Bull.*, 10:529–537.

40. Penfield, W. (1952): Epileptic automatism and the centrencephalic integrating system. *Res. Publ. Assoc. Res. Nerv. Ment. Dis.*, 30:513–528.

41. Penfield, W. (1969): Epilepsy, neurophysiology, and some brain mechanisms related to consciousness. In: *Basic Mechanisms of the Epilepsies*, edited by H. H. Jasper, A. A. Ward, Jr., and A. Pope, pp. 791–806. Little, Brown and Co., Boston.

42. Pinel, J. P. J., and Rovner, L. I. (1978): Electrode placement and kindling-induced experimental epilepsy. *Exp. Neurol.*, 58:335–346.

43. Pinel, J. P. J., and Van Oot, P. H. (1975): Generality of kindling phenomenon: Some clinical implications. *Can J. Neurol. Sci.*, 2:467–475.

44. Post, R. M., and Kopanda, R. T. (1976): Cocaine, kindling and psychosis. *Am J. Psychiatry*, 133:627–634.

45. Racine, R. J. (1972a): Modification of seizure activity by electrical stimulation—I. After-discharge threshold, *Electroencephalogr. Clin. Neurophysiol.*, 32:269–279.

46. Racine, R. J. (1972b): Modification of seizure activity by electrical stimulation—II. Motor seizures. *Electroencephalogr. Clin. Neurophysiol.*, 32:281–294.

47. Racine, R. J., Burnham, W. M., Gartner, J. G., and Levitan, D. (1973): Rates of motor seizure development in rats subjected to electrical brain stimulation: Strain and interstimulation interval effects. *Electroencephalogr. Clin. Neurophysiol.*, 35:553–556.

48. Racine, R. J. (1975): Modification of seizure activity by electrical stimulation: Cortical areas. *Electroencephalogr. Clin. Neurophysiol.*, 38: 1–12.

49. Racine, R., Tuff, L., and Zaide, J. (1975): Kindling unit discharge patterns and neural plasticity. *Can. J. Neurol. Sci.*, 2:395–405.

50. Rial, R. V., and Gonzalez, J. (1978): Kindling effect in the reptilian brain: Motor and electrographic manifestations. *Epilepsia*, 19:581–589.

51. Savage, D. D. S., Dasheiff, R., and McNamara, J. O. (1983): Kindled seizure induced reduction of muscarinic cholinergic receptors in rat hippocampal formation: Evidence for localization to dentate granule cells. *J. Comp. Neurol.*, 221:106–112.

52. Sramka, M., Sedlak, P., and Nadvornik, P. (1977): Observation of kindling phenomenon in treatment of pain by stimulation in thalamus. In: *Neurosurgical Treatment in Psychiatry, Pain, and Epilepsy*, edited by W. H. Sweet, pp. 651–654. University Park Press, Baltimore.

53. Sutula, T., and Steward, O. (1983): Quantitative analysis of synaptic potentiation during kindling. *Neurology* (Suppl. 1) 33:188.

54. Tanaka, A. (1972): Progressive changes of behavioral and electroencephalographic responses to daily amygdaloid stimulation in rabbits. *Fukuoka Acta Med.*, 63:152–163.

55. Tanaka, T., Kaijima, M., Daita, G., Ohgami, S., Yonemasu, Y., and Riche, D. (1982): Electroclinical features of kainic acid-induced status epilepticus in freely moving cats. Microinjection into the dorsal hippocampus. *Electroencephalogr. Clin. Neurophysiol.*, 54:288–300.

56. Tuff, L. P., Racine, R. J., and Adamec, R. (1983): The effects of kindling on GABA-mediated inhibition in the dentate gyrus of the rat. I. Paired-pulse depression. *Brain Res.*, 277:79–90.

57. Valdes, F., Dasheiff, R. M., Birmingham, F., Crutcher, K. A., and McNamara, J. O. (1982): Benzodiazepine receptor increases following repeated seizures: Evidence for localization to dentate granule cells. *Proc. Natl. Acad. Sci. USA*, 79:193–197.

58. Vosu, H., and Wise, R. A. (1975): Cholinergic seizure kindling in the rat: Comparison of caudate, amygdala, and hippocampus. *Behav. Biol.*, 13:491–495.

59. Wada, J. A., and Sato, M. (1974): Generalized convulsive seizures induced by daily electrical stimulation of the amygdala in cats. *Neurology*, 24:565–574.

60. Wada, J. A., Sato, M., and Corcoran, M. E. (1974): Persistent seizure susceptibility and recurrent spontaneous seizures in kindled cats. *Epilepsia*, 15:465–478.

61. Wada, J. A., Osawa, T., and Mizoguchi, T. (1975): Recurrent spontaneous seizure state induced by prefrontal kindling in Senegalese baboons *Papio papio*. *Can. J. Neurol. Sci.*, 2:477–492.

62. Wada, J. A. (1977): Pharmacological prophylaxis in the kindling model of epilepsy. *Arch. Neurol.*, 34:389–395.

63. Wada, J. A., Mizoguchi, T., and Osawa, T. (1978): Secondarily generalized convulsive seizures induced by daily amygdaloid stimulation in rhesus monkeys. *Neurology*, 28:1026–1036.

64. Walker, J. E., Mikeska, J. A., and Crawford, I. L. (1981): Cyclic nucleotides in the amygdala of the kindled rat. *Brain Res. Bull.*, 6:1–3.

65. Waquier, A., Ashton, D., and Melis, W. (1979): Behavioral analysis of amygdaloid kindling in beagle dogs and the effects of clonazepam, diazepam, phenobarbital, diphenylhydantoin, and flunarizine on seizure manifestation. *Exp. Neurol.*, 64:579–586.

66. Wasterlain, C. G., and Farber, D. B. (1982): A lasting change in protein phosphorylation associated with septal kindling. *Brain Res.*, 247:191–194.

67. Waszczak, B. L., Eng, N., and Walters, J. R. (1980): Effects of muscimol and picrotoxin on single unit activity of substantia nigra neurons. *Brain Res.*, 188:185–197.

68. Yakovlev, P. I. (1928): Epilepsy and parkinsonism. *N. Engl. J. Med.* 198:620.

Advances in Neurology, Vol. 44, edited by
A. V. Delgado-Escueta, A. A. Ward, Jr.,
D. M. Woodbury, and R. J. Porter.
Raven Press, New York © 1986.

15

Failure of GABAergic Inhibition: A Key to Local and Global Seizures

Eugene Roberts

*Department of Neurobiochemistry, Beckman Research Institute of the City of Hope,
Duarte, California 91010*

SUMMARY Current working models of nervous system function based on
many experimental observations are presented, often supported by extensive immunocytochemical findings, and partly by extrapolation of such findings into
reasonable potentialities. Particular emphasis is placed on consideration of the
roles of inhibitory GABAergic neurons in normal and abnormal information processing in the CNS.

For several years after its discovery (72), the
unique presence of relatively large amounts of
GABA in the tissue of the CNS of various species remained a puzzle. In the first review on
the subject in 1956 (57), I concluded in desper-
ation:

> Perhaps the most difficult question to an-
> swer would be whether the presence in the
> gray matter of the CNS of uniquely high
> concentrations of γ-aminobutyric acid and
> the enzyme which forms it from glutamic
> acid has a direct or indirect connection to
> conduction of the nerve impulse in this
> tissue.

However, later that year, the first suggestion
that GABA might have an inhibitory function in
the vertebrate nervous system came from
studies in which it was found that topically applied solutions of GABA exerted inhibitory effects on electrical activity in the brain (29,30).
In 1957, from studies with convulsant hydrazides (39,40), the suggestion was made that
GABA might have an inhibitory function in the
CNS. Evidence for an inhibitory function for
GABA also came from studies in 1957 that established GABA as the major factor in brain ex-

tracts responsible for the inhibitory action of
these extracts on the crayfish stretch receptor
system (5). Within a brief period, activity in this
field increased greatly so that the research being
carried out ranged from the study of the effects
of GABA on ionic movements in single neurons
to clinical evaluation of the role of the GABA
system in, for example, epilepsy, schizophrenia,
and various types of mental retardation. Much
of the early work on GABA was summarized in
1959 (74) at the first truly interdisciplinary neuroscience conference. The subject of neural inhibition finally had returned to center stage after
many years of languishing in the wings (for background and history on concepts of neural inhibition, see refs. 16,20,74,86, and 87).

For a number of years many researchers
doubted that GABA was a true neurotransmitter. Florey (23) stated that "All available evidence speaks, however, against it (GABA)
playing a role as inhibitory transmitter in vertebrates." Curtis and Watkins (11) concluded
that GABA was not a "specialized inhibitory
substance." Even as late as 1964, the following
quotation appeared in a textbook (14):

> Thus GABA may be ruled out as the trans-
> mitter in those situations where its identity

with the transmitter seemed best proved; it is not surprising, therefore, that in the mammalian central nervous system its depressant action is not analogous with inhibitory activity, its action being non-specific on all responses of the motor neurone. . . .

It was remarked that GABA entered the 1959 conference (74) as a proud transmitter candidate and left it as a poor metabolite.

Because I was not a neurophysiologist, it made no difference to me whether or not GABA was a neurotransmitter. My goal was the elucidation of its function in the nervous system, whatever it might be. However, I did sense that the "transmitter question" seemed to upset some people. There was much initial scepticism regarding transmitter function of GABA because of the large quantities of GABA present in brain, three to four orders of magnitude higher than those of ACh, then the only proven neurotransmitter. It would have been more acceptable to some researchers if the first identified inhibitory neurotransmitter had had a more exotic chemical structure than that of GABA. Neither was glycine, the simplest amino acid, acceptable; it was identified as a putative inhibitory neurotransmitter in the spinal cord (88).

The most convincing early evidence for the role of GABA as an inhibitory neurotransmitter was obtained from studies at crustacean neuromuscular junctions (see refs. 41,47,49, and 81 for summaries). The postsynaptic action of applied GABA mimics exactly that which is found on stimulating inhibitory nerves. Inhibitory axons contain enormous concentrations of GABA (0.1 M), whereas <1% of these levels can be detected in excitatory nerves. GABA is released from lobster inhibitory nerves in amounts proportional to the number and frequency of stimuli applied to the nerve and is not released by stimulation of excitatory nerves. The enzyme that forms GABA from L-glutamate, glutamic acid decarboxylase (GAD), is preferentially distributed in inhibitory nerves. Synaptically released GABA probably is inactivated by a Na^+-dependent uptake mechanism that is capable of acting against large concentration gradients. Picrotoxin, a convulsant agent, blocks the inhibitory action of GABA and the natural inhibitory transmitter similarly. Thus, in the crustacean peripheral nervous system, GABA is an excellent inhibitory transmitter, and perhaps is more convincingly documented as such than is any other known transmitter at any site of action. Over the years, strong evidence had been adduced from physiological and pharmacological studies for an inhibitory neurotransmitter role for GABA in the vertebrate CNS (10,42). However, the necessary definitive chemical correlative work and release experiments are much more difficult to achieve in the tightly packed vertebrate CNS than in the crustacean peripheral nervous system; tissue culture systems have also had some severe limitations.

A critical examination of our own work and that of others almost 20 years ago made it clear that none of the "classical" neurochemical approaches could clarify the manner in which GABA neurons might participate in information-processing in different regions of the vertebrate CNS. It was clear that direct visualization of components of the GABA system, particularly GABA neurons and their terminals, was necessary to obtain unequivocal proof of the existence of GABA function at specific synaptic sites in neural tissues. The most likely approaches to achieve this goal appeared to be those that might lead to visualization of the pertinent proteins GAD, GABA transaminase (GABA-T), and the GABA transport and receptor proteins) at the light and electron microscopic levels. Early in 1968, I decided with great trepidation to begin with GAD, the rate-limiting enzyme in GABA formation, since it was known to be present in an easily solubilized form and in high concentration in synaptosomes. We first made many attempts to develop chemical procedures for the visualization of GAD, but all failed because of the difficulties in demonstrating histochemically the products of the enzymatic reaction, GABA and CO_2. The difficult alternative approach was to locate GABA neurons by immunocytochemical procedures. This required the preparation of pure GAD from brain, development of antibodies to the enzyme, and visualization of the antibodies by a suitable labeling technique specifically at those cellular and subcellular sites where GAD, the antigen, is located. It is to this task that we have dedicated ourselves for the past 16 years. The basic strategy and chronology of the achievement of these goals in our laboratories has been summarized (61,63,67,68,70). Much subsequent work from our own laboratories and those of others is appearing at an ever-accelerating rate.

A continuing dialogue with Arthur Ward during the years of development of the immunocytochemical techniques eventually led to their application to the study of alumina cream epileptic lesions in monkey cortex (51,52). It now appears that a major cause of seizures may be the loss of inhibitory GABAergic nerve terminals at sites of focal cortical epilepsy.

More than 30 years of work were needed to

move from an unknown ninhydrin-reactive spot on a two-dimensional paper chromatogram of an extract of mouse brain to the establishment of GABA as a major inhibitory transmitter, to the visualization of GABA-releasing neurons in nervous system structures, and to the establishment of the beginnings of a rational pharmacology of the GABA system. Even this relatively modest degree of progress has been possible only because of the participation in these studies of scientists from the several pertinent disciplines world wide. The recent coalescence of these separate disciplines into the single discipline of "neurosciences" has made it possible for us to begin to share techniques, vocabularies, and outlooks as exemplified in this book. And yet, there is a sense of uneasiness among us. Who can master all of the pertinent facts and technologies, or even keep up with a small portion of the literature? I believe that one must strive constantly to establish valid core positions from which to view meaningfully *both* phenomena of major human interest—such as seizures, memory, consciousness, various aspects of normal and abnormal behavior, aging, etc.—and the molecular and submolecular events that constantly are taking place at the level of excitable membranes. In making my own continuing integrative efforts (58–60,62,64,66,68–71,73,75, 76). I have taken heart from Einstein's statement (21), "Man seeks to form for himself in whatever manner is suitable for him, a simplified and lucid image of the world, and so to overcome the world of experience by striving to replace it to some extent by this image." This has given me the courage to face the critical barbs that inevitably arise.

GABA-RELATED PHENOMENA AND MODELS OF NERVOUS SYSTEM FUNCTION

General Statement

Seizures are a final common path taken by central nervous tissue when excitatory activity exceeds the capacity of the tissue to modulate the activity. This article will be restricted largely to consideration of the roles of GABAergic neurons in seizures, assuming that in the mammalian nervous system the neural effects of release of GABA from them usually are inhibitory. From the earliest physiologic and pharmacologic observations of the GABA system more than 30 years ago, it was conjectured that decreases in the efficacy of the GABA system could result in convulsive seizures (61,62,66,69,74). However,

it had proved impossible in most instances to establish cause-and-effect relationships because of inadequate knowledge of the microanatomy, microphysiology, and microchemistry of information transmission in the mammalian CNS. Only recently have the tools become sufficiently well developed. A few "organizing principles" based on my current understanding of nervous system function follow.

What Are Neuronal Circuits Like in Principle?

The functional units of the nervous system are the cells that make up its structures (neurons and glia), the endothelial cells of the blood vessels that supply the regions in which these cells are found, and the chemically transmitting synapses and gap junctions through which the neurons communicate. Much of the communication that takes place between sensory transducer and neuron, between neuron and neuron, and between neuron and effector cell is believed to occur via the extracellular liberation of a substance or combinations of substances which interact with specialized regions of membranes of neurons or of muscle and gland cells to produce either excitatory or inhibitory effects. The key to the action of transmitter substances lies in the nature of the changes they cause in the conformation of receptive regions of excitable membranes. A transmitter is neither excitatory nor inhibitory in itself, but only in relation to a specific membrane region with which it interacts. Thus, the particular transmitter that a given neuron may liberate from its axonal terminals onto the membranes of many other neurons may exert excitatory effects in some instances and inhibitory effects in others. ACh is always excitatory when it interacts with nicotinic receptors at neuromuscular junctions, but it is inhibitory when liberated from brainstem neurons onto muscarinic receptors of cells in the reticular nucleus of the thalamus.

Electrotonic interactions through gap junctions as well as field effects may be of key importance in neural information processing. The formation and dissolution of effective electrotonic junctions between neuronal processes may be occurring continuously, and alterations of numerous factors, e.g., intracellular pH, levels of calcium ions, and membrane potential may play roles in determining the extent, efficacy, and stability of such junctions and the numbers and types of neurons that are linked through such junctions at any time (18,36,45).

In the case of a given neuron, substances that are liberated upon its dendrites, soma, and initial axon segment from specialized endings of other neurons may exert excitatory, inhibitory, or modulatory effects. There probably are many voltage-sensitive and passive cation and anion currents that can traverse excitable membranes, of which several have been identified to date. Synaptic excitatory effects upon a neuron may occur most frequently on dendrites. The action of an excitatory transmitter is believed to result in configurational changes in membranes upon which it impinges, increasing permeability to cations and in turn decreasing the potential across the membrane (depolarization). An inwardly directed sodium current is probably responsible for most of the observed depolarization of postsynaptic membranes. Increases of free intracellular calcium ions that may occur from inward flow or from release from mitochondria during nerve activity activate the opening of potassium channels and may have far-reaching metabolic effects. The outward potassium current then serves to repolarize the cell and, in many instances, to produce a hyperpolarization. The calcium balance then is restored through the action of Ca^{2+}-Mg^{2+} ATPase and mitochondrial reuptake, and the potassium channels are closed. The action of Na^+-K^+ ATPase restores the mono-cation balance. The latter ion pump may sometimes overshoot the mark and cause hyperpolarization of the membrane, which results in neural inhibition. Increase in free intracellular calcium mentioned above, brief as it may be, also is believed to trigger the sequence of events that is important for the release of neurotransmitters from nerve terminals, for the initiation of the metabolic reactions required for recovery from nerve activity, and for the retention at pre- and postsynaptic sites of a biochemical "memory" of the experience. During this period, changes occur in activation states of various enzymes related to cyclic nucleotide metabolism and of proteases, phosphoprotein phosphatases, and phosphokinases. As a result, there are alterations in degrees of phosphorylation of enzymes and cell structural components, release of cascades of metabolic recovery reactions, and alterations in affinities of membranes for transmitters and modulators and in their permeabilities for anions and cations. The profound cellular reorganization that can occur may result in short-term or long-term changes in activities of neurons (27).

Inhibitory transmitters, which most often are liberated on dendrites close to the cell body, on the cell body itself, or on initial axon segments, increase the permeability to anions (particularly chloride), thereby making excitable membranes more resistant to depolarization, accelerating the rate of return of the resting potential of all depolarized membrane segments that the transmitter contacts, and decreasing the sensitivity to stimulation of undepolarized membrane segments. GABA, the major inhibitory neurotransmitter in vertebrate organisms, typically produces an increase in membrane permeability to chloride ions that is measured as an increase in membrane conductance. When GABA contacts membranes that have specific receptors for it, chloride ions tend to distribute across the membrane according to the chloride equilibrium potential, which usually is similar to the resting potential of the cell. Thus, by opening appropriate ionic channels, inhibitory transmitters act on postsynaptic sites essentially like chemical voltage clamps, allowing shunting ionic currents and often, in the presence of suitably set anionic pumps, hyperpolarization of excitable membranes to occur. The action of inhibitory neurotransmitters obviously is an important counterbalance to the depolarizing influences exerted on neuronal membranes by passive cation leakage and by impinging excitatory influences (61,74).

Excitatory and inhibitory influences constantly interact on the membrane of a neuron. At a particular time, many factors determine whether or not the spatially and temporally summated effects are sufficient to reduce membrane potential to the critical level at which the all-or-none propagation of a spike discharge takes place or, in nonspiking neurons, to reduce the potential to an extent that would result in an increase in transmitter release from its terminals.

All neurons possess an innate capacity to fire spontaneously (62,69). If a particular neuron were isolated from its biologic context and maintained under suitable environmental conditions, it would exhibit a characteristic firing pattern close to its maximal potential rate, which would be paced by inward ionic currents and their inactivating processes. For each neuron, this pattern would be a unique result of the interaction of its genetic potential with the environmental influences that had acted on it up to the moment of observation. Each neuron would "speak with its own voice," since multiple environmental gradients exist from the time of earliest development. No two neurons in an organism, although similar, could be identical in every respect.

Most neurons in their normal environments in

intact organisms are members of neuronal groupings or circuits and have largely ceded their autonomy while becoming participants in an integrated neuronal community. Many neurons do not fire spontaneously at all (56). Glial cells can serve as one major restraining influence on spontaneous activity of neurons by decreasing intrinsic excitatory levels of neuronal membranes below their spontaneous firing levels. This would be done by removing substances from the extraneuronal environment in the regions of synapses (e.g., K^+ ions or protons), by adding substances to it, or by regulating diffusion of substances from it or to it in such a way as to shunt depolarizing ionic currents. Major inhibitory influences are exerted by the effects of neurotransmitters liberated onto neurons from inhibitory neurons. Such inhibitory neurons might be only phasically active, with their activity depending on the inputs to them, or they might be tonically active, spontaneously firing cells. Some inhibitory neurons might release inhibitory transmitter constantly without an action potential, the rate of release being determined by the degree of membrane polarization. Release from inhibition could be achieved by direct depolarization of the inhibited cell, by inhibition of the inhibitory neurons, or, most commonly, by a combination of both.

Disinhibition, a Major Organizing Principle: The Whip and the Reins

Inhibitory and excitatory neurons participate together in information processing in nervous systems in such a way as to make it possible for particular organisms to respond adaptively to their environments. The ubiquity and extent of immunocytochemically visualized presynaptic endings of inhibitory GABAergic neurons on various structures in the vertebrate nervous system is striking. One seems to be looking at a highly restrained nervous system, the inhibitory neurons acting like reins that serve to keep the neuronal "horses" from running away (62, 66,69). I believe that in coherent behavioral sequences, innate or learned, preprogrammed circuits are *released* to function at varying rates and in various combinations. This is accomplished largely by the disinhibition of pacemaker neurons whose activities are under the dual tonic inhibitory controls of local circuit GABAergic neurons and of GABAergic projection neurons coming from neural command centers. According to this view, disinhibition (relaxation of reins) is permissive, and excitatory input to pacemaker neurons (the whip) would have mainly a modulatory role. Disinhibition, acting in conjunction with intrinsic pacemaker activity and often with modulatory excitatory input, appears to be one of the major organizing principles in nervous system function. For example, cortical and hippocampal pyramidal neurons are literally studded with terminals from inhibitory GABAergic neurons. Not only are the endings of the local circuit GABAergic aspinous stellate neurons densely distributed around the somata and dendrites of the cortical pyramidal cells, but they also are located on initial axon segments, where they may act as frequency filters. In addition, GABA neurons have terminals from other GABAergic neurons impinging upon them (Fig. 1) (69). This gives a picture consistent with the idea that the pyramidal cells are tightly inhibited by local circuit inhibitory neurons which, themselves, may be inhibited by the action of other inhibitory neurons in such a way that disinhibition of the pyramidal neurons may occur. Local circuit GABAergic neurons also participate in processes that result in producing feedforward, feedback, surround, and presynaptic inhibition and presynaptic facilitation. In addition, command centers, e.g., the cerebellum, exert high-frequency tonic inhibition in various brain regions via GABAergic projection neurons, e.g., Purkinje cells, which, when decreased, release neural activity at the projection sites (see Neural Command Centers section below). The profuse cerebellar GABAergic projection to neurons in the lateral vestibular nucleus is illustrated in Fig. 2.

Both inhibition and disinhibition probably play key roles in information processing in all neural regions. Normally, the principal cells in particular neural sectors, which possess the capacity for spontaneous firing or great sensitivity to excitatory input, or both, may be held tightly in check by constant tonic action of inhibitory neurons. Through disinhibition, neurons in one neural sector may be released to fire at different rates and sequences and, in turn, serve to release circuits at other levels of the nervous system. Communication between neural stations and substations, I believe, takes place largely by throwing of disinhibitory neural "switches," and the activities within them take place largely through preprogrammed, hard-wired circuitry. This may be the way in which information flows from sense organ to cerebral sensory area, through associative areas to the motor cortex, and by way of the pyramidal paths to the final motor cells of the medulla and spinal cord.

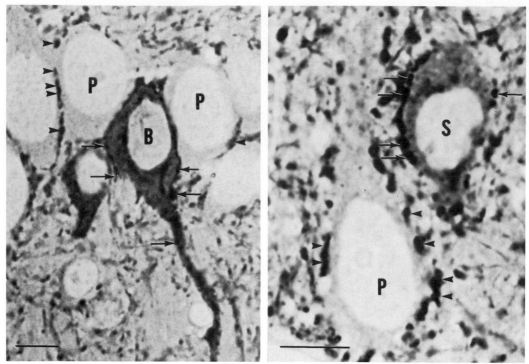

FIG. 1. GABA neurons and terminals in rat hippocampus and cortex. **Left:** A presumptive basket cell (B) in rat hippocampus that stains positively for L-glutamic acid decarboxylase (GAD) and is, therefore, a GABAergic neuron. It is studded with numerous GAD-positive terminals (arrows). **Right:** Soma of a GAD-positive stellate cell (S) in layer V of the rat visual cortex that also is studded with GAD-positive terminals. In both micrographs, it is seen that somata of pyramidal neurons (P), which are not GAD-positive, are contacted by numerous GAD-positive terminals. Bar represents 10 μm. (Courtesy of C. E. Ribak and J. E. Vaughn.)

Basic Neural Unit (Oversimplified and Partly Hypothetical)

The principal or pacemaker neuron (P) for the operation of a particular neural unit is shown to be under the restraint of the tonically active inhibitory interneuron, I_t (Fig. 3). A phasically active local circuit inhibitory neuron I_{pl}, when activated by excitatory afferent input from circuits in preceding neural sectors, would inhibit I_t. This would make it possible for the P neuron to fire by relieving it of the tonic inhibition exerted by I_t, i.e., by disinhibiting it. Excitatory input also could help release the P neuron by direct depolarization, in some instances via dendritic spikes propagated electrotonically to the soma. In reality, there would be multiple excitatory and inhibitory inputs onto both the P and I_t neurons. A particular I_t neuron might inhibit a number of P neurons, as probably occurs in the case of hippocampal basket cells or some retinal amacrine cells. The model requires that decrease or cessation of inhibitory signals from an I_t neuron would be a necessary, but not always sufficient, condition for the firing of a P neuron.

The latter might begin to fire spontaneously when partially or completely relieved of inhibition exerted by the I_t neuron, or excitatory input to the P neuron might be required for it to depolarize to the firing level, even when the tonic inhibitory influence on it has been decreased or completely removed. In the latter instance, less excitatory input would be required to fire the P neuron in the absence of inhibition by the I_t neuron than in its presence.

After an initial stimulus pattern is experienced by an organism, many neurons in various through-put sectors of the CNS are affected, either activated or inhibited. My concept of such sectors does not necessarily correspond exactly to a particular classically designated anatomic structure, but rather includes excitatory projection neurons and the excitatory interneurons upon which they impinge. For example, I propose that specialized thalamo-cortical cells and the intrinsic excitatory interneurons onto which they synapse be considered members of a neural sector. Cortical spinous stellate cells which receive excitatory thalamic inputs, and which in turn depolarize dendrites of cortical pyramidal

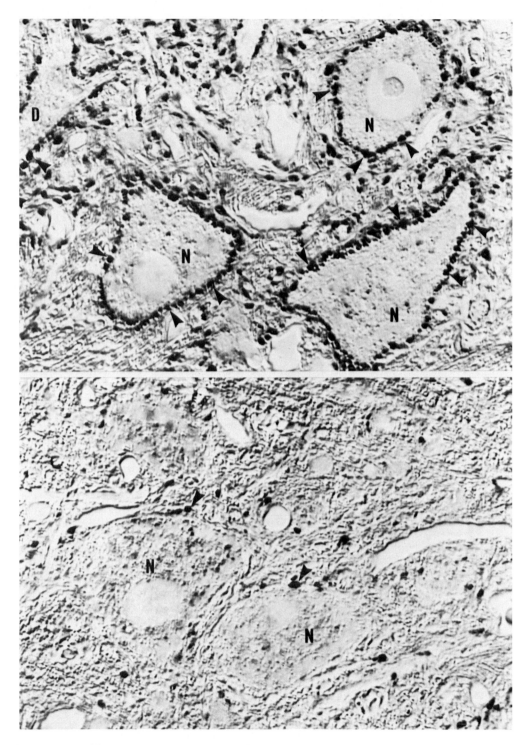

FIG. 2. Nomarski photomicrographs of normal (*a*) and partially deafferented (*b*) dorsal lateral vestibular nuclei from sections incubated in anti-GAD serum. In the normal specimen, neuronal cell bodies (N) and proximal dendrites (D) are surrounded by numerous GAD-positive axon terminals (arrowheads). In the deafferented specimen, such axon terminals are extremely sparse. Bar represents 15 μm. From CRC Press, Inc., C. Houser, and R. Barber, with permission (85).

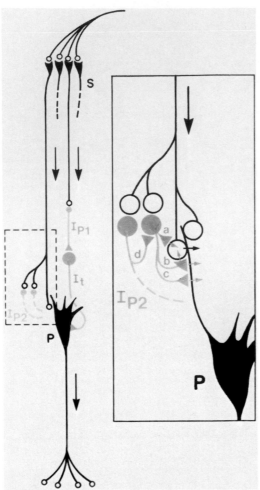

FIG. 3. Communication between neural sectors. Although not shown in the figure, the P neurons of preceding sectors are believed to make connections similar to those shown for the S neurons. Dark neurons, excitatory; gray neurons, inhibitory. I_t, tonically inhibitory; I_p, phasically inhibitory.

tant largely for extremely rapid communication, also may synapse on P and I_p neurons (not shown in Fig. 3) in a given sector (80).

The frequency of firing of the P neurons could at any given moment determine the exact details of S neuron activity, since the presynaptic impulses of the main axons of P neurons invade axonal branches, the activities of which vary with the frequency of firing of the main axon. Frequency-dependent differential channeling of information may take place at points of axonal branching (28,38,78). Although the terminals of all of the branches of a particular neuron probably liberate only one true neurotransmitter, the effects of this liberation might either be excitatory or inhibitory, depending on the nature of the postsynaptic receptors that are affected by the particular transmitter (38). Much recent data suggest that terminals of some neurons may contain a true transmitter and also a modulator, e.g., GABA or ACh and one of several neuropeptides. The frequency dependence of liberation of transmitter and modulator from inhibited nerve terminals containing both of them may not be the same. For example, a modulator that amplifies the postsynaptic efficacy of a true transmitter, or prolongs its action, may only begin to be liberated in graded amounts when the frequency of firing exceeds a certain level. Up to the latter frequency, there could be a regular relationship between firing frequency, number of quanta of true transmitter released, and extent and time of postsynaptic effect. Above that frequency, the liberation of an amplifying modulator might result in a progressively increasing degree of enhancement of the postsynaptic quantal efficacy of the neurotransmitter and/or a temporal expansion of its effect. In a similar manner, it can be envisioned how a deamplifying or desensitizing modulator might operate. I would like to suggest the possibility that in the terminals of some of the primary afferents to the spinal cord (viz., pain fibers) substance P may play the role of amplifying modulator of the effects of the excitatory transmitter. If glutamate were the transmitter, substance P and glutamate would be expected to show synergistic effects.

The P neurons integrate incoming signals, from dendritic endings to initial axon segment, and through their activities express frequency-dependent aspects of genetically coded neural programs that are communicated to the neurons onto which they synapse. Fibers from excitatory nerves synapse directly on dendrites of P neurons and also send branches to GABAergic interneurons (I_{p2}), which through their terminals can modulate and sculpt the activity generated by the direct excitatory input (Fig. 3, insert).

cells, can be considered to be examples of S neurons indicated in Fig. 3. The consequence of effective afferent neural input to any sector from any other sector of the nervous system, starting with receptors, is the change in activity caused by combinations of disinhibition and excitation of groups of excitatory P neurons. The individual P neurons in these groups control, through their activities, programs of activity in excitatory satellite neurons (S), which in turn signal P neurons in other neural sectors and/or effectors (muscles, glands). Although S neurons of active circuits can serve as the means of effective communication with other neural sectors, P neuron axons from other sectors, impor-

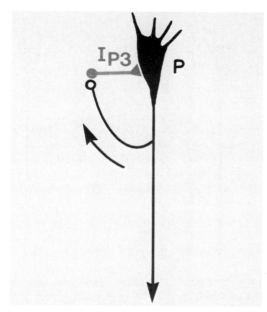

FIG. 4. Recurrent inhibition that can result in inhibitory phasing of its own activity by a neuron. Dark neurons, excitatory; gray neurons, inhibitory.

Terminals from such interneurons may form axoaxonic synapses (a) with the excitatory terminals, producing presynaptic inhibition. They may form axodendritic synapses (c) with dendrites in close proximity to the excitatory synapses, giving feed-forward postsynaptic inhibition that could short-circuit some of the excitation (1). In some instances, particularly potent inhibition might be exerted by individual inhibitory terminals that form both axoaxonic and axodendritic synapses (b). Finally, there can be synaptic inhibition of one I_{p2} interneuron by another (d) in such a manner as to decrease the above-described types of inhibition and result in presynaptic facilitation. Some phasically active inhibitory interneurons (I_{p3}), activated by excitatory recurrent collaterals of the P neurons, can furnish synaptic recurrent inhibition (Fig. 4), thereby exerting hyperpolarizing postsynaptic inhibition on the same P neurons by which they are activated. Such arrangements may result in the inhibitory phasing by a neuron of its own activity (see Discussion section below and Fig. 11 in ref. 1).

Inhibitory interneurons (I_{p4}) may be activated by collaterals coming from neurons in other sectors (Fig. 5). Reflecting activity occurring in succeeding neural sectors, such collaterals would furnish the links for feedback inhibition between neural sectors.

Neural Modules

Aggregates of mutually interrelated neurons, ranging from a few up to ~100 in number, in the cortex and elsewhere in the CNS, may serve as modules. In each neural sector, from receptor to cortex and cortex to effector, there may be redundant, functionally similar (but not identical) groups of neural modules. At each functional level in the CNS, I presume that there are classes of modules that respond to given inputs which are first determined at the level of receptor transduction and first-order neurons. In turn, these modules signal the frequency and intensity of input received by them in a manner interpretable by related modules in other sectors. Collaterals from their active P cells are presumed to synapse on inhibitory interneurons lying between the neural elements of different modules in such a manner that, after the onset

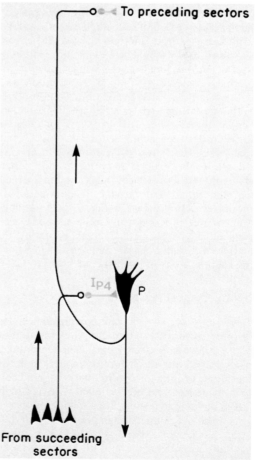

FIG. 5. Feedback inhibition from succeeding to preceding neural sectors. Dark neurons, excitatory; gray neurons, inhibitory.

of activity, each module would have a tendency to create an inhibitory surround by lateral inhibition in which adjacent or interpenetrating modules would tend to be held in a state of inactivity or reduced activity (Fig. 6). An active cortical "column" could consist of vertically communicating modules and might be surrounded by inhibited "columns." Units for different, or even antagonistic, functions frequently might be located side by side, exerting an influence upon one another. Thus, the activities of modules subserving a particular organismic function might inhibit some functionally redundant modules as well as some modules involved in parallel processing or in incompatible responses, viz., flexion–extension, eating–satiety, waking–sleeping, warming–cooling, attacking–fleeing.

A module is postulated to have, among its various cellular components, groups of spatially distributed, functionally redundant P neurons, as shown in Fig. 7. Let us assume that, as a result of existing patterns of connectivity, a particular class of impulses would begin to arrive from other sectors and that the two P neurons shown in Fig. 7 would be capable of responding to the arriving input. The P neurons within the module are depicted in Fig. 7 as communicating with each other via axon collaterals that produce both excitation and disinhibition in a manner similar to that suggested in Fig. 3 for communication between neural sectors. In Fig. 7, mutual excitation between P neurons can be considered to be exerted by release of chemical transmitters, by electrotonic coupling through gap junctions, and through field effects. Although it is not shown in Fig. 7, it is assumed that the direct depolarizing influences of P neurons on each other could be modified by the activities of inhibitory interneurons, as indicated for such neurons in the insert of Fig. 3.

Neural Command Centers

Nervous systems do not operate in a linear fashion. Minimally, a bifurcation of the flow of neural information from a particular sector takes place into direct through-put channels and also into those leading to coordinating command centers, which at rest are believed to exert high-frequency, monosynaptic tonic inhibition in various brain regions through inhibitory GABAergic projection (discussed in Disinhibition section above) (Figs. 8 and 9). Information arriving from several sources is integrated in the specialized neural command centers, which, for example, through inhibitory GABAergic projec-

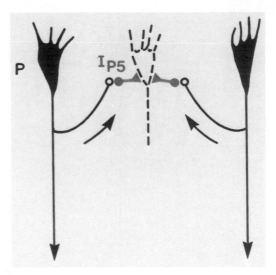

FIG. 6. Lateral inhibition of neurons belonging to other modules by P neurons in a given module. Dark neurons, excitatory; grey neurons, inhibitory.

tion neurons from the cerebellar cortex, the substantia nigra, the globus pallidus, and the reticular nucleus of the thalamus, exert high-frequency, monosynaptic tonic inhibition in various brain regions. Analysis of the inputs to the command centers is reflected, with variable time delays, in *decreased* frequencies of firing of appropriate combinations of their inhibitory output neurons (Fig. 9b), facilitating the *release* of neural activity at sites to which they project in such a manner that it becomes optimally compatible temporally and spatially with activity elsewhere in the CNS. The latter principle recently has been illustrated most convincingly in the monkey for the GABAergic projection neurons from the substantia nigra pars reticulata, which relay information from striatal command centers to the intermediate layers of the superior colliculus (32). The results were ". . . consistent with the idea that the substantia nigra cells discharge rapidly and inhibit superior colliculus cells tonically. A release of the tonic inhibition resulting from a decrease in substantia nigra cell activity would contribute to the generation of the burst of activity in the colliculus cells and, consequently, would contribute to the initiation of saccadic eye movements (32)."

The Basic Neural Unit as a Switch and the Module as the Quantifier

The net depolarizing effect of the combination of disinhibition and excitation occurring at any particular moment on the P neurons would be

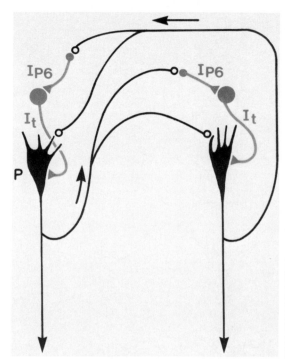

FIG. 7. Communication between P neurons in the same module in a given neural sector. It is presumed (not shown) that interneuronal inhibitory neurons are involved in a manner similar to that shown in insert in Fig. 3. Dark neurons, excitatory; gray neurons, inhibitory.

analogous to pressure applied to spring switches. When it is sufficiently great, contact is established, and the circuit is completed. In the biological situation, many modulatory metabolic, hormonal, and microenvironmental factors could affect the probabilities of neural switch closure. For example, the endogenous release or exogenous administration of an agent that decreases the efficacy of the tonically inhibitory interneurons (I_t neurons in Figs. 3–7) would decrease neural inhibition and would, by the analogy I am using, decrease the resistance of the springs in the neural switches. Thus, many more neural switches might be closed and pathways might be opened by a given input than would otherwise occur. The I_t neurons are presumed to restrain the activities of P neurons by tonic liberation of the inhibitory neurotransmitter GABA. Decreases in the rate of release of GABA or efficacy of such GABAergic neurons, or the effects of endogenously occurring or exogenously administered substances that block the postsynaptic action of GABA, desensitize postsynaptic receptor sites, or decrease in rates of release of GABA from GABA neurons

would increase the ease with which neural switches would be closed and circuits activated. The endogenous opioids, the enkephalins, markedly decrease the efficacy of a number of GABAergic pathways in the vertebrate nervous system (19,43,46). They have been shown specifically to depress inhibitory interneurons in the hippocampus, thereby increasing the firing rates of the pyramidal cells through disinhibition. On the other hand, the release of endogenous enhancers of GABA action or the administration of substances, such as diazepam, some barbiturates, diphenylhydantoin, and valproic acid amplify the efficacy of GABA at postsynaptic sites and have the opposite effects. Some of the latter and related substances and local anes-

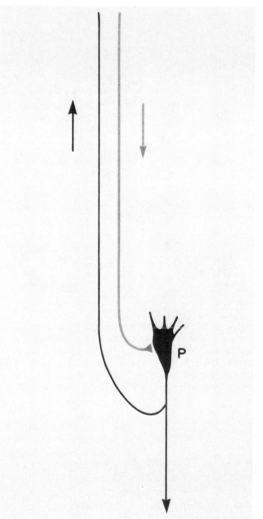

FIG. 8. Inhibition of P neurons in a given sector by projection neurons coming from command centers. Dark neurons, excitatory; gray neurons, inhibitory.

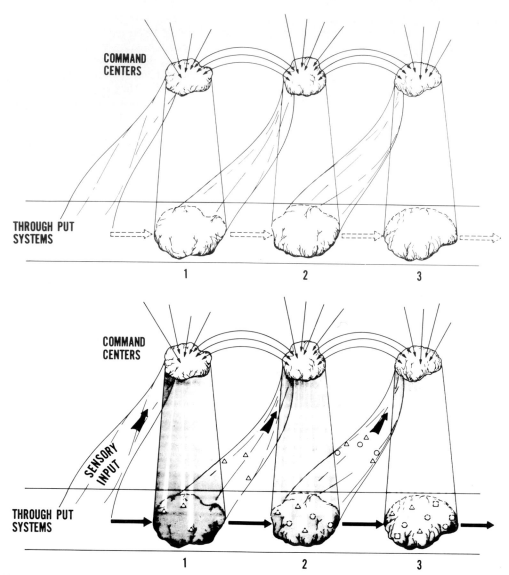

FIG. 9. A model for relationships between through-put systems and command centers. Minimally, a bifurcation of the flow of neural information from a particular sector takes place into direct through-put channels and also into those leading to command centers. **A:** Inactive state of system, in which tonic inhibition is maximally exerted by the output cells from the command centers. **B:** Active state of system, in which selective disinhibition of neural activity in the through-put systems is achieved by decreases in tonic inhibition exerted by the output cells of the command centers.

thetics also can increase the resistance of the neural switches by decreasing the conductile properties of the P neurons themselves (69). Thus, in the analogy I have made between neural and mechanical spring switches, the resistance of the springs can vary from moment to moment, depending on internal conditions, and it can be influenced in the biological situation by many endogenous factors and by the exogenous administration of drugs.

Modulatory Neural and Endocrine Systems

When an organism perceives that a problem exists, the stimuli reflecting the problem simultaneously release through-put and coordinative command circuits as well as auxiliary modulatory neural circuits. The through-put and command center neural circuitry may be considered to consist of cascades of serially aligned neuronal assemblies in which coded patterns of information entering originally from sensory transducers are progressively refined by the reduction of redundancy and the selection of particular features. The transformations of coded patterns in different neural sectors are achieved to a considerable extent by negative feedback loops that exist between and within the sectors and their temporal and spatial integration is achieved by activity of the command centers. The "hard-wired" neuronal elements of the through-put and command neuronal circuits, the blueprints for the construction of whose framework largely are inherited by the organism, are surrounded by local circuit neurons whose specific commitments may be made during development, as well as later in life, and which not only participate in virtually all phases of information processing, but also may undergo the plastic changes that must be involved in longterm retention of experience (69). Communications between the neural elements in these circuits takes place through synaptic and gap junctions on a millisecond or submillisecond time scale. A minimal scheme of such an arrangement assembled from Figs. 3–9 is shown in Fig. 10. Attention should be given to the great role assigned to inhibitory neurons in the information processing, rather than to the details of the circuitry, which certainly must vary from one instance to another.

ACh, the catecholamines, serotonin, neuroactive peptides, prostaglandins, and steroids in many instances may serve to optimize regional nervous system activity in relation to functional demands without themselves being involved in specific information transmittal. Upon release from nerve terminals, they exert chemical actions that influence the efficacy of the information-transmitting junctions in the mainline and command circuits. Some peptide or steroid hormones, for example, may temporarily line-label neural pathways, differentially facilitating behavioral options related to consummatory activities such as eating, drinking, and sex (77). Specific modulators may exert relatively longlasting effects on the cellular elements, possibly setting the gain on the efficacy of individual synapses, on specific types of synapses, or on all of the synapses in given regions or specific circuits. An inappropriate balance between availability and distribution of neural modulators with the activities in through-put neural and analyzer circuits could result in gross malfunction of the CNS.

When an organism first perceives that a problem exists, the stimuli reflecting the problem release through-put, command, and modulator neural circuits simultaneously, creating a general state of readiness at the outset so that all of the neural machinery is available for solving the problem at hand. At this early stage, some of the modulators may act as general sensory and response amplifiers. In addition to the neurally released modulators, a variety of hypothalamic, pituitary, and adrenal hormones (catecholamines, peptides and steroids) may be released into the bloodstream on signals originating in the CNS, in this way altering membrane properties and metabolic states of cells in various tissues, including those of the nervous system. The endocrine and neural events also are mutually interactive at all times. The cores of the neural modulator systems largely are probably located in brainstem and basal forebrain regions. For example, cholinergic pathways from magnocellular nuclei of the basal forebrain and noradrenergic pathways from the LC fan out similarly to terminate in various cortical and subcortical loci, often after long traverses away from their cell bodies. Coordinated readjustments between activities of all of the above systems take place at all stages during problem-solving by organisms.

The points at which structural or functional lesions or both can occur—lesions that would impair the cyberneticity of such a system as that outlined above—are legion. It is therefore no surprise that every known transmitter candidate and every potential modulator, under one circumstance or another, has been thought to be involved in various types of neural dysfunction including seizures.

SEIZURES

Consequences of Incoordination Between Inhibition and Excitation

When incoordination between the GABA system and other neurotransmitter and modulator systems persists, for whatever reason, the defect might involve a local brain region, several brain regions, or the entire CNS. A critically placed local incoordination might have drastic reverberations in the whole nervous system, as found in grand mal seizures arising from focal cortical lesions. Under relatively simple environmental conditions in individuals with such incoordinations, the nervous system could function in an apparently adequately adaptive manner, which might appear to be in the normal range. As the complexity and intensity of environmental inputs are increased, there would be a correlated increased degree of incoordination.

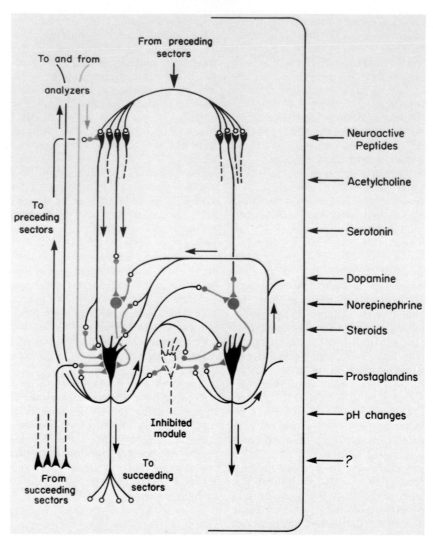

FIG. 10. A composite scheme illustrating some of the relationships suggested in Figs. 3–9. Attention should be focused on the complexity of relations involving inhibitory interneurons. A variety of neuromodulatory influences may affect the communications at all points. Dark neurons, excitatory; gray neurons, inhibitory.

Let us suppose that for some reason tonically active projection and local circuit (Figs. 3–10) inhibitory GABA neurons in the entire brain or in specific regions, have considerably lower than normal effectiveness on their recipient neurons which themselves are normally effective. Alternatively, let us suppose that the GABA neurons are normal and the neurons they ordinarily control are less than normally responsive to GABA or are potentially hyperactive because of intrinsically arising or extrinsically produced membrane changes. With increasing excitatory input, there would be an increased tendency to release pacemaker neurons. Abnormal or inappropriate behavior might be released (e.g., unprovoked vi-

olence, mania, schizophrenia); choreic movements, seizures, or spasticity might occur; there might be hypersensitivity to visual, auditory, tactile, olfactory, gustatory, or pain stimuli. GABA neurons play important roles in control mechanisms in various hypothalamic and brainstem centers. Thus, if specific regions within these latter structures were affected in a particular situation, abnormally enhanced responses might be observed, for example, in emotional reactivity, cardiac and respiratory functions, blood pressure, food and water intake, sweating, insulin secretion, liberation of gastric acid, motility of the colon, etc.

The permissive element in the activity of the

P neurons in a module is postulated to be the release from local and remote tonic inhibition. In various regions of the nervous system, the activity is largely determined by varying combinations of local and centrally generated disinhibitory commands. Direct excitation probably is not sufficient by itself to release the P neurons for activity during normal nervous system function. As the intensity of a particular input is increased from some low basal level, there is a corresponding increase of excitatory influences on the I_p neurons and directly on the P neurons in a given neural module, resulting in release of correspondingly greater numbers of P neurons. Inputs from their excitatory axon collaterals to each other would add to the excitatory and disinhibitory influences on P neurons in the same module, eventually recruiting them into synchronized discharge patterns (37). There is recurrent excitation between hippocampal pyramidal cells in the CA3 region (45). Spikes in one pyramidal cell can evoke spikes in another pyramidal cell. This could continue until virtually all available P neurons in the modules of a given sector were involved in responding to a pertinent input. Neither the models presented nor current data necessarily require the presence of abnormalities in membranes of particular neurons for this to occur. The giant EPSPs of local hippocampal seizures can result from the synchronous activity of normal neurons (37,82).

Enhanced synchrony of neuronal firing may arise in several ways: increased rate of release of synaptic excitatory transmitters; blockade of inhibitory transmitter receptor mechanisms; desensitization of receptors to inhibitory transmitters; decreased availability of inhibitory transmitter; decreased activity of inhibitory neurons; and increased formation or activation of electrotonic junctions. Decreases in rate of formation or release of inhibitory transmitter could result from decreased function or actual destruction of inhibitory neurons. A model applicable to such altered interactions within a population of affected cells is given in Fig. 10, which depicts active neural circuitry during a paroxysmal discharge. There are many experimental observations relevant to one or another of the above mechanisms (69). In the following section, I will concern myself only with a few of the items related to the GABA system, since the extensive immunocytochemical studies in many regions of the vertebrate CNS have shown that the vast majority of inhibitory neurons probably are GABAergic.

The Elementary Case: Loss of Inhibitory, GABAergic Nerve Terminals at Sites of Focal Cortical Epilepsy

Initially, it was necessary to determine whether or not GABA neurons decreased in number or whether their relationships to other neurons or to each other were disturbed morphologically in the CNS of organisms with various types of naturally occurring and experimentally induced seizures. If numbers of GABA neurons decreased, the restraints on excitatory pacesetter neurons in a given region of the CNS might be weakened and they would more easily recruit each other into the runaway activities characteristic of seizures, as in Fig. 11.

Identification of GABAergic neurons by immunocytochemical techniques allowed us to answer the morphologic questions (50,66,69). The GABA-synthesizing enzyme, GAD, was observed in somata, proximal dendrites, and axon terminals of nonpyramidal neurons in the rat visual cortex in all cortical layers, including the immediately subjacent white matter (50). All GAD-positive neurons observed were nonpyramidal cells. GAD-positive terminals formed symmetric synaptic junctions most commonly with dendritic shafts and somata of pyramidal and stellate neurons and less frequently with dendritic spines and with initial axon segments of pyramidal neurons in layers 3 and 4. The immunocytochemical localization of GAD in combination with physiologic and pharmacologic data indicates that these local circuit neurons mediate GABAergic inhibition and disinhibition in the neocortex and probably play key roles in information processing. Morphological data in rat cortex cited above and in normal monkey sensory-motor cortex (33) are consistent with the possibility that virtually all of the types of inhibitory neurons depicted schematically on the diagram in Figs. 3 and 10 are GABAergic. The several different morphological classes of intrinsic neurons that comprise the population of GABAergic neurons include small basket cells, spider-web cells, and chandelier cells (33).

Immunocytochemical studies of the sensorimotor cortex obtained from five epileptic monkeys treated with alumina cream correlated epileptic activity with numbers of GABAergic terminals (51). Highly significant reductions in numbers of GAD-positive terminals were found at the electrographically proven epileptogenic sites of alumina gel application by comparison with the contralateral nonepileptic homotopic cortex and at ipsilateral sections farther away

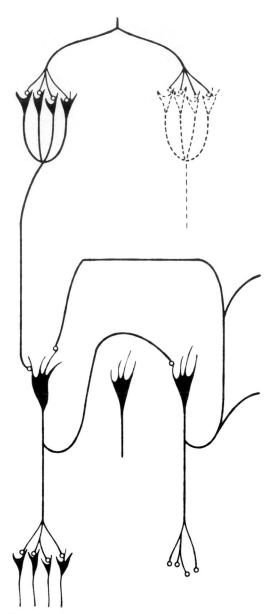

FIG. 11. Representation of a module or basic neural circuit without inhibition, depicting active neural circuitry during a paroxysmal discharge. The inhibitory neurons may become ineffective in ways discussed in the text. Inhibitory neurons are not shown in the diagram.

tors, to engage each other in paroxysmal, seizure-like discharges.

The latter observations are particularly pertinent since many epilepsies in human beings are caused by lesions in the brain resulting from trauma, such as head injuries, tumors, and cerebral angiomas. The above conditions may interfere with the normal blood supply to a particular region. Probably inhibitory GABAergic neurons (and glycinergic ones) have a high metabolic rate and are more sensitive to anoxia than are other types of cells (3,12,13,19,24). Their function may be disturbed differentially even by relatively slight degrees of anoxia (19), and degenerative changes and cell destruction take place rapidly if anoxia persists. This vulnerability also may extend to anoxia resulting from excessive functional demands and the large increases in metabolic activity and changes in physical state that occur in febrile states. An extraordinarily heavy excitatory bombardment to a particular brain sector, whatever its source, might create conditions in the vicinity of the local circuit neurons, such as too great elevation of cyclic GMP level (44) and depletion of glucose and oxygen and ATP in the affected region, which would adversely affect the function and possibly even the existence of the GABA interneurons in the region. Pathological processes, of whatever nature, that damage the microcapillaries, alter their permeability properties, cause prolonged local vasoconstriction, or in some more direct way induce mitochondrial malfunction, can result in destruction of the inhibitory GABA neurons with the replacement of their largely axosomatic synapses on pyramidal cells by processes of reactive astrocytes. This could sensitize the affected neural sector to epileptiform discharge. Electron microscopic observations on the monkey cortical material discussed above showed that there was a marked loss of axosomatic synapses on the pyramidal cells and a replacement of synaptic appositions with astrocytic processes in the alumina cream-treated animals. However, the symmetric, presumably excitatory, synapses on the dendrites of these pyramidal cells appeared to be largely intact (51).

In recent comprehensive biochemical studies of material from monkey cortical material complementary to the above morphological observations, a significant correlation with seizure frequency was found only with losses in GABAergic receptor-related binding and decrease in GAD activity (4).

Taken together, the above observations strongly support the notion that actual destruction of inhibitory GABA interneurons may be

from the alumina gel. These results support the idea that a relatively selective loss of inhibitory GABAergic neurons could be responsible for susceptibility to epileptic activity observed at seizure foci. Loss of adhering GABAergic neurons by excitatory projection neurons leads to poor inhibitory control of these neurons. This allows such projection neurons to fire excessively individually and, in particular neural sectors, to engage each other in paroxysmal, sei-

one of the major cerebral defects predisposing to seizures, at least in the case of focal epilepsy.

Inhibition and Seizures in Hippocampus

The hippocampus is the region in the brain that is most susceptible to seizures. Because of its key role in memory formation and retrieval and in establishing orientation in space and time, this brain structure recently has been subjected to a remarkable barrage of multidisciplinary investigations. In particular, physiological investigations have established the importance of inhibition in the function of the hippocampus, and immunocytochemical studies showed that the function of GABA neurons (basket and horizontal cells and other short-axon neurons) probably is decisive in maintenance of normal function of this structure. GAD-positive terminals forming axosomatic synapses on pyramidal cells correspond in location to the endings of basket cells, known indigenous inhibitory interneurons. GAD-positive basket cell somata have many GAD-positive boutons on them, again emphasizing the potential importance of disinhibition in central information processing (Fig. 1). The morphological observations, taken together with the possibility of recruitment of pyramidal cells by recurrent collaterals, are compatible with the view that seizures would occur in the hippocampus if the efficacy of GABA neurons were somehow impaired (see Fig. 10). When the afferent inputs to the hippocampus are stimulated at a sufficiently high frequency, the seizures that result probably can be attributed to diminution of the postsynaptic effectiveness of GABA released from inhibitory nerves and not to a suppression of their firing (6). This may be caused by desensitization of the receptors or the release of endogenous substances which block the receptor-recognition sites and/or the associated anion channels or pumps (6,69). On the other hand, the augmentation of pyramidal neuron activity and evocation of epileptiform activity by enkephalins appears to be achieved by the depression of the firing of inhibitory neurons—a direct demonstration of disinhibition (19,43,46). Finally, a variety of drugs that affect GABA-mediated postsynaptic inhibition can produce epileptiform discharges in the hippocampus, as well as in other brain structures (25).

Key Role for Basal Ganglia in Seizures

We reach another level of complexity when we attempt to understand the recent observations that expression of motor and limbic seizures in the rat requires the active participation of the substantia nigra (SN) (35). Seizures produced by maximal electroshock, PTZ, bicuculline, or kindling can be suppressed by elevating the GABA content in the zona reticulata of the SN by blockade of GABA transaminase with an irreversible inhibitor or by microinjection of muscimol, a potent GABA agonist.

The striato-nigropallidal command system coordinates a number of the mechanisms involved in the physical orientation of an organism in its perceived space-time continuum. The caudate nucleus, putamen, and SN exchange fibers with each other, as do the SN and globus pallidus (GP). The GP and SN receive inputs from the caudate and putamen and appear to have two-way communication with the subthalamic nucleus. There also are thalamic, cortical, septal, and midbrain inputs to the caudate and putamen. Normal relations within and between the above structures must involve minimally a coordinated functioning of different groups of intra- and intersystem neurons whose transmitters and/or modulators may be GABA, ACh, dopamine, serotonin, norepinephrine, glutamate, and substance P.

Neurons in the pars reticulata of the SN and from the internal segment of the GP (entopeduncular nucleus in the rat and cat) are the output neurons of the basal ganglia. Through their branching axons, GABA-mediated inhibition is exerted tonically on neurons in regions of the thalamus, superior colliculus, and midbrain tegmentum (17,55). The results of the computations of the extrapyramidal system are expressed, I believe, by selective *decreases* in tonic inhibition exerted in the recipient regions, which facilitate activation of neurons in these regions (Fig. 9). Our immunocytochemical studies of distribution of GABA neurons and their terminals in the basal ganglia (52,54) support the idea that the inhibitory projection neurons from the SN and GP may, themselves, be inhibited by GABAergic terminals of axons originating from neurons in the striatum, whereas excitatory striatonigral information may be communicated via fibers of substance P-releasing neurons. Pallidal and nigral inputs to the ventrolateral and ventroanterior thalamic nuclei are GABAergic and monosynaptically inhibitory (2,15,22,48,83,84). It may be presumed that the tonically inhibitory input from the SN restricts the information flowing from thalamic motor nuclei to the cortex and provides fine-tuning of posture and movement (55). Thus, thalamic inputs to the motor cortex importantly reflect the results of both nigral and pallidal inputs. It is of considerable interest in this regard that facilitation of gamma motor neurons can be achieved by stimulation of a midbrain region close to termination of the fibers from the GP, as well as by the stimulation of the caudate nucleus.

The above formulation may help explain why an epileptic focus in the motor cortex, for example, requires the participation of a normally functional SN for the propagation of generalized seizures. The enhanced cortico-striatal input from an epileptic cortical focus would cause correspondingly increased activity in appropriate regions of the striatum. This would result in increase of the striatal GABAergic inhibition of the GABAergic projection neurons originating in the SN and the GP. A major decrease in the input from the SN and GP during a cortical seizure would result in an increased tendency to release activity in other regions of the CNS, since there would be loss of tonic inhibitory restraints from the basal ganglia command center. This would predispose to paroxysmal discharges in other parts of the neuroaxis as well as in the epileptic cortical focus.

Neurons of the reticular nucleus of the thalamus (NR) probably exert a major tonic restraint on the flow of thalamic information to the cortex. This nucleus consists mainly of GABAergic neurons sending inhibitory projections into the thalamus (see ref. 34 and references cited therein). The NR, by its major projections to the thalamus, probably gates the output of the thalamic nuclei to the cortex. Regulation of NR activity would, in turn, influence the level of activity in the underlying thalamus. Excitation of reticularis neurons could increase the level of inhibition in the thalamic nuclei in either a generalized or selective manner, *whereas inhibition of the inhibitory neurons of the NR, through a process of disinhibition, could increase the responsiveness of thalamic relay neurons.* A potential system for producing disinhibition within the thalamus through the inhibition of reticularis neurons involves an extrinsic projection from the mesencephalic reticular formation. Reticularis neurons are inhibited both by stimulation of the mesencephalic reticular formation and the iontophoretic application of ACh. Activation of an inhibitory cholinergic pathway from the midbrain reticular formation to the NR, for which there is histochemical and biochemical evidence, may lead to facilitation of thalamocortical transmission.

Particularly pertinent to the present discussion is that there are GABAergic projections from the SN both to the motor nuclei of the thalamus (17) and to regions of the mesencephalic reticular formation. Let us suppose that GABAergic inputs from the SN tonically inhibit the cholinergic neurons of the brainstem reticular formation, which in turn, when released, directly inhibit the NR neurons. If there were a decreased SN output when there is increased activity in the striatum arising from a paroxysmally discharging cortical region, the SN neurons would cease to inhibit both the cholinergic neurons of the mesencephalic reticular formation and the thalamic motor nuclei. This would result in the release of thalamocortical inputs both from the inhibition of the direct SN inputs and from the restraints of the more closely lying GABAergic neurons of the NR. The situation then becomes circular. Paroxysmal discharges from an epileptic focus in the sensory-motor cortex would disinhibit the flow of thalamic information to the already poorly controlled focus and thus further loosen the controls on motor activity everywhere in the organism. Enhanced outputs by way of the cortical pyramidal cells to final motor cells in the medulla and spinal cord eventually would result in tonic-clonic convulsions of grand mal epilesy.

QUESTIONS ABOUT THERAPIES

If the point of view presented in this article generally is correct, a search for "causes" of epilepsy might be viewed as somewhat naive. In some instances, as in the case of focal cortical lesions, the original initiating event can be identified. However, there may be inherited or acquired deficiencies or susceptibilities to deficiencies that result in seizures. These may cover the whole gamut of metabolic or structural variables, from a tendency of a given region of the brain to become ischemic to a failure to produce essential cell membrane components by neurons, glia, or endothelial cells. Whatever its nature, by the time of observation, the active, acute pathological process usually has subsided, and numerous physiologic adjustments have been made by the organism, from compensatory plastic changes in neuronal circuitry to development of adaptive or maladaptive behavioral patterns. It is apparent that interference with GABAergic function can lead to local paroxysmal discharges in neural tissue, such as cortex. However, it also is true that GABAergic striatal translation of the abnormal cortical events and its transmission by decreased activity of GABAergic fibers from the SN and GP also seem necessary for the full expression of motor and limbic seizures. In view of the above, the complexity of interneuronal circuitry at all levels, and the differences in pharmacology of pre- and postsynaptic GABA receptors, it is difficult to arrive at a logical devising of *specific* synaptically targeted GABAergic pharmacotherapies of the epilepsies, although empirically derived substances, such as diphenylhydantoin, barbiturates, and diazepam sometimes become available and solve many practical problems.

To date, administration of GABA, itself, or a variety of GABA-mimetic substances has not proven to be as efficacious in seizure control as are a number of the standard, empirically derived drugs in use today. However, eventually a general GABAergic approach may be developed and be useful in seizure therapy. This is based upon the numerous observations that have shown GABA receptive sites to exist on neuronal membranes (ganglia, tissue culture, unmyelinated axons) that have no GABAergic synapses. Therefore, there may be hormones (hypothalamic, pituitary, or adrenal), peptidic or steroidal, which may act extrasynaptically at such sites to exert global damping effects on CNS function. Currently, we are looking for such substances among the known hormones as well as among extracts of the above-mentioned endocrine tissues. It is also worthwhile to search for substances or conditions that may cause up-regulation of components of the GABAergic synaptic apparatus as well as those of extra-synaptic GABA receptive sites.

In the study of any pathologic phenomenon, one aim is to identify the rate-limiting steps, bottlenecks at which tools presently available may be used to choke off the spread of the manifestations of the pathologic state. Often the best strategy is to try to focus on key events as close to the origin of the problem as possible, because the consequential, ever-widening ripples at every point of advance of the pathologic process create subsidiary problems that often are unpredictable and may eventually require additional therapies far removed from the original problem. There are multiple causations and many overt manifestations of epileptiform phenomena. What do all of them have in common? The most apparent common denominator and the hallmark of seizures is that principal neurons, which normally are involved largely as individuals or in small groups in highly specific aspects of information processing in a given neural sector, first begin to fire abnormally, frequently, when engaged in performing their regular assignments and then join other neurons in the same sector in a series of relatively simultaneous impulses at high frequency in a manner irrelevant to their role in information processing.

The most salient feature that emerges is that at the origin of seizures some neurons are firing

with maladaptively high frequencies. The firing mechanisms probably are similar in most neurons that show an action potential. If a substance could be administered or a procedure performed that could serve as a low-pass frequency filter with a cut-off point that would still allow neurons to perform their normal functions at the lower frequencies of firing ordinarily required, events close to the source of origin of seizures might be affected. Furthermore, it is possible that such an approach may also have differential effects on through-put principal neurons and on inhibitory projection neurons and local circuit interneurons. At lease some of the latter may not use action potentials but instead may release transmitter as a continuous function of membrane potentials that fluctuate within the release portion of their input–output curves and may maintain transmitter release indefinitely (26). These nonspiking interneurons could be much more resistant to procedures with a relatively specific effect on the spike-generating mechanism. The finding that a number of local anesthetics possess anticonvulsant properties at low levels but are convulsants at higher concentrations suggests that these substances may exert such differential effects. The most general approach that may be applicable to the treatment and/or prevention of epileptiform discharges in the nervous system may be to affect the conductile properties of those nerves that generate action potentials in such a way as to set a ceiling on the frequencies with which they could fire, while having little or no effect on inhibitory interneurons, many of which may not have a spike-generating mechanism. It is known that local anesthetics exert their action by producing a conduction block in peripheral nerves by blocking transmembrane sodium current (8). In addition, quite aside from knowledge of their mechanisms of action, local anesthetics have been used to prevent or abort a variety of seizures in animals and in humans, suppressing spike generation in cortical epileptic foci and even afterdischarges in electrically stimulated isolated brain slabs (7).

Frequency-dependent nerve block by local anesthetics has been shown in voltage clamp experiments to be attributable to a blockade of the sodium channels responsible for generation of the action potential (31). There appears to be a preferential, reversible binding of these drugs to some structural component of open sodium channels; and, therefore, the efficacy of blockade of nerve excitability by these substances is greatly enhanced when a nerve is firing rapidly as opposed to that observed with low-frequency firing. The degree of block depends on the rate of opening of sodium channels (9). Substances that exert such effects have also been found to have antiarrhythmic pharmacologic effects. Phenytoin has widespread therapeutic use as an antiarrhythmic drug as well as an anticonvulsant (9). It can block dangerous high-frequency myocardial activity through a frequency-selective effect that is similar to that on nerve. Several antiarrhythmic drugs, including propranolol, which also has β-adrenergic blocking and antipsychotic effects (61), have been shown to block myocardial excitability in a frequency-dependent manner, an action that probably contributes importantly to their anti-fibrillatory efficacy.

It seems to me that a systematic search could be made for new antiepileptic drugs among those substances that can produce frequency-selective nerve block in the CNS. Ideally, such substances also should be absorbed into the blood transdermally or intestinally and should have a high degree of specificity. If the incentive were sufficiently great, current technologies probably could find new antiepileptic drugs among this class of substances.

ACKNOWLEDGMENT

This work was supported in part by grant Nos. NS18858 and NS18859 from the National Institute of Neurological and Communicative Diseases and Stroke.

REFERENCES

1. Alger, B. E., and Nicoll, R. A. (1982): Feed-forward dendritic inhibition in rat hippocampal pyramidal cells studied in vitro. *J. Physiol.*, 328:105–123.
2. Anderson, M., and Yoshida, M. (1977): Electrophysiological evidence for branching nigral projections to the thalamus and the superior colliculus. *Brain Res.*, 137:361–364.
3. Arregui, A., and Barer, G. R. (1980): Chronic hypoxia in rats: Alterations of striatonigral angiotensin converting enzyme, GABA, and glutamic acid decarboxylase. *J. Neurochem.*, 34:740–743.
4. Bakay, R. A. E., and Harris, A. B. (1981): Neurotransmitter receptor and biochemical changes in monkey cortical epileptic foci. *Brain Res.*, 206:387–404.
5. Bazemore, A. W., Elliott, K. A. C., and Florey, E. (1957): Isolation of Factor I. *J. Neurochem.*, 1:334–339.
6. Ben-Ari, Y., Krnjevic, K., and Reinhardt, W. (1979): Hippocampal seizures and failure of inhibition. *Can. J. Physiol. Pharmacol.*, 57:1462–1466.
7. Bernhard, C. G., and Bohm, E. (1965): Local anaesthetics as anticonvulsants. Almqvist Wiksell, Stockholm.
8. Courtney, K. R. (1975): Mechanism of frequency-dependent inhibition of sodium currents in frog myelinated nerve by the lidocaine derivative GEA 968. *J. Pharmacol. Exp. Ther.*, 195:225–236.
9. Courtney, K. R., Kendig, J. J., and Cohen, E. N. (1978): The rates of interaction of local anesthetics with sodium channels in nerve. *J. Pharmacol. Exp. Ther.*, 207:594–604.
10. Curtis, D. R. (1979): GABAergic transmission in the mammalian central nervous system. In: *GABA-Neurotransmitters*, edited by P. Krogsgaard-Larsen, J. Scheel-Kruger, and H. Kofod, pp. 17–27. Munksgaard Press, Copenhagen.
11. Curtis, D. R., and Watkins, J. C. (1960): Investigations upon the possible synaptic transmitter function of gamma-aminobutyric acid and naturally occurring amino acids. In: *Inhibition in the Nervous System and Gamma-Aminobutyric Acid*, edited by E. Roberts, C. F. Baxter, A. Van Harreveld, C. A. G. Wiersma, W. R. Adey, and K. F. Killam, pp. 424–444. Pergamon Press, Oxford.
12. Davidoff, R. A., Graham, L. T., Jr., Shank, R. P., Werman, R., and Aprison, M. H. (1967): Changes in amino acid concentrations associated with loss of spinal interneurons. *J. Neurochem.*, 14:1025–1031.
13. Davidoff, R. A., Shank, R. P., Graham, L. T., Aprison, M. H., and Werman, R. (1967): Association of glycine with spinal interneurons. *Nature* 214:680–681.
14. Davson, H. (1964): *A Textbook of General Physiology*, 3rd ed. Churchill, London.
15. Deniau, J. M., Lackner, D., and Feger, J. (1978): Effect of substantia nigra stimulation on identified neurons in the VL-VA thalamic complex: Comparison between intact and chronically decorticated cats. *Brain Res.*, 176:273–284.
16. Diamond, S., Balvin, R. S., and Diamond, F. R. (1963): *Inhibition and Choice*. Harper and Row, New York.
17. DiChiara, G., Porceddu, M. L., Morelli, M., Mulas, M. L., and Gessa, G. L. (1979): Evidence for GABAergic projection from the substantia nigra to the ventromedial thalamus and to the superior colliculus of the rat. *Brain Res.*, 176:273–284.
18. Dudek, F. E., Andrew, R. D., MacVicar, B. A., Snow, R. W., and Taylor, C. P. (1983): Recent evidence for and possible significance of gap junctions and electrotonic synapses in the mammalian brain. In: *Basic Mechanisms of Neuronal Hyperexcitability*, edited by H. H. Jasper and N. M. van Gelder, pp. 31–73. Alan R. Liss, New York.
19. Dunwiddie, T., Mueller, A., Palmer, M., Stewart, J., and Hoffer, B. (1980): Electrophysiological interactions of enkephalins with neuronal circuitry in the rat hippocampus. I. Effects on pyramidal cell activity. *Brain Res.*, 184:311–330.
20. Eccles, J. C. (1969): *The Inhibitory Pathways of the Central Nervous System*. Charles C Thomas, Springfield.

21. Einstein, A., cited in Brecher, K. (1979): A guide for the perplexed. *Nature,* 278:215–218.

22. Feger, J., Deniau, J. M., Hammond-Le Guyader, C., and Ohye, C. (1976–1977): Connections from the basal ganglia to the thalamus. Proceedings of the 15th Annual Meeting of the Japanese Society of Stereotactic and Functional Neurosurgery, Maebashi, 1976. *Appl. Neurophysiol.,* 39:272–284.

23. Florey, E. (1960): Physiological evidence for naturally occurring inhibitory substances. In: *Inhibition in the Nervous System and Gamma-Aminobutyric Acid,* edited by E. Roberts, C. F. Baxter, A. Van Harreveld, C. A. G. Wiersma, W. R. Adey, K., and F. Killam, pp. 72–84. Pergamon Press, Oxford.

24. Francis, A. J., and Pulsinelli, W. (1982): Selective ischemic damage to striatal GABAergic neurons. *Brain Res.,* 243:271–278.

25. Glaser, G. H., Penry, J. K., and Woodbury, D. M. (1980): *Antiepileptic Drugs: Mechanisms of Action.* Raven Press, New York.

26. Graubard, K. (1978): Synaptic transmission without action potentials: Input–output properties of a non-spiking presynaptic neuron. *J. Neurophysiol.,* 41:1014–1025.

27. Greengard, P. (1981): *Intracellular Signals in the Brain.* The Harvey Lectures, Series 45, pp. 277–331. Academic Press, Orlando, Fla.

28. Grossman, Y., Spira, M. E., and Parnas, I. (1973): Differential flow of information into branches of a single axon. *Brain Res.,* 64:379–386.

29. Hayashi, T., and Suyhara, R. (1956): Substances which produce epileptic seizures when applied on the motor cortex of dogs, and substances which inhibit the seizure directly. In: 20th International Physiology Congress, Brussels, 1956, Abstracts of Reviews: Abstracts of Communications, p. 410.

30. Hayashi, T., and Nagai, K. (1956): Action of g-amino acids on the motor cortex of higher animals, especially γ-amino-β-oxy-butyric acid as the real inhibitory principle in brain. In: 20th International Physiology Congress, Brussels, 1956, Abstracts of Reviews: Abstracts of Communications, p. 410.

31. Hille, B. (1977): Local anesthetics: Hydrophilic and hydrophobic pathways for the drug-receptor reaction. *J. Gen. Physiol.,* 69:497–515.

32. Hikosaka, O., and Wurtz, R. H. (1983): Visual and oculomotor functions of monkey substantia nigra pars reticulata. IV. Relation of substantia nigra to superior colliculus. *J. Neurophysiol.,* 49:1285–1301.

33. Houser, C. R., Hendry, S. H. C., Jones, E. G., and Vaughn, J. E. (1983): Morphological diversity of immunocytochemically identified GABA neurons in the monkey sensory-motor cortex. *J. Neurocytol.,* 12:617–638.

34. Houser, C. R., Vaughn, J. E., Barber, R. P., and Roberts, E. (1980): GABA neurons are the major cell type of the nucleus reticularis thalami. *Brain Res.,* 200:341–354.

35. Iadarola, M. J., and Gale, K. (1982): Substantia nigra: Sites of anticonvulsant activity mediated by γ-aminobutyric acid. *Science,* 218:1237–1240.

36. Jefferys, J. G. R., and Haas, H. L. (1981): Synchronized bursting of CA1 hippocampal pyramidal cells in the absence of synaptic transmission. *Nature,* 300:448–450.

37. Johnston, D., and Brown, T. H. (1981): Giant synaptic potential hypothesis for epileptiform activity. *Science,* 211:294–297.

38. Kandel, E. R., and Gardner, D. (1972): The synaptic actions mediated by the different branches of a single neuron. In: *Neurotransmitters. Res. Publ. Assoc. Res. Nerv. Ment. Dis.,* vol. 50, edited by I. J. Kapin, pp. 91–146. Williams & Wilkins, Baltimore.

39. Killam, K. F., and Bain, J. A. (1957): Convulsant hydrazides I: In vitro and in vivo inhibition of vitamin B_6 enzymes by convulsant hydrazides. *J. Pharmacol. Exp. Ther.,* 119:255–262.

40. Killam, K. F. (1957): Convulsant hydrazides II: Comparison of electrical changes and enzyme inhibition induced by the administration of thiosemicarbazide. *J. Pharmacol. Exp. Ther.,* 119:263–271.

41. Kravitz, E. A., Iversen, L. L., Otsuka, M., and Hall, Z. W. (1966): Gamma-aminobutyric acid in the lobster nervous system: Release from inhibitory nerves and uptake into nerve-muscle preparations. In: *Structure and Function of Inhibitory Neuronal Mechanisms,* edited by C. von Euler, S. Skoglund, and U. Soderberg, pp. 371–376. Pergamon Press, New York.

42. Krnjevic, K. (1976): Inhibitory action of GABA and GABA-mimetics on vertebrate neurons. In: *GABA in Nervous System Function,* edited by E. Roberts, T. N. Chase, and D. B. Tower, pp. 269–281. Raven Press, New York.

43. Lee, H. K., Dunwiddie, T., and Hoffer, B. (1980): Electrophysiological interactions of enkephalins with neuronal circuitry in the rat hippocampus. II. Effects on interneuron excitability. *Brain Res.,* 184:331–342.

44. Lolley, R. N., Farber, D. B., Rayborn, M. E., and Hollyfield, J. G. (1977): Cyclic GMP accumulation causes degeneration of photoreceptor cells: Simulation of an inherited disease. *Science,* 196:664–666.

45. MacVicar, B. A., and Dudek, F. E. (1980): Local synaptic circuits in rat hippocampus: Interactions between pyramidal cells. *Brain Res.,* 184:220–223.

46. Nicoll, R. A., Alger, B. E., and Jahr, C. E. (1980): Enkephalin blocks inhibitory pathways in the vertebrate CNS. *Nature,* 287:22–25.

47. Otsuka, M. (1976): GABA in the crustacean nervous system: A historical review. In: *GABA in Nervous System Function,* edited by E. Roberts, T. N. Chase, and D. B. Tower, pp. 245–249. Raven Press, New York.

48. Penney, J. B., Jr., and Young, A. B. (1981): GABA as the pallidothalamic neurotransmitter: Implications for basal ganglia function. *Brain Res.,* 207:195–199.

49. Potter, D. D. (1966): The chemistry of inhibition in crustaceans with special reference to gamma-aminobutyric acid. In: *Structure and Function of Inhibitory Neuronal Mechanisms,* edited by C. von Euler, S. Skoglund, and U. Soderberg, pp. 359–370. Pergamon Press, New York.

50. Ribak, C. E. (1978): Aspinous and sparsely-spinous stellate neurons in the visual cortex of rats contain glutamic acid decarboxylase. *J. Neurocytol.*, 7:461–478.

51. Ribak, C. E., Harris, A. B., Vaughn, J. E., and Roberts, E. (1979): Inhibitory GABAergic nerve terminals decrease at sites of focal epilepsy. *Science*, 205:211–214.

52. Ribak, C. E., Harris, A. B., Vaughn, J. E., and Roberts, E. (1981): Immunocytochemical changes in cortical GABA neurons in a monkey model of epilepsy. In: *Neurotransmitters, Seizures, and Epilepsy*, edited by P. L. Morselli, K. G. Lloyd, W. Löscher, B. Meldrum, and E. H. Reynolds, pp. 11–22. Raven Press, New York.

53. Ribak, C. E., Vaughn, J. E., and Roberts, E. (1979): The GABA neurons and their axon terminals in rat corpus striatum as demonstrated by GAD immunocytochemistry. *J. Comp. Neurol.*, 187:261–284.

54. Ribak, C. E., Vaughn, J. E., and Roberts, E. (1980): GABAergic nerve terminals decrease in the substantia nigra following hemitransections of the striatonigral and pallidonigral pathways. *Brain Res.*, 192:413–420.

55. Rispal-Padel, L., Massion, J., and Grangetto, A. (1973): Relations between the ventrolateral thalamic nucleus and motor cortex and their possible role in the central organization of motor control. *Brain Res.*, 650:1–20.

56. Roberts, A., and Bush, B. M. H., editors (1981): Neurones without impulses. *Society for Experimental Biology Seminar*, series 6. Cambridge University Press, Cambridge.

57. Roberts, E. (1956): Formation and utilization of γ-aminobutyric acid in brain. In: *Progress in Neurobiology. 1. Neurochemistry*, edited by S. R. Korey and J. I. Nurnberger, pp. 11–25. Hoeber-Harper, New York.

58. Roberts, E. (1966): Models for correlative thinking about brain, behavior, and biochemistry. *Brain Res.*, 2:109–144.

59. Roberts, E. (1966): The synapse as a biochemical self-organizing microcybernetic unit. *Brain Res.*, 2:117–166.

60. Roberts, E. (1974): γ-Aminobutyric acid and nervous system function—A perspective. *Biochem. Pharmacol.*, 23:2637–2649.

61. Roberts, E. (1975): GABA in nervous system function—An overview. In: *The Nervous System, The Basic Neurosciences*, vol. I, edited by D. B. Tower, pp. 541–552. Raven Press, New York.

62. Roberts, E. (1976): Disinhibition as an organizing principle in the nervous system—The role of the GABA system. Application to neurologic and psychiatric disorders. In: *GABA in Nervous System Function*, edited by E. Roberts, T. N. Chase, and D. B. Tower, pp. 515–539. Raven Press, New York.

63. Roberts, E. (1976): Immunocytochemistry of the GABA system—A novel approach to an old transmitter. In: *Society for Neuroscience Symposia*, vol. 1. edited by J. A. Ferrendelli, B. S McEwen, and S. H. Snyder, pp. 123–138. Society for Neurosciences, Bethesda.

64. Roberts, E. (1977): The γ-aminobutyric acid system and schizophrenia. In: *Neuroregulators and Psychiatric Disorders*, edited by E. Usdin, D. A. Hamburg, and J. D. Barchas, pp. 347–357. Oxford University Press, New York.

65. Roberts, E. (1978): Interrelationships of GABA neurons explored by immunocytochemical techniques. In: *Interactions Between Putative Neurotransmitters in the Brain*, edited by S. Garattini, J. F. Pujol, and R. Samanin, pp. 89–107. Raven Press, New York.

66. Roberts, E. (1978): Roles of GABA neurons in information processing in the vertebrate CNS. In: *Neuronal Information Transfer*, edited by A. Karlin, V. M. Tennyson, and H. J. Vogel, pp. 213–239. Academic Press, Orlando, Fla.

67. Roberts, E. (1979): New directions in GABA research. I: Immunocytochemical studies of GABA neurons. In: *GABA-Neurotransmitters*, edited by P. Krogsgaard-Larsen, J. Scheel-Kruger, and H. Kofod, pp. 28–45. Munksgaard Press, Copenhagen.

68. Roberts, E. (1979): Status and perspective. In: *GABA-Neurotransmitters*, edited by P. Krogsgaard-Larsen, J. Scheel-Kruger, and H. Kofod, pp. 533–545. Munksgaard Press, Copenhagen.

69. Roberts, E. (1980): Epilepsy and antiepileptic drugs: A speculative synthesis. In: *Antiepileptic Drugs: Mechanisms of Action*, edited by G. H. Glaser, J. K. Penry, and D. M. Woodbury, pp. 667–713. Raven Press, New York.

70. Roberts, E. (1980): γ-Aminobutyric acid (GABA): A major inhibitory transmitter in the vertebrate nervous system. In: *Nerve Cells, Transmitters and Behaviour*, edited by R. Levi-Montalcini, pp. 163–213. Pontifical Academy of Sciences, Rome.

71. Roberts, E. (1981): A speculative consideration on the neurobiology and treatment of senile dementia. In: *Strategies for the Development of an Effective Treatment for Senile Dementia*, edited by T. Crook and S. Gershon, pp. 247–320. Mark Powley, New Canaan.

72. Roberts, E. (1983): γ-Aminobutyric acid (GABA): From discovery to visualization of GABAergic neurons in the vertebrate nervous system. In: *Actions and Interactions of GABA and Benzodiazepines*, edited by N. G. Bowery, pp. 1–25. Raven Press, New York.

73. Roberts, E. (1984): GABA-related phenomena, models of nervous system function, and seizures. *Ann. Neurol.*, 16 (Suppl.):S77–S89.

74. Roberts, E., Baxter, C. F., Van Harreveld, A., Wiersma, C. A. G., Adey, W. R., and Killam, K. F., editors (1960): *Inhibition in the Nervous System and Gamma-Aminobutyric Acid*. Pergamon Press, Oxford.

75. Roberts, E., and Matthysse, S. (1970): Neurochemistry: At the crossroads of neurobiology. *Annu. Rev. Biochem.*, 39:777–820.

76. Roberts, E., Wein, J., and Simonsen, D. G. (1964): γ-Aminobutyric acid (γ-GABA), Vitamin B$_6$, and neuronal function—A speculative synthesis. *Vitam. Horm.*, 22:503–559.

77. Scheller, R. H., Jackson, J. F., McAllister, L. B., Rothman, B. S., Mayeri, E., and Axel, R.

(1983): A single gene encodes multiple neuropeptides mediating a stereotyped behavior. *Cell*, 32:7–22.

78. Shinoda, Y., Arnold, A. P., and Asanuma, H. (1976): Spinal branching of corticospinal axons in the cat. *Exp. Brain Res.*, 26:215–234.

79. Sisken, B., Roberts, E., and Baxter, C. F. (1960): γ-Aminobutyric acid and glutamic decarboxylase activity in the brain of the chick. In: *Inhibition in the Nervous System and γ-Aminobutyric Acid*, edited by E. Roberts, C. F. Baxter, A. Van Harreveld, C. A. G. Wiersma, W. R. Adey, and K. Killam. Pergamon Press, Oxford.

80. Sloper, J. J. (1973): An electron microscope study of the termination of afferent connections to the primate motor cortex. *J. Neurocytol.*, 2:361–368.

81. Takeuchi, A. (1976): Studies of inhibitory effects of GABA in invertebrate nervous systems. In: *GABA in Nervous System Function*, edited by E. Roberts, T. N. Chase, and D. B. Tower, pp. 255–267. Raven Press, New York.

82. Traub, R. D., and Wong, R. K. S. (1982): Cellular mechanism of neuronal synchronization in epilepsy. *Science*, 216:745–747.

83. Ueki, A., and Yoshida, M. (1976/77): Some physiological aspects of the basal ganglia. Excitation of the neurons of the globus pallidus by the brain stem structures. Proceedings of the 15th Annual Meeting of the Japanese Society of Stereotactic and Functional Neurosurgery, Maebashi, 1976. *Appl. Neurophysiol.*, 39:296–301.

84. Uno, M., and Yoshida, M. (1975): Monosynaptic inhibition of thalamic neurons produced by stimulation of the pallidal nucleus in cats. *Brain Res.*, 99:377–380.

85. Vaughn, J. E., Barber, R. P., Ribak, C. E., and Houser, C. R. (1981): Methods for the immunocytochemical localization of proteins and peptides involved in neurotransmission. In: *Current Trends in Morphological Techniques*, Volume III, edited by J. E. Johnson, Jr., pp. 34–70. CRC Press, Inc., Boca Raton, Florida.

86. von Bekesy, G. (1967): *Sensory Inhibition*. Princeton University Press, Princeton.

87. von Euler, C., Skoglund, S., and Soderberg, U. (1968): *Structure and Function of Inhibitory Neuronal Mechanisms*. Pergamon Press, Oxford.

88. Werman, R., and Aprison, M. H. (1966): Glycine: The search for a spinal cord inhibitory transmitter. In: *Structure and Function of Inhibitory Neuronal Mechanisms*, edited by C. von Euler, S. Skoglund, and U. Soderberg, pp. 473–486. Pergamon Press, New York.

Advances in Neurology, Vol. 44, edited by
A. V. Delgado-Escueta, A. A. Ward, Jr.,
D. M. Woodbury, and R. J. Porter.
Raven Press, New York © 1986.

16

Role of the Substantia Nigra in GABA-Mediated Anticonvulsant Actions

Karen Gale

Department of Pharmacology, Georgetown University, Schools of Medicine and Dentistry, Washington, D.C. 20007

SUMMARY The relationship between cerebral GABA content and suscepti-bility to seizures is addressed from the point of view of specific brain loci at which GABA synapses may control convulsive activity. The substantia nigra (SN) has been identified as a critical site at which GABA-agonist drugs act to reduce susceptibility to a number of types of experimentally induced generalized sei-zures. Moreover, the ability of GABA-elevating agents to protect against seizures in the maximal electroshock model is directly correlated with increases in GABA specifically in the *nerve-terminal* compartment of SN. Studies with 2-deoxyglu-cose indicate that a marked increase in metabolic activity in SN is a common feature of several types of generalized seizures; it is possible that some of this increased activity is associated with GABAergic nerve terminals that become activated in an attempt to suppress seizure spread. Because GABA has been shown to inhibit nigral efferents, it is likely that GABA terminals inhibit nigral projections that are permissive or facilitative to seizure propagation. In support of this, bilateral destruction of SN attenuated clonic and tonic chemoconvulsant and electroshock seizures. Other treatments capable of reducing nigral output, namely opiate agonists (morphine and D-Ala-Met-enkephalin), and substance P antagonist analogs, were also found to have anticonvulsant effects when ap-plied bilaterally into SN. Thus, the seizure-facilitating nigral efferents may be subject to inhibition by both GABA and opiates and may normally be driven by substance P.

Of the various outputs from SN, the GABAergic projections to thalamus, re-ticular formation and/or superior colliculus are most likely responsible for influ-encing seizure propagation. Experimental evidence does not indicate a significant role of pars compacta nigrostriatal dopamine neurons for controlling the various types of seizures subject to nigral influence. We propose that the inhibition of the GABAergic outputs from SN pars reticulata can suppress the progression of seizure discharge through circuits involving the target areas of these outputs. Because chemical or electrical stimulation of SN does not *initiate* convulsions, it appears that seizure activity generated elsewhere in the brain may be amplified or sustained by activity in these nigral outputs.

Recently, new selectively-acting compounds with GABA agonist activity have been devel-oped for their possible therapeutic potential. These compounds have in turn stimulated basic research aimed at defining the role of GABA in numerous physiological processes. This reci-procity between GABA-related drug develop-ment and the understanding of basic mechanisms has been particularly productive with respect to epilepsy. Although an association between seizures and brain GABA was initially demonstrated during the 1950s (5,6,15,37,48,81), an appreciation of specific GABAergic mechanisms responsible for seizure control has had to await the selective pharmacological tools of the last decade.

A major problem that emerged from the early research on GABA was the lack of a constant quantitative relationship between brain GABA and susceptibility to seizures in animals treated with various GABAergic drugs. Although seizure protection and convulsive activity resulted from increases and decreases, respectively, in GABA levels (5,6,15,48,62,74), no specific prediction concerning seizure susceptibility could be made based on a given value of whole-brain GABA. This suggested that whole-brain GABA was not an indication of GABA available to those systems important for the control of seizures. In our laboratory, we became interested in using some of the newly available GABAergic compounds to identify GABA-related systems responsible for seizure control. We felt that this information was crucial to solving the problem of relating GABA content to anticonvulsant activity. We therefore designed a series of studies to address the issue of *localization* of GABA-mediated anticonvulsant action. The results of these studies will be described below in terms of: (a) an area of the brain that is critical for the influence of GABA on seizure sensitivity; and (b) the cellular compartment in which changes in GABA have an impact on seizure susceptibility. In addition, some other pathways and transmitters that may locally interact with GABA will be considered for their potential role in seizure control.

ANATOMICAL SITE OF GABA-MEDIATED ANTICONVULSANT ACTION

Ventral Midbrain Involvement

Because there was no basis *a priori* for selecting any particular brain areas as likely candidates for sites where GABA elevation would be anticonvulsant, we initially had to scan large portions of the brain. The elevation of GABA in major subdivisions of the brain was accomplished by microinjecting an irreversible inhibitor of GABA-transaminase, γ-vinyl-GABA (GVG), at the locations indicated in Fig. 1. Because GVG acts irreversibly, large volumes of brain tissue can be affected as the drug spreads from the injection site. As a result, GABA levels

can be elevated several-fold over distances of several millimeters.

To assess anticonvulsant activity, we selected the maximal electroshock (MES) seizure model because it is nonspecific and relatively unselective with respect to the neural circuitry activated. In addition, we had previously determined that systemically administered GVG had anticonvulsant activity in this model (26). We used the customary endpoint of tonic hindlimb extension (THE) for the evaluation of anticonvulsant activity.

At 6 hr after the GVG injections, significant protection from THE was obtained only in the group that had received GVG into the ventral midbrain (Table 1). Consistent with the irreversible action of GVG, complete blockade of THE was again found at 24 hr in the rats that had received GVG in the midbrain. In addition, at this later time, the group that had received GVG in the tectum showed significant, but not complete, seizure protection. No significant effects were observed in the remaining groups of rats.

GABA levels were measured in several areas after the various GVG injections in another group of rats. All injections caused a several-fold elevation of GABA in the vicinity of the injection site. Figure 2 shows net increases in GABA in various regions measured 6 hr after GVG. Maximal elevation was observed to extend over an area within a 2.0-mm radius of the microinjection site. By 24 hr, all tissues within a 3-mm radius were maximally elevated (2.4- to 4-fold more GABA than controls). It is evident from Fig. 2 that the injections (midbrain site) associated with anticonvulsant effects did not significantly alter GABA levels in medulla and cerebellum (we also found no change in spinal cord); we can therefore conclude that GABA elevation in the latter areas was not required for the anticonvulsant effect of GVG which we were measuring. Conversely, a several-fold elevation of GABA in forebrain (including thalamus, hippocampus, and cortex) or in hindbrain areas, was evidently not sufficient to confer protection in the MES test. Seizure protection appears most closely associated with GABA elevation in the midbrain tegmentum, including the substantia nigra (SN) and midbrain reticular formation.

Further localization of the active site in a dorsoventral plane was obtained by examining the effect of injections placed in the superior colliculi. At 6 hr after these injections, no antiseizure activity was obtained, thus eliminating the tectum and the more dorsal aspects of the tegmentum as potential candidates for mediating

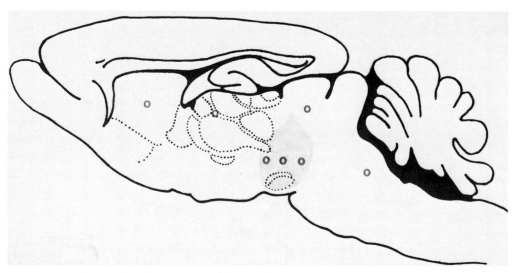

FIG. 1. Parasagittal section of rat brain illustrating sites at which microinjections of GVG were placed stereotaxically. Injection sites (○); for each site, a separate group of rats was used. GVG was dissolved in saline and injected in a volume of 1 μl over 5 min while the animal was under ether anesthesia.

the anticonvulsant effects of midbrain GVG injections (see Table 1). At 24 hr, significant seizure protection was obtained; at this time, there was marked elevation of GABA in the ventral midbrain.

The duration of seizure protection after a single midbrain injection of GVG was determined in another group of rats. Complete blockade of THE was observed for up to 72 hr after a single injection. Partial recovery of THE was obtained on the fourth day, and recovery of normal THE durations took place in all rats by the fifth day after injection. GABA levels in the vicinity of the injection site closely correlated with the duration of seizure protection (Fig. 3).

In another series of experiments, we injected GVG bilaterally (5 μg) into the ventral mesencephalic tegmentum, just dorsal to the SN, and tested the rats 6 hr later in one of four seizure models: (a) MES; (b) pentylenetetrazol (PTZ) 40 mg/kg intravenously (i.v.); (c) PTZ, 90 mg/kg subcutaneously (s.c.); and (d) bicuculline, 0.25 mg/kg i.v. The results shown in Table 2 demonstrate marked protection in all seizure tests; comparisons were made with controls receiving intracerebral saline injections.

Throughout the course of these studies, GVG-injected rats exhibited no overt alterations in motor function. All animals were alert and active; rats receiving midbrain injections of GVG were found to be somewhat more active (with respect to spontaneous locomotor activity), whereas rats receiving forebrain injections of GVG were slightly less active than controls.

These data demonstrate that the irreversible inhibition of GABA degradation in the ventral midbrain tegmental region provides long-lasting seizure protection. This protection is associated with marked increases in GABA, comparable to those observed when GVG is administered systemically in anticonvulsant doses (26). It is noteworthy that the intracerebral dose required for anticonvulsant effects is less than 0.01% of that required systemically. This may reflect the relatively poor penetration of GVG across the blood–brain barrier, a factor which is also probably responsible for the different time course observed for anticonvulsant activity following systemic GVG injection (as will be seen later in Fig. 7).

IDENTIFICATION OF THE SN AS THE MIDBRAIN SITE OF GABA-MEDIATED ANTICONVULSANT ACTIVITY

Having narrowed our search to the ventral midbrain tegmentum, we next had to identify the specific structure(s) within this region responsible for the GABA-mediated effects on seizures. For this purpose, we utilized muscimol, a directly-acting GABA receptor agonist. This compound has the advantage of a relatively rapid onset of action and does not spread as rapidly from the site of injection as does GVG. To compare the effectiveness of muscimol with that of GVG, we microinjected nanogram amounts bilaterally into the midbrain site where GVG had been effective and evaluated MES- or PTZ-in-

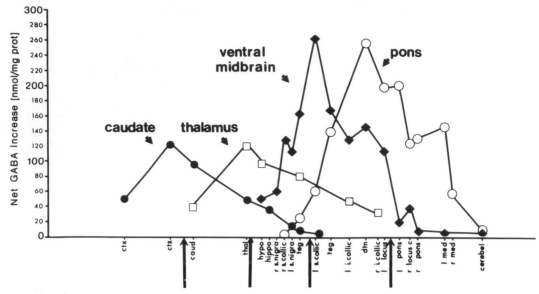

FIG. 2.   Net increase in GABA (over respective control value for each region) in several brain regions 6 hr after GVG (20 μg) microinjection in caudate (●); thalamus (□); ventral midbrain tegmentum (◆); or pontine tegmentum (○). Vertical arrows indicate the relative position of injection sites, which are located 3–4 mm apart. Brain areas, placed in proportion to relative distances from injection sites, are (*left to right*): frontal cortex, motor cortex, caudate, thalamus, hypothalamus, hippocampus, r. substantia nigra, r. superior colliculus, l. substantia nigra, rostral midbrain tegmentum, l. superior colliculus, caudal midbrain tegmentum, l. inferior colliculus, dorsal tegmental nucleus, r. inferior colliculus, l. locus coeruleus, l. pons, r. locus coeruleus, r. pons, l. and r. medulla, cerebellum. From Iadarola and Gale (40), with permission.

duced seizure activity. As shown in Table 3, midbrain application of muscimol (25–75 ng) significantly attenuated both MES- and PTZ-induced seizures. Complete blockade of THE in the MES test was obtained with 50 ng. The duration of seizure protection was dose-dependent. Significant protection was present to 5 hr after 50 ng; by 8 hr after this dose, seizure activity was not different from controls.

At all doses tested, muscimol caused hyperactivity, accompanied by stereotyped sniffing and gnawing. The duration of this behavior ranged from 2 hr (following 25 ng) to 6 hr (following 75 ng). When muscimol was placed in other injection sites in forebrain or in pons, doses as high as 500 ng were without anticonvulsant activity, despite marked depression of motor activity.

In the next series of experiments, the spread of drug from the microinjection site was further minimized by performing the microinjections in unanesthetized animals via chronically im-

TABLE 1. *Intracerebral GVG: Effect on duration and incidence of THE*

		THE duration (sec)		Incidence		Protected (%)	
Treatment group	N	6 hr	24 hr	6 hr	24 hr	6 hr	24 hr
1 Forebrain	5	5.4 ± .8	5.5 ± .6	5/5	5/5	0	0
2 Diencephalon	5	5.3 ± .9	4.6 ± 1.0	5/5	4/5	0	20
3 Midbrain	10	0.7 ± .6[a]	0[a]	2/10	0/10	80	100
4 Tectum	6	5.2 ± .9	2.5 ± 1.5[a]	6/6	3/6	0	50
5 Hindbrain	6	5.0 ± .9	4.8 ± 1.6	5/6	4/6	17	34
6 Sham midbrain	6	5.5 ± .6	5.8 ± .5	6/6	6/6	0	0
7 Control	6	6.1 ± .4	6.3 ± .5	6/6	6/6	0	0

Each value represents the mean ± SE for each treatment group.
[a] Significantly different from treatment group ($p < 0.01$). Incidence of THE: Number of rats showing THE over number of rats tested. Rats were tested at 6 hr and again 24 hr after GVG (see ref. 40).

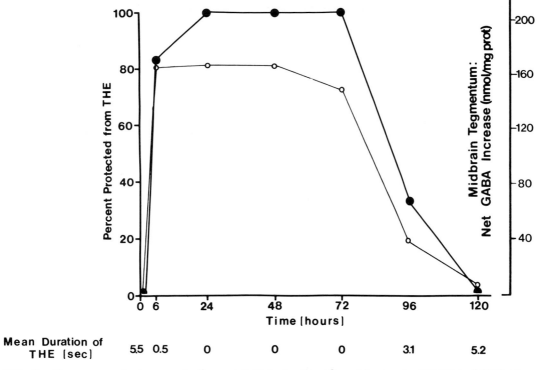

FIG. 3. Time course of seizure protection and GABA elevation after midbrain microinjection of GVG. Percentage of rats protected from THE in the MES test (●) (N = 6); net increase in GABA measured in the midbrain tegmentum in the vicinity of the injection site from separate groups of rats (○).

planted intracerebral guide cannulae. This preparation allowed us to use a very low dose of muscimol (5 ng) and test for anticonvulsant effects within a very short time (20 min) after microinjection.

Two groups of animals were tested: In the first group, injections were placed into the SN, whereas in the second group, injections were placed approximately 1.5 mm dorsal to the SN. We chose the SN as our initial target because of its exceptionally high GABA content, and density of GABA synapses.

Microinjection of a 5-ng dose of muscimol bilaterally into the SN suppressed seizures produced by i.v. bicuculline (Table 4). Injections of muscimol dorsal to the SN did not attenuate seizure activity. In two animals in which only one SN was injected (the contralateral injection was too dorsal), no protection was observed. It appeared essential that muscimol application be placed into the SN bilaterally in order to obtain seizure protection.

After midbrain application of muscimol, no deficits in motor function were observed in any rats. Neurological function (reflexes, gait, responsiveness) was normal and there was no se-

dation. Behaviorally, rats treated with intranigral muscimol exhibited hyperactivity accompanied by stereotyped sniffing and gnawing. Thus, the anatomical substrate mediating the anticonvulsant action of muscimol is clearly distinct from those mediating other characteristic GABA agonist effects such as sedation and ataxia.

INFLUENCE OF GABA TRANSMISSION IN SN ON SUSCEPTIBILITY TO A VARIETY OF EXPERIMENTAL SEIZURES

Using other experimental seizure models, various investigators have confirmed and extended our observations with intranigral application of GABA agonists. In animals with amygdala-kindled seizures, MacNamara et al. (61) found that bilateral intranigral application of muscimol (50 ng) markedly shortened the duration of the kindled motor seizure, from a mean of 39 ± 8 sec in controls to a mean of 3 ± 3 sec in muscimol-pretreated rats. In contrast, application of muscimol dorsal to the SN was without significant effect on seizure duration. In addition to decreasing the duration of the motor seizure, the

TABLE 2. *Seizure protection following bilateral injection of GVG into ventral midbrain tegmentum*

Intracerebral microinjection	MES	PTZ 40 mg/kg i.v.	PTZ 90 mg/kg s.c.	Bicuculline .25 mg/kg i.v.
Saline	6.3 ± .4	2.6 ± .2	8.7 ± .4	2.1 ± .3
GVG (5 μg)	0.6 ± .6[a]	1.2 ± .4[a]	4.2 ± .4[a]	0.5 ± .2[a]

[a] Significantly different from saline-treated controls. Values are mean ± SE of six to eight rats. Pentylene-tetrazol and bicuculline seizure severity was scored using either a 3-point (for i.v. injections) or a 10-point (for s.c. injections) rating scale. MES seizures were measured using duration of THE. Testing was done 6 hr after GVG.

intranigral muscimol treatment decreased the duration of the electrical afterdischarge recorded on the electroencephalogram (EEG) (61). Le Gal La Salle (53) obtained similar results after intranigral application of GVG, observing a marked decrease in afterdischarge duration and a concomitant shortening of the motor seizures in amygdala-kindled animals.

Moshe and Albala (70) found that bilateral injections of muscimol (100 ng) into SN raised the threshold for seizures induced by inhalation of fluorothyl in adult rats. These authors found that the intranigral muscimol treatment did not decrease fluorothyl seizure susceptibility in immature (15-day-old) rat pups, indicating that the nigral GABAergic system involved in seizure control is not yet fully developed. These investigators suggested that the apparent lack of nigral GABA-mediated seizure protection in the 15-day-old rat pups may be related to the increased susceptibility of these animals to seizures.

Intranigral muscimol injections (30 ng) also protected against tonic seizures induced by acoustic stimulation of rats during ethanol withdrawal (23,33a). In these studies, muscimol was also placed into other brain regions known to participate in audiogenic seizures. It was found that injections of muscimol into the inferior colliculus resulted in seizure protection considerably more dramatic than that obtained from injections in SN. These results raise an important point concerning the site of action of GABAergic agents with respect to seizure control. Although GABA-mediated transmission in SN may influence several different types of generalized seizures, for certain seizures this nucleus is probably not the *only* site at which GABAergic synapses can exert an anticonvulsant effect. Where specific neural circuits are involved in the initiation of a seizure, it is likely that enhancing GABA-mediated inhibition in such a circuit could suppress seizure generation. With respect to audiogenic seizures, the inferior colliculus is an important component of the circuitry required for initiating seizures. Although the inferior colliculus may do no more than passively relay acoustic sensory stimulation, enhancing inhibition at this site could interfere with the transmission of the sensory input required for triggering convulsive activity. A similar situation may obtain with respect to the involvement

TABLE 3. *Seizure protection following injection of muscimol into ventral midbrain tegmentum*

		Treatment								
	Control (not injected)	Saline (hr)			Muscimol					
		2.5[d]	5.0	8.0	2.5[d]		5.0			8.0
					25 ng[e]	50 ng	25 ng	50 ng	75 ng	50 ng
MES[b]	6.6	4.8	6.5	6.1	1.8[a]	0[a]	4.8	3.8[a]	.7[a]	6.0
PTZ[c] (40 mg/kg i.v.)	2.9	2.3	2.5	2.8	1.0[a]		1.6			2.6

[a] Significantly different from saline, $p < 0.05$; N = 4 to 6 per group. SEM were all <20% of the respective means for each group.
[b] THE duration (sec).
[c] Seizure rating on 3-point scale. Data from Iadarola and Gale (40), with permission.
[d] Pretreatment time (in hours) before seizure testing.
[e] Dose of muscimol.

TABLE 4. *Protection against seizures induced by bicuculline (0.4 mg/kg i.v.) after bilateral microinjection of muscimol into SN*

Microinjection[a]	Seizure score
Saline	3.0
Muscimol into SN	0.6[b]
Muscimol 2 mm dorsal to SN	2.8

SN, substantia nigra.

[a] Applied to awake, unrestrained rats 20 min prior to seizure test.

[b] Significantly different from saline-injected controls, $p < 0.01$.

Data from Iadarola and Gale (40), with permission.

of GABA in circuits involved in limbic seizure generation. Le Gal La Salle found that injections of GVG into the amygdala could suppress seizures induced by kindling in hippocampus (54). The latter author suggested that the amygdala is an essential component of the circuitry responsible for the initial development of a seizure provoked by stimulation of hippocampus. In contrast, it is unlikely that MES seizures depend upon a specific neural circuit for initiation; this may be the reason that GABA elevation

only in SN was effective in controlling these seizures (40).

SN AS A "COMMON DENOMINATOR" FOR THE CONTROL OF GENERALIZED CONVULSIONS?

The results discussed above indicate that the SN may contain synapses capable of modifying the development and propagation of a seizure regardless of the neural mechanisms responsible for the seizure initiation. In support of a participation of the SN in a variety of seizures, studies with 2-deoxyglucose (2-DG) accumulation have suggested that the SN is one of the most consistently altered brain regions in terms of 2-DG metabolism during convulsions. A marked increase in nigral glucose uptake has been seen in almost every seizure model examined, including amygdala kindling (17), PTZ and bicuculline (9,71a), kainic acid (2,9), penicillin, and cholinergic chemoconvulsants (71a). Although overall patterns of cerebral 2-DG uptake vary significantly between the different seizure models (particularly with respect to forebrain structures), activation of the SN appears to be a stable feature. However, the involvement of SN

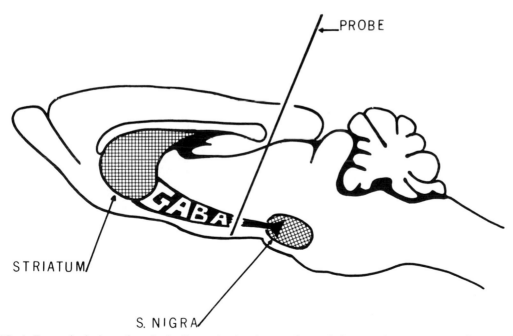

FIG. 4. Parasagittal view of rat brain illustrating hemitransection technique used to remove the GABAergic afferents to substantia nigra. A blunt probe, mounted in a stereotaxic electrode carrier, was inserted through the brain to the base of the skull and moved laterally from the midline (perpendicular to the plane of the drawing) in order to sever all fibers passing between the nigra and the forebrain. See Gale and Iadarola (25) for details.

may be limited to cases of fully *generalized* convulsions. This possibility is suggested by the fact that in *partially* kindled animals, no increase in nigral accumulation of 2-DG was observed; increased nigral metabolism was present only in animals showing fully generalized seizures (17). Thus, as discussed previously, although seizures may be initiated by a variety of different circuits not necessarily involving SN, the generalization of the seizures may utilize a common circuitry subject to nigral regulation.

The results of Ackerman et al. (1) and Albala et al. (2) indicate that the association between increased 2-DG metabolism and seizure activity may be specific to adult animals. Immature rats (15–16 days old) showed no increase in metabolic activity in SN during seizures induced by amygdala kindling or kainic acid. Because these rats appear to have a lower seizure threshold than adults have (2), it would seem that increased metabolic activity in SN is not necessary for the development and expression of seizures. Instead, increased metabolic activity in SN during seizures in adult animals may represent a compensatory increase in the activity of presynaptic GABA terminals in this nucleus in an attempt to suppress or control the propagation of the seizure.

CELLULAR COMPARTMENTATION OF GABA WITHIN SN

Based on our findings that the SN is a key site for GABA-mediated anticonvulsant activity, it might be expected that measurements of GABA levels in this nucleus would provide us with a consistent predictor of seizure susceptibility. Unfortunately, this is not the case, owing to the fact that several anatomically and functionally distinct compartments of GABA exist within the nucleus. The synthetic and degradative enzymes, as well as uptake mechanisms for GABA are present in both GABAergic terminals and cell bodies, as well as in glia and non-GABAergic neurons (4,7,46,52,69,86). In the SN, almost all of the glutamic acid decarboxylase (GAD) and GABA-transaminase can be accounted for by GABAergic afferent terminals and the perikarya of GABAergic efferents (25,28,85). We therefore questioned whether different GABA-elevating agents might exert differential effects on these two compartments of GABA. A relatively small increase in GABA in GABAergic nerve terminals would be expected to have a greater functional impact on nigral synaptic transmission than would a large increase in GABA in GABAergic perikarya. Thus, we explored the possibility that the extent of GABA

elevation specifically associated with GABAergic nerve terminals in SN could be more consistently correlated with seizure protection.

Deafferented SN as a Model for Examining Cellular Compartments of GABA

At least 80% of the GABA content of the nigra is associated with GABAergic nerve terminals that arise from cell bodies located several millimeters away in the forebrain. This anatomical arrangement makes it possible to sever the GABA-containing projections to the nigra without causing direct injury to the nucleus itself (see Fig. 4). By mechanically transecting these projections on one side of the brain (i.e., hemitransecting), we can therefore render one SN "nerve-terminal-poor," whereas the intact SN on the contralateral side retains its normally dense supply of GABA nerve terminals. Because no damage is done to the nigral cells on the lesioned side, both nigras are assumed to contain similar amounts of non-nerve-terminal GABA and associated enzymes. This represents between 10 and 20% of the total GABA of the intact nucleus (25). Thus, any differences between the nigras of the two hemispheres can be attributed to the "nerve-terminal" compartment. In this way, we can examine the relative impact of a drug treatment on the nerve-termi-

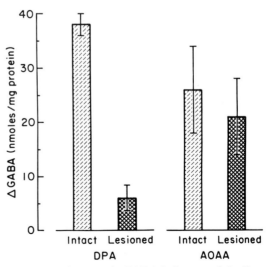

FIG. 5. Net increase in GABA in intact and deafferented (lesioned) substantia nigra after DPA (300 mg/kg i.p.) or AOAA (30 mg/kg i.p.). Control GABA levels (nmol/mg protein): intact, 103 ± 1.8; lesioned 21 ± 1.2. Transections were made 7–10 days prior to drug treatment. All values are significantly different from control ($p < 0.05$); N = eight rats. Data from Iadarola and Gale (39,41), with permission.

nal versus non-nerve terminal pools of nigral GABA.

Comparison Between Amino-Oxyacetic Acid (AOAA) and *n*-Dipropylacetate (DPA)

It has been repeatedly noted that functional effects of DPA are accompanied by much smaller changes in brain GABA than those that accompany the effects of AOAA. In fact, using AOAA, it is possible to elevate GABA to levels equivalent to those obtained with anticonvulsant doses of DPA, without producing significant seizure protection. In rat SN, an elevation of GABA equivalent to that obtained with an ED_{100} dose of DPA in the MES test (300 mg/kg) is obtained following doses of AOAA (30–35 mg/kg) that afford only minimal (ED_{25}) protection against MES. We were therefore interested in testing the hypothesis that a significant portion of the GABA increase produced by AOAA might be sequestered in a pool that does not directly participate in GABA-mediated synaptic transmission. Thus, we examined the effects of DPA and AOAA in hemitransected rats.

The effects of DPA [300 mg/kg intraperitoneally (i.p.)] and AOAA (30 mg/kg i.p.) on GABA in the SN from intact and transected hemispheres are presented in Fig. 5. In the intact SN, both drugs produced significant and similar increases in GABA. In the GABA-deafferented SN, AOAA produced a significant increase in GABA, the net value of which (21 nmol/mg protein) was similar to that obtained in the intact SN (26 nmol/mg protein). Consequently, only a small portion of the overall increase in GABA after AOAA could be attributed to the nerve terminal compartment. In contrast, DPA failed to increase the GABA content of the deafferented SN significantly; more than 90% of the GABA increase after DPA was found to depend on the presence of GABA nerve terminals. Thus, in the relative absence of GABAergic nerve terminals, the GABA-elevating effect of DPA appears to be lost, whereas the effect of AOAA is retained. This observation is consistent with the subcellular fractionation studies of Sarhan and Seiler (76) which demonstrated a selective effect of DPA on synaptosomal GABA. Thus, although the total GABA increase after DPA is modest (in contrast to AOAA), it appears to be almost exclusively nerve-terminal associated.

Effects of Systemically Administered GVG on Nigral Nerve Terminal GABA During First 12 hr

Increases in nigral GABA after systemic application of GVG are even more dramatic than

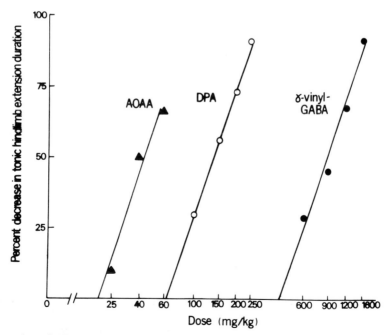

FIG. 6. Suppression of THE as a function of dose of AOAA, DPA, or GVG. Drugs were given i.p. at the following times before testing: AOAA, 2 hr; DPA, 30 min; GVG, 60 hr. N = 10–12 per point. MES was applied via corneal electrodes. Mean duration of THE for each group was subtracted from that of vehicle-injected controls and expressed as a percentage of control mean (8 sec). From Gale and Iadarola (26), with permission.

those observed with DPA and AOAA. By 6 hr after GVG (600–1,600 mg/kg i.p.) nigral GABA levels are increased by more than 50%; by 12 hr, nigral GABA reaches a maximum of 150–200% of control. Despite this marked elevation of nigral GABA, at 6 or 12 hr after these doses of GVG, there is no significant attenuation of electroshock seizures (26,78).

When changes in nigral GABA produced by GVG were examined in hemitransected rats, it was found that *12* hr after GVG (900 mg/kg) the net increase in GABA in the SN on the intact side (80 nmol/mg protein) was no larger than the net increase in the SN on the transected side, indicating that GABAergic nerve terminals were not necessary for the elevation of GABA produced by GVG at this time (26).

These data suggest that, as with AOAA, a large portion of the GABA elevation seen with GVG is associated with compartments other than GABAergic nerve terminals. Our observations are consistent with studies that have demonstrated marked effects of GABA-transaminase inhibition in tissues that are not known to contain GABA terminals (7,86), as well as with subcellular fractionation studies (76). Because compounds such as AOAA and GVG probably influence nerve-terminal GABA only after other compartments of GABA have been elevated several-fold, it is understandable that relatively large increases in total GABA are required to elicit GABA-related physiological effects with these drugs (8,34,51).

Correlation Between Increases in GABA in Nerve-Terminal Pool and Anticonvulsant Activity

To verify whether changes in GABA in a particular nigral compartment correlate with anticonvulsant activity, we examined the ability of DPA, AOAA, and GVG to reduce the duration of the THE phase of MES seizures. Fig. 6 shows the dose–response functions.

The effects of GVG were examined over several days following a single injection. The time course of action of GVG in the MES test is shown in Fig. 7; 12 hr after GVG no blockade or reduction in THE duration was observed. However, at 36 hr, a reduction in THE was obtained with the high dose (1,600 mg/kg) of GVG, and by 60 hr, the reduction in THE duration was maximum (see Fig. 6 for dose–response at this time). At 60 hr after GVG we also observed protection against seizures induced by PTZ and bicuculline; this was in contrast to previous studies which found GVG to be inactive in these seizure models when testing was done within 12 hr after GVG (78).

Because the anticonvulsant activity of GVG

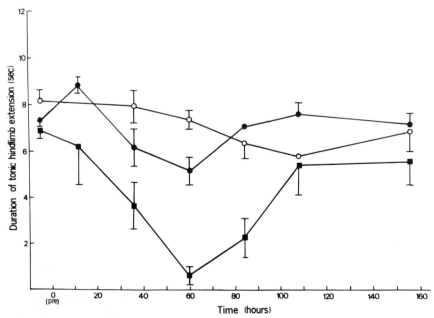

FIG. 7. Suppression of THE as a function of time (hr) after GVG. Values are means ± S.E. of 12 rats per group. Treatments (i.p. at T = 0): GVG 600 mg/kg, ●; GVG 1600 mg/kg, ■; saline (control) ○. Data from Gale and Iadarola (26), with permission.

was maximal at a time (60 hr) when brain GABA levels were starting to decline, the question of compartmentation of GABA seemed to be especially pertinent. By analyzing GABA levels in the intact and deafferented SN at various times after GVG (900 mg/kg), we were able to estimate the elevation in the nerve-terminal–associated compartment of GABA (26). At 36 hr after GVG, a greater net increase in GABA occurred in the intact SN than in the deafferented SN (~20% of the net increase on the intact side could not be accounted for by the increase in the lesioned SN). The increase in nerve-terminal GABA was more apparent at 60 hr; at this time, approximately one-half of the GABA increase in the intact SN was associated with the presence of nerve terminals (26).

Our data can, therefore, resolve some of the inconsistencies that we chose to examine. It appears that an effect on nerve-terminal GABA may be the critical feature shared by anticonvulsant doses of DPA and GVG. Moreover, the lack of anticonvulsant effects of moderate doses of AOAA, or of large doses of GVG within the first 12 hr, can be explained by their lack of effect on GABA associated with nerve terminals.

To examine the correlation between changes in nigral nerve-terminal GABA and anticonvulsant activity in the MES test, data from rats with transections were used to estimate the proportional changes in GABA in the two compartments. We have made the assumption that the difference in GABA content between the deafferented and intact SN represents nigral GABA associated with nerve terminals. These values are presented in Table 5, along with the percentage of reduction in THE duration associated with each treatment. The values reveal that the percent increase in the nerve-terminal pool is positively correlated ($r = +0.93$) with anticonvulsant activity in the MES test (Fig. 8). On the other hand, GABA increases in the nigra as a whole (intact SN) or in the non-nerve-terminal compartment, do not positively correlate with seizure protection. These data demonstrate that changes in GABA that occur in the non-nerve-terminal pool may actually conceal the degree of change in GABA in the functionally relevant (nerve-terminal) compartment. Moreover, the relatively undramatic effect of DPA on GABA levels assumes a different meaning when we realize that this is simply owing to its lack of effect on the non-nerve-terminal compartment. Although we cannot exclude the possibility that DPA may have anticonvulsant effects mediated by mechanisms other than GABA, our data suggest that the DPA-induced increase in nigral nerve-terminal GABA is sufficient to predict marked anticonvulsant activity in the electroshock seizure model.

It seems to be a general characteristic of "classical" GABA-transaminase inhibitors that they have their most marked effects on compartments of GABA other than those in GABAergic nerve terminals. We have found this to be true not only for AOAA and GVG, but also for gabaculine and ethanolamine-*o*-sulfate, both of which irreversibly inhibit GABA-transaminase and elevate GABA to an extent similar to that obtained after GVG application. Of all the GABA-elevating agents that we have studied, DPA appears to be unique in its relative lack of effect on non-nerve-terminal GABA. As a result, most or all of the GABA elevation that occurs after DPA can probably be used to influence synaptic transmission. An understanding of the mechanism by which DPA exerts its influence on nerve-terminal GABA metabolism would be especially useful as a basis for the design of additional agents with similar selectivity of action.

TABLE 5. *Relationship between suppression of THE and GABA elevation in SN*

Treatment[a]	Suppression of THE (%)	Increase in GABA (% over control)		
		Total	Non-nerve terminal	Nerve terminal
GVG (12 hr)[b]	0	98	646	0
GVG (36 hr)	28	85	373	19
GVG (60 hr)	45	57	160	33
DPA (30 min)	90	36	28	39
AOAA (2 hr)	18	25	100	7

THE, tonic hindlimb extension; GVG, γ-vinyl GABA; DPA, *n*-dipropylacetate; AOAA, amino-oxyacetic acid.

[a] Drugs were given i.p.: GVG, 900 mg/kg; AOAA, 30 mg/kg; DPA, 300 mg/kg.

[b] Time after treatment at which measurements were made.

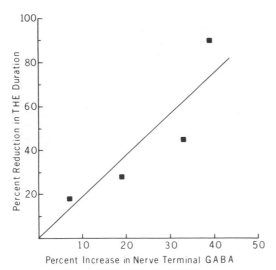

FIG. 8. Relationship between percentage of reduction in THE duration in the MES test and percentage of increase in GABA associated with nigral nerve terminals. Derived from values in Table 5. Correlation coefficient = 0.93.

Intracerebral Application of GVG: Effect on Nerve-Terminal GABA

Our next series of studies were aimed at characterizing the effect of the direct microinjection of GVG into SN with respect to GABA elevation in nigral nerve terminals. We therefore examined the time course of GABA elevation after microinjecting GVG (5 μg) directly into the intact and deafferented SN. The results, shown in Fig. 9, reveal a significant difference between the net increase in GABA in the intact versus deafferented SN, indicating that a portion of the GABA elevation following direct intracerebral application of GVG was associated with nerve terminals. This nerve-terminal related increase in GABA (i.e., the difference between the net increases in GABA in the intact and lesioned SN) was maximal by 6 hr and remained constant for at least an additional 24 hr. Thus, it appears that, unlike the long latency required for nerve-terminal GABA elevation following systemic injection of GVG, a rapid elevation of nerve-terminal GABA occurs following direct intracerebral application of GVG. At 6 hr after the intranigral injection of GVG, the increase in nigral nerve terminal GABA was comparable to that found at 60 hr following a high dose of GVG given sytemically. Because both treatments (6 hr after 5 μg intranigral GVG and 60 hr after 1,600 mg/kg i.p. GVG) are similar with respect to an-

ticonvulsant effect, this provides additional evidence for the close association between elevation of nerve terminal GABA in SN and anticonvulsant activity.

The faster onset of action of intracerebral GVG injections as compared with systemic GVG injections is most likely related to the fact that this compound crosses the blood–brain barrier poorly; therefore, with systemic treatment it is difficult to achieve concentrations of drug equivalent to those obtained after direct intracerebral injection. It appears that only in the presence of high local concentration of GVG is the GABA-transaminase associated with nerve terminals inactivated by GVG. This does not explain, however, the delay in the functional effects of systemically applied GVG, since the concentration of drug in the brain reaches a peak and starts to decline over the first 24 hr of drug administration. It is possible, on the other hand, that after systemic GVG treatment, most of the GABA-transaminase inactivation occurs in cell bodies and that the inactivated enzyme is then transported to the nerve-terminals. The delay in the impact on nerve terminals would then result from the amount of time it takes to replace the nerve-terminal GABA-transaminase with inactivated transaminase transported from the cell body. This would be expected to occur more rapidly in short-axon neurons than in long-distance pathways such as those projecting to SN.

Short-Latency Anticonvulsant Actions of Systemically-Administered GVG

Although protection against tonic-clonic seizures induced in rats by MES, bicuculline, and PTZ is obtained only after a latency of more than 12 hr following systemically injected GVG, this treatment has also been demonstrated to exert *short*-latency anticonvulsant actions. Within 6 hr after systemic GVG treatment, seizure protection has been observed in the following seizure models: (a) myoclonic activity induced by i.v. bicuculline in mice (10); (b) tonic seizures induced by i.v. or i.p. strychnine in mice (47,77,78); (c) isoniazid-induced convulsions in mice (47,77,78); (d) photic-induced seizures in baboons (64); (e) amygdala-kindled seizures in rats (45); and (f) audiogenic seizures in mice (77,78). In several of these cases, the peak action of GVG occurred between 3 and 8 hr and started to decline by 24 hr. In contrast, no effect of GVG was obtained within this time period (3 to 8 hr) with respect to protection against seizures induced by s.c. bicuculline, PTZ, or MES in mice (47,77,78).

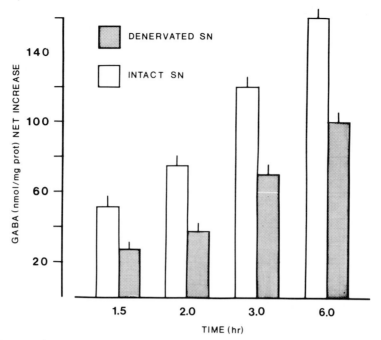

FIG. 9. Net increase (over respective controls) in GABA at various times after microinjection of GVG (5 μg) into intact or deafferented substantia nigra. Each value is mean ± S.E. of four to six rats; all values are significantly different from each other and from untreated controls. Data from Casu and Gale (11).

Thus, it appears that GVG may exert anticonvulsant actions by two distinct and independent mechanisms, giving rise to a biphasic time course of pharmacological activity. Our data suggest that only those actions that are present after a significant delay (i.e., at 24 hr or later, depending upon the species) following administration of systemic GVG, are likely to be related to an augmentation of nigral GABAergic neurotransmission. This is further supported by the observations of Gale and Casu (23a) that the ability of GVG to augment GABA-mediated actions on nigral neurons started to be evident at 24 hr and was maximally effective at 60 hr after an i.p. injection. On the other hand, the mechanism responsible for the short-latency, short-duration actions of GVG is not clear. The profile of these actions suggests that the underlying mechanism is distinct from that responsible for the longer-latency, longer-duration actions. It is quite likely, in fact, that the short-latency effects are unrelated to nigral GABA, since systemically administered GVG fails to augment GABA-mediated actions in SN at 6 hr (23a).

Some of the short-latency effects of GVG could be related to actions at synapses in regions other than SN. For example, the short-latency anticonvulsant effect of GVG in the audiogenic seizure model may be related to GABAergic effects in the inferior colliculus (23), a region that responds especially rapidly to the GABA-elevating action of systemically administered GVG (unpublished observations). If part of the rapid elevation of GABA occurs in GABAergic terminals of the inferior colliculus (e.g., in short intrinsic neurons) this could conceivably account for protection from audiogenic seizures during the first 24 hr following administration of GVG. The continued protection from audiogenic seizures beyond 24 hr after GVG administration may then result from the combined effects of nigral as well as collicular GABA elevation. It is difficult, however, to extend this explanation to most of the other short-latency anticonvulsant effects of GVG, because these effects start to diminish by 24 hr despite the fact that the inhibition of GABA-transaminase remains virtually constant during this time period (78). This raises the possibility that those actions of GVG that occur within several hours of systemic administration may be related to direct, reversible actions of this compound which are dependent upon the presence of free drug in the system. A significant portion of the non-protein-bound GVG found in the brain at 4 hr is still present at 24 hr, but is no longer detectable by 48 hr (unpublished observations). Whatever the mechanism of the short-term actions of GVG, it is important to recognize the possibility that this compound may produce transient anticonvulsant actions that are unrelated to its more sustained enhancement of GABA-mediated neurotransmission in SN.

Relationship Between Decreases in Nigral Nerve-Terminal GABA and Convulsions

We were interested in using our deafferented SN model to determine whether a loss of nerve-terminal GABA could account for convulsions occurring after combined treatment with a GABA synthesis inhibitor and GABA-elevating agent. We selected isonicotinic acid hydrazide (isoniazid) (INH) as the inhibitor of GABA synthesis, and evaluated INH-induced seizures and decreases of GABA in the presence and absence of pretreatment with DPA or GVG. Under the conditions of this experiment (Fig. 10, legend), DPA completely prevented INH-induced seizure activity, whereas GVG did not prevent the seizures induced by INH.

In control animals, or in the intact hemisphere of hemitransected rats, INH treatment (600 mg/kg i.p., 50 min before killing) caused a net decrease of 37 nmol/mg protein in the SN. A significant decrease also took place following INH in the intact SN of rats that had been pretreated with DPA or GVG (Fig. 10). When we examined the deafferented SN, we found INH to be without effect on GABA levels following GVG pretreatment suggesting that the INH-induced decrease (following GVG) in the intact SN was

entirely associated with nerve terminals. This situation is shown in Fig. 10, in which the non-nerve-terminal GABA content represents that measured in the deafferented SN, and the nerve-terminal GABA content represents the net difference between the intact and deafferented SN. From this analysis, we can see that the seizure protection afforded by DPA was associated with an attenuation of the effect of INH on nigral nerve-terminal GABA, whereas GVG was unable to prevent either the convulsion or loss of nerve-terminal GABA produced by INH. Thus, neither the marked inhibition of GABA-transaminase (>80%) nor the marked GABA increase that occurs 12 hr after GVG pretreatment, appear able to influence the rate of decline of nerve-terminal GABA following GABA synthesis inhibition. We have extended this observation by examining GABA levels at various times following INH administration (20, 40, 60 min.); the INH-induced rate of decline in GABA in several regions (superior colliculus, cortex, and cerebellum) was not altered by 12-hr pretreatment with GVG (2,000 mg/kg, i.p.) (46a). These results suggest that seizures and depletion of GABA in nerve terminals are related to one another and that these two phenomena can be manipulated independently of alterations in GABA metabolism that take place in non-nerve-terminal compartments. Furthermore, nerve terminals may represent a critical site for the degradation of GABA in circumstances in which there is less than complete inhibition of GABA-transaminase.

It appears from our results that a critical level of nerve-terminal GABA must be maintained in

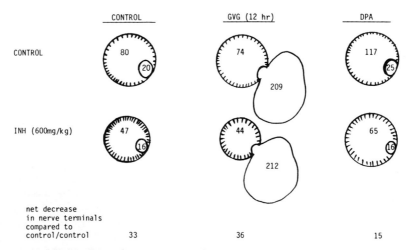

FIG. 10.   Nerve-terminal ( ) and non-nerve-terminal ( ) GABA (nmol/mg protein) in substantia nigra following isoniazid (INH), in the presence of GVG (2,000 mg/kg i.p., 12 hr before INH) or *n*-dipropylacetate (DPA, 300 mg/kg i.p., 5 min before INH).

SN in order to protect against INH-induced seizures. However, it is important to recognize that INH-induced seizures do not *originate* in SN. Bilateral application of INH directly into SN does not cause seizures, even when nigral GABA levels are decreased by over 50% (unpublished observations). Likewise, application of bicuculline, picrotoxin (71) or other convulsant stimuli (19,32,50) into SN does not induce seizures. It appears that seizure activity is initiated elsewhere in the brain and is then subject to nigral control during the process of propagation. For agents that act by decreasing GABA transmission, their effectiveness as convulsants may therefore depend upon their *combined* action at a seizure initiation site as well as in SN. A GABA-elevating agent would then be able to attenuate convulsions induced by GABA antagonists by acting at either or both of these sites. Because a seizure initiation site has not yet been identified for the GABA antagonists, we cannot at present determine the degree of nerve-terminal GABA depletion required for seizure initiation (however, see 90).

ANTICONVULSANT EFFECT OF NIGRAL LESIONS

Because GABA has been shown to inhibit nigral efferents, it is likely that GABA terminals inhibit nigral projections that normally facilitate seizure propagation. If, in fact, SN output can facilitate the manifestation of seizures, destruction of this nucleus should reduce seizure susceptibility.

To test this hypothesis, discrete bilateral lesions in the vicinity of SN were evaluated for their effect on experimentally-induced seizures (31). Lesions were produced either by electrocoagulation or by microinjection of the neurotoxin, kainic acid, the latter used to spare axons passing through the lesion site.

As shown in Table 6, the bilateral electrolytic as well as kainic acid lesions of SN significantly attenuated bicuculline-induced clonic and tonic seizures. A consistent feature of effective lesions was the nearly complete bilateral destruction of SN pars reticulata. When destruction of SN was unilateral only, there was no protection; this is similar to the lack of seizure protection seen when GABA agonists are microinjected into only one SN. Electrolytic lesions involving damage to only the ventral border of SN that bilaterally interrupted corticospinal tracts in the cerebral peduncle were also without significant effect. Electrolytic lesions 2 mm dorsal to the SN site, involving medial lemniscus and portions of posterior, ventral, and posterolateral nuclei of the thalamus, did not reduce seizure activity. Kainic acid lesions of midbrain tegmentum (2–3 mm in diameter) just dorsal to SN that did not bilaterally destroy SN also were without significant effect on seizures induced by bicuculline. It therefore appears that integrity of SN, and not of tissue adjacent to or axons passing through SN, is required for normal expression of generalized seizures with bicuculline.

As shown in Fig. 11, the mild facial and forepaw clonus (score = 1) elicited by low doses of bicuculline in control rats was not seen in rats with bilateral SN lesions; tonic forelimb extension (score = 3) associated with higher doses of bicuculline was also eliminated by these lesions. However, a dose of bicuculline two to four times that required to induce tonic seizures in control

TABLE 6. *Effects of mesencephalic lesions on bicuculline-induced seizures*

	Seizure score	N
Sham	2.8 ± 0.2	8
Lesions of SN		
Kainic acid	1.3 ± 0.2[a]	4
Electrolytic	1.4 ± 0.5[a]	4
Lesions of tegmentum not involving SN		
Kainic acid	2.5 ± 0.2	4
Electrolytic 2 mm dorsal to SN	2.6 ± 0.3	9
Electrolytic 2 mm caudal to SN	2.7 ± 0.3	3
Electrolytic 2 mm dorsal and caudal to SN	2.6 ± 0.4	4

SN, substantia nigra.

Values are seizure scores, mean ± SE; N, number of rats in each group. Bicuculline (0.3 mg/kg) was injected i.v.

[a] Significantly different from sham and from lesions not involving SN, as analyzed by the Mann-Whitney U-test for nonparametric grouped data, $p < 0.05$.

Data from Garant and Gale (31), with permission.

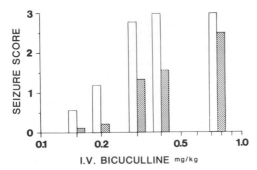

FIG. 11. Effect of nigral lesions on seizures induced by i.v. bicuculline. Data from sham-lesioned rats (open bars); data from rats with bilateral lesions of substantia nigra (shaded bars). Values are means of three to eight rats; the means for lesioned rats are significantly lower than controls at all but the highest dose, as analysed by the Mann-Whitney U-test for nonparametric grouped data, $p \leq 0.05$. Data from Garant and Gale (31), with permission.

animals elicited explosive clonic and/or tonic seizures in animals with bilateral SN lesions. This indicated that the protective effect of these lesions is caused by a shift in the dose–response for bicuculline, and not by a selective blockade of certain motor components of the seizures. In other experiments, we found that bilateral lesions of SN also protected rats from MES seizures (31).

We can conclude from our data that the destruction of nigral efferents results in a decreased susceptibility to generalized seizures, similar to the effects of augmentation of GABA transmission in SN. This suggests that inhibition of nigral efferents is anticonvulsant, or, conversely, that activity in nigral efferents permits or facilitates seizure generalization.

ROLE OF NEUROACTIVE PEPTIDES IN SN

If activity in nigral efferents is permissive or facilitative to seizure propagation, it should be possible to alter seizure sensitivity by manipulating a variety of neural inputs to the nigra. In addition to GABA, the SN receives projections containing substance P, opiate peptides, serotonin, glutamate, and possibly aspartate. All of these substances have effects on the activity of nigral efferents, and as such may play a role in seizure propagation.

Application of opiate receptor agonists into the SN produces behavioral (43) and biochemical (24) effects that resemble those produced by GABA agonists injected into this nucleus. This suggests that opiates may inhibit some of the

same nigral cells that are inhibited by GABA. On this basis, we examined the effects of bilateral intranigral application of morphine sulfate and [D-Ala^2]-Met-enkephalin on MES seizures.

Morphine sulfate (20 μg) injected into each nigra protected 87% of the rats from THE (Table 7). The degradation-resistant opiate agonist [D-Ala^2]-Met-enkephalin also reduced the incidence of THE. The opiate antagonist naloxone (1 mg/kg i.p., given at 20 min and again at 5 min prior to seizure testing) completely abolished the anticonvulsant effect of intranigral morphine (29). Anatomical specificity of the opiate agonist action was indicated by the lack of seizure protection following injection of the drugs into sites 1.5 to 4.0 mm rostral to the SN (29).

In contrast to these effects on MES seizures, we found that opiate microinjection into the SN was not effective against i.v. bicuculline seizures (29). This result is surprising, since the intranigral application of GABA agonists is effective against both electroshock and bicuculline-induced seizures (40). The disparity in opiate efficacy indicates that electroshock and bicuculline seizure propagation may involve different circuitry at the level of the SN, especially with regard to opiate neuron involvement. However, this dissociation of the anticonvulsant actions of intranigral morphine *is* consistent with the observation that systemically administered morphine is anticonvulsant in the electroshock test but is not anticonvulsant against bicuculline, PTZ, or picrotoxin seizures (20,21). Thus, opiate terminals in SN can exert an inhibitory influence on the seizure-facilitating nigral efferent cells, which may be similar but not identical to the inhibition produced by GABA.

The best-documented excitatory input to the SN is the substance P (SP)-containing projection deriving from the striatum. Studies by Melis and Gale (65,66), using antagonist analogs of SP, have indicated that both dopaminergic and nondopaminergic nigral efferents are controlled by GABA inhibition and SP-mediated excitation. This suggests that the seizure facilitating nigral efferents might be subject to excitatory control by SP. If this hypothesis is correct, blockade of SP excitation in the nigra should prove anticonvulsant.

Bilateral intranigral injection of a stable SP antagonist, [D-Pro^2-D Trp 7,9]-SP, significantly reduced the incidence of THE in the MES test (Table 7). On the other hand, injection of a degradation-resistant agonist analog of SP, [pGlu^5-, MePhe^8,Sar^9]-substance P$^{5-11}$ did not significantly alter the seizure response as compared with matched saline controls (Table 7). Thus, exogenous SP-like excitation in SN is not procon-

TABLE 7. *Effects of bilateral manipulations of SN neurons on the incidence of THE in the maximal electroshock seizure test*

Presumed effect on nigral outflow	Treatment	N	Percentage protected
No effect (controls)	Saline (1 μl)	16	0
	Lesions of ventral midbrain tegmentum *not* involving SN	10	10
Inhibition			
Gaba receptor stimulation	Muscimol (50 ng)	8	100[a]
Opiate receptor stimulation	Morphine sulfate (20 μg)	8	87[a]
Neuron destruction	Electrolytic lesion	10	100[a]
Disfacilitation			
SP receptor blockade	[D-Pro^2,D-Trp^{7,9}]-SP (antagonist, 20 μg)	8	87[a]
Excitation			
SP receptor stimulation	[pGLU^5,MePhe^8,Sar^9]-SP [5–11] (agonist, 20 μg)	7	29

SN, substantia nigra; THE, tonic hindlimb extension; SP, substance P.

All manipulations are bilateral; doses are per each nigra, delivered in 1 μl of saline. Seizure testing was performed 90–150 min after microinjection, or 24 hr after lesioning. Seizures were induced by administering 150 mA current for 200 msec via corneal electrodes to 80–120 g male Sprague-Dawley rats.

[a] THE significantly less than control, $p < 0.05$.

vulsant, perhaps because the endogenous substance P system is maximally active. Because blockade of SP excitation in the SN by specific antagonists is anticonvulsant (30), we tentatively conclude that the seizure-facilitating efferent neurons of the SN may normally be driven by SP.

The role of other putative nigral transmitters for regulating seizure susceptibility has yet to be examined. Because serotonin may exert a predominantly inhibitory influence in SN, it is possible that serotonergic agonists may be anticonvulsant at this site. The excitatory amino acids, on the other hand, may participate in driving the seizure facilitating nigral outputs; in this case, antagonists might exert anticonvulsant actions in the nigra (91). It should be recognized, however, that the ability of a substance to protect against seizures when applied directly to SN does not necessarily mean that the substance will be anticonvulsant when given systemically or intracerebroventriculary. In addition, an anticonvulsant action of a compound given intranigrally cannot be interpreted to indicate that the nigra is the exclusive or major site of action of that compound, unless numerous other brain areas have been examined as well. Thus, the conclusions that we have reached concerning GABAergic compounds cannot be generalized to drugs acting on other nigral transmitter systems until additional studies are completed.

NATURE OF THE SEIZURE FACILITATING NIGRAL EFFERENTS

The efferent pathways from SN include the nigrostriatal, nigrothalamic, nigrotectal, and nigrotegmental projections. The first of these is dopaminergic, originating in the pars compacta, whereas the others arise in the pars reticulata and contain GABA (12,13,49,60,84). The dopaminergic nigral projection is probably not responsible for the seizure modification obtained from intranigral treatments, since we have found dopaminergic agonists and antagonists to be ineffective against the various seizure models that we have studied. Moreover, virtually complete lesions of the dopamine neurons did not afford protection against seizures induced by kindling, fluorothyl, bicuculline, or electroshock in rats (C. Wasterlain, personal communication). Additional evidence against a critical role for the nigrostriatal dopaminergic projection in the nigral control of seizures derives from our nigral lesion studies. When we measured striatal tyrosine hydroxylase to determine the extent of damage to the nigrostriatal dopamine pathway, we found that this parameter did not correlate with the extent of seizure protection. In fact, seizure protection appeared to be dependent upon the extent of damage to the *pars reticulata* region, from which the *non*dopaminergic nigral efferents originate.

GABA has been demonstrated to inhibit the

nigral projections from pars reticulata based on both electrophysiological (35,60) and biochemical (67) criteria. Because these projections are themselves GABAergic (12,13,49,60,84), the net effect of GABA activity in nigral synapses is *disinhibition* of target neurons in thalamus, tectum, and tegmentum. Two important predictions can be derived from the knowledge of this circuitry: (a) Activity of neurons located in one or more of the nigral projection targets is anticonvulsant; and (b) GABA inhibition in one or more of these target areas is *pro*convulsant. This, of course would mean that the ability of a systemically administered GABA agonist to confer seizure protection would depend on the relative impact of the drug on "anticonvulsant" sites of action such as the nigra, and "proconvulsant" sites of action such as the nigral target areas. We are currently investigating the action of GABA in these target areas in an attempt to identify which one(s) may mediate the anticonvulsant actions elicited from SN.

The data presented earlier in this review indicate that the inhibition of nigral outflow reduces seizure susceptibility but that it does not preclude the animal's ability to exhibit any or all of the motor components of a seizure. Increasing the dose of chemoconvulsant to two times that normally required for inducing tonic seizures can elicit a full tonic seizure in an animal with intranigral application of GABA agonists or nigral lesions. It is therefore possible that the SN is part of a "preferred path" for seizure propagation; at higher levels of convulsant stimuli, however, structures other than those in the "preferred circuit" are recruited. This possibility was originally suggested by electrophysiological studies that implicated the SN and/or associated basal ganglia structures in the propagation of seizures. Heath noted a consistent spread of seizure activity to SN after electrical stimulation of hippocampus or implantation of cobalt into septum or hippocampus (38). Moreover, the studies of Jinnai and associates (44) and Hayashi (37), in which ablation of various cortical and subcortical regions was used to examine the course of cortically-induced seizure activity, concluded that the globus pallidus and SN were integral relay stations for seizure activity generated by chemical stimulation of either cortical or thalamic sites. Indeed, in both investigations, the SN was viewed as the last relay station "from whence the attack is propagated to the final common pathway." (18).

If we consider the nigra as an essential-link in a preferred path for seizure propagation, enhancing inhibition on nigral efferent neurons in pars reticulata could act as a barrier to the progress of seizure activity from rostral to caudal

levels. Alternatively, it is not necessary that the convulsive activity actually funnel through SN in order for GABA transmission in this nucleus to interfere with seizure spread. Convulsive activity may be propagated through other structures which receive, either directly or indirectly, projections from SN. In this scheme, thalamic, tectal and/or tegmental neurons might be part of a "seizure circuit" which can be regulated by nigral projections. Because augmentation of GABA tone in SN results in a net disinhibition of cells in the nigral efferent target areas, we can speculate that the firing of cells in these target areas may cause a desynchronization of convulsive activity that impedes further propagation (33).

Based on our results, we favor the latter view of the SN—i.e., as a regulator of seizure propagation, and not necessarily a relay for the transmission of seizure activity itself. If the nigra were in fact a critical relay in the preferred path for seizure propagation, lesions of this structure would be expected to qualitatively alter seizure expression. We find however, that although the sensitivity to seizure-inducing stimuli is decreased following nigral lesions, the temporal and spatial pattern of motor seizure activity is unchanged. We therefore propose that the nigra functions as a gating mechanism for seizure propagation, and possibly for brain excitability in general. According to this view, the outputs of the nigral would modulate the excitability of both rostral and caudal brain regions that participate in seizure development. Inhibition or destruction of nigral outputs would not actually interrupt the progression of seizure activity, but rather would dampen the responsiveness of the entire circuitry responsible for sustaining the propagated seizure.

SUMMARY AND CONCLUSIONS

By enhancing GABA transmission in anatomically restricted areas of the brain from the pontine level forward, we have been able to localize GABA-mediated anticonvulsant effects to the SN in rats. Moreover, the ability of GABA elevation to protect against maximal electroshock seizures appears to be exclusively associated with actions in SN, as marked elevations of GABA in all other brain regions examined were without significant effect in this seizure model.

Enhancement of GABA transmission in SN, either as a consequence of GABA transaminase inhibition (following GVG) or the direct stimulation of GABA receptors by muscimol, is also effective in attenuating seizures induced by bicuculline and PTZ (40), amygdala kindling (53,61), flurothyl (70), and audiogenic seizures during ethanol withdrawal (23,33a). In general, these anticonvulsant effects require *bilateral* nigral GABA receptor stimulation and appear to result from a reduction in sensitivity to the seizure stimulus, rather than from impairment of the rat's ability to manifest any specific motor component of the seizure. In the presence of enhanced nigral GABA transmission, a higher dose of chemoconvulsant or a more intense electrical stimulus is required to reinstate a normal seizure profile.

By comparing drug-induced changes in nigral GABA content in the presence and absence of GABAergic nerve terminals, we have been able to evaluate the relative effectiveness of a variety of drug treatments for elevating GABA in nigral nerve terminals. Our analysis revealed that protection against experimentally induced generalized seizures in rats is directly correlated with the ability of a GABA-elevating treatment to increase GABA associated specifically with nigral nerve terminals. This relationship extends across drug treatments (AOAA, GVG, DPA), across time for a given drug treatment, and across routes of drug administration (systemic versus intracerebral). Systemic injection of DPA and intranigral application of GVG were the treatments we found to be most effective for elevating GABA in nigral nerve terminals (by 39 and 60%, respectively) and were also the treatments that provided 100% protection against MES seizures. Conversely, large elevations of nigral GABA in non-nerve-terminal compartments (e.g., GABAergic perikarya) unaccompanied by significant increases in nerve terminal GABA, are not predictive of seizure protection.

Based on our studies with GABAergic agents in SN, we have proposed the following working model: GABA afferents to SN inhibit efferent neurons that normally permit or facilitate the generalization of maximal seizures. This proposal is supported by the fact that bilateral lesions of SN, which destroy nigral efferent cells, are also anticonvulsant. As with GABA agonists, nigral lesions caused a shift to the right in the dose–effect curve for chemoconvulsant seizures.

The nigral outputs that influence seizure sensitivity appear to be subject to the influence of other transmitters in addition to GABA (Table 7). Our data suggest that these outputs can be inhibited by opiates, which exert anticonvulsant actions in SN that are similar but not identical to those obtained with GABA agonists. SP, on the other hand, may provide an excitatory drive on the seizure-facilitating nigral efferents, based on our observation that antagonist analogues of this peptide have anticonvulsant actions when applied to the SN.

Although the precise relationship of the SN to seizure propagating circuits remains to be defined, we do not view the nigra as a necessary relay through which convulsive activity must propagate. It is more likely that the SN sends projections to other structures that are an integral part of the circuitry involved in sustaining generalized seizures. Any of several pathways may participate in this scheme. Because neither dopamine agonists nor antagonists produced significant anticonvulsant actions in the tests that we have used, it is unlikely that the anticonvulsant effects we have observed are mediated by nigrostriatal dopamine neurons. It is more likely that the diverse efferent (GABAergic) projections from pars reticulata are the critical linkages for controlling seizure propagation. In this case, inhibition of nigral efferent output (much of which is also inhibitory) to thalamus, tectum, and reticular formation could modulate the progression of seizure discharge through these systems. Because stimulation of nigral efferents does not generate convulsions, the SN is not a site for *initiation* of seizures. Rather, it appears that seizure activity generated elsewhere in the brain is amplified or sustained by activity in nigral efferents. Thus, the nigral outputs may act as a gating mechanism: the bilateral suppression of their activity causing a decrease in susceptibility to generalized seizures, regardless of the mechanism of seizure initiation.

It is tempting to speculate that a loss of inhibitory tone in SN (or conversely, augmentation of excitatory transmission at this site) might enhance the probability of obtaining generalized seizures. Although a decrease in GABAergic transmission in SN would not generate seizures, it could be responsible for facilitating the generalization of seizure activity emanating from more rostral loci. Thus, the SN must be considered as a possible site at which pathology could alter the susceptibility to generalized convulsions. Perhaps the appearance of overt clinical seizures depends upon both an epileptogenic focus (e.g., in forebrain) as well as a compromised inhibitory control mechanism at critical synapses in SN.

REFERENCES

1. Ackerman, R. F., Moshe, S. L., Albala, B. J., Engel, J. Jr. (1982): Anatomical substrates of amygdala kindling in immature rats demonstrated by 2-deoxyglucose autoradiography. *Epilepsia,* 23:494–495.
2. Albala, B. J., Moshe, S. L., and Okada, R. (1984): Kainic acid induced seizures: A developmental study. *Develop. Brain Res.,* 13:139–148.
3. Anlezark, G., Horton, R. W., Meldrum, B. S., and Sawaya, M. C. W. (1976): Anticonvulsant action of ethanolamine-*o*-sulphate and di-*n*-pro-

pylacetate and the metabolism of gamma-aminobutyric acid (GABA) in mice with audiogenic seizures. *Biochem. Pharmacol.*, 25:413–417.

4. Barber, R., and Saito, K. (1976): Light microscopic visualization of GAD and GABA-T in immunocytochemical preparations of rodent CNS. In: *GABA in Nervous System Function*, edited by E. Roberts, T. N. Chase, and D. B. Tower, p. 113. Raven Press, New York.

5. Baxter, C. F., and Roberts, E. (1959): Elevation of gamma-aminobutyric acid in rat brain with hydroxylamine. *Proc. Soc. Exp. Biol. Med.*, 101:811–815.

6. Baxter, C. F., and Roberts, E. (1960): Demonstration of thiosemicarbazide-induced convulsions in rats with elevated brain levels of gamma-aminobutyric acid. *Proc. Soc. Exp. Biol. Med.*, 104:426–427.

7. Beart, P. M., Kelly, J. S., and Schon, F. (1974): Gamma-aminobutyric acid in the rat peripheral nervous system, pineal and posterior pituitary. *Biochem. Soc. Trans.*, 2:266–268.

8. Bell, J. A., and Anderson, E. G. (1974): Dissociation between amino-oxyacetic acid-induced depression of spinal reflexes and the rise in cord GABA levels. *Neuropharmacology*, 13:885–894.

9. Ben Ari, Y., Tremblay, E., Riche, D., Ghilini, G., and Naquet, R. (1981): Electrographic clinical and pathological alterations following systemic administration of kainic acid, bicuculline or pentetrazole: Metabolic mapping using the deoxyglucose method with special reference to the pathology of epilepsy. *Neuroscience*, 6:1361–1391.

10. Buckett, W. R. (1981): Intravenous bicuculline test in mice: Characterization with GABA drugs. *J. Pharmacol. Methods*, 5:35–41.

11. Casu, M., and Gale, K. (1981): Intracerebral injection of gamma-vinyl-GABA: Method for measuring rates of GABA synthesis in specific brain regions *in vivo*. *Life Sci.*, 29:681–688.

12. Childs, J. A., and Gale, K. (1983): Neurochemical evidence for a nigrotegmental GABA-ergic projection. *Brain Res.*, 258:109–114.

13. DiChiara, G., Porceddu, M. L., Morelli, M., Mulas, M. L., and Gessa, G. L. (1979): Evidence for a GABAergic projection from the substantia nigra to the ventromedial thalamus and to the superior colliculus of the rat. *Brain Res.*, 176:273–284.

14. Da Vanzo, J. P., Greig, M. E., and Cronin, M. A. (1961): Anticonvulsant properties of amino-oxyacetic acid. *Am. J. Physiol.*, 201:833–837.

15. Eidelberg, E., Baxter, C. F., Roberts, E., and Saldias, C. A. (1960): *Inhibition in the Nervous System and Gamma-Aminobutyric Acid*, edited by E. Roberts, C. F. Baxter, A. Van Harreveld, C. A. G. Wiersma, R. Adey, and K. F. Killam, pp. 365–370. Pergamon Press, New York.

16. Emson, P. C., and Joseph, M. H. (1975): Neurochemical and morphological changes during the development of cobalt-induced epilepsy in the rat. *Brain Res.*, 93:91–110.

17. Engel, J., Wolfson, L., and Brown, L. (1978): Anatomical correlates of electrical and behavioral events related to amygdaloid kindling. *Ann. Neurol.*, 3:538–544.

18. Faeth, W. H., Walker, A. E., and Andy, O. J. (1954): The propagation of cortical and subcortical epileptic discharge. *Epilepsia*, 3:37–48.

19. Fariello, R. G., and Hornykiewicz, O. (1979): Substantia nigra and pentylenetetrazol threshold in rats: Correlation with striatal dopamine metabolism. *Exp. Neurol.*, 65:202–208.

20. Foote, F., and Gale, K. (1983): Morphine potentiates seizures induced by GABA antagonists and attenuates seizures induced by electroshock in the rat. *Eur. J. Pharmacol.*, 95:259–264.

21. Foote, F., and Gale, K. (1984): Proconvulsant effect of morphine on seizures induced by pentylenetetrazol in the rat. *Eur. J. Pharmacol.*, 105:179–184.

22. Fowler, L. J., Beckford, J., and John, R. A. (1975): An analysis of the kinetics of the inhibition of rabbit brain gamma-aminobutyrate aminotransferase by sodium *n*-dipropylacetate and some other simple carboxylic acids. *Biochem. Pharm.*, 24:1267–1270.

23. Fry, G. D., McCown, T. J., and Breese, G. R. (1983): Characterization of susceptibility to audiogenic seizures in ethanol-dependent rats after microinjection of GABA agonists into the inferior colliculus, substantia nigra or medial septum. *J. Pharmacol. Exp. Ther.*, 227:663–670.

23a. Gale, K., and Casu, M. (1981): Dynamic utilization of GABA in substantia nigra: Regulation by dopamine and GABA in striatum, and its clinical and behavioral implications. *Mol. Cell. Biochem.*, 39:369–405.

24. Gale, K., Moroni, F., Kumakura, K., Guidotti, A. (1979): Opiate receptors in substantia nigra: Role in the regulation of striatal tyrosine hydroxylase activity. *Neuropharmacology*, 18:427–430.

25. Gale, K., and Iadarola, M. J. (1980): GABAergic denervation of rat substantia nigra: Functional and pharmacological properties. *Brain Res.*, 183:217–223.

26. Gale, K., and Iadarola, M. J. (1980): Seizure protection and increased nerve terminal GABA: Delayed effects of GABA transaminase inhibition. *Science*, 208:288–291.

27. Gale, K., and Iadarola, M. J. (1980): Drug-induced elevation of GABA after intracerebral microinjection: Site of anticonvulsant action. *Eur. J. Pharmacol.*, 68:233–235.

28. Gale, K., Sarvey, C., Stork, J., Childs, J. A., Yalisove, B. L., and Dayhoff, R. E. (1984): Quantitative histochemical measurement of GABA-transaminase: Method for evaluation of intracerebral lesions produced by excitotoxic agents. *Brain Res.*, 307:255–262.

29. Garant, D. S., and Gale, K. (1985): Infusion of opiates into substantia nigra protects against maximal electroshock seizures in rats. *J. Pharmacol Exp. Therap.*, 234:45–48.

30. Garant, D. S., Iadarola, M. J., and Gale, K. (1982): Pharmacologic manipulation of peptide-mediated transmission in rat substantia nigra: Anticonvulsant effects. *Soc. Neurosci. Abstr.*, 281:2.

31. Garant, D. S., and Gale, K. (1983): Lesions of substantia nigra protect against experimentally induced seizures. *Brain Res.*, 273:156–161.

32. Gibbs, F. A., and Gibbs, E. L. (1936): The convulsion threshold of various parts of the cat's brain. *Arch. Neurol. Psychiatry*, 35:109–116.

33. Gloor, P. (1968): Generalized corticoreticular epilepsies. Some considerations on the pathophys-

iology of generalized bilaterally synchronous spike and wave discharge. *Epilepsia (Amst)*, 9:249–263.

33a. Gonzalez, L. P., and Hettinger, M. K. (1984): Intranigral muscinol suppresses ethanol withdrawal seizures. *Brain Res.*, 298:163–166.

34. Gottesfeld, Z., Kelly, J. S., and Renaud, L. P. (1972): The *in vivo* neuropharmacology of aminooxyacetic acid in the cerebral cortex of the cat. *Brain Res.*, 42:319–335.

35. Grace, A. A., and Bunney, B. S. (1979): Paradoxical GABA excitation of nigral dopaminergic cells: Indirect mediation through reticulata inhibitory neurons. *Eur. J. Pharmacol.*, 59:211–218.

36. Hayashi, T. (1953): A physiological study of epileptic seizures following cortical stimulation in animals and its application to human clinics. *Jpn. J. Physiol.*, 3:46, 306.

37. Hayashi, T. (1959): The inhibitory action of β-hydroxy-gamma-aminobutyric acid upon the seizure following stimulation of the motor cortex of the dog. *J. Physiol.*, 145:570–578.

38. Heath, R. G. (1976): Brain function in epilepsy: Midbrain, medullary, and cerebellar interaction with the rostral forebrain. *J. Neurol. Neurosurg. Psychiatry*, 39:1037–1051.

39. Iadarola, M. J., and Gale, K. (1979): Dissociation between drug-induced increase in nerve terminal and non-nerve terminal pools of GABA *in vivo*. *Eur. J. Pharmacol.*, 59:125–129.

40. Iadarola, M. J., and Gale, K. (1982): Substantia nigra: Site of anticonvulsant activity mediated by gamma-aminobutyric acid. *Science*, 218:1237–1240.

41. Iadarola, M. J., and Gale, K. (1980): Evaluation of increases in nerve terminal-dependent vs. nerve terminal-independent compartments of GABA *in vivo*. *Brain Res. Bull.* (Suppl. 2), 5:13–19.

42. Iadarola, M. J., Raines, A., and Gale, K. (1979): Differential effects of *n*-dipropyl-acetate and amino-oxyacetic acid on gamma-aminobutyric acid levels in discrete areas of rat brain. *J. Neurochem.*, 33:1119–1123.

43. Iwamoto, E. T., and Way, E. L. (1977): Circling behavior and stereotypy induced by intranigral opiate microinjections. *J. Pharmacol. Exp. Ther.*, 203:347–359.

44. Jinnai, D., Yoshida, T., Souji, T., and Kosaka, F. (1954): Experimental studies on the march of spasm during epileptic convulsion. *Acta Med. Okayama*, 8:26.

45. Kalichman, M. W., Burnham, W. M., and Livingston, K. E. (1982): Pharmacological investigation of gamma-aminobutyric acid (GABA) and fully developed generalized seizures in the amygdala-kindled rat. *Neuropharmacology*, 21:127–131.

46. Kanazawa, I., Iversen, L. L., and Kelly, J. S. (1976): Glutamate decarboxylase activity in pituitary and pineal glands, dorsal root ganglion and superior cervical ganglion. *J. Neurochem.*, 27:1267–1269.

46a. Keating, R. F., and Gale, K. (1981): Depletion of GABA and seizures produced by isoniazid after irreversible inhibition of GABA-transaminase. *Soc. Neurosci.*, 7:337.

47. Kendall, D. A., Fox, D. A., and Enna, S. J. (1981): Effect of gamma-vinyl GABA on bicu-culline-induced seizures. *Neuropharmacology*, 20:351–355.

48. Killam, K. F., and Bain, J. A. (1957): Convulsant hydrazides I: *In vitro* and *in vivo* inhibition of vitamin B_6 enzymes by convulsant hydrazides. *J. Pharmacol. Exp. Therap.*, 119:255–262.

49. Kilpatrick, I. C., Starr, M. S., Fletcher, A., James, T. A., and MacLeod, N. K. (1980): Evidence for a GABAergic nigrothalamic pathway in the rat. I. Behavioral and biochemical studies. *Exp. Brain Res.*, 40:45–54.

50. Kreindler, A., Zukermann, E., Steriade, M., and Chimion, D. (1958): Electroclinical features of convulsions induced by stimulation of brain stem. *J. Neurophysiol.*, 21:430–436.

51. Krnjevic, K., and Schwartz, S. (1968): The inhibitory transmitter in the cerebral cortex. In: *Structure and Function of Inhibitory Neural Mechanisms*, edited by C. Von Euler, and S. Skoglund, p. 419. Pergamon Press, New York.

52. Kuriyama, K. (1976): Subcellular localization of the GABA system in brain. In: *GABA in Nervous System Function*, edited by E. Roberts, T. N. Chase, and D. B. Tower, p. 187. Raven Press, New York.

53. Le Gal La Salle, G., Kijima, M., and Feldblum, S. (1983): Abortive amygdaloid kindled seizures following microinjection of gamma-vinyl-GABA in the vicinity of substantia nigra in rats. *Neurosci. Lett.*, 36:69–74.

54. Le Gal La Salle, G., and Feldblum, S. (1983): Role of the amygdala in development of hippocampal kindling in the rat. *Exp. Neurol.*, 82:447–455.

55. Lippert, B., Metcalf, B. W., Jung, M. J., and Casara, P. (1977): 4-Amino-hex-5-enoic acid, a selective catalytic inhibitor of 4-aminobutyric acid aminotransferase in mammalian brain. *Eur. J. Biochem.*, 74:441–445.

56. Loscher, W. (1980): Effect of inhibitors of GABA transaminase on the synthesis, binding, uptake and metabolism of GABA. *J. Neurochem.*, 34:1603–1608.

57. Loscher, W. (1981): A comparative study of the pharmacology of inhibitors of GABA-metabolism. *Naunyn Schmiedebergs Arch. Pharmacol.*, 315:119–128.

58. Loscher, W., and Frey, H. H. (1978): Amino-oxyacetic acid: Correlation between biochemical effects, anticonvulsant action and toxicity in mice. *Biochem. Pharmacol.*, 27:103–108.

59. Loscher, W., and Frey, H. H. (1977): Effect of convulsant and anticonvulsant agents on level and metabolism of gamma-aminobutyric acid in mouse brain. *Naunyn Schmiedebergs Arch. Pharmacol.*, 296:263–269.

60. MacLeod, N. K., James, T. A., Kilpatrick, I. C., and Starr, M. S. (1980): Evidence for a GABAergic nigrothalamic pathway in the rat. Electrophysiological studies. *Exp. Brain Res.*, 40:55–61.

61. MacNamara, J. O., Rigsbee, L. C., and Galloway, M. T. (1983): Evidence that substantia nigra is crucial to the neural network of kindled seizures. *Eur. J. Pharmacol.*, 86:485–486.

62. Maynert, E. W., and Kaji, H. K. (1962): On the relationship of brain gamma-aminobutyric acid to convulsions. *J. Pharmacol. Exp. Ther.*, 137:114–121.

63. Meldrum, B. S. (1975): Epilepsy and gamma-aminobutyric acid-mediated inhibition. In: *International Review of Neurobiology,* edited by C. C. Pfeiffer, and J. R. Smythies, p. 1. Academic Press, New York.

64. Meldrum, B. S., and Horton, R. (1978): Blockade of epileptic responses in the photosensitive baboon, *Papio papio,* by two irreversible inhibitors of GABA-transaminase, gamma-acetylenic GABA (4-amino-hex-5-enoic acid) and gamma-vinyl GABA (4-amino-hex-5-enoic acid). *Psychopharmacology,* 59:47–50.

65. Melis, M. R., and Gale, K. (1984): Evidence that nigral substance P controls the activity of the nigrotectal GABAergic pathway. *Brain Res.,* 295:389–293.

66. Melis, M. R., and Gale, K. (1984): Intranigral application of substance P antagonists prevents the haloperidol-induced activation of striatal tyrosine hydroxylase. *Naunyn Schmiedebergs Arch. Pharmacol.,* 326:83–86.

67. Melis, M. R., and Gale, K. (1983): Effect of dopamine agonists on GABA turnover in the superior colliculus: Evidence that nigrotectal GABAergic projections are under the influence of dopaminergic transmission. *J. Pharmacol. Exp. Ther.,* 226:425–431.

68. Metcalf, B. W. (1979): Inhibitors of GABA metabolism. *Biochem. Pharmacol.,* 28:1705–1712.

69. Minchin, M. C. W., and Beart, P. M. (1975): Compartmentation of amino acid metabolism in the rat dorsal root ganglion; a metabolic and autoradiographic study. *Brain Res.,* 83:437–449.

70. Moshe, S. L., and Albala, B. J. (1984): Nigral muscimol infusions facilitate the development of seizures in immature rats. *Dev. Brain Res.,* 13:305–308.

71. Olianas, M. C., DeMontis, G. M., Concu, A., Tagliamonte, A., and DiChiara, G. (1978): The striatal dopaminergic function is mediated by the inhibition of a nigral, non-dopaminergic neuronal system via a strionigral GABAergic pathway. *Eur. J. Pharmacol.,* 49:223–232.

71a. Pazdernik, P. L., Cross, R. S., Giesler, M., Samson, F. E., and Nelson, S. R. (1985): Changes in local cerebral glucose utilization induced by convulsants. *Neuroscience,* 14:823–825.

72. Rando, R. R. (1974): Chemistry and enzymology of Kcat inhibitors. *Science,* 185:320–324.

73. Ribak, C. E., Harris, A. B., Vaughn, J. E., and Roberts, E. (1979): Inhibitory, GABAergic nerve terminals decrease at sites of focal epilepsy. *Science,* 205:211–214.

74. Roa, D. P., Tews, J. K., and Stone, W. E. (1964): A neurochemical study of thiosemicarbazide seizures and their inhibition by amino-oxyacetic acid. *Biochem. Pharmacol.,* 13:477–487.

75. Roberts, E., Wein, J., and Simonsen, D. G. (1964): Gamma-aminobutyric acid (GABA), vitamin B6, and neuronal function—A speculative synthesis. *Vitam. Horm.,* 22:503–559.

76. Sarhan, S., and Seiler, N. (1979): Metabolic inhibitors and subcellular distribution of GABA. *J. Neurosci. Res.,* 4:399–421.

77. Schechter, P. J., Tranier, Y., Jung, M. J., and Bohlen, P. (1977): Audiogenic seizure protection by elevated brain GABA concentration in mice: Effect of gamma-acetylenic GABA and gamma-vinyl GABA, two irreversible GABA-T inhibitors. *Eur. J. Pharmacol.,* 45:319–328.

78. Schechter, P. J., and Tranier, Y. (1978): The pharmacology of enzyme-activated inhibitors of GABA-transaminase. In: *Enzyme-Activated Irreversible Inhibitors,* edited by N. Seiler, M. J. Jung, and J. Koch-Weser, p. 149. Elsevier/North-Holland.

79. Simler, S., Ciesielski, L., Maitre, M., Randrianarisoa, H., and Mandel, P. (1973): Effect of sodium *n*-dipropylacetate on audiogenic seizures and brain gamma-aminobutyric acid level. *Biochem. Pharmacol.,* 22:1701–1708.

80. Tower, D. B. (1976): GABA and seizures: Clinical correlates in man. In: *GABA in Nervous System Function,* edited by E. Roberts, T. N. Chase, and D. B. Tower, p. 461. Raven Press, New York.

81. van Gelder, N. M., and Elliott, K. A. C. (1958): Disposition of gamma-aminobutyric acid administered to mammals. *J. Neurochem.,* 3:139–143.

82. van Gelder, N. M., Sherwin, A. L., and Rasmussen, T. (1972): Amino acid content of epileptogenic human brain: Focal versus surrounding regions. *Brain Res.,* 40:385–393.

83. van Gelder, N. M., and Courtois, A. (1972): Close correlation between changing content of specific amino acids in epileptogenic cortex of cats, and severity of epilepsy. *Brain Res.,* 43:477–484.

84. Vincent, S. R., Hattori, T., and McGeer, E. G. (1978): The nigrotectal projection: A biochemical and ultrastructural characterization. *Brain Res.,* 151:159–164.

85. Vincent, S. R., Lehmann, J., and McGeer, E. G. (1980): The localization of GABA-transaminase in the striatonigral system. *Life Sci.,* 127:595–601.

86. Waniewski, R. A., and Suria, A. (1977): Alterations in gamma-aminobutyric acid content in the rat superior cervical ganglion and pineal gland. *Life Sci.,* 21:1129–1142.

87. Waszczak, B., Eng, N., and Walters, J. R. (1980): Effects of muscimol and picrotoxin on single unit activity of substantia nigra neurons. *Brain Res.,* 188:185–197.

88. Wood, J. D., Durham, J. S., and Peesker, S. J. (1977): Effect of di-*n*-propylacetate and gamma-acetylenic GABA on hyperbaric oxygen-induced seizures and GABA metabolism. *Neurochem. Res.,* 2:707–715.

89. Wood, J. D., Kurylo, E., and Newstead, J. D. (1978): Aminooxyacetic acid induced changes in gamma-aminobutyrate metabolism at the subcellular level. *Can. J. Biochem.,* 56:667–676.

90. Note added in proof: We have recently located a discrete site in the rat deep prepiriform cortex from which bilateral clonic seizures can be initiated with pmol amounts of the GABA antagonist bicuculline. Piredda, S., and Gale, K. (1985): A crucial epileptogenic site in the deep prepiform cortex. *Nature,* 317:623–625.

91. Note added in proof: In fact, an excitatory amino acid antagonist has recently been reported to exert anticonvulsant effects after microinjection into substantia nigra. De Sarro, G., Meldrum, B. S., and Reavill, C. (1985): Anticonvulsant action of 2-amino-7-phosphonoheptanoic acid in the substantia nigra. *J. Pharmacol.,* 106:175–179.

Advances in Neurology, Vol. 44, edited by
A. V. Delgado-Escueta, A. A. Ward, Jr.,
D. M. Woodbury, and R. J. Porter.
Raven Press, New York © 1986.

17

Benzodiazepine/Barbiturate/GABA Receptor–Chloride Ionophore Complex in a Genetic Model for Generalized Epilepsy

*R. W. Olsen, **J. K. Wamsley, *R. J. Lee, and *P. Lomax

*Department of Pharmacology, School of Medicine, and Brain Research Institute, University of California, Los Angeles, California 90024; and **Department of Psychiatry, University of Utah School of Medicine, Salt Lake City, Utah 84132*

SUMMARY   The inhibitory neurotransmitter γ-aminobutyric acid (GABA) acts through postsynaptic receptor sites which regulate membrane chloride ion channels. The GABA receptor–ionophore complex also contains modulatory receptor sites for two classes of centrally acting drugs, one for the benzodiazepines, and a second for both barbiturates and related depressants and for picrotoxin and related convulsants. The presence of these drug modulatory sites, directly on the GABA receptor protein, is consistent with other experimental observations; blocking GABA function can cause seizures, and augmenting GABA function can afford protection against seizures. This, and other circumstantial evidence, has suggested the possibility that a functional GABA deficit may be involved in some kinds of human epilepsy. Some neurochemical markers for GABA synapses have been reported to be altered in certain animal models as well as in human temporal lobe epilepsy. We have examined the postsynaptic GABA receptor complex using receptor binding assays for GABA, benzodiazepine (BZ), and barbiturate receptor sites in the seizure-susceptible gerbil, a genetic model of generalized epilepsy. A 30% deficit in BZ receptor binding was observed in the midbrain of seizure-sensitive animals relative to normal controls. This was shown by quantitative brain-slice binding autoradiography to involve a decrease in the number of binding sites in the substantia nigra (SN) and periaqueductal gray regions. A deficit in membrane receptors for BZs (which are linked to a subtype of postsynaptic GABA receptors) in a crucial region of brain might therefore contribute to seizure susceptibility in some kinds of epilepsy.

GABA RECEPTOR–IONOPHORE COMPLEX

Radioactive ligand binding to brain membrane homogenates allows *in vitro* assay of receptor sites for neurotransmitters and drugs. Specific receptor binding sites for GABA have been defined on the basis of tissue and subcellular localization, ligand affinity, and pharmacological specificity (16,26,27,33,58,100). In particular, sensitivity to the agonist muscimol and the antagonist bicuculline defines the GABA receptors (sometimes called type "A") which are coupled to chloride channels and modulated by barbiturates and benzodiazepines (BZs) (20,51,53).

High-affinity BZ binding sites in brain have been found to show a specificity for a series of BZs and related drugs consistent with their activity as anticonvulsants, anxiolytics, sedatives, and muscle relaxants (10,46,78,86). The discovery of "valium receptors" has touched off an explosion of research in the hope of utilizing this tool to gain new insights into normal and abnormal brain function.

The convulsant natural product picrotoxin has also been shown to have specific binding sites in brain membranes related to its action as an antagonist of GABA-activated chloride channels at a site distinct from the GABA recognition site. These sites are assayed with a radioactive analog [³H]α-dihydropicrotoxinin ([³H]DHP) (53, 55,93) or a related cage convulsant compound [³⁵S]t-butyl bicyclophosphorothionate [³⁵S](TBPS) (32,69,80). Picrotoxin binding sites are inhibited by convulsant picrotoxin analogs, cage convulsants, the convulsant BZ Ro5-3663, benzyl penicillin, bemegride, and pentylenetetrazol (PTZ), all of which can block GABA responses at the cellular level; [³H]DHP binding sites are also inhibited by certain depressant drugs, including barbiturates, the anxiolytic pyrazolopyridines, and some others, all of which can potentiate GABA responses at the cellular level (52–54,69,80,90–92). [³H]DHP binding sites are also inhibited by high concentrations of depressant BZs (52–55), a finding of possible relevance to the toxicity of these drugs.

These three classes of drug binding sites all appear to be closely coupled in a single protein complex (Fig. 1). Reciprocal allosteric interactions between the three receptor classes have been observed in membranes as well as in detergent-solubilized extracts (51,53,61,62,90). A modulation of binding and site–site interactions by chloride and other anions capable of permeating GABA-regulated chloride channels suggests that the chloride channel is likely to be a part of this receptor complex as well (13,51,79).

Table 1 summarizes the allosteric interactions between the various components of the "donut model" shown in Fig. 1. That GABA and BZ receptors are tightly coupled was shown by observations that GABA receptor ligands protect BZ receptor sites from heat inactivation (79), that GABA receptor ligands (agonists) enhance BZ binding (31,86) and possibly vice versa (28,96), and that GABA and BZ binding sites reside on the same partially purified macromolecule (3,25,75,82). There is no convincing evidence that any of the brain BZ binding sites are not associated with GABA receptors (53). However, only a subpopulation of bicuculline-sensitive GABA receptors seem to be coupled to BZ receptors as described in Fig. 1. The GABA receptors in this category seem to have a low af-

finity for GABA agonists, but can be assayed with the radioactive antagonist [³H]bicuculline methochloride (57,59).

A direct link between the convulsant/barbiturate sites and the BZ/GABA receptors was provided by the observation that the anxiolytic pyrazolopyridine compounds like etazolate (SQ 20009) enhanced, rather than inhibited, BZ receptor binding, and that this allosteric effect was inhibited by picrotoxin and was chloride-dependent (84). We observed that picrotoxin not only reversed the etazolate enhancement of BZ receptor binding at concentrations similar to those inhibiting radioactive [³H]DHP binding, but that etazolate and related compounds inhibited [³H]DHP binding at concentrations similar to those effective in enhancing BZ binding (38,55). Furthermore, other depressants which act like etazolate in inhibiting [³H]DHP binding, such as barbiturates, also showed a chloride-dependent, picrotoxin-sensitive enhancement of BZ binding owing to an increased affinity (37,55). This observation was quickly confirmed by several groups (2,77,89).

The barbiturate modulation was chemically specific, was blocked by picrotoxin and related GABA-antagonist convulsants which bind to [³H]DHP sites, and was absolutely dependent on the presence of physiological concentrations of chloride or other anions that are capable of carrying inhibitory currents in GABA-sensitive neurons (37). Furthermore, it was allosterically blocked by the GABA antagonist bicuculline (38,89). The same barbiturates and pyrazolopyridines were able to inhibit allosterically (by lowering the affinity) the binding of BZ receptor "inverse agonists" (excitatory ligands) such as [³H]β-carboline-3-carboxylate methyl ester (62,98).

Likewise, the observation of a chloride-dependence for barbiturate–BZ interactions led to the discovery that pyrazolopyridines and barbiturates enhanced GABA receptor binding in a chloride-dependent and picrotoxin-sensitive manner (2,56,61,67,85,87,95,96). Again, the same compounds inhibited allosterically the binding of the GABA receptor antagonist [³H]bicuculline methochloride (62,98). The action of barbiturates on GABA receptor binding involves an *apparent* increase in the *number* of high- and intermediate-affinity binding sites, which we interpret as an actual increase in *affinity* for low-affinity sites that normally are not detected, or are detected with difficulty, by radioactive agonists (56,61), but which can be assayed with [³H]bicuculline methochloride (57,59,98).

Most important, barbiturate interactions with

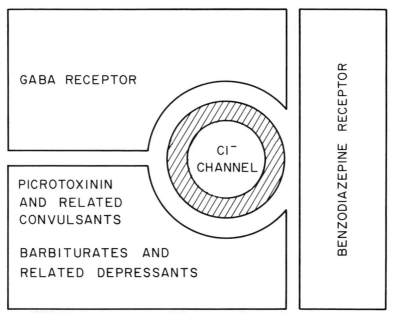

FIG. 1. Theoretical model of the GABA receptor–ionophore complex. The complex is envisioned as containing three drug receptor sites: the GABA receptor, the benzodiazepine receptor, and the picrotoxinin/barbiturate receptor. Associated with, or part of, these receptors is the chloride ion channel, the opening of which is regulated by GABA agonists binding to the GABA receptor. The activity of the chloride ion channel may also be modulated in a positive manner (depressant drugs) to potentiate the chloride ion permeability (and inhibition in the central nervous system) (CNS), or in a negative manner (excitatory agents) to block the chloride ion channel (and block CNS inhibition). Modulatory agents may be exogenous or endogenous substances. The presence of all these receptor–ionophore components in all GABA receptor systems in every part of the brain is not "obligatory," and some of the components may also exist in an uncoupled state. From Olsen, ref. 51, with permission.

the GABA/BZ receptor complex show a chemical specificity and stereospecificity (dimethylbutyl barbituric acid (DMBB) > secobarbital > (−)pentobarbital = (−)mephobarbital > (+)hexobarbital = (+)pentobarbital = amobarbital > (−)N^1-methyl, 5-phenyl, 5-propyl barbituric acid (MPPB) > cyclohexylidene-ethyl barbituric acid (CHEB) = (−)hexobarbital = phenobarbital = (+)mephobarbital > metharbital = (+)MPPB (36,37,53–55), which corre-

TABLE 1. *BZ and barbiturate receptors are associated with the postsynaptic GABA receptor–chloride ion channel complex*

1. GABA receptor agonists enhance BZ receptor binding and allosterically inhibit antagonist binding *in vitro* (and vice versa?).
2. Barbiturates and pyrazolopyridines enhance BZ receptor binding and inhibit inverse agonist binding *in vitro* in a stereospecific, chloride-dependent, and picrotoxinin-sensitive manner. These interactions are also allosterically inhibited by GABA receptor antagonists.
3. Barbiturates and pyrazolopyridines in a similar manner enhance GABA receptor agonist binding and allosterically inhibit antagonist binding.
4. Picrotoxinin-like convulsants allosterically modulate BZ and GABA receptor binding, and vice versa.
5. BZ binding sites throughout the brain are enhanced by GABA and pentobarbital; BZ binding sites and low-affinity GABA sites (bicuculline binding but not muscimol binding to high-affinity sites) show an indistinguishable brain regional distribution.
6. The reciprocal interactions between the three drug receptors in the complex persist in a partially purified detergent-solubilized protein species.
7. Anticonvulsant barbiturates and nonbarbiturates interact with the GABA/BZ receptor complex in a manner somewhat different from the sedative/hypnotic analogs.

BZ, benzodiazepine.

late well with the ability of these agents to reverse GABA antagonist action and with the enhancement of GABA agonist postsynaptic responses (8,63,83,97). A reasonably good correlation with anesthetic/hypnotic potency was obtained (36,37,53), and, while some of the effective agents are used as sedatives, anticonvulsants, and anxiolytics, and while some of them have *additional* excitatory activities, all of the drugs that enhance GABA/BZ receptor binding *in vitro* have been found to enhance GABA responses at the cellular or tissue level (7,8,21,29,49,63,74,76,83,97). All of these agents inhibit, at similar concentrations, the binding of [^{3}H]DHP and [^{35}S]TBPS to brain membranes (32,53–55,69). The ability of these barbiturates to enhance the affinity of GABA and BZ binding sites would be consistent with observations that these drugs prolong the lifetime of chloride channels activated by GABA receptor agonists (83). Thus, a barbiturate receptor site has been defined on the GABA receptor–ionophore complex.

The intimate relationship of the three-receptor complex for GABA, barbiturates, and BZs has been further demonstrated by the solubilization in mild detergent of a macromolecular species which retains the reciprocal chloride-dependent allosteric interactions at the three sites and which can be purified several hundred-fold by chromatographic procedures in which the various binding activities comigrate (61,62,75,81). This complex has a MW estimated at 215,000–355,000 in solutions of the detergent Triton X-100 and contains a 55,000 MW subunit photoaffinity labeled with [^{3}H]flunitrazepam, as well as one to three additional subunits (62,75,82). Purification of the GABA receptor complex will allow the application of the powerful tools of modern molecular biology to the analysis of a possible role for this protein in seizure disorders of a genetic origin.

DO MODULATORY SITES FOR BZs AND BARBITURATES ON THE GABA RECEPTOR–IONOPHORE COMPLEX MEDIATE ANTICONVULSANT ACTIVITY?

It is highly probable that [^{3}H]DHP and [^{35}S]TBPS binding sites on the GABA receptor–ionophore complex are involved in the convulsant actions of picrotoxin-like compounds and the cage convulsants (9,53–55,80,90), acting as antagonists of GABA postsynaptic inhibitory chloride channels. There are no other significant proposed mechanisms of action or receptors for

these agents. This site also appears to mediate the convulsant activity of PTZ (68) and bemegride (90).

Similarly, the interaction of depressant drugs with these convulsant receptor sites appears to reflect their ability to potentiate GABA function at the postsynaptic membrane level (discussed above). The most potent substances in this category are the anxiolytic pyrazolopyridines (such as etazolate) and etomidate (38,84,87,96), and those barbiturates that are most effective as anesthetics, hypnotics, and sedatives (3,36,37,77,89,95,96,98). The active compounds are also anticonvulsant, but those used clinically as anticonvulsants, such as phenobarbital and the nonbarbiturate chlormethiazole, not only are weaker inhibitors of convulsant binding sites but they do not enhance equilibrium BZ and GABA receptor binding (36,39,54). However, these anticonvulsants at high but still relevant concentrations (0.2–0.3 mM) decrease allosterically the *rates* of association and dissociation of BZ and GABA receptor binding (36). Unlike the more potent barbiturates, like pentobarbital, the modulation of on- and off-rates by phenobarbital balances out, with no resulting change in equilibrium constant such as is seen with pentobarbital (36). Because phenobarbital acts at the same picrotoxin-sensitive site as pentobarbital, phenobarbital or chlormethiazole in excess is able to prevent the enhancement of BZ binding by compounds such as pentobarbital (36,39,54). Other barbiturates such as hexobarbital appear to produce an enhancement similar to pentobarbital, but with a lower maximal effect. Thus, this *in vitro* receptor interaction of barbiturates appears to show variable efficacy (36) reminiscent of the partial agonist phenomenon seen in more physiological responses to drugs.

Several other anticonvulsants at 0.2–2 mM also block pentobarbital enhancement of benzodiazepine binding; these include metharbital, diphenylhydantoin, ethosuximide, primidone, trimethadione, and carbamazepine, but not sodium valproate (52,54). Table 2 lists the CNS depressant compounds with potential anticonvulsant activity that have been reported to have *some* interaction with the GABA receptor system (we do not comment on the validity of the claims). Included in the list is ethanol which, like pentobarbital, enhances BZ binding and inhibits picrotoxin binding under certain conditions (52,90). Ethanol withdrawal seizures respond well to the anticonvulsant activity of the BZs (11).

Nevertheless, it cannot be stated that *in vivo antiepileptic* action of any of these drugs is owing to their interaction with GABA receptor binding or the enhancement of GABA function. It is difficult to assign unambiguously a receptor site for these drugs, partly because of their low potency and partly because they have several other actions on the nerve membrane at almost the same concentrations (see Chapter 36).

The case of the BZs is not nearly so ambiguous. The GABA-linked high-affinity BZ receptor sites are generally believed to mediate the anticonvulsant as well as other pharmacological actions of these drugs. Consistent with the effectiveness of the BZs against some types of human seizure disorders (11) and in a variety of animal models (73), the occupancy of high-affinity BZ receptors in brain correlates highly with potency of protection against several types of drug-induced seizures, such as those induced by PTZ (10,19,45,66). It is important to note that the effective concentrations for binding *in vivo* (about 1 μM) are in agreement with therapeutic tissue levels and higher than the artificially low concentrations (1–10 nM) required for binding *to the same sites* seen under nonphysiological *in vitro* conditions such as 0°C (10,19,66), even though the anticonvulsant activity of the BZs apparently requires only a small percentage of occupancy of brain receptor sites (10,19,66). The correlation between binding potency and protection against electroshock seizures was not as good, but it could be argued that electroshock seizures involve a less specific hyperexcitability of numerous brain regions. Nevertheless, high-affinity BZ receptors are probably involved in all these animal tests, since antagonists for the

binding sites such as Ro15-1788 are able to reverse the anticonvulsant actions (10,73). Another link to the GABA system is provided by the observation that the anticonvulsant BZs decrease the rate of GABA turnover in brain; this, too, is reversed by the BZ receptor antagonists (73), showing that the high affinity receptors are involved.

GABA HYPOTHESIS OF SEIZURE DISORDERS

If, as we have just argued, drugs that augment GABA-mediated inhibition are active as anticonvulsants, and if this mechanism applies to at least some agents used in the clinical treatment of epilepsy, it follows that a functional GABA deficit might be responsible for some forms of epilepsy. This possibility is supported by considerations of the pharmacology of other convulsant and anticonvulsant drugs which can be related to GABA. Seizures can result from a block of the biosynthesis of GABA, a block of synaptic release of GABA, or a block of the postsynaptic response to GABA, at the level of the GABA receptor sites, the associated chloride channel, or at the modulatory drug sites for BZs or barbiturates/picrotoxin (52,54). Convulsants acting at all these sites, including certain β-carboline ligands for the BZ receptors (10,14), have been described.

Enhancement of GABA function can be effective in protecting against some types of seizure, not only at the postsynaptic modulatory drug sites, but also at the receptors, using GABA

TABLE 2. In vitro *interactions of CNS depressant agents with the GABA/BZ receptor–ionophore complex*

Agent	Interaction
Benzodiazepines	GABA receptor via BZ receptor
Barbiturates	GABA and BZ receptors via barbiturate/picrotoxinin site
Phenytoin	BZ receptor? B/P site?
Valproate	None (B/P site?)
Chlormethiazole	BZ receptor via B/P site
Carbamazepine	BZ receptor? B/P site?
Ethosuximide	BZ receptor? B/P site?
Trimethadione	BZ receptor via B/P site?
Ethanol	BZ receptor via B/P site
Meprobamate	B/P site?
Methaqualone	B/P site?
Etazolate	GABA and BZ receptors via B/P site
Etomidate	GABA and BZ receptors via B/P site

BZ, benzodiazepine; B/P = barbiturate/picrotoxinin
From Olsen, ref. 52; Squires et al. ref. 80; Stephenson et al., ref. 84; Tallman et al., ref. 86; and Ticku and Maksay, ref. 90, with permission.

mimicking agents (agonists or pro-drugs). Likewise, anticonvulsant activity has been observed for blockers of GABA uptake into cells, and for the well-known inhibitors (such as γ-vinyl GABA) of the GABA catabolic enzyme, GABA transaminase (52). Most of the GABA agonists and uptake inhibitors do not readily cross the blood–brain barrier, but this problem has been solved, at least partially, with hydrophobic and nonmetabolizable analogs (48). Although the clinical usefulness of these agents is still under investigation, it is clear that several examples of all these categories of GABA-enhancing agents have anticonvulsant activity.

Table 3 summarizes the five major points supporting a possible role of GABA in seizure disorders. The largely circumstantial evidence does actually demonstrate true impairment of GABA function in any type of human epilepsy, or even in any animal model. However, there are reports of altered GABA synaptic markers in some types of seizure disorders. GABA levels were found to be low in the cerebrospinal fluid (CSF) of patients with certain types of epilepsy, but they were also low in many other neurological conditions (99). Decreased GABA levels could *not* be correlated in general with hyperexcitable brain regions (94). However, in experimental epilepsy induced by alumina cream in the monkey, electron microscopy revealed a decrease in the levels of the GABA synthetic enzyme, L-glutamic acid decarboxylase (GAD), by immunocytochemistry, as well as a decrease in the density of synapses of symmetric morphology which are associated with GAD-positive nerve endings (70). The same animals showed lower levels of GABA, GAD, and GABA receptor binding in homogenates of the lesioned tissue, and lowered levels of GABA in CSF in the subarachnoid space on the lesioned side only (6). Other neurotransmitter receptor binding sites were also diminished in the lesioned epileptic tissue, but the decrease in GABA receptor binding was more substantial (6). A similar decrease in GAD was observed in epileptic foci produced by cobalt in rat brain (71). This study also reported a small *increase*

in GABA receptor binding in the same area, perhaps a result of denervation supersensitivity (71). In a preliminary study of human temporal lobe epilepsy, surgically removed focal tissue identified by stereo-EEG was found to contain lower GAD activity than nonfocal tissue from the same individual (40) (see Chapter 52). Further, a subset of these surgical biopsy samples showed *lower* GABA receptor binding in the foci than in nonfocal regions; the levels of the GABA catabolic enzyme, GABA-transaminase, and another receptor marker, kainic acid binding, were not altered (40). These studies suggest the possibility of impaired GABA synaptic function in some types of epilepsy.

In other animal models, GABA receptor binding was reported by two groups to be lower in a mouse strain (DBA/2J) that is susceptible to audiogenic seizures, as compared with other nonsusceptible strains (C57 B1/6 or T0). Ticku (88) found lower GABA binding, especially to high-affinity sites, in some brain regions of adult DBA/2 mice. However, the animals at that age do not show seizure susceptibility; such susceptibility is limited to 21–28 days of age. Horton et al. (30) also observed a decrease in high-affinity but not in low-affinity GABA binding in several brain regions, especially the pons/medulla of DBA/2J mice, at various ages including the susceptible times. The GABA-related benzodiazepine receptors were found lower in certain brain regions of the genetically epilepsy-prone rats (22).

BZ receptor binding (B_{max}) was shown to increase transiently in rat hippocampus following chemically or electrically induced seizures, the effect lasting only for several minutes (65). A transient increase in BZ receptor binding (affinity) was reported for Mongolian gerbils following seizures induced by unusual (but mild) handling of the animals (1). Repeated seizures induced by electroshock or kindling resulted in an increase in the number of BZ receptor sites in the dentate granule cell layer of rat hippocampus, assayed 24 hr after the last seizure (44) (see Chapter 14). The same group also observed a decrease in hippocampal muscarinic acetyl-

TABLE 3. *Role of gamma-aminobutyric acid in seizure disorders*

1. Seizures result from impaired GABA function (synthesis, release, receptor–ionophore action).
2. Seizure protection results from enhanced GABA function (agonists, uptake blockers, degradation blockers, indirect potentiators).
3. Some anticonvulsants potentiate GABA function.
4. The GABA postsynaptic membrane receptor–ionophore protein complex contains drug receptor sites for the benzodiazepines and for the barbiturates and picrotoxinin.
5. GABA synapses are altered in some types of epilepsy.

choline (ACh) receptors (18) and an increase in glutamate binding sites (72). Electrical kindling in the amygdala also produced a long-lasting *decrease* of 20% (assayed at 14 days) in the number of BZ binding sites in the ipsilateral cortex and hypothalamus (50). Electroshock seizures in pregnant rats resulted in decreased BZ receptor binding in brain membranes of pups assayed postnatally (24), and neonatal febrile seizures resulted in an altered BZ receptor binding curve assayed in the adult (12). In a related study, kindling of seizures could be produced by norharman, an excitatory β-carboline ligand of the BZ receptors (47). These studies suggest that BZ receptor deficits in certain brain regions could contribute to hyperexcitability, and that increased BZ receptor binding might be involved in a postictal increase of seizure threshold and/or a compensatory increase in inhibitory mechanisms. Our studies on a genetic model, the seizure-sensitive gerbil, also show a deficit in BZ receptors and therefore a possible functional GABA deficit.

SEIZURE-SUSCEPTIBLE GERBIL AS A GENETIC MODEL OF GENERALIZED EPILEPSY

The Mongolian gerbil *Meriones unguiculatus* shows a natural tendency to have generalized seizures in response to simple but novel sensory stimuli, such as being placed in a strange cage

(43). The seizures have been graded on a scale of increasing severity from 0 to 6. Animals with grade 4–5 seizures have been inbred at UCLA to produce a genetic strain with reproducible seizure susceptibility (SS). Animals with no seizures (grade 0) are maintained as seizure-resistant (SR) controls. The seizures develop at 50–80 days of age and are present throughout life (43).

The gerbil represents by various criteria a genetic model for generalized epilepsy in the human. Electrophysiological recordings show an involvement of parietal and sensorimotor cortex in the seizures, and in some cases a possible focus was recognizable (42). SS has been correlated with low brain dopamine levels in these gerbils (15). In addition, the parietal cortex and thalamus of SS animals had lower GABA levels than SR (15). However, a twofold *increase* in GAD-positive neurons and terminals was seen in the septal half of the hippocampus of SS as compared with SR gerbils (see Chapter 37). An abnormally low level of dendritic spines in the hippocampus of SS gerbils was seen in adult gerbils of >100 days of age (64), but this difference from SR was not present in younger animals, even at ages after seizures had developed (see Chapter 39). The number of hippocampal neuronal cell bodies was also shown to be diminished in seizing gerbils and the extent of the deficit was related to the severity of seizures [Grades 1–5, (17)]. Gerbil seizures have been

TABLE 4. *GABA receptor binding in homogenized membranes of SS and SR gerbils*[a]

Brain Region	[³H]GABA binding (pmol/g wet tissue)	
	SS (preseizure)	SR
Brain stem	2.3 ± 1.5[b]	4.7 ± 2.0
Cerebellum	32.8 ± 10	31.4 ± 11
Cortex	7.9 ± 2.5	8.2 ± 1.4
Rest of brain	2.7 ± 1.3	3.1 ± 1.0
Rest of brain	2.4 ± 0.9	2.4 ± 0.3
	[³H]Muscimol Binding	
	SS (post seizure)	SR
Pons/medulla	0.32 ± 0.05	0.34 ± 0.08
Cerebellum	5.74 ± 0.82	5.72 ± 1.2
Cortex	2.07 ± 0.48	2.0 ± 0.37
Thalamus/midbrain	0.60 ± 0.17	0.56 ± 0.13

SS, seizure susceptible; SR, seizure resistant.

[a] All values are means ± SD of six animals in triplicate. Dissected brain regions were frozen in 0.32 M sucrose and stored for up to 7 days. The tissue was thawed and homogenized and membranes prepared as previously described (56,58), with freeze-thawing and multiple washings. The binding of [³H]GABA (4 nM, 50 Ci/mmol) or [³H]muscimol (1 nM, 20 Ci/mmol) was measured by centrifugation, following 20-min equilibration at 0°C in 10 mM potassium phosphate, 50 mM KCl, pH 7.5. Background was estimated with 0.1 mM GABA. SS gerbils were sacrificed 60 sec after a seizure (postseizure) or after at least 2 hr without visible seizures (preseizure).

[b] $p < 0.1$ vs. SR.

TABLE 5. *Benzodiazepine receptor binding in homogenized membranes of SS and SR gerbils*

| Brain region | [³H]Diazepam binding (pmol/g tissue)[a] | | |
	SS (preseizure)	SR	Difference (%)
Preseizure			
Pons/medulla (6)	2.91 ± 0.81	3.18 ± 0.70	—
Cerebellum (6)	5.17 ± 0.59	5.83 ± 1.44	—
Cortex (6)	7.66 ± 1.56	8.38 ± 1.47	—
Thalamus/midbrain (6)	3.95 ± 0.61	5.31 ± 0.50	−26[b]
Hippocampus (6)	14.24 ± 2.96	16.80 ± 5.24	−15
Hippocampus (6)	11.98 ± 2.0	12.50 ± 4.36	—
Striatum (6)	12.90 ± 2.95	13.50 ± 4.67	—
Thalamus (6)	3.46 ± 0.72	3.65 ± 0.56	—
Rostral midbrain (6)	0.88 ± 0.2	1.08 ± 0.3	−23
Caudal midbrain (6)	1.08 ± 0.24	1.56 ± 0.51	−45[b]
Postseizure (N = 6)			
Pons/medulla	2.94 ± 0.84	3.84 ± 0.76	−28
Cerebellum	4.12 ± 0.54	3.94 ± 0.54	—
Cortex	9.88 ± 4.4	9.82 ± 1.8	—
Thalamus/midbrain	5.98 ± 1.28	5.28 ± 0.46	+12
Hippocampus	15.06 ± 3.52	14.38 ± 2.16	—
Striatum	13.86 ± 4.48	16.94 ± 3.22	−22
Preseizure	[³H]Flunitrazepam binding[c]		
Midbrain (3 animals pooled, 7 points)			
B_{max} (pmol/g tissue)	60	64	
K_D (nM)	2.3	2.3	
Linear coefficient	0.97	0.91	

SS, seizure susceptible; SR, seizure resistant.

[a] All values are the mean ± SD for the number of animals listed in parentheses, in triplicate. Brain regions were frozen in 0.32 M sucrose for up to 7 days, thawed, and homogenized. Washed membranes were prepared and assayed as previously described (38), with 1 μM clonazepam to estimate background. [³H]Diazepam (1 nM, 76.8 Ci/mmol) or [³H]flunitrazepam binding (0.25–20 nM, 86 Ci/mmol) were assayed by filtration following 60-min incubation at 0°C in 10 mM sodium phosphate, 0.2 M NaCl, pH 7.0. Preseizure and postseizure SS and SR are defined in Table 4.

[b] $p < 0.01$, Student's t-test. The other differences were not significant at 95% levels.

[c] Binding parameters were computed from linear regression Scatchard plots.

found to respond to the usual antiepileptic drugs used for generalized seizures (diphenylhydan-toin, phenobarbital) (42,43). A recent study on gerbils from the general population revealed that many of the animals could be induced to seize by a blast of air. These seizures were uniquely sensitive to GABA-augmenting anticonvulsants and BZs (41). Gerbil seizures have also been found to be altered by endogenous neuropep-tides (see Chapter 25). The seizures were blocked by ACTH, arginine vasopressin (34), β-endorphin (4), and opioid agonists (35), whereas thyrotropin releasing hormone (TRH) (5) increased SS.

The current study examines levels of BZ/GABA receptors in brain regions of the SS gerbil. Radioactive ligand binding to both membrane homogenates and to unfixed cryostat sections have been used to determine the density and distribution of receptors.

Gerbil brains were divided into four regions (brainstem, cerebellum, cortex, and "the rest of the brain") for GABA receptor binding assays. Six animals in each category (SS and SR) were not identified by the experimentalist until after completion of the assays. Membrane homogenates were assayed for [³H]GABA binding and barbiturate enhancement (by 1 mM pentobarbital) and the results are shown in Table 4. It should be noted that under these assay conditions a mixture of high- and low-affinity GABA receptor sites, primarily high-affinity sites, are measured (58). No significant difference in GABA binding or barbiturate enhancement was observed for cortex, cerebellum, and "rest of brain" regions between SS and SR gerbils. A marginal deficit in SS pons/medulla was observed (50%, $p < 0.1$). This region shows high variability owing to low receptor density. The SS animals were killed at a time when they had not had recent visible seizures. Another set of animals was compared, this time using

[³H]muscimol binding to assay GABA receptors, and killing the SS animals within 5 min after the onset of their seizure. No differences from SR were observed in any of the four areas, including the pons/medulla.

BZ receptors were assayed on these same animals. In this case, the brains were divided into seven areas, and the washed membranes were assayed, without further freezing and thawing, on the same day as the frozen tissue was thawed out and homogenized. Table 5 shows the [³H]diazepam binding at one ligand concentration to membranes from SS and SR gerbils. Although no significant difference was seen in the cerebellum, cortex, striatum, and pons/medulla, *lower* binding was observed in SS gerbil hippocampus (15%, not significant) and in the thalamus/midbrain region (26%, $p < 0.01$). Similar results were obtained if the data were calculated in terms of pmol bound per milligram of membrane protein (60).

Another set of animals was examined in hippocampus and in the thalamus/midbrain, divided into three parts. There was no difference in hippocampus; however, there was lower binding in SS thalamus (5%, not significant); rostral midbrain (23%, not significant) and caudal midbrain/colliculus (45%, $p < 0.05$). However, a Scatchard plot of [³H]flunitrazepam binding to total midbrain, pooled from three animals in each category for seven ligand concentration points, revealed no significant difference between SS and SR in either K_D (2.3 nM) or number of sites B_{max} (60 and 64 pmol/per gram of wet tissue, respectively).

Another set of animals was assayed with SS gerbils killed 5 min after a seizure. In these animals, no deficit in SS thalamus/midbrain was observed (SS binding was 12% higher, not significant). The SS gerbils did have lower binding in striatum (22%, not significant), and pons/medulla (28%, $p < 0.1$). Thus, there is a trend toward lower BZ and GABA receptor binding in brainstem of SS gerbils.

Because small differences in receptor binding of a discrete brain region could be diluted by a large volume of normal tissue in these grossly dissected samples, the method of brain-slice autoradiography (59) was used to provide finer localization of the density and distribution of BZ receptor binding sites in the gerbils, concentrating on the mesencephalon (60). [³H]-Flunitrazepam binding to slide-mounted sections is shown in an example in Fig. 2, and data from numerous sections are summarized in Table 6. These data confirm the differences in BZ receptor binding in SS and SR gerbil mid-

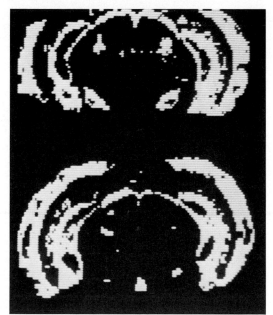

FIG. 2. Autoradiography of benzodiazepine (BZ) receptor binding in the gerbil. Cryostat sections of gerbil midbrain were labeled with [³H]flunitrazepam using conditions known to result in specific labeling of BZ receptors. Autoradiograms were generated on LKB Ultrofilm, and the film grain density was measured with a Leitz Orthoplan microscope and an MPV microphotometer interfaced with a DADS model 560 computer as described in Table 6. The grain density (and therefore BZ receptors) is shown in gray. **Upper trace:** a seizure-resistant animal; **lower trace:** a seizure-susceptible animal. Note the decreased density in the lower scan in regions corresponding to the substantia nigra and periaqueductal gray, and the increased density in the interpeduncular nucleus.

brain, showing a 20% *deficit* in autoradiographic grain density in the substantia nigra (SN) and a 12% *deficit* in the periaqueductal gray region of preseizure SS gerbils. No difference was seen in examined areas of retrosplenial cortex, hippocampus, and superior colliculus, and 19% *higher* binding was seen in the SS interpeduncular nucleus. Postseizure SS gerbils showed a significant increase in binding as compared with preseizure SS in several areas (SN, interpeduncular nucleus, and retrosplenial cortex). The postseizure gerbils still had significantly lower binding than SR in the nigra and periaqueductal gray. The increase in binding following a seizure may explain the lack of a difference in homogenate binding (Table 5) between *postseizure* SS and SR gerbils in thalamus/midbrain. It may also be related to the literature reports of similar increases in BZ binding observed following seizures in rats (44,65) and gerbils (1). It should be noted that

TABLE 6. *Benzodiazepine receptor binding in brain slices of gerbils using autoradiography*[a]

Brain region	SS (preseizure)	SS (postseizure)	SR
Retrosplenial cortex	64.8 ± 3.8	72.3 ± 1.3^b	66.0 ± 1.2
Hippocampus	74.0 ± 1.4	73.3 ± 1.7	75.9 ± 2.1
Periaqueductal gray	64.4 ± 0.7^c	65.5 ± 2.6	73.4 ± 1.0
Superior colliculus	75.4 ± 2.0	75.1 ± 1.5	78.1 ± 2.4
Interpeduncular nucleus	63.6 ± 3.4^c	68.8 ± 2.4^b	53.3 ± 2.5
Substantia nigra	59.3 ± 3.6^c	63.8 ± 0.6^b	74.5 ± 0.6
Substantia nigra[d]			
B_{max} (pmol/g tissue)	143^c		183
K_D (nM)	7.04		7.12
Linear coefficient	0.98		0.95

SS, seizure susceptible; SR, seizure resistant.

[a] Slide-mounted tissue sections (10 μm) were incubated with [³H]flunitrazepam (1 nM, 86 Ci/mmol) for 60 min at 0°C in 0.17 M Tris-HCl, pH 7.4. Background nondisplaceable binding was determined with 1 μM clonazepam. The rinsed and dried slides were apposed to ³H-sensitive LKB Ultrofilm for 14 days at 4°C. Autoradiographic grain densities on the developed films were measured as percentage of transmission by an MPV compact microphotometry system using a Leitz Orthoplan microscope, interfaced with a DADS 560 computer. The numbers represent the mean ± SEM of three separate experiments with 12 different readings taken in the indicated brain area (250 μm²) of five animals per category.

[b] $p < 0.05$ vs preseizure SS.

[c] $p < 0.05$ vs SR.

[d] Binding in pmol/g tissue was measured by comparing the percentage of transmission in the tissue autoradiograms (minus that in the background) to a standard curve generated from sections of brain paste containing ³H standards in the same autoradiograms. Seven concentrations of [³H]flunitrazepam (0.1–10 nM) were used to generate a Scatchard plot for specific binding in the substantia nigra pars reticulata of one animal in each group.

increases in available endogenous GABA in the samples, which can enhance BZ binding (10,31,51,86), might contribute to increased BZ binding in samples which have not been thoroughly washed (26).

Figure 2 shows a computer printout of BZ receptor binding autoradiographic density in a frontal section through the midbrain of a SR and preseizure SS gerbil, demonstrating the lower binding in SS SN and periaqueductal gray regions. Quantitative analysis of the densities over the SN pars reticulata measured on 250-μm² sections was made for seven concentrations of radioactive ligand and compared with a standard curve for sections of brain paste containing [³H]flunitrazepam. A Scatchard plot of these data (Table 6) revealed a significant 22% decrease in the number of binding sites (143 versus 183 pmol/per gram of tissue in the case examined) for SS SN as compared with SR SN, with no change in binding affinity ($K_D = 7$ nM for both).

Thus, the number of BZ receptors and presumably low-affinity GABA receptors is low in mesencephalic areas of the SS gerbil. This deficit in the SN and periaqueductal gray area could result from a decrease in the number of GABA-receptive neurons in these regions or from a deficit in the number of receptor proteins per cell. In either event, a deficit in GABA-mediated in-

hibition is implied that could contribute to seizure susceptibility in these gerbils. This would be consistent with the efficacy of GABA-augmenting anticonvulsants (41). Current studies are examining the developmental time-course of this receptor difference with respect to the age of onset of seizures, the relationship to severity of seizures, and the receptor densities on other regions, including thalamus, midbrain, pons/medulla, and hippocampus. Low-affinity GABA receptors are being analyzed directly with a new ligand, [³H]bicuculline methochloride (57,59). It would also be of interest to study GABAergic inputs to these regions as well as the projections of the GABA-receptive neurons affected.

The role of the midbrain periaqueductal gray in SS is not known, but could play a role in the pathological response to sensory stimuli in the gerbils. The SN could be involved in the circuitry leading to the motor expression of the seizures. However, this structure has been found to be quite important in controlling seizures of several kinds, induced by electroshock, convulsant drugs, or by kindling (see Chapters 14 and 16). GABA-augmenting anticonvulsants injected into several brain regions are most effective in the SN; the action of GABA-augmenting anticonvulsants applied systemically can be correlated to the increase in nigral nerve-ending pools of GABA; GABA-mimicking agents are anticonvulsant when injected into the SN but not nearby; and lesions of the SN reduce motor and limbic seizures (23). Thus, a deficit of GABA/BZ receptor function in this area could contribute to SS. The observation of lower receptor binding in the gerbil genetic epilepsy model would be consistent with the GABA hypothesis, and increasing evidence for alterations in GABA-mediated inhibitory synaptic transmission in some kinds of epilepsy seems to be an important clue which might help us to understand the basic mechanisms of human epilepsy.

ACKNOWLEDGMENTS

We thank A. M. Snowman for technical assistance. This work was supported by a PMAF Fellowship (to R. J. L.) and National Institutes of Health contract No. N01-NS-0-2332.

REFERENCES

1. Asano, T., and Mizutani, A. (1980): Brain benzodiazepine receptors and their rapid changes after seizures in the Mongolian gerbil. *Jpn. J. Pharmacol.*, 30:783–788.
2. Asano, T., and Ogasawara, N. (1981): Chloride-dependent stimulation of GABA and benzodiazepine receptor binding by pentobarbital. *Brain Res.*, 225:212–216.
3. Asano, T., Yamada, Y., and Ogasawara, N. (1983): Characterization of the solubilized GABA and benzodiazepine receptors from various regions of bovine brain. *J. Neurochem.*, 40:209–214.
4. Bajorek, J. G., and Lomax, P. (1982): Modulation of spontaneous seizures in the Mongolian gerbil: effects of β-endorphin. *Peptides*, 3:83–86.
5. Bajorek, J. G., Lee, R., and Lomax, P. (1981): Thyrotropin releasing hormone (TRH) increases seizure susceptibility and arousal behaviors in the Mongolian gerbil. *Soc. Neurosci. Abstr.*, 7:813.
6. Bakay, R. A. E., and Harris, A. B. (1981): Neurotransmitter, receptor and biochemical changes in monkey cortical epileptic foci. *Brain Res.*, 206:387–404.
7. Barnes, D. M., White, W. F., and Dichter, M. A. (1983): Etazolate (SQ 20009): Electrophysiology and effects on [³H]flunitrazepam binding in cultured cortical neurons. *J. Neurosci.*, 3:762–772.
8. Bowery, N. G., and Dray, A. (1978): Reversal of the action of amino acid antagonists by barbiturates and other hypnotic drugs. *Br. J. Pharmacol.*, 63:179–215.
9. Bowery, N. G., Collins, J. F., and Hill, R. G. (1976): Bicyclic phosphorus esters that are potent convulsants and GABA antagonists. *Nature*, 261:601–603.
10. Braestrup, C., Schmeichen, R., Nielsen, M.,

and Petersen, E. N. (1982): Benzodiazepine receptor ligands, receptor occupancy, pharmacological effect and GABA receptor coupling. In: *Pharmacology of Benzodiazepines,* edited by E. Usdin, P. Skolnick, J. F. Tallman, D. Greenblatt, and S. M. Paul, pp. 71–85. Macmillan Press, London.
11. Browne, T. R. (1983): Benzodiazepines. In: *Epilepsy: Diagnosis and Management,* edited by T. R. Browne and R. G. Feldman, pp. 235–245. Little, Brown and Co., Boston.
12. Chisholm, J., Kellogg, C., and Franck, J. E. (1985): Developmental hyperthermic seizures alter hippocampal benzodiazepine binding and morphology. *Epilepsia,* 26:151–157.
13. Costa, T., Rodbard, D., and Pert, C. B. (1979): Is the benzodiazepine receptor coupled to a chloride anion channel? *Nature,* 277:315–317.
14. Cowen, P. J., Green, A. T., Nutt, D. J., and Martin, I. L. (1981): Ethyl β-carboline-3-carboxylate lowers seizure threshold and antagonizes flurazepam-induced sedation in rats. *Nature,* 290:54–55.
15. Cox, B., and Lomax, P. (1976): Brain amines and spontaneous epileptic seizures in the Mongolian gerbil. *Pharmacol. Biochem. Behav.,* 4:263–267.
16. Coyle, J. T., and Enna, S. J. (1976): Neurochemical aspects of the ontogenesis of GABAnergic neurons in the rat brain. *Brain Res.,* 111:119–133.
17. Dam, A. M., Bajorek, J. G., and Lomax, P. (1981): Hippocampal neuron density and seizures in the Mongolian gerbil. *Epilepsia,* 22:667–674.
18. Dashieff, R. M., Savage, D. D., and McNamara, J. O. (1982): Seizures down-regulate muscarinic cholinergic receptors in hippocampal formation. *Brain Res.,* 235:327–334.
19. Duka, T., Hollt, V., and Herz, A. (1979): In vivo receptor occupation by benzodiazepines and correlation with the pharmacological effect in mouse. *Brain Res.,* 179:147–156.
20. Enna, S. J., editor (1983): *The GABA Receptors.* Humana Press, Clifton, New Jersey.
21. Evans, R. H. (1979): Potentiation of the effects of GABA by pentobarbitone. *Brain Res.,* 171:113–120.
22. Franck, J. E., Hjeresen, D. L., Baskin, D. G., Jobe, P. C., and Schwartzkroin, P. A. (1985): Genetically epilepsy-prone rats show a deficit and developmental decline in medical geniculate benzodiazepine receptors. *Abstr. Soc. Neurosci.,* 11:1320.
23. Gale, K. (1984): The role of the substantia nigra in the anticonvulsant actions of GABAergic drugs. In: *Neurotransmitters, Seizures, & Epilepsy,* vol. 2, edited by R. G. Fariello, J. Engel, Jr., P. L. Morselli, and L. F. Quesney, pp. 57–79. Raven Press, New York.
24. Gallager, D. W., and Wakeman, E. A. (1982): Prenatal exposure to electroconvulsive seizures and phenytoin: Development of benzodiazepine binding sites, reflex behaviors, and seizure thresholds in exposed offspring. *Eur. J. Pharmacol.,* 85:143–153.

25. Gavish, M., and Snyder, S. H. (1981): γ-Aminobutyric acid and benzodiazepine receptors: Copurification and characterization. *Proc. Natl. Acad. Sci. USA*, 78:1939–1942.

26. Greenlee, D. V., Van Ness, P. C., and Olsen, R. W. (1978): Endogenous inhibitor of GABA binding in mammalian brain. *Life Sci.*, 22:1653–1662.

27. Greenlee, D. V., Van Ness, P. C., and Olsen, R. W. (1978): Gamma-aminobutyric acid binding in mammalian brain: Receptor-like specificity of sodium independent sites. *J. Neurochem.*, 31:933–938.

28. Guidotti, A., Corda, M. G., Wise, B. C., Vaccarino, F., and Costa, E. (1983): GABAergic synapses. Supramolecular organization and biochemical regulation. *Neuropharmacology*, 22:1471–1479.

29. Haefely, W., and Polc, P. (1983): Electrophysiological studies on the interaction of anxiolytic drugs with GABAergic mechanisms. In: *Anxiolytics: Neurochemical, Behavioral, and Clinical Perspectives*, edited by J. B. Malick, S. J. Enna, and H. I. Yamamura, pp. 113–145. Raven Press, New York.

30. Horton, R. W., Prestwich, S. A., and Meldrum, B. S. (1982): γ-Aminobutyric acid and benzodiazepine binding sites in audiogenic seizure-susceptible mice. *J. Neurochem.*, 39:864–870.

31. Karobath, M., Placheta, P., Lippitsch, M., and Krogsgaard-Larsen, P. (1979): Is stimulation of benzodiazepine receptor binding mediated by a novel GABA receptor? *Nature*, 278:748–749.

32. King, R. G., and Olsen, R. W. (1984): Solubilization of convulsant/barbiturate binding activity on the GABA/benzodiazepine receptor complex. *Biochem. Biophys. Res. Commun.*, 119:530–536.

33. Krogsgaard-Larsen, P., Hjeds, H., Curtis, D. R., Lodge, D., and Johnston, G. A. R. (1979): Dihydromuscimol, thiomuscimol and related heterocyclic compounds as GABA analogues. *J. Neurochem.*, 32:1717–1724.

34. Lee, R. J., and Lomax, P. (1983): Thermoregulatory, behavioral and seizure modulatory effects of AVP in the gerbil. *Peptides*, 4:801–805.

35. Lee, R. J., Bajorek, J. G., and Lomax, P. (1984): Similar anticonvulsant, but unique behavioral effects of opioid agonists in the seizure-sensitive Mongolian gerbil. *Neuropharmacology*, 23:517–524.

36. Leeb-Lundberg, F., and Olsen, R. W. (1982): Interactions of barbiturates of various pharmacological categories with benzodiazepine receptors. *Mol. Pharmacol.*, 21:320–328.

37. Leeb-Lundberg, F., Snowman, A., and Olsen, R. W. (1980): Barbiturate receptors are coupled to benzodiazepine receptors. *Proc. Natl. Acad. Sci. USA*, 77:7468–7472.

38. Leeb-Lundberg, F., Snowman, A., and Olsen, R. W. (1981): Perturbation of benzodiazepine receptor binding by pyrazolopyridines involves picrotoxinin/barbiturate receptor sites. *J. Neurosci.*, 1:471–477.

39. Leeb-Lundberg, F., Snowman, A., and Olsen, R. W. (1981): Interaction of anticonvulsants with the barbiturate/benzodiazepine/GABA receptor complex. *Eur. J. Pharmacol.*, 72:125–129.

40. Lloyd, K. G., Munari, C., Bossi, L., Stoeffels, C., Talairach, J., and Morselli, P. L. (1981): Biochemical evidence for the alterations of GABA-mediated synaptic transmission in pathological brain tissue (stereo EEG or morphological definition) from epileptic patients. In: *Neurotransmitters, Seizures, & Epilepsy*, edited by P. L. Morselli, K. G. Lloyd, W. Löscher, B. Meldrum, and E. H. Reynolds, pp. 325–338. Raven Press, New York.

41. Löscher, W. (1984): Evidence for abnormal sensitivity of the GABA system in gerbils with genetically determined epilepsy. In: *Neurotransmitters, Seizures, & Epilepsy*, vol. 2, edited by R. G. Fariello, J. Engel, Jr., P. L. Morselli, and L. F. Quesney, pp. 179–188. Raven Press, New York.

42. Loskota, W. J., and Lomax, P. (1975): The Mongolian gerbil (*Meriones unguiculatus*) as a model for the study of the epilepsies: EEG records of seizures. *Electroencephalogr. and Clin. Neurophysiol.*, 38:597–604.

43. Loskota, W. J., Lomax, P., and Rich, S. T. (1974): The gerbil as model for the study of the epilepsies. *Epilepsia*, 15:109–119.

44. McNamara, J. O., Peper, A. M., and Patrone, V. (1980): Repeated seizures induce long-term increase in hippocampal benzodiazepine receptors. *Proc. Natl. Acad. Sci. USA*, 77:3029–3032.

45. Möhler, H., and Okada, T. (1977): Benzodiazepine receptors: Demonstration in the central nervous system. *Science*, 198:849–851.

46. Möhler, H., and Richards, J. G. (1983): Receptors for anxiolytic drugs. In: *Anxiolytics: Neurochemical, Behavioral, and Clinical Perspectives*, edited by J. B. Malick, S. J. Enna, and H. I. Yamamura, pp. 15–40. Raven Press, New York.

47. Morin, A. M., Watson, A. L., and Wasterlain, C. G. (1983): Kindling of seizures with norharman, a β-carboline ligand of benzodiazepine receptors. *Eur. J. Pharmacol.*, 88:131–134.

48. Morselli, P. L., Lloyd, K. G., Löscher, W., Meldrum, B., and Reynolds, E. H., editors (1981): *Neurotransmitters, Seizures, & Epilepsy*. Raven Press, New York.

49. Nicoll, R. A., and Wojtowicz, J. M. (1980): The effects of pentobarbital and related compounds on frog motoneurons. *Brain Res.*, 191:225–237.

50. Niznik, H. B., Kish, S. J., and Burnham, W. M. (1983): Decreased benzodiazepine receptor binding in amygdala-kindled rat brains. *Life Sci.*, 33:425–430.

51. Olsen, R. W. (1981): GABA-benzodiazepine-barbiturate receptor interactions. *J. Neurochem.*, 37:1–13.

52. Olsen, R. W. (1981): The GABA postsynaptic membrane receptor-ionophore complex: Site of action of convulsant and anticonvulsant drugs. *Mol. Cell. Biochem.*, 39:261–279.

53. Olsen, R. W. (1982): Drug interactions at the GABA receptor ionophore complex. *Annu. Rev. Pharmacol. Toxicol.*, 22:245–277.

54. Olsen, R. W., and Leeb-Lundberg, F. (1981): Convulsant and anticonvulsant drug binding sites related to the GABA receptor/ionophore system. In: *Neurotransmitters, Seizures, & Epilepsy*, edited by P. L. Morselli, K. G. Lloyd, W. Löscher, B. S. Meldrum, and E. H. Reynolds, pp. 151–163. Raven Press, New York.

55. Olsen, R. W., and Leeb-Lundberg, F. (1981): Convulsant and anticonvulsant drug binding sites related to GABA-regulated chloride ion channels. In: *GABA and Benzodiazepine Receptors, Advances in Biochemistry and Psychopharmacology*, vol 26, edited by E. Costa, G. DiChiara, and G. L. Gessa, pp. 93–102. Raven Press, New York.

56. Olsen, R. W., and Snowman, A. M. (1982): Chloride-dependent enhancement by barbiturates of GABA receptor binding. *J. Neurosci.*, 2:1812–1823.

57. Olsen, R. W., and Snowman, A. M. (1983): [³H]Bicuculline methochloride binding to low affinity GABA receptor sites. *J. Neurochem.*, 41:1653–1663.

58. Olsen, R. W., Bergman, M. O., Van Ness, P. C., Lummis, S. C., Watkins, A. E., Napias, C., and Greenlee, D. V. (1981): γ-Aminobutyric acid receptor binding in mammalian brain: Heterogeneity of binding sites. *Mol. Pharmacol.*, 19:217–227.

59. Olsen, R. W., Snowhill, E. W., and Wamsley, J. K. (1984): Autoradiographic localization of low affinity GABA receptors with [³H]bicuculline methochloride. *Eur. J. Pharmacol.*, 99:247–248.

60. Olsen, R. W., Wamsley, J. K., Lee, R., and Lomax, P. (1984): Alterations in the benzodiazepine/GABA receptor–chloride ion channel complex in the seizure-sensitive gerbil. In: *Neurotransmitters, Seizures, & Epilepsy*, vol. 2, edited by R. G. Fariello, J. Engel, Jr., P. L. Morselli, and L. F. Quesney, pp. 201–213. Raven Press, New York.

61. Olsen, R. W., Wong, E. H. F., Stauber, G. B., and King, R. G. (1984): Biochemical pharmacology of the GABA/benzodiazepine receptor/ionophore protein. *Fed. Proc.*, 43:2773–2778.

62. Olsen, R. W., Wong, E. H. F., Stauber, G. B., Murakami, D., King, R. G., and Fischer, J. B. (1984): Biochemical properties of the GABA/barbiturate/benzodiazepine receptor–chloride ion channel complex. In: *Neurotransmitter Receptors, Mechanisms of Action and Regulation*, edited by S. Kito, T. Segawa, K. Kuriyama, H. I. Yamamura, and R. W. Olsen, pp. 205–219. Plenum, New York.

63. Owen, D., Study, R., Gratz, E., and Barker, J. L. (1982): Pharmacological modulation of GABA responses in cultured mouse spinal neurons. *Soc. Neurosci. Abstr.*, 8:833.

64. Paul, L. A., Fried, I., Watanabe, K., Forsythe, A. B., and Scheibel, A. B. (1981): Structural correlates of seizure behavior in the Mongolian gerbil. *Science*, 213:924–926.

65. Paul, S. M., and Skolnick, P. (1978): Rapid changes in brain benzodiazepine receptors after experimental seizures. *Science*, 202:892–894.

66. Paul, S. M., Syapin, P. J., Paugh, B. A., Moncada, A., and Skolnick, P. (1979): Correlation between benzodiazepine receptor occupation and anticonvulsant effects of diazepam. *Nature*, 281:688–689.

67. Placheta, P., and Karobath, M. (1980): In vitro modulation by SQ 20009 and SQ 65396 of GABA receptor binding in rat CNS membranes. *Eur. J. Pharmacol.*, 62:225–228.

68. Ramanjaneyulu, R., and Ticku, M. K. (1984): Interactions of pentamethylenetetrazole and tetrazole analogues with the picrotoxinin site of the benzodiazepine-GABA receptor-ionophore complex. *Eur. J. Pharmacol.*, 98:337–345.

69. Ramanjaneyulu, R., and Ticku, M. K. (1984): Binding characteristics and interactions of depressant drugs with [³⁵S]t-butyl bicyclophosphorothionate, a ligand that binds to the picrotoxinin site. *J. Neurochem.*, 42:221–229.

70. Ribak, C. E., Harris, A. B., Vaughn, J. E., and Roberts, E. (1981): Immunocytochemical changes in cortical neurons in a monkey model of epilepsy. In: *Neurotransmitters, Seizures, & Epilepsy*, edited by P. L. Morselli, K. G. Lloyd, W. Löscher, B. Meldrum, E. H. Reynolds, pp. 11–22. Raven Press, New York.

71. Ross, S. M., and Craig, C. R. (1981): γ-Aminobutyric acid concentration, L-glutamate-1-decarboxylase activity, and properties of the γ-aminobutyric acid postsynaptic receptor in cobalt epilepsy in the rat. *J. Neurosci*, 1:1388–1396.

72. Savage, D. D., Werling, L. L., Nadler, J. V., and McNamara, J. O. (1982): Selective increase in L-[³H]glutamate binding to a quisqualate-sensitive site on hippocampal synaptic membranes after angular bundle kindling. *Eur. J. Pharmacol.*, 85:255–256.

73. Schmutz, M. (1983): Benzodiazepines, GABA, and epilepsy—The animal evidence. In: *Benzodiazepines Divided*, edited by M. R. Trimble, pp. 149–166. John Wiley, Chichester.

74. Schulz, D. W., and Macdonald, R. L. (1981): Barbiturate enhancement of GABA-modulated inhibition and activation of chloride ion conductance: Correlation with anticonvulsants and anesthetic actions. *Brain Res.*, 209:177–188.

75. Sigel, E., Stephenson, F. A., Mamalaki, C., and Barnard, E. A. (1983): A γ-aminobutyric acid/benzodiazepine receptor complex of bovine cerebral cortex. *J. Biol. Chem.*, 258:6965–6971.

76. Simmonds, M. A. (1981): Distinction between the effects of barbiturates, benzodiazepines and phenytoin on responses to γ-aminobutyric acid receptor activation and antagonism by bicuculline and picrotoxinin. *Br. J. Pharmacol.*, 73:739–747.

77. Skolnick, P., Rice, K. C., Barker, J. L., and Paul, S. M. (1982): Interaction of barbiturates with benzodiazepine receptors in the central nervous system. *Brain Res.*, 233:143–156.

78. Squires, R. F. (1983): Benzodiazepine receptor multiplicity. *Neuropharmacology*, 22:1443–1450.

79. Squires, R. F., and Saederup, E. (1982): γ-Aminobutyric acid receptors modulate cation

binding sites coupled to independent benzodiazepine, picrotoxinin, and anion binding sites. *Mol. Pharmacol.*, 22:327–334.

80. Squires, R. F., Casida, J. E., Richardson, M., and Saederup, E. (1983): [^{35}S]*t*-Butylbicyclophosphorothionate binds with high affinity to brain-specific sites coupled to γ-aminobutyric acid-A and ion recognition sites. *Mol. Pharmacol.*, 23:326–336.

81. Stephenson, F. A., and Olsen, R. W. (1982): Solubilization by CHAPS detergent of barbiturate-enhanced benzodiazepine-GABA receptor complex. *J. Neurochem.*, 39:1579–1586.

82. Stephenson, F. A., Watkins, A. E., and Olsen, R. W. (1982): Physicochemical characterization of detergent-solubilized γ-aminobutyric acid and benzodiazepine receptor proteins from bovine brain. *Eur. J. Biochem.*, 123:291–298.

83. Study, R. E., and Barker, J. L. (1981): Diazepam and (−)-pentobarbital: Fluctuation analysis reveals different mechanisms for potentiation of γ-aminobutyric acid responses in cultured central neurons. *Proc. Natl. Acad. Sci. USA*, 78:7180–7184.

84. Supavilai, P., and Karobath, M. (1981): Action of pyrazolopyridines as modulators of [^{3}H]-flunitrazepam binding to the GABA/benzodiazepine receptor complex of the cerebellum. *Eur. J. Pharmacol.*, 70:183–193.

85. Supavilai, P., Mannonen, A., and Karobath, M. (1982): Modulation of GABA binding sites by CNS depressants and CNS convulsants. *Neurochem. Int.*, 4:259–268.

86. Tallman, J. F., Paul, S. M., Skolnick, P., and Gallager, D. W. (1980): Receptors for the age of anxiety: Pharmacology of the benzodiazepines. *Science*, 207:274–281.

87. Thyagarajan, R., Ramanyaneyulu, R., and Ticku, M. K. (1983): Enhancement of diazepam and γ-aminobutyric acid binding by (+) etomidate and pentobarbital. *J. Neurochem.*, 41:578–585.

88. Ticku, M. K. (1979): Differences in γ-aminobutyric acid receptor sensitivity in inbred strains of mice. *J. Neurochem.*, 33:1135–1138.

89. Ticku, M. K. (1981): Interaction of depressant, convulsant and anticonvulsant barbiturates with [^{3}H]diazepam binding site at the benzodiazepine-GABA-receptor–ionophore complex. *Biochem. Pharmacol.*, 30:1573–1579.

90. Ticku, M. K., and Maksay, G. (1983): Convulsant/depressant site of action at the allosteric benzodiazepine-GABA receptor–ionophore complex. *Life Sci.*, 33:2363–2375.

91. Ticku, M. K., and Olsen, R. W. (1978): Interaction of barbiturates with dihydropicrotoxinin binding sites related to the GABA receptor–ionophore system. *Life Sci.*, 22:1643–1651.

92. Ticku, M. K., and Olsen, R. W. (1979): Cage convulsants inhibit picrotoxinin binding. *Neuropharmacology*, 18:315–318.

93. Ticku, M. K., Ban, M., and Olsen, R. W. (1978): Binding of [^{3}H]α-dihydropicrotoxinin, a γ-aminobutyric acid synaptic antagonist, to rat brain membranes. *Mol. Pharmacol.*, 14:391–402.

94. van Gelder, N. M. (1981): The detection of cerebral dysfunction by disturbances in the compartmentalized metabolism of certain amino acids. In: *Neurotransmitters, Seizures, & Epilepsy*, edited by P. L. Morselli, K. G. Lloyd, W. Löscher, B. Meldrum, and E. H. Reynolds, pp. 129–139. Raven Press, New York.

95. Whittle, S. R., and Turner, A. J. (1982): Differential effects of sedative and anticonvulsant barbiturates on specific [^{3}H]GABA binding to membrane preparations from rat brain cortex. *Biochem. Pharmacol.*, 31:2891–2895.

96. Willow, M., and Johnston, G. A. R. (1983): Pharmacology of barbiturates: Electrophysiological and neurochemical studies. *Int. Rev. Neurobiol.*, 24:15–49.

97. Wong, E. H. F., Leeb-Lundberg, L. M. F., Teichberg, V. I., and Olsen, R. W. (1984): γ-Aminobutyric acid activation of ^{36}Cl$^-$ flux in rat hippocampal slices and its potentiation by barbiturates. *Brain Res.*, 303:267–275.

98. Wong, E. H. F., Snowman, A. M., Leeb-Lundberg, L. M. F., and Olsen, R. W. (1984): Barbiturates allosterically inhibit GABA antagonist and benzodiazepine inverse agonist binding. *Eur. J. Pharmacol.*, 102:205–212.

99. Wood, J. H., Hare, T. A., Glaeser, B. S., Ballenger, J. C., and Post, R. M. (1979): Cerebrospinal fluid GABA reductions in seizure patients. *Neurology*, 29:1203–1208.

100. Zukin, S. R., Young, A. B., and Snyder, S. H. (1974): Gamma-aminobutyric acid binding to receptor sites in rat central nervous system. *Proc. Natl. Acad. Sci. USA*, 71:4802–4807.

Advances in Neurology, Vol. 44, edited by
A. V. Delgado-Escueta, A. A. Ward, Jr.,
D. M. Woodbury, and R. J. Porter.
Raven Press, New York © 1986.

18

GABA Receptors, Lipids, and Gangliosides in Cobalt Epileptic Focus

Charles R. Craig and Brenda K. Colasanti

Department of Pharmacology and Toxicology, West Virginia University Medical Center, Morgantown, West Virginia 26506

SUMMARY The seizure state induced in the rat by cerebral cortical implantation of cobalt metal has been increasingly used to study a variety of neurochemical parameters. This experimental model of epilepsy affords the opportunity to study events prior to the development of seizures, during the period of intense seizure activity, and during the period when seizure activity has essentially terminated. The seizures that occur in this model are intermittent and paroxysmal and share many other similarities with human epilepsy. The crucial question with this model, and indeed with any experimental model of epilepsy, is whether the basic seizure-producing mechanism(s) is similar. This question remains to be answered.

There have been studies that show that changes in certain neurochemical parameters parallel the onset, intensity, and decline of seizure activity in cobalt-epileptic animals. Although extremely interesting, by themselves they do not prove a cause-and-effect relationship. Such parallelism is more apparent in the case of GABA than in the cases of lipids and gangliosides. GABA and its synthetic enzyme, glutamic acid decarboxylase (GAD), are both at normal levels prior to the development of seizures, are significantly decreased during the period of seizures, and return toward control values at a time when seizures are no longer apparent. On the other hand, there is no change in postsynaptic GABA binding sites (B_{max}) prior to seizures, a significant increase in B_{max} during seizure activity, and a return toward normal by 21 days (when seizure activity has terminated).

Studies that have been carried out on lipids and gangliosides in cobalt-induced epilepsy are not nearly as extensive nor are the results as positive as those that have been obtained in the case of GABA. They do, however, provide provocative findings that may well be related to the genesis of epilepsy.

Cobalt metal applied to the cerebral cortex of experimental animals has been frequently used as a means of producing a model of epilepsy. Cobalt ion has also been shown to be capable of producing seizures (33), and it is likely that ionic cobalt is the active species, even when the metal is applied. The laboratory rat has been the most widely studied species, although cobalt appears to produce an epileptogenic condition in all species studied.

Before considering GABA receptors, lipids, and gangliosides in cobalt-induced epilepsy, it is necessary to ask first whether the seizure state produced in rats by the cerebral placement of cobalt is a worthwhile model to study, and whether there are any significant similarities between the model and human epilepsy. The sei-zures produced by cobalt are paroxysmal and intermittent, and other than the appearance of convulsions and electroencephalogram (EEG) spiking, there appear to be few other untoward effects of the metal. Figure 1 is a diagrammatic representation of the preparation. Figure 2 shows the electrocorticogram (ECoG) and elec-tromyogram (EMG) tracings from control rats.

The seizures exhibited by cobalt-epileptic an-imals may take various forms. Frequently, there is EEG evidence of convulsive activity (high-voltage, low-frequency wave forms) with no motor component, i.e., the rat, behaviorally, as-sumes a frozen posture. At other times, clonic movements of the forelimbs occur, often with the rat rearing during the time the forelimbs are exhibiting clonic movements; the latter may per-sist for several seconds. During this behavior, the ECoG is showing seizure activity. Less fre-quently seen, but nevertheless well documented (12), are generalized tonic-clonic seizures af-fecting all limbs. These convulsions may or may not be followed by unconsciousness. A typical generalized seizure is shown in Fig. 3. The in-cidence of generalized tonic-clonic seizures is much greater if the cobalt is applied bilaterally. In addition to overt seizures, periods of contin-uous spiking activity, which persist for 16–48 hr, are also readily apparent (Fig. 4) [12]. The time

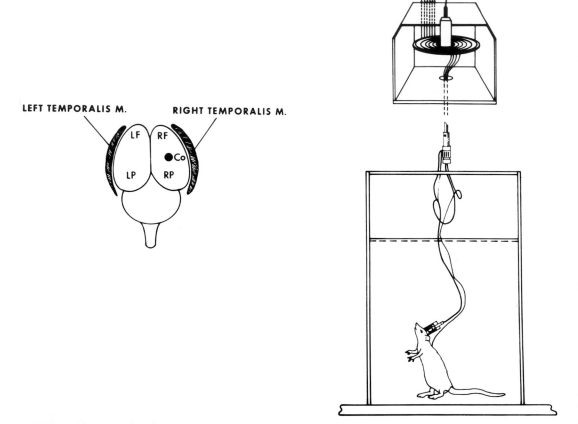

FIG. 1. Diagrammatic representation of rats treated with cobalt and prepared for recording of electrocorti-cogram (ECoG) and electromyogram (EMG). Screw electrodes are placed in cortex at left frontal (LF), right frontal (RF), left parietal (LP), and right parietal (RP) location. Muscle electrodes are inserted into left and right temporalis muscles. Cobalt is inserted into cortex at area indicated (Co). Following implantation of cobalt and recording electrodes, all electrodes are connected to an Amphenol connector, which is then held in position by acrylic dental cement. Two hours after completion of all surgical procedures, the rats are placed in individual recording cages and connected to a cable. The ECoG and EMG of these unrestrained and freely moving rats are then recorded continuously on four-channel polygraphs (Grass model 7C) over periods of 7–21 days. To reduce the volume of chart paper accumulated, the ECoG is usually recorded at the slow chart speed of 25 mm/min.

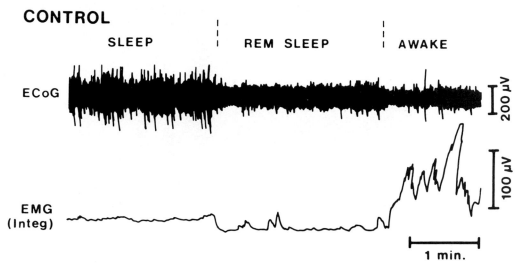

FIG. 2. ECoG and EMG tracings of the sleep-wakefulness cycle collected from a control rat. The ECoG during REM sleep resembles that during wakefulness but is paralleled by a marked reduction of the EMG activity surpassing that of NREM sleep.

course of cobalt epilepsy in the rat (Fig. 5) is such that there is initially a period of 4–5 days of very reduced seizure activity after cobalt implantation, and then a period of 6–7 days of intense epileptiform activity, which is followed by diminution of both seizures and spiking. By 21 days, seizure activity has essentially terminated, although the animals still have a lowered threshold to pentylenetetrazol-induced (PTZ) convulsions. The characteristic time course for the production of seizures permits the conducting of biochemical studies prior to the appearance of epileptiform activity, during the time of intense seizure activity, and after the seizures have essentially terminated.

Several studies have evaluated the ability of clinically useful anticonvulsant drugs to modify seizures produced in rats by cerebral cortical cobalt placement. Dow et al. (15) showed that ethosuximide at doses from 50 to 400 mg/kg, intraperitoneally (i.p.), markedly reduced the number of single spikes and abolished groups of spikes completely for up to 30 min. Craig et al. (13) studied the anticonvulsant effects of trimethadione and phenytoin in cobalt-epileptic rats. Both drugs were effective in decreasing the incidence of completely generalized seizures, but neither had any influence on incompletely generalized seizures. Chocholova (7) reported that diazepam was capable of decreasing spiking activity during sleep and wakefulness in the cobalt-epileptic rat. Chocholova and Radil-Weiss (8–10) demonstrated that chlordiazepoxide like-

wise decreased spike frequency, whereas high doses of phenytoin caused the suppression of typical episodes of spikes. Kästner et al. (24) reported that ethosuximide at doses of 100 mg/kg or higher suppressed cobalt-induced spike groups and reduced the spike amplitudes in rats. Scuvee-Moreau et al. (38) reported that single doses of ethosuximide of 400 mg/kg, i.p., produced a significant reduction in spike frequency for up to 1 hr in rats implanted with cobalt–gelatine rods. The latter authors were unable to show any anticonvulsant effect of phenytoin, but did show a marked suppression of spikes following carbidopa (a dopa decarboxylase inhibitor) and L-DOPA.

Other studies of importance with regard to drug therapy of epilepsy are those of Colasanti et al. (11) and DeVore et al. (14). It has been reported by Celesia et al. (5), Ferrer-Allado et al. (19), and others that the anesthetic, ketamine, enhances seizure discharges in human epileptic subjects. DeVore et al. (14) established that both nonanesthetic (30 mg/kg) and anesthetic (80 mg/kg) doses of ketamine were associated with activation of primary and projected focal electrical activity in the cobalt-epileptic rat. Therefore, a compound that exacerbates seizures in human epileptic subjects also increases electrical seizure activity in the cobalt-epileptic rat.

In summary, cobalt experimental epilepsy in the rat shares a large number of similarities with human epilepsy. It remains to be determined

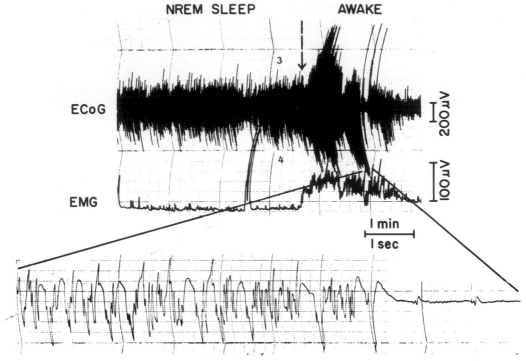

FIG. 3. Bipolar ECoG recordings collected from a cobalt-epileptic rat prior to and during a completely generalized tonic-clonic seizure at the end of sleep in a cobalt-epileptic rat. Note the electrical "silence" occurring after its termination. Effects of diphenylhydantoin and trimethadione on seizure activity during cobalt experimental epilepsy in the rat. From Craig et al., ref. 13, with permission.

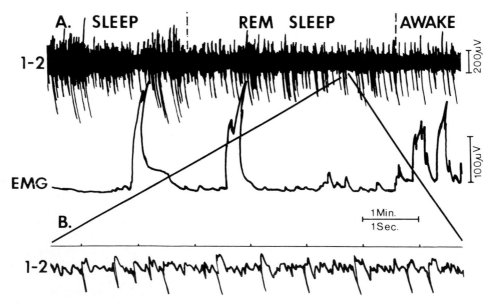

FIG. 4. The appearance of continuous spiking activity which occurs for prolonged periods in rats that have been implanted with cobalt. **A.** Appearance during sleep, REM sleep, and awake state recorded at a chart speed of 25 mm/min. **B.** A tracing of spiking activity during sleep at a chart speed of 25 mm/min.

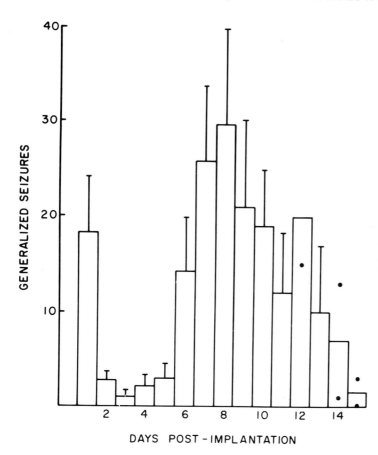

FIG. 5. Time course for the appearance of generalized seizure activity after bilateral cerebral implantation of cobalt. The values represent the means ± SEM for three to six rats except at days 12, 14, and 15, where the means are shown.

whether the biochemical abnormalities giving rise to epileptogenesis are the same in experimental animal models and in humans.

GABA RECEPTORS IN COBALT EPILEPSY

Gamma-aminobutyric acid (GABA) has clearly been shown to be a major inhibitory neurotransmitter in the mammalian nervous system, and there is a formidable amount of scientific literature relating GABA to seizure disorders.

The first evidence to suggest that GABA might be related to seizure disorders was the observation that a variety of inhibitors of glutamic acid decarboxylase (GAD) were convulsants (25). Because these inhibitors of GAD were also inhibitors of the degradative enzyme for GABA (GABA transaminase; GABA-T), and possibly other enzymes, the validity of the earlier observation was questioned (32). This led to a temporary loss of interest in the relationship between GABA and epilepsy. However, it soon became apparent with the development of more specific GABA-T inhibitors among these, ami-

nooxyacetic acid (AOAA), gabaculine, γ-acetylenic GABA, and γ-vinyl GABA (GVG) that elevation of brain GABA did provide anticonvulsant effects (29). Compounds that mimic GABA at its postsynaptic receptor are also anticonvulsants. These include progabide, homotaurine (18), and muscimol. The two classical antagonists of GABA, i.e., bicuculline and picrotoxinin, although differing in their mechanisms of antagonism (28) are both convulsants (Table 1).

Furthermore, brain GABA levels, as well as activities of GABA's synthetic enzyme, GAD, have been shown to be reduced in several types of experimental seizures. Van Gelder (42), as well as Van Gelder and Courtois (43), have shown that GABA levels are depressed in brains of cobalt-treated cats and mice. Emson and Joseph (16) showed in the rat that GABA and GAD were both significantly depressed in tissue surrounding the lesion 4–10 days following cobalt implantation with a return toward normal values by 24 days. GAD, but not GABA, was significantly reduced in the contralateral cortex as well. Ross and Craig (36) verified the above data for GABA and GAD in the ipsilateral cortex

TABLE 1. *Convulsant or anticonvulsant properties of agents with known effects on GABA*

Compound	Mechanism	Convulsant or anticonvulsant effects
Muscimol	GABA agonist	Anticonvulsant
THIP	GABA agonist	Anticonvulsant
Progabide	GABA agonist	Anticonvulsant
Aminooxyacetic acid	GABA-T inhibitor	Anticonvulsant
Gabaculine	GABA-T inhibitor	Anticonvulsant
Valproic acid	GABA-T inhibitor-?	Anticonvulsant
Bicuculline	GABA antagonist	Convulsant
Picrotoxinin	GABA antagonist	Convulsant
Penicillin	GABA antagonist	Convulsant

(Figs. 6 and 7), and furthermore showed that these were not nonspecific changes associated with cellular necrosis because copper, an element that produces extensive necrosis in the absence of seizures, did not cause alterations in GABA or GAD in any time period measured.

Balcar et al. (2) studied kinetic parameters of high-affinity uptake of L-glutamate and GABA in cobalt-induced cortical epileptogenic foci in rats and reported a decreased V_{max} for the uptake of GABA in the focal area with no change in the case of L-glutamate. Ross and Craig (35) reported that the high-affinity GABA synapto-somal transport system (a primary mechanism for removal of GABA following receptor occupation) was significantly depressed between 5 and 21 days following cobalt implantation (Fig. 8) with no change in the low-affinity uptake system. Another approach that has been used to demonstrate an alteration in the GABA system is the fluorescence procedure. Seidel et al. (39) demonstrated a decrease in GABA fluorescence in the pyramidal and granular layer of the hippocampus of the rat after cortical implantation of cobalt.

Receptor ligand binding studies have clearly

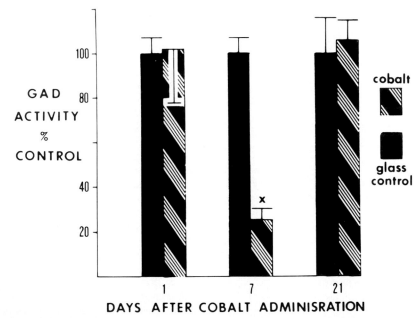

FIG. 6. Changes in glutamic acid decarboxylase activity in the rat frontal cerebral cortex adjacent to the cobalt lesion, relative to glass controls, 1, 7, and 21 days after cobalt implantation. Glutamic acid decarboxylase experiments were done in crude mitochondrial synaptosomal (P_2) fractions with 4 M [^{14}C]glutamic acid and excess cold glutamate and appropriate cofactors. The tissue was incubated for 30 min at 37°C in a shaking water bath. Each value represents the mean of at least eight but not more than 14 experiments. Vertical bar, SEM; X, $p < 0.01$. Gamma-aminobutyric acid (GABA) concentration, L-glutamate 1-decarboxylase activity, and properties of the GABA postsynaptic receptor in cobalt epilepsy in the rat. From Ross and Craig, ref. 36, with permission.

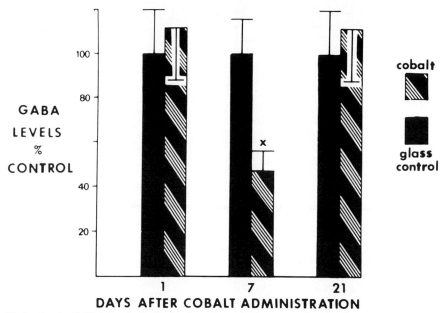

FIG. 7. Reduction in GABA levels in the rat frontal cerebral cortex adjacent to the cobalt lesion, relative to glass controls after 7 days. Each value represents the mean of 6–10 experiments. Each experiment was run in triplicate. Vertical bars, SEM; X, $p < 0.05$. GABA concentration, L-glutamate 1-decarboxylase activity, and properties of the GABA postsynaptic receptor in cobalt epilepsy in the rat. From Ross and Craig, ref. 36, with permission.

established the presence of GABA recognition sites on postsynaptic membranes (17). These recognition sites, when coupled with GABA or an appropriate GABA agonist, cause a shift in membrane permeability to inorganic ions, particularly chloride. This change in permeability results in hyperpolarization of the receptive neuron. GABA not only attaches to its own re-

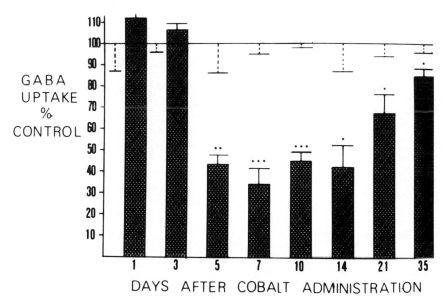

FIG. 8. Reduction of GABA uptake in rat frontal cerebral cortex adjacent to the cobalt implantation, relative to glass controls. Each value represents the mean of at least six experiments. Vertical bars indicate SE, •$p < 0.02$; ••$p < 0.01$; •••$p < 0.001$. Studies on GABA transport in cobalt experimental epilepsy in the rat. From Ross and Craig, ref. 35, with permission.

ceptor, but this amino acid can also interact at other sites, including GABA transport sites as well as several enzymes concerned with its synthesis and degradation. There are probably multiple forms of GABA recognition sites on postsynaptic receptors (hereafter referred to as GABA receptors) according to Browner et al. (4). There appear to be high- and low-affinity GABA receptors and, in addition, different classes of GABA receptors, based upon differing affinities for the GABA antagonist, bicuculline. At least some GABA receptors are part of a supramolecular entity that includes the GABA recognition site, a benzodiazepine recognition site, and the chloride ionophore, in addition to other unidentified components.

Ross and Craig (36) studied high-affinity postsynaptic GABA receptor binding characteristics K_d and B_{max}) in crude synaptic membranes from rats treated with cobalt, copper, or glass in tissue from the frontal cortex adjacent to the lesion but excluding any visually necrotic tissue. Copper was used as one control because it induces profound necrosis but no seizure activity. Studies were conducted at 1 day after surgery (before seizures ordinarily are seen), at 7 days (period of maximal seizures), and at 21 days (period of minimal seizure activity). No alteration in affinity (K_d) or the number of postsynaptic binding sites (B_{max}) was observed in the rats 1 day after cobalt implantation when compared with rats treated with glass or copper. However, at 7 days marked increases in postsynaptic GABA binding sites (B_{max}) occurred in cobalt-treated rats but not in copper- or glass-treated animals (Fig. 9). There was no change in affinity. By 21 days, the B_{max} was still elevated, although not significantly. These studies are summarized in Table 2.

The reason for an apparent increase in GABA receptor number is not clear, but may well represent an adaptive process (such as supersensitivity) as an attempt toward compensation for the lowered levels of GABA, the reduced GAD activity, and the lowered level of the high-affinity GABA transport mechanism resulting from cobalt implantation.

LIPIDS IN COBALT-EPILEPTIC FOCUS

The relationship of lipids to the epileptic process is unclear, even though it has been studied for decades. Wilder introduced specific diet therapy, high in fat and low in carbohydrate, for the treatment of human epilepsy in 1921. The classic ketogenic diet induces significant elevation in all plasma lipids, with steady state lipi-

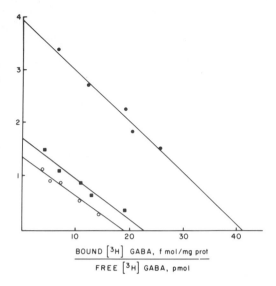

FIG. 9. Scatchard-plot analysis showing an increase in specific [³H]GABA binding to the frontal adjacent cortical preparations in cobalt-treated tissue (●) but not in copper treated tissue (■) relative to glass controls (○) 7 days after implantation. No change in affinity (K_D) occurs after any treatment. Each value represents the mean of six to nine separate experiments. Each experiment represents the frontal cerebral cortex pooled from seven rats and was run in duplicate. GABA concentration, L-glutamate 1-decarboxylase activity, and properties of the GABA postsynaptic receptor in cobalt epilepsy in the rat. From Ross and Craig, ref. 36, with permission.

demia occurring after 2–3 weeks. Plasma cholesterol may be increased by ~60% and total fatty acids by 80% (44). Success in treating human epilepsy with this regimen has been limited, at least in part because the ketogenic diet is unpalatable, making compliance a major problem.

An experimental study by Kopeloff and Alexander (26) suggested a role of lipids in the etiology of epilepsy. Their study demonstrated that increased levels of plasma cholesterol protected epileptic monkeys against PTZ-induced seizures. Alexander and Kopeloff (1) further showed that mice and rats fed cholesterol-rich diets had lowered susceptibility to PTZ-induced seizures.

Cenedella and Craig (6) measured total free fatty acids, free cholesterol, esterified cholesterol, triglycerides, and phospholipids in cerebral cortex samples from control and cobalt-epileptic rats. They reported that cobalt-induced epilepsy was associated with significant changes in cerebral cortical lipids in the area of the lesion as well as in the non-necrotic tissue adjacent to

TABLE 2. *Summary of kinetic parameters of GABA postsynaptic receptor binding at various times following application of metal to the frontal cerebral cortex*

		Days following metal application			
	Treatment	1	7	14	21
		nM			
K_D	Cobalt Glass	8.80 ± 0.42[a]	8.30 ± 0.67	15.40 ± 2.85	9.26 ± 1.15
	(control)	8.20 ± 0.36	5.56 ± 0.74	10.60 ± 3.4	9.36 ± 0.99
	Copper Glass		8.69 ± 1.92		
	(control)		9.55 ± 1.45		
		pmol/mg protein			
B_{max}	Cobalt Glass	1.68 ± 0.20[a]	3.97[b] ± 0.83	3.32 ± 0.79	2.64 ± 0.35
	(control)	1.52 ± 0.21[a]	1.36 ± 0.17	1.64 ± 0.32	1.41 ± 0.22
	Copper Glass		1.74 ± 0.25		
	(control)		1.55 ± 0.28		

[a] ± SEM.
[b] $p < 0.05$.

the lesion. The total lipid in the area of the lesion decreased sharply as a result of reductions in free cholesterol and total phospholipids. The levels of cholesterol esters and triglycerides increased in the area of the lesion, and cholesterol esters were also increased in the adjacent tissue. In addition, there were decreases in the proportion of phosphatidyl ethanolamine in the phospholipids from the lesion site and adjacent tissue and decreases in the proportions of oleic, arachidonic, and nervonic acids (unsaturated acids), and an increase in the proportions of lignoceric acid in the phospholipids.

In a related study, Lunt and Grove (30) measured unesterified fatty acids in an area of rat brain immediately surrounding the epileptic focus produced by cobalt powder. They reported an 81% increase in the content of unesterified fatty acids around the focal area. The predominant lipid was arachidonic acid. Bierkamper and Cenedella (3) conducted a very extensive investigation on cerebral cortical cholesterol change in cobalt-induced epilepsy in the rat. After implantation of cobalt (or other metals), measurements of cerebral cortical lipid concentrations were made in the direct area of metal implantation (i.e., lesion area) and in the non-necrotic tissue immediately adjacent to the lesion site. The cortical concentration of free cholesterol decreased in the adjacent and lesion site (Fig. 10), whereas the concentration of cholesterol esters greatly increased (Fig. 11) in the adjacent area from rats implanted with epileptogenic metals (cobalt and nickel) but not in those implanted with copper and stainless steel.

Differences in the fatty acid composition of the cholesterol esters from plasma and that from cobalt-lesioned cortex indicated that the accumulated cholesterol esters originated in the brain rather than in the plasma cholesterol ester pool. A time-course study revealed that changes in the cortical concentrations of free and esterified cholesterol precede the initial appearance of epileptiform activity as determined by electrocorticography. The conclusion of this study was that the reduction of free cholesterol levels probably reflected increased cholesterol metabolism in the cobalt-lesioned cortex. The increased metabolism of cholesterol could not be explained by changes in the activities of cholesterol ester synthetase and/or hydrolase(s).

Because cholesterol in the brain is localized almost exclusively in membranes, it is likely that the changes in brain sterols reflect losses in brain membranes. The resulting loss in membrane integrity could likely lead to increases in excitability associated with epileptiform states. Although not related to cobalt epilepsy per se, a study by Sarkar et al. (37) relates to the above study. It was shown that an experimental drug, U18666A, an inhibitor of desmosterol reductase, also produced chronic epileptiform activity in laboratory animals. In this study, the authors demonstrated that chronic administration of U18666A to rats, initiated at 1 day of age, produced marked decreases in the brain concentration of phospholipids. There were, however, no changes in concentration of cholesterol after 8 weeks of continuous treatment. It was at this time that epileptiform activity was greatest.

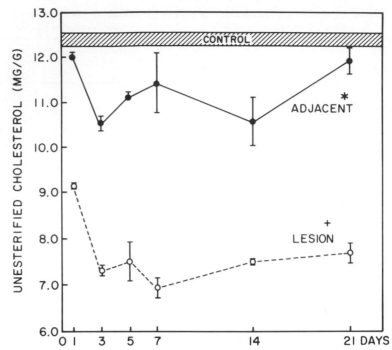

FIG. 10.   Free cholesterol concentrations in control cortex and in cortex from cobalt lesion (●) and adjacent (▲) areas of the implanted rats over a 21-day time course. Measurements were made by gas-chromatographic (GC) analysis. Each point represents the mean (with SE) of three samples, each sample being the pooled cortical tissue from three rats. Concentrations are given in milligrams of cholesterol per gram of cortex (wet wt); *p(t)<0.05 at days 3, 5, and 14 in the adjacent area; +p(t)<0.05 for days 1-21. Cerebral cortical cholesterol changes in cobalt-induced epilepsy. From Bierkamper and Cenedella, ref. 3, with permission.

ROLE OF BRAIN GANGLIOSIDES IN EPILEPSY

The finding that antiserum to a normal constituent of brain has epileptogenic properties when injected into the brain suggests the possibility of an immunological basis for epilepsy. An immunological basis for seizure disorders was first considered by Kopeloff et al. (27); this group serendipitously discovered the epileptogenic properties of alumina in monkeys when they tested the activity of egg-white precipitated by alumina cream and the alumina cream by itself as a control. More recently, brain gangliosides have been carefully considered for their role in maintaining neuronal membrane excitability.

Gangliosides are a class of sialoglycosphingo lipids that are highly concentrated in the ganglion cells of the central nervous system. Their exact role in the brain has not yet been established. It is established that they contribute to structures located at the outer cell surface, and they have been implicated in processes of membrane-mediated information transfer. Their role in seizure disorders is much less clear. Seyfried

et al. (40) reported a higher concentration of G_{M1} ganglioside in cerebrum, cerebellum, and brainstem from a seizure-susceptible strain of mice (DBA/2J) when compared with similar regions in a seizure-resistant (C57BL/6J) strain.

However, in another study (41), there were no significant or consistent abnormalities in gangliosides in cerebrum or brain stem in another mouse model of epilepsy, the tottering/leaner syndrome. The decreased concentration of total ganglioside that was reported in the cerebellum of these mutant mice is not considered to be a likely cause of the epilepsy since the changes in ganglioside were present at 21 days, whereas the seizures do not appear before 25 days of age. Another line of investigation into the role of gangliosides in seizure disorders has been followed by Rapport and co-workers (22–24). This group prepared antiserum to total brain gangliosides in rabbits, prepared immunoglobulin (Ig) fractions from the antisera, purified the antiganglioside antibodies (primarily to G_{m1} ganglioside) and, finally, tested the epileptogenic properties of all three preparations in rats. In general, they found recurrent EEG seizures which persisted for 1–3 weeks following the injection of 10 μl of anti-

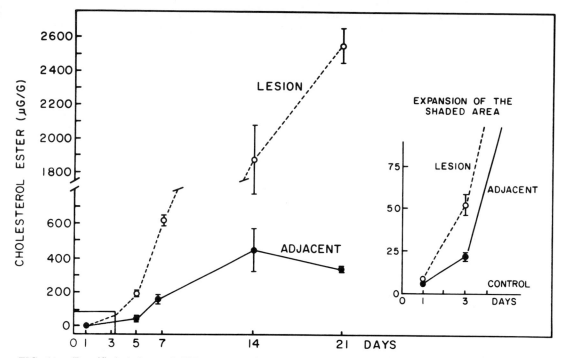

FIG. 11. Esterified cholesterol (CE) concentrations in cortex from cobalt lesion (○) and adjacent (●) areas of the implanted rats over a 21-day time course. Measurements were made by GC. Each point represents the mean (with SE errors) of three samples, each sample being from the pooled cortical tissue represented in Fig. 10. CE concentrations are given in gram of CE per gram of cortex (wet wt). The expanded scale insert on the right more readily demonstrates the CE changes occurring over the first three days of cobalt implantation; $p(t) < 0.01$ for all lesion and adjacent points from day 3 through day 21. Cerebral cortical cholesterol changes in cobalt-induced epilepsy. From Bierkamper and Cenedella, ref. 3, with permission.

serum into the sensorimotor cortex. Overt convulsions were rare, although abnormal EEG profiles were prominent (22). The relative specificity of the antiserum was established when it was further shown that, after absorption with pure G_{m1} ganglioside, the extract no longer produced EEG abnormalities. Overall, it was demonstrated that the epileptogenic effect of antiganglioside sera provided a positive correlation between titer (against pure G_{m1} ganglioside) and EEG response.

In the above studies, the Ig fractions were shown to be more effective in producing epileptic spiking than the antisera from which they were derived. In addition, the Ig fractions evoked EEG changes earlier than did the antisera (5–8 hr as compared with 24 hr). The purified antibodies were also effective, albeit they did not appear to induce EEG effects as intensive as those obtained with either native antisera or Ig fractions.

A subsequent study (20) was concerned with the ability of antibodies to G_{m1} ganglioside to affect neurotransmitter release from rat brain slices. In this report, the investigators were not able to show any effect of the antibody, after addition to slices, on the spontaneous release of GABA, norepinephrine, or serotonin, but they were able to demonstrate that depolarization-induced release of GABA (by either high K^+ or veratrine) was considerably enhanced by anti-G_{m1} ganglioside antibodies (Table 3). They detected only a slight enhancement of depolarization-induced release of norepinephrine and none in the case of serotonin.

In the most recent study on the importance of gangliosides in epilepsy, Frieder et al. (21) tested four anticonvulsant drugs against the immuno-

TABLE 3. *Release of neurotransmitters by*
G_{M1}-ganglioside antibody added to brain slices

Transmitter	Spontaneous release	Depolarization-induced release
GABA	No effect	↑ ↑
NE	No effect	Slight ↑
5HT	No effect	No effect

From data provided in Frieder and Rapport (1981): *J. Neurochem.*, 37:634–639.

TABLE 4. *Action of four anticonvulsants on two seizure models*

	Models	
Anticonvulsant	Immunological Model	Cobalt Model
Phenytoin	Decreased spiking	No effect
Ethosuximide	Decreased spiking	Decreased spiking
Diazepam	No effect	Decreased spiking
Aminooxyacetic acid	No effect	Decreased spiking

Results from Frieder, B. et al., (1982): *Exp. Neurol.*, 78:644–653, with permission.

logical model of epilepsy (induced by antiganglioside serum) and against cobalt-induced epilepsy. They reported that the two models differ in their response to anticonvulsant drugs (Table 4). Whereas phenytoin and ethosuximide were effective in reducing spike frequency in the antiganglioside serum model, diazepam and AOAA were not. In the cobalt model, on the other hand, these investigators found that AOAA, ethosuximide, and diazepam, but not phenytoin, were effective in reducing epileptiform spiking.

REFERENCES

1. Alexander, G. J., and Kopeloff, L. M. (1971): Induced hypercholesteremia and decreased susceptibility to seizures in experimental animals. *Exp. Neurol.*, 32:134–140.
2. Balcar, V. J., Pumain, R., Mark, J., Borg, J., and Mandel, P. (1978): GABA-mediated inhibition in the epileptogenic focus, a process which may be involved in the mechanism of the cobalt-induced epilepsy. *Brain Res.*, 154:182–185.
3. Bierkamper, G. G., and Cenedella, R. J. (1978): Cerebral cortical cholesterol changes in cobalt-induced epilepsy. *Epilepsia*, 19:155–167.
4. Browner, M., Ferkany, J. W., and Enna, S. J. (1981): Biochemical identification of pharmacologically and functionally distinct GABA receptors in rat brain. *J. Neurosci.*, 1:514–518.
5. Celesia, G. G., Bamforth, G. H., and Chen, K. R. (1974): Effects of ketamine in epileptics. *Neurology* (Minne.), 24:386.
6. Cenedella, R. J., and Craig, C. R. (1973): Changes in cerebral cortical lipids in cobalt-induced epilepsy. *J. Neurochem.*, 21:743–748.
7. Chocholova, L. (1976): Effect of diazepam on the electroencephalographic pattern and vigilance of unanesthetized and curarized rats with a chronic cobalt-gelatin focus. *Physiol. Bohemoslov.*, 25:129–137.
8. Chocholova, L., and Radil-Weiss, T. (1970): The level of vigilance and the EEG manifestations of cortical cobalt foci in rats. *Physiol. Bohemoslov.*, 19:385–396.
9. Chocholova, L., and Radil-Weiss, T. (1971): Effect of allobarbital on focal epilepsy in rats. *Physiol. Bohemoslov.*, 20:325–334.
10. Chocholova, L., and Radil-Weiss, T. (1973): Effect of diphenylhydantoin on paroxysmal EEG activity induced by cortical cobalt focus. *Act. Nerv. Super.* (Praha), 15:70–77.
11. Colasanti, B. K., Hartman, E. R., and Craig, C. R. (1973): Facilitative actions of vetamine on the EEG manifestations of cobalt experimental epilepsy. *Sleep Res.*, 2:146.
12. Colasanti, B. K., Hartman, E. R., and Craig, C. R. (1974): ECoG and behavioral correlates during the development of chronic cobalt experimental epilepsy in the rat. *Epilepsia*, 15:361–373.
13. Craig, C. R., Chiu, P., and Colasanti, B. K. (1976): Effects of diphenylhydantoin and trimethadione on seizure activity during cobalt experimental epilepsy in the rat. *Neuropharmacology*, 15:485–489.
14. DeVore, G. R., McQueen, J. K., and Woodbury, D. M. (1976): Ketamine hydrochloride and its effect on a chronic cobalt epileptic cortical focus. *Epilepsia*, 17:111–117.
15. Dow, R. C., Forfar, J. C., and McQueen, J. K. (1973): The effects of some anticonvulsant drugs on cobalt-induced epilepsy. *Epilepsia*, 14:203–212.
16. Emson, P. C., and Joseph, M. H. (1975): Neurochemical and morphological changes during the development of cobalt-induced epilepsy in the rat. *Brain Res.*, 93:91–110.
17. Enna, S. J., and Snyder, S. H. (1975): Properties of gamma-aminobutyric acid (GABA) receptor binding in rat brain synaptic membrane fractions. *Brain Res.*, 100:81–97.
18. Fariello, R. G. (1981): Neurophysiological investigations on direct GABA agonists. In: *Neurotransmitters, Seizures, and Epilepsy*, edited by P. L. Morselli, K. G. Lloyd, W. Loscher, B. Meldrum, and E. H. Reynolds, pp. 75–84. Raven Press, New York.
19. Ferrer-Allado, T., Brechner, U. L., Dymond, A., Cozen, H., and Crandall, P. (1973): Ketamine-induced electroconvulsive phenomena in the human limbic and thalamic regions. *Anesthesiology*, 38:333–344.
20. Frieder, B., and Rapport, M. M. (1981): Enhancement of depolarization-induced release of gamma-aminobutyric acid from brain slices by antibodies to ganglioside. *J. Neurochem.*, 37:634–639.
21. Frieder, B., Karpiak, S. E., and Rapport, M. M. (1982): Effect of antiepileptic drugs and an anticonvulsant on epileptiform activity induced by antibodies to ganglioside. *Exp. Neurol.*, 78:644–653.

22. Karpiak, S. E., Mahadik, S. P., Graf, L., and Rapport, M. M. (1981): An immunological model of epilepsy: Seizures induced by antibodies to G_{m1} ganglioside. *Epilepsia*, 22:189–196.

23. Karpiak, S. E., Graf, L., and Rapport, M. M. (1976): Antiserum to brain gangliosides produces recurrent epileptiform activity. *Science*, 194:735–737.

24. Kästner, I., Klingberg, F., and Muller, M. (1970): Zur wirkung des Ethosuximids auf die Kobalt-induzierte "Epilepsie" der Ratte. *Arch. Int. Pharmacodyn.*, 186:220–226.

25. Killam, K. F., and Bain, J. A. (1957): Convulsant hydrazides I. *In vitro* and *in vivo* inhibition by convulsant hydrazides of enzymes catalyzed by vitamin B_6. *J. Pharmacol. Exp. Ther.*, 119:255–262.

26. Kopeloff, L. M., and Alexander, G. J. (1971): Serum cholesterol in monkeys with chronic epileptic foci. *Life Sci.*, 10:869–876.

27. Kopeloff, L. M., Barrera, S. E., and Kopeloff, N. (1942): Recurrent convulsive seizures in animals produced by immunologic and chemical means. *Am. J. Psychiatry*, 98:881–902.

28. Krnjevic, K. (1983): GABA-mediated inhibitory mechanisms in relation to epileptic discharges. In: *Basic Mechanisms of Neuronal Hyperexcitability*, edited by H. H. Jasper and N. M. van Gelder, pp. 249–280. Liss, New York.

29. Löscher, W. (1981): Biochemical pharmacology of inhibitors of GABA metabolism and valproic acid. In: *Neurotransmitters, Seizures, and Epilepsy*, edited by P. L. Morselli, K. G. Lloyd, W. Löscher, B. Meldrum, and E. H. Reynolds, pp. 93–105. Raven Press, New York.

30. Lunt, G. G., and Grove, Y. K. (1975): The effects of cobalt-induced epilepsy on the unesterified fatty acid content of rat cerebral cortex. *Biochem. Soc. Proc.*, 3:701–702.

31. Massotti, M., Guidotti, A., and Costa, E. (1981): Characterization of benzodiazepine and gamma-aminobutyric recognition sites and their endogenous modulators. *J. Neurosci.*, 1:409–418.

32. Maynert, E. W., and Kaji, H. K. (1962): On the relationship of brain gamma-aminobutyric acid to convulsions. *J. Pharmacol. Exp. Ther.*, 137:114–121.

33. Pekoe, G. M., Craig, C. R., and Colasanti, B. K. (1978): Epileptogenic effects of cobaltous chloride after prolonged intraventricular infusion in the rat. *Fed. Proc.*, 37:2110.

34. Rapport, M. M., Karpiak, S. E., and Mahadik, S. P. (1979): Biological activities of antibodies injected into the brain. *Fed. Proc.*, 38:2391–2395.

35. Ross, S. M., and Craig, C. R. (1981): Studies on gamma-aminobutyric acid transport in cobalt experimental epilepsy in the rat. *J. Neurochem.*, 36:1006–1011.

36. Ross, S. M., and Craig, C. R. (1981): Gamma-aminobutyric acid concentration, L-glutamate 1-decarboxylase activity, and properties of the gamma-aminobutyric acid postsynaptic receptor in cobalt epilepsy in the rat. *J. Neurosci.*, 1:1388–1396.

37. Sarkar, C. P., Bierkamper, G. G., and Cenedella, R. J. (1982): Studies on mechanism of the epileptiform activity induced by U18666A. I. Gross alteration of the lipids of synaptosomes and myelin. *Epilepsia*, 23:243–255.

38. Scuvee-Moreau, J., Lepot, M., Brotchi, J., Gerebtzoff, M. A., and Dresse, A. (1977): Action of phenytoin, ethosuximide and of the carbidopa-L-dopa association in semi-chronic cobalt-induced epilepsy in the rat. *Arch. Int. Pharmacodyn.*, 230:92–99.

39. Seidel, J., Kastner, I., and Winkelmann, E. (1981): A loss of GABAergic hippocampus innervation in rats with cobalt-induced epilepsy demonstrated by Wolman fluorescence method. *Acta Histochem.*, 69:248–254.

40. Seyfried, T. N., Glaser, G. H., and Yu, R. K. (1978): Cerebral, cerebellar, and brainstem gangliosides in mice susceptible to audiogenic seizures. *J. Neurochem.*, 31:21–27.

41. Seyfried, T. N., Itoh, T., Glaser, G. H., Miyazawa, N., and Yu, R. K. (1981): Cerebellar gangliosides and phospholipids in mutant mice with ataxia and epilepsy: the tottering/leaner syndrome. *Brain Res.*, 216:429–436.

42. Van Gelder, N. M. (1972): Antagonism by taurine of cobalt induced epilepsy in cat and mouse. *Brain Res.*, 47:157–165.

43. Van Gelder, N. M., and Courtois, A. (1972): Close correlation between changing content of specific amino acids in epileptogenic cortex of cats and severity of epilepsy. *Brain Res.*, 43:477–484.

44. Wilder, B. J., and Bruni, J. (1981): Other drugs and therapies. In: *Seizure Disorders: A Pharmacological Approach to Treatment*, edited by B. J. Wilder and J. Bruni, p. 138. Raven Press, New York.

Advances in Neurology, Vol. 44, edited by
A. V. Delgado-Escueta, A. A. Ward, Jr.,
D. M. Woodbury, and R. J. Porter.
Raven Press, New York © 1986.

19

Roles of Biogenic Amines and Cyclic Nucleotides in Seizure Mechanisms*

James A. Ferrendelli

Division of Clinical Neuropharmacology, Departments of Pharmacology and Neurology, Washington University School of Medicine, St. Louis, Missouri 63110

SUMMARY Intercellular communication is an essential requirement for normal and abnormal functions of the mammalian central nervous system (CNS). Essentially all intercellular communication is accomplished by chemical substances which: (a) are released from cells; (b) act at various sites, usually at specific receptors, on cell surfaces; and (c) produce functional and metabolic effects by complex processes. Much of this book section is directed to discussion of the possible roles of various intercellular messengers (i.e., neurotransmitters, neuromodulators, and hormones) in basic mechanisms of epilepsy. This chapter focuses on the biogenic amines norepinephrine, dopamine, serotonin, and adenosine—substances which are putative neurotransmitters in the mammalian CNS and have been implicated in basic mechanisms in seizures. Also considered are relationships between seizure mechanisms and cyclic nucleotides (cyclic AMP and cyclic GMP), which are intracellular chemicals (or second messengers) that may mediate some of the effects of biogenic amines as well as other neurotransmitters.

Presently available data lead to the conclusion that norepinephrine, serotonin, adenosine, and perhaps dopamine appear to be involved in processes that inhibit or confine seizure activity. Cyclic AMP may also suppress initiation or spread of seizure activity. In contrast, cyclic GMP seems to have some role in initiating or maintaining seizure discharges.

Intercellular communication is an essential requirement for all normal and abnormal functions of the mammalian central nervous system (CNS). Essentially all intercellular communication is accomplished by chemical substances which: (a) are released from cells; (b) act at various sites, usually at specific receptors, on cell surfaces; and (c) produce functional and metabolic effects by complex processes. Much of this symposium is directed to discussion of the possible roles of various intercellular messengers (i.e., neurotransmitters, neuromodulators, and hormones) in basic mechanisms of epilepsy. This chapter focuses on the biogenic amines norepinephrine, dopamine, serotonin, and adenosine—substances which are putative neurotransmitters in the mammalian CNS and have been implicated in basic mechanisms in seizures. Also considered in this chapter are relationships between seizure mechanisms and cyclic nucleotides (cyclic AMP and cyclic GMP), which are intracellular chemicals (or second messengers) that may mediate some of the effects of biogenic amines as well as other neurotransmitters. No effort has been made to make this a comprehensive review of the above

---

* Reproduced from *Annals of Neurology*, 16:S98–S103 (1984).

subjects. Instead I hope to provide an overview which will serve as a guide for further consideration and investigation of these subjects.

RELATIONSHIPS BETWEEN BIOGENIC AMINES AND SEIZURES

Attempts to define the roles of specific neurotransmitters in the pathophysiological mechanisms of seizures face several inherent problems. Because of the nature of seizures, it is often necessary to perform experiments in the intact animal, a system which is obviously exceedingly complex. Most investigators have treated animals with various agents that purportedly increase or decrease the influence of an individual neurotransmitter system and then determine the effect on seizure activity. It is unfortunate that few, if any, of the agents tested under these conditions have a highly specific or even a single action on individual neurotransmitter systems in CNS. Many may affect other neurotransmitter system(s) as well, and some have additional different actions. Other approaches have included lesioning specific regions of brain to eliminate or reduce a specific population of cells and/or their contained neurotransmitter. Although this is often more specific than most systemically administered drugs, it is often impossible to evaluate other consequences of the lesions, particularly compensatory changes in other regions of brain. These problems do not invalidate experimental data, but do make their interpretation difficult; derived conclusions must necessarily be speculative.

NOREPINEPHRINE (NE)

The question of how seizures affect regional or whole-brain NE levels is not directly addressed in the literature. It is presumed that NE release occurs upon massive neuronal discharges during seizures and that synthesis and reuptake can, at least initially, compensate for that release; thus, it might be more appropriate to evaluate changes in NE turnover as a result of seizures. There are indications that NE turnover is modified by chemical convulsants (6,20). There is no correlation as yet of NE turnover with any particular phase(s) of the seizure.

The alternative approach to investigating the role of NE in seizures has been to produce either increases or decreases of NE influence pharmacologically, or by lesioning, and then to observe changes in seizure thresholds and characteristics. Diminishing the influence of NE in

brain clearly alters seizure activity. This was first reported by Chen et al. (4) in 1954, who demonstrated that reserpine-treated animals exhibited decreased thresholds to pentylenetetrazol (PTZ) seizures. Wenger et al. also showed effects on minimal electroshock seizures (40). Comparison of the effects of a tyrosine hydroxylase inhibitor with those of a dopamine (DA) β-hydroxylase inhibitor, both in reserpinized animals, suggests that decreases specifically in NE levels may result in decreases in minimal electroshock, maximal electroshock, and PTZ seizure thresholds (5,20). Mason and Corcoran produced regional CNS depletion of NE, without affecting serotonin (5-HT) or DA levels, by injecting 6-hydroxy dopamine (6-OHDA) into discrete areas of the brain (29,30). Their results demonstrated: (a) depletion of NE in the descending fibers that innervate the spinal cord increased the incidence of maximal electroshock seizures (MES) but not PTZ seizures; (b) depletion of cerebellar NE did not significantly alter thresholds for any seizures; and (c) depletion of NE in the ascending forebrain fibers increased susceptibility to PTZ seizures, as well as altered their characteristics (see below). Consistent with these results, Gross and Ferrendelli observed a decrease in the threshold for the tonic phase of PTZ seizure following depletion of brain NE produced by reserpine or 6-OHDA pretreatments (15).

Blockade of α- and β-adrenergic receptors can also alter seizure thresholds as well. Phentolamine and other α-antagonists lower the threshold for MES seizures, whereas propranolol, a β-antagonist, decreases thresholds of PTZ-induced seizures (20).

In addition to altering seizure threshold, NE also influences seizure characteristics. Gross and Ferrendelli examined the effects of several agents which purportedly reduce the influence of 5-HT on PTZ seizures (15). They demonstrated that depletion of brain NE, either with reserpine or 6-OHDA, markedly shortened the latency to tonic seizures after PTZ injection and increased their incidence. Propranolol or yohimbine, β- and α$_2$-adrenergic antagonists, respectively, had a similar action, but phentolamine, an α$_1$-antagonist, had little effect or may have diminished tonic seizure activity. The results reported by Mason and Corcoran showed that selective depletion of NE in the dorsal bundle by 6-OHDA also prolongs and increases the incidence of, but does not change the latency of, tonic seizures following PTZ injection (29). It has been difficult to demonstrate an effect of NE depletion on MES because of the rapidity of this seizure, but minimal electroshock seizures seem to be affected. Reserpine appears to increase the sensitivity of animals to minimal electroshock (4,40). This effect may be prolonged by treatment with combinations of reserpine and either a tyrosine hydroxylase inhibitor or disulfuram, a DA β-hydroxylase inhibitor (40).

It is much more difficult to demonstrate an effect resulting from elevated NE influence on seizure thresholds and activity. If elevated levels of NE are attained using precursors or uptake inhibitors, other monoaminergic neurotransmitter levels may be influenced. There are, however, some studies that have achieved an elevation of NE by using a combination of agents. L-DOPA pretreatment alone and in conjunction with a monoamine oxidase (MAO) inhibitor elevates seizure threshold for both electroshock and PTZ; however, this could be caused either by elevated DA or NE (5,19). Amphetamine produces equivocal results, depending on species and seizure model; however, parachloroamphetamine increases seizure threshold in mice for electroshock (20). Amphetamine and L-DOPA may decrease the incidence of tonic phase of PTZ seizures (20). It is well known that tricyclic antidepressant drugs can prevent MES and block the tonic phase of PTZ seizures. Whether this is owing to their ability to inhibit reuptake of biogenic amines or results from some other action is not known.

The preceding results lead to the conclusion that diminished NE influence in the CNS enhances seizure activity in the MES and PTZ seizure models, but it is difficult to establish that increased NE influence in CNS has an anticonvulsant effect. However, data from other experimental models of seizures support this concept. Using isolated tissues, usually the hippocampal slice, it is possible to produce epileptiform discharges with various agents (e.g., penicillin) and to determine the effects of direct addition of norepinephrine and related drugs. Using 2-fluoro-NE (α-agonist) and 6-fluoro-NE (β-agonist), Mueller et al. demonstrate that α-receptors suppress the population spike, β-receptors enhance the population spike, and selective depletion of NE in terminals eliminates the amphetamine-induced alterations in electrical activity (31). Recent work by Andersen shows that NE blocks slow, but not fast, inward currents and thus may suppress the synchronization that is associated with epileptiform activity in the slice (1). Hippocampal tissue transplanted to the anterior chamber of the eye becomes innervated by cholinergic and adrenergic nerve fibers (14). Iontophoretic application of NE or isoproterenol suppresses penicillin-induced epileptiform activity in these preparations, as does stimulation of the cervical sympathetic trunk (adrenergic input). This action can be prevented by pretreatment with reserpine or application of the β-adrenergic antagonist, dichloroisoproterenol. Some of these actions can be correlated with alterations in cyclic nucleotide levels (see below).

DA AND 5-HT

There are fewer data available which clearly establish roles of DA or 5-HT in seizures. A role for DA is suggested by the finding that increasing DA by administration of L-DOPA in combination with a dopamine β-hydroxylase inhibitor enhances seizure activity (5,23). Unfortunately, this elevates brain DA levels and also decreases NE levels; thus, the effects of this treatment could be a consequence of either or both changes. It has not been possible to show a direct correlation between either PTZ, MES, or ES seizure thresholds or characteristics and the DA agonist apomorphine, or the DA antagonists, haloperidol and fluphenazine (22). Kleinrok et al. were able to show a potentiation by DA of the anticonvulsant action of some GABA-ergic agonists, but not of the other anticonvulsants (21). DA iontophoresed onto the hippocampal slice can hyperpolarize and prolong the afterhyperpolarization which may or may not be associated with decreased epileptiform activity (2). A more convincing role for DA in seizure mechanisms is provided in other sections of this symposium.

Neurotransmission mediated by 5-HT also seems to have a role in seizure mechanisms. Parachlorophenylalanine (PCPA) depletion of 5-HT or blockade of 5-HT receptors with cyproheptadine results in a marked decrease in MES seizure thresholds, but only a slight drop in PTZ seizure threshold (20). Elevated MES and PTZ seizure thresholds can be achieved with 5-HTP, the precursor to serotonin. Additional study of this subject is surely needed.

ADENOSINE

Adenosine is a purine found in high concentrations in the brain and known to be released in reasonably large quantities under certain conditions (34). It is metabolized to inosine by adenosine deaminase and also taken up into cells by a high-affinity uptake system. There exist at least two external adenosine receptors (34). These are competitively blocked by theophylline and other methylxanthines in concentrations at least 100 times less than that which inhibits phosphodiesterase.

Maitre et al. demonstrated anticonvulsant actions of adenosine and nicotinamide against audiogenic seizures (26). Dunwiddie and Worth further defined the actions of adenosine which are as follows (7). Initially, adenosine produces sedation, hypothermia, and hypotension. These effects are dose-dependent and are blocked by low doses of theophylline. An anticonvulsant effect appears later and is also dose-dependent. Stable analogs of adenosine were observed to delay the onset of PTZ seizures. Theophylline enhanced the incidence of seizures with subconvulsant doses of PTZ.

Some effects of adenosine on MES in mice have been examined in our laboratory. The parameter that appeared most sensitive to this compound was the refractory time or the minimal time interval necessary before animals could have another seizure after an initial MES. Following a single MES, animals are refractory to a second maximal shock for a variable period. That time by which 50% of animals respond to the second shock is referred to as the RT_{50}. Intraperitoneal injections of 100–1,000 mg/kg of adenosine prolonged the RT_{50} as did similar doses of inosine. Guanosine was ineffective. An adenosine analog, 2-chloroadenosine, which is resistant to cellular uptake and metabolism, was significantly more potent in prolonging the RT_{50}. Dipyridamole, an adenosine-uptake inhibitor, was also very potent in extending the RT_{50}. Assessment of adenosine receptor blockade in the CNS by aminophylline was obscured by the high incidence of mortality in treated animals, presumably owing to the peripheral actions of the drug during or shortly after the initial MES. The above evidence suggests that adenosine plays a role in seizure mechanisms. Whether or not it is a neurotransmitter or modulator for these pathophysiological processes remains open to further investigation.

RELATIONSHIPS BETWEEN CYCLIC NUCLEOTIDES AND SEIZURES

Several different convulsant drugs and stimuli have been reported to elevate CNS levels of cyclic AMP, cyclic GMP, or both (3,9,10,12,13, 24,27,28,32,36,37). It appears that changes in cyclic nucleotide levels are associated with seizure activity or some closely related process and are independent of the processes that initiate the seizure activity. Moreover, seizures produce elevations of cyclic nucleotides in paralyzed,

ventilated animals, indicating that the biochemical changes are related to CNS processes and are not a result of systemic alterations such as increased motor activity or hypoxia. In addition, partial or focal seizures appear to alter cyclic nucleotide levels only in those regions of brain where seizure discharges occur, further indicating a direct relationship between the two phenomena (35,39).

Some studies have attempted to determine the temporal relationships between seizure discharges and changes in levels of cyclic nucleotides in brain *in vivo* (3,9,24,25,28,37). The results of these investigations have demonstrated that cyclic AMP increases only after the onset of clinically evident seizure activity or after the appearance of epileptiform EEG activity. In contrast, cyclic GMP levels have been reported to increase prior to the onset of clinical seizure, and subconvulsant doses (insufficient to produce clinically evident seizures or epileptiform EEG activity) as well as convulsant doses of drugs elevate cyclic GMP levels in brain. This indicates that cyclic AMP elevations are a consequence of seizure activity and that elevations of cyclic GMP are related to, but can occur independently of, seizure discharges.

Several drugs modify the effects of seizures on cyclic nucleotide levels in brain. Anticonvulsants such as phenytoin, phenobarbital, ethosuximide, valproic acid, and others attenuate or block seizure-induced accumulation of both cyclic AMP and cyclic GMP (10,12,25). However, these effects of anticonvulsant drugs are directly proportional to their ability to prevent seizures, indicating that the inhibitory effects of anticonvulsant drugs on seizure-induced accumulation of cyclic nucleotides are secondary to their antiepileptic action and are not a result of some direct effect on cyclic nucleotide formation or degradation.

Drugs other than anticonvulsants can modify cyclic nucleotide accumulation induced by seizures. Sattin (37) first demonstrated that theophylline or caffeine inhibited accumulation of cyclic AMP in mouse forebrain after maximal electroshock or after induction of seizures with hexafluorodiethyl ether. Lust et al. (24) reported that amphetamine, diphenhydramine, and trifluoroperazine all partially inhibited electroshock-induced elevation of cyclic AMP in mouse cerebral cortex. The increase in cyclic AMP levels in mouse cerebral cortex produced by seizures induced with 3-mercaptopropionic acid are reported to be attenuated by pretreatment of animals with propranolol (13). We examined the effects of several drugs, purported to alter noradrenergic influence in CNS, on PTZ-induced seizure activity and regulation of cyclic nucleotide levels in cerebral cortex and hippocampus in mice (15,16). Depletion of brain stores of NE with reserpine or treatment of neonatal mice with 6-OHDA decreases seizure latency and/or threshold and diminishes seizure-induced accumulation of cyclic AMP in brain. Propranolol, a β-adrenergic receptor antagonist, and yohimbine, an α_2-adrenergic receptor antagonist, have effects qualitatively similar to reserpine and 6-OHDA; however, phentolamine, an α_1-adrenergic antagonist increased seizure threshold and latency and did not reduce accumulation of cyclic AMP. Imipramine and D-amphetamine, drugs which increase noradrenergic influence in brain, had dissimilar actions. The former prevented tonic seizure but lowered the threshold and latency of clonic seizures; the latter worsened all seizure activity. Neither of these two drugs altered elevation of cyclic AMP levels. Aminophylline, a methylxanthine with multiple actions but most likely producing blockade of adenosine receptors in the CNS at the doses used in our experiments, also inhibited accumulation of cyclic AMP in several regions of brain and caused tonic seizures to develop sooner. None of the above drugs inhibited accumulation of cyclic GMP in PTZ-treated animals, and some augmented its increase slightly when seizure activity was more severe.

Thus, presently available data indicate that seizures increase cyclic AMP and cyclic GMP levels by two different mechanisms. With regard to cyclic AMP, it appears that biogenic amines, particularly NE, and perhaps adenosine, which are released from intracellular stores by the seizure discharge, activate adenylate cyclases and produce much, or perhaps all, of the increase of cyclic AMP levels. Furthermore, it appears that when the influence of NE or adenosine in CNS is diminished, seizure discharges spread and become sustained more rapidly and tonic seizures occur more quickly. An attractive possibility is that the reduction in cyclic AMP accumulation and the change in seizure activity are somehow related. The mechanism(s) responsible for the elevation of cyclic GMP levels has not been defined. However, we suggest that an increase in free intracellular concentration of calcium, which is known to occur during cellular depolarization and would certainly take place in brain tissue undergoing a seizure discharge, probably activates guanylate cyclase and produces at least some of the accumulation of cyclic GMP seen in epileptic brain. In support of this contention are the observations that cellular depolarization of brain tissue, *in vitro*, causes marked elevation of cyclic GMP levels, and this effect appears to be secondary to an augmented influx of calcium into cells (8,11). In addition, soluble guanylate cyclase in brain has been reported to be activated by calcium. Regardless of the mechanisms regulating cyclic GMP levels in epileptic brain, it is apparent that cyclic AMP and cyclic GMP are regulated differently, which suggests that the two cyclic nucleotides are involved in different pathophysiologic events during seizures.

There has been little attempt to assess directly the effects of cyclic nucleotides on seizure discharges, but the few studies reported have generated interesting data. Hoffer and colleagues have demonstrated that iontophoresis of cyclic GMP, or stable derivatives of this substance, powerfully excites and even produces epileptic activity in pyramidal neurons in hippocampus transplanted and maintained in the anterior chamber of the eye (17,18). These investigators also observed that phosphodiesterase inhibitors potentiated this response.

We have examined the effects of derivatives of cyclic AMP and cyclic GMP on evoked and spontaneous electrical activity in slices of guinea pig hippocampus maintained, *in vitro*. 8-Br-Cyclic GMP (0.03–0.1 μM) increased duration of evoked potentials two- to three-fold and markedly increased the amount of spontaneous activity in the slices, and, in some it produced spontaneous epileptiform activity. In contrast, 8-Br-cyclic AMP (0.1–10 μM) always depressed evoked potentials and spontaneous activity. Isobutylmethylxanthine (100 μM) or concentrations of K^+ between 6 and 9 mM which simultaneously elevated endogenous tissue levels of cyclic GMP and depressed cyclic AMP, also increased the duration of evoked potentials and markedly increased spontaneous activity.

CONCLUSIONS

The data reviewed above leads to the following conclusion concerning the relationship between seizures and some biogenic amines. It appears that NE is clearly involved in those processes that are responsible for the expression of tonic seizures, and it seems to suppress the development of these seizures. It may be involved in other aspects or phases of seizures, but this is less certain at present. This anticonvulsant action of NE may be mediated by β-adrenergic receptors. Forebrain NE systems appear to predominate in the anticonvulsant action. The roles of DA, particularly in MES and PTZ seizures, are less obvious and presently available data do not establish its involvement conclusively. Serotonergic systems do, however, appear to have some influence on seizures and may suppress the development of seizures, as expressed by increased thresholds to MES. Adenosine may contribute to the postictal depression following generalized convulsions and may also have some inhibitory action on initiation and maintenance of seizure discharges.

Although there is insufficient information to make any definitive statement concerning the roles of cyclic AMP and cyclic GMP in pathophysiologic mechanisms of epilepsy, presently available data do allow the formation of the following hypothesis. There is much evidence implicating cyclic AMP as the mediator of neurotransmitter-evoked changes in neuronal activity. Adenosine and the biogenic amines have been shown to be inhibitory when iontophoresed in the vicinity of most central neurons and also to elevate markedly cyclic AMP levels in incubated brain slices. Iontophoretically applied cyclic AMP also causes hyperpolarization of many central neurons. In addition, cyclic AMP depresses electrical activity in incubated hippocampal slices. All these data are consistent with the hypothesis that cyclic AMP may be the "second messenger" for biogenic amines and/or adenosine, and may in fact be responsible for the inhibitory action of these compounds. Our studies demonstrate that both reduction of NE influence in CNS, probably at β-receptors, and blockade of adenosine receptors in CNS inhibit seizure-induced cyclic AMP elevations and concomitantly hasten the appearance of tonic seizures after PTZ injection (see above). Together these data suggest a close relationship between neurotransmitter actions, accumulation of cyclic AMP, and seizure activity. We suggest that seizure discharges cause a release, from intracellular stores, of biogenic amines and adenosine, and that these substances then act at synaptic sites to increase intracellular cyclic AMP levels. Cyclic AMP, in turn, may act at membranes to alter ion permeability, as well as having other actions. Elevated cyclic AMP levels in brain may thus have an antiepileptic effect and perhaps have some role in mechanisms inhibiting the spread and/or duration of seizure discharges.

Cyclic GMP, unlike cyclic AMP, has not been definitely linked to any individual neurotransmitter system, but it has been shown to be related to neuronal activity. Many stimuli that produce cellular depolarization elevate levels of cyclic GMP in brain. Moreover, cyclic GMP has

been shown to alter neuronal activity in nervous tissue. Phillis (33) reported that iontophoretic application of cyclic GMP onto unidentified cat cerebral cortex cells increased their firing rate by 51%. A similar percentage of rat pyramidal tract neurons were activated by iontophoretically applied cyclic GMP (38). More recently, it has been demonstrated that cyclic GMP can produce seizure discharges in hippocampal explants and increase electrical activity in hippocampal slices. These results are particularly intriguing and, in association with the data on the effects of seizure on cyclic GMP levels, suggest that cyclic GMP may be involved in mechanisms responsible for initiating and/or maintaining seizure discharges.

REFERENCES

1. Anderson, P. (1983): Physiological and chemical control of hippocampal neurones. In: *Neurotransmitter Interaction and Compartmentation*, edited by H. F. Bradford, pp. 601–616. Plenum Press, New York.
2. Benardo, L. S., and Prince, D. A. (1982): Dopamine action on hippocampal pyramidal cells. *J. Neurosci.*, 2(4):415–423.
3. Berti, F., Bernareggi, V., Folco, G. C., Fumagalli, R., and Paoletti, R. (1976): Prostaglandin E₂ and cyclic nucleotides in rat convulsions and tremors. In: *First and Second Messengers—New Vistas, Advances in Biochemical Psychopharmacology*, vol. 15, edited by E. Costa, E. Giacobini, and R. Paoletti, pp. 367–377. Raven Press, New York.
4. Chen, G., Ensor, C. R., and Bohner, B. (1954): A facilitation action of reserpine on the central nervous system. *Proc. Soc. Exp. Biol. Med.*, 86:507–510.
5. Dadkar, V. N., Dahanukar, S. A., and Sheth, N. K. (1979): Role of dopaminergic and noradrenergic mechanisms in metrazole convulsions in mice. *Indian J. Med. Res.*, 70:492–494.
6. Doteuchi, M., and Costa, E. (1973): Pentylenetetrazole convulsions and brain catecholamine turnover rate in rats and mice receiving diphenylhydantoin or benzodiazepines. *Neuropharmacology*, 12:1059–1072.
7. Dunwiddie, T. V., and Worth, T. (1982): Sedative and anticonvulsant effects of adenosine analogs in mouse and rat. *J. Pharmacol. Exp. Ther.*, 220:70–76.
8. Ferrendelli, J. A. (1976): Cellular depolarization and cyclic nucleotide content in central nervous system. In: *First and Second Messengers-New Vistas, Advances in Biochemical Psychopharmacology*, vol. 15, edited by E. Costa, E. Giacobini, and R. Paoletti, pp. 303–313. Raven Press, New York.
9. Ferrendelli, J. A., Blank, A. C., and Gross, R. A. (1980): Relationships between seizure ac-

tivity and cyclic nucleotide levels in brain. *Brain Res.*, 200:93–103.

10. Ferrendelli, J. A., and Kinscherf, D. A. (1977): Cyclic nucleotides in epileptic brain: Effects of pentylenetetrazol on regional cyclic AMP and cyclic GMP levels *in vivo. Epilepsia*, 18:525–531.

11. Ferrendelli, J. A., Rubin, E. H., and Kinscherf, D. A. (1976): Influence of divalent cations on regulation of cyclic GMP and cyclic AMP levels in brain tissue. *J. Neurochem.*, 264:741–748.

12. Folbergrova, J. (1975): Cyclic 3′, 5′-adenosine monophosphate in mouse cerebral cortex during homocysteine convulsions and their prevention by sodium phenobarbital. *Brain Res.*, 92:165–169.

13. Folbergrova, J. (1977): Changes of cyclic AMP and phosphorylase a in mouse cerebral cortex during seizures induced by 3-mercaptopropionic acid. *Brain Res.*, 135:337–346.

14. Freedman, R., Taylor, D. A., Seeger, A., Olson, L., and Hoffer, B. J. (1979): Seizures and related epileptiform activity in hippocampus transplanted to the anterior chambers of the eye: Modulation by cholinergic and adrenergic input. *Ann. Neurol.*, 6:281–295.

15. Gross, R. A., and Ferrendelli, J. A. (1979): Effects of reserpine, propranolol and aminophylline on seizure activity and CNS cyclic nucleotides. *Ann. Neurol.*, 6:296–301.

16. Gross, R. A., and Ferrendelli, J. A. (1982): Relationships between norepinephrine and cyclic nucleotides in brain seizure activity. *Neuropharmacology*, 21:655–661.

17. Hoffer, B., Seiger, A., Freedman, R., Olson, L., and Taylor, D. (1977): Electrophysiology and cytology of hippocampal formation transplants in the anterior chamber of the eye. II. Cholinergic mechanisms. *Brain Res.*, 119:108–132.

18. Hoffer, B. J., Seiger, A., Taylor, D., Olson, L., and Freeman, R. (1977): Seizures and related epileptiform activity in hippocampus transplanted to the anterior chamber of the eye. I. Characterization of seizures, interictal spikes, and synchronous activity. *Exp. Neurol.*, 54:233–250.

19. Jobe, P. C., Picchioni, A. L., and Chin, L. (1973): Role of brain norepinephrine in audiogenic seizure in the rat. *J. Pharmacol. Exp. Ther.*, 184:1–10.

20. Kilian, M., and Frey, H. H. (1973): Central monoamines and convulsive thresholds in mice and rats. *Neuropharmacology* 12:681–692.

21. Kleinrok, Z., Czuczwar, S. J., Kozicka, M., and Zarkowski, A. (1981): Effect of combined GABA-ergic and dopaminergic stimulation on the action of some antiepileptic drugs in pentylenetetrazol-induced convulsions. *Pol. J. Pharmacol. Pharm.*, 33:13–23.

22. Kleinrok, F., Czuczwar, S., Wojak, A., and Przegalinski, E. (1978): On certain effects of dopaminergic agents in pentylenetetrazol convulsions. *Acta Physiol. Pharmacol. Bulg.*, 4:50–55.

23. Lazarova, M. B., and Roussinov, K. S. (1978): On certain effects of dopaminergic agents in pentylenetetrazol convulsions. *Acta Physiol. Pharmacol. Bulg.*, 4:50–55.

24. Lust, W. D., Goldberg, N. D., and Passonneau, J. V. (1976): Cyclic nucleotides in murine brain: The temporal relationship of changes induced in adenosine 3′,5′-monophosphate and guanosine 3′-5′-monophosphate following maximal electroshock or decapitation. *J. Neurochem.*, 26:5–10.

25. Lust, W. D., Kupferberg, H. J., Yonekawa, W. D., Penry, J. K., Passonneau, J. V., and Wheaton, A. B. (1978): Changes in brain metabolites induced by convulsants or electroshock: Effects of anticonvulsant agents. *Mol. Pharmacol.*, 14:347–356.

26. Maitre, M., Ciesielski, L., Lehmann, A., Kempf, E., and Mandel, P. (1974): Protective effect of adenosine and nicotinamide against audiogenic seizures. *Biochem. Pharmacol.*, 23:2807–2816.

27. Mao, C. C., Guidotti, A., and Costa, E. (1974): The regulation of cyclic guanosine monophosphate in rat cerebellum: Possible involvement of putative amino acid neurotransmitters. *Brain Res.*, 79:510–514.

28. Mao, C. C., Guidotti, A., and Costa, E. (1975): Evidence for an involvement of GABA in the mediation of the cerebellar cGMP decrease and the anticonvulsant action of diazepam.

29. Mason, S. T., and Corcoran, M. E. (1978): Forebrain noradrenaline and metrazol-induced seizures. *Life Sci.*, 23:167–172.

30. Mason, S. T., and Corcoran, M. E. (1979): Seizure susceptibility after depletion of spinal or cerebellar noradrenalin with 6-OHDA. *Brain Res.*, 166:418–421.

31. Mueller, A. L., Kirk, K. L., Hoffer, B. J., and Dunwiddie, T. V. (1982): Noradrenergic responses in rat hippocampus: Electrophysiological actions of direct- and indirect-acting sympathomimetics in the *in vitro* slice. *J. Pharmacol. Exp. Ther.*, 223:599–605.

32. Palmer, G. C., Jones, D. J., Medina, M. A., and Stavinoha, W. B. (1979): Anticonvulsant drug actions on *in vitro* and *in vivo* levels of cyclic AMP in the mouse brain. *Epilepsia*, 29:95–104.

33. Phillis, J. W. (1974): Evidence for cholinergic transmission in the cerebral cortex. *Adv. Behav. Biol.*, 10:57–77.

34. Phillis, J. W., and Wu, P. H. (1981): The role of adenosine and its nucleotides in central synaptic transmission. *Prog. Neurobiol.*, 16:187–239.

35. Raabe, W., Nicol, S., Gumnit, R. J., and Goldberg, N. D. (1978): Focal penicillin epilepsy increases cyclic GMP in cerebral cortex. *Brain Res.*, 144:185–188.

36. Rehncrona, S., Siesjo, B. K., and Westerberg, E. (1978): Adenosine and cyclic AMP in cerebral cortex of rats in hypoxia, status epilepticus and hypercapnia. *Acta Physiol. Scand.*, 104:453–463.

37. Sattin, A. (1971): Increase in the content of adenosine 3′.5′-monophosphate in mouse forebrain during seizures and prevention of the increase by methylxanthines. *J. Neurochem.*, 18:1087–1096.

38. Stone, T. W., Taylor, D. A., and Bloom, F. E.

(1975): Cyclic AMP and cyclic GMP may mediate opposite neuronal responses in the rat cerebral cortex. *Science,* 187:845–847.

39. Walker, J. E., Lewin, E., Sheppard, J. R., and Cromwell, R. (1973): Enzymatic regulation of adenosine 3′,5′-monophosphate (cyclic AMP) in the freezing epileptogenic lesion of rat brain and in homologous contralateral cortex. *J. Neurochem.,* 21:79–85.

40. Wenger, G. R., Stitzel, R. E., and Craig, C. R. (1973): The role of biogenic amines in the reserpine-induced alteration of minimal electroshock seizure thresholds in the mouse. *Neuropharmacology,* 12:693–703.

Advances in Neurology, Vol. 44, edited by
A. V. Delgado-Escueta, A. A. Ward, Jr.,
D. M. Woodbury, and R. J. Porter.
Raven Press, New York © 1986.

20

Long-Term Potentiation and Kindling: Similar Biochemical Mechanisms?

Michel Baudry

Department of Psychobiology, University of California at Irvine, California 92717

SUMMARY For years, the hypotheses concerning the physiological mechanisms of epilepsy and spreading depression have implicated failures in inhibitory mechanisms and, in particular, GABA-mediated responses. More recent experiments have focused on the participation of excitatory neurotransmitters and especially on glutamate-mediated responses in order to account for the long-lasting changes in the excitability of neurons found in epilepsy. Evidence supporting this view has been provided by the fact that two different types of manipulation resulting in long-lasting changes in synaptic excitability, namely kindling and long-term potentiation (LTP) of synaptic transmission, result in modification of excitatory amino acid receptors. Kindling represents the progressive development of generalized seizures generated by repeated low levels of electrical stimulation of various limbic structures, and is generally accepted as a good model of epilepsy; it is associated with an increase in excitatory mechanisms and, in particular, with an increase in the number of glutamate binding sites that are presumed to represent a category of glutamate receptors. Similarly, LTP is elicited by brief bursts of electrical stimulation in monosynaptic excitatory pathways and is also associated with an increase in the number of the same type of glutamate binding sites. The present review compares the similarities between these two long-lasting forms of synaptic plasticity, and proposes that similar biochemical mechanism might underlie the changes in glutamate receptors. In addition, it describes a molecular mechanism that involves a calcium-dependent protease associated with postsynaptic membranes, the activation of which results in the unmasking of glutamate receptors. Moreover, since this mechanism has been recently implicated in the storage of some types of information in the mammalian telencephalon, these studies raise the possibility that epilepsy may represent a dangerous side-effect of an efficacious learning mechanism.

Since its discovery in 1968 by Goddard (34), the kindling phenomenon has been widely used as a model to study the physiological, cellular, and molecular mechanisms related to human epilepsy (74). Thus, it was found that kindling is associated with an enhancement of monosynaptically evoked responses as well as a general increase in cell excitability in various regions of the brain depending on the sites of the stimulation selected to induce it (59). The former correlate of kindling in turn resembles the long-term potentiation (LTP) of synaptic transmission which follows bursts of high-frequency stimulation, initially discovered in 1974 by Bliss and Lomo (16) in the hippocampal formation and, more recently, in various circuits of the limbic system (60). LTP has received considerable attention because it is generally considered as a plausible mechanism used by the brain to store information and therefore to play a role in learning and memory (71). In addition, the effect can be elicited in the *in vitro* hippocampal slice preparation, allowing multidisciplinary approaches at the anatomical, electrophysiological, and biochemical levels (49). Thus, it seems that investigations of the mechanisms underlying the LTP effect can provide valuable information regarding first the kindling phenomenon and ultimately epilepsy. The idea that the emergence of a very efficient learning and memory mechanism was accompanied by the increase in likelihood of certain types of dysfunctions—epilepsy being one of them—will be developed in this chapter.

Because a key component of our work on LTP involves the synaptic receptor of various hippocampal pathways, the first part of this chapter will describe our efforts to characterize, classify, and quantify the different classes of excitatory amino acid receptors in hippocampus. In the second part, we will discuss the regulation of glutamate receptor binding by calcium ions, which involves a complex sequence of biochemical events, and then compare various properties of the LTP and kindling phenomena in order to discuss the possibility that they share similar biochemical mechanisms. Finally, we will propose some new ideas concerning the mechanisms of epilepsy, in particular the idea that epilepsy represents a side-effect of the learning and memory processes.

CLASSIFICATION AND PROPERTIES OF EXCITATORY RECEPTORS IN HIPPOCAMPUS

Although the evidence is fairly convincing that glutamate is the major excitatory neurotransmitter in various hippocampal pathways (69), definite conclusion has been hampered by the lack of a satisfactory description of the multiple receptors for excitatory amino acids and the lack of selective and specific agonists and antagonists. Based on physiological studies performed mainly on the spinal cord, Watkins and Evans (75) proposed the existence of three different classes of excitatory amino acid receptors: an *N*-methyl-D-aspartic acid (NMDA) receptor, preferentially stimulated by NMDA and blocked by D-α-aminoadipate and related compounds, a kainate receptor and a quisqualate receptor. Binding studies performed in several laboratories have indicated the existence of L-glutamate, L-aspartate, and kainate binding sites

with pharmacological properties distinct from those of the sites identified in electrophysiological studies (10,11,15,23,25,53,66). Because most of these studies involved different brain structures as well as different preparations, we decided to reinvestigate this question using various experimental approaches restricted to the hippocampus.

Physiological Studies

Antidromic and orthodromic electrical stimulation of the CA_1 pyramidal cells results in changes in extracellular field potentials, which can be easily quantified in the *in vitro* hippocampal slice preparation. The effects of bath-applied amino acid agonists or antagonists on this physiological response were used to classify the various populations of excitatory amino acid receptors in this preparation. Early in our research, we made the striking observation that, upon successive applications of L-glutamate, the decrease in evoked field potentials induced by millimolar concentrations of the amino acid exhibited a marked apparent desensitization, without a corresponding decrease in field potentials evoked by either orthodromic or antidromic stimulation (27). This apparent desensitization to the depolarizing effect of L-glutamate was not simply a nonspecific effect since neither the evoked potentials nor the physiological responses to other agonists such as kainate or D,L-homocysteate were altered. This suggested therefore that L-glutamate applied in the bath was stimulating a receptor different from the receptor activated by the endogenous neurotransmitter. This interpretation was reinforced by the finding that two antagonists which totally blocked synaptic transmission (D,L-α-aminoadipate and D,L-amino phosphonobutyrate) did not inhibit the L-glutamate-induced depolarization (28). An apparent desensitization was also obtained upon successive applications of D-glutamate, L-aspartate, or *N*-methyl-aspartate (NMA), but not of kainate of D,L-homocysteate. These observations thus provided a first subdivision of excitatory amino acids between those that exhibited the desensitization phenomenon and those that did not.

A second subdivision was provided by the differential blocking effects of two antagonists on the depolarizing effects of various excitatory amino acids. Thus, α-aminoadipate blocked the responses to *N*-methyl-aspartate, D-glutamate, or D,L-homocysteate, but not to L-glutamate or kainate. In addition, aminophosphonobutyrate blocked the responses to D,L-homocysteate, but not to *N*-methyl-aspartate, L-glutamate or kainate. In order to account for this collection of observations, a minimum of four receptor classes was needed; the classes were designated as follows:

1. A G_1 receptor that does not exhibit the desensitization phenomenon, that is stimulated preferentially by D,L-homocysteate, and that is blocked by both α-amino adipate and D,L-aminophosphonobutyrate.
2. A G_2 receptor that exhibits the desensitization phenomenon, is stimulated by L-glutamate, and is not blocked by α-aminoadipate and D,L-aminophosphonobutyrate.
3. An NMA receptor that exhibits the desensitization phenomenon, is stimulated by NMA and is blocked by α-aminoadipate.
4. A kainate receptor, that does not exhibit the desensitization phenomenon, is stimulated by kainate, and is not blocked by α-aminoadipate or aminophosphonobutyrate.

Because the synaptic receptor does not desensitize and is blocked by α-aminoadipate and aminophosphonobutyrate, it appears to be similar to the G_1 receptor, whereas the other three classes of receptors seem to represent extrasynaptic receptors.

Biochemical Studies

Confirmation of the classification of excitatory amino acid receptors into four classes was provided by the analysis of the properties of these receptors studied by the measurement of amino acid-induced stimulation of Na^+ efflux in hippocampal slices previously loaded with ^{22}Na, using a technique previously described by Luini et al. in striatal slices (44). We first confirmed the existence of the desensitization phenomenon for a number of excitatory amino acids; we then confirmed the differential blockade by α-aminoadipate of the effects of various amino acids. Moreover, the order of potency of a large number of excitatory amino acids determined by the Na efflux rate method closely paralleled that for their depolarizing effects, suggesting that most of these compounds induce depolarization by opening sodium channels (5).

By combining lesion experiments and pharmacological experiments, we obtained evidence for a presynaptic localization of at least part of the NMA and kainate types of receptors, whereas the G_1 and G_2 receptors seemed to represent mainly postsynaptic receptors (6). In addition, the G_2 receptors were shown to exhibit the phenomenon of supersensitivity either following lesions of afferent systems to the hippocampus or during the postnatal developmental period, suggesting that, as at the neuromuscular junction, the distribution of transmitter receptors can be dramatically altered in the central nervous system (CNS) depending on the state of activity of the target cells (6).

Binding Studies of Excitatory Amino Acid Receptors

Stimulated by the successful studies of a variety of receptors with binding techniques, various experimenters have tried to use various ligands to analyze excitatory amino acid receptors. Three classes of sites have been clearly identified with three different ligands: (a) a [³H]kainate binding site; (b) a [³H]L-glutamate binding site; and (c) a [³H]L-aspartate binding site (10,11,15,23,25,53,66). With the exception of the kainate site, none of these sites seems to correspond to any of the receptors defined by the electrophysiological studies of Watkins et al. In particular, despite intensive efforts, an NMDA site has never been detected in membrane preparation with any radiolabeled ligand, with the exception of a single brief report (67). As mentioned above, the characterization of the properties of the [³H]L-glutamate binding sites in hippocampal membranes offered a unique opportunity to compare these sites with the physiological receptors defined in hippocampal slices. This comparison strongly suggests that the [³H]L-glutamate binding site is associated with the G_1 postsynaptic transmitter receptor.

Ionic Sensitivity

Although the binding of [³H]L-glutamate to this site is independent of the presence of sodium ions, low concentrations of this cation result in a marked inhibition of the binding (8). This effect is relatively specific since sodium is 10 times more potent than lithium and almost 100 times more potent than potassium. By analogy with other neurotransmitter receptors associated with ionic channels [e.g., GABA and glycine with chloride (54,78)], we proposed that this inhibition of [³H]L-glutamate binding by sodium results from the association of a recognition site for glutamate and a sodium conductance channel in the glutamate receptor complex, and that the presence of sodium modifies the properties of the recognition site. As mentioned above, the G_1 site is indeed associated with a sodium conductance channel.

Localization

The developmental pattern as well as the subcellular localization of the [³H]L-glutamate binding sites fit with a synaptic localization (3, 29). Moreover, lesion of major afferent pathways to the hippocampus failed to induce a decrease in the number of these binding sites, suggesting a postsynaptic localization (6). A detailed regional distribution of the binding sites in rabbit hippocampus also indicated a preferential association with dendritic structures rather than with cell bodies (50).

Pharmacological Pattern

The order of potency for various excitatory amino acids to inhibit [³H]glutamate binding to hippocampal membranes (quisqualate > ibotenate > D,L-homocysteate > L-glutamate > L-aspartate > D-glutamate > D-aspartate) suggests that the site is associated with a receptor that preferentially recognizes the extended configuration of L-glutamate analogs, which is again compatible with the G_1 site (10). This idea is confirmed by the fact that α-aminoadipate and α-aminophosphonobutyrate, two blockers at the G_1 site, are able to inhibit glutamate binding site at micromolar concentrations, whereas NMA and kainate as well as glutamate diethylester are very poor inhibitors of the binding (10).

Thus, in terms of ionic sensitivity, localization, and pharmacological pattern, the [³H]L-glutamate binding sites in hippocampal membranes seem to be indistinguishable from the G_1 receptor evidenced by physiological and biochemical studies. The only paradoxical finding is that bath-applied L-glutamate does not activate the G_1 synaptic receptor, whereas [³H]L-glutamate can bind with high affinity to this site in isolated membranes, in the absence of sodium. However, in the presence of sodium (the situation normally occurring in physiological studies) no binding can be detected, suggesting that the effect of sodium is to shift the receptor allosterically towards a different configuration that exhibits a very low affinity for L-glutamate, and therefore cannot be detected with the binding technique. This, in association with the existence of very efficient uptake systems for glutamate, might well explain why exogenously-applied L-glutamate would not be able to reach the synaptic receptors at concentrations high enough to activate them, whereas endogenously-released glutamate might.

Thus, the [³H]glutamate binding site is likely to be a recognition site associated with the post-synaptic transmitter receptor in hippocampus; therefore, it is of considerable interest to study mechanisms implicated in the regulation of its properties.

REGULATION OF [³H]GLUTAMATE BINDING BY CALCIUM AND ITS MECHANISM

Although monovalent cations markedly inhibited [³H]L-glutamate to hippocampal membranes, several divalent cations were found to increase ³H-glutamate binding (8). In particular, calcium ions stimulated the binding two- to three fold, with an apparent EC_{50} of about 30 μM and a maximal effect at calcium concentration of 100–200 μM. The effect of calcium was strongly cooperative, with an apparent Hill coefficient of about 2.0. Manganese and strontium also stimulated [³H]glutamate binding, although higher concentrations were required; barium, magnesium, copper and iron were ineffective. The increase in binding was the result of an increase in the maximal number of sites without changes in the apparent affinity for glutamate; in addition, the pharmacological profile of the binding was similar in the presence or absence of calcium ions. These results indicated that the effect of calcium was to unmask binding sites normally present in the membranes and either inaccessible to the ligand or present under a configuration with a different affinity for glutamate and therefore normally not detected with the binding technique. Several arguments indicated that the stimulatory effect of calcium on the binding was not simply an ionic interaction but rather the result of a complex, enzymatically mediated chain of events. First, the effect of calcium was absent at temperatures below 20°C and was maximal at 37°C (13). The effect was also absent in membranes prepared from neonatal rat, and appeared between postnatal day 11 and 18 (3). Treatment of membranes with low concentrations of the detergent Triton X-100 resulted in the loss of the stimulatory effect of calcium (13). Finally, the effect of calcium was irreversible. After preincubation of membranes with calcium, calcium was removed by either dilution and centrifugation or by chelation with the calcium chelator EGTA; under these conditions, glutamate binding was still higher than in control membranes (7,8). By chelating calcium at various times after the start of the incubation, the time-course of the stimulatory effect of calcium on glutamate binding was found to be very rapid, being half-maximal at 1 min and maximal at about 5 min (7). All of these observations suggested that calcium stimulated a calcium-dependent enzyme present in the membrane preparation, the activation of which was responsible for the unmasking of glutamate binding sites. An important clue concerning the identity of this enzyme was provided by the finding that inhibitors of calcium-dependent thiol-proteinases totally prevented the calcium-induced increase in glutamate binding without altering basal glutamate binding (4,9). In particular, the relatively selective and potent thiol-proteinase inhibitor leupeptin (72), induced a dose-dependent inhibition of calcium stimulation of glutamate binding, with half-maximal inhibition obtained at about 20 μM and maximal inhibition at 80 μM (4,73). By adding leupeptin at various time intervals after starting incubation of membranes with calcium, we obtained a second determination of the time-course for the calcium stimulation of glutamate binding that was in very good agreement with that obtained with EGTA (7). Acquisition of further information concerning this mechanism required the identification of both the postulated calcium-dependent proteinase and its substrates.

Calcium-dependent proteinases had previously been studied and identified in cytosolic fractions of several tissues (35,56,58); recently, two forms of these enzymes have been characterized; one requiring micromolar calcium concentrations for activity was designated as calpain I, whereas the other, which required millimolar calcium concentrations, was called calpain II (24,31,51,56). Further studies have shown that these two enzymes differ in their MW and are immunologically distinct (52,70). By extracting synaptic plasma membranes in low ionic strength buffer, and separating the extracted material by ion-exchange chromatography, we obtained evidence that synaptic plasma membranes also possessed two forms of calcium-dependent proteinase activities differing in their calcium requirements. Comparing various properties of these two forms of proteinase activity with those of calpain I and II provided further evidence that synaptic plasma membranes contained these two enzymes, which appeared to be loosely associated with the membrane, quite possibly as part of the cytoskeleton (64).

Various laboratories have reported that endogenous substrates of calcium-dependent proteinase are proteins associated with the cytoskeleton of various cells. Thus, microtubule-associated protein 2 (MAP$_2$), neurofilament proteins, and tubulin have been shown to be degraded upon the addition of calcium, in a leupeptin-sensitive manner (37,58,79). By incubating synaptic plasma membranes in the presence of calcium and separating the different proteins by sodium dodecyl sulfate (SDS) gel electrophoresis, we showed that a high MW protein with an apparent MW of 240,000 daltons was also degraded in a leupeptin-sensitive manner (4). Because its migratory properties were similar to those of a protein called fodrin by Levine and Willard (40) and brain spectrin by a variety of researchers (14,18,22,32), we used various experimental approaches to determine that fodrin was indeed an endogenous substrate for calpain. First, we isolated calpain from rat erythrocytes and fodrin from rat brain and showed that purified fodrin was rapidly degraded in the presence of calpain and calcium, this degradation being totally blocked by the calpain inhibitor leupeptin (65).

Radiolabeling fodrin by reducing methylation enabled us to determine the apparent K_m of fodrin for calpain, about 50 nM, indicating the high affinity of fodrin for calpain, in the range of other substrates for this enzyme (79). Endogenous fodrin present in synaptic plasma membranes was also similarly degraded by isolated calpain from rat erythrocytes. Erythrocyte spectrin was also found to be a substrate for calpain, strengthening the similarities between spectrin and fodrin. In fact, the similarities between spectrin and fodrin have been the subject of extensive investigation. Both proteins consist of two subunits, α and β, with MW of 245,000–240,000, organized as a tetramer $(\alpha\beta)_2$ and exhibiting a high percentage of α-helicity; the α-subunits of both proteins are very closely related, since antibodies to α-spectrin cross-react with α-fodrin and their peptide maps are very similar (14,19,31,32). Both spectrin and fodrin bind actin and calmodulin and induce the gelation of F-actin (18,20,68). Finally, both proteins are involved in the capping of cell surface receptors in a variety of cell types (41,57). This latter property is interesting in view of the role of calcium and calpain in the regulation of glutamate receptor binding. Thus, we proposed that the calcium-induced degradation of fodrin through the activation of calpain is responsible for the unmasking of glutamate receptors either present in the membranes but inaccessible to the ligand, or present in the membrane under a configuration with a low-affinity for glutamate and therefore not measurable with the binding technique (45). In fact, considering the role of the cytoskeleton in the regulation of cell shape (21,61), we speculated that the function of this calcium-dependent proteinase associated with the cytoskeleton in a variety of cell types was to regulate not only the distribution of cell surface receptors but also the shape of the cell (in particular the shape of dendritic spines in neurons).

SIMILARITIES BETWEEN LTP AND KINDLING

As mentioned, kindling is associated with a long-term enhancement of synaptic responses quite similar to the LTP of synaptic efficacy obtained following brief bursts of high-frequency stimulation. Several types of experimental evidence suggest the possibility that kindling and LTP share similar cellular and biochemical mechanisms (Table 1). First, kindling and LTP are easily induced in limbic structures, but are rarely found in nontelencephalic structures (60). During postnatal development, LTP in the hippocampus is not observed before 10–12 days after birth (3), the time at which kindling also starts to develop (30). Once kindling is established in a given structure, it is not possible to induce LTP by brief bursts of high-frequency stimulation, indicating that these two processes are therefore nonadditive (60). Conversely, convulsant drugs such as picrotoxin facilitate the establishment of LTP (77). At the biochemical level, we showed that LTP in hippocampal slices is accompanied by an increase in the number of glutamate binding sites in synaptic membranes prepared from the stimulated slices; this increase in binding does not occur if the stimulation is performed under conditions preventing the establishment of LTP (such as low Ca^{2+}, high Mg^{2+}), or if the stimulation does not result in LTP (12,47). Because the establishment of LTP is critically dependent on the calcium concentration in the medium (26) and, more important because LTP can be blocked by the intracellular injection of the calcium chelator EGTA (48), we proposed that the high-frequency stimulation results in an influx of calcium in the postsynaptic cell, the activation of calpain inducing the degradation of fodrin, and finally in an increase in the number of glutamate receptors (45). The same mechanisms could also be responsible for the rounding of dendritic spines that has been found to accompany LTP both *in vivo* and *in vitro* (38,39). Kindling the entorhinal cortex in rats has been similarly shown to be accompanied by an increased number of glutamate binding sites in hippocampal synaptic membranes (63). Moreover, the calcium-induced stimulation of [³H]glutamate binding was reduced in hippocampal membranes from kindled rats, suggesting that the kindling-induced increase in binding is caused by the calcium stimulation of glutamate binding.

Thus, it is tempting to propose that in both LTP and kindling, repeated episodes of synaptic stimulation result in an influx of calcium in postsynaptic cells, an activation of calcium-dependent proteinase, the resulting degradation of fodrin, and the unmasking of glutamate receptors and eventually structural changes in dendritic spines. The main difference between kindling and LTP is that, in addition to enhancement of synaptic responses, kindling is accompanied by a general increase in cell excitability. Although the cellular basis for this increase in cell excitability is not understood, it is generally believed to result from a change in inhibitory mechanisms, possibly from changes in GABA receptors or in the relationships between GABA receptors and their associated "benzodiazepine" recognition sites (59). Considering that so little is known on the regulation of this complex association, it is possible that the same mechanisms previously discussed also modify the distribution or properties of other cell surface receptors and in particular of the GABA receptor-benzodiazepine receptors.

CONCLUSION: IS EPILEPSY A MALADAPTIVE SIDE-EFFECT OF A LEARNING MECHANISM?

It thus seems that a reasonable case can be made that kindling and LTP share similar cellular and biochemical mechanisms. If this is true, what kind of implications can we make concerning the relationships between learning— an obviously adaptive plastic property of the nervous system—and epilepsy, an obvious maladaptive property? Although it has not yet clearly been demonstrated that LTP plays a role in learning and memory, there are several suggestive indications. For example, during the learning of the classical conditioning response of the rabbit eyelid nictitating membranes, Thompson and associates have showed the development of a between-trial increase in the evoked perforant path to dentate granule cell response (76). Similarly, Carol Barnes has used various experimental approaches to provide evidence that LTP occurred as a result of a learning experience (2). Various groups have also described improvement or impairment of learning elicited by the establishment of LTP before or after the learning episode (see Morris and Baker, ref. 55 for a review). On the other hand, a wealth of publications has documented the

TABLE 1. *Comparison of various properties of LTP and kindling*

LTP	Kindling
Long-lasting increase in synaptic transmission	Long-term enhancement of synaptic transmission
Convulsant drugs enhance LTP	LTP does not occur following kindling
Primarily found in limbic structures	Primarily found in limbic structures
Develops after postnatal days 10–12	Develops after postnatal days 10–12
Is accompanied by an increase in number of glutamate receptor binding sites	Is accompanied by an increase in number of glutamate receptor binding sites

LTP, long-term potentiation.

utility of kindling as a model for the study of the processes resulting in human epilepsy (74). Moreover, epilepsy is often associated with impairments of learning and memory (43). It is thus possible to advance the hypothesis that epilepsy is associated with a disturbance in the normal learning processes such that instead of strengthening synaptic connections, repetitive episodes of neuronal activity result in abnormal enhanced cell excitability, leading to seizure development and progressive pathological damages such as loss of dendritic spines.

The increase in glutamate receptors produced by both LTP and kindling can be used to test the proposed linkages between the two physiological phenomenon; e.g., it would be particularly useful to determine if both utilize the calcium-dependent proteinase mechanism described above. If successful, these experiments would point the way to a novel type of pharmacology that might be of great value in the control of epilepsy. Moreover, they would reinforce the hypothesis that epilepsy represents a perturbation of cellular processes normally associated with neuronal and behavioral plasticity.

ACKNOWLEDGMENTS

This research was supported by National Science Foundation grant No. BNS-81-12156-01. The author wishes to express his profound gratitude to G. Lynch, whose constant friendship and support made this work an exciting endeavor.

REFERENCES

1. Anderson, D. R., Davis, J. L., and Carraway, K. L. (1977): Calcium-promoted changes of the human erythrocyte membrane. Involvement of spectrin, transglutaminase and a membrane-bound protease. *J. Biol. Chem.*, 252:6617–6623.
2. Barnes, C. A. (1979): Memory deficits associated with senescence: A neurophysiological and behavioral study in the rat. *J. Comp. Phys. Psychol.*, 93:74–104.
3. Baudry, M., Arst, D., Oliver, M., and Lynch, G. (1981): Development of glutamate binding sites and their regulation by calcium in rat hippocampus. *Dev. Brain Res.*, 1:37–48.
4. Baudry, M., Bundman, M., Smith, E., and Lynch, G. (1981): Micromolar levels of calcium stimulate proteolytic activity and glutamate receptor binding in rat brain synaptic membranes. *Science*, 212:937–938.
5. Baudry, M., Kramer, K., Fagni, L., Recasens, M., and Lynch, G. (1983): Classification and properties of excitatory amino acid receptor in hippocampus. II. Biochemical studies using the sodium efflux assay. *Mol. Pharmacol.*, 24:222–228.
6. Baudry, M., Kramer, K., and Lynch, G. (1983): Classification and properties of acidic amino acid receptors in hippocampus. III. Supersensitivity during the post-natal period and following denervation. *Mol. Pharmacol.*, 24:229–234.
7. Baudry, M., Kramer, K., and Lynch, G. (1983): Irreversibility and time-course of the calcium stimulation of ^{3}H-glutamate binding to rat hippocampal membranes. *Brain Res.*, 270:142–145.
8. Baudry, M., and Lynch, G. (1979): Regulation of glutamate receptors by cations. *Nature*, 282:748–750.
9. Baudry, M., and Lynch, G. (1980): Regulation of hippocampal glutamate receptors: Evidence for the involvement of a calcium-activated protease. *Proc. Natl. Acad. Sci. USA*, 77:2298–2302.
10. Baudry, M., and Lynch, G. (1981): Characterization of two ^{3}H-glutamate binding sites in rat hippocampal membranes. *J. Neurochem.*, 36(3):811–820.
11. Baudry, M., and Lynch, G. (1981): Hippocampal glutamate receptors. *Mol. Cell. Biochem.* 38:5–18.
12. Baudry, M., Oliver, M., Creager, R., Wieraszko, A., and Lynch, G. (1980): Increase in glutamate receptors following repetitive electrical stimulation in hippocampal slices. *Life Sci.*, 27:325–330.
13. Baudry, M., Smith, E., and Lynch, G. (1981): Influences of temperature, detergents and enzymes on glutamate receptor binding and its regulation by calcium in rat hippocampal membranes. *Mol. Pharmacol.*, 20:280–286.
14. Bennet, V., Davis, J., and Fowler, W. E. (1982): Brain spectrin, a membrane-associated protein related in structure and function to erythrocyte spectrin. *Nature*, 299:126–131.
15. Biziere, U., Thompson, H., and Coyle, J. T. (1980): Characterization of specific high-affinity

binding sites for L-^{3}H-glutamic acid in rat brain membranes. *Brain Res.*, 183:421–433.

16. Bliss, T. V. P., and Lomo, T. (1973): Long-lasting potentiation of synaptic transmission in the dentate area of the anaesthetized rabbit following stimulation of the perforant path. *J. Physiol.* (*Lond.*), 232:331–356.

17. Branton, D., Cohen, C. M., and Tyler, J. (1981): Interaction of cytoskeletal proteins on the human erythrocyte membrane. *Cell*, 24:24–32.

18. Brenner, S. L., and Korn, E. D. (1979): Spectrin-actin interaction: Phosphorylated and dephosphorylated spectrin tetramer cross-link F-actin. *J. Biol. Chem.*, 254:8620–8627.

19. Burridge, K., Kelly, T., and Mangeat, P. (1982): Nonerythrocyte spectrins: Actin-membrane attachment proteins occurring in many cell types. *J. Cell Biol.*, 95:478–486.

20. Carlin, R. K., Bartelt, D. C., and Siekevitz, P. (1983): Identifications of fodrin as a major calmodulin-binding protein in postsynaptic density preparations. *J. Cell Biol.*, 96:443–448.

21. Crick, F. (1982): *Do dendritic* spines twitch. *Trends Neurosci.*, 5:44–46.

22. Davis, J., and Bennett, V. (1983): Brain spectrin. Isolation of subunits and formation of hybrids with erythrocytes spectrin subunits. *J. Biol. Chem.*, 258:7757–7766.

23. De Barry, J., Vincendon, G., and Gombos, G. (1980): High affinity glutamate binding during postnatal development of rat cerebellum. *FEBS Lett.*, 109:175–179.

24. De Martino, G. N. (1981): Calcium-dependent proteolytic activity in rat liver: Identification of two proteases with different calcium requirements. *Arch. Biochem. Biophys.*, 211:253–257.

25. DiLauro, A., Meek, J. L., and Costa, E. (1982): Specific high-affinity binding of L-^{3}H-aspartate to rat brain membranes. *J. Neurochem.*, 38:1261–1267.

26. Dunwiddie, T. V., and Lynch G. (1979): The relationship between extracellular calcium concentrations and the induction of hippocampal long-term potentiation. *Brain Res.*, 169:103–110.

27. Fagni, L., Baudry, M., and Lynch, G. (1983): Desensitization to glutamate does not affect synaptic transmission in rat hippocampal slices. *Brain Res.*, 261:167–171.

28. Fagni, L., Baudry, M., and Lynch, G. (1983): Classification and properties of excitatory amino acid receptors in hippocampus. I. Electrophysiological studies of an apparent desensitization and interactions with drugs which block transmission. *J. Neurosci.* 3:1538–1546.

29. Foster, A., Mena, E., Fagg, G., and Cotman, C. (1981): Glutamate and aspartate binding sites are enriched in synaptic junctions isolated from rat brain. *J. Neurosci.*, 1:620–626.

30. Gilbert, M. E., and Cain, D. P. (1981): A developmental study of kindling in the rat. *Dev. Brain Res.*, 2:321–328.

31. Glenney, J. R., Glenney, P., Osborn, M., and Weber, K. (1982): An F-actin and calmodulin-binding protein from isolated intestinal brush borders has a morphology related to spectrin. *Cell*, 28:843–854.

32. Glenney, J. R., Glenney, P., and Weber, K. (1982): Erythroid spectrin, brain fodrin, and intestinal brush border proteins (TW-260/240) are related molecules containing a common calmodulin-binding subunit bound to a variant cell-type-specific subunit. *Proc. Natl. Acad. Sci. USA*, 79:4002–4005.

33. Goddard, G. V., and Douglas, R. M. (1976): Does the engram of kindling model the engram of normal long-term memory? In: *Kindling*, edited by A. J. Wada, pp. 1–18. Raven Press, New York.

34. Goddard, G. V., McIntyre, D. C., and Leech, C. U. (1969): A permanent change in brain function resulting from daily electrical stimulation. *Exp. Neurol.*, 25:295–330.

35. Guroff, G. (1964): A neutral, calcium-activated proteinase from the soluble fraction of rat brain. *J. Biol. Chem.*, 239:149–155.

36. Kishimoto, A., Kajikawa, J., Tabuchi, J., Shiota, M., and Nishizuka, Y. (1981): Calcium-dependent neutral proteases, widespread occurrence of a species of protease active a lower concentrations of calcium. *J. Biochem.*, 90:889–892.

37. Klein, I., Lehotay, D., and Godek, M. (1981): Characterization of a calcium-activated protease that hydrolyzes a microtubule-associated protein. *Arch. Biochem. Biophys.*, 208:520–527.

38. Lee, K., Schottler, F., Oliver, M., and Lynch, G. (1980): Brief bursts of high-frequency stimulation produce two types of structural change in rat hippocampus. *J. Neurophysiol.*, 44:247–258.

39. Lee, K., Oliver, M., Schottler, F., and Lynch, G. (1981): Electron microscopic studies of brain slices: The effects of high frequency stimulation on dendritic ultrastructure. In: *Electrical Activity in Isolated Mammalian CNS Preparations*, edited by G. Kerkut, pp. 189–212. Academic Press, Orlando, Fla.

40. Levine, J., and Willard, J. (1981): Fodrin: Axonally transported polypeptides associated with the internal periphery of many cells. *J. Cell Biol.*, 90:631–643.

41. Levine, J., and Willard, J. (1983): Redistribution of fodrin (a component of the cortical cytoplasm) accompanying capping of cell surface molecules. *Proc. Natl. Acad. Sci. USA*, 80:191–195.

42. London, E. D., and Coyle, J. T. (1979): Specific binding of ^{3}H-kainic acid to receptor sites in rat brain. *Mol. Pharmacol.*, 15:492–505.

43. Luczywek, E., and Mempel, E. (1980): Memory and learning in epileptic patients treated by amygdalotomy and anterior hippocampotomy. *Acta Neurochirurg.*, 30:169–175.

44. Luini, A., Goldberg, D., and Teichberg, V. (1981): Distinct pharmacological properties of excitatory amino acid receptors in the rat striatum: Study by the Na$^+$ efflux assay. *Proc. Natl. Acad. Sci. USA*, 78:3250–3254.

45. Lynch, G., and Baudry, M. (1981): Rapid structural modification in rat hippocampus: Evidence for its occurrence and an hypothesis concerning how it is produced. In: *Changing Concepts of the Nervous System*, edited by A. Morrison and P. Strick, pp. 21–31. Academic Press, Orlando, Fla.

46. Lynch, G., and Baudry, M. (1984): The biochemical intermediates in memory formation: A new specific hypothesis. *Science*, 224:1057–1063.

47. Lynch, G., Halpain, S., and Baudry, M. (1982): Effects of high-frequency synaptic stimulation on glutamate receptor binding studies with a modified *in vitro* hippocampal slice preparation. *Brain Res.*, 244:101–111.

48. Lynch, G., Larson, J., Kelso, S., Barrionuevo, G., and Schottler F. (1983): Intracellular injections of EGTA block the induction of hippocampal long-term potentiation. *Nature*, 305:719–721.

49. Lynch, G., and Schubert, P. (1980): The use of in vitro brain slices for multidisciplinary studies of synaptic function. *Ann. Rev. Neurosci.*, 3:1–22.

50. Mamounas, L., Thompson, R. F., Lynch, G., and Baudry, M. (1984): Classical conditioning of the rabbit eyelid response increases glutamate receptor binding in hippocampal synaptic membranes. *Proc. Natl. Acad. Sci. USA*, 81:2548–2552.

51. Mellgren, R. L. (1980): Cannine cardiac calcium-dependent proteases: Resolution of two forms with different requirements for calcium. *FEBS Lett.*, 109:129–133.

52. Mellgren, R. L., Repetti, A., Muck, T. C., and Easly, J. (1982): Rabbit skeletal muscle calcium-dependent protease requiring multimolar Ca^{2+}, purification, subunit structure, and Ca^{2+}-dependent autoproteolysis. *J. Biol. Chem.*, 257:7203–7209.

53. Michaelis, E. U., Michaelis M. L., and Boyarsky, L. L. (1974): High affinity glutamic acid binding to brain synaptic membranes. *Biochem. Biophys. Acta*, 367:338–348.

54. Mohler, H., and Okada, T. (1978): Properties of γ–Aminobutyric acid receptor binding with $(+)$–^{3}H-bicuculline methiodide in rat cerebellum. *Mol. Pharmacol.*, 14:256–265.

55. Morris, R., and Baker, M. (1984): Does long-term potentiation–synaptic enhancement have anything to do with learning or memory. In: *The Neuropsychology of Memory*, edited by N. Butters and L. Squire, pp. 521–535. Guilford Press, New York.

56. Murachi, T., Hatanaka, M., Yasumoto, Y., Nakayata, N., and Tanaka, K. (1981): A quantitative distribution study on calpain and calpastatin in rat tissues and cells. *Biochem. Int.*, 2:651–656.

57. Nelson, W. J., Colaco, C. A. L. S., and Lazarides, E. (1983): Involvement of spectrin in cell-surface receptor capping in lymphocytes. *Proc. Natl. Acad. Sci. USA*, 80:1626–1630.

58. Pant, H. C., and Gainer, H. (1980): Properties of a calcium-activated protease in squid axoplasm which selectively degrades neurofilament proteins. *J. Neurobiol.*, 11:1–12.

59. Racine, R., Kairiss, E., and Smith, G. (1981): Kindling mechanisms: Postactivation potentiation vs. the burst response. In: *Kindling II*, edited by J. Wada, pp. 15–29. Raven Press, New York.

60. Racine, R. J., Milgram, N. W., and Hafner, S.

(1983): Long-term potentiation phenomena in the rat limbic forebrain. *Brain Res.*, 260:217–231.

61. Ralston, G. B. (1978): The structure of spectrin and the shape of the red blood cell. *Trends Biochem. Sci.*, 3:195–198.

62. Roberts, P. J. (1974): Glutamate receptors in rat central nervous system. *Nature*, 252:399–401.

63. Savage, D. D., Werling, L. L., Nadler, J. V., and McNamara, J. O. (1982): Selective increase in L-^{3}H-glutamate binding to a quisqualate-sensitive site in hippocampal synaptic membranes after angular bundle binding. *Eur. J. Pharmacol.*, 85:255–256.

64. Siman, R., Baudry, M., and Lynch, G. (1983): Purification from synaptosomal plasma membranes of calpain I, a thiol-protease activated by micromolar calcium concentrations. *J. Neurochem.*, 41:950–956.

65. Siman, R., Baudry, M., and Lynch, G. (1984): Brain fodrin: Substrate for the endogenous calcium-activated protease calpain I. *Proc. Natl. Acad. Sci.*, 81:3572–3576.

66. Simon, J. P., Contrera, J. F., and Kuhar, M. J. (1976): Binding of ^{3}H-kainic acid, an alalogue of L-glutamate to brain membranes. *J. Neurochem.* 26:141–147.

67. Snodgrass, S. R. (1979): In vitro binding studies with ^{3}H-methyl-aspartate. *Soc. Neurosci. Abstr.*, 5:572.

68. Sobue, K., Kanda, K., Invi, M., Morimoto, K., and Kakiuchi, S. (1982): Actin polymerization induced by calpspectin, a calmodulin-binding spectrin-like protein. *FEBS Lett.*, 168:221–225.

69. Storm-Mathisen, J. (1977): Localization of transmitter candidates in the brain: The hippocampal formation as a model. *Prog. Neurobiol.* 8:119–181.

70. Suzuki, K., Ishiura, S., Tsuji, S., Katamoto, T., Sugita, H., and Imahori, K. (1979) Calcium-activated neutral protease from human skeletal muscle. *FEBS Lett.*, 104:355–358.

71. Swanson, L. W., Teyler, T. J., and Thompson, R. F. (1982): Properties and functional implications of long-term potentiation. *Neurosci. Res. Prog. Bull.*, 20:5.

72. Toyo-oka, T., Shimizu, T., and Masaki, T. (1978): Inhibition of proteolytic activity of calcium-activated neutral protease by leupeptin and antipan. *Biochem. Biophys. Res. Commun.*, 82:484–491.

73. Vargas, F., Greenbaum, L., and Costa, E. (1980): Participation of cysteine proteinase in the high-affinity Ca^{2+} dependent binding of glutamate to hippocampal synaptic membranes. *Neuropharmacology*, 19:791–794.

74. Wada, J., editor (1982): *Kindling II.* Raven Press, New York.

75. Watkins, J. C., and Evans, R. H. (1981): Excitatory amino acid transmitters. *Annu. Rev. Pharmacol. Toxicol.*, 21:165–204.

76. Weisz, D. J., Clark, G. A., Yang, B., Solomon, P. R., Berger, T. W., and Thompson, R. F. (1982): Activity of dentate gyrus during NM conditioning in rabbit. In: *Conditioning: Representation of Involved Neural Function*, edited by

C. D. Woody, pp. 131–145. Plenum Press, New York.

77. Wigstrom, H., and Gustafsson, B. (1983): Facilitated induction of long-lasting potentiation during blockade of inhibition. *Nature*, 701:603–605.

78. Young, A. B., and Snyder, S. H. (1974): The gly-cine synaptic receptor: Evidence that strychnine binding is associated with the ionic inductance mechanism. *Proc. Natl. Acad. Sci. USA*, 71:6002–6005.

79. Zimmerman, V. J. P., and Schlaepfer, W. W. (1982): Characterization of a brain calcium-activated protease that degrades neurofilament proteins. *Biochemistry*, 21:3977–3983.

Advances in Neurology, Vol. 44, edited by
A. V. Delgado-Escueta, A. A. Ward, Jr.,
D. M. Woodbury, and R. J. Porter.
Raven Press, New York © 1986.

21

Synaptic Mechanisms in the Kindled Epileptic Focus: A Speculative Synthesis

*Claude G. Wasterlain, **†Debora B. Farber, and *‡M. David Fairchild

*The Epilepsy Research Laboratory, VA Medical Center, Sepulveda, CA 91343, and the Brain Research Institute, **The Jules Stein Eye Institute, and *the Departments of Neurology, †Ophthalmology and ‡Pharmacology, UCLA School of Medicine*

SUMMARY   This chapter reviews the chemical kindling model of epilepsy and speculates on its significance. Both human and experimental epilepsies are extremely heterogeneous, and it is unlikely that a single molecular or cellular mechanism can account for such a diversity of behavioral manifestations. Recent studies of chemical kindling favor the view that in this model, epilepsy is a property of neuronal networks that can take place in a structurally intact brain and does not depend on the presence of gross or microscopic brain damage. Kindling can be obtained by daily injections of nanomolar amounts of multiple muscarinic agonists in selective brain regions such as the amygdala and, once acquired, it is very persistent and frequently accompanied by spontaneous seizures. No evidence exists for creation of a novel pathway, and studies of seizure threshold suggest the need for a critical mass of neurons even on initial stimulation. The amounts of muscarinic agents injected are small enough to have little recordable effect initially, and the number of stimulations needed varies directly with the dose and inversely with the interstimulus interval. Carbachol kindling is inhibited by picomolar amounts of muscarinic antagonists, and the relative potencies of drugs on the kindling behavior *in vivo* parallel their affinity for muscarinic receptors *in vitro*. The (+) isomer of acetyl-β-methylcholine, with good affinity for the muscarinic receptor, can induce kindling, whereas the (−) stereo isomer with poor affinity for the receptor cannot. No morphological differences are observed between animals injected with the (+) or the (−) isomer. These experiments suggest that the development of chronic focal epilepsy can take place in a structurally intact brain, be independent of the production of brain damage, and totally dependent on synaptic excitation. In other words, in this model, epilepsy may be a disease of cell–cell communication in which structurally normal neurons develop epileptiform responses as their interactions are modified through synaptic activation.

   A study of the relationships between carbachol and electrical kindling of the same site gave different results depending on the site of stimulation. In the amygdala, no interaction was found, but when both stimuli were aimed at the cholinoceptive hippocampal cells, a strong facilitation in both directions was observed. Thus, it appears that chemical and electrical kindling share similar mechanisms and that cross-facilitation depends on the existence of a common anatomy. The same anticonvulsants that block electrical kindling also inhibit chemical kindling. Diphenylhydantoin again was relatively ineffective. Interaction between neurotransmitter candidates showed a strong inhibitory effect of GABA and its agonists, a minor action of dopaminergic and β-adrenergic agents, and no significant effect of naloxone or glutamate in this location. Attempts to kindle with GABA antagonists met with limited success. A small increment in local seizure intensity was observed upon repeated injection, but neither the electrographic nor the clinical seizures ever generalized.

2-Deoxyglucose studies showed unilateral or bilateral enhancement of uptake in the amygdala in naive rats and in the early stages of kindling. During stages 3 to 5, dramatic increases in 2-deoxyglucose uptake were observed in the substantia nigra pars reticulata, hippocampus, entorhinal cortex, pyriform cortex, inferior frontal cortex, and septal nuclei; lesser increases were seen in neocortex, caudate, and putamen, and in some thalamic nuclei and brainstem areas. Rats injected with carbachol mixed with atropine or other muscarinic blockers resembled untreated controls.

A possible relevance of these models to human epilepsy is discussed. It has been speculated that the long delay which frequently separates injury and post-traumatic epilepsy may reflect a kindling-like phenomenon. We suggest that normal inhibitory mechanism act as a filter that prevents physiologically bursting neurons from inducing kindling. Brain lesions, particularly in hippocampus, may disturb this filter function and make the subject susceptible to progressive kindling by random environmental stimuli occurring over a period of weeks to months.

A number of biochemical abnormalities have been associated with the kindling phenomenon, but at present none of them has been shown to have an etiological role. Changes in calcium and calmodulin kinase activity associated with septal kindling are reviewed briefly and a speculative model of their significance is presented.

It may be true that epilepsy is the illness that has taught us most about the brain and its function, but in the process we have not learned very much about epilepsy. Table 1 summarizes some of the leading hypotheses regarding the cellular mechanism of epilepsy. The list of structures thought to be responsible for epilepsy includes every component of the brain from extracellular space to neuronal membrane, and the presumed abnormalities range from a massive destruction of inhibitory circuitry to a total absence of structural lesions. In other words, we all agree with Hippocrates that epilepsy comes from the brain, but the consensus does not go much beyond that statement. After decades of major investigative efforts, and some notable therapeutic successes, many, simple, basic questions concerning the pathogenesis of the epilepsies remain unanswered. Does the epileptic focus require local structural damage? Are the basic properties of the cells within the focus intrinsically abnormal, or is it just the interaction between cells that is abnormal? Does the abnormality involve neurons or glia, inhibitory or excitatory systems? Can we identify at least one transmitter involved in one particular form of chronic epilepsy? What are the key first and second messengers involved in seizure generation? Why is the abnormality expressed only at times, permitting normal brain function interictally? When epilepsy follows a cerebral insult, why is its onset so frequently delayed by months or years?

The remarkable diversity of the epilepsies implies a diversity of etiologies. There is little in common between a benign familial illness with age-dependent penetrance experienced in childhood and adolescence, characterized by mul-

TABLE 1. *Postulated pathogenic sites in epilepsy*

Extracellular space (narrowed, enlarged)
Glia (inadequate K + sponge)
Neurons
  pacemakers
    abnormal membrane
    release from inhibition
    denervation supersensitivity
  inhibitory interneurons
    reduced number
    reduced function (GAD)
Neuronal networks
  structurally abnormal
  functionally abnormal

tiple daily absences, which are easily induced by hyperventilation and have a characteristic electroencephalogram (EEG) (40,111) (petit mal), a serious and progressive brain disease with myoclonus and dementia (89,109,144), and the delayed occurrence of focal seizures with secondary generalization following a cortical trauma. Although some of the pathogenic mechanisms might be shared, one would expect that etiologies and cellular mechanisms of epileptogenesis would differ greatly between these and other epilepsies. Therefore, it may be overly optimistic to seek a single mechanism of epileptogenesis. In this review, we will focus on one particular model (chemical kindling) and will only discuss a small portion of the literature, with the full realization that the mechanisms elucidated in this model may well not be applicable to other seizure types.

CELLULAR MECHANISMS OF FOCAL EPILEPSY

Several of the cellular mechanisms listed in Table 1 imply a mediation by increased extracellular K^+ ion concentration of seizure initiation or seizure spread. For example, the narrowed extracellular space formations observed in an epileptic focus with a glial scar (73,74) might result in a decrease of the amount of space available for the diffusion of K^+ flowing out of neurons during depolarization, resulting in increased $[K^+]_0$ and in increased excitability. The same might occur if glial cells proved inadequate to their task as potassium sponges or buffers (13,61,115). Increased extracellular $[K^+]$ has indeed been repeatedly observed during neuronal firing and during seizures (110), and a sufficiently high $[K^+]_0$ can apparently induce seizure activity under favorable circumstances (164). However, studies of penicillin foci with ion-sensitive electrodes have cast a doubt on the role of these K^+-mediated mechanisms. The ictal rise in $[K^+]_0$ is much slower and often less marked at the periphery of the focus than in its center (102,158,159). Therefore, it is unlikely that the spread of epileptic seizures in penicillin foci is mediated by extracellular $[K^+]$. Similarly, when recording $[K^+]_0$, $[Ca^{2+}]_0$, and cell firing in an epileptic focus, it is clear that rises in $[K^+]_0$ follow and never precede neuronal discharges, whereas a clear fall in $[Ca^{2+}]_0$ occurs before the onset of most seizures and predicts their occurrence (76). As a result, theories based on changes in extracellular potassium as the mediator of serine initiation are probably not valid for most seizure foci. Cannon's hypothesis that partially isolated cortex might become hyperexcitable as a result of denervation supersensitivity (24) is now considered an unlikely mechanism of epileptogenesis, in part because the predicted supersensitivity of undercut cortex to acetylcholine has not been found (88,136).

Most recent theories of epileptogenesis have considered epilepsy to be a property of neuronal networks rather than a property of individual neurons. Ribak et al. (129) has demonstrated a decrease in immunoreactive glutamate decarboxylase, the rate-limiting enzyme of γ-aminobutyric acid (GABA) synthesis, in alumina cream foci. More recently, those data have been extended to other types of epilepsy (128). This hypothesis has the attraction of offering a simple and logical explanation of the known involvement of GABA in seizure and in anticonvulsant mechanisms. Future work will undoubtedly address the question of the specificity of this decline as compared with other transmitter mechanisms and will test directly the changes in GABA turnover and release in these foci and the possible occurrence of increased GABA inhibition in some types of epilepsy, as suggested by studies of long-term potentiation and kindling (12,99,123).

The "misdirected regeneration" hypothesis suggests that, following a cerebral lesion, misdirected central regeneration is responsible for an enhanced excitability, and therefore for epilepsy. Evidence of morphologically aberrant regenerative efforts has been obtained by Golgi studies of ablated human epileptic temporal lobes (39), but so far no direct evidence is available for a link between these aberrant Golgi stains and a change in excitability. In addition, the "free interval" between lesion and seizure onset is sometimes considerably longer than the duration of post-lesion sprouting.

In chronic alumina cream foci, many neurons (of types that do not burst spontaneously in a healthy brain) fire in bursts (22,160). One type of neurons fires regularly in bursts, regardless of the animal's behavior. Electrical stimulation of surrounding cortex does not modify this bursting pattern. Monkeys can, to some extent, control by operant conditioning the interval between bursts, but not the interval within bursts, that is, they act as if bursting were inherent in their basic membrane properties rather than a result of synaptic input. These cells have been termed "epileptic neurons", "group 1" or "pace-makers." A second group of cells, called "followers" or "group 2 neurons," also burst, but their bursting frequencies are highly dependent on behavioral state, can be influenced by cortical stimulation, and respond to operant conditioning. It has been proposed that a seizure is triggered when the pacemaker neurons recruit a sufficient number of follower neurons (160). It should be noted, however, that the postulated abnormal membrane properties have never been demonstrated directly, and that this theory rests entirely on indirect evidence. If correct, it does not apply to all types of epilepsy, since similar cells have not been found in kindled epileptic foci. Nonetheless, it provides a rational hypothesis to explain cell interactions in the alumina and in some human cortical foci; as we saw earlier there is little likelihood that all types of epileptic foci involve the same cellular mechanisms.

The "aggregate" hypothesis, e.g., the postulate that epilepsy does not require structural brain damage and is the result of abnormal interactions between networks of structurally normal neurons, will be the focus of our review, since the chemical kindling model permits a relatively direct test of that hypothesis.

CHEMICAL KINDLING: A MODEL OF FOCAL EPILEPSY

Description

We induced chemical kindling by once daily injections of 2.7 nmoles of carbachol or other muscarinic agonists in 0.2–1 μl of sterile isotonic fluid into the basolateral amygdala (62,145,152). The initial injection produced no behavioral or electrographic response in a few rats. Most animals developed mild spiking from the injection site, while a few had behavioral seizures and a widespread electrographic paroxysmal response. Once daily repetition of the same injection produced a gradually increasing response; electrographically (Fig. 1), the paroxysmal discharge increased in duration and complexity and rapidly spread to distant brain regions, while clinically most animals developed twitching of vibrissae and mouth (stage 1), then head jerks (stage 2), followed by synchronous forepaw clonus (stage 3) and finally by rearing (stage 4); they then fell backwards with clonic activity of all extremities (stage 5). Once initiated, seizures progressed rapidly over a 5- to 10-day period. Completed kindling (defined by

three consecutive stage 5 seizures) was very persistent, and was undiminished after 2, 4, and 8 weeks and even 6 months (N = 3) without further stimulation (152; C. G. Wasterlain, *unpublished observations*). The number of stimulations needed to reach full kindling varied inversely with the interstimulus interval, a property shared with electrical kindling (64,120) and with some types of learning (64). Surprisingly, the interval between injection and clinical seizures remained long in fully kindled rats (with 2.7 nmoles, 1.67 min, N = 161) and was not significantly correlated with either carbachol dosage or kindling stage. This very long interval suggests the existence, during that interval, of a complex and dynamic balance between excitatory and inhibitory circuits, which eventually results in kindled animals in the establishment of sufficient synchrony to produce alternating bursts of excitatory and inhibitory motor activity, that is, in clonic seizures. In that view, the long interval between stimulation and seizure activity observed in chemical kindling would be used to establish synchrony of neuronal output, which in electrical kindling is established from the start by a discreetly timed stimulus.

Is Brain Damage Necessary for the Creation of an Epileptic Focus?

Many patients who undergo temporal lobectomy for uncontrolled epilepsy (often with partial complex seizures) have evidence of gross structural damage at the site of the focus (14,45,127,141). When no cell loss or other structural damage is found, the results of surgery are less favorable, suggesting that in some of those patients the focus may have been located outside the ablated area (45,48). The limited data available from autopsy studies also suggest a high incidence from pathology in human epileptic foci (57,106). Similarly, many animal models of chronic focal epilepsy, such as those induced by alumina cream, cobalt, freeze lesions, and kainic acid, involve a considerable amount of cell loss and brain damage (90,118). In the biochemical investigation of those models or of surgically ablated human foci, it is exceedingly difficult to separate the epileptogenic from the nonspecific effects of cell loss. However, the kindling model of epilepsy is associated with only trivial amounts of brain damage, and offers an opportunity to test the aggregate hypothesis, e.g., the theory that epilepsy can result from abnormal functional interactions between struc-

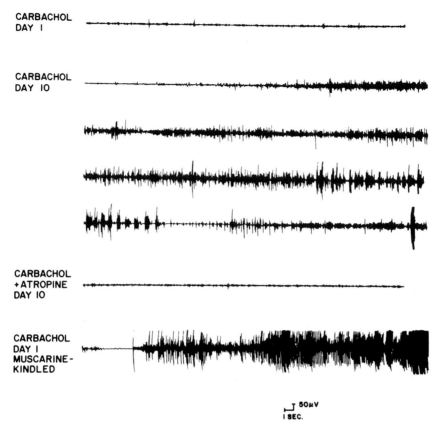

CARBACHOL
DAY I

CARBACHOL
DAY IO

CARBACHOL
+ATROPINE
DAY IO

CARBACHOL
DAY I
MUSCARINE-
KINDLED

50μV
I SEC.

FIG. 1. Electrographic record from the basolateral amygdala of male Holtzman rat following the first injection of carbachol (2.7 nmoles, 1 μl) shows minimal occasional spiking (*top line*). The same animal on its tenth stimulation shows prolonged seizure activity. A paired animal treated in the same way, except that each injection contained equimolar atropine (2.7 nmoles) mixed with carbachol, had a normal EEG after 10 injections. *Bottom trace,* a full seizure in response to the first injection of carbachol (2.7 nmoles) in an animal previously kindled with muscarine. Compare this response with that of a similarly injected naive rat (*top line*).

turally normal groups of neurons. Extensive morphological studies by Goddard and collaborators (65) both at the light- and at the electron-microscopic level, have suggested that no specific structural damage was associated with electrically kindled epilepsy. What damage was present resulted from the electrode implantation and was also observed in unkindled implanted controls. However, chemical kindling allowed a more rigorous test of that conclusion.

Because our animals were implanted with Teflon cannulas and the whole implant was free of metal in order to permit good microwave fixation, no iron salts or peroxides able to generate free radicals could be involved. The light microscopic appearance of the brain was similar in kindled rats injected with carbachol and in unkindled controls injected with a solution containing carbachol mixed with equimolar atropine. No difference in injectate osmolarity,

volume, pH, or sterility was found between groups, suggesting that in this experimental model the development of epilepsy does not depend upon the existence of focal brain damage.

Is a Novel Pathway Established?

In carbachol kindling of the amygdala, some animals develop seizures on the first day of stimulation. In our first series of 24 rats, nine experienced a stage 1 or 2 seizure on first injection of 2.7 nmoles of carbachol. Subsequent experiments showed that even stage 5 seizures can result on day 1, rarely after injection of 2.7 nmoles, but more frequently with larger amounts of carbachol. These seizures are undistinguishable from those seen in fully kindled rats. Therefore, there is no evidence that a new pathway was created, merely that the intensity of a response was enhanced. By contrast, in electrical kindling of the amygdala, it has been claimed that typical kindled-like seizures cannot be obtained on first stimulation, even with a large increase in current intensity (64,122).

Need for a Mass Effect

Kindling is clearly dose-dependent, since progressively increasing quantities of carbachol produced full kindled seizures in a progressively decreasing number of trials (Fig. 2). Concentration may be equally important, since nine rats which received 1 nmole daily in a volume of 0.2 μl kindled significantly faster than a similar group receiving 1 nmole daily in a volume of 1 μl. However, injections of 0.27 nmoles in 1 μl consistently failed to elicit kindling. In order to relate these effective quantities to concentrations at the receptor site, we studied autoradiographically the extent of diffusion of 1 μCi of [³H]-QNB (quinuclidinylbenzylate), a muscarinic antagonist injected in the amygdala in a 1 μl volume. After 5, 15, or 30 min, the bulk of radioactivity was localized to sphere of <2 mm in diameter. If the diffusion of carbachol, which on physical grounds alone would be expected to be similar to that of QNB, reached a sphere of 4-mm diameter in 30 min, its concentration in that sphere would be in the micromolar range; it would be sufficient to saturate all muscarinic receptors in that sphere, yet insufficient to induce kindling. Three possible explanations are offered: the first, that carbachol kin-

dling is not mediated by muscarinic receptors, is not tenable, as we will see below. The second explanation is that, by analogy with the nicotonic receptor, the "physiological" state of the muscarinic receptor is a low-affinity state, which is only stimulated by very high agonist concentrations. The third, and more likely, explanation is that a "mass effect" is required, e.g., that a sufficient concentration of agonist must reach a sufficient number of neurons within a short time in order to establish synchrony of firing in a critical mass of neurons necessary for seizure induction. This critical mass would then be able to recruit additional neurons and eventually to reach seizure threshold. This hypothesis emphasizes that the key abnormality of the seizure process is not so much the amount of neuronal firing as its hypersynchrony, and is quite compatible with the "aggregate" theory of epileptogenesis. In both electrical amygdaloid kindling and long-term potentiation, a "critical mass" of neurons is similarly required, as shown by McNamara et al., McNaughton and Barnes, and Pinel et al. (97,98,113), and a critical density of action potentials can be generated by cooperativity, for example, between median and lateral perforant paths stimulated synchronously.

Specificity of Seizure Pathways

Extensive cross-facilitation exists between different models of epilepsy (20,56,79,105, 114,116) and has suggested to many investiga-

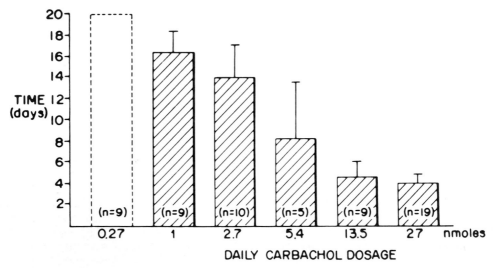

FIG. 2. Relationship between carbachol dosage and time needed to reach the first stage 5 seizure. Rats were injected once daily. If the injection failed to produce seizures, stimulation was discontinued after 20 trials, and that animal received a score of 20. All animals injected with 0.27 nmoles of carbachol belonged to that "failure" category.

tors that seizures involve nonspecific pathways. However, other results demonstrate much specificity in individual seizure types (65,122). For example, the enhanced afterdischarges and evoked potentials observed in many brain sites in amygdaloid-kindled rats on amygdaloid stimulation cannot be obtained by direct stimulation of these sites, suggesting that changes in excitability were highly specific for the pathway stimulated (122). Several lines of evidence in the chemical kindling experiments similarly suggest a high degree of both neurochemical and anatomical specificity. First, injections of 2.7 nmoles of carbachol in amygdala once daily easily induced kindling, but similar injections in motor cortex failed completely (152), although it should be noted that previous investigators using larger amounts of carbachol reported some success (145). Second, repeated amygdaloid injections of carbachol or other muscarinic agonists resulted in a decrease in seizure threshold for amygdaloid injections of carbachol (from 15.7 ± 3.7 nmoles Ca to 2.4 ± 1.1 nmoles Ca, $p < 0.01$) but not of bicuculline. Third, once-daily intracortical injections of small amounts of the putative GABA antagonists bicuculline, picrotoxin and penicillin produced very limited but significant increases of ictal responses and decreases in local seizure threshold for those compounds, whereas intraamygdaloid injections of the same compounds failed to do so. Fourth, the complex interactions between electrical and chemical kindling described below are most easily explained by assuming a high degree of pathway specificity. Taken together, these results suggest that simple "neurochemical" explanations such as "denervation supersensitivity" or "receptor down regulation" cannot fully explain the facts. Indeed, the remarkable thing about the differences in chemical kindling responses between cortex and amygdala is that both contain large amounts of muscarinic receptors and of GABA receptors. Yet one location kindles easily in response to muscarinic agents but not to putative GABA antagonists; the other location does the opposite. Clearly, if the kindled phenomenon reflected simple adaptive changes due to receptor occupancy by a ligand, it would occur regardless of location. Similarly, if epileptogenicity was only the result of local anatomy and circuitry, all excitatory agents at that site should kindle successfully. Admittedly, one category of agents was probably directly excitatory, whereas the other group presumably released neurons from inhibition, but this difference cannot explain the complete reversal of results between neocortex and amygdala. Our re-

sults suggest that the mechanisms of kindling must take into account both the chemical specificity of neural pathways and the complexities of their local circuitry.

Testing the Aggregate Hypothesis: Evidence for the Obligatory Generation of the Carbachol-Kindled Focus Through Muscarinic Synapses

Because carbachol can stimulate both nicotinic and muscarinic receptors, we mixed highly specific antagonists of those receptors with carbachol in a single injection of unchanged volume and osmolarity. The extent of diffusion of carbachol, tubocurarine, and atropine should be similar, since their MWs are in the same range, therefore, they should reach approximately the same target cells, minimizing the risk that blockade might occur at distant sites as could be the case with a systemic injection of antagonist. Large amounts of nicotinic blockers failed to have any influence upon carbachol-induced seizures, whereas very small amounts of the muscarinic antagonists atropine, QNB, or scopolamine significantly inhibited the seizures induced by carbachol (Fig. 3). For example, one molecule of atropine mixed with 5,000 molecules of carbachol was sufficient to reduce seizure intensity significantly (107). Moreover, kindling could be induced by other muscarinic agonists such as muscarine or (+)acetyl-β-methylcholine, and the latter showed potentiation by the cholinesterase inhibitor physostigmine.

(+)Acetyl-β-methylcholine has a (−)stereoisomer, with poor affinity for the muscarinic receptor, which failed to kindle (Fig. 4). Animals kindled for one agonist showed full transfer to other agonists (Fig. 5). Finally, the potency of muscarinic agonists or antagonists *in vivo* was proportional to their affinity for the muscarinic receptor *in vitro* (152). Extensive microscopic studies could not distinguish between animals kindled with carbachol and their unkindled littermates injected with carbachol mixed with atropine. These data provide strong evidence that an increase in activity through a group of muscarinic synapses in or around the amygdala is sufficient to induce a long-lasting kindled state characterized not only by a change in excitability but also, in some animals, by spontaneous seizures. It is sufficient to generate epilepsy in some animals. These results strongly support the aggregate hypothesis and the view that, in this model, epilepsy is a disease of cell–

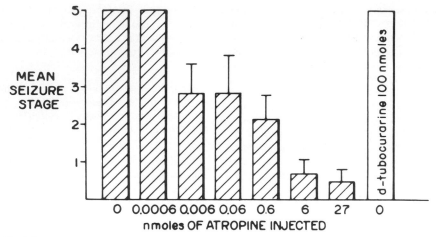

FIG. 3. Six fully kindled rats received 1-μl injections containing 27 nmoles of carbachol mixed with varying amounts of atropine (0.006–27 nmoles) or D-tubocurarine (up to 100 nmoles). The animals were rested for 1 week between stimulations and were their own controls. Bars indicate the mean ± SEM seizure stages following injections.

cell communication that can occur in the absence of any brain damage and in which key abnormalities lie in the (presumably synaptic) relationships between structurally normal neuronal networks.

Relationships Between Electrical and Chemical Kindling: An Indirect Look at the Problem of Pathway Specificity

The interactions between electrical and carbachol kindling were studied in rats implanted in the basolateral amygdala with a chemitrode, so that closely adjacent sites could be stimulated chemically (2.7 nmoles of carbachol once daily in 1 μl of sterile, isotonic fluid) or electrically (400 μA, 1 sec, 60 Hz, AC, through bipolar stainless steel electrodes in the wall of the cannula or chemitrode). In the first experiment,

group A (six rats) received daily carbachol injections and developed kindled seizures, whereas group B (six rats) received daily carbachol mixed with equimolar atropine, which blocked kindling. After 20 injections and 1 week of rest, both groups were stimulated electrically once a day and kindled at similar rates (Table 2). Two additional groups received electrical or sham stimulations, so that the former were kindled and the latter were not, followed after a week of rest by daily carbachol injections. Carbachol kindling proceeded at similar rates in both groups, and again no transfer between the two types of kindling was observed. Another group of six rats was injected with 27 nmoles of atropine solution (1 μl) 15 min before electrical stimulation. Its control group was similarly injected with 1 μl of isotonic sodium chloride solution 15 min prior to electrical stimulation. No

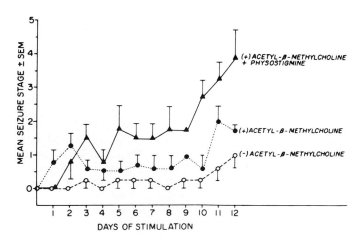

FIG. 4. Time course of kindling with stereoisomers of acetyl-β-methylcholine (3 nmoles in 1 μl), and with the (+) isomer (3 nmoles) mixed with physostigmine (10 nmoles). Note that the abscissa is below the zero line (baseline). Further trials did not confirm the upward trend shown on day 11 and 12 with the (−) isomer. The effects of physostigmine alone are described in the text. Differences between the (+) groups and (−) groups were significant on days 1, 2, 4, 6, 8, 9, and 11–20 ($p < 0.05$, Student's t-test). Physostigmine significantly enhanced seizure responses on days 3, 5, 6, 7, 8, and 10–20 ($p < 0.05$).

TABLE 2. *Interactions between chemical and electrical kindling in amygdala and hippocampus*

Stimulus/region	Status	Latency (No. of trials)	Progression to stage 5
Electrical K, amygdala	Naive, carbachol kindled	2.3 ± 2.3 1.7 ± 1.5	11.6 ± 4.1 10.2 ± 5.6
Chemical K, amygdala	Naive, electrically kindled	5.6 ± 3.2 4.3 ± 3.7	15.9 ± 4.7 14.2 ± 6.1
Electrical K, Septal–hippocampal	Naive, carbachol kindled	2.5 ± 2.1 1.2 ± 0.8	13.5 ± 3.5 1.7 ± 0.5
Carbachol K, hippocampus	Naive, electrically kindled	3.3 ± 2.8 2.3 ± 2.3	15.3 ± 3.9 2.2 ± 1.0

difference in the rate of development of kindled seizures was observed between the two groups on any day of stimulation. The mean number of trials necessary to reach the first stage 5 seizure was 11.5 ± 2.2 in atropine-treated and 13.2 ± 3.4 in saline-injected rats (152). Because the amount of atropine used was 10 times greater than that needed to block chemical kindling completely, it is clear that muscarinic blockade around the amygdaloid injection site does not inhibit electrical kindling. The lack of transfer observed in the previous experiments suggests a similar conclusion. On the other hand, Cain (21), testing transfer from carbachol kindling on one side of the brain to electrical kindling in the opposite hemisphere and reciprocally, found positive transfer in both directions. Other evidence in favor of a muscarinic role in electrical amygdaloid seizures includes their clinical and electrographic resemblance to carbachol seizures (152), the possible alteration in the rate of electrical kindling by systemic muscarinic agents (3,4,11,33), the occurrence of short-term changes in muscarinic receptors following kindling (95), and the supersensitivity of hippocampal pyramidal cells to iontophoresed acetylcholine (ACh) following kindling stimuli (15,60). Because our autoradiographic studies showed that muscarinic blockers injected into the amygdala remained localized within 2 mm of the site of injection after 30 min, it seemed possible that atropine may not have reached the target cells of electrical stimulation. Indeed, Kaneko et al. (81) observed that rats whose stimulated amygdala was nearly fully depleted of neurons by kainic acid treatment kindled faster than animals with an intact amygdala, suggesting that electrical amygdaloid kindling is mediated primarily through stimulation of fibers of passage which synapse at a distance. Similarly, Engel et al. (49) demonstrated that, in fully kindled rats, 2-deoxyglucose uptake in the stimulated amygdala is not increased during seizures.

We tested this hypothesis by investigating the interactions between electrical kindling of medial septum and carbachol kindling of the CA3-CA4 region of dorsal hippocampus. The projection from medial septum to hippocampus has been extensively studied (30,55,131,137,139); its neurotransmitter is ACh, acting on muscarinic receptors. This projection is the source of at least 90% of the cholinergic muscarinic synapses in hippocampus, an anatomically and physiologically well-defined limbic structure. Septal stimulation elicits prominent hippocampal afterdischarges and easily induces kindling (149); therefore, it appears likely that both electrical stimulation of medial septum and carbachol injection into hippocampus share a common stimulation of some hippocampal cholinoceptive cells. A group of six animals previously kindled by septal stimulation, and a control group exposed only to sham stimulation, were subjected to daily hippocampal injections of 2.7 nmoles of carbachol. The septal-kindled animals took significantly less time than the control group to reach seizure stages 2,3,4, and 5 (p < .05) (Table 2). The number of trials needed to obtain the first seizure was 2.3 ± 2.3 for septal-kindled rats and 3.3 ± 2.8 for control rats (NS), but the number of subsequent trials needed to reach the first stage 5 seizure was 2.2 ± 1 for septal-kindled rats and 15.3 ± 3.9 for control rats (p < .01). Significant transfer was also observed in the opposite direction when groups of hippocampal carbachol-kindled rats and saline-injected controls were kindled by medial septal stimulation: the chemically kindled group displayed accelerated electrical kindling compared to its control.

We interpret these results to mean that chemical and electrical kindling involve similar mechanisms, and that this results in transfer when they share a common chemical anatomy. In our amygdala experiments, it is likely that the injected carbachol or atropine did not diffuse far enough to reach the target cells of electrical stimulation, whereas in the septal–hippocampal system, a common pathway (presumed to be the cholinoceptive hippocampal pyramidal cells) was stimulated by both methods. These experiments suggest that many of the conclusions of chemical kindling experiments can apply to the electrical kindling model and illustrate the remarkable degree of pathway specificity involved in the kindling model of epilepsy.

Role of Other Putative Neurotransmitters and Effects of Anticonvulsants in Carbachol Kindling

Atropine fully inhibited the development of kindling in naive rats, but did not completely prevent carbachol seizures in previously kindled animals (152), suggesting that in fully kindled animals carbachol seizures are no longer a purely muscarinic phenomenon. To investigate the role of other putative neurotransmitters, agonists or antagonists, groups of 6–14 fully carbachol-kindled rats received intraamygdaloid injections of 2.7 nmoles of carbachol mixed with appropriate agents. Muscimol (3 nmoles) and GABA (150 nmoles) completely abolished seizure activity. Animals experienced more intense seizures when receiving haloperidol (3 nmoles) than dopamine (3 nmoles), and the same seizure enhancement was observed after propanolol (3 nmoles) as compared with isoproterenol (3 nmoles), suggesting a mild inhibitory role for dopaminergic and β-adrenergic systems, respectively. Glutamate and naloxone had no effect. These results confirm the known importance of GABAergic mechanisms in seizure expression and suggest an inhibitory influence of some catecholaminergic pathways.

The effects of anticonvulsants on carbachol kindling were similar to their described effects on electrical amygdaloid kindling (19,66,78,121, 142,146,157). In fully kindled animals, seizure expression after injection of 2.7 nmoles of carbachol was blocked by high-dose diazepam (20 mg/kg), valproate (240 mg/kg), and phenobarbital (30 mg/kg) injected intraperitoneally. Diphenylhydantoin (150 mg/kg i.p.) only reduced mean seizure intensity from stage 2.8 ± 0.8 to 1.8 ± 0.7 ($N = 5$, $p > 0.05$). The development of carbachol-kindled seizures in naive animals was delayed by valproate at moderate doses (120 mg/kg) and blocked by high-dose valproate (240 mg/kg) and diazepam (20 mg/kg). The latter resulted, at the time of stimulation, in serum levels

of 0.67 µg/ml $\pm$ 0.09 for diazepam, 0.12 µg/ml $\pm$ 0.03 for methyldiazepam, and in brain levels of 2.7 µg/per gram of tissue $\pm$ 0.6 for diazepam and 0.7 µg/per gram tissue $\pm$ 0.1 for desmethyldiazepam.

Effects of Repeated Injections of Putative GABA Antagonists

Attempts at kindling with the putative GABA antagonists bicuculline, picrotoxin, and penicillin have so far met with only limited success (156). Low nanomolar amounts of bicuculline (e.g., 0.1 nmole, 1 µl, sterile, isotonic, pH 6.5 suspension) or picrotoxin were injected once daily into motor cortex. These injections were initially subconvulsive in most animals, but after 10–20 trials the injections produced mild contralateral motor twitching involving the vibrissae, face, and forelimb in most rats. Occasional rats displayed mild hemiconvulsive activity; however, the seizures rarely spread to the other side and never became generalized even after > 100 trials. In fact, they remained quite mild in most rats. However, this slight increase in seizure susceptibility persisted after 1 or 2 weeks without stimulation.

Penicillin seizure threshold was tested once daily by injecting 1-µl volumes containing increasing amounts of penicillin into motor cortex, and assessing the response behaviorally by the appearance of contralateral facial or forepaw clonic activity. We assumed that this repetition would be akin to a chemical kindling paradigm. Penicillin seizure thresholds thus measured were generally quite stable. There was a mild but significant decrease in threshold on repeated testing, with precisely one-half of the animals showing a decrease, one-half remaining the same, and none showing an increase. Again, repeated injections never produced the generalized seizures so easily observed upon amygdaloid carbachol injection. Limited attempts to induce kindling by daily bicuculline injections into amygdala failed.

Norharman, an unsubstituted β-carboline, is a mixed "reverse agonist" of benzodiazepines such as diazepam. It is an effective, albeit relatively low-affinity, ligand of benzodiazepine receptors. Thirty minutes after i.p. injections of subconvulsive amounts (20 mg/kg) of this compound, high micromolar concentrations are found in brain (202 µM after 30 min); this does not change with repeated once-daily injections. After 10–15 trials, seizures begin to appear and occur in most animals after 20 trials. This kindling-like change persists after 1 week without stimulation (103). The seizures are blocked by large doses of diazepam.

In conclusion, repeated intracortical injection of putative GABA antagonists produced a mild local increase in seizure response and/or decrease in seizure threshold, but failed to produce full kindling in either cortex or amygdala, suggesting that when neuronal hyperactivity is induced by antagonists of inhibitory transmitters, some component needed for full kindling is missing. Because intense neuronal firing can be obtained, we speculate that the generation of hypersynchrony may require a functional GABA filter that is inhibited by these agents. Because the natural ligand of benzodiazepine receptors is unknown, our success in kindling with a "reverse agonist" of those receptors is more difficult to interpret. The electrographic and behavioral responses appear to fit the definition of kindling, but its generation through inhibitory synapses still lacks solid proof. In any case, it suggests a possible role in the genesis of kindling for the GABA receptor–benzodiazepine receptor–barbiturate binding site–chloride ionophore complex.

Metabolic Anatomy of Carbachol Kindling

Autoradiographic studies using [^{14}C]-deoxyglucose (2-DG) were carried out by the method of Sokoloff et al. (135). Carbachol seizures offer a more favorable model for 2-DG studies than electrical kindling, because of the long half-life ($t^{1/2}$) of carbachol and of the long duration of its effects (45 min to 2 hr). As a result, animals cycle in and out of seizures for the entire 45 min of 2-DG incorporation. An autoradiogram that averages 1 min of seizure activity with 44 min of postictal state is not obtained; the animals spend a large percentage of the 45 min in a seizure state instead; moreover, our animals were continuously recorded so that the duration spent in each seizure stage was known. The few rats that did not show electrographic seizures for at least 25 minutes (in 45) were eliminated from the study. Nevertheless, several seizure stages were frequently represented; arbitrarily, we classified animals in the highest seizure stage in which they spent at least 10% of their total time. Calculations of mean seizure stages over the 45 min did not alter the "rank order" of the animals. However, it is likely that fine gradations are not possible with this method. Animals in seizure stages 3–5 show little overlap with those in

stages 0–1 and with controls, but intermediates are easily defined.

Interictally, kindled rats were undistinguishable from untreated controls. During seizures, it was clear that autoradiograms (ARs) reflected the seizure stage rather than the kindling stage. For example, the ARs of a fully kindled rat that would have a stage 1 seizure could not be differentiated from the ARs of a naive animal having a stage 1 ictus. ARs showed the expression of kindling but did not reveal its underlying basis.

Most carbachol-injected rats having only an afterdischarge without behavioral manifestations showed an enhanced uptake of 2-DG at the site of the amygdaloid injection. Animals in stage 1 seizures (N = 2 only) showed unilateral (1) or bilateral (1) enhancement of 2-DG uptake in the amygdala region. Rats in stages 3–5 seizures showed dramatic bilaterally symmetrical increases in 2-DG uptake in many areas, the most striking being: the substantia nigra pars reticulata; the hippocampi; entorhinal cortex; pyriform cortex; inferior frontal cortex; septal nuclei. Less striking increases were seen in many areas of neocortex, particularly anteriorly; and increases were seen in caudate nuclei, putamen, many thalamic nuclei, and some brainstem areas (Fig. 7). Rats injected with carbachol + atropine generally resembled untreated controls (Fig. 5).

These data support the notion that amygdaloid-kindled seizures involve predominantly the limbic system and are a model of human partial complex seizures with limbic foci. Indeed, we have commented that the behavioral appearance of the ictal animals has many features in common with that seen in humans during absence-like partial complex seizures. However, the usefulness of the kindling model in selecting drugs with particular potency against human partial complex seizures remains to be established.

POSSIBLE RELEVANCE OF KINDLING TO HUMAN EPILEPSY

Does Kindling Occur in Humans?

Kindling has been demonstrated in many species, ranging from frog to monkey. The possible occurrence of human mirror foci (104) and the frequent occurrence of multiple foci, usually in synaptically connected sites, in the temporal lobes of epileptic subjects (148) raised the question of the possible occurrence of kindling in humans; recently, Stramka et al. (138) reported a

FIRST   CARBACHOL   CHALLENGE

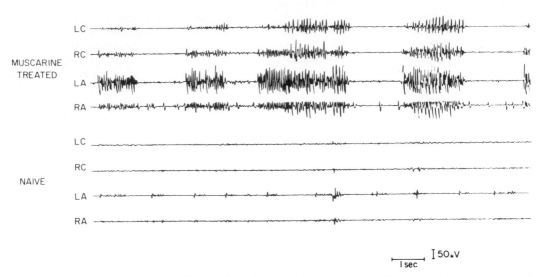

FIG. 5. Representative electrographic recordings from the L basolateral amygdala (LA), right amygdala (RA), left (LC), and right cortex (RC) of rats injected for the first time with carbachol (2.7 nmoles). One group received 20 previous injections of muscarine (3 nmoles in 1 μl of sterile isotonic saline), the other received 20 injections of isotonic saline alone.

47-year-old woman who suffered from intractable phantom pain for which she received daily electrical stimulation of the left thalamus. She was stimulated at 4 Hz and 50 Hz, 1 msec, up to 10 volts, 3 min daily, with some pain relief. On the 20th day of stimulation, she developed a partial elementary motor seizure with appropriate EEG changes. Stimulation was discontinued and the electrodes were removed, but on the following day she had a generalized seizure. Although her seizures are reported to be controlled by medication, her EEG shows epileptiform activity maximal on the left. However, her epilepsy could have been coincidental rather than kindled, and she had an old electrolytic lesion in the thalamus. No other example of human kindling has been reported.

The temporal profiles of some types of human epilepsy have also raised the possibility of a kindling-like phenomenon taking place in the silent period between insult and the development of epilepsy. Posttraumatic epilepsy is a common aftermath of head injuries, frequently developing 6 months to 2 years after the insult (5,25, 28,53,112,132). Hippocampal sclerosis may derive from a perinatal injury (43) or from febrile convulsions (50,51,107); frequently, however, the epileptic manifestations first take place years after these insults. A major difference between human idiopathic epilepsy and kindled epilepsy in animals has been the presence, in the vast majority of human brains sampled, of lesions, consisting predominantly of hippocampal sclerosis (14,44,45,52,59,94,126,141) which have not been demonstrated in kindled epilepsy (63–65,151,152). Based on the work of Cotman (34), DeLorenzo et al. (39) have proposed that after hippocampal insults, regeneration could be misdirected, possibly transforming some inhibitory pathways into excitatory pathways, and have shown some evidence for a change in direction of dendritic growth in human temporal lobes with hippocampal sclerosis. Such misdirected regrowth, presumed to be a regenerative effort following various insults, might be the basis of an epileptic condition. However, the time course of axonal regeneration in the central nervous system is usually much shorter than the time course of posttraumatic epileptogenesis. Active regrowth of axons or dendrites following a lesion proceeds for days to weeks (34,39,80) and is completed long before the common time of onset of posttraumatic epilepsy.

Why Does Kindling Not Occur Spontaneously?

Kindling has been shown to be a widespread and common phenomenon throughout the animal kingdom, yet spontaneous occurrence is rarely or never observed. In studies of the optimal frequency of firing needed to induce kindling, Goddard and Douglas (64) concluded that it was close to the natural bursting frequencies of some hippocampal neurons. If kindling is easily obtained from the hippocampus of most species, and if the optimal frequencies that produce it occur naturally in the healthy animal, one may wonder why kindling is not a common clinical phenomenon, and why most animals and humans do not seize in response to many sensory stimuli that are repeated with an appropriate frequency. Surely such stimulus frequencies do occur in life. Similarly, if agonists of the excitatory transmitter ACh, released in sufficient amounts with the proper interstimulus interval into the limbic system, cause kindling (153,154), one may wonder why release of ACh in response to natural stimuli does not induce kindling.

The "Filter" Hypothesis

The following unitary hypothesis reconciles those seemingly contradictory data and suggests a possible mechanism for both the association of epilepsy with hippocampal sclerosis or other cell damage in humans and its delayed development following trauma or other insults.

We speculate that within prehippocampal or hippocampal neuronal networks, an effective "filter" modulates sensory inputs so that either the critical mass or the critical frequencies needed to obtain kindling are never generated under normal circumstances. At least part of the filtering system should be located within the hippocampus itself, and probably within the CA1 region, so that lesions resulting in hippocampal sclerosis would effectively impair its function. GABAergic interneurons such as hippocampal basket cells and cortical aspinous stellate neurons, which distribute their projections around the soma or even on the initial axon segment of pyramidal cells, have been suggested to act as frequency filters (see Chapter 15), and are possible candidates for this filtering function. Misdirected regeneration of the type observed in Golgi preparations of ablated human temporal lobes (39) might weaken the effectiveness of that filter or reverse its function. The role of lesions then would be abolishment or reversal of the function of the prehippocampal filter; in essence, they would make the hippocampus vulnerable to kindling from routine daily neuronal input. Depending on the nature, intensity, and frequency of remaining excitatory inputs into hippocampus, a kindling-like phenomenon would then occur over the ensuing months to years, a period similar to that needed to kindle the hippocampus of non-human primates (147).

The rarity of stimulus-bound, sensory-induced epilepsies would simply reflect the paucity of direct sensory input into hippocampus. This model would also predict that hippocampal sclerosis would facilitate kindling, and would explain the frequency of emotional precipitants of seizures in patients with a temporal lobe focus. The area of hypometabolism observed by positron emission tomography (PET) of 18F deoxyglucose uptake in the temporal lobes of many human epileptics (46) came as a surprise to many investigators. It may reflect local cell loss (44); however, in many patients, the same area when recorded during a seizure can show very large increases in metabolic activity (47), demonstrating that its low basal metabolic rate is not a fixed condition. If our hypothesis of a presynaptic filter were correct, this hypometabolism might simply reflect the removal of the metabolic efforts devoted to the filter function, resulting in vulnerability of the area to incoming excitatory volleys. Alternatively, it might represent a constant effort by surrounding networks to suppress unfiltered input into hippocampus, and the resulting lowering of firing rates.

The most easily testable part of this hypothesis is that chronic anticonvulsants might prevent posttraumatic epilepsy. The incidence of posttraumatic epilepsy following open head injuries was the same in the Korean war (28), in which most victims received no anticonvulsants, as in the Vietnam war (27) in which phenytoin was used routinely. No controlled trials of sufficient scale have been reported. The military experience is insufficient to allow us to draw any conclusions, since the type of injuries and medical care differed vastly, particularly regarding severe head injuries, and since phenytoin is of doubtful efficacy in preventing kindling. A trial in Czechoslovakia (134) was reportedly successful in reducing the incidence of posttraumatic epilepsy with prophylactic phenytoin and phenobarbital but, like the military studies, it was uncontrolled and therefore requires confirmation.

SOME BIOCHEMICAL CHANGES IN MEMBRANE PHOSPHOPROTEINS ASSOCIATED WITH THE KINDLING PHENOMENON

Importance of Calcium as a Second Messenger

The regulation of function of specialized cells is coordinated by a variety of extracellular agents; those agents that do not penetrate the cell act on its membrane to generate a limited number of intracellular "second messengers," which in turn act on a large number of cell-specific components that provide the response characteristic of a particular cell type. In the central nervous system (CNS), there is a large number of neurotransmitters or neuromodulators, which act on specific receptors on the cell membrane. One result of that interaction is modification of the intracellular concentration of a second messenger such as a cyclic nucleotide or calcium ion (67,87,130). Because the concentration of calcium ion inside the neuron is less than one-thousandth of its extracellular concentration, the opening of calcium channels provides a rapid and effective amplification signal that has been shown to regulate a number of important cellular processes (10,70,127). In neurons, various extracellular neurotransmitters, neuromodulators, or neurohormones, and electrical activity which activates voltage-sensitive calcium channels, can effect a major increase in calcium concentration through the opening of highly regulated calcium channels (71,72). In some neurons, the intracellular concentration of calcium can regulate the conductance of potassium (100) or calcium (71,72) through specific membrane channels. In turn, the intracellular calcium concentration is lowered, and its action is terminated by sodium–calcium exchange or by active pumping out of the cell against a concentration gradient by a specific ATPase. Calcium is required for transmitter release, and may mediate the flow of information along neuronal networks in several ways (71,72). In the absence of extracellular calcium, major adaptive mechanisms of neurons, such as posttetanic potentiation or long-term potentiation, cannot take place, presumably because they depend on neurotransmitter release (7,42,54,143).

A raise in intracellular calcium concentration has different effects in different types of neurons, probably because the ultimate effectors of its action are relatively cell-specific. As is also the case with cyclic nucleotides, the "second messenger" effects a "message," which is expressed largely in terms of phosphoproteins (70). Cyclic AMP and cyclic GMP exert their physiological actions largely, if not exclusively, by activating specific protein kinases that phosphorylate specific cell proteins and thereby modify their function. These phosphoproteins thus represent the expressed "message" of the extracellular neurotransmitters, neuromodulators, or neurohormones. By contrast, calcium can regulate cell function by a wide variety of mechanisms (29). However, one of these mechanisms

is the activation of calcium-dependent protein kinases of several types (1,9,31,32,58,68,70,84–86,108,148,163). In one type of protein kinase which is of particular interest to us, the actions of calcium are mediated by the ubiquitous protein calmodulin (9,58,68,69,84–86,161); the activity of a particulate calcium- and calmodulin-dependent protein kinase in hippocampal synaptic plasma membranes apears modified in septal-kindled rats.

Change in Calcium- and Calmodulin-Dependent Phosphorylation of Hippocampal Synaptic Plasma Membranes Associated with Septal Kindling

Calcium and calmodulin greatly enhance ^{32}P incorporation *in vitro* from γ-[^{32}P]-ATP into many soluble and particulate proteins from rat brain, including a number of particulate proteins from synaptic plasma membranes. Although the phosphorylation of soluble proteins did not seem to be influenced by kindling, both the baseline and the calcium- and calmodulin-stimulated phosphorylation of several proteins from hippocampal synaptic plasma membranes (HSPM) were reduced in septal-kindled rats as compared with implanted or untreated controls (150). This reduced response to calcium and calmodulin was most important in a protein of MW~50,000 which is quite abundant in hippocampus but scarce in cerebellum, and may be identical to the major protein of postsynaptic densities (PSDs) (83,85), and in a doublet of MW 58,000–60,000 (Fig. 6). These proteins are not the only ones affected by kindling, and a similar trend was present in several additional membrane proteins. However, the 50,000 and 58,000–60,000 MW proteins have been identified as subunits of a calcium- and calmodulin-dependent protein kinase (see below) that autophosphorylates and phosphorylates a number of other synaptic proteins, implying that this calmodulin kinase may modulate the rate of phosphorylation of many synaptic proteins, including those affected by kindling, and through them may alter synaptic excitability.

The following evidence, obtained in collaboration with Goldenring and DeLorenzo, with Kennedy and collaborators, and with Oestreicher and Gispen (*unpublished observations*) suggests that the 50,000 and 58,000–60,000 MW proteins modified by kindling in HSPM are subunits of a calcium- and calmodulin-dependent protein kinase (calmodulin-kinase): Co-migration in 2-dimensional (2-D) (isoelectric focusing–

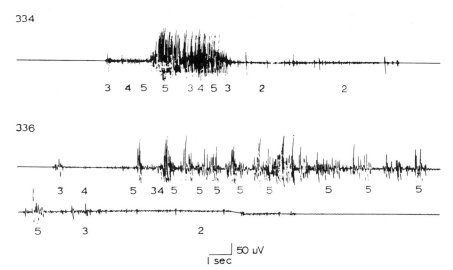

FIG. 6. Spontaneous seizures recorded from the basolateral amygdala of carbachol-kindled rats. Seizure stages are indicated under the respective electrographic tracings from rats 334 and 336. Note that in rat 336 widespread (stage 4) seizures preceded any sustained electrographic seizure activity from the amygdaloid electrode.

polyacrylamide gel electrophoresis (PAGE) gels, similar MW and isoelectric points, similar binding of ^{125}I-calmodulin in 2-D gels, similar peptide maps of trypsin digests and staphylococcal V8 protease digests, cross-reaction with monoclonal antibody to the 50K subunit of calmodulin kinase II, separation from B50 and from tubulin on gels, and lack of cross-reactivity with antibodies to B50 or to β tubulin.

The following controls showed that this change is closely associated with kindling behavior: (a) kindled rats sacrificed 8 weeks after their last stimulation had retained the associated biochemical changes, which therefore are long-lasting, as is the kindling behavior; (b) stimulated controls that received 100 stimulations 1 min apart showed neither kindling nor associated changes in HSPM protein phosphorylation; (c) a group of animals stimulated daily 15 min after injection with a large dose of diazepam showed neither kindling nor associated biochemical changes, and brain concentrations of diazepam (9.5 μM) and of its active metabolite N-desmethyldiazepam (2.4 μM) at the time of stimulation were in the range in which diazepam *in vitro* inhibits calcium- and calmodulin-dependent phosphorylation of the 50,000 and 58,000–60,000 MW HSPM proteins (IC_{50} = 20–34 μM and 19-25 μM, respectively).

Biochemical changes were prominent in hippocampus, in a region including amygdala, some entorhinal cortex, and most pyriform cortex; less prominent in cortex, basal ganglia and brainstem; and absent in cerebellum and spinal cord. Thus, the distribution of these changes showed a rough parallelism to that of kindling susceptibility. They were high in kindling-prone limbic structures and absent from regions that are incapable of kindling (cerebellum and spinal cord) (Fig. 8).

A Speculative Model of Septal Kindling

The functions of calmodulin kinase and its roles (if any) in the kindling phenomenon are unknown, and no solid evidence demonstrates a cause–effect relationship between biochemical and physiological changes. However, we can formulate a highly speculative but testable hypothesis relating these changes to epileptogenesis.

In interpreting the significance of these changes, several basic properties of calmodulin kinase should be noted. First, calmodulin kinase appears designed to respond to changes in $[Ca^{2+}]_i$ resulting from fine, physiological stimulation. Its response is maximal with low micromolar concentrations of Ca^{2+}, i.e., a very subtle stimulus would be sufficient to activate the enzyme maximally. Large increases such as those that may occur during seizures or ischemia are unnecessary or may even have an opposite effect. Second, the autophosphorylation of calmodulin kinase (observed with pure enzyme as well as with subcellular fractions) has no known function. It could represent an amplification

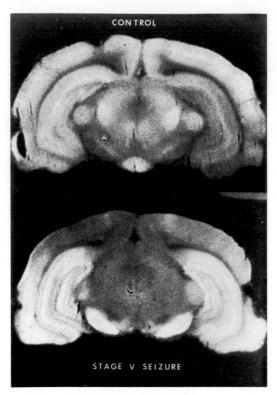

FIG. 7. Autoradiograms of ^{14}C-deoxyglucose uptake during kindled seizures induced by intraamygdaloid carbachol (2.7 nmoles). Higher rates of uptake of ^{14}C-deoxyglucose are shown in white. Note the prominent involvement of substantia nigra, hippocampus, and entorhinal cortex during kindled seizures.

signal, since an increase in $[Ca^{2+}]_i$ could trigger autophosphorylation, possibly modifying kinase activity, and thereby the phosphorylation and activity of many membrane proteins. Autophosphorylation could also provide a mechanism for increasing the duration of an adaptive change. If partial phosphorylation of the enzyme modified its rate of autophosphorylation (e.g., increased it when a minimum number of sites are occupied) the effects of intense stimulation would be long-lasting, since removal of a phosphate moiety would be quickly compensated by the increased likelihood of autophosphorylation. It is doubtful that this mechanism could account for the persistence of the kindling trace over years, but it could provide a lasting intermediate step. Third, calmodulin kinase may have both presynaptic and postsynaptic roles.

Presynaptically, there is evidence that a calmodulin kinase with subunits in the 50,000–60,000 MW range is present in brain synaptic

vesicles and synaptic cytosol (17,18) and in vesicles from *Torpedo* electric organ (35). Enriched vesicle fractions contain synapsin I and an endogenous kinase that phosphorylates it in the same sites as synapsin I (calmodulin) kinase. Diazepam and diphenylhydantoin inhibit both the release of neurotransmitters from synaptic vesicles and the calcium- and calmodulin-dependent phosphorylation of those vesicles (37,38). In summary, it is possible that the phosphorylation of synaptic vesicle proteins by calcium and calmodulin kinase modulates transmitter release. In addition, calmodulin-dependent phosphorylation controls the assembly or disassembly of microtubules (16,36,93) and may regulate cytoskeleton assembly and/or other functions of microtubules. Postsynaptically, there is strong evidence that the major protein of PSDs is a subunit of calmodulin kinase (82,85) that calmodulin kinase activity is abundant in PSDs (69), that particles close in size to calmodulin kinase (180 A) are seen by electron microscope in PSDs, crosslinked by S-S bonds (32). Calmodulin kinase therefore must have an important but as yet undefined role. Anticonvulsant drugs may exert some of their major action through their inhibition of calmodulin kinase (36–38). It is now evident that the proteins DPH-L and DPH-M were heterogeneous bands, a major component of which is made of calmodulin kinase subunits. Their calcium-dependent phosphorylation was inhibited by the most commonly used anticonvulsants (diphenylhydantoin, carbamazepine, and diazepam) at therapeutic concentrations.

Hypothesis

Kindling stimuli would induce Ca^{2+} entry (7) into both presynaptic and postsynaptic apparatus; the resulting rise in $[Ca^{2+}]_i$ would stimulate calmodulin kinase to autophosphorylate to the point where its activity would be enhanced (Fig. 9). Kindling stimuli would differ from nonkindling stimuli by inducing a higher level of autophosphorylation (above threshold for stimulation of enzyme function), either because of cooperativity between stimuli or because of the intensity, duration, and frequency of afterdischarge.

Enhanced autophosphorylation would lead to a higher level of endogenous phosphorylation of calmodulin kinase and of its target proteins *in vivo*. As a result, they would incorporate less ^{32}P from γ-[^{32}P]-ATP *in vitro*, resulting in an ap-

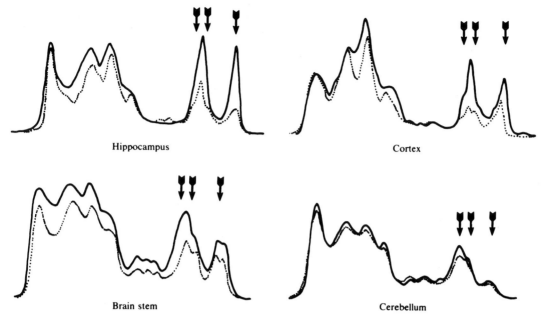

FIG. 8. Densitometric scans of autoradiograms obtained from brain regions of controls (—) and kindled rats (····). *Pair of arrows,* phosphoproteins of MWs 58,000–60,000, sometimes fused in a single band; *single arrow,* phosphoproteins of MW 50,000, which are prominently altered in kindled animals.

parent decrease in activity such as that observed by us in the posthoc assay.

Presynaptically, this increased level of endogenous calmodulin kinase activity would result in increased phosphorylation of synaptic vesicle proteins in response to Ca^{2+} influx and, as a result, might increase transmitter release (36). Postsynaptically, a lasting increase in calmodulin kinase activity might alter the response of PSDs to calcium entry in tissues such as hippocampus, in which this enzyme is a major component of PSDs (83,85). Tissues such as cerebellum, in which the 50,000 MW subunit of calmodulin kinase is not found, would be unable to kindle because of the absence of this putative link between calcium entry and synaptic response.

Stimulated controls that received kindling-like stimuli with very short interstimulus intervals would fail to show changes in calmodulin kinase because of failure to generate afterdischarges. In animals pretreated with diazepam, pharmacological inhibition of the Ca^{2+} stimulation of calmodulin kinase would keep changes below the critical threshold so that enzyme activity would remain the same. Because autophosphorylation of calmodulin kinase is unlikely to maintain itself beyond the lifespan of the enzyme (unless its

subunits turn over one by one), this scheme requires involvement of gene expression for its very long-term maintenance and to explain the effects of inhibitors of brain protein synthesis on kindling (78).

Other Biochemical Changes Associated with Kindling

Because changes in first (transmitter) or second messengers frequently find their ultimate expression in terms of phosphoproteins, the changes described above are by no means exclusive of a number of other biochemical changes recently found in association with kindling. For example, the decrease in concentration of a calcium-binding protein in hippocampus of kindled rats (8) and the increased permeability of hippocampal slices to ^{45}Ca after long-term potentiation (7,143) could represent other aspects of a change in response to calcium that altered synaptic responses. Ribak (see Chapter 37) reported a decrease in immunoreactive glutamate decarboxylase, the rate-limiting enzyme of GABA synthesis, in brains of kindled rats. This could result in failure of GABA inhibition and thereby in seizures, although it should be noted that such a failure has not been sug-

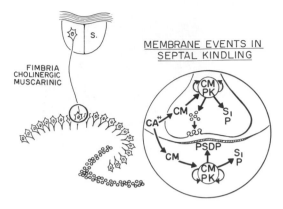

FIMBRIA
CHOLINERGIC
MUSCARINIC

MEMBRANE EVENTS IN
SEPTAL KINDLING

FIG. 9. Hypothesis outlining a possible role of calcium acting through the enzyme calmodulin kinase (both presynaptically and postsynaptically) in septal kindling. The presumed autophosphorylation of the enzyme when calcium enters the cell as a result of kindling stimulation modifies its activity, resulting in increased endogenous phosphorylation of presynaptic and postsynaptic membrane proteins, possibly altering transmitter release and postsynaptic function, resulting in enhanced responses of the target cell.

gested by physiological investigations (41,123). The many changes in numbers of various receptors for putative neurotransmitters (9,91–92,95–97) could also be proximal to changes in phosphoproteins. Problems related to the short-term nature of some of those changes and to the lack of physiological correlates (92,96,154) have been noted previously.

A number of other biochemical changes have been described in the kindled amygdala (see 96). Their significance is uncertain, since destruction of amygdala neurons facilitates kindling, suggesting that they are unlikely to harbor its engram (81).

CONCLUSIONS

Strong pharmacological evidence suggests that kindling can result solely from "plastic" changes in cerebral neuronal circuitry. In this model, epileptogenesis does not require any structural damage and can be induced through chemical or electrical stimulation of excitatory muscarinic synapses. Efforts to establish kindling through stimulation or blockage of inhibitory synapses have so far not been fully successful. The neurochemical basis for the kindling phenomenon remains elusive. A number of neurochemical changes have been found in association with some types of kindling, some testable models have been proposed, and the role

of calcium and of calcium-dependent processes has been emphasized, but the evidence for an etiological link between these phenomena and kindling is entirely indirect.

ACKNOWLEDGMENTS

Supported by the Research Service of the Veteran's Administration.

REFERENCES

1. Ahmad, Z., De Paoli-Roach, A. A., and Roach, P. J. (1982): Purification and characterization of a rabbit liver calmodulin-dependent protein kinase able to phosphorylate glycogen synthetase. *J. Biol. Chem.,* 257:8348–8355.
2. Ajmone Marsan, C., and Gumnit, R. J. (1974): Neurophysiological aspects of epilepsy. In: *Handbook of Clinical Neurology, The Epilepsies,* Vol. 15, edited by P. J. Vinken and G. W. Bruyn, pp. 30–59. Elsevier, New York.
3. Albright, P. S., Burnham, W. M., and Okazaki, M. (1979): Effect of atropine sulfate on amygdaloid kindling in the rat. *Exp. Neurol.,* 66:409–412.
4. Arnold, P. S., Racine, R. J., and Wise, R. A. (1973): Effects of atropine, reserpine, 6-hydroxydopamine, and handling on seizure development in the rat. *Exp. Neurol.,* 40:457–470.
5. Ascroft, P. B. (1941): Traumatic epilepsy after gunshot wounds of the head. *Br. Med. J.,* 1:739–744.
6. Ayala, G. F., Dichter, M., Gumnit, R. J., Matsumoto, H., and Spencer, W. A. (1973): Genesis of interictal spikes. *Brain Res.,* 52:1–17.
7. Baimbridge, K. G., and Miller, J. J. (1981): Calcium uptake and retention during long-term potentiation of neuronal activity in the rat hippocampal slice preparation. *Brain Res.,* 221:299–305.
8. Baimbridge, K. G., and Miller, J. J. (1982): Immunohistochemical loss of calcium-binding protein from dentate granule cells during kindling-induced epilepsy. *Soc. Neurosci. Abstr.,* 8:457.
9. Bennett, M. K., Erondu, N. E., and Kennedy, M. B. (1983): Purification and characterization of a calmodulin-dependent protein kinase that is highly concentrated in brain. *J. Biol. Chem.,* 258:12735–12744.
10. Berridge, M. J. (1975): The interaction of cyclic nucleotides and calcium in the control of cellular activity. *Adv. Cyclic Nucleotide Res.,* 6:1–98.
11. Blackwood, H. R., Martin, M. J., and Howe, J. G. (1982): A study of the role of the cholinergic system in amygdaloid kindling in rats. *Psychopharmacologia,* 76:66–69.
12. Bliss, T. V. P., and Dolphin, A. C. (1982): What is the mechanism of long-term potentiation in the hippocampus? *Trends Neurosci.,* 5:289–290.
13. Brotchi, J. (1978): The activated astrocyte. A histochemical approach to the epileptic focus. In: *Dynamic Properties of Glial Cells,* edited by

E. Schoffeniels, G. Franck, D. B. Towers, and L. Hertz, pp. 429–433. Pergamon, Oxford.

14. Brown, W. J. (1973): Structural substrates of seizure foci in the human temporal lobe. In: *Epilepsy: Its Phenomena in Man*, edited by M. A. B. Brazier, pp. 339–374. Academic Press, Orlando, Fla.

15. Burchfield, J. L., Duchowny, M. S., and Duffy, F. H. (1979): Neuronal supersensitivity to acetylcholine induced by kindling in the rat hippocampus. *Science*, 204:1096–1098.

16. Burke, B. E., and DeLorenzo, R. J. (1981): Ca^{2+}- and calmodulin-stimulated endogenous phosphorylation of neurotubulin. *Proc. Natl. Acad. Sci. USA*, 78:991–995.

17. Burke, B. E., and DeLorenzo, R. J. (1982): Ca^{2+} and calmodulin-regulated endogenous tubulin kinase activity in presynaptic nerve terminal preparations. *Brain Res.*, 236:393–415.

18. Burke, B. E., and DeLorenzo, R. J. (1982): Ca^{2+} and calmodulin-dependent phosphorylation of endogenous synaptic vesicle tubulin by a vesicle-bound calmodulin kinase protein. *J. Neurochem.*, 38:1205–1218.

19. Burnham, W. M., Livingstone, K. E., Lychacz, B., and Avila, J. (1977): Anticonvulsant effects of amytryptyline, diazepam, phenobarbital and procaine on "kindled" seizures. *Electroencephalogr. Clin. Neurophysiol.*, 43:777.

20. Cain, D. P. (1980): Effects of kindling or brain stimulation on pentylenetetrazol-induced convulsion susceptibility. *Epilepsia*, 21:243–249.

21. Cain, D. P. (1983): Bidirectional transfer of electrical and carbachol kindling. *Brain Res.*, 260:135–138.

22. Calvin, W. H. (1980): Normal repetitive firing and its pathophysiology. In: *Epilepsy: A Window to Brain Mechanisms*, edited by J. S. Lockard and A. A. Ward, Jr., pp. 97–121. Raven Press, New York.

23. Calvin, W. H., Ojeman, G. A., and Ward, A. A., Jr. (1973): Human cortical neurons in epileptogenic foci: Comparison of interictal firing patterns to those of "epileptic neurons" in monkeys. *EEG Clin. Neurophysiol.*, 34:337–351.

24. Cannon, W. B., and Rosenbluth, A. (1949): *The Supersensitivity of Denervated Structures*. Macmillan, New York.

25. Caveness, W. F. (1963): Onset and cessation of fits following craniocerebral trauma. *J. Neurosurg.*, 20:570–583.

26. Caveness, W. F. (1974): Etiological and provocative factors: Trauma. In: *Handbook of Clinical Neurology, Vol. 15, The Epilepsies*, edited by P. J. Vinken and G. W. Bruyn, pp. 274–294.

27. Caveness, W. F. (1976): Sequelae of cranial injury in the armed forces. In: *Handbook of Clinical Neurology, Vol. 24, Injuries of the Brain and Skull*, edited by P. J. Vinken and G. W. Bruyn, pp. 455–476. North-Holland, Amsterdam.

28. Caveness, W. F., Walker, A. E., and Ascroft, P. F. (1962): Incidence of posttraumatic epilepsy in Korean veterans as compared with those from World War I and World War II. *J. Neurosurg.*, 19:122–129.

29. Cheung, W. Y. (1980): Calmodulin plays a pivotal role in cellular regulation. *Science*, 207:19–27.

30. Functions of the Septo-Hippocampal System. *CIBA Foundation Symposium 58*, Elsevier, Amsterdam, 1978.

31. Cohen, P. (1982): The role of protein phosphorylation in neural and hormonal control of cellular activity. *Nature Lond.*, 296:613–620.

32. Cohen, R. S., Blomberg, F., Berzins, K., and Siekevitz, P. (1977): The structure of postsynaptic densities isolated from dog cerebral cortex. Overall morphology and protein composition. *J. Cell. Biol.*, 74:181–203.

33. Corcoran, M. E., Wada, J. A., Wake, A., and Urstad, H. (1976): Failure of atropine to retard amygdaloid kindling. *Exp. Neurol.*, 51:271–275.

34. Cotman, C. (1979): Neuronal plasticity in the rat hippocampus. *Fed. Proc.*, 57:46.

35. DeCamilli, P., Harris, S. M., Huttner, W. B., and Greengard, P. (1983): Synepsin I (protein I), a nerve terminal-specific phosphoprotein. II. Its specific association with synaptic vesicles demonstrated by immunochemistry in agarose-embedded synaptosomes. *J. Cell. Biol.*, 96:1355–1373.

36. DeLorenzo, R. J. (1981): The calmodulin hypothesis of neurotransmission. *Cell Calcium*, 2:365–385.

37. DeLorenzo, R. J., and Freedman, S. D. (1977): Calcium-dependent phosphorylation of synaptic vesicle proteins and its possible role in mediating neurotransmitter release and vesicle function. *Biochem. Biophys. Res. Commun.*, 77:1036–1043.

38. DeLorenzo, R. J., Freedman, S. D., Yohe, W. B., and Maurer, S. C. (1981): Stimulation of Ca^{2+}-dependent neurotransmitter release and presynaptic nerve terminal protein phosphorylation by calmodulin and a calmodulin-like protein isolated from synaptic vesicles. *Proc. Natl. Acad. Sci. USA*, 76:1838–1842.

39. DeLorenzo, R. J., Glaser, G. H., DeLucia, P., and Schwartz, D. (1982): The role of neuronal plasticity in epilepsy. *Neurology*, 32:492.

40. Doose, H., Gerken, H., Leonhart, L. R., et al. (1970): Centrencephalic myoclonic-astatic petit mal: Clinical and genetic investigations. *Neuropediatrie*, 2:59–78.

41. Douglas, R. M., McNaughton, B. L., and Goddard, B. V. (1983): Commissural inhibition and facilitation of granule cell discharge in fascia dentata. *J. Comp. Neurol.*, 219:285–294.

42. Dunwiddie, T. V., and Lynch, G. (1979): The relationship between extracellular calcium concentrations and the induction of hippocampal long-term potentiation. *Brain Res.*, 169:103–110.

43. Earle, K. M., Baldwin, M., and Penfield, W. (1953): Incisural sclerosis and temporal lobe seizures produced by hippocampal herniation at birth. *Arch. Neurol.*, 69:27–42.

44. Engel, J., Jr., Brown, W. J., Kuhl, D. E., Phelps, M. E., Mazziotta, J. C., and Crandall, P. H. (1982): *Ann. Neurol.*, 12:518–528.

45. Engel, J. Jr., Driver, V. M., and Falconer, M. A. (1975): Electrophysiological correlates of

pathological findings and surgical results in temporal lobe epilepsy. *Brain*, 98:124–156.

46. Engel, J. Jr., Kuhl, D. E., and Phelps, M. E. (1982): Interictal cerebral glucose metabolism in partial epilepsy and its relation to EEG changes. *Ann. Neurol.*, 6:510–517.

47. Engel, J. Jr., Kuhl, D. E., and Phelps, M. E. (1982): Patterns of human local cerebral glucose metabolism during epileptic seizures. *Science*, 218:64–66.

48. Engel, J. Jr., Rausch, R., Leib, J. P., Kuhl, D. E., and Crandall, P. H. (1981): Correlation of criteria used for localizing epileptic foci in patients considered for surgical therapy of epilepsy. *Ann. Neurol.*, 9:215–224.

49. Engel, J., Jr., Wolfson, L., and Brown, L. (1978): Anatomical correlates of electrical and behavioral events related to amygdaloid kindling. *Ann. Neurol.*, 3:538–544.

50. Falconer, M. A., Serafitinides, E. A., and Corsellis, J. A. N. (1964): Etiology and pathogenesis of temporal lobe epilepsy. *Arch. Neurol.*, 10:233–248.

51. Falconer, M. A. Genetic and related aetiological factors in temporal lobe epilepsy. A review. *Epilepsia*, 12:13–31.

52. Falconer, M. A. (1973): Reversibility by temporal-lobe resection of the behavioral abnormalities of temporal-lobe epilepsy. *N Engl. J. Med.*, 289:451–455.

53. Feeney, D. M., and Walker, A. E. (1979): The prediction of posttraumatic epilepsy—A mathematical approach. *Arch. Neurol.*, 36:8–12.

54. Finn, R. C., Browning, M., and Lynch, G. (1980): Trifluoperazine inhibits hippocampal long-term potentiation and the phosphorylation of a 40,000 dalton protein. *Neurosci. Lett.*, 19:103–108.

55. Fonnum, F. (1970): Topographical and subcellular localization of choline acetyltransferase in rat hippocampal region. *J. Neurochem.*, 17:1029–1037.

56. Freeman, F. G. (1978): Effects of alcohol on kindled seizure thresholds in rats. *Pharmacol. Biochem. Behav.*, 8:641–644.

57. Freytag, E., and Lindenberg, R. (1964): 294 medicological autopsies on epileptics. *Arch. Pathol.*, 78:274–286.

58. Fukunaga, K., Yamamoto, H., Matsui, K., Higashi, K., and Miyamoto, E. (1982): Purification and characterization of a Ca^{2+} and calmodulin-dependent protein kinase from rat brain. *J. Neurochem.*, 39:1607–1617.

59. Gastaut, H., Toga, M., Roger, J., and Gibson, W. C. (1959): A correlation of clinical electroencephalographic and anatomical findings in nine autopsied cases of temporal lobe epilepsy. *Epilepsia*, 1:56–85.

60. Girgis, M. (1981): Neuronal hypersensitivity to acetylcholineesterase inhibitors induced by a kindling stimulus in the rabbit brain. *Brain Res.*, 208:379–386.

61. Glotzner, F. L. (1973): Membrane properties of neuroglia in epileptogenic gliosis. *Brain Res.*, 55:159–171.

62. Goddard, G. V. (1969): Analysis of avoidance conditioning following cholinergic stimulation of amygdala. *J. Comp. Physiol. Psychol.* 2(Monograph):1–18.

63. Goddard, G. V. (1981): The continuing search for mechanism. In: *Kindling 2*, edited by J. Wada, pp. 1–14. Raven Press, New York.

64. Goddard, G. V., and Douglas, R. M. (1975): Does the engram of kindling model the engram of normal long-term memory? *Can. J. Neurol. Sci.*, 2:385–394.

65. Goddard, C. V., McIntyre, D. C., and Leech, C. K. (1969): A permanent change in brain function resulting from daily electrical stimulation. *Exp. Neurol.*, 25:295–330.

66. Goff, D., Miller, A. A., and Webster, R. A. (1978): Anticonvulsant drugs and folic acid on the development of epileptic kindling in rats. *Br. J. Pharmacol.*, 64:406.

67. Goldberg, N. D., and Haddox, M. K. (1977): Cyclic GMP metabolism and involvement in biological regulation. *Annu. Rev. Biochem.*, 46:823–896.

68. Goldenring, J. R., Gonzalez, B., McGuire, J. S., and DeLorenzo, R. J. (1983): Purification and characterization of a calmodulin-dependent kinase from rat brain cytosol able to phosphorylate tubulin and microtubule-associated proteins. *J. Biol. Chem.*, 258:23632.

69. Grab, D. J., Carlin, R. K., and Siekevitz, P. (1981): Function of calmodulin in postsynaptic densities. II. Presence of a calmodulin-activable protein kinase activity. *J. Cell Biol.*, 89:440–448.

70. Greengard, P. (1981): Intracellular signals in the brain. *Harvey Lecture*, 75:277–331.

71. Hagiwara, S., and Byerly, L. (1983): The calcium channel. *Trends Neurosci.*, 6:189–194.

72. Hagiwara, S., and Byerly, L. (1981): The calcium channel. *Annu. Rev. Neurosci.*, 4:69–125.

73. Harris, A. B. (1980): Structural and chemical changes in experimental epileptic foci. In: *Epilepsy: A Window to Brain Mechanisms*, edited by J. S. Lockard and A. A. Ward, Jr., pp. 149–164. Raven Press, New York.

74. Harris, A. B., and Jenkins, D. P. (1975): Intercellular space in epileptic brain. *Neurosci. Abstr.*, 1:719.

75. Heinemann, U., and Louvel, J. (1983): Changes in $[Ca^{2+}]_0$ and $[K^+]_0$ during repetitive electrical stimulation and during pentylenetetrazol-induced seizure activity in the sensory motor cortex of cats. *Pflugers Arch.*, 398:310–317.

76. Heinemann, U., Lux, H. D., and Gutnick, M. J. (1977): Extracellular free calcium and potassium during paroxysmal activity in the cerebral cortex of the cat. *Exp. Brain Res.*, 27:237–243.

77. Jefferys, J. G. R., and Haas, H. L. (1982): Synchronized bursting of CA_1 hippocampal cells in the absence of synaptic transmission. *Nature*, 300:448–450.

78. Jonec, V., and Wasterlain, C. G. (1981): Anticonvulsants block chemical kindling. *Neurology*, 31:157.

79. Kalichman, M. W., and Burnham, W. M. (1980): Locomotor and convulsive responses to

picrotoxin in amygdala-kindled rats. *Exp. Neurol.*, 70:167–172.

80. Kameyama, M., Wasterlain, C. G., Ackermann, R., Finch, D., and Kuhl, D. E. (1983): Neuronal response of the hippocampal formation to injury: Blood flow, glucose metabolism and protein synthesis. *Exp. Neurol.*, 79:329–346.

81. Kaneko, Y., Wada, J. A., and Kimura, H. (1981): Is the amygdaloid neuron necessary for amygdaloid kindling? In: *Kindling 2*, edited by J. A. Wada, pp. 249–264. Raven Press, New York.

82. Kelly, P. T., and Cotman, C. W. (1978): Synaptic proteins. Characterization of tubulin and actin and identification of a distinct postsynaptic density polypeptide. *J. Cell. Biol.*, 79:173–183.

83. Kelly, P. T., McGuinness, T. L., and Greengard, P. (1984): Evidence that the major postsynaptic density protein is a component of a Ca^{2+}/calmodulin-dependent protein kinase. *Proc. Natl. Acad. Sci. USA*, 81(3):945–949.

84. Kennedy, M. B., and Greengard, P. (1981): Two calcium/calmodulin-dependent protein kinases, which are highly concentrated in brain, phosphorylate protein 1 at distinct sites. *Proc. Natl. Acad. Sci. USA*, 78:1293–1297.

85. Kennedy, M. B., Bennett, M. K., and Erondu, N. E. (1983): Biochemical and immunochemical evidence that the "major postsynaptic density protein" is a subunit of a calmodulin-dependent protein kinase. *Proc. Natl. Acad. Sci. USA*, 80:7357–7361.

86. Kennedy, M. B., McGuinness, T., and Greengard, P. (1983): A calcium/calmodulin-dependent protein kinase from mammalian brain that phosphorylates synapsin I: Partial purification and characterization. *J. Neurosci.*, 3:818–831.

87. Kretsinger, R. H. (1979): The information role of calcium in the cytosol. *Adv. Cyclic Nucleotide Res.*, 11:1–26.

88. Krnjevic, K., Pumain, R., and Renaud, L. (1971): The mechanism of excitation by acetylcholine in the cerebral cortex. *J. Physiol.*, 215:247–268.

89. Lafora, G. R., and Gluck, B. (1911): Beitrag zur Histopathologie der myoklonischen Epilepsie. *Z. Ges. Neurol. Psychiat.*, 6:1–14.

90. Lancaster, B., and Wheal, H. V. (1984): Chronic failure of inhibition of the CA$_1$ area of the hippocampus following kainic acid lesions of the CA$_{3/4}$ area. *Brain Res.*, 295:317–324.

91. Lloyd, K. G., Munari, C., Bossi L., Stoeffels C., Talairach, J., and Morselli, P. L. (1981): Biochemical evidence for the alterations of GABA-mediated synaptic transmission in pathological brain tissue (stereo EEG and morphological definition) from epileptic patients. In: *Neurotransmitters, Seizures and Epilepsy*, edited by P. L. Morselli, pp. 325–338. Raven Press, New York.

92. Lynch, G. S., Gribkoff, V. K., and Deadwyler, S. A. (1976): Long-term potentiation is accompanied by a reduction in dendritic responsiveness to glutamic acid. *Nature*, 263:151–153.

93. Marcum, J. M., Dedman, J. R., Brinkley, B. R., and Means, A. R. (1978): Control of microtubule assembly-disassembly by calcium-dependent regulator protein. *Proc. Natl. Acad. Sci. USA*, 75:3771–3775.

94. Margerison, J. H., and Corsellis, J. A. N. (1966): Epilepsy and the temporal lobes: A clinical, electroencephalographic and neuropathological study of the brain in epilepsy, with particular references to the temporal lobes. *Brain*, 89:499–530.

95. McNamara, J. O. (1978): Muscarinic cholinergic receptors participate in the kindling model of epilepsy. *Brain Res.*, 154:415–420.

96. McNamara, J. O., Byrne, M. C., Dasheiff, R. M., and Fitz, J. G. (1980): The kindling model of epilepsy: A review. In: *Progress in Neurobiology*, Vol. 15, edited by J. W. Phillis and G. Kerkut, pp. 139–159. Pergamon, United Kingdom.

97. McNamara, J. O., Peper, A. M., and Patrone, V. (1980): Repeated seizures induce long-term elevation of hippocampal benzodiazepine receptors. *Proc. Natl. Acad. Sci. USA*, 77:3029–3032.

98. McNaughton, B. L., and Barnes, C. A. (1977): Physiological identification and analysis of dentate granule cell responses to stimulation of the medial and lateral perforant pathways in the rat. *J. Comp. Neurol.*, 175:439–453.

99. McNaughton, B. L., Douglas, R. M., and Goddard, G. V. (1978): Synaptic enhancement in fascia dentata: Cooperative among co active afferents. *Brain Res.*, 157:277–293.

100. McNaughton, B. L. (1983): Activity dependent modulation of hippocampal synaptic efficiency: Some implication for memory processes. In: *Molecular, Cellular and Behavioral Neurobiology of the Hippocampus*, edited by W. Seifert, pp. 233–249. Academic Press, Orlando, Fla.

101. Meech, R. W. (1978): Calcium-dependent potassium activation in nervous tissues. *Annu. Rev. Biophys. Bioeng.*, 7.1–18.

102. Moody, W. J., Futamachi, K. J., and Prince, D. A. (1974): Extracellular potassium activity during epileptogenesis. *Exp. Neurol.*, 42:248–263.

103. Morin, A. M., Watson, A. L., and Wasterlain, C. G. (1983): Kindling of seizures with norharman, a β-carboline ligand of benzodiazepine receptors. *Eur. J. Pharmacol.*, 88:131–134.

104. Morrell, F. (1979): Human secondary epileptogenic lesions. *Neurology*, 29:558.

105. Mucha, R. P., and Pinel, J. P. J. (1979): Increased susceptibility to kindled seizures in rats following a single injection of alcohol. *J. Stud. Alcohol.*, 40:258–271.

106. Norman, R. M., Sandry, S., and Corsellis, J. A. N. (1974): Pathoanatomical change in the epileptic brain. In: *Handbook of Clinical Neurology, Vol. 15, The Epilepsies*, edited by P. J. Vinken and G. W. Bruyn, pp. 611–620. Elsevier, New York.

107. Ounsted, C., Lindsay, J., and Norman, R. (1966): *Biological Factors in Temporal Lobe Epilepsy*. Heinemann, London.

108. Payne, M. E., Schworer, C. M., and Soderling, T. R. (1983): Purification and characterization of rabbit liver calmodulin-dependent glycogen synthase kinase. *J. Biol. Chem.*, 258:2376–2382.

109. Pedersen, E., Grynderup, V., Kissmeyer-Nielsen, F., Nielsen, J., Poulsen, J. H., and Reske-Nielsen, E. (1982): Familial progressive myoclonic epilepsy. *J. Neurol. Sci.*, 53:305–320.

110. Pedley, T. A., Fisher, R. S., Futamachi, K., and Prince, D. A. (1976): Regulation of extracellular potassium concentration in epileptogenesis. *Fed. Proc.*, 35:1254–1259.

111. Penry, J. K., Porter, R. J., and Dreyfuss, F. E. (1975): Simultaneous recording of absence seizures with videotape and electroencephalography: A study of 374 seizures in 48 patients. *Brain*, 98:427–440.

112. Phillips, G. (1954): Traumatic epilepsy after closed head injury. *J. Neurol. Neurosurg.*, 17:1–10.

113. Pinel, J. P. J., Phillips, A. G., and Deol, G. (1974): Effects of current intensity on kindled motor seizure activity. *Behav. Biol.*, 11:59–68.

114. Pinel, J. P. J., Van Oot, P. H., and Mucha, R. F. (1975): Intensification of the alcohol withdrawal syndrome by repeated brain stimulation. *Nature Lond.*, 254:510.

115. Pollen, D. A., and Trachtenberg, M. C. (1970): Neuroglia: Gliosis and focal epilepsy. *Science*, 67:1252–1253.

116. Post, R. M., Squillace, K. M., Pert, A., and Sass, W. (1981): The effect of amygdala kindling on spontaneous and cocaine-induced motor activity and lidocaine seizures. *Psychopharmacology*, 72:189–196.

117. Prince, D. A., and Futamachi, K. J. (1970): Intracellular recordings from chronic epileptogenic foci in the monkey. *EEG Clin. Neurophysiol.*, 29:496–510.

118. Purpura, D. P., Penry, J. K., Tower, D., Woodbury, D. M., and Walter, R. (1972): *Experimental Models of Epilepsy*. Raven Press, New York.

119. Racine, R. F. (1978): Kindling: The first decade. *Neurosurgery*, 3:234–252.

120. Racine, R. J., Burnham, W., Gartner, J., and Levitan, D. (1973): Rates of motor seizure development in rats subjected to electrical brain stimulation. Strain and interstimulation interval effects. *Electroencephalogr. Clin. Neurophysiol.*, 35:553–556.

121. Racine, R. J., Burnham, W. M., and Livingston, K. (1979): The effect of procaine hydrochloride and diazepam, separately or in combination, on corticogeneralized kindled seizures. *Electroencephalogr. Clin. Neurophysiol.*, 47:204–212.

122. Racine, R., Gartner, J., and Burnham, W. (1972): Epileptiform activity and neural plasticity in limbic structures. *Brain Res.*, 47:262–268.

123. Racine, R. J., Tuff, L. P., and Adamec, R. (1983): The effects of kindling on GABA-me-

124. Racine, R., Tuff, L., and Zaide, L. (1975): Kindling, unit discharge patterns and neural plasticity. *Can. J. Neurol. Sci.*, 2:395–405.

125. Racine, R., and Zaide, J. (1978): A further investigation into the mechanism of the kindling phenomenon. In: *Limbic Mechanisms: The Continuing Evolution of the Limbic System Concept*, edited by K. Livingston and O. Hornykiewicz, pp. 475–493. Plenum, New York.

126. Rasmussen, T. (1979): Cortical resection for medically refractory focal epilepsy: Results, lessons, and questions. In: *Functional Neurosurgery*, edited by T. Rasmussen and R. Marino, pp. 253–269. Raven Press, New York.

127. Rasmussen, R., and Goodman, D. B. P. (1977): Relationships between calcium and cyclic nucleotides in cell activation. *Physiol. Rev.*, 57:421–509.

128. C. E. Ribak, Chapter 37.

129. Ribak, C. E., Harris, A. B., Vaughn, J. E., and Roberts, E. (1979): Inhibitory GABAergic nerve terminals decrease at sites of focal epilepsy. *Science*, 205:211–214.

130. Robison, G. A., Butcher, R. W., and Sutherland, E. W. (1968): Cyclic AMP. *Annu. Rev. Biochem.*, 37:249.

131. Rose, A. M., Hattori, T., and Fibiger, H. C. (1976): Analysis of the septohippocampal pathway by light and electron microscope autoradiography. *Brain Res.*, 108:170–174.

132. Russell, W. R., and Whitty, C. W. M. (1952): Studies in traumatic epilepsy, factors influencing incidence of epilepsy after brain wounds. *J. Neurol. Neurosurg. Psychiatry*, 15:93–98.

133. Schwartzkroin, P. A. (1983): Mechanisms of cell synchronization in epileptiform activity. *Trends Neurosci.*, 6:157–160.

134. Servit, Z., and Musil, F. (1981): Prophylactic treatment of posttraumatic epilepsy: Results of a long-term follow-up in Czechoslovakia. *Epilepsia*, 22:315–320.

135. Sokoloff, L., Reivich, M., Kennedy, C., Des Rosiers, M. H., Patlake, S., Pettigrew, K. D., Sakurada, O., and Shirohara, M. (1977): The [^{14}C]-deoxyglucose method for the measurement of local cerebral glucose utilization: Theory, procedure and normal values in the conscious and anesthetized albino rat. *J. Neurochem.*, 28:897–916.

136. Spehlman, R., Daniels, J. C., and Chang, C. M. (1971): The effects of eserine and atropine on the epileptiform activity of chronically isolated cortex. *Epilepsia*, 12:123–132.

137. Storm-Mathisen, J. S., and Blackstadt, T. W. (1964): Cholinesterase in the hippocampal region. Distribution and relation to architectonics and afferent systems. *Acta Anat.*, 56:216–253.

138. Stramka, M., Sedlak, P., and Nadvornik, P. (1977): Observation of kindling phenomenon in treatment of pain by stimulation in thalamus. In: *Neurosurgical Treatment in Psychiatry*,

Pain and Epilepsy, edited by Sweet, Obrador, and Martin-Rodriguez, pp. 651–656. University Press, Baltimore.

139. Swanson, I. W., and Cowan, W. M. (1979): The connection of the septal region in the rat. *J. Comp. Neurol.,* 106:621–656.

140. Taylor, C. P., and Dodek, F. E. (1982): Synchronous neural afterdischarges in rat hippocampal slices without active chemical synapses. *Science,* 218:810–812.

141. Turner, D. A., and Wyler, A. R. (1981): Temporal lobectomy for epilepsy: Mesial temporal herniation as an operative and prognostic finding. *Epilepsia,* 22:623–629.

142. Turner, I. M., Newman, S. M., Louis, S., and Kutt, H. (1977): Pharmacological prophylaxis against the development of kindled amygdaloid seizures. *Ann. Neurol.,* 2:221–224.

143. Turner, R. W., Baimbridge, K. G., and Miller, J. J. (1982): Calcium-induced long-term potentiation in the hippocampus. *Neuroscience,* 7:1411–1416.

144. Unverricht, H. (1891): *Die Myoklonie.* F. Deuticke, Leipzig.

145. Vosu, H., and Wise, R. A. (1975): Cholinergic seizure kindling in the rat: Comparison of caudate, amygdala, and hippocampus. *Behav. Biol.,* 13:491–495.

146. Wada, J. A. (1977): Pharmacological prophylaxis in the kindling model of epilepsy. *Arch. Neurol.,* 34:389–395.

147. Wada, J. A. (1978): The clinical relevance of kindling: Species, brain sites and seizure susceptibility. In: *Limbic Mechanisms,* edited by K. E. Livingston and D. Hornykiewicz, pp. 369–388. Plenum, New York.

148. Waisman, D. M., Singh, T. J., and Wang, J. H. (1978): The modulator-dependent protein kinase. *J. Biol. Chem.,* 253:3387–3390.

149. Wasterlain, C. G., and Farber, D. (1982): A lasting change in protein phosphorylation associated with septal kindling. *Brain Res.,* 247:191–194.

150. Wasterlain, C. G., and Farber, D. B. (1984): Kindling alters the calcium/calmodulin-dependent phosphorylation of synaptic plasma membrane proteins in rat hippocampus. *Proc. Natl. Acad. Sci. USA,* 81:1253–1257.

151. Wasterlain, C. G., and Jonec, V. (1980): Muscarinic kindling: Transsynaptic generation of a chronic seizure focus. *Life Sci.,* 26:387–391.

152. Wasterlain, C. G., and Jonec, V. (1983): Chemical kindling by muscarinic amygdaloid stimulation in the rat. *Brain Res.,* 271:311–323.

153. Wasterlain, C. G., Masuoka, D., and Jonec, V. (1981): Chemical kindling: A study of synaptic pharmacology. In: *Kindling 2,* edited by J. A. Wada, pp. 315–329. Raven Press, New York.

154. Wasterlain, C. G., Morin, A. M., and Jonec, V. (1982): Kindling: A pharmacological approach. *EEG Clin. Neurophysiol.* 36 (Suppl.):264–273.

155. Wasterlain, C. G., Morin, A. M., and Jonec, V. (1982): Interactions between chemical and electrical kindling of the rat amygdala. *Brain Res.,* 247:341–346.

156. Wasterlain, C. G., Morin, A. M., Jonec, V., and Billawalla, T. (1979): Kindling with blockers of inhibitory synapses. *Neurology,* 29:346.

157. Wauquier, A., Ashton, D., and Melis, W. (1981): Behavioral analysis of amygdaloid kindling in beagle dogs and the effects of clonazepam, diazepam, phenobarbital, diphenylhydantoin, and flunarizine on seizure manifestations. *Science,* 213:546–549.

158. Wong, R. K. S., and Prince, D. A. (1979): Dentric mechanisms underlying penicillin-induced epileptiform activity. *Science,* 204:1228–1231.

159. Wong, R. K. S., and Prince, D. A. (1978): Participation of calcium spikes during intrinsic burst firing in hippocampal neurons. *Brain Res.,* 159:385–390.

160. Wyler, A. R., Fetz, E. E., and Ward, A. A., Jr. (1975): Firing patterns of epileptic and normal neurons in neocortex of undrugged monkeys during different behavioral states. *Brain Res.,* 98:1–20.

161. Yamauchi, T., and Fujisawa, H. (1980): Evidence for three distinct forms of calmodulin-dependent protein kinases from rat brain. *FEBS Lett.,* 116:141–144.

162. Yaari, Y., Konnerth, A., and Heinemann, U. (1983): Spontaneous epileptiform activity of CA_1 hippocampal neurons in low extracellular calcium solutions. *Exp. Brain Res.,* 51:153–156.

163. Yamauchi, T., and Fujisawa, H. (1982): Phosphorylation of microtubule-associated protein 2 by calmodulin-dependent protein kinase (kinase II) which occurs only in the brain tissues. *Biochem. Biophys. Res. Commun.,* 109:975–981.

164. Zuckermann, E. C., and Glaser, G. H. (1968): Hippocampal epileptic activity induced by localized ventricular perfusion with high-potassium cerebrospinal fluid. *Exp. Neurol.,* 20:89–110.

Advances in Neurology, Vol. 44, edited by
A. V. Delgado-Escueta, A. A. Ward, Jr.,
D. M. Woodbury, and R. J. Porter.
Raven Press, New York © 1986.

22

A Molecular Approach to the Calcium Signal in Brain: Relationship to Synaptic Modulation and Seizure Discharge

Robert John DeLorenzo

Department of Neurology, Medical College of Virginia, Richmond, Virginia 23298

SUMMARY   The synapse is a major regulatory site that has been implicated in modulating neuronal excitability and seizure discharge. Voltage-dependent calcium (Ca^{2+}) entry at the synapse plays a major role in initiating neurotransmitter release and in regulating synaptic function. Thus, obtaining a molecular understanding of the effects of Ca^{2+} on synaptic modulation would provide important insights into the regulation of synaptic activity and, possibly, the biochemical basis for some forms of epilepsy. Calmodulin is a major Ca^{2+}-binding protein in brain that has been implicated in mediating many of the second messenger effects of Ca^{2+} on neuronal function. The evidence implicating calmodulin in modulating synaptic excitability will be presented. Calmodulin was shown to be present at the synapse in association with synaptic vesicles and in the postsynaptic density. In addition, several calmodulin-regulated synaptic biochemical processes have been identified, including Ca^{2+}- and calmodulin-regulated protein phosphorylation, vesicular neurotransmitter release, vesicle–membrane interactions, and neurotransmitter turnover. These results indicate that calmodulin may play an important role in synaptic modulation and provide a molecular approach to investigating the Ca^{2+} signal in brain.

Several anticonvulsants have been shown to regulate some of calcium's effects on neuronal function. These anticonvulsants include phenytoin, carbamazepine, and the benzodiazepines. All of these compounds are effective against maximal electric shock (MES) seizure models in animals. Anticonvulsants were tested on several of the Ca^{2+}–calmodulin-regulated synaptic biochemical systems. The results demonstrate that phenytoin, carbamazepine, and the benzodiazepines were effective in inhibiting calcium calmodulin protein kinase activity in membrane and purified kinase preparations, vesicle neurotransmitter release, vesicle–membrane interactions, and voltage-sensitive calcium uptake in intact synaptosomes. Phenobarbital, ethosuximide, trimethadione, valproic acid, and vinyl γ-aminobutyric acid (GABA) were not effective in inhibiting these calcium-regulated processes. Thus, the effects of anticonvulsants on calcium-regulated processes were selective to a group of anticonvulsants that had been shown in several electrophysiological systems to antagonize some of the actions of calcium on neuronal excitability.

These observations suggested the existence of specific membrane receptors that might mediate the effects of these anticonvulsants on neuronal function through the regulation of calcium–calmodulin-regulated processes. To test this possibility, specific binding studies were performed with synaptic membranes by means of benzodiazepines. A saturable, stereospecific micromolar affinity membrane binding site has been identified for the benzodiazepines. The potency of the benzodiazepines to bind to the micromolar affinity receptors correlates with the potency of these compounds to inhibit MES-induced seizures. In addition, binding to the micromolar affinity receptors has been shown to regulate calcium calmodulin protein kinase activity in synaptic membrane preparations and depolarization-dependent calcium uptake in intact synaptosomes. These results provide evidence that specific saturable receptors exist in brain membrane that modulate the effects of the benzodiazepines on some of the calcium-regulated biochemical processes described in this presentation. Phenytoin and carbamazepine also displaced benzodiazepine binding from these receptor sites. However, benzodiazepine binding was not displaced by phenobarbital, ethosuximide, or trimethadione. Thus, the anticonvulsants that interact with these specific membrane sites are the same group of compounds that inhibit calcium–calmodulin-regulated processes and some of the effects of calcium on synaptic function.

The evidence presented in this chapter provides a molecular insight into the biochemical processes that mediate some of the actions of calcium on synaptic modulation. The identification of specific membrane binding sites that mediate some of the effects of specific anticonvulsants on calcium-regulated biochemical events provides the identification of molecular processes that play a role in regulating neuronal excitability and seizure discharge. These findings provide the ability to study these specific systems in clinical settings and obtain a molecular insight into the nature of seizure discharges.

EPILEPSY AND THE CA^{2+} SIGNAL AT THE SYNAPSE

The name epilepsy refers to the many varieties of recurrent seizures produced by paroxysmal excessive neuronal discharges in different parts of the brain (52,53,61). Status epilepticus represents an extreme situation in which seizures occur so frequently that there is little if any time between seizures (51,101). Seizures can be generalized in their presentation or can involve focal regions of the brain. There are many conditions that cause epilepsy, and the possible causes of seizures are numerous (57). Thus, no one approach to elucidating the causes of this complex clinical phenomenon will account adequately for the varieties of seizure disorders.

In developing a molecular approach to epilepsy, it is important to focus on an important regulatory system of neuronal function that may be related to the control of neuronal excitability and seizure initiation and to study it in detail. The synapse is a major site for modulating neuronal communication. Excitatory and inhibitory synaptic transmissions are believed to regulate ongoing neuronal discharges in brain (45). Thus, the synapse is a major regulatory site in the central nervous system (CNS), in which genetic alterations or pharmacological manipulations could produce changes in the baseline firing of a population of neurons and possibly initiate seizure discharge (44–46).

Recent advances in the study of synaptic systems in the peripheral CNS have provided a significant understanding of many of the properties of synaptic function, such as the identification of excitatory and inhibitory neurotransmitter substances, electromicroscopic characterization of synaptic structures, and electrophysiological characterization of synaptic activity. Although there are many aspects of synaptic function that could regulate synaptic excitability, a central regulating force at the synapse is the calcium ion and the various processes regulated by this cellular messenger (64,65,82,83). This chapter will focus on the role of calcium in regulating synaptic excitability and on how calcium-regulated synaptic processes may mediate the effects of anticonvulsants and the modulation of seizure discharge.

CALCIUM: A MAJOR SECOND MESSENGER AT THE SYNAPSE

The Ca^{2+} ion plays a major role in modulating the activity and function of nervous tissue (91,93). One of the most widely recognized roles of Ca^{2+} in synaptic function is its action on neurotransmission. Earlier studies demonstrated that the release of neurotransmitter substances by vertebrate neuromuscular junctions was dependent on the Ca^{2+} ion concentration in the media (16,93). Elegant studies at the synaptic level demonstrated that the effects of Ca^{2+} on neurotransmission were not secondary to effects of Ca^{2+} on the presynaptic action potential, but were directly dependent on the entry of Ca^{2+} into the nerve terminal (64,65,82,83). The action of Ca^{2+} in stimulus–secretion coupling has also been demonstrated in various secretory processes in several tissues (42).

The role of Ca^{2+} in synaptic function is well established. However, one of the major questions in neuroscience research at present is directed at discovering the molecular mechanism mediating the effects of Ca^{2+} on synaptic activity. Research since the 1970s has attempted to provide a molecular approach to studying the biochemistry of the Ca^{2+} signal in neurotransmitter release and synaptic modulation. *In vitro* and *in vivo* preparations were developed and used to study simultaneously the effects of Ca^{2+} on neurotransmitter release, synaptic protein phosphorylation, and synaptic membrane–synaptic vesicle interactions (4,19–25,36).

The results of these studies provided experimental evidence that Ca^{2+} regulates several biochemical and morphological events in synaptic preparations. Therefore, these experimental systems could be used to investigate the molecular mechanism mediating some of the effects of Ca^{2+} at the synapse. This research formed the foundation for studying the effects of anticonvulsants and convulsants on Ca^{2+}-regulated synaptic processes.

A MOLECULAR APPROACH TO EPILEPSY: FOCUS ON THE CALCIUM SIGNAL

Understanding the molecular basis for some of calcium's effects at the synapse may provide an insight into biochemical processes that regulate neuronal excitability. Because Ca^{2+} is a major second messenger in modulating neuronal function (91,93), it is reasonable to assume that alterations in the normal function of Ca^{2+}-regulated processes may underlie some of the abnormalities of neuronal excitability seen in seizure disorders (13,21,27). Accumulating evidence suggests that abnormalities in major Ca^{2+}-regulated enzymatic processes may underlie alterations in neuronal excitability (27).

Experiments in this laboratory have been directed at understanding specific biochemical processes that relate to synaptic function (8–11,17–39,54–57,97). Calcium ions play a major role in regulating synaptic activity (64,65, 82,83,91,93), and several of the excitatory effects of Ca^{2+} on synaptic function have been shown to be antagonized by the anticonvulsant phenytoin (20,21,27,29). Thus, synaptic biochemical processes that are stimulated by Ca^{2+} and inhibited by phenytoin are of considerable interest, because they may represent a molecular process that modulates neuronal excitability.

Numerous enzyme systems were studied in our laboratory in the early 1970s in an attempt to find a Ca^{2+}-stimulated, phenytoin-inhibited process. We identified a unique Ca^{2+}-stimulated protein phosphorylation system in brain that was also inhibited by phenytoin (17,18). It is important to emphasize that this Ca^{2+} kinase system is a protein phosphorylation system distinct from the well-described brain cyclic AMP protein kinases. Thus, efforts have been directed at determining the role of Ca^{2+}-dependent protein phosphorylation in modulating synaptic function and neuronal excitability. Furthermore, several anticonvulsant compounds have been shown to block Ca^{2+} uptake into cells (24,25,48,49,75,97) and to regulate several Ca^{2+}-dependent enzyme systems (24,25). This work provided the basis for further experimentation on these specific Ca^{2+}-regulated processes that were modulated by anticonvulsant compounds. We have also gained insights into the regulation of voltage-sensitive Ca^{2+} channels in brain (38,39,97). Studies from this laboratory have identified an "anticonvulsant" binding site on neuronal membrane that may play an important role in regulating Ca^{2+} currents and Ca^{2+}–calmodulin-regulated synaptic events (38,39,97).

This chapter will focus on the molecular basis for regulating the Ca^{2+} signal at the synapse. Although the precise mechanism mediating calcium's actions are not completely understood, significant advances have been made over the past 5 years in the identification of specific Ca^{2+}-regulated synaptic processes and in discovering how they may regulate synaptic excitability and seizure discharge.

CALMODULIN: A PROTEIN RECEPTOR FOR THE CALCIUM SIGNAL

Calmodulin is a major Ca^{2+} receptor protein in brain (7,14,15,72). It has been suggested that some effects of Ca^{2+} on nerve function may be modulated by the heat-stable, Ca^{2+}-dependent regulator protein, calmodulin, because the Ca^{2+}-dependent activation of several important enzyme systems in brain require calmodulin (15). Calmodulin has been purified and characterized from many sources and appears to be a Ca^{2+} receptor protein with a specific and strong binding affinity for Ca^{2+}. These results, and the presence of calmodulin-like proteins in a wide variety of mammalian and invertebrate tissues, have suggested that many of the physiological functions of Ca^{2+} may be mediated by Ca^{2+} receptor proteins such as calmodulin (15,72).

One of the major effects of Ca^{2+} in the nervous system is its action on synaptic function. It is of great importance to determine if calmodulin or calmodulin-like proteins mediate the effect of Ca^{2+} on depolarization-dependent neurotransmitter release and other aspects of synaptic modulation. Accumulating evidence suggests that calmodulin mediates many of the effects of Ca^{2+} on synaptic function (19–25). These results have led to the calmodulin hypothesis of neurotransmission (22). This hypothesis is shown diagrammatically in Fig. 1, and states that as Ca^{2+} enters the presynaptic and postsynaptic nerve terminals during depolarization, it binds to a high-affinity Ca^{2+} receptor protein, calmodulin, and initiates several Ca^{2+}–calmodulin-dependent biochemical processes that mediate synaptic activity.

Evidence for the role of calmodulin in synaptic activity will be presented in this chapter with a focus on the role of calmodulin systems in regulating neuronal excitability and on how these systems may be involved in seizure initiation. Many calmodulin-regulated processes are being identified at the synapse, and these Ca^{2+}-regulated systems provide a biochemical basis for studying the regulatory effects of Ca^{2+} on synaptic activity. An understanding of the function of these calmodulin-regulated systems may provide an insight into the molecular basis of some forms of epilepsy.

CALMODULIN AT THE SYNAPSE

Calmodulin represents approximately 1% of the total protein in brain cytoplasm and thus is found in relatively high concentrations in neuronal tissue (15). To implicate this major Ca^{2+} receptor protein in synaptic modulation, it is important to demonstrate that calmodulin is present at the synapse. The ability of calmodulin to bind to specialized synaptic organelles such as synaptic vesicles and to postsynaptic densities would further suggest that calmodulin may be involved in synaptic regulation. Thus, studies were initiated to determine if calmodulin could be isolated from brain fractions enriched in synaptic structures.

A synaptic vesicle-bound, heat-stable protein was isolated from highly enriched preparations of synaptic vesicles from rat cortex that had the same MW as calmodulin (19,21,25,36). This ves-

icle-bound protein could be removed from the vesicles in the presence of EGTA and was found to bind Ca^{2+} at micromolar concentrations. Calmodulin isolated from whole rat brain was shown to be identical to the vesicle Ca^{2+}-binding protein (19,21,25,36). Approximately 80–90% of the protein in this synaptoplasm preparation was shown to originate in the presynaptic terminal (2). The Ca^{2+}-binding protein in synaptoplasm was found to be identical to whole-brain calmodulin in MW, isoelectric point, amino acid composition, and ability to stimulate protein kinase and phosphodiesterase activity (19). Synaptic calmodulin constituted 0.71% of the total protein in the synaptoplasm preparation. Because the concentration of calmodulin in whole-brain fractions is ~1% of the total brain protein, the high percentage of calmodulin in synaptoplasm and synaptic vesicle fractions strongly indicates the presence of this Ca^{2+} receptor protein in the presynaptic nerve terminal. Calmodulin has also been isolated and characterized from postsynaptic density preparations (58,59).

The ability to isolate calmodulin from highly enriched preparations of presynaptic and postsynaptic fractions strongly indicates that calmodulin is a transsynaptic protein. Therefore, calmodulin is very well suited to mediate the effects of Ca^{2+} on both the presynaptic and postsynaptic sides of the synapse. Because calmodulin represents ~1% of the total protein in these subfraction preparations, it is unlikely that the calmodulin in these isolated fractions was derived from cytoplasmic contamination. Therefore, partial contamination of the synaptic cytoplasm, vesicle, and postsynaptic density preparations with whole-brain cytoplasm could not account for the high percentage of calmodulin found in these fractions.

Immunohistochemical studies of brain sections using antisera to calmodulin with light microscopy showed that calmodulin was localized in nerve processes and cell bodies, but not in nuclei (102). Electron microscopy showed heavy labeling in postsynaptic densities, but not in presynaptic elements. This observation was confirmed (77) using anticalmodulin F_{ab} fragments coupled to horseradish peroxidase. These reports did not mean that calmodulin existed in the presynaptic terminals. Calmodulin may be present in amounts below the detection limits of the procedure or may be sequestered so that its antigenic sites are masked.

Wood et al. (102) also found anticalmodulin labeling of dendritic microtubules. Such a result is in agreement with reports of the ability of calmodulin to prevent tubulin polymerization *in*

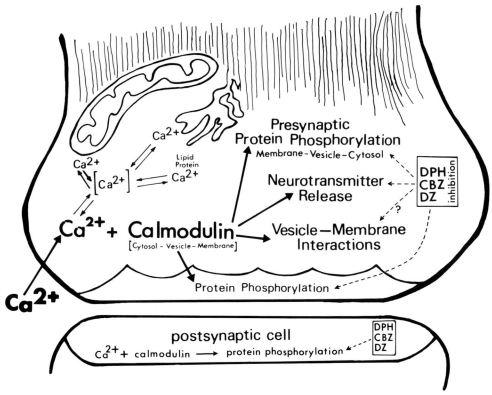

FIG. 1. Schematic model showing the roles of calcium and calmodulin in regulating synaptic protein phosphorylation, neurotransmitter release and turnover, and vesicle–membrane interactions and the inhibitory effect of phenytoin (DPH), carbamazepine (CBZ), and diazepam (DZ), on these calcium–calmodulin-stimulated processes. The inhibitory effects of these anticonvulsants on synaptic membrane protein phosphorylation may also modulate the depolarization-dependent entry of calcium into the nerve terminal (38). The importance of calmodulin in mediating the effects of calcium on synaptic activity is becoming more evident (24), and the effects of major anticonvulsants compounds on calcium–calmodulin systems provide an exciting area for further investigation (from ref. 38, with permission).

vitro (79). However, Lin et al. (77) did not find any labeling on microtubules; they noted only "granular labeling" in neurites. Differences in fixation procedures or simply regional differences in the brain may account for these discrepancies, because Lin et al. (77) used rat cerebellum and Wood et al. (102) used mouse basal ganglia. The latter explanation is more likely because Carlin et al. (13) have demonstrated that, at least in postsynaptic densities, the cerebellum has a much lower amount of calmodulin than do other brain regions.

Both Wood et al. (102) and Lin et al. (77) noted labeling of mitochondrial membranes and of smooth endoplasmic reticulum and plasma membrane. Neither detected any labeling of the nucleus. Lin et al. (77) also found labeling of free and attached ribosomes, but no labeling of the endoplasmic reticulum cisternae. This supports

the idea that calmodulin is synthesized and released into the cytoplasm, where it then associates with various membrane systems. Recent immunohistochemical studies in this laboratory using ultrathin frozen sections of rat brain synaptosomes have demonstrated that calmodulin antiserum decorates the presynaptic nerve terminal. This finding indicates that when the antibody has direct access to the presynaptic terminal, it recognizes calmodulin within the terminal. Thus, calmodulin appears to be a major Ca^{2+}-binding protein at the synapse.

CALCIUM–CALMODULIN SYNAPTIC SYSTEMS

Calmodulin has been shown to regulate numerous Ca^{2+}-mediated processes in both animal and plant tissues, suggesting that many, if not all, of the effects of Ca^{2+} on cellular function are regulated by calmodulin (15,72). The list of calmodulin-regulated biochemical systems is expanding rapidly. Several review articles (15, 24,72) have summarized the numerous effects of calmodulin on cellular function.

Demonstrating the existence of Ca^{2+}–calmodulin processes in neuronal tissue does not insure that these calmodulin-regulated biochemical processes are modulating synaptic activity. Thus, it is necessary to determine which calmodulin processes are present at the synapse and how these calmodulin biochemical systems may regulate synaptic function. Research from this laboratory and the work from several other groups has clearly documented that calmodulin is regulating many transsynaptic biochemical processes (25).

Phenytoin, the benzodiazepines, and carbamazepine have been shown to regulate several calmodulin-regulated processes (20,27,29,38,39). These compounds have been utilized to study calmodulin-modulated synaptic process, especially Ca^{2+} and calmodulin-regulated protein phosphorylation. Phosphorylation of synaptosomal proteins DPH-L and DPH-M were also enriched in synaptic vesicle fractions (Fig. 2) prepared from intact synaptosomes (33–35). These results demonstrated that the Ca^{2+}-stimulated phosphorylation observed in synaptosome fractions was occurring within the synaptosomes and not in some other membrane contaminations in the preparation.

A hypothesis was developed from these findings, suggesting that Ca^{2+}-dependent protein phosphorylation (a new phosphorylation system distinct from cyclic AMP kinases) may regulate the effects of Ca^{2+} on synaptic function and possibly some aspects of neurotransmitter release (17,33). The Ca^{2+}-dependent pattern of endogenous protein phosphorylation has been confirmed by other researchers in several isolated brain fractions (43) and in preparations of other tissues such as the adrenal medulla (1) and the electric organ of *Torpedo* (81).

Depolarization-dependent Ca^{2+} uptake in intact synaptosomes was shown to stimulate the phosphorylation of an 80,000 dalton protein (protein I) in intact synaptosomes (74). The levels of phosphorylation of proteins with identical MWs to proteins DPH-L and DPH-M were also shown to be stimulated in intact synaptosomes by depolarizing conditions that stimulated Ca^{2+} entry and simultaneously initiated neurotransmitter release from intact synaptosomes (19,21–25, 36) (Tables 1 and 2). The phos-

phorylation of these proteins in intact preparations was also shown to be occurring in the synaptic vesicle, synaptic membrane, and synaptic junctional complex preparations from these intact fractions (19,36) (Table 3). These results provided the first evidence that the depolarization-dependent phosphorylation of specific proteins in intact synaptosome preparations was actually occurring within the synaptosomes and was not associated with other contaminations in the synaptosome preparations. The level of phosphorylation of 50,000–60,000 dalton proteins also correlates with norepinephrine (NE) release in intact adrenal medulla cells (1).

The Ca^{2+}-stimulated endogenous phosphorylation pattern first described in synaptosomes (17) was known to be calmodulin dependent in crude preparations of brain membrane and in several other tissues (94,95). Calmodulin was subsequently demonstrated to mediate the effect (Fig. 3) of Ca^{2+} on the phosphorylation of specific synaptic vesicle proteins (36). Calmodulin was also shown to modulate the effects of Ca^{2+} on the endogenous phosphorylation of highly enriched synaptic membrane (19–21), synaptic junctional complex (19–21) and postsynaptic density (19,58,59) preparations. Thus, depolarization-dependent Ca^{2+} uptake in intact synaptosomes was shown to stimulate simultaneously the release of neurotransmitter substances and the phosphorylation of specific synaptic vesicle, synaptic membrane, synaptic junctional, and postsynaptic density proteins isolated from the intact synaptosomes following depolarization-dependent Ca^{2+} uptake (19,21) (Tables 2 and 3).

In summary, evidence from several laboratories has confirmed, with both intact and broken synaptosome fractions, the initial observations in isolated synaptosome fractions (17) that Ca^{2+} stimulated the phosphorylation of synaptic proteins. Phosphorylation of DPH-L and DPH-M, and possibly of other 50,000–60,000 dalton proteins, appears to be consistently observed and correlates with neurotransmitter release. In addition, protein I (74), low MW proteins (43), and several high MW proteins (36,43) have also been described as serving as endogenous substrates for the Ca^{2+}–calmodulin kinase and have been shown to phosphorylate in intact synaptosomes in response to Ca^{2+} uptake. The fact that Ca^{2+} and calmodulin stimulate the phosphorylation of specific proteins in highly enriched synaptic vesicle, synaptic membrane, synaptic junction, and postsynaptic density preparations strongly indicates that the Ca^{2+} kinase is indeed present at the synapse.

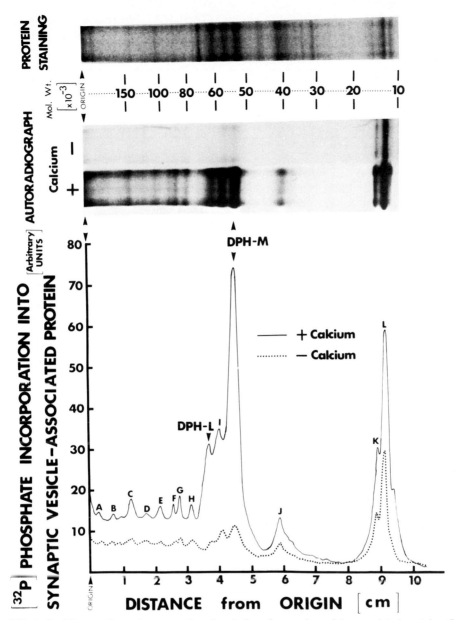

FIG. 2. Effect of calcium on the endogenous phosphorylation of synaptic vesicle-associated proteins. Synaptic vesicles were obtained and incubated under standard conditions in the presence of Mg Cl$_2$ (4 mM) and [γ-^{32}P]ATP (25 μM) plus or minus Ca Cl$_2$ (50 μM) under identical conditions to those described in Table 1 for norepinephrine release. Following the isolation of the vesicles after the reaction by centrifugation, the vesicle pellets were subjected to sodium-dodecyl sulfate-polyacrylamide gel electrophoresis, protein staining, autoradiography, and quantitation, as described previously (18,31). The results shown are representative of 12 individual experiments. Each arbitrary unit equals ~38.6 cpm. MW determinations were performed as described previously (18,31) (from ref. 34, with permission).

PURIFICATION OF CALMODULIN-DEPENDENT KINASE SYSTEMS

Calcium–calmodulin protein kinases have re-

cently been isolated and purified from rat brain cytoplasm (3,50,54–55,68,69,96). A calmodulin kinase has been isolated and purified in this laboratory using microtubule-associated protein 2

TABLE 1. *Effects of Ca^{2+} uptake on neurotransmitter release in intact synaptosomes in the presence or absence of trifluoperazine, phenytoin, and diazepam*

| | | Neurotransmitter release | |
Condition	$^{45}Ca^{2+}$ uptake	Norepi- nephrine	Acetyl- choline
Control	42	55	58
Ca^{2+}		61	64
Ca^{2+}, K, plus	100	100	100
Trifluoperazine	78	64	69
Phenytoin	75	69	63
Diazepam	79	67	68
Ca^{2+}, A23187, plus	95	91	96
Trifluoperazine	89	76	73
Phenytoin	91	74	78
Diazepam	93	76	71

Intact synaptosomes were incubated under various conditions after preincubation with ^{32}P followed by quantitation of $^{45}Ca^{2+}$-uptake and neurotransmitter release as described previously. Concentration of trifluoperazine, phenytoin, and diazepam were 20 μM, 80 μM, and 20 μM, respectively. Data give means of 10 determinations and are expressed as percentages of the maximally stimulated condition (100%). The largest ± SEM was 5.8. The concentration of the Ca^{2+} ionophore (A23187) was 2 μg/ml (from ref. 22, with permission).

TABLE 2. *Effects of Ca^{2+} uptake on protein phosphorylation in intact synaptosomes in the presence or absence of trifluoperazine, phenytoin, and diazepam*

| | Protein DPH-M phosphorylation | |
Condition	Whole synaptosomes	Synaptic vesicles
Control	56^a	37^a
Ca^{2+}	58^a	46^a
Ca^{2+}, K^+, plus	100	100
Trifluoperazine	64^a	56^a
Phenytoin	70^a	68^a
Diazepam	62^a	63^a
Ca^{2+}, A23187, plus	97	93
Trifluoperazine	72^b	66^b
Phenytoin	76^b	73^b
Diazepam	66^b	69^b

Intact synaptosomes were incubated under various conditions after preincubation with ^{32}P followed by quantitation of protein DPH-M phosphorylation in the whole synaptosome and in synaptic vesicles isolated from the synaptosomes as described previously. Data were modified from DeLorenzo (22). Concentrations of trifluoperazine, phenytoin, and diazepam were 15 μM, 80 μM, and 20 μM, respectively. Data give means of 10 determinations and are expressed as percentages of the maximally stimulated condition (100%).

[a] Statistically significant difference from the Ca^{2+}, K^+ condition, with $p < 0.001$.

[b] Statistically significant difference from the Ca^{2+}, A23187 condition, with $p < 0.001$.

and tubulin as major substrates (54,55). This kinase contains two calmodulin-binding subunits, designated rho (ρ) and sigma (σ) (Fig. 4). The ρ subunit of this kinase has an apparent MW of 52,000–53,000 daltons, and has been shown to be identical to the major postsynaptic density protein by multiple criteria (56). The σ subunit of the kinase has an apparent MW of 64,000 daltons. The subunits of this calmodulin kinase demonstrate autophosphorylation in a calmodulin-dependent manner (55) (Fig. 5). The autophosphorylation of the kinase subunits represents a significant component of phosphoprotein bands DPH-L and DPH-M. Thus, this kinase system represents a major portion of these important phosphoproteins that have been shown to be phosphorylated in response to voltage-sensitive Ca^{2+} uptake in intact synaptosomes.

Independently, calmodulin kinases have also been isolated from rat brain cytoplasm that phosphorylate protein I as a major substrate (3,68,69). These kinase preparations also contain two major subunits of 52,000 and 64,000 daltons, respectively, and have been designated type II calmodulin kinase. The 52,000-dalton subunit of this kinase system has also been

shown to be identical to the major postsynaptic density protein (67,70), indicating a similarity between this kinase system and the calmodulin kinase that phosphorylates microtubule associated proteins. Recently, a calmodulin kinase that phosphorylates microtubule-associated protein 2 as its major substrate has also been characterized from rat brain cytoplasm (96). This kinase system is also very similar to those described above (3,55). Thus, these studies provide a molecular insight into the nature of specific calmodulin kinase systems in brain that may represent a major site for converting the Ca^{2+} signal into a molecular change.

CALMODULIN REGULATION OF NEUROTRANSMISSION

Because the evidence strongly indicates that calmodulin is present at the synapse, this Ca^{2+} receptor protein is an attractive presynaptic protein for modulating the effects of calcium on neurotransmitter release. As calcium enters the presynaptic ending, it can bind to this high-af-

TABLE 3. *Effects of high K^+ and veratridine in the presence and absence of tetrodotoxin on intact synaptosome Ca^{2+} uptake and protein phosphorylation*

Condition	Ca^{2+} Uptake (%)	Protein phosphorylation (cpm)			
		Whole synaptosome	Synaptic vesicles	Synaptic membrane	Synaptic junctional complex
Control	—	381	858	419	782
Ca^{2+}	51	432	881	443	751
Ca^{2+}, K^+	100^a	721^a	2310^a	507^a	1935^a
Ca^{2+}, K^+, TTX	99^a	706^a	2166^a	516^a	1611^a
Ca^{2+}, V	87^a	698^a	1967^a	512^a	1431^a
Ca^{2+}, V, TTX	59	427	878	408	710

V, veratridine; TTX, tetrodotoxin.
Synaptosomes were incubated under various conditions after preincubation with ^{32}P. Following the reactions, synaptic vesicles, synaptic membrane, and synaptic junctional complexes were isolated from each reactions mixture. Data give mean values of four determinations and are representative of three separate experiments. [^{32}P]Phosphate incorporation is quantitated for protein DPH-M (cpm per 500 µg of protein) and were representative of several other synaptosomal phosphoproteins. Ca^{2+} uptake was determined as described in Table 1 and is presented for comparison (from DeLorenzo, ref. 19).
[a] $p < 0.001$.

finity receptor and initiate several biochemical processes involved in synaptic function (22,24). The first evidence that calcium-stimulated neurotransmitter release may be calmodulin-dependent was obtained from studies on isolated synaptic vesicles (36).

A more physiological procedure for isolating synaptic vesicles was developed (32,35,36); vesicles from this isolation procedure were shown to be much more responsive to calcium than were vesicles prepared under the standard hypotonic isolation methods (21). Calcium, in the presence of ATP and Mg^{2+}, simultaneously initiated the release of vesicle neurotransmitter substances, vesicle protein phosphorylation, and vesicle–membrane interactions (19–27,36). The calcium-responsive synaptic vesicle preparation was then studied to determine if calmodulin mediated the effects of calcium on vesicle neurotransmitter release.

The vesicles prepared under more physiological conditions also contained calmodulin (19). The calmodulin in the vesicle preparation was tightly bound to the vesicle surface and could be selectively removed by washing the vesicles with calcium-chelating agent, EGTA (19,36). Thus, it was possible to obtain preparations of calmodulin-containing (plain vesicles) and calmodulin-depleted (treated vesicles) vesicles. These vesicle fractions were then studied for neurotransmitter release (Table 4).

Calcium, in the presence of calmodulin, stimulated the release of norepinephrine (NE) and acetylcholine (ACh) from calmodulin-depleted vesicles (Table 4). Calcium or calmodulin alone,

however, had no significant effect on neurotransmitter release. Trifluoperazine, a phenothiazine that inactivates calmodulin, also inhibited Ca^{2+}–calmodulin-stimulated vesicle neurotransmitter release (Table 4). The calmodulin kinase inhibitors, phenytoin (17,20) and diazepam (8), were also found to inhibit Ca^{2+}-calmodulin-stimulated vesicle neurotransmitter release (Table 4). The calcium–calmodulin stimulation of release was also shown to be dependent on Mg^{2+} and ATP (21), and vesicles prepared under hypotonic conditions (21) did not show significant calcium–calmodulin-stimulated release of neurotransmitter substances. These results demonstrate that the effects of calcium on vesicle neurotransmitter release were mediated by calmodulin and required an intact biological system that was dependent on Mg^{2+} and ATP.

Although vesicle preparations offer several advantages for studying the effects of calcium on neurotransmitter release, it is important to correlate the results from the isolated vesicle fractions with data obtained from neurotransmitter release studies on intact nerve terminal preparations. Isolated intact nerve terminals (synaptosomes) have been shown to be an excellent preparation for studying the effects of calcium and membrane depolarization on neurotransmitter release (1).

Studies in this laboratory have used the intact synaptosome system (11,12,19) to study the role of calmodulin in neurotransmitter release as summarized in Tables 1–3. The disadvantage of the synaptosome system for studying the effects of calmodulin on the release process is that it is

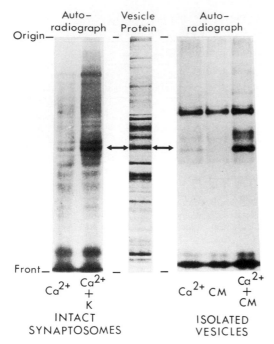

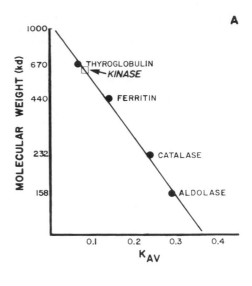

FIG. 3. Effects of calmodulin (CM) and Ca^{2+} on protein phosphorylation in isolated calmodulin-depleted synaptic vesicles (*right*) and of depolarization-dependent Ca^{2+} uptake on protein phosphorylation of synaptic vesicles isolated from ^{32}P-labeled intact synaptosomes (*left*). For experiments with isolated vesicles [γ-^{32}P]-ATP was added to the reaction mixture and incubated for 1 min in the presence and/or absence of Ca^{2+} (free [Ca^{2+}] 10 μM) and CM (5 μg). For experiments with intact synaptosomes, synaptosomes were preincubated with ^{32}P and were then incubated with Ca^{2+} (1 mM) or Ca^{2+} (1 mM) plus K^+ (65 mM). Following incubation, synaptic vesicles were rapidly isolated from each incubated synaptosome reaction and were analyzed for vesicle protein phosphorylation (from ref. 38, with permission). *Arrows:* protein DPH-M.

not yet possible to remove calmodulin from the synaptosome without destroying the viability of the preparation. However, various inhibitors of calmodulin (trifluoperazine) and calcium–calmodulin protein kinase activity (phenytoin and diazepam) that were shown to inhibit calcium–calmodulin release in vesicle preparations were used to probe the possible involvement of calmodulin in neurotransmitter release from intact nerve terminals (19–25). The effects of trifluoperazine on depolarization-dependent neurotransmitter release are shown in Table 1. Conditions that induce calcium entry by the depolarization of the synaptosome membrane (high K^+ or veratridine) or by using the calcium ionophore A 23187 caused significant synaptosomal release of NE and ACh. The increased release of neurotransmitter substances produced by

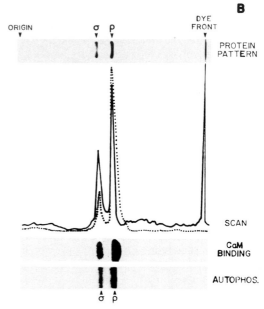

FIG. 4. Chromatography on Sephacryl S-300 Superfine. **(A)** Fractogel-purified TACK chromatographed on Sephacryl S-300 with an apparent MW of ~600,000 daltons. **(B)** The kinase fraction obtained from chromatography on Sephacryl displayed only two silver-staining protein components of 52,000 (rho, ρ) and 63,000 (sigma, σ) daltons, respectively, when resolved on one-dimensional sodium dodecyl sulfate-polyacrylamide gel electrophoresis. Both the ρ and σ subunits of TACK bound calmodulin in denaturing gels and displayed characteristic autophosphorylation. The densitometric scan demonstrates that the protein staining (—) and calmodulin binding (• • •) coincide (from ref. 55, with permission).

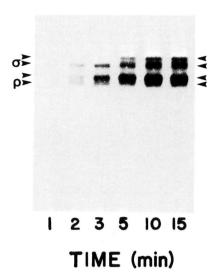

TIME (min)

FIG. 5. Autoradiographic patterns of autophosphorylation and calmodulin binding of TACK on one-dimensional and two-dimensional gels. **(A)** TACK phosphorylated in the absence of substrate under standard conditions for 1 min was resolved on one-dimensional sodium dodecyl sulfate-polyacrylamide gel electrophoresis (SDS-PAGE) and two-dimensional isoelectric focusing/SDS-PAGE. Both the phosphorylated rho (ρ) and sigma (σ) subunits of TACK focus at pIs between 6.7 and 7.2. **(B)** TACK (10 μg) preparations were resolved in one-dimensional and two-dimensional electrophoresis and processed for calmodulin binding. In both systems, the ρ and σ subunits of TACK bound calmodulin. The autophosphorylation and calmodulin binding patterns coincided with the protein staining of these subunits (data not shown) (from ref. 55, with permission).

both elevated K^+ and A 23187 was significantly inhibited by trifluoperazine (Table 1) in micromolar concentrations. These results suggest that inhibition of calmodulin by trifluoperazine blocks the release process. However, it is not possible from these experiments to determine if trifluoperazine is inhibiting release by blocking calcium uptake or by inhibiting a specific calcium-regulated process within the nerve terminal.

To test these possibilities, the effects of trifluoperazine on calcium uptake was investigated. It was shown that trifluoperazine inhibits the depolarization-dependent uptake of calcium into intact synaptosomes induced by either elevated K^+ or veratridine (19,21) (Table 1). However, the calcium uptake produced by A 23187 was not inhibited by trifluoperazine (19–25). Thus, trifluoperazine inhibits release in two ways: (a) by inhibiting depolarization-dependent

calcium uptake, and (b) by blocking a calcium-regulated process that modulates release even when calcium is entering the nerve terminal in the presence of A 23187.

The anticonvulsant, phenytoin, and the benzodiazepine, diazepam, also blocked NE and ACh release from intact synaptosomes produced by elevated K^+ and A 23187 (19–25) (Table 1). These calmodulin-kinase inhibitors, also inhibited K^+-stimulated Ca^{2+} uptake; however, like trifluoperisone, they did not significantly inhibit synaptosomal Ca^{2+} uptake induced by A 23187. Thus, this evidence indicates that phenytoin and diazepam inhibit release by blocking Ca^{2+} uptake and by antagonizing the effects of Ca^{2+} in the nerve terminal. Thus, studies from both isolated vesicles and intact synaptosome preparations suggest that calmodulin may act as the calcium receptor mediating the effects of calcium on neurotransmission.

CALCIUM–CALMODULIN-STIMULATED SYNAPTIC PROTEIN PHOSPHORYLATION AND NEUROTRANSMISSION

The evidence presented above suggests that Ca^{2+}–calmodulin-regulated synaptic biochemical processes may regulate the effect of Ca^{2+} on synaptic activity. Thus, it would be important to determine which calmodulin-regulated enzyme systems are involved in specific aspects of synaptic function. Calmodulin has been shown to mediate the activation of specific kinase systems in nonneuronal tissues (95), crude brain membrane (95), and highly enriched synaptic preparations, including synaptic vesicle (36), synaptic membrane (19), synaptic junction (19,21), and postsynaptic density fractions (19,58,59). Thus, Ca^{2+}-regulated protein kinase activity is a major enzyme system that may mediate the effects of calmodulin on synaptic function.

Experiments in this laboratory (21) demonstrated that the Ca^{2+}-calmodulin-dependent release of neurotransmitter substances from synaptic vesicles was also dependent on Mg^{2+} and ATP, suggesting that utilization of ATP by synaptic protein kinases may be involved in the release process. Experiments that simultaneously studied calcium–calmodulin-stimulated neurotransmitter release and protein phosphorylation in isolated vesicles and intact synaptosomes led to the hypothesis that calcium–calmodulin-regulated synaptic protein phosphorylation, a distinct phosphorylation system from the cyclic AMP protein kinases, may play a role in syn-

TABLE 4. *Effects of calmodulin and Ca^{2+}–calmodulin kinase inhibitors on Ca^{2+}–calmodulin-stimulated protein phosphorylation and neurotransmitter release in isolated synaptic vesicles*

	Neurotransmitter release (%)		Protein DPH-M
Condition	Acetylcholine	Norepinephrine	Phosphorylation (%)
Control	34	38	21
Ca^{2+}	41	44	25
Calmodulin	36	39	22
Ca^{2+} and calmodulin	100	100	100
Ca^{2+} and calmodulin, plus			
Trifluoperazine	62	68	55
Phenytoin	69	72	49
Diazepam	61	63	47

Calmodulin-depleted synaptic vesicles were isolated and studied for neurotransmitter release as described previously. Data give means of nine determinations and are expressed as percentages of the maximally stimulated condition (100%). The largest SEM was 6.1%. The effects of trifluoperazine (15 μM), phenytoin (80 μM), and diazepam (15 μM) were found to be statistically significant in comparison to the maximally stimulated values, with $p < 0.001$ (from DeLorenzo, ref. 19).

aptic modulation (19–25). The evidence supporting this hypothesis is summarized below.

Studies on calmodulin-depleted synaptic vesicles showed that protein phosphorylation (Fig. 3) and neurotransmitter release (Table 4) were both simultaneously stimulated by Ca^{2+} and calmodulin (19–25). In addition, it was shown that vesicle protein phosphorylation and neurotransmitter release had the same requirements for Mg^{2+}, ATP, Ca^{2+}, and calmodulin (21). Various incubation conditions, such as pH and buffer solutions that produced maximal Ca^{2+}-stimulated release, also gave maximal levels of phosphorylation (21). Phenytoin and diazepam, which specifically inhibit the vesicle Ca^{2+}–calmodulin kinase system, were also shown to inhibit neurotransmitter release significantly (Table 4). Trifluoperazine also simultaneously inhibited vesicle protein phosphorylation and neurotransmitter release (Table 4).

Vesicles prepared under conditions that inactivated the labile Ca^{2+}–calmodulin kinase system also showed no significant Ca^{2+}–calmodulin-stimulated release (21). Thus, in the isolated vesicle preparation, there is convincing evidence that protein phosphorylation and neurotransmitter release from vesicles are simultaneously activated by Ca^{2+} and calmodulin. The release of neurotransmitter substances in this vesicle system is directly dependent on Ca^{2+} and calmodulin, and proteins DPH-M and DPH-L (Fig. 3) were the most consistently observed phosphoproteins that showed the greatest Ca^{2+}–calmodulin-stimulated incorporation of ^{32}P-phosphate and the most significant inhibition by phenytoin (21–25).

In intact synaptosome preparations, depolar-

ization of the synaptosome membrane in the presence of Ca^{2+} stimulated the phosphorylation of an 80,000 dalton protein, designated protein I (74). Depolarization-dependent Ca^{2+} uptake was also shown to stimulate the phosphorylation of proteins DPH-L and DPH-M in intact synaptosomes (19–21). Because synaptosome preparations are not pure, it was important to demonstrate that the depolarization-dependent increase in protein phosphorylation was actually occurring within the synaptosomes. Experiments were conducted to isolate synaptic vesicle, synaptic membrane, synaptic junction, and postsynaptic density fractions from ^{32}P-labeled synaptosomes incubated under various conditions (21). These experiments demonstrated that the depolarization-stimulated phosphorylations of proteins DPH-L and DPH-M was occurring in specific synaptosome fractions (21) (Table 3).

It was subsequently shown that depolarization-dependent Ca^{2+} uptake simultaneously stimulated protein phosphorylation and neurotransmitter release in intact synaptosome preparations (Tables 1–3). The phosphorylation of proteins DPH-L, DPH-M, and several other proteins correlated with release in these studies. Furthermore, the level of phosphorylation of protein DPH-M in synaptic vesicles, synaptic junction, and postsynaptic density fractions from intact synaptosomes was also shown to correlate with neurotransmitter release (Tables 1–3). Because the Ca^{2+}-stimulated levels of phosphorylation of proteins DPH-L and DPH-M and several other proteins were shown to be dependent on calmodulin in vesicle, membrane, and synaptic junction preparations (19–25), it is reasonable to conclude that depolarization-dependent Ca^{2+}-uptake simultaneously stimulates Ca^{2+}–calmodulin-dependent protein phosphorylation and neurotransmitter release in intact synaptosome preparations.

Although it has been shown that Ca^{2+} entry into the nerve terminal simultaneously stimulates neurotransmitter release and protein phosphorylation, a more definitive correlation is needed to implicate Ca^{2+}-calmodulin kinase activity clearly in the process of neurotransmission. Studies in this laboratory using trifluoperazine, diazepam, and phenytoin demonstrated a more direct relationship between phosphorylation and release (Tables 1 and 2).

Trifluoperazine inhibited both synaptic protein phosphorylation and neurotransmitter release in intact synaptosome preparations (Tables 1 and 2). The effect of trifluoperazine on protein phosphorylation was exactly the same as its effects on neurotransmitter release (Table 2). Trifluoperazine inhibited phosphorylation by both inhibiting depolarization-dependent Ca^{2+} uptake induced by high K^+ and by directly inactivating the calmodulin kinase system, as seen in the presence of A 23187. Phenytoin and diazepam also inhibited the activation of calmodulin kinase activity in intact synaptosomes while simultaneously inhibiting neurotransmitter release (Tables 1 and 2). Thus, direct inactivation of calmodulin and the calmodulin kinase system was simultaneously occurring with the inhibition of the Ca^{2+}-dependent neurotransmitter release process in intact synaptosomes. Combining the direct studies on the isolated synaptic vesicle systems with the pharmacologic data obtained in the intact synaptosome preparation, it is reasonable to suggest that synaptic Ca^{2+}–calmodulin kinase activity may play an important role in modulating some of the effects of Ca^{2+} on synaptic transmission (19–25).

CALCIUM–CALMODULIN SYNAPTIC VESICLE AND SYNAPTIC MEMBRANE INTERACTIONS

Accumulating evidence suggests that vesicle and membrane interactions during exocytosis may be the fundamental step in neurotransmission. The possible role of calmodulin in mediating Ca^{2+}-stimulated membrane interactions should be studied. The following studies indicate that calmodulin may be involved in modulating vesicle–membrane interactions at the synapse (21–25).

Under conditions that stimulate vesicle and membrane protein phosphorylation and neurotransmitter release, it has been shown that ves-

icles interact with each other (Table 5) and also can become attached to and possibly interact with synaptic membrane (Table 6). Calcium combined with calmodulin caused a statistically significant increase in vesicle membrane interactions. Calcium or calmodulin alone did not significantly affect membrane interactions (Tables 5 and 6). Vesicle–membrane interactions were also found to be dependent on Mg^{2+} and ATP (21). In addition, vesicle–membrane interactions were also inhibited by phenytoin and diazepam (21–25).

These results indicate that, as are neurotransmitter release and synaptic protein phosphorylation, vesicle–membrane interactions may be mediated by calmodulin. The requirements of ATP and the inhibition by the Ca^{2+} kinase in-

TABLE 5. *Effects of calmodulin and Ca^{2+} on synaptic vesicle interactions*

Condition	Free vesicles (%)
Plain synaptic vesicles	
Control	51.3 ± 3.1
Ca^{2+}	$11.6^a \pm 1.3$
Calmodulin	52.8 ± 2.6
Ca^{2+} and calmodulin	$10.7^a \pm 0.9$
Calmodulin-depleted synaptic vesicles	
Control	48.6 ± 1.8
Ca^{2+}	$31.2^a \pm 3.1$
Calmodulin	46.5 ± 2.7
Ca^{2+} and calmodulin	$13.4^{a,b} \pm 0.8$

Plain and calmodulin-depleted synaptic vesicles were incubated for 1 min under standard conditions in the presence or absence of Ca^{2+} and/or calmodulin, isolated by centrifugation (100,000 g) and prepared for electron microscopy (see text). Free vesicles were defined as vesicles that did not touch other vesicles. Free vesicles are expressed as the percentage of free vesicles in the preparation. The percentage of free vesicles was determined in 500 representative electron micrographs (each containing ~150 vesicle profiles); data give mean value and SEM of free vesicles from these 500 determinations. The results shown are representative of three separate experiments. The percentage of free vesicles in the control and stimulated conditions was inversely affected by the force of centrifugation. However, the effects of Ca^{2+} and calmodulin on percentage of free vesicles were still statistically significant at four other speeds of centrifugation. Electron micrographs were randomly selected from the top, middle, and bottom of the vesicle pellet (19). The effects of Ca^{2+} and calmodulin on vesicle aggregation observed in thin sections were also seen in negatively stained and freeze-dried preparations (from ref. 19, with permission).
^{a} $p < 0.001$ in comparison with control conditions.
^{b} $p < 0.001$ in comparison with Ca^{2+} conditions.

TABLE 6. *Effects of calmodulin and Ca²⁺ on synaptic vesicle and synaptic membrane interactions*

Conditions	Synaptic vesicle and synaptic membrane interactions (no. of vesicles per micron of membrane)
Plain synaptic vesicles	
Control	3.12 ± 0.41
Ca²⁺	$14.33^a \pm 0.98$
Calmodulin	4.21 ± 0.29
Ca²⁺ and calmodulin	$15.26^a \pm 1.01$
Calmodulin-depleted synaptic vesicles	
Control	2.77 ± 0.25
Ca²⁺	$5.16^a \pm 0.41$
Calmodulin	3.16 ± 0.12
Ca²⁺ and calmodulin	$10.21^{a,b} \pm 0.83$

Plain or calmodulin-depleted synaptic vesicles were incubated with synaptic membrane for 1 min under standard conditions in the presence or absence of Ca²⁺ and/or calmodulin. Following incubation, synaptic membranes were immediately isolated from each reaction mixture by centrifugation at 25,000 g for 10 minutes at 4 °C. The isolated membrane pellets were then fixed and prepared for electron microscopy (19). Random electron micrographs were taken from the top to the bottom of the pellet, and the number of synaptic vesicles on each membrane fragment was quantitated. The number of vesicles attached to synaptic membrane is expressed as vesicles per micron (μM) of membrane. Data give mean values of 600 determinations and are representative of three separate experiments (from ref. 19, with permission).

[a] $p < 0.001$ in comparison with control conditions.
[b] $p < 0.001$ in comparison with Ca²⁺ conditions.

hibitors, phenytoin and diazepam, suggest that Ca²⁺–calmodulin-stimulated phosphorylation of synaptic proteins may trigger physical changes in the surface properties of the synaptic vesicle and membrane, initiating interaction between these membrane structures.

ANTICONVULSANT REGULATION OF THE CALCIUM SIGNAL

Anticonvulsants are major clinically used compounds that regulate neuronal excitability (29). Research has been accumulating to indicate that a major site of action of phenytoin, carbamazepine, and some of the benzodiazepines is to inhibit Ca²⁺-regulated processes (20,27,29). This evidence will be presented below. In addition, recent studies in this laboratory demonstrate that these compounds specifically inhibit multifunctional calmodulin kinase systems in brain. Because these calmodulin kinase systems have

been implicated in mediating several of the effects of Ca²⁺ on neuronal tissue, these results provide a molecular mechanism for some of the antagonistic effects of phenytoin, carbamazepine, and the benzodiazepines on the Ca²⁺ signal in brain and other tissues.

PHENYTOIN INHIBITS SEVERAL CALCIUM-DEPENDENT PROCESSES

Phenytoin has numerous effects on neuronal tissue (29). However, this major anticonvulsant has been shown to be especially effective in inhibiting the actions of Ca²⁺ in several experimental systems. Phenytoin has been shown to antagonize several Ca²⁺-dependent release processes. The Ca²⁺-dependent release of insulin from islet cells (73) and of oxytocin (84) and antidiuretic hormone from the pituitary (60) has been shown to be inhibited by phenytoin. The Ca²⁺-dependent release of NE from brain slices (88) and intact synaptosomes (48,49) has also been shown to be antagonized by therapeutic concentrations of phenytoin. Direct electrophysiological evidence also indicates that phenytoin inhibits the Ca²⁺-dependent release of neurotransmitter from the presynaptic nerve terminal (106). The antagonistic effects of phenytoin and calcium on the release of neurotransmitter and other hormones in several investigations (48,49,60,73,84,88,106) strongly suggest that some of the actions of phenytoin on neuronal tissue and synaptic transmission are mediated by the inhibition of a calcium-dependent molecular process.

Another major action of phenytoin is its effect on posttetanic potentiation (PTP), which refers to the augmentation of the postsynaptic compound action potential elicited by presynaptic stimulation following a repetitive stimulus (tetanus) (44–47,89,90,99,103). The physiologic phenomenon, PTP, has been implicated in causing hyperexcitable areas in brain as the result of recurrent feedback circuits during seizure activity (99). It is thought to be an important mechanism in the development of high-frequency trains of impulses in excitatory brain circuits. Furthermore, PTP has been implicated in regulating the spread of this activity to adjoining neurons as well as in their propagation to distal neuronal aggregates, resulting in uncontrolled spread of excitation to the whole brain and a maximal tonic seizure discharge. Phenytoin suppresses both PTP (44,89,90) and the local spread of epileptiform discharge from the epileptic focus without significantly depressing the spontaneous activity from the focus itself (90,103).

An examination of the mechanism producing PTP may facilitate our understanding of the action of phenytoin on this important physiologic phenomenon.

During the repetitive presynaptic stimuli used to induce PTP, calcium ions may accumulate intracellularly in the presynaptic nerve terminal. This extra accumulation of intracellular calcium augments the amount of calcium-dependent neurotransmitter released from the nerve terminal by a given impulse following the tetanus, causing an increase in the postsynaptic potential. The development of PTP has also been shown to be dependent on the presence of calcium ions in the extracellular medium. The inhibition of the calcium-dependent release of neurotransmitter during PTP at both peripheral (106) and central synapses (89,90) by phenytoin suggests that this anticonvulsant inhibits the action of calcium on neurotransmitter release from the presynaptic nerve terminal.

Phenytoin also inhibits the voltage-dependent uptake of calcium ions into intact presynaptic nerve terminal preparations (48,49). These experiments indicate that phenytoin directly hampers the calcium signal by preventing calcium entry into the nerve cell during depolarization. These studies have recently been confirmed, and it has been shown that under conditions that inhibit depolarization-dependent calcium uptake into synaptosomes, phenytoin also simultaneously inhibits the calcium-dependent release of NE and ACh from the nerve terminals (21–25). In addition, phenytoin was also found to inhibit release of neurotransmitter substances from intact synaptosomes under conditions that were independent of the effects of this compound on calcium uptake (21–25). Thus, evidence suggests that phenytoin regulates transmitter release by both inhibiting Ca^{2+} entry and blocking some specific presynaptic biochemical processes that modulate release.

Because phenytoin is such a widely effective anticonvulsant, it is important to investigate the molecular mechanism mediating the effects of this drug on the Ca^{2+} signal. Calcium acts as a second messenger in mediating numerous neuronal and nonneuronal functions. Phenytoin modulation of the Ca^{2+} signal could explain why phenytoin has so many effects on neuronal and nonneuronal tissues. By modulating calcium's effects, phenytoin may be regulating numerous Ca^{2+}-dependent processes that may play an important role in regulating seizure discharge. Phenytoin can thus be utilized as a pharmacological probe to investigate the molecular events mediating the Ca^{2+} signal.

CALCIUM–CALMODULIN PROTEIN PHOSPHORYLATION: INHIBITION BY PHENYTOIN

As described above, experiments in this laboratory have been directed at understanding specific biochemical processes mediating the effects of Ca^{2+} on synaptic function. Calcium plays a major role in regulating synaptic activity (91,93), and several of the excitatory effects of Ca^{2+} on synaptic function have been shown to be antagonized by the anticonvulsant phenytoin (44–46,60,73,84,88–90,99). Thus, synaptic biochemical processes that are stimulated by Ca^{2+} and inhibited by phenytoin are of considerable interest, because they may represent a molecular process that modulates neuronal excitability.

Numerous enzyme systems were studied in our laboratory in an attempt to find a Ca^{2+}-stimulated phenytoin-inhibited process that might provide an initial insight into the molecular events mediating the interactions of Ca^{2+} and phenytoin. We identified a unique Ca^{2+}-stimulated protein phosphorylation system in brain that was also inhibited by phenytoin (17–18,30–32,37). The effects of phenytoin on Ca^{2+}-stimulated synaptic vesicle protein phosphorylation are presented in Fig. 6. This Ca^{2+} kinase system is a protein phosphorylation system distinct from the well-described brain cyclic AMP protein kinases (21–25). Thus, efforts in this laboratory have been directed at determining the role of Ca^{2+}-dependent protein phosphorylation in modulating synaptic function and neuronal excitability.

This initial work set the foundation for studying several Ca^{2+}-regulated processes that might relate to neuronal excitability and anticonvulsant drug action. Because the effects of Ca^{2+} on many biochemical systems has been shown to be mediated by a Ca^{2+} binding protein calmodulin, we are now gaining insights into the molecular nature of the Ca^{2+} signal in brain. This biochemical and physiological data will be reviewed, since it is essential in developing a molecular insight into synaptic excitability.

EFFECTS OF OTHER ANTICONVULSANTS ON CALCIUM–CALMODULIN SYSTEMS

The effects of phenytoin on Ca^{2+}–calmodulin processes have been implicated in mediating some of the anticonvulsant effects of this compound on neuronal tissue. Phenytoin's effects on several seizure models and electrophysiological

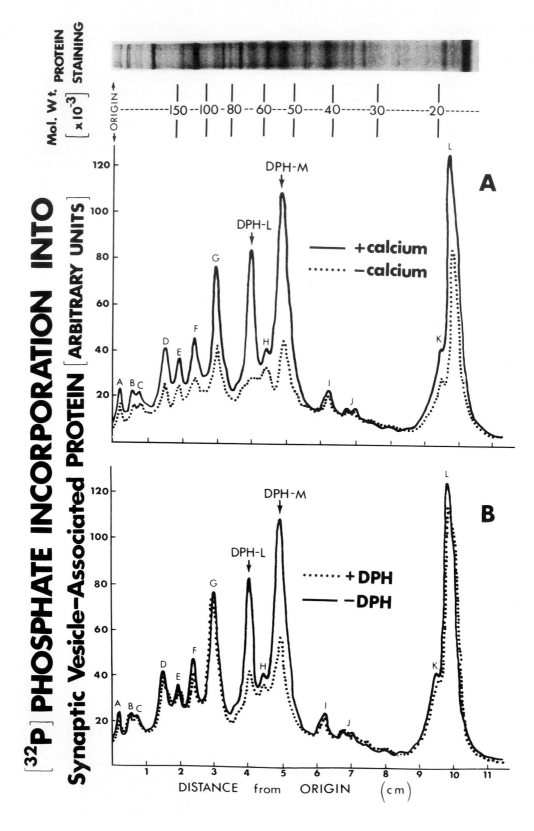

preparations are also produced by carbamazepine and some of the benzodiazepines (BZs). However, phenobarbital, ethosuximide, valproic acid, and trimethadrone have very different properties than phenytoin. Thus, it is important to determine the effects of these anticonvulsant compounds on Ca^{2+}–calmodulin systems.

The BZs are anticonvulsants that have membrane-stabilizing effects similar in some respects to those of phenytoin (103–105). Diazepam (Valium) has been shown to have remarkable structural similarities to phenytoin (12). Diazepam, like phenytoin, also significantly inhibits MES-induced seizures. It has been demonstrated that the BZs also inhibit Ca^{2+}–calmodulin-stimulated protein phosphorylation in brain membrane preparations (29).

The effects of the BZs (Fig. 7) on protein phosphorylation are stereospecific and are produced by membrane-bound BZ (29). The potency of BZ kinase inhibition correlated with the ability of the BZs to inhibit electric shock-induced convulsions (29). These results provided evidence that some of the anticonvulsant and neuronal stabilizing effects of BZs may be modulated by the Ca^{2+}–calmodulin protein kinase system. The potency correlation of the effects of the BZs to inhibit kinase activity with their ability to inhibit MES-induced seizures further suggested that regulation of Ca^{2+}–calmodulin kinase activity may play a role in mediating some of the anticonvulsant properties of these drugs.

Carbamazepine (Tegretol) is a major clinically useful anticonvulsant drug that has also been shown to inhibit PTP and antagonize the action of Ca^{2+} at the synapse (62). Thus, carbamazepine, like phenytoin, would be expected to inhibit Ca^{2+}–calmodulin protein phosphorylation and vesicle neurotransmitter release if these Ca^{2+}-modulated processes mediate the effects of these drugs on synaptic activity. As shown in Table 7, carbamazepine significantly inhibits the phosphorylation of synaptic proteins in whole synaptosomes, synaptic membrane, and synaptic vesicle fractions (27). This anticonvulsant also inhibits the Ca^{2+}–calmodulin-stimulated release of neurotransmitter substance from synaptic vesicles (Table 8). Thus, carbamazepine

has the same effects as phenytoin on both physiological and biochemical processes.

Esplin (46) has shown that phenobarbital has different effects than phenytoin on synaptic transmission. Experiments from this laboratory demonstrated that phenobarbital also had no significant effect on Ca^{2+}-calmodulin protein phosphorylation (Table 7) or vesicle neurotransmitter release (Table 8) in concentrations in excess of its therapeutic range (27). Trimethadione (47,103) has been shown to have no effect on PTP; neither did this useful anticonvulsant have any effect on protein phosphorylation or transmitter release (Tables 7 and 8). Nor did ethosuximide (Zarontin), a useful anticonvulsant in treating absence seizures, or sodium valproate (Depakene) have any significant effect on synaptic protein phosphorylation or neurotransmitter release (27).

These results indicate that the effects of phenytoin on Ca^{2+} systems is specific to a class of anticonvulsant compounds that have been shown to regulate Ca^{2+} processes in various electrophysiological and intact preparations. Because phenytoin, carbamazepine, and the BZs are very important clinical compounds that are very useful in treating epilepsy in humans, it is reasonable to suggest that regulation of calmodulin kinase systems and possibly other Ca^{2+}-regulated processes may account for some of the major effects of these compounds in modulating neuronal excitability. Thus, alterations in Ca^{2+}-regulated biochemical processes may represent a molecular mechanism for producing some forms of seizure activity.

ANTICONVULSANT RECEPTORS

BZs are important therapeutic agents with significant anticonvulsant actions (71). However, the exact molecular events associated with BZ anticonvulsant activity remain largely unknown. A specific binding site has been described that binds BZs in the nanomolar concentration range (6,85,98). This nanomolar BZ receptor (nM BZR) has been the object of intense study, and its binding has been shown to correlate with several pharmalogical effects of the BZs, including the inhibition of pentylenetetrazol (PET)-induced seizure activity. However, binding to this

---

FIG. 6. Effects of calcium and DPH on the endogenous phosphorylation of synaptic vesicle fraction proteins: synaptic vesicle protein was incubated under standard conditions for 1 min in the presence or absence of calcium ions, 1 mM **(A)**, or in the presence of calcium ions with or without DPH, 0.1 mM **(B)**, and subjected to polyacrylamide gel electrophoresis, protein staining, and quantitation. The results shown are representative of 15 individual experiments. Each arbitrary unit equals ~11.6 cpm (from ref. 34, with permission).

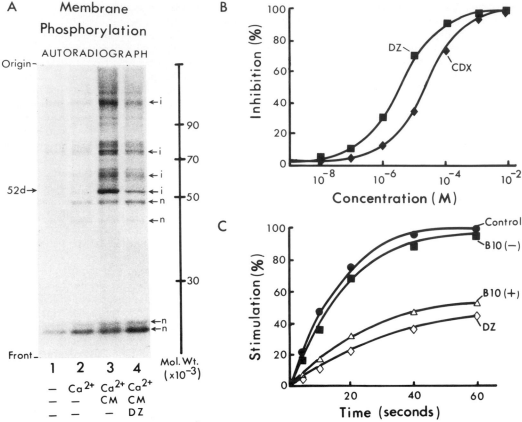

FIG. 7. **(A)** Effects of diazepam on Ca^{2+}–calmodulin (CM) stimulated protein phosphorylation in brain membrane. The standard reaction mixture for studying endogenous protein phosphorylation (final vol, 100 µl) contained 100 µg membrane protein, 50 mM PIPES buffer (pH 7.4), 5 mM $MgCl_2$, 0.2 mM EGTA (without Ca^{2+}) or 0.2 mM EGTA + 0.5 mM $CaCl_2$ (with Ca^{2+}), 11 µM [γ-^{32}P]P-ATP (5–10 Ci/mmole, New England Nuclear), with or without 5 µg calmodulin (CM), and 2 µl dimethyl sulfoxide (DMSO) or 2 µl diazepam dissolved in DMSO giving a final concentration in the reaction tube of 15 µM diazepam. Reactions were incubated for 1 min under standard conditions and prepared for autoradiography as described previously (31). The autoradiograph shown was representative of 20 independent experiments. **(B)** Drug concentration curves of diazepam (DZ) and chlordiazepoxide (CDX) for inhibition of Ca^{2+}–calmodulin membrane protein phosphorylation. Percentage of inhibition of incorporation of [^{32}P]phosphate into the 52 dalton (52d) protein is expressed as the percentage of the maximally inhibited condition, which was designated 100%. The data give the means of 10 determinations: largest SEM was ±5.5%. **(C)** Time course of the Ca^{2+}-calmodulin-stimulated phosphorylation of the 52d protein in the absence (control) or presence of DZ (10 µM), and the pharmacologically active and inactive benzodiazepine enantiomers (40 µM), B10(−) and B10(+). The data present the means of 10 determinations: largest SEM was ±4.2% (from ref. 29, with permission).

receptor does not correlate with BZ inhibition of MES-induced seizures. Furthermore, on a molecular level, the nM BZR has been associated with GABA receptor and the activation of the choloride ion (Cl^-) channel (98).

A second specific BZ binding site has been described which binds BZs in the micromolar concentration range (5). Binding of this micromolar BZ receptor (µM BZR) can be readily distinguished from nM BZR binding on the basis of kinetic and pharmacological properties. Furthermore, µM BZR binding correlates well with BZ inhibition of MES-induced seizures but not with anti-PET activity. Phenytoin, another potent inhibitor of MES-seizures, blocks [^{3}H]-diazepam (DZ) binding to the µM BZR (5), suggesting that the two anticonvulsant drugs act at the same membrane site.

TABLE 7. *Effects of anticonvulsants on calcium–calmodulin-stimulated synaptic protein phosphorylation*

Conditions	Synaptic protein phosphorylation			
	Synaptosome (%)	Synaptic vesicle (%)	Synaptic membrane (%)	Postsynaptic density (%)
Control	100	100	100	100
Phenytoin	45[a]	52[a]	67[a]	57[a]
Carbamazepine	56[a]	55[a]	63[a]	61[a]
Diazepam	41[a]	52[a]	59[a]	49[a]
Phenobarbital	97	94	98	96
Ethosuximide	99	93	97	94
Trimethadione	96	97	95	98
Sodium valproate	95	98	99	97

Synaptosomes (40), synaptic vesicles (35), synaptic membrane (40), and postsynaptic densities (66) were prepared by established procedures and incubated for 30 sec under standard conditions for studying calcium–calmodulin-stimulated protein phosphorylation in the presence of 10 μM calcium and 5 μg calmodulin (control) with or without phenytoin (50 μM), carbamazepine (100 μM), diazepam (8 μM), phenobarbital (500 μM), ethosuximide (500 μM), trimethadione (500 μM), or sodium valproate (500 μM). The incorporation of [^{32}P]phosphate into protein DPH-M, a major 52,000–53,000 dalton protein band in each fraction, was quantitated by standard procedures (31). The effects of each anticonvulsant on the calcium–calmodulin-stimulated phosphorylation of protein DPH-M were representative of their effects on the phosphorylation of several other protein bands in the different fractions. Data give mean values from 10 determinations and are representative of four separate experiments. Results are expressed as percentages of control condition (control = 100%). The largest SEM was ± 11% (from ref. 27, with permission).

[a] $p < 0.001$ in comparison to control condition, using Student's t-test. Drugs not producing significant effects on protein phosphorylation at therapeutic concentrations were tested at 10- to 50-fold higher concentrations and were found to have no significant effect on phosphorylation even at those concentrations.

Several investigators have shown that micromolar levels of diazepam inhibit calcium uptake in brain synaptosome fractions (24,39,48,75,97). In this study, we will describe BZ inhibition of depolarization-induced calcium uptake and will show that this inhibition is correlated with μM BZR binding. Modulation of depolarization-dependent calcium uptake (and subsequent calcium-dependent phenomena in the nerve terminal) may prove to be a major molecular effect of μM BZR activation and the mechanism of anti-MES seizure activity. These observations, together with other results given here, indicate that the μM BZR may represent a specific "anticonvulsant receptor" in rat brain membrane that plays a role in regulating calcium channels and calmodulin kinase activity.

MICROMOLAR AFFINITY BZ RECEPTORS

[^{3}H]DZ binding in rat brain membrane saturates in both the nanomolar and micromolar concentration ranges, corresponding to binding to nanomolar affinity and micromolar affinity binding sites (Fig. 8). Binding data analyzed by the method of Scatchard yields a curvilinear plot consistent with the existence of two distinct populations of specific binding sites. The apparent K_D for DZ binding at the micromolar site is 45 μM, and the receptor density (B_{max}) obtained from the plot is 360 pmole/mg. [^{3}H]DZ binding is stereospecific, has defined kinetic parameters, and has the characteristics of a general BZ receptor. A wide variety of BZs displace specific [^{3}H]DZ binding in a concentration-dependent fashion, including clonazepam (CNZ), flunitrazepam (FNZ), medazepam (MDZ), and Ro5-4864. The order of potency (K_I) of BZs at micromolar affinity binding sites is markedly different from the potency series at the nanomolar affinity site, indicating that the two receptor populations are pharmacologically distinct.

The apparent K_D for DZ binding at the nanomolar site is 1–2 nM, and the receptor density (B_{max}) is in the range of 1 pmole/mg. These pharmacological characteristics clearly distinguish the nM BZ receptor from the μM BZ binding site. In addition, the relative potency of DZ and the peripheral BZ, Ro5-4864, varies significantly at the two sites. At the nanomolar binding site, DZ is 10,000-fold more potent than ·Ro5-4864,

TABLE 8. *Effects of anticonvulsants on calcium–calmodulin-stimulated neurotransmitter release from synaptic vesicles*

	Neurotransmitter release	
Conditions	Norepinephrine (%)	Acetylcholine (%)
Control	100	100
Phenytoin	61[a]	65[a]
Carbamazepine	67[a]	62[a]
Diazepam	53[a]	54[a]
Phenobarbital	97	95
Ethosuximide	95	97
Trimethadione	98	99
Sodium valproate	94	96

Synaptic vesicles were isolated and studied under standard conditions for calcium–calmodulin-stimulated norepinephrine and acetylcholine release in the presence or absence of phenytoin (50 μM), carbamazepine (100 μM), diazepam (8 μM), phenobarbital (500 μM), ethosuximide (500 μM), trimethadione (500 μM), and sodium valproate (500 μM). Release is expressed as percentages of maximal stimulation in the presence of calcium and calmodulin (control = 100%). Data give the mean values of six determinations (from ref. 27, with permission).
[a] $p < 0.001$.

whereas at the micromolar binding site, the two compounds are essentially equipotent. The two classes of BZ receptors also differ functionally. The nanomolar affinity BZ receptor has been shown to exist in a supramolecular structure with the GABA receptor and the Cl^- ion channel, and its binding is influenced by GABA ligands. It has been suggested that a function of the nanomolar affinity receptor is to regulate the Cl^- ion channel. In contrast, concentrations of GABA ligands which modulate nM BZ binding and Cl^- fluxes have no effect on μM BZ binding (5). Thus, the μM BZ binding site does not function in a similar fashion to the activated nM affinity site. Due to the observation that μM BZs block Ca^{2+} uptake in synaptosomes, it is of considerable interest to elucidate the cellular functions associated with μM BZ binding (24,39, 48,75,97).

MICROMOLAR BZ RECEPTOR CHARACTERIZATION

The study of binding of a lipophilic drug in micromolar concentration ranges presents some interesting technical challenges. We have developed a reproducible assay by adjusting reaction conditions to minimize technical difficulties. The principal problems encountered with studies of this type are low aqueous solubility of the drugs, high nonspecific binding, and high cost of the radioligand used in micromolar concentrations. First, to reduce solubility problems, stock solutions of all BZs are prepared in absolute ethanol immediateley prior to use. Aliquots of the BZs in ethanol are added first to reaction tubes and are then diluted to final concentrations with aqueous buffer containing the receptor–membrane preparation. Final ethanol concentration routinely ranges from 5 to 10%. Increasing final ethanol concentrations dramatically reduces specific BZ binding and should be avoided. Second, high nonspecific binding to membrane preparations is expected when dealing with micromolar radioligand concentrations. Approximately 25–30% of total [³H]DZ or [³H]CNZ binding is specific. As a consequence, it is necessary to improve the reproducibility of the assay by minimizing the variable nonspecific binding of the radioligand to filters. Therefore, only glass fiber filters presoaked in aqueous buffer are used, and we routinely dilute (100× with ice-cold aqueous buffer) all radioactive samples immediately prior to filtration. This technique effectively reduces free radioligand concentration at the moment of filtration and lowers nonspecific filter binding. In addition, to reduce the costs associated with binding assays using micromolar radioligand concentrations, a displacement assay is used to measure micromolar BZ binding. Using this technique, radioligand (5–10 Ci/mmol) binding is compared in a series of samples containing identical concentration of radioligand (usually 1–10 μM) and increasing concentrations of unlabeled ligand. Maximum displacement can be defined as nonspecific binding and is generally 70–75% of total binding. Specific [³H]DZ binding is then calculated by subtracting nonspecific binding from each data point and correcting for the dilution of [³H]DZ specific activity. The displacement data can then be directly replotted according to Scatchard for comparison and analysis.

To increase the reproducibility of this assay, and to improve its value as a molecular probe of the μM BZ binding site, a photoactive BZ binding assay, with the formation of irreversible bonds, has been developed (38,39,97). Nitrocontaining BZs, such as CNZ and FNZ, form covalent linkages with their binding sites when exposed to short-wave ultraviolet (UV) light (86). Samples are then equilibrated with [³H]CNZ and CNZ under the conditions described above, and exposed uniformly to UV illumination (10 min at 5 cm) prior to filtration. The formation of irreversible bonds between [³H]CNZ and its binding sites allows increased

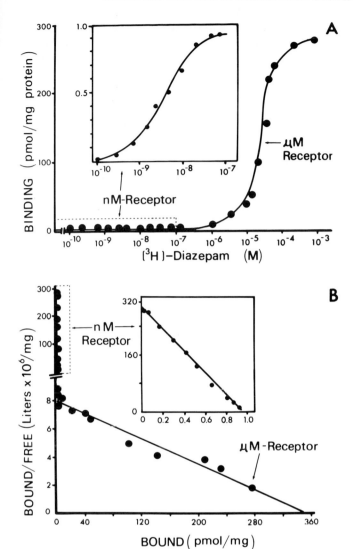

FIG. 8. (A) Saturation curve demonstrating the presence of two distinct classes of saturable benzodiazepine receptors. Binding assays were performed using [³H]diazepam concentrations in the 100 pM–800 μM range. For the nanomolar receptor, our binding assay yielded results similar to those obtained by Braestrup and Squires (6). Thirty micrograms of protein were used for each measurement, and each point is representative of at least 10 separate determinations. (B) Scatchard transformation of the saturation data showing markedly different binding parameters for the two receptors. Statistical analysis of the data in the Scatchard plot indicated a K_D of 45.0 μM, a B_{max} of 360.4 pmole/mg protein, and r = 0.969 for the micromolar receptor; and a K_D of 3.1 nM, a B_{max} of 0.893 pmole/mg protein, and r = 0.997 for the nanomolar receptor (from ref. 5, with permission).

dilution of samples prior to filtration and more complete washing of the filters without risking dissociation of bound radioligand-receptor complexes. Using this technique, saturable UV-induced micromolar [³H]CNZ binding that has similar pharmacological properties to that observed with the standard reversible [³H]DZ binding assay is obtained. Although we are pursuing the pharmacological relationship between reversible BZ binding and irreversible UV-induced BZ binding, the photoaffinity assay shows considerable promise as a technique for reproducible analysis of μM BZ binding sites and investigation of the molecular nature of the receptor.

PHENYTOIN AND CARBAMAZEPINE DISPLACE DIAZEPAM FROM THE MICROMOLAR BZ RECEPTOR

Phenytoin has been shown to displace diazepam from the μM BZR in therapeutic concentration ranges (5), suggesting that this membrane binding site may be modulated by several anticonvulsants. To test this possibility, we determined the ability of several anticonvulsants to displace diazepam from the μM BZR. Carbamazepine was effective in displacing diazepam, but phenobarbital and trimethadione were not good antagonists at this membrane site. In addition, ethosuximide, valproic acid, and vinyl GABA were not effective in displacing diazepam in therapeutic concentrations.

These results indicate that the μM BZR, by interacting with the anticonvulsants described above, is effective in antagonizing the actions of calcium and calmodulin kinase activity. Anticonvulsants that do not inhibit these calcium systems do not bind in therapeutic concentrations to the μM BZR. Based on these observations, a hypothesis has been developed that the μM BZR represents a membrane binding site that plays a role in regulating the calcium signal and thus may modulate neuronal excitability.

FUNCTION OF ANTICONVULSANT RECEPTORS

The ability of phenytoin, carbamazepine, and the BZs to interact at a binding site on brain membrane suggests that this site may play a role in regulating some of the anticonvulsant and neuronal stabilizing properties of these compounds. All three of these drugs are effective in inhibiting MES-induced seizures, posttetanic potentiation, calmodulin kinase activity, and calcium uptake in intact nerve terminal preparations. Thus, studies were initiated to determine if these specific membrane receptors were responsible for some of the effects of these compounds on calcium uptake and calmodulin kinase activity. The following data indicate that regulation of depolarization-dependent calcium uptake and calmodulin kinase activity are major functions regulated by this class of anticonvulsant binding sites.

BZ INHIBITION OF CALCIUM UPTAKE

To investigate the effects of BZs on synaptosomal Ca^{2+} uptake (Fig. 9), $^{45}Ca^{2+}$ flux was monitored under both depolarized and nondepolarized conditions (97). Calcium uptake is time-dependent and is dramatically stimulated by depolarizing concentrations of K^+ (70 mM) (4,87). BZs inhibit the depolarization-dependent component of Ca^{2+} uptake, suggesting that the Ca^{2+} uptake inhibited by BZs enters the nerve terminal through the voltage-sensitive Ca^{2+} channel (Fig. 10). BZ inhibition was concentration-dependent in the micromolar range and stereospecific.

Calcium influx due to synaptosomal depolarization occurs predominantly through voltage-sensitive Ca^{2+} channels, but it may also occur through tetrodotoxin (TTX)-sensitive voltage-dependent Na^+ channels. To determine whether BZs inhibit Ca^{2+} uptake by blocking Ca^{2+} and/ or Na^+ channels, we studied the effects of DZ on high K^+-induced Ca^{2+} uptake in the presence of a concentration of TTX that was shown to block veratridine-induced depolarization (4). Several lines of evidence confirm that BZ-sensitive Ca^{2+} uptake is mediated by the voltage-sensitive Ca^{2+} channel (Table 9). Veratridine, which induces depolarization by opening Na^+ channels, effectively stimulates Ca^{2+} uptake. Veratridine-induced Ca^{2+} uptake is also blocked by BZs, demonstrating that BZs block depolarization-induced Ca^{2+} flux. The Na^+ channel blocker, TTX, is effective at blocking veratridine-stimulated depolarization, but does not inhibit high K^+-induced Ca^{2+} uptake. Furthermore, DZ (150 μM) is equally effective at inhibition of high K^+-induced Ca^{2+} uptake in the presence or absence of TTX (50 μM).

These results indicate that Ca^{2+} uptake induced by high K^+, and its inhibition by BZs, are not mediated by the TTX-sensitive Na^+ channel. In addition, the organic Ca^{2+} antagonist verapamil (100 μM) and the dihydropyridine nitrendipine (200 μM) had some effect as Ca^{2+} channel inhibitors. In summary, these investigations indicate that BZ inhibition of Ca^{2+} accumulation in synaptosomes occurs through blockage of Ca^{2+} uptake induced by depolarization and may be mediated by voltage-sensitive Ca^{2+} channels.

BZs ACT AS CALCIUM CHANNEL ANTAGONISTS

Voltage-sensitive Ca^{2+} channels in synaptosomes and other neuronal preparations are blocked by Mn^{2+} (87,92). Under our experimental conditions (Table 10), Mn^{2+} characteristically blocked depolarization-induced Ca^{2+} uptake by >90%. Micromolar concentrations of DZ also blocked Ca^{2+} uptake by >95%. In addition, BZ inhibition was additive with that of Mn^{2+} (Table 10). These results indicate that BZs act as Ca^{2+} channel antagonists in nerve terminal preparations.

IRREVERSIBLE RECEPTOR BINDING BLOCKS CALCIUM UPTAKE

BZ inhibition of voltage-sensitive Ca^{2+} uptake in synaptosomes appears to be mediated by μM BZ binding sites (38,39,97). Inhibition and binding are concentration-dependent, saturable in micromolar concentration ranges, and stereospecific. The potency of Ro5-4864 was similar to that of DZ in both Ca^{2+} uptake and BZ binding studies.

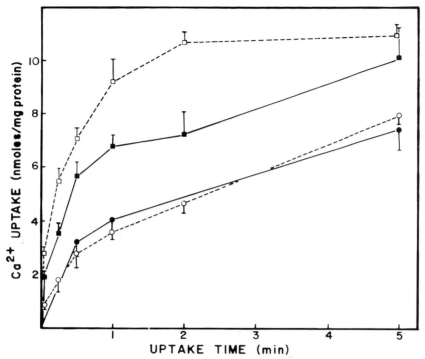

FIG. 9. Effects of DZ on synaptosomal Ca^{2+} uptake. Data represent $^{45}Ca^{2+}$ uptake into synaptosomes in the presence of low K^+ (5 mM K^+, ○) and high K^+ (70 mM K^+, □). The effect of DZ (150 μM) on Ca^{2+} uptake in the presence of low K^+ (●) and high K^+ (■) is also illustrated. Values represent means of eight determinations and are representative of three experiments (error bars, ±SEM) (from ref. 97, with permission).

The effect of irreversible BZ binding initiated by UV irradiation on Ca^{2+} flux was also examined. Intact synaptosomes were equilibrated with CNZ or FNZ and were then exposed uniformly to UV light (38,97). The photoaffinity-labeled synaptosomes were then washed free of unbound BZ and examined for $^{45}Ca^{2+}$ uptake properties. Synaptosomes with UV-induced BZ binding showed markedly reduced depolarization-induced $^{45}Ca^{2+}$ uptake in comparison to control preparations (Fig. 11). This effect of membrane-bound BZs on Ca^{2+} influx occurred in the absence of free BZ in the reaction media. This observation indicates that the Ca^{2+} channel antagonist properties of the BZs are mediated by the interaction of these compounds with a population of μM BZ binding sites. In addition, the data strongly suggest that UV-induced BZ binding may serve as an effective probe into the molecular nature of the voltage-sensitive Ca^{2+} channel in brain.

MANGANESE INHIBITION OF μM BZ BINDING

Mn^{2+} is a well-established Ca^{2+} channel blocker (87,92). Furthermore, Mn^{2+} is believed to interact directly with the Ca^{2+} channel and actually to insert and bind to the pore of the channel. Thus, it would be important to determine if Mn^+ affects BZ binding to the μM BZ receptor. Recent experiments in this laboratory have demonstrated that 2 mM Mn^{2+} significantly inhibits μM BZ receptor binding. The effect of Mn^{2+} is dose-dependent and reversible. These observations suggest that the μM BZ receptor may be closely linked or part of the Ca^{2+} channel. However, further studies are necessary to determine the exact relationship of this μM BZ receptor and the voltage-gated Ca^{2+} channel.

TISSUE DISTRIBUTION OF μM BZ RECEPTORS

By means of the UV-activated BZ binding assay (38,97), specific CNZ binding was determined in heart, spleen, kidney, and liver (Fig. 12). Brain had the highest specific binding per milligram of membrane. However, all tissues tested manifested specific μM BZ binding. These

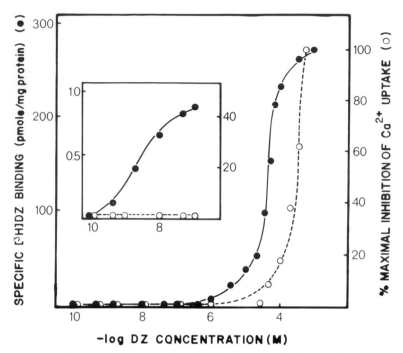

FIG. 10. Comparison of the saturation curve for [³H]DZ membrane binding and DZ inhibition of high K⁺-induced Ca²⁺ uptake. [³H]DZ binding (●) was performed by filtration assay with 300 µg brain membrane protein. Data represent specific binding and are the means of 10 determinations. DZ inhibition of ⁴⁵Ca²⁺ uptake (○) was determined by quantitation of high K⁺-stimulated synaptosomal ⁴⁵Ca²⁺ uptake in the presence or absence of DZ at varying concentrations. Data represent means of 12 determinations. *Inset:* expansion of [³H]DZ binding curve and DZ inhibition of Ca²⁺ uptake at low DZ concentrations (from ref. 97, with permission).

results suggest that µM BZ receptors are widely distributed in body tissues. Because many cell types contain voltage-sensitive Ca²⁺ channels, it is interesting to speculate that these µM BZ binding sites in peripheral tissues may also play a role in regulating Ca²⁺ currents. Further investigations of the effects of BZs on Ca²⁺ currents in nonneuronal tissue may provide insights into voltage-regulated Ca²⁺ channels.

TABLE 9. *Effect of veratridine, tetrodotoxin, and diazepam on synaptosomal Ca²⁺ uptake*

Condition	⁴⁵Ca Uptake (% of maximum)
Low K⁺	41 ± 6
High K⁺	100
High K⁺ + DZ (200 µM)	52 ± 3
Low K⁺ + V (50 µM)	91 ± 4
Low K⁺ + V (50 µM) + DZ (200 µM)	64 ± 7
Low K⁺ + V (50 µM) + TTX (50 µM)	61 ± 5
High K⁺ + TTX (50 µM)	96 ± 4
High K⁺ + TTX (50 µM) + DZ (200 µM)	58 ± 6

V, veratridine; TTX, tetrodotoxin; DZ, diazepam. From ref. 39, with permission.

BZs SIMULTANEOUSLY INHIBIT DEPOLARIZATION-DEPENDENT CALCIUM UPTAKE AND NEUROTRANSMITTER RELEASE

It is important to demonstrate that inhibition of voltage-gated Ca²⁺ uptake in synaptosomes also inhibits voltage-sensitive neurotransmitter release. Release of neurotransmitter substances is tightly associated with Ca²⁺ uptake in neurons. The data presented in Table 1 demonstrate that diazepam significantly inhibits NE and ACh release in intact synaptosomes under conditions that simultaneously inhibit Ca²⁺ uptake. These results indicate that the BZs act like Mn²⁺ in neurons, since they inhibit both Ca²⁺ uptake and neurotransmitter release.

ANTICONVULSANT RECEPTORS REGULATE CALCIUM–CALMODULIN PROTEIN KINASE ACTIVITY

Phosphorylation experiments demonstrate that membrane-bound BZs inhibit membrane-bound calcium–calmodulin-stimulated protein kinase activity in micromolar concentrations

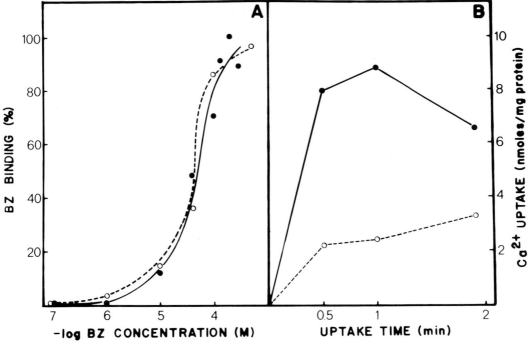

FIG. 11. (A) Comparison of the saturation curves for specific [³H]DZ membrane binding (○) and irreversible specific [³H]FNZ binding (●). Data give means of six determinations and represent percentages of maximal binding. **(B)** High K⁺-induced ⁴⁵Ca²⁺ uptake in control (●) and FNZ irreversibly labeled synaptosomes (○). Data give means of four determinations (from ref. 97, with permission).

(8,29). The ability of membrane-bound BZs to inhibit calcium–calmodulin kinase activity does not correlate with BZ binding to the nM BZR, but does correlate very significantly with binding to the micromolar affinity receptor (29). Irreversible binding to the μM BZR irreversibly inactivated membrane calmodulin kinase activity. These results indicate that both calmodulin kinase activity and voltage-dependent calcium uptake are regulated by these membrane receptors. Although the exact mechanism of regulation must still be determined, these find-

ings provide a direct insight into a membrane regulatory site on brain synaptic membrane that modulates two major calcium-mediated processes.

Recent studies in this laboratory have investigated the effects of the BZs and phenytoin on the purified calcium–calmodulin kinase system. Diazepam inhibited the purified kinase with a K_I of ~80 μM. The kinase was also inhibited by phenytoin. These results demonstrate that the BZs and phenytoin can directly interact with and inhibit the subunits of purified calmodulin kinase, suggesting that the kinase may represent a component of the μM BZR. Further studies are being directed at the molecular mechanism mediating the inhibitory effects of these compounds on the purified kinase system.

TABLE 10. *Comparison of the effects of BZs and Ca²⁺ channel antagonists on K-induced synaptosomal Ca uptake*

Agent	K⁺-Induced Ca²⁺ uptake (% inhibition)
DZ (0.2)	56 ± 5.3
DZ (0.6)	95 ± 4.6
Mn²⁺ (1.0)	63 ± 4.1
Mn²⁺ (10)	93 ± 3.3
Mn²⁺ (1.0) and DZ (0.2)	86 ± 4.8

BZs, benzodiazepines; DZ, diazepam.
From ref. 39, with permission.

CALCIUM SYSTEMS IN REGULATING SEIZURE DISCHARGE

Seizure activity involves the overstimulation of numerous synaptic contacts, causing the characteristic electroencephalographic evidence of neuronal excitability (45,53,99). During a seizure, excessive amounts of Ca²⁺ enter the synapse (45), activating Ca²⁺–calmodulin and other

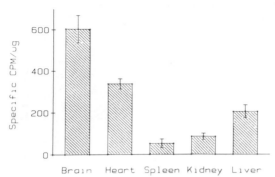

FIG. 12. Tissue distribution of specific UV-induced [^{3}H]CNZ binding in membrane preparations. Data give means of three determinations (from ref. 39, with permission).

Ca^{2+}-regulated processes. Thus, the Ca^{2+} channel and specific Ca^{2+}-regulated processes play an important role in modulating neuronal activity during a seizure discharge.

Regulation of Ca^{2+}–calmodulin enzyme systems by specific anticonvulsant compounds may underlie the molecular action of these drugs in modulating neuronal excitability. The evidence presented in this chapter demonstrates that phenytoin, carbamazepine, and the BZs in therapeutic levels inhibit: (a) Ca^{2+}–calmodulin-regulated protein phosphorylation in synaptosome, synaptic membrane, synaptic vesicle, postsynaptic density, and synaptic junctional complex preparations; (b) Ca^{2+}–calmodulin-stimulated synaptic vesicle and synaptic membrane interactions *in vitro;* (c) neurotransmitter release in isolated vesicle and intact nerve terminal preparations; (d) voltage-gated Ca^{2+} channels in synaptosomes; and (e) [^{3}H]diazepam binding to the μM BZRs. In contrast, the anticonvulsants, phenobarbital, ethosuximide, trimethadione, and sodium valproate had no significant effect even at high levels on these Ca^{2+} processes. These results also parallel the effects of these anticonvulsants on PTP and their actions in several models used to study epilepsy (103–105). The findings have generated the hypothesis that some of the anticonvulsant effects of phenytoin, carbamazepine, and the BZs are mediated by the effects of these compounds on voltage-sensitive Ca^{2+} channels and specific Ca^{2+}–calmodulin-regulated synaptic processes.

The involvement of Ca^{2+} in regulating seizure activity and the inhibition of specific Ca^{2+} processes by a group of anticonvulsants that regulate the Ca^{2+} signal in various neuronal preparations indicate that specific Ca^{2+}-regulated synaptic processes are involved in generating

and maintaining seizure discharges. It is now possible to study each of these Ca^{2+}-regulated molecular systems and determine their role in neuronal excitability. Elegant studies in the kindling model of epilepsy (100) have indicated that the activity of a hippocampal membrane Ca^{2+}–calmodulin kinase system is regulated by kindling, producing a long-term change in the activity of this kinase. These findings further implicate the possible involvement of the Ca^{2+}–calmodulin kinase systems in modulating neuronal excitability.

A MOLECULAR GENETIC APPROACH TO EPILEPSY

Although more research is necessary to implicate Ca^{2+} systems clearly in the modulation of seizure activity, the evidence reviewed here indicates that specific calcium systems are activated during the activity produced during seizure discharges. Calmodulin kinase systems (54–56,68,69) are considered to be a major regulating site for mediating the "Ca^{2+} signal" in brain. A major calmodulin kinase system has now been purified from brain (54–56). It is now possible to study the genetic expression of this important enzyme system. Furthermore, studies are being initiated in this laboratory to determine the possibility of isozyme variations of this laboratory to determine the possibility of isozyme variations of this kinase system in genetic models of epilepsy and in human epilepsy.

The ability to bind irreversibly radioactive analogues (97) to the μM BZR will facilitate the isolation and characterization of the molecular components of this receptor. Because binding to this receptor has been shown to regulate voltage-sensitive Ca^{2+}-channels (38,39,97), this major receptor in brain may play an important role in modulating neuronal excitability. Alterations in the level of this receptor or isozyme variation in the components of the receptor molecules could provide a molecular mechanism for altering the Ca^{2+} signal at the synapse. Thus, this receptor will be studied in various animal models of epilepsy and in human cases.

Currently, there are no biochemical tests that can be used to diagnosis epilepsy, mainly because of lack of an identifiable molecular defect underlying the seizure state. It is reasonable to assume that isozyme variants or altered levels of one or more of the components in the synaptic Ca^{2+}–calmodulin kinase system, the μM BZR, or other Ca^{2+}-regulated processes could produce altered neuronal excitability. These types of alterations may represent the molecular sub-

strate underlying inheritable seizure susceptibility in animals and humans. It is now possible
to determine the role of altered forms of this
important enzyme system in genetic epilepsy.
Recent studies in our laboratory have detected
a more active Ca^{2+}–calmodulin kinase system
in certain strains of epileptic mice that appears
to be genetically linked to seizure susceptibility.
It is hoped that our studies will provide some
insight into the molecular basis of epilepsy and
provide better methods for developing new anticonvulsant drugs and specific laboratory tests
for some forms of epilepsy.

ACKNOWLEDGMENT

The helpful discussions for W. Taft, J. Goldenring, M. Vallano, and A. Kleinhaus were
greatly appreciated. This research was supported by Research Career Development Award
NSI-EA 1 K04 NS 245, U.S. Public Health Service Grants NS 13632 and NS 06208, and grant
AFOSR-0284.

REFERENCES

1. Amy, C. M., Kirshner, N. (1981): Phosphorylation of adrenal medulla cell proteins in conjunction with stimulation of catecholamine secretion. *J. Neurochem.*, 3:847–854.

2. Barondes, S. H. (1974): Synaptic macromolecules: Identification and metabolism. *Annu.
Rev. Biochem.*, 43:147–194.

3. Bennett, M. K., Erondu, N. E., and Kennedy,
M. B. (1983): Purification and characterization
of a calmodulin-dependent protein kinase that
is highly concentrated in brain. *J. Biol. Chem.*,
258:12735–12744.

4. Blaustein, M. P., Johnson, E. M., and Nee-
dleman, P. (1972): Calcium-dependent norepinephrine release from presynaptic nerve endings *in vitro. Proc. Natl. Acad. Sci. USA*,
69:2237–2240.

5. Bowling, A. C., and DeLorenzo, R. J. (1982):
Micromolar benzodiazepine receptors: Identification and characterization in central nervous
system. *Science*, 216:1247–1250.

6. Braestrup, C., and Squires, R. F. (1978): Pharmacological characterization of benzodiazepine
receptors. *Eur. J. Pharmacol.*, 48:263–270.

7. Brostrum, C. O., Huang, Y. C., Breckenridge,
B., and Wolff, D. J. (1975): Identification of a
calcium-binding protein as a calcium-dependent
regulator of brain adenylate cyclase. *Proc.
Natl. Acad. Sci. USA*, 72:64–68.

8. Burdette, S., and DeLorenzo, R. J. (1980): Benzodiazepine inhibition of calcium-dependent
protein phosphorylation in synaptosomal and
synaptic vesicle preparations. *Neurology (Minneap.)*, 30:449.

9. Burke, B., and DeLorenzo, R. J. (1981): Ca^{2+}
and calmodulin-stimulated endogenous phos-

10. Burke, B. E., and DeLorenzo, R. J. (1982):
Ca^{2+} and calmodulin regulated endogenous tubulin kinase activity in presynaptic nerve terminal preparations. *Brain Res.*, 236:393–415.

11. Burke, B. E., and DeLorenzo, R. J. (1982):
Ca^{2+} and calmodulin-dependent phosphorylation of endogenous synaptic vesicle tubulin by
vesicle-bound calmodulin kinase system. *J.
Neurochem.*, 38:1205–1218.

12. Camerman, A., and Camerman, N. (1970): Diphenylhydantoin and diazepam: Molecular
structure similarities and steric basis of anticonvulsant activity. *Science*, 168:1457–1458.

13. Carlin, R. K., Grab, D. J., Cohen, R. S., and
Siekevitz, P. (1980): Isolation and characterization of postsynaptic densities from various brain
regions: Enrichment of different types of postsynaptic densities. *J. Cell Biol.*, 86:831.

14. Cheung, W. Y. (1970): Cyclic $3',5'$-nucleotide
phosphodiesterase: Demonstration of an activator. *Biochem. Biophys. Res. Commun.*,
38:533–538.

15. Cheung, W. Y. (1980): Calmodulin role in cellular regulation. *Science*, 207:19–27.

16. DelCastillo, J., and Stark, L. (1952): The effects
of calcium ions on the motor end-plate potentials. *J. Physiol. Lond.*, 124:553–559.

17. DeLorenzo, R. J. (1976): Calcium-dependent
phosphorylation of specific synaptosomal fraction proteins: Possible role of phosphoproteins
in mediating neurotransmitter release. *Biochem. Biophys. Res. Commun.*, 71:590–597.

18. DeLorenzo, R. J. (1977): Antagonistic action of
diphenylhydantoin and calcium on the level of
phosphorylation of particular rat and human
brain proteins. *Brain Res.*, 134:125–138.

19. DeLorenzo, R. J. (1980): Role of calmodulin in
neurotransmitter release and synaptic function.
Ann. N.Y. Acad. Sci., 356:92–109.

20. DeLorenzo, R. J. (1980): Phenytoin: Calcium–
calmodulin-dependent protein phosphorylation
and neurotransmitter release. In: *Antiepileptic
Drugs: Mechanisms of Action*, edited by G. H.
Glaser, J. K. Penry, and D. M. Woodbury, pp.
399–414. Raven Press, New York.

21. DeLorenzo, R. J. (1981): Calcium, calmodulin,
and synaptic function: Modulation of neurotransmitter release, nerve terminal protein
phosphorylations, and synaptic vesicle morphology by calcium and calmodulin. In: *Regulatory Mechanisms of Synaptic Transmission*,
edited by R. Tapia and C. W. Cotman, p. 205.
Plenum Press, New York.

22. DeLorenzo, R. J. (1981): The calmodulin hypothesis of neurotransmission. *Cell Calcium*,
2:365–385.

23. DeLorenzo, R. J. (1982): Calmodulin modulation of the calcium signal in synaptic transmission. In: *Compartmentation and Interaction of
Neurotransmitters*, edited by H. Bradford, pp.
101–120. Plenum Press, New York.

24. DeLorenzo, R. J. (1982): Calmodulin in neurotransmitter release and synaptic function. *Fed.
Proc.*, 41:2275.

25. DeLorenzo, R. J. (1982): Calmodulin in syn-
     aptic function and neurosecretion. In: *Calcium
     and Cell Function,* edited by W. Y. Cheung, pp.
     271–309. Academic Press, Orlando, Fla.
26. DeLorenzo, R. J. (1983): Calcium-calmodulin
     systems in psychopharmacology and synaptic
     modulation. *Psychopharmacol Bull.,* 19:393–
     397.
27. DeLorenzo, R. J. (1983): Calcium-calmodulin
     protein phosphorylation in neuronal transmis-
     sion: A molecular approach to neuronal excit-
     ability and anticonvulsant drug action. In: *Ad-
     vances in Neurology, Vol. 34, Status Epilep-
     ticus,* edited by A. V. Delgado-Escueta, C. G.
     Wasterlain, D. M. Treiman, and R. J. Porter,
     pp. 325–338. Raven Press, New York.
28. DeLorenzo, R. J. (1984): Calmodulin systems in
     neuronal excitability: A molecular approach to
     epilepsy. *Ann. Neurol.* (*in press*).
29. DeLorenzo, R. J., Burdette, S., and Holder-
     ness, J. (1981): Benzodiazepine inhibition of the
     calcium-calmodulin protein kinase system in
     brain membrane. *Science,* 213:546–549.
30. DeLorenzo, R. J., and Dashevsky, L. (1984):
     Anticonvulsants In: *Handbook of Neurochem-
     istry,* Vol. 9 edited by A. Lajtha. Plenum Press,
     New York (*in press*).
31. DeLorenzo, R. J., Emple, G. P., and Glaser,
     G. H. (1976): Regulation of the level of endog-
     enous phosphorylation of specific brain proteins
     by diphenylhydantoin. *J. Neurochem.,* 28:21–
     30.
32. DeLorenzo, R. J., and Freedman, S. D. (1977):
     Possible role of calcium-dependent protein
     phosphorylation in mediating neurotransmitter
     release and anticonvulsant action. *Epilepsia,*
     18:357–365.
33. DeLorenzo, R. J., and Freedman, S. D. (1977):
     Phenytoin inhibition of calcium-dependent pro-
     tein phosphorylation in synaptic vesicles. *Neu-
     rology,* 27:375.
34. DeLorenzo, R. J., and Freedman, S. D. (1977):
     Calcium-dependent phosphorylation of synaptic
     vesicle proteins and its possible role in me-
     diating neurotransmitter release and vesicle
     function. *Biochem. Biophys. Res. Commun.,*
     71:590–597.
35. DeLorenzo, R. J., and Freedman, S. D. (1978):
     Calcium-dependent neurotransmitter release
     and protein phosphorylation in synaptic vesi-
     cles. *Biochem. Biophys. Res. Commun.,*
     80:183–192.
36. DeLorenzo, R. J., Freedman, S. D., Yohe,
     W. B., and Maurer, S. C. (1979): Stimulation of
     Ca^{2+}-dependent neurotransmitter release and
     presnaptic nerve terminal protein phosphoryla-
     tion by calmodulin and a calmodulin-like pro-
     tein isolated from synaptic vesicles. *Proc. Natl.
     Acad. Sci. USA,* 76:1838–1842.
37. DeLorenzo, R. J., and Glaser, G. H. (1976): Ef-
     fect of diphenylhydantoin on the endogenous
     phosphorylation of brain protein. *Brain Res.,*
     105:381–386.
38. DeLorenzo, R. J., and Taft, W. C. (1984): An-
     ticonvulsant receptors: Regulation of depolar-
     ization-induced calcium uptake. In: *Advances
     in Epileptology: XVth Epilepsy International*

Symposium, edited by R. J. Porter, pp. 221–
230. Raven Press, New York.
39. DeLorenzo, R. J., Taft, W. C., and Andrews,
     W. T. (1984): Regulation of voltage-sensitive
     calcium channels in brain by micromolar af-
     finity benzodiazepine receptors. In: *Calcium,
     Neuronal Function and Transmitter Release,*
     edited by R. Rahamimoff, Martinus Nijhoff,
     Boston (in press).
40. DeRobertis, E., and DeLores, Arnaiz, G. R.
     (1969): Structural components of the synaptic
     region: In: *Handbook of Neurochemistry,* Vol.
     2, edited by A. Laftha, pp. 365–392. Plenum
     Press, New York.
41. Dodge, R. A., and Rahamimoff, R. (1967): Co-
     operative action of calcium ions in transmitter
     release at the neurotransmitter junction. *J. Phys-
     iol.* (*Lond.*), 193:419–432.
42. Douglas, W. W. (1968): Stimulus-secretion cou-
     pling: The concept and clues from chromaffin
     and other cells. *Br. J. Pharmacol.,* 34:451–474.
43. Ehrlich, Y. H. (1978): Phosphoproteins as spe-
     cifiers for mediators and modulators in neuronal
     function. In: *Modulators, Mediators and Spe-
     cifiers in Brain Function,* edited by Y. H. Ehr-
     lich, J. Volarka, L. O. Davis, and E. G. Brunn-
     graber, pp. 75–101. Plenum Press, New York.
44. Esplin, D. W. (1957): Effects of diphenylhydan-
     toin on synaptic transmission in cat spinal cord
     and stellate ganglion. *J. Pharmacol. Exp. Ther.,*
     120:301–323.
45. Esplin, D. W. (1972): Synaptic systems models.
     In: *Experimental Models of Epilepsy—A
     Manual for the Laboratory Worker,* edited by
     D. P. Purpura, J. K. Penry, D. P. Tower, D. M.
     Woodbury, and R. D. Walter, pp. 223–248.
     Raven Press, New York.
46. Esplin, D. W. (1963): Criteria for assessing ef-
     fects of depressant drugs on spinal cord syn-
     aptic transmission, with examples of drug se-
     lectivity. *Arch. Int. Pharmacodyn. Ther.,* 143:
     479–497.
47. Esplin, D. W., and Curto, E. M. (1957): Effects
     of trimethadione on synaptic transmission in the
     spinal cord: Antagonism of trimethadione and
     pentylenetetrazol. *J. Pharmacol. Exp. Ther.,*
     121:457–467.
48. Ferrendelli, J. A., and Daniels-McQueen, S.
     (1982): Comparative actions of phenytoin and
     other anticonvulsant drugs on potassium- and
     veratridine-stimulated calcium uptake in syn-
     aptosomes. *J. Pharmacol. Exp. Ther.,* 220:29–
     34.
49. Ferrendelli, J. A., and Kinocherf, D. A. (1977):
     Phenytoin: Effects on calcium flux and cyclic
     nucleotides. *Epilepsia,* 18:331–336.
50. Fukunaga, K., Yamamoto, H., Matsui, K., Hi-
     gashi, K., and Miyamoto, E. (1983): Purifica-
     tion and characterization of a Ca and calmod-
     ulin-dependent protein kinase from rat brain. *J.
     Neurochem.,* 39:1607–1617.
51. Gastaut, H. (1970): Properties antiepileptiques
     exceptionnelles d'une benzodiazepine nouvelle.
     Vie Med., 38:5175–5188.
52. Gastaut, H., Jasperr, H., Bancaud, J., and Wal-
     tregny, A., editors (1969): *The Physiopathogen-*

esis of the Epilepsies. Charles C Thomas, Springfield, Illinois.

53. Glaser, G. H. (1975): Epilepsy. In: *Recent Advances in Clinical Neurology,* edited by W. B. Matthews, pp. 23–66. Churchill Livingston, London.

54. Goldenring, J. R., Gonzalez, B., and DeLorenzo, R. J. (1982): Isolation of a brain Ca-calmodulin tubulin kinase containing calmodulin binding proteins. *Biochem. Biophys. Res. Commun.,* 108:421–428.

55. Goldenring, J. R., Gonzalez, B., McGuire, J. S., Jr., and DeLorenzo, R. J. (1983): Purification and characterization of a calmodulin-dependent kinase from rat brain cytosol able to phosphorylate tubulin and microtubule-associated proteins. *J. Biol. Chem.,* 258:12632–12640.

56. Goldenring, J. R., McGuire, J. S., and DeLorenzo, R. J. (1984): Identification of the major postsynaptic density protein as homologous with the major calmodulin-binding subunit of a calmodulin-dependent protein kinase. *J. Neurochem.,* 42:1077–1084.

57. Goldenring, J. R., Vallano, M. L., and DeLorenzo, R. J. (1985): Phosphorylation of microtubule-associated protein 2 at distinct sites by calmodulin-dependent and cyclic-AMP-dependent kinases. *J. Neurochem.,* 45:900–905.

58. Grab, D. J., Berzins, K., Cohen, R. S., and Siekevitz, P. (1979): Presence of calmodulin in postsynaptic densities isolated from canine cerebral cortex. *J. Biol. Chem.,* 254:8690–8696.

59. Grab, D. J., Carlin, R. K., and Siekevitz, P. (1980): The presence and functions of calmodulin in the postsynaptic density. *Ann. N.Y. Acad. Sci.,* 356:55–72.

60. Guzek, J. W., Russell, J. T., and Thorn, N. A. (1947): Inhibition by diphenylhydantoin of vasopressin release from isolated rat neurohypophyses. *Acta Pharmacol. Toxicol.,* 34:1–4.

61. Jasper, H. H., Ward, A. A., Jr., and Pope, A., editors (1969): *Basic Mechanisms of the Epilepsies.* Little, Brown and Co., Boston.

62. Julien, R. M., and Hollister, R. P. (1975): Carbamazepine: Mechanism of action. In: *Advances in Neurology, Vol. II, Complex Partial Seizures and Their Treatment,* edited by J. K. Penry and D. D. Daly, pp. 263–277. Raven Press, New York.

63. Kakiuchi, S., and Yamazaki, R. (1970): Calcium dependent phosphodiesterase activity and its activating factor (PAF) from brain. *Biochem. Biophys. Res. Commun.,* 41:1104–1110.

64. Katz, B., and Miledi, R. (1969): Tetrodotoxin-resistant electric activity in presynaptic terminals. *J. Physiol. (Lond.),* 203:459–487.

65. Katz, B., and Miledi, R. (1970): Further study of the role of calcium in synaptic transmission. *J. Physiol. (Lond.),* 207:789–801.

66. Kelly, P. T., and Cotman, C. W. (1978): Synaptic proteins: Characterization of tubulin and actin and identification of a distinct postsynaptic density polypeptide. *J. Cell Biol.,* 79:173–183.

67. Kelly, P. T., McGuinness, T. L., and Greengard, P. (1984): Evidence that the major postsynaptic density protein is a component of a Ca^{++}/calmodulin dependent protein kinase. *Proc. Natl. Acad. Sci. USA,* 81:945–949.

68. Kennedy, M. B., and Greengard, P. (1981): Two calcium/calmodulin-dependent protein kinases, which are highly concentrated in brain, phosphorylate protein I at distinct sites. *Proc. Natl. Acad. Sci. USA,* 78:1293–1297.

69. Kennedy, M. B., McGuinness, T. L., and Greengard, P. (1983): A calcium/calmodulin-dependent protein kinase from mammalian brain that phosphorylates synapsin I: Partial purification and characterization. *J. Neurosci.,* 3:818–826.

70. Kennedy, M. B., Bennett, M. K., and Erondu, N. E. (1983): Biochemical and immunochemical evidence that the "major PSD protein" is a subunit of a calmodulin-dependent protein kinase. *Proc. Natl. Acad. Sci. USA,* 80:7357–7361.

71. Killiam, E. K., and Suria, A. (1980): Benzodiazepines. In: *Antiepileptic Drugs: Mechanisms of Action,* edited by G. H. Glaser, J. K. Penry, and D. M. Woodbury, pp. 597–616. Raven Press, New York.

72. Klee, C. B., Crouch, T. H., and Richman, P. G. (1980): Calmodulin. *Annu. Rev. Biochem.,* 49:489–515.

73. Knopp, R. H., Sheini, J. C., and Freinkel, N. (1972): Diphenylhydantoin and an insulin-secreting islet adenoma. *Arch. Intern. Med.,* 130:904–908.

74. Krueger, B., Forn, J., and Greengard, P. (1977): Depolarization-induced phosphorylation of specific proteins, mediated by calcium influx, in rat brain synaptosomes. *J. Biol. Chem.,* 252:2764–2773.

75. Leslie, S. W., Friedman, M. B., and Coleman, R. R. (1980): Effects of chlordiazepoxide on depolarization-induced calcium influx into synaptosomes. *Biochem. Pharmacol.,* 29:2439–2443.

76. Lin, Y. M., Lin, Y. P., and Cheung, W. Y. (1974): Cyclic $3':5'$-nucleotide phosphodiesterase: Purification, characterization, and active forms of the protein activator from bovine brain. *J. Biol. Chem.,* 249:4943–4954.

77. Lin, C., Dedman, J. R., Brinkley, B. R., and Means, A. R. (1980). Localization of calmodulin in rat cerebellum by immunoelectron microscopy. *J. Cell Biol.,* 85:473–480.

78. Llinas, R., Steinburg, I. Z., and Walton, K. (1976): Presynaptic calcium currents and their relation to synaptic transmission: Voltage clamp study in squid giant synapse and theoretical model for the calcium gate. *Proc. Natl. Acad. Sci. USA,* 73:2918–2922.

79. Marcum, J. M., Dedman, J. R., Brinkley, B. R., and Means, A. R. (1978): Control of microtubule assembly and dissassembly by calcium-dependent regulator protein. *Proc. Natl. Acad. Sci. USA,* 75:3771–3775.

80. Merritt, H. H., and Putnam, T. J. (1938): Sodium diphenylhydantoinate in the treatment of convulsive disorders, *JAMA,* 111:1068–1073.

81. Michaelson, D. M., and Avissar, S. (1979): Ca^{2+}-dependent protein phosphorylation of purely cholinergic *Torpedo* synaptosomes. *J. Biol. Chem.,* 254:12542–12546.

82. Miledi, R. (1973): Transmitter release induced

by injection of calcium ions into nerve terminals. *Proc. R. Soc. Lond. Biol.*, 183:421–425.

83. Miledi, R., and Slater, C. R. (1966): The action of calcium on neuronal synapses in the squid. *J. Physiol. (Lond.)*, 184:473–478.

84. Mittler, J. C., and Glick, S. M. (1972): Radioimmunoassayable oxytocin release from isolated neural lobes: Response to ions and drugs. In: *Abstracts of the Fourth International Congress on Endocrinology, 47.*

85. Mohler, H., and Okada, T. (1977): Properties of [^{3}H]-diazepam binding to benzodiazepine receptors in rat cerebral cortex. *Life Sci.*, 20:2102–2110.

86. Mohler, H., Battersby, M. K., and Richards, J. G. (1980): Benzodiazepine receptor protein identified and visualized in brain tissue by a photoaffinity label. *Proc. Natl. Acad. Sci. USA*, 77:1666–1670.

87. Nachshen, D. A., and Blanstein, M. P. (1979): The effects of some organic calcium antagonists on calcium influx in presynpatic nerve terminals. *Mol. Pharmacol.*, 16:579–586.

88. Pincus, J. H., and Lee, S. H. (1973): Diphenylhydantoin and calcium: Relation to norepinephrine release from brain slices. *Arch. Neurol.*, 29:239–244.

89. Raines, A., and Standaert, F. G. (1967): An effect of diphenylhydantoin on post-tetanic hyperpolarization of intramedullary nerve terminals. *J. Pharmacol. Exp. Ther.*, 156:591–597.

90. Raines, A., and Standeart, F. G. (1966): Pre- and postjunctional effects of diphenylhydantoin at the soleus neuromuscular junction. *J. Pharmacol. Exp. Ther.*, 153:361–366.

91. Rasmussen, H., and Goodman, D. B. P. (1977): Relationships between calcium and cyclic nucleotides in cell activation. *Physiol. Rev.*, 57:421–509.

92. Reuter, H. (1973): Divalent ions as charge carriers in excitable membranes. *Prog. Biophys. Molec. Biol.*, 26:1–43.

93. Rubin, R. P. (1972): The role of calcium in the release of neurotransmitter substances and hormones. *Pharmacol. Rev.*, 22:389–428.

94. Schulman, H., and Greengard, P. (1978): Stimulation of brain membrane protein phosphorylation by calcium and an endogenous heat-stable protein. *Nature*, 271:478–479.

95. Shulman, H., and Greengard, P. (1978): Ca^{2+}-dependent protein phosphorylation system in membranes from various tissues, and its activation by "calcium-dependent regulator." *Proc. Natl. Acad. Sci. USA*, 75:5432–5436.

96. Shulman, H. (1984): Phosphorylation of microtubule-associated proteins by a Ca^{2+}/calmodulin-dependent protein kinase. *J. Cell Biol.*, 99:11–19.

97. Taft, W. C., and DeLorenzo, R. J. (1984): Micromolar-affinity benzodiazepine receptors regulate voltage-sensitive calcium channels in nerve terminal preparations. *Proc. Natl. Acad. Sci. USA*, 81:3118–3122.

98. Tallman, J. F., Paul, S. M., Skolnick, P., and Gallagher, D. W. (1980): Receptors for the age of anxiety: Pharmacology of the benzodiazepines. *Science*, 207:274–281.

99. Toman, J. E. P. (1969): Discussion: Further observations on dephenylhydantoin. In: *Basic Mechanisms of the Epilepsies*, edited by H. H. Jasper, A. A. Ward, Jr., and A. Pope, pp. 682–688. Little, Brown and Co., Boston.

100. Wasterlain, C. G., and Farber, D. B. (1984): Kindling alters the calcium/calmodulin-dependent phosphorylation of synaptic plasma membrane proteins in rat hippocampus. *Proc. Natl. Acad. Sci. USA*, 81:1253–1257.

101. Wilder, B. J., Ramsay, R. E., Willmaore, L. J., Feussner, G. F., Perchalski, R. J., and Shumate, J. B. (1977): Efficacy of intravenous phenytoin in the treatment of status epilepticus: Kinetics of central nervous system penetration. *Ann. Neurol.*, 1:511–518.

102. Wood, J. G., Wallace, R. W., Whitaker, J. N., and Cheung, W. Y. (1980): Immunocytochemical localization of calmodulin in regions of rodent brain. *Ann. N.Y. Acad. Sci.*, 365:75–82.

103. Woodbury, D. M. (1972): Applications to drug evaluations. In: *Experimental Models of Epilepsy*, edited by D. P. Purpura, J. K. Penry, D. B. Tower, D. M. Woodbury, and R. D. Walter, pp. 557–583. Raven Press, New York.

104. Woodbury, D. M., and Kemp, J. W. (1970): Some possible mechanisms of action antiepileptic drugs. *Pharmakopsychiatr. Neuropsychopharmakol.*, 3:201–226.

105. Woodbury, D. M., Penry, J. K., and Schmidt, R. P., editors (1972): *Antiepileptic Drugs.* Raven Press, New York.

106. Yaari, Y., Pincus, J. H., and Argov, Z. (1977): Depression of synaptic transmission by diphenylhydantoin. *Ann. Neurol.*, 1:334–338.

107. Yamauchi, T., and Fujisawa, H. (1980): Evidence for three distinct forms of calmodulin-dependent protein kinases from rat brain. *FEBS Lett.*, 166:141–144.

Advances in Neurology, Vol. 44, edited by
A. V. Delgado-Escueta, A. A. Ward, Jr.,
D. M. Woodbury, and R. J. Porter.
Raven Press, New York © 1986.

23

Cerebral Methylations in Epileptogenesis

O. Z. Sellinger, R. A. Schatz, and P. Gregor

Laboratory of Neurochemistry, Mental Health Research Institute, University of Michigan Medical Center, Ann Arbor, MI 48109

SUMMARY This chapter deals with the neurochemical consequences of the administration of the chemical convulsant agent L-methionine-*dl*-sulfoximine (MSO) on the brain of rodents. The principal notion is that this convulsant agent differs qualitatively from most quick-acting and predominantly lethal convulsant agents, commonly used in laboratory studies in epilepsy modeling because it has a preconvulsant latency period of several hours and also because it need not be fatal to the animals receiving it if they are properly managed during the preconvulsant period and following the first seizure attack. The historical profile of MSO as a useful and unique laboratory tool for neurochemical and molecular studies is briefly recounted, and the point is made that MSO is a close derivative of the amino acid L-methionine, which is used by each and every brain cell as a protein building block and as a precursor of the universal cellular methyl donor molecule, S-adenosyl-L-methionine. The importance of methylations, a set of reactions which consist in the transfer of the methyl group of S-adenosyl-L-methionine to several dozens of endogenous methyl acceptor molecules, small and large, is stressed and reviewed both historically and as this process relates to MSO epileptogenesis. The multiple effects of MSO on the methylation of small MW compounds, histamine being the working example, are reviewed. The involvement of phospholipid, nucleic acid, and protein methylations, all apparent targets of MSO action, in that they respond to the MSO challenge by a significant rate increase is elucidated. Finally, the effects of MSO at the functional level of brain receptor action are presented. It is pointed out that other investigators have recently also related methylation of synaptic membrane phospholipids with an increased ability of the benzodiazepine receptor proteins to recognize and bind ligands. Our own observations are consistent with the notion that the convulsant effect of MSO is mediated through changes in methylation which, unfortunately, are not yet precisely identified, either as to where they must occur in the brain to be of critical importance or as to whether specific molecular systems must be affected before serious functional alterations are communally propagated and epileptogenesis ensues.

The biochemical approach to the study of seizures, or better yet, the study of seizure models by neurochemists has been (over the years and if one examines the literature critically) a rather thankless chore, providing no valid answer to the question of what goes wrong, biochemically, in the nerve cell that causes it to lose control over its firing rate, and that leads it to explode at seizure time in an enormous burst of ionic, electrical, and metabolic hyperactivity. Although, over time, devotees of laboratory rodent epilepsy have injected millions of rats, mice, etc.

with convulsant and often lethal doses of count-less toxic substances, known in the jargon as "effective" convulsant agents, or, by pressing a button, have zapped the brains of these animals with megavolts, acutely or chronically, they have not elucidated the reasons of why seizures occur when they do in the epileptic patient. Moreover, although neurochemists and other re-searchers have excised the brains from the ro-dents' heads and have measured the most assorted metabolites, enzymes, receptor sites, inhibitors, activators, factors, etc. in their membranes, and cytosols, synaptosomes, ves-icles, etc., are they closer to solving the basic mystery? Indeed, upon examining the evidence critically, one may ask how they could be if most of the convulsant agents they administer seize the rodents to death and, conversely, if testing of anticonvulsant agents only aims at estab-lishing a rank-order of "potency" in regard to the standard killer convulsants? The question then arises as to the scope and rationale of a biochemical approach to the study of epilepto-genic mechanisms. Do neurochemists actually wish to know only how to rank a synthetic series of chemicals or do they aspire to understand the nature of the alterations of the molecular system or the process brought about by the agent under study? It is clearly impossible from one's limited perspective to assess what the relatively few neurochemists working with rodent seizure models wish to accomplish as a group. It is my impression, however, that for most of them, it is becoming increasingly difficult to persevere in exploring a given mechanism. On the other hand, some researchers, including the authors of this chapter, have persevered in working with a particular convulsant agent and have been un-willing to abandon the struggle, because they believe that their work contributes to the eluci-dation of the biochemical/molecular events gen-erated by the agent of their affection and to the understanding of the underlying biochemical/molecular basis of the seizure itself. The deep-rooted conviction shared by these few re-searchers (17,51) is that they must test several different experimental situations in their efforts to uncover multiple mechanisms of action of their agent. Only by doing this will they be in a favorable position to assess intelligently the nat-ural likelihood that biochemical/molecular alter-ations analogous to those observed in their model system mark the seizure-susceptible neu-rons in the epileptic patient's brain. Their find-ings may also assist in developing ways to transfer relevant information to the clinical level of inquiry.

The convulsant agent that has been the prin-cipal focus of our research efforts for the past many years is L-methionine-dl-sulfoximine (MSO) (2,3,24). My colleagues and I have written about MSO on several occasions (9,17,43,45,49,51). The purpose of the present chapter is not, therefore, to provide a detailed chronological overview of what is known, but rather to accentuate the positive and try to ex-plain why, even today, this drug remains an agent of choice for the study of seizures in lab-oratory rodents. There are two basic reasons for this; first MSO action has a convenient period of latency (4–5 hr), during which time its effects are obviously generated de novo, and are re-cruited, cascaded, amplified, and ultimately manifested in seizure form. Second, MSO has a well-documented stimulatory effect on cerebral methylation processes (46), which may turn out to be of crucial relevance for an interpretation of its convulsant action and for the transfer of the information gained to human epilepsy.

Recently, methylation and seizure-related phenomena (25) have also been associated by workers who do not use MSO. Because some of this research is tangential to our own recent ef-forts directed at documenting effects of MSO at the level of the cerebral benzodiazepine (Bz) re-ceptor sites (5,15), and since the Bz receptor complex is known to be involved in the media-tion of convulsant–anticonvulsant mechanisms (5), the relevant findings will also be briefly de-scribed.

WHAT IS MSO?

MSO is a derivative of the natural and essen-tial amino acid L-methionine, the word essential being used here not in the nutritional sense but reflecting rather the inability of brain tissue to synthesize sufficient amounts of methionine from homocysteine (30), a conversion taking place principally in the liver. Methionine must, therefore, be brought into the brain from the pe-riphery (52). Once there, its principal functions are: (a) to be incorporated into brain tissue pro-teins and (b) to serve as the only source of the universal methyl donor molecule S-adenosyl-L-methionine (AdoMet) (6,50). The latter pathway plays a very significant role in cerebral metab-olism (50), because this tissue carries out methyl transfer reactions very efficiently, both at the level of small MW methyl acceptors (31,33,36), such as the biogenic amines and peptides, and at the level of large MW methyl acceptors, in-cluding proteins (35), phospholipids (18,23,35), and nucleic acids (9,41,47). Among the latter, methylation is known to target DNA, mRNA, rRNA, and tRNA; among proteins it affects basic and acidic amino acids (50). Chemically, MSO may be synthesized from methionine in two steps (3): the first step is an oxidation to the sulfoxide, and the second step is the reaction of the sulfoxide with hydrazoic acid. In protein-bound form, methionine may be converted to MSO as well. In the 1940s, this reaction resulted from the commercial bleaching wheat flour with nitrogen trichloride (2,3,24). The bleaching process was banned when it was discovered that commercial products made from flour so bleached gave dogs who ate them "fits" and "hysteria." The toxic principle was quickly identified as MSO, and an effective convulsant agent for use in the laboratory was born (16,20,21,45).

MSO, A TOOL IN RODENT EPILEPSY RESEARCH

By the late 1960s, the trail of research that postulated a mechanism of action for MSO through inhibition of the cerebral enzyme glutamine synthetase had come to a dead end (29,42); in 1968, it could be demonstrated that a severe inhibition of this enzyme could be maintained in animals that also received methionine and were hence protected from MSO seizures. Subsequently, we found that following joint administration of methionine and MSO, and under properly chosen scheduling conditions, methionine effectively retarded the accumulation of MSO in the brain, yet did not appear to alter its regional disposition (13,33). Regarding its subcellular distribution, several clues indicated the effects of methionine administration on the binding of MSO to brain membrane fractions (13), particularly in the cerebellum. Investigations of the cellular fate of MSO in brain were undertaken; by 1971, we had described a trypsin-free bulk procedure for the separation of neuronal cell bodies from astroglial cells (44). These studies showed that, on a time scale of 3 hr following its i.p. administration, MSO traversed the glial compartment ahead of the neuronal one, but that, at the time of its maximal tissue concentration, i.e., at 3 hr, the neuronal compartment contained more of the drug per milligram of cellular protein than did the glial one. All of these observations, although admittedly far from being thoroughly investigated, thus did not point to a highly localized and specific interaction of MSO with specialized morphological compartments or cell types of brain tissue. Because of this, the conclusion was reached in the early 1970s that MSO acts on or affects, directly or indirectly, a general "household" process operating in all brain cells at physiological levels, and that its action was therefore unlike that of a neurotoxic agent, seeking out specific nerve tracts, receptor sites or target cells, such as 6-hydroxydopamine (6-OHDA), muscimol, or kainate.

Finding such a general metabolic process which would be targeted by MSO and whose role in cellular physiology of brain cells was undisputed became the next objective of the MSO research. Methylation appeared to be the best candidate, given the close chemical relationship between MSO, methionine, and AdoMet, and thus, the numerous and biologically highly important AdoMet-dependent methyl transfer reactions (6,50). It should be remembered that, at the time (mid-1970s), the physiological role of the methylation of biogenic amines was being actively researched by many luminaries of biochemical neuroscience.

WHOLE-ANIMAL MSO STUDIES AND BRAIN METHYLATION

Over the years, many compounds have been tested for anti-MSO action. The protective effect of L-methionine was first reported in 1956 (22). Derivatives of L-methionine which "the body" is able to convert to L-methionine rapidly and effectively, such as L-methionine methyl ester, L-methionine amide and the N-formyl and N-acetyl derivatives, were added to the list of effective compounds subsequently (42). D-methionine was found to be effective as well, and we reported that brain tissue is able to racemize it to the L-form "in time" for protection against the seizure (14). The α-methyl derivative of methionine, in which the hydrogen attached to the carbon that also carries the amino group is replaced by a methyl group, proved ineffective in protecting against the MSO seizure (42), although its joint administration (i.p.) with a convulsant dose of MSO, did result in a marked reduction of MSO in the brain, relative to levels seen after administration of MSO alone. However, since 0.02 μmoles per brain are apparently sufficient to elicit seizures, the reduction seen after α-methyl methionine must not have been effective enough for seizure protection to ensue. More recently, cycloleucine (0.5–1 g/kg), a specific inhibitor of the AdoMet-forming enzyme (ATP: L-methionine S-adenosyltransferase, EC 2.5.1.6) has been shown to retard the onset of the MSO seizure (38) and to improve the 24-hr survival time of the injected mice greatly. Similarly, the coadministration of MSO with DL-homocysteine thiolactone (0.5 g/kg) had the identical effect (40). Although the administration of MSO + adenosine (1 g/kg) was found to have no ameliorative effects on either seizure latency or survival rates (40), combining MSO with both adenosine (Ado) and DL-homocysteine thiolactone (HcyT) (200 mg/kg of each) achieved the desired effect by assuring survival of all the mice tested. An important set of observations, made during the course of the whole animal studies, was that the administration of the combination Ado + HcyT to mice receiving MSO earlier, afforded protection against MSO seizures, but only when given at least 3 and no later than 4 hr after MSO, i.e., within 1 hr before seizure onset. When the brains of the animals receiving Ado + HcyT 4 hr after MSO were examined for S-adenosyl-L-homocysteine (AdoHcy) levels, a 200% increase over control values was noted (40). In the same experiment, the levels of AdoHcy in the brains of mice receiving MSO alone fell to ~30% of control levels. A useful clue was thus obtained, namely that cerebral AdoHcy levels could act as indicators of whether MSO seizures would ensue. It became possible to assess the relevance of brain methylations to the MSO seizure biochemically, by testing the assumption that high levels of AdoHcy, indicating low methylation rates, reflected a "no go" seizure mode, whereas low levels of AdoHcy, reflecting "over"-methylation, indicated a "go" seizure mode (39).

MSO AND THE METHYLATION OF SMALL MW BRAIN ACCEPTOR MOLECULES

The key discovery, and one that led to the extensive subsequent investigations of cerebral methylation rates during MSO epileptogenesis, was the marked reduction of cerebral AdoMet levels, which reached their lowest values 3 hr after i.p. administration of MSO (31), i.e., at a time when brain MSO levels are at their highest levels as well (13,33). An additional and positive correlation was the finding that the levels of AdoMet decreased uniformly in all brain regions tested, just as (several years earlier) MSO was shown to accumulate in brain tissue (13). Furthermore, it could be shown that the AdoMet reductions were not the result of the inhibition of the AdoMet-forming enzyme (38), a possibility that appeared attractive at first, given that this enzyme, like the strongly MSO-inhibited glutamine synthetase (16), also uses ATP and Mg^{2+} ions in the catalytic reaction. It was also demonstrated that the reduction of AdoMet could not be accounted for by decreased cerebral methionine pools (28). Other researchers have shown that cerebral ATP levels remain unchanged after MSO (11). Therefore, by elimination, the most likely explanation for reduced AdoMet levels after administration of MSO was that transfer of the methyl groups of AdoMet becomes accelerated, exceeding its synthetic rate (34). This notion was subjected to several tests, first by studying the effect of MSO on the methylation of brain histamine (34) *in vivo* and on histamine N-methyltransferase *in vitro* (4,32). The single-step methylation of histamine was targeted for study for two reasons: first, the metabolism of histamine in brain proceeds almost exclusively by the methylation pathway; and second, unlike a catecholamine, histamine methylates to a single, easily identifiable product, N-methylhistamine. The specific radioactivity of N-methylhistamine was therefore monitored over time in the brains of control and MSO-treated mice, following the injection of an intraventricular pulse of ^{3}[H]histamine and was found to exhibit significantly higher values in the MSO animals. *In vitro* studies also showed that, after administration of MSO, the activity of histamine N-methyltransferase assayed as elevated over control values (32). More recently, effects of the anti-MSO combination (Ado plus HcyT) on the conversion of ^{3}[H]histamine to ^{3}[H]-N-methylhistamine *in vivo* were examined (36) and opposite results were obtained, namely a considerable decrease in the specific radioactivity of the newly formed ^{3}[H]methyl N-methylhistamine, indicating effective inhibition of its formation by the high levels of cerebral AdoHcy generated following the administration of its two precursors, Ado and HcyT or, for that matter, of L-homocysteine alone (12). Table 1 illustrates typical effects of MSO and of Ado plus HcyT on the *in vivo* synthesis of N-methylhistamine in mouse brain. It may be seen that the conversion index, as defined in the legend to Table 1, increased by 105% after MSO, while decreasing by 66% after Ado plus HcyT. As expected, the activity of histamine N-methyltransferase, as measured in an *in vitro* assay, was also significantly reduced after Ado plus HcyT, yet control activity levels could be restored by dialyzing the appropriate brain extracts, a procedure which, in all likelihood, caused the removal of most of the AdoHcy. Additional evidence in support of a relationship between the methylation of histamine and seizures was obtained when this process was compared in the brain of the audiogenic seizure-susceptible and seizure-resistant deer-

TABLE 1. *Effect of MSO and of adenosine + DL-homocysteine thiolactone (Ado + HcyT) on the N-methylhistamine conversion index in mouse brain*

Experiment	Treatment	Conversion index[a] (nmoles/g)	Change (%)
1	Control	2.2	
	MSO	4.5	+ 105
2	Control	7.3	
	Ado + HcyT	2.5	− 66

[a] dpm/g (^{3}[H]methyl histamine)/dpm/nmole (^{3}[H]histamine). Two microcuries of ^{3}[2,5-H]histamine diHCl (7.7 Ci/mmol) were injected intraventricularly in each animal, 15 and 5 min before death, respectively, in experiments 1 and 2.

MSO, 170 mg/kg, 3 hr before death; Ado + HcyT: 200 mg/kg of each, 40 min before death.

mice (*Peromyscus maniculatus, var. bairdii*) (10). The results indicated that, following the administration of a short pulse of intracerebral ^{3}[H]histamine, the genetically seizure-susceptible individuals mobilized the amine by converting it to the methylated metabolite at significantly higher rates than did their genetically seizure-resistant littermates. It is noteworthy that the acceleration took place in the face of significantly lower brain levels of histamine, routinely found in the seizure-susceptible deermice.

Before describing additional effects of MSO and of the anti-MSO combination Ado plus HcyT on brain methylation reactions, two separate but related observations should be briefly mentioned. The first one relates to the theory that under normal conditions, in the absence of MSO, an increase in rates of cerebral methylation can be achieved by producing higher than control brain levels of AdoMet. Although this result may be readily achieved by administering massive loads of L-methionine (1,30), no concomitant acceleration of methylations is known to ensue. The capability of AdoMet itself to produce such an effect in this context was therefore tested. Mice were injected i.p. with up to 500 mg/kg of the free base-equivalent of the water-soluble AdoMet derivative, AdoMet disulfate di-*p*-toluenesulfonate (26). It was assumed that this would lead to marked increases in cerebral methylation, including that of histamine to *N*-methylhistamine. The results (37), however, refuted this theory, inasmuch as they revealed a marked reduction of histamine methylation in the brain, despite significant increases (41%) in brain AdoMet levels. The second observation is that the administration of MSO results not only in a faster than normal utilization of AdoMet for methyl transfer reactions, but it also appears to result in a faster than normal utilization of methionine (presented as ^{14}[3,4-C]-L-methinine) as a precursor of the polyamines, spermidine and

spermine (27,28). Table 2 displays the results of experiments in which MSO and Ado plus HcyT were used to achieve opposite effects in this context. These findings represent further evidence that both the polyamine-yielding moiety of methionine and that of its methyl group are utilized more efficiently in the MSO-epileptogenic brain than in the control brain.

MSO AND THE METHYLATION OF HIGH MW BRAIN ACCEPTOR MOLECULES

Although it has not been investigated in great detail, the altered formation of ^{3}[H]methylated brain phospholipids following administration of MSO or Ado plus HcyT was originally reported in 1981 (35). While it was noted then that this process is markedly inhibited by the super-high levels of brain AdoHcy arising after administration of Ado plus HcyT, the selective stimulation of this process after administration of MSO is a more recent finding (40). Particularly striking, in retrospect, is the preferential reduction of ^{3}[H]methyl-phosphatidyl *di-* and *tri-*methyl-ethanolamines following administration of Ado plus HcyT (35), as opposed to the selective enhancement of the formation of ^{3}[H]methyl-phosphatidyl *mono*methylethanolamine following MSO (40). The distinct topographic localizations of the two enzymes concerned with the overall process of membrane phospholipid methylation (7,8,18,19) in brain tissue and the relative difference in access to these enzymes of, respectively, AdoHcy and AdoMet have been invoked to explain this unexpected and, admittedly, nonreplicated finding. Yet we believe that it is highly likely that if the kind of specificity already encountered at the level of membrane phospholipid methylation (7,8,18,23) is corroborated by further research, the theory that methylation is an indispensable process in the mediation of the convulsant effects of MSO and of the anticon-

TABLE 2. *Effect of MSO and of adenosine* + DL-*homocysteine thiolactone (Ado* + *HcyT) on the conversion of* $^{14}[3,4\text{-}C]$*methionine to* $^{14}[C]$*spermidine and* $^{14}[C]$*spermine in mouse brain*

Experiment	Treatment	$^{14}[C]$spermidine (dpm/nmole)	Change (%)	$^{14}[C]$spermine (dpm/nmole)	Change (%)
1	Control	28.4 ± 1.0 (7)		40.1 ± 1.2 (7)	
	MSO	42.7 ± 3.9 (11)[a]	+50	60.6 ± 4.3 (11)[b]	+50
2	Control	12.3 ± 0.7 (6)		16.8 ± 0.9 (6)	
	Ado + HcyT	8.84 ± 0.67 (6)[a]	−28	13.0 ± 1.19 (6)[c]	−23

Two and one microcuries of $^{14}[C]$methionine were injected intraventricularly, in experiments 1 and 2, respectively. The pulse time was 1 hr in both experiments.
[a] $p < 0.005$; [b] $p < 0.001$; [c] $p < 0.05$.
MSO, 150 mg/kg, 3 hr before death; Ado + HcyT: 500 mg/kg of each, 40 min before death.

vulsant effects of Ado plus HcyT will be greatly strengthened.

The involvement of phospholipid methylation in the function of the Bz-receptor of brain has recently also been reported (25). It was noted in these studies that AdoMet stimulates $^3[H]$methyl incorporation into cerebellar membrane phospholipids and enhances the binding of $^3[H]$-diazepam to the membrane-bound Bz receptor by increasing the apparent B_{max} value (pmoles per milligram), *viz* the number of receptor sites. Conversely, inhibition of the methyl transfer from $^3[H]$AdoMet to phospholipids by preincubation with AdoHcy abolished the increased ligand binding. A further effect (25) was generation of high-affinity GABA binding sites following incubation of the cerebellar membranes with AdoMet, a property that is absent in membranes preincubated without AdoMet. The possible relevance of these findings to those involving both methylation and MSO epileptogenesis stems from two recent observations. First, the binding of $^3[H]$muscimol (Table 3) and of $^3[H]$flunitrazepam (data not shown), two Bz–GABA receptor-specific ligands, becomes differentially altered in the cerebral cortex, the cer-

ebellum, and the hippocampus of MSO-treated rats; some of the MSO effects are counteracted by the subsequent administration of Ado plus HcyT. Second, methylation of the Bz receptor complex and/or of the phospholipids integrated into the membrane system (25) which holds it in place, may be part of an ongoing mechanism controlling the specific physiological responses of this "plurivalent" receptor complex. Table 3 shows lower than control K_d (nM) (affinity) values for $^3[H]$muscimol in the cortex, higher values in the cerebellum, and unchanged values in the hippocampus after administration of MSO. The administration of Ado plus HcyT reversed the decrease in K_D in the cortex but not in the cerebellum, whereas in the hippocampus the K_D value remained unchanged. Changes in the B_{max} (pmoles per milligram) values after MSO also occurred in an opposite direction in the cortex and cerebellum, whereas the hippocampus showed a net tendency towards higher than normal values, resembling the cortex. In both cortex and hippocampus, B_{max} values returned to normal after the administration of Ado plus HcyT, a trend that was absent in the cerebellum. It is difficult to assess the full functional

TABLE 3. *Effect of MSO and of MSO* + *adenosine and* DL-*homocysteine thiolactone (Ado* + *HcyT) on the binding of* $^3[H]$*muscimol to benzodiazepine receptor of rat cerebral cortex, cerebellum, and hippocampus*

Treatment	Cortex		Cerebellum		Hippocampus	
	K_d	B_{max}	K_d	B_{max}	K_d	B_{max}
Control	7.08	1.082	3.87	1.178	4.48	0.454
MSO	4.07[a]	0.719[b]	5.34[c]	1.601[d]	4.04	0.569[e]
MSO + Ado + HcyT	7.22	0.874	5.82	1.556[b]	4.99	0.459

MSO, 150 mg/kg, 3 hr before death; adenosine + DL-homocysteine thiolactone, 200 mg/kg of each 40 min before death. K_d, nM; B_{max}: pmoles/mg of protein. Binding was determined using exhaustively washed membranes, prepared in 20 mM of Tris-citrate, pH 7.2. The centrifugation and washing procedure included six wash cycles and two freeze–thaw cycles, to ensure removal of endogenous GABA.
[a] $p < 0.01$; [b] $p < 0.005$; [c] $p < 0.05$; [d] $p < 0.001$; [e] $p < 0.025$, as compared with control.

significance of these varied and regionally different changes in ligand binding but, as noted previously when effects of MSO on the cerebral metabolism of 5-hydroxytryptamine were studied (48), the combined presence of multiple and regionally opposite metabolic and biochemical alterations appears to be a feature of MSO epileptogenesis. The Bz receptor-related findings (Table 3) support the hypothesis advanced previously (48), namely that MSO is able to elicit time-dependent, regional, and biochemically diverse perturbations in brain function, and that the epileptogenic state which results as a consequence of the administration of MSO must be the sum total of a vast array of disinhibiting "mini-events" occurring in a concerted sequence and culminating in seizure onset.

Finally, we reported recently that one acute dose of Ado plus HcyT greatly diminishes the incorporation of ^{3}[H]methyl groups into the carboxylmethyl groups of brain proteins (35) and that protein carboxylmethylation, a process that accomplishes the removal of the negative charges on the free carboxyl groups of the aspartyl and glutamyl residues of proteins, appears to be maximally inhibited when the brain levels of AdoHcy become maximal; it is unclear what the physiological consequences of such an impairment of protein carboxylmethylation may be for overall or specific neuronal function. Similarly, the converse was recently noted, i.e., a marked enhancement of the rate of brain protein carboxylmethylation after one convulsant dose of MSO (15); a precise delineation of the physiological significance of this finding is still needed. Indirect evidence also points to the possibility that the proteins making up the Bz receptor complex undergo carboxylmethylation under normal physiological conditions and at a particularly active rate, during early postnatal development (15), when most functionally active proteins mature by undergoing intense and highly specific posttranslational modifications. Experiments are currently in progress to show that chronically administered MSO and/or Ado plus HcyT perturb the normal maturation of the Bz receptor complex. The consequences of such an event may be of crucial importance for the understanding of that facet of MSO action which almost certainly affects the methylation of synaptic macromolecules.

ACKNOWLEDGMENTS

The research described in this chapter was partly supported by grants from the National Institutes of Health and the Epilepsy Foundation of America.

REFERENCES

1. Baldessarini, R. J., and Kopin, I. J. (1966): S-adenosylmethionine in brain and other tissues. *J. Neurochem.*, 13:769–777.
2. Bentley, H. R., McDermott, E. E., Moran, E., Page, J., and Whitehead, J. K. (1950): Action of nitrogen trichloride on certain proteins. I. Isolation and identification of the toxic factor. *Proc. R. Soc. Lond.*, 137:402–417.
3. Bentley, H. R., McDermott, E. E., and Whitehead, J. K. (1951): Action of nitrogen trichloride on certain proteins. II. Synthesis of methionine sulphoximine and other sulphoximines. *Proc. R. Soc. (Lond.)*, 138:265–272.
4. Bowsher, R. R., Verburg, K. M., and Henry, D. P. (1983): Rat histamine *N*-methyltransferase. Quantification, tissue distribution, purification and immunologic properties. *J. Biol. Chem.*, 258:12215–12220.
5. Braestrup, C., and Nielsen, M. (1983): Benzodiazepine receptors. In: *Handbook of Psychopharmacology, Vol. 17. Biochemical Studies of CNS Receptors*, edited by K. L. Iversen, S. D. Iversen, and S. H. Snyder, pp. 285–384. Plenum, New York.
6. Cantoni, G. L. (1982): S-adenosylamino acids: Thirty years later. 1950–1981. In: *Biochemistry of S-adenosylmethionine and Related Compounds*, edited by E. Usdin, R. T. Borchardt, and C. R. Creveling, pp. 5–10. Macmillan, London.
7. Crews, F. T., Hirata, F., and Axelrod, J. (1980): Identification and properties of methyltransferases that synthesize phosphatidylcholine in rat brain synaptosomes. *J. Neurochem.*, 34:1491–1498.
8. Crews, F. T., Hirata, F., and Axelrod, J. (1980): Phospholipid methyltransferase asymmetry on synaptosomal membranes. *Neurochem. Res.*, 5:983–991.
9. Der, O., and Sellinger, O. Z. (1980): Transfer ribonucleic acids in the developing brain: The effect of the convulsant methionine sulfoximine on tRNA function. In: *Circulatory and Developmental Aspects of Brain Metabolism*, edited by M. Spatz, B. B. Mrsulja, Lj. Rakic, and W. D. Lust, pp. 261–278. Plenum, New York.
10. Doyle, R. L., Schatz, R. A., and Sellinger, O. Z. (1981): Differences in the methylation of brain histamine *in vivo* between audiogenic seizure-sensitive and resistant deermice. *Life Sci.*, 28:2805–2810.
11. Folbergrova, J., Passonneau, J. V., Lowry, O. H., and Schulz, D. W. (1969): Glycogen, ammonia and related metabolites in the brain during seizures evoked by methionine sulphoximine. *J. Neurochem.*, 16:191–203.
12. Gharib, A., Chabannes, B., Sarda, N., and Pacheco, H. (1983): *In vivo* elevation of mouse brain S-adenosyl-L-homocysteine after treatment with L-homocysteine. *J. Neurochem.*, 40:1110–1112.
13. Ghittoni, N. E., Ohlsson, W. G., and Sellinger, O. Z. (1970): The effect of methionine on the regional and intracellular disposition of ^{3}[H]-

methionine sulphoxine in the rat brain. *J. Neurochem.*, 17:1057–1068.

14. Ghittoni, N. E., and Sellinger, O. Z. (1971): Effect of the convulsant methionine sulfoximine on the *in vivo* uptake and metabolism of D-methionine in the brain. *J. Neurobiol.*, 2:153–168.

15. Gregor, P., and Sellinger, O. Z. (1983): Developmental changes in protein carboxylmethylation and in the benzodiazepine receptor proteins in rat brain. *Biochem. Biophys. Res. Commun.*, 116:1056–1063.

16. Griffith, O. W., and Meister, A. (1978): Differential inhibition of glutamine and gamma-glutamylcysteine synthetase by alpha-alkyl analogs of methionine sulfoximine that induce convulsions. *J. Biol. Chem.*, 253:2333–2338.

17. Hevor, T. K., and Gayet, J. (1979): Cyclic nucleotides in the brain of mice and rats submitted to the convulsant methionine sulfoximine. *Biochem. Pharmacol.*, 28:3507–3512.

18. Hirata, F. (1982): Overviews on phospholipid methylation. In: *Biochemistry of S-adenosylmethionine and Related Compounds*, edited by E. Usdin, R. T. Borchardt, and C. R. Creveling, pp. 109–117. Macmillan, London.

19. Hirata, F., Viveros, O. H., Diliberto, E. J., Jr., and Axelrod, J. (1978): Identification and properties of two methyltransferases in conversion of phosphatidylethanolamine to phosphatidylcholine. *Proc. Natl. Acad. Sci. USA*, 75:1718–1721.

20. Hrebicek, J., and Kolousek, J. (1968): Preparoxysmal changes of spontaneous and evoked electrical activity of the cat brain after administration of methionine sulphoximine. *Epilepsia*, 9:145–162.

21. Lodin, Z. (1958): An electroencephalographic study of the changes produced by the administration of methionine sulfoximine in dogs and rats. *Physiol. Bohemoslov.*, 7:95–101.

22. Lodin, Z., and Kolousek, J. (1956): Metabolism of methionine and methionine sulphoximine in relation to function of the central nervous system. *Physiol. Bohemoslov.*, 5:43–53.

23. Mato, J. M., and Alemany, S. (1983): What is the function of phospholipid *N*-methylation? *Biochem. J.*, 213:1–10.

24. Mellanby, E. (1946): Diet and canine hysteria. Experimental production by treated flour. *Br. Med. J.*, 2:885–890.

25. di Perri, B., Calderini, G., Battistella, A., Raciti, R., and Toffano, G. (1983): Phospholipid methylation increases ³[H]diazepam and ³[H]GABA binding in membrane preparations of rat cerebellum. *J. Neurochem.*, 41:302–308.

26. Pezzoli, C., Stramentinoli, G., Galli-Kienle, M., and Pfaff, E. (1978): Uptake and metabolism of S-adenosyl-L-methionine by isolated rat hepatocytes. *Biochem. Biophys. Res. Commun.*, 85:1031–1038.

27. Porta, R., Doyle, R. L., Tatter, S. B., Wilens, T. E., Schatz, R. A., and Sellinger, O. Z. (1981): The biosynthesis of polyamines in the brain of audiogenic seizure-susceptible and resistant deermice. *J. Neurochem.*, 37:723–729.

28. Porta, R., Schatz, R. A., Tatter, S. B., and Sellinger, O. Z. (1983): The biosynthesis of polyamines in mouse brain: Effects of methionine sul-

29. Rowe, W. B., Ronzio, R. A., and Meister, A. (1969): Inhibition of glutamine synthetase by methionine sulfoximine. Studies on methionine sulfoximine phosphate. *Biochemistry*, 8:2674–2680.

30. Rubin, R. A., Ordonez, L. A., and Wurtmen, R. J. (1974): Physiological dependence of brain methionine and S-adenosylmethionine concentrations on serum amino acid patterns. *J. Neurochem.*, 23:227–231.

31. Schatz, R. A., and Sellinger, O. Z. (1975): Effect of methionine and methionine sulfoximine on rat brain S-adenosylmethionine levels. *J. Neurochem.*, 24:63–66.

32. Schatz, R. A., and Sellinger, O. Z. (1975): The elevation of cerebral histamine-*N*- and catechol-*O*-methyltransferase activities by L-methionine-*d,l*-sulfoximine. *J. Neurochem.*, 25:73–78.

33. Schatz, R. A., Harris, R., and Sellinger, O. Z. (1976): The effect of methionine on the uptake, distribution and binding of the convulsant methionine sulfoximine in the rat. *Neurochem. Res.*, 1:53–63.

34. Schatz, R. A., Frye, K., and Sellinger, O. Z. (1978): Increased *in vivo* methylation of ³[H]histamine in the methionine sulfoximine epileptogenic mouse brain. *J. Pharmacol. Exp. Ther.*, 207:794–800.

35. Schatz, R. A., Wilens, T. E., and Sellinger, O. Z. (1981): Decreased cerebral protein carboxyl- and phospholipid-methylation after *in vivo* elevation of S-adenosylhomocysteine. *Biochem. Biophys. Res. Commun.*, 98:1097–1107.

36. Schatz, R. A., Wilens, T. E., and Sellinger, O. Z. (1981): Decreased transmethylation of biogenic amines after *in vivo* elevation of brain S-adenosyl-L-homocysteine. *J. Neurochem.*, 36:1739–1748.

37. Schatz, R. A., Stramentinoli, G., and Sellinger, O. Z. (1981): Decreased cerebral catabolism of ³[H]histamine *in vivo* after S-adenosylmethionine administration. *J. Pharmacol. Exp. Ther.*, 216:118–124.

38. Schatz, R. A., Tatter, S. B., and Sellinger, O. Z. (1982): Cycloleucine, methylation and MSO seizures. *Trans. Am. Neurochem.*, 13:205.

39. Schatz, R. A., Wilens, T. E., Tatter, S. B., and Sellinger, O. Z. (1982): Hypermethylation in the MSO-epileptogenic brain; reversal by dilantin or phenobarbital. In: *Biochemistry of S-Adenosylmethionine and Related Compounds*, edited by E. Usdin, R. T. Borchardt, and C. R. Creveling, pp. 6756–6778. Macmillan, London.

40. Schatz, R. A., Wilens, T. E., Tatter, S. B., Gregor, P., and Sellinger, O. Z. (1983): Possible role of increased brain methylation in methionine sulfoximine epileptogenesis. *J. Neurosci. Res.*, 10:437–447.

41. Sellinger, O. Z. (1982): Methionine sulfoximine *in vivo* modifies the tRNA^lys pool of developing rat brain. *J. Neurochem.*, 38:1676–1685.

42. Sellinger, O. Z., Azcurra, J. M., and Ohlsson, W. G. (1968): Methionine sulfoximine seizures. VIII. The dissociation of the convulsant and glutamine synthetase inhibitory effects. *J. Pharmacol. Exp. Ther.*, 164:212–222.

43. Sellinger, O. Z., and Azcurra, J. M. (1970): The breakdown of polysomes and the stimulation of protein synthesis as cerebral mechanisms of defense against seizures. In: *Protein Metabolism of the Nervous System*, edited by A. Lajtha, pp. 517–532. Plenum, New York.

44. Sellinger, O. Z., Azcurra, J. M., Johnson, D. E., Ohlsson, W. G., and Lodin, Z. (1971): Independence of protein synthesis and drug uptake in nerve cell bodies and glial cells isolated by a new technique. *Nature (New Biol)*, 230:253–256.

45. Sellinger, O. Z., Azcurra, J. M., Ohlsson, W. G., Kohl, H. H., and Zand, R. (1972): Neurochemical correlates of drug-induced seizures: Selective inhibition of cerebral protein synthesis by methionine sulfoximine. *Fed. Proc.*, 31:160–165.

46. Sellinger, O. Z., and Schatz, R. A. (1979): Cerebral utilization of adenosylmethionine and adenosylhomocysteine: Effects of methionine sulfoximine. In: *Biochemical and Pharmacological Roles of Adenosylmethionine and the Central Nervous System*, edited by V. Zappia, E. Usdin, and F. Salvatore, pp. 89–103. Pergamon, New York.

47. Sellinger, O. Z., and Der, O. (1981): Effect of methionine sulfoximine on methylation of guanine residues in astroglial transfer ribonucleic acids. *Neurochem. Res.*, 6:153–162.

48. Sellinger, O. Z., and Dietz, D. D. (1981): The metabolism of 5-hydroxytryptamine in the methionine sulfoximine epileptogenic rat brain. *J. Pharmacol. Exp. Ther.*, 216:77–82.

49. Sellinger, O. Z., Schatz, R. A., Porta, R., and Wilens, T. E. (1984): Brain methylation and epileptogenesis: The case of methionine sulfoximine. *Ann. Neurol.*, 16(Suppl.):S115–S120.

50. Usdin, E., Borchardt, R. T., and Creveling, C. R., editors. (1982): *Biochemistry of S-adenosylmethionine and Related Compounds*. Macmillan, London.

51. Woodbury, D. M. (1980): In *Antiepileptic Drugs: Mechanisms of Action*, edited by G. H. Glaser, J. K. Penry, and D. M. Woodbury, pp. 294–304. Raven, New York.

52. Wurtman, R. J. (1979): In: *Biochemical and Pharmacological Roles of Adenosylmethionine and the Central Nervous System*, edited by V. Zappia, E. Usdin, and F. Salvatore, pp. 71–80. Pergamon, New York.

Advances in Neurology, Vol. 44, edited by
A. V. Delgado-Escueta, A. A. Ward, Jr.,
D. M. Woodbury, and R. J. Porter.
Raven Press, New York © 1986.

24

Role of Noradrenergic Ascending System in Extinction of Epileptic Phenomena

Patrick Chauvel and Suzanne Trottier

Epilepsy Research Unit, INSERM U97, F-75014 Paris, France

SUMMARY   This chapter reviews results which show that in electroshock-induced and chemically induced convulsions, audiogenic seizures of genetic epilepsy-prone rats and mice, in the kindling focus and the cobalt lesion seizure, susceptibility is modulated by a noradrenergic mechanism. In general, mechanisms that increase or decrease norepinephrine activities decrease or increase seizures, respectively, in these models. In the kindling phenomenon, since the seizure itself provokes an increase in norepinephrine (NE) turnover, with decreased β-adrenoceptor binding and hyposensitivity to ionophoretic catecholamine application, down regulation could be the cause of hyperexcitability or a consequence of it. In the cobalt focus, supersensitivity to NE appeared when NE-containing terminal density decreased (denervation supersensitivity) and β-receptor sites increased >50%. Perfusion experiments with NE support the hypothesis that the cortical NE system inhibits the spread of chronic epileptogenic activities in the cobalt focus. In the quaking mouse and in the tottering mouse, noradrenergic dysfunction underlying epileptogenesis may be expressed as a hyperinnervation.

In the 1960s, advances in neurochemistry and histology identified catecholamines as neurotransmitters in the central nervous system (CNS). Histofluorescence studies visualized the morphology of specific catecholaminergic fiber systems, distributed diffusely in the brain, and originating from a small number of nuclei located mainly in the brainstem (32,68,84). Functional neurochemical experiments, on the other hand, showed that norepinephrine (NE) and dopamine (DA) could be measured in synaptosomal fractions, that they both could be released by electrical stimulation or K^+ stimulation (see ref. 59 for review), that specific receptors existed in postsynaptic membranes (see ref. 100 for review), and that termination of their activity was achieved by reuptake into the presynaptic

terminals and enzymatic inactivation by catechol-*O*-methyltransferase (COMT) and monoamine oxidase (MAO) (78).

Thus, based on these anatomical and biochemical criteria, separate systems were described, namely: (a) a nigro–striatal dopaminergic pathway; (b) a mesocortical dopaminergic system originating from the ventral tegmental area of the mesencephalon, with projections localized in precise cortical and rhinencephalic areas; and (c) a noradrenergic ascending system arising primarily from the locus coeruleus (LC) and projecting widely to many different parts of the cerebellum, diencephalon, and telencephalon. This third system has a general rostrocaudal orientation at the cerebral cortical level, and various patterns of organization depend on the cerebral cortical area involved. An important noradrenergic projection to the spinal cord also originates from neighboring areas in the brainstem and influences spinal motoneuronal activity (7,8,32,38,49,84,86–88,98,109,118).

Numerous studies have been devoted to the characterization of these specific catecholaminergic systems in the CNS. In particular, specific exclusion of one system or the other can be achieved by stereotaxic electrolytic lesions or by local or general injections of specific neurotoxins, such as 6-hydroxydopamine (6-OHDA) and 4 *N*-(2 chloroethyl)-*N*-ethyl-2-bromobenzylamine or DSP-4 (30,116). Moreover, many pharmacological tools have been developed based on previous studies of the autonomic nervous system. There are drugs that act upon different steps of catecholamine metabolism, such as synthesis inhibition (α-methylparatyrosine [α-MPT], FLA 63, disulfiram), storage impairment (reserpine), release inhibition (guanethidine), and degradation impairment (monoamine oxydase inhibitors [IMAO]). There are other drugs that are more or less specific receptor agonists or antagonists. According to their sites of action, they act preferentially on either presynaptic uptake mechanisms or postsynaptic activations. These actions in turn may be mediated by specific receptors, classified as α- and β-receptors (100). Most investigators agree that β-receptors mediate one type of postsynaptic activation, whereas α-1 receptors mediate another type of postsynaptic activation. Uptake mechanisms are controlled by α_2-receptors. However, one can not exclude the possibility that some drugs have both presynaptic and postsynaptic sites of action, especially when they act on α-receptors, which may be located in both sites.

The physiological consequences of the various interactions between catecholamines and receptors are not fully understood. It is likely that their action depends on the type of receptor activated, just as it does in the autonomic nervous system. Microionophoretic studies of NE and antagonist or agonist drugs in the mammalian cortex suggest that β-receptor activation is inhibitory and α-receptor activation is excitatory (110). LC electrical stimulation coupled with ionophoretic application of NE and NE-antagonists on the same neuron demonstrate that the influence of LC neurons on target cells in the cortex is inhibitory and β-receptor mediated. However, it seems clear from both physiological and biochemical experiments that the mode of action of catecholamines in the CNS is not only that of a neurotransmitter but more generally that of a neuromodulator. Indeed, it is well established that NE and DA activate postsynaptic adenylcyclases (78). Furthermore, ultrastructural studies of NE-containing terminals in the rat cortex have suggested that, in addition to conventional asymmetrical synapses, NE release can be directly achieved in the extracellular space at the level of the so-called varicosities (27,28,61,91).

An immediate consequence of these advances in catecholamine biochemistry was the recognition that dopamine was depleted in the nigro–striatal pathways of Parkinsonian patients. This discovery was made very soon after recognition of DA as a neurotransmitter (separate and independent of NE transmission) and identification of the nigro-striatal pathway as dopaminergic. This recognition led to the successful therapeutic correction of DA depletion by L-DOPA. Investigators were thus encouraged to search for similar defects in neurotransmission in other brain diseases such as epilepsy.

Although epilepsy has been long suspected to be a functional disorder of neuronal excitability, experiments testing this suspicion have only recently been done through cellular–neuronal and glial studies. Because of the widespread distribution of catecholaminergic systems in the brain, two working catecholamine hypotheses on epilepsy can be put forward: (a) epilepsy is a diffuse alteration of neuronal excitability as in the generalized epilepsies; here a global alteration of catecholamine systems would be responsible for seizures; or (b) focal alterations of aminergic afferents are related to the development of partial epilepsy; here the epileptogenic process is localized (epileptic focus) in cerebral cortical and hippocampal structures where catecholaminergic projections exist.

Using pharmacological, biochemical, histological, and physiological tools mentioned above, two main problems can be approached in acute and chronic experimental models of epilepsy. The first questions whether epileptic phenomena can be modulated by altering the efficiency of catecholaminergic transmission in the CNS. The second searches for a primary defect in catecholamine transmission which could lead to the genesis of epilepsies. Considering the great diversity of experimental models of epilepsy, the following corollary questions should be addressed: Can the type of modulation exerted by catecholamines be common (or not) to the different models of epilepsy? If a primary defect can be detected, would it be expressed with similar or different distributions in different experimental models of epilepsy? Are various defects in catecholamine metabolism present in the different experimental models?

GENERAL EFFECTS OF MONOAMINES IN MODELS OF GENERALIZED EPILEPSIES

Pharmacological manipulations of monoamine metabolism influence the convulsive threshold in various models of epilepsy. Drugs that decrease brain monoamine concentrations in rats and mice by inhibiting monoamine synthesis (α-MPT, FLA 63), NE release (guanethidine), or monoamine storage (reserpine, tetrabenazine) lower the convulsive threshold of chemically induced convulsions (22,92), electroshock seizures (56,64), and genetically determined convulsions (12,45,104). Conversely, drugs that increase brain monoamine concentrations by inhibiting monoamine destruction (IMAO) protect against electroshock convulsions, audiogenic seizures (57), and chemically induced convulsions (70,104). These results can be interpreted in two different ways. Epileptogenesis may be due to a deficiency in monoaminergic transmission or to a modulation by the catecholaminergic system of the subthreshold epileptogenic process.

SPECIFIC INVOLVEMENT OF NE IN MODULATION OF ACUTE GENERALIZED EPILEPSIES

Experiments using 6-OHDA have provided strong and highly specific evidence for the anticonvulsant function of NE in generalized models of epilepsies. After uptake by catecholaminergic terminals, the neurotoxin 6-OHDA is transformed into a quinone derivative which produces fiber degeneration. The more or less specific effect of this drug is conditioned by the way it is administered. As predicted, fiber degeneration of catecholaminergic terminals by 6-OHDA lowered convulsive threshold to Metrazol injections. When 6-OHDA was injected intraventricularly in rats, clinical seizure patterns changed. Marked tonic extensions contrasted with clonic manifestations of control animals, and the duration of seizures was longer. 6-OHDA injected into the ventricular system depleted both NE and DA. Mason and Corcoran (66,67) stereotaxically injected 6-OHDA into the ascending noradrenergic bundle arising from the LC and significantly reduced NE levels in the cerebral cortex, hippocampus, and hypothal-

amus. DA brain concentration was not affected. They then observed clinical seizure patterns after one subcutaneous (s.c.) injection of Metrazol. The latency of the first generalized seizure was unaffected, but the duration and number of convulsions were greatly increased when compared with those of controls.

To further differentiate the respective role of NE and DA in the control of maximal electroconvulsive thresholds, the same authors compared rats whose NE was depleted by 6-OHDA injections into the dorsal bundle with rats whose DA was depleted by 6-OHDA injections into the nigro-striatal bundle. No alteration in any parameter of ECS-induced convulsions was observed in DA-depleted rats. In contrast, duration of convulsions was significantly increased in NE-depleted rats as compared with controls; latency and clinical pattern were unchanged (67).

These results show that NE depletion alone is sufficient to increase seizure susceptibility. Furthermore, the data argue in favor of the specificity of NE depletion in exacerbation of these convulsive states. It could mean that when external factors, e.g., toxic or metabolic disorders, induce convulsions in normal brain, catecholamines may protect against seizures and in that function, NE is more efficient than dopamine, i.e., NE may act as an endogenous anticonvulsant.

CATECHOLAMINES AND CHRONIC MODELS OF GENETICALLY DETERMINED GENERALIZED EPILEPSIES

The modulatory effects of catecholamines have also been extensively studied in genetically determined epilepsies of rats and mice. In these animals, clinically generalized seizures are reflexly precipitated through the audiogenic mode.

Subcutaneous injections of 6-OHDA in newborn rats, who subsequently acquire susceptibility to audiogenic seizures, produced a further increase in audiogenic response scores when the animals reached 60 days. The increase in severity of audiogenic seizures coincided with a significant reduction of NE concentrations in the cerebral cortex, spinal cord, and pons medulla without any concomitant change in DA concentrations (12). Furthermore, drugs that interfered with storage (reserpine, Ro-1284), or synthesis (α-MPT) of catecholamines increased severity of audiogenic seizures. Conversely, Desipramine, a drug that inhibits NE reuptake without effect on DA uptake (39), protected rats against sound-induced seizures (45). Moreover, pharmacological studies that have used drug combinations to increase NE or DA brain concentrations selectively have supported the above observations. The drug combination of L-dihydroxyphenylalanine plus Iproniazid, which increases NA and DA, produces a significant decrease in audiogenic seizures; however, pretreatment with diethyldithiocarbamate, then with L-dihydroxyphenylalanine plus Iproniazid, which increases only DA, has no effect against audiogenic convulsions in genetic epilepsy-prone rats (GEPR) (57). All these results suggest that in this natural model of epilepsy (GEPR), seizure susceptibility is also modulated by a noradrenergic mechanism, as earlier hypothesized in studies of chemically or electrically induced convulsions.

Questions then arise whether these artificial manipulations of catecholamine (and more precisely NE) metabolism reveal an innate dysfunction of catecholaminergic systems or whether they influence nonspecifically an epileptogenic neuronal activity of another origin. To answer these questions, aminergic function and epileptogenicity have been correlated in different strains of epilepsy-susceptible animals.

Observations at different stages of development of DBA/2J (audiogenic seizure-susceptible mice), C57BL/6J (nonsusceptible mice), and the F1 hybrid between these strains, have shown that the lowest brain NE and 5-hydroxytryptamine (5-HT) concentrations occurred at the period of maximal susceptibility (21 days) (103,104). The degree of susceptibility was related to the relative level of brain monoamine concentrations. The sensitivity of these strains to drugs acting on monoamine metabolism and storage is strikingly different; the greatest susceptiblity to seizures occurred in those mice with the highest sensitivity to depleting drugs (54). Baseline NE concentrations were decreased in many areas of the CNS in epilepsy-prone rats. Abnormal drops in baseline 5-HT concentrations were also present in many areas of the CNS except cerebellum and spinal cord. In contrast, endogenous DA concentrations were normal (24,48).

Similar results have been observed in other models of generalized epilepsy. NE brain concentrations were decreased in parathyroidectomized and pinealectomized rats, whereas 5-HT and DA concentrations were not altered (95). Similar observations have been reported for pinealectomy-induced convulsions in the gerbil (96,97). NE and DA contents are also reduced in cerebral cortex and thalamus following withdrawal of barbital-dependent rats (85).

Investigators questioned whether the NE defect was (a) a primary etiological factor for seizures, (b) one of multiple alterations, or (c) just a epiphenomenon. Jobe et al. (47) wondered if it was possible to transform nonsusceptible rats into epileptic ones by depleting brain monoamines. Ro4-1284, a benzoquinolizine that inhibits the vesicular storage mechanism of monoamines, induced audiogenic seizures in nonsusceptible progeny from epilepsy-prone (audiogenic seizure susceptible) parents (NSPSP). In control rats (non-seizure susceptible progeny of non–epilepsy-prone rats) only a negligible fraction of animals exhibited sound-induced convulsions. Both types of rats showed a profound reduction of NE and 5-HT in the CNS, immediately after Ro-1284 injection. Nineteen days after Ro-1284 administration, NE and 5-HT brain contents of the two groups returned to normal values, even though audiogenic seizures persisted in the NSPSP group. Thus, Jobe et al. suggested that a deficiency in monoaminergic function is an important modulatory factor in audiogenic seizure susceptibility of rats that also carry some other genetically determined susceptibility factor(s). Jobe et al. further suggested that a monoaminergic deficit is necessary for appearance of susceptibility but not for its continuation (46).

IS THE ABNORMALITY IN NE THE SINGLE DEFECT OR ONE AMONG MULTIPLE DEFECTS INVOLVED IN EPILEPTOGENESIS?

It is apparent from the above discussion that whatever the model and the experimental conditions, an additional factor must be associated with the catecholamine (or NE) alteration in order to generate epilepsy. The catecholamine deficit may be considered as either a predisposing or a trigger factor (46).

As neurochemical data progressively accumulate in experimental models of epilepsy, the following general statement emerges. If epileptogenesis is linked with an alteration in chemical neurotransmission, it would probably result from a combination of several neurotransmission system disorders. Whether multiple combinations are used in different models to lead finally to epilepsy remains to be elucidated. If the alternative hypothesis is considered, abnormalities in chemical neurotransmission would not be causally involved, as in the case of a primary neuronal membrane alteration. In this hypothesis, the various abnormalities that have been described could represent consequences rather than causes of epileptic activity. Thus, in experiments which produced fiber degeneration pharmacologically or increased functions of neurotransmitter systems, NE would be considered a modulator or an anticonvulsant.

At present, it is fair to say that no evidence exists to support the concept that catecholamines are at the origin of epilepsy.* On the other hand, it is fairly well established that catecholamines modulate and reduce epileptic discharges. One of the remaining questions is whether they exert an overall control upon the epileptogenic process. In the models of generalized epilepsies mentioned above, duration, intensity, and repetition of convulsions were exaggerated if NE was depleted. It was difficult to discern if NE exerted a more precise control on mechanisms of onset, spread, or arrest of generalized epileptic discharges.

NE AND MODULATION OF PARTIAL CHRONIC EPILEPSIES

Kindling Phenomenon: Control of Discharge Spread by Noradrenergic Mechanisms

Daily repetition of low-intensity electrical stimulations of discrete forebrain structures may provoke a permanent change in responses evolving from localized afterdischarge to generalized convulsions (40). Five successive stages of kindling development have been described, ranging from hyperactivity and exploring behavior (stage 1) to generalized tonic-clonic convulsion with postictal depression (stage 5). Kindling rate is defined as the number of stimulation sessions inducing an afterdischarge necessary to reach the stage 5 convulsion.

Initial studies reported that reserpine or intraventricular 6-OHDA facilitated amygdaloid kindling (3,25). Pharmacological manipulations of brain monoamine levels and adrenoceptors suggested that NE rather than DA was the modulating factor. α-MPT, disulfiram, and propranolol augmented the kindling rate (the two latter drugs also increasing the afterdischarge duration), whereas apomorphine and pimozide, phenoxybenzamine, and clonidine had no effect

(16). More direct arguments in favor of this suggestion were then brought forward. When intraventricular injections of 6-OHDA are associated with s.c. injections of desmethylimipramine (DMI), a drug that protects NE fibers against 6-OHDA, kindling facilitation is suppressed (71). Furthermore, selective lesions stereotaxically made by 6-OHDA, either in the NE dorsal bundle or in the ascending DA pathway, show that only NE depletion influences kindling development (26). In the same way, acute DMI administration delays kindling; chronic DMI administration, which leads to a desensitization of receptors (by diminution of NE-binding sites), increases kindling rate (73). The same predominant role of NE in the control of kindling effect is observed after stimulations of other target structures such as the dorsal hippocampus (2) or the frontal cortex (1). There are, therefore, striking similarities between the kindling data and those obtained from generalized models, suggesting that the modulatory role of the noradrenergic system is roughly analogous in these models.

The clinical and electrical effects of NE depletion on the kindling development have been carefully analyzed. In amygdaloid kindling, it is generally admitted that the first afterdischarge threshold and its duration are not modified. The kindling rate at the primary site is always increased such that the first convulsion may be obtained with the first afterdischarge (26,72,81). Moreover, afterdischarge bilateralization and kindling rate at the secondary site are also facilitated (26). In contrast, once tonic-clonic seizures appear (stage 5), noradrenergic depletion has no more effect (81). Furthermore, in dorsal hippocampus (74) and frontal cortex (1) kindling, NE depletion has the same effect (no afterdischarge modification and facilitation of the kindling rate). In summary, this kind of facilitation of the kindling phenomenon is interpreted as a disinhibition of the spread of paroxysmal activity from the stimulated structure but not as an increased epileptogenicity of the structure itself (26).

Although there is no controversy about the present role of NE in modulation of paroxysmal discharges in the kindling phenomenon, the existence of a specific functional lesion of monoaminergic systems in this model is far from being established. Tyrosine hydroxylase activity is permanently decreased at the amygdaloid stimulation site (34). Engel and Sharpless (33) noted NE and DA decrease in amygdala, but only DA levels were significantly different from

---

* Editors' note: Except perhaps in the spike wave producing tottering mice (see Chapter 4) where an increased number of NE terminals have been demonstrated.

electrode-implanted (nonstimulated) sham animals. However, Callaghan and Schwark (16) found that NE and not DA concentrations are decreased in both limbic lobes, in hippocampus, frontal cortex, and mesencephalon. On the other hand, McIntyre-Burnham et al. (76), measuring levels of NE, DA, and 3,4-dihydroxyphenylacetic acid (DOPAC) in extrafocal sites, observed an increase of both NE and DA (and not DOPAC) in hypothalamus. Stock et al. (107) were unable to demonstrate any modification of NE, DA, and DOPAC in amygdala, hippocampus, hypothalamus, brainstem, neostriatum, and neocortex.

Recent studies have provided further data on noradrenergic alterations in kindling. Three weeks after kindling completion, NE and DA release is unchanged (51). At the same time, there is a down regulation of β-adrenoceptors as measured by a reduction in the number of β-binding sites (75). The same result was found by McNamara 3 days after kindling completion (77). These β-adrenoceptor alterations seem to be selective, since there is no modification of other neurotransmitter receptor binding sites (4). The kindling effect is probably not related to presynaptic noradrenergic disturbances, but rather to a long-term β-adrenoceptor hyposensitivity.

Hypothetically then, if an abnormal paroxysmal discharge occurs in an intact brain, the forebrain NE mechanisms may prevent its spread and avoid generalization. However, if the discharge recurs periodically, a permanent change may be induced in brain response, resulting in a lower threshold for generalization, and at least partially consisting of a β-adrenoceptor down regulation. However, since the seizure itself is able to provoke an increased NE turnover (55,65) with decreased β-adrenoceptor binding (9,106), and hyposensitivity to ionophoretic catecholamine application (105), it is not definitely known whether this down regulation is the cause of hyperexcitability or a consequence of it (even if experiments are done three weeks after the last seizure).

Chronic Cobalt Focus: Limiting Action of Noradrenergic Cortical Projections

We studied the biochemical, histological, and physiological parameters of the cerebral cortical noradrenergic projections in the chronic cobalt focus of rats because of the reliability of correlations between electrical and clinical events. In addition, the limited duration of epilepsy allowed us to follow the entire evolution of epileptogenic discharges. Finally, the cortical le-

sion caused by cobalt (112) allowed us to correlate structural and functional abnormalities in specific neurotransmitter systems.

Dow et al. (31) were the first to describe the epileptogenic action of cobalt powder. Our technique consists in depositing a very small quantity of metallic cobalt (0.5 mg) onto the sensorimotor cortex. According to electrocorticographic and clinical signs, four stages of cobalt focus development are delineated: stage 1—before any clinical or electrical epileptic manifestations are present; stage 2—when maximal EEG spikes are associated with myoclonic jerks of the contralateral forelimb; stage 3—when steadily firing EEG spikes appear without clinical signs; and stage 4—when progressive extinction of the epileptic syndrome occurs. The total duration rarely exceeds 30 days.

There was no significant change in focal NE content at stage 1; it then dropped to nearly 60% of the control values at stage 2 and stage 3; afterwards, it was slowly restored at stage 4. No significant alteration was observed in the contralateral homotopic cortex (102,114). These results corroborate those of Clayton and Emson who measured tyrosine hydroxylase activity during evolution of a cobalt focus (23).

We also studied the structural variations of noradrenergic fibers as epileptic activities evolved in the cobalt focus. We used the glyoxylic acid histofluorescence method (8,63). The fluorescence pictures in the perifocal area (cortical region surrounding the cobalt deposit and outside the cobalt necrosis) might be summarized as follows. At stage 1, the density of NE-containing terminals appeared to have diminished; remaining fibers appeared normal or were distorted with swollen varicosities. At stage 2, the decrease in the NE-containing terminal density was maximal and was more evident in the molecular layer when compared with the normal noradrenergic innervation of the first layer. At stage 3, the NE-containing terminal density was further reduced. At stage 4, new noradrenergic fibers had sprouted and invaded the perifocal area. These fibers appeared to be more delicate than normal ones and more numerous. They were randomly distributed and were not oriented parallel to the pial surface as is typical in the molecular layer. These histochemical data indicated that local destruction of NE-containing terminals preceded the onset of epileptic seizures; maximal destruction of NE terminals occurred when epilepsy developed. Regeneration of these NE fibers coincided with arrest of paroxysmal discharges (82,83,113).

We also measured the biochemical indices of noradrenergic terminal density by assaying NE high-affinity uptake in crude synaptosomal preparations, prepared from the perifocal area. At stage 1, NE uptake was unchanged; at stage 2, it was decreased by 50%; it remained at low values, then progressively increased in the course of stage 3; it had returned to normal values at the end of the syndrome. Uptake kinetics analysis showed a diminution of V_{max} (i.e., a reduction in number of uptake sites) without a change of K_m (affinity). The 3,4-dihydroxyphenylglycol (DOPEG)-NE concentration ratio (NE turn-over index) did not vary, whatever the stage of evolution. The concomitant occurrence of decreased cortical noradrenergic projections and of a partial epilepsy does not necessarily imply that they are causally related. In addition to fiber degeneration, cobalt is responsible for some neuronal loss (35). If the area of fiber destruction and of neuronal loss were overlapping, it could be assumed that noradrenergic deafferentation would have a limited effect upon neuronal excitability. To solve this question, microionophoretic studies of cortical neurons situated in the perilesional area were performed to detect changes in neuronal adrenoceptor sensitivity during the development of the cobalt focus.

The results show that cobalt application and/or subsequent induced epilepsy lead to an alteration of NE receptor sensitivity in the cortex. This alteration varies according to the stage of development of the focus. It evolves from a hyposensitivity state before the beginning of epilepsy (stage 1) to a supersensitivity when epilepsy fully develops (stage 2). NE receptors reverse to a subsensitive state when paroxysmal events decrease and vanish (stages 3 and 4).

Supersensitivity to NE during stage 2 can be interpreted as a "denervation supersensitivity" (19,89). Indeed in other experimental conditions in which noradrenergic fibers were destroyed (LC lesion, 6-OHDA injections), supersensitivity of postsynaptic cortical neurons to ionophoretically applied NE was demonstrated (119). However, NE receptor sensitivity decreased in stage 3 although NE-containing terminals had not yet sprouted, possibly because of postsynaptic adaptation mechanisms linked with the epileptic activity itself. Different models of convulsive seizures are known to provoke postsynaptic hyposensitivity as measured by a decreased number of β-adrenoceptor binding sites (9,77). The identity of β-adrenoceptor binding sites and of ionophoretically activated NE receptors have not been fully demonstrated.

We also performed binding studies of α-adrenoceptors (^{3}H-Prazosin, ^{3}H-clonidine) and β-ad-

renoreceptors ([^{3}H]Dihydroalprenolol) in the cortex surrounding the cobalt deposit. There is no modification of α-adrenoceptor binding throughout the evolution of epileptic paroxysm. In constrast, a reversible modulation of the number of β-receptor sites is observed. At stage 2, it is increased by >50% in the epileptogenic cortex as well as in the contralateral cortex; afterwards, it is decreased to normal values at stage 3. These results indicate a selective and reversible modulation (in the sense of up regulation) of β-adrenoceptors that is closely correlated with the evolution of epilepsy and of noradrenergic denervation. Changes of affinity and density of β-adrenoceptors support the results of previous ionophoretic studies. They confirm that the inhibitory effect of ionophoretically applied NE in the cortex is probably mediated by β-adrenoceptor activation.

On the other hand, it is tempting to compare the change of β-receptor binding (from the period of maximal seizure activity to that of epilepsy extinction in the cobalt focus model) to the down regulation that occurs after kindling completion (75). If both sets of data depend on the same underlying phenomenon, this down regulation would represent a secondary rather than a primary determining factor of a convulsive state (13,14).

The data concerning neuronal adrenoceptors in cobalt foci support the idea that the NE fiber destruction and subsequent regeneration influence cortical neurons involved in epileptogenesis. As yet there is no clear proof that the deficit of NE transmission in the cortex specifically causes seizures in the cobalt focus. However, we can propose the hypothesis that cortical NE system limits the spread of chronic epileptogenic activities.

If that is the case, a prior suppression of the noradrenergic input to the cortex would modify the electrical and/or clinical features of the focus. An electrolytic lesion of the LC ipsilateral to the motor focus produces an exacerbation of the paroxysmal activity in all its characteristics: reduced latency of spiking, increased intensity, duration of partial seizures (stage 2), and longer duration of stage 3. Therefore, it produces a prolonged duration of the overall epileptic syndrome. If the LC lesion is contralateral to the focus, a marked development of a spiking mirror focus occurs in the contralateral homotopic cortex, whereas it is rarely observed in the control experiments (17,50). If the lesion is bilateral (bilateral LC lesion, 6-OHDA intraperitoneally injected in newborn animals), in addition to the previous modifications, a marked prolongation of paroxysmal events is especially noted.

In order to obtain a confirmation of the previous hypothesis, we sought to reverse these phenomena by artificially recovering NE content in the epileptogenic cortex. A perfusion inside the CNS of a NE-containing solution with a mini-osmotic pump able to ensure a constant flow (52) for a period of 2 weeks was used. The perfusion catheter was placed in the lateral ventricle of rats with a cobalt focus, associated or not with an ipsilateral or contralateral lesion of the LC (13,53).

In animals with a cobalt focus, ipsilateral perfusion induces a decrease of the epileptogenic focal activity (frequency of spiking as well as motor signs), but there is no significant effect on the latency of focal spike appearance. In animals with an ipsilateral lesion of the LC, the NE perfusion does not modify the electrical and clinical evolution of the cobalt focus. On the contrary, if NE is perfused on the same side as the contralateral LC lesion, there is a nearly suppressing effect on the secondary focus.

Consequently, these data clarified the role of the cortical noradrenergic system. It is less involved in the onset of the focal epileptic syndrome than in restriction of its development. Alterations of this system potentiate the spread of paroxysmal activities from the primary focus, whereas its regenerative properties contribute to limit or even to stop their evolution (18).

EVIDENCE AGAINST THE CONCEPT OF A COMMON OR UNIVERSAL DEFECT IN NORADRENERGIC TRANSMISSION IN EXPERIMENTAL EPILEPSIES

From the analysis of the previous models of partial epilepsies, a general concept of the role of noradrenergic mechanisms in epilepsy could emerge. Roughly applying this concept to the understanding of generalized epilepsies would risk paradoxical statements. In the case of DBA/2J mice, it would be reasonable to attribute their temporary seizure susceptibility to an abnormal ontogenesis of monoaminergic systems. As noted above, maximal susceptibility (at 21 days of postnatal age) would correspond to an immature organization of these systems; the progressive recovery from epilepsy would correspond to the limiting effect of the developing aminergic systems (54,104). If this is a valid hypothesis, one would expect that increased availability of NE at synapses would limit seizure intensity. In fact, α_2-adrenoceptor antagonist yohimbine administration has no effect, whereas α_2-adrenoceptor agonist clonidine protects mice against audiogenic seizures. Moreover, the anticonvulsant effect of clonidine is reversed by yohimbine

(44,54). In light of the previous hypothesis, these results are unexpected, since clonidine is supposed to decrease noradrenergic transmission (provided that α_2-receptors are only presynaptically localized in CNS) (60).

Quaking mice, a mutant of the C57BL/6J strain, exhibit tonic as well as audiogenic seizures (6,18). Pharmacological experiments have shown that seizures could be inhibited by yohimbine; this protective effect was selectively reversed by clonidine (21). This apparent discrepancy between the studies might indicate that the presynaptic or postsynaptic adrenoceptors are abnormally distributed in DBA/2J mice. Indeed in quaking mice, as in control animals, clonidine delays the FLA 63-induced disappearance of NE, and yohimbine increases the rate of utilization of NE. This suggests a normal distribution and functioning of adrenoceptors in quaking mouse (69). Because pharmacological studies of this mutant mouse have clearly shown a selective involvement of noradrenergic mechanisms (especially α-adrenoceptors) (21), a search for a basic alteration of these mechanisms was undertaken. An increase of NE content and electrically induced [^{3}H]NE release was observed in the brainstem (69).

Furthermore, a study of the mutant mouse tottering demonstrated a coexistence of a convulsive disorder (focal motor and absence seizures) with an increased number of noradrenergic axons in remote areas innervated by the LC, associated with a marked elevation of NE content (100–200% increase) (62). This peculiar observation remains unique. It is important to remember that the noradrenergic dysfunction underlying epileptogenesis may be expressed as a hyperinnervation as well as a hypoinnervation.

PATHOPHYSIOLOGICAL HYPOTHESIS OF A NORADRENERGIC DYSFUNCTION: EXCITATION/INHIBITION DUALITY, SYNCHRONIZATION, AND RESISTANCE TO EXTINCTION

Some explanations about the mode of action of NE in modulation of generalized or partial epilepsies could be derived from what is known about its synaptic mechanisms. There is general agreement that ionophoretic application of NE depresses spontaneous neuronal discharges in many central structures (particularly the cerebral cortex and cerebellum) (58,93). This inhibitory action is related to membrane hyperpolarization and increased resistance (42). It is reproduced by electrical stimulation of the LC and antagonized by β-adrenoceptor antagonists (29,90,94). However, it has been demonstrated that NE has clear-cut excitatory effects in other structures (particularly the brainstem) (111), as well as in those central structures in which inhibitory actions have been reported (101). It was first interpreted as a disinhibition through an inverting interneuronal path; however, it was proven that NE had opposite effects on the same neuron (10). Excitatory effects would be mediated by α-receptor activation and inhibitory ones would be mediated by β-receptor activation (110). Their differential distribution could account for the various types of action.

In light of these physiological data, it seems impossible to support any simplistic view (a lack of inhibition for instance) of a noradrenergic defect in epilepsies. This conclusion was predicted by the analysis of apparent paradoxical results in experimental models. It has recently been shown that, in hippocampal slices, the frequency of low-calcium–induced field bursts (depolarization shifts) of pyramidal cell populations is enhanced by bath-applied low concentrations of NE; this effect is mediated by β-receptor activation (41). It must be remembered that at higher concentrations, ionophoretic application of NE on the same cells is usually inhibitory. It is quite plausible that such drastic conditions (low extracellular calcium, reduced NE release) could be achieved in chronic epileptogenic foci at the time of maximal spiking. In the focal area, NE would reinforce the epileptogenic activity; however, other noradrenergic mechanisms [linked with the plastic properties of the catecholaminergic systems (11,108)], peripheral to the focus, could be simultaneously working, helping to circumscribe and then to reduce the extent of its activity. The subsequent increase of NE release (due to the regenerative process) could secondarily reverse the net effect of NE-mediated synaptic activation to a predominant overall inhibitory modulation.

In addition to the proper action of NE on postsynaptic neurons, interactions with other neurotransmitters must be considered. In cerebellum, afferent excitatory as well as inhibitory influences upon Purkinje cell discharge are enhanced by ionophoretic application of NE or by LC stimulation (36,43). In the same way, excitatory effect of glutamate and inhibitory effect of GABA are potentiated (79,80). If this modulatory role of the noradrenergic pathway is a general one, it would lead to an increased afferent signal to noise ratio in a given cerebral area (117). It is difficult to imagine which function is lost when this action is impaired in epilepsy. However, it may be that a decrease in the influence of external impinging inputs on the individual elements of a neuronal pool would result in enhanced synchrony of discharges between them, a major factor of epileptogenesis.

Finally, the most common feature of the noradrenergic system alteration, especially apparent in partial epilepsies, is the resistance of paroxysmal activities to extinction. Psychophysiological studies showing that selective NE depletion causes resistance to extinction of previously learned responses must be emphasized. In a large number of different behavioral tests, such lesioned animals continue to respond even in nonreward situations. It is interpreted as the inability "to filter out or to learn to ignore irrelevant stimuli" (68). Indeed, a general function of the central noradrenergic systems would be to delete long-lasting traces of abnormal neuronal discharges. Ontogenetic or acquired dysfunctions of these systems would result in the so-called predisposition to epilepsy.

REFERENCES

1. Altman, I. M., and Corcoran, M. E. (1983): Facilitation of neocortical kindling by depletion of forebrain noradrenaline. *Brain Res.,* 270:174–177.
2. Araki, H., Aihara, H., Watanabe, S., Chta, H., Yamamoto, T., and Euki, S. (1983): The role of noradrenergic and serotonergic systems in the hippocampal kindling effect. *Jpn. J. Pharmacol.,* 33:57–64.
3. Arnold, P. S., Racine, R. J., and Wise, R. S. (1973): Effects of atropine, reserpine, 6-hydroxydopamine and handling on seizure development in the rat. *Exp. Neurol.,* 40:457–570.
4. Ashton, D., Leysen, J. E., and Wauquier, A. (1980): Neurotransmitters and receptor binding in amygdaloid kindled rats: Serotonergic and noradrenergic modulatory effects. *Life Sci.,* 27:1547–1556.
5. Barbeau, A., and McDowell, F. H., editors (1970): *L-DOPA and Parkinsonism.* F. A. Davis, Philadelphia.
6. Baumann, N., Maurin, Y., Puech, A., Chauvel, P. and Simon, P. (1980): Approche biochimique et pharmacologique des troubles fonctionnels observes chez des mutants dysmyeliniques (systemes gabaergique et noradrenergique). *C.R. Soc. Biol.,* 174:437–445.
7. Berger, B., Tassin, J. P., Blanc, G., Moyne, M. A., and Thierry, A. M. (1974): Histochemical confirmation for dopaminergic innervation of the rat cerebral cortex after destruction of the noradrenergic pathway. *Brain Res.,* 81:332–337.
8. Berger, B., and Glowinski, J. (1978): Dopamine uptake in the serotoninergic terminals in vitro: A valuable tool for histochemical differentiation of catecholaminergic and serotoninergic terminals in rat cerebral structures. *Brain Res.,* 147:29–45.

9. Bergstrom, D. A., and Kellar, K. J. (1979): Effect of electroconvulsive shock on monoaminergic receptor binding sites in rat brain. *Nature,* 278:464–466.

10. Bevan, P., Bradshaw, C. M., Roberts, M. H. T., and Szabadi, E. (1973): The excitation of neurons by noradrenaline. *J. Pharm. Pharmacol.,* 25:309–314.

11. Björklund, A., and Stenevi, U. (1979): Regeneration of monoaminergic and cholinergic neurons in the mammalian central nervous system. *Physiol. Rev.,* 59:62–100.

12. Bourn, W. M., Chin, L., and Picchioni, A. L. (1977): Effect of neonatal 6-hydroxydopamine treatment on audiogenic seizures. *Life Sci.,* 21, 5:701–705.

13. Bregman, B., Dedek, J., Nassif, S., Trottier, S., and Chauvel, P. (1983): Noradrenergic mechanisms control propagation of chronic cobalt focus activities in the rat. In: *Cerebral Blood Flow, Metabolism and Epilepsy,* edited by M. Baldy-Moulinier, D. H. Ingvar, and B. S. Meldrum, pp. 351–356. John Libbey Eurotext, London.

14. Bregman, B., Le Saux, F., Trottier, S., Chauvel, P., and Maurin, Y. (1985): Chronic cobalt-induced epilepsy: Noradrenaline ionophoresis and adrenoceptor binding studies in the rat cerebral cortex. *J. Neural Transm.,* 63:109–118.

15. Bregman, B., Chauvel, P., and Maurin, Y. (1985): Modulation of cortical β-adrenoceptor binding sites during the evolution of a chronic cobalt-induced epilepsy in the rat. *J. Neurochem. (submitted for publication).*

16. Callaghan, D. A., and Schwark, W. S. (1979): Involvement of catecholamines in kindled amygdaloid convulsions in the rats. *Neuropharmacology,* 18:541–545.

17. Chauvel, P., Boucher, R., and Poirier, L. J. (1977): Exacerbation of cobalt focus by lesions of catecholaminergic systems. *Electroencephalogr. Clin. Neurophysiol.,* 43:563.

18. Chauvel, P., Louvel, J., Kurcewicz, I., and Debono, M. (1980): Epileptic seizures of the quaking mouse: Electroclinical correlations. In: *Neurological Mutations Affecting Myelination,* edited by N. Baumann, pp. 513–516. Elsevier/North-Holland, Amsterdam.

19. Chauvel, P., Trottier, S., Nassif, S., and Bregman, B. (1982): Alterations of cortical noradrenergic mechanisms in cobalt foci. In: *Advances in Epileptology: XIIIth Epilepsy International Symposium,* edited by H. Akimoto, H. Kazamatsuri, M. Seino, and A. Ward, pp. 531–535. Raven Press, New York.

20. Chauvel, P., Trottier, S., Nassif, S., and Dedek, J. (1982): Une alteration des afferences noradrenergiques est-elle en cause dans les epilepsies focales? *Rev. E.E.G. Neurophysiol.,* 12:1–7.

21. Chermat, R., Doare, L., Lachapelle, F., and Simon, P. (1981): Effects of drugs affecting the noradrenergic system on convulsions in the quaking mouse. *Naunyn Schmiedebergs Arch. Pharmacol.,* 318:94–99.

22. Chimote, K. V., and Moghe, P. S. (1977): Putative neurotransmitters in central nervous system and chemoconvulsions. *Arch. Inst. Pharmacodyn. Ther.,* 228:304–313.

23. Clayton, P. R., and Emson, P. C. (1975): Changes in monoamines related enzymes in cobalt-induced epilepsy. *Biochem. Soc. Trans.,* 3:261–263.

24. Consroe, P., Picchioni, A., and Chin, L. (1979): Audiogenic seizure susceptible rats. *Fed. Proc.,* 38:2411–2416.

25. Corcoran, M. E., Fibiger, H. C., McCaughran Jr., J. A., and Wada, J. A. (1974): Potentiation of amygdaloid kindling and Metrazol-induced seizures by 6-hydroxydopamine in rats. *Exp. Neurol.,* 45:118–133.

26. Corcoran, M. E., and Mason, S. T. (1980): Role of forebrain catecholamines in amygdaloid kindling. *Brain Res.,* 190:473–484.

27. Descarries, L., and Lapierre, Y. (1973): Noradrenergic axon terminals in the cerebral cortex of rat. I. Radioautographic vizualisation after topical application of DL-(^{3}H) norepinephrine. *Brain Res.,* 51:141–160.

28. Descarries, L., Watkins, K. C., and Lapierre, Y. (1977): Noradrenergic axon terminals in the cerebral cortex of rat. III. Topometric ultrastructural analysis. *Brain Res.,* 133:197–222.

29. Dillier, N., Lazlo, J., Muller, B., Koela, W. P., and Olpe H. R. (1978): Activation of an inhibitory noradrenergic pathway projecting from the locus coeruleus to the cingulate cortex of the rat. *Brain Res.,* 154:61–68.

30. Dooley, D. J., Bittiger, H., Hauser, K. L., Bishoff, S. F., and Waldmeier, P. C. (1983): Alteration of central alpha- and beta-adrenergic receptors in the rat after DSP-4, a selective noradrenergic neurotoxin. *Neuroscience,* 9:889–898.

31. Dow, R. S., Fernandez-Guardiola, A., and Manni, E. (1962): The production of cobalt experimental epilepsy in the rat. *Electroencephalogr. Clin. Neurophysiol.,* 14:399–407.

32. Emson, P. C., and Lindvall, O. (1979): Distribution of putative neurotransmitters in the neocortex. *Neuroscience,* 4:1–30.

33. Engel, J. J., and Sharpless, N. S. (1977): Long-lasting dopamine depletion in the rat amygdala induced by kindling stimulation. *Brain Res.,* 136:381–386.

34. Farjo, I. B., and Blackwood, D. H. R. (1978): Reduction in tyrosine hydroxylase activity in the rat amygdala induced by kindling stimulation. *Brain Res.,* 153:423–426.

35. Fischer, J., Holubar, J., and Malik, E. (1967): The production of cobalt experimental epilepsy in the rat. *Electroencephalogr. Clin. Neurophysiol.,* 14:399–407.

36. Freedman, R., Hoffer, B. J., Woodward, D. J., and Puro, D. (1977): A functional role for the adrenergic input to the cerebellar cortex: Interaction of norepinephrine with activity evoked by mossy and climbing fibers. *Exp. Neurol.,* 55:269–288.

37. Fuxe, K., Hamberger, B., and Hokfelt, T. (1968): Distribution of noradrenaline nerve terminals in cortical areas of the rat. *Brain Res.,* 8:125–131.

38. Fuxe, K., Hokfelt, T., Johansson, D., Lidbrink, P., and Ljungdahl, A. (1974): The origin of the dopamine nerve terminals in limbic and frontal cortex. Evidence for meso-cortical dopamine neurons. *Brain Res.*, 82:349–355.

39. Glowinski, J., Axelrod, J., and Iversen, L. I. (1966): Regional studies of catecholamines in the rat brain. IV. Effects of drugs on the disposition and metabolism of H-norepinephrine and H-dopamine. *J. Pharmacol. Exp. Ther.*, 153:30–41.

40. Goddard, G. V., McIntyre, D., and Leech, C. K. (1969): A permanent change in brain function resulting from daily electrical stimulation. *Exp. Neurol.*, 25:295–330.

41. Haas, H. L., Jefferys, J. G. R., Slater, N. T., and Carpenter, D. O. (1984): Modulation of low calcium induced field bursts in the hippocampus by monoamines and cholinomimetics. *Pflugers Arch.*, 400:28–33.

42. Heinemann, U., Lux, H. D., and Zander, K. J. (1978): Effects of norepinephrine and DB-c-AMP on active uptake of K in the cerebral cortex of cats. In: *Ionophoresis and Transmitter Mechanisms in the Mammalian Central Nervous System*, edited by R. W. Ryall and J. S. Kelly, pp. 419–428. Elsevier North Holland, Amsterdam.

43. Hoffer, B. J., Siggins, G. R., Oliver, A. P., and Bloom, F. E. (1973): Activation of the pathway from the locus coeruleus to rat cerebellar Purkinje neurons: Pharmacological evidence of noradrenergic central inhibition. *J. Pharmacol. Exp. Ther.*, 184:553–569.

44. Horton, R., Anlezark, G., and Meldrum, B. (1980): Noradrenergic influences on sound-induced seizures. *J. Pharmacol. Exp. Ther.*, 214:437–442.

45. Jobe, P. C., Picchioni, A. L., and Chin, L. (1973): Role of brain norepinephrine in audiogenic seizures in the rat. *J. Pharmacol. Exp. Ther.*, 184:1–10.

46. Jobe, P. C., and Laird, H. E. (1981): Neurotransmitter abnormalities as determinants of seizure susceptibility and intensity in the genetic models of epilepsy. *Biochem. Pharmacol.*, 30:3137–3144.

47. Jobe, P. C., Brown, R. D., and Dailey, J. W. (1981): Effect of Ro 4-1284 on audiogenic seizure susceptibility and intensity in epilepsy-prone rats. *Life Sci.*, 28:2031–2038.

48. Jobe, P. C., Laird, H. E., Ko, K. H., Ray, T., and Dailey, J. W. (1982): Abnormalities in monoamine levels in the central nervous system of the genetically epilepsy-prone rat. *Epilepsia*, 23:359–366.

49. Jones, B., and Moore, R. Y. (1977): Ascending projections of the locus coeruleus in the rat. II. An autoradiographic study. *Brain Res.*, 127:23–53.

50. Kafiluddin, E. A., Trottier, S., and Chauvel, P. (1978): Increased focal epileptic activity in rats after lesions of the locus coeruleus. *Neurosci. Lett.* 1 (*Suppl.*):64.

51. Kant, G. J., Meyerhoff, J. L., and Corcoran, M. E. (1980): Release of norepinephrine and do-pamine from brain regions of amygdaloid-kindled rats. *Exp. Neurol.*, 70:701–705.

52. Kasamatsu, T., Pettigrew, J. D., and Ary, M. (1979): Restoration of visual cortical plasticity by local microperfusion of norepinephrine. *J. Comp. Neurol.*, 185:163–182.

53. Kasamatsu, T., Pettigrew, J. D., and Ary, M. (1981): Cortical recovery from effects of monocular deprivation. Acceleration with norepinephrine and suppression with 6-hydroxydopamine. *J. Neurophysiol.*, 45:254–266.

54. Kellog, C. (1976): Audiogenic seizures: Relation to age and mechanisms of monoamine neurotransmission. *Brain Res.*, 106:87–103.

55. Kety, S. S., Javoy, F., Thierry, A. M., Julou, L., and Glowinski, J. (1967): A sustained effect of electroconvulsive shock on the turn-over of norepinephrine in the central nervous system of the rat. *Proc. Natl. Acad. Sci. (Wash)*, 58:1249–1254.

56. Killian, M., and Frey, H. H. (1973): Central monoamines and convulsive thresholds in mice and rats. *Neuropharmacology*, 12:681–692.

57. Ko, K. H., Dailey, J. W., and Jobe, P. C. (1982): Effect of increments in norepinephrine concentrations on seizure intensity in the genetically epilepsy-prone rat. *J. Pharmacol. Exp. Ther.*, 222:662–669.

58. Krnjevic, K., and Phillis, J. W. (1963): Iontophoretic studies of neurons in the mammalian cerebral cortex. *J. Physiol.*, 165:274–304.

59. Krnjevic, K. (1974): Chemical nature of synaptic transmission in vertebrates. *Physiol. Rev.*, 54:418–540.

60. Langer, S. Z. (1977): Presynaptic receptors and their role in the regulation of transmitter release. *Br. J. Pharmacol.*, 60:481–497.

61. Lapierre, Y., Beaudet, A., Demianczuk, N., and Descarries, L. (1973): Noradrenergic axon terminals in the cerebral cortex. II. Quantitative data revealed by light and electron microscopic radioautography of the frontal cortex. *Brain Res.*, 63:175–182.

62. Levitt, P., and Noebels, J. L. (1981): Mutant mouse tottering: Selective increase of locus ceruleus axons in a defined single-locus mutation. *Proc. Natl. Acad. Sci. USA*, 78:4630–4634.

63. Lindvall, O., Björklund, A., Hokfelt, T., and Ljungdahl, A. (1973): Application of the glyoxylic acid method to vibratome sections for improved visualization of central catecholamine neurons. *Histochemie*, 35:31–38.

64. London, E. D., and Buterbaugh, G. G. (1978): Modification of electroshock convulsive responses and thresholds in neonatal rats after brain monoamine reduction. *J. Pharmacol. Exp. Ther.*, 206:81–90.

65. Masserano, J. M., Takimoto, G. S., and Weiner, N. (1981): Electroconvulsive shock increases tyrosine hydroxylase activity in the brain and adrenal gland of the rat. *Science*, 214:662–664.

66. Mason, S. T., and Corcoran, M. E. (1978): Forebrain noradrenaline and metrazol-induced seizures. *Life Sci.*, 23:167–172.

67. Mason, S. T., and Corcoran, M. E. (1979): Cat-

echolamines and convulsions. *Brain Res.,* 170:497–507.

68. Mason, S. T., and Iversen, S. D. (1979): Theories of the dorsal bundle extinction effect. *Brain Res. Rev.,* 1:107–137.

69. Maurin, Y., Arbilla, S., Dedek, J., Lee, C. R., Baumann, S., and Langer, S. Z. (1982): Noradrenergic neurotransmission in the brain of a convulsive mutant mouse: Differences between the cerebral cortex and the brain stem. *Naunyn Schmiedeberg Arch. Pharmacol.,* 320:26–33.

70. Maynert, E. W., Marczynski, T. J., and Browning, R. A. (1975): The role of the neurotransmitters in the epilepsies. In: *Advances in Neurology,* edited by W. J. Friedlander, pp. 79–147. Raven Press, New York.

71. McIntyre, D. C., Saari, M., and Pappas, B. A. (1979): Potentiation of amygdala kindling in adult or infant rats by injections of 6-Hydroxydopamine. *Exp. Neurol.,* 63:527–544.

72. McIntyre, D. C., and Edson, N. (1981): Facilitation of amygdala kindling after norepinephrine depletion with 6-hydroxydopamine in rats. *Exp. Neurol.,* 74:748–757.

73. McIntyre, D. C., Edson, N., Chao, G., and Knowles, V. (1982): Differential effect of acute vs chronic desmethylimipramine on the rate of amygdala kindling in rats. *Exp. Neurol.,* 78:158–166.

74. McIntyre, D. C., and Edson, N. (1982): Effect of norepinephrine depletion on dorsal hippocampus kindling in rats. *Exp. Neurol.,* 77:700–704.

75. McIntyre, D. C., and Roberts, D. C. S. (1983): Long-term reduction in beta-adrenergic receptor binding after amygdala kindling in rat. *Exp. Neurol.,* 82:17–24.

76. McIntyre Burnham, W., King, G. A., and Lloyd, K. G. (1981): Extra-focal catecholamine levels in "kindled" rat forebrains. *Prog. Neuropsychopharmacol.,* 5:537–541.

77. McNamara, J. O. (1978): Selective alterations of regional beta-adrenergic receptor binding in the kindling model of epilepsy. *Exp. Neurol.,* 61:582–591.

78. Meyer, S. E. (1980): Neurohumoral transmission and the autonomic nervous system. In: *The Pharmacological Basis of Therapeutics,* edited by A. Goodman Gilman, L. S. Goodman, and A. Gilman, pp. 56–90, Macmillan, New York.

79. Moises, H. C., Woodward, D. J., and Hoffer, B. J. (1979): Interactions of norepinephrine with Purkinje cell responses to putative amino acid neurotransmitters applied by microiontophoresis. *Exp. Neurol.,* 64:493–515.

80. Moises, H. C., and Woodward, D. J. (1980): Potentiation of GABA inhibitory action in cerebellum by locus coeruleus stimulation. *Brain Res.,* 182:327–344.

81. Mohr, E., and Corcoran, M. E. (1981): Depletion of noradreline and amygdaloid kindling. *Exp. Neurol.,* 72:507–511.

82. Moore, R. Y. (1974): Central regeneration and recovery of function: The problem of collateral innervation. In: *Plasticity and Recovery of Function in CNS,* edited by D. G. Stein, J. J.

Rosen, and N. Butters, pp. 111–129. Academic Press, Orlando, Fla.

83. Moore, R. Y. (1974): Growth of adrenergic neurons in the adult mammalian nervous system. In: *Dynamics of Degeneration and Growth in Neurons,* edited by K. Fuxe, L. Olson, and Y. Zotterman, pp. 379–388, Pergamon, Oxford.

84. Moore, R. Y., and Bloom, F. E. (1979): Central catecholamine neuron systems: Anatomy and physiology of the dopamine systems. *Annu. Rev. Neurosci.,* 1:129–166.

85. Morgan, W. W., Pfeil, K. A., and Gonzales, E. G. (1977): Catecholamine concentration in discrete brain areas following the withdrawal of barbital dependent rats. *Life Sci.,* 20:493–499.

86. Morrison, J. H., Grzanna, R., Molliver, M. E., and Coyle, J. T. (1978): The distribution and orientation of noradrenergic fibers in the neocortex of the rat: An immunofluorescence study. *J. Comp. Neurol.,* 181:17–40.

87. Morrison, J. H., Molliver, M. E., and Grzanna, R. (1979): Noradrenergic innervation of cerebral cortex: Widespread effects of local cortical lesions. *Science,* 205:313–316.

88. Morrison, J. H., Molliver, M. E., Grzanna, R., and Coyle, J. T. (1981): The intracortical trajectory of the coeruleo-cortical projection of the rat: A tangentially organized cortical afferents. *Neuroscience,* 6:139–158.

89. Nassif, S., Bregman, B., Kurcewicz, I., Trottier, S., and Chauvel, P. Microionophoretic studies of the cortical NA system alterations in the rat cobalt focus. (*manuscript in preparation*).

90. Olpe, H. R., Glatt, A., Laszlo, J., and Schellenberg, A. (1980): Some electrophysiological and pharmacological properties of the cortical noradrenergic projection of the locus coeruleus in the rat brain. *Brain Res.,* 186:9–20.

91. Olschowka, J. A., Molliver, M. E., Grzanna, R., Rice, F. L., and Coyle, J. T. (1981): Ultrastructural demonstration of noradrenergic synapses in the rat central nervous system by dopamine-β-hydroxylase immunocytochemistry. *J. Histochem. Cytochem.,* 29:271–280.

92. Pfeifer, A. K., and Galambos, E. (1967): The effect of reserpine α-methyl-M-tyrosine, phenylamine and guanethidine on metrazol-convulsions and the brain monoamine level in mice. *Arch. Int. Pharmacodyn.,* 165:201–211.

93. Phillis, J. W. (1976): An involvement of calcium and Na-K-ATPase in the inhibitory actions of various compounds on central neurons. In: *Taurine,* edited by R. Huxtable and A. Barbeau, pp. 209–223. Raven Press, New York.

94. Phillis, J. W., and Kostopoulos, G. P. (1977): Activation of a noradrenergic pathway from the brain stem to rat cerebral cortex. *Gen. Pharmacol.,* 8:379–384.

95. Philo, R. and Reiter, R. J. (1978): Brain amines and convulsions in four strains of parathyroidectomized, pinealectomized rat. *Epilepsia,* 19:133–137.

96. Philo, R., and Reiter, R. J. (1981): The involvement of brain amines in pinealectomy-induced

convulsions in the gerbil: I. Serotonin. *Behav. Brain Res.*, 3:71–82.

97. Philo, R. (1982): Catecholamines and pinealectomy-induced convulsions in the gerbil (*Meriones unguiculotus*). *Prog. Clin. Biol. Res.*, 92:233–241.

98. Pickel, V. M., Segal, M., and Bloom, F. E. (1974): A radioautography study of the efferent pathway of the nucleus coeruleus. *J. Comp. Neurol.*, 155:15–42.

99. Purpura, D. P., Penry, J. K., Tower, D. B., Woodbury, D. M., and Walter, R. D., editors (1972): *Experimental Models of Epilepsy.* Raven Press, New York.

100. Reisine, T. (1981): Adaptative changes in catecholamine receptors in the central nervous system. *Neuroscience*, 6:1471–1502.

101. Roberts, M. H. T., and Straughan, D. W. (1968): Actions of noradrenaline and mescaline on cortical neurons. *Naunyn Schmeidbergs Arch. Pharmacol.*, 259:191–192.

102. Scatton, B., Dedek, J., Zivkovic, B., Liegeois, C., Trottier, S., Chauvel, P., and Bancaud, J. (1981): Alterations of catecholamines, serotonine, acetylcholine and cyclic nucleotides in brain regions after cobalt induced epilepsy in the rat: Influence of anticonvulsant treatment. In: *Neurotransmitters, Seizures and Epilepsy,* edited by P. Morselli, K. Lloyd, W. Loscher, and E. H. Reynolds, pp. 215–226. Raven Press, New York.

103. Schlesinger, K., and Boggan, W. (1965): Genetics of audiogenic seizures: I. Relation to brain serotonin and norepinephrine in mice. *Life Sci.*, 4:2345–2351.

104. Schlesinger, K., Boggan, W., and Freedman, D. X. (1968): Genetics of audiogenic seizures: II. Effects of pharmacological manipulation of brain serotonin, norepinephrine and gamma-aminobutyric acid. *Life Sci.*, 7:437–447.

105. Spehlmann, R., and Norcross, K. (1984): Decreased sensitivity of neurons in the basolateral amygdala to dopamine and noradrenaline iontophoresis after a kindling stimulus. *Exp. Neurol.*, 83:204–210.

106. Stanford, S. C., and Nutt, D. J. (1982): Comparison of the effects of repeated electroconvulsive shock on α 2- and β-adrenoceptors in different regions of rat brain. *Neuroscience*, 7:1753–1757.

107. Stock, G., Kummer, P., Stumpf, H., Zeener, K., and Sturm, V. (1983): Involvement of dopamine in amygdaloid kindling. *Exp. Neurol.*, 80:439–450.

108. Svendgaard, N. A., Bjorklund, A., and Stenevi, U. (1975): Regenerative properties of central monoamine neurons. *Adv. Anat. Embryol. Cell Biol.*, 51:1–77.

109. Swanson, L. W., and Harman, B. K. (1975): The central adrenergic system. An immunofluorescence study of the location of cell bodies and their efferent connections in the rat utilizing dopamine-β-hydroxylase as marker. *J. Comp. Neurol.*, 163:467–506.

110. Szabadi, E. (1979): Adrenoceptors on central neurons: Microelectrophoretic studies. *Neuropharmacology*, 18:831–843.

111. Tebecis, A. K., editor (1974): *Transmitters and Identified Neurons in the Mammalian Central Nervous System.* Scientechnica, Bristol.

112. Trottier, S., Truchet, M., and Laroudie, C. (1980): Secondary ion microanalysis in the study of cobalt-induced epilepsy in the rat. *Exp. Neurol.*, 76:231–245.

113. Trottier, S., Berger, B., Chauvel, P., Dedek, J., and Gay, M. (1981): Alterations of the cortical noradrenergic system in chronic cobalt epileptogenic foci in the rat: A histofluorescent and biochemical study. *Neuroscience*, 6:1069–1080.

114. Trottier, S., Claustre, Y., Caboche, J., Dedek, J., Chauvel, P., Nassif, S., and Scatton, B. (1983): Alterations of noradrenaline and serotonin uptake and metabolism in chronic cobalt-induced epilepsy in the rat. *Brain Res.*, 272:255–262.

115. Ungerstedt, U. (1971): Stereotaxic mapping of the monoamine pathways in the rat brain. *Acta Physiol. Scand.*, 367 (*Suppl.*):1–48.

116. Uretsky, N. J., and Iversen, L. L. (1970): Effects of 6-hydroxydopamine on catecholamine-containing neurons in the rat brain. *J. Neurochem.*, 17:269–278.

117. Waterhouse, D. J., Moises, H. C., and Woodward, D. J. (1980): Noradrenergic modulation of somatosensory cortical neuronal responses to ionophoretically applied putative neurotransmitters. *Exp. Neurol.*, 69:30–49.

118. Waterhouse, B. D., Lin, C. S., Burne, A., and Woodward, D. J. (1983): The distribution of neocortical projection neurons in the locus coeruleus. *J. Comp. Neurol.*, 217:418–431.

119. Yarbrough, G. C., and Phillis, J. W. (1975): Supersensitivity of central neurons. A brief review of an emerging concept. *Can. J. Neurol. Sci.*, 2:147–152.

Advances in Neurology, Vol. 44, edited by
A. V. Delgado-Escueta, A. A. Ward, Jr.,
D. M. Woodbury, and R. J. Porter.
Raven Press, New York © 1986.

25

Neuropeptides: Anticonvulsant and Convulsant Mechanisms in Epileptic Model Systems and in Humans

*‡Joseph G. Bajorek, **†Randall J. Lee, and **†Peter Lomax

*Departments of Neurology and **Pharmacology and †the Brain Research Institute, UCLA School of Medicine, and ‡Department of Neurology, Veterans Administration Hospital (Wadsworth), Los Angeles, CA 90024

SUMMARY Neuropeptides represent a new class of compounds with important implications for the understanding of the mechanisms and treatment of epileptic disorders. Several systems of peptide modulators—in particular the opioid-like peptides, vasopressin, somatostatin, thyrotropin-releasing hormone (TRH) and ACTH—have partially demonstrated endogenous roles in some forms of epilepsy. Seizures and stressful situations may release endogenous opioid peptides and mediate postictal depression and postictal seizure refractoriness. Vasopressin is believed to increase susceptibility to convulsions and may be involved in the pathogenesis of febrile convulsions. Derangements in TRH regulation may lower thresholds for seizure expression by regulating arousal systems; however, some TRH analogs have proven to be effective anticonvulsants. Long-term alterations in somatostatin regulation could be components of focal epilepsies. ACTH is particularly useful in the treatment of infantile spasms. Pharmacological effects of these and other peptides have potentials for defining new classes of anticonvulsants. Cholecystokinin (CCK) and its analogs, the opioid peptides β-endorphin and FK33824, TRH analogs, and several dipeptides exhibit potent anticonvulsant properties in chemical, electroshock, and genetic model screens. Convulsant actions of CRF, somatostatin, TRH, vasopressin, and high doses of endorphin or enkephalins may provide new tools to study regulatory mechanisms of cerebral excitability. The enkephalin epileptogenic effect is being developed as a predictive tool for new anti-petit mal anticonvulsants. Advances in molecular biology have identified the genes of particular peptide families. A concept has developed that the large propeptide precursors, coded by these genes, whose processing leads to functional peptide formation and release, regulate peptidergic humoral responses to external stimuli. This idea may have particular applications in the understanding of the genetic basis of some seizure states. Techniques for amplification of mRNA expression have identified specific neuronal proteins and peptides. Knowledge of protein and propeptide structural cleavage sites has suggested previously unknown candidates for modular systems in epileptic states. Technological advances in automated peptide sequencing and synthesis have allowed the development of metabolically resistant analogs and antagonist peptides. The anticonvulsant potencies of CCK, TRH, and opioid peptides have been defined more clearly with these methods. The mingling of these new technologies with traditional pharmacological and physiological methods in the comprehensive study of each peptide system is expected to advance the understanding of peptide regulation in many of the epilepsies.

The relationship of steroidal hormones to the pathophysiology of the epilepsies was studied in detail in the years prior to 1970. The focus was an outgrowth of interest in the function and mechanism of action of the newly synthesized steroid and thyroid hormones, in particular, the glucocorticoids, mineralocorticoids, gonadal steroids, and thyroid hormones. The possible role of these hormones in regulating epileptic excitability was expounded in the hypothesis, derived from clinical observations, that stressful events that mobilize hormonal release could act as precipitators of seizure states in particular forms of epilepsy. Studies on animal models of epilepsy and in human epilepsy established a modulatory role for the corticosteroids, gonadal steroids, and thyroid hormones. These studies are reviewed by Woodbury and Vernadakis (106). A more recent review emphasizes the role of the pituitary–thyroid axis (96). Understanding of the regulatory phenomena of pituitary release led to the isolation and characterization of peptidergic extrapituitary hormones and hypothalamic releasing factors. Sites of feedback and feedforward regulation in hypothalamic–pituitary–target axes were defined in the central nervous system (CNS). However, the pituitary peptides and hypothalamic peptides thus isolated were found to have additional effects. deWeid (17) determined that the hypophyseal hormone ADH or vasopressin could modulate memory consolidation, whereas Nemeroff et al. (72) established the effect of TRH as a profound antagonist of pentobarbital-induced sedation. In addition, Krivoy et al. (54) had already described transmitter-type and modulatory-type actions for substance P. These findings established the concept of specific complex roles for neuropeptides in behavioral physiology and the biochemistry of the nervous system. Techniques for immunochemical measurement of the peptides resulted in their localization over extensive areas of the CNS and peripheral nervous system (PNS) (53). In a similar manner, the availability of antibodies specific to small peptides from intestinal tissues or from the skin of amphibians permitted investigators to demonstrate their presence in the CNS. More than 100 peptides have been clearly identified in the CNS and more are being studied. It is now proposed that neurons may harbor multiple forms of modulators, transmitters, and messenger proteins, although there is considerable debate on this score (63). One outcome of increased complexity is the example presented by the endogenous opioid peptides. Since the discovery of the enkephalins in 1975 (42) they have been implicated indirectly in psychiatric disorders, the epilepsies, endogenous pain modulation, and stress responses (53). However, the mechanisms responsible for these effects are unclear and interactions with traditional transmitter systems, endocrine responses, and feedback circuitry have only recently been studied. Similarly, their relationship to the pathophysiology of the epilepsies has been superficially determined.

Our purpose is to identify peptidergic systems functionally related to the epilepsies and to suggest how the special techniques of different disciplines can be utilized to study the mechanisms that lead to changes in excitability. Three major concepts are discussed. First, endogenous peptides may be neuroregulators with inhibitory or stimulatory properties. The clearest evidence is seen in the opioid and the vasopressin peptides. Second, the posttranslational processing of propeptides into functional peptides may also play a large role in the regulation of excitability. This processing is tightly controlled and could lead to the production of varying amounts of peptide. Finally, identification and cloning of peptide genes has generated cDNA probes with which to test gene expression, methods for producing purified peptides in large quantities and knowledge about the structure and organization of peptide genes and their processing. Novel peptides have been identified as possible modulators by this approach. The direct application of techniques from molecular biology to the study of the epilepsies will occur in the near future.

ENDOGENOUS OPIOID-LIKE PEPTIDES

The most extensively documented role for a family of peptides in epileptic mechanisms concerns peptides related to the opiate alkaloids, based on shared affinity at similar receptor subtypes, and on similar pharmacological effects. Originally, these peptides were envisioned as possible endogenous convulsants, since intraventricular administration of large quantities of β-endorphin or Met-enkephalin or Leu-enkephalin (but not dynorphin) in rats resulted in electrographic discharges in the cortical electroencephalogram (EEG) (35,36,100). Behavioral motor convulsions were not associated with the electrographic activity in these rats, although wet dog shakes and catatonia were evident. Analysis of the discharges revealed that they originated primarily in the limbic system, especially from hippocampal pyramidal cells, an area that is susceptible to epileptogenic disorders. Because extracellular application of the opioid peptides on most neuronal elements is inhibitory, it was postulated that the mechanism of excitation specific to hippocampal areas was due to an action on inhibitory interneurons that modulate pyramidal cells (111). The resulting disinhibition increased pyramidal discharges. Direct effects on dendritic processes have also been described, leading to a current debate over the precise mechanism for these effects (18). β-Endorphin and Met-enkephalin and Leu-enkephalin have similar effects in these areas. Naloxone hydrochloride, a specific opioid antagonist active at μ- receptors, blocked most of the electrographic effects of the peptides and all of the behaviors indicating that these were specific receptor-mediated events with possible physiological relevance (35,100). However, the generalization of the effect to other species was not upheld, since in cats (26), baboons (67), and gerbils (3,6) different results were seen. Electrographic changes in cats were accompanied by motor disturbances (26). In the gerbil (6) and photosensitive baboon (67), genetic models of epilepsy, the primary effect, especially at doses that did not elicit toxic effects (catatonia, behavioral stereotypy), was anticonvulsant activity against natural seizures. In addition, when opioid peptides were evaluated against ongoing seizures in a chemical convulsant model (fluorothyl seizures) or electroshock (ECS) they suppressed rather than potentiated the seizures (7,97). Naloxone blocked the anticonvulsant effects in the gerbil, baboon, and fluorothyl models, suggesting a link to specific opioid receptors (6,67,97). Thus, the pharmacological profile of the opioid peptides in epileptic systems depends upon dose and species specificity. This complexity prevents the simple categorization of functional roles for these peptidergic systems.

Naloxone and naltrexone, a related opioid antagonist with prolonged activity, provided the means to test the hypothesis that epileptogenic or anticonvulsant effects of opioid peptides were integral components of endogenous epileptic mechanisms in model systems or of epilepsy in humans. Attempts to block endogenous opioid actions with these antagonists in models of epilepsy characterized by spontaneous seizures— such as the baboon or gerbil—failed (5,31,67). We interpret this as a lack of mediation by endogenous opioids of seizure initiation and spread. However, if natural seizures are induced in gerbils (5,57,62,95) or if seizures are induced in rats by ECS (78), or if kindled rats are seized (12,30,50), a reduced susceptibility to further seizures follows that can be partially blocked by

naloxone or naltrexone. This may indicate a release of naloxone-sensitive endogenous opioid-like peptides during the seizure that mediate postictal seizure inhibition. The inhibition may be specific for seizure state. In the gerbil model, natural seizures induced prior to testing shift the convulsant dose–response for seizures induced by pentylenetetrazole (PTZ) in a manner consistent with antiepileptic properties, an effect antagonized by naltrexone, whereas no effect was noted on maximal electroshock seizures (60). Release of enkephalins following massive seizures has been demonstrated (41) and supports the contention that the naloxone-sensitive postictal anticonvulsant effects of seizures may be mediated by endogenous opioids. Other treatments which may release endogenous opioids, such as restraint or injection stress, also produce naloxone-sensitive anticonvulsant actions (5). In a different type of experiment in which opioid withdrawal is modeled, withdrawal seizures were partially suppressed by injection of peptidase inhibitors, indicating an involvement of endogenous anticonvulsant peptidergic factors, possibly opioid-like, since opioids specifically inhibit many withdrawal signs (75). Postictal effects on electrographic discharges, possibly mediated by endogenous opioids, were demonstrated by Frenk et al. (30) following kindled seizures. Naloxone blocked postictal EEG inhibitory afterdischarges whereas morphine enhanced them. Direct evidence as to which endogenous opioid(s) are released by ictal or stressful events must await refinement of techniques for assaying these peptides. Mechanisms responsible for the postictal effects include a spreading depression induced by the release of endogenous opioids (90), or a γ-aminobutyric acid (GABA)-mediated inhibition induced by high levels of endogenous peptides (19,83,105). The inhibitory effect of opiates or opioid peptides applied to individual neuronal elements (28,105) may also result in general inhibition of seizure spread and development. In one genetic model system, the audiogenic mouse, naloxone was shown to exacerbate seizure severity, indicating a role for endogenous opioids in the processes mediating the convulsions (86).

Evidence for an endogenous role for opioid-like peptides in human epilepsy is derived from two studies which demonstrated the effects of naloxone administration to epileptic patients with intractable complex partial seizures. If an epileptogenic action of endorphins or enkephalins were part of the underlying mechanisms in partial complex seizures, naloxone administration should block the seizures. In one study, no effects were seen (69); in the other, no direct anticonvulsant effects of naloxone on the seizures occurred; paradoxically, some patients may have had components of their seizures enhanced (25). Further study of effects in humans are required.

Kindled seizures represent a unique model system in which the opioid peptides have been tested. In contrast to the effects of convulsant drugs or ECS, a permanent change in seizure susceptibility is expressed in this model, in which a genetic component is absent. However, contradictory evidence has emerged. No endogenous role in the development of kindling or in kindled seizures is evident in three studies (14,30,77) in which naloxone had no effect. In other studies, naloxone decreased the time for kindling and increased the severity of the seizures (34). Different groups have demonstrated that naloxone had anticonvulsant activity against kindled seizures and that opioids potentiate kindling (61,91). Multiple injections of β-endorphin kindled rats in site-specific areas of the amygdala and hippocampus (9). These animals exhibited motor convulsions and showed no tolerance to the peptide injections, suggesting that this may be a mediating mechanism for the kindling process. Permanent increases in dynorphin and enkephalins levels in amygdala following kindling indicate that they may have a role in maintainance of the condition (78,103). The interpretation of such studies requires further experiments to delineate these different and contradictory data. The implication that opioid peptides contribute to mechanisms that establish permanent changes in epileptic excitability is very important and requires that these experiments be replicated and their results verified.

Another aspect of the opioid peptides is their usefulness in the development of pharmacological tools to study epilepsy. Analogs of the peptides have been shown to possess anticonvulsant properties at several opioid receptor subtypes (16,29). Studies with opiate alkaloids in the gerbil have determined that μ, κ, and σ agonists are anticonvulsant, but that naloxone blocks only the effects at the μ- and κ-receptors (58). In fluorothyl seizures, a range of opioid agonists with μ and σ activity has anticonvulsant properties, whereas other receptor agonists are convulsants (15). The effects and interactions of the opiate alkaloids on seizures were reviewed recently (29). Antagonistic systems, in which μ-agonists are antiepileptic whereas δ-agonists are epileptic, are hypothesized. Opioid peptides may be a useful developmental tool since anticonvulsants specific for petit mal epilepsy are active in blocking the electrographic discharges seen in rats following administration of large doses of the peptides Met-enkephalin and Leu-enkephalin (87,88). This is proposed as a specific model system for developing new drugs against petit mal epilepsy (87). It may also have functional relevance, since anticonvulsant drugs decrease β-endorphin levels in the hypothalamus (66) and may reflect mechanisms in the action of these anticonvulsants.

Opioid peptide mechanisms in the epilepsies can be summarized to involve three areas of current and future study. First, the primary effect of low doses of exogenously administered peptides is an anticonvulsant action against induced seizures in various model systems. Higher doses may be convulsant through different mechanisms or by altered regulation of similar mechanisms. However, the high doses are associated with stereotypic and abnormal behaviors, possibly indicating nonspecific toxic effects. Second, the mediation of postictal depression and of seizure termination may be specific actions for the opioid peptides, particularly in the case of mechanisms for preventing status epilepticus. They do not appear to play a role in initiation or spread of seizures in most model systems. Kindling and audiogenic mouse models may be an exception, but current information about those effects is sparse and contradictory. Third, opioid peptide epileptogenic actions provide an apparent model for petit mal drug development.

Metabolically stable analogs may provide a new class of anticonvulsant agents against some seizure classes.

Thyrotropin-Releasing Hormone

Thyrotropin-releasing hormone (TRH), aside from its hypothalamic-pituitary action, is widely distributed in the CNS. A pharmacological property noted initially was the antagonism of barbiturate anesthesia and drowsiness (72). Iontophoretic application on CNS neurons was primarily excitatory. Species-specific behavioral effects are obtained if TRH is administered centrally or peripherally. Rats exhibit wet dog shakes (104). Gerbils exhibit stereotypic hindlimb foot stomping (5). Wild excitation and gyration is seen in fowl (74). The excitatory nature of these effects has led to the hypothesis that TRH is a component of a general arousal system. One hypothesis we entertain envisions TRH as an excitatory component of a group of peptides that up regulate or down regulate central excitability. In fact, effects of exogenous and endogenous opioids are counteracted by TRH (40) and, as discussed above, the opioid peptides seem to be an endogenous system that limits excitability.

Tested directly in epileptic model systems, TRH had no effect on ECS seizures, but did potentiate the anticonvulsant action of barbiturates, contrary to its antagonism of barbiturate sedation (73). In the gerbil, we found an increase in seizure severity following central administration of TRH; however, it was coupled with stereotypic foot stomping linked to behavioral excitation (5). Peripheral administration resulted in identical foot stomping behavior, but had no effect on any of the seizure parameters. The interpretation of these conflicting results awaits further experiments. Kindled rats exhibit an increase in TRH levels in amygdala, hippocampus, nucleus accumbens, and cortex 48 hr following their last seizure (68), indicating that the peptide may be involved in long-term modulation related to kindling maintenance. Multiple electroshock convulsions have similar long-term effects in elevating TRH levels in rats 48 hr following the last convulsion (56). A direct link to human epilepsy may exist. When TRH is used to assess thyroid function in patients with neurologic disorders, there are case reports of exacerbation of convulsive disorders (20,64). Two of four patients had seizures in one report (64).

However, a completely different hypothesis has been advanced (84) from studies in which anticonvulsive actions occurred against kindled seizures in cats administered TRH or a potent analog (DN-1417), with little TSH-releasing activity. The anticonvulsive effect is variable and transient, which is interpreted as evidence for mediation by, or interaction with, catecholaminergic systems. Clinical trials with DN-1417 have been attempted with partial success in Lennox syndrome (42). Further such studies may expose a new class of antiepileptic drugs specific for certain refractory epilepsies.

Arginine Vasopressin

In addition to its antidiuretic properties, the hypophyseal peptide, arginine vasopressin (AVP) has clear actions on CNS function. It induces resistance to extinction of passive avoidance behaviors (17). Early in the testing of AVP for behavioral effects, barrel rotation convulsions were observed, associated with electrographic epileptiform discharges (1,55). The convulsant action could be blocked by low doses of oxytocin or partially by β-MSH (1). In the seizure-sensitive gerbil, central vasopressin administration had no effects on the natural seizures, but peripheral administration effectively prevented convulsions (59). Whether this was mediated by the antidiuretic or by vasoconstrictive properties of the peptide is unknown. An AVP analog, vasotocin, has a similar antiepileptic effect on pentylenetetrazole (PTZ)-induced convulsions following peripheral administration (47).

A disorder in AVP regulation has been hypothesized as a mechanism underlying febrile convulsions (48,101). Vasopressin administered intraventricularly in low doses induced convulsions in rats. Multiple injections sensitized the animals to these convulsive effects (48,107). In addition, the convulsive threshold for febrile seizures in AVP-treated animals was significantly lower than in untreated animals. By taking advantage of the genetic lack of AVP in the Brattleboro rat strain, it was shown that these animals possess an increased threshold for febrile seizures as compared with normal controls. These results led to the postulate that AVP can modulate the responsiveness of an animal to febrile convulsions and that a defect in AVP processing may be part of the mechanism of febrile convulsions (48,101). Production of endogenous AVP release by hemorrhage or hypertonic saline treatment was effective in sensitizing rats to AVP-induced convulsions (8). This supports a possible role for endogenous AVP in epileptic states. Other evidence questions these results. Brattleboro rats kindled at slower rates, especially at stage 1 and 2 levels, than do control rats (33). Moreover, this group failed to duplicate the sensitization or kindling-like phenomena of multiple AVP injections (13,33). Further experiments will determine whether endogenous AVP plays a role in other models of epilepsy.

Somatostatin

Somatostatin was originally evaluated in behavioral paradigms in concert with AVP and oxytocin peptides. It has no effects on memory acquisition, but did produce stereotyped behaviors (55). The most interesting behavior was its induction of barrel rotation "convulsions" (12). Recent evidence indicates that levels of somatostatin increase in limbic cortex of rats following the development of fully kindled seizures (49). This effect appears to be permanent, lasting over a 2-month period following the last kindled seizure. The number and affinity of somatotropin inhibitory factor (SRIF) receptors remains the same in these areas, although there is a decrease in receptor number in the hippocampus of these kindled rats when there are no changes in SRIF content. Further support for an endogenous function for somatostatin in reducing seizure thresholds in kindled animals is the effectiveness of cystamine, which reduces somatostatin levels, in blocking kindled convulsions (39). In the same study, intraventricular administration of antibodies to SRIF likewise blocked kindled seizure induction. Similar protective effects of somatostatin antiserum were previously demonstrated against strychnine toxicity (11).

Interaction of the effects of somatostatin with opioid systems may also occur. Somatostatin injected intraventricularly blocks the development of electroshock-induced amnesia in rats (102). Release of endogenous opioid-like peptides following ECS is well known and may be the mechanism antagonized by somatostatin. Direct somatostatin injection also produces opioid-like actions that are antagonized by naloxone (79).

A theoretical construct for SRIF mechanisms in seizure initiation and spread is still far off, but there are indications that it may have a role in human disorders, since levels of SRIF are altered in psychiatric and epileptic states (52). A suggestion that this agent may be involved in the development of focal seizures has been proposed (24). This integrates well with the preliminary evidence from kindled animals, especially since kindling may be one of the better models of permanent focal epilepsy. The anatomical distribution of somatostatin pathways and the exact mechanisms of its seizure induction must be defined. It would help to test this agent in other epileptic model systems.

ACTH

Contributions by the hypothalamic–pituitary–adrenal axis to the development of epileptic disorders is well established (106). However, the extent of direct extrapituitary actions of ACTH or its analogs in relation to epilepsies is unknown. Related regulatory peptides such as corticotropin-releasing factor (CRF) are currently being investigated.

Original reports described ACTH therapy as a useful treatment for several seizure disorders (51). However, the subjects of those studies were young patients whose seizures were particularly amenable to ACTH regimens (51). Recent clinical trials have determined that infantile spasms should be treated preferentially with ACTH (44,81,87). The mechanism by which amelioration of these seizures occurs is currently incompletely defined (80).

Animal models of epilepsy respond to ACTH injection in varying ways. In the seizure-sensitive gerbil, ACTH and the fragment ACTH 4–10 administered intraventricularly had no effect except for a slight anticonvulsant and sedative action (4,5). In kindled rats, ACTH had some anticonvulsant properties (82). In general, when ACTH is administered to most species, no behavioral or electrographic alterations occur other than excessive grooming. One exception is a report of convulsant effects in rabbits following central injection of ACTH fragments 1–10, 4–10, and 4–9 (94).

A hypothalamic-releasing factor for ACTH has recently been isolated. Evaluation of its pharmacological profile following central administration uncovered a potent convulsant action (23). Four or more hours after central administration of CRF, rats underwent electrographic and behavioral seizures. Speculation about its mechanism of seizure induction centered on a kindling hypothesis (23). Considering the prolonged interval between administration and convulsions, it is unclear whether direct effects on excitability or effects mediated by ACTH, endorphins, or adrenal steroids are involved. CRF does excite hippocampal cells directly (2). It is more difficult to discover how feedback or feedforward regulation between hypothalamic, pituitary, adrenal, and CNS ACTH, CRF, and glucocorticoid receptor sites are affected by this treatment. These regulatory loops are difficult to study since interruption leads to compensatory effects. This area, and especially the function of CRF in other epileptic model systems, may be particularly productive in the future. Most genetic models of spontaneous seizures—such as the baboon, gerbil, audiogenic mouse and rat, or *el* mouse—seize following a severe stimulus, which may activate this system.

Other Neuropeptides

Preliminary reports (often mentioned in passing) on other neuropeptides indicate that an extensive number of compounds may have varying roles in seizure disorders.

CCK fragments and analogs possess potent anticonvulsant activity in several chemical convulsant models, including strychnine-, picrotoxin-, and harman-induced convulsions (108, 110). The mechanism does not appear to be related to benzodiazepine anticonvulsant actions, since the specificity differs from the anticonvulsant effects of diazepam, and the benzodiazepine antagonist RO-15-1788 does not block the CCK actions (109,110). Many analogs have been synthesized, and structure activity relationships have been determined (46). Only a specific fragment of CCK is responsible for the anticonvulsant action and may lead to the development of new anticonvulsant agents. The role of these endogenous peptides in seizure models has not been evaluated.

Two small dipeptides, which were synthesized to take advantage of the protective action of added amino groups, also have anticonvulsant effects. One group is active against audiogenic seizures in DBA2 mice by antagonizing aspartic acid receptors (45). The other is a dipeptide analog of GABA effective against PTZ seizures (32). It is tempting to speculate about the existence of similar endogenous peptides.

Screens for peptidergic compounds have shown anticonvulsant properties by LHRH, TRH, and MSH against audiogenic seizures (76). Fluorothyl seizures decrease the release of prolactin, LH, and FSH, whereas ECS increases prolactin release. The release of LHRH or prolactin may mediate many of the postictal disruptions seen following seizures, such as in reproductive function (27,38). These singular reports may identify many new important relationships between peptidergic systems and epileptic disorders; therefore, they must be confirmed and completed with further study.

APPROACHES FOR VERIFYING PEPTIDERGIC PARTICIPATION IN EPILEPTIC MECHANISMS

A common thread linking current studies of peptidergic function is the order in which experimental information is derived. Initial identification and isolation leads to the study of effects on behavioral and electroencephalographic variables after intraventricular, intracerebral, or systemic administration. Extracellular and intracellular recordings of effects on individual neuronal elements often exposes possible electrophysiological mechanisms. The pharmacology of peptide interaction with existing transmitter or modulator systems is studied. Peptide biochemistry concurrently suggests possible neurochemical mechanisms of action. Anatomical localization by immunohistochemical techniques defines some of the pathways involved. Peptide physiology under situations expected to mobilize release or activity indicates possible endogenous function. The difficulty lies in the integration of these diverse results. Catecholamines have been studied in a similar manner for 40 years, and a complete understanding of their mechanism of action in any one disease state or behavioral paradigm is still unclear. Peptides add the complexity of several hundred new

candidates, often localized in the same structures, and released under similar conditions. In fact, an effective integration of peptide mechanisms in the epilepsies, defined by existing techniques, would provide a theoretical construct for epileptogenic mechanisms. New approaches provided by the interdisciplinary application of techniques derived from molecular biology suggest several mechanisms and tools that will add to such an understanding.

Regulatory control of peptide production and release may occur at the phase of pre- and post-translational processing. One of the most interesting developments has been the identification of large precursor proproteins containing one or more peptides. This was known earlier to be true of many large proteins, but now appears to be a general principle. The proteolytic processing of these precursors produces functional peptides (99). Propiomelanocortin (POMC), proenkephalin, prodynorphin, provasopressin, prosomatostatin, and proCRF are of particular relevance since they appear to be good candidates in epileptogenic systems. Especially important is the evidence that many of these precursors contain multiple peptides. As an example, POMC includes α, β, and γ MSH, ACTH and β-endorphin (37). The cleavage of these peptides from their precursor may result in release of several different peptides, which produces an integrated response. Although we do not understand how this may act in different epileptic states, in an example from an invertebrate, the sea slug *Aplysia,* the processing of proELH leads to a complex coordinated behavioral egg-laying response mediated by a group of peptides resident on the same prohormone (85). A similar type of coordinated response could be envisioned for β-endorphin, ACTH, and MSH in regulating postictal or ictal changes in cerebral excitability. These peptides may form a coordinated response to stress or seizures. Likewise, the presence of AVP and neurophysin II on provasopressin suggests that processing of the precursor simultaneously produces the active peptide and a carrier or binding protein. In addition, much of the processing of these precursors may be specific to cell type and even cellular localization. The expression of the precursor may differ in synaptic terminals from cell bodies and differ in expression between pituitary and extrapituitary cells. The processing of the precursor includes many possible biochemical modifications, including phosphorylation, acetylation, methylation, amidation, or sulfonation. These specify precursor sites of translocation or action. One outcome of the intense study of these agents is that specific cleavage sites, defined by pairs of basic amino acid residues, have exposed segments representing previously unknown peptides including γ-MSH, Synenkephalin, and Leumorphin (21,70). More candidate peptides are possible. Cloning of peptide genes has allowed the production of cDNA probes and the testing of the expression of specific mRNA products. Douglass et al. (22) have described how these techniques could be utilized on genetic models of epilepsy. One could assess the level of regulation and response that is linked to genetically predisposed seizures. Furthermore, having cDNA probes for the peptidergic genes, one could measure directly mRNA expression and regulation under stressful conditions. In models with identified chromosomal abnormalities leading to seizures, one could test for the viability of specific peptidergic systems and whether they contribute to the epileptic condition.

An outgrowth of these genetic engineering techniques has been the attempt to identify and classify all neuronal-specific proteins. Extraction of mRNAs may allow as much as 40% of brain proteins to be isolated by current techniques. Sutcliffe et al. (92,93) have already produced part of such a library and have in fact identified several novel proteins and peptides whose function in the CNS is being studied. Cleavage sites on many of these proteins may reveal more new modulatory peptides. These techniques offer several advantages over traditional protein extraction methods: purity, direct sequence information, and sufficient source material for monoclonal antibody production. The coupling of these techniques with pharmacological and physiological studies will permit the isolation of more peptidergic regulators.

In addition to these techniques, improvements in the synthesis and structural analysis of peptides by use of automatic sequencing and synthesis instrumentation permits the rapid development of analogs for identified endogenous peptides. These methods can be used to produce new pharmacological agonists and antagonists with specialized activity and metabolic stability. Usefulness of antagonist availability is exemplified by the opioid antagonist, naloxone. Without it, endogenous relationships of opioid peptides to seizure states in the gerbil or rat postictal phase could not have been determined. In addition, the availability of a range of opioid agonists permitted clarification of receptor specificity of convulsant and anticonvulsant properties.

In most instances, peptidergic families do not have such an extensive pharmacopeia available. However, AVP pharmacology highlights ways in which the problem of studying peptidergic mechanisms in the epilepsies may in future experiments be augmented by deriving *peptide* agonists and antagonists. Families of vasopressin and oxytocin peptides have been synthesized with agonist and antagonist activity at multiple receptor subtypes (65). Structural modifications that identify active sites with antidiuretic, vasopressor, oxytocic, behavioral, and memory consolidation properties are available. One analog, vasotocin, antagonizes PTZ convulsions, which may signify a AVP mechanism in the seizure expression of that model (47).

It is obvious that antagonist and agonist peptides for all peptides with possible links to particular forms of epilepsy will be extensively tested in the near future in all epileptic model systems.

CONCLUSIONS

The number of possible peptide modulators appears incalculable. The relationship of any one system to epileptic disorders is still very sketchy, due simply to the lack of sufficient research. However, several candidate peptides families have been identified, especially the opioid peptides, somatostatin, AVP, TRH, and ACTH. The following list provides an overview of future directions that may define how these peptidergic systems fit into mechanisms responsible for the epilepsies. First, the testing of peptidergic actions in model systems at macrocellular and extracellular levels can delineate the effectiveness of a peptide in a specific form of epilepsy. Parameters of dose–response relationships and species or cell type specificity will provide guides to fruitful study areas. Second, development of effective antagonists is vital to determining endogenous relationships, as exemplified by the use of naloxone in testing endogenous opioid actions. Third, peptide production and release are tightly regulated by complex interactions at genomic, transcriptional, translational, and posttranslational levels. Techniques from molecular biology for cloning peptide genes, generating cDNA probes, and for testing mRNA expression provide some new tools to evaluate these aspects of regulation. An application to the study of epileptogenic mechanisms appears imminent. Finally, propeptide precursors may be a clue as to how some CNS functions are integrated. In some instances, a single propeptide such as POMC may release several active segments that simultaneously affect multiple physiological variables.

REFERENCES

1. Abood, L. G., Knapp, R., Mitchell, T., Booth, H., and Schwab, L. (1980): Chemical requirements of vasopressins of barrel rotation convulsions and reversal by oxytocin. *J. Neurosci. Res.*, 5:191–199.

2. Aldenhoff, J. B., Gruol, D. L., Rivier, J., Vale, W., and Siggins, G. R. (1983): Corticotropin releasing factor decreases postburst hyperpolarization and excites hippocampal neurons. *Science.*, 221:875–877.

3. Bajorek, J. G., Chesarek, W., Felmar, M., and Lomax, P. (1978): Effects of Met5-enkephalin and naloxone on spontaneous seizures in the mongolian gerbil. *Proc. West. Pharmacol. Soc.*, 21:365–370.

4. Bajorek, J. G., Felmar, M., and Lomax, P. (1980): Effects of beta-endorphin, ACTH, and cortisol on seizures in the Mongolian gerbil. *Fed. Proc.*, 39:981.

5. Bajorek, J. G., Lee, R. J., and Lomax, P. (1984): Neuropeptides: A role as endogenous mediators or modulators of epileptic phenomena. *Ann. Neurol.*, 16(suppl):S31–S38.

6. Bajorek, J. G., and Lomax, P. (1982): Modulation of spontaneous seizures in the mongolian gerbil: Effects of beta-endorphin. *Peptides.*, 3:83–86.

7. Berman, E. F., and Adler, M. W. (1981): The effects of opioids and beta-endorphin on maximal electroconvulsive (MES) seizures in rats. *Fed. Proc.*, 40:281.

8. Burnard, D. M., Pittman, Q. J., and Veale, W. L. (1983): Increased motor disturbances in response to arginine vasopressin following hemorrhage or hypertonic saline evidence for central arginine vasopressin release in rats. *Brain Res.*, 273:59–66.

9. Cain, D. P., and Corcoran, M. E. (1984): Intracerebral β-endorphin, Met-enkephalin and morphine: Kindling of seizures and handling-induced potentiation of epileptiform effects. *Life Sci.*, 34:2535–2542.

10. Caldecott-Hazard, S., Shavit, Y., Ackermann, R. F., Engel, J. Jr., Frederickson, R. C., and Liebeskind, J. C. (1982): Behavioral and electrographic effects of opioids on kindled seizures in rats. *Brain Res.*, 251:327–333.

11. Chihara, K., Arimura, A., Chihara, A., and Schally, A. V. (1978): Effect of intraventricular administration of antisomatostatin gamma globulin on the LD50 of strychnine and pentobarbital in rats. *Endocrinology.*, 103:912–916.

12. Cohn, M. L., and Cohn, M. (1975): Barrel rotation induced by somatostatin in the non-lesioned rat. *Brain Res.*, 96:138–141.

13. Corcoran, M. E., Cain, D. P., Finlay, J. M., and Gillis, B. J. (1984): Vasopressin and the kindling of seizures. *Life Sci.*, 35:947–952.

14. Corcoran, M. E., and Wada, J. A. (1979): Nal-oxone and the kindling of seizures. *Life Sci.*, 24: 791–795.

15. Cowan, A., Geller, E. B., and Adler, M. W. (1979): Classification of opioids on the basis of change in seizure threshold in rats. *Science*, 206:465–467.

16. Cowan, A., Tortella, F. C., and Adler, M. W. (1981): A comparison of the anticonvulsant effects of two systemically active enkephalin analogues in rats. *Eur. J. Pharmacol.*, 70:117–121.

17. deWeid, D. (1977): Peptides and behavior. *Life Sci.*, 20:195–204.

18. Dingledine, R. (1981): Possible mechanisms of enkephalin action on hippocampal CA1 pyramidal neurons. *J. Neurosci.*, 1:1022–1035.

19. Dingledine, R., Iversen, L. L., and Breuker, E. (1978): Naloxone as a GABA antagonist: Evidence from iontophoretic, receptor binding and convulsant studies. *Eur. J. Pharmacol.*, 47:19–27.

20. Dolva, L. O., Riddervold, F., and Thorsen, R. K. (1983): Side effects of thyrotropin releasing hormone. *Br. Med. J.*, 287:532.

21. Douglass, J., Civelli, O., and Herbert, E. (1984): Polyprotein gene expression: Generation of diversity of neuroendocrine peptides. *Annu. Rev. Biochem.*, 53:665–715.

22. Douglass, J. O., Civelli, O., Birnberg, N., Comb, M., Uhler, M., Lissitzky, J. C., and Herbert, E. (1984): Regulation of expression of opioid peptide genes. *Ann. Neurol.*, 16(Suppl.): S22–S30.

23. Ehlers, C. L., Henriksen, S. J., Wang, M., Rivier, J., Vale, W., and Bloom, F. E. (1983): Corticotropin releasing factor produces increases in brain excitability and convulsive seizures in rats. *Brain Res.*, 278:332–336.

24. Elomaa, E., Lehtovaara, R., Johansson, G., and Kukkola, L. (1980): Local somatostatin of the brain an agent in the genesis of focal epilepsy?. In: *Monographs in Neural Sciences, Vol. 5. Epilepsy: A Clinical and Experimental Research: Procceedings of the 2nd European Regional Conference on Epilepsy*, edited by J. Majkowski, pp. 30–31. S. Karger, Basel.

25. Engel, J. Jr., Ackermann, R. F., Caldecott-Hazard, S., and Chugani, H. T. (1984): Do altered opioid mechanisms play a role in human epilepsy? In: *Neurotransmitters in Seizures and Epilepsy II*, edited by R. G. Fariello et al., pp. 263–274. Raven Press, New York.

26. Ervin, F. R., Palmour, R. M., Flores, C. G. C. J. K., and Fong, B. (1978): Behavioral and electrophysiological effects of endorphins and enkephalins. In: *Characteristics and Function of Opioids*, edited by J. M. vanRee and L. Terenius, pp. 417–420. *Elsevier North Holland, Amsterdam.*

27. Franceschi, M., Perego, L., Cavagnini, F., Cattaneo, A. G., Invitti, C., Caviezel, F., Strambi, L. F., and Smirne, S. (1984): Effects of long-term antiepileptic therapy on the hypothalamic pituitary axis in man. *Epilepsia*, 25:46–52.

28. French, E. D., and Siggins, G. R. (1980): An iontophoretic survey of opioidpeptide actions in the rat limbic system: In search of opiate epi-

leptogenic mechanisms. *Regulatory Peptides*, 1:127–146.

29. Frenk, H. (1983): Pro- and anticonvulsant actions of morphine and the endogenous opioids: Involvement and interactions of multiple opiate and non-opiate systems. *Brain Res. Rev.*, 6:197–210.

30. Frenk, H., Engel, J. Jr., Ackermann, R. F., Shavit, Y., and Liebeskind, J. C. (1979): Endogenous opioids may mediate postictal behavioral depression in amygdaloid-kindled rats. *Brain Res.*, 167:435–440.

31. Frenk, H., Paul, L., Diaz, J., and Bailey, B. (1978): The effects of opiate antagonists on the seizure patterns of an animal model of epilepsy. *Soc. Neurosc. Abstr.*, 4:142.

32. Galzigna, L., Bianchi, M., Bertazzon, A., Barthez, A., and Quadro, G. (1984): An amino protected gamma amino butyric acid dipeptide with anticonvulsant action. *J. Neurochem.*, 42:1762–1766.

33. Gillis, B. J., and Cain, D. P. (1983): Amygdala and pyriform cortex kindling in vasopressin deficient rats Brattleboro strain. *Brain Res.*, 271:375–378.

34. Hardy, C., Panksepp, J., Rossi, J. III, and Zolovick, A. J. (1980): Naloxone facilitates amygdaloid kindling in rats. *Brain Res.*, 194:293–297.

35. Henriksen, S. J., Bloom, F. E., McCoy, F., Ling, N., and Guillemin, R. (1978): Beta-endorphin induces nonconvulsive limbic seizures. *Proc. Natl. Acad. Sci. USA*, 75:5221–5225.

36. Henriksen, S. J., Chouvet, G., McGinty, J., and Bloom, F. E. (1983): *Neuropeptides and the Epilepsies: Current Perspectives. Epilepsy: An Update on Research and Therapy*. Alan R. Liss, New York, 105–120.

37. Herbert, E., Birnberg, N., Lissitsky, J. C., Civelli, O., and Uhler, M. (1981): Pro-opioimelanocortin: A model for the regulation of expression of neuropeptides in pituitary and brain. *Neurosci. Commentaries*, 1:16–27.

38. Herzog, A. G., Russell, V., Vaitukaitis, J. L., and Geschwind, N. (1982): Neuroendocrine dysfunction in temporal lobe epilepsy. *Arch. Neurol*, 39:133–135.

39. Higuchi, T., Sikand, G. S., Kato, N., Wada, J. A., and Friesen, H. G. (1983): Profound suppression of kindled seizures by cysteamine, possible role of somatostatin to kindled seizures. *Brain Res.*, 288:359–362.

40. Holaday, J. W., Tseng, L. F., Loh, H. H., and Li, C. H. (1978): Thyrotropin releasing hormone antagonizes beta-endorphin hypothermia and catalepsy. *Life Sci.*, 22:1537–1544.

41. Hong, J. S., Gillin, J. C., Yang, H. Y., and Costa, E. (1979): Repeated electroconvulsive shocks and the brain content of endorphins. *Brain Res.*, 177:273–278.

42. Hughes, J., Smith, T. W., Kosterlitz, H. W., Fothergill, L. A., Morgan, B. A., and Morris, H. R. (1975): Identification of two related peptapeptides from the brain with potent opiate agonist activity. *Nature*, 258:577–579.

43. Inanaga, K., Ueda, S., Inoue, Y., and Imatoh, N. (1982): Clinical trial of TRH analog on refractory epilepsies. *Folia Psychiatr. Neurol. Jpn.*, 36:316.

44. Izumi, T., and Fukuyama, Y. (1984): Influence of ACTH on serum hormone content and its anticonvulsant action towards infantile spasms. *Life Sci.*, 34:1023–1028.

45. Jones, A. W., Croucher, M. J., Meldrum, B. S., and Watkins, J. C. (1984): Suppression of audiogenic seizures in DBA2 mice by two new dipeptide *n* methyl-D aspartic acid receptor antagonists. *Neurosci. Lett.*, 45:157–162.

46. Kadar, T., Pesti, A., Penke, B., Toth, G., Zarandi, M., and Telegdy, G. (1983): Structure activity and dose effect relationships of the antagonism of picrotoxin induced seizures by cholecystokinin fragments and analogs of cholecystokinin in mice. *Neuropharmacology*, 22:1223–1230.

47. Kasting, N. W., Veale, W. L., and Cooper, K. E. (1983): Vasotocin protects rats against convulsions induced by pentylentetrazol. *Experientia*, 37:1001–1002.

48. Kasting, N. W., Veale, W. L., Cooper, K. E., and Lederis, K. (1981): Vasopressin may mediate febrile convulsions. *Brain Res.*, 213:327–333.

49. Kato, N., Higuchi, T., Friesen, H. G., and Wada, J. A. (1982): Changes in immunoreactive somatostatin and beta-endorphin content in rat brain after amygdaloid kindling. *Life Sci.*, 32:2415–2422.

50. Kelsey, J. E., and Belluzzi, J. D. (1982): Endorphin mediation of post-ictal effects of kindled seizures in rats. *Brain Res.*, 253:337–340.

51. Klein, R. (1970): Effects of ACTH and corticosteroids on epileptiform disorders. In: *Progress in Brain Research, Pituitary, Adrenal and the Brain*, vol. 32, edited by D. de Weid and J. A. W. M. Weijen, pp. 263–269. New York, Elsevier.

52. Kohler, J., Schroeter, E., and Cramer, H. (1982): Somatostatin-like immunoreactivity in the cerebrospinal fluid of neurological patients. *Arch. Psychiatry. Nervenkr.*, 231:503–508.

53. Krieger, D. T. (1983): Brain peptides, what, where and why?. *Science*, 222:975–985.

54. Krivoy, W. A., Lane, M., and Kroeger, D. C. (1963): The actions of certain polypeptides on synaptic transmission. *Ann. N.Y. Acad. Sci.*, 104:312–329.

55. Kruse, H., van Wimersa Greidanus, T. B., and deWeid, D. (1977): Barrel rotation induced by vasopressin and related peptides in rats. *Pharmacol. Biochem. Behav.*, 7:311–313.

56. Kubek, M. J., and Sattin, A. (1984): Effect of electroconvulsive shock on the content of thyrotropin-releasing hormone in rat brain. *Life Sci.*, 34:1149–1152.

57. Lee, R. J., Bajorek, J. G., and Lomax, P. (1983): Opioid peptides and seizures. *Life Sci.* 33(Suppl. 1):567.

58. Lee, R. J., Bajorek, J. G., and Lomax, P. (1984): Similar anticonvulsant but unique behavioral effects of opioid agonists in the seizure sensitive Mongolian gerbil. *Neuropharmacology*, 23:517–524.

59. Lee, R. J., and Lomax, P. (1983): Thermoregulatory, behavioral and seizure modulatory effects of arginine vasopressin in the gerbil *Meriones unguiculatus. Peptides,* 4:801–806.

60. Lee, R. J., and Lomax, P. (1984): The effect of spontaneous seizures on pentylenetetrazole and maximum electroshock induced seizures in the mongolian gerbil. *Eur. J. Pharmacol.,* 106:91–96.

61. Le Gal La Salle, G., Calvino, B., and Ben-Ari, Y. (1977): Morphine enhances amygdaloid seizures and increases interictal spike frequency in kindled rats. *Neurosci. Lett.,* 6:255–260.

62. Loskota, W. J., Lomax, P., and Rich, S. T. (1974): The gerbil as a model for the study of the epilepsies. *Epilepsia* 15:109–119.

63. Lundberg, J. M., and Hokfelt, T. (1983): Coexistence of peptides and classical neurotransmitters. *TINS,* 6:325–333.

64. Maeda, K., and Tanimoto, K. (1981): Epileptic seizures induced by thyrotropin releasing hormone. *Lancet,* 1:1058–1059.

65. Mains, R. E., Eipper, B. A., Glembotski, C. C., and Dores, R. M. (1983): Strategies for the biosynthesis of bioactive peptides. *TINS,* 229–235.

66. Martini, A., Sacerdote, P., Mantegazza, P., and Panerai, A. E. (1984): Antiepileptic agents affect hypothalamic β-endorphin concentrations. *J. Neurochem.,* 43:871–873.

67. Meldrum, B. S., Menini, C., Stutzmann, J. M., and Naquet, R. (1979): Effects of opiate-like peptides, morphine and naloxone in the photosensitive baboon, *Papio-papio. Brain Res.,* 170:333–348.

68. Meyerhoff, J. L., Bates, V. E., and Kubek, M. J. (1982): Increases in brain thyrotropin releasing hormone (TRH) following kindled seizures. *Soc. Neurosci. Abstr.,* 8:457.

69. Montplaisir, J., Saint-Hilaire, J. M., Walsh, J. T., Laverdi'ere, M., and Bouvier, G. (1981): Naloxone and focal epilepsy: A study with depth electrodes. *Neurology,* 31:350–352.

70. Mutt, V. (1983): New approaches to the identification and isolation of hormonal polypeptides. *TINS,* 357–360.

71. Nakamura, J., Inokuchi, H., Nishi, S., and Inanaga, K. (1983): The effects of a TRH analog on the electrical activity of the CA1 hippocampal pyramidal neurons. *Folia Psychiatr. Neurol. JPN.,* 37:350–351.

72. Nemeroff, C. B., Loosen, P. T., Bisset, G., Manberg, P. J., Wilson, I. C., Lipton, M. A., Prange, A. J. Jr., and (1979): Pharmaco-behavioral effects of hypothalamic peptides in animals and man: Focus on thyrotropin releasing hormone and neurotensin. *Psychoneuroendocrinology.,* 3:279–310.

73. Nemeroff, C. B., Prange, A. J. Jr., Bissette, G., Breese, G. R., and Lipton, M. A. (1975): Thyrotropin-releasing hormone (TRH) and its beta-alanine analogue: Potentiation of the anticonvulsant potency of phenobarbital in mice. *Psychopharmacol. Commun.,* 1:305–317.

74. Nistico, G., Rotiroti, D., DeSarro, A., and Stephenson, J. D. (1978): Behavioral, electrocort-

ical and body temperature effects after intracerebral infusion of TRH in fowls. *Eur. J. Pharmacol.,* 50:253–260.

75. Pinsky, C., Dua, A. K., and LaBella, F. S. (1982): Peptidase inhibitors reduce opiate narcotic withdrawal signs, including seizure activity, in the rat. *Brain Res.,* 243:301–307.

76. Plotnikoff, N. P., and Kastin, A. J. (1977): Neuropharmacological review of hypothalamic releasing factors. In: *Neuropeptide Influences on the Brain and Behavior,* edited by L. H. Miller, C. A. Sandman, and A. J. Kastin, pp. 81–107. Raven Press, New York.

77. Post, R. M., Davenport, S., Pert, A., and Squillace, K. M. (1979): Lack of effect of an opiate agonist and antagonist on the development of amygdala kindling in the rat. *Commun. Psychopharmacol.,* 3:185–190.

78. Przewlocki, R., Lason, W., Stach, R., and Kacz, D. (1983): Opioid peptides, particularly dynorphin, after amygdaloid-kindled seizures. *Regulatory Peptides,* 6:385–392.

79. Rezek, M., Havlicek, V., Leybin, L., LaBella, F. S., and Friesen, H. (1978): Opiate-like naloxone reversible actions of somatostatin given intracerebrally. *Can. J. Physiol. Pharmacol.,* 56:227–231.

80. Riikonen, R. (1983): Infantile spasms: Some new theoretical aspects. *Epilepsia,* 24:159–168.

81. Riikonen, R. (1982): A long-term follow-up study of 214 children with the syndrome of infantile spasms. *Neuropediatrics.,* 13:14–23.

82. Rose, R. P., and Bridger, W. H. (1982): Hormonal influences on seizure kindling: The effects of post-stimulation ACTH or cortisone injections. *Brain Res.,* 231:75–84.

83. Sagratella, S., and Massotti, M. (1982): Convulsant and anticonvulsant effects of opioids: Relationship to GABA-mediated transmission. *Neuropharmacology,* 21:991–1000.

84. Sato, M., Morimoto, K., and Wada, J. A. (1984): Antiepileptic effects of thyrotropin-releasing hormone and its new derivative, DN-1417, examined in feline amygdaloid kindling preparation. *Epilepsia,* 25:537–544.

85. Scheller, R. H., Kaldany, R. R., Kreiner, T., Mahon, A. C., Nambu, J. R., Schaefer, M., and Taussig, R. (1984): Neuropeptides: Mediators of behavior in *Aplysia. Science,* 225:1300–1308.

86. Schreiber, R. A. (1979): The effect of naloxone on audiogenic seizures. *Psychopharmacology,* 66:205–206.

87. Snead, O. C. III, and Bearden, L. J. (1980): Anticonvulsants specific for petit mal antagonize epileptogenic effect of leucine enkephalin. *Science,* 210:1031–1033.

88. Snead, O. C. III, and Bearden, L. J. (1982): The epileptogenic spectrum of opiate agonists. *Neuropharmacology,* 21:1137–1144.

89. Snead, O. C. III, Benton, J. W., and Myers, G. J. (1983): ACTH and prednisone in childhood seizure disorders. *Neurology,* 33:966–970.

90. Sprick, U., Oitzl, M. S., Ornstein, K., and Huston, J. P. (1981): Spreading depression induced by microinjection of enkephalins into the

hippocampus and neocortex. *Brain Res.*, 210:243–252.

91. Stone, W. S., Eggleton, C. E., and Berman, R. F. (1982): Opiate modification of amygdaloid-kindled seizures in rats. *Pharmacol. Biochem. Behav.*, 16:751–756.

92. Sutcliffe, J. G., and Milner, R. J. (1984): Brain specific gene expression. *TIBS*, 9:95–99.

93. Sutcliffe, J. G., Milner, R. J., Shinnick, T. M., and Bloom, F. E. (1983): Identifying the protein products of brain-specific genes with antibodies to chemically synthesized peptides. *Cell*, 33: 671–682.

94. Tartara, A., Bo, P., Maurelli, M., and Savoldi, F. (1983): Centrally administered amino terminal fragments of ACTH 1-10, 4-10, 4-9 display convulsant properties in rabbits. *Peptides*, 4:315–318.

95. Thiessen, D. D., Lindzey, G., and Friend, H. C. (1968): Spontaneous seizures in the Mongolian gerbil (*Meriones unguiculatus*). *Psychon. Sci.*, 11:227–228.

96. Timiras, P. S., and Hill, H. F. (1980): Hormones and epilepsy. In: *Antiepileptic Drugs: Mechanisms of Action,* edited by G. H. Glaser, J. K. Penry, and D. M. Woodbury, 655–666. Raven Press, New York.

97. Tortella, F. C., Cowan, A., and Adler, M. W. (1981): Comparison of the anticonvulsant effects of opioid peptides and etorphine in rats after icy administration. *Life Sci.*, 10:1039–1045.

98. Tortella, F. C., Cowan, A., Belenky, G. L., and Holaday, J. W. (1981): Opiate-like electroencephalographic and behavioral effects of electroconvulsive shock in rats. *Eur. J. Pharmacol.*, 76:121–128.

99. Turner, A. J. (1984): Neuropeptide processing enzymes. *TINS*, 7:258–260.

100. Urca, G., Frenk, H., Liebeskind, J. C., and Taylor, A. N. (1977): Morphine and enkephalin: Analgesic and epileptic properties. *Science,* 197:83–86.

101. Veale, W. L., Cooper, K. E., and Ruwe, W. D. (1984): Vasopressin: Its role in antipyresis and febrile convulsions. *Brain Res. Bull.*, 12:161–165.

102. Vecsei, L., Bollock, I., and Telegdy, G. (1983): Intracerebroventricular somatostatin attenuates electroconvulsive shock induced amnesia in rats. *Peptides,* 4:293–296.

103. Vindrola, O., Briones, R., Asai, M., and Fernandez-Guardiola, A. (1981): Amygdaloid kindling enhances the enkephalin content in the rat brain. *Neurosci. Lett.*, 21:39–43.

104. Wei, E., Sigel, S., Loh, H., and Way, E. L. (1975): Thyrotropin releasing hormone and shaking behavior in rat. *Nature*, 253:739–740.

105. Werz, M. A., and Macdonald, R. L. (1982): Opiate alkaloids antagonize postsynaptic glycine and GABA responses: Correlation with convulsant action. *Brain Res.*, 236:107–119.

106. Woodbury, D. M., and Vernadakis, A. (1967): Influence of hormones on brain activity. In: *Neuroendocrinology,* vol. 2, edited by L. Martini and W. F. Ganong, pp. 335–375. Academic Press, New York.

107. Wurpel, J., Balaban, C., Barbella, Y., Dundore, R., Keil, L., and Severs, W. (1984): Seizure activity, barrel rotation after intracerebroventricular vasopressin. *Fed. Proc.*, 43:4004.

108. Zetler, G. (1982): Ceruletide analogs and cholecystokinin octapeptide CCK-8 effects on motor behavior, hexobarbital induced sleep and harman induced convulsions. *Peptides,* 3:701–704.

109. Zetler, G. (1982): Caerulein and cholecystokinin octa peptide sedative and anticonvulsive effects in mice unaffected by the benzodiazepine antagonist RO-15-1788. *Neurosci. Lett.*, 28:287–290.

110. Zetler, G. (1980): Anticonvulsant effects of caerulein and cholecystokinin octapeptide, compared with those of diazepam. *Eur. J. Pharmacol.*, 65:297–300.

111. Zieglgansberger, W., French, E. D., Siggins, G. R., and Bloom, F. E. (1979): Opioid peptides may excite hippocampal pyramidal neurons by inhibiting adjacent inhibitory interneurons. *Science,* 205:415–417.

Advances in Neurology, Vol. 44, edited by
A. V. Delgado-Escueta, A. A. Ward, Jr.,
D. M. Woodbury, and R. J. Porter.
Raven Press, New York © 1986.

26

Opioid Peptides and Epileptogenesis in the Limbic System: Cellular Mechanisms

George Robert Siggins, Steven Jon Henriksen, Charles Chavkin, and Donna Gruol

Scripps Clinic and Research Foundation, La Jolla, California 92037

SUMMARY The localization of opioid peptides in the rat hippocampal formation and the epileptogenic action of β-endorphin and certain enkephalin analogues have led to speculations that opioids may play a role in limbic seizures. These immunochemical and electroencephalographic data are compatible with single-unit electrophysiological studies showing predominant excitations of hippocampal pyramidal neurons in CA1 and CA3 fields produced by iontophoresis of endorphins or enkephalins. These excitations are naloxone sensitive and appear to arise from a disinhibitory mechanism due to inhibition of inhibitory interneurons. Thus, intracellular recordings in *in vitro* preparations of hippocampus usually show opioid-induced reduction of inhibitory postsynaptic potentials.

However, more recent studies suggest that a major opioid-containing pathway in the hippocampus, the mossy fiber projection from the dentate gyrus to CA3 pyramidal neurons, contains more pro-dynorphin–derived peptides than pro-enkephalin. Intracerebroventricular dynorphin does not induce epileptiform activity in the rat, and single-unit and field-potential studies show mixed effects on CA3 neuronal excitability, with more inhibitory responses than are seen with the enkephalins. Selective inactivation of μ opioid receptors reveals that dynorphin, which was previously shown to express specificity for κ receptors, can act on δ receptors in CA1. Furthermore, a specific κ agonist, U50,488H, has inhibitory actions when applied directly to CA3 neurons. These data suggest the presence of multiple opioid receptor types in the hippocampus. These multiple receptors may point to heterogeneous functions of the different families of opioid peptides in various regions of the hippocampus, and could explain the divergent effects reported for the various opioids and naloxone to promote or prevent paroxysmal activity.

The responsiveness of individual neurons to numerous putative neurotransmitters has been an area of intense study (see refs. 9,42,45,47), yet very little is known regarding the possible role of these substances in epileptiform activity (see refs. 4,10,24,29,30,32,36,43,59). In addition, the role of central synaptic or neurochem- ical processes in the *recurrent* nature of paroxysmal activity also remains an enigma. Yet it is just this property that is diagnostic of epilepsy. Several studies have demonstrated that experimental epileptogenesis may occur as a result of altered synaptic as well as nonsynaptic processes (see refs. 24,43). For example, intracellular recordings from central nervous system (CNS) neurons have revealed that large prolonged depolarization shifts (PDSs) and high-frequency spike activity are coincident with the paroxysmal discharges observed in the electroencephalogram (EEG) during epileptic events (34,43). This suggests that normal mechanisms underlying single neuron excitability, and synchronization with other neurons, are likely substrates for generation of at least some of the abnormal events seen in the epileptic EEG. It also follows that various abnormalities in synaptic events, variously distributed over the neuraxis, could be pathognomonic of the different types of epilepsies.

Clinically, an estimated 50% of epilepsies are not fully controlled by presently available drug therapy. This suggests that effective drug regimens require further knowledge of brain function and the neuropharmacological substrates critical for the development or control of seizures. The fact that the epileptic symptomatologies are differentially sensitive to various antiepileptic drug treatments further suggests multiple neurobiological substrates of these syndromes.

A substantial proportion of epilepsies are of limbic distribution, including the partial-complex seizures and certain focal seizures of the frontal pole. These epilepsies have proven particularly resistant to drug therapy. To date, experimental studies of these limbic seizures have dealt primarily with the general hyperexcitability of this brain area as demonstrated by the use of exogenous epileptogenic agents and brain stimulation. Although these studies have generated understanding of some aspects (e.g., time course) of epileptic phenomena, they have provided little insight into the details of *endogenous* epileptogenic processes, and have not led to development of adequate antiepileptogenic agents for the treatment of the limbic seizures.

As suggested above, it seems likely that synaptic processes are involved in certain epilepsies (see refs. 43 and 59). Recent immunohistochemical and immunoassay studies indicate the presence in the limbic system of numerous neuropeptides, including various types of opioid peptides, that may play some synaptic role. Moreover, these neuropeptides provide a fresh neurochemical substrate for the investigation of epileptic phenomena. Recently, one particular limbic brain area, the hippocampus, has been extensively surveyed immunohistochemically and biochemically, and a variety of neuroactive opioid peptides have been identified and tested physiologically (see ref. 9 for review). Interest in the possible role of endogenous opioids in

limbic seizures gained further impetus from reports that intraventricular administration of minute amounts of endorphins elicited dramatic limbic seizures in rats (21,54) (Fig. 1). As far as we are aware, this was the first demonstration of limbic epileptiform activity produced by apparently "physiological" amounts of an endogenous transmitter candidate.

DISTRIBUTION OF HIPPOCAMPAL OPIOIDS

To date, there appear to be three major groups of opioid peptides, based upon the structure of the three separate prohormones and their individual patterns of cellular origin (Table 1). Early immunohistochemical investigations of endogenous opioids in rodents demonstrated broad distribution in most limbic structures, but sparse labeling of cells in the hippocampus (2,26,46, 53,57). Regional studies also indicated low levels of Leu^5-enkephalin (ENK)-immunoreactivity (IR) in the CA1 pyramidal cell field (3). However, more recent radioimmunoassay studies have revealed that the highest concentration of ENK-IR resides in the dentate-CA3 fields with only half as much ENK-IR in CA1 and the subiculum (1,27).

Considerable interest has centered on the hippocampal mossy fiber pathway that originates in the dentate granule cells and projects through the hilus to innervate CA3 pyramidal cell dendrites. In the rat, these fibers (and the granule cell sources), were originally thought to contain primarily enkephalin (2,17). However, enkephalin antisera used in these earlier immunochemical studies also cross-react with dynorphin. Subsequent histochemical studies in our laboratory using more specific antisera (35) have shown that these fibers primarily possess immunoreactivity for dynorphin(s), and a much lower level of pro-enkephalin–derived opioids (5,28). This pathway was previously thought to be exclusively excitatory, likely to involve release of an acidic amino acid such as glutamate or aspartate. The presence of pro-dynorphin–derived peptides and such an excitatory amino acid in the same pathway has aroused speculation that these substances may be co-transmitters within the same mossy fiber terminals.

In addition, more recent histochemical studies of the rat CA1 hippocampal field demonstrate scattered dynorphin-IR and enkephalin-IR cells and fibers (1,2,17,24,35,48). Enkephalin-IR, but not dynorphin-IR, is also observed in the rat entorhinal cortex, in cells that project to the hippocampus and dentate gyrus. Thus, we believe the opioid immunoreactivity in the three opioid

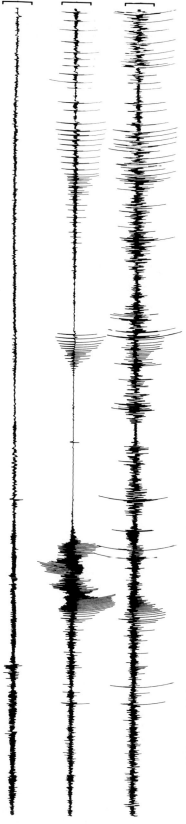

FIG. 1. Multitrace electroencephalographic record of β-endorphin induced epileptiform activity in the rat. β-Endorphin was administered intracerebroventricularly in a total dose of 3 nmoles at the beginning of the trace. *Top trace*, bipolar recording taken from a deep electrode in dorsal hippocampus; *middle trace*, bipolar recording of cortical EEG; *lower trace*, taken from a deep bipolar electrode in the amygdala. Calibration bars to the right of the traces represent 1 mV. The total time of the recording is 4.4 min. Behavioral convulsions were not seen after the endorphin injection, but wet dog shakes and exploratory behavior were noted during the epileptiform events. Note the high-voltage paroxysmal spikes followed by a prolonged isoelectric period prominent in the hippocampal trace and the lack of epileptiform events in the cortical trace.

TABLE 1. *Families of endogenous opioid neuropeptides*

Opioid precursor	Identified products[a]	Receptor specificity[b]
Pro-opiomelanocortin	β-Endorphin, α-endorphin, γ-endorphin (ACTH, α-MSH, β-MSH, γ-MSH)	μ > δ = κ
Pro-enkephalin	Met-enkephalin, Leu-enkephalin, and other slightly extended forms	δ > μ > κ
Pro-dynorphin	Dynorphin-A, dynorphin-(1–8), dynorphin-B, α-neoendorphin, β-neoendorphin (Leu-enk?)	κ > μ > δ

[a] Other intermediate processing products have also been identified.
[b] Provisional assignment of relative receptor selectivities based on *in vitro* bioassays and membrane-binding studies.

peptidergic systems of the hippocampal formation represents the presence of two different prohormonal systems: (a) predominantly pro-dynorphin–derived peptides in the dentate-CA3 mossy fiber pathway; (b) predominantly pro-enkephalin–derived peptides in scattered interneurons in CA1 and CA3; and (c) pro-enkephalin–derived peptides in the entorhinal to dentate/hippocampal perforant path.

The localization of the opioid peptides in nerve cells and fibers of the hippocampus suggest that they are likely transmitter candidates. This possibility is supported by recent biochemical studies showing that at least five related prodynorphin/neoendorphin-derived peptides can be released from hippocampal slices by high K^+ in a Ca^{2+}-dependent manner (6): these include dynorphin-A(1–17), dynorphin-A(1–8), dynorphin-B, α-neoendorphin and β-neoendorphin. Pro-enkephalin–derived peptides are also released in this preparation (5,6).

FUNCTION OF LIMBIC OPIOIDS

Enkephalins and β-Endorphin

Early investigations of endogenous opioid peptides in the CNS suggested a role in the regulation of neuronal excitability. Intraventricular administration in rodents of nanomole amounts of β-endorphin and several enkephalin analogues elicited a variety of subcortical and cortical electrographic signs of epileptogenesis (21, 54) (Fig. 1). A major aspect of these opioid-induced electrographic abnormalities is the development of repetitive paroxysmal sharp EEG waveforms primarily confined to limbic brain areas and particularly observable in the hippocampus (21,54) (Fig. 1). This suggests that one of the primary pharmacological sites of action of this naloxone-reversible epileptogenic effect could be the rat limbic system, and that a major

role for opioid peptides could be the regulation of limbic excitability (21).

These early encephalographic studies are compatible with microelectrophoretic cellular investigations suggesting a unique excitatory effect of opioid peptides in the rat hippocampus (25,41,60). In extracellular single-unit recordings, the preponderant stereospecific action of opiate alkaloids or opioid peptides in the majority of brain regions is depression of spontaneous, glutamate-evoked or acetylcholine (ACh)-evoked discharge. The depressions are generally blocked by naloxone and are qualitatively similar throughout the mammalian central and peripheral nervous systems (see refs. 13, 42, and 61 for review). A few exceptions exist, such as the naloxone-reversible excitatory responses seen in hippocampal pyramidal cells (25,41,60). Large iontophoretic currents of β-endorphin during single-unit recording also can occasionally trigger repetitive large potentials suggestive of epileptiform activity (14). The single-unit excitations and epileptiform activity are intrinsic to the hippocampus, since they can also be evoked by superfusion of opioids into intraocular transplants of hippocampus (51).

However, early *in vivo* studies of hippocampus in our laboratory, using GABA blockade by bicuculline and blockade of transmitter release by Mg^{2+} ions indicate that the excitatory responses of hippocampal pyramidal neurons may be viewed as indirect, resulting from a primary inhibitory effect of the opioid on neighboring inhibitory interneurons, leading to excitation of pyramidal cells by disinhibition (60). Nonetheless, extracellular studies cannot reveal the exact details of the mechanisms behind this unique opioid excitation. Therefore, several laboratories embarked on intracellular studies using recently developed *in vitro* preparations such as hippocampal slices or explant cultures.

Such intracellular studies of pyramidal cells

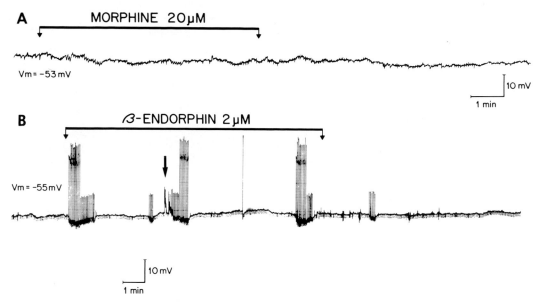

FIG. 2. Morphine and β-endorphin have little effect on membrane potential of two different CA1 pyramidal cells in the hippocampal slice preparation: intracellular recording. Polygraph tracings of membrane potential (Vm, resting membrane potential for each cell) taken during superfusion of artificial CSF (see ref. 49 for composition) or of artificial cerebrospinal fluid with opioid added (*arrowed brackets:* duration of opioid application). **(A)** Slight changes in Vm occurred spontaneously throughout the recording and were not related to the period of morphine application; **(B)** small downward deflections from Vm are calibration pulses triggered every 3 sec; large upward deflections (and associated slow hyperpolarizations) represent the artifacts, spikes (attenuated by the slow rise time of the polygraph), and postsynaptic potentials evoked by stimulation (0.33 Hz) of the Schaffer collateral afferents (stratum radiatum) to CA1. *Large arrow:* onset of two abrupt potential shifts (PDSs) likely to represent paroxysmal activity elicited by the opioid peptide. In this and all subsequent figures of voltage records, up is positive.

of the hippocampus CA1 have shown little or no direct effects on membrane potential (Fig. 2) or input resistance of morphine or several opioid peptides (Leu^5-enkephalin; Met^5-enkephalin; D-Ala^2, D-Leu^5-enkephalin; D-Ala^2, D-Leu^5-enkephalin amide; β-endorphin), in concentrations up to 50 μm (11,15,16,19,20,37–39,48,49). When such direct effects do occur, they usually appear as epileptiform activity such as the PDSs seen with β-endorphin (49) (Fig. 2); these may arise from changes in synaptic efficacy (see below). The lack of a direct membrane effect on pyramidal cells is predicted by the disinhibition hypothesis. Much lower opioid concentrations (10^{-7}–10^{-6}M) are capable of altering synaptic responses to afferent stimulation (11,15,16,19,20, 33,37–39,44,45,48,49,55). Unfortunately, there has not been complete agreement as to the mechanism by which the opioids alter synaptic potentials. Most studies on the hippocampal slice indicate that the enkephalins and β-endorphin primarily reduce the size of recurrent and feed-forward inhibitory postsynaptic potentials (IPSPs) in both CA1 and CA3 fields (19,33,37–39,48,49). This also supports the hypothesis of a disinhibitory mechanism. This disinhibition

appears to be exerted presynaptically to the pyramidal cell, since pyramidal cell responses to γ-aminobutyric acid (GABA), the likely transmitter for these IPSPs, were not reduced by the opioids (11,37–39).

However, two other hippocampal slice studies (11,20) have shown only enhanced excitatory postsynaptic potentials (EPSPs) without change in the IPSP, whereas a third (49) noted a reduction of EPSPs (as well as IPSPs and depolarizing glutamate responses) in about one-half of the pyramidal neurons studied. *In vitro* studies using explant cultures of rat hippocampus have observed both reduced IPSPs and enhanced EPSPs; both effects developed prior to, and perhaps triggered, PDSs suggestive of epileptiform activity.

It is still uncertain whether the observed hippocampal opioid effects are due to direct hyperpolarization of the interneurons, to a true modulation of transmitter release, or to a more remote action. However, the bulk of the extracellular (see 12,31,37,38,40,44,60) and intracellular (see 44 and above) data still seem to support a disinhibitory mechanism of action for the single-unit excitatory and epileptigenic effect of

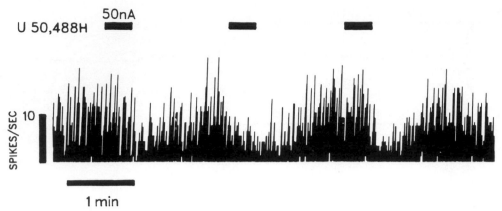

FIG. 3. The κ agonist U50,488H depresses the spontaneous discharge activity of an extracellularly recorded CA3 neuron *in vivo*. This ratemeter polygraph record was taken from a rat anesthetized with halothane (1%) and immobilized in a stereotaxic frame (see refs. 22–24 for methods). U50,488H was applied to this neuron by iontophoresis from a multibarrel micropipette for the durations indicated by the bars above the record. Note the profound reduction in discharge rate elicited by this opioid.

these opioid peptides in hippocampus (see ref. 9 for review). Still, a facilitation of excitatory transmission has not been ruled out entirely. Some of the discrepancies between laboratories might be ascribed to: (a) different methods of afferent stimulation and the difficulties in selectively stimulating pure excitatory or inhibitory pathways; (b) the use of different opioid agonists acting on different opiate receptors; (c) the method of drug administration; and (d) the fact that the hippocampal pyramidal cell is usually the subject of these intracellular recordings, yet the primary site of opioid action appears to be presynaptic to this cell. However, a recent preliminary intracellular study by Nicoll and Madison (40) of hippocampal interneurons suggests that they are hyperpolarized by enkephalin analogues, thus directly supporting the disinhibition hypothesis.

Dynorphins

As described above, it is becoming increasingly apparent that one or more of the prody-

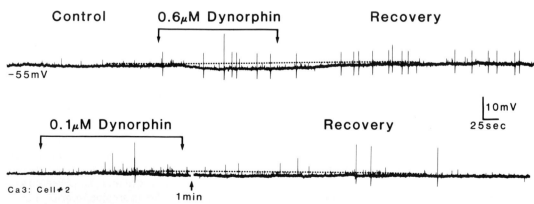

FIG. 4. Dynorphin-B hyperpolarizes a CA3 pyramidal neuron in the hippocampal slice: intracellular recording with a K-acetate–filled micropipette. The traces indicate membrane potential, as in Fig. 2. The Vm of this cell was −55 mV. *Arrowed brackets:* duration of the dynorphin superfusion. Other methods and features are as in Fig. 2. The brief deflections in the records are spontaneous synaptic potentials, spikes, and associated after-potentials that are attenuated by the slow rise time of the polygraph. Note that dynorphin accelerates this spontaneous activity in spite of the hyperpolarizations elicited. *Dotted line:* Vm. Note the 1-min break in the lower record.

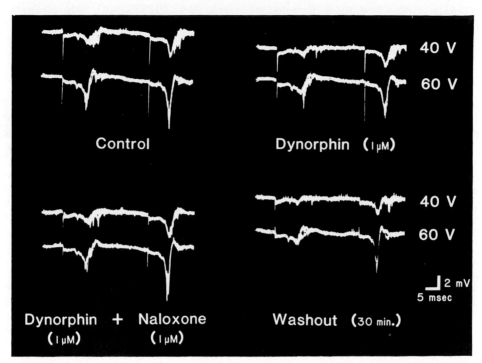

FIG. 5. Inhibitory effect of dynorphin-B on CA3 field potentials evoked by stimulation of the hilar mossy fiber area in the hippocampal slice preparation. Multiple oscilloscope sweeps at two different stimulus strengths (40 and 60 V) were used to generate the two tracings for each condition. A paired-pulse stimulus paradigm was used; as a result of frequency facilitation, the second response of each pair is bigger than the first. The stimulus (0.1-msec pulse duration) is indicated by the brief downward deflection preceding the slower field potential response by 3–5 msec. The widening of the traces at certain points is a result of evoked single-unit activity riding on the field potentials. Note that dynorphin appears to reduce the size of the population spike (large negative response), especially that of the second response of the pair, and that naloxone reverses this effect of dynorphin.

norphin-derived opioid peptides such as dynorphin-A or dynorphin-B, dynorphin-A(1–8), α-neoendorphin, or β-neoendorphin, may contribute a significant proportion of mammalian central opioid peptides in hippocampus as well as other brain areas (see 1,6,18 and above). However, to date, only a few electrophysiological studies on the pro-dynorphin–derived peptides have been reported. Preliminary studies in rats injected intraventricularly with microgram amounts of dynorphin-A(1–13) demonstrated a variety of behavioral effects but no epileptogenic response, thus pharmacologically differentiating dynorphin from other epileptogenic opioids (S. J. Henriksen, *unpublished observations*). Prompted by our recent observations of the apparent predominance of dynorphin in the rat hippocampal mossy fibers innervating CA3 neurons (6,23,24,35), we and others (56) have recently investigated the response of hippocampal neurons to iontophoretically administered dynorphin.

Extracellular single-unit *in vivo* studies using iontophoresis of dynorphin-B(1–13) or dynorphin-A(1–17) have shown both depressant and facilitatory actions on presumed CA3 hippocampal pyramidal neurons. In the study by Walker et al. (56) the predominantly depressant actions of dynorphin A(1–13) were not antagonized by intraperitoneal (i.p.) naloxone. The studies by Henriksen et al. (22–24) noted naloxone antagonism of the more predominant excitations, but not the inhibitions less frequently observed. However, a more recent analysis has shown that some of the inhibitions are also antagonized by naloxone (S. J. Henriksen, G. Chouvet, and F. E. Bloom, *unpublished observations*). The studies of Henriksen et al. (22–24) indicate both similarities to, and differences from, the excitatory actions of iontophoretically applied enkephalins described above, with respect to both field-potential and single-unit recordings. For example, dynorphin elicits more prolonged excitations than do the enkephalins

(22–24). These data, and those showing predominantly depressant effects (Fig. 3) of selective κ opiate agonists (22–24) suggest the involvement of several types of opioid receptors in hippocampus (see ref. 7).

Preliminary intracellular studies of dynorphin effects on CA3 pyramidal neurons in the hippocampal slice are somewhat consistent with these extracellular findings: depending on the particular cell studied, either slow hyperpolarizing (Fig. 4) or depolarizing responses are seen with low concentrations of dynorphin A and B (19). The changes in membrane potential were occasionally associated with changes in discharge activity in a direction opposite to that expected (19) (see Fig. 4), thus raising the possibility of indirect action of dynorphin. Neither were the depolarizing responses of the type expected of mossy fiber activation, being slow and not always capable of activating spikes. Similar mixed or weak effects in CA3 were seen with respect to the action of dynorphins on extracellular field potentials evoked by mossy fiber stimulation (19), although inhibitory dynorphin action was sometimes observed (Fig. 5).

These dynorphin effects contrast with the effects of enkephalins on these CA3 neurons, where few inhibitory effects are seen (41,60) and excitatory effects appear to be due primarily to reduction of IPSPs, with little direct change in membrane potential or resistance (19,33). Further studies will be required to determine: (a) if these dynorphin-induced potential changes are due to remote effects on other input neurons; (b) if they are naloxone sensitive; and (c) if multiple opiate receptor subtypes (see Table 1) are involved.

Indeed, we have recently performed field-potential studies of hippocampal slices that suggest that dynorphins act, like morphine, on the μ receptors in CA1 (7), rather than on κ receptors as expected from data obtained in smooth muscle bioassays and brain membrane binding assays (8). Thus, dynorphin-A(1–17) and dynorphin-B increased the evoked field-potential response recorded in the hippocampal CA1 pyramidal layer, as did several other opioids tested (7). Treatment of the hippocampal slice with β-funaltrexamine, an irreversible antagonist selective for μ receptors, blocked the effects of normorphine, dynorphin-A, and dynorphin-B, but did not change the response to D-Ala^2, D-Leu^5-enkephalin (7). κ Receptors were not detected in CA1, as judged by potency ratios for the opioids and the lack of effect of ethylketocyclazocine and U-50,488H, both selective κ agonists. Furthermore, preliminary intracellular recordings of CA1 pyramidal cells show that 1

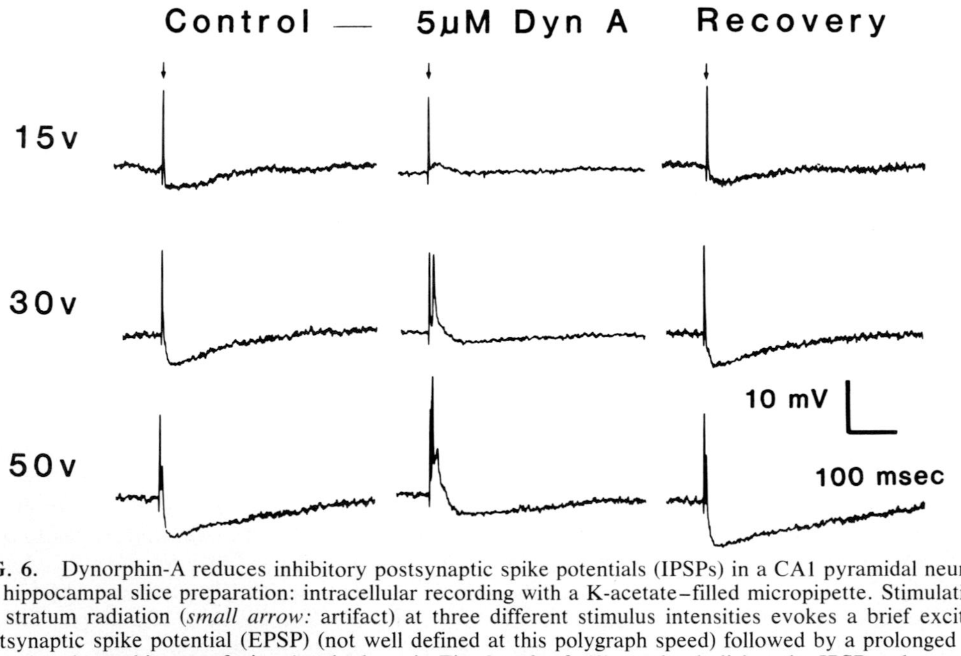

FIG. 6. Dynorphin-A reduces inhibitory postsynaptic spike potentials (IPSPs) in a CA1 pyramidal neuron in the hippocampal slice preparation: intracellular recording with a K-acetate–filled micropipette. Stimulation of the stratum radiation (*small arrow:* artifact) at three different stimulus intensities evokes a brief excitatory postsynaptic spike potential (EPSP) (not well defined at this polygraph speed) followed by a prolonged IPSP. Note that dynorphin superfusion (methods as in Fig. 2 and ref. 49) nearly abolishes the IPSP and appears to enhance the EPSP, probably by removing the "shunting" effect of the IPSP. There was no dynorphin effect on membrane potential or resistance in this cell. Thus, this data is consistent with a disinhibitory action of dynorphin in CA1, as postulated for the action of other opioids in this region.

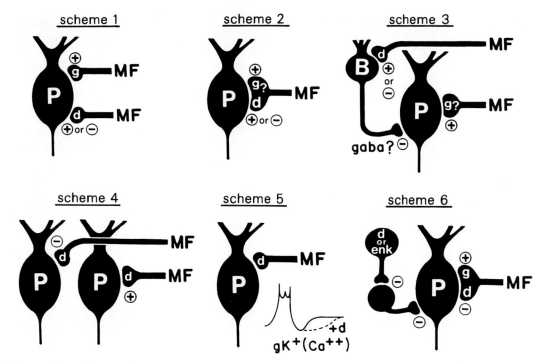

FIG. 7. Several hypothetical schemes for the function of dynorphin in the CA3 hippocampus. Dynorphin (d) may be contained within mossy fibers (MF) in the CA3 fields, either in mossy fibers separate from those containing glutamate (g) as in scheme 1 or as a co-transmitter with glutamate (scheme 2). In the latter case, it may act presynaptically to alter release of glutamate from the same or other terminals, perhaps through a voltage-dependent mechanism (see scheme 5). It may have either direct excitatory (+) or inhibitory (−) actions on pyramidal (P) cells in these two schemes. Dynorphin may also exist in mossy fibers projecting to inhibitory interneurons that may be either inhibited or excited by dynorphin (scheme 3). Dynorphin may have different direct effects on different pyramidal cells in CA3 (scheme 4), or may alter voltage-dependent conductances (e.g., Ca^{2+} or Ca^{2+}-dependent K^+ conductances) such as those responsible for the afterhyperpolarization following bursts of spikes (scheme 5; see ref. 58). Finally, dynorphin in interneurons may act like enkephalin by inhibiting other interneurons, whereas its release from mossy fibers could directly affect pyramidal cells or the MF terminals (scheme 6).

μM dynorphin-A(1–17) dramatically reduces the amplitude of evoked IPSPs (Fig. 6) without effect on resting membrane properties (C. Chavkin and G. R. Siggins, *unpublished observations*) as previously shown for other opioids acting at μ receptors and δ receptors (15,16, 33,38,48,49). It remains for future research to establish whether multiple opiate receptor subtypes also exist in the CA3 fields, as suggested by the single-unit *in vivo* studies showing different response types to different opiate agonists (22–24, 41; see above).

DISCUSSION

It is clear from the foregoing discussion that opioid peptides exist in the hippocampus and can dramatically influence neuronal excitability.

The question still remains as to whether endogenous opioids are actually involved in limbic epilepsies. However, in light of the data described, the presence of multiple opiate receptors in the hippocampus could explain the complex cellular and EEG effects of the various opioid peptides. These multiple receptors could therefore clarify a possible role of opioid peptides in limbic epilepsy. Hence, opioid peptides of the endorphin–enkephalin groups and morphine-like opiate alkaloids, which act at μ receptors and δ receptors, appear to be predominantly excitatory in the hippocampus. The dynorphins exhibit both excitatory and inhibitory effects, perhaps through actions at both μ receptors and κ receptors. It seems likely that the predominant receptors involved in opioid effects in the CA1 hippocampus are of the μ and δ subtypes, whereas κ receptors also may be involved in CA3 opioid responses.

Such an arrangement of opioid receptors may also help to explain the immunohistochemical and immunoassay data. Thus, whereas dynorphin has been detected in a few scattered cells and fibers in CA1, the predominant opioid peptides here appear to be derived from pro-enkephalin and contained in interneuron-like cells. In contrast, pro-dynorphin–related peptides predominate in CA3 hippocampus in apparent mossy fibers projecting from dentate gyrus, although there are scattered enkephalin-IR–containing interneurons in CA3 as well. There seem to be relatively low levels of pro-enkephalin–derived peptides in the mossy fiber pathway per se; therefore, their possible role in this system is currently unclear.

Our speculation is that the enkephalin-containing cells in CA1 (and perhaps also in CA3) project to inhibitory interneurons and provide inhibitory control of these neurons. The enkephalin-containing neurons could thus be strategically situated to regulate the degree of recurrent and feed-forward inhibition exerted on the major output cell, the pyramidal neuron, by the other inhibitory interneurons. Therefore, any condition that selectively increased the tonic discharge of these enkephalin-containing cells could reduce the degree of recurrent and feed-forward inhibition of pyramidal cells, resulting in their exhanced excitability. Given the feed-forward excitatory nature of the collateral connections between pyramidal cells in the hippocampus, it is easy to see how such reduced inhibition could result in recurrent epileptiform activity.

In contrast, although research in this area is still incomplete, the dynorphin-containing mossy fiber projection to CA3 pyramidal cells may be at least partially inhibitory. Activation of these dynorphin fibers could effectively dampen excitatory or even epileptic transmission through this important link in the trisynaptic loop through the hippocampus (50). However, exogenous dynorphin may have dual actions in this area, directly inhibiting pyramidal neurons through κ receptors and indirectly exciting them by inhibiting neighboring inhibitory interneurons through μ receptors. Another avenue to be explored is the possibility that dynorphin, acting on presynaptic κ receptors, could alter voltage-dependent ionic conductances and/or transmitter release, perhaps by the reduction of calcium currents entering synaptic terminals (e.g., mossy fiber endings) during an action potential. Such a dynorphin mechanism

(reduction of the duration of calcium-dependent action potentials) has been proposed for dorsal root ganglia and their primary afferent fibers (58). By so acting at mossy fiber endings, dynorphin would again have a net inhibitory effect on the CA3 pyramidal cells. Such multiple actions could account for the mixed and inconsistent effects of dynorphin in field potential studies of CA3 in the hippocampal slice (19). Several alternative roles for dynorphin in CA3 are schematized in Fig. 7.

The inhibitory effects of dynorphin might also explain why this peptide does not have epileptogenic EEG effects when injected intraventricularly, whereas β-endorphin and the enkephalins do. Although dynorphin can exert excitatory actions on CA1 pyramidal cells (by disinhibition), it may inhibit enough CA3 pyramidal cells to prevent spread of this excitation. In contrast, β-endorphin and the enkephalins excite all pyramidal neurons, allowing recurrent excitation to spread throughout the hippocampus.

Recent studies by Tortella et al. (52) support the idea of the inhibitory influence of dynorphin acting at κ receptors. Thus, subcutaneous (s.c.) or intracerebroventricular (i.c.v.) injection of the specific κ agonist, U50,488, provides protection against certain electroshock-induced seizures in rats (52). These and other studies also suggest that certain seizures (perhaps those of limbic origin) may be treated by some κ-selective opiate-related drugs. The possibility that postictal depression results from release into cerebrospinal fluid of an opioid-like substance (32) may be a related finding. These new directions in opioid research could provide hope for future understanding and treatment of the limbic epilepsies.

ACKNOWLEDGMENTS

We thank Drs. R. Valentino, J. McGinty, and G. Chouvet for allowing us to summarize portions of our collaborative work and Drs. N. Ling and R. Guillemin for providing the opioid peptides. We also thank Ms. Nancy Callahan for typing the manuscript. Our original data reported here were supported by grant Nos. (DA 03665 and AA 06420) from the U.S. Public Health Service and the Klingenstein Foundation.

REFERENCES

1. Bayon, A., Shoemaker, W. J., McGinty, J. F., and Bloom, F. E. (1983): Immunodetection of endorphins and enkephalins: A search for reli-

ability. In: *International Review of Neurobiology*, Vol. 24, pp. 51–92. Academic Press, Orlando, Fla.

2. Bloom, F. E., and McGinty, J. (1981): Cellular distribution and functions of endorphins. In: *Endogenous Peptides and Learning and Memory Processes*, edited by J. McGaugh and J. Martinez, pp. 199–229. Academic Press, Orlando, Fla.

3. Bloom, F. E., Segal, D., Ling, N., and Guillemin, R. (1976): Endorphins: Profound behavioral effects in rats suggest new etiological factors in mental illness. *Science*, 194:630–632.

4. Burley, E. S., and Ferrendelli, J. A. (1984): Regulatory effects of neurotransmitters on electroshock and pentylenetetrazol seizures. *Fed. Proc.* 43:2521–2524.

5. Chavkin, C., Bakhit, C., and Bloom, F. E. (1983): Evidence for dynorphin-A as a neurotransmitter in rat hippocampus. *Life Sci.*, 33:13–16.

6. Chavkin, C., Bakhit, C., Weber, E., and Bloom, F. E. (1983): Relative contents and concomitant release of prodynorphin/neoendorphin-derived peptides in rat hippocampus. *Proc. Natl. Acad. Sci. USA*, 80:7669–7673.

7. Chavkin, C., Henriksen, S. J., Siggins, G. R., and Bloom, F. E. (1985): Selective inactivation of opioid receptors in rat hippocampus demonstrates that dynorphin A and B act on mu receptors in CA1. *Brain Res.*, 331:366–370.

8. Chavkin, C., James, F. F., and Goldstein, A. (1982): Dynorphin is a specific endogenous ligand of the kappa opioid receptor. *Science*, 215:413–415.

9. Corrigall, W. A. (1983): Opiates and the hippocampus: A review of the functional and morphological evidence. *Pharmacol. Biochem. Behav.* 18:255–262.

10. Craig, C. R. (1984): Evidence for a role of neurotransmitters in the mechanism of topical convulsant models. *Fed. Proc.*, 43:2525–2528.

11. Dingledine, R. (1981): Possible mechanisms of enkephalin action on hippocampal CA1 pyramidal neurons. *J. Neurosci.* 1:1022–1035.

12. Dunwiddie, T., Mueller, A., Palmer M., Stewart, J., and Hoffer, B. (1980): Electrophysiological interactions of enkephalins with neuronal circuitry in the rat hippocampus. I. Effects on pyramidal cell activity. *Brain Res.*, 184:311–330.

13. Frederickson, R. C. A. (1977): Enkephalin pentapeptides—A review of current evidence for a physiological role in vertebrate neurotransmission. *Life Sci.*, 21:23–40.

14. French, E. D., and Siggins, G. (1980): An iontophoretic survey of opioid peptide actions in the rat limbic system: In search of opiate epileptogenic mechanisms. *Reg. Peptides*, 1:127–146.

15. Gähwiler, B. H., and Herrling, P. L. (1981): Effects of opioid peptides on synaptic potentials in explants of rat hippocampus. *Reg. Peptides*, 1:317–326.

16. Gähwiler, B. H. (1980): Excitatory action of opioid peptides and opiates on cultured hippocampal pyramidal cells. *Brain Res.*, 194:193–203.

17. Gall, C., Brecha, N., Karten, H. J., and Chang, K. (1981): Localization of enkephalin-like immunoreactivity to identified axonal and neuronal populations of the rat hippocampus. *J. Comp. Neurol.*, 198:335–350.

18. Goldstein, A., Tachibana, S., Lowney, L. I., Hunkapiller, M., and Hood, L. (1979): Dynorphin-(1-13), an extraordinarily potent opioid peptide. *Proc. Natl. Acad. Sci. USA*, 76:6666–6670.

19. Gruol, D. L., Chavkin, C., Valentino, R. J., and Siggins, G. R. (1983): Dynorphin-A alters the excitability of pyramidal neurons of the rat hippocampus in vitro. *Life Sci.*, 33:533–536.

20. Haas, H. L., and Ryall, R. W. (1980): Is excitation by enkephalins of hippocampal neurones in the rat due to presynaptic facilitation or to disinhibition? *J. Physiol.*, 308:315–330.

21. Henriksen, S. J., Bloom, F. E., McCoy, F., Ling, N., and Guillemin, R. (1978): β-endorphin induces nonconvulsive limbic seizures. *Proc. Natl. Acad. Sci. USA*, 75:5221–5225.

22. Henriksen, S. J., Chouvet, G., and Bloom, F. E. (1982): *In vivo* cellular responses to electrophoretically applied dynorphin in the rat hippocampus. *Life Sci.*, 31:1785–1788.

23. Henriksen, S. J., Chouvet, G., McGinty, J., and Bloom, F. E. (1982): Opioid peptides in the hippocampus: Anatomical and physiological considerations. *Ann. N.Y. Acad. Sci.*, 398:207–220.

24. Henriksen, S., Chouvet, G., McGinty, J., and Bloom, F. E. (1983): Neuropeptides and the epilepsies: Current perspectives. In: *Epilepsy: An Update on Research and Therapy*. Alan R. Liss, New York, pp. 105–120.

25. Hill, R. G., Mitchell, J. F., and Pepper, C. M. (1977): The excitation and depression of hippocampal neurons by iontophoretically applied enkephalins. *J. Physiol.*, 272:50–51P.

26. Hökfelt, T., Elde, R., Johansson, O., Terenius, L., and Stein, L. (1977): The distribution of enkephalin-immunoreactive cell bodies in rat central nervous system. *Neurosci. Lett.*, 5:25–31.

27. Hong, J. S., and Schmid, R. (1981): Intrahippocampal distribution of Met-enkephalin. *Brain Res.*, 205:415–418.

28. Khachaturian, H., Lewis, M., Hollt, V., and Watson, S. (1983): Telencephalic enkephalinergic systems in the rat brain. *J. Neurosci.*, 3:844.

29. Killam, E. K., and Killam, K. F., Jr. (1984): Evidence for neurotransmitter abnormalities related to seizure activity in the epileptic baboon. *Fed. Proc.*, 43:2510–2515.

30. Laird, H. E. II, Daily, J. W., and Jobe, P. C. (1984): Neurotransmitter abnormalities in genetically epileptic rodents. *Fed. Proc.*, 43:2505–2509.

31. Lee, H. K., Dunwiddie, T., and Hoffer, B. (1980): Electrophysiological interactions of enkephalins with neuronal circuitry in the rat hippocampus. II. Effects on interneuron excitability. *Brain Res.*, 184:331–342.

32. Long, J. B., and Tortella, F. C. (1984): Cerebrospinal fluid from convulsed rats causes a naloxone-reversible increase in the seizure threshold of recipient animals: Regulation of

postseizure inhibition by endogenous opioid systems. *Soc. Neurosci. Abstr.*, 10:929.

33. Masukawa, L. M., and Prince, D. A. (1982): Enkephalin inhibition of inhibitory input to CA1 and CA3 pyramidal neurons in the hippocampus. *Brain Res.*, 249:271–280.

34. Matsumoto, H. (1964): Intracellular events during the activation of cortical epileptiform discharges. *Electroencephalogr. Clin. Neurophysiol.*, 17:294–307.

35. McGinty, J. F., Henriksen, S. J., Goldstein, A., Terenius, L., and Bloom, F. E.: Dynorphin is contained within hippocampal mossy fibers: Immunochemical alterations after kainic acid administration and colchicine-induced neurotoxicity. *Proc. Natl. Acad. Sci. USA*, 90:589–593.

36. McNamara, J. O. (1984): Role of neurotransmitters in seizure mechanisms in the kindling model of epilepsy: *Fed. Proc.*, 43:2516–2520.

37. Nicoll, R. A. (1982): Responses of central neurons to opiates and opioid peptides. In: *Regulatory Peptides: From Molecular Biology to Function*, edited by E. Costa and M. Trabucchi, pp. 337–346. Raven Press, New York.

38. Nicoll, R. A., Alger, B. E., and Jahr, C. E. (1980): Enkephalin blocks inhibitory pathways in the vertebrate CNS. *Nature*, 287:22–25.

39. Nicoll, R. A., Alger, B. E., and Jahr, C. E. (1980): Peptides as putative excitatory neurotransmitters: Carnosine, enkephalin, substance P and TRH. *Proc. R. Soc. (Lond.) B.*, 210:133–149.

40. Nicoll, R. A., and Madison, D. V. (1984): The action of enkephalin on interneurons in the hippocampus. *Soc. Neurosci. Abstr.*, 10:660.

41. Nicoll, R. A., Siggins, G. R., Ling, N., Bloom, F. E., and Guillemin, R. (1977): Neuronal actions of endorphin and enkephalin among brain regions: A comparative microiontophoretic study. *Proc. Natl. Acad. Sci. USA*, 74:2584–2588.

42. North, R. A. (1979): Opiates, opioid peptides and single neurones. *Life Sci.*, 24:1527–1546.

43. Prince, D. (1978): Neurophysiology of epilepsy. In: *Annu. Rev. Neurosci.*, edited by M. W. Cowan, Z. W. Hall, and E. R. Kandel, pp. 395–415. Annual Review, Palo Alto.

44. Robinson, J. H., and Deadwyler, S. A. (1981): Intracellular correlates of morphine excitation in the hippocampal slice preparation. *Brain Res.*, 224:375–387.

45. Ryall, R. W., and Kelly, J. S., eds. (1978): *Iontophoresis and Transmitter Mechanisms in the Mammalian Central Nervous System*. Elsevier North Holland, Amsterdam.

46. Sar, M., Stumpf, W. E., Miller, R. J., Chang, K-J, and Cuatracasas, P. (1978): Immunohistochemical localization of enkephalin in the rat brain and spinal cord. *J. Comp. Neurol.*, 187:17–38.

47. Siggins, G. R., and Gruol, D. L. (1985): Synaptic mechanisms in the vertebrate central nervous system. In: *Handbook of Physiology, Volume on Intrinsic Regulatory Systems of the Brain*, edited by F. E. Bloom. The American Physiological Society (*in press*).

48. Siggins, G. R., McGinty, J. F., Morrison, J. H., Pittman, Q. J., Zieglgänsberger W., Magistretti, P. J., and Gruol, D. L. (1982): *The Role of Neuropeptides in the Hippocampal Formation*, edited by E. Costa and M. Trabucchi, pp. 413–422. Raven Press, New York.

49. Siggins, G. R., and Zieglgänsberger, W. (1981): Morphine and opioid peptides reduce inhibitory synaptic potentials in hippocampal pyramidal cells *in vitro* without alteration of membrane potential. *Proc. Natl. Acad. Sci. USA*, 78:5235–5239.

50. Swanson, L. W., Teyler, T. J., and Thompson, R. F. (1982): Hippocampal long-term potentiation: Mechanisms and implications for memory. In: *Neuroscience Research Program Bulletin*, Vol. 20, MIT Press, Cambridge, Massachusetts.

51. Taylor, D., Hoffer, B., Zieglgänsberger, W., Siggins, G., Ling, N., Seiger, A., and Olson, L. (1979): Opioid peptides excite pyramidal neurons and evoke epileptiform activity in hippocampal transplants *in oculo*. *Brain Res.*, 176:135–142.

52. Tortella, F. C., Robles, L., and Holaday, J. W. (1984): Seizure-specific, dose- and time-dependent anticonvulsant profile for U50,488, a novel κ opioid agonist, in rats. *Soc. Neurosci. Abstr.*, 10:408.

53. Uhl, G., Goodman, R., Childers, S., and Snyder, S. (1978): Immunohistochemical mapping of enkephalin containing cell bodies and nerve terminals in the brain stem of the rat brain. *Brain Res.*, 166:75–94.

54. Urca, G., Frenk, H., Liebeskind, J. C., and Taylor, A. N. (1977): Morphine and enkephalin: Analgesic and epileptic properties. *Science*, 197:83–86.

55. Valentino, R. J., and Dingledine, R. (1982): Pharmacological characterization of opioid effects in the rat hippocampal slice. *J. Pharmacol. Exp. Ther.*, 223:502–509.

56. Walker, J. M., Moises, H. C., Coy, D. H., Baldrighi, G., and Akil, H. (1982): Nonopiate effects of dynorphin and des-tyr-dynorphin. *Science*, 218:1136–1138.

57. Wamsley, J., Young, W., and Kuhar, M. (1980): Immunohistochemical localization of enkephalin in rat forebrain. *Brain Res.*, 190:153–174.

58. Werz, M. A., and Macdonald, R. L. (1984): Dynorphin decreases a voltage-dependent Ca conductance in mouse dorsal root ganglion neurons in cell culture. *Neurosci. Lett.*, 46:185–190.

59. Woodbury, D. M. (1984): Neurotransmitters and epilepsy: Distinguishing characteristics and unifying precepts. *Fed. Proc.*, 43:2529–2531.

60. Zieglgänsberger, W., French, E. D., Siggins, G. R., and Bloom, F. E. (1979): Opioid peptides may excite hippocampal pyramidal neurons by inhibiting adjacent inhibitory interneurons. *Science*, 205:415–417.

61. Zieglgänsberger, W., and Fry, J. (1976): Actions of enkephalins on cortical and striatal neurones of naive and morphine/tolerant dependent rats. In: *Opiates and Endogenous Opioid Peptides*, edited by H. Kosterlitz, pp. 213–238. Elsevier, Amsterdam.

Section 5

SPREAD AND ARREST
OF SEIZURES

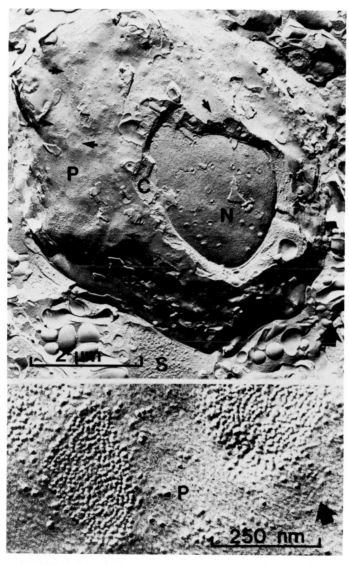

Gap junction in freeze-fracture replica of a dentate granule cell in the rat hippocampus. A: soma of the granule cell; B: two gap junctions. (From the data of B. A. MacVicar and F. E. Dudek, ref. 73 of Chapter 30; reprinted from ref. 22, Chapter 30, with permission.)

Advances in Neurology, Vol. 44, edited by
A. V. Delgado-Escueta, A. A. Ward, Jr.,
D. M. Woodbury, and R. J. Porter.
Raven Press, New York © 1986.

27

Spread and Arrest of Seizures: The Importance of Layer 4 in Laminar Interactions During Neocortical Epileptogenesis

John S. Ebersole and Allen B. Chatt

*Epilepsy Center, Neurology Service, Veterans Administration Medical Center, West Haven, Connecticut
06516 and Department of Neurology, Yale University School of Medicine, New Haven, Connecticut 06510*

SUMMARY   Much of the past investigation of epileptogenesis has centered on characterizing the paroxysmal depolarization shift (PDS) and postulating its origin. Spatial as well as functional analyses of cortical epileptic foci have been few in number, and in nearly all of them fully evolved drug foci, which were used for their stability, probably obscured differences in the responsivity among constituent neuronal populations at earlier stages of epileptic evolution. Proportionately little attention has been directed at determining where penicillin acts within the cortex. For the past 12 years, we have addressed both issues. Specific questions have included, for both individual neurons and neuronal aggregates: (a) what are the initial abnormalities of responsiveness in an acute epileptic focus; (b) how do these abnormalities evolve as the focus develops; (c) is there a differential susceptibility of various neocortical layers to epileptogenesis; (d) how do the various cortical laminar populations interact during epileptogenesis; (5) how do the resultant response abnormalities propagate within and between cortical columns; and (f) what are the effects of anticonvulsants on the various spatial and temporal features of epileptogenesis?

In pursuit of this information, we have recorded the evolution of discrete and temporary epileptic foci in cat striate cortex, which were induced by the microinjection or iontophoresis of penicillin into the different cortical layers. Simultaneous, multilaminar responses of individual neurons and of neuronal aggregates to selective visual stimulation have been characterized before, during, and after focus development using multibarrel micropipettes. Correlations between drug diffusion and these multilaminar recordings were made periodically by using ^{14}C-labeled penicillin.

Stages: Using these techniques, new characteristics of focal epilepsy come to light that are not apparent in the spontaneous spiking of the typical established penicillin focus. Three successive stages of penicillin-induced epileptogenic abnormality were noted in the responses of isolated neurons: (a) an initial graded enhancement of the primary latency response to field-specific stimuli into a burst discharge (the EPR burst); (b) the subsequent graded development of a longer latency burst in response to field-specific and nonspecific stimuli (the LR burst); and (c) the evolution of a single stereotyped burst discharge (IIS) as the latency separating EPR and LR bursts declined (PDS or LR discharge). Each type of neuronal burst was accompanied by a local field potential of similar latency, but of progressively increasing amplitude, with each successive stage of epileptogenesis.

It is our belief that the EPR neuronal burst and its counterpart field potential reflect an action of penicillin upon the responsiveness of individual neurons that does not require population interactions. The EPR is an abnormal response to a normal input, which is usually monosynaptic and in this case geniculocortical. The LR burst, on the other hand, represents the early stage of the more commonly described PDS, just as its associated LR field potential represents the early graded form of the interictal spike. We believe that the different characteristics of the late response is a reflection of a neuronal population origin. Feedback and feedforward interactions may elaborate the EPRs of a smaller pacemaker population of neurons into an amplified synaptic drive for themselves and other follower members of the aggregate whose responsiveness has also been enhanced by penicillin's disinhibitory action. Unlike the EPR, the LR burst is an abnormal neuronal response to an already enlarged, recurrent, or collateral input. Penicillin epileptogenesis in striate cortex is dependent upon both types of abnormality.

Laminar Susceptibility: Microinjection of penicillin into various cortical laminae is not equally effective in inducing epileptogenesis. Layer 4 of striate visual cortex was found to be the most sensitive. Successive stages of epileptiform abnormalities, both evoked and spontaneous, were induced more rapidly and more fully with injection into layer 4 than with comparable injections in the other laminae. In the case of a layer 4 focus, both EPR and LR abnormalities originated from the injection site and resulted solely from penicillin's effect within that layer. Although late responses could be induced independently at more superficial or deeper injection sites, latency to the onset of response abnormality was significantly longer, and a penicillin-induced enhancement of the layer 4 primary response was always an initial abnormality. Autoradiography of sections from a cortical biopsy removed at the onset of LR abnormalities verified that ^{14}C-labeled penicillin confined to layer 4 was sufficient for epileptogenesis, whereas tissue removed at the same stage from superficial and deep foci revealed penicillin infiltration into layer 4. The decreased sensitivity of the pyramidal layers to epileptogenic alteration may be related to different types and/or increased levels of inhibitory modulation present within them, that are less easily overcome by penicillin's partial GABA blockade than that in stellate layer 4.

Laminar Interactions: Functional relationships among cortical layers were assessed by observing the development of epileptiform response abnormalities in one layer and their concomitant expression in the others. Most impressive was the close response coupling between the development of LR abnormalities in stellate layer 4 and their immediate reflection in pyramidal layers 2–3. Recruitment of these superficial layers was shown autoradiographically not to be a function of penicillin diffusion, but more likely a result of LR burst propagation from layer 4. Other close functional associations were noted between deep pyramidal layers 5–6 and layer 4 and, to a lesser extent, between layers 2–3 and 5–6. In these foci, LRs evolving in the former layers were preferentially propagated to the latter. In both these instances, however, response alterations evolved more slowly than with microinjection into layer 4, thereby allowing for additional penicillin diffusion. Significantly, the initial abnormality in both was the development of EPRs in layer 4. We assume that these provided the evolving foci in the pyramidal layers with an enhanced, but otherwise normal, synaptic trigger which synchronized epileptogenic neuronal interactions there. It is of considerable interest that these close functional relationships exist only between cortical layers with subpopulations of neurons known to possess direct anatomical connections by means of axon collaterals. Where normal connectivity is sparse or absent, however, epileptiform response abnormality spreads more slowly and appears to be dependent upon the diffusion of penicillin, i.e., the development of response abnormalities in layer 4 with a layer 2–3 focus, in layer 5–6 with a layer 4 focus, and perhaps in layers 2–3 with a layer 5–6 focus.

Anticonvulsant Effects: A differential laminar action of intravenous phenytoin (PHT) upon the evolution of discrete penicillin foci induced in striate layer 4 has also been characterized. At therapeutic serum levels, spontaneous LRs and IISs from all cortical layers were suppressed, but remained elicitable by physiologic stimulation. The evoked epileptiform responses from superficial layers 2–3, however, were disproportionately delayed in development and reduced in amplitude as compared to those from the layer 4 focus. This differential effect of PHT upon those layers which normally can both elaborate and then disseminate epileptiform discharges to surrounding cortex may be the reason for PHTs purported clinical effect in preventing seizure spread. Preliminary data from similar experiments utilizing phenobarbital showed instead a more uniform translaminar suppression of evoked epileptiform potentials. Phenobarbital seems to act to control epileptogenesis at the pacer level within the focus proper and not (preferentially) its spread to follower populations.

Since the demonstration approximately 20 years ago that a paroxysmal depolarization shift (PDS) was the neuronal discharge underlying the electrocorticographic interictal spike in penicillin focal epilepsy (50), there has been a continuing controversy over its origin. For the first 10 years, the concept of abnormal cellular interaction within the "epileptic aggregate" dominated thinking as a result of *in vivo* intracellular experiments which suggested that PDSs were giant, probably recurrent, excitatory postsynaptic potentials (EPSPs) (see ref. 4 for review). The enhanced synaptic barrage of this theory necessitated an initial response abnormality somewhere in the proposed feedback loops. A candidate for this abnormality was later identified by us as an enhancement of normal neuronal responsivity to cell-specific input—the enhanced physiologic response (EPR)—which preceded PDS development (17). The effect of penicillin was thought probably to be directed at synapses on dendrites since earlier investigations showed normal soma membrane characteristics between discharges (1,14).

The identification of nonsynaptic factors in epileptogenesis, namely axonal antidromic bursting (the "backfiring" phenomenon) (31,81) and extracellular potassium changes accompanying the development of an epileptic focus (23,57,72) added to our understanding of epileptic phenomena. These factors could not resolve the etiology question, however, since both phenomena tended to follow rather than precede PDSs and were accordingly thought to be related to ictal development (32,59).

Within the past 6 years, with the advent of *in vitro* recordings from hippocampal slices, there was a resurgence of interest in the idea of "intrinsic" cellular abnormalities in spike generation, i.e., the "epileptic neuron" (69,80). It was suggested that PDSs induced by penicillin arise from a calcium-mediated current at distant dendritic sites, and that the synaptic input to affected neurons during epileptogenesis, even if recurrent and enhanced, provides only a synchronous trigger for the abnormal mechanism by which they generate their own PDSs (69). In their 1980 general hypothesis on the mechanisms underlying epileptiform discharges, Schwartzkroin and Wyler (80) similarly concluded that burst firing is an intrinsic neuronal property that may be released or triggered by a variety of external influences. In the case of penicillin, a reduction of γ-aminobutyric acid (GABA)-mediated inhibition, which usually dissipates current before reaching the soma, would give excitatory afferents the enhanced effectiveness necessary to trigger intrinsic epileptiform bursts.

Based on *in vivo* field potential and cellular observations, we continued to believe that the two basic theories of focal penicillin epilepsy were not mutually exclusive, but that both intrinsic neuronal and population interaction abnormalities were requisite for neocortical epileptogenesis (19). Current *in vitro* experimentation with the neocortex slice preparation is now also tending to support this concept, as will be discussed later (33).

It is our belief that the divergent observations, which prevented the two basic theories of epileptogenesis from being unified sooner, was a function of the experimental models used. Much of the previous *in vivo* experimentation used the topical application of penicillin by various strategies. All depended upon diffusion of penicillin into the cortex, and most awaited the development of spontaneous interictal spike potentials as their measure of epileptogenesis. Early changes in the normal responsiveness of neurons from a direct effect of penicillin or that resultant from the early stages of population interaction cannot be appreciated easily in these relatively large, fully developed epileptic foci, especially if only spontaneous activity or that evoked by nonphysiologic stimuli is recorded. Any consideration of a differential epileptogenic sensitivity of the various cortical laminae and their constituent cellular elements is necessarily biased toward the superficial layers, which are affected first and with higher drug concentrations.

In vitro slice preparations of cortex can pro-

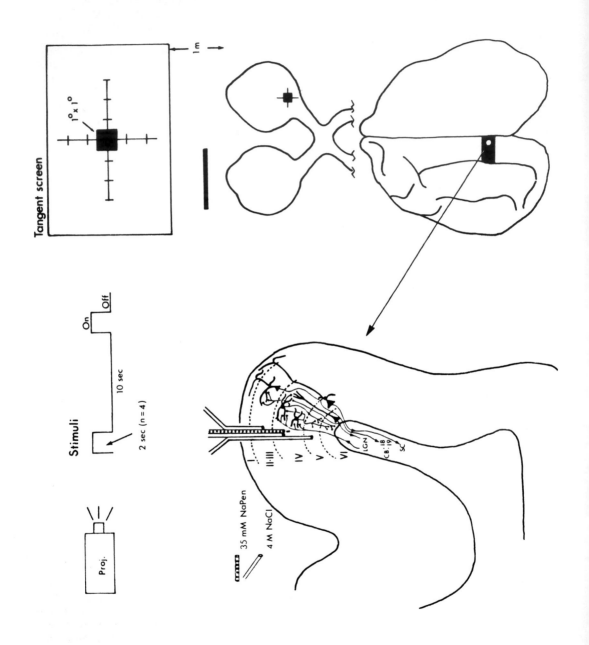

Tangent screen

1°x1°

1 m

Stimuli

On   Off

10 sec

2 sec (n=4)

Proj.

35 mM NaPen

4 M NaCl

I

II-III

IV

V

VI

LGN

CB:18

19

SC

vide detailed information on individual cells and their membrane properties, but the normal local circuit or more distant interactions cannot be assured in the reduced cell population of a slice. Bathing solutions of drugs, nonphysiologic electrical stimulation of afferent pathways and intracellular recordings from single neurons do not facilitate an understanding of the complexities involved in the relationships between the abnormalities of individual neurons and neuronal populations in epileptogenesis. The same limitations apply to a greater degree in studies using isolated cultured neurons.

In the original 1969 volume of basic mechanisms of the epilepsies (37), Jasper began his chapter on seizure propogation by stating that "an understanding of basic mechanisms of the epilepsies can never be achieved by considering properties of single cells alone." This thought remains valid today, for although we have learned much about the basic chemistry and membrane physiology of neurons engaged in burst activity, we also recognize that it is only in the context of intact brain that any of these potential mechanisms for abnormality achieve, or fail to achieve, operational significance. We feel that it is particularly important to have an appreciation for this larger perspective when discussing basic mechanisms, especially as they relate to the spread of seizures. It is the role of *in vivo* research to proceed to the next logical level in complexity and to address questions involving the interaction of populations of neurons.

AN *IN VIVO* MODEL OF NEOCORTICAL EPILEPTOGENESIS

Over the past 10 years, our laboratory has directed its attention toward problems at the level of individual neurons and neuronal aggregates. This chapter will involve a discussion of the background surrounding these problems as well as the status of our current understanding. A number of specific questions have been asked. What are the initial abnormalities of responsiveness in an acute epileptic focus? How do these abnormalities evolve as the focus develops? Is there a differential susceptibility of various neocortical layers to epileptogenesis? Do specific neocortical subpopulations participate differently in epileptogenesis? How do resultant response abnormalities propagate within and between cortical columns? Finally, what are the effects of various anticonvulsant drugs on these spatially and temporally fractionated abnormalities?

We have chosen to sacrifice the intracellular knowledge of membrane potentials and currents within individual cells for the larger perspective provided by the extracellular recording of neurons and neuronal populations. The experimental model we used involved several basic departures from most of the previous investigations of mammalian epileptic phenomena (Fig. 1). First, cat visual cortex was chosen for study rather than the more customary motor, somatosensory, or hippocampal cortex. Visual neurons offer distinct advantages since their responses are easily elicitable and consistent and require very specific stimuli. Subtle alteration in a neuron's normal response can be readily detected, therefore, with recurrent testing of its receptive field. Second, physiologic stimulation in the cat's visual field with bars of light of appropriate configuration and location was used instead of clearly nonphysiologic shocks to white or grey matter. The precision and variability of this type of stimulation provided the specificity needed to activate individual cells or small populations of cells selectively. Third, in addition to the responses of isolated units, regional field potentials were recorded from small populations of neurons within cortical laminae rather than just from the brain's surface. Fourth, microinjection or microiontophoresis of penicillin, rather than topical application, produced an epileptic focus that was discrete, temporary, and repeatable. These methods allow involved neurons or neuron populations to be characterized before, during, and after the development of an epileptic focus. Fifth, instead of looking at only one cortical area, simultaneous two- and three-lamina monitoring of both local field potentials and multiple-unit activity was accomplished by means of multiple-barreled micropipettes fabricated with longitudinal tip separations. At one of the three levels, penicillin can be microinjected through a second barrel of a twin pipette. By this method, responses from

FIG. 1. A schematic representation of the most recent stimulation and recording techniques utilized in the cat visual cortex model of acute penicillin epileptogenesis. Note the recurrent field-specific photic stimuli and four-barrel microelectrodes that were used. The latter, fabricated in several configurations, provided simultaneous monitoring of response activity in three different layers plus the capability of microinjecting penicillin into any one of them. A 10-sec interval between stimulus trains of 4 on–off alterations provided a period in which spontaneous spike development could be evaluated.

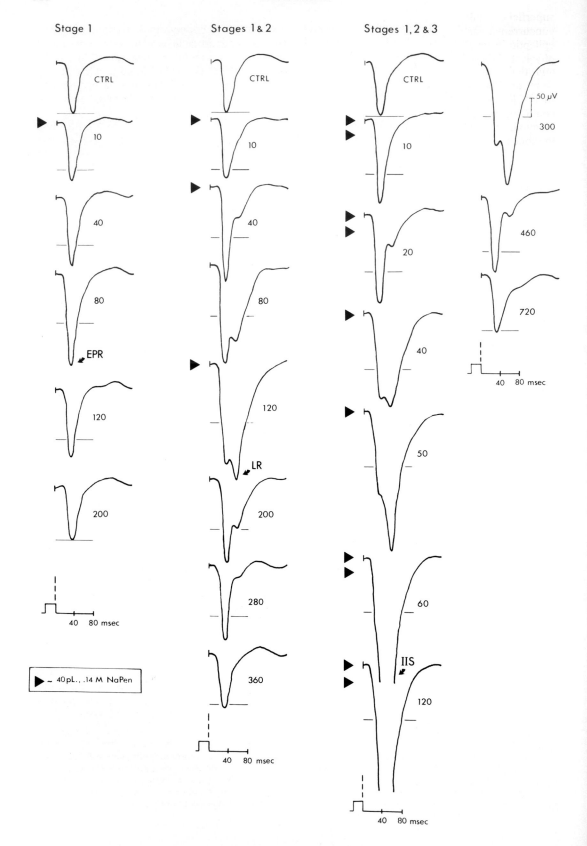

Stage 1

Stages 1 & 2

Stages 1, 2 & 3

CTRL

CTRL

CTRL

50 μV

10

10

10

300

40

40

20

460

80

80

40

720

EPR

120

40   80 msec

120

120

LR

50

200

200

40   80 msec

280

60

~ 40 pL., .14 M NaPen

360

IIS

120

40   80 msec

40   80 msec

superficial, middle, and deep laminae can be concurrently sampled during the evolution of an epileptic focus at one of these sites. Finally, the physical distribution of penicillin with the cortex and the histologic location of injection sites were documented by means of dye marking or [^{14}C]penicillin autoradiography. Correlations could be made between epileptic pathophysiology and the extent of penicillin diffusion from the focus origin.

Evolution of Epileptiform Abnormalities: Intracortical Field Potentials

Initial Response Alterations

Using the techniques just described, new characteristics of focal epilepsy have come to light (7,19,20) that were not apparent in the spontaneous spiking of the typical penicillin focus. A punctate 1°-square stimulus in the visual field will activate a small region of striate cortex and elicit therein a simple negative field potential that has its maximum at a depth of approximately 1,000 μm, which corresponds to layer 4 (see Fig. 12). Microiontophoresis or microinjection of penicillin in picoliter to nanoliter quantities at this depth induces a consistent and systematic sequence of changes in local responsiveness. The earliest and most elemental effect of penicillin is an enhancement in the amplitude of the primary latency evoked potential (Fig. 2, stage 1). This effect is graded, temporary, and related in a quantitative fashion to the amount of penicillin injected. This EPR can be seen in isolation with small injections of penicillin early in the development of a penicillin epileptic focus or as the last remaining effect during the decline of a focus. It can be seen without any evidence of change in the surface electrocorticogram (ECoG) and without any longer latency potentials. Because it is both the first and last effect and can be seen separately, the EPR must require the lowest penicillin concentration and/or

the smallest population of cells affected by penicillin.

Late Response Alterations

Repeated small microinjections or a larger introduction of penicillin induces, in addition to the EPR, the development of a new potential with properties clearly different from the EPR (Fig. 2, stage 2). We have called these potentials, late responses or LRs, since they arise at a latency longer than the EPR and do not evolve directly from them. These LRs are not initially stereotyped, but are graded with both development and decline of the penicillin focus and are somewhat variable in both amplitude and latency at any one stage. Only at the height of such foci are LRs relatively stereotyped and do LRs take on the form of the traditional interictal spike (IIS). At this level of development, the early latency EPR component is obscured, although it can be shown to be still present by manipulations of stimulus rate and intensity. It is this response (Fig. 2, stage 3), which does not reveal what has gone before it, that is likely to be seen with topical penicillin application or larger intracortical injections of convulsant. The LR has a longer refractory period than the EPR. At rates >1/sec, LRs often fail to be elicited with every stimulus and display increased variability in amplitude and latency. Spontaneous interictal activity occurs only at the later stages of LR development, when it is becoming more stereotyped. The configuration of these spontaneous potentials is the same as the evoked response minus the early latency EPR component.

These observations at a field potential level suggested that separate stages of epileptogenesis were available for analysis during the development and decline stages of an epileptic focus, in addition to the stereotyped IIS present at the steady state peak of focus evolution. A closer look at the neuronal response counterparts of these field potentials was clearly indicated.

FIG. 2. Tracings of computer-averaged responses (n = 4) to 1° off stimuli presented to the receptive field center of a striate cell population (P0.5, L2.0; 1,000 μm deep). Responses are recorded before (CTRL), during, and after microejection of 140 mM sodium penicillin (NaPen) from one barrel of a two-barrel micropipette. Three stages of abnormality were dependent on the amount of NaPen injected. Stage 1: a short-lived enhancement of the primary, physiologic response (EPR; latency, 40 msec), which regressed to normal within 200 sec after the microinjection. Stages 1 and 2: additional microinjections following the development of the EPR induced a new response component (late response, LR) at a longer, 60–80 msec latency. Return to normal responses from a stage 2 abnormality required more time (240 sec) following the last microinjection. Stages 1 + 2 + 3: the intracortical-interictal spike (IIS) evolved from the LR component with further microinjection of NaPen. During this stage, the large amplitude of the IIS obscured the EPR. Return to normal activity took 10 min. Right-directed triangles (▶) indicate microinjection of NaPen. Numbers next to responses denote seconds from the first microinjection (from ref. 19).

Evolution of Epileptiform Abnormalities: Isolated Unit Recordings

Initial Neuronal Bursting

Comparable effects were demonstrated by iontophoresis of penicillin in the immediate vicinity of an isolated, striate cortical neuron (17,21). The initial abnormality is an enhancement of the cell's normal or physiologic response to a stimulus appropriate to its receptive field. Advances in the rate of iontophoresis induce a progressive increase in the number and frequency of spikes to form an "EPR burst" (Fig. 3). The nonpreferred stimulus continues to elicit no response discharges. The local intracortical field potential does enlarge somewhat, although to a lesser extent than shown previously, since less penicillin is introduced. No change is evident at the cortical surface, however. A field potential is also evoked by the nonpreferred stimulus, and it too is modestly enlarged, presumably from a penicillin effect on those neighboring cells for which this stimulus was specific.

A similar enhancement of responses from both individual neurons and neuronal populations has been documented as the initial effect of penicillin iontophoresis in cat somatosensory cortex (49). Although more easily appreciated as an alteration of the response to physiologic stimulation, a progressive increase in the spontaneous firing rate of neurons in rat frontal-parietal cortex, unaccompanied by epileptiform burst discharges, was also the first effect of penicillin iontophoresis there (2).

Late Neuronal Bursting

Longer latency spikes with properties distinct from the EPR burst become apparent at higher rates of penicillin iontophoresis into visual cortex (Fig. 4). These LR bursts develop only after an enhancement of the neuron's physiologic response and routinely continue to enlarge after the EPR bursts have stopped increasing. In addition, they are associated with field potentials that progressively increase in amplitude and eventually outstrip the primary latency potentials. In the case of simple cells with responses that are tonic or quasitonic, the new spike bursts typically develop in the previously spike-free period separating the initial from later parts of the response. As these LR bursts evolve, a period of reduced responsiveness follows them, such that one or more of the other bursts with a longer latency are suppressed.

Significantly, the LR bursts are also evoked by a wide variety of nonpreferred stimuli. Stimuli not specific for a neuron's receptive field evoke only the LR burst, but this is preceded by an early field potential, presumably from the enhanced primary responses of neighboring cells for which the stimulus was specific (Fig. 5). Occasionally, simultaneous recordings are made of two or more nearby neurons with their responses being differentiated by their amplitude. In these instances EPRs are elicited from both cells before LRs are evoked in either. When LR bursts do develop, they tend to be synchronous. The neuron preferentially stimulated responds with a combined EPR and LR burst, whereas the neighboring neuron for which the stimulus was not specific responds only with an LR burst. Therefore, at a cellular level, just as at a population level, epileptiform responses are not triggered without preceding local activity.

Spontaneous LR bursts have the same configuration as those evoked by nonpreferred stimulation; i.e., they are unaccompanied by a preceding EPR response (Fig. 6). In addition, the latency between EPR and LR bursts decreases as a focus evolves so that the two appear as one. As in the case of the field potentials, LR neuronal bursts also have a longer refractory period than do EPR bursts.

Unified Theory of Epileptogenesis

It is our belief that the EPR burst and its counterpart field potential reflect an action of penicillin upon the responsiveness of individual neurons that does not require population interactions. The EPR is an abnormal response of neurons to a normal input, which is usually monosynaptic and, in this case, geniculocortical. To this extent, it may be called an intrinsic abnormality, although the basic mechanism is probably a reduction of GABA inhibitory modulation rather than a direct increase in excitatory synaptic input or neuronal responsivity. The LR burst, on the other hand, represents the earliest stage of the more commonly described PDS or depolarization shift (DS), just as its associated LR field potential represents the early graded form of the interictal spike. We believe that the different characteristics of the LR burst are a reflection of a neuronal population origin. This response is most likely based upon excitatory synaptic coupling among the neurons affected by penicillin. Feedback and feed-forward interactions may elaborate the EPRs of a smaller pacemaker population of neurons into a longer latency-amplified synaptic drive for themselves

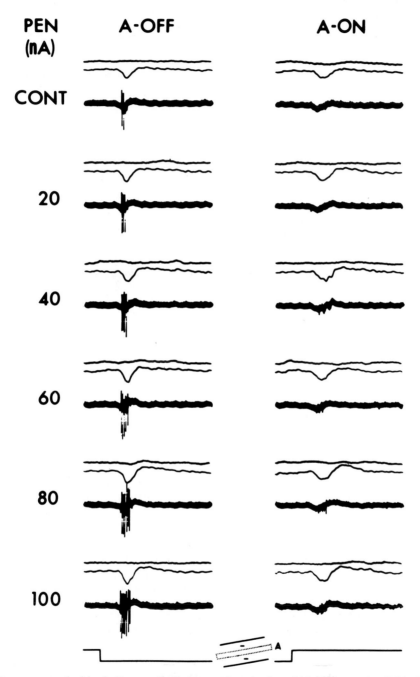

FIG. 3. Responses evoked by both on and off phases of a stimulus within the receptive field of a complex cell. The top trace in each group of three responses is the surface electrocorticogram (ECoG); the second trace is the depth ECoG; and the bottom trace is the microelectrode unit record. Positivity is up for all traces. Note the progressive increase in the number of unit spikes in the response to the preferred off stimulus with advances in the iontophoresis rate, the lack of unitary responses to the nonpreferred stimulus, and the absence of surface interictal potentials. Calibrations ECoG, 125 μV/division; depth ECoG, 1.0 mV/division; microelectrode record, 0.5 mV/division; visual receptive field, 0.5°/division; sweep duration, 200 ms.

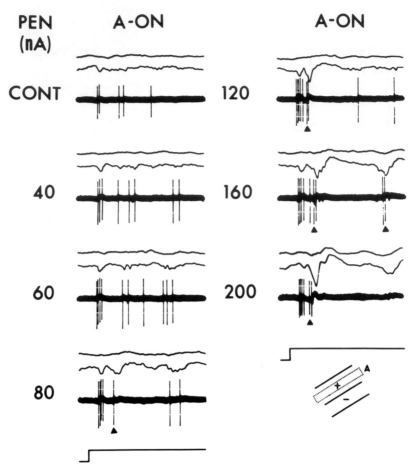

FIG. 4. Responses to a preferred n stimulus in the receptive field of a simple cell. With increases in penicillin iontophoresis (A-on, 80–200 nA) note the development of a late response (▶) in the previous spike-free interval following the initial EPR burst. This LR is associated with a progressively enlarging depth ECoG potential and subsequent period of unit-response suppression. Calibration: ECoG, 125 μV/division; depth ECoG, 1.0 mV/division; microelectrode record, 1.0 mV/division; visual receptive field, 0.4°/division; sweep duration, 500 msec (from ref. 17).

and other follower members of the aggregate whose responsiveness has also been enhanced by the drug. As shown above, the role of a neuron as pacemaker or follower will vary with the specifics of the triggering thalamocortical afference. Unlike the EPR, the LR burst is thus an abnormal neuronal response to an already en-

larged, multisynaptic recurrent or collateral input. In striate cortex at least, penicillin epileptogenesis is dependent on both abnormalities in the response of individual neurons and upon abnormalities of interactions among populations of neurons—a unification of both the epileptic neuron and epileptic aggregate theories.

FIG. 5. Responses to both phases of two stimuli which differ in position. Stimulus A is of preferred orientation within the neuron's receptive field; S is parallel to A, but outside the receptive field. Note the development of LRs and associated ECoG potentials to the surround stimuli (S-off, S-on) with penicillin iontophoresis (~100nA), and to the nonpreferred stimulus (A-on) at a higher rate (~150nA). Only the preferred stimulus (A-off) evoked both EPR and LR (e.g., 200nA; ▷ EPR; ▶, LR). Small-amplitude, early latency responses (e.g., ○) of another neuron(s) are evoked by two of the three stimuli not preferred by the prominent cell (A-on, S-off). Late responses (e.g., ●) are elicited by all three. LRs of the prominent cell which are evoked by nonpreferred stimuli during high rates of iontophoresis follow the EPRs and are synchronous with the LRs of the other neuron(s) (e.g., A-on, S-off; 200 nA). Calibrations: ECoG, 250 V/division; depth ECoG, 1.0 mV/division; microelectrode record, 1.0 mV/division; visual receptive field, 0.5°/division; sweep duration, 500 msec (from ref. 21, with permission).

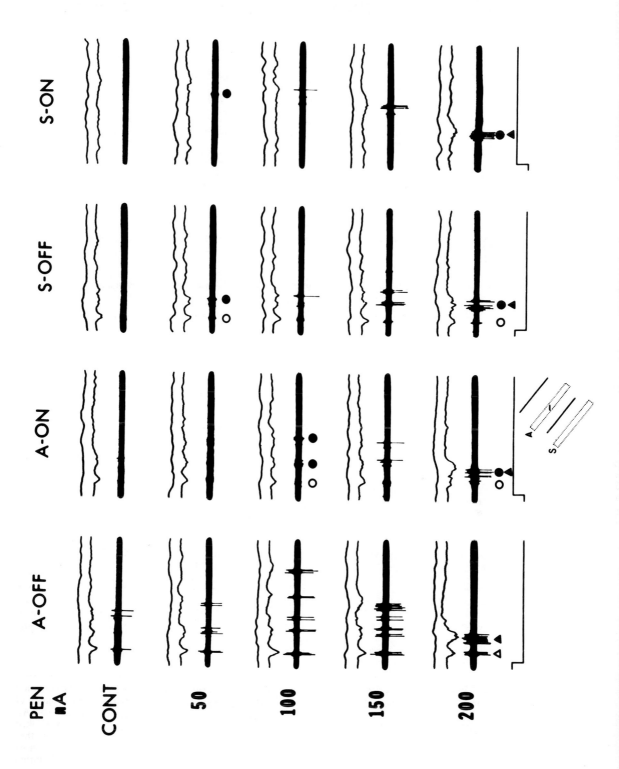

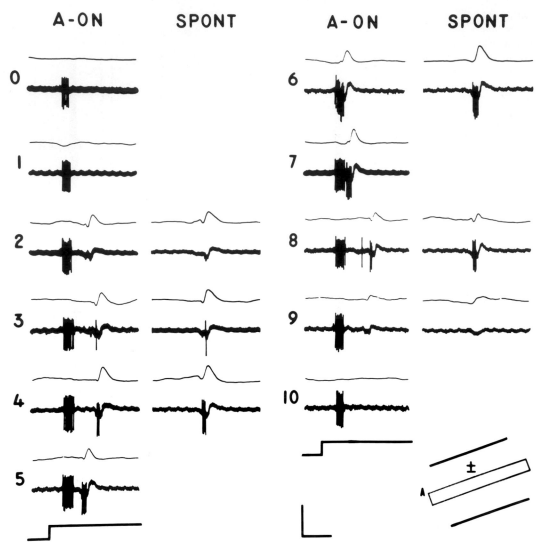

FIG. 6. Comparison of spontaneous activity and responses evoked by a preferred on stimulus during penicillin iontophoresis from a second electrode approximately 500 μm from the neuron. Each row represents responses at approximately the same stage of focus development. *Upper trace:* ECoG; *lower trace:* microelectrode recording. Row 0 illustrates the physiologic response before penicillin was applied. Responses in rows 1 through 3 occurred, respectively, 3, 4, and 5 min after iontophoresis (lasting 7 min) was begun, and those in rows 4 through 10 occurred 2, 4, 5, 9, 17, 33, and 35 min after iontophoresis was ended. Note that evoked activity included an EPR during all stages of the focus evolution. LR (PDS) discharges appeared the same whether spontaneous or evoked, except when their latency approached that of the physiologic response and an elongated burst resulted. Calibration: vertical = 3 mV for microelectrode; 300 V for ECoG; horizontal = 60 msec for A-on columns, 48 msec for spontaneous columns, and 0.75° for receptive field (from ref. 21, with permission).

LAMINAR DISTINCTIONS DURING NEOCORTICAL EPILEPTOGENESIS

Laminar Sensitivity to Convulsants

Penicillin

Much of the experimentation that originally characterized the interictal spike potential and

its cellular counterpart, the PDS, utilized penicillin as the convulsant agent (50,71). Investigations over nearly 20 years have continued to concentrate on characterizing the physiologic effects of penicillin (for review, see refs. 19,69,80). Comparatively little attention, however, has been directed toward determining where penicillin exerts its convulsant effects within this functionally diverse and morphologically layered structure (8,22,44,58). Identifying whether the action of penicillin is uniform across cortical depths or whether epileptogenic effects of penicillin vary with the type of neurons and/ or their location among the cortical laminae would seem critical to understanding this model of epileptogenesis.

Methods commonly used in the study of acute epileptic foci do not lend themselves to the analysis of the effects of penicillin on a laminar basis. Most *in vivo* experiments have utilized the topical application of penicillin solution by various strategies. All depend upon diffusion of penicillin into the cortex, and most await the development of spontaneous interictal spike potentials, frequently minutes later, as their measure of epileptogenesis. These techniques bias any conclusions concerning laminar effects toward the superficial layers that are affected first and with higher drug concentrations. Furthermore, the monitoring of spontaneous spiking cannot provide an accurate estimate of the differentiation of effect among the cortical laminae because of the long latency to onset, which allows for the widespread diffusion of penicillin.

In this section, we present the details of our investigations in cat striate cortex, which show a selective susceptibility of layer 4 to the epileptogenic effects of penicillin (7). In these studies, we have attempted: (a) to overcome the deficiencies of topical application by using selective intracortical microinjection of penicillin in picoliter and low nanoliter quantities; and (b) to improve on the resolution of other laminar studies (22,44,58) by monitoring, directly at the convulsant injection site, abnormalities induced in the intracortical field potentials evoked by physiologic visual stimulation specific for the region of cortex being monitored. As discussed previously, these evoked potentials have been shown to be a more sensitive indicator of altered responsivity secondary to penicillin than spontaneous IIS potentials, with response alterations occurring within seconds instead of minutes (17,19,21). In fact, the first two of the three distinct stages of epileptogenesis (EPR and LR) are noted *before* spontaneous IIS potentials are seen. This early detection of epileptic abnormalities after penicillin injection permits a more precise measurement of laminar sensitivity due to lessened diffusion time. A histologic analysis of the extent and location of penicillin diffusion by means of radioautography has supplemented conclusions drawn from the physiologic data.

Figure 7 summarizes the results obtained from microinjections of relatively large volumes of NaPen (200–300 pl/4 sec to a total volume of 1.5–2.0 nl). These injections produced epileptiform abnormalities at three of five depths tested within striate cortex (stereotaxic coordinates: P2.0, L1.5); 500–600, 1,000–1,250 and 1,400–1,600 μm. The degree of abnormality induced at these cortical depths was assessed by: (1) the *final stage* of epileptogenesis attained (EPR, LR, or IIS); (b) the *amplitude increase* within a given stage; and, most important, (3) by the *rate of abnormality onset* following the introduction of NaPen. Initial response alterations (EPR) developed more quickly (<10 sec versus 30 sec) and more completely (IIS versus LR) at the 1,000–1,250 μm site than at the 1,400–1,600 μm site. Evoked epileptiform abnormalities evolved completely to interictal spikes *only* at the 1,000–1,250 μm site, and LRs were initiated there within 30 sec of NaPen injection. At 500–600 μm, abnormalities developed only after a longer time (>60 sec) and did not evolve to the levels achieved at either of the deeper induction sites. Utilization of the same NaPen microinjection parameters at 100–200 μm or at 2,000 μm and deeper produced no epileptiform abnormalities within 10–15 min. Larger microinjections (500 pl/4 sec), however, presented for a longer period of time (>60 sec) did produce epileptiform activity recordable at these depths, but only after a considerable delay. Smaller microinjections totaling in the mid-picoliter range (300–500 pl) induced response abnormalities only in layer 4, as can be seen in Fig. 8.

In every animal in which a depth of maximal NaPen sensitivity was isolated electrophysiologically and marked with labeled penicillin or fast green dye, the site was located in layer 4. Because the onset of epileptiform abnormalities is considerably delayed when penicillin is injected at depths other than 1,000 μm, it was possible that this delay represented the time needed for the convulsant to diffuse into layer 4. This supposition has been supported by recent combined *multilaminar* electrophysiologic, autoradiographic, and radioassay data that lend further credence to the importance of this layer in providing a natural trigger in the development of penicillin-induced neocortical epileptiform abnormalities (8).

In this series of experiments, ^{14}C-labeled penicillin was injected into different cortical layers, and tissue surrounding the micropipette tract was excised and frozen within 30 sec of the onset of intracortical LR abnormalities. In some animals in which superficial or deep injections were made, tissue was excised prior to the development of these epileptiform responses. In all

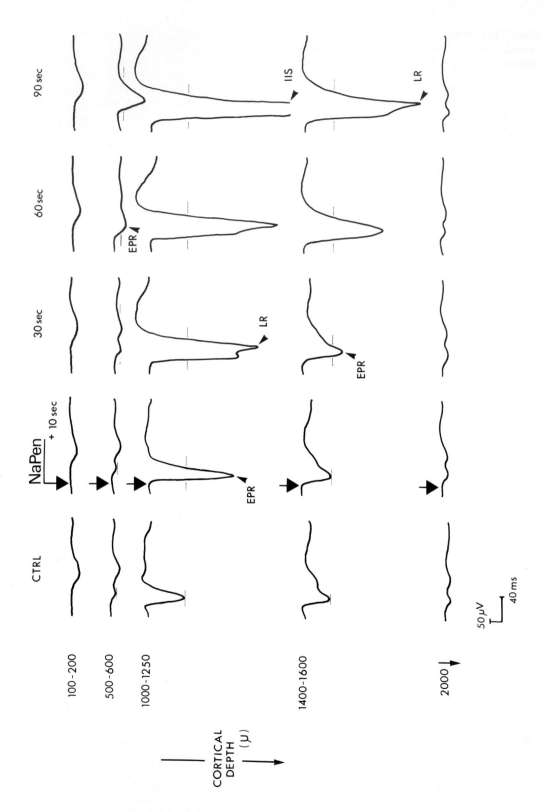

cases, the tissue was then sectioned in a cryostat, freeze-dried, exposed for 12 hr to a separate emulsion-coated slide, and counterstained with cresyl violet. This technique allowed us to monitor the movement of penicillin across cortical laminae and to correlate the extent of tissue involvement with multisite, cortical electrophysiology. Because diffusion from the point-source injection was nearly symmetrical, the injection site could be identified as the center of the autoradiographic exposure pattern. Additional verification of the size of the diffusion pattern was obtained in the sagittal plane from alternate sections processed for liquid scintillation counting (LSC).

The pattern of response alterations across cortical laminae varies with the site of penicillin microinjection. These patterns will be discussed in detail in the next section. The data of Fig. 9A, however, are representative of the progression of penicillin-induced epileptogenesis seen in five animals when maximally sensitive layer 4 was injected. If tissue is excised and preserved for histological analysis when the first LR potential develops at 30 sec, as can be seen in Fig. 9B, the labeled penicillin from the injection site is almost completely confined to layer 4. In Fig. 9C, LSC measurements in the sagittal plane confirm the nearly symmetrical nature of the 600-μm spread of the convulsant.

When penicillin is injected into the most superficial cortical layers, the onset and development of epileptic abnormalities are somewhat different, as seen in Fig. 10A. Alterations in normal responses are slow to become apparent. Fig. 10B shows heavy labeling in the injected layers (2–3) when tissue is removed at the LR stage of epileptogenesis. The migration of labeled penicillin into granular cell layer 4, however, is also unmistakable. Tissue removed from animals prior to the development of these initial epileptiform abnormalities (<40 sec) showed no evidence of penicillin diffusion beyond the borders of the injected supragranular layers. Figure 10C illustrates the diffusion in the plane orthogonal to the cross-section. A similar 800 μm of tissue exhibits high radioactive levels, whereas 1,200 μm of tissue has levels clearly above background.

The progression of epileptiform abnormalities translaminarly when penicillin was microinjected into the deeper cortical layers is characterized in Fig. 11A. Again, the first noticeable change in normal activity occurs after considerable delay. Though the injected layers are densely labeled in Fig. 11B, heavy labeling can also be seen in layer 4, where tissue was removed at the LR stage of epileptogenesis. In tissue excised from two other animals prior to initial response abnormalities (<80 sec), the spread of labeled penicillin was limited to the deep injection layers. Extensive diffusion within the sagittal plane is reflected in high radioactive counts over 1,000 μm of tissue with lesser levels extending over 1,400 μm, as can be seen in Fig. 11C.

Latency to the onset of epileptiform abnormalities recorded from the pyramidal cell layers did vary across animals. Those injections made closer to layer 4 produced more rapid response alterations and, consequently, a smaller amount of penicillin labeling than did more distal injections. As monitored by radioautography and LSC radioassay techniques, however, the diffusion of penicillin into layer 4 correlated well with the onset of epileptiform response abnormalities in all experimental animals regardless of the injected depth.

Although nongranular cortex may be capable of independently initiating penicillin-induced epileptiform activity under different conditions, these conditions must involve either a greater drug concentration or a much larger mass of affected tissue than we can involve before layer 4 is infiltrated. We have utilized penicillin concentrations of from 35 mM to 1.7 M and have not seen epileptogenesis in the superficial and deep pyramidal cell layers when there were no effects on layer 4 responsiveness. Furthermore, using topical application directly involving a much larger superficial tissue mass than we have shown, other investigators (58) have found that labeled penicillin was still not confined to the supragranular layers at the onset of interictal activity, ~5% having penetrated into layer 4.

In related work, Holmes and Lockton (35,44,45) have assessed the laminar sensitivity of rat somatosensory cortex to penicillin's influ-

---

FIG. 7. Averaged responses (n = 4) to 1° square off stimuli presented ¼ sec. A sequence of responses before, during, and after the injection of NaPen was recorded at each of five cortical depths. Response sequences within rows describe the response profile over time at the depth into which penicillin was injected. Time intervals between NaPen injections at different depths (rows) were of at least 15 min, or until responses returned to normal. Response abnormalities rapidly followed injections totaling 1.5–2.0 nl (200–300 pL/4 sec) of 140 mM NaPen at the 1,000–1,250-μm site, but were delayed 30 sec at the 1,400–1,600-μm site. At 500–600 μm, the response alteration began 60 sec following NaPen injection. No effect was seen at either the most superficial or the deepest injection sites. Negativity: down (from ref. 7).

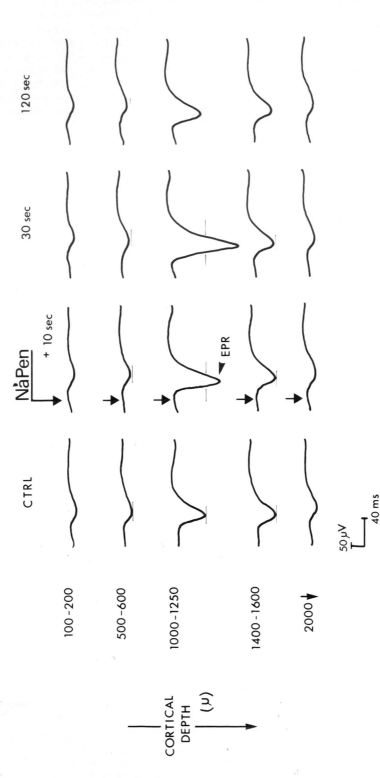

ence by means of selective intracortical microiontophoresis. They concluded that deep layer 3 is the most susceptible neocortical stratum. This divergence from our results may be accurate and related to intrinsic differences in the lamination, organization, and afference of rat somatosensory cortex (16,90,92) as compared with cat striate cortex (27,47). These results may also reflect differences in methodology, however. Distinguishing penicillin's effects on deep layer 3 from those on layer 4 is technically difficult in the rat preparation, since layer 4 is only a thin, 100^+ micron-wide band of tissue. It is easily encompassed within the radius of their calculated, critical cortical mass for epileptogenesis (450 μm), when centered in layer 3. This problem of resolution is compounded by the use of spontaneous IIS potentials, whose longer delay to onset is associated with more extensive penicillin diffusion, and by the use of separately positioned electrodes for penicillin administration and recording. By contrast, cortical layer 4 in cat striate cortex is 500–600 μm wide, which is sufficient for our techniques to resolve true laminar differences. Our accuracy is enhanced by the use of evoked epileptiform response alterations, rather than spike rate or amplitude. The former develop earlier than spontaneous IISs and provide definite stages of epileptogenesis to monitor. As will be shown later in our multilaminar recordings, LR or IIS amplitude is not a good measure of epileptogenic sensitivity, since potentials recorded from a more superficial layer may be as large as or larger than from the focus origin.

Bicuculline

This convulsant agent is also a GABA-blocker, differing from penicillin by being more complete in its action. Although we know of no systematic investigations concerning bicuculline's laminar effectiveness in inducing epileptogenesis in the intact brain, George and Connors (26) have recently presented preliminary data from the neocortical slice on the effects of this agent which confirms the unique susceptibility of layer 4 and our observations on its importance in the development of epileptiform activity.

Mechanisms for Epileptogenic Susceptibility

The heightened sensitivity of layer 4 to penicillin, and perhaps to bicuculline, may be related to many factors. Layer 4 has been shown to be anatomically distinct as: (a) the major terminus of primary geniculocortical afferents; (2) the lamina within which essentially all spiny stellate cells (the neocortical excitatory interneuron) are found; and (c) the branch-point for serial cortical processing of information (27,47,85). Although penicillin has been shown to be a partial GABA-blocker with demonstrated disinhibitory influences (15,55,89,93), morphological evidence suggests that the potential for at least certain types of inhibitory control within layer 4 may not be as great as in nongranular cortex. For instance, although most pyramidal neurons in the striate neocortex receive symmetric, inhibitory synaptic connections onto the axonal initial segment, these connections are rarely found on the spiny stellates which are exclusive to layer 4, although other inhibitory contacts do occur on the soma and dendrites (47). Furthermore, no evidence of the potentially influential, "cartridge-type" inhibitory array surrounding the axon hillock has been found on spiny stellates (47), whereas they are found on pyramidal cells in both supra- and infragranular cortex (47,82).

In addition to this comparatively weak inhibition, the granular cell layer receives a dense sensory-specific, excitatory projection from the lateral geniculate nucleus (27,47), and excitation from intrinsic spiny stellate cell collateralizations within layer 4 and from deep (layer VI) pyramidal cell recurrent projections (27,47). These substantial excitatory contacts may be more influential on spiny stellate cells, with their relatively circumscribed dendritic trees, than are excitatory contacts on pyramidal cells which receive much of their excitatory activity over widely distributed apical trees. Furthermore, neurons in this layer have recently been identified that respond to depolarization and synaptic activation with a burst discharge rather than isolated spikes (11).

Numerous hypotheses can be generated by combining these characteristics of layer 4 and its various constituents with the demonstrated disinhibitory action of penicillin (13,15,55,89). A selective reduction of the purportedly weak re-

FIG. 8. Experimental protocol similar to Fig. 7 except that smaller volumes of NaPen were used (0.3–0.5 nl presented 40–60 pl/4s). Response abnormalities followed injection at 1,000–1,250 m but were not observed at any of the other sites. Negativity: down (from ref. 7).

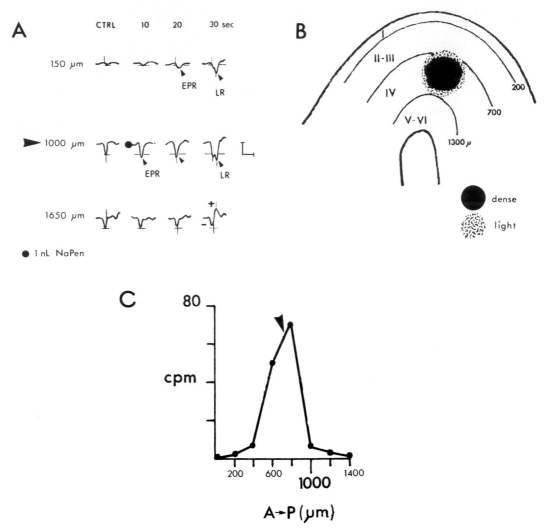

FIG. 9. (A) Response profiles recorded simultaneously from three different depths in cat striate cortex before (CTRL) and after penicillin microinjection at the 1,000-μm site. Initial abnormalities (EPRs) develop in layer IV with epileptiform activity (LRs) evolving subsequently in IV and at the superficial site. Amplitude, 50 μV; time, 50 msec in all figures. (B) Camera lucida drawing from a ^{14}C autoradiograph of this penicillin focus (P + 4.5). The diffusion of penicillin is nearly completely confined to layer IV with only sparse label migrating 50 μm into deep layer III despite postbiopsy tissue handling. (C) Alternate sections subjected to LSC analysis compare favorably with the extent of diffusion above. *Arrow:* site at which the tissue section was taken in each figure (from ref. 8).

current and collateral inhibition in the local circuit interactions among stellate cells of layer 4 may dramatically accentuate the discharge of neurons responsive to our specific excitatory synaptic input. Further elaboration of this enhanced response by local synaptic integration within a population of neurons devoid of normal inhibitory influences might lead to the longer latency epileptiform discharge of a larger neuronal population as described by us here (the LR and IIS) and previously (17,19,20), by Gutnick et al. (33) in the neocortical slice, and as computer-modeled recently by Traub and Wong (88). It will remain for future investigations, however, to determine definitively whether layer 4 sensitivity to convulsant-induced epileptogenesis is truly a function of the intrinsic properties of spiny stellate cells, of other layer 4 neurons (70), of qual-

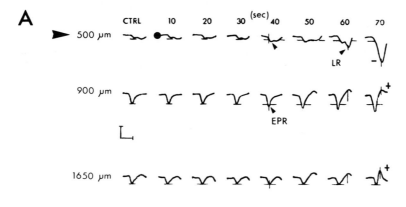

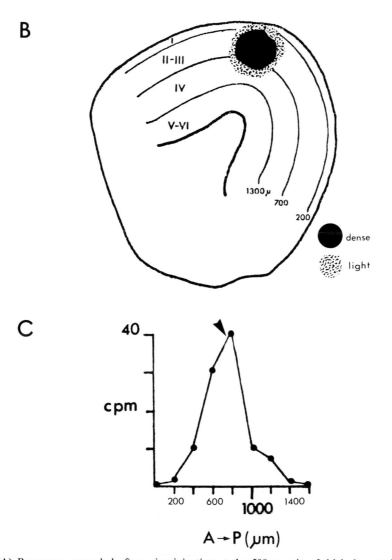

FIG. 10. **(A)** Responses recorded after microinjection at the 500-μm site. Initial abnormalities develop in layers IV and II–III with epileptiform activity evolving later in the injected layer. **(B)** Camera lucida drawing taken from a ^{14}C autoradiograph of this focus (P + 2.5). Note that penicillin has penetrated 300–400 μm into layer IV (densely for 200 μm). **(C)** The LSC analysis sagittally again corresponds well to coronal labeling (from ref. 8).

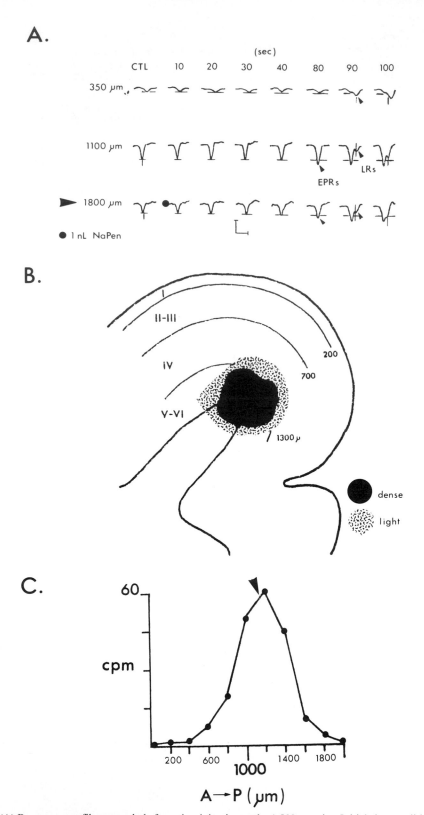

FIG. 11. **(A)** Response profiles recorded after microinjection at the 1,800-μm site. Initial abnormalities develop in layers IV and VI, with epileptiform activity evolving later in all layers. **(B)** Camera lucida drawing of a ^{14}C autoradiograph (P + 4.5). Penicillin has again penetrated 300 μm into layer IV with 150 μm of tissue in deep IV densely labeled. **(C)** Diffusion here was larger than in previous figures, but again corresponds closely to that in the tissue section above (from ref. 8).

itatively or quantitatively different inhibition, of differences in population connectivity within the lamina, or of some combination of these factors.

SPREAD OF SEIZURES: INTERLAMINAR PROPAGATION OF RESPONSE ABNORMALITIES DURING EPILEPTOGENESIS

Many advances in characterizing the cellular and field potential correlates of epilepsy have come from the *in vivo* study of acute focal epilepsy in animal models (for review, see refs. 4,19,62,69,80). Much of this experimentation utilized the topical application of convulsants, the principal one being penicillin. All of these studies depended upon the gradual diffusion of drug into the cortex, and most awaited the resultant spontaneous interictal spiking to begin analysis. Understandably, these relatively large and fully-evolved foci yielded recordings showing a rather uniform involvement of neurons in the pathologic, PDS process (50). Perhaps due in part to this assumed homogeneity within the epileptic aggregate, most of the past investigation has been centered upon characterizing the PDS and postulating its origin. Proportionately little attention has been directed at determining how neuronal aggregates among the various cortical layers interact. Although we now know that layer 4 in visual cortex is most susceptible to convulsant agents, what is the nature of its role in epileptogenesis? Do certain neurons or groups of neurons in the other laminae also have specific roles? Does the interaction among all these aggregates result in standard patterns of epileptic recruitment within and between cortical columns?

Spatial as well as functional analyses of cortical epileptic foci are few in number. Topographical examination of spontaneous interictal potentials from the cortical surface has characterized systematic changes in the amplitude and polarity of epileptic potentials when recordings are made from regions progressively more distant from the center of the focus (29). Laminar recordings after the topical application of penicillin to cat neocortex have revealed negative interictal potentials or seizure-associated DC shifts of varying amplitudes at all depths through the center of the focus. Although maximum negativity was recorded from depths corresponding to layers 4 and 5, little could be said concerning the functional relationships among the layers, given the uniformity that was seen (30). More recent laminar studies of small topical penicillin foci began to reveal the differences present at

earlier stages of epileptogenesis. Focal interictal epileptiform discharges (FIED) of negative polarity could be restricted to the upper layers of motor cortex, whereas synchronous positive potentials were noted from the deeper laminae (22). Responses were recorded from the spinal cord, however, only when negative interictal potentials spread to layer 5, where cells of origin for the pyramidal tract are located. The finding of synchronous hyperpolarizations in cells outside of the focus, rather than the massive depolarization of the PDS, has led additionally to the theory of an "inhibitory surround" (14,67,68). Ectopic spike generation was shown to delineate the central, interictally active portion of a focus from the ictally recruitable surround (24). In nearly all these endeavors, however, fully evolved foci, which were used for their stability, may have obscured differences in the responsivity of constituent neuronal populations that existed at earlier stages of development.

In order to clarify the functional relationships among laminar neuronal subpopulations during epileptogenesis, we have recorded the evolution of temporary epileptic foci induced by microinjection of penicillin into the different cortical layers. Multiple simultaneous perspectives were gained by recording local field potentials and multiunit extracellular activity from multibarreled microelectrodes with longitudinal tip separations (Fig. 2). Although such recordings cannot offer detailed information on membrane physiology, they do provide useful information about the aggregate activity of neuronal populations, including those of smaller stellate neurons that are difficult to record intracellularly.

These investigations demonstrated that epileptiform responses recorded from different layers within a cortical column evolve in stereotyped patterns depending upon the level at which penicillin is introduced (8,20). Significant new information concerning the functional relationships among these layers was gained by observing associations between the development of response abnormalities in one layer and their expression in another. In addition, these spatiotemporal patterns of epileptogenesis were found to correlate well with known intracortical circuitry. These data all support the idea that identifiable neuronal subpopulations do have specific roles in the onset and spread of epileptiform abnormalities within the cortex.

Laminar Interactions During Epileptogenesis

These multilaminar data will be presented and

discussed in terms of three cortical subdivisions: supragranular pyramidal layers 2–3, stellate or granular layer 4, and infragranular pyramidal layers 5–6, which correspond in area 17 to cortical depths of ~200–700, 700–1,300, and 1,300–2,000 μm, respectively. The rationale for this laminar division into cortical bands of 500–700 μm is based upon differing predominant cell types, neuronal receptive field characteristics, and stages of input processing. These bands are well within the depth resolution of the techniques used. Furthermore, laminar analysis of field potentials recorded every 100 μm during electrode withdrawal revealed no additional potentials either before or during focus evolution that were not monitored by our standard recording configuration (see Fig. 12). Among the six possible permutations for interlaminar communication within these subdivisions, electrophysiologic evidence for three were clearly evident and two of the three interactions were particularly prominent.

Epileptic Foci Induced in Layer 4

Most significant was the close response coupling that existed between stellate layer 4 and pyramidal layers 2–3 (Fig. 13). Following penicillin injection, the early EPR of layer 4 was associated with an increase in the normally small and longer latency response of layers 2 and 3. In a dramatic fashion, however, the layer 4 LR was associated with a large synchronous potential from the superficial laminae. Note as well the degree of increase in this pyramidal layer response in relation to its control. The EPRs of layer 4 are routinely 2–3 times the amplitude of its control response; the LRs are 10–15 times this size, but the LRs of layers 2 and 3 are often ≧20 times the amplitude of its control response. The entire evolution of the late epileptiform potentials in layer 4 was closely paralleled by similar potentials from the superficial pyramidal layers; however, these later responses never appeared independently of the layer 4 LR. Simul-

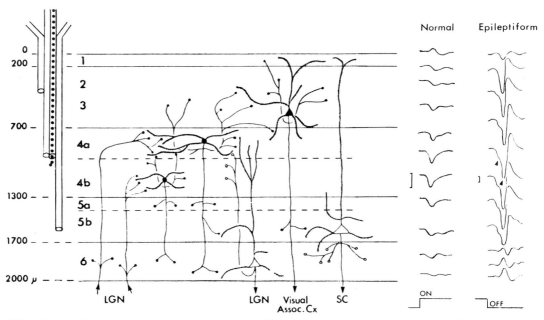

FIG. 12. A schematic representation of the cytoarchitectonics of cat striate cortex using information developed by Lund et al. (47) and Gilbert and Wiesel (27). Predominant cell types together with their principal afferent and efferent connections are illustrated. The configuration of a typical four-barrel drug injection/recording electrode spanning the layers is shown, *left. Right:* representative field potentials which were recorded every 200 μm during the withdrawal of an electrode array from striate cortex. These were evoked by punctate photic stimuli before (normal) and after (epileptiform) the microinjection of approximately 1 nl of 35 mM of penicillin into layer 4. Note that the largest primary potentials are seen in layer 4 *before* penicillin injection, and the largest enhanced primary (EPRs) and late responses (LRs) are also seen in layer 4 *after* penicillin injection (*arrowheads*). A reversal of polarity of the LR potential in the deeper cortical layers (positive; upward-going) and an absence of EPRs in both superficial and deep layers are shown. Calibrations: 50 μV, 110 msec sweep time (from ref. 20).

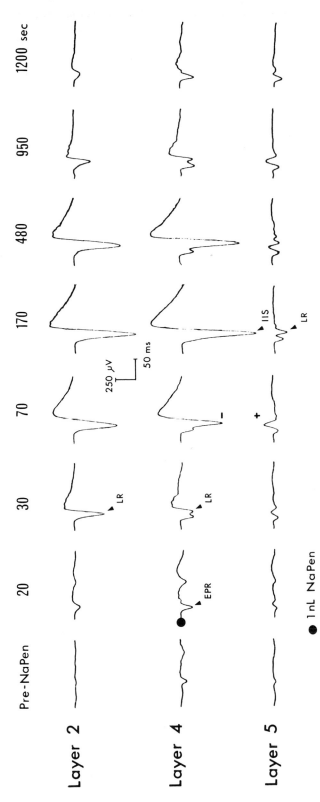

FIG. 13. Simultaneous three-layer recording during the development of an epileptic focus originating in layer 4 induced by the microinjection of 1 nl of penicillin. Note the rapid onset of response alterations (EPR and LR) from layer 2, and the slower spread of epileptiform activity into layer 5. Separate EPR and LR components from layer 4 are only obliterated at the height of the focus (interictal spike potential, IIS). The layer 2 LR response faithfully follows the layer 4 LR throughout the evolution. Layer 5 LR potentials deteriorate more rapidly, leaving behind only a positive potential at the same latency, which was also apparent during early focus development. Recording depths were approximately 300, 900 and 1,450 µm, respectively. Elapsed time following the onset of penicillin is given on the top line of this and subsequent figures (from ref. 20).

taneous multiunit extracellular recordings from a layer 4 focus revealed the typical sequence: EPR burst, followed by dual EPR–LR bursts, which eventually fuse into a PDS burst at the interictal spike stage (Fig. 14). Unit recordings from superficial layers typically showed only a single burst discharge, which was synchronous with the LR bursts of layer 4. This relationship persisted during the decline of focus.

It is unlikely that the superficial LR potentials

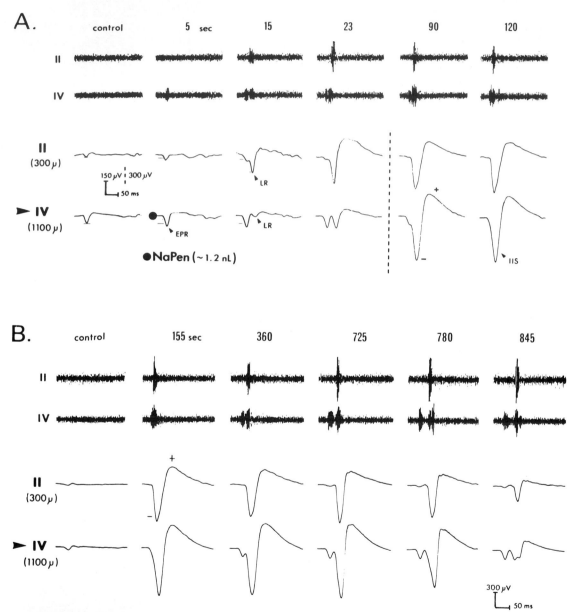

FIG. 14. (A) Simultaneous field potential and multiunit recordings from layers 2 and 4 during the onset of an epileptic focus originating in layer 4 induced by the microinjection of approximately 1.2 nanoliters of penicillin. Note cellular burst discharges associated with both EPR and LR potentials from layer 4, and with LR potentials from layer 2. LR bursts from layer 2 are synchronous with those from layer 4. Double, EPR-LR bursts from layer 4 unite into one prolonged burst at the interictal spike (IIS) stage, seen here (120 sec) and in B (155 sec). A gain change follows the vertical dashed line. (B) Note the separation of layer 4 EPR and LR burst discharges and their counterpart field potentials with regression of the focus. Layer 2 LR bursts remain synchronous with those from layer 4. Multiple cellular bursts are seen to underlie the layer 4 LR potential toward the end of the focus decline (from ref. 20).

are a far-field reflection of activity in layer 4, since simultaneous cellular bursts are also recorded from layers 2–3. Both LR potentials and neuronal bursts were, however, dependent upon layer 4 and appear to be due to the rapid propagation of abnormal activity from it. Recruitment of layers 2–3 did not seem to be a function of penicillin diffusion into the upper layers, since LRs were elicited within 20–30 sec of the injection, which is too short a time for significant physical spread of the drug out of layer 4, as we have demonstrated autoradiographically. Furthermore, penicillin injection directly into the superficial layers cannot induce LRs as rapidly or as well. Because comparable potentials were not seen in the deep pyramidal layers at a similar distance from the injection site, penicillin spread through capillary action along the electrode track is also an improbable explanation for this association. It is more likely that epileptiform LR bursting within layer 4 provides the superficial pyramidal layers with an intense synaptic barrage that is carried by existing interlaminar pathways.

By contrast, there is much less of a close association between a layer 4 focus and the response alterations of deep pyramidal layers (Fig. 13). Often there was little or no change in the normal layer 5–6 response until an LR was generated in layer 4, and then only a positive "mirror" image potential of moderate amplitude was noted. Gradually an EPR developed in the deep layers; the positive potential would decline in the amplitude and be replaced by a negative LR potential. Note that these changes in layer 5–6 responses required minutes to evolve as compared to seconds for the superficial abnormalities and thus may be related to penicillin diffusion.

Epileptic Foci Induced in Layers 2–3

The functional relationship between layer 4 and layers 2–3 is not reciprocal, however (Fig. 15). Following the microinjection of comparable amounts of penicillin into the superficial pyramidal layers, the development of response abnormalities proceeds more slowly, and their interlaminar progression is different from that seen with layer 4 injections. In this case, initial effects were noted only after a minute and consisted of increases in the amplitude of the layer 2–3 and the layer 4 primary response. Usually, within 2 min, longer latency LR potentials were recorded from the superficial injection site. Initially, these were not associated with comparable potentials from the underlying layers, but

rather with a positive mirror image potential. Eventually, synchronous LR potentials did evolve in layers 4 and 5–6. During the decline of epileptic foci originating in the superficial layers, the LR potentials from the deep pyramidal layers often persisted beyond those from layer 4.

Extracellular recording of multiunit activity showed cellular bursts in the superficial layers synchronous with the initial LR potentials, whereas EPR bursting was usually only seen from layer 4. LR bursts were finally noted from all three recording sites, and a double EPR–LR burst was noted from layer 4 only. LR bursting persisted longer in layers 5–6 than in layer 4 during the decline of superficial foci.

Although epileptiform activity can develop in superficial pyramidal layers without comparable LR potentials existent in the underlying laminae, this activity does not appear to be entirely independent of layer 4 responses. In fact, little or no change was seen in any response from layers 2–3 before a layer 4 EPR developed—a sure sign that penicillin had begun to diffuse into the granular lamina. We feel that the EPRs of layer 4 provide the developing superficial focus with an enhanced but otherwise normal synaptic input to trigger epileptogenic neuronal interaction. In contrast, the gradual development of LRs in layer 4 has a time frame consistent with the physical spread of penicillin from the superficial injection site.

There appears to be a closer functional association between the superficial and deep pyramidal layers. Even though separated by the stellate layer, LR field potentials and neuronal bursts often appeared in layers 5–6 sooner and/or persisted there longer than in layer 4 during the evolution of a superficial focus.

Epileptic Foci Induced in Layers 5–6

The second prominent response association existed between the deep pyramidal laminae and layer 4 (Fig. 16). Microinjection of penicillin into layers 5–6 is also accompanied by response alterations that evolve more slowly than those following a layer 4 injection. After ~30–45 sec, EPRs were evident in both layers 5–6 and 4; within 60–90 sec, LRs developed at the injection site. When deep pyramidal LRs appeared in this case, a counterpart LR rapidly developed in layer 4. In fact, the layer 4 LR was commonly of larger amplitude than that from the focus proper. Response alterations from layer 4 otherwise paralleled those from 5–6. Multiunit recordings (Fig. 17) showed EPR bursts from both

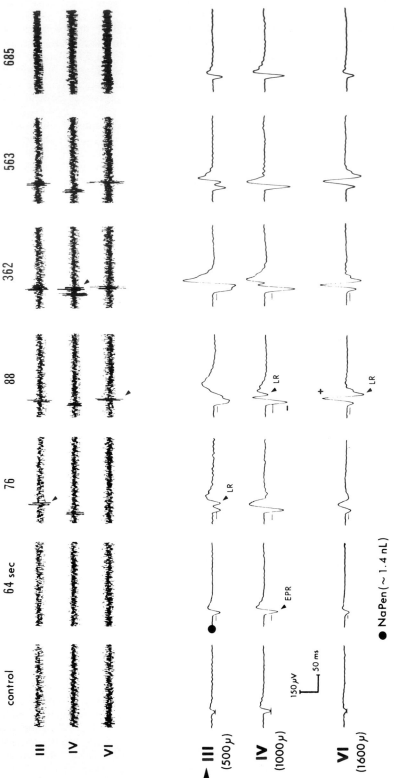

FIG. 15. Simultaneous field potential and multi-unit recordings from layers 3, 4, and 6 during the evolution of an epileptic focus originating in layer 3 induced by the microinjection of approximately 1.4 nanoliters of penicillin. Note the development of a layer 4 EPR potential prior to that of a layer 3 LR, and the relatively longer time to the onset of both when compared to Fig. 14. EPR cellular bursting from layer 4 is recorded at the same time that LR bursts develop in layer 3. Layer 3 LRs are initially accompanied only by positive potentials from deeper laminae (76 sec). Layer 4 and 6 LRs evolve gradually with additional time. Synchronous LR unit bursts are recorded from layer 6 soon after their onset in layer 3 (88 sec) and before their appearance in layer 4. At the height of the focus (362 sec), EPR-LR double bursts are seen in layer 4, while only LR bursts are recorded from layers 3 and 6. LR field potentials and unit bursts decline in layer 4 before those of layer 6, while EPR potentials and bursts, and a positive potential unassociated with cellular discharge remain (563 sec) (from ref. 20).

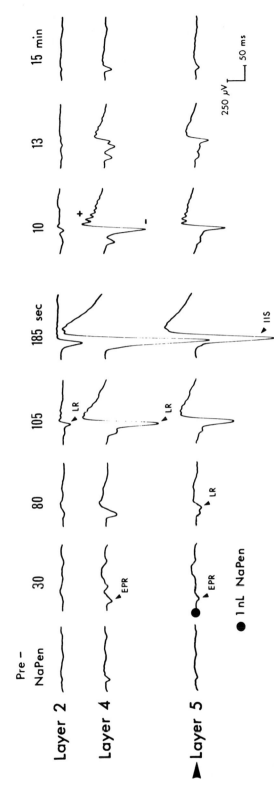

FIG. 16. Simultaneous three-layer recording during the development of an epileptic focus originating in layer 5 after the microinjection of ~1 nl of penicillin. Note the appearance of EPRs in both layers 4 and 5 prior to the onset of LR responses in the deeper layer. LR activity is soon reflected in the layer 4 response and, to a lesser extent, superficially. Interictal spike potentials principally from layers 4 and 5 are evident 3 min after injection. Note the continued close association of layer 4 on layer 5 LR responses during the decline of the focus. Multiple, long latency LRs with some degree of amplitude independence between laminae are seen in the 13-min responses. Recording depths were approximately 300, 850 and 1,400 m, respectively (from ref. 20).

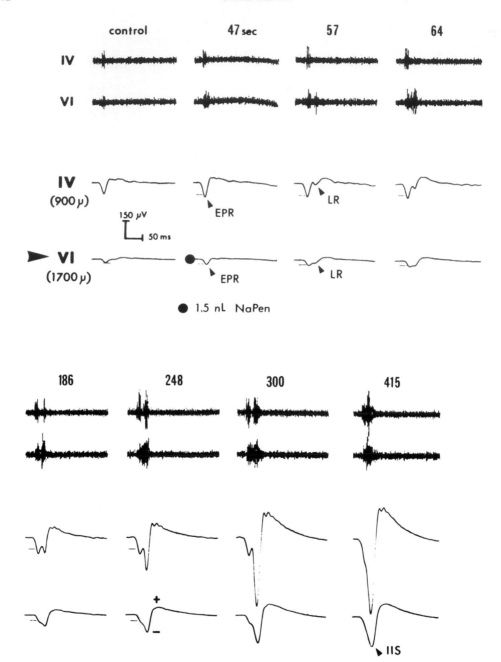

FIG. 17. Simultaneous field potential and multiunit recordings from layers 4 and 6 during the development of an epileptic focus originating in layer 6 induced by the microinjection of ~1.5 nl of penicillin. Note that EPR bursts and field potentials appear in both layers prior to the development of LR activity. LR cellular burst discharges from layer 4 develop after those from layer 6. Double EPR–LR bursts are recorded from both layers 6 and 4 during much of the evolution of the focus. Amplitude of the LR field potentials from layer 4 surpasses that of layer 6 at the height of development (from ref. 20).

deep pyramidal and granular layers as the initial abnormality. The development of LR bursts from layers 5–6 preceded those from layer 4, although dual EPR–LR bursts were seen from both sites during much of the focus evolution.

Thus, a deep pyramidal focus may provide excitatory synaptic input for the overlying stellate layer. However, in the case of such deep foci, as with superficial foci, a contribution to epileptogenesis from penicillin diffusion into layer 4 cannot be ruled out, since the development of LRs in layers 5–6 takes ⩾ 1 min; by that time, EPRs are noted in layer 4. As noted previously, the functional relationship between layers 5–6 and 4 is not reciprocal. In addition, only relatively small LR potentials were usually recorded from superficial pyramidal layers in association with a layer 5–6 focus (Fig. 16) and LR bursts were seldom seen. The translaminar projection of response abnormalities thus appears to be limited in extent as well as in direction.

Spontaneous Epileptiform Potentials

Spontaneous LRs were also noted after penicillin injection, but they appeared later in the evolution of a given focus than did their evoked counterparts. A differential laminar susceptibility to spontaneous events was evident and often *more* pronounced than a comparison of onsets of evoked LRs. Spontaneous LRs from layer 4 foci routinely appeared within 1 min of the first evoked LR and had a recurrence rate of 5–20/min during stimulus-free periods. Spontaneous LRs from a layer 2–3 focus were slower to develop, even relative to the prolonged onset of their evoked epileptiform activity, and had a slower intrinsic frequency. Layer 5–6 foci were somewhat more capable of producing spontaneous LR activity than were layer 2–3 foci in terms of latency to onset, frequency, and amplitude. Layer 4 seems to play a significant role in the expression of epileptogenesis in those other layers. The more layer 4 becomes involved through diffusion of penicillin, as measured by changes in its primary evoked potential, the more likely spontaneous LRs are to appear from superficial and deep foci. As the primary receiving lamina, layer 4 is well situated to relay, in an enhanced fashion, intrinsic thalamocortical activity, which may act as a trigger for foci in other layers.

The laminar profiles of these spontaneous LR and IIS potentials were the same as those that were evoked, minus the primary latency EPR component, as illustrated in Fig. 18. The eventual form of an epileptiform response seemed more closely related to the location and size of the penicillin focus rather than to whether triggering was internal (spontaneous) or external (evoked). Although called spontaneous, these potentials probably result from response synchronization and integration within a neuronal population that is initiated by internal thalamocortical triggers. Spontaneous activity would occur later in the evolution of a focus than would evoked epileptiform potentials because the visual stimulus is a more powerful initial synchronizer of the neuronal population, which in turn would facilitate LR generation.

Critical Mass for Neocortical Epileptogenesis

These multilaminar studies have confirmed our previous conclusion that layer 4 of striate cortex is most sensitive to the epileptogenic effects of penicillin (7,18). Epileptiform abnormalities, both evoked and spontaneous, were induced more rapidly and more fully with injection into layer 4 than with comparable injections in the other laminae. Unlike our previous sensitivity study, in which recordings were made from the injection site only, multilaminar monitoring verified the degree and temporal sequence of involvement of adjacent layers as well. The possibility of distant rather than local effects occurring first could be ascertained.

In the case of a layer 4 focus, both EPR and LR abnormalities originate from the injection site. The same cannot be said of foci from more superficial or deeper injections. The action of penicillin within layer 4 appears to be *sufficient* for epileptogenesis, a conclusion that has been confirmed experimentally by utilizing ^{14}C-labeled penicillin (6,8), as reviewed above. The direct involvement of cellular elements within striate layer 4 with penicillin appears to be *important,* if not necessary, for the initiation of epileptogenesis in other laminae, under our experimental conditions. Although initial LR epileptiform activity can be generated locally when superficial and deep cortical injections are made, the onset is delayed significantly in comparison to layer 4 injections. Our present data confirm that this delay represents a time during which penicillin diffuses into layer 4 and induces an EPR there. We suggest that this enhanced response provides adjacent layers with an increased, but otherwise normal, afferent input which synchronizes their neuronal aggregates (20). Without such a natural trigger, penicillin confined to either of the nongranular layers does not induce complete epileptogenesis *in vivo.*

The concept of the epileptogenic "critical mass" has been long debated, i.e., the smallest volume of cortex and/or the smallest neuronal population that can support IIS generation. Progressively smaller penicillin-soaked pledgets or other applicators were initially used. A surface area of 0.7 mm² was finally proposed in experiments that also included surgical division of larger foci (74). Other experimenters using small applicators and discrete physiologic stimuli concluded that a single cortical column was the

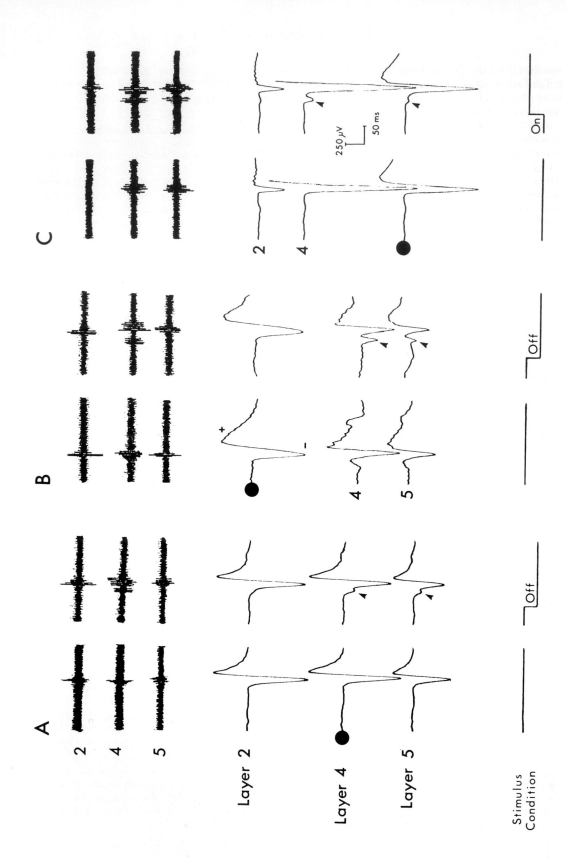

A

2
4
5

B

C

Layer 2

Layer 4

Layer 5

250 μV

50 ms

Off

Off

On

Stimulus
Condition

smallest functioning epileptogenic unit (25). Penicillin foci as small as 650 μm in diameter have been observed by radioactive [^{14}C]deoxyglucose measurements of increased metabolic activity (10). All of these experiments had the same basic limitations, however, namely topical drug application and surface monitoring of responses. By using multicontact laminar recording and a delivery of topical penicillin controlled in its distribution by penicillinase, epileptiform potentials limited to the upper cortex were later shown (22). Laminar epileptic foci have now been demonstrated in the present investigations. The critical mass for epileptogenesis is thus even smaller than a neocortical column, and may be as small as a single layer within a column in the case of lamina 4 in visual cortex.

Circuitry Mediating Laminar Interactions During Epileptogenesis

The closest functional relationships during the translaminar evolution of epileptiform abnormalities exist between cortical layers with subpopulations of neurons known to possess anatomical connections by means of axon collaterals (27,47) (see Fig. 12). The principal efferents from the spiny stellate cells of layer 4, which are the major recipients of geniculocortical input, are directed to the more superficial pyramidal layers. This normal pathway is probably utilized in the rapid projection of layer 4 response abnormalities to layers 2–3. The close association between the responses of layers 5–6 and layer 4 is likewise probably related to ascending axon collaterals of layer 6 pyramidal cells that are known to terminate in layer 4. Completing a potential loop within the cortex are collaterals of axons of superficial pyramidal neurons, which terminate in the deep pyramidal layers before exiting the cortex. This latter circuit may explain why the responses of layers 5–6 often show a closer relationship to those of layers 2–3 than do those of intervening layer 4 in the presence of a superficial focus.

In general, it would appear that abnormalities from discrete intracortical foci spread rapidly in the direction of known interlaminar connections, surpassing that attributable to penicillin diffusion. On the other hand, when normal connectivity is sparse or absent, epileptiform response abnormality spreads more slowly and appears to be dependent upon the diffusion of penicillin and the intrinsic sensitivity of the layers being infiltrated.

Complementing the above anatomical findings, and consistent with our position concerning the major laminar interactions during epileptogenesis, are current source density (CSD) analyses of normal and epileptiform potentials from visual cortex reported by other investigators (56,64–66). This mathematical transformation of laminar-evoked response data can be used to determine the sites and polarities of gross transmembrane currents (extracellular sinks and sources) which generate field potentials. CSD profiles are thought to reveal principally the basic pattern of excitatory postsynaptic activity in terms of extracellular active current sinks and passive current sources (56). Excitatory activity underlying the normal visual evoked potential was found to flow along several intracortical pathways, all of which start in layer 4 (56). The most prominent was from layer 4, through strong local connections to layer 3, and from there through longer and more widespread connections to layer 2. Similar CSD analyses of penicillin-induced IIS (65,66) or tonic seizures (64) routinely have shown major and initial current sinks at cortical depths corresponding to layer 4 with subsequent spread of excitatory activity into the superficial layers. Other visual cortex excitatory pathways, determined by CSD methods to be of lesser magnitude, involve polysynaptic activity within layer 4 itself prior to projection to layer 3, and spread from layer 4 to deeper pyramidal layers (56). The former may be involved in the rapid elaboration of epileptiform response abnormalities within layer 4 as well as in the spread of these abnormalities to the superficial pyramidal layers that we have shown here.

Positive "mirror" potentials that were found deep to a more superficial focus or occasionally

---

FIG. 18. Simultaneous three-layer recordings of spontaneous *and* evoked epileptiform spike potentials and associated cellular discharges recorded during the evolution of epileptic foci induced at three different levels (● in **A**, **B** and **C**). Note that the response configurations for the spontaneous events are similar to those for the evoked events minus the EPR components in the middle and deep laminae. Time to onset of the first spontaneous potential was routinely longer than that for the first evoked LR, regardless of injection site, and was always shortest in a layer 4 induction. Responses similar to those in **A** occurred between 1 and 1.5 min following penicillin injection, in **B** between 5 and 8 min, and in **C** between 2 and 3 min. Recording depths for conditions A and C were the same as in Fig. 13 and 16, respectively; those for condition B were 200, 800, and 1,400 μm (from ref. 20).

in superficial layers with deep foci appeared to result when major connections between layers did not exist or occurred before these connections became fully functional. When recorded in isolation, without an accompanying LR, it was evident that they were not associated with cellular discharges. These positive potentials are probably passive current sources for the active sinks of the epileptic focus. CSD analysis of an early stage of a topical penicillin focus supports this (65). The most likely carriers of this current flow are the long apical dendrites of deep pyramidal cells, which are known to span all neocortical laminae (27,47). These positive potentials have been noted by other investigators using superficial foci, but they were thought, incorrectly we believe, to be an active expression of inhibition (22).

EPR and LR (PDS) Neuronal Bursts: Laminar Correlates

Two forms of multiunit burst discharge have been repeatedly observed in both our isolated unit and multilaminar investigations. Prior to the latter studies, these two discharge types were distinguishable by their latency, association with specific field potential waveforms, order of appearance and disappearance during the evolution of a focus, requirement for stimulus specificity, and response to alterations in stimulus rate. The presence of a differential laminar prominence has additionally been demonstrated in the more recent data (20). The primary latency EPR burst induced by penicillin has already been shown to be an exaggeration of the normal response of neurons to a physiologic stimulus in both visual and somatosensory cortex (17,21,49). The present results support, at least for layer 4, the additional previously held conclusion that EPR bursts occur in a population of neurons before LR or PDS bursts are evoked in any neuron (17).

These data further demonstrate that this ability to respond in an enhanced fashion to normal levels of synaptic input is not uniform among neocortical laminar subpopulations when they are exposed to penicillin. EPR discharges and field potentials were noted principally in those layers that received monosynaptic geniculocortical input, namely layer 4 and to a lesser extent the deep pyramidal laminae. Substantially less penicillin-induced enhancement was noted in the earliest latency response of populations in the superficial pyramidal layers, whose input originated in layer 4. It is unclear whether this difference in response to the drug

is related to intrinsic properties of the predominant cell type (stellate versus pyramidal), differences in intralaminar circuitry, type or abundance of synaptic input (particularly inhibition), or some combination of the three. Layer 4 neurons appear to play an important initiating role in epileptogenesis by being able to respond in this enhanced fashion better than any other neocortical neuronal population. Indeed, since layer 4 is also more sensitive to low penicillin concentrations, EPR bursts of cells in this layer may be an initial effect of the drug, regardless of where it is injected into the cortex.

The second type of neuronal discharge was the LR burst. It has been shown to be the early stage of the more commonly described PDS or DS (17,21), and it almost certainly has a neuronal population origin. Unlike the EPR, multiunit LR discharges and field potentials were recorded nearly as well from all cortical layers in one or another experimental condition. Typically, both more penicillin and a longer time period were needed before LRs became evident. These longer latency bursts were never seen in isolation without being preceded by EPR activity locally *or* at least in layer 4.

The degree of GABA-mediated disinhibition induced by penicillin in our model does not seem to be sufficient for independent epileptogenesis among the neuronal aggregates of all cortical layers, however. Development of epileptic foci in the pyramidal layers, particularly those that are superficial, appears to need or at least to benefit from enhanced external triggering, which is probably provided by layer 4 EPR activity. A similar relationship has been shown in hippocampal slice preparations (54,94). CA1 pyramidal cells in contact with penicillin will not, under normal conditions, burst spontaneously, although they readily follow a triggering burst from the CA2–3 region, which has spontaneous bursting capability. Hippocampal granule cells, at the other extreme, will not generate bursts when exposed to penicillin even if triggered.

A more complete or differently mediated disinhibition, which might be supplied by higher concentrations or volumes of penicillin or by other GABA antagonists such as bicuculline (61) or picrotoxin (60), or by glycine inhibitors such as strychnine (12), may enable cortical laminae other than layer 4 to develop epileptic foci independently (34), as noted below. These more powerful convulsive agents may induce such extensive change, however, that early or subtle differences in response among the laminae are masked, thereby obscuring the basic mechanisms underlying these alterations.

Although layer 4 has now been unequivocally identified as being most sensitive to the convulsant effects of the GABA antagonists (7,8, 18,20,26) questions concerning the necessity of its involvement in epileptogenesis are now arising. In a recent preliminary report, PDS activity was evoked from superficial layers which had been severed from layer 4 in a guinea pig neocortical slice preparation (34). Although the results of this experiment are no doubt accurate, we disagree with the basic conclusion that layer 4 is not normally required for the generation of PDS in other cortical layers. When penicillin is utilized *in vivo,* response abnormalities appear initially in layer 4 regardless of the injection site (8,20) and these are followed rapidly by alterations in other layers known to receive normal interlaminar projections from layer 4. Layer 4 provides adjacent layers with a *natural trigger* for epileptogenesis in the *in vivo* model. The epileptiform spikes induced by picrotoxin reported above were evoked by electrical current applied to the cortical surface. In this case, a trigger was nonetheless still required, albeit a nonphysiologic and a nonspecific one.

Correlations with *In Vitro* Recordings

In vitro experimentation with the hippocampal slice, and more recently with the neocortical slice, has added much to our understanding of neuronal membrane properties in epileptogenesis (11,33,39,40,54,69,70,78–80,94). Although the presence of intrinsic neuronal membrane properties that can lead to burst generation was stressed as the most important factor in epileptogenesis after the initial studies of hippocampal neurons (69,80), analysis of neocortical neurons has confirmed the importance of enhanced synaptic input to members of a neuronal aggregate by means of excitatory interactions (33). Three interrelated factors have now been proposed by Prince (70) as being important for epileptogenesis: (a) the presence of intrinsic neuronal membrane properties that can lead to burst generation, (b) the loss of normal inhibitory control mechanisms, *and* (c) the degree of excitatory synaptic coupling among neurons of an aggregate.

The recent *in vitro* investigations of *neocortex* have generally supported our work in the intact animal (11,26,33). In addition to intrinsic membrane events, excitatory synaptic currents from interactions within the cell population have been shown to underlie a major portion of the slow envelope of the PDS recorded from these neurons. Neocortical neurons do not possess many of the voltage-dependent membrane mechanisms which predispose hippocampal pyramidal cells to bursting. The DSs or, in our terminology, LR bursts of neocortical neurons *in vitro* have most of the properties of their *in vivo* counterparts. Neurons with reduplicative bursts have been observed, but spontaneous DS bursting is not seen in the reduced and isolated cell populations of the neocortical slice preparation. Although the EPSP preceding a DS burst has been demonstrated in most of these neurons, the lack of cell-specific, physiologic stimulation has made the consistent recognition of an EPR burst and its development prior to that of DS generation understandably difficult *in vitro*. In addition to verifying that neocortical layer 4 is most susceptible to the epileptogenic effects of the GABA antagonists (in this case, bicuculline), George and Connors (26) have also confirmed by means of CSD analysis that epileptogenesis in this slice preparation originated in layer 4 and propagates into adjacent pyramidal layers, principally those that are more superficial.

Neurons with an unusually increased responsivity and the ability to burst to intracellular depolarization under normal conditions have been noted in neocortical slices in the middle layers (11), where we and now others have demonstrated an increased epileptogenic susceptibility. The role of these neurons as potential "pacemakers" has been posited, although they have not been separately identified in preparations in which epileptogenesis was induced with convulsant drugs, nor, in order to confirm this suspected role, have they been observed during the transformation from the normal to epileptic state. Intracellular dye marking of these peculiar neurons has shown them to be pyramidal in form (70).

From the data and discussions above, it should be apparent that we also believe that layer 4 neurons function as pacemakers. EPR bursts of a selective neuronal aggregate, responding to normal thalamocortical input, provide the initial trigger for population synchronization. We feel, however, that this role is not limited to an unusual population of cells within layer 4, but that it is a more general property of neurons within this lamina. The composition of the "pacemaker" aggregate for any given larger population discharge will not necessarily always be the same, but will vary with the specific distribution of the initiating thalamocortical input. Consequently, our data emphasize differences in neuronal connectivity, especially inhibitory modulation, and intralaminar circuitry, rather than intrinsic membrane variations between individual neurons, as the more significant factors that determine laminar sensitivity and define the roles played by neuronal populations in epileptogenesis.

A distinction between EPR and LR neuronal bursts, which have been recorded from both striate and somatosensory (49) cortex *in vivo,* has not usually been made *in vitro.* In neocortical slice preparations, this may be related to methodological considerations, such as nonphysiologic stimulation. In the hippocampus, intrinsic differences in both neuron properties and connectivity may be additional factors. Wong and Traub attest in a recent report (94) that the synchronized PDS burst of a population of hippocampal pyramidal neurons, whether evoked or spontaneous, is initiated by the output of a small number of pacer neurons through a local synaptic integration process, particularly in the CA2 region. The role of afferents is not to elicit delayed burst discharges from the aggregate directly, but to evoke initial bursts from the pacemaker cells. The exact nature of the *initial* burst of the CA2–3 pacemaker neurons, however, has not been well defined experimentally (87,94). In computer simulations in these reports (87,94) it was assumed that both pacer and follower bursts are alike and of the DS or LR type. Penicillin disinhibition in the model provides the mechanism by which mutual excitation can evoke synchronous responses from a population of neurons each capable of intrinsic bursting. Neocortical neurons, on the other hand, do not appear to have this capacity. When inhibition has been reduced, initial afferent excitation evokes EPR, not LR, bursts even from the pacer cells. Mutual excitatory interactions among the aggregate provide both synchronization and further amplification of the synaptic input needed to elicit LR bursts.

Johnston and Brown (39,40) have maintained that there are two classes of burst discharges recordable from hippocampal pyramidal cells as well. Although they are similar in appearance, appropriate criteria based on quantitative physiological tests can distinguish them as separate phenomena. The "endogenous" burst is an independent single cell event based upon voltage-sensitive membrane properties. The "network" or PDS burst is dependent on synaptic interactions among a group of neurons and is evoked from individual cells by a "giant" EPSP. Confusion may arise when recordings are made from hippocampal CA2–3 region, since both endogenous and network bursts that are either spontaneous or triggered can be seen in the same neuron. Johnston and Brown conclude that

burst discharges should not be termed PDS unless shown to be "network" in character. Although these data are derived from a different cell population and experimental model, the conceptual relationship between these burst types and our EPR and LR appears similar.

A LAMINAR THEORY OF NEOCORTICAL EPILEPTOGENESIS

Any general theory of epileptogenesis in neocortex must take into account the various roles of specific neuronal subpopulations. Consideration in this regard justifiably begins with those of the granular layer, because it is unusual in both its anatomy and physiology. Layer 4 is composed chiefly of stellate cells with spiny dendrites, which are unique to this region (47). Layer 4 neurons receive monosynaptic excitation from primary geniculocortical inputs, for which they are the major terminus, and phasic disynaptic inhibition through interneurons within their own lamina (86). Spiny stellate cells in turn make only excitatory contracts on other neurons. Dendritic branches, and particularly the axon arborizations of these spiny cells, form a complex network within the granular layer (27,47), which is compounded by the high packing density of neurons. The major outflow from layer 4 is to the superficial pyramidal layers 3 and 2.

Another category of stellate cells have dendrites that are smooth or sparsely spined (47,63). Aspinous neurons make up only 3–4% of the population of stellate cells in layer 4 but, unlike spiny stellate neurons, they can be found in all the major cortical laminae. Cells of this type are presumably the interneurons within layer 4 that mediate, by means of GABA, inhibition upon the spiny stellate neurons (63,83). We will postulate at this point that the inhibitory modulation of layer 4 stellate responses is significantly different from that found in the pyramidal layers. This difference may be one either of type and/or quantity, and may be a crucial factor in the heightened susceptibility of layer 4 to epileptogenesis. Neuromorphological evidence supports this presumption. Although aspiny stellate cells are found in all layers, more types are found in the pyramidal layers and certain types, such as the "chandelier" cells, are rarely found in layer 4 (47,63).

The initial result of penicillin-induced disinhibition in layer 4 is an exaggeration of the normal neuronal response, i.e., the EPR burst. This initial increase in responsiveness is limited in degree, since the excitatory, thalamocortical input is normal, and is limited in extent, because it is evoked only from a select population of neurons whose receptive fields respond to the stimulus, whether externally or internally derived. These activated neurons within the penicillin-affected population act as epileptogenic "pacemakers". Rich interconnections among the stellate cells of layer 4 provide a network in which excitatory synaptic coupling can now become even more effective. Feed-forward and feedback excitation initiated by EPR activity forms the basis for large recurrent and collateral synaptic drives on members of the population. Pacemaker neurons will typically be observed to fire doubly with both EPR and LR bursts, whereas follower neurons will respond only with the latter. Early or late in the evolution of a focus, when population synchrony is incomplete, reduplicative LR bursts may be noted. With a slightly different stimulus, the roles of pacemaker and follower within the population change. Because layer 4 stellate neurons have the greatest capacity for EPR generation, they may be the only subpopulation within which such dual and reversible roles are likely.

Not only are layer 4 populations most capable of initiating and elaborating epileptiform responses independently, but they also play a key role in epileptogenesis in the other cortical laminae by providing them with needed triggering. Translaminar pacing from layer 4 takes two forms. First, enhanced but otherwise physiologic driving may be supplied by EPR burst activity to pyramidal populations to assist in the epileptogenesis of superficial or deep penicillin-induced foci. Although these populations may be in contact with more penicillin, they are less susceptible to its epileptogenic effects than are the layer 4 stellate cells. Second, synchronous LR bursting within the neuronal aggregate of a layer 4 focus can furnish layers 3 and 2 with a substantially more intense afferent barrage. The location of layer 4 at the origin and branch-point of serial cortical processing aides in the dissemination of both types of pacemaker activity over existing interlaminar pathways.

The pyramidal neurons of the superficial cortical layers have abundant interconnections and a wide horizontal spread of their axon arborizations (27). The major outflow from layers 2 and 3 is to related cortical areas both ipsilaterally and contralaterally. Axons from these pyramidal cells on their way out of the cortex give off collaterals into layer 5, where they terminate on the deep pyramidal cells in that layer. Many types of aspiny stellate cells, presumably with inhibitory interneuron function, are also found in the pyramidal layers. In general, they have a wide separation of their axon arborizations, particularly in the vertical direction. They may span two layers, providing perhaps interlaminar inhibitory links, which modulate the usual excitatory connections (27,47). Certain of these aspiny neurons, perhaps the chandelier cells with cartridge synapses, are thought to act as tonic inhibitors of pyramidal neuron activity. Other interneurons may act as phasic inhibitors or may act on the tonic inhibitors as "disinhibitor" cells. The latter have been hypothesized by Roberts in his theory of the functional organization of cortex (76).

A potentially important subpopulation of pyramidal neurons are the "border" or "star" pyramids, which are located at the layer 3–4 interface and whose basal dendrites extend into layer 4 (47). These neurons are positioned to receive various synaptic inputs, such as disynaptic excitation from layer 4 spiny stellate cells, disynaptic inhibition from layer 4 aspiny stellate cells, trisynaptic inhibition from layer 3 aspiny stellate cells, and perhaps even trisynaptic disinhibition. The epileptogenic effects of penicillin in layer 4 could quickly augment the responsiveness of these pyramidal neurons, not only secondary to increased excitatory input from the EPR and LR bursts of spiny stellate neurons, but also from a blockade of GABA inhibition on their proximal basal dendrites due to an early direct effect of penicillin. Such twin actions can rapidly lead to response exaggeration. Burst discharges from this population of pyramidal neurons may supplement those of the spiny stellate neurons in forming a large synchronous projection into more superficial layers 3 and 2, as can be seen in the evolution of a layer 4 focus.

Even when penicillin has only begun to diffuse into the superficial layers after a layer 4 injection, large epileptiform responses may be evoked from the pyramidal neurons located there. If one accepts Roberts' idea that tonic inhibitors of pyramidal cells are themselves inhibited by other interneurons that receive stellate input, the enhanced afference from layer 4 stellate cells engaged in LR bursting would be doubly excitatory. Dual mechanisms of increased excitatory input and decreased tonic inhibition would allow these superficial pyramidal neurons to express a greater augmentation in activity than seen in stellate counterparts. Subpopulations in laminae 2 and 3 can thus be thought of as powerful elaborators of response abnormality originating in layer 4.

These pyramidal neuron populations are, however, less susceptible to direct penicillin epileptogenesis, perhaps because of the increased inhibitory control placed upon them by interneurons. Penicillin's partial blockade of GABA may be less effective due to the different types and/or the increased quantity of inhibition present. Consequently, EPR bursting is less well developed in the superficial pyramidal layers. Even when disinhibition has occurred, an exaggerated afference may be needed to synchronize the population sufficiently initially. Diffusion of penicillin into layer 4 from a topical or layer 2–3 injection results in the stellate EPR responses that can provide the necessary triggering to facilitate further epileptogenic development. Although clearly capable of generating their own epileptiform responses eventually, pyramidal neurons of layers 2 and 3 are dependent upon layer 4 for pacing and as such are principally followers.

In addition, blockade of inhibition by penicillin may have opposing effects if disinhibitory neurons exist in the circuitry of the pyramidal layers. Although increased responses would result from a lessening of direct inhibitory influences, a concurrent blockade of disinhibitor cells would lead to decreased pyramidal cell responsivity. This mixed effect of penicillin may be another reason why the pyramidal layers are less susceptible to epileptogenesis and would explain at the same time why the LR response of layers 2–3 is often of greater amplitude with a layer 4 focus than when penicillin is placed directly into the superficial layers.

The same principles of functional organization may hold true for layers 5–6. Additional inhibitory restraints and a reduction of disinhibitory function may explain as well the lessened susceptibility of deep pyramidal neurons to penicillin epileptogenesis. EPR bursting is present, but is not as well developed as in stellate populations. Because these layers do receive some direct geniculate input, unlike the superficial laminae, they are somewhat less dependent upon layer 4 pacing for the generation of local epileptiform responses.

ARREST OF SEIZURES: LAMINAR DIFFERENCES IN ANTICONVULSANT ACTION

The treatment of epilepsy remains empirical to this day. Our understanding of its pathophysiology is rudimentary, and we know even less about the actions of drugs used in the attempt to control seizures. The search for fundamental mechanisms of anticonvulsant action has been limited by the experimental models available and by our incomplete understanding of the complexities of epileptogenesis. Investigation using mammalian brain *in vivo* has the advantage that extrapolation to human disease is relatively straightforward. Many of the disadvantages inherent in an analysis of neuronal function within such a complex system may be minimized if sufficient experimental control is provided by the model chosen.

In recent years, there have been significant advances in documenting the actions of antiepileptic drugs upon cellular biochemical processes, membranes, isolated neurons, axons, and neuromuscular junctions. Most of these investigations noted effects on normal physiology, however. Most reported an association between anticonvulsants and either decreased neuronal firing, reduced nerve impulse transmission, or some membrane alteration that would be expected to lead to such a result. That these actions represented clinical antiepileptic mechanism of drugs, rather than a nonspecific or toxic effect, could only be inferred rather than demonstrated. It has not been established for a single anticonvulsant which, if any, of its documented effects is its antiepileptic action.

The study of the effects of anticonvulsants on neurons within intact mammalian cortex is poorly represented in current research, particularly since this model provides an improved setting for observing true antiepileptic action. All stages and levels of epileptiform abnormality, from neuronal burst discharges to seizures, can be induced in cortex and are available for analysis. More important, most epileptiform phenomena require interactions among organized and interconnected cell populations that exist, for the most part, only in intact brain. Theories of anticonvulsant action based on *in vitro* data have seldom taken into account the diversity of cellular elements, aggregates, and local circuit actions that play specific roles in normal as well as pathologic epileptiform functioning and may be specifically acted on by these drugs. Interpretations suggesting that antiepileptic drugs must necessarily produce a general depressant effect on neuronal firing do not fit well with the recent appreciation of inhibition as a basic organizing principle of cortical functioning and disinhibition as a major factor in, at least, experimental epilepsy. Indeed, if antiepileptic agents possess selectivity of action and influence only certain types of neurons, almost any effect could be anticonvulsant—even increased responsiveness, if the drug affected principally inhibitory interneuron action. It is therefore only in the context of intact cortical circuitry and cellular interactions that physiologic responses to drug action can be definitively interpreted as being antiepileptic and achieve, or fail to achieve, operational significance.

PHT

The multiple theories concerning the antiepileptic effects of PHT are a testimony to the remaining uncertainty as to which of them are clinically significant. PHT has been shown to have several actions on membranes and synapses, particularly on the function of ion channels, which are inferred to possess antiepileptic potential (see ref. 95). In simple neuronal systems, PHT significantly affects synaptic mechanisms. A decrease in EPSPs (3,48) and prolongation of inhibitory postsynaptic potentials (IPSPs) mediated by GABA have been observed. These depressant actions may be antiepileptic.

Direct assessments of PHT's anticonvulsant actions of the PHTs *in vitro* have shown less evidence of direct effects on neuronal excitability than were posited above. Although PHT suppressed the bursting response of *Aplysia* cells exposed to pentylenetetrazol (38), in a culture of mammalian spinal cord neurons it did not abolish epileptiform burst discharges induced by picrotoxin or augment GABA or glycine inhibition (51). At concentrations appropriate for cerebrospinal fluid (CSF), PHT only limited repetitive firing (52). PHT did suppress spontaneous, but not evoked, penicillin-induced neuronal bursts or interictal population spikes from guinea pig hippocampal slices (77). However, no effects were observed on resting membrane potentials, input resistance, action potential parameters, or threshold intensity for intracellular stimulation. The significance of these effects in altering the development and spread of epileptiform abnormalities *in vivo* remains a subject of speculation.

In mammalian brain *in vivo,* the antiepileptic actions of PHT are also limited. It is very effective in the MES seizure test in blocking the cortical spread of seizure activity, but has little effect in elevating seizure threshold to pentylenetetrazol or bicuculline (84). PHT given intravenously shortens the duration, decreases the high-frequency components, and suppresses the spread of focal electrically induced seizures in cats (36). In experiments with topical penicillin foci in cats, PHT abolished clinical (motor) seizure activity despite persistent focal EEG spiking (42). It has been shown to *increase* IIS frequency, decrease spike duration, and suppress afterdischarges (5). Spiking from weak foci was eliminated by high PHT concentrations.

Antiepileptic actions directed mainly against longer polysynaptic pathways were suggested.

If an investigation of the mechanisms of anticonvulsant action on mammalian brain is to extract basic information from such a complex system, it will require a well-documented and well-controlled epilepsy model. The model discussed in this chapter provides a means for studying epileptiform response abnormalities at the level of both neurons and neuronal aggregates involving neocortical intralaminar, interlaminar, and intercolumnar population interactions. The potential, therefore, exists to test anticonvulsants against epileptic pathophysiology at these same levels. Because epilepsy is both a local and a propagated phenomenon, the ability to make these distinctions may be crucial in understanding the differing actions of antiepileptic drugs.

We have characterized the action of intravenous (I.V.) PHT upon the evolution of discrete neocortical epileptic foci induced by the injection of sodium penicillin in nanoliter volumes into striate cortical layer 4 (9). The evolution of temporary penicillin epileptic foci originating from layer 4 (Fig. 19) was compared before and after the I.V. infusion of PHT. Several effects were noted following the establishment of therapeutic serum levels. Most striking was the suppression of spontaneous IIS from all cortical layers monitored (Fig. 20). The duration of these foci following phenytoin, as measured from the onset to the termination of spontaneous spiking, was dramatically shortened, as compared to similarly induced foci before PHT. Despite nearly complete cessation of spontaneous discharges, PHT did not suppress the ability of the penicillin-treated cortex to generate epileptiform potentials, since they remained elicitable by physiologic stimuli specific for the region. When the amplitudes of epileptiform LR and IIS potentials were measured (Fig. 19), however, additional differential laminar effects became evident. Potentials from superficial layers 2–3 were disproportionately reduced relative to those from other layers (Fig. 21). Delays in the development of response abnormalities and a reduction in their rate of amplitude increase were demonstrated as well.

All of the demonstrated effects of PHT depressed epileptogenesis and would have contributed to diminished levels of abnormal activity at subsequent synaptic relays. The degree of suppression was consistently and substantially greater in the more superficial laminae, since it is layers 2–3 of the striate cortex which: (a) receive their input from layer 4, (b) have been

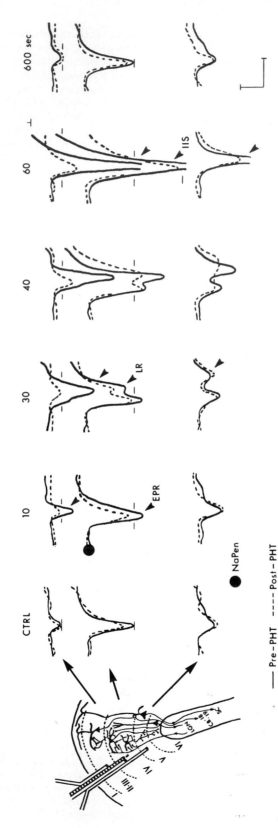

FIG. 19. Simultaneous recordings from three neocortical layers evoked by visual flash stimuli before, during, and after the microinjection of 1 nl of sodium penicillin (NaPen) into layer 4. Typical alterations in response profiles across laminae are seen before PHT injection. Epileptiform response suppression can be seen across all recorded laminae following intravenous PHT administration. Recording depths were 400, 1,000, and 1,600 μm. *Top line:* elapsed time following the onset of penicillin. Calibrations: 50 μV, 40 msec (from ref 9, with permission).

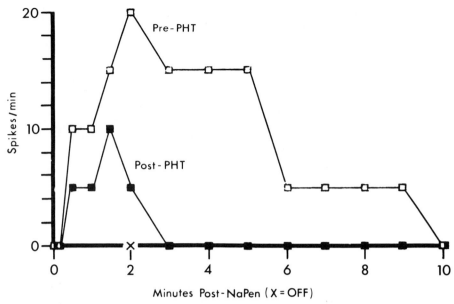

FIG. 20. *Pre-PHT* illustrates the development of spontaneous epileptiform spike frequencies following the injection of penicillin into striate layer 4. *Post-PHT* describes the effect of intravenous injection of phenytoin on the same response parameter after similar penicillin injection. Serum blood levels were measured at 14 μg/ml. At these concentrations, PHT did not protect completely against the onset of spontaneous spiking, but did limit its frequency and duration significantly (from ref. 9).

shown to follow closely and even to elaborate epileptiform responses projected from layer 4, and which in turn (c) send their principal axonal projections into adjacent areas of the visual cortex (20,27,28,47). Preliminary evidence from our laboratory suggests that epileptiform activity levels are even further reduced at these more distant sites. This differential effect of PHT on layers that can both elaborate and widely disseminate epileptiform discharges may be the way its basic membrane mechanisms act within intact cortex and may be the reason for the purported clinical effectiveness of PHT in preventing seizure spread.

The marked differential effect of PHT on spontaneous versus evoked epileptiform responses is also provocative. With I.V. doses that result in therapeutic blood levels, PHT suppressed spontaneous IIS of all laminae, but did not suppress the *ability* of the penicillin-treated cortex to generate these epileptiform potentials, since they could still be evoked by a physiologic stimulus specific for the region. The synchronous excitation of a sufficiently large population of neurons within the penicillin focus may overcome this antiepileptic effect of PHT in our model and enable neuronal response integration within the local population to proceed to the generation of an interictal potential. The

limited action of PHT in this regard suggests that it may also be more effective at the initial and, therefore, weaker stages of local circuit interactions, in which response abnormalities of individual neurons (subthreshold population events) coalesce or fail to coalesce into longer latency population discharges as described by Traub and Wong (87) in their computer models.

These data at the level of small neuronal populations within distinct cortical layers support the contention of past *in vivo* and *in vitro* studies (5,77) that epileptiform responses mediated by longer polysynaptic pathways appear to be more effectively suppressed by PHT than by those of the focus itself. An understanding of the mechanisms mediating this effect in the *intact organism* may be clearer now than previously if one considers the morphology and synaptology of the cortical layers in which the differential effects were demonstrated. Layer 4 is believed to be dominated by excitatory processes because of its large excitatory input from many brain nuclei (47,63), and because there is evidence that inhibition may be less effective here than in other layers of the cortical column (8,46,47,82). If the mechanism by which PHT exerts its anticonvulsive effect *in vivo* is principally a nonspecific depression of synaptic activity (see ref. 95 for review) one might expect

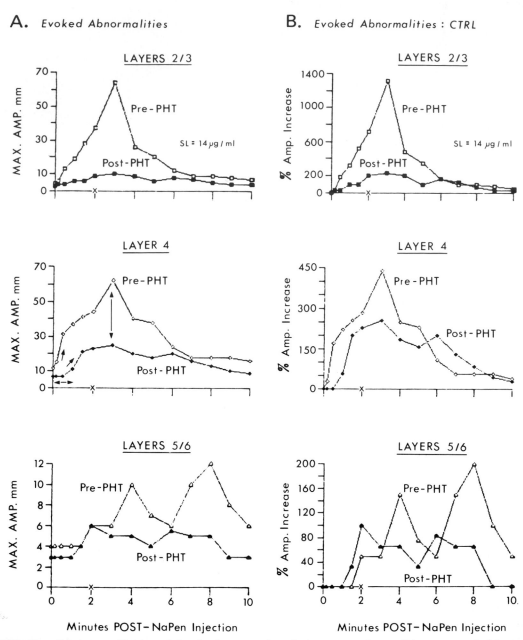

A. *Evoked Abnormalities*

B. *Evoked Abnormalities : CTRL*

Minutes POST–NaPen Injection   Minutes POST–NaPen Injection

FIG. 21. **(A)** A quantification of the development of evoked response abnormalities over cortical layers following penicillin injection before and after PHT administration. Generalized amplitude suppression and deficits in the onset of response abnormalities (delayed *and* reduced rate of increase) can be seen *Post-PHT* (*arrows* in layer 4). In addition, the prepenicillin normal response is attenuated by PHT. Amplitudes were measured directly from paper records with 10 μm equaling 1 mm of deflection. Penicillin injection discontinued at X. **(B)** Data from *A* presented as a percentage of amplitude increase from normal, prepenicillin activity levels. This figure demonstrates that evoked abnormalities induced by penicillin are still substantial, even following PHT administration. PHT does have a significant impact on epileptogenesis, however, with epileptiform response onset interrupted and response abnormalities dramatically suppressed in layers 2 and 3 (from ref. 9).

the greatest influence of PHT to be within the layer 4 focus, in which excitatory synaptic activity is substantial. This was not the case. The effectiveness of PHT was maximal in the supragranular layers, in which abundant influential inhibitory connections, including cartridge-type synapses surrounding the initial segments of pyramidal cells, have been demonstrated morphologically (47,82) and in which inhibitory control over pyramidal cell output is thought to be considerable (75). It is possible that this differential laminar effectiveness may be a population manifestation of a local prolongation of postsynaptic inhibition seen previously in isolated extracellular recordings from the cat cortex by Raabe and Ayala (73).

These correlations could also be interpreted as lending some support to position of White et al. and Woodbury that the *predominant* generalized effect of PHT may be stimulatory and not depressive (91,95), since the anticonvulsant effects demonstrated in this study were manifested principally in laminae in which inhibitory processes are believed to dominate over excitatory events. The excitatory effects of PHT, however, are most often seen at high dose levels —a condition that we have tried to avoid in this experiment. A final possible explanation for our results involves some recent studies showing a selective suppressive effect of PHT on high-frequency neuronal firing (41,43,52,53). This mechanism may help to explain the differential laminar effects of PHT that we have reported *if* the discharge frequencies of neuronal PDSs that underlie LR or IIS field-potentials are greater in layers 2–3 than in layer 4.

Phenobarbital

We have recently begun complementary experiments utilizing phenobarbital (PB) as the anticonvulsant agent. To date, two observations are noteworthy. Intravenous PB resulting in therapeutic serum levels also suppresses spontaneous IISs. Unlike phenytoin, however, phenobarbital induces a generalized translaminar suppression of evoked epileptiform potentials. PB may act to control epileptiform responsivity at the pacer level within the focus proper and not preferentially on the spread of epileptiform activity to follower populations. Utilization of the more refined physiologic measures provided by this model has thus already begun to reveal subtle, but potentially significant, differences in the character and distribution of antiepileptic actions within the cortex.

CONCLUSION

By means of simultaneous multilaminar recordings during the evolution of discrete epileptic foci, we have demonstrated among the various layers of cat visual cortex a diversity of (a) susceptibilities to epileptogenesis, (b) patterns of response alteration across both space and time, and (c) associations between the activity of specific neuronal subpopulations. We have further demonstrated laminar actions of anticonvulsant drugs. Differentiation across the cortical layers, rather than homogeneity, appears to be the rule in the functional organization of these discrete epileptic foci. There is evidence that these distinctive characteristics are a reflection both of differences in intrinsic responsivity among cell types and of variation in connectivity within the layers. The respective roles for laminar neuronal subpopulations in the onset, propagation, and control of epileptiform response abnormalities can now be better understood. These laminar distinctions among neocortical subpopulations can be summarized as follows. First, layer 4 of striate neocortex is the most susceptible to penicillin epileptogenesis. This may be related to inhibitory modulation within layer 4 that may be quantitatively or qualitatively different from that in the pyramidal layers. Second, EPR bursts of a selective layer 4 neuronal aggregate, responding to normal thalamocortical input, provide the initial trigger for population synchronization. Although layer 4 neurons probably function as epileptogenic pacemakers, we feel that this role is not limited to certain unusual cells, but is a general property of this laminar population. Third, neuronal interactions within layer 4 appear to be sufficient for epileptogenesis. Cellular and circuitry conditions are favorable for the elaboration of pacemaker EPR bursts into network-driven LR or PDS bursts in a larger follower population. Fourth, penicillin action within layer 4, resulting in EPR activity there, may be necessary for, or is at least supportive of, epileptic foci originating in pyramidal layers. Due to their decreased susceptibility, pyramidal aggregates seem to require a larger than normal synaptic trigger. Fifth, propagation of epileptiform LR burst activity, as well as the more modest interlaminar pacing by EPRs, preferentially follows existing interlaminar pathways. The most significant pathway appears to be between stellate layer 4 and pyramidal layers 2–3. Finally, antiepileptic drugs may possess differential laminar activity. Phenytoin, for example, appears to suppress epileptiform responses propagated to pyramidal layers 2–3 disproportionately.

REFERENCES

1. Ajmone-Marsan, C. (1969): Effects of topical epileptogenic agents. In: *Basic Mechanisms of the Epilepsies,* edited by Jasper, H. H., Ward, A. A., and Pope, A., pp. 299–319. Little Brown and Co., Boston.
2. Avoli, M., Brancati, A., Pacitti, C., and Barra, P. F. A. (1982): Neuronal responses to putative neurotransmitters during penicillin epileptogenesis. *Neuroscience,* 7:1955–1961.
3. Ayala, G. F., Johnston, D., Lin, S., and Dichter, H. N. (1977): The mechanisms of action of diphenylhydantoin on invertebrate neurons: II. Effects on synaptic mechanisms. *Brain Res.,* 121:259–270.
4. Ayala, G. F., Dichter, M., Gunnit, R. J., Matsumoto, H., and Spencer, W. A. (1973): Genesis of epileptic interictal spikes. New knowledge of cortical feedback systems suggests a neurophysiological explanation of brief paroxysms. *Brain Res.,* 52:1–17.
5. Bustamante, L., Leuders, H., Pippenger, C., and Goldensohn, E. S. (1980): The effects of phenytoin on the penicillin-induced spike focus. *Electroencephalogr. Clin. Neurophysiol.* 48:90–97.
6. Chatt, A. B., and Ebersole, J. S. (1981): Evidence of the neocortical microcircuitry involved in epileptogenesis. *Neurosci. Abstr.,* 7:812.
7. Chatt, A. B., and Ebersole, J. S. (1982): The laminar sensitivity of cat striate cortex to penicillin induced epileptogenesis. *Brain Res.,* 241:382–387.
8. Chatt, A. B., and Ebersole, J. S. (1984): Identification of penicillin diffusion at the onset of epileptogenesis in the cat striate cortex following differential laminar microinjection. *Brain Res.,* 290:361–366.
9. Chatt, A. B., and Ebersole, J. S. (1984): Phenytoin preferentially suppresses epileptiform response activity in the superficial cortical layers. *Brain Res.,* 295:394–400.
10. Collins, R. C., and Caston, T. V. (1979): Activation of cortical circuits during interictal spikes. *Ann. Neurol.,* 6:117–125.
11. Connors, B. W., Gutnick, M. J., and Prince, D. A. (1982): Electrophysiological properties of neocortical neurons in vitro. *J. Neurophysiol.,* 48:1302–1320.
12. Curtis, D. R., Duggan, A., Felix, D., Johnston, G. A. R., and McLennan, H. (1971): Antagonism between bicuculline and GABA in the cat brain. *Brain Res.,* 33:57–73.
13. Curtis, D. R., Game, C. J. A., Johnston, G. A. R., McCulloch, R. R., and Maclachlan, R. M. (1972): Convulsant action of penicillin. *Brain Res.,* 43:242–245.
14. Dichter, M., and Spencer, W. A. (1969): Penicillin-induced interictal discharges from the cat hippocampus. I. *J. Neurophysiol.,* 32:649–662.
15. Dingledine, R., and Gjerstad, L. (1979): Penicillin blocks hippocampal IPSPs, unmasking prolonged EPSPs. *Brain Res.,* 168:205–209.
16. Donoghue, J. P., Kerman, K., and Ebner, F. (1979): Evidence for two organizational plans within somatic sensory-motor cortex of the rat. *J. Comp. Neurol.,* 183:647–664.
17. Ebersole, J. S. (1977): Initial abnormalities of neuronal responses during epileptogenesis in visual cortex. *J. Neurophysiol.,* 40:514–526.
18. Ebersole, J. S., and Chatt, A. B. (1980): The laminar susceptibility of cat visual cortex to penicillin-induced epileptogenesis. *Neurology,* 30: 355.
19. Ebersole, J. S., and Chatt, A. B. (1981): Toward a unified theory of focal penicillin epileptogenesis: An intracortical evoked potential investigation. *Epilepsia,* 22:347–361.
20. Ebersole, J. S., and Chatt, A. B. (1984): Laminar interactions during neocortical epileptogenesis. *Brain Res.,* 298:253–271.
21. Ebersole, J. S., and Levine, R. A. (1975): Abnormal neuronal responses during evolution of a penicillin epileptic focus in cat visual cortex. *J. Neurophysiol.,* 38:250–266.
22. Elger, C. E., Speckmann, E. J., Prohaska, O., and Caspars, H. (1981): Pattern of intracortical potential distribution during focal interictal epileptiform discharges (FIED) and its relation to spinal field potentials in the rat. *Electroencephalogr. Clin. Neurophysiol.,* 51:393–402.
23. Fisher, R. S., Pedley, T. A., and Moody, W. J. (1976): The role of extracellular potassium in hippocampal epilepsy. *Arch. Neurol.,* 33:76–83.
24. Gabor, A. J., and Scobey, R. P. (1975): Spatial limits of epileptogenic cortex: Its relationship to ectopic spike generation. *J. Neurophysiol.,* 38: 395–404.
25. Gabor, A. J., and Scobey, R. P. (1977): Epileptogenicity and the cortical column. *Electroencephalogr. Clin. Neurophysiol.,* 43:461–462.
26. George, C. P., and Connors, B. W. (1983): Initiation of synchronized bursting in neocortex. *Neurosci. Abstr.,* 9:396.
27. Gilbert, C. D., and Wiesel, T. N. (1979): Morphology and intracortical projections of functionally characterized neurones in the cat visual cortex. *Nature,* 280:120–125.
28. Gilbert, C. D., and Wiesel, T. N. (1981): Laminar specialization and intercortical connections in cat primary visual cortex. In *The Organization of the Cerebral Cortex,* edited by F. O. Schmitt, F. G. Worden, G. Adelman, and S. G. Dennis, pp. 163–191. MIT Press, Cambridge, MA.
29. Goldensohn, E. S., Zablow, L., and Salazar, A. (1977): The penicillin focus: I. Distribution of potential at the cortical surface. *Electroencephalogr. Clin. Neurophysiol.,* 42:480–492.
30. Gumnit, R. J., Matsumoto, H., and Vasconetto, C. (1970): DC activity in the depth of an experimental epileptic focus. *Electroencephalogr. Clin. Neurophysiol.,* 28:333–339.
31. Gutnick, M. J., and Prince, D. A. (1974): Effects of projected cortical epileptiform discharges on neuronal activities in cat VPL. I. Interictal discharge. *J. Neurophysiol.,* 37:1310–1327.
32. Gutnick, M. J., and Prince, D. A. (1975): Effects

of projected cortical epileptiform discharges on neuronal activities in ventrolateral thalamus of the cat: Ictal discharge. *Exp. Neurol.*, 46:418–431.

33. Gutnick, M. J., Connors, B. W., and Prince, D. A. (1982): Mechanisms of neocortical epileptogenesis in vitro. *J Neurophysiol.*, 48:1321–1335.

34. Gutnick, M. J., Grossman, Y., and Carlen, P. (1982): Epileptogenesis in subdivided neocortical slices. *Neurosci. Lett.*, 10(*Suppl.*):226.

35. Holmes, O., and Lockton, J. W. (1982): Penicillin epileptogenesis in the rat: Diffusion and differential laminar sensitivity of the cortex cerebri. *Brain Res.*, 231:131–141.

36. Ito, T., Hori, M. Yoshida, K., and Shimizu, M. (1977): Effect of anticonvulsant on cortical focal seizures in cats. *Epilepsia*, 18:63–71.

37. Jasper, H. (1969): Mechanisms of propagation: Extracellular studies. In: *Basic Mechanisms of the Epilepsies*, edited by H. H. Jasper, A. A. Ward, Jr., and A. Pope, pp. 421–451. Little Brown, Boston.

38. Johnston, D., and Ayala, G. F. (1975): Diphenylhydantoin: The action of a common anticonvulsant on bursting pacemaker cells in *Aplysia*. *Science*, 189:1009–1011.

39. Johnston, D., and Brown, T. H. (1981): Giant synaptic potential hypothesis for epileptiform activity. *Science*, 211:294–297.

40. Johnston, D., and Brown, T. H. (1983): Mechanisms of neuronal burst generation. In: *Electrophysiology of Epilepsy*, edited by P. Schwartzkroin and H. Wheal, pp. 277–301. Academic Press, London.

41. Kendig, J. L., Courtney, K. R., and Cohen, E. N. (1979): Anesthetics: Molecular correlates of voltage and frequency sensitive sodium channel block in nerve. *J. Pharmacol. Exp. Ther.*, 210:446–452.

42. Kutt, H., Louis, S., and McDowell, F. (1968): Intravenous diphenylhydantoin in experimental seizures. *Arch. Neurol.*, 18:465–471.

43. Lewis, D. V., Zbicz, K. L., Nepp, M. E., Colmers, W. F., and Wilson, W. A. (1979): Diphenylhydantoin enhances early adaptation in *Aplysia* giant neurons. *J. Pharmacol. Exp. Ther.*, 218:41–45.

44. Lockton, J. W., and Holmes, O. (1980): Site of the initiation of penicillin-induced epilepsy in the cortex cerebri of the rat. *Brain Res.*, 190:301–304.

45. Lockton, J. W., and Holmes, O. (1983): Penicillin epilepsy in the rat: The responses of different layers of the cortex cerebri. *Brain Res.*, 258:79–89.

46. Lund, J. S. (1981): Intrinsic organization of the primate visual cortex, area 17, as seen in golgi preparations. In: *The Organization of the Cerebral Cortex*, edited by F. O. Schmitt, F. G. Worden, G. Adelman, and S. G. Dennis, pp. 105–124. MIT Press, Cambridge, Massachusetts.

47. Lund, J. S., Henry, G. H., MacQueen, C. L., and Harvey, A. R. (1979): Anatomical organization of the primary visual cortex (area 17) of the cat. *J. Comp. Neurol.*, 184:599–618.

48. MacDonald, R. L., and Barker, J. L. (1977): Studies of the mechanism of action of convulsants and anticonvulsants in cultured mammalian neurons. *Ann. Neurol.*, 2:264.

49. Macon, J. B., and King, D. W. (1979): Penicillin iontophoresis and the responses of somatosensory cortical neurons to amino acids. *Electroencephlogr. Clin. Neurophysiol.*, 47:52–63.

50. Matsumoto, H., and Ajmone-Marsan, C. (1964): Cortical cellular phenomena in experimental epilepsy: Interictal manifestations. *Exp. Neurol.*, 9:286–304.

51. McLean, M. S., and MacDonald, R. L. (1982): Multiple effects of phenytoin on action potentials of mouse spinal cord neurons in cell culture. *Neurology*, 32:A223.

52. McLean, M. J., and MacDonald, R. L. (1983): Phenytoin and carbamazapine selectively limit sustained high frequency repetitive firing of cultured mouse neurons. *Neurosci. Abstr.*, 9:398.

53. McLean, M. J., and MacDonald, R. L. (1983): Selective effects of anticonvulsant drugs on high frequency repetitive firing of action potentials in mouse spinal cord neurons in cell culture. *Neurology*, 33 (Suppl. 2):213.

54. Mesher, R. A., and Schwartzkroin, P. A. (1980): Can CA3 epileptiform discharge induce bursting in normal CA1 hippocampal neurons? *Brain Res.*, 183:472–476.

55. Meyer, H., and Prince, D. A. (1973): Convulsant actions of penicillin: Effects on inhibitory mechanism. *Brain Res.*, 53:477–482.

56. Mitzdorf, U., and Singer, W. (1978): Prominent excitatory pathways in the cat visual cortex (A17 and A18): A current source density analysis of electrically evoked potentials. *Exp. Brain Res.*, 33:371–394.

57. Moody, W. J., Futamachi, K. J., and Prince, D. A. (1974): Extracellular potassium activity during epileptogenesis. *Exp. Neurol.*, 42:248–263.

58. Noebels, J. L., and Pedley, T. A. (1977): Anatomic localization of topically applied [14C] penicillin during experimental focal epilepsy in cat neocortex. *Brain Res.*, 125:293–303.

59. Noebels, J. C., and Prince, D. A. (1978): Development of focal seizures in cerebral cortex: Role of axon terminal bursting. *J. Neurophysiol.*, 41:1267–1281.

60. Olsen, R. W., and Leeb-Lundberg, F. (1981): Convulsant and anticonvulsant drug binding sites related to the GABA receptor/ionophore system. In: *Neurotransmitters, Seizures and Epilepsy*, edited by P. L. Morselli, W. Loscher, K. G. Lloyd, B. Meldrum, and E. H. Reynolds. Raven Press, New York.

61. Olsen, R. W., Ticku, M. K., Greenlee, D. and Van Ness, P. (1979): GABA receptor and ionophore binding sites: Interaction with various drugs. In: *GABA Neurotransmitters: Pharmacochemical, Biochemical and Pharmacological Aspects*, edited by P. Krogsgaard-Larsen, J. Scheel-Kruger, and H. Kofod. Academic Press, Orlando, Fla.

62. Pedley, T. A. (1978): The pathophysiology of focal epilepsy: Neurophysiologic considerations. *Ann. Neurol.*, 3:2–9.

63. Peters, A., and Fairen, A. (1978): Smooth and sparsely-spined stellate cells in the visual cortex of the rat: A study using a combined Golgi-electron microscope technique. *J. Comp. Neurol.*, 181:129–172.

64. Petsche, H., Pockberger, H., and Rappelsberger, P. (1982): Current source density studies of epileptic phenomena and the morphology of the rabbit's striate cortex. In: *Physiology and Pharmacology of Epileptogenic Phenomena*, edited by M. R. Klee, H. D. Lux, and E. J. Speckmann, pp. 53–63. Raven Press, New York.

65. Pockberger, H., Petsche, H., and Rappelsberger, P. (1981): Die beeinflussung von interiktalen penicillin-spitzen durch clonazepam. *Z. EEG EMG*, 12:69–75.

66. Pockberger, H., Petsche, H., and Rappelsberger, P. (1982): The action of benzodiazepines on focal penicillin induced interictal activity. In: *Physiology and Pharmacology of Epileptogenic Phenomena*, edited by M. R. Klee, H. D. Lux, and E. J. Speckmann. Raven Press, New York.

67. Prince, D. A., and Wilder, B. J. (1967): Control mechanisms in cortical epileptogenic foci. *Arch. Neurol.*, 16:194–202.

68. Prince, D. A. (1968): Inhibition in "epileptic" neurons. *Exp. Neurol.*, 21:307–321.

69. Prince, D. A. (1978): Neurophysiology of epilepsy. *Annu. Rev. Neurosci.*, 1:395–415.

70. Prince, D. A. (1983): Ionic mechanisms in cortical and hippocampal epileptogenesis. In: *Basic Mechanisms of Neuronal Hyperexcitability*, edited by H. H. Jasper and N. M. van Gelder, pp. 217–243. Alan R. Liss, New York.

71. Prince, D. A. (1968): The depolarization shift in "epileptic neurons." *Exp. Neurol.*, 21:467–485.

72. Prince, D. A., Lux, H. D., and Neher, E. (1973): Measurement of extracellular potassium activity in cat cortex. *Brain Res.*, 50:489–495.

73. Raabe, W., and Ayala, G. F. (1976): Diphenylhydantoin increases cortical postsynaptic inhibition. *Brain Res.*, 105:597–601.

74. Reichenthal, E., and Hocherman, S. (1979): A critical epileptic area in the cat's cortex and its relation to cortical columns. *Brain Res.*, 47:147–152.

75. Ribak, C. E. (1983): A loss of inhibitory GABA terminals that synapse axon initial segments of pyramidal cells in epileptic focus. *Neurosci. Abstr.*, 13:627.

76. Roberts, E. (1980): Epilepsy and antiepileptic drugs: A speculative synthesis. In: *Antiepileptic Drugs: Mechanisms of Action*, edited by G. H. Glaser, J. K. Penry, and D. M. Woodbury, pp. 667–713. Raven Press, New York.

77. Schneiderman, J. H., and Schwartzkroin, P. A. (1982): Effects of phenytoin on normal activity and on penicillin-induced bursting in the guinea pig hippocampal slice. *Neurology*, 32:730–738.

78. Schwartzkroin, P. A., and Prince, D. A. (1977): Penicillin-induced epileptiform activity in the hippocampal in vitro preparation. *Ann. Neurol.*, 1:463.

79. Schwartzkroin, P. A., and Prince, D. A. (1978): Cellular and field potential properties of epileptogenic hippocampal slices. *Brain Res.*, 147:117–130.

80. Schwartzkroin, P. A., and Wyler, A. R. (1980): Mechanisms underlying epileptiform burst discharge. *Ann. Neurol.*, 7:95–107.

81. Schwartzkroin, P. A., Mutani, R., and Prince, D. A. (1975): Orthodromic and antidromic effects of a cortical epileptiform focus on ventrolateral nucleus of the cat. *J. Neurophysiol.*, 38:795–811.

82. Somogyi, P. (1977): A specific axo-axonal interneuron in the visual cortex of the rat. *Brain Res.*, 136:345–350.

83. Somogyi, P., Freund, T. F., Halasz, N., and Kisvarday, Z. F. (1981): Selectivity of neuronal [3H]GABA accumulation in the visual cortex as revealed by Golgi staining of the labeled neurons. *Brain Res.*, 225:431–436.

84. Swinyard, E. A., Brown, W. C., and Goodman, L. S. (1952): Comparative assays of antiepileptic drugs in mice and rats. *J. Pharmacol Exp. Ther.*, 106:47–59.

85. Szentagothai, J. (1973): Synaptology of the visual cortex. In: *Handbook of Sensory Physiology*, Vol. VII, 3B, edited by R. Jung, pp. 269–324. Springer, New York.

86. Toyama, K., Matsunami, K., Ohno, T., and Tokashiki, S. (1974): An intracellular study of neuronal organization in the visual cortex. *Exp. Brain Res.*, 21:45–66.

87. Traub, R. D., and Wong, R. K. S. (1982): Cellular mechanism of neuronal synchronization in epilepsy. *Science*, 216:745–747.

88. Traub, R. D., and Wong, R. K. S. (1983): Synchronized burst discharge in disinhibited hippocampal slice. II. Model of cellular mechanism. *J. Neurophysiol.*, 49:459–471.

89. Van Duijn, H., Schwartzkroin, P. A., and Prince, D.A. (1973): Action of penicillin on inhibitory processes in the cat's cortex. *Brain Res.*, 53:470–476.

90. Welker, C., and Woolsey, T. (1974): Structure of layer IV in the somato-sensory neocortex of the rat. *J. Comp. Neurol.*, 158:437–454.

91. White, H. S., Anderson, R. E., Kemp, J. W., and Woodbury, D. M. (1983): Mechanism of action of phenytoin: Differential effect on neuronal and glial cell Na^+,K^+-ATPase. *Neurosci. Abstr.*, 13:1106.

92. Wise, S. P. (1975): The laminar organization of certain afferent and efferent fiber systems in rat somatosensory cortex. *Brain Res.*, 90:139–142.

93. Wong, R. K. S., and Prince, D. A. (1978): Penicillin blocks inhibitory control of dendrite burst generation in hippocampal neurons. *Neurosci. Abstr.*, 4:239.

94. Wong, R. K. S., and Traub, R. D. (1983): Synchronized burst discharge in disinhibited hippocampal slice. I. Initiation in CA2-CA3 region. *J. Neurophysiol.*, 49:442–458.

95. Woodbury, D. M. (1982): Phenytoin: Mechanisms of action. In: *Antiepileptic Drugs*, edited by D. M. Woodbury, J. K. Penry, and C. E. Pippenger, pp. 269–282. Raven Press, New York.

Advances in Neurology, Vol. 44, edited by
A. V. Delgado-Escueta, A. A. Ward, Jr.,
D. M. Woodbury, and R. J. Porter.
Raven Press, New York © 1986.

28

Temporal and Spatial Distribution of Intracellular Potentials During Generation and Spread of Epileptogenic Discharges

*Eli S. Goldensohn and **Alfred M. Salazar

*Albert Einstein College of Medicine, Bronx, New York 10467, and College of Physicians and Surgeons, Columbia University, New York 10032; and **Department of Neurology, College of Physicians and Surgeons, Columbia University, New York, New York 10032*

SUMMARY This chapter addresses the characteristics and spatial distribution of intracellular potentials, the spread of paroxysmal depolarization shifts (PDSs) through the cortex, the extracellular field potentials in three dimensions, and the concentrations of penicillin in direct contact with elements in the epileptogenic focus. Data are presented that show that (a) there are several types or gradations of PDS intensities within each focus; (b) PDS types are distributed in groups related to their distance from the center of the focus and to the concentration of the epileptogenic drug; (c) the morphology and repetition rate of electroencephalogram (EEG) spikes are related to features of the intracellular potentials; (d) a mathematical model can estimate the distribution of concentrations of penicillin within the focus over long periods; (e) no barriers impede diffusion of penicillin either at the cortical surface or at the boundary between gray and white matter; (f) the potential field of the EEG spike is defined in three dimensions; and (g) PDSs spread through the focus at the rate of 0.25 m/sec.

The characteristic electroencephalographic (EEG) feature indicating the presence of epilepsy is the EEG spike (41,77,101). Intracellular recording has shown that the spike itself is a reflection of shifts in the polarization of neurons within the cerebral cortex (28,60,61). In experimental epileptogenic foci, paroxysmal depolarization shifts (PDSs) are the main generators of EEG spikes, and PDSs with related postsynaptic potentials and other transmembranal potential shifts constitute the bulk of epileptogenic electrical activity. This chapter deals principally with the epileptogenic focus in the intact mammalian neocortex. It describes the spatial distribution of intracellular potentials during spike generation, estimates the rate of spread of epileptiform activity, and relates the electrical events to the concentration distribution of the epileptogenic agent penicillin.

Topical application of penicillin is particularly suited for investigating the mechanisms underlying the development and spread of epileptiform activity because it can be made to involve a limited aggregate of chemically affected neurons (30,77,81,98) and because the resulting interictal and ictal corticographic activity closely resembles that seen in human focal epilepsy (31). Other reasons that penicillin has been favored for the production of experimental foci include (a) techniques of application to the cortex either topically or by microinjection are relatively uncomplicated (8,19,30); (b) penicillin produces epileptiform activity in a wide variety of vertebrates from fish (91) to humans (99); (c) the onset of paroxysmal activity occurs promptly following application and continues spontaneously at regular intervals for hours (30); (d) focal discharges can be triggered by afferent stimulation physiologically (69) and electrically (59); (e) gross cytoarchitectural changes following application are uncommon (66); (f) the rate of spread is related to the amount applied (21,55); (g) epileptiform activity induced is sensitive to anticonvulsants (7,21); (h) the epileptiform activity induced is reversible, allowing an animal to be used as its own control (21).

The PDSs which are the principal generators of recurrent negative EEG spikes found at the epileptogenic focus are of much greater amplitude and longer in duration than usual excitatory postsynaptic potentials (EPSPs). Interictal paroxysmal activity, however, also includes the synchronous participation of organized interconnected populations of cortical neurons whose usual functions are altered to contribute to the production of recurrent synchronous discharges. The mechanisms underlying the generation of interictal EEG spike paroxysms are discussed in detail in other chapters in this volume. Currently two major hypotheses concerning the origin of the PDS are being merged (42,75). The first holds that the PDS is a giant excitatory postsynaptic potential (EPSP) (43). The input for the giant EPSP is ascribed to a number of mechanisms including excessive recurrent excitation (1,5,18), bursting of axon terminals (4,65,78), facilitation of EPSPs (3,25, 74,100), and suppression of inhibition (3, 9,14,97). Further strong direct evidence in favor of the giant EPSP hypothesis is found in hippocampal slices models using penicillin and D-tubocurarine (42,43,48). The second hypothesis suggests that the PDS is the result of intrinsic membrane properties of the neurons and that synaptic events serve only to either synchronize or trigger PDSs rather than to generate them (34,74,86). Support for this hypothesis includes the finding that PDS-like bursts can be evoked nonsynaptically by brief intracellular current pulses in mouse hippocampal membrane in tissue culture (108) and in molluscan neurons isolated from synaptic influence (102). Also, spontaneous PDS-like bursts observed in hippocampal pyramidal cells *in vitro* have been attributed to endogenous properties (75,84,105). An early phase of the PDS has been attributed to membrane depolarizations which generate sodium spikes and the later phase which follows (85,94,105) to depolarization which reaches

threshold for calcium spike activation (88). Summations of calcium spikes or other voltage-dependent calcium potentials, possibly located on dendrites (50,106), contribute to the maintenance of the depolarization envelope during the late phase of the PDS (105,106). A synthesis of the two hypotheses has now been made by recognizing that some hippocampal PDSs depend mainly on intrinsic properties and others in the neocortex and hippocampus are principally synaptic (42,43,75).

The PDS is followed by an hyperpolarizing afterpotential (HAP) lasting several hundred milliseconds (60,72,82,107). The HAP is associated with suppression of spontaneous unit activity in the focus. Early studies indicated that the HAP was generated by inhibitory postsynaptic potentials (IPSP) triggered by recurrent inhibition from interneurons that had been activated by axon collaterals of the pyramidal cells exhibiting PDSs (71). More recently, a nonsynaptic mechanism has been proposed for the HAP which involves a Ca^{2+} or Ca^{2+}-Na^+-activated slow increase in K^+ conductance at pyramidal-cell dendrites (38,39). The HAP serves to limit the frequency of epileptiform EEG spikes, since the population of neurons that produce the spikes remains hyperpolarized and resistant to generating action potentials for up to more than 500 msec.

Another type of neuronal activity that occurs in association with spontaneous interictal spike discharges is the prominent prolonged IPSP found in cortical neurons over a relatively large area of cortex at the periphery of the focus (2,44,60,72). The term "surround inhibition" (76) is used to describe activity of this population of neurons. Surround inhibition impedes the propagation of epileptiform activity into adjacent cortex by providing an encircling field of strong inhibition coincident with the central focal excitation.

Many of the important observations cited above on generation and termination of the PDS were made from *in vitro* experiments on hippocampal tissue slices. The use of tissue-slice techniques has provided a simplified mammalian preparation suitable for detailed studies, but the relation of their concentrations of penicillin to those present in the intact brain during epileptogenesis had been largely unexplored. Prior to this report, only one previous study supplied information for estimating the concentration of penicillin at a focus in the intact brain (64), and only minimal information has been available on either the distribution profile (10) or the kinetics of movement of penicillin (64) within the cortex during the development and spread of focal epileptogenic discharges.

A mathematical model (82) is described in this chapter that estimates tissue concentrations and the rate at which boundaries of neuronal populations exposed to concentrations greater than specified threshold values change with time during the development and spread of epileptiform activity. In other models used in which penicillin enters the brain by diffusion from the cortical surface, the areas of cortex exposed to the drug vary widely (33,64,80). These and other variables affect the size of the epileptogenic zone directly by determining the extent of diffusion and the concentration profile of penicillin. As a consequence, the interrelationships among neurons participating in focal epileptogenic activity have been limited. A needed, well-characterized experimental model that can serve as a standard was developed (82).

Since hippocampal as well as neocortical pyramidal cells receive a majority of their excitatory synaptic contacts on both apical and basal dendritic spines while inhibitory synapses predominate at or near the soma and initial segment, experiments aimed at differentiating between the two hypothesized primary sites of action of penicillin are difficult in the brain-slice preparations because all parts of the neuron are in contact with the same concentration of the drug. Furthermore, it has not been determined to what extent similar mechanisms underly epileptiform activity in the more simply organized hippocampus as compared to the vertically oriented columnal organization of the neocortex (40,96). Although hippocampal slices *in vitro* display many characteristics of the intact hippocampus, neocortical slices do not (89). An appropriate neocortical model that is well characterized electrically and in which concentrations of the convulsant drug are known and can be manipulated conveniently was developed and is described next.

The separation of the generation of an epileptiform discharge from its spread requires an operational definition of the terms. In the studies discussed here, the epileptogenic generator is signaled by spontaneous recurrent spikes which are derived from and confined to a minimal aggregate of neurons which is capable from time to time of recruiting larger and more remote regions into an epileptogenic process. There are two types of spread. One is within the epileptogenic generating area that results in the recurrent confined spike and the second type is activity outside of the generating area. The method of examining and separating these processes ex-

perimentally requires a focus that is small, discrete, stable, and reproducible, that can be maintained for long periods without spread, but that nevertheless is capable of producing involvement of larger and more remote regions.

Production of such a focus requires controlled delivery of an epileptogenic agent in order to establish the spatial distribution of concentration of the agent in contact with the cell populations. The concentration dependence of responses in more simplified *in vitro* systems is known for mammalian tissues (15,56) and has provided much information on the mechanisms of action of penicillin on excitable membranes, but is of limited use in interpreting processes of initiation and spread because normal structural relationships have been disrupted. Knowing the concentrations of penicillin in the intact brain, however, allows transfer of useful information between *in vitro* and *in vivo* experimental data.

The following sections describe the spatial distribution of intracellularly recorded electrical activity during interictal spiking and the distribution of penicillin concentration within and surrounding an epileptogenic focus. It then correlates the activity with local penicillin concentrations. It also gives estimates of the rate of spread of the electrical fields and intracellularly recorded PDSs during spike generation.

TECHNIQUES FOR PRODUCING A SMALL DISCRETE FOCUS, RECORDING FROM IT, AND DEVELOPING A PENICILLIN DIFFUSION MODEL

Reproducible foci are made in the sensorimotor cortex of cats by diffusion of 840 mM penicillin G in lactated Ringer's solution from the lumen of 1.0 mm O.D. glass capillary tubes with fire-polished tips with a lumen of 450 to 550 μm. Applied to the pial surface, the tip forms a reasonably tight seal without causing injury. A gelled suspension of Ringer–agar prevents leakage of penicillin from the tube, which also serves as the recording electrode at the site of spike generation.

1. Surface electrical activity is recorded from both the penicillin-containing capillary and a 1.0-mm-diameter silver–silver chloride ball electrode approximately 2 mm lateral to the focus. A pressure plate is used to dampen cortical pulsation. Intracellular recordings were obtained using glass micropipette electrodes filled with 1.25 M potassium citrate.

2. Intracellular recordings are obtained using glass micropipette electrodes filled with 1.25 M potassium citrate and having resistances of 15–40 megohms. Standard amplification and recording techniques were used.

3. For measuring the diffusion of penicillin in the focus, glass capillary electrodes are prepared essentially as described above and a 50-μl aliquot of the prepared penicillin G sodium solution was added to a vial containing 50 μCi of ^{14}C-labeled penicillin G potassium, giving a tracer concentration of 1.0 μCi/μl.

The penicillin-containing capillary is kept in contact with the cortex for three different periods: (a) 5 min, a time when fully developed interictal negative sharp waves are seen at the focus; (b) 15 min, a time prior to electrographic stability when, in addition to negative sharp waves at the focus, the activity of the surrounding area is characterized by simultaneous high amplitude positive sharp waves; (c) 60 min, a time well after the focus has stabilized electrographically.

After each alloted time has elapsed, the electrode at each site is lifted. The animal is then given an overdose of pentobarbital i.v. and killed with saturated KCl solution i.v. Three 8 × 8 × 6 mm blocks excised within 1 min using the dye spots as guides. Quick freezing is done and the tissue is freeze-dried at $-60°C$ for 3 days before embedding.

4. In developing a theoretical model for diffusion of penicillin, the 0.5 mm diameter lumen of the capillary from which diffusion takes place is best described as a disc source. The concentration distribution which develops can be approximated by that from a spherical source. The model assumes that the concentration of penicillin at the source remains constant, that diffusion takes place in a homogeneous medium, and that a fraction of the diffusing penicillin is removed from the cortex by a process obeying first-order kinetics. The solution of the diffusion equation for a spherical source can be modified to account for the removal process and written

of removal where $k = (\ln 2)/\tau$ is the half-time removal. The error associated with this approximation decreases from approximately 10% to 1% as r increases from $1.6a$ to $5.0a$. Since fitting as well as calculation of extracellular penicillin concentrations using Eq. 1 were performed with r within the range $2a$ to $16a$ this solution was adequate. A complete treatment of the derivation of this equation is available (82).

Tissue blocks were sectioned sequentially at 20 μm, either normal to or tangential to the surface. Five successive 20-μm sections were pooled for liquid scintillation counting. Equation 1 was fitted to the data from each cortical block using a nonlinear regression program on an IBM System/360. Parameters used were source residence time (t), distances from the sample plane to the source (d), the disappearance half-time (τ), and source radius (a). The best-fit values for the diffusion coefficient (D) and the effective source concentration (C) were computed.

The source radius, $a = 0.25$ mm, was that of the lumen of the penicillin-containing capillary. The dimensions of the dye spots in the shorter periods of source residence had a similar radius. After 60 min, however, the size of the dyespots were up to two times larger and fitting at 60 min used a source radius of 0.5 mm.

The disappearance half-time (τ) $= 2$ hr was determined in separate experiments on 15 animals. In each animal, three foci 8 to 9 mm apart are made along the suprasylvian gyrus, allowing 15 min of contact for the ^{14}C-penicillin source. To determine the rate of disappearance, separate blocks of brain ($7 \times 7 \times 6$ mm) containing the labeled foci are excised at the end of different intervals following removal of the source and the amount of radioactivity remaining is measured. One group of samples is taken immediately after removal of the penicillin capillary, the second group after 60 min, and the third after 120 min. Placement of the penicillin-containing capillaries by intervals allows all three foci to be excised at the same time. The location of the foci assigned to each time interval is randomized.

$$ C = \frac{C_0 a}{\pi r}\left\{ \text{erfc}\left[\frac{(r - a)}{2\sqrt{Dt}}\sqrt{kt}\right]\exp\sqrt{k/D}(a - r) - \text{erfc}\left[\frac{(r - a)}{2\sqrt{Dt}} + \sqrt{kt}\right]\exp\sqrt{k/D}(r - a)\right\} \quad (1) $$

where C is the concentration at any time t and radius r from the source, C_0 is the source concentration, a is the source radius, D is the diffusion coefficient, and $k = \tau$ is the rate constant

5. For surface potential mapping, recordings are made using a 3×4 electrode array of 12,500 μm I.D. Ringer–agar-filled capillaries spaced 2 mm apart. One of the inner electrodes of the

array contains the penicillin. Sixteen successive, temporally aligned interictal spikes are averaged from each of the 12 electrodes to a reference on neck muscle. By interpolating potentials between the 12 known values, computerized displays of the surface potential distributions are made at 4-msec epochs.

6. For laminar field potential mapping, recordings of extracellular fields are made using low-resistance glass microelectrodes filled with 1.25 M potassium citrate. Single microelectrodes record from 12 standard depths at four standard distances from the center of the focus. Sixteen interictal spikes are averaged at each of up to 48 locations. The stability of the spikes at the surface of the cortex for periods up to 1½ hr, which allows definition of the two-dimensional fields, implies that the underlying activity was similarly stable for three-dimensional field analysis. Continuous potential surfaces at 4-msec epochs are generated by interpolating between the points where recordings are made and presented as intensity modulated oscilloscope displays.

The onset of focal spiking usually occurs within 1 min after penicillin application and is signalled by quasiperiodic monophasic negative spikes confined to a surface area of less than 2 mm in diameter. Spread of epileptiform potentials into the surrounding cortex usually becomes evident within 5 min and appears predominantly as positive spikes coincident with the negative spikes at the center of the focus. At 30 min later the negative spikes at the center and the positive spikes in the surrounding areas stabilize in amplitude and duration for several hours, excepting occasional periods of decreases in amplitude.

Female cats weighing 2.5 to 3.5 kg, pretreated with atropine sulphate (0.2 mg i.m.), are anesthetized using an ether–oxygen–room air mixture. The animals are maintained on this mixture while tracheotomy and right femoral vein cannulation is performed. A single dose of pentobarbital sodium (15 mg/kg i.p.) was then administered and the ether eliminated from the respiratory mixture. A posterior fossa craniectomy provides spinal fluid drainage and exposed spinous processes allow anchorage for suspension. A craniectomy is performed through the left frontal sinus and the anterior sigmoid, anterior aspect of the posterior sigmoid, and coronal gyri are exposed. Skin incision sites and pressure points are infiltrated with lidocaine and the animal is then immobilized with succinylcholine chloride. Positive pressure respiration is used, and body temperature is maintained using a heat lamp.

TYPE AND DISTRIBUTION OF INTRACELLULAR POTENTIALS FOUND WITHIN AND SURROUNDING THE FOCUS

Intracellular records from neurons within neocortical epileptogenic foci created by penicillin show the abrupt, large, prolonged decreases in the transmembrane potential which characterize PDSs. The PDSs are coincident with high amplitude predominantly negative spikes seen in the electrocorticogram (28,60,61,70). PDSs are induced by a variety of other pharmacological and physical epileptogenic agents applied to the neocortex (28,83,104), hippocampus (73), and spinal cord (45).

Surrounding the regions of PDSs is a population of neurons that show mainly increased transmembrane potentials during the surface discharge (32,33,76). The spatial distribution and contribution of these hyperpolarized neurons to generation of the surface epileptiform activity seen at the cortex and scalp had not been clearly defined. Some data indicate that the activity of cells at all depths along a single electrode track tends to be similar within the focus with either PDSs predominant or IPSPs predominant (76).

Incomplete forms of PDS have been reported during stimulation of the cortex (59) and thalamus (58), as well as spontaneously during developing and waning foci (12,60,61,71). Intermediate forms of the surrounding inhibited neurons, characterized by early excitation with or without action potentials, have also been reported during spontaneous focal discharges (13,59,76).

The foci used in the work reported below are based on a method (30) in which several hours of continuous recording of focal interictal spiking is obtained at and around a penicillin source of 0.2 mm² area by a 3 × 4 electrode array covering a rectangular area of 4 × 6 mm on the surface of the anterior sigmoid gyrus of the cat. The method is designed to minimize and control the cortical area exposed to the drug in order to make a small, discrete, highly reproducible focus. The distributions of potential for averaged focal spikes display a strong central symmetry with high voltage negativity at the peak of the interictal spike confined to a region of radius less than 2 mm from the center of the focus. At the same time, the surrounding surface shows a lower voltage positivity.

The intracellular recordings from neurons in cats are temporally related to the interictal EEG spiking, and the relationship remained consistent in a given neuron during successive spikes.

Distinct characteristics of shape and timing suggest four classes of cellular behavior (Fig. 1). Each class of discharges has a separate axial symmetrical distribution within the region of the focus (Fig. 2). Fully developed paroxysmal depolarization shifts are found in a radius of approximately 1.5 mm from the center of the penicillin source. Shorter duration transitional forms, termed truncated and larval PDSs, predominate at radial distances between 1.5 and 2.5 mm.

Those with prolonged depolarizations having durations similar to the associated negative EEG spikes are called sustained PDSs (29). They usually begin with a short burst of action potentials and terminate with a rapid depolarization followed by a long-lasting hyperpolarizing afterpotential. The action potentials in the initial burst have decreasing peak amplitudes, and complete spike inactivation occurs with maximum depolarization. Paroxysmal depolarizations of similar amplitude, which begin with the same sequence as sustained PDSs but which began repolarizing before the end of the negative EEG spike, had occurred are characterized by truncated PDSs (82). The term larval PDS is applied when depolarizations are of lower amplitude and briefer and the bursts of action potentials decrease in peak amplitude but do not become fully inactivated. Repolarizations of both larval and truncated PDSs are also followed by HAPs (Fig. 3). Neurons without PDSs, which showed only long-lasting hyperpolarizations coincident with negative EEG spikes with suppression of spontaneous action potentials, are classified as prolonged IPSPs (82). Some prolonged IPSPs contained an early, brief, depolarizing hump. The depolarization is of low amplitude and is not accompanied by action potentials. The bursts of action potentials in both the initial portions of the PDS and the early depolarization humps seen at the onset of prolonged IPSPs are coincident with a brief positive EEG spike component that precedes the larger negative EEG spike (Fig. 4). Both the action potential bursts and the early depolarizations are complete before the EEG negative spike reaches its maximum.

Arbitrary standards for measurement of surface and intracellular activity were chosen. The duration of the focal spike includes both the major negative wave and the prepositivity when present. In 7 animals, focal spikes did not have prepositivity, and in 4, prepositivity was present early in the development of the focus and later disappeared. The PDS duration includes the de-

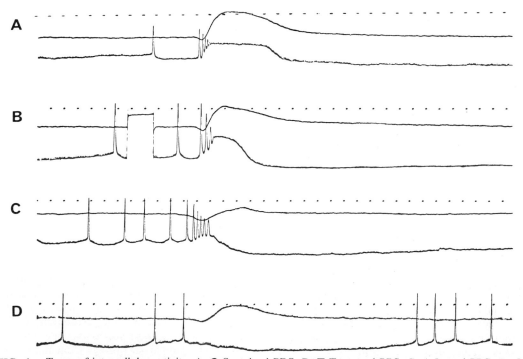

FIG. 1. Types of intracellular activity. **A:** ● Sustained PDS. **B:** ■ Truncated PBS. **C:** △ Larval PDS. **D:** ○ Prolonged IPSP. *Upper traces:* Electrocorticogram recorded from the penicillin-containing electrode (negative up). *Lower traces:* Intracellular record (positive up). Time marker 10 msec at the extracellular baseline. Common voltage calibration in **B**, 50 mV. Modified from ref. 29.

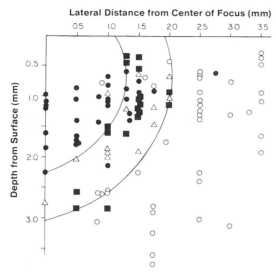

Lateral Distance from Center of Focus (mm)

FIG. 2. Distribution of PDSs and IPSPs in and around penicillin focus: ●, sustained PDS, ■, truncated PDS, △, larval PDS, ○, prolonged IPSP. The *solid curved lines* delineate the zone of transition between the region of maximum sustained PDS density near the center of the focus and that of prolonged IPSP activity in the inhibitory surround (see statistical procedures for explanation). (Modified from ref. 29.)

polarization phase and the rapid repolarization phase preceding the HAP. On the average, the onset of the surface spike at the penicillin electrode, whether or not prepositivity was present, coincided with the onset of each of the three types of PDS. To measure the duration of prolonged IPSPs, which often lack clearly recognizable onsets, the onset of the EEG spike at the penicillin electrode is used. Because of uncertainty in determining the moment that the HAP is over, the point of maximum HAP amplitude is used as an index of HAP duration. The mean EEG focal spike duration was 79 ± 22 msec with a mean amplitude of 4 ± 2 mV. A summary of the intracellular data is presented in Table 1. While the amplitudes of both sustained and truncated PDSs do not differ (combined mean 18 ± 7 mV), that for the larval form is significantly lower (6 ± 4 mV). Repolarization following the plateau phase of sustained PDSs coincides with the end of the interictal high-voltage surface negative wave recorded from the focus. However, repolarization following truncated and larval PDSs occurs significantly sooner, preceding the end of the EEG spike by approximately 30 and 50 msec, respectively. The time elapsed from PDS onset of the point of maximum HAP am-

plitude is longest for cells with sustained PDSs (201 ± 50 msec). Cells showing truncated and larval PDSs begin to return to predischarge resting conditions significantly sooner, after 141 ± 54 and 103 ± 35 msec, respectively. The amplitude and time course of the hyperpolarizations produced by cells showing prolonged IPSPs are similar to the amplitude and time course of HAPs following truncated and larval PDSs. Each reaches a maximum hyperpolarizing potential of about 9 mV by about 80 msec, with the return of spontaneous action potentials at about 500 msec after onset of hyperpolarization. However, the durations of the HAPs following sustained PDSs are significantly longer. They take about 120 msec to reach their maximum amplitude (6 mV), and spontaneous action potentials return much later at about 1000 msec (Table 1).

Correlation between the duration of each type of PDS and the duration of the associated surface spike discharge is shown in Table 2. There is a strong correlation between the durations of both sustained and truncated PDSs and the duration of the corresponding surface focal spikes, indicating that both make large contributions to the generation of the focal spike.

In a given animal, the length of sustained PDSs and the length of the negative surface spikes are remarkably consistent throughout an experiment. Although the means of sustained PDSs and associated focal spike durations were very close, 71 ± 16 msec and 74 ± 11 msec, respectively, the range in durations among different animals was between 50 and 110 msec. Organization or intrinsic cellular differences may account for the differences in durations of the sustained PDSs among animals.

Figure 2 shows the distribution of each type of the four types of cellular activity in depth and lateral distance from the center of the penicillin contact. The mean radial distance for each type of cellular activity was calculated, and Table 3 and Fig. 2 show that each type of intracellular activity occupies a distinct region of cortex surrounding the site of the applied penicillin. Sustained PDSs are nearest the center of the focus and are rarely found at distances greater than 1.5 mm lateral to the center of the penicillin capillary. Truncated PDSs are intermingled at the periphery of the distribution of the sustained PDSs. Larval PDSs are also found within this area. The region more than 2.0 mm lateral to the penicillin capillary is occupied almost exclusively by cells with prolonged IPSPs.

Examples of a sustained and a truncated PDS are shown in Fig. 3 recorded from two neurons

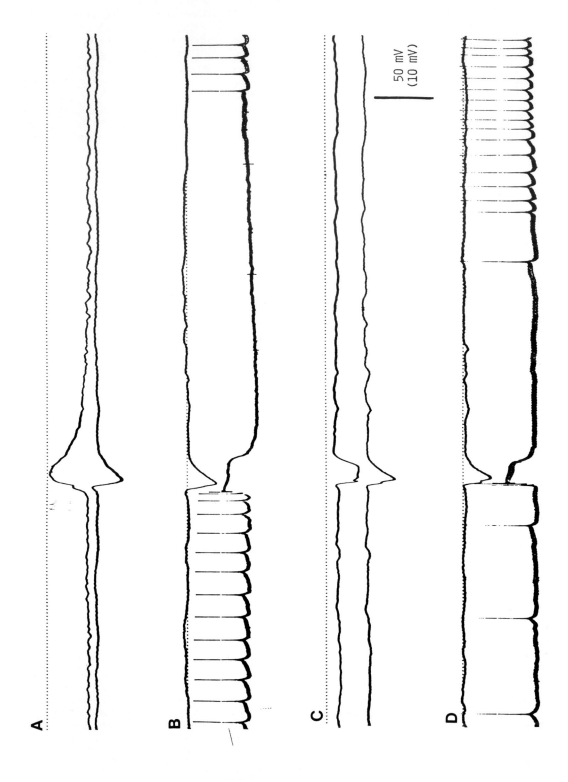

50 mV
(10 mV)

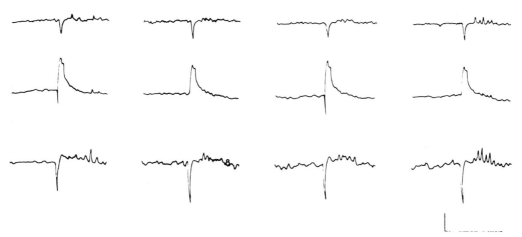

FIG. 4. Instability of the early positivity at the penicillin electrode alone (*middle row*). *Upper and lower rows* 2 mm from penicillin electrode, laterally and medially, respectively. Negativity up. Note the prominent positivity prior to the negative spike in columns 1 and 3, which is absent in 2 and 4. All spikes within a 30-sec period. Calibration, 1 mV, 1 sec. (From ref. 30, with permission.)

at different locations within the same focus. Simultaneous with the PDSs there is a surface positive sharp wave being recorded from 2 mm lateral to the center of the focus. The relative constancy of the amplitude and duration of the EEG positive waves over time indicates that both intracellular recordings were obtained during a period in which the focus was stable. As demonstrated in Fig. 3, both repolarization and recovery of spontaneous action potentials begin later in the sustained PDS near the center of the focus than for the truncated PDS 1.5 mm away.

In one experiment, a single neuron in the anterior sigmoid gyrus was impaled prior to creating the focus. The penicillin-containing electrode was then carefully lowered so that its center on the surface was 0.6 mm lateral to the microelectrode. Simultaneous recordings were obtained both from the surface and intracellularly as the penicillin focus developed. Evolution of the focal EEG spike recorded from the penicillin electrode showed the usual progression of EEG changes (30). The changes were characterized initially by a reversal in the polarity of spindle bursts from surface negative to surface positive. Enhancement of several spindles in the burst occurred next, followed by focal spiking within the burst. The focal spikes then increased in amplitude and duration over the next 20 min before relative electrical stability was attained. The intracellularly recorded activity coincident with the focal spikes went through successive stages, beginning with prolonged IPSPs similar to those depicted in Fig. 2. With spindle enhancement, there were slightly deeper hyperpolarizations following action potentials associated with the spindles. By the time the spindles inverted and the negative focal EEG spike emerged, the hyperpolarizations were considerably deeper and the interval between spontaneous firings of the cell lengthened. As the focal EEG spike increased in duration and amplitude, a transition occurred from pure prolonged IPSPs to ones containing a brief, early,

FIG. 3. Examples of a sustained and a truncated PDS recorded during microelectrode penetrations in two different locations within the same focus. Figure also demonstrates prolonged hyperpolarizing afterpotentials (HAP). **A and C.** Electrical activity recorded from the cortical surface. **A,** *upper trace:* Focal negative spike recorded from a microelectrode positioned on the pial surface at the center of the dye spot marking the location of the focus. **C,** *upper trace:* Positive spike recorded from the same microelectrode repositioned on the surface 1.5 mm lateral to the center of the focus. **A and C,** *lower traces:* Positive spike recorded from a 1 mm diameter silver–silver chloride ball electrode located in a fixed position on the pial surface approximately 2 mm lateral to the center of the focus. **B and D.** Intracellular electrical activity during focal interictal spiking. time marker 10 msec at the extracellular baseline (positive up). **B,** *lower trace:* Sustained PDS underlying the negative spike in **A** (*upper trace*) at a depth of 1.62 mm. **D,** *lower trace:* Truncated PDS underlying the positive spike in **C** (*upper trace*) at a depth of 1.14 mm. **B and D,** *upper traces:* Positive spikes coincident with the intracellular events recorded from the same fixed-position macroelectrode as in **A** and **C** (*lower traces*). Voltage calibration: intracellular recordings 50 mV, surface recordings 10 mV. (From F. M. Salazar and E. S. Goldensohn, *in preparation.*)

TABLE 1. *Mean values of the measured parameters for each type of intracellular activity[a]*

Type of neuronal activity	PDS duration (msec)	Onset to maximum hyperpolarization (msec)	Onset to first action potential (msec)	PDS amplitude (mV)	Maximum amplitude hyperpolarization (mV)	N
Sustained PDS	82 ± 22[b]	201 ± 50[c]	1240 ± 438[c]	18 ± 8	6 ± 3[d]	28[e]
Truncated PDS	55 ± 15[b]	141 ± 54[d]	645 ± 360	18 ± 7[a]	9 ± 5	19[f]
Larval PDS	35 ± 10	103 ± 35	475 ± 150	6 ± 4	10 ± 3	13
Prolonged IPSP	—	82 ± 27	365 ± 214	—	9 ± 3	34

[a] Mean ± SD.
[b] Level of significance of the difference between the superscripted mean and the mean immediately below, $p < 0.001$.
[c] As in b, but $p < 0.01$.
[d] As in b, but $p < 0.05$.
[e] Five cells of the 35 showing sustained PDSs had no HAP and two cells had a depolarizing afterpotential. These were excluded from the averages.
[f] One cell of the 20 showing truncated PDSs had no HAP and was excluded from the averages.

low-amplitude depolarization. Following this, larval, then truncated, and finally sustained PDSs appeared.

THE DISTRIBUTION OF CONCENTRATIONS OF PENICILLIN WITHIN THE FOCUS

A number of previous studies attempted to determine the size and location of the neuronal pools in contact with convulsant agents at the first appearance of focal spiking or when electrical seizure patterns developed (11,21,27,35, 46). However, they did not directly approach the problem of the distribution of concentrations until Noebels and Pedley (64) attempted to quantify the distribution and determine the diffusional kinetics of penicillin in epileptogenic foci. They derived their diffusion coefficient from measurements of the distribution of ^{14}C-labeled penicillin following a 3-min application. Their data indicated that penicillin enters the cortex primarily by passive diffusion during that period, but they could not state whether later in time this would continue to be the primary process. Also, since they assumed an infinite plane sheet diffusion source, their diffusion coefficient applies only for penicillin movement in a direc-

tion normal to the surface. Recently a method for continuous measurement of penicillin activity in the brain has been described (92).

The concentration dependence of responses in more simplified in vitro systems is known for mammalian (15,57,63,87) and nonmammalian (37,103) tissues and has provided information on the mechanisms of action of penicillin on excitable membranes. That data, however, has a limited use interpreting processes within the intact brain, as normal structural relationships have been disrupted. Knowing the concentrations of penicillin in the intact brain, however, allows useful transfer between *in vivo* and *in vitro* experimental data.

In the previous section in this chapter on techniques a three-dimensional mathematical model is described that estimates the concentrations of penicillin within the cortex as a function of time. The model permits correlation between cellular and field electrical phenomena with local concentrations of penicillin in a variety of experimental cortical foci.

For estimating the spatiotemporal distribution of concentrations of penicillin in the extracellular space, ^{14}C-labeled penicillin was applied to the supra sylvian gyrus using the techniques described earlier in this chapter. Distribution was

TABLE 2. *Correlation between focal spike duration and the duration of each category of depolarizing intracellular activity*

Category	PDS duration (msec)	Focal spike duration (msec)	Correlation coefficient		N
			r	p	
Sustained PDS	71.0 ± 16.3	74.1 ± 11.0	0.843	<0.001	15
Truncated PDS	48.6 ± 14.1	74.2 ± 13.6	0.689	<0.01	12
Larval PDS	36.7 ± 7.8	71.3 ± 11.2	0.298	NS	7

TABLE 3. *Mean radial distance from the center of the penicillin source to the cells displaying each type of intracellular activity during the focal electrocorticograph spike*

Category	Radial distance (mm)	N	IPSP type[a]		
			Tru	Lar	Pro
Sustained PDS	1.601 ± 0.415	30	$p < 0.01$	$p < 0.001$	$p < 0.001$
Truncated PDS	1.999 ± 0.465	18		NS[b]	$p < 0.001$
Larval PDS	2.100 ± 0.339	13			$p < 0.001$
Prolonged IPSP	3.098 ± 0.768	37			

[a] Tru, truncated; Lar, larval; Pro, prolonged.
[b] NS, $p > 0.05$.

determined at intervals during the development and stabilization of epileptogenic activity using liquid scintillation counting of 100-μm serial sections through brain blocks containing the labeled foci. A mathematical model for the diffusional kinetics of penicillin in the neocortex was constructed for a disk source in an infinite homogeneous medium, assuming that the labeled penicillin molecule remains intact. A first-order process for clearance of penicillin from the cortex via routes other than diffusion was found. A clearance half-time of 2 hr was determined. Analysis of the distribution profiles using nonlinear regression indicate that penetration of penicillin into the cortex occurs passively with a diffusion coefficient of 0.72 ± 0.09 mm/hr and that the pial membrane does not impede free passage of penicillin. Similar distributions of penicillin in three separate foci at 1 hr of diffusion demonstrate the reproducibility of the method. Assuming a lower limit of 1 mM penicillin for detectable effects of cortical neurons on the basis of *in vitro* experiments, calculations using the model indicate that the dimensions of the population of neurons in contact with 1 mM or more increases rapidly within the first hour. After an hour it is less rapid and is less than 30% over the next 4 hr. A relatively slow rate of increase in the dimensions of the neuronal pool in contact with significant concentrations of epileptogenic agent correlates well with the stability of waveform, amplitude, duration, and frequency of EEG spikes that occur at the focus.

One-way analysis of variance on the results of the clearance study indicate that similar foci from different locations on the gyrus could be treated comparably. A disappearance half-time of 111 min was calculated from the data in Fig. 5. Evidence that up to 10% of the reduction in counts after 120 min could be attributed to diffusion of labeled penicillin beyond the boundaries of the sample blocks suggested that our data underestimated the value of T. Therefore,

$T = 2$ hr was used as a parameter in the diffusion model.

The values of the diffusion coefficients (D) and the effective surface concentrations (C_s) giving the best fit to the individual distribution of counts in 23 sectioned foci are summarized in Table 3. The diffusion coefficients for the three source residence times were not significantly different from one another and averaged $D = 0.72 ± 0.09$ mm/hr (mean ± SD, $n = 31$). The mean effective surface concentration at the 60-min source residence time was significantly lower than at the shorter times and may have been related to lower penicillin concentration of an adherent ring of penicillin solution that often formed at the tip of the electrode at this time. The parameter C_s can be used to estimate the

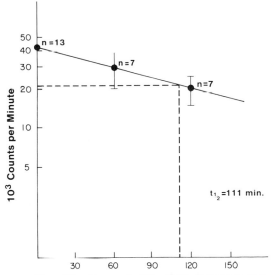

FIG. 5. Semi-log plot of disappearance of counts from the focus with time. Plotted values are means (SD, vertical bars) of the recovered counts at each of the source-free intervals. (From ref. 82, with permission.)

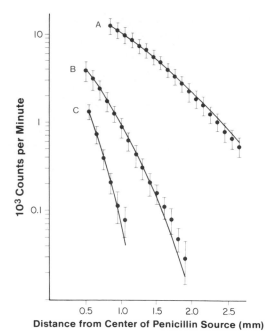

FIG. 6. Averaged distributions from each of the three source-residence times. Plotted values are the means (SD, vertical bars) of the counts recovered from sections at equivalent distances from the center of the penicillin source. **A:** $t = 60$ min ($n = 10$). **B:** $t = 15$ min ($n = 10$). **C:** $t = 5$ min ($n = 5$). *Solid lines* represent the theoretical best-fit curves. (From ref. 82, with permission.)

percent extracellular volume (% ECV). The data from all three groups were averaged, yielding $C_s = 309{,}551 \pm 97{,}182$ cpm (mean ± SD, $n = 31$). Dividing C_s by the concentration of counts present in the penicillin-containing capillaries ($\times 100$) gives an ECV of 15.1 ± 4.7%.

The expected distribution of penicillin beyond twice the radius of the source is nearly spherically symmetric. Thus, sections tangential to the surface should contain twice the amount of material found in sections normal to the surface at the same distance from the source. As expected, a factor of nearly two separates the best-fit curves for the two planes of section. Averaged distributions for the three source residence times are shown in Fig. 6.

The pial membrane does not appear to present a significant surface barrier to the diffusion of penicillin. This is indicated by the closeness of fit between the theoretical and observed distributions in Figs. 5 and 6.

The data indicate the extent to which individual neurons within a focus are in direct contact with penicillin. The rate of increase in the size of the neuronal population exposed to effective concentrations of penicillin as diffusion continues has also been measured. Most earlier studies on the spatial distribution of penicillin (10,21,95) and other topical convulsants (11,104) did not quantitate the concentration of the drug within the focus. The population boundaries reported earlier did not define the true extent of their foci, since minimal concentrations of the epileptogenic agent were unknown. The data show the spatial distribution and concentration profile of penicillin as a function of time and distance from the source (Fig. 6).

The diffusion model developed uses three groups of assumptions. The first group consists of those concerning the movement of penicillin in the cortex from any source geometry. They include the assumption that penicillin distributes itself in neocortex by passive diffusion confined to the extracellular space; that the cortex represents a homogeneous and isotropic medium; that any binding to fixed membrane alters only the value of the diffusion coefficient; and that clearance of penicillin from the extracellular space occurs by a first-order process. This last assumption was later tested experimentally and confirmed a first-order removal with a half-time of about 2 hr. The other assumptions were confirmed reasonably well by the closeness of fit of the model to the data from the three different planes of section through the focus.

The second group of assumptions is specific to the experimental design: that the loss of penicillin from the source by diffusion into the brain does not significantly reduce the concentration of the solution at the cortical surface; that the osmotic effect of the entering penicillin molecules does not significantly change the proportions of intracellular and extracellular space; and that distortion of cortical blocks is minimal during excision, freezing, and paraffin embedding. The amount of label remaining in the source after an experiment compared to the total amount of label contained in each brain block indicates that the concentration of the source is not significantly reduced even after an hour of diffusion. The finding that the model fits equally well close to the source, where high concentrations of penicillin exerted a maximal osmotic effect, and up to 2.0 mm distant suggests that the osmotic effects are not significant. However, one cannot ignore the possibility that the lowered value of the effective source concentration found after 60 min may be partly the result of local edema produced by increased osmolarity. The spherical symmetry of the distribution of ^{14}C-penicillin recovered from the cortical blocks indicates that effects from distortion of the tissue were minimal.

Although information on the metabolism of penicillin in the cat is lacking, it is assumed that most of the penicillin in the brain during the experiment remains in the active form. In cases of renal failure in humans, the half-life of biologically active benzylpenicillin can reach 30 hr, and it seems likely that the labeled molecule rather than a metabolic fragment is measured.

Noebels and Pedley (64) attempted to quantify the distribution of penicillin in neocortex and to determine its diffusion coefficient. Following a 3-min application of a large rectangular pledget containing ^{14}C-penicillin, whole brain sections cut tangentially were counted. Their results apply to the movement of penicillin in one direction only, i.e., normal to the surface. They concluded that penetration of penicillin into neocortex occurred by passive diffusion during the 3 min it was applied. The three-dimensional model described here confirms that movement occurs by passive diffusion and indicates that it continues for longer periods. The isotropy found here shows that penicillin moves equally well in all directions, despite the predominant cytoarchitectonic organization of densely packed, vertically oriented neurons that lie in the diffusion path.

The diffusion coefficient of 0.72 mm^2/hr · 1 described here (82) is considerably smaller than the 1.5 mm^2/hr · 1 reported by Noebels and Pedley (64). Methodological differences can account for the discrepancy. With their diffusion of only 3 min, continued diffusion for as little as 15 sec during excision could have resulted in overestimation of the value of the diffusion coefficient. This possibility prompted us to select 5 min as the minimum diffusion interval. Although Noebels and Pedley ascribed the deviation between their theoretical and observed distributions to a surface barrier restricting entry of penicillin, they did not include the factor of confinement of the movement of penicillin to the extracellular space. This is within the range of 7 to 20% for cortical extracellular volume as reported elsewhere (23,49,79). If included it eliminates the need to postulate a surface barrier. Our results, which account for the extracellular volume by making the effective surface concentration an unknown parameter, also suggest that penicillin entry into the cortex is unrestricted at the surface. This view is well supported (49), although there have been other considerations (6,24, 36,68). Had there been significant restriction of penicillin entry into the brain, a divergence between the theoretical and observed distributions would have occurred. This would have been most noticeable near the surface, where the effects of a diffusion barrier on penicillin would be most pronounced.

An approximate value for the diffusion coefficient was calculated from molecular theory. Assuming that penicillin diffuses in the extracellular space as if it were an uncharged spherical molecule, the Stokes–Einstein relation yields an estimate of a diffusion coefficient for penicillin in free solution at 25°C of 1.9 mm^2/hr · 1. An empirical modification of the Stokes relation that accounts for molecular asymmetry and hydration (53) reduces this to 1.7 mm^2/hr · 1. Penicillin molecules in aqueous solution appear to assume a disk-like conformation (17). The Stokes relation corrected for oblate ellipsoids of rotation further reduces the value of D to 1.6 mm/hr. The effective viscosity of water increased by a factor depending on the ratio of the radius of the diffusing particle to the radius of the channel (67). Because the approximately molecular radius of penicillin is 5 Å (17), and the accepted width of the intercellular space in neocortix is 100 to 150 Å, an estimated 20% reduction of the diffusion coefficient in free solution would be expected. Binding of penicillin molecules to fixed membrane would produce a further decrease. The value of D for penicillin of 1.5 mm/hr reported by Noebels and Pedley is similar to that expected for penicillin in free solution. The D of 0.72 mm/hr reported here represents a reduction on the order expected. This value for D is supported by the finding that the value of the parameter C_s, obtained by fitting to the same data, yields an estimated ECV of 15%, which is in the range of 7 to 20% for neocortical ECV reported elsewhere (23,49,79).

The value for the diffusion coefficient we obtained was used to calculate the extent of diffusion at the onset of focal EEG spiking at 1.6 ± 0.3 min after placement of the penicillin. We assumed a lower limit of 1 mM penicillin for detectable effects on cortical neurons on the basis of *in vitro* experiments (16,37,56,62). The results indicate that at the onset of focal spiking, the population of cells expected to be in contact with concentrations greater than 1 mM extends not more than 0.78 mm from the source. The change with time of the population in contact with a minimum of 1 mm correlates well with the development of interictal spiking (30). At 10 min after the first appearance of EEG spikes, the radial distance to the 1 mM penicillin limit doubles to 1.5 mm, and the population of cells in contact with this concentration extends into the deeper levels of the cortex. This is a time when predominantly negative spikes at the center of the focus begin to stabilize in form and surface positive spikes are established in surrounding cortex up to 4 mm away (30). The next doubling of the radial distance to the 1 mM penicillin limit occurs 75 min later. At this time the concentration distribution begins to approach a steady state with electrographic stability of waveform, amplitude, duration, and frequency of EEG spikes at the center of the focus and in the surrounding cortex (7,30).

The changes with time of the radii of the spherical surfaces at several different constant concentrations for several hours are shown in Fig. 7. A rapid increase in the extent of brain in contact with a concentration of penicillin of 1 mM or more occurs within the first hour. After this time, the rate of increase diminishes. Between the first and second hour, the size of the 1 mM contour increased by 26% while the increase is less than 30% during the subsequent 4 hr.

The theoretical model presented here can be applied directly to experiments using other source concentrations. Lueders et al. (55), using the same technique of penicillin application used in the present study, found that 34 mM penicillin was the minimal source concentration necessary to produce focal spiking consistently in the cat. The EEG spikes they recorded became relatively stable roughly within the same time as our 840-mM focus. The 30-mM curve in Fig. 7 for the 840mM focus corresponds to 1.12 mM for a 34-mM focus. During the period between 1½ and 6 hr the radius of the cellular population exposed to 1.2 mM penicillin in the 34-mM focus increases only slightly less than 10%. If regions where penicillin concentrations are less than 1.2 mM do not participate in neuronal responses that gen-

erate EEG spikes, the model predicts the electrographic stability after 90 min observed by Lueders et al. (55).

This study on the diffusional kinetics of penicillin enables determination of extracellular concentration as a function of time and distance from a source during the formation of the focus. It provides a basis for correlation of penicillin concentration with cell and population activities in epileptogenesis. The model provides a relatively stable volume of neurons involved in epileptogenic activity for periods of time long enough to allow detailed electrical investigation such as follows in the next part of this chapter.

RELATIONSHIP BETWEEN LOCAL CONCENTRATIONS AND INTRACELLULAR POTENTIALS AT A FOCUS

Attempts to probe the mechanisms involved in the generation of epileptiform electrical activity resulting from the topical application of penicillin must consider the direct action of local concentrations of the drug surrounding the neurons. The intrinsic properties of the neurons, the local concentration of penicillin, and the location of the cell within the organized neural networks of the cerebral cortex all determine the way a particular neuron behaves. Analysis of focal epileptiform activity from a single cell must consider its position relative to the center of the focus (which determines the concentration of penicillin) and the effect of that cell's location for interaction among existing complex synaptic organizations of the brain.

In the preceding section of this chapter, a mathematical model was developed character-

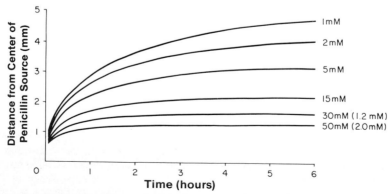

FIG. 7. Radii of hemispherical contours of constant concentration resulting from the continuous diffusion of penicillin from the source. The values assigned to each curve are those for diffusion from an 840-mM source concentration with a lumen of radius 0.25 mm located on the surface of the cortex. (From ref. 82, with permission.)

izing the distribution of penicillin in the cortex during topical applications and the diffusion coefficient for penicillin in the cortex was determined. In an earlier section it was shown that the electrical activities of neurons participating in focal epileptogenesis exhibit progressive decreases in excitation as distance increases from the center of the focus. Prolonged IPSPs are found at the periphery, larval and truncated PDSs are found in a zone of transition, and highly excited neurons evincing sustained PDSs occur near the center of the focus.

The elapsed time from the placement of the penicillin source to the time of impalement of the neuron (source residence time) was recorded for 58 of the 102 cells whose electrical activity was described in the preceding section. The times and measurements of the radial distances from the center of the source allow calculation of estimated local concentrations of penicillin in contact with the cells. The calculated concentrations are shown in Table 4, together with the averaged electrical parameters for each category of intracellular activity. Good concurrence between concentration and individual cell electrical activity is indicated in Table 4.

That distribution of intracellular activity within and surrounding the focus reflects the geometry of the concentration distribution of penicillin underlying the source may be seen in Fig. 8. Here, the four categories of intracellular activity are plotted as a function of radial distance and source residence time. The concentrations at which each category of cellular activity is found are plotted on the same coordinates. While possible, columnar and/or laminar effects upon the intracellular activity may play a role. The fact that the form of the concentration curves fits well with the distributions of two markedly different types of activity (i.e, prolonged IPSPs and truncated PDSs) would seem to imply that the instantaneous local concentration of penicillin is more important than location or organization in determining the type of activity exhibited by each of the cells impaled. The

relationship is weaker between penicillin concentration and distribution of larval PDSs. This may be the result of both the small sample size and the relatively short interval over which recordings from these cells were obtained.

Although Prince and Wilder (76) emphasized the utilization of existing columnar organization in the neocortex during focal epileptogenesis because the activity they encountered along a single electrode track tended to be similar in both the focus itself and in the inhibitory surround, our data (Fig. 2) show differences in activity along an electrode track in the zone of transition between the focus and the inhibitory surround. This indicates that intracortical penicillin concentrations are determinant in our foci.

Calculation of the concentration at any point in the focus depends on knowledge of the depth of the recording electrode and its horizontal distance from the center of the source. Although the exact location of the electrode tip is rarely known, most stable recordings are probably obtained at or near the soma of the cell. Therefore, the relationship of concentration and cellular electrical activity with mechanism of action applies only to the region at or near the soma. For the pyramidal cells impaled, the concentrations of penicillin can be very much higher at the terminal branches of their apical dendrites, which lie closer to the penicillin source. Therefore, a concentration gradient of penicillin of unknown magnitude can exist along the cell, and its action may be considerable. Histological location and three-dimensional reconstruction of the intracellularly labeled neurons would enable the necessary measurements to estimate the concentration of penicillin in any part of the cell.

In various *in vitro* preparations, the major effects of increasing penicillin concentration is to decrease progressively the effectiveness of inhibitory processes while augmenting those of excitation. Significant depression of inhibition occurs at relatively low penicillin concentrations (2–7 mM) (37,56,57,62), although the actual threshold for a measurable effect may be much

TABLE 4. *PDS and IPSP characteristics at different local concentrations of penicillin*[a]

Type of neuronal activity	Local concentration (mM)	PDS duration (msec)	Onset to maximum hyperpolarization (msec)	Onset to first action potential (msec)	PDS amplitude (mV)	Maximum amplitude hyperpolarization (mV)	N
Sustained PDS	28 ± 11	73 ± 16	243 ± 201	1026 ± 418	17 ± 7	6 ± 3	14
Truncated PDS	14 ± 3	51 ± 8	139 ± 23	475 ± 143	19 ± 3	8 ± 3	9
Larval PDS	10 ± 7	33 ± 6	107 ± 23	548 ± 151	8 ± 4	9 ± 3	7
Prolonged IPSP	5 ± 4	—	79 ± 23	350 ± 210	—	8 ± 4	28

[a] Mean ± SD.

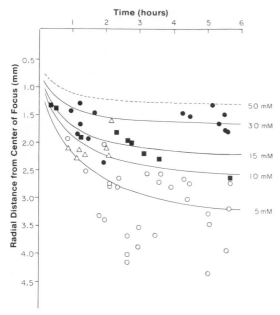

FIG. 8. Scatter diagram of PDS categories and prolonged IPSPs plotted against radial distance from the focus and time of cell penetration. *Solid and dashed curves* are radii of hemispherical contours of constant penicillin concentration. ● Sustained PDS (309 mM), ■ truncated PDS (15 mM), △ larval PDS (10 mM), ○ prolonged IPSP (5 mM). The concentration of each solid curve is the mean value (rounded to the nearest 5 mM) at which each category of intracellular activity was found. At concentrations above 50 mM (*dashed curve*), most cells encountered were completely depolarized. (From ref. 82, with permission.)

lower. Augmentation of excitation may begin at somewhat higher concentrations (6–8 mM) (4,25,26,65). The mean estimated local concentrations of penicillin in the vicinity of neurons displaying each category of electrical activity reported here at 5–28 mM are within the range of concentrations used in the *in vitro* studies cited (1.0–84 mM). Furthermore, the concentration of penicillin related to each of the categories of electrical activity is consistent with the effects found in *in vitro* preparations that indicate the emergence of net excitation with increasing penicillin concentration. Although penicillin concentration as low as 2 mM reliably produce depolarization shifts and epileptiform field potentials in hippocampal slices *in vitro,* the higher range of concentration related to these events in this neocortical study may reflect intrinsic differences between hippocampus neocortex in both membrane properties and synaptic organization.

While the concentration of penicillin related to each of the categories of electrical activity

reported here is generally consistent with the effects found *in vitro* preparations that indicate the emergence of net excitation with increasing penicillin concentrations, our findings are not sufficient to establish similar actions *in vivo*. They do, however, provide a basis for testing hypotheses relating mammalian epileptogenesis in the intact brain to mechanisms of action of a convulsant drug in simpler *in vitro* systems.

The data have shown the spatial distribution and concentration profile of penicillin as a function of time and distance from the source. This data also indicate the extent to which the abnormal potentials generated by individual neurons are direct responses to contact with penicillin. The rate of increases in the size of the neuronal population exposed to effective concentrations of penicillin as diffusion continues (Fig. 9) has also been measured. Most earlier studies on the spatial distribution of penicillin (10,95) and other topical convulsants (104) did not succeed in quantitating the concentration of the drug within the focus, and the population boundaries at minimal effective concentrations of the epileptogenic agent were not known.

TWO- AND THREE-DIMENSIONAL EXTRACELLULAR FIELDS

The surface negative EEG spike is the consistent indicator of an epileptogenic focus. As was shown (Fig. 3) (28,60), there are close temporal and spatial relationships between the surface negative focal spike and the PDS. Because both the PDS and the surface spike are negative, it has been suggested that most PDSs are generated from superficial layers of the cortex (30). The surface positive EEG wave in the surround of our model focus overlies cellular IPSPs that are found at all levels in the cortex extending from 2.0 mm to at least 3.5 mm from the center of the focus. Gumnit and Takahashi (33) and Gumnit et al. (32) in laminar studies suggested that both deep excitation and deep inhibition occur in the depth of the surround and may be responsible for the surface positivity.

In strong penicillin foci, an early EEG positivity lasting 10 to 30 msec (Fig. 4) precedes the negative EEG surface wave generated by the PDSs. The location of the generators of this early positivity and the character of the cellular activity that generates it is as yet unexplained. The variability in its amplitude and relative size in relation to the negative spike is puzzling (30), because the early positivity at the strong epileptogenic focus is the initial event preceding the longer but more spatially delimited high-voltage

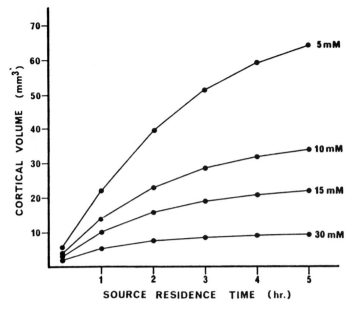

FIG. 9. Growth volumes bounded by contours of known concentrations. (From ref. 82, with permission.)

negativity at each focal interictal spike. As it is, the earliest recognizable event locating its extracellular field and current generators is essential to understanding spike generation. The early positivity has a relatively widespread distribution and could reflect EPSPs that trigger the next PDSs by overcoming waning inhibition from HAPs and IPSPs. Thus early positivity may be a part of a mechanism involved in triggering or synchronizing the epileptogenic aggregate of neurons to generate the intermittent interictal negative spikes. It is less likely, but also possible, that the early positivity is a part of the inhibitory surround. The fact that two adjacent penicillin foci can interact and become synchronous when separated by less than 4 mm but become asynchronous when 6 mm apart (54) suggests that the surround positivity when separated by more than 2.5 mm from the center of the focus is composed of a number of populations, some of which reflect deep excitation as well as inhibition.

There is a reversal of negative spindle polarity by penicillin that precedes the appearance of the negative surface spike (Fig. 10). This may reflect depolarization inactivation of the superficial sink for type II spindles described by Spencer and Brookhart (93). As the spindles reverse and penicillin penetrates further within the next 60 sec, pyramidal cells produce PDSs, perhaps by depolarization activation of apical dendrites to produce PDSs. Another possibility is that the penicillin alters the superficial laminar distribution of synaptic activity by interfering with inhibitory afferent synapses (16,56). Recent evidence by Kistopoulos et al. (47) shows that spindles and spike and wave discharges have rather similar fields in the vertical dimension and that polarity of the individual waves of both reverses between a depth of 200 and 400 μm. Elger and Speckman (22) report that in developing foci in which penicillin penetrates only the superficial layers of the cortex, full-blown PDSs are found at depths of 150 to 200 μm below the surface, and even after 15 or 20 min of recording prolonged PDSs are found in the superficial layers. Less complete PDSs of shorter duration and forms without depolarization inactivation were seen in the deeper layers. Nevertheless, according to Schwartzkroin and Wyler (90) and Lockton and Holmes (51,52), is the cell bodies residing near layer IV, considerably farther below the surface, that produce the PDSs. Also, Ebersole and Chatt (19,20) found layer IV of the cortical lamina of cats to be the most sensitive level of the cortex of penicillin. In their study of epileptogenic activity in the visual cortex, layer IV was 1,000 μm deep.

These conflicting data and unresolved questions indicate that further definition of the three-dimensional spatial and temporal distributions of extracellular fields and current generators is essential for understanding the generation and spread of epileptiform activity.

THREE-DIMENSIONAL FIELD ANALYSIS

Potentials at the cortical surface surrounding a discrete penicillin focus during the course of

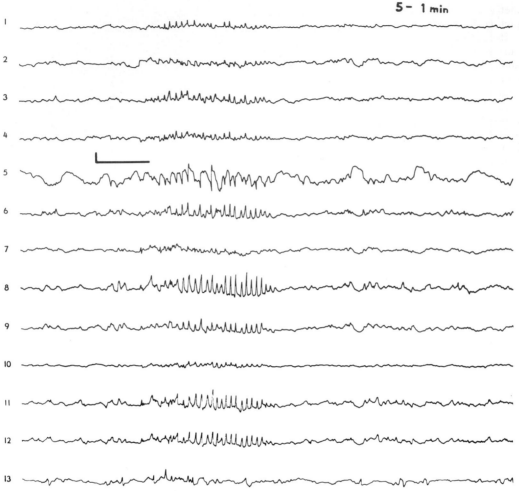

FIG. 10. Inversion of spindles at the penicillin-containing capillary (channel 5) 1 min after its placement and just before spiking starts. Calibration, 500 μV, 1 sec. Negative up. Reference is neck muscle. (From ref. 30, with permission.)

established interictal electrocortigraphic spiking show similar configurations from spike to spike over periods up to several hours (30). Because of this, information recorded at different depths and horizontal distances from the focus over an extended period of time can describe essentially the same field. The reproducible measurements made during and timed by the EEG spike recorded at the penicillin electrode during an experiment permit the collection of synchronized extracellularly recorded potentials from several cortical locations at different times by positioning a microelectrode with respect to the center of the penicillin-containing electrode. Spikes were averaged at each location to insure that minor variations would not be given undue significance. This procedure was used to determine the extracellular potential distribution at multiple depths, from the cortical surface to a depth of 3.5 mm. Several plunges at different lateral distances are completed in each experiment, enabling the determination of a composite field-potential distribution from multiple locations within the focus during the equivalent of a single interictal spike. Focal discharges were stable for sufficient periods after the removal of the penicillin-containing electrode to allow plunges into the region directly under the applied penicillin.

A computer program used continuous functions of position to interpolate the potential between the points measured. This was done at 4-msec epochs throughout the duration of the interictal spike. The surface potential during such a spike was found to be axially symmetric around the center of the focus, and axial symmetry was assumed to hold for the depth in depicting the potential field in three dimensions.

Because the surface potential distribution during an interictal spike is radially symmetric about the axis of the penicillin source, the three-dimensional extracellular potential field can be characterized geometrically by describing the recording sites in terms of two coordinates, depth from the pial surface and radius from the axis of the penicillin electrode. Data for the fields were obtained by averaging 16 successive interictal spikes at standard depths and distances from the center of the focus. Data from a typical experiment are shown in Fig. 11. The negative spike at the surface near the center of the focus has the same polarity throughout the depth of the cortex, and it peaks at 0.5 to 1.0 mm below the surface. The positive spikes in the surround, however, invert at a depth of about 0.3 mm, becoming negative spikes that

peak in amplitude at depths between 0.5 and 1.0 mm below the surface, as do the negative spikes recorded near the center of the focus (Fig. 11).

To facilitate analysis of the spatial and temporal relationships of the field, continuous functions of position were used to interpolate the potential between the discrete points at which the measurements were made to produce intensity-modulated displays of the field in a plane normal to the surface at 4-msec epochs throughout the interictal spike, as shown in Fig. 12. Initiation of the major negative phase of the surface interictal spike is preceded by the rise of a wave of negativity at a depth of 0.5 to 1.0 mm below the penicillin source in most foci examined. A lower-amplitude negativity occurs almost simultaneously but at a greater depth, 2.0 to 2.5 mm. Occasionally the earliest potential change from baseline occurs at the periphery of the focus but at this same depth.

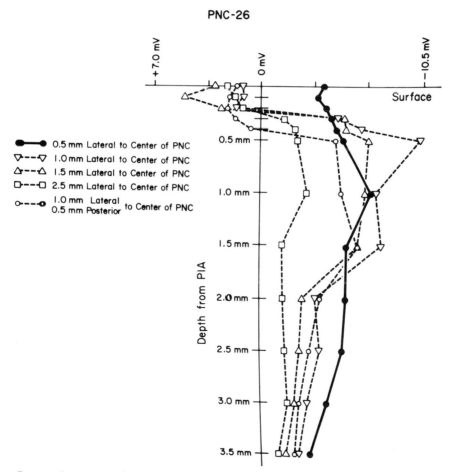

FIG. 11. Computed averages of relative amplitudes and of polarity of spikes at the surface and at various depths in the cortex. The negative surface spike near the center of the focus remains negative through all depths peaking in amplitude at between 0.5 and 1.0 mm. Surface spikes are positive in the surround and invert at depths between 0.2 and 0.3 mm, with a negative peak between 0.5 and 1.0 mm. (From ref. 29, with permission.)

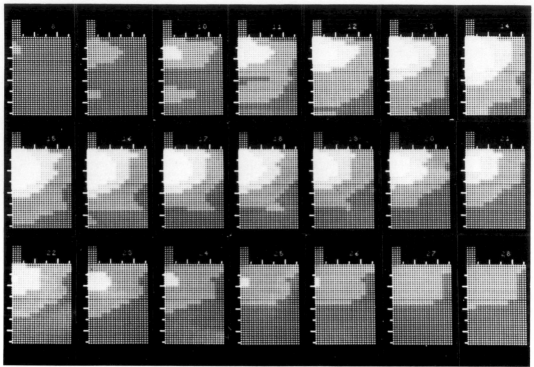

FIG. 12. Spread of the field potential in the cortex during an interictal spike. Successive computed intensity modulated displays represent changes in the distribution of potential in a plane normal to the cortical surface during a single composite spike. Time increases from *left to right, top to bottom.* Whiteness indicates negativity. The rectangle at the *upper left* of each display shows the location of the penicillin source and its shading represents zero potential. The absolute value of the potential at any point is scaled relative to the maximum negativity attained during the spike. *Ordinate:* axis of the penicillin capillary; depth in 0.5 mm steps from surface. *Absissa:* lateral distance in 0.5-mm steps from axis of the focus. The initial and later most intense negativity occurs at about 0.6 mm and spreads in all directions during the first 36 msec to involve a relatively large cortical volume before receding. Surface positivity in surrounding cortex occurs but is not resolved in these displays because of scaling techniques; 4-msec epochs. (From L. Zablow, A. M. Salazar, and E. S. Goldensohn, *in preparation.*)

INTRACELLULAR CHANGES DURING SPREAD OF POTENTIAL FIELD IN THE FOCUS

In a stable focus, the latencies of PDS onsets in individual cells can be measured with reference to the interictal spike on the cortical surface after selecting suitable features of the intracellular and population potentials to define the moment of their onsets. The dependence of these latencies on the location of the cells in the focus was examined by an analysis of the multiple linear regression of latencies on the distances of the cells from the axis through the center of the focus and on their depths in the cortex.

Statistically significant relationships to both coordinates were found. The dependence of onset times of the PDSs on their lateral distance from the axis of the focus is shown in Fig. 13

for 47 cells. The portions of the latencies contributed by the depth dependency have been removed by the statistical analysis. The reciprocal of the slope of the regression line, which is in effect the lateral velocity of propagation of PDS initiation from cell to cell, is 0.25 m/sec.

There are less precise features for recognizing the developing negative extracellular potential in the depths during an interictal spike. An arbitrary chosen fraction of the maximum negativity attained is represented by the edge of the lightest white contour in a sequence of potential distributions. This allows measurement of the velocity of lateral spread of the negative field in the depth during the developing spike. For the data plotted in Fig. 13B, the rate of development of negative potential outward from the axis of the focus is also approximately 0.25 m/sec. The close correspondence of the rates of spread of PDSs provides evidence that the development

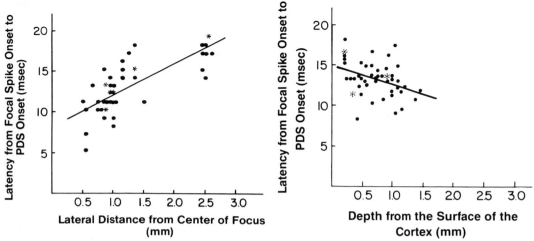

FIG. 13. **A:** Scatter plot of PDS onset latencies relative to focal spike onsets as a function of horizontal distance from the axis of a stable focus. PDS onset latencies are shortest near the center of the focus, increasing from about 8 msec at a distance of 0.5 mm to 18 msec at 2.5 mm. The outward velocity of propagation of PDS activity from cell to cell is 0.25 m/sec. The portion of the PDS onset latency contributed by the depth dependency has been removed by the multiple linear regression analysis. Each point represents the average PDS onset latency of 10 successive interictal spikes. *Asterisks* denote pairs of cells with the same values. *Solid lines* are best linear fit. **B:** PDS onset latencies relative to focal spike onsets as a function of depth. This also occurs at the rate of approximately 0.25 m/sec.

of the negative extracellular potential is due to a sequential onset of PDSs that occur progressively more distant from the axis of the focus at a velocity of about 0.25 m/sec.

REFERENCES

1. Ayala, G. F., Dichter, M., Gumnit, R. J., Matsumoto, H., and Spencer, W. A. (1973): Genesis of epileptic interictal spikes: New knowledge of cortical feedback systems suggests a neurophysiological explanation of brief paroxysms. *Brain Res.,* 52:1–17.
2. Ayala, G. F., Matsumoto, H., and Gumnit R. J. (1970): Inhibitory mechanisms during tonic clonic seizures. *Electroencephalogy Clin. Neurophysiol.,* 28:96.
3. Ayala, G. F., Matsumoto, H., and Gumnit, R. J. (1970): Excitability changes and inhibitory mechanisms in neocortical neurons during seizures. *J. Neurophysiol.,* 33:73–85
4. Ayala, G. F., Spencer, W. A., and Gumnit, R. J. (1971): Penicillin as an epileptogenic agent: Effect on an isolated synapse. *Science,* 171:915–917.
5. Ayala, G. F. and Vasconetto, C. (1972): Role of recurrent excitatory pathways in epileptogenesis. *Electroencephalogy Clin. Neurophysiol.,* 33:96–98.
6. Bayleydier, C., Biscone, J. C., and Quoex, C. (1973): Etude radioautoraphique de la barriere hemo-encephalique a la penicilline dans l'epilepsie experimentale chronique. *Acta Neuropathol. (Berlin),* 24:321–330.
7. Bustamente, L., Lueders, H., Pippenger, C.,

and Goldensohn, E. S. (1980): The effects of phenytoin on the penicillin-induced spike focus. *Electroencephalogy Clin. Neurophysiol.,* 48: 90–97.
8. Calvin, W. H., Ojemann, G. A., and Ward, A. A., Jr. (1973): Human cortical neurons in epileptogenic foci: Comparison of interictal firing patterns to those of "epileptic" neurons in animals. *Electroencephalogy Clin. Neurophysiol.,* 34:337–351.
9. Clarke, G. and Hill, R. G. (1972): Effects of a local lesion in responses of rabbit cortical neurons to putative neurotransmitters. *Br. J. Pharmacol.,* 44:435–441.
10. Collins, R. D. (1976): Metabolic response to focal penicillin seizures in rat: Spike discharge vs. after discharge. *J. Neurochem.,* 27:1473–1482.
11. Cornblath, D. R., and Ferguson, J. H. (1976): Distribution of radioactivity from topically applied ^{3}H-acetylcholine in relation to seizures. *Exp. Neurol.,* 50:495–504.
12. Courtney, K. R., Noebels, J. L., and Prince, D. A. (1976): Neuronal events in the area surrounding penicillin foci in cat neocortex. *Neurosci. Abstr.,* 2:258.
13. Courtney, K. R. and Prince, D. A. (1977): Epileptogenesis in neocortical slices. *Brain Res.,* 127:191–196.
14. Curtis, D. R., Game, C. J. A., Johnson, G. A. R., McCulloch, R. M., and MacLachlan, R. M. (1972): Convulsive action of penicillin. *Brain Res.,* 43:242–245.
15. Cutler, R. W. P. and Young, J. (1979): The effect of penicillin on the release of γ-aminobutyric acid from cortex slices. *Brain Res.,* 170:157–163.

16. Davidoff, R. A. (1972b): Penicillin and inhibition in the cat spinal cord. *Brain Res.,* 45:638–642.

17. Dexter, D. D. and van der Veen, J. M. (1978): Conformations of penicillin G: Crystal structure of procaine penicillin G monohydrate and a refinement of the structure of potassium penicillin G. *J. Chem. Soc.(Perkin I),* 3:185–190.

18. Dichter, M. and Spencer, W. A. (1969): Penicillin-induced interictal discharges from the cat hippocampus. I. Characteristics and topographical features. *J. Neurophysiol.,* 32:649.

19. Ebersole, J. S. and Chatt, A. B. (1980): The laminar susceptability of cat visual cortex to penicillin-induced epileptogenesis. *Neurology,* 30:355.

20. Ebersole, J. S. and Chatt, A. B. (1981): Toward a unified theory of focal penicillin epileptogenesis: An intracortical potential investigation. *Epilepsia,* 22:347–361.

21. Edmonds, H. L., Stark, L. G. and Hollinger, M. A. (1974): The effects of diphenylhydantoin, phenobarbital and diazepam on the penicillin-induced epileptogenic focus in the rat. *Exp. Neurol.* 45:377–386.

22. Elger, C. E., and Speckmann, E. J. (1983): Penicillin-induced epileptic foci in the motor cortex: vertical inhibition. *Electroencephalogy Clin. Neurophysiol.,* 56:604–622.

23. Fenstermacher, J. D., Li, C. L., and Levin, V. A. (1970): The extracellular space of the cerebral cortex of normothermic and hypothermic cats. *Exp. Neurol.,* 27:101–114.

24. Fisher, R. S., Pedley, T. A., and Prince, D. A. (1976): Kinetics of potassium movement in normal cortex. *Brain Res.,* 101:223–237.

25. Futamachi, K. J. and Prince, D. A. (1975): Effect of penicillin on an excitatory synapse. *Brain Res.,* 100:589–597.

26. Futamachi, K. J. and Prince, D. A. (1971): The effects of penicillin on crayfish neuromuscular junction. *Fed. Proc.,* 30:323 (abstr.).

27. Gabor, A. J. and Scobey, R. P. (1975): Spatial limits of epileptogenic cortex: Its relationship to ectopic spike generation. *J. Neurophysiol.,* 38:395–404.

28. Goldensohn, E. S. and Purpura, D. P. (1963): Intracellular potentials of cortical neurons during focal epileptogenic discharges. *Science,* 139:840–842.

29. Goldensohn, E. S., and Ward, A., Jr. (1975): Pathogenesis of epileptic seizures. In *The Nervous System, Vol. 2: The Clinical Neurosciences,* edited by D. B. Tower, pp. 249–260. Raven Press, New York.

30. Goldensohn, E. S., Zablow, L., and Salazar, A. M. (1977): The penicillin focus. I. Distribution of potential at the cortical surface. *Electroencephalogy Clin. Neurophysiol.,* 42:480–494.

31. Goldensohn, E. S., Zablow, L., and Stein, B. (1970): Interrelationships of form and latency of spike discharge from small areas of human cortex. *Electroencephalogy Clin. Neurophysiol.,* 29:321–322.

32. Gumnit, R. J., Matsumoto, H., and Vasconetto, C. (1970): DC activity in the depth of an experimental epileptic focus. *Electroencephalogy Clin. Neurophysiol.,* 28:333–339.

33. Gumnit, R. J. and Takahashi, T. (1965): Changes in direct current activity during experimental focal seizures. *Electroencephalogy Clin. Neurophysiol.,* 19:63–74.

34. Gutnick, M. J., Connors, B. W., and Prince, D. A. (1982): Mechanisms of neocortical epileptogenesis *in vitro. J. Neurophysiol.,* 48:1321–1335.

35. Gutnick, M. J., and Prince, D. A. (1972): Thalamocortical relay neurons: Antidromic invasion of spikes from the cortical epileptogenic focus. *Science,* 176:424–426.

36. Haug, H. (1971): Die membrane limitans gliae superficialis der schrinde der Katze. *Z. Zellforsch,* 115:79–87.

37. Hochner, B., Spira, M. E., and Werman, R. (1976): Penicillin decreases chloride conductance in crustacean muscle: A model for the epileptic neuron. *Brain Res.,* 107:85–103.

38. Hotson, J. R., Prince, D. A., and Schwartzkroin, P. A. (1979): Anomalous inward rectification in hippocampal neurons. *J. Neurophysiol.,* 42:889–895.

39. Hotson, J. R., Schwartzkroin, P. A., and Prince, D. A. (1977): Calcium activated after hyperpolarization in hippocampal slices maintained *in vitro. Soc. Neurosci. Abstr.,* 3:218.

40. Hubel, D. H., and Wiesel, T. N. (1965): Receptive fields and functional architecture in two nonstriate visual areas (18 and 19) of the cat. *J. Neurophysiol.,* 28:229.

41. Jasper, H. H. (1972): Application of experimental models to human epilepsy. In *Experimental Models of Epilepsy,* edited by D. P. Purpura, J. K. Penry, D. Tower, D. M. Woodbury, and R. Walter, pp. 585–601. Raven Press, New York.

42. Johnston, D., and Brown, T. H. (1984): The synaptic nature of the paroxysmal depolarizing shift in hippocampal neurons. *Ann. Neurol.* 16(suppl):S65–S71.

43. Johnston, D., and Brown, T. H. (1981): Giant synaptic potential hypothesis for epileptiform activity. *Science,* 211:294–297.

44. Jordan, J. E. (1983): Changes in the inhibitory surround associated with penicillin spike. *Electroencephalogy Clin. Neurophysiol.,* 56:6P.

45. Kao, L. I., and Crill, W. E. (1972): Penicillin-induced segmental myoclonus. I. Motor responses and intracellular recording from motoneurons. *Arch. Neurol. (Chicago),* 261:156–161.

46. Kennedy, C., Des Rosiers, M. H., Jehle, J. W., Reivich, M., Sharpe, F., and Sokoloff, L. (1975): Mapping of functional neural pathways by autoradiographic survey of local metabolic rate with ^{14}C-deoxyglucose. *Science,* 187:850–851.

47. Kostopoulos, G., Avoli, M., Pellegrini, A., and Gloor, P. (1982): Laminar analysis of spindles and of spikes of the spike and wave discharge of feline generalized penicillin epilepsy. *Electroencephalogy Clin. Neurophysiol.,* 53:1–13.

48. Lebeda, F. J., Hablitz, J. J., and Johnston, D. (1982): Antagonism of GABA-mediated responses by *d*-tubocurarine in hippocampal neurons. *J. Neurophysiol.*, 48:622–632.

49. Levin, V. A., Fenstermacher, J. D., and Patlak, C. S. (1970): Sucrose insulin space measurement of cerebral cortex in four mammalian species. *Am. J. Physiol.*, 219:1528–1533.

50. Llinas, R., and Hess, R. (1976): Tetrodotoxin-resistant dendritic spikes in avian purkinje cells. *Proc. Natl. Acad. Sci. U.S.A.*, 73:2520–2523.

51. Lockton, J. W., and Holmes, O. (1980): Site of initiation of penicillin-induced epilepsy in the cortex cerebri of the rat. *Brain Res.*, 190:301–304.

52. Lockton, J. W., and Holmes, O. (1983): Penicillin epilepsy in the rat: The responses of different layers of the cortex cerebri. *Brain, Res.*, 184:220–223.

53. Longsworth, L. D. (1953): Diffusion measurements, at 25, of solutions of amino acids, peptides and sugars. *J. Am. Chem. Soc.*, 75:5705–5709.

54. Lueders, H. Bustamante, L. A., Zablow, L., and Goldensohn, E. S. (1981): The independence of closely spaced discrete experimental spike foci. *Neurology*, 31:846–851.

55. Lueders, H., Bustamante, L., Zablow, L., Krinsky, A. and Goldensohn, E. S. (1980): Quantitative studies of spike foci induced by minimal concentrations of penicillin. *Electroencephalogy Clin. Neurophysiol.*, 48:80–89.

56. Macdonald, R. L., and Barker, J. L. (1978): Specific antagonism of GABA-mediated postsynaptic inhibition in cultured mammalian spinal cord neurons: A common mode of convulsant action. *Neurology*, 28:325–330.

57. MacDonald, R. D., and Barker, J. L. (1978): Different actions of anticonvulsant and anesthetic barbiturates revealed by use of cultured mammalian neurons. *Science*, 200:775–777.

58. Matsumoto, H., Ayala, G. F., and Gumnit, R. J. (1969): Neuronal behavior and triggering in cortical epileptic focus. *J. Neurophysiol.*, 32:688–703.

59. Matsumoto, H. (1964): Intracellular events during the activation of cortical epileptiform discharges. *Electroencephalogy Clin. Neurophysiol.*, 17:294–307.

60. Matsumoto, H., and Ajmone-Marsan, C. (1964a): Cortical cellular phenomena in experimental epilepsy: Interictal manifestations. *Exp. Neurol.*, 9:286–304.

61. Matsumoto, H., and Ajmone-Marsan, C. (1964b): Cortical cellular phenomena in experimental epilepsy. Ictal manifestations. *Exp. Neurol.*, 9:305–326.

62. Meyer, H. and Prince, D. A. (1973): Convulsant actions of penicillin: Effects on inhibitory mechanisms. *Brain Res.*, 53:447–482.

63. Nicoll, R. A., Eccles, J. C., Oshima, T., and Rubia, F. (1975): Prolongation of hippocampal inhibitory postsynaptic potentials by barbiturates. *Nature (Lond.)*, 258:625–627.

64. Noebels, J. L., and Pedley, T. A. (1977): Anatomic localization of topically applied ^{14}C penicillin during experimental focal epilepsy in cat neocortex. *Brain Res.*, 125:293–303.

64a. Noebels, J. L., and Prince, D. A. (1977): Presynaptic origin of penicillin after-discharges at mammalian nerve terminals. *Brain Res.*, 138:59–74.

65. Noebels, J. L., and Prince, D. A. (1978): Development of focal seizures in cerebral cortex: Role of axon terminal bursting. *J. Neurophysiol.*, 41:1267–1281.

66. Okada, K., Ayala, G. F. and Sung, J. H. (1971): Ultrastructure of penicillin-induced epileptogenic lesion of the cerebral cortex in cat. *J. Neuropathol. Exp. Neurol.*, 30:337–353.

67. Paine, P. L., and Scherr, P. (1975): Drug coefficients for the movement of rigid spheres through liquid-filled cylindrical pores. *Biophys. J.*, 15:1087–1091.

68. Pape, L. G., and Katzman, R. (1972): Response of glia in cat sensorimotor cortex to increased extracellular potassium. *Brain Res.*, 38:71–92.

69. Prince, D. A. (1966): Modification of focal cortical epileptogenic discharge by afferent influences. *Epilepsia*, 7:181–201.

70. Prince, D. A. (1974): Neuronal correlates of epileptiform discharges and cortical DC potentials. In *Handbook of Electroencephalography and Clinical Neurophysiology*, edited by O. Creutzfeldt, pp. 56–76. Elsevier, Amsterdam.

71. Prince, D. A. (1968): The depolarization shift in 'epileptic' neurons. *Exp. Neurol.*, 21:467–485.

72. Prince, D. A. (1968): Inhibition in "epileptic" neurons. *Exp. Neurol.*, 21:307–332.

73. Prince, D. A. (1971): Topical convulsant drugs and metabolic antagonists. In *Experimental Models of Epilepsy*, edited by D. P. Purpura, J. K. Penry, D. Tower, D. M. Woodbury, and R. Walker, pp. 51–83. Raven Press, New York.

74. Prince, D. A. (1978): Neurophysiology of epilepsy. *Ann. Rev. Neurosci.*, 1:395–415.

75. Prince, D. A., and Connors, B. W. (1984): Mechanisms of epileptogenesis in cortical structures. *Ann. Neurol.* 16(suppl.):S59–S64.

76. Prince, D. A., and Wilder, B. J. (1967): Control mechanisms in cortical epileptogenic foci: 'Surround' inhibition. *Arch. Neurol.*, 16:194–202.

77. Purpura, D. P., Penry, J. K., Tower, D. B., Woodbury, D. M., and Walter, M. D. (eds.) (1971): *Experimental Models of Epilepsy—A Manual for the Laboratory Worker*, p. 615. Raven Press, New York.

78. Rains, A. and Dretchen, K. L. (1975): Neuroexcitatory and depressant effects of penicillin at the cat soleus neuromuscular junction. *Epilepsia*, 16:469–476.

79. Rall, D. P., Oppelt, W. W. and Patlak, C. S. (1962): Extracellular space of brain as determined by diffusion of insulin from the ventricular system. *Life. Sci.*, 2:43–48.

80. Rampton, D. S., and Ramsay, D. J. (1974): The effects of pentobarbitone anesthesia on the volume and composition of the extracellular fluid of dogs. *J. Physiol.*, 237–533.

81. Reichenthal, E., and Hocherman, S. (1979): A critical epileptic area in the cat's cortex and its

relation to the cortical columns. *Electroenceph. Clin. Neurophysiol.*, 47:147–152.

82. Salazar, A. M. (1980): Penicillin as an epileptogenic agent. Ph.D. thesis, State University of New York, Stony Brook, New York.

83. Sawa, M., Kaji, S., and Usuki, K. (1964): Intracellular phenomena in electrically induced seizures. *Electroencephalogy Clin. Neurophysiol.*, 19:248–255.

84. Schwartzkroin, P. A. (1975): Characteristics of CA1 neurons recorded intracellulary in the hippocampal *in vitro* slice preparation. *Brain Res.*, 85:423–436.

85. Schwartzkroin, P. A., and Pedley, T. A. (1979): Slow depolarizing potentials in "epileptic" neurons. *Epilepsia*, 20:267–277.

86. Schwartzkroin, P. A., and Prince, D. A. (1977): Penicillin-induced epileptiform activity in the hippocampal *in vitro* preparation. *Ann. Neurol.*, 1:463–469.

87. Schwartzkroin, P. A., and Prince, D. A. (1978): Cellular and field potential properties of epileptogenic hippocampal slices. *Brain Res.*, 147:117–130.

88. Schwartzkroin, P. A., and Slawsky, M. (1977): Probable calcium spikes in hippocampal neurons. *Brain. Res.*, 135:157–161.

89. Schwartzkroin P. A., and Wheal H. V. (1984): *Electrophysiology of Epilepsy*. Academic, London.

90. Schwartzkroin, P. A., and Wyler, A. R. (1980): Mechanisms underlying epileptiform burst discharge. *Ann. Neurol.*, 7:95–107.

91. Servit, Z., and Strejckova, A. (1970): An electrographic epileptic focus in the fish forebrain. Conditions and pathways of propagation of focal and paroxysmal activity. *Brain Res.*, 17:103–113.

92. Speckmann, E. J., Elger, C. E., and Lehmenkuehler, A. (1983): Penicillin activity in brain tissue: A method for continuous measurement. *Electroencephalogy Clin. Neurophysiol.*, 56:664–667.

93. Spencer, W. A., and Brookhart, J. M. (1961): A study of spontaneous spindle waves in sensorimotor cortex of the cat. *J. Neurophysiol.*, 24:50–66.

94. Spencer, W. A. and Kandel, E. R. (1969): Synaptic inhibition in seizures. In *Basic Mechanisms of the Epilepsies*, edited by H. H. Jasper, A. A. Ward, Jr., and A. Pope, pp. 575–603. Little, Brown, Boston.

95. Stark, L. G., Edmonds, H. L., and Holinger, M. A. (1974): The distribution of ^{14}C-penicillin in rat brain following the induction of an epileptogenic focus. *Proc. West. Pharm. Soc.*, 17:51–54.

96. Szentagothai, J. (1969): Architecture of the cerebral cortex. In *Basic Mechanisms of the Epilepsies*, edited by H. H. Jasper, A. A. Ward, Jr., and A. Pope, pp. 13–28. Little, Brown, Boston.

97. Van Duijn, H., Schwartzkroin, P. A., and Prince, D. A. (1976): Action of penicillin on inhibitory processes in the cat's cortex. *Brain Res.*, 53:470–476.

98. Walker, A. E., and Johnson, H. C. (1946): *Penicillin in Neurology*, p. 204. Charles C. Thomas, Springfield, Illinois.

99. Walker, A. E., Johnson, H. C. and Lollros, J. J. (1945): The convulsive effects of penicillin applied to the cerebral cortex of monkey and man. *Surg. Gynecol. Obstet.*, 81:692.

100. Walsh, G. O. (1971): Penicillin iontophresis in neocortex of cat: Effects on the spontaneous and induced activity of single neurons: *Epilepsia*, 12:1–11.

101. Watkins, J. C. (1976): A general view of possible causative factors in epilepsy and their investigation by means of pharmacological agents. In *Biochemistry and Neurology*, edited by H. F. Bradford and C. D. Marsden, pp. 253–259. Academic, London.

102. Williamson, T. L. and Crill, W. E. (1976): The effects of pentylenetetrazol on molluscan neurons. I. Intracellular recordings and stimulation. *Brain Res.*, 116:217–224.

103. Wilson, W. A., and Escueta, A. V. (1974): Common synaptic effects of pentylenetetrazol and penicillin. *Brain Res.*, 72:168–171.

104. Willmore, L. J., Fuller, P. M., Butler, A. B., and Bass, N. H. (1975): Neuronal compartmentation of ionic cobalt in rat cerebral cortex during initiation of epileptiform activity. *Exp. Neurol.*, 47:280–289.

105. Wong, R. K. S., and Prince, D. A. (1978): Participation of calcium spikes during intrinsic burst firing in hippocampal neurons. *Brain Res.*, 159:385–390.

106. Wong, R. K. S., and Prince, D. A. (1979): Dendritic mechanisms underlying penicillin-induced epileptiform activity. *Science*, 204:1228–1231.

107. Wong, R. K. S., and Prince, D. A. (1981): Afterpotential generation in hippocampal pyramidal cells. *J. Neurophysiol.*, 45:86–97.

108. Zipser, B., Crain, S. M., and Bornstein, M. B. (1973): Directly evoked paroxysmal depolarization of mouse hippocampal neurons in synaptically organized explants in long term culture. *Brain Res.*, 60:489–495.

Advances in Neurology, Vol. 44, edited by
A. V. Delgado-Escueta, A. A. Ward, Jr.,
D. M. Woodbury, and R. J. Porter.
Raven Press, New York © 1986.

29

Cellular Basis of Neuronal Synchrony in Epilepsy

*Robert K. S. Wong, **,†Roger D. Traub, and *Richard Miles

*Department of Physiology and Biophysics, University of Texas Medical Branch, Galveston, Texas 77550;
**IBM T. J. Watson Research Center, Yorktown Heights, New York 10598; and †Neurological Institute,
New York, New York 10032

SUMMARY Synchronized discharge of populations of cortical neurons are often observed to underly both the interictal spikes and tonic seizures generated in experimental epilepsy studies. Recently it has been shown that similar synchronized discharges occur in cortical brain slices treated with convulsants such as penicillin, picrotoxin, or bicuculline. The favorable experimental conditions offered by the *in vitro* preparation have facilitated a detailed examination on the cellular basis for the generation of the epileptic neuronal synchrony. In this chapter we shall review some experimental observations on the neuronal synchronization and describe a mechanism for its generation based on the computer simulation approach. Three factors are considered to be essential for epileptic synchronization observation *in vitro*. First, cortical neurons may intrinsically generate bursts of action potentials. Second, recurrent excitatory connections exist that are sufficiently powerful that bursting activity may spread between synaptically connected neurons. Third, inhibition within the local neuronal circuit must be adequately attenuated to allow excitation to spread through the recurrent excitatory connections. Computer simulation studies have been based on these assumptions, using neuronal networks where each cell is connected to more than one postsynaptic neuron. Bursting initiated in one cell excites all its follower cells, and the sequential recruitment of an increasing number of cells eventually leads to a simultaneous discharge of the population.

A number of recent experimental observations lend credence to the proposed scheme for neuronal synchrony. Simultaneous paired intracellular recordings provided direct evidence that a burst of action potentials in a presynaptic cell can activate action potentials postsynaptically. Furthermore, it is shown that the rhythm of spontaneous discharge in a neuronal population can be influenced by the activity of one neuron within the population.

At least two important types of epileptiform events, interictal spikes and tonic seizures with 10- to 20-Hz electrocorticograph (ECoG) waves, consist of the synchronized neuronal bursting of a population of cortical nerve cells (5). Experimentally, the electroencephalogram (EEG) or ECoG paroxysmal waves defining the epileptiform event are observed to occur simultaneously with a depolarization and/or an increase in firing rate in at least some neurons in the cortical region where the paroxysmal waves are of maximum amplitude. These experimental data have been obtained from both the hippocampus (8) and neocortex during focal penicillin-induced and electrically induced seizure events (16,17, 21,22) and also during generalized penicillin epilepsy (10). A similar type of simultaneity seems likely to occur during human interictal discharges (37). These observations suggest that synchronized neuronal bursting is the common factor underlying many clinically described forms of epilepsy. Clearly, knowledge of the cellular mechanisms underlying synchrony is crucial to our understanding of epilepsy in general.

Analogues of both interictal spikes and seizures can be produced in hippocampal slices treated with convulsant agents (19,23,24,36) and indeed in microdissected segments of the CA3 region of the slice containing as few as about 1,000 cells (19) (Fig. 1). The small size of the neuronal population generating this behavior has permitted detailed investigations of the cellular mechanisms underlying synchronized neuronal activity. These studies have involved both experimental electrophysiology and computer simulations. Using results derived *in vitro,* we can now simulate in detail both single synchronized bursts (the analogue of interictal spikes) and synchronized afterdischarges (the analogue of tonic seizure).

Before proceeding, we must comment on how we define synchronization. Electrical events within the slice can be synchronized on different time scales. Since a burst in a hippocampal neuron lasts about 50 to 100 msec, bursting can be "synchronized" if bursts in different neurons occur within tens of milliseconds of one another. It is this kind of synchrony that will be considered here. Synchronization of action potentials within such an event can also occur, probably being mediated in part by electrical interactions (27). We shall not discuss these interactions here.

The critical components of epileptic synchronization observed *in vitro* in the presence of convulsant agents are the following:

1. Pyramidal cells can generate intrinsic bursts. These bursts occur spontaneously in the CA2–CA3 region, which is the pacemaker region for synchronized activity.

2. Convulsant agents, such as penicillin and picrotoxin, act by blocking synaptic inhibition.

3. Local chemical excitatory connections exist between pyramidal cells in the CA2–CA3 region. Large excitatory synaptic conductance

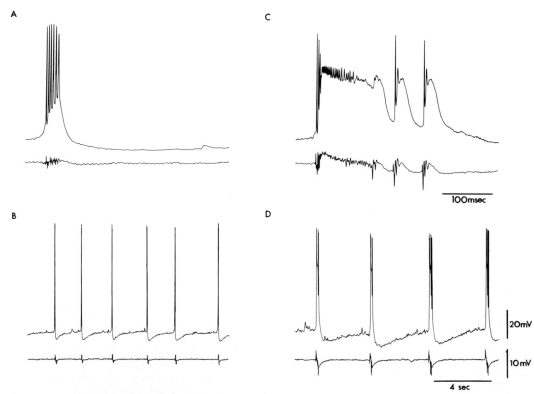

FIG. 1.   Spontaneous interictal **(A, B)** and ictal **(C, D)** activity recorded from isolated CA3 segments prepared from a hippocampal slice (19). Upper trace of each record is obtained by intracellular recording, lower trace record is the extracellular population activity. Time calibrations are the same for **A** and **C**, and for **B** and **D**.

changes occur in pyramidal cells during synchronized bursts. Blockade of chemical synapses prevents the occurrence of synchronized bursts.

These experimental observations are sufficient to account for the initiation of interictal discharges. Furthermore, the additional assumption that neurons become refractory after high-frequency activation allows synchronized after-discharges to be explained. We shall now illustrate and amplify these major points.

INTRINSIC BURSTING

Hippocampal pyramidal cells have the property that a brief (2 msec) excitatory stimulus can evoke a neuronal response lasting 30 to 50 msec (Fig. 2). This response, called a burst, consists of a series of three or more action potentials, riding on a depolarizing wave. Experiments carried out using the hippocampal slice preparation suggest that these bursts are "intrinsic" in the sense that they can be generated by membrane conductances in individual cells, without participation of any other neurons (33). A direct demonstration of the intrinsic bursting capability has been possible using isolated pyramidal cells enzymatically dissociated from the hippocampus of adult guinea pigs. Here we observe that burst firing can be triggered by short pulse depolarizations (Fig. 3) and can occur spontaneously. Data from the slice also show that both somatic and dendritic regions of an individual CA3 pyramidal cell can function as independent sites for burst firing (34). A computer model describing this firing behavior of CA3 neurons has been proposed (28). The generation of action potentials

in CA1 neurons is even more interesting in that the dendrites and somata of individual neurons can exhibit differential firing patterns (35). Thus the apical dendrites of CA1 neurons have intrinsic bursting capabilities, whereas depolarizing current delivered to the soma of CA1 pyramidal cells usually evokes only repetitive firing that does not outlast the stimulus.

ACTION OF CONVULSANT AGENTS

There is considerable evidence that the inhibitory transmitter in the hippocampus is gamma-aminobutyric acid (GABA). The epileptiform events which we have studied occur in the presence of the convulsant agents penicillin, bicuculline, and picrotoxin. A common action of these agents is that they antagonize the postsynaptic action of GABA (7,9,32). When GABA actions are blocked, epileptiform activity appears in all pyramidal cell regions of the hippocampus. It has been demonstrated that synchronized bursts originate in the CA2–CA3 region and propagate to the CA1 region (19,24,36). This has been shown by cutting the connection from CA2–CA3 to CA1, and by cutting segments of CA2 or CA3 regions which themselves can generate synchronized bursts. The CA1 region, when isolated, shows a much higher threshold for the generation of these spontaneous synchronized bursts and usually does not show any activity at all (but see ref. 12).

The most important action of convulsants in inducing epileptiform action appears to be in blocking inhibition so that intrinsic bursts, generated by pyramidal cells, can be recruited by excitatory synaptic input from other pyramidal cells (32). In the absence of convulsant agents,

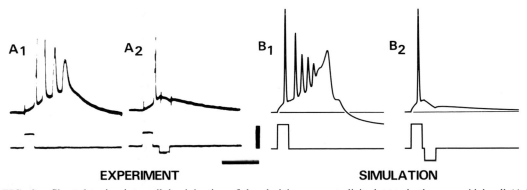

EXPERIMENT　　　　　　　　　　　　**SIMULATION**

FIG. 2. Short duration intracellular injection of depolarizing current elicits bursts in the pyramidal cell (A_1) and in the simulated pyramidal cell (B_1). A hyperpolarizing pulse applied subsequently abolished the burst and revealed the underlying depolarizing afterpotential in both cases (A_2, B_2). **Top traces:** intracellular record. **Bottom traces:** intracellularly injected current; depolarizing current is up. Horizontal calibration, 30 msec; vertical calibration, 15 mV.

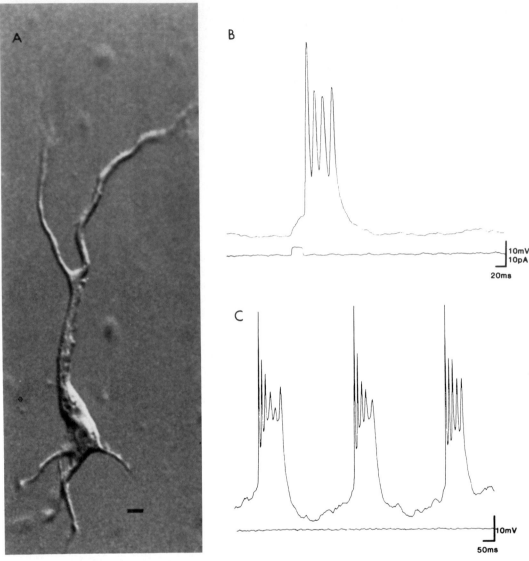

FIG. 3. **A:** A pyramidal-type neuron obtained from the hippocampus of adult guinea pig using an enzymatic-mechanical dissociation procedure. Calibration is 10 μm. **B, C:** Intracellular records obtained from this type of cell with the single suction pipette technique. **B:** Burst triggered by short duration depolarizing pulse. **C:** Spontaneous pacemaker bursting behavior. (From R. Numann and R. K. S. Wong, *unpublished*.)

activation of pyramidal cells by an afferent volley also elicits feedback (4) or feedforward (2) inhibition which acts to suppress burst firing (32).

EXCITATORY CHEMICAL CONNECTIONS BETWEEN NEURONS IN THE CA2–CA3 REGION

The existence of local excitatory connections is essential for the generation of spontaneous synchronized bursting in the CA2–CA3 region.

The properties of these connections have been examined by simultaneous intracellular recordings from pairs of cells in the CA3 region (15,18). We have now demonstrated monosynaptic connections between neurons in the CA2–CA3 region (Fig. 4) that have the important property that a burst elicited in the presynaptic neuron can elicit a burst in the follower cell. These connections, although powerful, occur only rarely. The data of MacVicar and Dudek (15) also showed that, even including polysynaptic connections, excitatory interactions occurred in

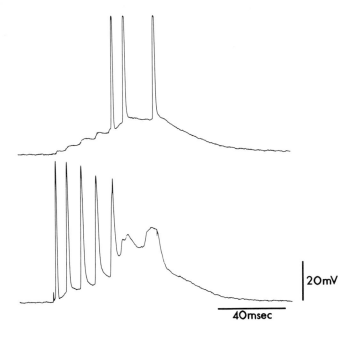

FIG. 4. Intracellular records from two monosynaptically connected CA3 neurons. **Top trace:** postsynaptic cell. **Bottom trace:** presynaptic cell. Each action potential of the presynaptic cell burst elicited an excitatory postsynaptic potential in the postsynaptic cell, which eventually reached threshold and fired a burst of action potentials.

20mV

40msec

only five of 88 paired recordings. We have now used computer simulations to show that a low density of synaptic connections is sufficient to explain the experimental data on synchronization.

Several experimental results suggest that chemical excitatory synapses are important for epileptiform synchronization. In the presence of low Ca^{2+} and high Mg^{2+}, synchronized discharge is suppressed. Blockade of chemical synapses by the excitatory amino acid antagonist γ-D-glutamyl glycine also completely suppresses synchronized activity and at lower concentrations causes afterdischarges to disappear one by one, resulting in the occurrence of a single synchronized burst (19). Furthermore, by hyperpolarizing neurons during an interictal discharge, a synaptically induced depolarization may be revealed. Johnston and Brown (14) have voltage-clamped individual pyramidal cells during synchronized bursts to demonstrate a reversal potential for this depolarization underlying the burst and thus show that it is a chemical postsynaptic excitatory event. Our studies show that the synaptic input arises from recurrent excitatory synapses between CA3 cells (18,30,31).

MODEL OF EPILEPTIFORM SYNCHRONIZED BURSTING

Computer simulations based on experimental data show that the intrinsic bursting capability

of pyramidal cells and the recurrent connections between them will function to generate a synchronized discharge when inhibition is blocked by convulsants. The computer model accounts for a number of other observations on the synchronized bursts that had previously been puzzling: (a) the long and variable latency (50–150 ms) from a localized stimulus to the occurrence of a synchronized population burst, (b) the appearance of double bursts, and (c) the "all-or-none" properties of the evoked synchronized bursts and their long refractory period (Fig. 5).

Our model consists of a population of neurons (100–400) as described previously (28), each able to generate intrinsic bursts. These neurons are interconnected randomly with a sparse network of excitatory synapses. There are two critical assumptions: First, each cell is connected, on the average, to more than one follower cell, so that *growth* of a population response can occur; second, the synaptic connections are sufficiently strong that a burst in a given neuron can evoke bursting in its follower neurons and *propagation* of activity through the system can occur (Fig. 5). In this way, a localized stimulus (to four cells in Fig. 5) can rapidly grow into a population response. During the initial period of recruitment, the number of neurons involved is small, and in experiments the extracellular population recording is expected to be below noise level. This factor can explain the long latency of evoked synchronized bursts. Also, double bursts occur due to closed loops in the neuronal

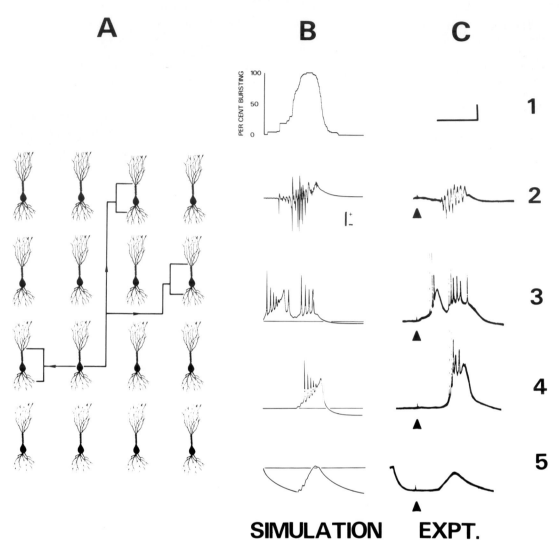

FIG. 5. Simulation of epileptiform synchronized bursting in a network of hippocampal neurons. **A:** Schematics of the neuronal network. For clarity, a 4 × 4 array is shown, although a 10 × 10 array is used in the simulation. Every cell sends an output to an average of five other cells (only three connections are shown). There are no inhibitory synaptic connections. **B:** Simulated interictal spike, obtained with steady depolarizing current of 1.5 nA to four cells in the population. B1, percent of total cells in the network bursting. B2, field potential. B3, simulated soma membrane potential of cell receiving stimulus (an initiating cell). Note double burst caused by the reflected EPSP resulting from activities in the follower cells. B4, membrane potential of another more typical cell. B5, membrane potential of the same cell as in B4, with injection of 1.5 nA hyperpolarizing current revealing the underlying EPSP. **C:** Experimental interictal spikes recorded from the hippocampal slice. C2, field potential. C3 to C5, intracellular recording from CA2 neurons during interictal spike. Cell in C5 is hyperpolarized by an injected current. Calibration: 50 msec in **B** and 60 msec in **C**; 25 mV for intracellular records in **A**, 4 mV in B2, and 20 mV in B3 to B5. (Parts **B** and **C** from ref. 30, with permission.)

network. Thus, a cell whose initial burst is early can be restimulated by the excitatory projections from neurons activated during the major population response.

In accordance with the experimental data, the population event is in part terminated by a Ca^{2+}-mediated K^+ conductance in individual cells (1,13). Recent studies have shown that this con-

ductance may not be the only one involved in terminating the synchronized bursts (11,25). Another K^+ conductance of slow kinetics and long duration must also be involved (3). The data obtained by Newberry and Nicoll (20) further suggest a possible involvement of a second type of GABA action which is insensitive to convulsants.

The model makes the important prediction that stimulation of a single neuron within the synchronized population may influence the spontaneous rhythm of the population event. As shown in Fig. 6 this prediction has since been confirmed (18). The data show that intracellular depolarizing currents injected into one cell to produce burst firing can entrain the rhythm of the spontaneous synchronized bursts. The timing of this stimulus is important for its influence on the population rhythm, since there is a refractory period of the neuronal population, which appears to outlast that of individual cells, following a synchronized discharge (18,30,36).

AFTERDISCHARGES

The basic model described above can account also for the occurrence of picrotoxin induced afterdischarges in the hippocampal slice. Afterdischarges may also be generated in segments of the hippocampus containing about 1,000 cells and involve the repeated activation of all members of the neuronal population. In other words, afterdischarges do not arise from activity reverberating between two neuronal populations (19). In attempts to simulate afterdischarge in our modeling studies, we discovered that a stronger refractory period of the simulated neu-

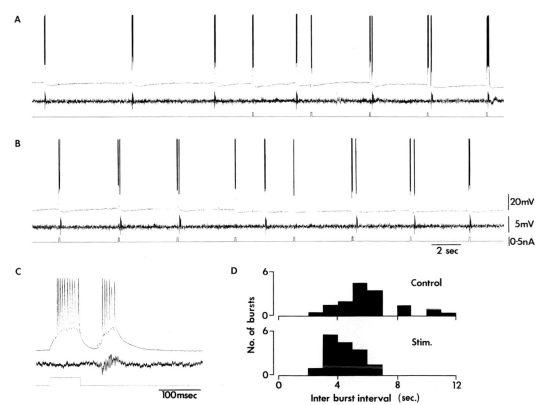

FIG. 6. Repetitive intracellular stimulation of a single neurone in a CA3 segment partially entrains synchronized population activity. To test for entrainment, the mean control interval between population bursts, in this case 6.23 ± 2.20 sec (mean ± SD, n = 36), was established. Repetitive intracellular stimulation was then applied with intensity sufficient to elicit a burst of action potentials and with interval shorter than control, here once every 4 sec. **A:** Intracellular stimulation began approximately halfway through the record. Although the first two stimuli had no effect on the population, synchronized population bursts at higher frequency than before stimulation closely followed the intracellular bursts elicted by the next three stimuli shown. **B:** Cellular activation was followed closely by a population burst on six out of eight occasions showing that entrainment was not complete. **C:** Current injection elicited a burst of action potentials with no field potential correlate followed, with a latency of 90 msec, by a synchronized population burst reflected in both intracellular and field potential records. During this period of repetitive intracellular stimulation 22 of 36 population bursts followed a stimulus with latency of less than 200 msec. If stimulation has no effect on the population rhythm, two population bursts would have been expected to occur with this latency. **D:** Distribution of intervals between population bursts preceding (control) and during (stimulus) repetitive stimulation. The mean control interval was 6.23 ± 2.20 sec (mean ± SD, n = 36). During stimulation once every 4 sec, the mean interval was 4.35 ± 1.10 sec (n = 36), significantly (p < 0.01) lower than control. (From ref. 18, with permission.)

rons was needed than in simulations of interictal discharges. Thus neurons will burst until refractoriness sets in and then may no longer be excited regardless of the afferent input. The consequence of the refractoriness is as follows: neurons that become active during the beginning of the synchronized event also stop firing before the synchronized population discharge terminates. Thus, although there is overall synchrony of bursting on a time scale of tens of milliseconds, subtle phase differences are introduced and, importantly, some cells "shut off" before

others. This phenomenon allows recovery of these "early" neurons before the activity in the synchronized burst ends. They are then reexcited and in turn excite the follower neurons to reinitiate a second population discharge resulting in several afterdischarges (29) (Fig. 7). The mechanism thus represents a form of reentry; however, the sequence of cell recruitment during each afterdischarge need not be stereotypically repeated.

Thus the essential conditions in our hypothesis for afterdischarge generation are the same

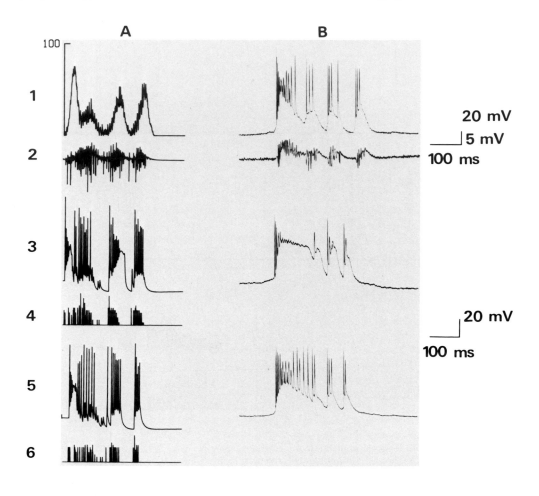

SIMULATION   EXPERIMENT

FIG. 7.   A: Synchronized afterdischarges in a model that includes axonal refractoriness. There are 100 cells, an average of 2.5 inputs/cell, synaptic delays are randomly scattered between 3.5 and 5.5 msec, and synaptic strength is 0.3 µS. The stimulus was an intracellulary injected current of 2.5 nA for 100 msec into four cells (not shown), starting at time 0. A1, the number of cells with soma membrane potential ≥20 mV relative to resting potential. A2, estimated field potential (positive up). A3, A5, intracellular soma membrane potentials of two cells. A4, A6, their respective synaptic inputs. The cell of A3 receives input from four other cells, while the cell of A5 receives input from two other cells. Note the rhythmical oscillations with period about 75 msec. Synchronization is relative rather than absolute. B: Top traces, intracellular (B1) and extracellular (B2) recordings during afterdischarges. B3, B5, comparison of the intracellular events in two neurons recorded simultaneously during afterdischarge.

as those required for single synchronized bursts: (a) intrinsic bursting capability, (b) disinhibition, and (c) mutual excitation. We expect that the cellular mechanism we propose for epileptiform events in the hippocampus is also relevant to the neocortex. We are aware that the intrinsic bursting capability of neocortical cells is more limited than that for hippocampus (6,26). Nevertheless it is possible that weak intrinsic bursting capability may be compensated, in epileptic foci, by a sufficiently dense or powerful excitatory network to allow for obligatory signal transmission between neocortical neurons.

In summary, we can say that the hippocampal slice model continues to expand our understanding of the basic mechanisms of epilepsy. It is possible to study the relevant properties of individual neurons and, with the success of the dissociated neuron preparation, even individual ionic channels in hippocampal neurons. At the same time, the limited size of the slice may allow an eventual quantitative description of the collective neuronal behavior underlying epilepsy.

ACKNOWLEDGMENTS

Supported in part by Department of Health and Human Services grant NS 18464 and a Klingenstein Fellowship Award. We wish to thank Dr. W. D. Knowles, Dr. P. E. Seiden, and Dr. L. Schulman for helpful discussions.

REFERENCES

1. Alger, B. E., and Nicoll, R. A. (1980): Epileptiform burst after hyperpolarization: Calcium-dependent potassium potential in hippocampal CA1 pyramidal cells. *Science,* 210:1122–1124.
2. Alger, B. E., and Nicoll, R. A. (1982): Feedforward dendritic inhibition in rat hippocampal pyramidal cells studied in vitro. *J. Physiol.,* 328:105–123.
3. Alger, B. E. (1984): Characteristics of a slow hyperpolarizing synaptic potential in rat hippocampal pyramidal cell. *J. Neurophysiol.,* 52:892–910.
4. Andersen, P., Eccles, J. C., and Loyning, Y. (1964): Pathway of postsynaptic inhibition in the hippocampus. *J. Neurophysiol.,* 27:608–619.
5. Brenner, R. P., and Atkinson, R. (1982): Generalized paroxysmal fast activity: electroencephalographic and clinical features. *Ann. Neurol.,* 11:386–390.
6. Connors, B. W., Gutnick, M. J., and Prince, D. A. (1982): Electrophysiological properties of neocortical neurons in vitro. *J. Neurophysiol.,* 48:1302–1320.
7. Curtis, D. R., Game, C. J. A., Johnston, G. A. R., McCulloch, R. M., and MacLachlan, R. M. (1972): Convulsive action of penicillin. *Brain Res.,* 43:242–245.
8. Dichter, M., and Spencer, W. A. (1969): Penicillin-induced interictal discharges from the cat hippocampus. II. Mechanisms underlying origin and restriction. *J. Physiol.,* 305:297–313.
9. Dingledine, R., and Gjerstad, L. (1980): Reduced inhibition during epileptiform activity in the *in vitro* hippocampal slice. *J. Physiol.,* 305:297–313.
10. Fisher, R. S., and Prince, D. A. (1977): Spikewave rhythms in cat cortex induced by parenteral penicillin. I. Electroencephalographic features. *Electroencephalogy Clin. Neurophysiol.,* 42:608–624.
11. Hablitz, J. J. (1981): Effects of intracellular injections of chloride and EGTA on postepileptiform burst hyperpolarizations in hippocampal neurons. *Neurosci. Lett.,* 22:159–163.
12. Hablitz, J. J. (1983): Mechanisms underlying picrotoxin-induced epileptiform activity in the hippocampus. *Neurosci. Abstr.,* 9:397.
13. Hotson, J. R., and Prince, D. A. (1980): A calcium-activated hyperpolarization follows repetitive firing in hippocampal neurons. *J. Neurophysiol.,* 43:409–419.
14. Johnston, D., and Brown, T. H. (1981): Giant synaptic potential hypothesis for epileptiform activity. *Science,* 211:294–297.
15. MacVicar, B. A., and Dudek, F. E. (1980): Local synaptic circuits in rat hippocampus: Interactions between pyramidal cells. *Brain Res.,* 184:220–223.
16. Matsumoto, H., and Ajmone Marsan, C. (1964): Cortical cellular phenomena in experimental epilepsy: Interictal manifestations. *Exp. Neurol.,* 9:286–304.
17. Matsumoto, H., and Ajmone Marsan, C. (1964): Cortical cellular phenomena in experimental epilepsy: Ictal manifestations. *Exp. Neuron.,* 9:305–326.
18. Miles, R., and Wong, R. K. S. (1983): Single neurones can initiate synchronized population discharge in the hippocampus. *Nature (Lond.),* 306:371–373.
19. Miles, R., Wong, R. K. S., and Traub, R. D. (1984): Synchronized afterdischarges in the hippocampus: Contribution of local synaptic interaction. *Neuroscience,* 12:1179–1189.
20. Newberry, N. R., and Nicoll, R. A. (1984): Baclofen directly hyperpolarizes hippocampal pyramidal cells. *Nature (Lond.),* 308:450–452.
21. Prince, D. A. (1968): The depolarization shift in "epileptic" neurons. *Exp. Neurol.,* 21:467–485.
22. Sawa, M., Nakamura, K., and Naito, H. (1968): Intracellular phenomena and spread of epileptic seizure discharges. *Electroencephalogy Clin. Neurophysiol.,* 24:146–154.
23. Schwartzkroin, P. A., and Prince, D. A. (1977): Penicillin-induced epileptiform activity in the hippocampal *in vitro* preparation. *Ann. Neurol.,* 1:463–469.
24. Schwartzkroin, P. A., and Prince, D. A. (1978): Cellular and field potential properties of epileptogenic hippocampal slices. *Brain Res.,* 147:117–130.
25. Schwartzkroin, P. A., and Stafstrom, C. E. (1980):

Effects of EGTA on the calcium-activated after-hyperpolarization in hippocampal CA3 cells. *Science*, 210:1125–1126.

26. Stafstrom, C. E., Schwindt, P. C., and Crill, W. E. (1982): Negative slope conductance due to a persistent subthreshold sodium current in cat neocortical neurons *in vitro*. *Brain Res.*, 236:221–226.

27. Taylor, C. P., and Dudek, F. E. (1982): Synchronous neural afterdischarges in rat hippocampal slices during blockade of chemical synapses. *Science*, 218:810–812.

28. Traub, R. D. (1982): Simulation of intrinsic bursting in CA3 hippocampal neurons. *Neuroscience*, 7:1233–1242.

29. Traub, R. D., Knowles, W. D., Miles, R., and Wong, R. K. S. (1984): Synchronized afterdischarges in the hippocampus: Simulation studies of the cellular mechanism. *Neuroscience*, 12:1191–1200.

30. Traub, R. D., and Wong, R. K. S. (1982): Cellular mechanism of neuronal synchronization in epilepsy. *Science*, 216:745–747.

31. Traub, R. D., and Wong, R. K. S. (1983): Synchronized burst discharge in disinhibited hippo-

campal slice. II. Model of cellular mechanism. *J. Neurophysiol.*, 49:442–458.

32. Wong, R. K. S., and Prince, D. A. (1979): Dendritic mechanisms underlying penicillin-induced epileptiform activity. *Science*, 204:1228–1231.

33. Wong, R. K. S., and Prince, D. A. (1981): Afterpotential generation in hippocampal pyramidal cells. *J. Neurophysiol.*, 45:86–97.

34. Wong, R. K. S., Prince, D. A., and Basbaum, A. I. (1979): Intradendritic recordings from hippocampal neurons. *Proc. Natl. Acad. Sci. U.S.A.*, 76:986–990.

35. Wong, R. K. S., and Traub, R. D. (1982): The dendrites and somata of hippocampal pyramidal cells generate different action potential patterns. *Neurosci. Abstr.*, 8:412.

36. Wong, R. K. S., and Traub, R. D. (1983): Synchronized burst discharge in the disinhibited hippocampal slice. I. Initiation in the CA2–CA3 region. *J. Neurophysiol.*, 49:459–471.

37. Wyler, A. R., Ojemann, G. A., and Ward, A. A., Jr. (1982): Neurons in human epileptic cortex: Correlation between unit and EEG activity. *Ann. Neurol.*, 11:301–308.

Advances in Neurology, Vol. 44, edited by
A. V. Delgado-Escueta, A. A. Ward, Jr.,
D. M. Woodbury, and R. J. Porter.
Raven Press, New York © 1986.

30

Role of Electrical Interactions in Synchronization of Epileptiform Bursts

*F. Edward Dudek, *Robert W. Snow, and **Charles P. Taylor

*Department of Physiology, Tulane University School of Medicine, New Orleans, Louisiana 70112; and
**Department of Pharmacology, Warner-Lambert/Parke-Davis Research, Ann Arbor, Michigan 48105

SUMMARY   Four general mechanisms can hypothetically contribute to or mediate localized synchronization of neuronal activity: (a) recurrent excitatory chemical synapses, (b) electrotonic coupling via gap junctions, (c) electrical field effects (ephaptic interactions), and (d) changes in the concentration of extracellular ions (e.g., K^+). It has generally been believed that synchronization of epileptiform bursts derives primarily, if not exclusively, from recurrent excitatory chemical synapses. Dual intracellular recordings from the CA3 area of the hippocampus have been used to demonstrate the existence of recurrent synaptic excitation, and computer simulations have provided a theoretical framework for the idea that relatively sparse interactions through recurrent excitatory chemical synapses can generate synchronized bursting after inhibitory pathways are blocked with convulsant agents. Additional experimental studies have supported the hypothesis that a model for seizure discharge, the penicillin-induced paroxysmal depolarization shift (PDS), is associated with a large increase in excitatory synaptic conductance. However, recent studies have suggested that electrical interactions are also likely to play an important role in spike synchronization during epileptic discharges.
      Several research groups have used in vitro preparations to show that afterdischarges and spontaneous bursts of population spikes (which represent synchronized action potentials) can occur after chemical synaptic transmission has been blocked in solutions containing low $[Ca^{2+}]$. Although this result was first observed in the CA1 area, it has recently been confirmed in other regions of the hippocampus. These experiments indicate that mechanisms other than chemical synaptic transmission are capable of synchronizing action potentials in the hippocampus. In this chapter, two forms of electrical interaction that could mediate synchronization will be considered: (a) electrotonic coupling through gap junctions and (b) electrical field effects through extracellular space. Changes in the concentration of extracellular ions are another mechanism not involving chemical synapses. However, it seems unlikely that ionic changes act on the rapid time scale of electrical interactions, and their contribution is discussed elsewhere in this volume. We review evidence for the existence of electrotonic coupling and electrical field effects in the hippocampus and neocortex, and discuss their possible involvement in the synchronization of epileptiform events.
      Although electrotonic junctions have been observed in many mammalian tissues and have been studied extensively in the nervous systems of nonmammalian preparations, the presence and possible significance of electrotonic coupling via gap junctions between mammalian cortical neurons have largely been ignored until recently. Several lines of evidence now support the hypothesis that electrotonic coupling does exist between some neurons in hippocampus and neocortex.

1. Intracellular injection of the fluorescent dye Lucifer yellow (MW 457) into a single neuron frequently caused small groups of neurons to be stained.

2. In a small percentage of intracellular recordings, antidromic stimulation revealed collision-resistant, short-latency depolarizations suggestive of weak electrotonic coupling.

3. In a small fraction of simultaneous dual intracellular recordings from the CA3 area of the hippocampus, intracellular current injection provided evidence for weak electrotonic coupling. There is also the possibility of strong coupling between some pairs of cells.

4. Freeze-fracture and thin-section electron microscopy have shown gap junctions between neocortical neurons and in the hippocampus between pyramidal cells and among granule cells. However, gap junctions between neurons in these structures are rare.

Taken together, these data strongly support the hypothesis that electrotonic coupling exists in the hippocampus and neocortex. All of the studies indicate that relatively few electrotonic junctions exist and coupled cells are only connected to, at most, a few nearby neurons. The possible contribution of such limited electrotonic synapses to synchronization is discussed. Finally, we discuss the idea that the strength or number of electrotonic junctions could be enhanced under certain pathophysiological conditions.

Electrical field effects occur when the electrical current produced by neural activity changes the excitability of other unconnected neurons. Field effects (ephaptic interactions) were once considered a prime candidate for the mechanism of synchronization and spread of epileptiform events. However, the physiological research of the last two decades has largely ignored the possibility of such interactions in the mammalian brain. Recent data using differential recording (intracellular minus extracellular) of transmembrane potential in hippocampal neurons have provided evidence for excitatory electrical field effects during large population spikes. These depolarizing events had a waveform similar to population spikes and were too fast to be electrotonic or chemical synaptic potentials. Field effect depolarizations were recorded in nearly every hippocampal neuron whenever population spikes occurred: after antidromic or orthodromic activation either *in vitro* or *in vivo,* during synchronous bursts in the CA1 area with chemical transmission blocked by low-$[Ca^{2+}]$ solutions, and finally during PDSs in picrotoxin-treated hippocampal slices. These experiments provide strong evidence that electrical field effects contribute to synchronization of hippocampal neurons during seizures. However, the number of neurons that must fire synchronously in order for an electrical field to have a significant effect on nearby inactive neurons has yet to be determined. It is also unknown whether similar electrical field effects occur in the neocortex. Conditions that might modify the strength of electrical field effects are discussed.

Recently, computer simulations of an array of hypothetical CA1 hippocampal neurons, which were not connected by chemical synapses, have duplicated the experimental results on synchronization via electrical interactions. In the model system, electrical field effects alone could recruit and synchronize neighboring hyperexcitable neurons. Restricted, weak electrotonic coupling could enhance synchronization in the model. Further computer simulations should give a quantitative theoretical basis for evaluating how electrotonic coupling and electrical field effects synchronize neurons.

The relative contribution of electrical field effects and electrotonic coupling to the synchronization of epileptiform bursts is unknown. Ultimately the quantitative contribution of each hypothetical mechanism of seizure synchronization should be specified with particular reference to the time course of each type of interaction. This is important because factors that enhance or depress these synchronizing effects may modulate the ability of neuronal populations to participate in seizures. Perhaps such factors could be exploited in the future to help control seizures.

HISTORICAL INTRODUCTION

In the 15 years since the publication of the first edition of *Basic Mechanisms of the Epilepsies,* a large body of research has been aimed at the causes of hyperexcitability and burst discharges. It is generally accepted that bursts of action potentials superimposed on a paroxysmal depolarization shift (PDS) in almost all of the neurons generate the interictal spike, which is usually considered the simplest epileptiform event. Much less effort has been expended on the mechanisms for synchronization of epileptiform events. The large field potentials recorded during seizures result from synchronization of neuronal activity. At the outset, we must distinguish between projected and localized synchronization; if a region of the central nervous system discharges synchronously, excitatory projections to other regions would be expected to recruit synchronous firing in the area receiving the excitatory synapses. Although such projected synchronization is presumably of importance in epilepsy, we will only discuss mechanisms of *localized* synchronization. We will primarily consider electrotonic junctions and electrical field effects.

Excitatory Recurrent Chemical Synapses

Recurrent excitation is likely to mediate synchronization with a delay between individual neurons ranging from a millisecond to tens of milliseconds. The general conclusion of Jasper (41) and Purpura (84) in the original edition of this volume was that chemical synaptic transmission is probably the primary mechanism of synchronization of interictal and ictal events. Probably the most influential paper to elaborate this view was by Ayala and co-workers (5). Following on the work of Dichter and Spencer (18,19), these authors emphasized the possible importance of recurrent chemical synapses in triggering and synchronizing the PDS. A large body of subsequent research has essentially accepted a chemical synaptic mechanism of synchronization and has focused on the issue of whether the inward current of the PDS is the result of giant synaptic conductances or of intrinsic voltage-dependent conductance changes (45–47). Dual intracellular recordings have shown that a small percentage of pyramidal cell pairs in the CA3 area of the hippocampus are interconnected, either directly or through inter-

neurons, by local recurrent excitatory chemical pathways (70,78). These data and the recently obtained knowledge of the electrical properties of hippocampal neurons have been combined and elaborated into computer simulations that strongly support the possibility that chemical synapses synchronize the slow depolarizations associated with the PDS (119).

Electrical Interactions

Our position in this chapter is *not* that chemical recurrent excitatory synapses and changes in the concentration of the extracellular ions are unimportant; instead, we wish to elaborate the evidence for electrical interactions between mammalian cortical neurons, and we propose that they may also be important in synchronization and spread of seizures. We must emphasize the differences between the two mechanisms of electrical interaction. (a) Specific channels in gap junctions connecting some adjacent cells are thought to mediate electrotonic coupling. (b) Electrical field effects (ephaptic interactions) involve current flow through extracellular space independent of specialized structural connections. The problem of electrical and chemical mediation of neuronal communication is one of the oldest issues in neurobiology, and it has always involved controversy. It is difficult to review this field with any degree of justice to the many investigators that have contributed. We have selected references and data that we feel are particularly relevant to our recent experimental results.

Electrotonic Coupling

During the 1950s and 1960s, it became clear that some neurons were electrotonically coupled through specialized membrane structures (gap junctions). Furshpan and Potter (26) showed rectifying electrotonic coupling to be the basis for transmission at the giant motor synapse in the crayfish. Bennett and colleagues (9–11) subsequently provided electrophysiological and ultrastructural evidence for electrotonic coupling through gap junctions in spinal and medullary neurons of fish. Subsequent electron microscopic and electrophysiological studies in rat mesencephalic nucleus (6), rat lateral vestibular nucleus (61), and cat inferior olive (66,67,103) have provided data supporting the hypothesis of electrotonic transmission through gap junctions in certain subcortical areas of the mammalian brain. Early work on coupling in the vertebrate nervous system has been summarized (7,8,59, 102). Reviews on the general characteristics of intercellular communication through gap junctions are also available (e.g., 68,82).

Electrical Field Effects

There were numerous early studies suggesting the presence of electrical field effects, but probably the most important were the papers of Jasper and Monnier (42) and Arvanitaki (4). In the former work, two crustacean nerve fibers were placed in contact and it was shown that electrical transmission could occur at this "artificial synapse" (42). Similarly, Arvanitaki (4) showed that under certain conditions, transmission could occur from one squid axon to another; in this paper the term "ephapse" was proposed for the site of close apposition of two neuronal membranes. Other studies have incorporated similar artificial models, where two separate nerves are placed next to each other and electrical transmission can occur across extracellular space (e.g., ref. 86). Furthermore, there is a long record of studies showing that fibers can interact with each other electrically within a single nerve (29,34,50,54,76). Nelson (81) showed electrical interactions among antidromically activated spinal motoneurons in the cat. Furthermore, electrical field effects are thought to occur under certain pathological conditions of peripheral nerve (87,93). Other studies with weak applied electrical fields have also supported the hypothesis that electrical fields from neuronal activity can modify membrane excitability (43,48,114). Probably the most convincing evidence that electrical field effects play a role in neuronal integration under normal conditions has been obtained with the Mauthner cell system of the goldfish (23,25,27,58). These studies were also the first to provide a firm theoretical framework for electrical field effects. In the model put forth by Furukawa and Furshpan (27), it was clearly shown how electrical current caused by neural activity could polarize nearby passive membranes in a way that would change excitability, and theoretical predictions were matched with experimental findings. Furthermore, inhibitory electrical field effects have recently been demonstrated in the rat cerebellum (56). Electrical field effects, particularly inhibitory interactions, have been reviewed by Korn and Faber (57,59,60).

Early researchers had shown that drug-induced epileptiform activity could remain synchronized across a knife-cut in neural tissue, but that a small gap blocked the synchronization (12,28,64,65). Nonetheless, observations that neocortical seizure foci could be subdivided and made asynchronous with a knife-cut were taken as evidence against the importance of electrical fields in synchronization (for review, see ref. 84). Primarily because of this type of experiment, the possibility of significant electrical field effects in normal or abnormal brain function has been under considerable disfavor (e.g., ref. 40). However, *positive data* for synchronization across knife-cuts must be viewed as evidence for the importance of electrical field effects. Negative results in this experiment are weak evidence, because a knife-cut necessarily disrupts the very substrate upon which electrical field effects would operate. The original argument from the anatomical literature that field effects might be important during hippocampal seizures was premised on the observation of tightly packed neurons without intervening glia in stratum pyramidale (and to some extent in dendritic layers) (30–33). Since knife-cuts would interrupt the tight packing of pyramidal somata and increase extracellular space by over an order of magnitude, negative data with this technique cannot rule out a potentially important role of electrical field effects in undamaged brain tissue. Nonetheless, Jasper (41) and Purpura and co-workers (84,85) did propose a possible role of electrical field effects in the synchronization of epileptiform bursts. Only in the last few years, however, have physiological experiments directly approached this problem. After discussing the evidence for electrotonic coupling between hippocampal and neocortical neurons, we will review recent electrophysiological experiments from our laboratory and by other groups supporting the hypothesis that electrical field effects are a rapid mechanism of synchronization in the hippocampus.

Changes in Concentration of Extracellular Ions

It is well established that intense synchronous activity in the hippocampus and neocortex is associated with increases in extracellular $[K^+]$, decreases in extracellular $[Ca^{2+}]$, and changes in the concentration of other ions. Such electrical activity is also likely to be associated with substantial movements of water, so that the size and resistance of the extracellular space would be modified. Changes in the concentration of extracellular ions can affect excitability. It is unclear how fast these fluctuations actually occur, but the general view seems to be that the changes in extracellular ionic concentrations are slow, ranging from hundreds of milliseconds to minutes (55,120). Theoretically, however, a point source of ions that was insulated from large areas of diffusion could cause a rapid accumulation of ions. This particular question—the time course of changes in extracellular ionic concentrations—is one that deserves further research, particularly in light of the recent paper by Yarom and Spira (121) showing rapid excitation between closely apposed cockroach neurons through changes in extracellular $[K^+]$. However, others discuss these mechanisms in this volume (39,69,101).

RESULTS AND DISCUSSION

Synchronous Bursts Without Active Chemical Synapses in Hippocampus

With four hypothetical mechanisms, it is difficult to evaluate the potential contribution and relative importance of each mechanism to synchronization. For an initial experimental approach to this issue, the problem can conceptually be reduced to the involvement of chemical synapses versus electrical and ionic interactions. It is generally agreed that recurrent chemical synapses contribute to synchronization of the slow depolarization of the PDS, but are chemical synapses necessary for synchronization? Can electrical and ionic interactions synchronize hippocampal neurons without chemical synapses?

We blocked chemical synapses with the Ca^{2+}-antagonist, Mn^{2+}, and then increased excitability by incubating hippocampal slices in a low-$[Ca^{2+}]$ solution (24). Chemical synaptic transmission in the CA1 area was rapidly blocked in this medium. In our studies this blockade was routinely monitored by stimulation of one or two orthodromic pathways while recording extracellularly and intracellularly from the cell body layer. The CA1 pyramidal cells progressively became more excitable (110,112). Immediately after changing to the low-$[Ca^{2+}]$ solution, alvear stimulation evoked single antidromic spikes; over the next hour, however, stimulation of the alveus triggered progressively longer afterdischarges of population spikes. The observation of population spikes under these conditions indicated that action potentials of the

CA1 pyramidal cells were occurring synchronously (2). Simultaneous intracellular and extracellular recordings also supported this conclusion. The afterdischarges sometimes lasted for seconds, and bursts of spikes were separated by silent periods. Therefore it seemed unlikely that spike synchronization occurred simply because the population of cells had the same intrinsic electrophysiological properties and thus responded identically to the electrical stimulus. Furthermore, we were able to block early spikes in an afterdischarge with hyperpolarizing current pulses and still observe synchronous firing of the impaled cell with later population spikes in the afterdischarge (112). More convincing, however, is that under some conditions the CA1 population fired *spontaneous* bursts of population spikes (Fig. 1A). Each intracellular action potential was synchronous with a population spike, although not all population spikes were associated with intracellular action potentials. Thus the synchronization was not absolute. Jefferys and Haas (44) independently showed that in a similar solution with low $[Ca^{2+}]$ and slightly elevated $[Mg^{2+}]$, CA1 cells could fire regular bursts at approximately 20-sec intervals (Fig. 2A; cf. Fig. 3A). As with many of our evoked afterdischarges, each burst of repetitive population spikes was superimposed on a slow extracellular negativity (Fig. 2B and C). Because population spikes were present, a fast synchronizing mechanism other than chemical synapses had to be operative under these experimental conditions. In some of the spike bursts, intracellular recordings showed slow depolarizations of over 10 mV that were associated with partial spike inactivation (Fig. 2D), similar to what has been observed during the PDS. Therefore, chemical synapses are not necessary for regular repetitive bursting, nor for the rapid synchrony underlying population spikes (2–5 msec duration).

During the experiments in CA1 (44,110,112), synchronous activity did not occur in or spread to the CA3 area. It is well known that the CA1 and CA3 areas differ substantially in cell size, electrophysiological properties, and neuronal packing density. The lack of synchronous afterdischarges of population spikes and spontaneous bursts could have been due to differences in excitability of the different populations in these solutions and/or to a lack of appropriate synchronizing mechanisms in the CA3 area. As shown in Fig. 3, however, we found that if the concentration of divalent cations was decreased further, both the dentate gyrus and the CA3 area were capable of firing spontaneous bursts of

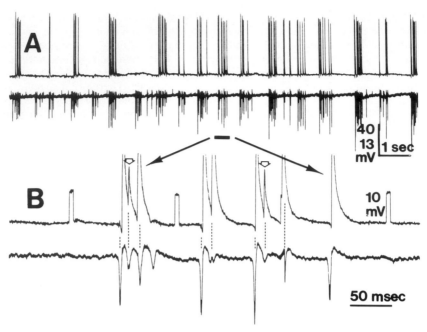

FIG. 1. Intracellular and extracellular recordings of spontaneous bursts of synchronous action potentials in an isolated slice of hippocampus while chemical synapses were blocked with a solution containing Mn^{2+} (2.3 mM) and lowered $[Ca^{2+}]$ (0.5 mM). **A:** On a slow time scale, bursts of intracellular action potentials (*upper trace*) occurred synchronously with many of the spontaneously recurring bursts of extracellularly recorded population spikes (*lower trace*). **B:** Expanded time scale of region indicated by bar in **A**. *Vertical dashed lines* indicate the synchronous occurrence of intracellular action potentials and population spikes. Note the presence of subthreshold depolarizations (*open arrows*), which were also synchronous with population spikes. (From ref. 110, with permission.)

population spikes (98). A variety of spontaneous firing patterns have been observed. In one type of discharge, a slow extracellular negativity lasting many seconds was associated with intense firing on the intracellular electrode; at the end of the extracellular negativity (Fig. 3B), spontaneous population spikes occurred that were synchronous with the intracellular recordings (98). Figure 3C and D shows spontaneous population spikes in both the CA2 and CA3 areas. It should be noted that although CA3 could fire spontaneous bursts, the amplitude of the population spikes was generally smaller and spontaneous population spikes were less likely to occur than in the dentate gyrus, which in turn was less susceptible than the CA1 area. The decreased likelihood of obtaining spontaneous bursts of population spikes in the CA3 area, and the smaller amplitude of population spikes that were observed in this area could be due to lower tolerance of this region to the trauma of slice preparation, since much larger population spikes have been observed *in situ* (113). Nonetheless, these data indicate that all hippocampal sub-

fields are capable of firing spontaneous population spikes, occasionally in a bursting mode, without chemical synapses.

The slow negativity and changes in excitability that have been observed under these conditions are presumably associated with changes in the concentration of extracellular ions, such as K^+. At this point, it is difficult to rule out the possibility that during intense repetitive firing in low-$[Ca^{2+}]$ solution, a gradual leakage of neurotransmitter contributes to the slow spread of these epileptiform events. One must emphasize the importance of carefully monitoring the blockade of chemical synapses during this type of experiment. More recently, however, Konnerth et al. (55) used multiple K^+-sensitive microelectrodes to correlate the spread of the slow negative shifts in extracellular potential with changes in extracellular $[K^+]$. On the other hand, the rapid synchronization necessary to obtain population spikes is probably obtained with electrical interactions alone (see discussion of ionic effects below). It is highly likely that extracellular ion shifts and electrical interactions

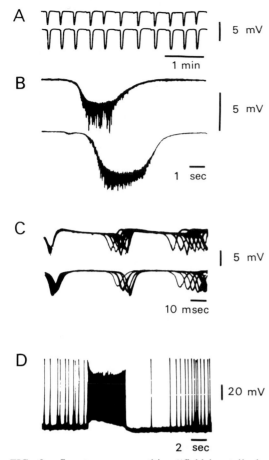

FIG. 2. Spontaneous repetitive "field bursts" observed in hippocampal slices while incubated in a low-[Ca^{2+}] (0.2 mM) solution with elevated [Mg^{2+}] (4 mM). **A:** Extracellular recordings from two locations separated by 1 mm and within the cell body layer of CA1. On a slow time scale, a negative shift in extracellular potential occurred regularly at about three per minute. **B:** On a faster time scale, population spikes could be seen during the negative shifts in potential. **C:** Fast superimposed traces during a burst showing synchronous population spikes on two extracellular electrodes separated by 0.5 mm. **D:** Intracellular recording during a "field burst" revealed high-frequency burst of action potentials superimposed on a slow depolarization. (From ref. 44, with permission.)

are also operative when chemical synapses are present, and these effects would be quite significant if the neurons were sufficiently excitable. Since electrotonic coupling and electrical field effects may synchronize neuronal firing on the time-scale of a population spike, the evidence for each of these forms of intercellular communication and the data indicating that they may be involved in synchronization will be reviewed below.

Electrotonic Coupling in Hippocampus and Neocortex

We have recently reviewed studies of dye coupling, electrotonic coupling, and gap junctions in hippocampus and neocortex (22), and therefore we will briefly summarize previous results and suggest future avenues of investigation.

Dye Coupling

Previous experiments on a wide variety of preparations have shown that when the fluorescent dye Lucifer yellow (LY) (107,108) is injected into a single cell, those cells that are coupled by gap junctions to the injected cell are also frequently stained (8,68,82). The rationale of this experiment is that gap junctions are thought to contain channels that connect the cytoplasm of coupled cells. Molecules of less than about 1,000 molecular weight, including LY (molecular weight 457), have been shown to diffuse between coupled cells through these channels. Intracellular injection of LY into CA1 (Fig. 4A) (3) and CA3 hippocampal pyramidal cells (71), dentate granule cells (73), and neocortical neurons (Fig. 4B) (37) is associated with multiple staining (dye coupling) in two thirds to three-quarters of the injections. These studies have all been performed *in vitro* using brain slice preparations, but comparable data have been obtained in rat hippocampus after *in vivo* injections (74). Coupling appears to be soma–somatic, dendro–somatic, and/or dendro–dendritic (Fig. 4). In some dye-coupled neocortical neurons, the cells are oriented in a columnar fashion (i.e., a row of neurons aligned perpendicular to the pial surface). In these examples of neuronal dye-coupling, little or no extracellular dye or staining of glia was observed. Intracellular injections of LY into glial cells also showed extensive dye coupling, which was restricted to other glial cells (35). Extracellular ejections rarely, but occasionally, stained cells. Dye coupling among rat neocortical neurons was found to be most extensive in the first days after birth and less common in adulthood (15).

This method has drawn criticism because of the possibility (1,51) that multiple staining could result from dye leakage as the micropipette simultaneously impaled two or more cells (49; cf. ref. 3). However, it seems difficult to attribute the high rate of dye coupling seen after intracellular injection of LY to such an artifact, since extracellular ejections rarely stained cells. Similarly, cells with apparent dendro–dendritic dye coupling (when the microelectrode was known

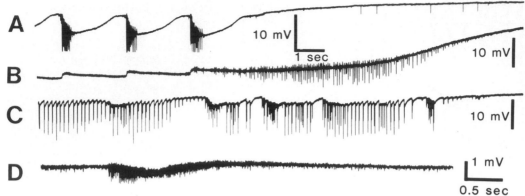

FIG. 3. Spontaneous bursts of synchronous action potentials recorded extracellularly from the cell body layer in each area of the hippocampus after chemical synaptic transmission was blocked in a low-$[Ca^{2+}]$ solution containing Mn^{2+}. **A:** CA1. **B:** Dentate granule cells. **C:** CA2. **D:** CA3. The trace in **B** was recorded near the termination of a slow negative shift in extracellular potential. The bursts had different waveforms in each area of the hippocampus. Bursts of population spikes were infrequent and smaller in amplitude in the CA3 area. Population spikes were usually observed in the dentate gyrus near the end of a prolonged, extracellularly recorded negativity. (From ref. 98, with permission.)

to be in the cell body layer) and columnar dye coupling (when the electrode was known to pass in a different orientation) are difficult to reconcile with an electrode track artifact. Nonetheless, the potential for this type of artifact is real, and it is important that adequate precautions be taken (3). Future studies could benefit by directly visualizing the temporal sequence of dye movement during the injection and the spatial relationship between dye-coupled neurons and the electrode track. Similarly, it would be useful if both large (>2,000 molecular weight) and small (<1,000 molecular weight) dyes could be injected into the same cell; one would expect dye transfer through gap junctions to be selective to small molecules, whereas an electrode track artifact would allow passage of both small and large molecules. A more difficult but elegant approach would be to examine the injected cells with the electron microscope to determine if gap junctions are present at the site of apparent contact among dye-coupled cells.

Lowered intracellular pH (8) and/or raised intracellular $[Ca^{2+}]$ (68; cf. ref. 106) are thought to uncouple cells by a direct closure of gap-junction channels. Thus, one should be able to treat brain slices in a manner expected to alter intracellular pH and/or intracellular $[Ca^{2+}]$ and show that dye coupling is reduced or eliminated. Recent studies indicate that exposure of neocortical slices to CO_2 leads to total elimination of dye coupling among glia (16) and significant reduction in the amount of dye coupling among neurons (16,36). In the study of Gutnick and Lobel-Yaakov (36), the decrease in dye coupling

was observed without apparent changes in electrophysiological properties (e.g., action potential amplitude) and evidence was also presented that treatment with membrane-impermeant acid (HCl) did not affect the incidence of dye coupling. In contrast, extracellular exposure to membrane-permeant acid (propionate), which acidified the cytoplasm, significantly reduced dye coupling among hippocampal pyramidal cells (73a). These studies strongly support the hypothesis that pH-regulated gap junction channels mediate most of the dye coupling observed in hippocampal and neocortical slices.

Electrophysiological Evidence

Antidromic stimulation has been widely used in the vertebrate nervous system to test for electrotonic coupling. The rationale behind this experiment is that antidromic activation of a population of neurons should excite the axons of cells coupled to an impaled neuron. If the axon of the impaled neuron has a higher threshold than the axon of its coupled cell(s), low-intensity antidromic stimuli should yield short-latency depolarizations (SLDs) in the impaled neuron. If blockade of axonal spikes caused the antidromic SLDs, a preceding somatic action potential should collide with the axonal spike (or make the axon refractory) and occlude the SLD. If orthodromic action potentials do not block the antidromic SLDs, they are considered to be electrotonic coupling potentials. This test was performed successfully in about 27% of neocor-

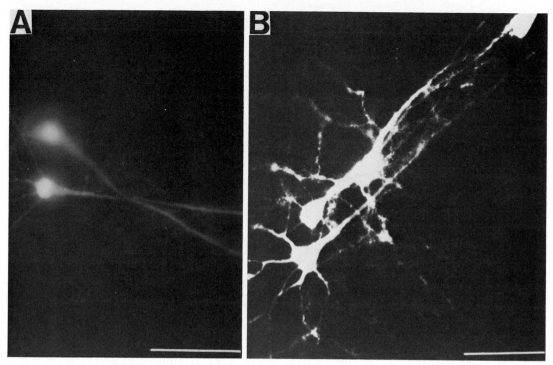

FIG. 4. Dye coupling in hippocampus and neocortex. One neuron was injected with Lucifer yellow and two or more neurons were filled with dye. **A:** Two dye-coupled CA1 pyramidal cells with clearly separated somata from a slice of rat hippocampus. Apparent sites of contact included the proximal apical dendrite. **B:** Dye-coupled neurons in a neocortical slice preparation from an adult guinea pig. Four dye-coupled neurons were stained in a columnar pattern perpendicular to the pia. Bars in **A** and **B** are 50 μm. (**A** from ref. 22, with permission; **B** from ref. 37, with permission.)

tical neurons (Fig. 5A1) (37) and in approximately 5% of CA1 pyramidal cells (Fig. 5A2) (109). A positive result from this test is unlikely to be artifactual. However, a negative result does not necessarily rule out the existence of coupling. For example, there are at least two conditions when coupled cells will fail this test. First, if the impaled cell was coupled *strongly* enough to another cell so that an action potential was transmitted in either direction between the cells, the test would necessarily fail. An antidromic SLD that collides with an orthodromic spike (51,53) could either be a blocked axon spike or a coupling potential from a strongly coupled cell. Second, if the coupling was very weak, the coupling potential would be too small to distinguish and one would obtain another type of false-negative result. Despite the possibility of these false-negative results, it has been difficult to explain the wide disparity between the relatively large fraction of cells that show dye coupling after intracellular injection of LY and the smaller percentage of cells that yield a positive result with the antidromic test. If one could

rapidly and reversibly increase and decrease the strength of electrotonic coupling among mammalian neurons, one could better evaluate the data from these tests.

The most rigorous and direct method for analyzing the electrophysiological properties of an electrotonic junction is with dual intracellular recordings. This technique, however, is substantially more difficult than the antidromic test, particularly if one is to provide morphological evidence that the two electrodes were in different cells. Contrary to published reports (51,52), it is impossible on electrical criteria alone to distinguish between (a) two intracellular electrodes in strongly coupled cells and (b) two electrodes within the same cell, but with larger surface area. The equivalent electrical circuits for these two conditions are identical. MacVicar and Dudek (72) presented evidence that 5 to 7% of their pairs of impaled CA3 hippocampal pyramidal cells were electrotonically coupled (Fig. 5B). Depolarizing and hyperpolarizing current pulses injected through one electrode caused small voltage changes in the other cell and vice

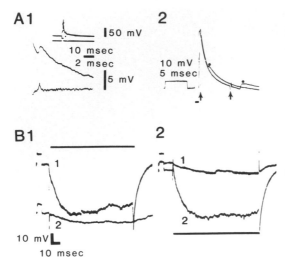

FIG. 5. Electrophysiological tests for electrotonic coupling. **A:** Indirect evidence for coupling in neocortex and hippocampus. A1, Antidromic test in neocortical neuron of the guinea pig. The two upper traces shown as an inset are at low gain and slow·sweep speed; the first record shows an action potential from a depolarizing current pulse (2 msec, 0.75 nA, second record) followed by a short-latency depolarization (SLD) in response to an antidromic stimulus (*closed circle*) presented during the repolarization phase of the action potential. The two enlarged traces shown below are at higher gain and faster sweep speed. The upper record in the enlarged traces shows the waveform of the SLD that was evoked on the falling phase of the action potential; the lower trace is an electrically differentiated record of the upper trace. A2, antidromic test in a CA1 pyramidal cell from a rat hippocampal slice preparation after chemical synaptic transmission was blocked in a low-[Ca^{2+}] (0.5 mM) solution containing Mn^{2+} (2.3 mM). The short bar at the bottom of the figure indicates a brief depolarizing current pulse through the intracellular electrode, and the arrows show the occurrence of two antidromic stimuli. Superimposed traces show two SLDs (*closed circles*) that were not blocked by the preceding action potentials. The SLD was still present after short interstimulus intervals. The SLDs in A1 and A2 were probably electrotonic coupling potentials, because they were not blocked at short interstimulus intervals. **B:** Direct evidence for electrotonic coupling between CA3 pyramidal cells of rat hippocampus using dual intracellular recording. The two high-resistance electrodes contained horseradish peroxidase, and two neurons were subsequently stained after these recordings. Injection of 3-nA hyperpolarizing current pulses (indicated by *bars*) into either cell caused small hyperpolarizations in the other coupled pyramidal cell. The beginning of each trace shows a 10-mV, 5-msec calibration pulse. See original report for description of recording and staining controls. (A1 from ref. 37, with permission; A2 from ref. 109, with permission; **B** from ref. 72, with permission.)

versa (Fig. 5B) (72). When action potentials occurred in one CA3 pyramidal cell, rapid depolarizations (fast prepotentials) were seen on the other intracellular recording. This finding suggests that some fast prepotentials (104) are actually electrotonic coupling potentials rather than dendritic spikes. Two lines of evidence were presented that under these conditions the two microelectrodes were not in the same cell (72). After the data illustrated in Fig. 5B were obtained, horseradish peroxidase (HRP) was injected separately through each of the two intracellular electrodes with an injection protocol that had previously only stained single cells. Subsequent histological examination revealed two pyramidal cells stained with HRP that were in apparent contact. Recently, Miles and Wong (77) have observed weak electrotonic coupling in approximately 5% of dual intracellular recordings in the CA3 area. A similar result was also obtained with granule cells in the dentate gyrus (73). Comparable experiments in the CA1 area by Knowles and Schwartzkroin (51,52) revealed no examples of weak coupling between intracellular electrodes, but several (approximately 10%) pairs of nearly isopotential recordings were interpreted to be simultaneous recording from a single cell. In the study of MacVicar and Dudek (72) on CA3 pyramidal cells, several pairs (approximately 5%) of nearly isopotential recordings were also seen. It is unclear whether these recordings were from cells that were strongly coupled or from dual impalements of a single neuron. In summary, these data support the hypothesis of weak electrotonic coupling (and maybe strong coupling) between a small fraction of *pairs* of hippocampal neurons, but dual recordings from single neurons in the mammalian brain have revealed a low probability of recording from the appropriate pairs for both electrotonic and chemical synapses.

Although these electrophysiological experiments do support the hypothesis of restricted electrotonic coupling among some hippocampal neurons, further studies are needed. It would be useful to determine the electrical frequency transfer characteristics and the electrotonic distance from the somata to the electrotonic junctions and also to correlate the strength of electrotonic coupling between cell pairs with the morphological size and location of the gap junctions (see below). However, these experiments are extremely difficult because of the small percentage of cell pairs that show electrotonic interaction. It should be emphasized that the same technical problem of few interacting pairs of recordings also exists for recurrent excitatory chemical synaptic interactions. For both types of synapses, each neuron is connected to only a small fraction of its neighbors. Nonetheless, the only method for *directly* analyzing the characteristics of electrotonic junctions is dual intracellular recording. An important improvement that could be incorporated into this type of study is to use two different types of intracellular stain to confirm that the electrodes were actually in two different cells. Another approach would be to view penetration of two independent cells directly under a compound microscope (the thickness of the slices makes this difficult). It is only with these methods, however, that we can hope to obtain accurate data on the fraction of cell pairs that show electrotonic coupling and the strength of that coupling.

It has been argued that dye coupling is largely artifactual because of the disparity between the percentage of LY injections that yield dye-coupling and those that demonstrate electrotonic coupling (1,51). However, a potential artifact of the electrode track would also lead to coupling of electrical signals from adjacent cells. That is, an artifactual pathway for dye transfer would also allow passage of electrical current. Therefore, this proposed artifact could not explain the observed disparity. Furthermore, in identified neurons of the snail *Helisoma*, Murphy et al. (80) have shown directly that dye coupling is only associated with strong electrotonic coupling and is not present between cells with low electrotonic coupling ratios; a similar situation among mammalian cortical neurons could hypothetically explain the disparity between dye coupling and electrotonic coupling, as determined with the antidromic test, since cells that were coupled strongly enough to pass dye might necessarily fail the antidromic test (as described above). Additional work is required to reconcile the differences obtained with these techniques.

Gap Junctions

Electron microscopic observation of hippocampal and neocortical neurons has revealed the presence of gap junctions between some cells, but they have been difficult to find and are therefore relatively rare. The easiest method for observing gap junctions is the freeze-fracture technique, because one can examine large areas of membrane much more rapidly and can more easily recognize gap junctions (clusters of particles on the protoplasmic membrane face, and pits on the extracellular face). When gap junctions among various cell types are frequent, it has been possible to see them in thin sections,

but unequivocal evidence for gap junctions is harder to obtain with this method because of the much smaller percentage of membrane area that can be examined along with the added difficulty of demonstrating that close membrane appositions have the properties of gap junctions. Schmalbruch and Jahnsen (91) examined the CA3 area with freeze-fracture replicas and were able to find gap junctions on somata and proximal dendrites of cells that received chemical synapses and were tentatively identified as pyramidal cells (Fig. 6) (see also Figs. 8 and 9 of ref. 22). Similarly, freeze-fracture replicas of the granule cell body layer and proximal dendrites revealed gap junctions (Fig. 7), although they were also rare (73). In both of these studies it was pointed out that positive identification of gap junctions on pyramidal and granule cells respectively was extremely difficult compared to the identification of gap junctions on glial cells. Some of the gap junctions were rather large (0.6 μm diameter) and contained hundreds of particles, thus suggesting a high junctional conductance and relatively strong electrotonic coupling (see ref. 109 for discussion). Schmalbruch and Jahnsen (91) also examined the CA3 area with thin-section electron microscopy and were unable to find unequivocal evidence of gap junctions between CA3 pyramidal cells with this technique, although they were recognizable between glial cells. Examination of thin sections of the CA1 area has revealed evidence that gap junctions may be present, but again they were extremely difficult to find (see Fig. 11C in ref. 92). Recently, Kosaka (62,63) has examined all areas of the hippocampus with thin sections and was unable to find gap junctions between granule cells or among pyramidal cells, but did apparently find them among various interneurons.

Collectively, these data confirm that gap junctions are present on both pyramidal and granule cells in hippocampus, but they are relatively rare compared to the numbers of gap junctions on glia and in other types of mammalian tissues. Long-standing evidence from studies using thin sections and freeze-fracture shows that gap junctions exist in the neocortex of various mammals (79,83,94,95). One of the basic issues that must be examined now is whether gap junctions are found at the apparent sites of dye-coupling and electrotonic coupling.

Possible Role of Electrotonic Coupling in Synchronization

Although several lines of evidence support the hypothesis of electrotonic coupling through gap

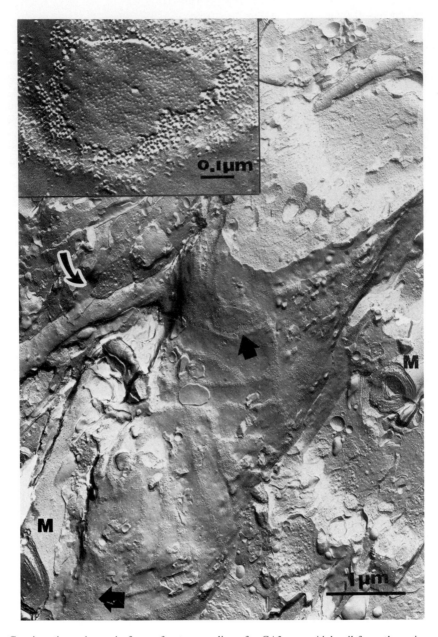

FIG. 6. Gap junctions shown in freeze-fracture replica of a CA3 pyramidal cell from the guinea pig hippocampus. The P-face of an apical dendrite is shown; the cell body was below. *Straight arrows* show two gap junctions on the apical dendrite. The *curved arrow* shows a thin dendritic branch with a synaptic bouton. Two myelinated axons (M) are present. The inset is a higher magnification of a gap junction that illustrates the irregular array of particles on the P-face and the corresponding pits in the attached E-face. (From ref. 91, with permission.)

junctions among small groups of hippocampal and neocortical neurons, the evidence argues against extensive "syncytial" coupling. Without widespread connectivity, it would be impossible to get synchronization of an entire population by electrotonic coupling alone. However, re-

stricted coupling could lead to localized synchronization of small groups of cells. A group of synchronous cells would be expected to generate a larger field potential than a single neuron, and would thus be more likely to recruit and synchronize other neurons through electrical

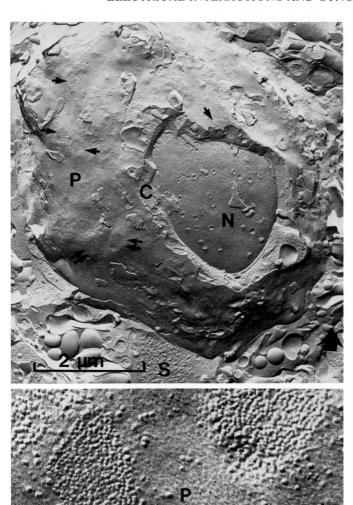

FIG. 7. Gap junctions in freeze-fracture replica of a dentate granule cell in the rat hippocampus. **Top:** Soma of granule cell. The fracture shows the P-face of the somatic membrane. The nuclear membrane (N), which contains nuclear pores, is also shown because the cytoplasm of the neuron is cross-fractured. The process (S) synapsing on the granule cell body is also cross-fractured. *Arrows* indicate gap junctions. **Bottom:** Two gap junctions (indicated by *double arrows* in top photograph) on the P-face of the granule cell body. (From the data of ref. 73; reprinted from ref. 22, with permission.)

field effects (see below). Data from invertebrate and lower vertebrate preparations (7) have indicated that weakly coupled neurons can fire asynchronously when their membrane potentials are well below spike threshold, but the coupled neurons fire synchronously if the group is all close to firing threshold. Convulsant agents can indirectly enhance transmission through weak electrotonic synapses in the sea hare *Aplysia* (88). Synaptic inhibition would tend to uncouple neurons by shunting their junctions (105), so blockade of chemical synaptic inhibition (e.g., with convulsant drugs) would increase the effectiveness of electrotonic junctions. The presence of both chemical and electrotonic synapses in a neuronal population can cause complex inter-

actions: the addition of electrotonic junctions to the Traub and Wong (118) model leads to shunting of the excitatory synapses early in the cascade and to subsequent blockage of the epileptiform bursts. Under these conditions the electrotonic junctions still synchronize electrical activity of the coupled neurons, but because of changes in neuronal input resistance they alter the relationship between strength of chemical synaptic input and probability of synchronous population bursting.

During the synchronous afterdischarges and bursts described above, we have seen partial spikes that could represent electrotonic coupling potentials from spikes in other cells (Fig. 8). However, electrotonic coupling is impossible to

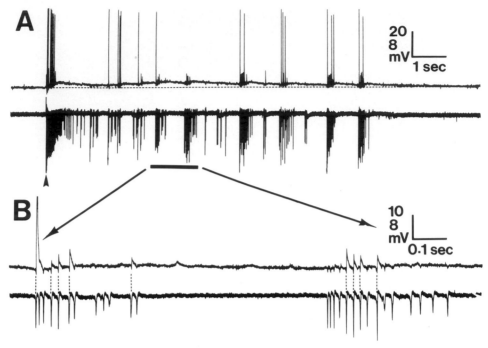

FIG. 8. Small, spike-like depolarizations synchronous with population spikes during an afterdischarge of repetitive bursts. **A:** An alvear stimulus (*arrow*) triggered an afterdischarge lasting 10 sec, which is shown at slow time scale. Upper traces are intracellular records; lower traces are extracellular recordings. Note that some population spikes are associated with subthreshold depolarizations on the intracellular record. The dashed line shows resting potential. **B:** Expansion of the underlined period in **A.** Small subthreshold depolarizations occurred synchronously with population spikes (see *vertical dashed lines*). Such events are not field effect depolarizations (see above) and may be either electrotonic synaptic potentials or remote action potentials within the impaled cell. (From the data of 110, reprinted from ref. 22, with permission.)

prove with a single intracellular electrode. Therefore, these data are consistent with the hypothesis that restricted electrotonic coupling contributes to localized synchronization, but additional studies are needed to determine the contribution of electrotonic coupling to synchronization of epileptiform bursts. Experimental manipulation of the strength of electrotonic coupling is one approach that could provide information on the contribution of electrotonic junctions to synchronization.

Although it seems likely that relatively few electrotonic junctions exist between neurons in cortical areas of the normal adult brain, it is possible that some conditions that enhance the epileptogenicity of cortical tissue may do so by increasing the number and/or strength of electrotonic junctions. One condition worthy of further consideration is neuronal damage (e.g., axotomy or dendrotomy). Several recent studies on identified neurons in the snail *Helisoma* have shown that axotomy can cause the formation of new electrotonic junctions (13) and increase the strength of existing ones (14). In the latter situ-

ation, the enhanced strength of electrotonic coupling is associated with an increased likelihood of dye coupling (80). Damage to axons or dendrites of mammalian cortical neurons might also lead to an increase in electrotonic coupling and in this way increase synchronous activity. It is also possible that neuronal damage during the preparation of brain slices for neurophysiology experiments may lead to the formation or strengthening of electrotonic junctions; recent studies on neocortical slices suggest this may occur (36a). Although there is evidence for coupling in hippocampus and neocortex independent of the slice preparation, the possibility that cutting or crushing neuronal processes modifies coupling could have important ramifications concerning trauma-induced epilepsy.

Another pathological condition that could increase electrotonic coupling between cortical neurons is viral infection. Traub and Pedley (117) have hypothesized enhancement of electrotonic coupling as a possible mechanism for sharp waves in the electroencephalogram during Creutzfeldt–Jakob disease. In several similar spongiform virus encephalopathies, electron micrographs suggest that neuronal membranes may fuse or form gap junctions, which would effectively allow transmission of electrical signals between these neurons. Electrophysiological studies at the single-cell level are now required to evaluate whether pathologically enhanced electrotonic coupling is the basis of epileptiform synchronization in this class of viral infection.

Electrical Field Effects in Hippocampus

The voltage-dependent channels responsible for the excitable properties of neuronal membranes are sensitive to the potential difference between the inside of the neuron and the *extracellular space immediately outside the neuron*. Intracellular recordings from mammalian neurons are generally referenced to a distant ground electrode, which explains why the effects of localized electrical fields were not observed in most previous studies. This recording arrangement includes the implicit assumption that the extracellular space at the site of impalement is at ground potential. However, active neurons can generate electrical fields of sufficient amplitude in the extracellular space to affect the excitability of nearby neurons. Intracellular recordings referenced to ground cannot accurately record the contribution of localized electrical fields. The *transmembrane potential* of a neuron in the presence of electrical fields can be experimentally estimated with a differential voltage recording made by two microelectrodes located on each side of the neuronal membrane; that is, the local extracellular potential is subtracted from the intracellular potential. As previously demonstrated in the Mauthner cell system of teleost fishes, this technique can reveal the effects of the electrical field produced by activity of a single large neuron on other nearby neurons (23,57,59). In the hippocampus, the laminar and parallel orientation of neurons and the small extracellular space (with associated high extracellular impedance) cause unusually large field potentials during synchronous activity.

Differential Recording

In order to demonstrate the presence of electrical field effects in the hippocampus, differential recordings were used in which each intracellular recording was referenced to an equivalent recording from immediately outside the impaled pyramidal cell. In our initial studies,

chemical synapses were blocked with low-$[Ca^{2+}]$ solutions containing Mn^{2+} in order to eliminate complications associated with chemical synaptic transmission (111). The rationale was that if electrical field effects were present during population spikes, we should be able to detect them during antidromic activation. Figure 9A shows differential recordings during an antidromic population spike that was evoked with a stimulation intensity below threshold for the axon of the impaled cell. Note that the population spike recorded from the intracellular electrode referenced to ground was smaller than the population spike observed in the adjacent extracellular recording. Therefore, differential recording showed that during the population spike, a transmembrane depolarization actually occurred instead of the apparent intracellular "negativity" (Fig. 9A). The waveform of antidromic transmembrane depolarizations (particularly the lack of a slow repolarization) was too fast to be caused by either electrotonic or chemical synapses. For the remainder of this discussion, similar depolarizations that were not observable in conventional intracellular recordings with a single microelectrode referenced to ground will be referred to as "transmembrane depolarizations." After this type of recording, a control procedure was used to determine that the extracellular electrode was indeed close to the impaled neuron. The intracellular electrode was dislodged by overcompensating the negative capacitance feedback (or withdrawing the micropipette 5–10 µm), and then a similar antidromic stimulus was applied (111). A flat differential recording with both electrodes extracellular indicated that the previous experiment was a good estimate of actual transmembrane potential.

When transmembrane depolarizations were elicited during a subthreshold depolarizing current pulse, the two depolarizations summated to evoke action potentials. This result indicates that the transmembrane depolarizations revealed with differential recording actually increase neuronal excitability. During the summation experiment, action potentials occurred simultaneously with population spikes, suggesting that transmembrane depolarizations could be the result of a synchronizing mechanism underlying the large population spikes in the hippocampus. Antidromically activated transmembrane depolarizations were finely graded with stimulus intensity, were not changed by injected hyperpolarizing current, and were not occluded by a previous orthodromic action potential. These properties are consistent with the hy-

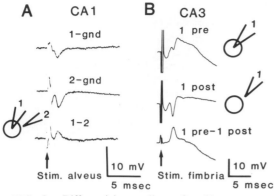

FIG. 9. Differential recordings of rapid transmembrane depolarizations from pyramidal cells. **A:** Transmembrane depolarization in CA1 during antidromic activation after chemical synapses were blocked with a low-[Ca^{2+}] (0.5 mM) solution containing Mn^{2+} (2.3 mM). An alvear stimulus (*arrow*) evoked a small negative-going population spike in the intracellular recording referenced to bath ground (1-gnd) and a larger population spike in a similar extracellular recording (2-gnd). When the extracellular field potential (2-gnd) was subtracted from the intracellular potential (1-gnd), a brief transmembrane depolarization was seen in the differential recording (1 − 2). When both microelectrodes were extracellular, the control differential recording was relatively flat after an alvear stimulus, thus showing that the transmembrane recording was accurate (other control records are shown in ref. 111). **B:** Transmembrane depolarization in normal solution during orthodromic activation of CA3. Action potentials were blocked with injection of QX-314. Each trace is the average of four responses to a fimbrial stimulus (*arrow*). A series of intracellular records referenced to bath ground (1 pre) were obtained and then the microelectrode was withdrawn from the neuron. Another series of recordings were made with the same microelectrode immediately outside the previously impaled neuron (1 post). The differential recording shows a rapid transmembrane depolarization (1 pre − 1 post). Note that, because of extracellular positivity during the synaptic response, the transmembrane recording revealed a reduced EPSP amplitude. Control extracellular recordings using separate electrodes were made simultaneously with the illustrated records (not shown), and no significant change in the field potential occurred between the times of the intracellular (1 pre) and extracellular (1 post) recordings. (**A** from the data of ref. 111; **B** from the results of ref. 97.)

pothesis that an excitatory field effect during the population spike causes these transmembrane depolarizations. The spatial distribution of sinks and sources during a population spike in the CA1 area was determined with current source density analysis and used to develop a relatively simple model of electrical current flow thought to cause hippocampal field effects (111) (see below). Similar studies in the CA1 area by an

independent group have recently corroborated these data and this interpretation (89).

In the normal brain and in most epileptic models, excitatory chemical synaptic transmission is clearly operative. Furthermore, on the basis of neuronal packing density, one would expect the CA3 area to be the least likely area in the hippocampus for electrical field effects to be important. However, differential recording of transmembrane potential in CA3 pyramidal cells has revealed field-effect depolarizations that were synchronous with antidromic population spikes *in vivo* (113) and during orthodromic population spikes *in vitro* (Fig. 9B) (97). It is also apparent in Fig. 9B that the population excitatory postsynaptic potential (EPSP) recorded in stratum pyramidale affects the amplitude of transmembrane depolarization during the EPSP recorded intracellularly at the soma. The field effect associated with synaptic potentials would be more complicated to study than those of the population spike, but this is worthy of further investigation.

Conceptual Model

A model for the hypothetical mechanism of electrical field effects during a hippocampal population spike is shown schematically in Fig. 10. In this model, the major driving force for the field effect is the inward active current from a population of synchronously firing hippocampal pyramidal somata. The active current of the pyramidal cells is recorded extracellularly as a negative-going population spike, which can be tens of millivolts in amplitude and which represents a current sink in the cell body layer. The inward somatic current must complete an electrical circuit, and the passive return path is through distal dendrites of the active population back into the extracellular medium. This passive limb of the circuit causes an electrical current source in the dendritic extracellular space. Although much of the current flows back to the somatic sink through the extracellular space, a fraction flows within the dendrites and passively out the somata of nonfiring pyramidal cells. The current flow outward across the impedance of passive neural somatic membranes generates a transmembrane depolarization across the somatic membrane. The waveform of the transmembrane depolarization is expected to be similar to that of the population spike (both are caused by electrical current flowing in the same circuit). The anatomical features necessary for the electrical field effect are (a) the parallel arrangement of pyramidal cells at right angles to the extracellular voltage gradient and (b) the tight neu-

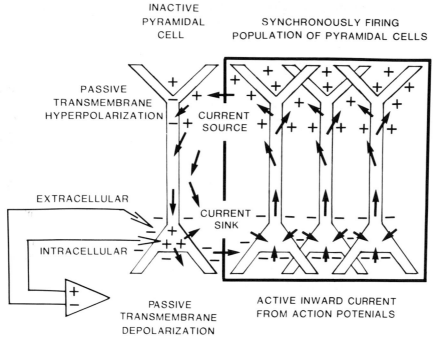

INACTIVE PYRAMIDAL CELL

SYNCHRONOUSLY FIRING POPULATION OF PYRAMIDAL CELLS

PASSIVE TRANSMEMBRANE HYPERPOLARIZATION

CURRENT SOURCE

EXTRACELLULAR

CURRENT SINK

INTRACELLULAR

PASSIVE TRANSMEMBRANE DEPOLARIZATION

ACTIVE INWARD CURRENT FROM ACTION POTENIALS

FIG. 10. Schematic diagram of model for electrical field effects. The box at the right contains a population of synchronously firing pyramidal cells. The active inward spike current at the cell bodies of these neurons creates a current sink or negativity in the extracellular space around the soma of the inactive pyramidal cell, which is shown to the left. The somatic sink and dendritic source are associated with current flow, which is indicated by arrows. Differential recording with intracellular and extracellular microelectrodes reveals a rapid transmembrane depolarization in the soma of a nearby passive pyramidal cell.

ronal packing with high extracellular impedance relative to the intracellular impedance. Radially symmetrical glial cells would therefore be expected to experience little or no electrical field effect measured at their somata. The diagram shows a synchronous population of pyramidal cells as the generator of the current sink (Fig. 10), but an action potential in a single neuron might also exert a small electrical field effect on an adjacent passive pyramidal cell. Theoretical models of adjacent axons (75) have indicated that if two cells were firing spontaneously, an electrical field effect would tend to synchronize their action potentials. Because a relatively small population of synchronously active neurons could hypothetically recruit adjacent inactive pyramidal cells that were near threshold, this mechanism could result in a regenerative self-exciting cascade of synchronized firing. In fact, multiple extracellular records (112) showed that in some cases population spikes did appear to propagate without decrement across a large population of cells.

Finally, a similar model may apply to the neocortex, although presently no electrophysiological evidence exists for electrical field effects in any neocortical area. However, the dendritic

bundles frequently reported for neocortex and other brain areas have provided the anatomical basis for speculations on electrical interactions (e.g., 90,96).

Contribution of Electrical Field Effects to Synchronization

The transmembrane depolarizations shown to occur during antidromic and orthodromic population spikes would tend to excite inactive neurons when part of the population was firing synchronous afterdischarges and spontaneous bursts. Because electrotonic coupling does not appear to be extensive enough to synchronize action potentials throughout the population when chemical synapses are blocked, electrical field effects probably represent a critical synchronizing mechanism. We tested this hypothesis with differential recording during afterdischarges and spontaneous bursts in the CA1 area and showed that most spikes in nearly every pyramidal cell were triggered by brief transmembrane depolarizations similar to those that have been attributed to electrical field effects during antidromic and orthodromic population spikes (110,112). In intracellular recordings referenced to ground, an apparent negativity preceded the action potential while differential transmembrane recordings revealed a rapid depolarizing prepotential. These brief transmembrane depolarizations, as indicated above, were too rapid to be caused by electrotonic or chemical synapses or by rapid fluctuations in extracellular [K$^+$] (see below). These events represent field-effect depolarizations, which would be expected to exert a powerful synchronizing influence on the cells.

Although the preceding data provide strong evidence that electrical field effects contribute significantly to the synchronization of epileptiform discharges when chemical synapses are not present, it has not been previously demonstrated that electrical field effects synchronize action potentials during the PDS after exposure to GABA-blocking convulsant agents that leave recurrent excitatory synapses functional. Therefore, recent experiments in our laboratory were designed to measure the influence of field-effect depolarizations during the PDS in picrotoxin-treated slices (99). When hippocampal slices were exposed to 200 μM picrotoxin, large depolarizations associated with inactivating spikes began to occur spontaneously (Fig. 11, inset). When steady hyperpolarizing current or the anesthetic QX-314 (17) was injected into the cell to block action potentials during the PDS, differential recording revealed rapid transmembrane depolarizations (Fig. 11) that appeared similar to those described above during blockade of chemical synapses. The intracellular transmembrane recordings of Figure 11 provide direct evidence that electrical fields generate synchronizing depolarizations in convulsant-treated brain tissue with active chemical synapses.

At this point it is appropriate to consider the possibility that rapid changes in the concentration of extracellular ions (primarily K$^+$) contribute to the synchronization of action potentials and are responsible for the brief transmembrane depolarizations revealed with differential recording. If fast, transient increases in extracellular [K$^+$] were occurring during afterdischarges of population spikes, they should be detected with intracellular recordings from glial cells in the cell body layer. The membrane potential of glial cells has been shown to be a Nernstian function of extracellular [K$^+$] (100) and would be expected to respond to changes in extracellular [K$^+$] just as quickly as an impaled pyramidal cell. Intraglial recordings during synchronous afterdischarges revealed a slow depolarizing envelope without significant rapid transmembrane depolarizations (112), thus supporting the hypothesis that changes in extracellular [K$^+$] occur on a time scale of several milliseconds to seconds and do not generate the rapid transmembrane depolarizations that we have attributed to electrical field effects. In Fig. 8A, it may be seen that in addition to the rapid subthreshold depolarizations described previously, a superimposed slow depolarization followed each burst of population spikes. Because of the similarity of these slow depolarizations to those seen in glial recordings and the absence of chemical synaptic potentials, we have attributed such slow depolarizations to extracellular accumulation of K$^+$ (see ref. 112 for discussion). It would be surprising if K$^+$ accumulation provided a rapid synchronizing influence upon single action potentials during hippocampal bursts and afterdischarges. Because the brief transmembrane depolarizations can be attributed positively to field effects and because they can be detected routinely during synchronous firing of hippocampal population spikes, they imply a significant contribution of intrinsic electrical fields to the synchronization process during epileptiform bursts.

Relatively few electrophysiological data are available concerning physiological changes that might modulate the strength of electrical field effects. On theoretical grounds, any treatment or condition that caused cellular swelling or reduced extracellular space (i.e., increased extracellular resistance relative to cytoplasmic resistance) would be expected to augment the effect of intrinsically generated electrical fields on adjacent neurons. It has been shown that repetitive activation and seizures reduce the size of the extracellular space and increase extracellular resistance in cat neocortex (20,21). One can thus hypothesize a positive feedback during seizures whereby repetitive synchronous activity increases extracellular resistance, which then enhances the excitatory effect of electrical fields and recruits additional neurons into seizure activity. Reduced myelination in spinal nerves of dystrophic mice causes electrical transmission between axons (87), and a similar phenomenon could occur between cortical neurons. The earliest ultrastructural changes in Creutzfeldt–Jakob disease include cellular swelling (see ref. 117), which could promote electrical interactions through field effects. Therefore, similar to electrotonic coupling through gap junctions, certain neurological disorders could hypothetically enhance the epileptogenicity of cortical tissue by altering cellular morphology and the neuronal microenvironment in a manner that strengthens

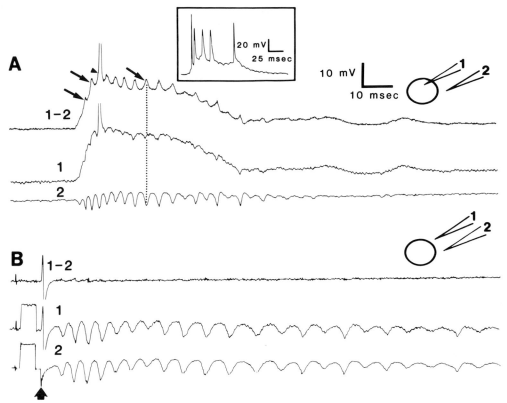

FIG. 11. Field effect depolarizations during a spontaneous paroxysmal depolarization shift (PDS) in 200 μM picrotoxin. **A:** Intracellular recording in second trace (electrode 1, see diagram) and nearby extracellular recording in third trace (electrode 2) were made with respect to bath ground. The difference between these recordings (1 − 2, first trace) is the actual transmembrane potential during the PDS. Field effect depolarizations (some marked by *arrows*) were correlated with the extracellularly recorded population spikes (*dotted line*). The cell was hyperpolarized to reduce spiking. One action potential arises from a field effect depolarization (at *triangle*). Box encloses a spontaneous PDS without hyperpolarizing current. **B:** Extracellular control recordings after impalement was lost. The previously intracellular electrode (electrode 1, see diagram) recorded the extracellular field potential just outside the cell in response to stimulation of stratum radiatum (at *arrow*). The differential recording (1 − 2) showed that the electrodes were electrically close. The square deflection before the stimulus is a 10-mV, 5-msec calibration. Recordings were made in the CA1 region of hippocampus.

the excitatory effects of endogenous electrical fields.

Computer Simulations of Synchronous Hippocampal Afterdischarges

One problem with analyzing the relative contribution of electrotonic coupling and electrical field effects to synchronization is that it is difficult experimentally to regulate the strength of these electrical interactions and observe the resulting changes in synchronization. Furthermore, it is presently difficult to evaluate quantitatively the amount of electrotonic coupling and the relative strength of field effects in any population of cortical neurons. On the other hand, the model of epileptiform discharges in

low-[Ca^{2+}] solutions without active chemical synapses is a simplified system of network interactions, because the relatively unknown characteristics of excitatory and inhibitory recurrent pathways and also of Ca^{2+} currents and Ca^{2+}-activated K^+ currents can be reduced significantly or eliminated. Traub and co-workers (116) have used computer simulation methods in an attempt to model electrical interactions as a basis for the synchrony of these afterdischarges. The model consists of a 10 × 10 array of hippocampal pyramidal cells where each neuron contains 28 compartments. The membrane of each neural element has voltage-dependent Na^+ current, voltage-dependent K^+ current, and an M current (38) similar to previous models (115). The Ca^{2+} equilibrium potential has been lowered and the voltage-dependent rate functions have been shifted along the voltage axis, as would be expected in a low-[Ca^{2+}] solution. The extracellular space is simulated with a network of resistors connecting extracellular "nodes" in 19 positions along the extracellular longitudinal axis of each neuron (i.e., 1,900 extracellular nodes in the network). In this computational model, considerable synchronization was obtained with electrical field effects alone, if the resistance of the extracellular space was assumed to be high and the cells were near threshold. In some simulations electrotonic junctions (resistors) were added between the 100 neurons with a probability $p = 0.25$ for a junction to occur between any adjacent pair of cells in the two-dimensional lattice of cells. The addition of electrotonic coupling to the network enhanced synchronization (Fig. 12). These computer simulations are extremely useful because (a) they provide theoretical support for the model elaborated by Taylor and Dudek (111); (b) they explicitly indicate those parameters that need to be measured in order to provide a more complete understanding of the synchronization process when chemical synapses are not present; and (c) they allow evaluation of the effects of changing the strength of electrical fields and/or the extent and strength of electrotonic coupling on synchronization. As described above, experimental modification of real electrical field effects or electrotonic coupling may be difficult to perform and will certainly be difficult to evaluate theoretically; the computer simulations thus provide important insights into how these two synchronizing mechanisms may interact to generate epileptiform bursts. Ultimately, this model of electrical interactions may be combined with one containing recurrent excitatory chemical synapses plus normal Ca^{2+} currents and Ca^{2+}-activated K$^+$ currents to model network behavior underlying generation of the PDS by convulsant agents such as picrotoxin.

CONCLUSIONS

The experimental results reviewed here support the hypothesis that electrical interactions contribute to synchronization of epileptiform bursts in the hippocampus. Chemical synapses and changes in the concentration of extracellular ions are expected to be important, but electrotonic coupling and electrical field effects may also synchronize neurons and can act on a particularly rapid time scale. Electrophysiological evidence from recordings of transmembrane po-

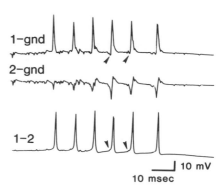

FIG. 12. Records of an afterdischarge from computer simulation of 100-neuron model. Details of the model are described in text. The stimulus that triggered the afterdischarge was a brief current pulse to 16 neurons. Intracellular (1-gnd) and extracellular (2-gnd) records were from the somatic compartment and were referenced to ground; the transmembrane recording (1 − 2) was the difference between the intracellular and extracellular records. Note that the intracellular recording referenced to ground (1-gnd) shows a brief negativity (*arrows*) before each action potential, while the transmembrane recording (1 − 2) reveals that field effect depolarizations (*arrows*) actually trigger the action potentials (cf. Fig. 11). (From the data of 116, reprinted with permission from R. D. Traub.)

tential changes during synchronous activity support the hypothesis that electrical field effects are important. Presently, the actual contribution of electrotonic coupling to synchronization is unknown, but it would be expected to contribute to synchronization whenever it is present.

Several conceptual questions still need to be answered, however. Can one specify in a quantitative manner the contribution of each hypothetical mechanism to synchronization of epileptiform bursts? This analysis would have to consider the time course of each mechanism and also the type of epileptic model. Our best estimates for the time course of various synchronizing influences are summarized in Fig. 13. In this regard, electrical interactions would have a latency of less than a millisecond. A quantitative description of the time course of synchronizing mechanisms for a particular epileptic model should specify the minimum latency and the maximum duration of the interaction between two communicating neurons. Such a quantification of interactions would be important for simulation studies. It would be useful to know whether any one mechanism can support regenerative activity without the contribution of other mechanisms, or whether several mechanisms must act together to evoke epileptiform bursts. Are electrical mechanisms involved in the initi-

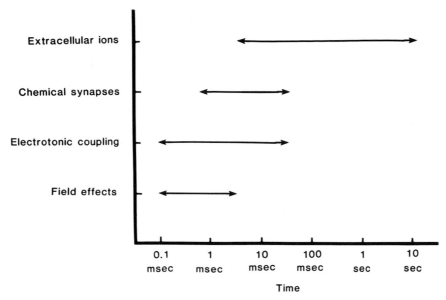

FIG. 13. Diagram illustrating hypothetical time scale of interaction of each synchronizing mechanism. For each type of communication between two neurons, the *arrowed line* represents the approximate range of times between the minimum latency and the maximum duration for the effects of a single population spike in the hippocampus. The times are only approximations, but they are estimated from actual data on hippocampal neurons. The latency for an electrical field-effect depolarization is practically instantaneous and the duration is comparable to a population spike (111). For an electrotonic coupling potential, latency should also be virtually instantaneous, but duration is prolonged because of the slow time course of the depolarizing afterpotential (109). Latency for a chemical synaptic potential from a recurrent excitatory pathway is estimated at 0.5–1.0 msec and the passive properties determine duration (70). The effects of changes in the concentration of extracellular ions are estimated from differential intracellular recording of the glial cell depolarization after a population spike (111). Note that the time axis is logarithmic.

ation of synchrony between small groups of cells that would not normally fire synchronously? In this way, could such mechanisms contribute to the onset of seizures? What are the spatial dimensions of communication for the various synchronizing mechanisms? What factors might potentiate or suppress each synchronizing effect? Are the mechanisms "plastic"? Do the strength of electrotonic coupling or electrical field effects change as a causative factor in certain forms of epilepsy? It should be obvious that much work remains to be done, but future research should eventually be able to answer many of these questions.

ACKNOWLEDGMENTS

Several of the figures in this chapter represent the research of other investigators; we are grateful to Dr. M. J. Gutnick, Dr. H. L. Haas, Dr. H. Jahnsen, Dr. J. G. R. Jefferys, Dr. D. A. Prince, Dr. H. Schmalbruch, and Dr. R. D. Traub for allowing us to publish figures from their work. Dr. R. D. Andrew and Dr. B. A.

MacVicar were instrumental in our research on electrotonic coupling in the hippocampus, and some of the figures published here are from work with them. We thank Dr. B. W. Connors, Dr. M. J. Gutnick, Dr. U. Heinemann, Dr. K. Krnjević, Dr. B. A. MacVicar, Dr. J. J. Miller, and Dr. R. D. Traub for helpful discussions and sharing unpublished data with us. Dr. E. P. Christian, Dr. N. R. Kreisman, and Dr. R. D. Traub provided constructive criticisms of a previous draft of this article. We are also grateful to B. Farmer for preparing the manuscript and R. Granier for photographic work. This manuscript was prepared under the support of National Institutes of Health grant NS 16683.

REFERENCES

1. Alger, B. E., McCarren, M., and Fisher, R. S. (1983): On the possibility of simultaneously recording from two cells with a single microelectrode in the hippocampal slice. *Brain Res.*, 270:137–141.
2. Andersen, P., Bliss, T. V. P., and Skrede, K. K. (1971): Unit analysis of hippocampal population spikes. *Exp. Brain Res.*, 13:208–221.

3. Andrew, R. D., Taylor, C. P., Snow, R. W., and Dudek, F. E. (1982): Coupling in rat hippocampal slices: dye transfer between CA1 pyramidal cells. *Brain Res. Bull.*, 8:211–222.

4. Arvanitaki, A. (1942): Effects evoked in an axon by the activity of a contiguous one. *J. Neurophysiol.*, 5:89–108.

5. Ayala, G. F., Dichter, M., Gumnit, R. J., Matsumoto, H., and Spencer, W. A. (1973): Genesis of epileptic interictal spikes. New knowledge of cortical feedback systems suggests a neurophysiological explanation of brief paroxysms. *Brain Res.*, 52:1–17.

6. Baker, R., and Llinás, R. (1971): Electrotonic coupling between neurons in the rat mesencephalic nucleus. *J. Physiol. (Lond.)*, 212:45–63.

7. Bennett, M. V. L. (1977): Electrical transmission: A functional analysis and comparison to chemical transmission. In: *Handbook of Physiology, Section I: The Nervous System, Vol. 1, Cellular Biology of Neurons, Part 1,* edited by E. R. Kandel, pp. 357–416. American Physiology Society, Bethesda, Maryland.

8. Bennett, M. V. L., and Goodenough, D. A. (1978): Gap junctions, electrotonic coupling, and intercellular communication. *Neurosci. Res. Program Bull.,*16:373–486.

9. Bennett, M. V. L., Nakajima, Y., and Pappas, G. D. (1967): Physiology and ultrastructure of electrotonic junctions. III. Giant electromotor neurons of *Malapterurus electricus. J. Neurophysiol.*, 30:209–235.

10. Bennett, M. V. L., Pappas, G. D., Aljure, E., and Nakajima, Y. (1967): Physiology and ultrastructure of electrotonic junctions. II. Spinal and medullary electromotor nuclei in mormyrid fish. *J. Neurophysiol.*, 30:180–208.

11. Bennett, M. V. L., Pappas, G. D., Gimenez, M., and Nakajima, Y. (1967): Physiology and ultrastructure of electrotonic junctions. IV. Medullary electromotor nuclei in gymnotid fish. *J. Neurophysiol.*, 30:236–300.

12. Bremer, F. (1941): L'activité "spontanée" de la moelle épinière. *Arch. Int. Physiol.*, 51:51–84.

13. Bulloch, A. G. M., and Kater, S. B. (1981): Selection of a novel connection by adult molluscan neurons. *Science*, 212:79–81.

14. Bulloch, A. G. M., Kater, S. B., and Murphy, A. D. (1980): Connectivity changes in an isolated molluscan ganglion during in vivo culture. *J. Neurobiol.*, 11:531–546.

15. Connors, B. W., Benardo, L. S., and Prince, D. A. (1983): Coupling between neurons of the developing rat neocortex. *J. Neurosci.*, 3:773–782.

16. Connors, B. W., Benardo, L. S., and Prince, D. A. (1984): Carbon dioxide sensitivity of dye-coupling among glia and neurons of the neocortex. *J. Neurosci.*, 4:1324–1330.

17. Connors, B. W., and Prince, D. A. (1982): Effects of local anesthetic QX-314 on the membrane properties of hippocampal pyramidal neurons. *J. Pharmacol. Exp. Ther.*, 220:476–481.

18. Dichter, M., and Spencer, W. A. (1969): Penicillin-induced interictal discharges from the cat hippocampus. I. Characteristics and topographical features. *J. Neurophysiol.*, 32:649–662.

19. Dichter, M., and Spencer, W. A. (1969): Penicillin-induced interictal discharges from the rat hippocampus. II. Mechanisms underlying origin and restriction. *J. Neurophysiol.*, 32:663–687.

20. Dietzel, I., Heinemann, U., Hofmeier, G., and Lux, H. D. (1980): Transient changes in the size of the extracellular space in the sensorimotor cortex of cats in relation to stimulus-induced changes in potassium concentration. *Exp. Brain Res.*, 40:432–439.

21. Dietzel, I., Heinemann, U., Hofmeier, G., and Lux, H. D. (1982): Stimulus-induced changes in extracellular Na^+ and Cl^- concentration in relation to changes in the size of the extracellular space. *Exp. Brain Res.*, 46:73–84.

22. Dudek, F. E., Andrew, R. D., MacVicar, B. A., Snow, R. W., and Taylor, C. P. (1983): Recent evidence for and possible significance of gap junctions and electrotonic synapses in the mammalian brain. In: *Basic Mechanisms of Neuronal Hyperexcitability*, edited by H. H. Jasper and N. M. van Gelder, pp. 31–73. Alan R. Liss, New York.

23. Faber, D. S., and Korn, H. (1983): Field effects trigger post-anodal rebound excitation in vertebrate CNS. *Nature (Lond.)*, 305:802–804.

24. Frankenhaeuser, B., and Hodgkin, A. L. (1957): The action of calcium on the electrical properties of squid axons. *J. Physiol. (Lond.)*, 137:218–244.

25. Furshpan, E. J., and Furukawa, T. (1962): Intracellular and extracellular responses of the several regions of the Mauthner cell of the goldfish. *J. Neurophysiol.*, 25:732–771.

26. Furshpan, E. J., and Potter, D. D. (1959): Transmission at the giant motor synapse of the crayfish. *J. Physiol. (Lond.)*, 145:289–325.

27. Furukawa, T. and Furshpan, E. J. (1963): Two inhibitory mechanisms in the Mauthner neurons of goldfish. *J. Neurophysiol.*, 26:140–176.

28. Gerard, R. W. and Libet, B. (1940): The control of normal and "convulsive" brain potentials. *Am. J. Psychol.*, 96:1125–1152.

29. Granit, R., and Skoglund, C. R. (1945): Facilitation, inhibition and depression at the "artificial synapse" formed by the cut end of a mammalian nerve. *J. Physiol. (Lond.)*, 103:435–448.

30. Green, J. D. (1960): The hippocampus. *Handbook of Physiology, Section 1: Neurophysiology, vol. II,* edited by J. Field, pp. 1373–1389. American Physiology Society, Washington D.C.

31. Green, J. D. (1964): The hippocampus. *Physiol. Rev.*, 44:561–608.

32. Green, J. D., and Maxwell, D. S. (1961): Hippocampal electrical activity I. Morphological aspects. *Electroenc. Clin. Neurophysiol.*, 13:837–846.

33. Green, J. D., and Petsche, H. (1961): Hippocampal electrical activity IV. Abnormal electrical activity. *Electroenc. Clin. Neurophysiol.*, 13:868–879.

34. Grundfest, H., and Magnes, J. (1951): Excitability changes in dorsal roots produced by electrotonic effects from adjacent afferent activity. *Am. J. Physiol.*, 164:502–508.

35. Gutnick, M. J., Connors, B. W., and Ransom, B. R. (1981): Dye-coupling between glial cells

in the guinea pig neocortical slice. *Brain Res.*, 213:486–492.

36. Gutnick, M. J., and Lobel-Yaakov, R. (1983): Carbon dioxide uncouples dye-coupled neuronal aggregates in neocortical slices. *Neurosci. Lett.*, 42:197–200.

36a. Gutnick, M. J., Lobel-Yaakov, R., and Rimon, G. (1985): Incidence of neuronal dye-coupling in neocortical slices depends on the plane of section. *Neuroscience*, 15:659–666.

37. Gutnick, M. J., and Prince, D. A. (1981): Dye coupling and possible electrotonic coupling in the guinea pig neocortical slice. *Science*, 211:67–70.

38. Halliwell, J. V., and Adams, P. R. (1982): Voltage-clamp analysis of muscarinic excitation in hippocampal neurons. *Brain Res.*, 250:71–92.

39. Heinemann, U. et al., Chapter 32.

40. Hubel, D. H. (1982): Cortical neurobiology: A slanted historical perspective. *Ann. Rev. Neurosci.*, 5:363–370.

41. Jasper, H. H. (1969): Mechanisms of propagation: Extracellular studies. In: *Basic Mechanisms of the Epilepsies*, edited by H. H. Jasper, A. A. Ward, Jr., and A. Pope, pp. 421–438. Little, Brown & Co., Boston.

42. Jasper, H. H., and Monnier, A. M. (1938): Transmission of excitation between excised non-myelinated nerves. An artificial synapse. *J. Cell. Comp. Physiol.*, 11:259–277.

43. Jefferys, J. G. R. (1981): Influence of electric fields on the excitability of granule cells in guinea-pig hippocampal slices. *J. Physiol. (Lond.)*, 319:143–152.

44. Jefferys, J. G. R., and Haas, H. L. (1982): Synchronized bursting of CA1 hippocampal pyramidal cells in the absence of synaptic transmission. *Nature (Lond.)*, 300:448–450.

45. Johnston, D., and Brown, T. H. (1981): Giant synaptic potential hypothesis for epileptiform activity. *Science*, 211:294–297.

46. Johnston, D., and Brown, T. H. (1984): Mechanisms of neuronal burst generation. In: *Electrophysiology of Epilepsy*, edited by P. A. Schwartzkroin and H. V. Wheal, pp. 277–301. Academic, New York.

47. Johnston, D., and Brown, T. H., Chapter 12.

48. Kaczmarek, L. K., and Adey, W. R. (1974): Weak electric gradients change ionic and transmitter fluxes in cortex. *Brain Res.*, 66:537–540.

49. Kaneko, A., Nishimura, Y., Tauchi, M., and Shimai, K. (1981): Morphological observation of retinal cells presumably made syncytial by an electrode penetration. *J. Neurosci. Meth.*, 4:299–303.

50. Katz, B., and Schmitt, O. H. (1942): A note on interaction between nerve fibres. *J. Physiol. (Lond.)*, 100:369–371.

51. Knowles, W. D., Funch, P. G., and Schwartzkroin, P. A. (1982): Electrotonic and dye coupling in the hippocampal slice. *Neuroscience*, 7:1713–1722.

52. Knowles, W. D., and Schwartzkroin, P. A. (1981): Local circuit synaptic interactions in hippocampal brain slices. *J. Neurosci.*, 1:318–322.

53. Knowles, W. D., and Schwartzkroin, P. A. (1981): Axonal ramifications of hippocampal CA1 pyramidal cells. *J. Neurosci.*, 1:1236–1241.

54. Kocsis, J. D., Ruiz, J. A., and Cummins, K. L. (1982): Modulation of axonal excitability mediated by surround electrical activity: An intra-axonal study. *Exp. Brain Res.*, 47:151–153.

55. Konnerth, A., Heinemann, U., and Yaari, Y. (1984): Slow transmission of neural activity in hippocampal area CA1 in absence of active chemical synapses. *Nature (Lond.)*, 307:69–71.

56. Korn, H. and Axelrad, H. (1980): Electrical inhibition of Purkinje cells in the cerebellum of the rat. *Proc. Natl. Acad. Sci. U.S.A.*, 77:6244–6247.

57. Korn, H. and Faber, D. S. (1975): Mechanisms and functions of electrically mediated inhibition in the vertebrate central nervous system. In: *Sensory Physiology and Behavior*, edited by R. Galun, P. Hillman, I. Parnas, and R. Werman, pp. 289–305. Plenum, New York.

58. Korn, H., and Faber, D. S. (1975): An electrically mediated inhibition in goldfish medulla. *J. Neurophysiol.*, 38:452–471.

59. Korn, H., and Faber, D. S. (1979): Electrical interactions between vertebrate neurons: Field effects and electrotonic coupling. In: *The Neurosciences: Fourth Study Program*, edited by F. O. Schmitt and F. G. Worden, pp. 333–358. MIT Press, Cambridge.

60. Korn, H., and Faber, D. S. (1980): Electrical field effect interactions in the vertebrate brain. *Trends Neurosci.*, 3:6–9.

61. Korn, H., Sotelo, C., and Crepel, F. (1973): Electrotonic coupling between neurons in the rat lateral vestibular nucleus. *Exp. Brain Res.*, 16:255–275.

62. Kosaka, T. (1983): Gap junctions between non-pyramidal cell dendrites in the rat hippocampus (CA1 and CA3 regions). *Brain Res.*, 271:157–161.

63. Kosaka, T. (1983): Neuronal gap junctions in the polymorph layer of the rat dentate gyrus. *Brain Res.*, 277:347–351.

64. Libet, B., and Gerard, R. W. (1939): Control of the potential rhythm of the isolated frog brain. *J. Neurophysiol.*, 2:153–169.

65. Libet, B., and Gerard, R. W. (1941): Steady potential fields and neurone activity. *J. Neurophysiol.*, 4:438–455.

66. Llinás, R., Baker, R., and Sotelo, C. (1974): Electrotonic coupling between neurons in cat inferior olive. *J. Neurophysiol.*, 37:560–571.

67. Llinás, R. and Yarom, Y. (1981): Electrophysiology of mammalian inferior olivary neurones in vitro. Different types of voltage-dependent ionic conductances. *J. Physiol. (Lond.)*, 315:549–567.

68. Loewenstein, W. R. (1981): Junctional intercellular communication: the cell-to-cell membrane channel. *Physiol. Rev.*, 61:829–913.

69. Lux, H. D., Heinemann, U., and Dietzel, I., Chapter 31.

70. MacVicar, B. A., and Dudek, F. E. (1980): Local synaptic circuits in rat hippocampus: In-

teractions between pyramidal cells. *Brain Res.*, 184:220–223.

71. MacVicar, B. A., and Dudek, F. E. (1980): Dye-coupling between CA3 pyramidal cells in slices of rat hippocampus. *Brain Res.*, 196:494–497.

72. MacVicar, B. A., and Dudek, F. E. (1981): Electrotonic coupling between pyramidal cells: A direct demonstration in rat hippocampal slices. *Science*, 213:782–785.

73. MacVicar, B. A., and Dudek, F. E. (1982): Electrotonic coupling between granule cells of rat dentate gyrus: Physiological and anatomical evidence. *J. Neurophysiol.*, 47:579–592.

73a. MacVicar, B. A., and Jahnsen, H. (1985): Uncoupling of CA3 pyramidal neurons by propionate. *Brain Res.*, 330:141–145.

74. MacVicar, B. A., Ropert, N., and Krnjevic, K. (1982): Dye-coupling between pyramidal cells of rat hippocampus in vivo. *Brain Res.*, 238:239–244.

75. Maeda, K., Yagi, T., and Noguchi, A. (1980): Induced excitation and synchronization of nerve impulses in two parallel unmyelinated fibers. *IEEE Trans. Biomed. Engineer.* BME-27:139–145.

76. Marrazzi, A. S., and Lorente de Nó, R. (1944): Interaction of neighboring fibres in myelinated nerve. *J. Neurophysiol.*, 7:83–101.

77. Miles, R., and Wong, R. K. S. (1982): The origins of primary and secondary synchronized bursts in disinhibited hippocampal slices. *Soc. Neurosci. Abstr.*, 8:910.

78. Miles, R., and Wong, R. K. S. (1983): Single neurones can initiate synchronized population discharge in the hippocampus. *Nature (Lond.)*, 306:371–373.

79. Møllgard, K. and Møller, M. (1975): Dendro-dendritic gap junctions: A developmental approach. In: *Physiology and Pathology of Dendrites*, edited by G. W. Kreutzberg, pp. 79–89. Raven, New York.

80. Murphy, A. D., Hadley, R. D., and Kater, S. B. (1983): Axotomy-induced parallel increases in electrical and dye coupling between identified neurons of *Helisoma*. *J. Neurosci.*, 3:1422–1429.

81. Nelson, P. G. (1966): Interaction between spinal motoneurons of the cat. *J. Neurophysiol.*, 29:275–287.

82. Peracchia, C. (1980): Structural correlates of gap junction permeation. *Int. Rev. Cytol.*, 66:81–146.

83. Peters, A. (1980): Morphological correlates of epilepsy: Cells in the cerebral cortex. In: *Antiepileptic Drugs: Mechanisms of Action*, edited by G. H. Glaser, J. K. Penry, and D. M. Woodbury, pp. 21–48. Raven, New York.

84. Purpura, D. P. (1969): Mechanisms of propagation: Intracellular studies. In: *Basic Mechanisms of the Epilepsies*, edited by H. H. Jasper, A. A. Ward, Jr., and A. Pope, pp. 441–451. Little, Brown & Co., Boston.

85. Purpura, D. P., McMurtry, J. G., Leonard, C. F., and Malliani, A. (1966): Evidence for dendritic origin of spikes without depolarizing prepotentials in hippocampal neurons during

and after seizure. *J. Neurophysiol.*, 29:954–977.

86. Ramón, F., and Moore, J. W. (1978): Ephaptic transmission in squid giant axons. *Am. J. Physiol.*, 234:C162–169.

87. Rasminsky, M. (1980): Ephaptic transmission between single nerve fibres in the spinal nerve roots of dystrophic mice. *J. Physiol. (Lond.)*, 305:151–169.

88. Rayport, S. G., and Kandel, E. R. (1981): Epileptogenic agents enhance transmission at an identified weak electrical synapse in *Aplysia*. *Science*, 213:462–464.

89. Richardson, T. L., Turner, R. W., and Miller, J. J. (1984): Extracellular fields influence transmembrane potentials and synchronization of hippocampal neuronal activity. *Brain Res.*, 294:255–262.

90. Roney, K. J., Scheibel, A. B., and Shaw, G. L. (1979): Dendritic bundles: Survey of anatomical experiments and physiological theories. *Brain Res. Rev.*, 1:225–271.

91. Schmalbruch, H., and Jahnsen, H. (1981): Gap junctions on CA3 pyramidal cells of guinea pig hippocampus shown by freeze-fracture. *Brain Res.*, 217:175–178.

92. Schwartzkroin, P. A. (1983): Local circuit considerations and intrinsic neuronal properties involved in hyperexcitability and cell synchronization. In: *Basic Mechanisms of Neuronal Hyperexcitability*, edited by H. H. Jasper and N. M. van Gelder, pp. 75–108. Alan R. Liss, New York.

93. Seltzer, Z., and Devor, M. (1979): Ephaptic transmission in chronically damaged peripheral nerves. *Neurology*, 29:1061–1064.

94. Sloper, J. J. (1972): Gap junctions between dendrites in the primate neocortex. *Brain Res.*, 44:641–646.

95. Sloper, J. J. and Powell, T. P. S. (1978): Gap junctions between dendrites and somata of neurons in the primate sensori-motor cortex. *Proc. R. Soc. Lond. [Biol.]*, 203:39–47.

96. Shaw, G. L., Harth, E., and Scheibel, B. (1982): Cooperativity in brain function: assemblies of approximately 30 neurons. *Exp. Neurol.*, 77:324–358.

97. Snow, R. W., and Dudek, F. E. (1986): Evidence for neuronal interactions by an electrical field effect in CA3 and dentate regions of rat hippocampal slices. *Brain Res.* (in press).

98. Snow, R. W., and Dudek, F. E. (1984): Synchronous epileptiform bursts without chemical transmission in CA2, CA3 and dentate areas of the hippocampus. *Brain Res.*, 298:382–385.

99. Snow, R. W., and Dudek, F. E. (1984): Electrical fields directly contribute to action potential synchronization during convulsant-induced epileptiform bursts. *Brain Res.*, 323:114–118.

100. Somjen, G. C. (1979): Extracellular potassium in the mammalian central nervous system. *Ann. Rev. Physiol.*, 41:159–177.

101. Somjen, G. C., Aitken, P. G., Giacchino, J. L., and McNamara, J. O., Chapter 33.

102. Sotelo, C., and Korn, H. (1978): Morphological correlates of electrical and other interactions

through low-resistance pathways between neurons of the vertebrate central nervous system. *Int. Rev. Cytol.*, 55:67–107.

103. Sotelo, C., Llinàs, R., and Baker, R. (1974): Structural study of inferior olivary nucleus of the cat: morphological correlates of electrotonic coupling. *J. Neurophysiol.*, 27:541–559.

104. Spencer, W. A., and Kandel, E. R. (1961): Electrophysiology of hippocampal neurons. IV. Fast prepotentials. *J. Neurophysiol.*, 24:272–285.

105. Spira, M. E., and Bennett, M. V. L. (1972): Synaptic control of electrotonic coupling between neurons. *Brain Res.*, 37:294–300.

106. Spray, D. C., Stern, J. H., Harris, A. L., and Bennett, M. V. L. (1982): Gap junctional conductance: Comparison of senstivities to H and Ca ions. *Proc. Natl. Acad. Sci. U.S.A.*, 79:441–445.

107. Stewart, W. W. (1978): Functional connections between cells as revealed by dye-coupling with a highly fluorescent naphthalimide tracer. *Cell*, 14:741–759.

108. Stewart, W. W. (1981): Lucifer dyes—Highly fluorescent dyes for biological tracing. *Nature (Lond.)*, 292:17–21.

109. Taylor, C. P., and Dudek, F. E. (1982): A physiological test for electrotonic coupling between CA1 pyramidal cells in rat hippocampal slices. *Brain Res.*, 235:351–357.

110. Taylor, C. P., and Dudek, F. E. (1982): Synchronous neural afterdischarges in rat hippocampal slices without active chemical synapses. *Science*, 218:810–812.

111. Taylor, C. P., and Dudek, F. E. (1984): Excitation of hippocampal pyramidal cells by an electrical field effect. *J. Neurophysiol.*, 52:126–142.

112. Taylor, C. P., and Dudek, F. E. (1984): Synchronization without active chemical synapses during hippocampal afterdischarges. *J. Neurophysiol.*, 52:143–155.

113. Taylor, C. P., Krnjević, K., and Ropert, N. (1984): Facilitation of CA3 pyramidal cell firing by electrical fields generated antidromically. *Neuroscience*, 11:101–109.

114. Terzuolo, C. A., and Bullock, T. H. (1956): Measurement of imposed voltage gradient adequate to modulate neuronal firing. *Proc. Natl. Acad. Sci. U.S.A.*, 42:687–694.

115. Traub, R. D. (1982): Simulation of intrinsic bursting in CA3 hippocampal neurons. *Neuroscience*, 7:1233–1242.

116. Traub, R. D., Dudek, F. E., Taylor, C. P., and Knowles, W. D. (1985): Simulation of hippocampal afterdischarges synchronized by electrical interactions. *Neuroscience*, 14:1033–1038.

117. Traub, R. D., and Pedley, T. A. (1981): Virus-induced electrotonic coupling: hypothesis on the mechanism of periodic EEG discharges in Creutzfeldt-Jakob disease. *Ann. Neurol.*, 10:405–410.

118. Traub, R. D., and Wong, R. K. S. (1983): Synaptic mechanisms underlying interictal spike initiation in a hippocampal network. *Neurology*, 33:257–266.

119. Wong, R. K. S., Traub, R. D., and Miles, R., Chapter 29.

120. Yaari, Y., Konnerth, A., and Heinemann, U. (1983): Spontaneous epileptiform activity of CA1 hippocampal neurons in low extracellular calcium solutions. *Exp. Brain Res.*, 51:153–156.

121. Yarom, Y., and Spira, M. E. (1982): Extracellular potassium ions mediate specific neuronal interaction. *Science*, 216:80–82.

Advances in Neurology, Vol. 44, edited by
A. V. Delgado-Escueta, A. A. Ward, Jr.,
D. M. Woodbury, and R. J. Porter.
Raven Press, New York © 1986.

31

Ionic Changes and Alterations in the Size of the Extracellular Space During Epileptic Activity

H. D. Lux, U. Heinemann, and I. Dietzel

Abteilung Neurophysiologie, Max-Planck-Institut fuer Psychiatrie, D 8033 Planegg-Martinsried, Federal Republic of Germany

SUMMARY Experiments with ion-selective microelectrodes revealed that a considerable activity of K ions appears temporarily in the extracellular space (ES) during enhanced neuronal activity and is removed from the ES by diffusion, active uptake, and entry into glial cells. The glial uptake results from the preferential glial K permeability and spatial glial K buffering. The glia responds to the local extracellular accumulation by a depolarization of the exposed part of its membrane. This depolarization will spread along the glial syncytium or extended glial cells. At sites where the extracellular K concentration has not yet increased, the membrane potential will thus be depolarized with respect to the K diffusion potential. Here K will move from the intra- into the extracellular space, in order to restore the electrochemical equilibrium. This induces a current that carries K into glial cells at sites of maximal K accumulation and that transports K out of glial cells at remote areas. In this way K is spatially redistributed. The corresponding current loop in the ES is predominantly carried by Na and Cl, the majority ions. Thus, Na and Ca are transported to the site of K accumulation while Cl moves away. The Cl and K ions are only partially replaced by Na. Hence, a decrease of extracellular osmolarity results, which leads to a water flux from the ES into the cells, inducing a shrinkage of the ES at sites of maximal K accumulation. At remote sites, the opposite effect is expected due to K flow out of glia and Cl transport to these sites. Thus, remote from the area of maximal neuronal activity, an increase of the ES is expected. This mechanism can explain the measured depth profile of the changes in the ES.

At sites of maximal neuronal activity, the extracellular space undergoes a reduction by more than 30%. The ionic changes are accompanied by slow negative potential shifts. An increase in intracellular osmolarity due to enhanced metabolic activity and possibly KCl uptake mechanisms contributes to the changes in volume and ionic concentration. Model calculations of the after-effects of the loss of positive charges from the extracellular space and the K-specific glial buffering could predict size and time course of these changes. Experimental tests of this view include observations during epileptiform activity in gliotic scar foci as well as in hippocampal slices with depressed synaptic transmission.

The extra- and intracellular ionic changes influence the generation, spread, and termination of seizure activity. Thus, the increased extracellular K activity and the decreased free Ca will increase the neuronal excitability. A gain in intracellular Cl due to the osmotic changes could shift the Cl equilibrium potential in a depolarizing direction and consequently decrease the efficacy of postsynaptic inhibition, while an increase in intracellular Na concentration is assumed to activate an electrogenic transport process that helps to repolarize the nerve cell membrane potentials during and after a seizure.

Early studies on the ionic interrelationship of extracellular and intracellular spaces in invertebrate preparations suggested an increase of the extracellular potassium concentration during enhanced neuronal activity (30,133). Because of scarce information about the *in vivo* anatomy of brain spaces, it was difficult to extrapolate such data to pathophysiological processes during epilepsy. A survey of the actual ionic changes during epilepsy was only made possible by the use of ion-selective (160,161) microelectrodes (ISM). Such studies showed that the extracellular microenvironment undergoes temporal changes. Indeed, increases of neuronal activity, in particular those that are characteristic for epileptiform activity, result in considerable alterations of the ionic constitution and the size of the extracellular space. Thus, epileptiform activity is regularly associated with increases in extracellular potassium concentration ($[K^+]_o$) (35,40, 77,137,151) and most often also with increases (21,22) in extracellular chloride concentration ($[Cl^-]_o$), while extracellular sodium ($[Na^+]_o$) (20,22,23,108) and calcium concentration ($[Ca^{2+}]_o$) tend to decrease during seizure activity (see Chapter 32) (50,64,65,66,147). At the same time, the size of the extracellular space decreases by about 30% at sites of maximal neuronal activity (20,158). This effect counteracts to some degree possible larger decreases in $[Na^+]_o$, $[Ca^{2+}]_o$, and $[Cl^-]_o$ and may help to preserve neuronal functioning under conditions of excessive activity. On the other hand, the swelling of cells that underlies the reductions of extracellular space may eventually impair local microcirculation, and thereby oxygen supply, and thus contribute to cell damage during epilepsy (130).

These extra- and intracellular ionic changes influence the generation, spread, and termination of seizure activity (66,136). Thus, increases in $[K^+]_o$ (27,45,54,131) and decreases in $[Ca^{2+}]_o$ (31,126) will increase neuronal excitability. Increases in intracellular chloride concentration will shift the chloride equilibrium potential in a depolarizing direction and consequently decrease the efficacy of postsynaptic inhibition (1,80,112,118), while an increase in intracellular Na^+ concentration is assumed to activate an electrogenic transport process (81,87) that contributes to re- and even hyperpolarization of nerve cell membrane potentials during and after a seizure.

CHARACTERISTICS OF THE EXTRACELLULAR SPACE

The size of the extracellular space (ES) varies between 10 and 50 nm (157). It consists of an electrolyte-filled matrix of mainly glycoproteins. Membrane-bound receptors face the ES (for review see ref. 125), providing the sites for neurotransmitters, neuromodulators, and hormones and also for substances that have to reach the intracellular space by active or coupled transport (3) in order to serve their role in anabolic or catabolic metabolism.

The volume fraction of the ES with respect to brain volume was estimated with various methods to range from 5 to 20% (34,109,156, 157). A recently developed method (128) uses the sensitivity of the Corning K^+ ion exchange resin to choline and tetramethylammonium (TMA) and other tetraalkylated ammonium ions (124). With these electrodes, it is possible to compare the diffusional distribution of TMA released in constant amounts from a nearby iontophoresis electrode both in nervous tissue and in free solution. Since TMA—and also choline—uptake can be neglected during the time of measurement (55,105,128), the volume fraction and the tortuosity of the extracellular space can be estimated from a comparison of the diffusional equilibration in free solutions and in the tissue. In the cerebellum (125,128) and neocortex of rats (105), the volume fraction of the ES was estimated to be about 18%. Although there appears to be a certain scatter in the size of the ES (73,132), there is so far little indication that the ES varies systematically with cortical depth. However, in rat hippocampal slices (68; U. Heinemann and W. J. Wadman, *in preparation*), variations of the ES with respect to different layers and areas were found. While the ES of the dentate area appeared to be comparable to that in other structures, it was smaller in area CA1. In the stratum radiatum, moleculare, and oriens, the volume fraction was found to range from 12 to 16%, while it was only 2 to 7% in stratum pyramidale of area CA1. This confirms previous observations that cellular elements are particularly densely packed in the stratum pyramidale of area CA1 (45). This low extracellular volume fraction could render the hippocampal area CA1 very suited for ephaptic interactions, since the same transmembrane currents will result in a higher extracellular current density and larger and steeper potential gradients than in other areas of the brain.

The diffusion measurements suggest that most molecules can diffuse freely in the ES. The observation that Ca^{2+} diffusion may be slowed (123) could be explained by the Ca^{2+} buffering capacity of the ES. The extracellular free Ca^{2+} at 1.2 mM is 25% lower than the total 1.6 mM Ca^{2+} content of the cerebrospinal fluid (2). This discrepancy may reflect buffering of Ca^{2+} by bicarbonate and proteins and a constant clearance of Ca^{2+} into the vascular system.

CHANGES IN THE SIZE OF THE EXTRACELLULAR SPACE

Changes in extracellular space were inferred from concentration changes of TMA^+ or choline$^+$. Constant amounts of these ions were iontophoretically injected into the ES (Fig. 1). If the neocortex was superfused with a hyperosmotic solution containing sucrose, iontophoretically evoked TMA^+ or choline$^+$ signals were reduced (20). This indicated a widening of the ES consequent to a water flow from the intraosmotic into the hyperosmotic extracellular space.

As is illustrated in Fig. 2, repetitive electrical stimulation leads to increases in TMA^+ signals by up to 50%. This depends on stimulus intensity, frequency, and train duration. Such increases in TMA^+ signals were observed during

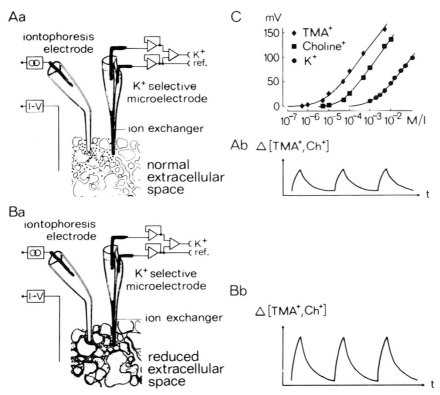

FIG. 1. Monitoring of extracellular space size changes and of extracellular potassium concentration with a nominally K$^+$-selective electrode. **Aa:** Arrangements of electrodes. A double-barreled ion-selective/reference microelectrode is used to measure changes in extracellular potassium concentration and iontophoretically induced concentration increases of tetramethylammonium (TMA) or choline (calibration curves in **C**). The marker substance for the extracellular space is regularly released in constant amounts from the iontophoresis electrode by means of a current pump. The applied current is monitored through a current voltage converter (I–V). **Ab:** Schematic illustration of iontophoretically induced changes in TMA or choline concentrations at resting conditions. **Ba, Bb:** Illustration of alterations in the size of the extracellular space (ES). A reduction of ES size results in an increase of iontophoretically induced TMA or choline signals.

iontophoretic elevations of $[K^+]_o$ or when cells died after the movement of the electrode assembly within the cortex, which led to large transient rises in $[K^+]_o$ (20,57). It can thus be assumed that the ES shrinks under these conditions. A similar activity-dependent shrinkage of ES size was also observed in the developing optic nerve (15).

Figure 2 shows the depth dependence of changes in the ES in relation to the laminar profile of stimulus-induced changes in $[K^+]_o$. The shrinkage of the ES is largest in middle cortical layers, at sites of maximal K^+ accumulation, while expansions of the ES can be observed in deep cortical layers and sometimes also in upper cortical layers. The average reduction of the ES during stimulus-induced seizure activity was 30% in middle cortical layers. A reduction of the ES could be caused by metabolically induced increases in intracellular osmolarity leading to a subsequent water entry into cells. By summating measured increases (Fig. 4) in $[Cl^-]_o$, $[Na^+]_o$, and $[K^+]_o$ (20,22,23,105) at the end of seizure activity, an increase in tissue osmolarity by 10 to 30 mM was estimated. This, however, only accounts for a reduction of the ES by about 8% (20,22). Therefore, additional mechanisms are required, which should also explain why the decreases of the ES are largest at the site of maximal K^+ elevations and why a widening of the ES occurs at remote areas.

Epilepsy is not the only condition during which the size of the ES can decrease. Changes in ES have also been observed during spreading depression (55,125) and hypoxia (55). There, they amount to about 50 and 60%, respectively. Even larger reductions in the ES are observed during local application of excitatory amino acids, where the ES can shrink by up to 80% (25,70a).

SEIZURE-RELATED CHANGES IN EXTRACELLULAR POTASSIUM CONCENTRATION

Kinetics and Laminar Distributions of Changes in $[K^+]_o$

Electrical stimulation of the cortex (16,77, 113,118,146,152), thalamus (52,58), spinal cord (8,92,93,148), dorsal-column nuclei (95,96,97), and hippocampus (5,28), or of appropriate fiber systems to and from these areas, leads, in most cases, to considerable rises in $[K^+]_o$ from baseline levels of about 3 mM (Figs. 2 and 3). Their amplitudes depend on stimulus intensity, frequency, and train duration and are limited by "ceiling levels" of between 10 and 12 mM (28,29,52,63) in different preparations and structures. Only rarely, when a predominantly inhibitory pathway is stimulated, such stimulations can cause decreases in $[K^+]_o$, presumably resulting from decreases in neuronal discharge rate below resting level (52,62,144). Large rises in $[K^+]_o$ are also associated with seizures induced by drugs such as penicillin (122), pentetrazol (61,113,114), oenanthotoxin (111), 4-aminopyridine (37,59), and picrotoxin (59).

After termination of stimulation (and eventually evoked self-sustained epileptiform afterdischarges, SAD), $[K^+]_o$ delines to subbaseline levels (Figs. 2 and 3) and then slowly returns to previous resting level (62,92,108). The amplitudes and durations of these undershoots in $[K^+]_o$ are directly related to the amplitude of the preceding rise in $[K^+]_o$ (58,62,96,97,108,152).

Elevations in $[K^+]_o$ are not uniformly distributed throughout a given structure, and they correlate closely with the increase in activity of nearby neurons. Therefore, measurements of changes in $[K^+]_o$ can help to localize a focus in an epileptic tissue. In cat neocortex, the largest rises in $[K^+]_o$ are usually found in layer III/IV (16,67), irrespective of the area studied and irrespective of the convulsant used to elicit epileptiform activity. In the thalamic relay nucleus (52), they are greatest in those areas that are actually activated. In hippocampus, the largest increases in $[K^+]_o$ are observed in the pyramidal cell layer (5,68,98).

Most potassium appears to stem from unmyelinated parts of a neuron such as somatas and dendrites of nerve cells and from terminal fiber systems. In the cerebellum, 40 to 60% of K^+ elevations during stimulation of the parallel fibers were estimated to result from presynaptic release (127). Postsynaptic intracellular stimulation revealed that activation of Ca^{2+}-dependent K^+ conductances (94,99,100) is most effective in causing elevations of $[K^+]_o$ (78). This is due to the large permeability of these channels (129). Hyperpolarizing current injection into nerve cells did not lead to measurable changes in $[K^+]_o$, while de- and hyperpolarizing current injection into glial cells elicited increases and decreases in $[K^+]_o$, respectively (78). This suggests that deviations from the electrochemical equilibrium in glia could result in changes of $[K^+]_o$. Part of the $[K^+]_o$ rises could also result from an increase in concentration due to a shrinkage of the ES. A shrinkage of the ES by 50% would, however, increase $[K^+]_o$ by only 1.5 mM.

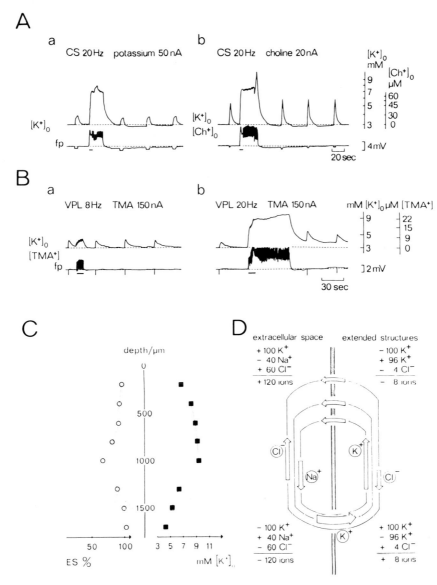

FIG. 2. Stimulus-induced changes in extracellular potassium concentration and in extracellular space size. **Aa:** Iontophoretically induced and stimulus-induced rises in extracellular K^+ concentration and simultaneously recorded negative potential shift in the field potential recording during stimulation of the cortical surface with 20 Hz. Train duration indicated by horizontal bars. Field potentials (fp) in this and subsequent figures recorded with negativity upward. Note that iontophoretically induced K^+ signals are smaller during and subsequent to seizure activity. **Ab:** Same experiment, but iontophoretically induced changes in extracellular choline concentration. Note the increase in choline signals subsequent to seizure activity. Note also that field potential transients induced by current injection from the phoresis pipette are increased in amplitude in both **Aa** and **Ab**, indicating that the resistivity of the ES increased following seizure activity. **Ba, Bb:** Rises in $[K^+]_o$ induced by weak (**a**) and moderate (**b**) stimulation of the nucleus ventroposterolateralis and iontophoretically induced TMA signals. Note that the more intense stimulation induced changes in TMA signals, indicating a shrinkage of the ES. **C:** Laminar profile of reductions in ES size and of increases in $[K^+]_o$ elicited by repetitive electrical stimulation in cat somatosensory cortex. Note that the shrinkage of ES size is largest in the area of maximal K^+ accumulation. Numbers on the vertical axis refer to recording depth below cortical surface. **D:** Illustration of the ionic movements that accompany spatial K^+ buffering by extended passive structures (glia and passive neurons). For details see text.

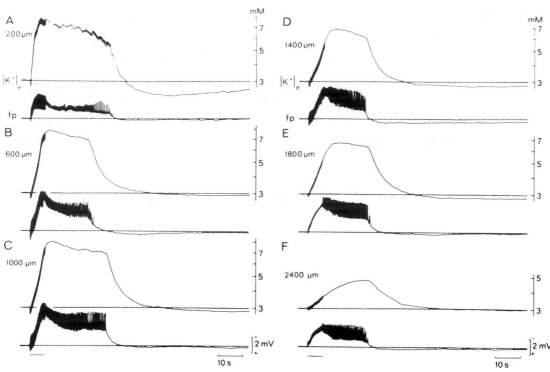

FIG. 3. Laminar profile of stimulus-induced changes in extracellular potassium concentration and simultaneously recorded field potentials (fp). Numbers refer to recording depth below cortical surface. Rises in $[K^+]_o$ were elicited by reptitive electrical stimulation of the cortical surface. Time calibration in **F** applies also to the other recordings.

An important question is what percentage of the K^+ released from neuron does actually appear in the ES. A significant fraction could immediately be cleared away into neurons and glia. An approximation can be obtained by correlating the initial rise in $[K^+]_o$ during a stimulus train to the number of extracellularly recorded action potentials. This gives an estimate of an increase in $[K^+]_o$ by 0.01 to 0.04 mM per action potential (21), which is close to estimates obtained by correlating $[K^+]_o$ baseline fluctuations to spontaneous discharge activity (150). If this K^+ release is multiplied by the number of action potentials generated during a tonic clonic seizure, an increase of $[K^+]_o$ to between 25 and 50 mM would be expected. Since the ceiling level is between 10 and 12 mM, about 70% of the released K^+ should have disappeared from the ES by some K^+ regulation mechanism. Similar estimates were obtained in the hippocampus when the generation of population spikes was related to the rise in $[K^+]_o$ (68).

Additional information about such clearance mechanisms stems from comparisons of extra-cellular and intracellular recordings in the isolated frog spinal cord and in the drone retina. If all the K^+ released from neurons remained in the ES, the kinetics of the extracellular K^+ concentration should mirror the intracellular $[K^+]$ change. Since the neurons occupy at least twice as much volume as the ES, the extracellular $[K^+]_o$ rise should be twice as large as the intracellular $[K^+]$ decrease. However, extracellular and intracellular $[K^+]$ changes reached about the same values (44), and intraneuronal $[K^+]$ continued to drop during repetitive stimulation while extracellular $[K^+]$ had already reached its peak level (44). Such measurements revealed that only a fraction of the neuronally released K^+ appears in the ES. That glial K^+ uptake plays a role in K^+ regulation is suggested by observations in the drone retina, which demonstrated that $[K^+]$ increased within glial cells during stimulation with light (12,13). Such mechanisms effectively prevented excessive increases in $[K^+]_o$ that would otherwise result in a depolarizing inactivation of action potential-generating mechanisms (for review, see ref.

115). Larger rises in $[K^+]_o$ and inactivation of neuronal firing are, however, observed during spreading depression.

Undershoots in $[K^+]_o$ and Termination of Seizure Activity

To finally restore the normal electrolyte concentration in the tissue, active K^+ reuptake into neurons is necessary. Various lines of evidence indicate that active K^+ uptake is involved in the generation of the undershoots in $[K^+]_o$ that occur in some preparations after enhanced neuronal activity. Thus, O_2 consumption is increased during and after increases in $[K^+]_o$, and the enzymes of the respiratory chain are activated (108; for review see ref. 146). Additional evidence for K^+ uptake during this period stems from experiments in which iontophoretically evoked K^+ signals were studied (5,62,63,66,68). It was found (Fig. 2Aa) that externally introduced constant amounts of K^+ resulted in smaller K^+ signals during stimulus-induced rises and subsequent undershoots as compared to resting conditions (5,63,68). An interesting point in this finding is that increased K^+ uptake persists after $[K^+]_o$ has decayed to subbaseline levels. This could be explained by a maintained elevation in intracellular $[Na^+]$, which is the main activating factor for K^+ uptake. Indeed, recent intracellular measurements in frog spinal cord have shown that intracellular $[Na^+]$ is elevated much longer than is extracellular $[K^+]_o$ and that the membrane potential is much more hyperpolarized than the K^+ equilibrium potential at that time (44). All these findings indicate that undershoots are generated by the activation of an Na^+-K^+ exchange pump. The pumping can, however, only cause a decrease in $[K^+]_o$ below baseline levels if the locally available amount of K^+ has previously been reduced by other K^+ clearance mechanisms such as K^+ uptake into glial cells (7,47,48) and spatial redistribution of K^+ by diffusion (119) and glial buffering (19,21).

The duration of the undershoots is related to the duration of the postictal depression of the electroencephalograph (EEG) (58,65) and of the intracerebral field potentials (fp) in all experimental epilepsies so far investigated. During the undershoots, the frequency and the amplitude of interictal discharges were reduced and the neuronal discharge rate declined to below resting frequency. In the thalamic relay nucleus ventroposterolateralis (VPL), the probability of antidromic invasion of action potentials and the efficacy of orthodromic synaptic transmission were reduced (58). Similarly, the threshold to induce self-sustained afterdischarges was found to be elevated (58).

Intracellular studies revealed that the membrane potential often declined before the end of repetitive stimulation (110) or seizure activity (129). The same pattern of membrane potential changes could be induced by intracellular Na^+ injection (81,87). This suggests that activation of an electrogenic pump mechanism, with a net outward transport of positive charges (153,154), participates in the termination of seizure activity. In addition, the membrane conductance was found to be increased early during repolarization and undershoots of membrane potentials. This is probably due to seizure-related intracellular accumulation of Ca^{2+} and a subsequent activation of a Ca^{2+}-dependent K^+ conductance (74,76,78,94). How much these two factors contribute quantitatively to termination of seizure activity and which other factors are involved is yet unknown. Such factors could be extracellular adenosine accumulation (104) and increases in PCO_2 (9), which both can suppress development of ictal activity.

Changes in Extracellular Sodium Concentration

Since Na^+ and K^+ are expected to exchange in about a 1:1 ratio during action potentials (72,86), considerable reductions of $[Na^+]_o$ are expected during seizure activity. Indeed, reductions in $[Na^+]_o$ by up to 9 mM in neocortex (22,23,106) and by more than 15 mM in hippocampus (166) have been measured during repetitive electrical stimulation (Fig. 4) and drug-induced seizures (Fig. 8) (20). The kinetics of the $[Na^+]_o$ changes mirror the $[K^+]_o$ increases only initially. After a decline for 1 to 5 sec during stimulation or seizures, $[Na^+]_o$ rises again, and in deeper cortical layers it may even increase above resting level still during the enhanced neuronal firing (Fig. 4). That $[Na^+]_o$ decreases less than $[K^+]_o$ rises does not mean, however, that more K^+ enters the ES than Na^+ leaves the cells. A 30% reduction of the ES in middle cortical layers should have elevated the initial $[Na^+]_o$ to near 200 mM from about 145 mM under resting conditions. Hence, the amount of Na^+ leaving the ES is comparable to the amount of 25 to 50 mM released K^+. Similar estimates of extracellular Na^+ loss are also obtained when the initial reduction in $[Na^+]_o$ is extrapolated

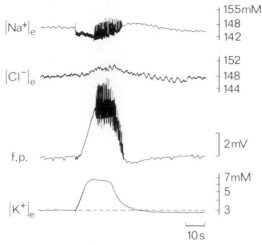

FIG. 4. Comparison of stimulus-induced changes in extracellular Na⁺, Cl⁻, and K⁺ concentration during repetitive electrical stimulation and subsequent self-sustained seizure activity in the sensorimotor cortex of cat. The Na⁺ recording was not corrected for simultaneously occurring changes in extracellular Ca^{2+} concentration. Field potential (fp) is also shown.

over the number of action potentials generated during a seizure.

Changes in Extracellular Chloride Concentration

The results reported so far indicate that extracellular Na⁺ and K⁺ concentrations can increase at the end of seizure activity in middle cortical layers, where the largest activation of neuronal elements occurs. This points to a simultaneous increase in tissue osmolarity, which should also reflect in a rise of the extracellular anion concentrations. Measurements of $[Cl^-]_o$ changes (Figs. 4 and 8) revealed that $[Cl^-]_o$ increases during seizure activity by up to 7 mM, which was in some experiments preceded by a small reduction in $[Cl^-]_o$ (20–22,106). The sum of changes in $[Na^+]_o$, $[K^+]_o$, and $[Cl^-]_o$ in middle cortical layers indicates an increase in osmolarity by maximally 28 mOsm. Such an increase in tissue osmolarity could for instance be explained by an increase in intracellular osmotic pressure caused by cleavage of larger molecules during the time of enhanced neuronal and metabolic activity (6,79). This in turn would cause a water flux out of the extracellular space into the hyperosmotic cells until the osmotic pressure is equal in adjacent compartments. At the same time, a shrinkage of the ES would occur. An estimated increase in tissue osmolarity by 28

mOsm can, however, only explain a decrease in the size of the ES by about 8%. This is a quarter of the actually observed shrinkage.

Because of the shrinkage of the ES, the increases in $[Cl^-]_o$ do not mean that Cl⁻ is released during neuronal activity. With an initial $[Cl^-]_o$ of 150 mM, a decrease of the ES by 30% would increase $[Cl^-]_o$ to near 200 mM. The actually observed $[Cl^-]_o$ rises are much smaller and suggest that about 35 mM Cl⁻ could leave the ES during a seizure of some 30 sec. If some of this chloride would enter neurons (17,114) and if it is assumed that the neuronal compartment is twice as large as the extracellular one, an increase in intracellular chloride concentration by maximally 17 mM is expected. Indeed, similar increases in intraneuronal $[Cl^-]$ have been observed during enhanced neuronal activity in cat spinal cord (114). Such $[Cl^-]_i$ rises could also be caused by ammonia, which is able to cause epileptiform activity (1,82). Thus it appears that chloride entry into neurons with a resulting reduction of IPSP amplitudes may well support seizure generation. However, it should also be considered that some Na⁺ (3) and Cl⁻ could enter glial cells in spite of low conductances for these ions in glial cell membranes (85). Cl⁻ could enter glial cells by means of a KCl cotransport (7,162), which explains the continued K⁺ uptake into glial cells under conditions of homogeneous K⁺ elevation in a given tissue (71,85).

SPATIAL BUFFERING OF POTASSIUM CAN ACCOUNT FOR SLOW POTENTIAL GENERATION DURING SEIZURES AND FOR SHRINKAGE OF THE EXTRACELLULAR SPACE SIZE

Since metabolic effects can only partially explain the shrinkage of the ES, additional mechanisms have to be taken into account. Experiments with K⁺-selective microelectrodes suggested that a considerable amount of K⁺ may be temporarily removed from the ES into glial cells during enhanced neuronal activity (12,85). Two mechanisms by which glial cells could remove extracellular K⁺ are also accompanied by water fluxes from the ES into the cells. These are uptake of KCl and spatial glial buffering.

Spatial K⁺ buffering (21,101,133) depends on local extracellular K⁺ accumulation and a subsequent depolarization of glial cells. This depolarization will spread along the glial syncytium or extended glial cells. At sites where the extracellular K⁺ concentration has not yet increased, the membrane potential will thus be depolarized with respect to the K^+ diffusion potential (36). Here K^+ will move from the intra- into the extracellular space, in order to restore the electrochemical equilibrium. This induces a current that carries K^+ into glial cells at sites of maximal K^+ accumulation and that transports K^+ out of glial cells at remote areas. In this way K^+ is spatially redistributed. This K^+ shift in turn causes an extracellular potential gradient, which leads to an extracellular current (10,145). This extracellular current is, however, not carried by potassium (4). According to their larger concentrations, Na^+ and Cl^- ions are the dominating charge carriers in the extracellular space. Thus, Na^+ is transported to the site of K^+ accumulation while Cl^- moves away. The Cl^- and K^+ ions are only partially replaced by Na^+. Hence, a decrease of extracellular osmolarity results, which leads to a water flux from the ES into the cells, inducing a shrinkage of the ES at sites of maximal K^+ accumulation. At remote sites, the opposite effect is expected due to K^+ flow out of glia and Cl^- transport to these sites (Fig. 2D). Thus, remote from the area of maximal neuronal activity, an increase of the ES is expected. This mechanism can thus explain the measured depth profile of the changes in the ES (Fig. 2C). In addition, it accounts for the generation of the slow field potentials. By such a mechanism, glial cells can also contribute to the homeostasis of extracellular Cl^-, Ca^{2+}, and Na^+ concentration (19,22,59).

This mechanism requires that glial-cell membranes are predominantly K^+ permeable and that the cells are spatially extended and/or to a certain degree electrically coupled. If glial membranes are exclusively permeable to K^+, then their membrane potential can only be influenced by changing the K^+ concentrations on both sides of the membrane. The relationship between changes in $[K^+]_o$ and glial membrane potentials has been studied in a number of preparations (36,85,102,103,110,133,135,141,142). In some preparations, smaller membrane potentials were measured than were predicted from the Nernst equation. The technical reasons for this, such as the precise determination of the K^+ elevation, the neglect of extracellular field potential changes associated with elevations in $[K^+]_o$, and inhomogeneities in the K^+ elevation around a glial cell, have been discussed (110). However, when such factors could be controlled experimentally by the precise measurement of extra- and intracellular K^+ concentration (85), an excellent agreement between the measured and predicted membrane potentials was found. Also, patch-clamp analysis of glial cells has demonstrated that glial cells possess only K^+ channels under physiological conditions (83). The K^+ conductance of glial membrane channels is rather large, displays little or no voltage sensitivity, and is associated with very long open states. These large conductances account for the low input resistance of glial cells. Consequently, intraglial current injection causes much more easily changes in $[K^+]_o$ than in intraneuronal current injection (78).

Both astrocytes and oligodendrocytes can have long processes, and some astrocytes may stretch throughout the cortical thickness (145). Evidence that glial cells are electrically coupled is based on several observations. Gap junctions by which glial cells can be electrically coupled have been found (163) in neocortex. Both *in situ* and *in vitro* investigations have suggested that oligodendrocytes and astrocytes are dye-coupled, since Lucifer yellow injected into one glial cell stained regularly more than one cell (51,84). However, the spatial K^+ buffer mechanism would also function in the absence of electrical coupling, as long as a spatial K^+ concentration gradient exists along the surfaces of a series of extended glial cells. K^+ released remote from the site of uptake would depolarize the neighboring cells, causing uptake at one site and release at remote sites etc., until the spatial K^+ gradient is homogeneous. This state is, however, only rarely reached during a single seizure, and even during prolonged status epilepticus a spatial K^+ gradient is preserved in neocortex (61).

SLOW FIELD POTENTIAL GENERATION, ELEVATION IN $[K^+]_o$, AND K^+-MEDIATED DEPOLARIZATION OF GLIAL CELLS

If spatial glial buffering occurs in a tissue, then local increases in $[K^+]_o$, which lead to transglial K^+ currents, should be accompanied by electrical potential changes. These potential changes should last as long as the current flows and the largest negative potential changes will indicate the site where K^+ leaves the ES. Since the current flows as long as the glial cells are depolarized by the extracellular K^+ elevation, the time course of the glial cell depolarization resembles the time course of the slow potential changes. Indeed, slow potentials show an intimate relationship to depolarizations of glial cells during interictal spikes, sustained seizures and during spreading depression (11,18,43,110,145,149,151), while the relationship is less close to the behavior of nerve cells. Negative field potential (fp) shifts have their largest amplitude at the site of maximal K^+ elevations, and they may reverse polarity at remote sites. Shortly after the end of seizure activity, the fp changes polarity and becomes positive at sites of maximal K^+ elevation. This relationship was established in neocortex, thalamus, spinal cord, hippocampus, and cerebellum (52,67,68,127). Similar slow field potential profiles were previously observed in a number of experimental epilepsies (26,49).

An interesting finding is that the slow field potentials change their polarity much faster than the $[K^+]_o$ elevations (52,93,110). This mismatch of slow field potential and $[K^+]_o$ changes at the end of seizure activity could be explained by a reversal of the direction of the K^+ current at that time. After the end of the seizure, K^+ is predominantly pumped back into those neurons that previously released the largest amount of K^+. The spatially unequal pumping rate of the neurons induces a positive change in the extracellular potential while reducing $[K^+]_o$. This in turn leads to a release of K^+ out of adjacent glial cells and a reversal of the glial buffer current. Since the K^+ flowing into neurons is partially replaced by K^+ coming out of glia, K^+ drops more slowly than the field potentials (57).

As expected from the spatial K^+ buffer hypothesis, artificial elevations of $[K^+]_o$ by means of superfusion or local application of K^+ induce negative field potential shifts, both in normal and gliotic tissue of alumina cream foci (29,38,39,57,63,67). Moreover, any pharmacological treatment that results in alterations of stimulus-induced K^+ elevations produces alterations of the accompanying slow field potentials (8,67,148). Thus, convulsants such as picrotoxin enhanced both slow negative field potentials and amplitudes of K^+ elevations (8), while anticonvulsants such as phenytoin, barbiturates, and diazepines had the opposite effect (67). Similar alterations of K^+ signals and slow field potentials were also reported when baseline K^+ levels were varied in an *in vitro* preparation (67). Moreover, slow field potentials also accompanied K^+ elevations elicited by local K^+ application and by antidromic stimulation under conditions of blocked chemical synaptic transmission (88,89) in the *in vitro* hippocampal slice (68,89). This indicates that slow potentials are not just a sum of synaptic potentials.

PREDICTIONS OF SPATIAL K^+ REDISTRIBUTION BASED ON A LAMINAR ANALYSIS OF SEIZURE-RELATED SLOW POTENTIALS

As described above, spatial K^+ buffer currents are reflected in characteristic extracellular

potential changes, with a potential minimum at locations where K^+ leaves the ES. The magnitude of the K^+ currents may be estimated from the spatial changes of the slow field potential gradients (14,19,20,24,46). For this purpose, laminar profiles of slow potential changes during seizure activity were measured in the neocortex (Fig. 5). Repetitive stimulation of the thalamus or the cortical surface induced negative potentials at the sites of maximal neuronal activity and positive slow potentials at remote areas. From these potential gradients, which amount on the average to 4 mV/mm tissue vertical to the cortical surface, a current source density profile can be reconstructed using techniques originally used in the analysis of synaptic potentials (32,33,53,121,134,143).

Such a current source density (CSD) (Fig. 5B and C) analysis revealed a large sink in about layer III/IV and sometimes a second smaller one in layer V, separated and surrounded by current sources. Under the assumption that this sink–source distribution arises from spatial K^+ buffer currents, the amount of K^+ moving out of or into the ES, respectively, can be estimated. These estimates yield K^+ movements of 0.1 to 0.5 mmol/sec · liter of brain tissue. Hence, over the time of a seizure of 10 sec, 3 to 5 mmol K^+ are transported by the spatial currents. If a volume fraction of 20% is assumed, it can be estimated that such a current should have reduced the extracellular K^+ concentration by 15 to 25 mM during the course of seizure activity. Since without K^+ regulation mechanisms an increase in $[K^+]_o$ to about 40 mM could be expected (see above), this reduction in $[K^+]_o$ due to glial buffering could explain why the actually observed $[K^+]_o$ increases amount to only 10 to 12 mM.

MODEL PREDICTIONS

From the measurements described so far, it becomes clear that the ionic changes, the field potentials, and the extracellular volume changes are interrelated. Therefore, it should be possible to predict most of these changes from a small set of basic measurements. In order to describe how the intraneuronal, intraglial, and extracellular Na^+, K^+, and Cl^- concentrations, as well as the changes in the relative volumes of glial, neuronal, and extracellular compartments, depend on each other, a mathematical model was developed (19,23).

Basically, the model uses generally valid principles such as conservation of mass and charge. In addition, specific properties of brain tissue were incorporated. Thus, it was assumed that

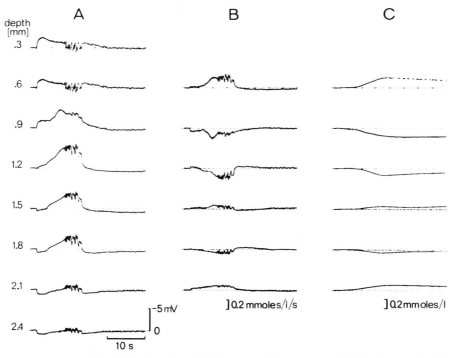

FIG. 5. **A:** Laminar profile of stimulus-induced field potential changes recorded simultaneously with an eight-contact glass microelectrode assembly inserted about perpendicularly to the cortical surface. The interval between electrode tips was 300 μm. **B:** Current source density profile calculated from the field potential recordings in **A**. Under the assumption that the current underlying generation of field potentials represents transmembraneous K⁺ currents, the calculated currents are expressed in K⁺ displacement per liter brain tissue per second by dividing the current through the Faraday number. Inward currents into cells are represented as downward deflections. **C:** Integrated displacement of potassium over time.

the total volume of the brain stays constant, there is no difference in osmolarity between adjacent cells, Na^+ is exchanged against K^+ during neuronal activity in a 1:1 ratio (86), and glial cells are exclusively permeable for K^+ (83,85,110). Using this model, all ionic concentration changes and the volume changes in the different compartments can be calculated, if the glial membrane potential, changes in osmolarity, and amount of K^+ transferred into glial cells via glial buffering or active uptake are known (Fig. 6).

CHANGES IN $[K^+]_o$ AND ES SIZE IN GLIOTIC FOCI INDUCED BY ALUMINA CREAM

Glial K^+ buffering is associated with the induction of slow potential shifts (39), decreases of the size of the ES at sites of maximal neuronal activity, and a widening of the ES at remote areas (21). To further investigate the possible role of glial buffering, a model preparation was used where K^+ release was limited to a re-

stricted active zone bordering passive tissue. Such a preparation is the chronic gliotic scar focus induced by topical application of alumina cream. Here the epileptogenic zone of neuronal tissue is bordering an area where the neurons are replaced by glial cells.

In this border zone between normal and gliotic tissue, spontaneous epileptic activity could be seen which was characterized by increases of 0.3 to 1 mM in $[K^+]_o$ (Fig. 7A and B) associated with relatively small reductions in $[Ca^{2+}]_o$ (57,60,68). Repetitive electrical stimulation induced maximal changes in $[K^+]_o$ and $[Ca^{2+}]_o$ in these areas. To test whether active K^+ uptake is impaired in these active zones, we measured the relationship between rises in $[K^+]_o$ and subsequent undershoots. These measures showed no statistically significant deviation from those in normal cortex. Measurements of changes in $[K^+]_o$ induced by iontophoretic application of K^+ before, during, and after seizure activity revealed that artificially induced K^+ elevations were reduced during undershoots in $[K^+]_o$ as was the case in normal cortex. Thus, we conclude that active K^+ uptake is not significantly

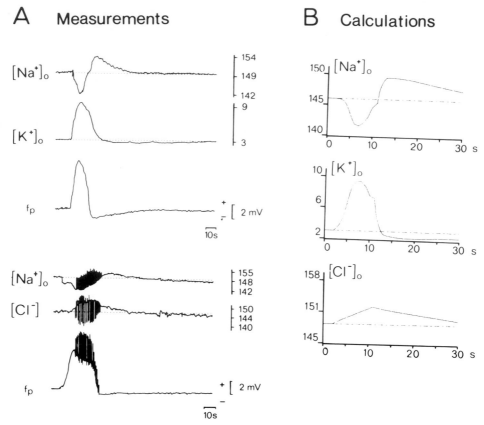

FIG. 6. Comparison of measured Na^+, Cl^-, and K^+ concentration changes with calculated ionic changes. The calculations were based on the assumption that spatial K^+ buffering contributes to electrolyte regulation and were based on field potential (fp) analysis as in Fig. 5, recordings of glial membrane potential taken from the literature, and the assumption that seizure activity is accompanied by a 10–30-mM increase in intracellular particle concentrations. The differences between calculated (20%) and measured (30%) ES size changes may be attributed to KCl uptake.

impaired in the area of epileptogenesis (57; see also 42,107,159), and epileptogenesis may be due to alterations in Ca^{2+}-dependent electrogenesis (60,138,139,140; see also 116,117).

Based on the spatial K^+ buffer hypothesis, a number of predictions can be made that can at least be qualitatively tested. These include that K^+ changes induced by stimulation should be recordable over a larger area than changes in $[Ca^{2+}]_o$. Indeed, this is the case, as revealed by recordings where a combined assembly of K^+- and Ca^{2+}-selective electrodes was used to monitor changes in $[K^+]_o$ and $[Ca^{2+}]_o$ at various intervals between the center of the scar and the epileptic focus at the border of the gliotic tissue. While rises in $[K^+]_o$ were observed as deep as 1.5 mm in the gliotic tissue, decreases in $[Ca^{2+}]_o$ were only observed at distances of less than 400 μm from the focus. In order to verify that no excitable elements are found within gliotic

tissue, we monitored changes in $[Ca^{2+}]_o$, $[K^+]_o$, and $[Na^+]_o$ during excitatory amino acid application within the gliotic tissue. No significant ionic changes were found at sites where also stimulus-induced changes in $[Ca^{2+}]_o$ were absent, suggesting that the stimulus-induced K^+ release in these areas does not stem from adjacent excitable elements.

Second, we expected that artificial application of K^+ should induce negative potential shifts in both normal and gliotic tissue. For normal cortical tissue it has been shown by various groups that superfusion with K^+-enriched solutions induced slow field potentials (29,38,39, 63). The same is the case when K^+ is microinjected into brain tissue by either iontophoresis (67) or pressure. Both superfusion and K^+ iontophoresis are also capable of eliciting slow negative potential shifts in gliotic tissue (57,67,68).

Third, we expected that constant current

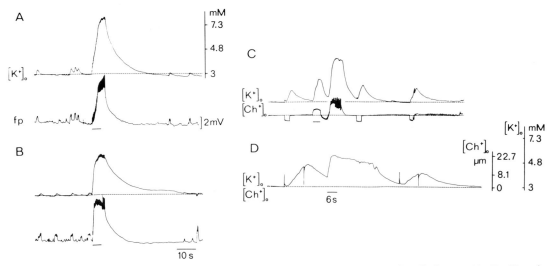

FIG. 7. Recording of stimulus-induced rises in $[K^+]_o$ in the bordering zone of a gliotic scar (**A, B, C**) and within gliotic tissue (**D**). **A, B**: Rises in $[K^+]_o$ during cortical surface stimulation and spontaneously occurring rises in $[K^+]_o$ during spontaneous interictal activity. Note the depression of spontaneous interictal discharges during the decay of $[K^+]_o$. **C, D**: Seizure related rises in $[K^+]_o$ following stimulation of the ventrobasal thalamic complex. Note the delay between seizure onset and stimulus-induced increase in $[K^+]_o$. Seizure in C is followed by an enhanced choline signal, while seizure in D is followed by a reduced choline signal. Recording in A from the border zone between normal and gliotic tissue, in D from inside gliotic tissue. Calibrations in A apply also to **B**, and calibrations in **D** also to recording in **C**.

through gliotic tissue should result in large alterations of $[K^+]_o$, which exceed those expected if the current were restricted to the ES. Indeed, a comparison of current transport effects on extracellular K^+ concentration between normal (41) and gliotic tissue (57) showed that similar alterations of $[K^+]_o$ are observed in gliotic and normal tissue, demonstrating that transcellular currents and even transglial currents are capable of redistributing potassium.

Further, we expected that stimulus-induced $[K^+]_o$ increases in the surrounding zone of an epileptic scar would be associated with reductions in the ES, while a widening of the ES should occur within the gliotic tissue. This is indeed the case as evidenced in Fig. 7C and D. This does not mean, however, that the ES cannot shrink within gliotic tissue. When K^+ is artificially elevated within gliotic tissue by means of local K^+ iontophoresis, it is observed that TMA or choline signals induced by constant current injections increase in amplitude, indicating a reduction of ES size.

CHANGES OF EXTRACELLULAR POTASSIUM CONCENTRATION AND EXTRACELLULAR SPACE IN THE HIPPOCAMPAL SLICE

In normal cortical tissue, K^+ release can be restricted to one particular cellular layer. This permits further investigations on the mechanisms underlying K^+ homeostasis. Such a situation can be met in the *in vitro* hippocampal slice under conditions of blocked chemical synaptic transmission (88,89). When axons from hippocampal pyramidal cells are antidromically stimulated, action potentials only invade into the soma and the proximal apical dendrites. Thus, K^+ release during repetitive stimulation is restricted to this area. Indeed, we found that K^+ release is maximal during antidromic stimulation in the pyramidal cell layer (SP), and K^+ signals decrease steeply towards the alveus and the stratum moleculare. This laminar profile is also preserved under conditions of blocked chemical synaptic transmission, i.e., when $[Ca^{2+}]_o$ was lowered to 0.2 mM and Mg^{2+} was increased to 6 mM. The associated slow potential shifts show a maximal negativity in SP and reverse to positive potentials at a distance of 100 to 150 μm from SP in stratum radiatum. Measurements of ES size changes in and outside SP reveal that the extracellular space size decreases in SP while it increases at remote sites, as expected from the spatial K^+ buffer hypothesis (68).

The voltage gradients of the antidromically induced population spikes and of the slow field potential changes are also of interest because they allow for an estimate of the current source

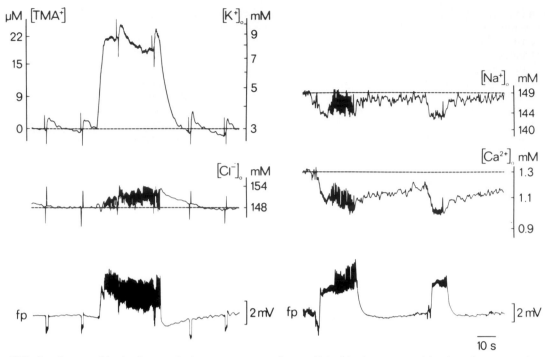

FIG. 8. Survey of ionic changes during spontaneous seizures elicited by intravenous injection of pentetrazole (40 mg/kg body weight). Recordings on the left side were performed with an assembly consisting of a K^+-selective, chloride-selective reference electrode with a nearby tetramethylammonium chloride-containing iontophoresis electrode. Note the alterations in field potentials (fp) induced by TMA current injection during and following seizure activity. Records on the right were obtained with a triple-barreled Ca^{2+}/Na^+/reference electrode.

density in the stratum pyramidale. The voltage gradients for the antidromically evoked population spikes are in the order of 100 mV/mm, which could create short but very intense currents in the order of 10 μA/mm². If only 1‰ of this current would flow through neuronal elements, a considerable depolarization would be expected (as much as 30 mV), which is sufficient to elicit action potentials. This illustrates that ephaptic interactions are very likely to occur in area CA1. A laminar analysis of slow field potentials revealed that a considerable amount of K^+ may be spatially redistributed during repetitive stimulation (68).

GENERALIZED CONVULSIONS, STATUS EPILEPTICUS, AND OTHER PATHOPHYSIOLOGICAL ALTERATIONS OF THE EXTRACELLULAR ENVIRONMENT

Similar investigations were also performed during repeated stimulations and during generalized convulsions induced by pentetrazol (20). When stimulations were repeated in middle cor-

tical layers every 30 to 50 sec, the decreases of the ES summated and the ES could decrease by up to 60% (61). While typically $[Na^+]_o$ and $[Ca^{2+}]_o$ would increase during the first stimulation, both ionic concentrations decreased during later stimulations (20,61). This could indicate that the extracellular osmolarity decreases during repeated seizure activity.

Figure 8 illustrates ionic changes during convulsions induced by pentetrazole (PTZ). These are comparable to those elicited by electrical stimulation, with the exception that decreases $[Na^+]_o$ and $[Ca^{2+}]_o$ occur in all cortical layers. Consequently, the increase in osmolarity is smaller than that during stimulus-induced seizures. The decreases in ES compared to those observed during repetitive stimulation. Analysis of the slow field potential changes during PTZ-induced seizures reveals that due to the longer duration of seizures, more K^+ was spatially dispersed (20). Preliminary data suggest that if the extracellular volume fraction is taken into account, 45 mM K^+ should appear in addition to the 7 mM actually observed.

PTZ often induced a series of ictal episodes,

and repeated injections of PTZ may even induce a status epilepticus (61). During such states a considerable summation of $[Ca^{2+}]_o$ and $[Na^+]_o$ changes can be observed (20,61). Later during status epilepticus also a constant elevation of baseline $[K^+]_o$ is seen (61). At present there are no data available on $[Cl^-]_o$ changes as well as on changes in ES under this condition, but it may be expected that $[Cl^-]_o$ decreases also under this condition in order to preserve extracellular electroneutrality. This reduction of extracellular osmolarity may in part result from a break in the blood-brain barrier with a subsequent entry of proteins and water into the ES. Under this condition, the brain tissue may swell to such an extent that local microcirculation is disturbed, with a resultant reduction of oxygen supply. Recent experiments in *in vitro* hippocampal slices have suggested that such a drop of oxygen supply may be sufficient to evoke seizure activity even near physiological levels of $[K^+]_o$ and $[Ca^{2+}]_o$ (165). These local factors, together with a considerable Ca^{2+} accumulation inside nerve cells and general disturbances of blood pressure and heart rate during status epilepticus, may account not only for the continuation of status epilepticus but also for the considerable cell damage associated with this situation. The ionic and ES size changes under these conditions are approximating those observed during excitatory amino acid application (25,69, 70), spreading depression, and hypoxia (55, 56,75,90,91). All these experimental conditions have in common that the decreases in $[Na^+]_o$, $[Cl^-]_o$, and $[Ca^{2+}]_o$ exceed the simultaneously observed rises in $[K^+]_o$, and these conditions may be associated with cell death.

We have shown in this chapter that epileptic activity is generally associated with considerable alterations of the extracellular ionic constitution and with reductions in the size of the ES. Model calculations also predict considerable alterations of the ionic constitution in the intracellular compartments. All these changes have profound effects on ictal activity. Thus, rises in $[K^+]_o$ and decreases in $[Ca^{2+}]_o$ support the development of seizure activity (54,89,131,164, 167). Increases in intracellular Cl^- concentration will impair inhibitory synaptic transmission (1,17,80,112,118). Accumulation of Ca^{2+} within cells (46) as well as disturbances in local O_2 supply may be factors involved in epilepsy related cell death. Spatial K^+ buffering by affecting the ES size helps to preserve transmembraneous ionic concentration gradients and appears to be an important physiological mechanism in electrolyte regulation without an immediate expense in energy. It will, however, spread potassium from active areas into yet inactive areas and thus contribute to the spread of ictal activity. The shrinkage of the ES will enhance extracellular current density and may thus contribute to synchronization of neuronal activity by ephaptic interactions. As yet unclear are the mechanisms that determine the initiation of status epilepticus, but continued research will facilitate our understanding of this condition.

ACKNOWLEDGMENTS

This research was supported by Deutsche Forschungsgemeinschaft (DFG) grants to U. Heinemann and H. D. Lux and by a Heisenberg fellowship to U. Heinemann. We thank Dr. J. Hablitz and Dr. J. D. C. Lambert for reading the manuscript. We gratefully acknowledge the technical help of U. Roessler, I. Borst, and G. Schuster in the preparation of the manuscript.

REFERENCES

1. Aickin, C. C., Deisz, R. A., and Lux, H. D. (1982): Ammonium action on postsynaptic inhibition in crayfish neurones: implications for the mechanism of chloride extrusion. *J. Physiol. (Lond.)*, 329:319–339.
2. Ames, A., Sakanoue, M., and Endo, S. (1964): Na, K, Ca, Mg and Cl concentrations in choroid plexus fluid and cisternal fluid compared with plasma ultrafiltrate. *J. Neurophysiol.*, 27:672–681.
3. Balcar, V. J., Borg, J., and Mandel, P. (1977): High affinity uptake of L-glutamate and L-aspartate by glial cells. *J. Neurochem.*, 28:87–93.
4. Barry, P. H., and Hope, A. B. (1969): Electroosmosis in membranes: effects of unstirred layers and transport numbers. I Theory. *Biophys. J.*, 9:700–728.
5. Benninger, C., Kadis, J., and Prince, D. A. (1980): Extracellular calcium and potassium changes in hippocampal slices. *Brain Res.*, 187:165–182.
6. Blennow, G., Folbergrova, J., Nilsson, B., and Siesjo, B. (1979): Cerebral metabolic and circulatory changes in the rat during sustained seizures induced by D,L-homocysteine. *Brain Res.*, 179:129–146.
7. Bourke, R. S., and Nelson, K. M. (1972): Further studies on the K^+-dependent swelling of primate cerebral cortex 'in vivo': The enzymatic basis of the K^+-dependent transport of chloride. *J. Neurochem.*, 19:663–685.
8. Bruggencate, G. ten, Lux, H. D., and Liebl, L. (1974): Possible relationships between extracellular potassium activity and presynaptic inhibition in the spinal cord of the cat. *Pfluegers Arch.*, 367:301–317.
9. Caspers, H., and Speckmann, E. J. (1972): Cerebral pO_2, pCO_2 and pH changes during con-

vulsive activity and their significance for spontaneous arrest of seizures. *Epilepsia*, 13:699–725.

10. Castellucci, V. F., and Goldring, S. (1970): Contribution to steady potential shifts of slow depolarization in cells presumed to be glia. *Electroencephalogy Clin. Neurophysiology*, 28:109–118.

11. Cohen, M. V. (1970): The contribution by glial cells to surface recordings from the optic nerve of an amphibian. *J. Physiol. (Lond.)*, 210:565–580.

12. Coles, J. A., and Orkand, R. K. (1983): Modification of potassium movement through the retina of the drone (*Apis mellifera*) by glial uptake. *J. Physiol. (Lond.)*, 340:157–174.

13. Coles, J. A., and Tsacopoulos, M. (1979): Potassium activity in photoreceptors, glial cells and extracellular space in the drone retina: Changes during photostimulation. *J. Physiol. (Lond.)*, 290:525–549.

14. Coles, J. A., Tsacopoulos, M., Robineau, P., and Gardner-Medwin, A. R. (1981): Movement of potassium into glial cells in the retina of the drone, apis mellifera, during photostimulation. In: *Ion-Selective Microelectrodes and Their Use in Excitable Tissue*, edited by E. Sykova, P. Hnik, and L. Vyklicky, pp. 345–349. Plenum, London.

15. Connors, B. W., Ransom, B. R., Kunis, B. M., and Gutnick, M. J. (1982): Activity-dependent K^+ accumulation in the developing rat optic nerve. *Science*, 216:1341–1343.

16. Cordingley, G. E., and Somjen, G. G. (1978): Dissipation of locally accumulated extracellular potassium in the cat cerebral cortex. *Brain Res.*, 151:291–306.

17. Deisz, R. A., and Lux, H. D. (1982): The role of intracellular Cl^- in hyperpolarizing post-synaptic inhibition of crayfish stretch receptor neurones. *J. Physiol. (Lond.)*, 326:123–138.

18. Dichter, M. A., Hermann, C. J., and Selzer, M. (1972): Silent cells during interictal discharges and seizures in hippocampal penicillin foci. Evidence for the role of extracellular K^+ in the transition from the interictal state to seizures. *Brain Res.*, 48:173–183.

19. Dietzel, I. (1983): Ladungsverschiebungen und Elektrolytaenderungen in der Hirnrinde. Untersuchungen waehrend erhoehter neuronaler Aktivitaet im sensomotorischen Kortex der Katze. Dissertation. RWTH Aachen.

20. Dietzel, I., and Heinemann, U. (1983): Extracellular electrolyte changes during enhanced neuronal activity can be explained by spatial glial K^+-buffering in addition to small increases in osmotic pressure—possibly induced by increases in metabolic activity. In: *Cerebral Blood Flow, Metabolism and Epilepsy*, edited by M. Baldy-Moulinier, D. Ingvar, and B. S. Meldrum, pp. 195–201. John Libbey, London.

21. Dietzel, I., Heinemann, U., Hofmeier, G., and Lux, H. D. (1980): Transient changes in the size of the extracellular space in sensorimotor cortex of cats in relation to stimulus induced changes in potassium concentration. *Exp. Brain Res.*, 40:432–439.

22. Dietzel, I., Heinemann, U., Hofmeier, G., and Lux, H. D. (1982): Changes in the extracellular volume in the cerebral cortex of cats in relation to stimulus induced epileptiform afterdischarges. In: *Physiology and Pharmacology of Epileptogenic Phenomena*, edited by M. R. Klee, H. D. Lux, and E.-J. Speckmann, pp. 5–12. Raven, New York.

23. Dietzel, I., Heinemann, U., Hofmeier, G., and Lux, H. D. (1982): Stimulus-induced changes in extracellular Na^+ and Cl^- concentration in relation to changes in the size of the extracellular space. *Exp. Brain Res.*, 46:73–84.

24. Dietzel, I., Heinemann, U., and Lux, H. D. (1985): Relation between slow potential changes and ionic movements during enhanced neuronal activity in cat brain. (*Submitted for publication.*)

25. Engberg, I., Flatman, J. A., Lambert, J. D. C., and Lindsay, A. (1983): An analysis of bioelectrical phenomena evoked by microiontophoretically applied excitotoxic amino-acids in the feline spinal cord. *Excitotoxins (Wenner-Gren Center International Symposium Series, Vol. 39)*, edited by K. Fuxe, E. Roberts, and R. Schwarcz, pp. 170–183. Macmillan Press Ltd., Basingstone.

26. Ferguson, J. H., and Jasper, H. H. (1971): Laminar DC studies of acetylcholine-activated epileptiform discharge in cerebral cortex. *Electroencephalogy Clin. Neurophysiol.*, 30:377–390.

27. Fertziger, A. P., and Ranck, J. B., Jr. (1970): Potassium accumulation in the interstitial space during epileptiform seizures. *Exp. Neurol.*, 26:571–585.

28. Fisher, R. S., Pedley, T. A., Moody, W. J., Jr., and Prince, D. A. (1976): The role of extracellular potassium in hippocampal epilepsy. *Arch. Neurol.*, 33:76–83.

29. Fisher, R. S., Pedley, T. A., and Prince, D. A. (1976): Kinetics of potassium movement in normal cortex. *Brain Res.*, 101:223–237.

30. Frankenhaeuser, B., and Hodgkin, A. L. (1956): The after-effects of impulses in the giant fibres of loligo. *J. Physiol. (Lond.)*, 131:341–376.

31. Frankenhaeuser, B., and Hodgkin, A. L. (1957): The action of calcium on the electrical properties of squid axons. *J. Physiol. (Lond.)*, 137:218–244.

32. Freeman, J. A., and Nicholson, C. (1975): Experimental optimization of current-source density technique for anuran cerebellum. *J. Neurophysiol.*, 38:369–382.

33. Freeman, J. A., and Stone, J. (1969): A technique for current density analysis of field potentials and its application to frog cerebellum. In: *Neurobiology of Cerebellar Evolution and Development*, edited by R. Llinas, pp. 421–430. American Medical Association, Chicago.

34. Freygang, W. H., Jr., and Landau, W. M. (1955): Some relations between resistivity and electrical activity in the cerebral cortex of the cat. *J. Cell. Comp. Physiol.*, 45:377–392.

35. Futamachi, K. J., Mutani, R., and Prince, D. A.

(1974): Potassium activity in rabbit cortex. *Brain Res.*, 75:5–25.

36. Futamachi, K. J., and Pedley, T. A. (1976): Glial cells and extracellular potassium: Their relationship in mammalian cortex. *Brain Res.*, 109:311–322.

37. Galvan, M., Grafe, P., and Bruggencate, ten G. (1982): Convulsive actions of 4-aminopyridine on neurons and extracellular K^+ and Ca^{++} activities in guinea pig olfactory cortex slices. In: *Pharmacology and Physiology of Epileptogenic Phenomena*, edited by M. R. Klee, H. D. Lux, and E.-J. Speckmann, pp. 353–360. Raven, New York.

38. Gardner-Medwin, A. R. (1980): Membrane transport and solute migration affecting the brain cell microenvironment. In: *Dynamics of the Brain Cell Microenvironment*, edited by C. Nicholson, pp. 208–226. Neuroscience Research Program Bulletin, MIT Press, Cambridge.

39. Gardner-Medwin, A. R. (1983): A study of the mechanisms by which potassium moves through brain tissue in the rat. *J. Physiol. (Lond.)*, 335:353–374.

40. Gardner-Medwin, A. R., Coles, J. A., and Tsacopoulos, M. (1981): Clearance of extracellular potassium: evidence for spatial buffering by glial cells in the retina of the drone. *Brain Res.*, 209:452–457.

41. Gardner-Medwin, A. R., and Nicolson, C. (1983): Changes of extracellular potassium activity induced by electric current through brain tissue in the rat. *J. Physiol. (Lond.)*, 335:375–392.

42. Gloetzner, F. L. (1973): Membrane properties of neuroglia in epileptogenic gliosis. *Brain Res.*, 55:159–171.

43. Gloetzner, F., and Gruesser, O. J. (1968): Membranpotential und Entadungsformen cortikaler Zellen, EEG und cortikales DC-Potential bei generalisierten Krampfanfaellen. *Arch. Psychiatr. Nervenkrankenh.*, 210:313–339.

44. Grafe, P., Rimpel, J., Reddy, M. M., and Bruggencate, ten G. (1982): Changes of intracellular sodium and potassium ion concentration in frog spinal motoneurons induced by repetitive synaptic stimulation. *Neuroscience*, 7:3213–3220.

45. Green, J. D. (1964): The hippocampus. *Physiol. Rev.*, 44:501–608.

46. Griffith, T., Evans, M. C., and Meldrum, B. S. (1982): Intracellular sites of early Ca^{2+} accumulation in the rat hippocampus during status epilepticus. *Neurosci. Lett.*, 30:329–334.

47. Grisar, T., Franck, G., and Schoffeniels, E. (1978): K^+-activation mechanisms of the (Na^+, K^+)-ATPase of bulk-isolated glia and neurons. In: *Dynamic Properties of Glia Cells*, edited by E. Schoffeniels, pp. 359–369. Pergamon, Oxford.

48. Grisar, T., Franck, G., and Schoffeniels, E. (1980): Glial control of neuronal excitability in mammals. II. Enzymatic evidence: Two molecular forms of the (Na^+, K^+)-ATPase in brain. *Neurochemistry Int.*, 2:311–320.

49. Gumnit, R. J., Matsumoto, H., and Vasconetto, C. (1970): DC activity in the depth of an experimental epileptic focus. *Electroencephalogy Clin. Neurophysiol.*, 28:333–339.

50. Gutnick, M. J. (1982): Ionic fluctuations and cyclic changes in epileptogenic excitability in hippocampal foci. In: *Physiology and Pharmacology of Epileptogenic Phenomena*, edited by M. R. Klee, H. D. Lux, and E.-J. Speckmann, pp. 105–111. Raven, New York.

51. Gutnick, M. J., Connors, B. W., and Ramson, B. R. (1981): Dye-coupling between glial cells in the guinea pig neocortical slice. *Brain Res.*, 213:486–492.

52. Gutnick, M. J., Heinemann, U., and Lux, H. D. (1979): Stimulus induced and seizure related changes in extracellular potassium concentration in cat thalamus (VPL). *Electroencephalogy Clin. Neurophysiol.*, 47:329–344.

53. Haberly, L. B., and Shepherd, G. H. (1973): Current-density analysis of summed evoked potentials in opossum prepyriform cortex. *J. Neurophysiol.*, 36:789–803.

54. Hablitz, J. J., and Lundervold, A. (1981): Hippocampal excitability and changes in extracellular K^+. *Exp. Neurol.*, 71:410–420.

55. Hansen, A. J., and Olsen, C. E. (1980): Brain extracellular space during spreading depression and ischemia in the rat brain cortex. *Acta Physiol. Scand.*, 108:355–365.

56. Hansen, A. J., and Zeuthen, T. (1981): Extracellular ion concentrations during spreading depression and ischemia in rat brain cortex. *Acta Physiol. Scand.*, 113:437–445.

57. Heinemann, U., and Dietzel, I. (1984): Extracellular potassium concentration in chronic alumina cream foci of cats. *J. Neurophysiol.*, 52:421–434.

58. Heinemann, U., and Gutnick, M. J. (1979): Relation between extracellular potassium and neuronal activities in cat thalamus (VPL) during projection of cortical epileptiform discharge. *Electroencephalogy Clin. Neurophysiol.*, 47:345–357.

59. Heinemann, U., Konnerth, A., Louvel, J., Lux, H. D., and Pumain, R. (1982): Changes in extracellular free Ca^{2+} in normal and epileptic sensorimotor cortex of cats. In: *Physiology and Pharmacology of Epileptogenic Phenomena*, edited by M. R. Klee, H. D. Lux, and E.-J. Speckmann, pp. 29–35. Raven, New York.

60. Heinemann, U., Konnerth, A., and Lux, H. D. (1981): Stimulation induced changes in extracellular free calcium in normal cortex and chronic alumina cream foci of cats. *Brain Res.*, 213:246–250.

61. Heinemann, U., and Louvel, J. (1983): Changes in $[Ca^{2+}]_o$ and $[K^+]_o$ during repetitive electrical stimulation and during pentetrazol induced seizures activity in the sensorimotor cortex of cats. *Pfluegers Arch.*, 398:310–317.

62. Heinemann, U., and Lux, H. D. (1975): Undershoots following stimulus-induced rises in extracellular potassium concentration in the cerebral cortex of cat. *Brain Res.*, 93:63–76.

63. Heinemann, U., and Lux, H. D. (1977): Ceiling of stimulus induced rises in extracellular potassium concentration in the cerebral cortex of cats. *Brain Res.*, 120:231–249.

64. Heinemann, U., and Lux, H. D. (1983): Ionic changes during experimentally induced epilepsies. In: *Progress in Epilepsy Research,* edited by F. C. Rose, pp. 87–102. Pitman Medical, London.

65. Heinemann, U., Lux, H. D., and Gutnick, M. J. (1977): Extracellular free calcium and potassium during paroxysmal activity in cerebral cortex of the cat. *Exp. Brain Res.,* 27:237–243.

66. Heinemann, U., Lux, H. D., and Gutnick, M. J. (1978): Changes in extracellular free calcium and potassium activity in the somatosensory cortex of cats. In: *Abnormal Neuronal Discharges,* edited by M. Chalazonitis, and M. Boisson, pp. 329–345. Raven, New York.

67. Heinemann, U., Lux, H. D., Marciani, M. G., and Hofmeier, G. (1979): Slow potentials in relation to changes in extracellular potassium activity in the cortex of cats. In: *Origin of Cerebral Field Potentials,* edited by E. J. Speckmann, and H. Caspers, pp. 33–48. George Thieme, Stuttgart.

68. Heinemann, U., Neuhaus, S., and Dietzel, I. (1983): Aspects of potassium regulation in normal and gliotic brain tissue. In: *Cerebral Blood Flow, Metabolism and Epilepsy,* edited by M. Baldy-Moulinier, H. D. Ingvar, and B. S. Meldrum, pp. 271–278. John Libbey, London.

69. Heinemann, U., and Pumain, R. (1980): Extracellular calcium activity changes in cat sensorimotor cortex induced by iontophoretic application of amino acids. *Exp. Brain Res.,* 40:247–250.

70. Heinemann, U., and Pumain, R. (1981): Changes in extracellular free Ca^{2+}, K^+ and Na^+ during iontophoretic application of excitatory amino acids in the neocortex of cat. *Pfluegers Arch.* 389:R18.

70a. Heinemann, U., and Pumain, R. (1986): Excitatory amino acid and epilepsy induced changes in extracellular space size. In: *Excitatory Amino Acids and Epilepsy,* edited by R. Schwarcz, and Y. Ben Ari. Plenum Press, New York (*in press*).

71. Hertz, L. (1978): An intense potassium uptake into astrocytes, its further enhancement by high concentrations of potassium, and its possible involvement in potassium homeostasis at the cellular level. *Brain Res.,* 145:202–208.

72. Hodgkin, A. L., and Huxley, A. F. (1952): A quantitative description of membrane current and its application to conduction and excitation in nerve. *J. Physiol. (Lond.),* 117:500–544.

73. Hoeltzell, P. B., and Dykes, R. W. (1979): Conductivity in the sensomotory cortex of the cat—Evidence for cortical anisotropy. *Brain Res.,* 177:61–82.

74. Hofmeier, G., and Lux, H. D. (1981): The time course of intracellular free calcium and related electrical effects after injection of $CaCl_2$ into neurons of the snail, *Helix pomatia. Pfluegers Arch.,* 391:242–251.

75. Hossmann, K. A., Sakaki, S., and Zimmermann, V. (1977): Cation activities in reversible ischemia of the cat brain. *Stroke,* 8:77–81.

76. Hotson, J. R., and Prince, D. A. (1980): A calcium-activated hyperpolarization follows repetitive firing in hippocampal neurons. *J. Neurophysiol.,* 43:409–419.

77. Hotson, J. R., Sypert, G. W., and Ward, A. A. (1973): Extracellular potassium concentration changes during propagated seizures in neocortex. *Exp. Neurol.,* 38:20–26.

78. Hounsgaard, J., and Nicholson, C. (1983): Potassium accumulation around individual Purkinje cells in cerebellar slices from the guinea-pig. *J. Physiol. (Lond.),* 340:359–388.

79. Howse, D. C., Caronna, J. J., Duffy, T. E., and Plum, F. (1974): Cerebral energy metabolism, pH, and blood flow during seizures in the rat. *J. Physiol. (Lond.),* 227:1444–1450.

80. Iles, J. F., and Jack, J. J. B. (1980): Ammonia: Assessment of its action on postsynaptic inhibition as a cause of convulsions. *Brain Res.,* 103:555–578.

81. Ito, M., and Oshima, T. (1964): The extrusion of sodium from cat spinal motoneurones. *Proc. Roy. Soc. B. (Lond.),* 161:109–131.

82. Jung, R., and Toennies, J. F. (1950): Hirnelektrische Untersuchungen ueber Entstehung und Erhaltung von Krampfentladungen: Die Vorgaenge am Reizort und die Bremsfaehigkeit des Gehirns. *Arch. Psych. Nervenkrankheiten,* 185:701–735.

83. Kettenmann, H., Orkand, R. K., Lux, H. D., and Schachner, M. (1982): Single potassium channel currents in cultured mouse oligodendrocytes. *Neurosci. Lett.,* 32:41–46.

84. Kettenmann, H., Orkand, R. K., and Schachner, M. (1982): Coupling among identified cells in nervous system cultures. *J. Neurosci.,* 3:506–516.

85. Kettenmann, H., Sonnhof, U., and Schachner, M. (1983): Exclusive K^+ dependence of the membrane potential in cultured oligodendrocytes. *J. Neurosci.,* 3:500–505.

86. Keynes, R. D. (1951): The ionic movements during nervous activity. *J. Physiol. (Lond.),* 114:119–150.

87. Koike, H., Mano, N., Okada, Y., and Oshima, T. (1972): Activities of the sodium pump in cat pyramidal tract cells investigated with intracellular injection of sodium ions. *Exp. Brain Res.,* 14:489–503.

88. Konnerth, A., and Heinemann, U. (1983): Effects of GABA on presumed presynaptic Ca^{2+} entry in hippocampal slice. *Brain Res.,* 270:185–189.

89. Konnerth, A., Heinemann, U., and Yaari Y. (1984): Slow transmission of neural activity in hippocampal area CA1 in absence of active chemical synapses. *Nature (Lond.),* 307:69–71.

90. Kraig, R. P., and Nicholson, C. (1978): Extracellular ionic variations during spreading depression. *Neuroscience,* 3:1045–1059.

91. Kraig, R. P., Ferreira-Filho, C. R., and Nicholson, C. (1983): Alkaline and acid transients in cerebellar microenvironment. *J. Neurophysiol.,* 49:831–850.

92. Kriz, N., Sykova, E., Ujec, E., and Vyklicky, L. (1974): Changes of extracellular K^+ concentrations induced by neuronal activity in the spinal cord of the cat. *J. Physiol. (Lond.),* 238:1–15.

93. Kriz, N., Sykova, E., and Vyklicky, L. (1975): Extracellular potassium changes in the spinal cord of the cat and their relation to slow poten-

tials, active transport and impulse transmission. *J. Physiol. (Lond.)*, 225:363–390.

94. Krnjevic, K., and Lisiewicz, A. (1972): Injections of calcium ions into spinal motoneurones. J. Physiol. (*Lond.*), 225:363–390.

95. Krnjevic, K., and Morris, M. E. (1972): Extracellular K^+ activity and slow potential changes in spinal cord and medulla. *Can. J. Physiol. Pharmacol.*, 50:1214–1271.

96. Krnjevic, K., and Morris, M. E. (1974): Extracellular accumulation of K^+ evoked by activity of primary afferent fibers in the cuneate nucleus and dorsal horn of cats. *Can. J. Physiol. Pharmacol.*, 52:852–871.

97. Krnjevic, K., and Morris, M. E. (1975): Factors determining the decay of K^+-potentials and focal potentials in the central nervous system. *Can. J. Physiol. Pharmacol.*, 53:923–934.

98. Krnjevic, K., Morris, M. E., and Reiffenstein, R. J. (1980): Changes in extracellular Ca^{2+} and K^+ activity accompanying hippocampal discharges. *Can. J. Physiol. Pharmacol.*, 58:579–583.

99. Krnjevic, K., Puil, E., and Werman, R. (1975): Evidence for Ca^{2+} activated conductance in cat spinal motoneurons from intracellular EGTA injections. *Can. J. Physiol. Pharmacol.*, 53:1214–1218.

100. Krnjevic, K., Puil, E., and Werman, R. (1978): EGTA and motoneural after-potentials. *J. Physiol. (Lond.)*, 275:199–223.

101. Kuffler, S. W., and Nicholls, J. G. (1966): The physiology of neuroglia cells. *Ergeb. Physiol.*, 57:1–90.

102. Kuffler, S. W., Nicholls, J. G., and Orkand, R. K. (1966): Physiological properties of glial cells in the central nervous system of amphibia. *J. Neurophysiol.*, 29:768–787.

103. Kuffler, S. W., and Potter, D. D. (1963): Glia in the leech central nervous system physiological properties and neuron-glia relationship. *J. Neurophysiol.*, 27:290–320.

104. Lee, K. S., Schubert, P., and Heinemann, U. (1984): The anticonvulsant action of adenosine. A postsynaptic, dendritic action by a possible endogenous anticonvulsant. *Brain Res.*, 321:160–164.

105. Lehmenkuehler, A., Caspers, H., and Kersting, U. (1984): Relations between DC-potentials, extracellular ion activities and extracellular volume fraction in the cerebral cortex with changes in pCO_2. In: *Recent Advances in Theory and Application of Ion Selective Electrodes in Physiology and Medicine*, edited by M. Kessler, D. K. Harisson, and J. Hoeper. Springer, Berlin. (*In press.*)

106. Lehmenkuehler, A., Zidek, W., and Caspers, H. (1982): Changes of extracellular Na^+ and Cl^- activity in the brain cortex during seizure discharges. In: *Physiology and Pharmacology of Epileptogenic Phenomena*, edited by M. R. Klee, H. D. Lux, and E.-J. Speckmann, pp. 37–45. Raven, New York.

107. Lewis, D. V., Matsuga, N., Schuette, W. H., and van Buren, J. (1977): Potassium clearance and reactive gliosis in the alumina gel lesion. *Epilepsia*, 18:499–506.

108. Lewis, D. V., and Schuette, W. H. (1975):

NADH fluorescence and $[K^+]_o$ changes during hippocampal electrical stimulation. *J. Neurophysiol.*, 38:405–417.

109. Li, C.-L., Bak, A. F., and Parker, L. O. (1968): Specific resistivity of the cerebral cortex and white matter. *Exp. Neurol*, 20:544–557.

110. Lothman, E. W., and Somjen, G. G. (1975): Extracellular potassium activity, intracellular and extracellular potential responses in the spinal cord. *J. Physiol. (Lond.)*, 252:115–136.

111. Louvel, J., and Heinemann, U. (1983): Changes in $[Ca^{2+}]_o$, $[K^+]_o$ and neuronal activity during oenanthotoxin induced epilepsy. *Electroencephalogy Clin. Neurophysiol.*, 56:457–466.

112. Lux, H. D. (1971): Ammonium and chloride extrusion: Hyperpolarising synaptic inhibition in spinal motoneurones. *Science*, 173:555–557.

113. Lux, H. D. (1974): Kinetics of intracellular potassium: Relation to epileptogenesis. *Epilepsia*, 15:375–393.

114. Lux, H. D. (1974): Fast recording ion specific electrodes. Their use in pharmacological studies in the CNS. *Neuropharmacology*, 13:509–517.

115. Lux, H. D. (1980): Ionic conditions and membrane behaviour. In: *Antiepileptic Drugs: Mechanisms of Action*, edited by G. H. Glaser, J. K. Penry, and D. M. Woodbury, pp. 63–83. Raven, New York.

116. Lux, H. D. (1983): An invertebrate model of paroxysmal depolarizing shifts. In: *Electrophysiology of Epilepsy*, edited by P. A. Schwartzkroin and H. V. Wheal, pp. 344–352. Academic, London.

117. Lux, H. D., and Heinemann, U. (1982): Consequences of calcium-electrogenesis for the generation of paroxysmal depolarization shift. In: *Epilepsy and Motor System*, edited by E.-J. Speckmann, and C. E. Elger, pp. 101–119. Urban und Schwarzenberg, Muenchen.

118. Lux, H. D., Loracher, C., and Neher, E. (1970): The action of ammonium on postsynaptic inhibition of cat spinal motoneurons. *Exp. Brain Res.*, 11:431–447.

119. Lux, H. D., and Neher, E. (1973): The equilibration time course of $[K^+]_o$ in cat cortex. *Exp. Brain Res.*, 17:190–205.

120. Lux, H. D., Neher, E., and Marty, A. (1981): Single channel activity associated with the calcium dependent outward current in *Helix pomatia*. *Pfluegers Arch.*, 389:293–295.

121. Mitzdorf, U., and Singer, W. (1978): Prominent excitatory pathways in the cat visual cortex (A17 and A18): A current source density analysis of electrically evoked potentials. *Brain Res.*, 33:371–394.

122. Moody, W., Futamachi, K. J., and Prince, D. A. (1974): Extracellular potassium activity during epileptogenesis. *Exp. Neurol.*, 42:248–263.

123. Morris, M. E., and Krnjevic, K. (1981): Slow diffusion of Ca^{2+} in the rat's hippocampus. *Can. J. Physiol. Pharmacol.*, 59:1022–1025.

124. Neher, E., and Lux, H. D. (1973): Rapid changes of potassium concentration at the outer surface of exposed single neurons during membrane current flow. *J. Gen. Physiol.*, 61:385–399.

125. Nicholson, C. (1980): Dynamics of the brain cell

microenvironment. *Neuroscience Research Programme Bulletin*, 18:177–322.

126. Nicholson, C. (1980): Modulation of extracellular calcium and its functional implications. *Fed. Proc.*, 39:1519–1523.

127. Nicholson, C., Bruggencate, G. ten, Stoeckle, H., and Steinberg, R. (1978): Calcium and potassium changes in extracellular microenvironment of cat cerebellar cortex. *J. Neurophysiol.*, 41:1026–1039.

128. Nicholson, C., and Phillips, J. M. (1981): Ion diffusion modified by tortuosity and volume fraction in the extracellular microenvironment of the rat cerebellum. *J. Physiol. (Lond.)*, 321:225–257.

129. Oakley, J. C., Sypert, G. W., and Ward, A. A., Jr. (1972): Conductance changes in neocortical propagated seizure: seizure termination. *Exp. Neurol.*, 37:300–311.

130. Olney, J. W., de Gubareff, T., and Sloviter, R. S. (1983): "Epileptic" brain damage in rats induced by sustained electrical stimulation of the perforant path. II. Ultrastructural analysis of acute hippocampal pathology. *Brain Res. Bull.*, 10:699–712.

131. Ogata, N., Hori, N., and Katsuda, N. (1976): The correlation between extracellular potassium concentration and hippocampal epileptic activity in vitro. *Brain Res.*, 110:371–375.

132. Organ, L. W., and Kwan, H. C. (1970): Electrical impendance variation along a track of brain tissue. *Ann. N.Y. Acad. Sci.*, 170:491–508.

133. Orkand, R. K., Nicholls, J. G., and Kuffler, S. W. (1966): Effect of nerve impulses on the membrane potential of glial cells in the central nervous system of amphibia. *J. Neurophysiol.*, 29:788–806.

134. Petsche, H., Pockberger, H., and Rappelsberger, P. (1984): On the search for the sources of the electroencephalogram. *Neuroscience*, 11:1–27.

135. Picker, S., and Goldring, S. (1982): Electrophysiological properties of human glia. *Trends Neurosci.*, 5:73–76.

136. Prince, D. A. (1978): Neurophysiology of epilepsy. *Ann. Rev. Neurosci.*, 1:395–415.

137. Prince, D. A., Lux, H. D., and Neher, E. (1973): Measurements of extracellular potassium activity in cat cortex. *Brain Res.*, 50:489–495.

138. Pumain, R. (1981): Intracellular studies in chronic epileptogenic foci reveal dendritic abnormalities. *Brain Res.*, 219:445–450.

139. Pumain, R., and Heinemann, U. (1982): Intracellular potential and extracellular calcium changes in chronic epilepsy. In: *Advances in Epileptology: XIIIth Epilepsy International Symposium*, edited by H. Akimoto, H. Kazamatzuri, M. Seino, and A. A. Ward, pp. 497–500. Raven, New York.

140. Pumain, R., and Heinemann, U. (1985): Stimulus-evoked and amino-acid induced ionic changes in rat neocortex. *J. Neurophysiol.*, 53:1–16.

141. Ransom, B. R., and Goldring, S. (1973): Ionic

determination of membrane potential of cells presumed to be glia in cerebral cortex of cat. *J. Neurophysiol.*, 36:855–868.

142. Ransom, B. R., and Goldring, S. (1973): Slow depolarization in cells presumed to be glia in cerebral cortex of cat. *J. Neurophysiol.*, 36:869–878.

143. Rappelsberger, P., Pockberger, H., and Petsche, H. (1981): Current source density analysis: methods and application to simultaneously recorded field potentials of the rabbit's visual cortex. *Pfluegers Arch.*, 389:159–170.

144. Singer, W., and Lux, H. D. (1975): Extracellular potassium gradients and visual receptive fields in the cat striate cortex. *Brain Res.*, 96:378–383.

145. Somjen, G. G. (1973): Electrogenesis of sustained potentials. *Progr. Neurobiol.*, 1:199–237.

146. Somjen, G. G. (1978): Metabolic and electrical correlates of the clearing of excess potassium in the cortex and spinal cord. In: *Studies in Neurophysiology*, edited by E. Porter, pp. 182–201. Cambridge University Press, London.

147. Somjen, G. G. (1980): Stimulus-evoked and seizure related responses of extracellular calcium activity in spinal cord compared to those in cerebral cortex. *J. Neurophysiol.*, 44:617–632.

148. Somjen, G. G., and Lothmann, E. W. (1974): Potassium sustained focal potential shifts and dorsal root potentials of the mammalian spinal cord. *Brain Res.*, 69:153–157.

149. Sugaya, E., Takato, M., and Noda, Y. (1975): Neuronal and glial activity during spreading depression in cerebral cortex of cat. *J. Neurophysiol.*, 38:822–841.

150. Sykova, E., Rothenberg, S., and Kreule, I. (1974): Changes of extracellular potassium concentration during spontaneous activity in the mesencephalic reticular formation of the rat. *Brain Res.*, 79:333–337.

151. Sypert, G. W. and Ward A. A., Jr. (1971): Unidentified neuroglia potentials during propagated seizures in neocortex. *Exp. Neurol.*, 33:239–255.

152. Sypert, G. W., and Ward, A. A., Jr. (1974): Changes in extracellular potassium activity during neocortical propagated seizures. *Exp. Neurol.*, 45:19–41.

153. Tang, C. M., Cohen, M. W., and Orkand, R. K. (1980): Electrogenic pumps in axons and neuroglia and extracellular potassium homeostasis. *Brain Res.*, 194:238–286.

154. Thomas, R. C. (1972): Electrogenic sodium pump in nerve and muscle cells. *Physiol. Rev.*, 52:563–594.

155. Tower, D. B. (1960): *Neurochemistry of Epilepsy*. Charles C. Thomas, Springfield, Illinois.

156. Van Harreveld, A., and Malhotra, S. K. (1967): Extracellular space in the cerebral cortex of the mouse. *J. Anat.*, 101:197–207.

157. Van Harreveld, A., Murphy, T., and Nobel, K. W. (1963): Specific impedance of rabbit's cortical tissue. *Am. J. Physiol.*, 205:203–207.

158. Van Harreveld, A., and Schade, J. P. (1962): Changes in the electrical conductivity of cere-

bral cortex during seizure activity. *Exp. Neurol.*, 5:383–400.

159. Vern, B. A., Schuette, W. H., and Thibault, C. E. (1977): [K$^+$]$_o$ clearance in cortex: A new analytical model. *J. Neurophysiol.*, 40:1015–1023.

160. Vyskocil, F., Kriz, A., and Bures, J. (1972): Potassium selective microelectrodes used for measuring the extracellular brain potassium during spreading depression and anoxic depolarization in rats. *Brain Res.*, 39:255–259.

161. Walker, J. C., Jr. (1971): Ion specific liquid ion exchanger microelectrodes. *Anal. Chem.*, 43:89A–92A.

162. Walz, W., and Hertz, L. (1982): Quabain-sensitive and quabain-resistant net uptake of potassium into astrocytes and neurons in primary cultures. *J. Neurochem.*, 39:70–77.

163. Williams, V., Grossman, R. G., and Edmunds, S. M. (1980): Volume and surface area esti-

mates of astrocytes in the sensorimotor cortex of the cat. *Neuroscience*, 5:1151–1159.

164. Yaari, Y., Konnerth, A., and Heinemann, U. (1983): Spontaneous epileptiform activity of CA1 hippocampal neurons in low extracellular calcium solutions. *Exp. Brain Res.*, 51:153–156.

165. Yaari, Y., Konnerth, A., and Heinemann, U.: Nonsynaptic epileptogenesis at the mamalian hippocampus in vitro: Role of extracellular potassium. *J. Neurophysiol. (in press)*.

166. Zanotto, L., and Heinemann, U. (1983): Aspartate and glutamate induce reductions in extracellular free calcium and sodium concentration in area CA1 of "in vitro" hippocampal slices of rats. *Neurosci. Lett.*, 35:79–84.

167. Zuckermann, E. C., and Glaser, G. H. (1968): Hippocampal epileptic activity induced by localized ventricular perfusion with high-potassium cerebrospinal fluid. *Exp. Neurol.*, 20:87–110.

Advances in Neurology, Vol. 44, edited by
A. V. Delgado-Escueta, A. A. Ward, Jr.,
D. M. Woodbury, and R. J. Porter.
Raven Press, New York © 1986.

32

Extracellular Calcium and Potassium Concentration Changes in Chronic Epileptic Brain Tissue

*U. Heinemann, *A. Konnerth, **R. Pumain, and ***W. J. Wadman

*Abteilung Neurophysiologie, Max-Planck-Institut fuer Psychiatrie, D 8033 Planegg-Martinsried, Federal Republic of Germany; **Unite de la recherche sur l'epilepsie, INSERM U97, Centre Paul Broca, 75014 Paris, France; and ***Dierfysiologisch Instituut, 1098 SM Amsterdam, The Netherlands*

SUMMARY Repetitive electrical stimulation and application of excitatory amino acids lead to decreases in extracellular Ca^{2+} concentration and to rises in extracellular K^+ concentration ($[Ca^{2+}]_o$, $[K^+]_o$) with a typical laminar distribution in a given neo- or allocortical structure. These ionic changes result from transmembrane ion fluxes along their respective electrochemical gradients. Epileptogenic drugs that impair repolarizing K^+ conductances or inhibitory synaptic transmission enhance such extracellular ionic changes, but they do not alter the laminar distribution of $[K^+]_o$ and $[Ca^{2+}]_o$ changes. Enhanced $[Ca^{2+}]_o$ concentration changes are also observed in chronic epilepsies such as the chronic alumina cream and cobalt focus, the kindling epilepsy, and during photically induced seizures in the baboon *Papio papio*. In chronic epilepsies, the sites of maximal $[Ca^{2+}]_o$ changes shift to other layers, suggesting changes in the distribution of ion channels over the surface of nerve cells that may be involved in epileptogenesis in chronic epilepsies. The K^+ and Ca^{2+} concentration changes associated with seizure contribute to the generation and spread of epileptic activity. This is demonstrated by the fact that lowering of extracellular free calcium concentration can induce spreading epileptiform activity in the absence of chemical synaptic transmission, with $[K^+]_o$ rises preceding epileptiform activity.

Based on observations of changes in ionic concentrations in chronic epileptic tissue and in particular on observations of changes in extracellular free calcium concentration ($[Ca^{2+}]_o$), we suggest that a reorganization of ionic channels over the membrane surface of neurons in chronic epileptogenic tissue may be important for the generation of epileptic activity. Research from many laboratories on different preparations has indicated that the intrinsic activity of central neurons is governed by various ionic conductances. Generation of depolarization shifts (119,120) that underlie paroxysmal activity may involve three depolarizing conductances:

slow Na^+ conductances (17,45,108,171), transient (13,107) and slow Ca^{2+} conductances (26,30,45,80,81,82,92,117,118), and unspecific cation conductances, activated by intracellular increases in Ca^{2+} (15,70) or cyclic adenosine monophosphate concentrations (2,174). A transient Ca^{2+} conductance released from inactivation by hyperpolarization of the nerve cell may underlie rhythmic firing in thalamic and other central neurons (13,76,77,110). This Ca^{2+} conductance can mediate Ca^{2+} entry into cells that are almost at resting membrane potentials. The depolarizing conductances related to epilepsy, particularly the Ca^{2+} conductances, appear to be normally under control of inhibitory transmitters such as gamma-aminobutyric acid (GABA) (24,57,66). Various repolarizing K^+ conductances determine, apart from synaptic activity, the extent by which slow possibly burst generating conductances can be activated. Of particular interest are the Ca^{2+}-mediated K^+ conductances (10,74,96,100,130), because they could be involved in the termination of ictal activity.

The density and surface distribution of ion channels vary from neuron to neuron and possibly also over time. Thus, Ca^{2+} conductances are present not only in presynaptic endings where Ca^{2+} entry is required for the depolarization secretion coupling but also in patches of apical dendrites of principal relay cells (106,109,165,191) and to a lesser degree at the soma level (11,17,81,82,110,167; see also 76,77,153). Ca^{2+} conductances in apical dendrites may be related to the occurrence of dendrodendritic synapses (105). Moreover, it was suggested that freshly explanted neurons in culture may possess more Ca^{2+} conductances than redifferentiated ones (36,37, see also 193). Lesions of the central nervous system may alter the distribution of ionic conductances. Thus axotomized motoneurons aquire the capability for dendritic action potential generation (101), and axonal growth cones possess Ca^{2+}-permeable membranes (43,131,147). Ectopic action potential generation and changes in the distribution of ionic conductances have also been reported in neuromas (187,188) and during demyelination processes (86,87). Similar alterations may take place in chronic epileptic tissue. We investigated the hypothesis that the pattern of Ca^{2+} conductances is altered in chronic epileptic tissue.

The problem of experimental analysis in such a study is that in chronic epileptic tissue most neurons could function normally. Nevertheless, a small number of abnormally behaving neurones may drive a large number of cells into abnormal behavior (136,180,182). Therefore, screening methods are required to uncover abnormalities in the distribution of ionic conductances in a given tissue. We took advantage of the fact that, due to the limited extracellular space (93,142,184), ionic currents across neuronal membranes lead to changes in the extracellular ionic concentrations. With ion-selective microelectrodes (122,144,148), we compared changes in $[Ca^{2+}]_o$ evoked by repetitive electrical stimulation or application of excitatory amino acids (40,163) in normal tissue to those elicited in chronic epileptic tissue. Our observations suggest that a redistribution of Ca^{2+}

conductances over the neuronal membrane has occurred in epileptic tissue. This redistribution may play an important role in the epileptogenic process, possibly together with alterations of the cytoarchitectonics of a given tissue such as loss of GABAergic neurons (5,111,159,160), changes in transmitter metabolism (179), and changes in other voltage or chemically gated channel distributions.

STIMULUS-INDUCED AND AMINO ACID-INDUCED REDUCTIONS IN EXTRACELLULAR FREE Ca^{2+} IN NORMAL NEOCORTEX OF RATS AND CATS

Repetitive electrical stimulation of the cortical surface (Fig. 3A) or of appropriate afferent pathways (60,64,114,140,141,153,170) as well as application of excitatory amino acids such as the putative neurotransmitters glutamate and aspartate (Fig. 1A) and their respective agonists *N*-methyl-D-aspartate and quisqualate (66,67,68, 95,138,151,152) induced decreases in $[Ca^{2+}]_o$ (ΔCa) in cat and rat neocortex. The ΔCa evoked by electrical stimulation could be as large as 0.45 mM. During application of excitatory amino acids, more than 90% (Fig. 1B) of extracellular Ca^{2+} may leave the extracellular space (ES). These ionic changes were associated with particular large negative extracellular potential shifts (29,31,67). The decreases of $[Ca^{2+}]_o$ were not uniformly distributed. In cat somatosensory cortex (Figs. 1C and 3A), one particularly large sink was present in layer II (66), while in rat motor cortex two sinks were found (Fig. 4B): one in layer II/III and one in layer V (151,153). Both stimulus- and amino acid-induced ΔCa could be blocked by inorganic Ca^{2+} antagonists such as Co^{2+}, Ni^{2+}, Mn^{2+} (Fig. 1A), and La^{3+}. Tetrodotoxin (TTX), which prevents generation and propagation of Na^+-dependent action potentials, blocked stimulus induced decreases in $[Ca^{2+}]_o$ but reduced amino acid induced ΔCa by at most 10% (67,154; see also 195). This suggests that activation of presynaptic endings due to excitation of interneurons and of recurrent collaterals contributes little to the extracellular Ca^{2+} loss. Ca^{2+} uptake into glia is probably neglectable (73,84). Simultaneous measurements of $[Na^+]_o$ and $[Ca^{2+}]_o$ (Fig. 1A) or in $[Ca^{2+}]_o$ and $[K^+]_o$ were performed in cat cortex in order to find out whether Ca^{2+} leaves the extracellular space through amino acid controlled ionophores which possess in other preparations a certain degree of Ca^{2+} permeability (12,149,176). All excitatory amino acids induced maximal reduc-

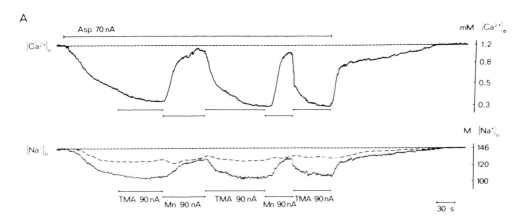

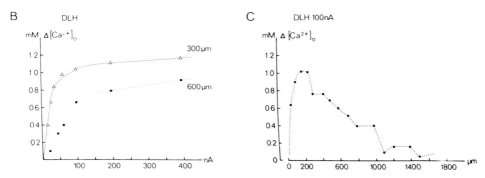

FIG. 1. Amino acid-induced changes in extracellular calcium and sodium concentration in the somatosensory cortex of cats. **A:** Simultaneous recording of $[Ca^{2+}]_o$ and $[Na^+]_o$ during iontophoretic application of aspartate. At time indicated by bars, tetramethylammonium (TMA) or manganese (Mn^{2+}) was applied. The Na^+ signal, due to the sensitivity of the Na^+ resin for changes in $[Ca^{2+}]_o$, had to be corrected for the Ca^{2+} interference (*dotted line*). Note that application of Mn^{2+} had little effect on the Na^+ response, while it depressed the Ca^{2+} response almost completely. **B:** Dose–response curve of DL-homocysteate (DLH) induced changes in $[Ca^{2+}]_o$ in two recording depths at 300 and 600 μm below cortical surface. The amplitudes of the Ca^{2+} responses are plotted as a function of iontophoresis current. **C:** Laminar profile of DLH-induced changes in $[Ca^{2+}]_o$. The amplitudes of changes in $[Ca^{2+}]_o$ are plotted as a function of recording depth below cortical surface.

tions in $[Na^+]_o$ by up to 35 mM (63). The amplitudes of amino acid-induced changes in $[Na^+]_o$ and in $[K^+]_o$ varied less than ΔCa with the recording depth in cortex. Large changes in these ionic concentrations could be observed at sites where $[Ca^{2+}]_o$ changes were small. Further, Ca^{2+} antagonists could prevent the amino acid-induced extracellular Ca^{2+} loss without affecting the simultaneously recorded decreases in $[Na^+]_o$ (Fig. 1A). GABA, which does not interfere with binding sites for excitatory amino acids, also depressed Ca^{2+} signals without any effect on changes in $[Na^+]_o$. This suggests that most Ca^{2+} leaves the ES through selective voltage-gated Ca^{2+} channels. However, quantitative differences existed between different excitatory amino acids. Thus, effects of GABA and of

Mn^{2+} were weaker on *N*-methyl-D-aspartate (NMDA) induced Ca^{2+} signals than on quisqualate (Quis) induced ones. Simultaneous recordings of Quis- and NMDA-induced Ca^{2+} and Na^+ signals revealed that comparable Na^+ signals were associated with larger reductions in $[Ca^{2+}]_o$ when evoked by NMDA than when evoked by Quis (U. Heinemann and R. Pumain, *in preparation*). This is in line with the assumption that the NMDA-controlled ionophores possess a larger Ca^{2+} permeability than Quis-activated ionophores. Alternatively, NMDA may directly activate Ca^{2+} channels (23) or depress K^+ channels (27,49, see 28). This discrepancy between NMDA and Quis actions may account for the larger convulsant action of NMDA (32,69; see also 124,125,126). Similar observations were also made in the dentate area of the *in vitro* hippocampal slice (U. Heinemann and L. Zanotto, *in preparation*).

In order to determine which cellular elements are responsible for the stimulus- and amino acid-induced $[Ca^{2+}]_o$ decreases, unilateral lesions of the pyramidal tract were performed in rats (153). One to four months later we compared the histology and the laminar distribution of Ca^{2+} sinks in the motor cortices of the "lesioned" and control side. The lesion of pyramidal tract fibers rostral to the decussation induced a rather selective degeneration of the pyramidal cell bodies in layer V of the neocortex (71,83,102). Figure 4 will show a comparison of laminar profiles of DL-homocysteate-induced Ca^{2+} decreases in the lesioned and the control side. In the lesioned side, the sinks for Ca^{2+} in layer II and V disappeared, indicating that the large decreases of $[Ca^{2+}]_o$ in these layers are associated normally with Ca^{2+} uptake into pyramidal cells (1). Similar observations were made for profiles of Ca^{2+} signals elicited by glutamate and aspartate (153). Stimulus- and amino acid-induced ΔCa in layer II were 60% smaller in the lesioned than in the control side. This suggests that about 60% of the extracellular Ca^{2+} enters specifically pyramidal tract neurons.

CHANGES IN $[Ca^{2+}]_o$ IN THE *IN VITRO* HIPPOCAMPAL SLICE PREPARATION

Repetitive electrical stimulations and application of excitatory amino acids (Fig. 2) induced stimulus- and dose-dependent reductions in $[Ca^{2+}]_o$ in area CA1 of the *in vitro* hippocampal slice (7,97–99,128,194). Upon repetitive antidromic stimulation of axons from hippocampal pyramidal cells (HPC) in the alveus and upon orthodromic stimulation of afferent Schaffer collaterals and commissural fibers in stratum radiatum (SR) and stratum moleculare (SM), $[Ca^{2+}]_o$ decreased from a baseline concentration of 1.6 mM by about 0.7 mM. The reductions in ΔCa were largest in the stratum pyramidale (SP) (7,57,85,99,128). When synaptic transmission was largely suppressed by increasing the Mg^{2+} concentration in the bath to 9 mM, antidromically induced Ca^{2+} decreases were 30% smaller (57; see also 9,42,75) whereas orthodromically induced Ca^{2+} signals were reduced by 90% (128). This suggests that between 70 and 90% of the stimulus-induced extracellular Ca^{2+} loss can be ascribed to postsynaptic Ca^{2+} entry (57). A similar conclusion was reached when stimulus-induced Ca^{2+} signals were analyzed in slices in which chemical synaptic transmission was sup-

pressed by lowering baseline $[Ca^{2+}]_o$ to 0.2 mM (89,90). Both orthodromic and antidromic stimulation still evoked reductions in $[Ca^{2+}]_o$, but while antidromically evoked ΔCa were still largest in SP, orthodromically induced maximal $[Ca^{2+}]_o$ changes were displaced towards SR and SM. At slightly higher baseline Ca^{2+} levels, chemical synaptic activity may not be completely blocked, and with large stimulus intensities or frequencies a noticeable synaptic transmission often developed during a train of high-frequency stimuli. With this reestablishment of synaptic transmission, reductions in $[Ca^{2+}]_o$ increased by a factor of three to four. Hence presynaptic Ca^{2+} entry contributes much less to extracellular Ca^{2+} loss than does postsynaptic Ca^{2+} entry. Moreover, the fact that Ca^{2+} leaves the ES during antidromic activation of HPC in the absence of chemical synaptic transmission suggests that Ca^{2+} enters HPC cells largely through voltage gated channels.

Excitatory amino acids (Asp, Glu, DLH, NMDA, and Quis; see ref. 137) induced dose-dependent reductions in $[Ca^{2+}]_o$ and in $[Na^+]_o$ (194). To test whether Ca^{2+} can move through chemically gated ionophores (8,12,176) we replaced increasing amounts of NaCl by Tris HCl. This treatment resulted in smaller Ca^{2+} signals (194). However, when more than 60% of Na^+ was replaced by Tris HCl, the ΔCa became larger again, and with complete replacement of Na by Tris, they became even larger than under control conditions. This suggests that amino acid operated ionophores possess a certain degree of Ca^{2+} permeability. NMDA- and Quis-induced changes in $[Na^+]_o$ and $[Ca^{2+}]_o$ differed with respect to their relative amplitudes, similar to what was observed in the neocortex. Under conditions that resulted in comparable reductions in $[Na^+]_o$ for the two amino acids, Quis responses were accompanied by smaller reductions in $[Ca^{2+}]_o$ than NMDA responses. Similarly, NMDA- and Quis-induced intracellularly recorded depolarizations of comparable amplitude were associated with smaller ΔCa when evoked by Quis (101a). The peculiar voltage dependence of the NMDA action (143), in addition to a divalent binding site regulation of the activity of the NMDA receptor site (4), may contribute to this effect. Since Ca^{2+} signals were depressed by inorganic Ca^{2+} antagonists such as Ni^{2+}, Co^{2+}, and Mn^{2+} by up to 80% and by GABA and baclofen by up to 60% (57), we conclude that more than 60% of amino acid-induced reductions in extracellular Ca^{2+} concentration can be ascribed to Ca^{2+} movement through voltage gated ionophores (Fig. 2).

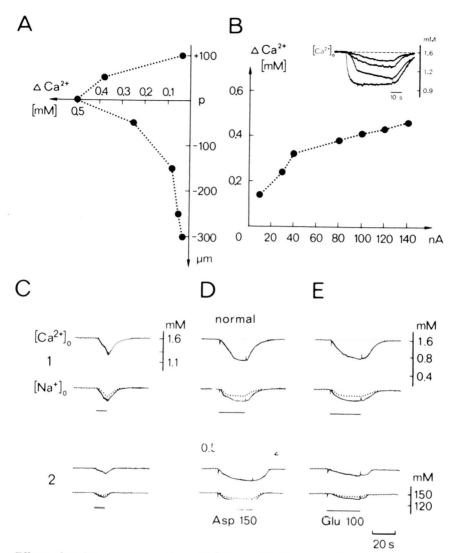

FIG. 2. Effects of excitatory amino acids on $[Ca^{2+}]_o$ and $[Na^+]_o$ in area Ca1 of the *in vitro* hippocampal slice. **A, B:** Effects of aspartate. The *inset* in **B** illustrates sample recordings of Ca^{2+} concentration changes induced by iontophoretic aspartate application with different iontophoresis currents. In **A** the amplitudes of the Ca^{2+} signals are plotted as a function of the recording site within hippocampal area CA1 and in **B** as a function of the applied iontophoresis currents. **C, D, E:** Effects of Ni^{2+} on stimulus (**C**) and amino acid-induced (**D, E**) changes in $[Na^+]_o$ and $[Ca^{2+}]_o$. Note that, unlike in neocortex and area dentata, Na^+ signals are affected by the inorganic Ca^{2+} antagonist Ni^{2+}.

During excitatory amino acid application, presynaptic entry of Ca^{2+} probably accounts for little of the ΔCa, since treatments with elevated Mg^{2+} concentration and TTX (which prevented stimulus-induced ΔCa almost completely) had little effect on amino acid-induced Ca^{2+} decreases (128). Further evidence for this conclusion stems from experiments in which relatively large distances between the tips of the iontophoresis and recording electrodes (150 to 300

μm) were employed. When such electrode assemblies were inserted with both tips into stratum pyramidale, we observed detectable reductions in Ca^{2+} only, when spreading depression was elicited. When the same electrode assembly was inserted parallel to the orientation of the dendritic tree, small doses of excitatory amino acids caused significant reductions in $[Ca^{2+}]_o$ at the tip of the electrode.

Amino acids-induced profiles of $[Ca^{2+}]_o$

changes were comparable to those elicited by ortho- and antidromic stimulation, with a maximum ΔCa in the pyramidal-cell layer (Fig. 2). The conclusion that pyramidal-cell somata have the highest density of Ca^{2+} channels is, however, premature, since estimates of the extracellular volume fraction in the hippocampus indicate that the extracellular space is approximately one third smaller (65; W. J. Wadman and U. Heinemann, *in preparation*) in the pyramidal-cell layer than in other layers of hippocampal area CA1. Therefore large reductions in $[Ca^{2+}]_o$ in SP could result from movements of relatively small amounts of Ca^{2+}, and it is likely that the largest density of Ca^{2+} channels is found on proximal parts of apical dendrites within stratum radiatum.

The question also arose as to whether the characteristic spatial profile of Ca^{2+} concentration changes is dependent on the action of inhibitory transmitters such as GABA, which is capable of preventing both stimulus- and amino acid-induced ΔCa. At Ca^{2+} concentrations of 2 mM, iontophoretic application of excitatory amino acids will excite inhibitory interneurons, provoke GABA release, and thereby affect the local Ca^{2+} uptake into cells. Therefore we investigated the laminar distribution of Quis- and NMDA-induced decreases in $[Ca^{2+}]_o$ in the presence of the GABA antagonist bicuculline (53). This treatment led to a shift of the site of maximal Ca^{2+} loss from SP towards SR. A similar shift of the laminar profiles of ΔCa was found when excitatory amino acid-induced ΔCa were studied in media containing low Ca^{2+}, high Mg^{2+} levels, where synaptic transmission was blocked (Fig. 6). These findings suggest both (a) that Ca^{2+} entry into cells is under GABAergic control and (b) that Ca^{2+} sinks may be more effective in SR where the proximal parts of apical dendrites are located.

Ca^{2+} AND K^+ CONCENTRATION CHANGES IN THE CHRONIC ALUMINA CREAM FOCUS IN CAT CORTEX

In normal cat cortex, changes in $[Ca^{2+}]_o$ evoked by repetitive stimulation of the cortical surface or by stimulation of the ventrobasal thalamic complex are largest in upper cortical layers (58,59,60), while stimulus-induced $[K^+]_o$ changes are greatest in middle cortical layers (IV) (18,19). This typical distribution of Ca^{2+} sinks and K^+ sources is altered in chronic epileptic foci induced by topical application of alumina cream. The foci were characterized by a scar surrounded by a zone of marked gliosis

(189). The epileptogenic area was always located at the transition zone between normal and gliotic tissue (54,59). The spontaneous interictal field potentials were associated with 0.1- to 0.8-mM increases in $[K^+]_o$ and with decreases in $[Ca^{2+}]_o$ by up to 0.2 mM. Sites at which these modifications were found varied considerably from experiment to experiment, and in spite of the fact that all investigated animals had displayed at least three clinically manifest tonic–clonic seizures, we were not always able to identify an area with ongoing epileptic activity. However, laminar analysis of changes in $[K^+]_o$ and $[Ca^{2+}]_o$ showed that the largest stimulus-induced changes of $[K^+]_o$ and $[Ca^{2+}]_o$ were found at sites of spontaneously occurring interictal activity, which could be found in any layer of the cortex (59). Stimulus-induced decreases in $[Ca^{2+}]_o$ were as large as 0.7 mM (Fig. 3B), in contrast to 0.45 mM in normal cortex, while rises in $[K^+]_o$ were maximally 8.6 mM, which is only slightly larger than in normal cortex (maximum 7.6 mM) (54,62). An analysis of K^+ regulation, which took spatial K^+ buffering into account, revealed that K^+ regulation is not impaired in this epileptogenic tissue (54). This suggests that the occurrence of large Ca^{2+} sinks at atypical sites is important for the epileptogenic process. Similar changes, but with a more regular laminar distribution, were found in the chronic cobalt focus.

THE COBALT FOCUS IN RAT MOTOR CORTEX

Seven to nine days after topical application of 0.3 mg metallic cobalt powder onto the sensorimotor cortex of rats, an epileptogenic focus developed, characterized in EEG recordings by epileptiform spikes most often associated with myoclonic jerks of the contralateral forelimb. The area of maximal epileptogenesis was usually found at distances of 0.3 to 1 mm from the edge of the cobalt induced lesion. The ionic cobalt concentration in this tissue was estimated to be on the order of micromolar (183), which is too small to cause blockade of Ca^{2+} channels (3). The lesion was restricted to layers I to III, and the perifocal area was histologically characterized by mild sponginess of the neuropile, shrinkage of cells, and gliosis (183).

We compared stimulus- and amino acid-induced changes in $[Ca^{2+}]_o$ in the epileptogenic cortex to those in the contralateral normal cortex. In the area immediately surrounding the cobalt lesion we found usually only one major Ca^{2+} sink (Fig. 4), which extended from layer III to layer V, while the large sink normally

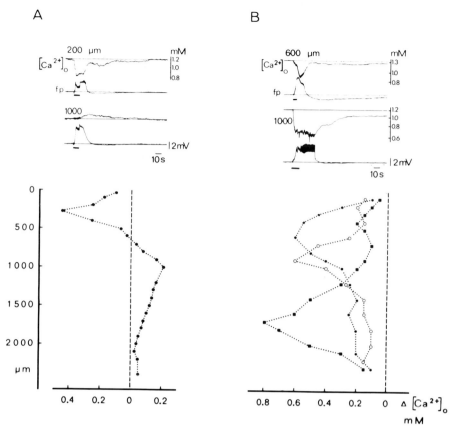

FIG. 3: Laminar profiles of stimulus induced changes in $[Ca^{2+}]_o$ in normal cat sensorimotor cortex and in the border zone of an alumina cream lesion. Numbers refer to depth below cortical surface. Bars indicate duration of stimulus trains. Note the enhancement of changes in $[Ca^{2+}]_o$ and the alterations in the laminar profiles. **A:** Average from three different experiments. **B:** Laminar profiles from three different experiments.

present in layer II was much less apparent. Spontaneous interictal discharges were associated with rises in $[K^+]_o$ by up to 1 mM, while decreases in $[Ca^{2+}]_o$ were always not detectable. Maximal rises in $[K^+]_o$ as well as kinetics of changes in $[K^+]_o$ indicated that K^+ regulation was not essentially impaired. Maximal reductions in $[Ca^{2+}]_o$ were somewhat larger in cobalt foci than in normal tissue.

Intracellular studies of neuronal activity during paroxysmal activity in the surface electrocorticogram revealed that about 59% of neurons behaved normally while 41% behaved abnormally (150). In 68% of the latter, depolarizing paroxysmal membrane potential shifts of up to 35 mV, which could last for 800 msec, were observed. These depolarizing shifts could neither be reversed nor elicited by depolarizing current injection. In the rest of the abnormally behaving neurons (32%), full action potentials were intermingled with partial spikes of varying amplitude, which were still present when depolarizing cur-

rent injection had inactivated action potential generation in the initial segment of the axon and in the somatodendritic transition zone. These findings indicate that both abnormalities are generated at a dendritic level. Moreover, most of the abnormally behaving neurons were found in layers III to V where particularly large Ca^{2+} decreases were found during electrical stimulation and application of excitatory amino acids.

Stimulus- and amino acid-induced Ca^{2+} signals were found to be increased also in acute cobalt foci, induced by superfusion of the sensorimotor cortex of cats with Co^{2+}-enriched artificial cerebrospinal fluid (Fig. 5) (88). Seizure activity developed only after Co^{2+} had been washed out and synaptic transmission had returned. When seizure activity developed, decreases in $[Ca^{2+}]_o$ induced either by excitatory amino acids or by repetitive stimulation were enhanced (Fig. 5D). These foci remained active for up to 10 hr after washout of cobalt, suggesting that the site of action is intracellular. The

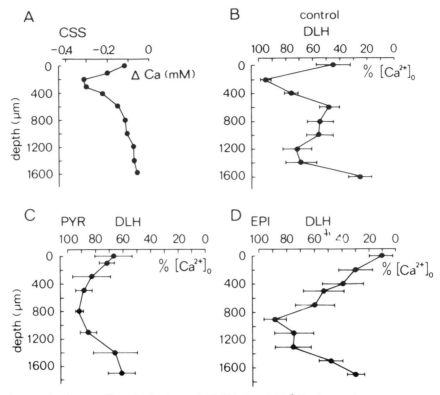

FIG. 4: Average laminar profiles of stimulus and DLH induced $[Ca^{2+}]_o$ changes in rat motor cortex. **A:** Plot of stimulus-induced $[Ca^{2+}]_o$ changes elicited by cortical surface stimulation (CSS; 10 sec, 20 Hz, 0.1 msec) as a function of recording depth below cortical surface. **B:** Laminar profile of DLH-induced decreases in $[Ca^{2+}]_o$ as a function of recording depth below cortical surface. **C:** Laminar profile of DLH-induced Ca^{2+} concentration changes in cortices from pyramidal-tract lesioned animals. **D:** Same in the border zone of a cobalt powder focus. For statistical analysis, the Ca^{2+} signals were normalized with respect to the largest response in a given experiment. *Dots* represent mean values and *bars* the respective standard deviations.

Ca^{2+} sinks were largest in layers II and III, with only a slight shift to deeper layers as compared to control and chronic cobalt foci, and remained in the zone of apical dendritic arborizations. At these sites the spontaneous paroxysmal discharges induced by Co^{2+} application were also largest, suggesting that this is the trigger zone of the acute Co^{2+} focus. It has been shown that intracellular injection of Co^{2+} impairs chloride extrusion (175) and thereby reduces the efficacy of postsynaptic inhibition (123). In addition, Co^{2+} disrupts axonal and possibly also dendritic transport processes (52). It may be speculated that an impairment of such dendritic transport processes may prevent the transport of Ca^{2+} channels into apical dendrites, with a resultant increase of Ca^{2+} channels at somanear portions of the dendrite and a possible increase in excitability.

THE KINDLING EPILEPSY

Repetitive electrical stimulation applied daily produces in many parts of the vertebrate brain a long term enhancement of neuronal excitability and epileptic activity of progressive severity and generalization (39). Eventually spontaneous interictal and ictal activity developed that originates from the kindled area (39,129, 157).

We performed experiments in area CA1 of the hippocampus. Rats were implanted under physiological control with a bundle of three stimulating electrodes positioned in the alveus, SR, and SM of the left dorsal hippocampus. Two recording electrodes were positioned nearby in SR and SO (184,185). This configuration of chronic implanted electrodes allowed possible electrode displacements to be controlled. Kindling stimuli

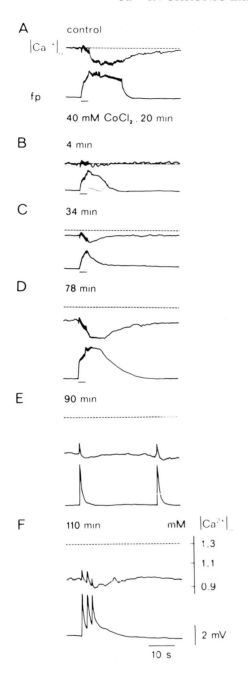

FIG. 5. Stimulus-induced changes in $[Ca^{2+}]_o$ during the development of an acute cobalt focus in cat sensorimotor cortex. **A:** Reduction of $[Ca^{2+}]_o$ elicited by repetitive cortical surface stimulation (indicated by *horizontal bars*). **B:** Soon after application of Co^{2+}, the Ca^{2+} signal is blocked. **D:** After washout, Ca^{2+} signals recover and become larger than control at about the time when the focus becomes active. **E, F:** Interictal and paroxysmal activity is also associated with reductions in $[Ca^{2+}]_o$.

were applied three times a day to SR/SM. The animals were kindled to stage V of Racine's scale (155,156), characterized by the appearance of generalized tonic–clonic convulsions associated with a loss of posture. In this state a second seizure often followed a few minutes after that induced by stimulation.

In the course of kindling, spontaneous interictal discharges developed. Analysis of the accompanying field potentials revealed an early form that had the same potential profile as that obtained during orthodromic stimulation, while a later form was characterized by a reversed potential profile suggesting a site of origin near the somata of hippocampal pyramidal cells (112,186). During kindling, the probability increased that population spikes were riding on interictal field potentials, indicating that more and more neurons became involved into the spontaneous paroxysmal activity.

In vivo experiments (W. J. Wadman and F. H. Lopes da Silva, *in preparation*) under well-defined experimental conditions showed that stimulus-induced long-term potentiation gradually increases during kindling, despite some irregularities (158). Studies on paired pulse stimulation with an interval of 20 msec revealed that the efficacy of inhibitory processes decreased as kindling progressed. This may result from a loss of GABAergic control or from a reduced efficacy of depolarizing Ca^{2+}-dependent K^+ conductances.

After reaching stage V of Racine's scale, hippocampal slices from the left implanted and right unimplanted side were prepared. The profile of orthodromically evoked potential revealed no major alterations, and no spontaneous interictal discharges were observed *in vitro*.

In the *in vitro* slices from kindled rats we not only investigated changes in $[Ca^{2+}]_o$ that could be induced by electrical and chemical means, but we also investigated K^+ regulation, since it has been suggested that these mechanisms may be impaired in other models of epilepsy (146,169). The relationship between the amplitude of stimulus induced rises in $[K^+]_o$ and that of subsequent undershoots was essentially unaltered (61,65), indicating that active K^+ uptake mechanisms are undisturbed in slices from kindled animals. Laminar profiles of stimulus-induced changes in $[K^+]_o$ also did not reveal marked alterations, suggesting that spatial K^+ buffering is not impaired in this stage of kindling.

The most striking alterations in slices from kindled rats (185) were found with respect to stimulus- and amino acid-induced changes in

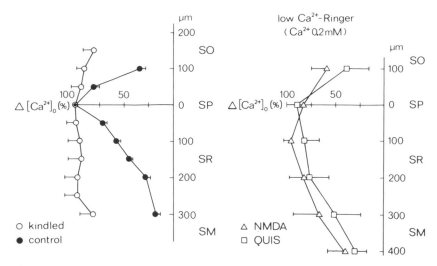

FIG. 6. **Left:** Laminar profiles of amino acid-induced Ca^{2+} concentration changes in the hippocampal slice area CA1 of normal and kindled animals. The data were normalized as in rat cortex. Data from experiments where Asp and where DLH were applied are included in the plots. Note the increase in the efficacy of Ca^{2+} sinks in the stratum radiatum/moleculare. **Right:** Laminar profile of Quis- and NMDA-induced Ca^{2+} concentration changes in media that contained 0.2 mM Ca^{2+} and 6 mM Mg^{2+} in order to suppress transmitter release from excited neurons. Note the shift of the maximal response from stratum pyramidale (SP) to stratum radiatum (SR).

$[Ca^{2+}]_o$. Figure 6 illustrates a comparison of laminar profiles of stimulus-induced changes in $[Ca^{2+}]_o$ in normal and in "kindled" slices. The signals in each individual experiment were, for the purpose of this analysis, normalized with respect to the largest signal (always found in SP), and data from various experiments were averaged. The data reveal that decreases in $[Ca^{2+}]_o$ are enhanced in SR and SM of kindled animals. These changes appear not to be simply a consequence of chronic electrode implantation, since they were also noted in slices obtained from the unimplanted hippocampus, which was kindled through the commissural pathway and showed *in vivo* the same ictal and interictal phenomena (186).

In order to define the underlying mechanisms more precisely, we also investigated the laminar profiles of amino acid-induced changes in $[Ca^{2+}]_o$. In kindled slices, large reductions in $[Ca^{2+}]_o$ could be observed in any layer of area CA1, and the relative extracellular Ca^{2+} loss in apical dendritic layers was five times larger than in normal slices. The amplitudes of Ca^{2+} signals were not reduced in SP with respect to those from normal slices. This finding suggests that the capacity for Ca^{2+} uptake has increased in the apical dendrites of hippocampal pyramidal cells.

The question also arose as to whether this increase in the amplitude of stimulus-dependent

and excitatory amino acid-dependent Ca^{2+} signals could be explained by a loss of GABAergic control, which is suggested by *in vivo* data. A comparison of Ca^{2+} profiles obtained from normal and kindled slices with those obtained from slices where chemical synaptic transmission was blocked or in the presence of bicuculline revealed that extracellular Ca^{2+} loss, particularly in SM, is larger in kindled slices. These results suggest that loss of GABAergic control alone cannot account for the observed alterations. Although our data point to an increase in postsynaptic Ca^{2+} conductances associated with the kindling process, they are not yet conclusive. Reductions in K^+ conductances and alterations in the laminar profiles of amino acid receptor distribution, which are thought to underlie long-term potentiation (6), may also be involved in the kindling epileptogenesis.

CHANGES IN $[Ca^{2+}]_o$ AND $[K^+]_o$ DURING SEIZURE ACTIVITY INDUCED BY INTERMITTENT LIGHT STIMULATION IN THE NEOCORTEX OF THE BABOON *PAPIO PAPIO*

Some of the baboons *Papio papio* respond to intermittent light stimulation (ILS) with EEG paroxysms accompanied by myoclonic jerks and eventually by tonic–clonic seizures (132,134, 135). This photosensitivity is reduced when the animals are immobilized with flaxedil but can be restored after injection of subconvulsive doses of allylglycine (133). The seizures probably originate in the frontal cortex, since light-induced paroxysmal evoked potentials and sustained seizure activity is largest and started first in this area (134,172).

ILS does not evoke significant reductions in $[Ca^{2+}]_o$, and rises in $[K^+]_o$ are smaller than 0.5 mM. After prolonged periods of repeated ILS, paroxysmal responses develop that can be associated with small reductions in $[Ca^{2+}]_o$ of less than 0.1 mM. When self-sustained afterdischarges developed, $[Ca^{2+}]_o$ fell by up to 0.2 mM and $[K^+]_o$ rose by 1 to 2 mM. However, when a generalized seizure finally developed, $[Ca^{2+}]_o$ decreased rapidly to very low extracellular levels of sometimes less than 80 μM and to about 0.25 mM on average (16). Such large reductions in $[Ca^{2+}]_o$ could occur in all cortical layers (Fig. 7), and they persisted throughout the seizures, i.e., for as long as 3 min. After the seizure it took several minutes for Ca^{2+} to return to baseline levels. Such light-induced seizures were associated with negative potential shifts of on average 7.3 mV and with rises in $[K^+]_o$ by up to

13 mM. These large reductions in $[Ca^{2+}]_o$ were reminiscent of spreading depression, but the moderate increases in $[K^+]_o$ and the amplitudes of the negative field potentials appeared to be too small for these observations to be ascribed to spreading depression. This conclusion is confirmed by the fact that spreading depression with a transient arrest of electrographic activity was observed in 4 animals. These spreading depressions could occur spontaneously or develop from seizures and were accompanied by increases in $[K^+]_o$ by on average 32 mM and by negative potential shifts of more than 22 mV.

The finding that seizure-related elevations in $[K^+]_o$ are limited to similar ceiling levels, as in rats and cats, suggests that K^+ regulation is not disturbed in these animals. However, a detailed analysis of this problem is at present not available.

The cause for the large reductions in $[Ca^{2+}]_o$ seen during light induced seizures is not definitely established, but it can be speculated that allylglycine, which is a blocker of endogenous GABA synthesis, plays an important role in this process. The reduction of GABAergic inhibition could contribute to the large reductions in

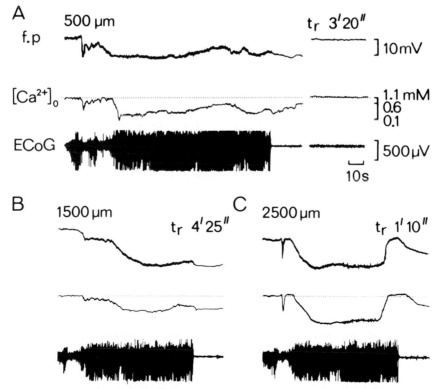

FIG. 7. Intermittent light stimulation-induced seizures in the frontal cortex of the baboon *Papio papio*. Traces marked ECoG represent surface electrocorticograms. Note the large decreases in $[Ca^{2+}]_o$.

$[Ca^{2+}]_o$. However, it is difficult to understand why, after seizure arrest, it took more than 1 hr until another seizure could be elicited. Also, the relative readiness of these monkeys in contrast to other species to develop spreading depression is not understood.

Another problem is raised by these observations: how can seizure activity be maintained and even spread at these low $[Ca^{2+}]_o$ levels at which synaptic transmission is normally blocked? This led us to study the effects of lowered Ca^{2+} concentration on neuronal activity in the hippocampal slice preparation.

EFFECTS OF EXTRACELLULAR CHANGES IN K^+ AND Ca^{2+} CONCENTRATION ON THE DEVELOPMENT OF SEIZURE ACTIVITY

Effects of changes in $[Ca^{2+}]_o$ and $[K^+]_o$ were studied in *in vitro* hippocampal slices. Perfusion with low-Ca^{2+} media increased the excitability of the hippocampal nerve cells, as indicated by the development of burst responses to ortho- and antidromic stimulation during washout of Ca^{2+} (25,177). At Ca^{2+} levels of about 0.2 mM, spontaneous epileptiform activity (SEA) develops (Fig. 8) predominantly in area CA1, and it persists at Ca^{2+} levels of below 10^{-6} M (79,192). Such spontaneous activity developed also in other parts of the brain under comparable conditions (14). SEA is characterized by prolonged slowly rising and decaying depolarizations of about 25 mV with trains of superimposed action potentials. The different spontaneous epileptiform discharges (SED) occur at a frequency of 2 to 9/min (192). SEA is extracellularly associated with negative potential shifts, rises in $[K^+]_o$ to about 11 mM, and reductions in $[Na^+]_o$ and $[Ca^{2+}]_o$ by up to 10 and 0.1 mM, respectively. This compares well with ionic changes during sustained seizures in intact neocortex (19,20,21,104). SEA reflects intrinsically generated epileptic activity, since synaptic transmission was found to be blocked at Ca^{2+} levels of below 0.2 mM (89). Most antiepileptic drugs (34,55,72; see also 47,103) prevent its development (carbamezipine, phenobarbital, and phenytoin at about therapeutic levels, valproate at 1 to 5 mM), while midazolam and the NMDA antagonists 2-APV and DL-aminoadipate were found to be ineffective (Fig. 8C).

Blockade of synaptic transmission is not a necessary condition for the induction of SEA, since it can already be induced at a Ca^{2+} level of about 0.8 mM when extracellular $[K^+]_o$ is elevated or when oxygen supply is reduced (192a).

Decrease of divalent cation concentration alone does not account for SEA, since reductions of Mg^{2+} alone will alter stimulus evoked responses into burst discharges and only rarely cause development of about 60 ms spontaneous burst discharges (U. Heinemann and J. D. C. Lambert, *submitted for publication*). A number of mechanisms may be involved in the generation of SEA. A reduced Ca^{2+} level may lead to a decreased Ca^{2+} entry and thereby to a diminished efficacy of repolarizing Ca^{2+}-dependent K^+ conductances, which would lose still more in efficacy because of extracellular K^+ accumulation (168). The reduction in efficacy of intrinsic and synaptic inhibitory control may free intrinsic capabilities of burst generation from normal control and therefore account for the induction of SEA.

Simultaneous recordings of spontaneous epileptiform discharges (SED) along pyramidal cell layer showed that they spread from the site of initiation (normally area CA1a) into neighboring regions (91,192). Negative potential shifts must not necessarily be superimposed by population spikes (192). However, when present, population spikes are closely time-locked but not perfectly synchronized (91a). These observations suggest that the mechanisms which cause synchronization of population spikes are different from those which cause the spread of SEA. SEDs could also be induced by electrical stimulation. The stimulus intensity required to elicit SEDs was much lower in the alveus and in the PC layer than in any other layer of the slice (91). Stimulation of PC layer can, in any part of area CA1, induce epileptiform activity, which then spreads with the same speed as SEA along the PC layer.

While SEA was associated at its site of origin with monophasic increases in $[K^+]_o$, diphasic rising slopes with an initial slow rate of rise were noted when SEDs were recorded at remote areas (91). In even more remote areas, increases in $[K^+]_o$ even preceded onset of SEA, suggesting that spatial redistribution of $[K^+]_o$ (19,20,21) was underlying spread of SEA. Consistent with this hypothesis are the observations that increases in baseline $[K^+]_o$ accelerated the frequency of SEA and that local applications of potassium by pressure ejection (Fig. 8A) induced SEA, which then spreads at a speed similar to that of spontaneous and stimulus-induced epileptiform discharges. Thus there is good evidence that spatial redistribution of $[K^+]_o$ underlies the spread of SEA (91).

This mechanism is obviously too slow to account for the synchronization of the population

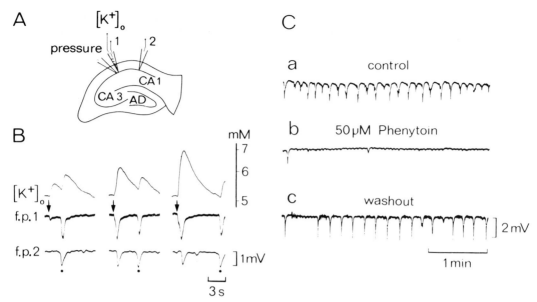

FIG. 8. A: Schematic representation of the experimental arrangement. **B:** Application of increasing amounts of potassium (marked by *arrows*) indicates the all-or-none nature of the K^+-evoked epileptiform discharges. Spontaneously occurring epileptiform discharges marked by dot spread in this experiment from electrode 2 to electrode 1. **C:** Phenytoin blocks reversibly spontaneous epileptiform activity, which develops in the absence of chemical synaptic transmission.

spikes superimposed on SEA. Ephaptic interactions may be involved in this synchronization process (78,161,178). Since the extracellular space is particularly small in area CA1 (65; see also 41,142), the hippocampus could be particularly liable for ephaptic interactions. The extracellular currents generated during population spikes in the extracellular medium as derived from the steep voltage gradient of approximately 100 mV/mm tissue are certainly large enough to account for such a synchronization mechanism (65). Since similar voltage gradients are also present in normal tissue, it is expected that ephaptic interactions play also an important role under normal conditions. The relatively slow spread of SEA is probably mediated by spatial redistributions of potassium. The associated shrinkage of extracellular space size found also in neocortex (19,20) may enhance the probability of ephaptic interactions during the course of the seizure. The chance for such ephaptic interactions is particularly large in the dendritic bundles formed in neocortex throughout layers II and III (33).

SIGNIFICANCE OF ALTERATIONS IN $[K^+]_o$ FOR SPREAD OF SEIZURE ACTIVITY IN INTACT NERVOUS TISSUE

Spread of seizure activity is known to occur in intact neocortex and in the thalamic relay nu-

cleus VPL (46,62). The propagation of seizure activity along anatomical pathways depends on the velocity of action potential propagation in the concerned pathway. However, a slower form of seizure spread can be observed, for example, in the course of the jacksonian march.

The possible role of potassium accumulation was previously tested in a study of seizure spread toward and within thalamic relay nuclei. After ablation of the whole somatosensory neocortex, repetitive electrical stimulation of the underlying white matter could induce seizure activity in the somatosensory relay nucleus VPL (46,56). Interestingly, this activity spreads from its site of initiation throughout the ventrobasal complex, and if a seizure is initiated by stimulation of cortical white matter underlying the hindpaw representation area, it also spreads within 1 to 5 sec to the forepaw representation area. Since at present there is no known anatomical pathway for excitatory synaptic coupling within the thalamus from one sensory channel to the next, this finding may indicate that K^+ redistribution is involved in this phenomenon. Indeed, as K^+ accumulates, burst discharges develop. While the rise in $[K^+]_o$ is monophasic at the site of initiation of seizure activity, it is diphasic with an initial slow rate of rise at sites where seizure activity starts later during the course of stimulation.

In neocortex itself, similar relationships were

found: while stimulus-induced rises in $[K^+]_o$ are monophasic at the site of seizure initiation close to the stimulation electrodes, they are diphasic when recorded at some distance. The onset of the secondary rise can be accelerated by local iontophoretic application of K^+ (62), lending further support to a role of potassium accumulation in spread of epileptic activity. This will depend both on the depolarizing effects of K^+ accumulation on neuronal membranes and on the reduced driving force for K^+ outward currents as a result of a depolarizing shift of the K^+ equilibrium potential (51,62,127,140,145). This recruitment may be further facilitated through the excitability-increasing effects associated with reductions of $[Ca^{2+}]_o$ (35,139,140). These include changes in surface charge screening and a reduced efficacy of repolarizing Ca^{2+}-dependent K^+ conductances as well as a disinhibitory effect.

DISCUSSION AND CONCLUSIONS

In the investigated chronic models of epilepsy, we have found that stimulus-induced and seizure-related Ca^{2+} signals are larger than in normal cortical tissue and that their laminar distribution is altered to a great extent. Increased Ca^{2+} signals (Table 1) were also observed in seizures induced by convulsants, which impaired either GABAergic synaptic transmission, such as penicillin (44,64,154; see also 164,190), picrotoxin (50,58), and bicuculline (53), or K^+ conductances, such as 4-aminopyridine (38,58; see also 162) and oenanthotoxin (113,115), as well as with convulsants which combine both effects such as pentetrazol (60,115). However, in all the drug-induced epilepsies, the sites of maximal reductions in $[Ca^{2+}]_o$ remained at the site where Ca^{2+} uptake into cells was largest also in normal tissue, suggesting that a diminution of GABAergic control or a reduced efficacy of repolarizing K^+ conductances cannot account alone for the observed alterations of Ca^{2+} profiles in chronic epilepsies. One explanation for our findings is therefore a long-term modification of the distribution and/or density of Ca^{2+} channels in the epileptogenic tissue. For instance, increased Ca^{2+} conductances at soma-near parts of the apical dendrites of pyramidal cells of layer V in chronic cobalt foci, could account for the depolarizing shifts of long duration recorded in such foci. However, other possibilities exist that can explain our findings. These include an increase in binding sites for excitatory amino acids, a shift from quisqualate and kainate to NMDA binding sites and changes in Na^+ or K^+ conductances.

The finding that epileptiform activity can, in area CA1 of the hippocampus, persist in an ethyleneglycol-bis-(β-aminoethylether) - N,N,N',N'-tetraacetic acid (EGTA)-buffered medium with a reduced driving force for Ca^{2+} inward currents suggests that Ca^{2+} currents are not in every case essential for the generation of epilepsy. However, the possibility has also to be considered that EGTA modifies the Ca^{2+} channels into sodium permeable ones (94). The resultant intracellular Na^+ accumulation may then lead to a

TABLE 1. *Comparison of $[Ca^{2+}]_o$ changes in different acute and chronic experimental epilepsies*[a]

$[Ca^{2+}]_o$, Δ[Ca]	PTZ	Pen	PTX	4-AP	CoCl₂	Al(OH)₃	Cobalt	Photos.
Baseline before seizures	↓	—	↓	↓	↓	—	—	—
Baseline between seizures	↓	↓	↓	↓	↓	—	—	—
Increase in stimulus-induced Δ[Ca] (%)	70%	50%	50%	40%	20%	70%	20 to 30%	—
Δ[Ca] interictal spikes	—	0.15 mM	—	—	0.20 mM	0.20 mM	0.15 mM	—
Depth of maximal Δ[Ca]	200 μm	200 μm	200 μm	200 μm	200 μm	unpredictable	700–900 μm	?
Depth extent of Δ[Ca]	1800 μm	1500 μm	1500 μm	1800 μm	1800 μm	All layers possible	All layers possible	All layers possible
Amplitude of maximal Δ[Ca]	0.7	0.7	0.7	0.7	0.6	0.7	0.7	1.15

[a] Abbreviations: PTZ, pentylenetetrazol, 25–40 mg i.v.; Pen, penicillin, 3000 IU topically applied; PTX, picrotoxin, 5 mg/kg i.v.; 4-AP, 4-aminopyridine, 50 μM topically applied; CoCl₂, 40 mM topically applied as a solution soaked cotton ball; Al(OH)₃, chronic alumina cream focus in cat induced 6 months to 6 years before the actual experiment; cobalt, cobalt powder focus in rats; photos., photosensitive baboon *Papio papio*.

release of Ca^{2+} from intracellular storage sites (9; but see 48,166). Indeed, a mobilization of intracellular Ca^{2+} has been observed in pentetrazole-treated snail neurons in the presence of low extracellular Ca^{2+} levels (173). Such intracellular increases in $[Ca^{2+}]_i$, like increases in intracellular cAMP concentration, may activate unspecific depolarizing conductances. Indirect evidence suggests that such a conductance may also be present in area CA1 of hippocampal slices, since amino acid evoked extracellular Na^+ losses are in this area, in contrast to other parts of the central nervous system, to a large extent dependent on Ca^{2+} entry into cells (194). Yet another explanation for the epileptogenesis in low-Ca^{2+} media is suggested by the recent finding of J. J. Hablitz, U. Heinemann, and H. D. Lux (51a) that lowering of extracellular Ca^{2+} concentration can induce a transient inward Na^+ current resistant to TTX. Our findings suggest that apart from remodeling of inhibitory control in chronic epileptic tissue also other mechanisms have to be taken into account. These could involve an increase in Ca^{2+} conductances within the epileptic tissue but also in other slow depolarizing conductances, as well as a loss of repolarizing K^+ conductances. The monitoring of ionic changes during epileptic or otherwise enhanced neuronal activity has proven to be helpful in such an analysis.

ACKNOWLEDGMENTS

This research was supported by Deutsche Forschungsgemeinschaft (DFG) grants He 1128/2 and He 1128/3 and by the SFB 220 to U. Heinemann and by European Training Program in Brain and Behavior Research (ETP) twinning grant to U. Heinemann and R. Pumain. We thank U. Roessler, I. Kurzciewicz, and G. Schuster for expert technical assistance in the experiments and I. Borst and U. Roessler for help in the preparation of the manuscript. Dr. J. Hablitz and Dr. J. D. C. Lambert provided helpful criticism of early drafts of this manuscript.

REFERENCES

1. Agnew, W. F., Yuen, T. G. H., Bullara, L. A., Jaques, D., and Pudensz, R. H. (1979): Intracellular calcium deposition in brain following electrical stimulation. *Neurol. Res.*, 1:187–202.
2. Aldenhoff, J. B., Hofmeier, G., Lux, H. D., and Swandulla, D. (1983): Stimulation of a sodium influx by cAMP in *Helix* neurons. *Brain Res.*, 276:289–296.
3. Alvarez-Leefmans, F. J., de Santis, A., and Miledi, R. (1979): Effects of some divalent cations on synaptic transmission in frog spinal neurones. *J. Physiol. (Lond.)*, 294:387–406.
4. Ault, B., Evans, R. H., Francis, A. A., Oakes, D. J., and Watkins, J. C. (1980): Selective depression of excitatory amino acid induced depolarizations by magnesium ions in isolated spinal cord preparations. *J. Physiol. (Lond.)*, 307:413–428.
5. Balcar, V. J., Pumain, R., Mark, J., Borg, J., and Mandel, P. (1978): GABA-mediated inhibition in the epileptogenic focus, a process, which may be involved in the mechanisms of the cobalt-induced epilepsy. *Brain Res.*, 154:182–185.
6. Baudry, M., Oliver, A., Creager, R., Wieraszko, A., and Lynch, G. (1980): Increase in glutamate receptors following repetitive electrical stimulation in hippocampal slices. *Life Sci.*, 27:325–330.
7. Benninger, C., Kadis, J., and Prince, D. A. (1980): Extracellular calcium and potassium changes in hippocampal slices. *Brain Res.*, 187:165–182.
8. Berdichevsky, E., Riveros, N., Sanches-Armass, S., and Orrego, (1983): Kainate, N-methylaspartate and other excitatory amino acids increase calcium influx into rat brain cortex cells in vitro. *Neurosci. Lett.*, 36:75–80.
9. Blaustein, M. P. (1974): The interrelationship between sodium and Ca^{2+} fluxes across cell membranes. *Rev. Physiol. Biochem. Pharmacol.*, 70:33–82.
10. Brown, D. A., and Griffith, W. H. (1983): Calcium-activated outward current in voltage-clamped hippocampal neurones of the guinea-pig. *J. Physiol. (Lond.)*, 337:287–301.
11. Brown, D. A., and Griffith, W. H. (1983): Persistent slow inward calcium current in voltage-clamped hippocampal neurones of the guinea-pig. *J. Physiol. (Lond.)*, 337:303–320.
12. Buhrle, C., and Sonnhof, U. (1983): The ionic mechanism of the excitatory action of glutamate upon the membranes of motoneurones of the frog. *Pfluegers Arch.*, 396:154–162.
13. Carbone, E., and Lux, H. D. (1984): A low voltage-activated calcium conductance in embryonic chick sensory neurons. *Biophys. J.*, 46:413–418.
14. Champagnat, J., Denavit-Saubie, M., and Siggins, G. R. (1983): Rhythmic neuronal activities in the nucleus of the tractus solitarius isolated in vitro. *Brain Res.*, 280:155–159.
15. Collquhoun, D., Neher, E., Reuter, H., and Stevens, C. F. (1981): Inward current channels activated by intracellular Ca in cultured cardiac cells. *Nature (Lond.)*, 294:752–754.
16. Pumain, R., Menini, C., Heinemann, U., Silva-Barrat, C., and Louvel, J. (1985): Chemical synaptic transmission is not necessary for epileptic activity to persist in the neocortex of the photosensitive baboon. *Exp. Neurol.*, 89:250–258.
17. Connors, B. W., Gutnick, M. J., and Prince, A. (1982): Electrophysiological properties of neocortical neurons in vitro. *J. Neurophysiol.*, 48:1302–1320.
18. Cordingley, G. E., and Somjen, G. G. (1978): Dissipation of locally accumulated extracellular potassium in the cat cerebral cortex. *Brain Res.*, 151:291–306.

19. Dietzel, I., and Heinemann, U. (1983): Extracellular electrolyte change during enhanced neuronal activity can be explained by spatial glial K$^+$-buffering in addition to small increases in osmotic pressure—Possibly induced by increases in metabolic activity. In: *Cerebral Blood Flow, Metabolism and Epilepsy,* edited by M. Baldy-Moulinier, D. Ingvar, and B. S. Meldrum, pp. 195–201. John Libbey, London.

20. Dietzel, I., Heinemann, U., Hofmeier, G., and Lux, H. D. (1980): Transient changes in the size of the extracellular space in the sensorimotor cortex of cats in relation to stimulus induced changes in potassium concentration. *Exp. Brain,* 40:432–439.

21. Dietzel, I., Heinemann, U., Hofmeier, G., and Lux, H. D. (1982): Stimulus-induced changes in extracellular Na$^+$ and Cl$^-$ concentration in relation to changes in the size of the extracellular space. *Exp. Brain Res.,* 46:73–84.

22. Dietzel, I., Lux, H. D., and Heinemann, U. (1984): Relations between slow cortical field potential changes and ionic movements during enhanced neuronal activity.

23. Dingledine, R., (1983): *N*-Methyl-D-aspartate activates voltage-dependent calcium conductance in rat hippocampal pyramidal cells. *J. Physiol. (Lond.),* 343:385–405.

24. Dunlap, K., and Fischbach, G. D. (1981): Neurotransmitter decrease the calcium conductance activated by depolarization of embryonic chick sensory neurones. *J. Physiol. (Lond.),* 317:519–535.

25. Dunwiddie, T. V. and Lynch, G. (1979): The relationship between extracellular calcium concentration and the induction of hippocampal longterm potentiation. *Brain Res.,* 169:103–110.

26. Eckert, R., and Lux, H. D. (1976): A voltage-sensitive persistent calcium conductance in neuronal somata of *Helix. J. Physiol. (Lond.),* 254:129–151.

27. Engberg, I., Flatman, J. A., and Lambert, J. D. C. (1979): The actions of excitatory amino acids on motoneurones in the feline spinal cord. *J. Physiol. (Lond.),* 288:227–261.

28. Engberg, I., Flatman, J. A., and Lambert, J. D. C. (1979): The action and interaction of calcium antagonists and DL-homocysteate on cat spinal motoneurones. *J. Physiol. (Lond.),* 296:96–97.

29. Engberg, I., Flatman, J. A., Lambert, J. D. C., and Lindsay, A. (1983): An analysis of bioelectrical phenomena evoked by microiontophoretically applied excitotoxic amino-acids in the feline spinal cord. *Excitotoxins (Wenner-Gren International Symposium),* edited by K. Fuxe, E. Roberts, and R. Schwarcz, pp. 170–183. Macmillan Press Ltd., Basingstone.

30. Erulkar, S. D., and Fine, A. (1979): Calcium in the nervous system. *Rev. Neurosci.,* 4:181–231.

31. Flatman, J. A., and Lambert, J. B. C. (1979): Sustained extracellular potentials in the cat spinal cord during the microiontophoretic application of excitatory amino acids. *J. Neurosci. Methods,* 1:205–218.

32. Flatman, J. A., Schwindt, P. C., Crill, W. E., and Stafstrom, C. E. (1983): Multiple actions of *N*-methyl-D-aspartate on cat neocortical neurons in vitro. *Brain Res.,* 266:169–173.

33. Fleischhauer, K., Petsche, H. and Wittkowsky, W. (1972): Vertical bundles of dendrites in the neocortex. *Z. Anat. Entwicklungesch.,* 136:213–223.

34. Franceschetti, S., Hamon, B., and Heinemann, U.: Effects of valproate on field potentials and evoked ionic changes in 'in vitro' hippocampal slices of rats. In preparation.

35. Frankenhaeuser, B., and Hodgkin, A. L. (1957): The action of calcium on the electrical properties of squid axons. *J. Physiol. (Lond.),* 137:218–244.

36. Fukuda, J., and Kameyama, M. (1979): Enhancement of Ca spikes in nerve cells of adult mammals during neurite growth in tissue culture. *Nature (Lond.),* 279:546–548.

37. Fukuda, J., and Kameyama, M. (1980): Tetrodotoxin-sensitive and tetrodotoxin-resistant sodium channels in tissue cultured spinal ganglion neurons from adult mammals. *Brain Res.,* 182:191–197.

38. Galvan, M., Grafe, P., and ten Bruggencate, G. (1982): Convulsive actions of 4-aminopyridine on neurones and extracellular K$^+$ and Ca^{++} activities in guinea-pig olfactory cortex slices. In: *Pharmacology and Physiology of Epileptogenic Phenomena,* edited by M. R. Klee, H. D. Lux and E. J. Speckmann, pp. 105–111. Raven, New York.

39. Goddard, G. V., McIntyre, P. C., and Leech, C. K. (1969): A permanent change in brain function resulting from daily electrical current through brain tissue in the rat. *Exp. Neurol.,* 25:295–330.

40. Gration, K. A. F., Lambert, J. J., Ramsey, R. L., Rand, R. P., and Usherwood, P. N. R. (1981): Agonist potency determination by patch clamp analysis of single glutamate receptors. *Brain Res.,* 230:400–405.

41. Green, J. D. (1964): The hippocampus. *Physiol. Rev.,* 44:501–608.

42. Griffiths, T., Evans, M. C., and Meldrum, B. S. (1982): Intracellular sites of early Ca^{2+} accumulation in the rat hippocampus during status epilepticus. *Neurosci. Lett.,* 30:329–334.

43. Grinvald, A., and Farber, I. C. (1981): Optical recording of calcium action potentials from growth cones of cultured neurones with a laser microbeam. *Science,* 212:1164–1177.

44. Gutnick, M. J. (1982): Ionic fluctuations and cyclic changes in epileptogenic excitability in hippocampal foci. In: *Physiology and Pharmacology of Epileptogenic Phenomena,* edited by M. R. Klee, H. D. Lux, and E. J. Speckmann, pp. 105–111. Raven, New York.

45. Gutnick, M. J., Connors, B. W., and Prince, D. A. (1982): Mechanisms of neocortical epileptogenesis in vitro. *J. Neurophysiol.,* 48:1321–1325.

46. Gutnick, M. J., Heinemann, U., and Lux, H. D. (1979): Stimulus induced and seizure related changes in extracellular potassium con-

centration in cat thalamus (VPL). *Electroencephalogr. Clin. Neurophysiol.*, 47:329–344.

47. Haas, H. L., Jefferys, J. G. R., Slater, N. T., and Carpenter, D. O. (1984): Modulation of low calcium induced field bursts in the hippocampus by monoamines and cholinomimetics. *Pfluegers Arch.*, 400:28–33.

48. Hablitz, J. J. (1981): Altered burst responses in hippocampal CA3 neurons injected with EGTA. *Exp. Brain Res.*, 42:483–485.

49. Hablitz, J. J. (1982): Conductance changes induced by DL-homocysteic acid and N-methyl-DL-aspartic acid in hippocampal neurons. *Brain Res.*, 247:149–153.

50. Hablitz, J. J. (1984): Picrotoxin-induced epileptiform activity in hippocampus: Role of endogenous versus synaptic factors. *J. Neurophysiol.*, 51:1011–1027.

51. Hablitz, J. J., and Lundervold, A. (1981): Hippocampal excitability and changes in extracellular K⁺. *Exp. Neurol.*, 71:410–420.

51a. Hablitz, J., Heinemann, U. and Lux, H. D.: Reductions in extracellular calcium activate a transient inward current in chick dorsal root ganglion cells. (*Submitted for publication.*)

52. Hammerschlag, R., Chia, A. Y., and Dravid, A. R. (1976): Inhibition of fast axonal transport of [H3] protein by cobalt ions. *Brain. Res.*, 114:353–358.

53. Hamon, B., and Heinemann, U.: Effects of bicuculline and GABA on extracellular free Ca²⁺ in 'in vitro' hippocampal slices. (*Submitted for publication.*)

54. Heinemann, U., and Dietzel, I. (1984): Extracellular potassium concentration in chronic alumina cream foci of cats. *J. Neurophysiol.*, 52:412–434.

55. Heinemann, U., Franceschetti, S., Hamon, B., Konnerth, A., and Yaari, Y. (1985): Effects of anticonvulsants on spontaneous epileptiform activity which develops in the absence of chemical synaptic transmission in hippocampal slices. *Brain Res.*, 325:349–352.

56. Heinemann, U., and Gutnick, M. J. (1979): Relation between extracellular potassium and neuronal activities in cat thalamus (VPL) during projection of cortical epileptiform discharge. *Electroencephalogr. Clin. Neurophysiol.*, 47:345–357.

57. Heinemann, U., Hamon, B. and Konnerth, A. (1984): GABA and baclofen reduce changes in extracellular free calcium in area CA1 of rat hippocampal slices. *Neurosci. Lett.*, 47:295–300.

58. Heinemann, U., Konnerth, A., Louvel, J., Lux, H. D., and Pumain, R. (1982): Changes in extracellular free Ca²⁺ in normal and epileptic sensorimotor cortex of cats. In: *Physiology and Pharmacology of Epileptogenic Phenomena*, edited by M. R. Klee, H. D. Lux, and E. J. Speckmann, pp. 29–35. Raven, New York.

59. Heinemann, U., Konnerth, A., and Lux, H. D. (1981): Stimulation induced changes in extracellular free calcium in normal cortex and chronic alumina cream foci of cats. *Brain Res.*, 213:246–250.

60. Heinemann, U., and Louvel, J. (1983): Changes in [Ca²⁺]ₒ and [K⁺]ₒ during repetitive electrical stimulation and during pentetrazol induced seizure activity in the sensorimotor cortex of cats. *Pfluegers Arch.*, 398:310–317.

61. Heinemann, U., and Lux, H. D. (1975): Undershoots following stimulus induced rises in extracellular potassium concentration in the cerebral cortex of cat. *Brain Res.*, 93:63–76.

62. Heinemann, U., and Lux, H. D. (1977): Ceiling of stimulus induced rises in extracellular potassium concentration in the cerebral cortex of cat. *Brain Res.*, 120:231–249.

63. Heinemann, U., and Lux, H. D. (1983): Ionic changes during experimentally induced epilepsies. In: *Progress in Epilepsy*, edited by F. C. Rose, pp. 87–102. Pitman Medical, London.

64. Heinemann, U., Lux, H. D., and Gutnick, M. J. (1977): Extracellular free calcium and potassium during paroxysmal activity in the cerebral cortex of cat. *Exp. Brain Res.*, 27:237–243.

65. Heinemann, U., Neuhaus, S., and Dietzel, I. (1983): Aspects of K⁺ regulation in normal and gliotic brain tissue. In: *Cerebral Blood Flow, Metabolism and Epilepsy*, edited by M. Baldy-Moulinier, D. H. Ingvar, and B. S. Beldrum, pp. 271–278. John Libbey, London.

66. Heinemann, U., and Pumain, R. (1980): Extracellular calcium activity changeB in cat sensorimotor cortex induced by iontophoretic application of aminoacids. *Exp. Brain Res.*, 40:247–250.

67. Heinemann, U., and Pumain, R. (1981): Effects of tetrodotoxin on changes in extracellular free calcium induced by repetitive electrical stimulation and iontophoretic application of excitatory amino acids in the sensorimotor cortex of cats. *Neurosci. Lett.*, 21:87–91.

68. Heinemann, U., and Pumain, R. (1981): Changes in extracellular free Ca²⁺, K⁺ and Na⁺ during iontophoretic application of excitatory amino acids in the neocortex of cat. *Pfluegers Arch.*, 389:R18.

69. Herrling, P. L., Morris, R., and Salt, T. E. (1983): Effects of excitatory amino acids and their antagonists on membrane and action potentials of cat caudate neurones. *J. Physiol. (London)*, 339:207–222.

70. Hofmeier, G., and Lux, H. D. (1981): The time course of intracellular free calcium and related electrical effects after injection of CaCl₂ into neurons of the snail, *Helix pomatia. Pfluegers Arch.*, 391:242–251.

71. Holmes, G., and May, W. P. (1909): On the exact origin of the pyramidal tracts in man and other mammals. *Brain*, 32:1–43.

72. Hood, T. W., Siegfried, J., and Haas, H. L. (1983): Analysis of carbamazepine actions in hippocampal slices of the rat. *Cell. Mol. Neurobiol.*, 3:213–222.

73. Hoesli, L., Hoesli, E., Andres, P. F., and Landolt, H. (1981): Evidence that the depolarization of glial cells by inhibitory amino acids is caused by an efflux of K⁺ from neurones. *Exp. Brain Res.*, 42:43–48.

74. Hotson, J. R., and Prince, D. A. (1980): A calcium-activated hyperpolarization follows repet-

itive firing in hippocampal neurons. *J. Neuro-physiol.*, 43:409–419.

75. Ichida, S., Tokunaga, H., Moriyama, M., Oda, Y., Tanaka, S., and Kita, T. (1982): Effects of neurotransmitter candidates on 45-Ca uptake by cortical slices of rat brain: Stimulatory effect of L-glutamic acid. *Brain Res.*, 248:305–312.

76. Jahnsen, H., and Llinas, R. (1984): Electro-physiological properties of guinea-pig thalamic neurones: An in vitro study. *J. Physiol. (Lond.)*, 349:205–226.

77. Jahnsen, H., and Llinas, R. (1984): Ionic basis for the electroresponsiveness and oscillatory properties of guinea-pig thalamic neurones in vitro. *J. Physiol. (Lond.)*, 349:227–247.

78. Jefferys, J. G. R. (1979): Initiation and spread of action potentials in granule cells maintained in vitro in slices of guinea-pig hippocampus. *J. Physiol. (Lond.)*, 289:375–388.

79. Jefferys, J. G. R., and Haas, H. L. (1982): Syn-chronized bursting of CA1 hippocampal pyra-midal cells in the absence of synaptic transmis-sion. *Nature (Lond.)*, 300:448–450.

80. Johnston, D. (1976): Voltage clamp reveals basis for calcium regulation of bursting pacemaker potentials in "*Aplysia*" neurons. *Brain Res.*, 107:418–423.

81. Johnston, D., and Brown, T. H. (1983): Inter-pretation of voltage-clamp measurements in hippocampal neurons. *J. Neurophysiol.*, 50:465–485.

82. Johnston, D., and Hablitz, J. J. (1980): Voltage clamp discloses slow inward current in hippo-campal burst-firing neurones. *Nature (Lond.)*, 286:391–393.

83. Kalil, K., and Schneider, G. E. (1975): Retro-grade cortical and axonal changes following le-sions of the pyramidal tract. *Brain Res.*, 89:15–27.

84. Kelly, J. S., Krnjevic, K., and Yim, G. K. W. (1967): Unresponsive cells in cerebral cortex. *Brain Res.*, 6:767–769.

85. King, G. L., and Somjen, G. G. (1981): Extra-cellular calcium and action potentials of soma and dendrites of hippocampal pyramidal cells. *Brain Res.*, 226:339–343.

86. Kocsis, J. D., Waxman, C., Hildebrand, C., and Ruiz, J. A. (1982): Regenerating mammalian nerve fibres: Changes in action potential wave-form and firing characteristics following blockage of potassium conductance. *Proc. R. Soc. B (Lond.)*, 217:77–87.

87. Kocsis, J. D., and Waxman, S. G. (1983): Elec-trophysiology of conduction in mammalian re-generating nerves. In: *Nerve Organ and Tissue Regeneration: Research Perspectives*, edited by F. J. Seil, pp. 89–107. Academic, New York.

88. Konnerth, A. (1982): Extrazellulaere Kalium-und Kalziumaenderungen der Hirnrinde. Dis-sertation, Ludwig Maximilians-Universitaet, Muenchen.

89. Konnerth, A., and Heinemann, U. (1983): Ef-fects of GABA on presumed presynaptic Ca^{2+} entry in hippocampal slices. *Brain Res.*, 270:185–189.

90. Konnerth, A., and Heinemann, U. (1983): Pre-synaptic involvement in frequency facilitation in the hippocampal slice. *Neurosci. Lett.*, 42:255–260.

91. Konnerth, A., Heinemann, U., and Yaari, Y. (1984): Slow transmission of neural activity in hippocampal area CA1 in absence of active chemical synapses. *Nature (Lond.)*, 307:69–71.

91a. Konnerth, A., Heinemann, U., and Yaari, Y.: Nonsynaptic epileptogenesis at the mammalian hippocampus in vitro. I. Development of sei-zure like activity in low extracellular calcium. *J. Neurophysiology (in press)*.

92. Kostyuk, F. G. (1980): Calcium ionic channels in electrically excitable membrane. *Neurosci-ence*, 5:945–959.

93. Kraig, R. P., and Nicholson, C. (1978): Ex-tracellular ionic variations during spreading depression. *Neuroscience*, 3:1045–1059.

94. Krishtal, O. A., Pidolpichko, V. I., and Shak-hovalov, Y. A. (1981): Conductance of the cal-cium channel in the membrane of snail neu-rones. *J. Physiol. (Lond.)*, 310:423–434.

95. Krnjevic, K. (1974): Chemical nature of syn-aptic transmission in vertebrates. *Physiol. Rev.*, 54:419–540.

96. Krnjevic, K., and Lisiewicz, A. (1972): Injec-tions of calcium ions into spinal motoneurones. *J. Physiol. (Lond.)*, 225:363–390.

97. Krnjevic, K., Morris, M. E., and Reiffenstein, R. J. (1980): Changes in extracellular Ca^{2+} and K^+ activity accompanying hippocampal dis-charges. *Can. J. Physiol. Pharmacol.*, 58:579–583.

98. Krnjevic, K., Morris, M. E., and Reiffenstein, R. F. (1982): Stimulation-evoked changes in ex-tracellular K^+ and Ca^{2+} in pyramidal layers of the rat's hippocampus. *Can. J. Physiol. Phar-macol.*, 60:1643–1657.

99. Krnjevic, K., Morris, M. E., Reiffenstein, R. J., and Ropert, N. (1982): Depth distribution and mechanism of changes in extracellular K^+ and Ca^{2+} concentrations in the hippocampus. *Can. J. Physiol. Pharmacol.*, 60:1958–1971.

100. Krnjevic, K., Puil, E., and Werman, R. (1975): Evidence for Ca^{2+} activated conductance in cat spinal motoneurons from intracellular EGTA in-jections. *Can. J. Physiol. Pharmacol.*, 53:1214–1218.

101. Kuno, M. and Llinas, R. (1970): Enhancement of synaptic transmission by dendritic potentials in chromatolysed motoneurones of the cat. *J. Physiol. (Lond.)*, 210:807–821.

101a. Lambert, J. D. C., and Heinemann, U. (1985): Aspects of the actions of excitatory amino acids on hippocampal CA1 neurones. In: *Calcium Electrogenesis and Neuronal Functioning*, ed-ited by U. Heinemann, M. Klee, E. Neher, and W. Singer. Springer, Heidelberg (*in press*).

102. Lasek, A. M. (1942): The pyramidal tract: a study of retrograde degeneration in the monkey. *Arch. Neurol. Psychiatry*, 48:561–567.

103. Lee, K. S., Schubert, P., and Heinemann, U. (1984): The anticonvulsant action of adenosine. A postsynaptic, dendritic action by a possible endogenous anticonvulsant. *Brain Res.*, 321:160–164.

104. Lehmenkuehler, A., Zidek, W., and Caspers, H. (1982): Changes of extracellular Na^+ and Cl^-

activity in the brain cortex during seizure discharges. In: *Physiology and Pharmacology in Epileptogenic Phenomena*, edited by M. R. Klee, H. D. Lux, and E. J. Speckmann, pp. 37–45. Raven, New York.

105. Llinas, R., Greenfield, S. A., and Jahnsen, H. (1984): Electrophysiology of pars compacta cells in the in vitro substantia nigra—A possible mechanism for dendritic release. *Brain Res.*, 294:127–132.

106. Llinas, R., and Hess, R. (1976): Tetrodotoxin-resistant dendritic spikes in avian Purkinje cells. *Proc. Natl. Acad. Sci. U.S.A.*, 73:2520–2523.

107. Llinas, R., and Jahnsen, H. (1982): Electrophysiology of mammalian thalamic neurones in vitro. *Nature (Lond.)*, 11:406–408.

108. Llinas, R., and Sugimori, M., (1980): Electrophysiological properties of in vitro Purkynje cell somata in mammalian cerebellar slices. *J. Physiol. (Lond.)*, 305:171–195.

109. Llinas, R., and Sugimori, M. (1980): Electrophysiological properties of 'in vitro' Purkinje cell dendrites in mammalian cerebellar slices. *J. Physiol. (Lond.)*, 305:197–213.

110. Llinas, R., and Yarom, Y. (1981): Electrophysiology of mammalian inferior olivary neurones 'in vitro'. Different types of voltage-dependent ionic conductances. *J. Physiol. (Lond.)*, 305:549–568.

111. Lloyd, K. G., Munari, C., Bossi, L., Stoeffels, C., Talairach, J., and Morselli, P. L. (1981): Biochemical evidence for the alterations of GABA-mediated synaptic transmission in pathological brain tissue (stereo-EEG or morphological definition) from epileptic patients. In: *Neurotransmitters, Seizures and Epilepsy*, edited by P. L. Morselli, K. G. Lloyd, W. Loscher, B. Meldrum, and E. H. Reynolds, pp. 325–338. Raven, New York.

112. Lopes da Silva, F. H., Wadman, W. J., Leung, L. S., and van Hulten, K. (1982): Long-term changes in EEG and evoked potentials during the development of an epileptic focus (by kindling) in the prepyriform cortex in the dog. *Electroencephalogr. Clin. Neurophysiol. Suppl.*, 36:274–287.

113. Louvel, J., Aldenhoff, J., Hofmeier, G., and Heinemann, U. (1982): Effects of the convulsant drug oenanthotoxin on snail neurones and on cat cortex. In: *Physiology and Pharmacology of Epileptogenic Phenomena*, edited by M. R. Klee, H. D. Lux, and E. J. Speckmann, pp. 47–52. Raven, New York.

114. Louvel, J., and Heinemann, U. (1980): Diminution de la concentration extracellulaire des ions calcium lors des crises epileptiques focales induites par l'eonanthotoxine dans le cortex du chat. *C. R. Acad. Sci. (Paris)*, 291:997–1000.

115. Louvel, J., and Heinemann, U. (1981): Mode d'action du pentetrazole au niveau cellulaire. *Rev. Electroencephalogr. Neurophysiol.*, 11:335–339.

116. Louvel, J., and Heinemann, U. (1983): Changes in $[Ca^{2+}]_o$, $[K^+]_o$ and neuronal activity during oenanthotoxin induced epilepsy. *Electroencephalogr. Clin. Neurophysiol.*, 56:457–466.

117. Lux, H. D. (1980): Ionic conditions and membrane behavior. In: *Antiepileptic Drugs: Mechanisms of Action*, edited by G. H. Glaser, J. K. Penry, and D. M. Woodbury, pp. 63–83. Raven, New York.

118. Lux, H. D. (1982): Observations of single Ca^{2+} channels. In: *Single Channel Recording*, edited by B. Sakmann and E. Neher, pp. 437–449. Plenum, New York.

119. Lux, H. D. (1983): An invertebrate model of paroxysmal depolarizing shifts. *Electrophysiology of Epilepsy*, edited by P. A. Schwartzkroin and H. V. Wheal, pp. 344–352. Academic, London.

120. Lux, H. D., and Heinemann, U. (1982): Consequences of calcium electrogenesis for the generation of paroxysmal depolarisation shift. In: *Epilepsy and Motor System*, edited by E. J. Speckmann, and H. Elger, pp. 101–119. Urban und Schwarzenberg, Muenchen.

121. Lux, H. D., Heinemann, U., and Dietzel, I., Chapter 31.

122. Lux, H. D., and Neher, E. (1973): The equilibration time course of $[K^+]_o$ in cat cortex. *Exp. Brain Res.*, 17:190–205.

123. Lux, H. D., and Schubert, P. (1969): Postsynaptic inhibition: Intracellular effects of various ions in spinal motoneurons. *Science*, 166:625–626.

124. MacDonald, J. F. (1978): A comparison of the action of glutamate, ibotenate and other related amino acids on feline spinal interneurones. *J. Physiol. (Lond.)*, 275:449–465.

125. MacDonald, J. F., and Wojtowicz, J. M. (1980): Two conductance mechanisms activated by applications of L-glutamic, L-aspartic, DL-homocysteic, N-methyl-D-aspartic, and DL-kainic acids to cultured mammalian central neurones. *Can. J. Physiol. Pharmacol.*, 58:1393–1397.

126. MacDonald, J. F., Porietis, A. V., and Wojtowicz, J. M. (1982): L-Aspartic acid induces a region of negative slope conductance in the current-voltage relationship of cultured spinal cord neurons. *Brain Res.*, 237:248–253.

127. Malenka, R. C., and Kocsis, J. D. (1982): Effects of GABA on stimulus-evoked changes in $[K^+]_o$ and parallel fiber excitability. *J. Neurophysiol.*, 48:608–621.

128. Marciani, M. G., Louvel, J., and Heinemann, U. (1982): Aspartate induced changes in extracellular free calcium in "in vitro" hippocampal slices of rats. *Brain Res.*, 238:272–277.

129. McNamara, J. O., Byrne, M. C., Dasheif, R. M., and Fitz, J. G. (1980): The kindling model of epilepsy: A review. *Progr. Neurobiol.*, 15:139–159.

130. Meech, R. W. (1974): Prolonged action potentials in Aplysia neurones injected with EGTA. *Comp. Physiol.*, 48:397–410.

131. Meiri, H., Spira, M. E., and Parnas, I. (1980): Membrane conductance and action potential of a regenerative axonal tip. *Science*, 211:707–722.

132. Meldrum, B. (1980): Photically-induced epilepsy in the baboon, *Papio papio*. In: *Animal Models of Neurological Disease*, edited by F. C. Rose, pp. 202–216. Pitman, Tunbridge-Wells.

133. Meldrum, B. S., Menini, C., Naquet, R., Laurent, H., and Stutzmann, J. M. (1979): Proconvulsant, convulsant and other actions of the D- and L-stereoisomers of allylglycine in the photosensitive baboon, *Papio papio. Electroencephalogr. Clin. Neurophysiol.*, 47:383–395.

134. Menini, C. (1976): Role du cortex frontal dans l'epilepsie photosensible du singe *Papio papio. J. Physiol.* (*Paris*) 72:5–44.

135. Menini, Ch., Stutzmann, J. M., Laurent, H. and Naquet, R. (1980): Paroxysmal visual evoked potentials (PVEP) in the *Papio papio*. I. Morphological and topographical characteristics. Comparison with paroxysmal discharges (DP). *Electroencephalogr. Clin. Neurophysiol.*, 50: 356–364.

136. Miles, R., and Wong, R. K. S. (1983): Single neurones can initiate synchronized population discharge in the hippocampus. *Nature* (*Lond.*), 304:371–373.

137. Monaghan, D. T., Holets, V. R., Toy, D. W., and Cotman, C. W. (1983): Anatomical distributions of four pharmacologically distinct 3H-L-glutamate binding sites. *Nature* (*Lond.*), 306:176–179.

138. Nadler, J. V., Vaca, K. W., White, W. F., Lynch, G. S., and Cotman, C. W. (1976): Aspartate and glutamate as possible transmitters of excitatory hippocampal afferents. *Nature* (*Lond.*), 260:538–540.

139. Nicholson, C. (1980): Modulation of extracellular calcium and its functional implications. *Fed. Proc.*, 39:1519–1523.

140. Nicholson, C. (1980): Dynamics of the brain cell microenvironment. *NRP Bull.* 18:177–322.

141. Nicholson, C., ten Bruggencate, G., Stockle, H., and Steinberg, R. (1978): Calcium and potassium changes in extracellular microenvironment of cat cerebellar cortex. *J. Neurophysiol.*, 41:1026–1039.

142. Nicholson, C., and Phillips, J. M. (1981): Ion diffusion modified by tortuosity and volume fraction in the extracellular microenvironment of the rat cerebellum. *J. Physiol.* (*Lond.*), 321:225–257.

143. Nowak, L., Bregestovski, P., Ascher, P., Herbet, A., and Prochiantz, A. (1984): Magnesium gates glutamate-activated channels in mouse central neurones. *Nature*, 307:462–465.

144. Oehme, M., Kessler, M., and Simon, W. (1976): Neutral carrier Ca^{2+} microelectrode. *Chimia*, 30:204–206.

145. Ogata, N., Hori, N., and Katsuda, N. (1976): The correlation between extracellular potassium concentration and hippocampal epileptic activity in vitro. *Brain Res.*, 110:371–375.

146. Oliver, A. P., Hoffer, B. J., and Wyatt, R. J. (1980): Kindling induces long-lasting alterations in response of hippocampal neurons to elevated potassium levels in vitro. *Science*, 208:1264–1265.

147. Prince, D. A. (1978): Neurophysiology of epilepsy. *Annu. Rev. Neurosci.*, 1:395–415.

148. Prince, D. A., Lux, H. D., and Neher, E. (1973): Measurement of extracellular potassium activity in cat cortex. *Brain Res.*, 50:489–495.

149. Puil, E. (1981): *S*-glutamate: Its interactions with spinal neurons. *Brain Res. Rev.*, 3:229–332.

150. Pumain, R. (1982): Intracellular potentials of cortical neurons in a chronic epileptogenic focus. In: *Physiology and Pharmacology of Epileptogenic Phenomena*, edited by M. R. Klee, H. D. Lux, and E. J. Speckmann, pp. 65–72. Raven, New York.

151. Pumain, R., and Heinemann, U. (1982): Extracellular free Ca^{2+} changes in normal neocortex and in chronic epileptogenic foci in rats. *Neuroscience*, 7:S172.

152. Pumain, R., and Heinemann, U. (1982): Intracellular potential and extracellular calcium changes in chronic epilepsy. In: *Advances in Epileptology: XIIIth Epilepsy International Symposium*, edited by H. Akimoto, H. Kazamatsuri, M. Seino, and A. Ward, pp. 497–500. Raven, New York.

153. Pumain, R., and Heinemann, U. (1985): Stimulus-evoked and amino-acid induced ionic changes in rat neocortex. *J. Neurophysiol.*, 53:1–16.

154. Pumain, R., Kurcewicz, I., and Louvel, J. (1983): Fast extracellular calcium transients: Involvement in epileptic processes. *Science*, 222:177–179.

155. Racine, R. J. (1972): Modification of seizure activity by electrical stimulation. I. Afterdischarge threshold. *Electroencephalogr. Clin. Neurophysiol.*, 32:269–279.

156. Racine, R. J. (1972): Modification of seizure activity by electrical stimulation. II. Motor seizure. *Electroencephalogr. Clin. Neurophysiol.*, 32:281–294.

157. Racine, R. (1978): Kindling: The first decade. *J. Neurosurg.*, 3:234–252.

158. Racine, R. J., and Hafner, S. (1983): Long-term potentiation phenomena in the rat limbic forebrain. *Brain Res.*, 260:217–231.

159. Ribak, C. E., Harris, A. B., Vaughn, J. E., and Roberts, E. (1979): Inhibitory, GABAergic nerve terminals decrease at sites of focal epilepsy. *Science*, 205:211–214.

160. Ribak, C. E., and Reiffenstein, R. J. (1982): Selective inhibitory synapse loss in chronic cortical slabs: A morphological basis for epileptic susceptibility. *Can. J. Physiol. Pharmacol.*, 60:864–870.

161. Richardson, T. L., Turner, R. W., and Miller, J. J. (1984): Extracellular field influence transmembrane potentials and synchronization of hippocampal neuronal activity. *Brain Res.*, 294:255–262.

162. Rogawski, M. A., and Barker, J. L. (1983): Effects of 4-aminopyridine on calcium action potentials and calcium current under voltage clamp in spinal neurons. *Brain Res.*, 280:180–185.

163. Sawada, S., Takada, S., and Yamamoto, C. (1982): Excitatory actions of homocysteic acid on hippocampal neurones. *Brain Res.*, 238:282–285.

164. Schwartzkroin, P. A., and Prince, D. A. (1978): Cellular and field potential properties of epilep-

togenic hippocampal slices. *Brain Res.*, 147: 117–130.

165. Schwartzkroin, P. A., and Slawsky, M. (1977): Probable calcium spikes in hippocampal neurons. *Brain Res.*, 135:157–161.

166. Schwartzkroin, P. A., and Stafstrom, C. E. (1980): Effects of EGTA on the calcium-activated afterhyperpolarization in hippocampal CA3 pyramidal cells. *Science*, 210:1125–1126.

167. Schwindt, P., and Crill, W. (1980): Role of a persistent inward current in motoneuron bursting during spinal seizures. *J. Neurophysiol.*, 43: 1296–1318.

168. Schwindt, P. C., and Crill, W. E. (1980): Properties of a persistent inward current in normal and TEA-injected motoneurons. *J. Neurophysiol.*, 43:1700–1724.

169. Somjen, G. G. (1979): Extracellular potassium in the mammalian central nervous system. *Annu. Rev. Physiol.*, 41:97–177.

170. Somjen, G. G. (1980): Stimulus-evoked and seizure-related responses of extracellular calcium activity in spinal cord compared to those in cerebral cortex. *J. Neurophysiol.*, 44:617–632.

171. Stafstrom, C. E., Schwindt, P. C., and Crill, W. E. (1982): Negative slope conductance due to a persistent subthreshold sodium current in cat neocortical neurons in vitro. *Brain Res.*, 236:221–226.

172. Stutzmann, J. M., Laurent, M., Valin, A., and Menini, C. (1980): Paroxysmal visual evoked potentials (PVEPs) in *Papio papio*. Evidence for a facilitatory effect of intermittent photic stimulation. *Electroencephalogr. Clin. Neurophysiol.*, 50:365–374.

173. Sugaya, E., Onuzuka, M., Furuichi, H., Sugaya, A., and Tsuda, T. (1982): Intracellular calcium and bursting activity. In: *Pharmacology and Physiology of Epileptogenic Phenomena*, edited by M. R. Klee, H. D. Lux, and E. J. Speckmann, pp. 325–334. Raven, New York.

174. Swandulla, D., and Lux, H. D. (1984): Changes in ionic conductances induced by cAMP in Helix neurons. *Brain Res.*, 305:115–122.

175. Sypert, G. W. and Bidgood, W. D. (1977): Effect of intracellular cobalt ions on postsynaptic inhibition in cat spinal motoneurones. *Brain Res.*, 134:372–376.

176. Takeuchi, N. (1963): Effects of calcium on the conductance change on the endplate membrane during the action of transmitter. *J. Physiol. (Lond.)*, 167:141–155.

177. Taylor, Ch.P., and Dudek, F. E. (1982): Synchronous neural afterdischarges in rat hippocampal slices without active chemical synapses. *Science*, 218:810–812.

178. Taylor, C. P., Krnjevic, K., and Ropert, N. (1984): Facilitation of hippocampal CA3 pyramidal cell firing by electrical fields generated antidromically. *Neuroscience*, 11:101–109.

179. Tower, D. B. (1960): *Neurochemistry of Epilepsy*. Charles C. Thomas, Springfield, Illinois.

180. Traub, R. D., and Llinas, R. (1979): Hippocampal pyramidal cells: significance of dendritic ionic conductances for neuronal function and epileptogenesis. *J. Neurophysiol.*, 42:476–496.

181. Traub, R. D., and Wong, R. K. S. (1982): Cellular mechanism of neuronal synchronisation in epilepsy. *Science*, 216:745–747.

182. Traub, R. G., and Wong, R. K. S. (1983): Synchronized burst discharge in disinhibited hippocampal slice. II. Model of cellular mechanism. *J. Neurophysiol.*, 49:459–471.

183. Trottier, S., Truchet, M., and Laroudie, C. (1982): Secondary ion microanalysis in the study of cobalt-induced epilepsy in the rat. *Exp. Neurology*, 76:231–245.

184. Van Harreveld, A., and Malhotra, S. K. (1967): Extracellular space in the cerebral cortex of the mouse. *J. Anat.*, 101:197–207.

185. Wadman, W. J., and Heinemann, U. (1983): Laminar profiles of changes in extracellular potassium and calcium concentration in slices obtained from kindled rats. In: *Cerebral Blood Flow, Metabolism and Epilepsy*, edited by M. Baldy-Mouliner, D. H. Ingvar, and B. S. Meldrum, pp. 315–323. John Libbey, London.

186. Wadman, W. J., Lopes da Silva, F. H., and Leung, L. S. (1983): Two types of interictal transients of reversed polarity in rat hippocampus during kindling. *Electroencephalogr. Clin. Neurophysiol.*, 55:314–319.

187. Wall, P. D. and Gutnick, M. J. (1974): Properties of afferent nerve impulses originating from neuroma. *Nature (Lond.)*, 248:740–743.

188. Wall, P. D., and Gutnick, M. J. (1974): Ongoing activity in peripheral nerves: the physiology and pharmacology of impulses originating from a neuroma. *Exp. Neurol.*, 43:580–593.

189. Wyler, A. R., and Ward, A. A. (1980): Epileptic neurons. In: *Epilepsy: A Window to Brain Mechanisms*, edited by J. Lockard and A. A. Ward, pp. 51–68. Raven, New York.

190. Wong, R. K. S., and Prince, D. A. (1978): Participation of calcium spikes during intrinsic burst firing in hippocampal neurons. *Brain Res.*, 159:385–390.

191. Wong, R. K. S., Prince, D. A., and Basbaum, A. I. (1979): Intradendritic recordings from hippocampal neurons. *Proc. Natl. Acad. Sci. U.S.A.*, 76:986–990.

192. Yaari, Y., Konnerth, A., and Heinemann, U. (1983): Spontaneous epileptiform activity of CA1 hippocampal neurons in low extracellular calcium solutions. *Exp. Brain Res.*, 51:153–156.

192a. Yaari, Y., Konnerth, and Heinemann, U.: Nonsynaptic epileptogenesis at the mammalian hippocampus in vitro. II. Role of extracellular potassium. *J. Neurophysiol. (in press)*.

193. Yoshida, S., Matsuda, Y., and Samejima, A. (1978): A tetrodotoxin-resistant sodium and calcium component of action potentials in dorsal root ganglion cells of the adult mouse. *J. Neurophysiol.*, 41:1096–1106.

194. Zanotto, L., and Heinemann, U. (1983): Aspartate and glutamate induced reductions in extracellular free calcium and sodium concentration in area CA1 of 'in vitro' hippocampal slices of rats. *Neurosci. Lett.*, 35:79–84.

195. Zieglgaensberger, W., and Puil, E. A. (1972): Tetrodotoxin interference of CNS excitation by glutamic acid. *Nature [New Biol.]*, 239:204–205.

Advances in Neurology, Vol. 44, edited by
A. V. Delgado-Escueta, A. A. Ward, Jr.,
D. M. Woodbury, and R. J. Porter.
Raven Press, New York © 1986.

33

Interstitial Ion Concentrations and Paroxysmal Discharges in Hippocampal Formation and Spinal Cord

*G. G. Somjen, *P. G. Aitken, **J. L. Giacchino, and **J. O. McNamara

*Department of Physiology, Duke University Medical Center, Durham, North Carolina 27710; and
**Epilepsy Research Laboratory, Veterans Administration Medical Center, Durham, North Carolina 27705

SUMMARY This chapter contains a summary of previous work, as well as some new data concerning the roles of potassium and calcium in electrically and chemically induced seizures. During tonic–clonic seizure discharges, the extracellular concentration of potassium, $[K^+]_o$, increases from its resting level of 3.0 to 3.5 mM to between 8.0 and 12.0 mM. The time course of the $[K^+]_o$ increase is such that it cannot play a part in causing either the onset or termination of paroxysmal firing, but its magnitude is in the range where K^+ ions have a profound influence on the functions of excitable membranes and synapses. During nonparoxysmal activation of central nervous system (CNS) tissue, $[Ca^{2+}]_o$ may decrease, increase, or remain unchanged. When the same stimulus train is repeated every few seconds, in time the $[Ca^{2+}]_o$ response may change polarity even if the experimental conditions have not deliberately been altered. Changes in cerebral pH can cause small changes in the level of free Ca^{2+} ions in the CNS interstitium, possibly contributing to the variability of its response. At the site of origin of seizure discharges, however, $[Ca^{2+}]_o$ does decrease in most or all cases.

Paroxysmal firing provoked in hippocampal formation by repetitive stimulation of an afferent pathway and recorded with extracellular microelectrodes in a cell-body layer consists of "giant" population spikes riding on a sustained negative shift of the baseline potential. The paroxysmal sustained potential (SP) shift appears to be generated by intense and sustained depolarization of the cell bodies of dentate granule cells, and of hippocampal pyramidal cells. This is different from spinal cord and cerebral neocortex, where paroxysmal SP shifts are generated mainly by depolarization of neuroglial cells. The giant population spikes are probably the result of lockstep firing of granule cells and of pyramidal cells.

DEFINING THE PROBLEM

Three questions can be asked concerning the relationship between seizure discharges and each of the inorganic ions in the interstitial fluid of central nervous system (CNS) tissue: (a) Does the interstitial concentration of the ion change before or during a seizure, and if so, to what degree? (b) What are the cellular processes that cause such a change, if one occurs? (c) What are the consequences of the change of ion concentration and what role do they play in the generation of seizures? Reliable information is available today to answer the first of these three questions, but not the other two. The changes of interstitial ion concentrations that occur during paroxysmal firing have been reviewed recently (e.g., 38,39), and therefore previous findings will not be discussed in detail again here. In this chapter we will only briefly sum up conclusions based on previous work, then describe more recent findings and relate them to older ones. We will attempt to come to a set of conclusions defining the present state of our knowledge. For the most part, in this chapter we will deal with tonic–clonic paroxysmal discharges, not the brief phasic events known as interictal discharges. In all of this we will concentrate on potassium and calcium, the two ions with which our laboratory has the most experience.

ROLE OF POTASSIUM

We know most about potassium. Findings reported by several laboratories over the past decade agree that interstitial potassium concentration, $[K^+]_o$, rises when cerebral neocortex, hippocampal formation, or spinal cord is seized by a paroxysm, no matter what caused the seizure. At the beginning of the paroxysmal discharge the rise of $[K^+]_o$ is slightly delayed relative to the storm of electric discharges. This fact suggests that the rise of $[K^+]_o$ does not initiate seizures, nor does it cause the transition from interictal to ictal firing. During an ictal event, $[K^+]_o$ increases from its "resting" level of 2.8 to 3.5 mM to a ceiling level somewhere between 8 and 12 mM. When a seizure ends, $[K^+]_o$ generally is not higher than during most of the tonic phase of the paroxysm, and therefore it probably is not responsible for bringing the paroxysmal discharge to a halt. During the postictal depressive phase, $[K^+]_o$ is at or below the "resting" control level. The low to normal $[K^+]_o$ during the postictal electric silence is in marked contrast to its behavior during spreading depression, when $[K^+]_o$ rises to levels that are much higher than those ever seen during seizures. This difference emphasizes that these two types of neuronal depression, the postictal and Leao's type, are caused by different biophysical mechanisms.

While it is thus generally agreed that the elevation of $[K^+]_o$ is not the cause either of initiating or of arresting a seizure, it is also clear that the level to which $[K^+]_o$ rises during a seizure is pathologic and that it cannot fail to influence neuronal functioning. Potassium ions must therefore be one of the components of the feedback that governs the course of a seizure. Its exact role, however, is not clear at present.

One reason for this uncertainty concerning the influence of $[K^+]_o$ is that K ions have several different effects on neurons and on the synapses connecting them. While in a qualitative sense the various ways in which K^+ affects neuronal function have been studied in great detail, the quantitative relationships between the concentration of K ions and their several different effects have not been defined, especially not for central nervous tissue of mammals.

Elevated $[K^+]_o$ causes, of course, depolarization of all excitable cells; to this point no doubt can be attached. The dependence of the membrane potential on $[K^+]_o$ has been determined for a variety of nerve fibers (e.g., 9,19), and for the dorsal-root ganglion cells of rats (6,41), but not for the neurons of the mammalian CNS. The functional consequences of K^+-induced depolarization cannot be accurately predicted. Generally speaking, it is known that moderate depolarization brings neuronal membranes closer to the firing threshold and thus enhances excitability; more severe depolarization causes firing; and further depolarization inactivates the mechanism responsible for excitation and hence suppresses the cell's ability to respond to stimuli. The $[K^+]_o$ levels at which these transitions from one functional effect to another occur are probably different for different types of cells, and they have not yet been determined. To complicate matters, there is the possibility that the K^+ content of cytoplasm may be influenced by the prevailing extracellular K^+ concentration. Since the influence exerted by $[K^+]_o$ on $[K^+]_i$ may increase with time, the consequences of prolonged exposure to high $[K^+]_o$ may be different from those of brief, transient increases.

Besides the effect of elevated $[K^+]_o$ on neuronal excitability, we also have to consider its possible significance for synaptic transmission. One long-held view is that elevated $[K^+]_o$ curtails the amount of transmitter released from presynaptic terminals, because afferent impulses arriving in a depolarized terminal would be of abnormally low amplitude (14,30,47). However, others found that, at the neuromuscular junction of the frog, elevated $[K^+]_o$ could cause an increase rather than a decrease of the amount of acetylcholine liberated by each motor nerve impulse (7,15,42). Reflex transmission in the spinal cord of frogs and excitatory synaptic transmission in the hippocampal formation and olfactory cortex of rats appear to be influenced by elevated $[K^+]_o$ in a manner similar to the frog neuromuscular junction (17,21,39,46,47,48). In all these cases, a moderate elevation of $[K^+]_o$ leads to enhancement of excitatory synaptic transmission, in part by increasing the output of transmitter and in part by mild depolarization of postsynaptic target cells. However, more severe elevation of $[K^+]_o$ blocks all synapses by inactivating the excitable machinery of cell membranes. How inhibitory synaptic transmission might be influenced by changes of $[K^+]_o$ is not clear at present.

ROLE OF CALCIUM

While the behavior of $[K^+]_o$ during intense neuronal excitation is predictable and uniform, not only in any one region of the CNS but also from one preparation to any other, that of $[Ca^{2+}]_o$ is less so. In the experiment illustrated in Fig. 1, in the initial hours of observation a train of afferent volleys caused a lowering of $[Ca^{2+}]_o$ in the dorsal horn of the spinal cord, but later a similar stimulus train evoked a rather large increase. Reversal of the polarity of $[Ca^{2+}]_o$ responses can also occur in cerebral cortex. For example, in one experiment, the surface of the cortex was stimulated by trains of pulses repeated at 40-sec intervals. In the course of about 45 min, while neither recording nor stimulating electrodes were moved, and while the electric response of the tissue remained unchanged, the response of $[Ca^{2+}]_o$ was converted from a decrease into an increase (A. Dray and G. G. Somjen, *unpublished results*). An example of $[Ca^{2+}]_o$ increasing during paroxysmal afterdischarge provoked by stimulating the surface of the cerebral neocortex is shown in Fig. 2D.

In the ventral horn of the spinal cord $[Ca^{2+}]_o$ is usually relatively stable, except after treatment with a convulsant dose of penicillin. After injection of penicillin, trains of afferent volleys invariably evoke large decreases of $[Ca^{2+}]_o$, and spontaneous seizure discharges are also accompanied by similar responses of $[Ca^{2+}]_o$ (Fig. 3). Heinemann et al. (18) first reported that in the cerebral cortex $[Ca^{2+}]_o$ often starts to decrease even before seizure discharges begin. They suggested that, unlike K^+, the movement of Ca^{2+} may in some direct manner be related to the initiation of paroxysmal activity. The observations made on spinal cord seemed to be in agreement with this idea (37). We knew from previous work that the paroxysmal activity induced by penicillin in the spinal cord originates in the ventral horn (8,25,26,27). The observations of $[Ca^{2+}]_o$ in the ventral horn have led to the tentative conclusion that in or near a seizure focus $[Ca^{2+}]_o$ is decreasing, whereas in the zones sur-

rounding the pacemaker of paroxysmal activity and in the parts of the gray matter into which seizure discharges are secondarily conducted, $[Ca^{2+}]_o$ is more likely to increase. Some additional support for this suggestion came from the report by Janus et al. (20), who induced focal seizures by topical application of penicillin to the motor area of the cerebral cortex and observed that each time when a seizure erupted $[Ca^{2+}]_o$ increased in the spinal segments to which the output of the cortex was addressed.

The fact that under seemingly similar conditions of excitation $[Ca^{2+}]_o$ might increase, decrease, or remain unchanged suggests that opposing processes are at work, some raising and others lowering it. It seems that, depending on circumstances as yet to be specified, sometimes the one and sometimes the other process dominates. It is easy to find a hypothetical mechanism for the lowering of $[Ca^{2+}]_o$. Since the intracellular concentration of free Ca^{2+} is only about 10^{-6} M whereas its extracellular concentration is 10^{-3} M, a steep gradient separates the two phases. Any increase in the permeability of cell membranes for Ca^{2+} would therefore cause an intense inward flow of the ion. It is less clear what it is that could raise the level of $[Ca^{2+}]_o$.

The theoretically possible mechanisms that could raise $[Ca^{2+}]_o$ include:

1. Outward transport of Ca ions from neurons or from glial cells. This is not very likely, because so little free Ca^{2+} exists in the cytoplasm.

2. Transport of Ca^{2+} from blood into interstitial fluid of the CNS. There is no evidence either in favor or against this possibility, and there is no known signal from neurons to endothelial cells that could initiate such transport.

3. Water might move from interstitial space into cytoplasm, leaving Ca ions behind and thus raising their concentration. Dietzel et al. (11) have shown that cells indeed can swell and consequently the interstitial space can shrink during intense neuronal activation. Reconciling the theoretical model of Dietzel (10) with the observed distribution of $[Ca^{2+}]_o$ responses during seizures presents however a difficulty. According to the computations of Dietzel (10,12), the interstitial space should shrink in the epicenter of neuronal activity and it should actually swell in the shell of tissue that surrounds the core of maximal neuronal activation. In fact, however, $[Ca^{2+}]_o$ usually decreases where seizures appear to be generated, and it is more likely to increase in the zone that surrounds the seizure generator. This, seemingly, is the opposite of what would be expected if the changes of

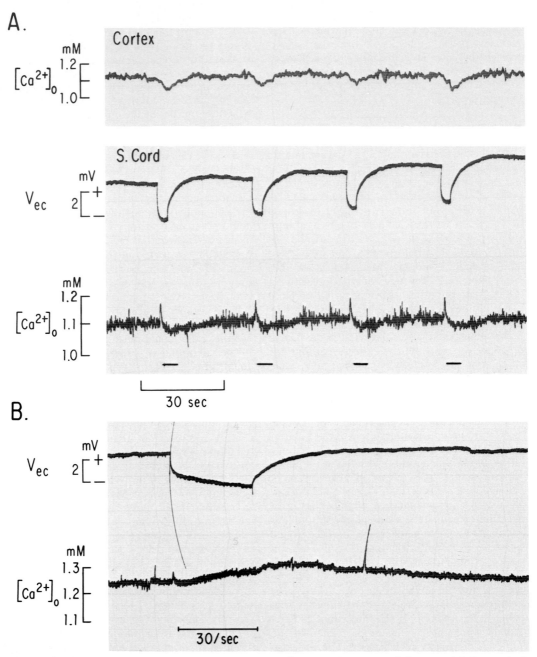

FIG. 1. Responses of interstitial calcium concentration, $[Ca^{2+}]_o$, and of the extracellular potential, V_{ec}, evoked by repetitive stimulation of the popliteal nerve of a cat. The animal was comatose due to bilateral lesion of the mesencephalic reticular formation. **A:** The *upper tracing* was recorded 0.2 mm below the pial surface of the leg area of the contralateral somatosensory receiving area of the cerebral cortex and the *second* and *third tracings* 1.5 mm below the dorsal surface of the ipsilateral side of the L1 segment of the spinal cord. At the four short unmarked horizontal bars, the popliteal nerve was stimulated at 300 Hz frequency. **B:** Recorded from the spinal cord about 10 hr later. (From ref. 37, with permission.)

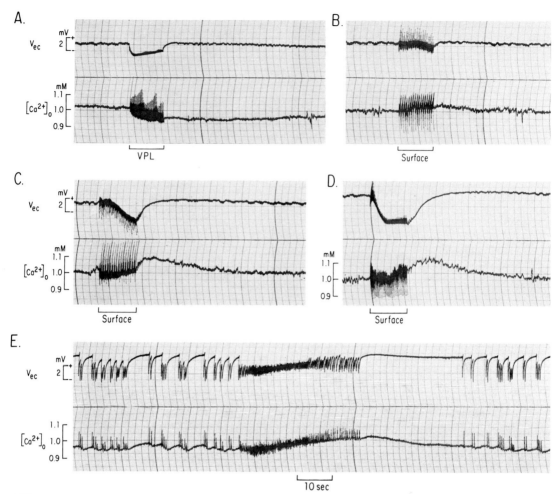

FIG. 2. Extracellular potential and interstitial calcium concentration recorded 1.0 mm under the surface of the somatosensory cortex of another cat. **A:** The ventroposterolateral nucleus of the thalamus was stimulated through stereotaxically placed electrodes. **B, C, D:** The cortical surface was stimulated with pulse trains of different frequency, intensity, and polarity. **E:** Spontaneous interictal activity and a seizure with postictal depressed period following the i.v. injection of a convulsant dose of penicillin. (From ref. 37, with permission.)

concentration could be attributed to movements of water according to the scheme of Dietzel (10). The results of recent experiments, to be discussed shortly, nevertheless suggest that movements of water may play an important part in changing $[Ca^{2+}]_o$ levels.

4. There is one more possible mechanism for the rise of $[Ca^{2+}]_o$. Ca^{2+} could be released from binding, or from sequestration. Figure 4 illustrates that changes of interstitial pH can indeed lead to changes of $[Ca^{2+}]_o$, albeit small ones. The recordings of Fig. 4 were taken from an anesthetized, paralyzed cat that was artificially hyperventilated. The gas inspired by the animal was alternated between room air and 90% oxygen with 10% CO_2. While the changes of $[Ca^{2+}]_o$ induced in the cerebral cortex by these manipulations were small compared to the changes of $[Ca^{2+}]$ in blood plasma, they were nevertheless reproducible and not negligible. It is unlikely that the rise and fall of cerebral $[Ca^{2+}]_o$ seen in Fig. 4 were the consequence of transfer of Ca ions between blood and brain. In other experiments when blood $[Ca^{2+}]$ was changed by intravenous infusion either of $CaCl_2$ or of Na citrate, changes of cerebral $[Ca^{2+}]_o$ were even more modest (when related to comparable changes in blood plasma) than those induced by respiratory alkalosis and acidosis (1,40; also G. Somjen and B. Allen, *unpublished*

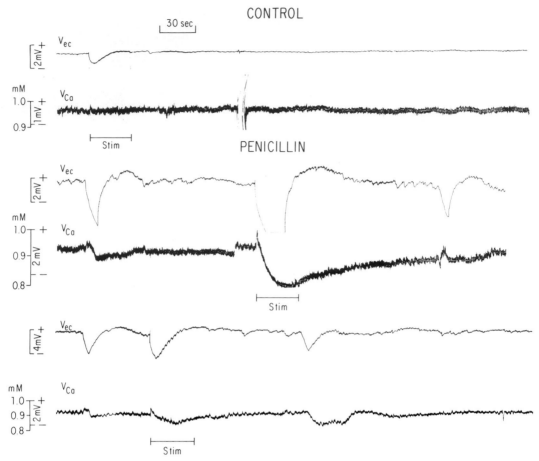

FIG. 3. Recordings from ventral horn of a spinal cord before and after the i.v. administration of a convulsant dose of penicillin. At bars marked "stim," the popliteal nerve was stimulated at 300 Hz; other responses are associated with spontaneous seizure discharges. Note lack of response of $[Ca^{2+}]_o$ to stimulation before penicillin administration, and marked responses thereafter. (From ref. 37, with permission.)

data). This suggests that cerebral acidosis and alkalosis alter cerebral $[Ca^{2+}]_o$ by varying the ratio of bound to free Ca in the tissue.

It is known that during seizures cerebral pH is acidified (e.g., refs. 5,45). If the increase of $[Ca^{2+}]_o$ seen in Fig. 4 seems too small to completely explain the rise of $[Ca^{2+}]_o$ during seizures, it still might be one factor contributing to it.

NEW FINDINGS

The variability of the behavior of $[Ca^{2+}]_o$ is further illustrated by comparing Figs. 5 and 6. These two sets of recordings were obtained in the hilus of the fascia dentata of the hippocampal formation of two rats, both under urethane anesthesia. In both, the afferent fibers of the per-

forant path were stimulated with bipolar electrodes placed in the region of white matter known as the angular bundle. Interstitial ion concentrations were measured with double-barreled ion selective microelectrodes and the extracellular potential was recorded from the reference barrels of the same electrodes. With stimulating and recording electrodes placed in these locations, single stimulus pulses evoke positive focal potential waves usually interpreted as summed synaptic potentials, or "population EPSPs", pEPSPs (2,3,22). The pEPSPs appear as the vertical upstrokes of the polygraph pen during the application of the stimulus train in tracing a of Fig. 5. This train of stimuli caused $[Ca^{2+}]_o$ to decrease in a smooth trajectory (Fig. 5b). Tracings c and d of Fig. 5 illustrate the responses to a train of slightly stronger stimuli

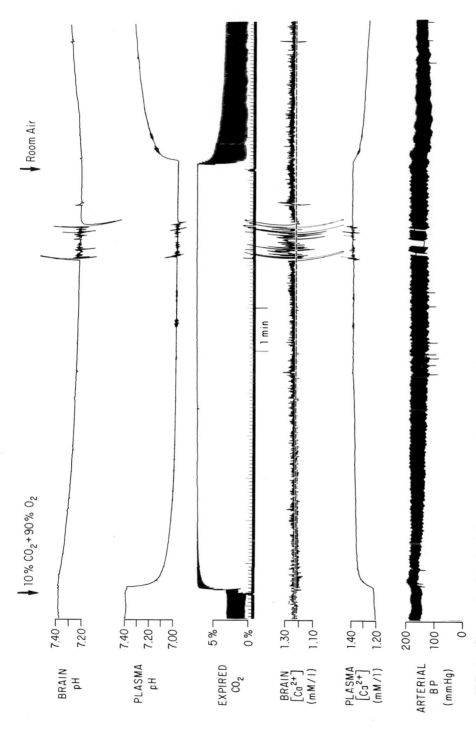

FIG. 4. Changes in pH and calcium concentration in circulating arterial blood and in the interstitial fluid of the cerebral cortex during forced hyperventilation of a cat under chloralose anesthesia. Plasma pH and [Ca²⁺] were measured with ion-selective electrodes built into a flow cell inserted in a closed loop in the common carotid artery. Interstitial ion concentrations in cortex were measured as for Figs. 1–3. At *arrows*, inspired gas changed as indicated. (Unpublished experiment of B. Allen and G. Somjen.)

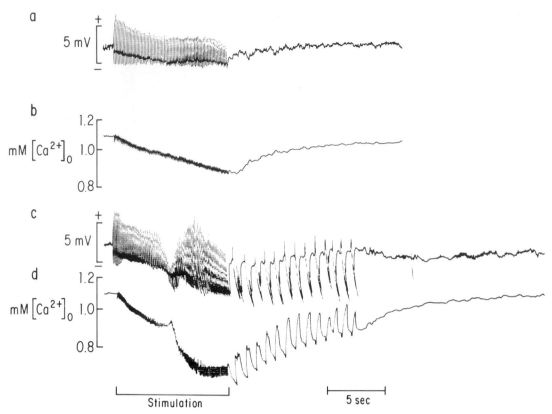

FIG. 5. Extracellular electric potential and interstitial calcium concentration in the hilus of fascia dentata of a rat under urethane anesthesia. At the horizontal mark, the angular bundle was stimulated. **a** and **b**: Recorded simultaneously, while the stimulus was 8 Hz with 0.1-msec, 0.4-mA pulses. **c** and **d**: 15-Hz, 0.6-mA pulses.

delivered at a higher frequency. This train provoked in its wake a series of burst discharges. These interrupted paroxysmal afterdischarges (PaADs) have the characteristics of clonic seizures. At a time about halfway during the stimulus train, an inflection downward is seen in both tracings C and D of Fig. 5, and at the end of stimulation $[Ca^{2+}]_o$ is at a very low level. During the bursts of PaAD, $[Ca^{2+}]_o$ oscillates between wide limits, to return to its resting level at the end of the paroxysm.

The recordings of Fig. 6 were made in another rat, but under conditions similar to those of Fig. 5, except that the frequency response of the polygraph was filtered to emphasize slow changes. In this case $[Ca^{2+}]_o$ changed little during the initial phase of stimulation (Fig. 6b), although the extracellular voltage showed the usual negative shift (Fig. 6a and c) and $[K^+]_o$ (Fig. 6d) did rise sharply. Halfway during the stimulation, $[Ca^{2+}]_o$ rose suddenly but transiently, and then decreased below the resting control level during the PaAD. In addition, the

PaAD was marked by oscillatory variations of $[Ca^{2+}]_o$.

Among the 20 rats studied so far under conditions similar to those illustrated in Figs. 5 and 6, in the majority of cases the course of $[Ca^{2+}]_o$ was more like that shown in Fig. 6 than in Fig. 5; that is, before the eruption of paroxysmal firing it either remained unchanged or it rose above baseline. Then, with the onset of IPaD, $[Ca^{2+}]_o$ usually began to suddenly decline. The unpredictability of the course of $[Ca^{2+}]_o$ becomes more understandable if it is considered to be the result of opposing processes. The process tending to raise its concentration—presumably the loss of water from extracellular to the intracellular compartment, and the release of Ca^{2+} from binding by the tide of acidification—initially may equal or even best the process that lowers its concentration. At the outburst of paroxysmal activity, however, it seems that the flux of Ca^{2+} into neurons becomes strong enough to take the upper hand.

Figure 7 illustrates the behavior of $[Ca^{2+}]_o$,

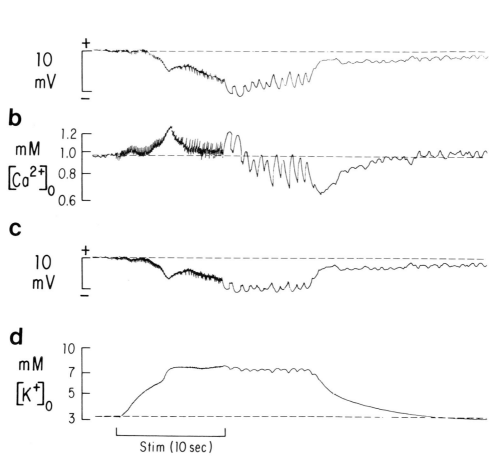

FIG. 6. Extracellular potential (**a** and **c**), interstitial calcium concentration (**b**), and potassium concentration (**d**) in granule-cell layer of fascia dentata of a rat anesthetized with urethane. **a**: Recorded from reference barrel of Ca^{2+}-selective electrode. **d**: From reference barrel of K^+-selective electrode. The two electrodes were separated by about 0.2 mm in the antero–posterior direction and by less than 0.05 mm laterally and dorso–ventrally. At the marker bar, the angular bundle was stimulated at 8 Hz for 10 sec. For all traces, the maximal frequency response of the pens was limited to 3 Hz by electronic filtering to emphasize slow changes.

$[K^+]_o$, and extracellular voltage in the same rat as Fig. 6, but in a slightly more dorsal location, in the dendritic field of dentate granule cells. The pEPSPs evoked by angular bundle stimulation were negative here. The "DC" component (SP shift) of the voltage response moved, initially, also in the negative direction, but it changed to a positive SP about halfway through the stimulus train (Fig. 7A and C). In this location in the tissue, $[Ca^{2+}]_o$ rose during the initial phase of the stimulus and decreased at the time when the SP shift reversed polarity. True to its consistent character, $[K^+]_o$ responded with an increase through all phases of the stimulus and the ensuing PaAD.

Figures 5, 6, and 7 show one feature in common. In all three sets of recordings there is a sharp inflection of all tracings at roughly the halfway point of the 10-sec stimulus train. On recordings made with an oscilloscope, it becomes clear that at the time when such discontinuities appear on polygraph tracings, the electric response of the tissue changes dramatically. Such responses are shown in Fig. 8, recorded with two tungsten microelectrodes placed in the cell body layers of fascia dentata and of CA3 zone of the hippocampus of another rat. Figure 8a shows the responses evoked by the first two pulses in a 10-sec, 6-Hz train of stimuli. In fascia dentata these responses consist of the ex-

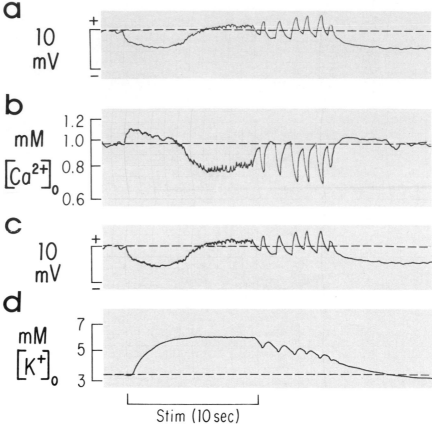

FIG. 7. Stimulating and recording conditions similar to those in Fig. 6, except that the pair of recording electrodes was placed 0.6 mm more dorsally, in the dendritic field of the granule cells.

pected positive pEPSPs, each with a single negative compound action potential ("population spike"). Figure 8b shows the responses evoked after 8.2 sec of stimulation: now each pulse evokes a burst of several population spikes and there is firing also in the intervals between stimulus pulses. We call the firing that occurs during a stimulus train but not locked to the stimulus pulses "intercurrent paroxysmal discharges" or IPaDs. Inflections on polygraph tracings, such as the ones illustrated in Figs. 5, 6, and 7, always occurred at the onset of IPaD, revealed by concurrent oscilloscope recording. The action potentials fired in IPaD have the same polarity and range of amplitudes as the population spikes evoked by the afferent stimuli. The PaADs that follow in the wake of a stimulus train are characterized by bursts of similar "spontaneous" population spikes (Fig. 8c).

For interpretations of the mechanism of these seizure discharges, the following features are worthy of note. (a) The compound action potentials recorded in the granule cell layer of fascia dentata by extracellular electrodes during IPaD and PaAD have unusually large amplitude (10–40 mV) and they are of short duration (2–3 msec at the "base" of the spike). (b) While the population spikes evoked by stimulation of the afferent fiber bundle are always grafted on a pEPSP, those fired "spontaneously" in IPaD or PaAD generally are not. A brief, small, positive deflection may precede the burst of negative spikes that make a PaAD, but the individual impulses within a PaAD or an IPaD seem to be triggered from a "flat" baseline. (c) In the granule-cell layer of fascia dentata, paroxysmal discharges "ride" on a negative shift of the baseline potential (negative SP shift). (d) In the dendritic field of the dentate granule cells, the SP shifts associated with paroxysmal discharges are either absent or of opposite polarity, that is, positive.

To further clarify the cellular mechanism of paroxysmal firing, we experimented with hippocampal tissue slices *in vitro*. It proved difficult to provoke paroxysmal firing in the fascia den-

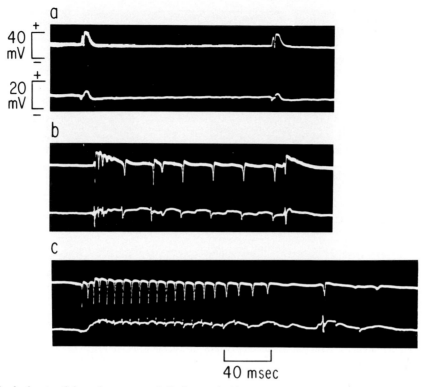

FIG. 8. Evoked potentials and paroxysmal discharges in hippocampal formation. In each pair of recordings, the *upper* was taken from the granule-cell layer of fascia dentata and the *lower* from the pyramidal-cell layer of the CA3 zone of the hippocampus. The angular bundle was stimulated at 6 Hz with 0.1-msec, 0.4-mA pulses for 10 sec. **a:** Responses evoked by the first two pulses in the train of stimuli. **b:** Responses to two identical pulses occurring after 8 sec of stimulation; note the intercurrent paroxysmal discharge (IPaD) during the time between the two stimulus pulses. **c:** Burst of paroxysmal afterdischarges (PaAD) following completion of the stimulus train.

tata region of the slice, but the pyramidal cells of CA1 region responded with both IPaD and PaAD to trains of afferent volleys of sufficient intensity and frequency. The threshold for paroxysmal firing decreased when the level of $[K^+]_o$ in the bathing solution was raised from the control level of 3.5 mM to a higher value. Figure 9A–C shows recordings of the electric activity in stratum pyramidale of CA1 zone of a slice in 3.5 mM $[K^+]_o$. The train of orthodromic stimuli provoked IPaD as well as PaAD. Unlike the PaAD in hippocampal formation of intact brains, the PaAD in this case consisted of continuous—i.e., tonic—firing, not clonic bursts. When $[K^+]_o$ was raised in the bath to 7.0 mM, more intense and longer PaADs were provoked, which now consisted of an initial tonic and a later clonic phase (Fig. 9D–F). Compared to the intense paroxysmal firing recorded in the cell body layer, there is relatively little paroxysmal acitivity in the dendritic field (stratum radiatum) of the pyramidal cells, even though large negative pEPSPs were evoked, as expected, by the afferent fiber volleys (compare Fig. 9D with Fig. 9F). Here, as in the intact brain, there were no pEPSPs preceding the individual population spikes during IPaD and PaAD.

The initiation of the action potentials during paroxysmal firing is further clarified by intracellular recording. Figure 10 illustrates such an experiment on another slice, maintained at the moderately elevated $[K^+]_o$ level of 5.5 mM. During the initial tonic phase of the PaAD, the extracellular potential showed a marked negative SP shift, and the membrane potential of the pyramidal cell shows a sustained depolarization. Note that the true membrane potential change is the sum of the extracellular negative and the intracellular positive shifts of potential, since both were recorded with reference to ground potential. The maximal transmembrane depolarization so determined amounts to 22.5 mV in this example.

Because of the limited frequency response of the polygraph, only partially compensated by playing back the recording tape in "slow mo-

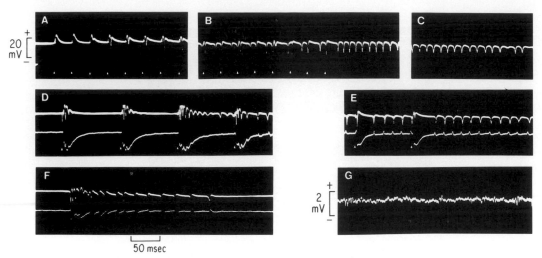

FIG. 9. Extracellular recordings from CA1 zone of a hippocampal tissue slice. All recordings made with condenser coupled amplifiers. **A, B,** and **C:** Bathing medium containing 3.5 mM K$^+$. **D–G:** In 7.0 mM K$^+$. The recordings in **A–C** and the *upper traces* in **D–F** are from the cell body layer (stratum pyramidale), and the *lower traces* in **D–F** are from the dendritic field (stratum radiatum). The *small triangles* indicate stimulus pulses (0.1 mA, 0.1 msec) applied to Schaffer collateral bundle in stratum radiatum. **A:** Beginning of stimulus train. **B:** End of stimulus train, showing IPaD and beginning of PaAD. **C:** End of PaAD. **D:** Beginning of other stimulus train, showing burst responses due to elevated [K$^+$] and the onset of IPaD. **E:** End of the stimulus train. **F:** Burst of PaAD following the stimulus train. **G:** Spontaneous firing in elevated [K$^+$] in the absence of stimulation; note change of gain, and small amplitude of impulses presumably attributable to sporadic firing of individual neurons.

tion," the action potentials shown in Fig. 10 suffered attenuation in recording. In spite of this attenuation it is apparent from Fig. 10 (and confirmed on oscilloscope recordings, not illustrated here), that the action potentials fired during the tonic paroxysmal depolarization are of abnormally low amplitude compared to those fired before the seizure-provoking stimulus train. These truncated impulses are reminiscent of those fired by spinal motor neurons during tonic paroxysmal depolarization induced by convulsant doses of penicillin (Fig. 11) (27). The partial failure of impulses is probably the result of the precipitous decrease of membrane resistance during tonic paroxysmal depolarization (Fig. 12) (13).

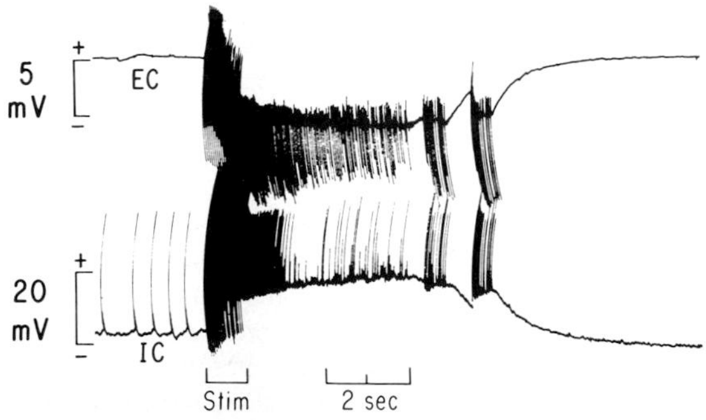

FIG. 10. The extracellular potential (EC) in stratum pyramidale and the intracellular potential (IC) of a pyramidal cell in CA1 zone of a hippocampal tissue slice *in vitro.* At horizontal mark, the Schaffer collaterals were stimulated in the stratum radiatum at 20 Hz for 1 sec. Polygraph tracing from magnetic tape recording; tape played back at one-fourth of recording speed to enhance frequency response (effective frequency response of pens 240 Hz).

DISCUSSION AND CONCLUSIONS

Over the last few years much attention has been paid in many laboratories to the brief phasic events known as interictal discharges and to the paroxysmal depolarizing shift (PDS) believed to be their cellular mechanism. Two major theories are current, one attributing PDSs to so-called "slow" voltage-dependent ion conductance changes, the other to "giant" excitatory synaptic potentials. Actually, the majority of investigators now seems to believe that both synaptic influences and self-regenerating membrane currents play a part, but they differ in the emphasis placed on these different factors (see Chapters 6, 10, 12, 13, and 29). The problem of the PDS is of course relevant to the general problems of epilepsy, but solving it will not lead, by itself, to a full understanding of the mechanism of the more prolonged paroxysmal discharges that can result in clinical seizures.

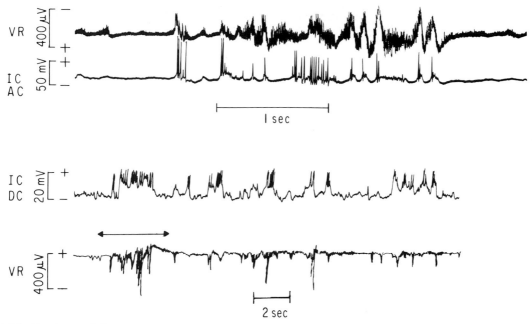

FIG. 11. Intracellular recordings (IC) from a motor neuron in L7 spinal segment of a cat, and the discharges recorded from the ventral root (VR) of the same segment. Spontaneous seizure activity induced by the i.v. administration of penicillin. The *upper* two recordings were made on moving film with AC-coupled amplifiers and an oscilloscope; the *lower* two were made with DC amplifiers on polygraph chart paper. The horizontal *double-headed arrow* placed between the lower two traces marks the time during which the recordings of the upper two traces were taken. Note sustained depolarization seen on the DC-coupled polygraph recording, not visible due to AC-coupling of the upper (oscilloscope) record. (From ref. 27, with permission.)

If we examine the tonic depolarization that appears to underlie tonic paroxysmal activity, two sets of questions emerge. One concerns the biophysical change of the membrane that leads to depolarization and the other the primary cause of that biophysical change. While we do not have the answers to these questions, there are certain clues in our observations worth examining. In the motor neurons of the spinal cord, the tonic paroxysmal depolarizations induced by penicillin are, as we have seen, associated with a very substantial decrease of the input resistance of the cells, so much so that sometimes the resistance became too small to measure. The paroxysmal discharges of the neurons in a spinal segment are usually preceded by widespread depolarization of primary afferent nerve fibers, detected as paroxysmal dorsal root potentials (Fig. 13) (16,25,26). It seems possible that depolarization of primary afferent terminals, with the consequent release of excitatory synaptic transmitter substance, is the event that initiates the tonic paroxysmal depolarization of these neurons.

In the hippocampal formation, we have no direct indication of involvement of presynaptic terminals in the initiation of paroxysmal depolarization. Some indirect support for such a mechanism comes however from certain observations made by Nadler et al. (31,32). These investigators found that the necrosis of granule and pyramidal cells caused by treatment with kainic acid can be prevented by placing experimental lesions into afferent tracts leading to the hippocampal formation, some time before the administration of the kainic acid. Moreover, Sloviter and Damiano (34) reported observations suggesting that the cytotoxic neuron loss caused by kainic acid is the result of excessive prolonged paroxysmal firing by the neurons. Taken together, these results suggest that, in order to induce suicidal paroxysmal firing of postsynaptic neurons, kainic acid must first act on presynaptic terminals.

The PaAD provoked in the CA1 zone of hippocampal tissue slices usually consisted of an initial tonic, followed by a clonic phase. Such PaAD were more readily provoked when the slice was bathed in a medium containing elevated $[K^+]_o$ than when $[K^+]_o$ was at the control level of 3.5 mM. It should be remembered however that the 5.5 or 7.0 mM $[K^+]_o$ levels we used

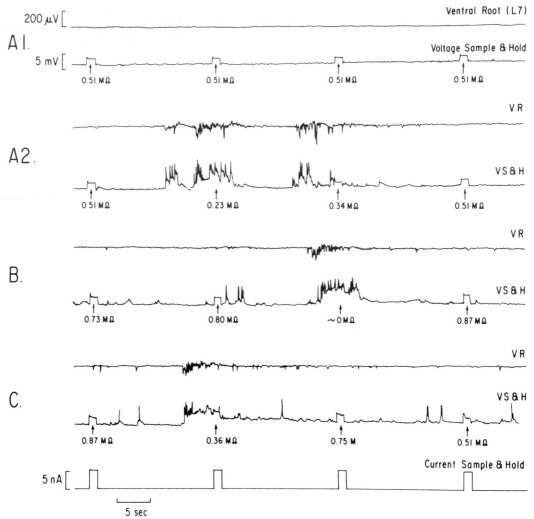

FIG. 12. Measurements of input resistance of motor neurons during seizure discharges induced by i.v. injection of penicillin. **A1:** From a motor neuron before penicillin treatment. **A2:** From the same cell after penicillin administration. **B** and **C:** From two other neurons after penicillin. Recordings were made with circuit designed for single-electrode voltage clamping (49), but in "current clamp" mode. Recordings from ventral root (VR) added to indicate times of seizure discharges in spinal segment. Tracing marked "voltage sample and hold" shows intracellular potential; "current sample and hold" shows the current pulses injected into the cells (identical for **A, B,** and **C**). Numbers below voltage tracings indicate calculated input resistances in megohms. The resting input resistance of the neurons was not altered by the penicillin treatment, but input resistance was drastically decreased during each tonic paroxysmal depolarization. (From ref. 13, with permission.)

as elevated levels in these experiments are not higher than those measured in intact brains during paroxysmal discharges (e.g., Fig. 6).

Ben Ari et al. (4) proposed that the cause of the seizures provoked by electrical stimulation in the hippocampal formation is the failure of synaptic inhibition during prolonged repetitive stimulation. While failure of inhibition may indeed play a part, it is unlikely to provide the complete explanation of IPaDs and PaADs. In order for failing inhibition to account for the tonic paroxysmal depolarization of hippocampal neurons, it would be necessary for "background" inhibition to maintain these neurons hyperpolarized by more than 20 mV in the "resting" control state, for that is the magnitude of the depolarization associated with the outbreak of paroxysmal discharge (e.g., Fig. 10). While not impossible, this seems unlikely, especially in the hippocampal slice preparation.

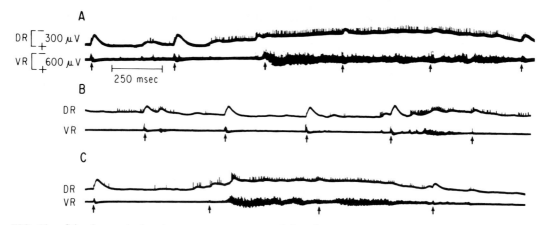

FIG. 13. Stimulus-evoked and spontaneous paroxysmal dorsal root potentials (DRPs) recorded from a dorsal root filament in a spinal cat treated with a convulsant dose of penicillin. At each arrow a stimulating pulse was delivered to the posterior biceps-semi-tendinosus (A and B) or to the sural (C) nerve. Recording on moving film with direct coupled amplifiers. Note that the paroxysmal DRP commences before onset of seizure discharge in ventral root; note "occlusion" of stimulus-evoked DRP during paroxysmal DRP, and note antidromic impulses in dorsal root recording during paroxysmal DRP. (From ref. 26, with permssion.)

Slices are missing much of the circuit that could conceivably maintain intense background inhibitory bombardment.

In the hippocampal formation of intact brains, PaADs consisted of clonic bursts only. While these PaADs did not have a tonic phase, the IPaD occurring during the stimulus train itself could be taken to be its equivalent. PaAD was never provoked without IPaD preceding it, although IPaD did occur without ensuing PaAD when the stimulus train was just below the threshold required for provoking PaAD. The reason for the *in vitro* slice's different response could be the different afferent path (angular bundle in the intact brain and Schaffer collaterals in slices) or the different neuronal network of the isolated slice preparation. Whatever its exact nature, the onset of IPaD was always clearly marked by a discontinuity in the tracings of extracellular electric potential and of ion concentrations. These discontinuities seem to signal the onset of a new process. There are certain similarities between the tonic depolarization of pyramidal cells in the hippocampal slice and the depolarization of spinal motor neurons, and also between the extracellular recordings made during tonic PaAD in the slice and those made in hippocampal formation in intact brains. These similarities lead us to suspect that there may be common features in the biophysical mechanism generating these tonic paroxysmal depolarizations.

During paroxysmal discharges the soma membrane of granule cells (in intact brains) and of CA1 pyramidal cells (of *in vitro* slices) appeared strongly depolarized, with little or no sign of dendritic depolarization. That the perikaryal region of the neurons is the primary site of paroxysmal depolarization, can be inferred from the extracellular sustained potential (SP) shifts that regularly accompanied IPaDs and PaADs (Figs. 5d, 6a and c, and Fig. 10, trace EC). The polarity of these paroxysmal SP shifts was negative in the cell-body layer, which is the opposite of the polarity of the pEPSPs evoked in the same locations by single pulse stimulation of the same afferent pathway. It is because the pEPSPs are positive in the cell-body layers and negative in the dendritic fields that they are believed to be generated by depolarization of the dendritic trees. By contrast, paroxysmal SP shifts either are not detectable or are positive in recordings made in the dendritic fields. (See the positive shift of potential in traces A and C of Fig. 7, about halfway during the applied stimulus, at the time of onset of the IPaD.)

The gray matter of the spinal cord is not built according to the regular laminar plan typical of the hippocampal cortex. Territories of dendrites and somata of motor neurons overlap, and therefore the current flow around them cannot be analyzed with the same ease. It nevertheless is noteworthy that the signs of maximal paroxysmal activity during seizures in the spinal cord were deep in the tissue, near the center of the ventral gray matter, where motor neuron perikarya are maximally concentrated (8,25,26, 27,37).

A note is in order here concerning the interpretation of the SP shifts in hippocampal formation. In the cerebral neocortex and in the gray matter of the spinal cord, the SP shifts evoked by trains of afferent volleys and those accompanying paroxysmal discharges are apparently generated mainly by the depolarization of glial cells (23,24,35,36). In the hippocampal formation, SP shifts seem to be generated mainly by membrane potential changes of granule cells and pyramidal cells. The reason for this different interpretation is best illustrated in Figs. 6 and 7, containing recordings from cell body and dendritic layers of fascia dentata. In both sets of recordings, $[K^+]_o$ is seen rising during afferent stimulation and rising even more during paroxysmal firing (traces D of Figs. 6 and 7). While $[K^+]_o$ behaves similarly, the SP shifts behave differently in the two layers. Traces A and C of Fig. 6 show the potential remaining close to the baseline level during the first few seconds of stimulation, while $[K^+]_o$ is already rising sharply. In Fig. 7A and C the extracellular potential does shift in the negative direction at the onset of stimulation, but then it turns positive when the IPaD erupts. This behavior is clearly different from that of the SP shifts associated with seizure discharges in the neocortex and spinal cord. Such SP shifts in the spinal cord and neocortex are consistently negative in all cytoarchitectonic layers, and their amplitudes "map" rather accurately the rise of $[K^+]_o$ in both time and space (8,23,24,26). The opposite polarities of the paroxysmal SP shifts recorded in dendritic and perikaryal layers of fascia dentata do not prove, but strongly suggest, that they are generated predominantly by the granule cells.

As a last point of discussion, the nature of the compound action potentials, or "population spikes," fired during IPaD and PaAD of hippocampal neurons merits some attention. Similar spontaneously fired spikes were first described by Purpura et al. (33) in hippocampal formation of cats treated with penicillin. Their unusually large amplitude, between 10 and 40 mV in our recordings, and their brief duration suggest that many tightly packed neurons fire action potentials that are very accurately time-locked. Similar population spikes are also evoked sometimes by afferent volleys (e.g., Fig. 8A). In those cases, synchronization is ensured by the simultaneous arrival of afferent impulses, experimentally evoked by the electric stimulus. But most of the "spontaneously" fired paroxysmal population spikes are not preceded by pEPSP waves that could explain the simultaneous firing of many neurons. We believe that the most likely

explanation of this precisely time-locked discharge is electric interaction between the neurons. Recent reports by MacVicar and Dudek (28,29) and by Taylor et al. (43) suggest that granule cells of fascia dentata and pyramidal cells of the CA1 region can interact both by way of electrotonically patent gap junctions and ephaptic current (see Chapter 30). We would like to suggest that this special type of unusually precise temporal coordination should be called *lock-step,* or *locked* firing, to distinguish it from those more usual forms of synchronization that are achieved by other mechanisms (e.g., ref. 44; also see Chapter 29).

If hippocampal neurons are communicating electrically, the question arises why they do not always fire in lock-step. Spontaneously fired "giant" population spikes have not been reported, except during paroxysmal firing. We did observe such spontaneous giant spikes during PaAD in unanesthetized, freely moving rats equipped with implanted electrodes. In these rats, dentate granule cells fired in lock-step during the PaAD provoked by 60-Hz stimuli before the animal was kindled, and also during the motor seizure provoked after kindling was completed. Not all paroxysmal discharges contain giant population spikes, however. The hippocampal electroencephalogram (EEG) of rats anesthetized with gamma-hydroxybutyrolactone is characterized by frequent large amplitude sharp waves with interspersed silent periods. These brief paroxysmal events resemble interictal discharges. Unlike the PaAD, they occur without signs of lock-step firing of neurons. It should be remembered, of course, that conventional EEG recordings would not display these action potentials, for their detection requires amplifier and recording systems capable of registering frequencies up to several thousand hertz. Even so, it is clear that lock-step firing is not common, although it can reliably be provoked under certain specifiable conditions. At this time we can only guess at the mechanism forcing hippocampal neurons into locked firing. There may be some specific stimulus that opens electrotonic communication between these neurons, or it may be sufficient if a critical number of neighboring cells is depolarized to a liminal level to cause the phase-locking of their firing.

ACKNOWLEDGMENT

Work published here first was supported by grants NS 17771 and NS 18670 of the National Institutes of Health.

REFERENCES

1. Allen, B. W., and Somjen, G. G. (1983): The influence of pH on Ca^{2+} in circulating blood. *Fed. Proc.*, 42:296.
2. Andersen, P., Bliss, T. V. P., and Skrede, K. K. (1971): Unit analysis of hippocampal population spikes. *Exp. Brain Res.*, 13:208–221.
3. Andersen, P., Holmquist, B., and Voorhoeve, P. E. (1966): Entorhinal activation of dentate granule cells. *Acta Physiol. Scand.*, 66:448–460.
4. Ben-Ari, Y., Krnjević, K., and Reinhardt, W. (1979): Hippocampal seizures and failure of inhibition. *Can. J. Physiol. Pharmacol.*, 57:1462–1466.
5. Caspers, H., and Speckmann, E.-J. (1972): Cerebral pO_2, pCO_2 and pH: Changes during convulsive activity and their significance for spontaneous arrest of seizures. *Epilepsia*, 13:699–725.
6. Connors, B. W. (1979): Physiological and pharmacological studies of the membrane properties of mammalian dorsal root ganglion cells. Doctoral dissertation, Duke University, Durham, N.C.
7. Cooke, J. D., and Quastel, D. M. J. (1973): The specific effect of potassium on transmitter release by motor nerve terminals and its inhibition by calcium. *J. Physiol.*, 228:435–458.
8. Cordingley, G. E., and Somjen, G. G. (1978): The clearing of excess potassium from extracellular space in spinal cord and cerebral cortex. *Brain Res.*, 151:291–306.
9. Curtis, H. J., and Cole, K. S. (1942): Membrane resting and action potentials from the squid giant axon. *J. Cell. Comp. Physiol.*, 19:135–144.
10. Dietzel, I. (1983): Ladungsverschiebungen und Elektrolytenänderungen in der Hirnrinde. Doctoral dissertation, Rheinisch-Westfälische Technische Hochschule, Aachen, Federal Republic of Germany.
11. Dietzel, I., Heinemann, U., Hofmeir, G., and Lux, H. D. (1980): Transient changes in the size of the extracellular space in the sensory motor cortex of cats in relation to stimulus-induced changes in potassium concentration. *Exp. Brain Res.*, 40:432–439.
12. Dietzel, I., Heinemann, U., Hofmeir, G., and Lux, H. D. (1982): Changes in the extracellular volume in the cerebral cortex of cats in relation to stimulus induced epileptiform afterdischarges. In: *Physiology and Pharmacology of Epileptogenic Phenomena*, edited by M. R. Klee, H. D. Lux, and E.-J. Speckmann, pp. 5–12. Raven Press, New York.
13. Dunn, P., and Somjen, G. G. (1977): Membrane resistance, monosynaptic EPSPs, and the epileptogenic action of penicillin in spinal motoneurons. *Brain Res.*, 128;569–574.
14. Erulkar, S. D., and Weight, F. F. (1977): Extracellular potassium and transmitter release at the giant synapse of squid. *J. Physiol.*, 266:209–218.
15. Gage, P. W., and Quastel, D. M. J. (1965): Dual effect of potassium on transmitter release. *Nature (Lond.)*, 206:625–626.
16. Gray, C., and Somjen, G. (1979): Paroxysmal activity in spinal cord of cats induced by focal microinjection of penicillin. *Fed. Proc.*, 38:897.
17. Hablitz, J. J., and Lundervold, A. (1981): Hippocampal excitability and changes in extracellular potassium. *Exp. Neurol.*, 71:410–420.
18. Heinemann, U., Lux, H. D., and Gutnick, M. J. (1977): Extracellular free calcium and potassium during paroxysmal activity in the cerebral cortex of the cat. *Exp. Brain Res.*, 27:237–243.
19. Huxley, A. F., and Stampfli, R. (1951): Effect of potassium and sodium on resting and action potentials of single myelinated nerve fibers. *J. Physiol.*, 112:496–508.
20. Janus, J., Speckmann, E. J., and Lehmenkuhler, A. (1981): Relations between extracellular K^+ and Ca^{++} activities and local field potentials in the spinal cord of the rat during focal and generalized seizure discharges. In: *Ion-Selective Microelectrodes and Their Use in Excitable Tissues*, edited by E. Sykova, P. Hnik, and L. Vyklicky, pp. 181–186. Plenum Press, New York.
21. King, G., and Somjen, G. (1981): Effects of variation of extracellular potassium activity ($[K^+]_o$) on snynaptic transmission and $[Ca^{2+}]$ responses in hippocampal tissue *in vitro*. *Neurosci. Abstr.*, 7:439.
22. Lomo, T. (1971): Patterns of activation in a monosynaptic cortical pathway: The perforant path input to the dentate area of the hippocampal formation. *Exp. Brain Res.*, 12:18–45.
23. Lothman, E., LaManna, J., Cordingley, G., Rosentha., M., and Somjen, G. (1975): Responses of electrical potential, potassium levels and oxidative metabolic activity of cerebral neocortex of cats. *Brain Res.*, 88:15–36.
24. Lothman, E. W., and Somjen, G. G. (1975): Extracellular potassium activity, intracellular and extracellular potential responses in the spinal cord. *J. Physiol.*, 252:115–136.
25. Lothman, E. W., and Somjen, G. G. (1976): Motor and electrical signs of epileptiform activity induced by penicillin in the spinal cord of decapitate cats. *Electroencephalogr. Clin. Neurophysiol.*, 41:237–252.
26. Lothman, E. W., and Somjen, G. G. (1976): Functions of primary afferents, and responses of extracellular K^+ during spinal epileptiform seizures. *Electroencephalogr. Clin. Neurophysiol.*, 41:253–267.
27. Lothman, E. W., and Somjen, G. G. (1976): Reflex effects and postsynaptic membrane potential changes during epileptiform activity induced by penicillin in decapitate spinal cords. *Electroencephalogr. Clin. Neurophysiol.*, 41:337–347.
28. MacVicar, B. A., and Dudek, F. E. (1981): Electrotonic coupling between pyramidal cells: A direct demonstration in hippocampal slices. *Science*, 213:782–785.
29. MacVicar, B. A., and Dudek, F. E. (1982): Electrotonic coupling between granule cells of rat dentate gyrus: Physiological and anatomical evidence. *J. Neurophysiol.*, 47:579–592.
30. Morris, M. E., and Krnjević, K. (1976): Extracellular K^+ accumulation and modulation of sensory transmission. In: *Advances in Pain Re-*

search and Therapy, Vol. 1, edited by J. J. Bonica and D. Albe-Fessard, pp. 117–122. Raven Press, New York.

31. Nadler, J. V., and Cuthbertson, G. J. (1980): Kainic acid neurotoxicity toward hippocampal formation: Dependence on specific excitatory pathways. *Brain Res.,* 195:47–56.

32. Nadler, J. V., Evenson, D. A., and Smith, E. M. (1981): Evidence from lesion studies for epileptogenic and non-epileptogenic neurotoxic interaction between kainic acid and excitatory innervation. *Brain Res.,* 205:405–410.

33. Purpura, D. P., McMurtry, J. G., Leonard, C. F., and Malliani, A. (1966): Evidence of dendritic origin of spikes without depolarizing prepotentials in hippocampal neurons during and after seizure. *J. Neurophysiol.,* 29:954–979.

34. Sloviter, R. S., and Damiano, B. P. (1981): Sustained electrical stimulation of the perforant path duplicates kainate-induced electrophysiological effects and hippocampal damage in rats. *Neurosci. Lett.,* 24:279–284.

35. Somjen, G. G. (1970): Evoked sustained focal potentials and the membrane potential of neurons and of unresponsive cells of the spinal cord. *J. Neurophysiol.,* 33:562–582.

36. Somjen, G. G. (1973): Electrogenesis of sustained potential shifts of the central nervous system. *Prog. Neurobiol.,* 1:199–237.

37. Somjen, G. G. (1980): Stimulus-evoked and seizure-related responses of extracellular calcium activity in spinal cord compared to those in the cerebral cortex. *J. Neurophysiol.,* 44:617–632.

38. Somjen, G. G. (1980): Influence of potassium and neuroglia in the generation of seizures and their treatment. In: *Antiepileptic Drugs: Mechanisms of Action,* edited by G. H. Glaser, J. K. Penry, and D. M. Woodbury, pp. 155–167. Raven Press, New York.

39. Somjen, G. G. (1984): Interstitial ion concentration and the role of neuroglia in seizures. In: *Electrophysiology of Epilepsy,* edited by H. V. Wheal and P. A. Schwartzkroin, pp. 303–341. Academic Press, London.

40. Somjen, G. G., and Allen, B. W. (1983): Does hyperventilation cause tetany? *Proc. Int. Union Physiol. Sci.,* 15:146.

41. Somjen, G., Dingledine, R., Connors, B., and Allen, B. (1981): Extracellular potassium and calcium activities in the mammalian spinal cord, and the effect of changing ion levels on mammalian neural tissues. In: *Ion-selective Microelectrodes and Their Use in Excitable Tissues,* edited by E. Sykova, P. Hnik, and L. Vyklicky, pp. 159–180. Plenum Press, New York.

42. Takeuchi, A., and Takeuchi, N. (1961): Changes in potassium concentration around motor nerve terminals produced by current flow and their effect on neuromuscular transmission. *J. Physiol.,* 155:46–58.

43. Taylor, C., Krnjević, K., and Ropert, N. (1983): Field interactions in CA3 hippocampal pyramidal layer in rats in vivo. *Can. J. Physiol. Pharmacol.,* 61:A32–33.

44. Traub, R. D., and Wong, R. K. S. (1983): Synaptic mechanisms underlying interictal spike initiation in a hippocampal network. *Neurology,* 33:257–266.

45. Tschirgi, R. D., Inanaga, K., Taylor, J. L., Walker, R. M., and Sonnenschein, R. R. (1957): Changes in cortical pH and blood flow accompanying spreading cortical depression and convulsion. *Am. J. Physiol.,* 190:557–562.

46. Voskuyl, R. A., and Keurs, ter H. E. D. J. (1981): Modification of neuronal activity in olfactory cortex slices by extracellular K^+. *Brain Res.,* 230:372–377.

47. Vyklický, L. (1978): Transient changes in extracellular potassium and presynaptic inhibition. In: *Iontophoresis and Transmitter Mechanisms in the Mammalian Central Nervous System,* edited by R. W. Ryall and J. S. Kelly, pp. 284–286. Elsevier, Amsterdam.

48. Vyklický, L., and Syková, E. (1980): The effects of increased extracellular potassium in the isolated spinal cord on the flexor reflex of the frog. *Neurosci. Lett.,* 19:203–207.

49. Wilson, W. A., and Goldner, M. M. (1975): Voltage clamp with a single microelectrode. *J. Neurobiol.,* 6:411–422.

Advances in Neurology, Vol. 44, edited by
A. V. Delgado-Escueta, A. A. Ward, Jr.,
D. M. Woodbury, and R. J. Porter.
Raven Press, New York © 1986.

34

Na$^+$,K$^+$-ATPase: Structure, Function, and Interactions with Drugs

*,**,***William L. Stahl and *,***Ward E. Harris

*Neurochemistry Laboratory, Veterans Administration Medical Center, Seattle, Washington 98108; and Departments of **Physiology and Biophysics and ***Medicine (Neurology), University of Washington School of Medicine, Seattle, Washington 98195

SUMMARY Na$^+$,K$^+$-ATPase is a key element for homeostasis of sodium, potassium, and calcium ions in the nervous system and may also play a role in neurotransmitter release. Transitory changes in Na$^+$,K$^+$-ATPase activity occur in epileptic tissue, but this may be due to secondary compensatory processes rather than to primary events leading to epilepsy. A special role for the Na$^+$,K$^+$-ATPase in glial cells for controlling the concentration of extracellular potassium in normal and epileptic states remains controversial. Studies that have utilized immunocytochemical and histochemical techniques generally do not support localization of high concentrations of Na$^+$,K$^+$-ATPase in glial cells. A precise delineation of the structure and conformations of the Na$^+$,K$^+$-ATPase and sites of interaction with drugs is an important major goal of current research. Studies with fluorescent probes indicate that phenytoin exerts a major fluidizing effect on lipids of membranes, and this effect may be related in part to association of the drug with intrinsic membrane proteins.

Pumps and Neurotransmitters

In resting cells, the permeability to K$^+$ is much greater than to Na$^+$, so that membrane resting potential responds mainly to the K$^+$ concentration gradient. The Na$^+$/K$^+$ pump rate is a major factor in determining the membrane resting potential, and this is achieved by coupled active transport of Na$^+$ and K$^+$ with expenditure of ATP (4,6). The Na$^+$/K$^+$ pump (Na$^+$,K$^+$-ATPase) is of obvious importance for maintenance and restoration of ion gradients that are necessary for initiation of the action potential, as well as for regulation of intracellular cation concentrations and for maintenance of constant cell volume (66). The concentrations of Na$^+$ and K$^+$ within the cell also will influence the rate of a variety of enzyme reactions (46).

A number of cation pumps have been found in nervous tissue (Fig. 1). In addition to the Na$^+$,K$^+$-ATPase, two Ca^{2+} transport systems, the calmodulin-sensitive Ca^{2+}-ATPase (37) and a reversible Na$^+$/Ca^{2+} exchange (2,73,75), have been described. The latter is inhibited by amiloride (61). The relative contributions of the latter two transporters in controlling intracellular Ca^{2+} are not certain, but recent work suggests that Na$^+$/Ca^{2+} exchange processes may act both at the cell's plasma membrane and at the mitochondrial outer membrane (76). The interplay of these processes is important for controlling intracellular Ca^{2+}. In particular, dissipation of the Na$^+$ gradient by the Na$^+$,K$^+$-ATPase inhibitor ouabain leads to a dramatic increase of intracellular Ca (71,72,75), since the Na$^+$/Ca^{2+} exchange process is greatly diminished. This relationship between the Na$^+$,K$^+$-ATPase and Ca^{2+} levels in cells has led to the

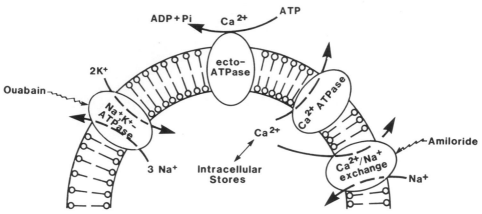

FIG. 1. Cation homeostasis in cells of the nervous system. Sodium and potassium are actively pumped by the Na^+,K^+-ATPase to maintain high K^+ and low Na^+ in cells with expenditure of ATP. The Na^+ gradient is important for driving Na^+/Ca^{2+} exchange, which in combination with the Ca^{2+}-ATPase is responsible for maintaining low levels of Ca^{2+} inside cells. Energy for the Na^+/Ca^{2+} exchange is derived from the Na^+ gradient and therefore is indirectly linked to the Na^+,K^+-ATPase. Intracellular mechanisms involving mitochondria and smooth endoplasmic reticulum are also involved in homeostasis (66), but relative contributions by plasma membrane versus intracellular mediated processes are uncertain. The ecto-Ca^{2+}-ATPase may utilize ATP released by exocytosis, but its function is unknown (81). The latter enzyme appears to be defective in seizure prone mice (80,81; see Chapter 5). Pi, inorganic phosphate.

hypothesis that the Na^+,K^+-ATPase may actually act as a trigger for neurotransmitter release (Fig. 2) (54,83). This is based in part on observations that drugs (e.g., ouabain) that inhibit the Na^+,K^+-ATPase tend to release putative neurotransmitters in a variety of preparations, including synaptosomes (42,44). Putative neurotransmitters that have been reported to stimulate the Na^+,K^+-ATPase tend to reduce release of these substances.[1] In a study of eight putative neurotransmitters present in synaptosomes, O'Fallon et al. (44) found that all were released, probably from the cytoplasmic compartment, by K^+ or ouabain. This is of interest since putative amino acid transmitters appear to be localized in the cytoplasmic rather than the vesicle compartments (11). The apparent stimulatory effect of putative neurotransmitters could involve direct interaction with a component of the Na^+,K^+-ATPase or indirect activation through interaction of neurotransmitter receptors (Fig. 2) closely associated and interacting

with the Na^+,K^+-ATPase within the plasma membrane (54). In effect, inhibition of the Na^+,K^+-ATPase should result in a decreased rate of removal of intracellular Na^+ and an increased rate of Ca^{2+} uptake. Stimulation of the Na^+,K^+-ATPase would reduce internal Na^+ and increase the inward directed Na^+ gradient, decreasing Ca^{2+} entry. It appears that this mechanism would be more important in regulating neurotransmitter release from the cytoplasmic than from the vesicular pool. In view of the uncertainties regarding the stimulatory effect of neurotransmitters on Na^+,K^+-ATPase activity, a role for the Na^+,K^+-ATPase in neurotransmitter release remains highly speculative.

Indirect modulation of the Na^+,K^+-ATPase or association with membrane proteins is suggested by several recent studies. Varon and Skaper (82) have found that nerve growth factor regulates neuronal Na^+,K^+-ATPase, perhaps via interaction with nerve growth factor receptors. Likewise, insulin (59) or the putative transmitters mentioned above (54,83) may modulate the Na^+,K^+-ATPase via specific membrane receptors (Fig. 2). Resch and his colleagues (58,78) have found that the Na^+,K^+-ATPase and lysolecithin acyl transferase are associated in membranes. Together, these studies suggest a functional mosaicism in the plasma membrane of many cells linking the Na^+,K^+-ATPase and several receptors and intrinsic membrane proteins and enzymes.

---

[1] Stimulation of Na^+,K^+-ATPase by putative neurotransmitters (66) and peptides (3) has been observed mainly in homogenates of brain, but the mechanism of this effect is controversial. Activation measured *in vitro* could be due to complexing inhibitors (87) or to disruption of membrane barriers of vesicles, giving substrates and ligands access to enzymatic sites in the interior of the vesicles. The peptide alamethicin and several detergents stimulate Na^+,K^+-ATPase activity by the latter mechanism (29).

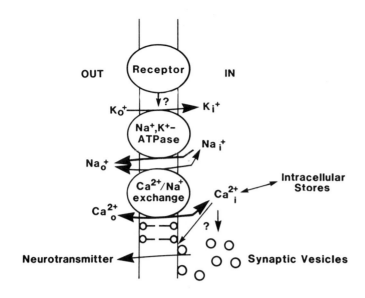

FIG. 2. Possible modulation of neurotransmitter release by the Na,K-ATPase. A functional mosaicism may exist in plasma membranes as suggested here by interaction with membrane receptors (R) or other membrane proteins.

Extracellular Potassium

The mechanism by which K^+ is cleared from the extracellular space is of great interest. Extracellular K^+ may increase by 1 to 3 mM after neuronal firing and during epileptic episodes it may be three to four times higher. Elevated K^+ may increase neuronal excitability, so control of $[K^+]_o$ in the CNS is of critical importance. Neurons reaccumulate K^+ by active transport exclusively by the Na^+/K^+ pump (Fig. 3). After neuronal discharge, the Na^+,K^+-ATPase in glia may be involved in clearing extracellular potassium (18), although this role for the pump remains controversial (46,69,84). Passive transport of K^+ into the glial cell is possible (Fig. 3, dashed line), since K^+ permeability is high and the electrochemical gradient across the glial membrane is close to equilibrium. The K^+ passively accumulated by glia could then be released to the extracellular fluid from a glial process at some distance from the original source. The K^+ released by glia may be reassimilated by neurons at a more distant site via the active Na^+/K^+ transport system. This proposed mechanism of passive K^+ transport in glia is called spatial buffering (36) and is favored by many neurophysiologists (see Chapters 31 and 32).

The role of *active* K^+ transport by glia is difficult to assess. Walz et al. (84) and Pentreath (46) have concluded that the Na^+,K^+-ATPase in invertebrates is not directly involved in active clearance of excess K^+ from the extracellular

space. Clearly, glia must possess a Na^+,K^+-ATPase to maintain Na^+/K^+ gradients, and this is essential for maintenance of the membrane potential. An important question is whether the Na^+,K^+-ATPase in glia is appreciably influenced by extracellular load. Studies *in vitro* with glia isolated from vertebrates and with vertebrate glial cell lines suggest that this may be the case. Franck et al. (18) reported that the maximum velocity of the Na^+,K^+-ATPase in bulk-isolated glia was found with 20 mM K^+, whereas the maximum activity for isolated neurons was found in 5 mM K^+. An important test used to support active transport of an ion (K^+) is to establish if significant deviation from the Nernst equation occurs (cf. ref. 34 for review). No deviation was found for leech glia in the original studies of Kuffler and his colleagues and work by Picker et al. (51) with identified astrocytes in mammalian brain slices supports this conclusion. Kimelberg (34) found a Nernstian response to K^+ in the mammalian glia in primary culture. On the other hand, Franck et al. (18) found non-Nernstian behavior of K^+ in cultured astrocytes. The bulk of neurophysiological evidence, however, does not appear to support active clearance of excess extracellular K^+.

One might predict high levels of Na^+,K^+-ATPase in glia if active transport of K^+ were an especially important function of these cells. Biochemical and physiological studies using isolated cells or cultured cells have reported higher levels of Na^+,K^+-ATPase in glia rather than neurons (18; also see Chapter 53). These studies

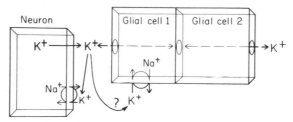

FIG. 3. Potassium transport into neurons and glia. Neurons reaccumulate K^+ by active transport via the Na^+,K^+-ATPase. Accumulation of K^+ by glia may involve spatial buffering (passive transport, *dashed line*) or the Na^+,K^+-ATPase

are not in accord with localization studies using histochemical and immunocytochemical approaches (28,45,69). The latter studies indicate low levels of Na^+,K^+-ATPase in glial membranes. Using rat primary retinal cultures of neurons and glia (Fig. 4), we were unable to demonstrate significant immunoreactive Na^+,K^+-ATPase associated with glial cells. High Na^+,K^+-ATPase-like immunoreactivity was associated with plasma membranes of neuronal cell bodies and their processes (Fig. 4A–D), but markedly lower immunoreactivity was found in underlying glial cells in mixed cultures (Fig. 4B). Staining was generally uniform over perikaryal plasma membranes (Fig. 4) and showed a bead-like appearance in neuronal processes. This supports previous findings in brain tissue that utilized histocytochemical procedures specific for Na^+,K^+-ATPase (69). Therefore, although the importance of the Na^+,K^+-ATPase in maintaining membrane potential in glia is certain, its role as a regulator of extracellular K^+ remains unresolved.

Na^+,K^+-ATPase Changes in Epilepsy

Research on the role of the Na^+,K^+-ATPase in epilepsy has centered on defects in transport that could involve reduced clearing of extracellular potassium released from depolarized neurons via passive mechanisms (spatial buffering) or reduced active transport mediated by the Na^+,K^+-ATPase in neurons or glia. Alternatively, it is possible that a defect in the Na^+,K^+-ATPase could modify the excitability level of cells by affecting calcium transport or neurotransmitter release by the mechanisms described by Vizi (83) and Powis (54).

Tower (79) proposed that defective Na^+/K^+ transport might contribute to spontaneous repetitive spiking, based in part on the decreased ability of human epileptic brain slices to accumulate potassium. Rapport et al. (55) examined Na^+,K^+-ATPase and acetylcholinesterase in

epileptic and nonepileptic human cerebral cortex. The tissue was taken from four epileptic patients suffering intractable generalized or psychomotor seizures. Controls were from normal tissues obtained as part of other neurosurgical procedures. A striking 60% decrease in Na^+,K^+-ATPase was found in the epileptic cortex by comparison to controls, and differences in acetylcholinesterase activity were not significant. These findings support Tower's thesis, but a deficiency in Na^+,K^+-ATPase might be secondary to a primary event triggering the epileptogenic process.

Studies using animal models have the advantages that the development of electroencephalograph (EEG) abnormalities and enzyme changes can be correlated. Focal epilepsy has been produced by implantation of cobalt (56) or by local freezing (40). In the latter case, Lewin and McCrimmon (40) examined Na^+,K^+-ATPase and EEG changes in rats at 8 and 24 hr after lesioning of the right somatosensory cortex. After 8 hr, a time roughly correlated with maximal EEG abnormalities in the rat, the Na^+,K^+-ATPase in the lesioned cortex was elevated approximately 26% compared to tissue from sham-operated animals. Changes in the left somatosensory cortex were not significantly different from controls, and after 24 hr EEG and Na^+,K^+-ATPase activities in the lesioned cortex were similar to controls.

Rapport and Ojemann (56) implanted cobalt-gelatin pellets over the sensorimotor cortex of cats and, in a carefully designed series of experiments, studied Na^+,K^+-ATPase in the primary focus and in the mirror focus of the animals for a period of up to 40 days after lesioning. Behavioral and EEG studies were carried out concurrently, and the effect of phenytoin treatment was also assessed. A transient increase of 190% occurred in Na^+,K^+-ATPase activity in the primary focal lesion as well as in the mirror focus (150% increase) (Fig. 5) and was maximal at 7–10 days. By 40 days no difference in

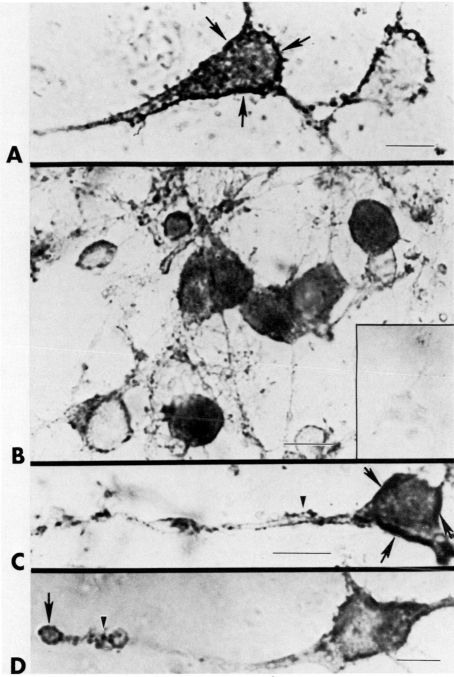

FIG. 4.   Localization of Na$^+$,K$^+$-ATPase in rat retinal primary cultures using the peroxidase–antiperoxidase method. A: Neuronal cultures (11 days) showing Na$^+$,K$^+$-ATPase-like immunoreactivity. *Arrows* indicate heavy reaction product on membranes that outline cell bodies. Antiserum dilution 1:200. B: Mixed cultures of neurons and flat cells (16 days) stained for Na$^+$,K$^+$-ATPase. Very immunoreactive neurons lie on relatively unreactive flat cells (glia). Antiserum dilution 1:500. **Inset,** same dilution but serum was preabsorbed with an excess of purified lamb kidney Na$^+$,K$^+$-ATPase. Neuronal cells and processes immunostained for Na$^+$,K$^+$-ATPase. C: *Arrows* identify very immunoreactive plasma membrane of cell body. Reaction product appears to be on cytoplasmic face of membrane. *Arrowhead:* bead-like appearance of reaction product in major process of cell. Antiserum dilution, 1:1,000. **D:** *Arrow,* growth cone; arrowhead, bead-like reaction product. Antiserum dilution 1:200. All magnification bars = 10 μm.

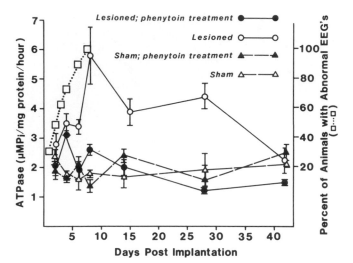

FIG. 5. Changes in Na,K-ATPase in primary epileptic focus in the cat. Animals were implanted with gelatin pellets (sham) or cobalt-gelatin pellets (lesioned), and in some cases animals were treated with phenytoin. EEG was monitored and Na,K-ATPase was measured on tissue excised from the primary and mirror foci; EEG response is shown for the lesioned animals. (Redrawn from ref. 56, with permission.)

Na^+,K^+-ATPase was observed between lesioned and control animals. This transient increase in Na^+,K^+-ATPase was blocked by phenytoin administration. The increase in enzyme activity paralleled but lagged behind development of EEG abnormalities in the lesioned animals (Fig. 5), suggesting that the involved cells first became hyperexcitable, and increased Na^+,K^+-ATPase activity was a response of the cells in the tissue to an intracellular electrolyte abnormality. This result is similar to that found by Lewin and McCrimmon (40), and in both cases the transient changes in Na^+,K^+-ATPase activity may be adaptive responses to abnormal ion fluxes.

Grisar et al. (22) produced freezing lesions in cats and studied kinetic characteristics of glial fractions and synaptosomal fractions isolated from cerebral cortex. Na^+,K^+-ATPase values for the cortex sample were not reported, but generally enzyme activity in these fractions was maximally decreased by at least 50% at 3 to 6 days after lesioning. K^+ sensitivity of the Na^+,K^+-ATPase glial fractions was decreased in the primary and mirror foci, whereas no change occurred in tissue around the primary focus.

Together, these studies confirm that changes, which are often transitory, occur in the Na^+,K^+-ATPase of epileptic tissue. The studies with different models may be giving insights into different aspects of the process, but at present it would seem that changes in the activity of the Na^+,K^+-ATPase may be cellular adaptations to abnormal ion fluxes or due to degenerative secondary changes in the cellular membranes of the affected cells. Further work is clearly needed with regard to the role of the Na^+,K^+-ATPase in neurons and glia.

Progress in delineating aberrations in pump function will require a better understanding of normal function of the Na^+,K^+-ATPase. In part, this will be achieved through determination of structure–function relationships of the pump.

STRUCTURE OF THE Na^+,K^+-ATPase

Polypeptides

The Na^+,K^+-ATPase has been purified from a variety of sources and has been successfully reconstituted into lipid vesicles, where it pumps Na^+ and K^+ with the same stoichiometry as in cells (21). This conclusively establishes that the Na^+,K^+-ATPase is indeed the Na^+/K^+ pump. In these experiments, vesicles were loaded with potassium and the stoichiometry of Na^+ and K^+ pumped to ATP hydrolyzed was 3:2:1, which is consistent with coupling ratios observed in erythrocytes and nerve. The use of systems of defined composition should be valuable for delineating transport mechanisms. The enzyme from brain has not been purified to the degree achieved in other tissues, e.g., kidney or electric eel electric organ. The basic enzymatic machinery of the enzyme from all sources is thought to be very similar. While work continues on purification of the brain enzyme, studies carried out on other more highly purified preparations would seem to be directly applicable to brain.

When purified preparations of the Na^+-ATPase are examined by sodium dodecyl sulfate

(SDS)–polyacrylamide gel electrophoresis, two major bands, one with an apparent M_r of 95,000 (the α subunit) and a glycopeptide with an apparent M_r of about 45,000 (the β subunit) are found. Sometimes a third component, a proteolipid (the γ polypeptide) of M_r 12,000 is also observed, but its specific function is unknown. The α polypeptide is the catalytic subunit for the enzyme containing the site for phosphorylation as well as the site for ouabain binding. The α and β subunits differ in amino composition, but the percentage of hydrophobic amino acids present in both species is relatively similar (39,48). Even less is known about the γ polypeptide. This low-molecular-weight proteolipid generally migrates near the dye front on electrophoresis gels (9). The involvement of the γ polypeptide in the holoenzyme structure (Fig. 6) is still controversial and is based in part on experiments where photolyzable derivatives of ouabain have been shown to covalently link to both the α and γ polypeptides (17,60).

Studies using cross-linking reagents (1,24, 25,38) suggest that the α and β (and perhaps the

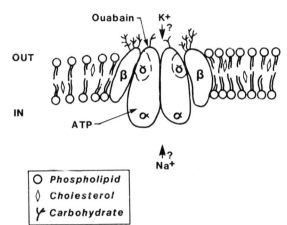

FIG. 6. Subunit structure of the Na⁺,K⁺-ATPase. The Na⁺,K⁺-ATPase contains the α polypeptide (catalytic subunit), β glycopolypeptide, and possibly a lower-molecular-weight γ polypeptide and is isolated in enzymatically active form as membrane particles containing phospholipid and cholesterol. The α and β components are transmembrane integral polypeptides, probably forming an $\alpha_2\beta_2$ oligomer. Enzyme activity is inhibited by the cardiac glycoside ouabain from the extracellular side of the membrane, and ATP binds at the cytoplasmic surface. It is uncertain whether ions are pumped through a channel between subunits (1) or through one of the subunits. However recent studies suggest that the $\alpha\beta$ asymmetric unit is fully capable of catalyzing Na⁺,K⁺-ATPase activity and would argue against transport of Na⁺ and K⁺ between subunits (10,50).

γ) polypeptide are in close contact, and changes in the conformation of the larger α subunit affects the susceptibility of the glycopeptide to proteolysis (30).

Nervous tissue, especially brain, appears to contain two molecular forms of the catalytic subunit designated α and $\alpha(+)$, while other tissues contain only α (77). The two forms differ in molecular weight, $\alpha(+)$ being slightly higher in molecular weight than the α form. The $\alpha(+)$ form may primarily be present in neurons and is more sensitive to ouabain inhibition than the α form (77). We have found that polyclonal antibodies against the lamb kidney Na⁺,K⁺-ATPase react with both α and $\alpha(+)$ from brain (62).

These findings are of interest, since other studies had shown that inhibition of the brain Na⁺,K⁺-ATPase by cardiac glycosides is complex and may involve two binding sites. On the other hand, only one inhibition site is generally implicated in nonnervous tissue. These data, as well as the differing K⁺ affinities of neuronal and glial preparations discussed earlier, are consistent with the idea that more than one functional Na⁺,K⁺-ATPase may exist in nervous tissue.

Molecular Weight

Considerable differences in subunit molecular weights have been reported which may be due to the different species and analytical conditions used (66). Recent calculations (48) mainly from sedimentation equilibrium studies suggest α and β molecular weights of 106,000 to 120,000 and 38,000 to 43,000 (protein only), respectively. The molecular weight of the detergent solubilized enzyme yields values of about 380,000. Since the α/β ratio for subunits is 1:1, the native enzyme is probably an $\alpha_2\beta_2$ tetramer as suggested in Fig. 6, with a calculated molecular weight of 330,000. Ultrastructural studies, especially using electron microscopy and freeze-fracture techniques, demonstrate that the holoenzyme preparations contain membrane-like fragments with a substructure of globular particles (66). Quadripartite particles with a diameter of about 100 Å have been observed using rotary shadowing, suggesting a subunit structure which may represent the α and β polypeptides described and represented in Fig. 6. The molecular weight estimated from these morphological studies is about 500,000, which is in reasonable agreement with the biochemical studies described above.

Conformational States

An important goal for biochemical studies on

the Na^+,K^+-ATPase is to relate conformational changes to the mechanism by which Na^+ and K^+ transport is accomplished.

Extensive *kinetic* studies, especially in the laboratories of Albers (15) and Post (53), support the presence of at least two phosphorylated (E_1-P and E_2-P) and two nonphosphorylated (E_1 and E_2) states of the enzyme. It is accepted that conformational transitions are associated with changes in state of the catalytic subunit ($\alpha,\alpha+$) of the enzyme (32,66,68), as suggested in Fig. 7, where E_1 has a higher affinity for Na^+ and ATP inside the cell (Figs. 6 and 7) and E_2 has a higher affinity for K^+ and is phosphorylated by inorganic phosphate (Pi) but not by ATP. Despite the evidence for these species and their modulation by specific ligands, there is controversy about which of the above reactions might be involved in cation translocation. The scheme (Fig. 7) relates the known enzymatic reactions and probable conformations involved in Na/K transport. Here E_1 exchanges K^+ for Na^+ in the cytoplasmic medium and the enzyme is phosphorylated by ATP. The E_2-P form exchanges Na^+ for K^+ in the extracellular medium. Magnesium is required for phosphorylation of the enzyme and for several of the enzymatic steps. The reactions involving E_1 may be primarily related to the mode of Na^+ transport, and the reactions involving E_2 may be related to K^+ transport.

An important direction for research in recent years has been to try to better understand transport and enzyme mechanisms by examining physicochemical properties of the enzyme. Unequivocal *structural* changes in the α subunit in the presence of ligands (e.g., ATP, Mg^{2+}, Na^+, K^+, ouabain) known to modify Na^+,K^+-ATPase

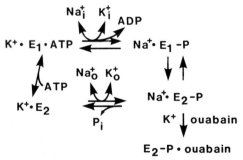

FIG. 7. Reaction scheme relating enzymatic reactions and principal conformations of the Na^+,K^+-ATPase. E_1 exchanges K^+ (inside) for Na^+ (inside) and is phosphorylated by ATP. The E_2 form is phosphorylated by Pi, but not by ATP, and the E_2 form of the enzyme exchanges Na^+ (outside) for K^+ (outside). Ouabain binds to the E_2-P form and is a specific inhibitor of Na,K-ATPase activity.

activity and Na/K pumping in cells have been clearly demonstrated. This has come in part from studies of (a) reactive sulfhydryl groups (23,24,27,63,68,70), (b) controlled proteolysis (30), and (c) changes in intrinsic tryptophan fluorescence (31) of the purified Na^+,K^+-ATPase in the presence of specific ligands. Examples of experimental approaches that relate structural/conformational changes in the Na^+,K^+-ATPase subunits with specific states of the enzyme are described in detail elsewhere (1,25,68). Work done in many laboratories using a variety of techniques has detected conformational changes in the α subunit of the Na^+,K^+-ATPase and tend to confirm the existence of nonphosphorylated and phosphorylated forms of the enzyme given in Fig. 7. These conformational changes may relate to transport by involving a channel with binding sites accessible from both sides of the bilayer (Fig. 6). Such a channel might pass through the space between α_2 subunits (1) or through a protomer unit such as $\alpha\beta$. At present, there is no compelling evidence to choose between these possibilities, but this should be possible when the details of the structure of the Na^+,K^+-ATPase are known.

Lipids

Purified preparations of the Na^+,K^+-ATPase contain 250 to 300 moles phospholipid/mole enzyme (based on the number of ouabain binding sites or phosphorylation sites (48,49,66), and most of this phospholipid is stripped from the enzyme when the latter are purified on columns in the presence of sodium dodecyl sulfate. The subunits are probably irreversibly denatured by this treatment since enzyme activity is absent after reconstitution of the enzyme from the purified subunits in the presence of exogenous phospholipid. There is loss of Na^+,K^+-ATPase enzyme activity (67) when membranes enriched in the Na^+,K^+-ATPase are treated with phospholipases, detergents, or organic solvents that substantially reduce phospholipid content. Many experiments have suggested that specific negatively charged phospholipids—e.g., phosphatidylserine (PS)—play a key role in modulating the enzyme's activity. DePont and co-workers (12) showed that by treating the Na^+,K^+-ATPase with enzymes to reduce total phospholipid content by 65% and phosphatidylserine by 100%, only an 18% loss of Na^+,K^+-ATPase activity occurred. This suggests that the general modulation of the activity of Na^+,K^+-ATPase by phospholipids is primarily mediated by the fluidity of the acyl chains of the fatty acids present in the phospholipids. The enzyme undergoes a large decrease in activation energy as temperature is increased beyond about 20 to 22°C, the point corresponding to "melting" of the fatty acid chains of the phospholipids. Replacement of native phospholipids with ones having more saturated acyl groups shifted the temperature transition point for the change in activation energy to higher values, while substitution of more highly unsaturated acyl groups shifted the transition point to lower values (35). These experiments suggest that the activity of the Na+,K+-ATPase is modified by the fluidity of the lipids in the membrane. However, maximum efficiency of the enzyme may require the presence of some negatively charged phospholipid (12). Electron spin resonance spectra of spin-labeled phospholipids show that protein influences the lipid composition at protein–lipid interfaces. Negatively charged species like PS or phosphatidylinositol may be preferentially immobilized in a lipid boundary layer closely associated with the Na+,K+-ATPase (5). It may be that optimum enzyme function requires that phospholipids in the bilayer segregate to match appropriate hydrophobic and hydrophilic portions of the enzyme subunits. Brothers et al. (5) suggested that basic amino acid residues— e.g., arginine and lysine—may be located near the surface boundary of the lipid bilayers. Therefore, charge as well as fluidity may modulate enzyme activity.

Studies (64) indicate that phospholipids are likely involved in the conversion of the E_1-P to E_2-P forms of the enzyme (Fig. 7). Affinity of the enzyme for Na+ and/or nucleotides are minimally affected by the removal of phospholipids (85). Ligands should approach sites on the extramembraneous portion of the enzyme from either the intra- or extracellular sides (Fig. 6) and would probably not directly involve the lipid bilayer. The E_1-P to E_2-P step, which involves a conformational change in the enzyme, could easily be modulated by the lipid bilayer in which the protein resides. This would be expected if the interaction of several of the enzymes subunits were required for full activity.

Cholesterol within the membrane has also been implicated in modifying the activity of the Na+,K+-ATPase, but it has been shown that all of the cholesterol could be removed from the purified Na+,K+-ATPase with little loss of enzyme activity (49). Cholesterol is probably not essential for activity of the Na+,K+-ATPase, but when present in the membrane it modifies the fluidity of the bilayer by disrupting the packing of the acyl chains of the phospholipids (8,33).

INTERACTIONS WITH ANTICONVULSANT DRUGS

The precise mechanisms of action of anticonvulsant drugs are not known, although direct interactions with specific membrane components are favored by many investigators. Woodbury (86) found a direct correlation between the ratio of extracellular to intracellular sodium concentrations and the electroshock seizure threshold in rats. He found that phenytoin increased the rate of sodium flux in normal rats and decreased the intracellular brain sodium concentrations in normal rats and in rats subjected to electroshock seizures. He proposed that the antiseizure activity of phenytoin results from its stimulation of the Na+ pump, thereby decreasing intracellular sodium. A number of studies have been done to test this hypothesis, but support has not been universal. Rawson and Pincus (57) used microsomal fractions of rat and guinea pig brain and human whole brain homogenates to study Na+,K+-ATPase activity assayed under optimal conditions (100 mM NaCl, 30 mM KCl, 3 mM MgCl$_2$, 3 mM ATP). In the presence of 100 μM phenytoin, Na+,K+-ATPase activity was inhibited 19 to 28%. Festoff and Appel (16) found inhibition of Na+,K+-ATPase activity in rat brain synaptosomes under similar assay conditions, but observed that the Na/K ratio in the assay system was a critical factor in eliciting a stimulatory effect. In the presence of 100 μM phenytoin, they observed a stimulation in enzymatic activity of approximately 50% at an Na/K ratio of 25 to 50:1 and optimal stimulation of 92% at a 250:1 ratio (50 mM Na, 0.2 mM K). Siegel and Goodwin (65) confirmed the stimulatory effect of phenytoin at high Na/K ratios and ascribed the results to a decrease of Na+ inhibition of the pump by the drug. These stimulatory effects of phenytoin have been ascribed by Deupree (13,14) to potassium contamination in the phenytoin solution and not to an effect of the drug. Such contamination would raise enzyme activity by decreasing the Na/K ratio toward more optimal values.

An alternative explanation has been made for the decreased intracellular sodium observed in the presence of phenytoin. This could be achieved by decreased passive inward movement of sodium, rather than by increased active transport of sodium out of cells. Pincus et al. (52) showed in lobster nerves that phenytoin is able to lower the intraneuronal sodium concentration without affecting potassium in the presence of ouabain, which would block Na+,K+-ATPase activity. Perry et al. (47) found that in squid axons phenytoin, like tetrodotoxin (TTX), blocked resting and excitable sodium channels as well as those held open by veratridine. They suggested that the phenytoin and TTX may be structural analogs and that phenytoin could exert its primary effects by specific inhibition of resting sodium permeability. Catterall (7) has recently found that phenytoin blocks sodium channel activation by an allosteric competitive mechanism. Swanson and Crane (74) examined the effects of phenytoin on ion transport and high energy phosphate levels in brain slices. In this system, electrical stimulation normally decreases intracellular K$^+$, increases intracellular Na$^+$, and decreases creatine phosphate and ATP. These investigators found that the expected changes were all substantially reduced in the presence of phenytoin. ^{22}Na exchanged into the intracellular space was reduced by phe-

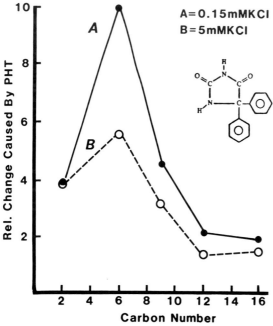

FIG. 8. Effect of phenytoin (PHT) on polarization of fluorescent fatty acids in synaptosomes. Synaptosomes (50 μg protein/ml) were preincubated in media containing either **(A)** 0.15 mM KCl, 100 mM NaCl, 2.5 mM MgCl$_2$, 2.5 mM CaCl$_2$, 40 mM Tris-HCl, pH 7.4, or **(B)** 5 mM KCl, 50 mM NaCl, 2.5 mM MgCl$_2$, 2.5 mM CaCl$_2$, 40 mM Tris-HCl, pH 7.4 ± phenytoin (20 μg/ml) for 30 min at 37°C. Fluorescent probe was then added (1 μM, final concentration). Polarization of fluorescence was measured after 0.5 hr (excitation 381 nm, emission 470 nm). The fluorescent probes used were: 2-, 6-, 9-, and 12-(9-anthroyloxy)stearic acid or 16-(9-anthroyloxy)palmitic acid. The structure of phenytoin is shown in the **inset.**

nytoin. These studies suggest that phenytoin acts by limiting the increase in sodium permeability that occurs on membrane depolarization rather than by stimulating the Na$^+$,K$^+$-ATPase. It is conceivable that the drug may modify Na translocation by several mechanisms. Which of these are important physiologically for control of seizures is uncertain. It seems very likely that a primary site of action of phenytoin is the plasma membrane.

The binding of phenytoin in brain subcellular organelles after either *in vivo* or *in vitro* administration of the drug has been investigated (43). Phenytoin bound reversibly to nearly all subcellular particles examined and most of the drug was found in soluble form. Significant amounts of drug were bound to membrane lipids. Studies by Goldberg and Todoroff (20) and Goldberg (19) provided further evidence for binding of phenytoin to membrane phospholipids, and it was postulated (19) that such interactions might have a major influence on membrane stabilization, perhaps by enhancing Ca^{2+} association with membranes.

We have recently studied the effects of phenytoin on fluidity of synaptosomal membranes. In these studies (26), fatty acids with a fluorescent reporter group on either the 2-, 6-, 9-, 12-, or 16-carbon atoms of stearic or palmitic acids were incorporated into synaptosomal membranes (Fig. 8). The preparations were incubated in high- (5 mM) or low- (0.15 mM) potassium media in the presence or absence of phenytoin. Since the probe penetrates to different depths of the bilayer, a measure of the molecular motion of the native fatty acids of the phospholipids of the bilayer can be assessed through examination of fluorescence parameters. The polarization of fluorescence reflects the rotation of the reporter group and theoretically can vary between 0 and 0.5 (rigid) and will depend on the probe's association with groups within the membrane and temperature. In this system, raising the temperature by 1°C would decrease the polarization by 0.003. When polarization of fluorescence of the probes in synaptosomes was examined (Fig. 8), a clear decrease in polarization was seen in each instance where phenytoin was preincubated with the synaptosomes. This in effect means that the probe rotates more in the presence of phenytoin and the fluidity in the vicinity of the probe is greater. The maximum effect (reported as an equivalent polarization change due to temperature change) was observed when the fluorescent probe was at the six-carbon position, suggesting that the greatest effect is exerted about 5 Å within the bilayer. Perhaps the most intriguing observation was that in the presence of 0.15 mM K$^+$, phenytoin had a more pronounced effect on polarization than did 5 mM K$^+$. In the former case, the ΔP was .0433, which could be achieved independently by raising the temperature of the preparation by 7°C. This represents a major effect on the fluidity of the membrane by phenytoin. At least a portion (up to 50%) of the fluidizing effect was also seen in sonicated lipids obtained from the same synaptosomal preparations (data not shown). Therefore, at least a part of the effect may be related to association of phenytoin with other membrane constituents, e.g., intrinsic proteins.

This approach will be useful in unraveling the mechanism of action of phenytoin and other anticonvulsant drugs. The present data suggests a modification of the fluidity of synaptosomal membranes by phenytoin, which is optimum at about 5 Å into the bilayer structure. A similar fluidizing effect has been observed with the anticonvulsant valproic acid by Lyon and Goldstein (41) using spin-labeled probes. The change in fluidity of the hydrocarbon region of the lipid bilayer reported here could also specifically modify the activity of many intrinsic membrane proteins, including the Na$^+$,K$^+$-ATPase or ion channels, and will require further study.

REFERENCES

1. Askari, A. (1982): Na$^+$,K$^+$-ATPase: Relation of conformational transitions to function. *Mol. Cell. Biochem.*, 43:129–143.
2. Baker, P. F. Blaustein, M. P., Hodgkin, A. L., and Steinhardt, R. A. (1969): The influence of calcium on sodium efflux in squid axons. *J. Physiol. (Lond.)*, 200:421–458.
3. Bernstein, H. G., Poeggel, G., Dorn, A., Luppa, H., and Ziegler, M. (1981): Insulin stimulates Na-K-activated ATPase in hippocampus. *Experientia*, 37:434–435.
4. Bonting, S. L., and Caravaggio, L. L. (1963): Studies on the sodium-potassium activated adenosine triphosphatase. V. Correlation of enzyme activity with cation flux in six tissues. *Arch. Biochem. Biophys.*, 101:37–46.
5. Brotherus, J. R., Jost, P. C., Griffith, O. H., Kena, J. F. W., and Hokin, L. E. (1980): Charge selectivity at the lipid-protein interface of membrane Na,K-ATPase. *Proc. Natl. Acad. Sci. U.S.A.*, 77:272–276.
6. Caldwell, P. D., Hodgkin, A. L., Keynes, R. D., and Shaw, T. I. (1960): The effect of injecting "energy-rich" phosphate compounds on the active transport of ions in the giant axons of *Loligo. J. Physiol. (Lond.)*, 152:561–570.
7. Catterall, W. A. (1981): Inhibition of voltage-sensitive sodium channels in neuroblastoma cells by antiarrhythmic drugs. *Mol. Pharmacol.*, 20:356–362.
8. Chapman, D. (1975): Phase transitions and fluidity characteristics of lipids and cell membranes. *Q. Rev. Biophys.*, 8:185–235.
9. Collins, J. H., Forbush, B., III, Lane, L. K., Ling, E., Schwartz, A., and Zot, A. (1982): Purification and characterization of an (Na$^+$ + K$^+$)-ATPase proteolipid labeled with a photoaffinity derivative of ouabain. *Biochim. Biophys. Acta*, 686:7–12.
10. Craig, W. S. (1982): Monomer of Na and K ion activated ATPase displays complete enzymatic function. *Biochemistry*, 21:5707–5717.
11. De Belleroche, J. S., and Bradford, H. F. (1977): On the site or origin of transmitter amino acids released by depolarization of nerve terminals in vitro. *J. Neurochem.*, 29:335–343.
12. De Pont, J. J. H. H. M., Van Prooijen-Van Eeden, A., and Bonting, S. L. (1978): Role of negatively charged phospholipids in highly purified (Na$^+$ + K$^+$)-ATPase from rabbit kidney outer medulla. Studies on the (Na$^+$ + K$^+$)-activated ATPase, XXXIX. *Biochim. Biophys. Acta*, 508:464–477.
13. Deupree, J. D. (1976): Evidence that diphenylhydantoin does not effect ATPases from brain. *Neuropharmacology*, 15:187–195.
14. Deupree, J. D. (1977): The role or non-role of ATPase activation by phenytoin in the stabilization of excitable membranes. *Epilepsia*, 18:309–315.
15. Fahn, S., Koval, G. J., and Albers, R. W. (1966): Na,K-activated ATPase of *Electrophorus* electric organ. I. An associated Na-activated transphosphorylation. *J. Biol. Chem.*, 241:1882–1889.
16. Festoff, B. W., and Appel, S. H. (1968): Effect of diphenylhydantoin on synaptosome sodium, potassium-ATPase. *J. Clin. Invest.*, 47:2752–2758.
17. Forbush, B., III, Kaplan, J. H., and Hoffman, J. F. (1978): Characterization of a new photoaffinity derivative of ouabain: Labelling of the large polypeptide and of a proteolipid component of the Na,K-ATPase. *Biochemistry*, 17:3667–3676.
18. Franck, G., Grisar, T., and Moonen, G. (1983): Glial and neuronal Na$^+$,K$^+$-pump. *Adv. Cell. Neurobiol.*, 4:133–159.
19. Goldberg, M. A. (1977): Phenytoin, phospholipids and calcium. *Neurology*, 27:827–833.
20. Goldberg, M. A., and Todoroff, T. (1976): Diphenylhydantoin binding to brain lipids and phospholipids. *Biochem. Pharmacol.*, 25:2079–2083.
21. Goldin, S. M. (1977): Active-transport of sodium and potassium-ions by sodium and potassium ion-activated adenosine-triphosphatase from renal medulla-reconstitution of purified enzyme into a well-defined in vitro transport system. *J. Biol. Chem.*, 252:5630–5642.
22. Grisar, T., Franck, G., and Delgado-Escueta, A. V. (1983): Glial contribution to seizure: K$^+$ activation of Na$^+$,K$^+$-ATPase in bulk isolated glial cells and synaptosomes of epileptogenic cortex. *Brain Res.*, 261:75–84.
23. Harris, W. E., and Stahl, W. L. (1977): Conformational changes of purified Na$^+$,K$^+$-ATPase

detected by a sulfhydryl fluorescence probe. *Biochim. Biophys. Acta*, 485:203–214.

24. Harris, W. E., and Stahl, W. L. (1980): Organization of thiol groups of electric eel electric organ sodium-plus-potassium ion-stimulated ATPase studied with bifunctional reagents. *Biochem. J.*, 185:787–790.

25. Harris, W. E., and Stahl, W. L. (1984): Conformational states of $(Na^+ + K^+)$-transporting ATPase. Formation of 240,000-M_r and 116,000-M_r polypeptides in the presence of a bifunctional thiol probe. *Biochem. J.*, 218:331–339.

26. Harris, W. E., and Stahl, W. L. (1984): Phenytoin modifies the polarization of fluorescent lipids in synaptosomes. (*Submitted for publication.*)

27. Hart, W. H., Jr., and Titus, E. D. (1973): Sulfhydryl groups of sodium-potassium transport ATPase. *J. Biol. Chem.*, 248:4674–4681.

28. Inomata, J., Mayahara, H., Fujimoto, K., and Ogawa, K. (1983): Ultrastructural localization of ouabain-sensitive potassium dependent p-nitrophenylphosphatase $(Na^+, K^+$-ATPase) activity in the central nervous system of the rat. *Acta Histochem. Cytochem.*, 16:277–285.

29. Jones, L. R., Maddock, S. W., and Besch, H. R., Jr. (1980): Unmasking effect of alamethicin on the (Na^+, K^+)-ATPase, β-adrenergic receptor-coupled adenylate cyclase and cAMP-dependent protein kinase activities of cardiac sarcolemmal vesicles. *J. Biol. Chem.*, 255:9971–9980.

30. Jørgensen, P. L. (1982): Mechanism of the Na^+, K^+-Pump. Protein structure and conformations of the pure $(Na^+ + K^+)$-ATPase. *Biochim. Biophys. Acta*, 694:27–68.

31. Karlish, S. J. D., and Yates, D. W. (1978): Tryptophan fluorescence of $(Na^+ + K^+)$-ATPase as a tool for study of the enzyme mechanism. *Biochim. Biophys. Acta*, 527:115–130.

32. Karlish, S. J. D., Yates, D. W., and Glynn, I. M. (1978): Conformational transitions between Na^+-bound and K^+-bound forms of $(Na^+ + K^+)$-ATPase, studied with formycin nucleotides. *Biochim. Biophys. Acta*, 525:252–264.

33. Kimelberg, K. H. (1975): Alterations in phospholipid-dependent $(Na + K)$ATPase activity due to lipid fluidity. Effects of cholesterol and Mg. *Biochim. Biophys. Acta*, 413:143–156.

34. Kimelberg, K. H. (1983): Primary astrocyte cultures—A key to astrocyte function. *Cell. Mol. Neurobiol.*, 3:1–16.

35. Kimelberg, K. H., and Papahadjopoulos, D. (1974): Effects of phospholipid acyl chain fluidity, phase transitions and cholesterol on $(Na^+ + K^+)$-stimulated-ATPase. *J. Biol. Chem.*, 25:1071–1080.

36. Kuffler, S. W. (1967): Neuroglial cells: Physiological properties and a potassium mediated effect of neuronal activity on the glial cell membrane potential. *Proc. R. Soc. Lond. [Biol.]*, 168:1–21.

37. Kuo, C.-H., et al. (1979): Regulation of ATP-dependent Ca uptake of synaptic plasma membranes by Ca-dependent modulator protein. *Life Sci.*, 25:235–240.

38. Kyte, J. (1972): Properties of two polypeptides of the Na,K-activated ATPase. *J. Biol. Chem.*, 247:7642–7649.

39. Lane, L. K., Potter, J. D., and Collins, J. H. (1979): Large-scale purification of Na,K-ATPase and its protein subunits from lamb kidney medulla. *Prep. Biochem.*, 9:157–170.

40. Lewin, E., and McCrimmon, A. (1967): ATPase activity in discharging cortical lesions induced by freezing. *Arch. Neurol.*, 16:321–325.

41. Lyon, R. C., and Goldstein, D. B. (1980): The comparative effect of sodium valproate, sodium octanoate and sodium valerate on spin-labeled synaptosomal plasma membranes from mouse brain. *Fed. Proc.*, 39:1100.

42. Meyer, E. M., and Cooper, J. R. (1981): Correlations between Na^+, K^+-ATPase activity and acetylcholine release in rat cortical synaptosomes. *J. Neurochem.*, 36:467–475.

43. Nielsen, T., and Cotman, C. (1971): The binding of diphenylhydantoin to brain and subcellular fractions. *Eur. J. Pharmacol.*, 14:344–350.

44. O'Fallon, J. F., Brosemer, R. W., and Harding, J. W. (1981): The Na^+, K^+-ATPase: A plausible trigger for voltage-independent release of cytoplasmic neurotransmitters. *J. Neurochem.*, 36:369–378.

45. Pech, I. V., and Stahl, W. L. (1984): Immunocytochemical localization of Na^+, K^+-ATPase in primary cultures of rat retina. *Neurochem. Res.*, 9:759–769.

46. Pentreath, V. W. (1982): Potassium signalling of metabolic interactions between neurons and glial cells. *Trends Neurol. Sci.*, 5:339–345.

47. Perry, J. G., McKinney, L., and DeWeer, P. (1978): The cellular mode of action of the anti-epileptic drug 5,5-diphenylhydantoin. *Nature (Lond.)*, 272:271–273.

48. Peters, W. H. M., De Pont, J. J. H. H. M., Koppers, A., and Bonting, S. L. (1981): Studies on $(Na^+ + K^+)$ activated ATPase XLVII. Chemical composition, molecular weight and molar ratio of the subunits of the enzyme from rabbit kidney outer medulla. *Biochim. Biophys. Acta*, 641:55–70.

49. Peters, W. H. M., Fleuren-Jakobs, A. H. M., De Pont, J. J. H. H. M., and Bonting, S. L. (1981): Studies on $(Na^+ + K^+)$-activated ATPase XLIX. Content and role of cholesterol and other neutral lipids in highly purified rabbit kidney enzyme preparation. *Biochim. Biophys. Acta*, 649:541–549.

50. Peters, W. H. M., Swarts, H. G. P., De Pont, J. J. H. H. M., Schuurmans Stekhoven, F. M. A. H., and Bonting, S. L. (1981): $(Na^+ + K^+)$-ATPase has one functioning phosphorylation site per α subunit. *Nature (Lond.)*, 290:338–339.

51. Picker, S., Pieper, C. F., and Goldring, S. (1981): Glial membrane potentials and their relationship to $[K^+]_o$ in man and guinea pig. *J. Neurosurg.*, 55:347–363.

52. Pincus, J. H., Grove, I., Marino, B. B., and Glaser, G. E. (1970): Studies on the mechanism of action of diphenylhydantoin. *Arch. Neurol.*, 22:566–571.

53. Post, R., Hegyvary, C., and Kume, S. (1972): Activation by ATP in the phosphorylation ki-

netics of Na and K transport ATPase. *J. Biol. Chem.*, 247:6530–6540.

54. Powis, D. A. (1981): Does Na,K-ATPase play a role in the regulation of neurotransmitter release by prejunctional α-adrenoceptors? *Biochem. Pharmacol.*, 30:2389–2397.

55. Rapport, R. L., II, Harris, A. B., Friel, P. N., and Ojemann, G. A. (1975): Human epileptic brain. Na,K-ATPase activity and phenytoin concentrations. *Arch. Neurol.*, 32:549–554.

56. Rapport, R. L., and Ojemann, G. A. (1975): Prophylactically administered phenytoin. Effects of the development of chronic cobalt-induced epilepsy in the cat. *Arch. Neurol.*, 33:539–548.

57. Rawson, M. D., and Pincus, J. H. (1968): The effect of diphenylhydantoin on Na,K,Mg-activated ATPase in microsomal fractions of rat and guinea pig and on whole homogenates of human brain. *Biochem. Pharmacol.*, 17:573–579.

58. Resch, K., Loracher, A., Mähler, B., Stock, M., and Rode, H. N. (1978): Functional mosaicism of the lymphocyte membrane. *Biochim. Biophys. Acta*, 511:176–193.

59. Resh, M. D. (1983): Insulin activation of (Na⁺,K⁺)-ATPase exhibits a temperature-dependent lag time. Comparison of the glucose transporter. *Biochemistry*, 22:2781–2784.

60. Rogers, T. B., and Lazdunski, M. (1979): Photoaffinity labeling of a small protein purified Na⁺,K⁺-ATPase. *FEBS Lett.*, 98:373–376.

61. Schellenberg, G. D., Anderson, L., and Swanson, P. D. (1983): Inhibition of Na⁺-Ca²⁺ exchange in rat brain by amiloride. *Mol. Pharmacol.*, 24:251–258.

62. Schellenberg, G. D., Pech, I. V., and Stahl, W. L. (1981): Immunoreactivity of subunits of the (Na⁺,K⁺)-ATPase: Cross-reactivity of the α, α(+) and β forms in different organs and species. *Biochim. Biophys. Acta*, 649:691–700.

63. Schoot, B. M., De Pont, J. J. H. H. M., and Bonting, S. L. (1978): Studies on (Na⁺+K⁺)-activated ATPase. XLII. Evidence for two classes of essential sulfhydryl groups. *Biochim. Biophys. Acta*, 522:602–613.

64. Schuurmans-Stekhoven, F., and Bonting, S. L. (1981): Transport adenosine triphosphatases: Properties and functions. *Physiol. Rev.*, 61:1–76.

65. Siegel, S. J., and Goodwin, B. B. (1972): Na,K-activated ATPase of brain microsomes: Modification of sodium inhibition by diphenylhydantoin. *J. Clin. Invest.*, 51:1164–1169.

66. Siegel, S. J., Stahl, W. L., and Swanson, P. D. (1981): Ion transport. In: *Basic Neurochemistry*, edited by G. J. Siegel, R. W. Albers, R. Katzman, and B. W. Agranoff, pp 107–143. Little, Brown, Boston.

67. Stahl, W. L. (1973): Role of phospholipids in the Na⁺,K⁺ stimulated adenosine triphosphatase system of brain microsomes. *Arch. Biochem. Biophys.*, 154:56–67.

68. Stahl, W. L. (1984): Na⁺,K⁺-ATPase: Function, structure and conformations. *Ann. Neurol.*, 16(Suppl):S124–S127.

69. Stahl, W. L., and Broderson, S. H. (1976): Localization of Na⁺,K⁺-ATPase in brain. *Fed. Proc.*, 35:1260–1265.

70. Stahl, W. L., and Harris, W. E. (1979): A fluorescent sulfhydryl probe for studying conformational changes of the Na,K-ATPase. In: *Na,K-ATPase Structure and Kinetics*, edited by J. C. Skou, and J. C. Nørby, pp. 157–167. Academic, New York.

71. Stahl, W. L., and Swanson, P. D. (1969): Uptake of calcium by subcellular fractions isolated from ouabain-treated cerebral tissues. *J. Neurochem.*, 16:1553–1563.

72. Stahl, W. L., and Swanson, P. D. (1971): Movements of Ca and other cations in isolated cerebral tissues. *J. Neurochem.*, 18:415–427.

73. Stahl, W. L., and Swanson, P. D. (1972): Calcium movements in brain slices in low Na or Ca media. *J. Neurochem.*, 19:2395–2407.

74. Swanson, P. D., and Crane, P. O. (1972): Diphenylhydantoin and movement of radioactive sodium into electrically stimulated cerebral slices. *Biochem. Pharmacol.*, 21:2899–2905.

75. Swanson, P. D., Anderson, L., and Stahl, W. L. (1974): Uptake of Ca ions by synaptosomes from rat brain. *Biochim. Biophys. Acta*, 356:174–183.

76. Swanson, P. D., Schellenberg, G. D., Clark, A. F., and Roman, I. J. (1981): Calcium buffering systems in brain. In: *Chemisms of the Brain*, edited by R. Rodnight, H. Bachelard, and W. L. Stahl, pp. 12–20. Churchill Livingstone, Edinburgh.

77. Sweadner, K. J. (1979): Two molecular forms of (Na⁺ + K⁺)-ATPase in brain. *J. Biol. Chem.*, 254:6060–6067.

78. Szamel, M., Schneider, S., and Resch, K. (1981): Functional interrelationship between (Na⁺ + K⁺)-ATPase and lysolecithin acyltransferase in plasma membrane of mitogen-stimulated rabbit thymocytes. *J. Biol. Chem.*, 256:9198–9204.

79. Tower, D. B. (1969): Neurochemical mechanisms. In: *Basic Mechanisms of the Epilepsies*, edited by H. H. Jasper, A. A. Ward, Jr., and A. Pope, pp. 611–646. Little Brown, New York.

80. Trams, E. G., and Lauter, C. J. (1978): Ecto-ATPase deficiency in glia of seizure-prone mice. *Nature (Lond.)*, 271:270–271.

81. Trams, E. G., and Lauter, C. J. (1978): A comparative study of brain Ca²⁺-ATPases. *Comp. Biochem. Physiol.*, 59B:191–194.

82. Varon, S., and Skaper, S. D. (1983): The Na⁺,K⁺ pump may mediate the control of nerve cells by nerve growth factor. *Trends Biochem. Sci.*, 8:22–25.

83. Vizi, E. S. (1978): Na⁺-K⁺-activated adenosinetriphosphatase as a trigger in transmitter release. *Neuroscience*, 3:367–384.

84. Walz, W., Wuttke, W., and Schlue, W. R. (1983): The Na⁺-K⁺ pump in neuropile glial cells of the medicinal leech. *Brain Res.*, 267:93–100.

85. Wheeler, K. P. (1975): Role of phospholipid in intermediate stops of Na,K-ATPase reaction. *Biochem. J.*, 146:729–738.

86. Woodbury, D. M. (1955): Effect of diphenylhydantoin on electrolytes and radiosodium turnover in brain and other tissues of normal, hyponatremic and postictal rats. *J. Pharmacol. Exp. Ther.*, 115:74–95.

87. Wu, P. H., and Phillis, J. W. (1979): Effects of vanadate on brain (Na⁺ + K⁺)-ATPase and *p*-nitrophenylphosphatase: Interactions with monovalent and divalent ions and with noradrenaline. *Int. J. Biochem.*, 10:629–635.

Advances in Neurology, Vol. 44, edited by
A. V. Delgado-Escueta, A. A. Ward, Jr.,
D. M. Woodbury, and R. J. Porter.
Raven Press, New York © 1986.

35

Role of Glial Cation and Anion Transport Mechanisms in Etiology and Arrest of Seizures

H. Steve White, Dixon M. Woodbury, C. F. Chen, John W. Kemp,
S. Y. Chow, and Y. C. Yen-Chow

Division of Neuropharmacology and Epileptology, Departments of Physiology and Pharmacology, University of Utah School of Medicine, Research Park, Salt Lake City, Utah 84108

SUMMARY   The intrinsic processes involved in the initiation and arrest of seizures are not completely understood. Cortical and cerebellar inhibitory mechanisms, accumulation of metabolic products, and glial uptake of extracellular potassium (K^+_o), anions, and released neurotransmitters are all important processes that limit focal firing and terminate a seizure once it has been initiated. Of these, the intrinsic cortical inhibitory mechanisms—i.e., recurrent and surround inhibition—appear to be the most important. Active cation and anion transport processes are two metabolic events that have yet to be elucidated but clearly could be involved in terminating a seizure discharge. For example, without an active mechanism to transport chloride, opening of the chloride channel by the inhibitory transmitter GABA would not result in increased chloride permeability.

The transient hypoxia and hypercapnia and lactic acidosis that follows a severe tonic–clonic seizure produces a mixed systemic metabolic and respiratory acidosis. In experimental animals, the hypercapnia that results is sufficient to block seizure discharges. Increasing the CO_2 concentration significantly reduces the extension to flexion (E/F) ratio of mice given maximal electroshock seizures (MES) and increases the time required for 50% of the animals to recover sufficiently from a first MES to be able to have another MES. The decreased E/F ratio and the increased recovery time (RT_{50}) are both indicative of a decrease in seizure activity. Since the extent to which CO_2 is allowed to accumulate in the brain is regulated by the glial specific enzyme carbonic anhydrase (CA), it follows that the glial cell has an integral role in the mechanisms involved in arresting seizure activity. In contrast, hypoxia increased the E/F ratio and decreased the RT_{50}, evidence that seizure activity was enhanced.

Another metabolic factor affecting duration of seizure activity, susceptibility to seizures, and recovery from seizures is glucose. Recovery from seizures depends in part on an adequate supply of this energy source. An inverse correlation ($R = 0.95$) between RT_{50} and blood sugar was found when the blood sugar was altered experimentally by treatments that altered the endocrine status (pancreatectomy, treatment with alloxan, cortisol, insulin, glucagon, and dextrose). Since glial cells contain (as glycogen) the small amount of glucose present in the brain, they probably hasten the ability of the brain to recover normal function following a seizure. Glycogenolysis and the subsequent release of glucose from glial cells not only hastens recovery from a seizure but also provides an energy source for maintaining active transport mechanisms concerned with the regulation of cation and anion concentrations in the extracellular fluid (ECF). The importance of these processes, which include Cl^- and HCO_3^- transport, mediated by CA and by HCO_3^--ATPase, and an $HCO_3^- - Cl^-$ exchange, is exemplified by the data on the Frings strain of the audiogenic mouse. The intensity of audiogenic seizures was found to be directly related to the activity of CA in these mice. Furthermore, when active Cl^- transport into glial cells was blocked by the monovalent anions, perchlorate and thiocyanate, an increase in brain excitability (increased E/F ratio) was observed. It is apparent that CA plays an important role in anion transport in the brain, which in turn regulates brain excitability.

In naive animals, the CA inhibitor, acetazolamide (ACZ) significantly increased the intracellular to extracellular K^+ (K^+_i/K^+_o) ratio, increased the intracellular HCO_3^- space, and slightly increased intracellular Na^+ and Cl^- spaces in the brain. These effects were accompanied by an anticonvulsant effect (abolishment of the extensor component of the MES). In rats rendered tolerant to ACZ, the MES pattern was normal and the K^+_i/K^+_o ratio was the same as in the controls, as was the intracellular HCO_3^- space.

ACZ also produces marked effects on the electrical properties of cultured glial cells that correlate with its inhibitory effects on CA and its effects on brain excitability. In low doses ACZ hyperpolarizes the glial cell membrane by increasing the total $[CO_2]$ and the K^+_i/K^+_o ratio, whereas in high doses, it depolarizes these cells by blocking $HCO_3^- - Cl^-$ exchange across the glial membrane. These studies further exemplify the important role that CA plays in anion (Cl^- and HCO_3^-) and cation (K^+) transport in glial cells and in regulating the level of excitability in the brain.

Additional evidence supporting the importance of glial and glial transport enzymes in seizures and seizure arrest mechanisms is provided by *in vivo* and *in vitro* drug studies that examined the effects of convulsant and anticonvulsant agents on electrolytes and transport enzymes. It appears from these studies that the seizure produced by the convulsant agent pentylenetetrazol initiates the recruitment of glial regulatory processes. Among these, an increase in the activity of the enzymes CA and HCO_3^--ATPase was observed in both the cerebral and cerebellar cortices. Thus, neuronal depolarization products such as CO_2, H^+, K^+, and NH_3 can cause marked changes in the glial enzymes that handle these products. This example serves to illustrate the integral relationship that exists between neuronal and glial cells within the central nervous system (CNS).

It is probable that, in addition to their effects on neuronal cells, anticonvulsants such as phenytoin also act by enhancing glial-cell protective mechanisms. Experiments conducted in this laboratory have demonstrated that therapeutic concentrations of phenytoin increase both the DNA and the CA activity of rat cerebral cortex. Since only the glial cell is capable of division after birth, an increase in DNA is indicative of an effect on this cell. Thus, we have demonstrated both *in vivo* and *in vitro* that therapeutic (micromolar) concentrations of phenytoin via an action on glial Na^+, K^+-ATPase provide the CNS with an enhanced ability to regulate K^+_o. Although an increase in K^+_o is probably not important in initiation of the seizure process, it is thought by some investigators to be involved in the transition from interictal to ictal firing and in the maintenance of the seizure discharge. These studies provide further insight into the role of glia in the brain, and into the mechanisms of anticonvulsant action of phenytoin.

From these and other studies, it is apparent that the glial cell plays an active role in the homeostasis of the brain extracellular environment, and that metabolic and drug induced alterations in their transport mechanisms can profoundly affect brain excitability.

Although a seizure focus or a genetic defect that causes seizures is always present, ictal episodes are only occasional and short-lived events in the behavior of an epileptogenic focus. It is essential, therefore, to consider the various processes that delimit focal firing and that terminate a seizure once it has been initiated. The most important processes appear to be inhibitory mechanisms, accumulation of metabolic products that inhibit seizure activity, and glial uptake of extracellular potassium (K^+_o), anions, and released neurotransmitters. The intrinsic cortical inhibitory mechanisms—i.e., recurrent and surround inhibition—appear to be the most important processes to restrain a focus from firing and to arrest an ongoing seizure discharge. However, the metabolic events accompanying inhibitory discharge have not been elucidated. They appear to involve active cation and/or anion transport processes that are regulated by inhibitory neurotransmitters, such as GABA and glycine. Extracortical inhibitory systems also exert some measure of control as well. For example, stimulation of portions of the cerebellum suppresses interictal spiking activity in the penicillin- or cobalt-induced cortical focus, and cerebellar ablations facilitate the spike activity (4,11). Also, stimulation of the caudate suppresses the acute cortical penicillin focus (see ref. 20 for summary). Whether the same or similar inhibitory systems are operative to terminate seizures in parts of the cortex other than the sensory motor areas is not known.

During severe tonic–clonic seizures, respiratory arrest occurs briefly and there is a transient hypoxia and hypercapnia. Also, since intense muscular activity takes place during the seizure, lactic acid accumulates in the plasma. This results in a mixed systemic metabolic and respiratory acidosis. In experimental animals, and possibly in humans, CO_2 accumulates in brain to a level sufficiently high to block seizure discharges (38,50). The extent to which CO_2 accumulates is regulated by the enzyme carbonic anhydrase (CA), which is exclusively located in glial cells, as discussed below. Thus, the glial system plays an integral role in the mechanisms involved in arresting seizure activity. This chapter will discuss the evidence for such a role of CA.

That CO_2 accumulation, as well as hypoxia and hyperoxia, does affect seizure arrest is demonstrated by the results shown in Fig. 1. The effects of hypoxia, hyperoxia and hypercapnia on the extension to flexion (E/F) ratio of mice given maximal electroshock seizures (MES) and on their ability to recover from MES are shown in this figure [plotted from the results of Woodbury et al. (51)]. The recovery time (RT_{50}) was measured as the time for 50% of the animals to recover sufficiently from a first MES to be able to have another MES. It is evident from this figure that CO_2 has a profound effect to decrease the E/F ratio and markedly increase RT_{50}. It can therefore effectively arrest seizure activity. Hypoxia, in contrast, increased E/F ratio and decreased RT_{50} in mice, evidence that seizure activity is enhanced. Hyperoxia had the opposite effect—i.e., decreased E/F ratio and slightly increased RT_{50}. Thus, higher concentrations of oxygen tend to enhance seizure arrest.

A number of other metabolic factors also af-

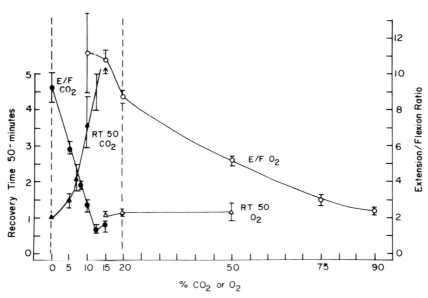

FIG. 1. Effects of various concentrations of CO_2 and oxygen (*abscissa*) on the RT_{50} (*left ordinate*) from maximal electroshock seizures (MES) and the extension/flexion ratio (*right ordinate*) in rats. The RT_{50} is the time (min) for 50% of rats to recover sufficiently from an initial MES to have a second MES. See text for explanation.

fect duration of seizure activity, susceptibility to seizures, and recovery from seizures. These factors are important in the control of epileptic seizures and will be discussed briefly. The rate of recovery from seizures depends most importantly on an adequate supply of its energy source, glucose. Since very little glucose is stored in the brain (mainly glial cells in adults as glycogen), the main source of glucose for the brain is from blood and from glycogenolysis from liver. Because of its dependence on glucose, we tested the effects of alteration in this parameter in blood on the RT_{50}. In Fig. 2 the relationship between RT_{50} and blood sugar is plotted. The points represent various procedures or treatments in rats that change the blood sugar by altering the endocrine status, such as pancreatectomy, and treatment with alloxan, cortisol, insulin, glucagon and dextrose. It is evident from the data in Fig. 2 (see ref. 49) that there is an inverse correlation ($r = 0.95$) be-

tween RT_{50} (ordinate) and the blood sugar level (abscissa). This curve is fitted as a power-function regression which is the expected fit, since at low blood sugar concentrations profound postictal depression and eventually coma occur, hence the RT_{50} goes to infinite values, and at high blood sugar concentration the RT_{50} values change little because the entrance of glucose into the brain is an active process that is saturated at these high levels. Thus, recovery is enhanced by a high blood sugar and slowed by a low level. Providing an adequate source of energy hastens the ability of the brain to recover normal function. Glial cells probably play a role in this process as well, because they contain the small amount of glycogen that is present in the brain. Potassium appears to play a key role in the regulation of glycogen synthesis in glia and in the formation of glucose by glycogenolysis. Thus, K^+ released from neurons during activity appears to promote glycogen synthesis in glia

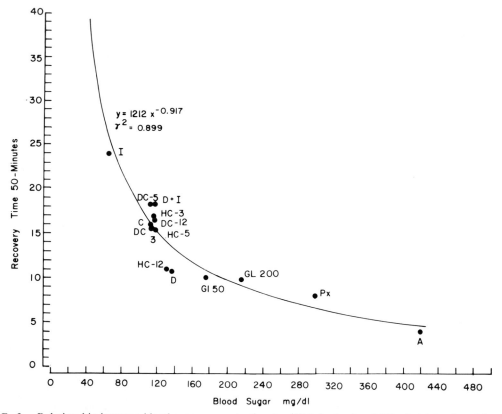

FIG. 2. Relationship between blood sugar concentration (mg/dl) (*abscissa*) and RT_{50} (min) (*ordinate*) in rats given various treatments or procedures that alter blood sugar. The solid line was fitted to the plotted points as a power-function regression with the equation $y = 1,212 \, x - 0.917$ ($r^2 = 0.899$). The abbreviations represent the following treatments or procedures: C, control; I, insulin; DC-3, DC-5, DC-12, deoxycorticosterene acetate, 1.5 mg/kg body weight, given for 3, 5, or 12 days, respectively; HC-3, HC-5, HC-12, hydrocortisone (cortisol) acetate, 1.5 mg/kg given for 3, 5, or 12 days, respectively; GL-50, GL-200, glucagon, 50 μg/100 g body weight and 200 μg/100 g body weight; Px, pancreatectomized; A, alloxan-treated rats. See text for discussion.

and cAMP released from neurons during activity (possibly via an effect of K^+) promotes glycogenolysis and release of glucose from these cells. Such released glucose thus provides an energy source for maintaining active transport mechanisms concerned with regulation of cation and anion concentrations in the extracellular fluid (see ref. 23).

ROLE OF GLIA IN SEIZURE ARREST

Evidence from many workers has shown that glial cells play an important role in modulating K_o^+, as well as the acid–base and anion balances of the interstitial fluid of the brain, a process that helps to ameliorate chronic neuronal hyperexcitability. Thus the K^+- and Cl^--modulating systems appear to be involved in arresting focal spread and on-going seizure activity. In addition, the active uptake by glia of those neurotransmitters that are associated with excessive neuronal activity (for example, glutamate) probably also contributes to the process of terminating seizures (10,29). It is important, therefore, to discuss the role of glia in modulating brain excitability and ameliorating seizures.

Carbonic anhydrase (CA) has a central role in the cooperative metabolism of neurons and closely contacting glia during regulation of anion and acid–base balance of brain cells and the interstitial and cerebrospinal fluids (CSF). It is located exclusively in glia and choroid plexus but depends for its substrate on metabolites that are mostly generated and released during neuronal discharge. CA is directly involved in maintenance of Cl^- concentration and indirectly that of K^+ concentrations in glial cells. In addition, the enzymes Na^+,K^+-ATPase and HCO_3^--ATPase are constituents of glia and are involved in regulation of Na^+ and K^+ and Cl^- and HCO_3^- concentrations, respectively. In view of the central role of CA and the two ATPases in cation and anion transport in glia, it is important to examine their role in CNS excitability and seizure arrest mechanisms and to ascertain the effects of convulsant and anticonvulsant drugs on these glial processes.

That CA activity is related to brain excitability is demonstrated by the data on the Frings strain of audiogenic seizure mice shown in Fig. 3 (see ref. 46). The intensity of audiogenic seizure— that is, the presence of running, submaximal, or maximal seizure activity— is directly related to the activity of CA. The largest change in the brainstem was between the control and running seizures groups. The increase in CA activity in the more intense seizure groups was much less. The same was true for the cerebellum, but in the cerebral cortex there appeared to be a linear relation in both left and right cortices between CA activity and intensity of seizure. Other data from this laboratory (see review in ref. 46) has also

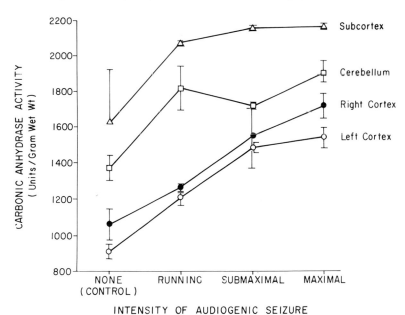

FIG. 3. Effect of seizure intensity on carbonic anhydrase activity in various areas of the brain in Frings strain audiogenic seizure mice. Carbonic anhydrase activity (units/g wet brain tissue) is plotted along the *ordinate* and the intensity of the audiogenic seizure is shown along the *abscissa*. Vertical bracketed lines are standard errors. See text for discussion.

demonstrated a relation between CA activity and excitability in cobalt-induced focal seizures in rats and with various convulsant drugs.

Before determining the role of glia in seizure arrest and of the effects of drugs on them, it is essential to understand the normal distribution of electrolytes in glial cells and neurons. Figure 4 shows the distribution of monovalent cations and anions in plasma and CSF and in neurons and glia of rat cerebral cortex. The data are derived from values determined in this laboratory by electrolyte analysis and by resolution of uptake curves for the various cations and anions and also from data in the literature (30,31). This analysis indicates that the volume of glial cells is 22% of the wet brain weight, neuronal volume 43%, and interstitial fluid volume 14% (30,31,52). Examination of the data on concentrations of electrolytes in neurons indicates that chloride is approximately in equilibrium with the membrane potential, assumed to be -70 mV, in this diagram. Iodide concentration and other anions are also assumed to be passively distributed. The concentrations of sodium and chloride are approximately the same as in other excitable tissues. In glial cells, a striking feature is the high chloride concentration of 46 mmol/l of glial cell water ($E_{Cl^-} = -25$ mv). The results show that chloride is actively transported into glial cells from the interstitial fluid, since E_{Cl^-} is considerably lower than the transmembrane potential of -80 or -90 mV. Others have demon-

strated active chloride transport into glia (6; see ref. 13 for review). Also, the glial concentration of sodium (76 mmol/l in water) is considerably higher than in the neurons. Thus, glial cells contain high concentrations of sodium and chloride. Potassium concentrations in the two compartments (glia and neuronal) are similar. The other striking feature is the high concentration of bicarbonate ion (18 mM in cell water) and the high pH (7.29) in the glial cells as compared with the neurons (8 mM and 6.97). These HCO_3^- concentrations and pH values were derived from data on the resolution of curves for $H^{14}CO_3^-$ and ^{14}C-dimethyloxazolidine-2,4-dione (^{14}C-DMO) uptake by rat cerebral cortex. These two methods yield similar values. The ratio of H^+ ion in glial cells (51.3 nM in cell water) to that in extracellular water (41.7 nM) is 1.23, whereas this ratio between neurons (107.2 nM) and extracellular water is 2.57. Thus, glial cells would appear to have a more active proton pump than do neurons, probably because of the presence of carbonic anhydrase. This mechanism would increase the ability of the glia to regulate the interstitial acid–base balance. This is supported by our observations that acetazolamide, a selective inhibitor of CA, reduces the ability of these cells to regulate interstitial and neuronal pH (see further discussion below). Measurements of the pH of glial cells in culture by ^{14}C-DMO also show that these cells have a higher pH than do neurons. Thus, in dibutyryl cyclic AMP-treated

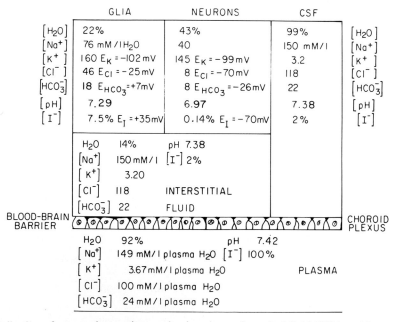

FIG. 4. Distribution of monovalent cations and anions in cerebrospinal fluid (CSF) and in neurons and glial cells of rat cerebral cortex. See text for explanation.

glial cell cultures the pH was 7.19 and, after treatment with phenytoin, 7.22. These values are close to those found *in vivo*.

Iodide ion is also transported actively into glia, as is the case with chloride. Thus, glial cells have an active inward anion transport mechanism that involves both chloride and iodide ions, a process that the evidence suggests involves a chloride–bicarbonate exchange system that appears to be mediated in part by the CA located in the glial cell membrane (13).

In Table 1 (see p. 712), taken from the data of Gill *et al.* (6), are shown the effects of acetazolamide (ACZ), monovalent anions and metabolic inhibitors on the active uptake of chloride ($^{36}Cl^-$) by isolated cultured astrocytes. Chloride transport is inhibited by 10 mM concentrations of perchlorate, thiocyanate, bromide, and iodide. Also, ACZ in concentrations of 5 and 10 mM inhibited $^{36}Cl^-$ uptake into these cultured glia by 66.2 and 41.2% of the control value, respectively. Thus, CA, by increasing HCO_3^- concentration in glial cells, provides the substrate necessary for exchange with interstitial Cl^- and therefore is involved in the Cl^- active uptake process. It is also energy-dependent, as is indicated by the inhibition of transport by 2,4-dinitrophenol and by fluoride.

Since inhibition of Cl^- transport into glial cells by low doses of the monovalent anions, perchlorate, and thiocyanate, which inhibit CA and HCO_3^--ATPase, results in an increase in brain excitability (increased E/F ratio) and since higher doses cause seizures, which can be enhanced by ACZ (48) it is evident that glial-cell active Cl^- transport is involved in regulation of brain excitability and that CA and HCO_3^--ATPase mediate this process.

Further support for a role of these enzymes is derived from our studies on the effects of ACZ on electrolyte and acid–base distribution in the cerebral cortex of normal rats and rats made tolerant to the anti-MES effects of ACZ. These data are depicted in Fig. 5, plotted from the data of Koch and Woodbury (15). A single dose of ACZ at 20 mg/kg significantly increased the intracellular to extracellular K^+ (K_i/K_o) ratio, increased the intracellular HCO_3^- space, and slightly increased intracellular Na^+ and Cl^- brain spaces. This dose also completely blocked the extensor component of the MES, an anticonvulsant effect. However, it only slightly elevated the electroshock seizure threshold. In rats rendered tolerant to ACZ by an i.p. injection of 20 mg/kg at 48-hr intervals for four doses, the MES pattern was normal and the K_i/K_o ratio was the same as that of the controls, as was also the

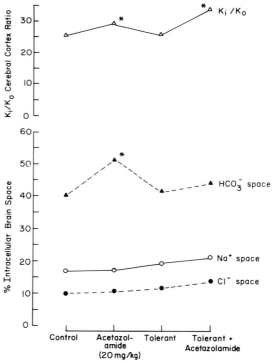

FIG. 5. Effects of acetazolamide on electrolyte and acid–base distribution in the cerebral cortex of control rats and rats made tolerant to the anti-MES effects of acetazolamide. *Upper ordinate:* Ratio (K_i/K_o) of intracellular (K_i) to extracellular (K_o) potassium in the cerebral cortex. *Lower ordinate:* Intracellular brain space (%) for Na^+, Cl^-, and HCO_3^-. The *abscissa* represents the various treatment schedules used: group 1, controls; group 2, acetazolamide given in a single dose of 20 mg/kg; group 3, the rats were rendered tolerant to acetazolamide by giving 20 mg/kg every 48 hr for four doses; group 4, tolerant rats given a single dose of acetazolamide at 20 mg/kg. See text for discussion. Data calculated from the results of Koch and Woodbury (15).

intracellular HCO_3^- space. The intracellular Na^+ and Cl^- spaces were increased above the values of both the controls and the ACZ-treated groups. When the ACZ-tolerant animals were given a single dose of ACZ at 20 mg/kg, K_i/K_o was significantly increased above the values of the three other groups. However, the intracellular HCO_3^- space in the cerebral cortex was only slightly increased. The intracellular Na^+ and Cl^- spaces were increased by ACZ given to the tolerant group, as compared with the tolerant group alone. It is evident from these studies that changes in K_i/K_o parallel those of the intracellular HCO_3^- space in the different treatment groups, whereas Na^+ and Cl^- intracellular space values change in parallel in the different groups. However, tolerant rats respond to a single dose of ACZ with a nonsignificant increase in HCO_3^- space but a marked increase in K_i/K_o that is greater than in the normal rats receiving ACZ. Tolerant rats receiving this dose of ACZ are still mostly tolerant to MES, but do show some response. Thus, the Na^+ and Cl^- responses to this drug are greater in the tolerant than in the nontolerant controls. It is evident that the ability of ACZ to abolish the extensor phase of the MES is directly related to the HCO_3^- concentration in the brain cells. Whether the increase in HCO_3^- space is in glial or neuronal cells is not known, but other data from our laboratory indicate that inhibition of CA in the glial cells by ACZ causes CO_2 to accumulate in glia and possibly in neurons. The accumulated CO_2 level in the brain on administration of ACZ is responsible for the anti-MES effects of this drug (47, see also ref. 14). It is apparent from these studies that CA plays an important role in anion transport in the brain, which in turn regulates brain excitability. The increase in the K_i/K_o ratio induced by ACZ in both groups of rats appears to be due to an ACZ-induced increase in Na^+,K^+-ATPase activity, which is more marked in the tolerant animals, and is probably a compensatory response to the inhibition of HCO_3^-–Cl^- exchange by ACZ.

To characterize further the role of glial CA in regulation of brain excitability, we measured the effects of ACZ on transmembrane potentials (E_m) of isolated astrocytes in culture. The results are shown in Figs. 6 and 7. ACZ at a dose of 1 $\times$ 10^{-7} M increased the membrane potential of the astrocytes by 17%, but at 1 $\times$ 10^{-6} M the cells were depolarized by 14%, at 1 $\times$ 10^{-5} M by 3%, at 1 $\times$ 10^{-4} M by 10%, and at 1 $\times$ 10^{-3} M, a dose that completely inhibits CA, by 55% (Fig. 6). If astrocytic cultures depolarized by 1 $\times$ 10^{-3} M ACZ are washed to remove the drug, the E_m returns to the control value (Fig. 7). Thus, the ACZ effect is reversible. It is evident that ACZ has marked effects on the electrical properties of glial cells that correlate with its inhibitory influence on glial CA and its effects on brain excitability. In low doses, this inhibitor hyperpolarizes glia, presumably by increasing total CO_2 concentrations in brain and increasing the K_i/K_o ratio. This results in an anti-MES effect and slight elevation of electroshock seizure threshold (14). The inhibition of CA at this concentration of ACZ probably involves only the cytosolic fraction which would cause CO_2 to accumulate in neurons. In high doses, ACZ depolarizes glial cells, probably by inhibiting both cytosolic and membrane-bound CA, the latter of

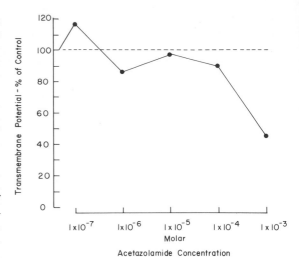

FIG. 6. Effects of various concentrations of acetazolamide on transmembrane potentials (E_m) of astrocytes isolated from the cerebral cortex of 3-day-old rats and grown in culture. *Ordinate* is transmembrane potential of acetazolamide-treated astrocytes as a percent of values obtained in untreated cultures of astrocytes. *Abscissa* is molar concentrations of acetazolamide. See text for discussion. (*Unpublished observations* of H. S. White, Y. C. Yen-Chow, S. Y. Chow, and D. M. Woodbury).

which, our evidence suggests, is involved in HCO_3^-–Cl^- exchange across glial membranes. This action blocks Cl^- and K^+ entry into glia and increases extracellular K^+ concentration. The result is an increase in excitability as measured by a decrease in electroshock seizure threshold (14). Thus, the effect of ACZ on astrocytes can explain its effects on brain excitability.

In Fig. 8 are summarized some of our experiments that indicate a role of HCO_3^--ATPase, a mitochondrial enzyme, in regulation of glial-cell membrane potential. The E_m of isolated astrocytes in culture is plotted along the abscissa and HCO_3^--ATPase activity along the ordinate. The points represent various treatments of the cell with phenytoin and/or dibutyryl cyclic adenosine monophosphate (see below). The correlation coefficient of the linear regression of these data is 0.966. Data from this laboratory suggest that HCO_3^--ATPase plays a role in anion transport in glia, as previously discussed. Thus, the anion transport mechanism appears to be an important determinant of membrane potential in glia, and alterations in its activity—i.e., with perchlorate, acetazolamide, etc.—can profoundly affect E_m and secondarily brain excitability, as discussed above.

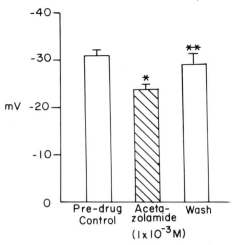

FIG. 7. Effect of acetazolamide (1×10^{-3} M) on transmembrane potential in millivolts (mV) (*ordinate*) of isolated astrocytes in culture as compared with untreated cells and with cells exposed to the same concentration of acetazolamide and then washed with the culture medium to remove the drug. See text for explanation. (*Unpublished observations* of H. S. White, Y. C. Yen-Chow, S. Y. Chow, and D. M. Woodbury).

EFFECTS OF CONVULSANT DRUGS ON GLIAL CELLS

Another approach to evaluating the role of glia and glial transport enzymes in seizures and seizure arrest mechanisms is to examine the effects of a convulsant agent, pentylenetetrazol (PTZ), on brain electrolytes and transport enzymes at various times after administration of threshold and maximal seizure doses at different stages of brain development. Some of the results of one such study performed by C. F. Chen and S. White in this laboratory are shown in Fig. 9. PTZ in doses of 45 and 90 mg/kg was injected into groups of rats 3, 15, and 23 days of age, and the animals were killed 10, 20, or 30 min later for removal of cerebellum, cerebral cortex, CSF, and plasma. The brain tissues were analyzed for protein, DNA, Na^+, K^+-ATPase, HCO^--ATPase, and CA activities and for electrolytes (Na^+, K^+, and Cl^-), and the CSF and plasma for electrolytes. In Fig. 9 are shown the effects of PTZ on CA activity (ordinate) in the cerebral cortex and cerebellum of rats at various times after injection (abscissa) and at different ages. The seizures with this drug generally occur within 3 to 5 min and usually end by 10 min in the case of threshold seizure doses (45 mg/kg) and by 20 to 30 min in the case of maximal seizure doses (90 mg/kg). Thus, at the 20- and 30-min intervals, the rats are in the postictal phase.

The curves show the events that are occurring during and following a seizure and therefore concern arrest mechanisms. The data demonstrate that PTZ induces time-dependent changes in CA activity in both cerebral cortex and cerebellum and that these effects are both dose- and age-dependent. Thus, in 3-day-old rats, cerebral cortical CA activity is increased at 10 but decreased at 20 and 30 min after injection of PTZ at 45 mg/kg, but decreased at all time periods after PTZ at 90 mg/kg, which causes intense seizure activity. In the cerebellum, PTZ at 45 mg/kg caused an increase in CA activity at all time periods, whereas at 90 mg/kg there was little change in the activity of this enzyme with time. At both dose levels, but much more markedly at 90 mg/kg, PTZ increased the ratio of cerebellar/cerebral cortical CA activity (cb/cc CA ratio) in 3-day-old rats. This appears to indicate enhanced inhibitory output by the cerebellum, a response that would ameliorate or arrest the seizures. However, since at this age CA activity (and consequently, glial cell activity) in both brain areas is extremely low and inhibitory

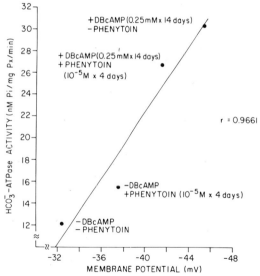

FIG. 8. Relationship between transmembrane potential (E_m) (mV) (*abscissa*) and HCO_3^--ATPase activity (nmol Pi/mg protein · min) (*ordinate*) in isolated cultures of astrocytes from cerebral cortex of 3-day-old rats. The various treatment schedules with phenytoin and/or dibutyl cyclic adenosine monophosphate (DBcAMP) used to alter enzyme activity and E_m are shown in the figure. The solid line is the linear regression fit of the data ($r = 0.9661$). P_i = inorganic phosphate; P_x = protein. See text for discussion. (*Unpublished observations* of H. S. White, Y. C. Yen-Chow, S.Y. Chow, and D. M. Woodbury).

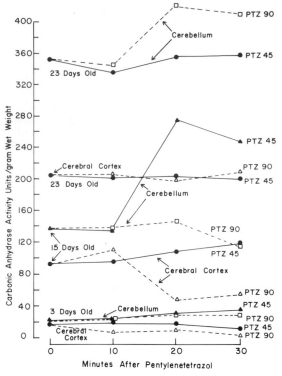

FIG. 9. Effects of pentylenetetrazol on cerebral cortical and cerebellar carbonic anhydrase activity at various times after administration of threshold convulsant (45 mg/kg) and maximal convulsant (90 mg/kg) doses to 3-, 15-, and 23-day-old rats. *Ordinate* is carbonic anhydrase activity (units/g wet brain weight) and *abscissa* is time (min) after injection of pentylenetetrazol (45 or 90 mg/kg). See text for explanation. (*Unpublished observations* of C. F. Chen, H. S. White, and D. M. Woodbury).

mechanisms in the cerebellum are poorly developed, the CA response to PTZ is small and the ability of the glial cell–CA system to protect against seizures is limited.

As the animals age, glial cells proliferate and CA activities in both the cerebral cortex and cerebellum progressively increase. Also, the differences between their two activities widen as the inhibitory mechanisms in the cerebellum mature. In 15-day-old rats, PTZ at 45 mg/kg increased CA activity in the cerebral cortex and even more markedly in the cerebellum at 20 and 30 min after injection. The minimal seizure activity occurring with this dose ceased during this period. Thus, the cerebellum is much more markedly stimulated by PTZ than is the cerebral cortex, such that the cb/cc CA ratio is markedly increased. At 90 mg/kg, after an initial slight increase in CA activity in the cerebral cortex at 10 min, PTZ markedly inhibited CA activity at

20 and 30 min post drug injection. In the cerebellum, CA activity slightly increased at 20 min and slightly decreased at 30 min after injection of PTZ at 90 mg/kg in 15-day-old rats. Thus, the cb/cc CA ratio was markedly increased by both doses of PTZ at 20 min after injection and was still elevated at 30 min, but the value was less than at 20, an indication that the glial CA response was returning to normal as the seizures dissipated. Thus, the glial arrest mechanisms, apparently initiated by the seizures per se, caused by PTZ, are powerfully brought into play as a result of increased neuronal activity. These PTZ-stimulated cerebellar inhibitory mechanisms appear to be CA-mediated active Cl⁻ transport processes, since the electrolyte data indicate that Cl^- concentrations in brain cells varied with CA activity. PTZ has been shown to act in part by inhibiting the postsynaptic effects of gamma-aminobutyric acid (GABA) (44). Since GABA receptors are present in cortex and to an even greater extent in cerebellum, the effect of PTZ on CA would appear to be mediated via its GABA effects. Thus, inhibition of the GABA effect would increase excitability of the cerebellum to a greater extent than in the cortex and the increase excitability would increase CA activity in glial cells of the cerebellum more than in the cortex. The effect of GABA to increase Cl^- permeability of the postsynaptic membrane depends on the establishment of active outward Cl^- transport across this membrane. Since Cl^- transport across glial cells, which involves CA, regulates interstitial Cl^- concentrations, it is possible that the PTZ-activated increase in CA as a result of the absence of a GABA effect may alter glial-cell Cl^- transport and indirectly regulate Cl^- transport across the postsynaptic membrane by maintaining homeostasis of Cl^- in the extracellular fluid. Thus, the protective effect of glia against seizures may be mediated through GABA. *In vitro,* both GABA and glycine, which increase Cl^- permeability of the postsynaptic membrane, inhibit CA activity in brain homogenates, and glycine blocks the effect of strychnine to increase CA activity. Thus, there appears to be a close relationship between CA, Cl^- transport, inhibitory neurotransmitters, and excitability.

In 23- as compared with 15-day-old rats, the CA activity in both the cerebellum and cerebral cortex increased, but the change was much more marked in the former. PTZ at 45 mg/kg had little stimulatory effect in 23-day-old rats on CA activity in both the cerebral cortex and the cerebellum. However, PTZ at 90 mg/kg, instead of inhibiting cerebral cortical activity, as it did at

15 days, had no effect on this tissue at 23 days; it actually enhanced CA activity in the cerebellum at 20 and 30 min after PTZ, instead of having little effect as it did at 15 days. Thus, higher doses of PTZ are necessary to produce the same CA responses in older as compared with younger animals, apparently because the glial cells are more mature and contain a higher activity of CA, which is actively responding to the seizure activity at a maximum rate and cannot therefore be much further enhanced by PTZ even at 90 mg/kg.

It is evident from these data that the cerebellar–cerebral cortical glial cell CA mechanism plays an important role in ameliorating seizure activity. Our previous studies (49) have shown that the increased CA response noted in glial cells and the increased polyspike activity in the electrocorticogram observed in rats with cobalt-induced focal epilepsy are decreased with age as the CA activity in the brain increases. These results also show that the ability to respond is progressively decreased as the rats age, because CA activity is maximal and cannot therefore be further stimulated to provide an additional protective response against seizures than is already present.

Similar seizure-protective adaptive changes to those occurring with CA also occur with Na^+,K^+-ATPase, which regulates Na^+–K^+ transport, and with HCO_3^--ATPase, which is involved in anion transport, following administration of PTZ at 45 and 90 mg/kg in 3-, 15-, and 23-day-old rats. Thus, neuronal depolarization products such as CO_2, H^+, K^+, and NH_3 cause marked changes in the glial enzymes that handle these products, such as to ameliorate their effects to increase excitability and to maintain the depolarized state. These responses play a large role in the various processes involved in seizure arrest.

EFFECTS OF PHENYTOIN ON GLIAL CELLS

One of the possible mechanisms by which anticonvulsant drugs can prevent or ameliorate seizures is to enhance the glial-cell protective mechanisms discussed above. Effects of these drugs can be directly on glial cells or indirectly through depolarization of neurons. Experiments in this laboratory depicted in Figs. 10 to 15 demonstrate that phenytoin (PHT) does indeed act on glial cells, both directly and indirectly. Evidence suggesting that PHT stimulates glial cells is provided by the observations shown in Fig. 10 that the prolonged administration (20 mg/kg

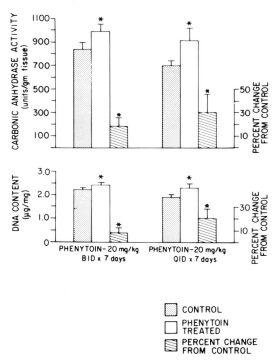

FIG. 10. Effect of chronic (20 mg/kg, i.p. bid and qid for 7 days) PHT treatment on cerebral cortical carbonic (CA) anhydrase activity **(top)** and DNA content **(bottom)** of the adult rat. All values are expressed as the mean + SEM. The absolute activity of CA (units/g tissue) and DNA content (μg/mg tissue) for vehicle-treated controls and PHT-treated animals is represented by the *stippled* (controls) and *open* (PHT-treated) *bars. Hatched bars* represent the percent change from control following PHT treatment. Asterisk, $p < 0.05$. (From ref. 41, with permission.)

bid for 7 days) of PHT increases both the DNA content and the carbonic anhydrase activity of the cerebral cortex (41).

In Fig. 11 are shown the effects of PHT at 20 mg/kg in single and multiple doses (two times or four times a day for 7 days) in 3-day-old and adult rats on Na^+ and K^+ concentrations and on Na^+,K^+-ATPase activity.

Three-day-old rats are an excellent model for studying *in vivo* the effects of a drug on neurons, since the brain at this age is comprised primarily of neurons and essentially no functional glial cells. The marked inhibition of Na^+,K^+-ATPase and the subsequent increase in total Na^+ and decrease in total K^+ (Fig. 11) after an acute dose of PHT given at this age reflect a direct action on neurons. An increase in total Na^+ of the magnitude shown in this figure, accompanied by a decrease in total K^+, would be expected to produce a substantial depolarization of the neuronal membrane. Because both anatomical and bio-

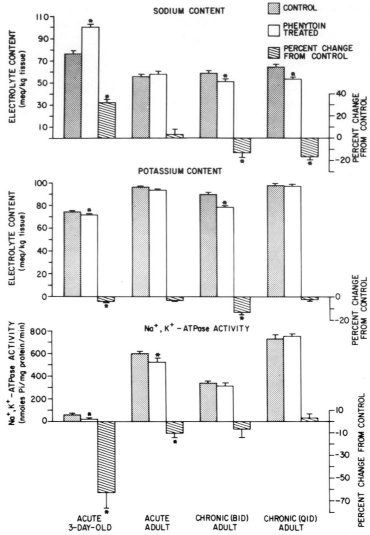

FIG. 11. Effect of acute (2 hr) and chronic (bid and qid for 7 days) PHT treatment (20 mg/kg, i.p.) on neonatal and adult rat cerebral cortical Na$^+$ and K$^+$ content and Na$^+$,K$^+$-ATPase activity. All values are expressed as the mean + SEM. The total cerebral cortical Na$^+$ and K$^+$ content and Na$^+$,K$^+$-ATPase activity of vehicle-treated controls and PHT-treated animals is represented by the *stippled* (controls) and *open* (PHT-treated) *bars*. *Hatched bars* represent the percent change from control following PHT treatment. Asterisk, $p < 0.05$. (From ref. 41, with permission.)

chemical evidence suggest that cerebral and cerebellar inhibitory circuits are poorly developed at this age, depolarization of neurons would lead not to protection against, but enhancement of, seizure activity. On the other hand, in adult animals PHT possesses anticonvulsant activity by virtue of its ability to depolarize (stimulate) the now predominating inhibitory pathways. These data provide not only an explanation of PHT's excitatory effects that have been observed in neonatal animals (36) and adult animals (9) and human patients (7,16,17,21,27,28,35) with high

doses but, when extrapolated to adults, provide new information pertaining to its often controversial mechanism of action. (For discussion, see ref. 41.)

PHT has been previously demonstrated to increase epithelial cell (toad bladder, frog skin, choroid plexus, and glial cells) Na$^+$ and K$^+$ transport (1,2,12,26,39,40) and thus decrease Na^+_i and increase K^+_i. Since this effect is opposite that described above for neurons, it might be anticipated that the effect of PHT, when it is administered to adult rats whose neuropil is comprised of both functional neurons and glia, would be lessened or even completely attenuated. Although, as depicted in Fig. 11, the acute administration of PHT to adult rats was found to inhibit Na$^+$,K$^+$-ATPase, increase total Na$^+$, and decrease total K$^+$, the magnitude of its effect was much less than that observed in 3-day-old animals. PHT's effect on Na$^+$,K$^+$ ATPase activity and total electrolyte content was further attenuated with prolonged administration (twice daily and four times a day treatment for 7 days). Both of these dosing regimens significantly reduced the total Na$^+$ content of the central nervous system (CNS) and increased the whole homogenate Na$^+$,K$^+$-ATPase activity to control levels. Although a decrease in total Na$^+$ without any change in enzyme activity would suggest that PHT is decreasing membrane permeability to Na$^+$ by blocking Na$^+$ channels, this is unlikely in the brain, since radioactive sodium turnover has been previously reported to be increased rather than decreased, a finding that Na$^+$ transport or efflux was increased (43). Thus, in adult rats, it would appear that chronic PHT enhances the activity or increases the synthesis of Na$^+$,K$^+$-ATPase in glial cells, and this increased activity masks the continuing inhibition of this enzyme in the neurons. That PHT is

differentially affecting neuronal and glial cells is supported by enzyme studies conducted on subcellular fractions obtained from the cerebral cortex of rats treated chronically four times a day for 7 days and shown in Fig. 12. Although there was no change in whole homogenate or microsomal Na$^+$,K$^+$-ATPase activity, a significant increase in myelin (a glial product) ATPase activity occurred. In contrast, there was a marked decrease in synaptosomal (neuronal fraction) enzyme activity. From these studies, it is apparent that a majority of the discrepancies in the literature with regard to the effects of phenytoin on Na$^+$,K$^+$-ATPase activity in adults (see ref. 45 for review) can be explained by a paucity of *in vivo* studies on subcellular fractions of brain during ontogenesis of the nervous system and of *in vitro* studies on isolated glia.

PHT's ability to enhance glial cell Na$^+$,K$^+$-ATPase activity could result either from a direct effect on the glial enzyme or indirectly through its action to depolarize neuronal cells. To determine whether PHT directly affects glial cell Na$^+$,K$^+$-ATPase, we have studied its effects on this enzyme in primary glial cell cultures (42). The results are shown in Fig. 13. The Na$^+$,K$^+$-ATPase activity of cultured cells was measured in the presence of increasing K^+_o concentration

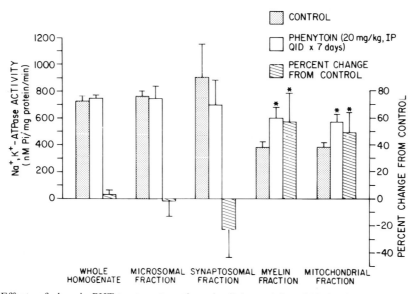

FIG. 12. Effects of chronic PHT treatment on the subcellular activity of Na$^+$,K$^+$-ATPase. Adult male rats were administered PHT (20 mg/kg, i.p.) four times a day for 7 days. At 2 hr after the last dose, animals were sacrificed and perfused with 0.32 M sucrose, and the cerebral cortex was removed. Subcellular fractions obtained by sucrose density centrifugations were assayed for Na$^+$,K$^+$-ATPase activity according to the procedures outlined in ref. 41. All values are expressed as the mean + SEM. Subcellular Na$^+$,K$^+$-ATPase activity of the vehicle-treated controls and PHT-treated animals is represented by the *stippled* (controls) and *open* (PHT-treated) *bars*, respectively. *Hatched bars* represent the percent change from control following PHT treatment. Asterisk, p < 0.05. (From ref. 41, with permission.)

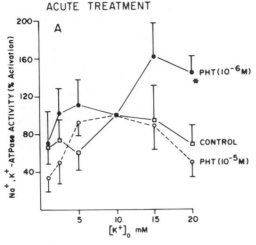

ACUTE TREATMENT

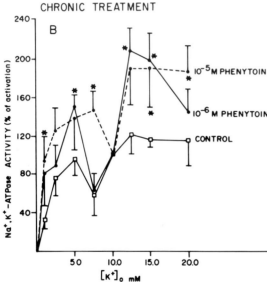

CHRONIC TREATMENT

FIG. 13. Influence of K^+ on the Na^+,K^+-ATPase activity of 22- to 26-day glial cultures acutely **(A)** and chronically **(B)** exposed to micromolar concentrations of PHT. Data are expressed in percent of activation of activities measured in the presence of 10 mM K^+ (considered 100%). Asterisk, $p < 0.05$ when compared to vehicle-treated controls. (From ref. 42, with permission.)

following acute and chronic treatment with PHT. The results are expressed as a percentage of the enzyme activity obtained at a K^+_o of 10 mM. Following acute exposure to 10^{-6} M PHT (Fig. 13A), a significant activation of Na^+,K^+-ATPase was observed at 20 mM K^+_o, but at all other K^+_o concentrations, the activation pattern of control and PHT-treated cells was not statistically different. However, it is of interest to point out that in the presence of 10^{-6} M PHT, the resulting K^+_o activation curve was defined

by two distinct peaks in enzyme activity. These peaks at 5 and 15 mM K^+_o were markedly higher than were the corresponding peaks of control cells. In sharp contrast, the K^+_o activation pattern of cells acutely exposed to 10^{-5} M PHT was characterized by one broad peak in enzyme activity that extended over a wide range of K^+_o concentrations (5–15 mM).

The Na^+,K^+-ATPase activity of cultured glial cells was also measured in the presence of increasing K^+_o following chronic exposure to similar concentrations of PHT for 4 days (Fig. 13B). In both control and treated cells, activation curves were characterized by two peaks in enzyme activity. The percent of enzyme activated at each K^+_o concentration examined was higher in cells chronically exposed to PHT as compared to control cells.

These results indicate that glial cultures chronically treated with PHT have increased their capacity to control by an active process the elevated K^+_o. As illustrated in Fig. 13B, the efficiency of glial Na^+,K^+-ATPase was substantially enhanced over a wide-range of K^+_o. The enhanced efficiency of PHT-treated cells at low K^+_o would presumably prevent extracellular fluid (ECF) K^+ concentrations from rising much above normal levels during excessive neuronal firing. In addition, these cells are also capable of enhanced regulation at high K^+_o in the event that levels should exceed the normal physiological range. Mechanistically, these results suggest that through an enhancement of glial regulatory processes, PHT may prevent the transition of interictal discharges to ictal episodes, an event that as suggested by Dichter et al. (3) results from elevated K^+_o. Furthermore, these results are consistent with the clinical ability of PHT to prevent the spread (ictal transition) from a seizure focus, but not the initiation process (interictal discharge). Because focal discharge is not prevented, it might be further reasoned that PHT is only able to enhance K^+_o regulation in perifocal areas and not able to influence the regulatory ability of glial cells in the primary focus.

Results of electrophysiological studies also support the hypothesis that PHT enhances regulation of K^+_o. Figure 14 clearly demonstrates that for any given level of K^+_o, cells chronically exposed to PHT are likely to be less depolarized than controls. These data, therefore, fit with the expectation that protected tissues are less depolarized than susceptible ones for an equivalent concentration of K^+_o (32). During normal physiological activity, ECF K^+ is maintained between 3 and 4 mM (25); however, it can rise as high as 12 mM during seizures and has been ob-

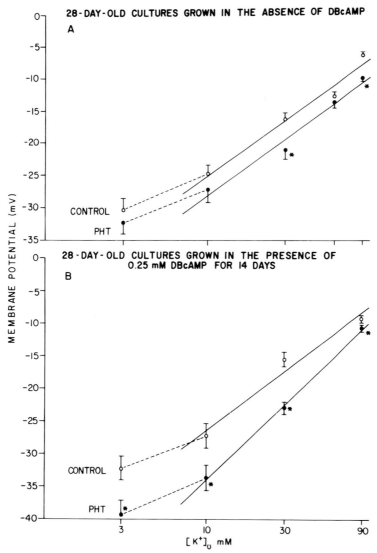

FIG. 14. Effect of chronic PHT treatment on the K^+_o depolarization of 28-day-old glial cells grown in the **(A)** absence and **(B)** presence of DBcAMP. Culture medium was replaced with HEPES buffered medium containing varying K^+ concentrations. Na^+ concentration of the buffer was reciprocally changed as the K^+_o was increased in order to maintain osmolality. The number of cells impaled at each K^+_o concentration ranged between 23 and 41. Each value shown is the mean ± SEM. Asterisk, $p < 0.05$ when compared to vehicle treated-controls. (From ref. 42, with permission.)

served to rise even higher (greater than 20 mM) during spreading depression (5,33,34,37). In light of the increasing evidence suggesting that increases in K^+_o could affect neuronal firing, Pollen and Trachtenberg (24) in 1970 proposed that epilepsy could be the result of inadequate spatial buffering of K^+_o by glial cells. Numerous studies have suggested that the subsequent removal of elevated K^+_o is via an active accumulation into adjacent astrocytes. However, following the failure of several electrophysiological

studies to demonstrate any difference in baseline K^+_o between normal and epileptogenic brains (19,22), it was concluded that an impairment of glial buffering was an unlikely cause of paroxymal depolarization shifts. Nevertheless, as pointed out by Lewis et al (18), the highly localized and transient nature of relatively large K^+_o electrodes could miss transient and localized increases in K^+_o induced by bursts of high frequency firing associated with alumina gel foci (18). These authors have also demonstrated, that within gliotic scars induced by local application of alumina gel, clearance of K^+_o was slowed despite no observable difference in the base-line potassium level of epileptogenic and normal brain areas. The insensitivity of the K^+ electrode in detecting fine kinetic characteristics of cation movement has been further discussed by Grisar et al. (8). This later report has examined in some detail the kinetic characteristics of Na^+,K^+-ATPase of synaptosomal and glial fractions isolated from normal and focal areas of epileptogenic brains. Results reported therein demonstrate that a significant defect in the ability of glial cells isolated from focal lesions to regulate elevated K^+_o does exist. In addition, glial cells isolated from brain areas surrounding the lesion appeared to have an increased ability to regulate K^+_o during periods of epileptiform discharges. The demonstration that exogenously administered compounds (i.e., PHT) are capable of enhancing the ability of the CNS to regulate not only K^+_o (Figs. 13B and 14) but also other neuroactive compounds through an interaction with glial cells provides important insight into the etiology and the arrest of seizures.

Acutely, concentrations of PHT greater than 10^{-5} M appeared to decrease the efficiency of glial Na^+,K^+-ATPase. One possible explanation for this apparent discrepancy is that PHT increases membrane permeability to Na^+ in glial cells. In so doing, Na^+_i increases and subsequently depolarizes the cell membrane. It has been demonstrated previously that PHT is capable of increasing the short-circuit current (SCC) across frog skin and toad bladder (39,40). In these models, the SCC is a direct measure of active Na^+ transport, and the increase in SCC is the result of enhanced permeability of mucosal-side membrane to Na^+ (for discussion see ref. 50). The link between glial cells, frog skin, and toad bladder is that all three are epithelial cells and would therefore be expected to respond to PHT in a similar manner. Thus, as the Na^+ concentration increases with increasing PHT concentrations, the cell membrane is depolarized. As shown in Fig. 15, PHT produced a marked membrane depolarization following acute exposure of cultured glial cells to concentrations exceeding 10^{-5} M. This observation provides one explanation for the excitatory effects often observed clincially when plasma PHT concentrations become too high. For example, in the presence of depolarizing concentrations of PHT, glial cells may have a reduced ability to regulate K^+_o. The resultant increase in K^+_o concentrations leads to a nonspecific depolarization of all surrounding neurons (inhibitory and exci-

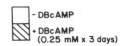

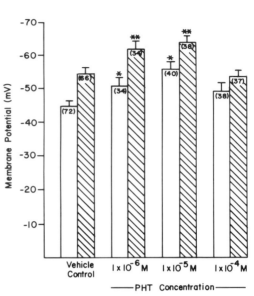

FIG. 15. Effect of acute PHT on the membrane potential of 17-day-old cultured glial cells grown in the absence and presence of DBcAMP. Cells plated on collagen-coated culture dishes were exposed to various concentrations of PHT for 1 hr prior to E_m measurement. *Open bars* represent cells grown in the absence of DBcAMP, and *hatched bars* represent cells grown in the presence of 0.25 mM DBcAMP for 3 days. Number in parenthesis represents the number of individual cells impaled at each point. Asterisk, $p < 0.05$ when compared to open-bar control. Double asterisk, $p < 0.05$ when compared to hatched-bar control. (From ref. 42, with permission.)

tatory) and a possible reduction in seizure control.

ACKNOWLEDGMENTS

The authors wish to thank Ms. Toni Gillett for typing this manuscript. Unpublished observations reported in this chapter were obtained by support from grant NS-15767 from the National Institute of Neurological and Communicative Disorders and Stroke (NINCDS). Dixon M. Woodbury was the recipient of a Research Career Award (5-K6-NB-13838) from NINCDS, National Institutes of Health, Bethesda, Maryland.

REFERENCES

1. Carroll, P. T., and Pratley, J. N. (1970): The effects of diphenylhydantoin on sodium transport in frog skin. *Comp. Gen. Pharmacol.* 1:365.

2. DeSousa, R. C., and Grosso, A. (1976): Effects of diphenylhydantoin on transport processes in frog skin (*Rana ridibunda*). *Experientia*, 29: 1097–1098.

3. Dichter, M. A., Herman, C. J., and Selser, M. (1972): Silent cells during interictal discharges and seizures in hippocampal penicillin foci. Evidence for the role of extracellular K^+ in the transition from the interictal state to seizures. *Brain Res.* 48:173–183.

4. Dow, R. C. (1965): Extrinsic regulatory mechanisms of seizure activity. *Epilepsia*, 6:122–140.

5. Futamachi, K. J., Mutani, R., and Prince, D. A. (1974): Potassium activity in rabbit cortex. *Brain Res.*, 75:5–25.

6. Gill, T. H., Young, O. M., and Tower, D. B. (1974): The uptake of ^{36}Cl into astrocytes in tissue culture by a potassium-dependent, saturable process. *J. Neurochem.*, 23:1011–1018.

7. Glaser, G. H. (1972): Diphenylhydantoin: toxicity. In: *Antiepileptic Drugs*, edited by D. M. Woodbury, J. K. Penry, and R. P. Schmidt, pp. 219–226. Raven Press, New York.

8. Grisar T., Franck, G., and Delgado-Escueta, A. V. (1983): Glial contribution to seizures: K^+ activation of (Na^+, K^+)-ATPase in bulk isolated glial cells and synaptosomes of epileptogenic cortex. *Brain Res.*, 261:75–84.

9. Gruber C. M., Haury V. G., and Drake, M. E. (1940): The toxic actions of sodium diphenylhydantoin (Dilantin) when injected intraperitoneally and intravenously in experimental animals. *J. Pharmacol. Exp. Ther.* 68:433–436.

10. Henn, F. A., Haljamae, H., and Hamburger, A. (1972): Glial cell function: Active control of extracellular K^+ concentration. *Brain Res.* 43:437–443.

11. Hutton, J. R., Frost, J. D., and Foster, J. (1972): The influence of the cerebellum in cat penicillin epilepsy. *Epilepsia*, 13:401–408.

12. Johanson, C., and Smith, Q. R. (1977): Phenytoin-induced stimulation of the Na–K pump in the choroid plexus-cerebrospinal fluid system. *Soc. Neurosci.*, 3:316(#102).

13. Kimelberg, H. K., and Bourke, R. S. (1980): Anion transport in the nervous system. In: *Handbook of Neurochemistry, 2nd ed., Vol. 1*, edited by A. Lajtha, pp. 31–67. Plenum Press, New York.

14. Koch, A. L., and Woodbury, D. M. (1958): Effects of carbonic anhydrase inhibition on brain excitability. *J. Pharmacol. Exp. Ther.*, 122:335–342.

15. Koch, A., and Woodbury, D. M. (1960): Carbonic anhydrase inhibition and brain electrolyte composition. *Am. J. Physiol.*, 198:434–440.

16. Lascelles, P. T., Kocen, R. S., and Reynolds E. H. (1970): The distribution of plasma phenytoin levels in epileptic patients. *J. Neurol. Neuorosurg. Psychiatry*, 33.501–505.

17. Levy, L. L., and Fenichel, G. M. (1965): Diphenylhydantoin activated seizures. *Neurology*, 15:716–722.

18. Lewis, D. V., Mutsuga, N., Schuette, W. H., and Van Buren, J. (1977): Potassium clearance and reactive gliosis in the alumina gel lesion. *Epilepsia*, 18(4):499–506.

19. Lux, H. D. (1974): The kinetics of extracellular potassium: Relation to epileptogenesis. *Epilepsia*, 15:375–393.

20. Merlis, J. (1974): Neurophysiological aspects of epilepsy. In: *Epilepsy, Proceedings of the Hans Berger Centenary Symposium*, edited by P. Harris and C. Mawdsley, pp. 5–19. Churchill Livingstone, Edinburgh.

21. Patel, H., and Crichton, J. V. (1968): The neurologic hazards of diphenylhydantoin in childhood. *J. Pediat.*, 73:676–684.

22. Pedley, T. A., Fisher, R. S., Futamachi, K. J., and Prince, D. A. (1976): Regulation of extracellular potassium concentration in epileptogenesis. *Fed. Proc.*, 35(6):1254–1259.

23. Pentreath, V. W. (1982): Potassium signaling of metabolic interactions between neurons and glial cells. *Trends Neurosci.*, 5:339–345.

24. Pollen, D. A., and Trachtenberg, M. C. (1970): Neuroglia: Gliosis and focal epilepsy. *Science*, 167:1252–1253.

25. Prince, D. A., Pedley, T. A., and Ransom, B. R. (1978): Fluctuations in ion concentrations during excitation and seizures. In: *Dynamic Properties of Glial Cells*, edited by E. Schoffeniels, G. Franck, L. Hertz, and D. B. Tower, pp. 281–303. Pergamon Press, Oxford.

26. Riddle, T. G., Mandel, L. J., and Goldner, M. M. (1975): Dilantin-calcium interaction and active Na transport in frog skin. *Eur. J. Pharmacol.* 33:189–192.

27. Roseman, E. (1961): Dilantin toxicity. A clinical and electroencephalographic study. *Neurology*, 11:912–921.

28. Schreiner, G. E. (1958): The role of hemodialysis (artificial kidney) in acute poisoning. *Arch. Intern. Med.*, 102:896–913.

29. Schrier, B. K., and Thomson, E. J. (1974): On the role of glial cells in the mammalian nervous system. Uptake, excretion and metabolism of putative neurotransmitters by cultured glial tumor cells. *J. Biol. Chem.*, 249:1769.

30. Smith, Q. R., Johanson, C. E., and Woodbury, D. M. (1981): Uptake of ^{36}Cl and ^{22}Na by the brain-cerebrospinal fluid system: Comparison of the permeability of the blood-brain and blood cerebrospinal fluid barriers. *J. Neurochem.*, 37:117–124.

31. Smith, Q. R., Woodbury, D. M., and Johanson, C. E. (1982): Kinetic analysis of ^{36}Cl, ^{22}Na and ^3H-mannitol uptake into the *in vivo* choroid plexus–cerebrospinal fluid–brain system: Ontogeny of the blood–brain and blood-CSF barriers. *Dev. Brain Res.*, 3:181–198.

32. Somjen, G. G. (1975): Electrophysiology of neuroglia. *Annu. Rev. Physiol.*, 37:163–190.

33. Somjen, G. G. (1979): Extracellular potassium ion in the mammalian central nervous system. *Annu. Rev. Physiol.*, 41:159–177.

34. Somjen, G. G., Rosenthal, M., Cordingley, G., Lamanna, J., and Lothman, E. (1976): Potassium, neuroglia and oxidative metabolism in central gray matter. *Fed. Proc.*, 35:1266–1271.

35. Troupin, A. S., and Ojemann, L. M. (1975): Paradoxical intoxication—A complication of anticonvulsant administration. *Epilepsia*, 16:753–758.

36. Vernadakis, A., and Woodbury, D. M. (1969): The developing animal as a model. *Epilepsia,* 10:163–178.

37. Viskocil, F., Kriz, N., and Bures, J. (1972): Potassium selective microelectrodes used for measuring the extracellular brain potassium during spreading depression and anoxic depolarization in rats. *Brain Res.,* 39:255–259.

38. Ward, J. R., and Call, L. S. (1949): Changes in blood chemistry in rats following electrically-induced seizures. *Proc. Soc. Exp. Biol. Med.,* 70:381–382.

39. Watson, E. L., and Woodbury, D. M. (1972): Effects of diphenylhydantoin on active sodium transport in frog skin. *J. Pharmacol. Exp. Ther.,* 180:767–776.

40. Watson, E. L., and Woodbury, D. M. (1973): Effects of diphenylhydantoin on electrolyte transport in various tissues. In: *Chemical Modulation of Brain Function,* edited by H. C. Sabelli, pp. 187–188. Raven Press, New York.

41. White, H. S., Chen, C. F., Kemp, J. W., and Woodbury, D. M. (1985): Effects of acute and chronic phenytoin on the electrolyte content and the activities of Na^+,K^+,Ca^{++},Mg^{++}-, HCO_3^--ATPases and carbonic anhydrase of neonatal and adult rat cerebral cortex. *Epilepsia,* 26(1):43–57.

42. White, H. S., Yen-Chow, Y. C., Chow, S. Y., Kemp, J. W., and Woodbury, D. M. (1985): Effects of phenytoin on primary glial cell cultures. *Epilepsia,* 26(1):58–68.

43. Woodbury, D. M. (1955): Effects of diphenylhydantoin on electrolytes and radiosodium turnover in brain and other tissues of normal, hyponatremic and postictal rats. *J. Pharmacol. Exp. Ther.,* 115:74–95.

44. Woodbury, D. M. (1980): Convulsant drugs: Mechanisms of action. *Adv. Neurol.,* 27:249–303.

45. Woodbury, D. M. (1980): Antiepileptic drugs. Phenytoin: Proposed mechanisms of anticonvulsant action. In: *Antiepileptic Drugs: Mechanisms of Action,* edited by G. C. Glaser, J. K. Penry, and D. M. Woodbury, pp. 447–471. Raven Press, New York.

46. Woodbury, D. M., Engstrom, F. L., White, H. S., Chen, C. F., Kemp, J. W., and Chow, S. Y. (1984): Ionic and acid-base regulation of neurons and glial during seizures. *Ann. Neurol.* 16 (Suppl.):S135–S144.

47. Woodbury, D. M., and Karler, R. (1960): Role of carbon dioxide in the nervous system. *Anesthesiology,* 21:686–703.

48. Woodbury, D. M., and Kemp, J. W. (1977): Basic mechanisms of seizures: Neurophysiological and biochemical etiology. In: *Psychopathology and Brain Dysfunction,* edited by C. Shagass, S. Gershon, and A. J. Friedhof, pp. 149–182. Raven Press, New York.

49. Woodbury, D. M., and Kemp, J. W. (1979): Initiation, propagation and arrest of seizures. In: *Pathophysiology of Cerebral Energy Metabolism,* edited by B. B. Mrsulja, Lj. M. Rakic, I. Klatzo, and M. Spatz, pp. 313–351. Plenum, New York.

50. Woodbury, D. M., Kemp, J. W., and Chow, S. Y. (1983): Mechanism of action of antiepileptic drugs. In: *Epilepsy,* edited by A. A. Ward, J. K. Penry and D. Purpura, pp. 179–223. Raven Press, New York.

51. Woodbury, D. M., Rollins, L. T., Henrie, J. R., Jones, J. C., and Sato, T. (1956): Effects of carbon dioxide and oxygen on properties of experimental seizures in mice. *Am. J. Physiol.* 184:202–208.

52. Woodward, D. L., Reed, D. J., and Woodbury, D. M. (1967): The extracellular space of rat cerebral cortex. *Am. J. Physiol.,* 212:367–370.

NOTE ADDED IN PROOF

TABLE 1. *Inhibition of ^{36}Cl uptake into astrocytes*

Inhibitor (10 mM)	5–8 mM K^+ control at 10 min (%)
Acetazolamide	$41 \cdot 2$ ($66 \cdot 2$)[a]
Perchlorate	$34 \cdot 1$
Thiocyanate	$28 \cdot 2$
Bromide	$25 \cdot 9$
Iodide	$41 \cdot 2$
2,4-Dinitrophenol	$12 \cdot 2$
Fluoride	$11 \cdot 4$

[a] Value for 5 mM acetazolamide given in parentheses. Cultured cells on small glass cover slips were incubated at 37°C for 10 min in media containing 144 mM Cl^- plus ^{36}Cl (2×10^6 cpm/ml), 5–8 mM K^+ and 142 mM Na^+, in the presence of [^3H]inulin as a measure of extracellular fluid (from ref. 6 with permission).

Advances in Neurology, Vol. 44, edited by
A. V. Delgado-Escueta, A. A. Ward, Jr.,
D. M. Woodbury, and R. J. Porter.
Raven Press, New York © 1986.

36

Anticonvulsant Drugs: Mechanisms of Action

Robert L. Macdonald and Michael J. McLean

Department of Neurology, University of Michigan Medical Center, Ann Arbor, Michigan 48109

SUMMARY   A variety of the anticonvulsant drugs, including carbamazepine, phenytoin, primidone, phenobarbital, clonazepam, valproic acid, and ethosuximide, are available for use in the treatment of patients with seizure disorders. These anticonvulsants vary in their efficacy against experimental seizures in animals and against seizures in humans. The mechanistic basis for this variability in anticonvulsant drug action remains uncertain, but numerous mechanisms of action have been proposed. We have used mouse neurons in primary dissociated cell culture to study the action of these anticonvulsant drugs on several aspects of membrane excitability and synaptic transmission. We have proposed that the anticonvulsant drugs can be classified according to their actions on sustained high frequency repetitive firing (SRF) of action potentials and on postsynaptic gamma-aminobutyric acid (GABA) responses. Phenytoin and carbamazepine were both effective against SRF but did not modify postsynaptic GABA responses at therapeutically relevant concentrations. Phenobarbital, benzodiazepines, and valproic acid modified both SRF and postsynaptic GABA responses. Ethosuximide had no effect on SRF or GABAergic mechanisms. Based on these results, we have proposed that blockade of SRF may underlie the action of phenytoin, carbamazepine, phenobarbital, valproic acid, and benzodiazepines against generalized tonic–clonic seizures in humans and maximal electroshock seizures in animals. Enhancement of GABAergic synaptic transmission may underlie efficacy of benzodiazepines and valproic acid drugs against generalized absence seizures in humans and pentylenetetrazol-induced seizures in experimental animals. The mechanism of action of ethosuximide against generalized absence seizures in humans and pentylenetetrazol-induced seizures in experimental animals may be by a third, as yet unknown, mechanism.

Administration of anticonvulsant drugs has been and will continue to be the primary method of therapy for the epilepsies. Since initial choice of anticonvulsant drug is usually governed by seizure diagnosis, anticonvulsant drugs are generally classified according to their effectiveness against specific seizure types. Thus, relatively selective drugs including phenytoin and carbamazepine are used to treat patients with generalized tonic–clonic or partial seizures, and etho-suximide and valproic acid are used to treat patients with generalized absence seizures (Table 1).

From an experimental point of view, it has been useful to identify the effectiveness of anticonvulsant drugs against seizures in experimental animals. The most discriminating seizure tests have been the maximal electroshock (MES) seizure test and pentylenetetrazol (PTZ) seizure threshold test (76,177). Anticonvulsants

TABLE 1. *Relative efficacy of anticonvulsant drugs*

Anticonvulsant	GTC[a]	GA[b]	MES ED_{50}[c]	PTZ ED_{50}[c]
Phenytoin	+	−	9.5	N.A.
Carbamazepine	+	−	8.8	N.A.
Primidone	+	−	12.1	N.A.
Phenobarbital	+	−	13.6	17.0
Valproic acid	+	+	271.7	148.6
Clonazepam	+/−	+	86.6	0.009
Ethosuximide	−	+	N.A.[d]	130.4

[a] Efficacy against generalized tonic–clonic seizures.
[b] Efficacy against generalized absence seizures.
[c] Mean effective dose (mg/kg, i.p., mice) in the maximal electroshock (MES) seizure and pentylenetetrazol (PTZ) seizure tests. Data from Krall et al. (76), except for phenobarbital and primidone (17).
[d] N.A., not active.

effective at nontoxic doses in abolishing the tonic hind-limb response in the MES seizure test are generally effective against generalized tonic–clonic seizures, while those effective at nontoxic doses in the PTZ seizure threshold test are generally effective against generalized absence seizures (Table 1). Using this approach, anticonvulsant drugs can be classified as those effective in MES but not PTZ seizures (phenytoin, carbamazepine, and primidone), those with mixed effectiveness (phenobarbital, valproic acid, and clonazepam), and those that are only effective against PTZ seizures (ethosuximide).

The potentially most useful classification of anticonvulsant drugs is one based on anticonvulsant mechanisms of action. Unfortunately, it has not been possible to develop such a classification, since the specific mechanisms of action of the major anticonvulsant drugs remain uncertain. In this chapter, the actions of the most commonly used anticonvulsant drugs, including phenytoin, carbamazepine, primidone, phenobarbital, clonazepam, valproic acid, and ethosuximide, will be reviewed. For each of these drugs, multiple biochemical and physiological actions have been described. Determination of which of these actions are clinically relevant as anticonvulsant actions requires satisfaction of at least two specific criteria: (a) the drug must act at clinically relevant concentrations and (b) the drug action must be directly demonstrated to be anticonvulsant. Of the two criteria, only the first is reasonably demonstrable at the present time. To satisfy the first criterion, it must be demonstrated that a drug action occurs at free serum concentrations, since it is the unbound drug that equilibrates with cerebrospinal fluid and central nervous system extracellular space. Thus, emphasis will be placed on those anticonvulsant actions produced at therapeutic free serum concentrations.

PHENYTOIN

Phenytoin (Dilantin®; 5,5-diphenylhydantoin) is essentially the only hydantoin in clinical use at the present time. Using animal seizure models, Merritt and Putnam (107) identified phenytoin as an anticonvulsant drug with reduced sedative–hypnotic actions. Phenytoin is effective in generalized tonic–clonic seizures and in all types of partial seizures (see ref. 33). Phenytoin is administered to adults at 5 to 7 mg/kg · day to achieve therapeutic serum concentrations of 10 to 20 μg/ml (40–80 μM). However, since phenytoin is about 90% protein bound, free serum and cerebrospinal fluid phenytoin concentrations are only 1 to 2 μg/ml (99,156,162). Phenytoin is effective against MES seizures but is ineffective against PTZ seizures (49,76,178).

Despite widespread use, the mechanism of anticonvulsant action of phenytoin has remained uncertain. Phenytoin has been shown to have multiple actions (for review, see ref. 195), including (a) *nonsynaptic* actions to reduce sodium conductance, enhance active sodium extrusion, block repetitive firing, and reduce posttetanic potentiation, (b) *postsynaptic* actions to enhance GABA-mediated inhibition and reduce excitatory synaptic transmission, and (c) *presynaptic* actions to reduce calcium entry and to block release of neurotransmitter. In the sections below, these actions of phenytoin will be reviewed, and it will be suggested that phenytoin anticonvulsant action is due, at least in part, to limitation of sustained, high-frequency, repetitive firing.

Phenytoin Reduction of Sustained, High-Frequency, Repetitive Firing

Nonsynaptic or direct membrane actions of phenytoin include (a) reduction of maximal rate of action potential depolarization (60,82,115, 155), (b) a use- or frequency-dependent reduction of inward sodium current (29,69,100,152), (c) reduction of posttetanic potentiation (36), (d) limitation of repetitive firing of sodium-dependent action potentials (7,22,75,103,137,142,183), and (e) reduction of ouabain- and veratridine-induced sodium influx (128). These data implicate regulation of Na^+ influx, a membrane process reflecting cellular excitability, as a mechanism of anticonvulsant action.

In spinal-cord neurons in cell culture, neither resting membrane potential nor input resistance was altered significantly by phenytoin at concentrations of 2 to 50 µg/ml (8–200 µM) (103). Phenytoin at 2 µg/ml did not alter single sodium-dependent action potentials, but at concentrations greater than 2 µg/ml, maximal rate of rise ($\dot{V}_{max}$)[1] of action potentials was reduced to about 50% of the control, with corresponding reduction of action potential overshoot and increase in duration. The $\dot{V}_{max}$ increased with membrane hyperpolarization but did not attain the values found in neurons hyperpolarized in control medium. These findings suggested (a) that the reduction in $\dot{V}_{max}$ was *voltage-dependent,* as well as *concentration-dependent;* (b) that there were at least two components to the reduction, one reversed by moderate hyperpolarization and the other not; and, (c) that, because of the voltage-dependent removal of part of the effect, this action of phenytoin was not like tetrodotoxin, a well-characterized blocker of inward sodium current (see ref. 112 for review).

In contrast, phenytoin altered repetitive firing of trains of action potentials at concentrations less that 2 µg/ml. Both spinal cord (Fig. 1, CONT) and neocortical (Fig. 3, CONT) neurons produced sustained trains of rapidly firing action potentials in response to long-duration (450 msec) depolarizing current steps. The $\dot{V}_{max}$ of successive action potentials diminished to a new steady-state value during the pulses, but all neurons were able to sustain repetitive firing throughout the pulses. When phenytoin was added to the medium at concentrations of 1–2 µg/ml, the first action potential in the trains was unchanged. However, action potential firing could be sustained only briefly (Fig. 1, PT), and steep reduction of $\dot{V}_{max}$,—i.e., more rapid adap

tation—preceded cessation of firing (see Fig. 4A). In effect, the evolution of the phenytoin effect was *use-dependent,* requiring the firing of several action potentials to reach maximal effect. The threshold concentration of phenytoin at which the limitation of repetitive firing began was 0.5 to 1.0 µg/ml. In a group of neurons whose membrane potentials ranged from −55 to −65 mV, the reduction of action potential firing was dose-dependent, with nearly maximal limitation of the number of action potentials during pulses of 500 msec duration and 15 to 20 mV amplitude achieved at about 2 µg/ml (Fig. 2, PT). Thus, the limitation of repetitive firing occurred at phenytoin concentrations equivalent to therapeutic cerebrospinal fluid (CSF) levels. Limitations of repetitive firing of neocortical and hippocampal neurons in cell culture and of pyramidal cells in hippocampal slices occurred over the same range of phenytoin concentrations (104,105).

The limitation of repetitive firing by phenytoin was *voltage-dependent* (Fig. 3). In phenytoin (2 µg/ml), when the membrane was hyperpolarized to −90 mV (Fig. 3, −90 mV), action potential firing was sustained, as in controls (Fig. 3, CONT). With membrane depolarization (Fig. 3, −68 mV), the ability to sustain rapid firing decreased and severe limitation was observed at the original resting potential (Fig. 3, 56 mV). Thus, the limitation became more severe with depolarization, and, conversely, protection against the phenytoin effect was afforded by hyperpolarization.

The limitation of repetitive firing by phenytoin was also *time-dependent* (Fig. 4B). Given the rapid return to basal sustained firing rates after cessation of the depolarizing test pulse, we investigated the time course of removal of phenytoin-induced limitation by comparing $\dot{V}_{max}$ of an action potential elicited at various intervals after a conditioning train to that of the first action potential of the train. In control medium, $\dot{V}_{max}$ had recovered nearly completely within 50 msec after the conditioning train. In the presence of phenytoin at 2 µg/ml, however, about 400 msec was required for recovery.

In summary, at concentrations known to produce clinically relevant anticonvulsant efficacy (1–2 µg/ml), phenytoin produced concentration-dependent limitation of rapid sustained firing of action potentials. This action was use-dependent, (i.e., it evolved with firing of several action potentials) and was time-dependent, slowing recovery of Na^+-dependent action potentials from inactivation. In addition, the degree of limitation was voltage-dependent, the effect being en-

---

[1] As long as the rising phase of the action potential is generated by Na^+ influx and not other cations, $\dot{V}_{max}$ reflects predominantly the inward Na^+ current. For further consideration, see ref. 65.

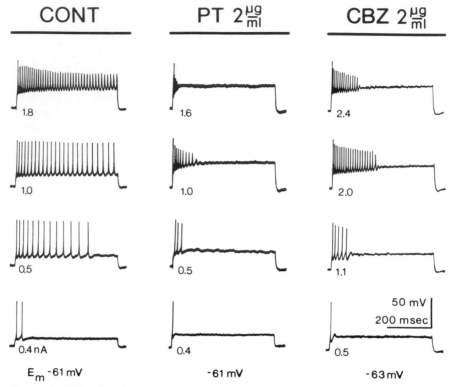

FIG. 1. Phenytoin (PT) and carbamazepine (CBZ) limited the ability of spinal-cord neurons to sustain repetitive firing of action potentials. CONT, controls. Each column shows four panels of action potentials recorded from a single spinal neuron in response to intracellularly applied current pulses (amplitude in nA given at *lower left* of each panel; pulse amplitude increased from *bottom* to *top*). Note inability of neurons in PT and CBZ (2 μg/ml)(equivalent to therapeutic cerebrospinal fluid levels) to sustain repetitive firing of action potentials. Resting membrane potentials (E_m) are shown at the bottom of each column. Calibration at lower right applies throughout.

hanced by membrane depolarization and reduced by membrane hyperpolarization.

The mechanism of the phenytoin block of repetitive firing is unclear. Voltage-clamp studies (29,69,100,152) have shown both voltage-dependent and use-dependent reductions of inward sodium current at higher concentrations of phenytoin. These actions correlate with the use and voltage dependence of limitation of repetitive firing and the parallel reduction of $\dot{V}_{max}$ of the sodium-dependent action potentials of the cultured neurons by phenytoin. The fact that the $\dot{V}_{max}$ of single action potentials or of the first action potential of a train (e.g., evoked by a long, depolarizing current pulse) was not reduced from the control value by phenytoin at a therapeutic concentration suggests that phenytoin binds reversibly (in a voltage- and time-dependent manner) to sodium channels inactivated following action potential initiation to produce frequency-dependent limitation. In effect, with the firing of each successive action potential in a train, more channels might accumulate

in the inactivated state until insufficient channels remain unbound by phenytoin to support further excitation. In such a model, phenytoin can be viewed as slowing the recovery from inactivation, as supported by the results described here (102,103) and in voltage-clamp studies (29,100,152). The rate of recovery appears to be voltage-sensitive: either phenytoin removal is faster or binding is decreased at higher membrane potentials, so that limitation is diminished (or protected against) with hyperpolarization. Enhanced affinity of phenytoin for the inactivated sodium channel with progressive depolarization from the resting potential could explain the ability of neurons to fire spontaneously at nearly the same rate as cells in control solution until they become depolarized. Extensive investigation of the use-dependent actions of local anesthetic/antiarrhythmics, such as lidocaine, has led to similar models (12,64,65,72,78,172,199). The actions of phenytoin described here are also similar to the previously described use-dependent phenomenon of slow inactivation induced

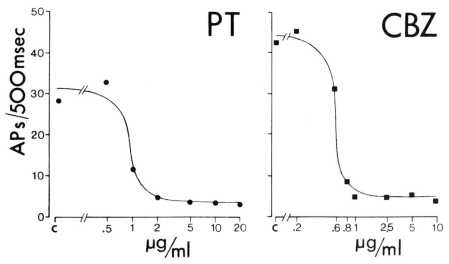

FIG. 2. Concentration dependence of limitation of repetitive firing of spinal cord neurons by phenytoin (PT) and carbamazepine (CBZ). Each data point shows the mean number of action potentials during 500-msec, 15–20-mV depolarizing current pulses for groups of 5–47 neurons with membrane potentials ranging from −55 to −65 mV. Reduction occurred at therapeutic CSF concentrations (1–2 μg/ml for PT; 0.8–5 μg/ml for CBZ).

by sulfhydryl reagents (158) and local anesthetics (73,172).

As an alternative mechanism, could phenytoin limit repetitive firing by affecting potassium conductances? The lack of effect of phenytoin on membrane potential and input resistance argues against effects on resting potassium conductance. Zbicz and Wilson (200) demonstrated a slowly generated outward potassium current in *Aplysia* neurons, which was enhanced by phenobarbital, but not by phenytoin. In addition, phenytoin has not been shown to augment voltage-activated potassium currents in *Xenopus* nerve (152) or neuroblastoma cells (100). Thus, it is unlikely that phenytoin exerts its anticonvulsant activity through effects on potassium conductance.

Other Phenytoin Actions

Postsynaptically, phenytoin has been shown to reduce the excitatory responses of rat cortical (145) and hippocampal (101) neurons to iontophoretically applied acetylcholine and glutamate, and to acetylcholine at the frog neuromuscular junction (41). Data concerning the effects of phenytoin on postsynaptic responses to the inhibitory neurotransmitter gamma-aminobutyric acid (GABA) have been contradictory, perhaps because of phylogenetic differences between preparations used. Phenytoin increased the responses in crayfish stretch receptors (2,31) and *Aplysia* abdominal ganglion neurons (6).

However, the GABA responses of mammalian dorsal root ganglion cells (28), hippocampal neurons (60), and frog motoneurons (120) were unaffected by phenytoin. Resolution of this apparent discrepancy seems to be important, since both reduction of excitation and augmentation of inhibition are potentially useful mechanisms of anticonvulsant action.

Phenytoin augmented postsynaptic responses of spinal cord neurons in cell culture to iontophoretically applied GABA, but only at concentrations above 5 μg/ml (103). Responses to iontophoretically applied glutamate were not reduced significantly at phenytoin concentrations as high as 50 μg/ml.

Presynaptically, phenytoin (2.5–25 μg/ml) has been shown to block transmitter release at the frog and mouse neuromuscular junction (22, 41,197,198) and potassium-evoked release of ^{3}H-norepinephrine from rat brain slices (130). This blockade may be effected by reducing calcium influx important for excitation-secretion coupling, as evidenced by decreased calcium influx into rat brain slices (130), lobster nerves (57), and rat brain synaptosomes (37,170). In addition, phenytoin decreased the amplitude of calcium-dependent potentials in mouse neuroblastoma cells (185) and reduced cyclic nucleotide concentrations in synaptosomes (32,38,173). Abbreviation of Ca^{2+}-dependent somatic action potentials, and thus calcium entry, of mouse spinal cord neurons in cell culture by phenytoin occurred at 5 μg/ml or more (103).

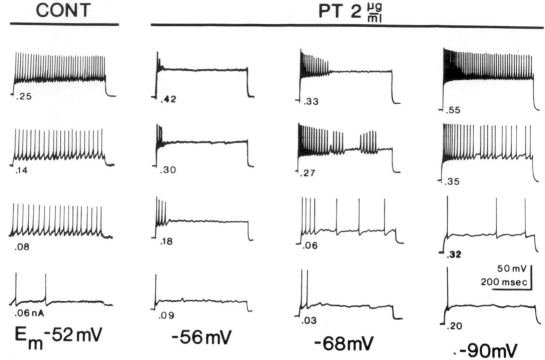

FIG. 3. Limitation of repetitive firing of neocortical neurons by phenytoin (PT) was voltage-dependent. Here limitation of firing of one neuron (E_m -56 mV) in medium containing PT (2 μg/ml) was limited in comparison with a neuron (E_m -52 mV) in control (CONT) solution. Progressive hyperpolarization of the neuron exposed to PT to -68 and -90 mV resulted in restoration of sustained, repetitive firing.

Phenytoin Anticonvulsant Action

On the basis of concentration dependence, only limitation of high frequency repetitive firing occurred at clinically useful concentrations. Effects in assays of pre- and postsynaptic mechanisms were observed at phenytoin concentrations known to produce clinical toxicity.

It must be borne in mind that phenytoin is ineffective against generalized absence seizures and affords only incomplete seizure control in some mixed forms of epilepsy. Presumably, the cellular activity that serves as a substrate for such seizures might not be dependent on high-frequency firing of sodium-dependent action potentials (the predominant activity of spinal cord and neocortical neurons) and, hence, might be resistant to phenytoin and other anticonvulsant drugs that share as a major mechanism of action the limitation of rapid repetitive firing. For example, hippocampal pyramidal neurons continue to fire penicillin-induced epileptiform bursts in the presence of high concentrations of phenytoin (149). Interestingly, in the hippocampal neurons the interspike interval between sodium-dependent action potentials increased in

phenytoin, suggesting early use-dependent inactivation, but calcium-dependent components of the burst were unaffected and interrupted the sodium-dependent activity. This illustrates how the coexistence of electrical activities with different ionic dependencies, even in the same cell type, might create epileptiform discharges resistant to certain classes of anticonvulsants.

CARBAMAZEPINE

Carbamazepine [Tegretol®, 5-carbamoyl-5H-dibenz(b,f)azepine] is chemically related to tricyclic antidepressants by virtue of the dibenzoazepine nucleus. First used to treat trigeminal neuralgia (16) and epilepsy in Europe, it was only approved for adult antiepileptic therapy in the United States in 1974. Clinically, carbamazepine is useful against partial seizures and generalized tonic–clonic seizures and is ineffective against generalized absence seizures (23), a spectrum similar to phenytoin (for review, see ref. 184). Carbamazepine is a lipid soluble anticonvulsant drug that is 70 to 80% protein-bound in serum. Anticonvulsant action is

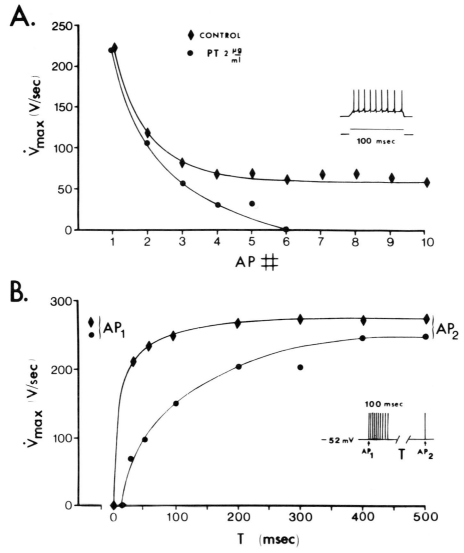

FIG. 4. Effects of phenytoin (PT) on maximal upstroke velocity ($\dot{V}_{max}$) of repetitively firing action potentials (APs). **A:** Use-dependent evolution of PT action. Progressive reduction of $\dot{V}_{max}$ during exposure to PT (2 µg/ml; *circles*) led to cessation of firing after five APs (abcissa shows ordinal number, AP#, during 100-msec pulse) in the same cell that fired 10 APs in control solution (*diamonds*). **B:** Time-dependent recovery from inactivation. Following a conditioning train of APs evoked by brief stimuli (0.1 msec) to induce the use-dependent reduction of $\dot{V}_{max}$, a test AP (AP$_2$) was elicited after an interval (T) and its $\dot{V}_{max}$ compared to that of the first AP of the conditioning train (AP$_1$). In PT-containing solution (*circles*), the interval to recover to control $\dot{V}_{max}$ was markedly prolonged in comparison to control (*diamonds*). Data were obtained from two neurons (one control and one exposed to PT) with matching resting potentials of −52 mV. *Insets* show experimental paradigms. (From ref. 103, with permission.)

produced in adults by doses of 10 to 20 mg/kg · day to achieve total serum levels of 4 to 12 µg/ml (16–48 µM). Thus, assuming 75% protein binding, free-serum and CSF levels are about 1.0 to 3.0 µg/ml (4.2–12.6 µM). In animals, carbamazepine protects against MES seizures, but not against PTZ seizures (68,76).

Carbamazepine Reduction of Sustained, High-Frequency, Repetitive Firing

The mechanisms by which carbamazepine exerts anticonvulsant activity are not as thoroughly studied as those of phenytoin (for review, see ref. 175). Carbamazepine inhibited antidromically propagated repetitive action potential discharges after tetanic stimuli (61) and reduced muscle spindle activity (static and stretch-induced) in spinal cats (62), suggesting direct membrane action.

To date, we have investigated principally direct membrane effects of carbamazepine (104). Like phenytoin, at therapeutic concentrations (0.8–2.4 µg/ml in CSF) carbamazepine limited high-frequency repetitive firing of action potentials elicited by long depolarizing current pulses of spinal cord neurons (Fig. 5) or of neocortical neurons. The value of $\dot{V}_{max}$ decreased as the action potential generation failed. This effect was concentration-dependent, with a threshold at about 0.6 to 0.8 µg/ml and maximal suppression at about 2 to 3 µg/ml (Fig. 2), voltage-sensitive (Fig. 5), and use-dependent (Figs. 1 and 5).

Other Actions of Carbamazepine

In spinal cats, polysynaptic, but not monosynaptic, reflexes were inhibited by intravenous anticonvulsant administration (180) suggesting an action on synaptic transmission. There is controversy over the possible role of catecholamines in the action of anticonvulsants including carbamazepine (135,143) and carbamazepine increased firing in locus coeruleus neurons, an action which was blocked by desmethylimipramine (121). Carbamazepine reduced binding of adenosine congeners to rat brain membranes and inhibited adenosine uptake into brain slices, suggesting a purinergic component to carbamazepines anticonvulsant efficacy (163). Carbamazepine also may interact with benzodiazepine receptors (164) to augment GABA-mediated inhibition, though this action requires confirmation. Schauf et al. (147) reported that carbamazepine reduced both inward sodium current (50%) and outward potassium current (40%) in *Myxicola* giant axons under voltage clamp conditions, but carbamazepine concentrations were high (0.25–1.0 mM or 58–235 µg/ml).

At concentrations up to 10 µg/ml (equivalent

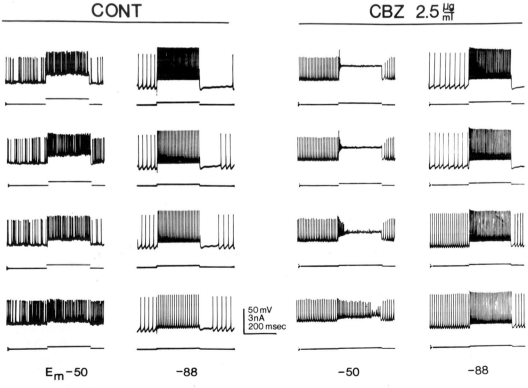

FIG. 5. Limitation of repetitive firing by carbamazepine (CBZ) occurred at a critical frequency above the spontaneous firing rate and was voltage-dependent. CONT, control. In medium containing CBZ (2.5 µg/ml), ability to sustain high-frequency, repetitive firing was limited during 450-msec depolarizing current pulses in a spontaneously firing spinal neuron (third column) at −50 mV (compare to another neuron in control solution at the same resting potential, as shown in the first column). When the neuron exposed to CBZ was hyperpolarized to −88 mV (fourth column), the ability to sustain high-frequency, repetitive firing during the applied current pulses was restored (compare to a third neuron at the same membrane potential in the second column). Note that all neurons could sustain spontaneous firing at slower rates than occurred during the interposed depolarizing current steps in both control and CBZ-containing neurons.

to total serum concentrations of 30–50 μg/ml), postsynaptic responses of spinal-cord neurons in cell culture to iontophoretically applied GABA and glutamate were unaffected (D. M. Rock and R. L. Macdonald, *unpublished data*).

These results suggest that carbamazepine, like phenytoin, limits sustained, high-frequency, repetitive firing at anticonvulsant free-serum concentrations and supports the suggestion, based on similarity of clinical spectra, that the two drugs may have similar anticonvulsant mechanisms.

DEOXYBARBITURATES

Primidone (Mysoline®; 5-ethyldihydro-5-phenyl-4,6(1*H*,5*H*)-pyrimidinedione) is a deoxybarbiturate that is metabolized to two active compounds, phenylethylmalonamide (PEMA) and phenobarbital. It was initially shown to be clinically effective by Handley and Stewart (54) and is currently used in treatment of generalized tonic–clonic seizures and all forms of partial seizures but is ineffective against generalized absence seizures. Primidone is administered to adults at 10 to 25 mg/kg · day to achieve a total serum level of 5 to 12 μg/ml (23–55 μM). Primidone is only 20% bound to serum proteins, and thus CSF concentrations are 80% of total serum concentrations. In mice, it is more effective against MES seizures than PTZ seizures (50,76). When metabolism of primidone to PEMA and phenobarbital is blocked, primidone is effective against MES seizures but not against PTZ seizures (17).

There has been uncertainty over whether primidone is an effective anticonvulsant or whether its anticonvulsant efficacy is due to its two metabolites, PEMA and phenobarbital (for review, see refs. 40 and 196). The issue appears to have been resolved by measuring the brain concentrations of primidone, PEMA, and phenobarbital that are effective against MES and PTZ seizures. These drug concentrations were determined with and without blockade of conversion of primidone to its metabolites by administration of SKF 525A (11,17). Primidone has independent action against MES seizures but is ineffective against PTZ seizures. Phenobarbital (see below) has efficacy against both seizure types, while PEMA is effective against both seizure types only at toxic doses. Furthermore, primidone and phenobarbital together are more effective than either drug alone. Thus, it is likely that the clinical efficacy of primidone is due to the combined and possibly synergistic actions of primidone and metabolically derived phenobarbital.

The anticonvulsant mechanism of action of primidone is uncertain. We have studied primidone action on amino acid responses and on sustained high-frequency firing of mouse neurons in cell culture. Primidone had no effect on postsynaptic GABA and glutamate responses at concentrations up to 200 μM (≈50 μg/ml) (J. H. Skerritt, D. M. Rock, and R. L. Macdonald, *unpublished data*) (Fig. 6). Primidone (and phenobarbital) limited sustained, high-frequency, repetitive firing at relatively high concentrations (>200 μM, or >50 μg/ml) (M. J. McLean and R. L. Macdonald, *unpublished data*) (Fig. 7). However, when primidone (12 μg/ml) and phenobarbital (20 μg/ml) were combined, they limited sustained, high-frequency, repetitive firing at clinically relevant concentrations. From these preliminary results, it would appear that primidone and metabolically derived phenobarbital may act synergistically to reduce sustained, high-frequency, repetitive firing.

BARBITURATES

Phenobarbital (Luminal®; 5-ethyl-5-phenylbarbituric acid) was one of the first anticonvulsant drugs used to treat seizures (58). Phenobarbital is useful in the management of generalized tonic–clonic seizures and all types of partial seizures but is ineffective against generalized absence seizures. At high serum concentrations, anticonvulsant barbiturates produce sedation and anesthesia. Therapeutic serum levels of phenobarbital are about 40 to 160 μM (10–40 μg/ml), but since phenobarbital is about 40% protein-bound, the therapeutic free-serum and CSF phenobarbital concentration range is about 25 to 100 μM. Barbiturates are effective against both MES and PTZ seizures (50,76,138).

Numerous barbiturate actions have been identified (91,118,134,154). Barbiturates have been demonstrated to act (a) *postsynaptically* to modify neurotransmitter action (enhancement of GABAergic inhibition and reduction of glutaminergic and cholinergic excitation) and to directly increase membrane chloride ion conductance, (b) *presynaptically* to reduce calcium entry and thus to block release of neurotransmitters, and (c) *nonsynaptically* to reduce voltage-dependent sodium and potassium conductances and to block repetitive firing. Despite identification of multiple barbiturate actions, the specific clinical anticonvulsant, sedative, and anesthetic actions of barbiturates remain uncertain. In the sections below, each of the identified barbiturate actions will be reviewed, and data obtained from mouse neurons in cell culture will be presented that suggest that barbiturate anti-

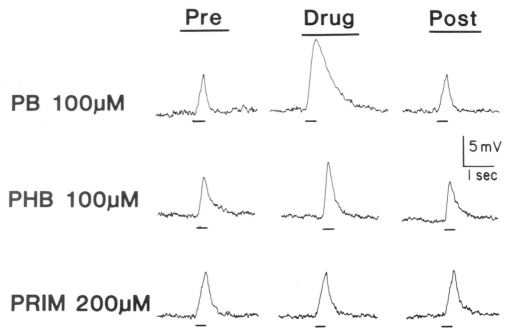

FIG. 6. Pentobarbital (PB) and phenobarbital (PHB) but not primidone (PRIM) enhanced GABA responses. GABA was applied by iontophoresis at the horizontal bars and PB, PhB, and PRIM were applied by local diffusion from large pipettes. Membrane potential was held more negative than −70 mV. (From J. H. Skerritt and R. L. Macdonald, *unpublished results.*)

convulsant action may be due, at least in part, to postsynaptic enhancement of inhibitory GABAergic synaptic transmission and postsynaptic reduction of excitatory synaptic transmission and to limitation of sustained, high-frequency, repetitive firing.

Barbiturate Modification of Postsynaptic Neurotransmitter Responses

Phenobarbital and pentobarbital enhanced GABA responses and reduced glutamate responses on spinal-cord roots (116,117) and on mouse spinal-cord neurons in cell culture (10, 92,94,95,140,150). The enhancement of GABA responses was selective, since the barbiturates did not enhance responses evoked by β-alanine, glycine, or taurine. Phenobarbital enhanced GABA responses at concentrations clinically relevant for anticonvulsant action (25–100 μM) (Fig. 6) (150; J. H. Skerritt and R. L. Macdonald, *unpublished data*).

The mechanism whereby barbiturates enhance GABA responses has now been partially clarified. It was postulated that barbiturates enhance GABA responses by enhancing GABA binding to GABA receptors and/or modifying chloride ion channel properties (increased mean unitary channel conductance or duration) (94).

However, barbiturates had not been demonstrated to modify high-affinity GABA binding (125) but had been demonstrated to interact with the picrotoxinin binding site on the GABA–receptor complex (123,182). It was postulated that barbiturates acted at the picrotoxinin binding site to modify chloride channel function. Recently, barbiturates have been shown to enhance binding of GABA to membranes prepared from rat brain (5,124,191). The enhancement of GABA binding was chloride-dependent. Whether the enhancement is due to an increased number of GABA binding sites (5,124) or to an increase in receptor affinity (191) is uncertain. The dose dependence of pentobarbital enhancement of GABA binding was similar to that for enhancement of GABA responses. However, phenobarbital has been shown to enhance GABA binding only in a single study (191). Olsen and Snowman (124) could not demonstrate an enhancement of GABA binding. However, as with pentobarbital, phenobarbital reduced the dissociation rate constants for ^{3}H-diazepam binding (79) and competitively inhibited the enhancement of benzodiazepine binding by pentobarbital (124). Thus, phenobarbital probably binds to the same sites as pentobarbital.

Enhancement of GABA binding by barbiturates may enhance postsynaptic GABA re-

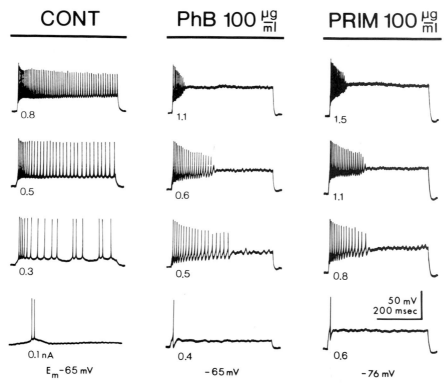

CONT   PhB 100 $\frac{\mu g}{ml}$ PRIM 100 $\frac{\mu g}{ml}$

FIG. 7. Phenobarbital (PhB) and primidone (PRIM) limited repetitive firing of spinal cord neurons at high concentrations. PhB and PRIM were bath applied, and comparisons were made to neurons recorded from in control bathing medium. Repetitive firing was evoked by applying a series of depolarizing current pulses (450 msec) from holding potentials at −80 to −55 mV.

sponses by altering chloride channel function. Barbiturates prolong GABAergic inhibitory postsynaptic potentials, presynaptic inhibition, and postsynaptic GABA responses (92,93,116, 117,119,140), suggesting that barbiturates may prolong the mean open lifetime of chloride channels. This was confirmed using noise analysis of GABA current fluctuations produced on mouse spinal-cord neurons in cell culture (9,174). Mean channel conductance was not altered significantly, but pentobarbital decreased the frequency of channel openings.

Thus, barbiturates appear to enhance postsynaptic GABA responses by binding to a site on GABA receptors that is distinct from the GABA binding site, and the enhancement of GABA binding results in a prolongation of mean open lifetime of chloride channels.

Barbiturate Actions on Repetitive Firing

Pentobarbital and phenobarbital have been demonstrated to reduce repetitive firing of *Aplysia* neurons by enhancing a slow outward potassium current (200). The barbiturate action

to reduce repetitive firing occurred over clinically meaningful concentrations, and therefore may have importance for anticonvulsant action. However, the barbiturate-sensitive potassium conductance has not been described in vertebrate neurons. Thus, its relevance to clinical anticonvulsant actions remains uncertain. Phenobarbital also limited sustained, high-frequency, repetitive firing of mouse spinal-cord and cortical neurons in cell culture at high concentrations (>200 μM) (Fig. 7) (104). It is unclear whether or not this action of the barbiturates contributes to its anticonvulsant action.

Other Barbiturate Actions

In addition to enhancing GABA responses on frog dorsal and ventral roots, pentobarbital directly depolarized the roots, and the depolarization was antagonized by the GABA antagonists bicuculline and picrotoxin (116,117). Similarly, pentobarbital (>100 μM) and phenobarbital (>500 μM) hyperpolarized mouse spinal-cord neurons in cell culture and increased membrane conductance, and the barbiturate action was reversed by GABA antagonists (94,95,150). Thus it was suggested that barbiturates bind to GABA receptors to activate chloride ion conductance.

In addition to postsynaptic actions, barbiturates act presynaptically to reduce release of neurotransmitter by reducing presynaptic calcium entry (see refs. 63,91, for review). Barbiturates reduced the calcium influx induced by potassium depolarization of mouse brain synaptosomes (15,126) and rat sympathetic ganglia (14) and by preganglionic stimulation of rat sympathetic ganglia (14). It is likely that the reduction of calcium entry into synaptosomes was due to a reduction of voltage-dependent calcium conductance (47,48,111).

The finding that barbiturates block calcium entry was directly tested using calcium-dependent action potentials evoked in mouse spinal-cord neurons in cell culture (63). Both phenobarbital and pentobarbital reduced calcium-dependent action potential duration, but pentobarbital (25–600 μM) was about five times more potent than phenobarbital (100–5,000 μM). Both barbiturates reduced membrane plateau conductance, suggesting that the barbiturates reduced calcium-ion conductance. This finding has been directly confirmed by recording inward calcium currents using the single-electrode voltage clamp from mouse neurons in cell culture in cesium-containing medium and with intracellular cesium ion injection (98). Cesium application blocked most potassium ion conductance. Both phenobarbital and pentobarbital reduced the inward calcium current without altering resting (leak) conductance. Thus, pentobarbital and phenobarbital block calcium entry through voltage-dependent calcium channels.

Pentobarbital and phenobarbital also have been demonstrated to reduce voltage-dependent sodium and potassium conductances (13,113, 114,151), but only at high drug concentrations (>250 μM).

Which Barbiturate Actions Are Anticonvulsant?

Barbiturates clearly have multiple actions on central nervous system neurons. However, each barbiturate produces these actions over different concentration ranges. Phenobarbital enhanced GABA responses (and antagonized glutamate responses) at anticonvulsant therapeutic free-serum concentrations (25–100 μM) but did not activate membrane chloride-ion conductance or reduce calcium-dependent action potentials below 100 μM. Therefore, it is likely that barbiturates produce anticonvulsant action, at least

in part, by enhancing postsynaptic GABA responses and possibly by antagonizing postsynaptic excitatory transmitter responses. Phenobarbital reduces repetitive firing at concentrations achieved in treatment of status epilepticus but not at concentrations achieved in ambulatory patients.

VALPROIC ACID

Valproic acid (Depakene®; di-*n*-propylacetic acid, 2-propylvaleric acid, 2-propylpentanoic acid) was identified as an anticonvulsant drug in 1963 (108) and was approved for use in the United States in 1978. Valproic acid has been shown to be effective in the management of generalized absence, myoclonic and generalized tonic–clonic seizures (20,131,161). When administered to adults at 30 to 60 mg/kg · day, valproic acid is active clinically at serum levels of about 0.33 to 1 mM (50–150 μg/ml) but is highly (85–95%) protein-bound. The extent of protein binding varies with total serum concentration and ranges from about 95% at total serum level of 50 μg/ml to about 80% at 150 μg/ml (30). Cerebrospinal fluid levels reflect free valproic acid levels, and therefore central nervous system concentrations of 2.5 to 30 μg/ml (17.5–210 μM) are likely to be relevant drug concentrations. It is effective against both MES and PTZ seizures (76,159,176).

Valproic Acid Action on GABAergic Synaptic Transmission

The mechanism of action of valproic acid remains uncertain, but may involve modification of GABAergic synaptic transmission (for review, see refs. 24,77). Valproic acid has been shown to increase brain GABA levels (46,160). The basis for the elevation in brain GABA may involve an interaction between valproic acid and several enzymes involved in the synthesis and degradation of GABA. Valproic acid has been shown to be a weak inhibitor of GABA-aminotransferase (GABA-T), the first enzyme in the degradative pathway for GABA, with K_i values ranging from 23 to 87 mM (84,160), and a stronger inhibitor of the next degradative enzyme, succinic semialdehyde dehydrogenase (SSA-DH), with K_i values between 0.5 and 1.0 mM (4,56,146,187). Furthermore, valproic acid has been shown to activate the major synthetic enzyme glutamic acid decarboxylase (GAD) (85,88,89).

The action of valproic acid on brain GABA

levels has recently been extended to an analysis of valproic acid induced alterations of GABA metabolism at the subcellular level. Valproic acid was demonstrated to selectively increase GABA levels in synaptosomes (66,85,86,87, 144,194). Furthermore, the enhancement of brain GABA levels was variable in different brain regions with the largest increases occurring in brain regions with high GAD and GABA levels (67), and an enhancement in GABA levels was not produced in substantia nigra after its GABAergic input had been surgically removed (66). These observations suggest that valproic acid increases GABA in nerve terminals. However, valproic acid did not increase release of GABA from synaptosomes (1) or from frog spinal-cord slices (52).

It has been demonstrated that valproic acid selectively enhances postsynaptic GABA responses evoked on mouse spinal cord neurons in cell culture (96). No alteration of glycine or glutamic acid responses were produced, and valproic acid had no direct action on membrane potential or conductance. This finding has been confirmed in rat brainstem (42), carp retina (59), rat cerebral cortex (8,70) and frog spinal cord

(52). The studies using mammalian preparations have employed iontophoretic application of valproic acid, and therefore it is unclear whether the action of valproic acid occurs at sufficiently low concentration. Subsequent studies have shown that valproic acid enhances GABA responses only above 1 mM (55,141). Furthermore, valproic acid displaced ^{3}H-dihydropicrotoxin from its binding site to GABA receptors at relatively high concentrations (>150 μM; IC_{50} of 500 μM) (18l).

Valproic Acid Action on Repetitive Firing

We have recently demonstrated that valproic acid and its sodium salt limited sustained, high-frequency, repetitive firing of spinal-cord neurons in cell culture (Fig. 8) (104,141). The effect was maximal at sodium valproate concentrations above 12 μM (2 μg/ml).

Correlation of Valproic Acid Actions and Anticonvulsant Effects

Valproic acid has been shown possibly to enhance GABAergic synaptic transmission and

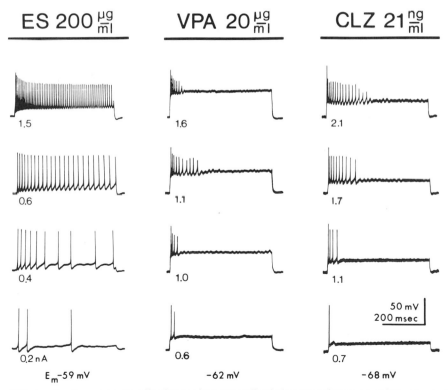

FIG. 8. Effects of anticonvulsants effective against generalized absence seizures on ability of spinal neurons to sustain high frequency repetitive firing of action potentials. Ethosuximide (ES) did not limit repetitive firing at a concentration above therapeutic range (200 μg/ml). Valproic acid (VPA) or its sodium salt limited repetitive firing at therapeutic concentrations. Clonazepam (CLZ) also limited repetitive firing.

to reduce sustained, high-frequency, repetitive firing. The increase in brain GABA levels by valproic acid correlated with the onset and duration of anticonvulsant action in some animal seizure models (83,86,88–90,160). However, in other animal seizure models, elevation of whole brain GABA did not correlate with anticonvulsant action (4,34,83,193,194). Despite the demonstration that valproic acid modifies brain GABA levels by modifying synthesis and/or degradation, several problems remain with accepting this as the anticonvulsant mechanism of action. First, the drug concentrations required are very high. It is not clear that valproic acid will activate GAD or antagonize GABA-T or SSA-DH at the lower, clinically relevant concentrations. Second, the increase in synaptosomal GABA may be too small to account for anticonvulsant activity (194). Third, the increase in synaptosomal GABA content did not correlate with anticonvulsant action against isonicotinic acid hydrazide seizures (194). Fourth, it has not been demonstrated that elevation of brain or synaptosomal GABA results in an enhancement of synaptically released GABA. Nonetheless, the finding that valproic acid enhancement of synaptosomal GABA correlates with anticonvulsant action against PTZ seizures supports the GABA metabolism hypothesis (86).

While valproic acid enhancement of GABAergic synaptic transmission may correlate with activity against PTZ seizures, the increase in synaptosomal GABA content did not correlate with anticonvulsant action against MES seizures (70,71,86). We suggest that the ability of valproic acid to limit sustained, high-frequency, repetitive firing may be the mechanism of action for activity against MES and generalized tonic–clonic seizures.

BENZODIAZEPINES

Benzodiazepines are used widely to treat anxiety, insomnia, spasticity, and seizures. Diazepam (Valium®; 7-chlor-1-methyl-5-phenyl-l,3 dihydro-2H-1,4-benzodiazepine-2-one) is used as an anticonvulsant primarily in the acute treatment of status epilepticus. While long-term anticonvulsant therapy is usually unsuccessful due to the development of tolerance, diazepam has been reported to have action against myoclonic, atonic, absence, photosensitive, and alcohol-withdrawal seizures (18). Clonazepam (Clonopin®; 7-nitro-5-(2-chlorophenyl)-1,3-dihydro-2H-1,4-benzodiazepine-2-on) is approved for therapy of myoclonic seizures, atonic seizures, absence seizures, and infantile spasms. Clonazepam is administered to adults at 0.05 to 0.2

mg/kg · day to achieve a total plasma level of 20 to 80 ng/ml (16–64 nM). Since clonazepam is highly protein bound (80%) (186), CSF levels should be lower than total serum levels. Diazepam and clonazepam are both effective against PTZ seizures and block MES seizures, but only at toxic doses (76,139,179).

Benzodiazepines have been demonstrated to alter synaptic transmission and membrane properties of neurons and muscle cells (for reviews, see refs. 53,74). Benzodiazepines have been shown to act: (a) *postsynaptically* to enhance GABAergic inhibition (26,93,95,132,136,192), (b) *presynaptically* to enhance presynaptic inhibition (132,133,148), to block presynaptic calcium uptake (80) and to enhance or reduce neurotransmitter release (109,122) and (c) *nonsynaptically* to reduce voltage-dependent sodium and potassium ion conductances (153,189), to increase chloride ion conductance (188), and to reduce repetitive firing of action potentials (168,188,189).

Benzodiazepine Enhancement of GABA Responses

Diazepam depressed mono- and polysynaptic spinal cord reflexes at doses that enhance GABA-mediated presynaptic inhibition in dorsal horn and cuneate nucleus (133,148). An interaction between GABA responses and benzodiazepines was directly demonstrated using chick (26,27) and mouse (93,95) spinal-cord neurons in cell culture. Chlordiazepoxide and diazepam both enhanced GABA responses evoked on spinal-cord neurons in a dose-dependent manner without altering resting membrane potential or conductance. The effect was selective since responses to glycine, taurine, β-alanine, and glutamic acid were unaffected by chlordiazepoxide. The enhancement of GABA responses was produced by diazepam and clonazepam above 1 nM, peaked at about 100 nM (165,166,167,168) (Fig. 9), and thus is produced at clinically relevant benzodiazepine concentrations.

The mechanism of benzodiazepine enhancement of GABA responses is likely to involve binding of benzodiazepines to specific benzodiazepine receptors, which are coupled to GABA receptors (110,171). Benzodiazepines have been shown to enhance GABA binding to brain membranes (51,106,169) by increasing the affinity of lower affinity GABA binding (169). Using fluctuation analysis, diazepam was shown to increase the frequency of GABA-coupled chloride channel openings on spinal-cord neurons in cell culture without altering the conductance or mean open lifetime of the channels (174). Thus,

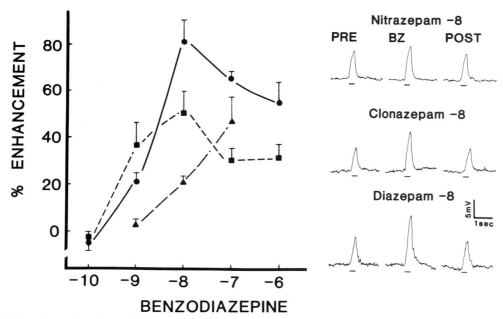

FIG. 9. Benzodiazepines enhanced GABA responses of spinal-cord neurons. Diazepam (*circles*), clonazepam (*squares*), and nitrazepam (*triangles*) applied locally from large diffusion pipettes enhanced iontophoretic GABA responses recorded with 3 M KCl-containing micropipettes. Drug concentrations are logarithm molar. Membrane potentials were held more negative than −70 mV. Data shown are means (±SEM). In specimen records on **right**, GABA was applied at *horizontal bars*, and post responses were obtained 2 min following removal of benzodiazepine pipettes. (From ref. 167, with permission.)

benzodiazepines may enhance GABA responses by increasing the affinity of GABA receptors and increasing the frequency of chloride channel openings.

Benzodiazepine Reduction of Repetitive Firing

In addition to enhancing GABA responses, benzodiazepines have been shown to reduce high-frequency, repetitive firing of action potentials in muscle (188,189) and neurons (168). Diazepam and clonazepam reduced sustained high-frequency, repetitive firing of some mouse spinal-cord neurons above 35 nM and reduced firing to a few action potentials of all neurons above 200 nM (Fig. 8) (168). These concentrations are above therapeutic free-serum concentrations achieved in ambulatory patients prior to developing tolerance but are within the range of free-serum concentrations achieved in patients treated for status epilepticus. The mechanism of the reduction in repetitive firing is uncertain.

Other Benzodiazepine Actions

Benzodiazepines have been shown to reduce potassium-stimulated neurotransmitter release (109) and to block uptake of calcium by synaptosomes (80). Similarly, diazepam reduced the duration of calcium-dependent action potentials of mouse dorsal-root ganglion neurons in cell culture (168). The reduction of action potential duration was produced following reduction of membrane potassium conductance by intracellular injection of cesium ion, suggesting that diazepam directly blocked calcium conductance rather than enhanced potassium conductance. In contrast to the high potency of diazepam in enhancing GABA responses (1–100 nM) and reducing repetitive firing (35–200 nM), diazepam did not modify calcium uptake or calcium-dependent action potential duration below 1 μM.

Benzodiazepines have also been shown to reduce sodium and potassium conductances at high concentrations (200 μM) (153,189). Flurazepam reduced the peak inward sodium current about 50%, induced a slow phase in recovery from sodium channel inactivation, and induced a frequency-dependent sodium channel block. Flurazepam also produced potassium channel inactivation.

Correlation of Benzodiazepine Pharmacological Actions with Clinical Effects

Benzodiazepines block generalized absence seizures and PTZ seizures at low doses and enhance GABA responses at low concentrations that are clinically relevant. Thus, we suggest that enhancement of GABA action at postsynaptic receptors is the main anticonvulsant action of benzodiazepines. However, at higher doses, benzodiazepines block generalized tonic–clonic seizures, status epilepticus, and MES. At concentrations higher than those enhancing GABA responses, benzodiazepines limit high-frequency, sustained, repetitive firing. Thus, we suggest that limitation of high frequency repetitive firing may underlie some anticonvulsant actions of benzodiazepines in humans and experimental animals. Finally, benzodiazepines have a high therapeutic index, and they produce sedation only at very high doses. Benzodiazepines block calcium entry into neurons at high concentrations, and this calcium channel block may be responsible for reduced release of neurotransmitter and sedation.

SUCCINIMIDES

Ethosuximide (Zarontin®; 2-ethyl-2-methylsuccinimide), methsuximide (Celontin®; N,2-dimethyl-2-phenylsuccimide), and phensuximide (Milontin®; N-methyl-2-phenylsuccimide) are anticonvulsant succinimide drugs with differing effectiveness against experimental and clinical seizures. Ethosuximide is the drug of choice in the management of generalized absence seizures (19) and, with rare exceptions, is not useful in treatment of other seizure types. Methsuximide is also effective in treatment of generalized absence seizures but also has effectiveness against generalized tonic–clonic and partial seizures (190). Phensuximide is rarely used, since it appears to be less effective than the other succinimides against generalized tonic–clonic seizures (190). Both methsuximide and phensuximide may also have more toxic side effects than ethosuximide, thus further limiting their usefulness. Ethosuximide is effective in adults at doses of 20 to 40 mg/kg · day and in children at 20 to 30 mg/kg · day. Therapeutic plasma levels range from 40 to 100 µg/ml (300–700 µM) (19). Since ethosuximide is not bound to protein in plasma, CSF and plasma levels are similar (157). Ethosuximide is effective against PTZ seizures at nontoxic doses but ineffective against MES seizures, except at highly toxic doses (25,76). Both methsuximide and phensuximide are more effective against PTZ seizures than MES seizures, but both drugs have efficacy against both seizure types at nontoxic doses (25,76).

Despite the widespread acceptance of the treatment of generalized absence seizures, the mechanism of action of ethosuximide is unknown (for a review, see ref. 39). Ethosuximide has been reported to inhibit cerebral cortical

Na^+,K^+-ATPase activity, and the inhibition of the Na^+,K^+-ATPase may be in synaptic terminal membranes (43–45,81). However, with chronic treatment, Na^+,K^+-ATPase was increased (81). In addition, ethosuximide slightly reduced the activities of succinate dehydrogenase (81) and aldehyde reductase (35). The significance of these biochemical changes is uncertain. Ethosuximide depressed veratridine-induced increases in cyclic GMP (ID_{50} = 2.4 mM) but not increases in cyclic AMP in mouse cortical slices, while methsuximide and phensuximide suppressed both cyclic GMP (ID_{50} = 2.4 or 6.2 mM, respectively) and cyclic AMP (ID_{50} = 1.4 or 8.0 mM, respectively) increases produced by veratridine (38).

Ethosuximide administration to rats for 10 days (150 mg/kg · day; plasma levels 98.6 µg/ml) had little effect on whole-brain or regional GABA or taurine levels but increased subcortical (but not cortical) glutamic and aspartic acid levels (127). In contrast, ethosuximide has been shown to reverse the isoniazid-induced reduction of glutamic acid dehydrogenase activity, the synthetic enzyme for conversion of glutamic acid to GABA, and reduction of brain GABA levels (89).

Ethosuximide has had variable effects on calcium fluxes and release of neurotransmitter. Ethosuximide did not alter calcium influx into depolarized synaptosomes at concentrations less than 0.4 mM but produced a small increase in (20%) calcium influx at 4 mM (170).

Finally, ethosuximide has been shown to have variable actions on synaptic transmission. Ethosuximide (200–400 mg/kg) did not alter the amplitude of single monosynaptic reflex responses recorded from cat lumbosacral ventral roots following hind-limb afferent-nerve stimulation; however, ethosuximide enhanced the decline of the ventral-root responses produced by 2 to 10 Hz repetitive stimulation (21). The effect was attributed to an enhanced depletion of neurotransmitter stores rather than as a primary effect on neurotransmitter release. In contrast, ethosuximide (200 µM) enhanced release of neurotransmitter from motor nerve terminals (129), an effect suggested to be due to increased presynaptic calcium entry. Ethosuximide did not enhance GABA responses recorded from mouse spinal cord or cortical neurons in cell culture (D. M. Rock and R. L. Macdonald, *unpublished results*). Ethosuximide (1 mM) was shown to have no effect on transmitter release at the frog neuromuscular junction but to reduce miniature end-plate potential amplitude (20%), a postsynaptic effect. Finally, ethosuximide did not alter sustained, high-frequency, repetitive firing of spinal-cord neurons at concentrations as high as 3.5 mM (500 μg/ml) (104).

It is clear that insufficient information is available to identify the anticonvulsant mechanism of action of ethosuximide, and thus no hypothesis will be advanced.

CONCLUSION

Based on the data presented in this chapter, we suggest that there are at least two mechanisms of anticonvulsant drug action: reduction of sustained, high-frequency, repetitive firing, and enhancement of GABAergic synaptic transmission (Table 2). Phenytoin, carbamazepine and valproic acid all limited high-frequency, repetitive firing at therapeutic free-serum concentrations. Primidone limited high-frequency, repetitive firing at concentrations that were above therapeutic free-serum concentrations but had increased potency when combined with low concentrations of phenobarbital and the benzodiazepines, clonazepam and diazepam, limited repetitive firing at concentrations that were above those in ambulatory patients but that are achieved clinically during the treatment of status epilepticus. Finally, ethosuximide did not limit repetitive firing even at very high concentrations. We suggest that the ability of anticonvulsant drugs to limit sustained, high-frequency, repetitive firing may correlate with their effectiveness against maximal electroshock seizures, and therefore that ethosuximide has no efficacy in that seizure test due to its inability to modify repetitive firing. We would suggest further that the ability of anticonvulsant drug to limit sustained, high-frequency, repetitive firing may also correlate with therapeutic efficacy against generalized tonic–clonic seizures and status epilepticus.

Phenobarbital and the benzodiazepines, diazepam and clonazepam, enhance postsynaptic GABA responses at therapeutic free-serum concentrations. While the mechanism of action of valproic acid remains uncertain, there is a suggestion that it may enhance GABAergic synaptic transmission by increasing presynaptic release of GABA. In contrast, phenytoin, carbamazepine, and primidone do not modify GABAergic synaptic transmission. We suggest that the ability of clinically used anticonvulsant drugs to enhance GABAergic synaptic transmission may be responsible for the efficacy against pentylenetetrazol seizures. Furthermore, we would suggest that the ability of these drugs to enhance GABAergic synaptic transmission may also correlate with their efficacy against generalized absence seizures.

With descriptions of the basic actions of these anticonvulsant drugs, it is clear that they can be divided in several subclasses. Phenytoin, carbamazepine, and primidone can be classed as drugs that modify sustained, high-frequency firing but do not modify GABAergic synaptic transmission. Phenobarbital, valproic acid, and clonazepam modify repetitive firing and GABAergic synaptic transmission. Finally, ethosuximide has not been demonstrated to modify either repetitive firing or GABAergic synaptic transmission. This classification again correlates well with the clinical efficacy of these drugs. The first class of drug, which is selective for repetitive firing and maximal electroshock seizures, has efficacy in generalized tonic–clonic seizures and in status epilepticus. The second class of drugs has mixed actions. For example, valproic acid has efficacy against generalized tonic–clonic seizures and generalized absence seizures. Finally, the third class of drug has selective action only against pentylenetetrazol seizures and generalized absence seizures.

While this approach to the classification of anticonvulsant drugs appears to have some merit, there are inconsistencies that remain. Primidone has been demonstrated to have action against electroshock seizures when its metabolic trans-

TABLE 2. *Relative effectiveness of anticonvulsant drugs in reducing repetitive firing, enhancing GABA responses, and in treatment of seizures in humans and experimental animals*

	RF[a]	MES[b]	GTC[c]	GABA[d]	PTZ[e]	GA[f]
PT	+ +	+ +	+ +	0	0	0
CBZ	+ +	+ +	+ +	0	0	0
PRM	+ +[a]	+ +	+ +	0	0	0
PhB	+	+ +	+	+ +[b]	+ +	0
VPA	+ +	+ +	+ +	+/?[c]	+ +	+ +
CLZ	+	+	+	+ +	+ +	+ +
ESM	0	0	0	0	+ +	+ +

[a] Reduction of repetitive firing.
[b] Block of maximal electroshock seizures.
[c] Block of generalized tonic-clonic seizures.
[d] Enhancement of GABA responses.
[e] Block of pentylenotetrazol seizures.
[f] Block of generalized absence seizures.

formation to phenobarbital has been blocked. We have not been able to demonstrate that it has effects on repetitive firing at therapeutic free-serum concentrations. However, it is possible that despite the blockade of metabolic transformation of primidone, there is some phenobarbital that is metabolically derived. Thus, it may be the synergistic action of phenobarbital and primidone that is responsible for the efficacy against MES seizures. Likewise, phenobarbital has effectiveness against MES seizures, but we have not been able to demonstrate thus far that phenobarbital limits repetitive firing at therapeutic free-serum concentrations. However, in the treatment of status epilepticus, free-serum phenobarbital levels are achieved that would be effective in limiting repetitive firing. The establishment of a role for valproic acid in enhancing GABAergic synaptic action remains unproven. Therefore this correlation remains tenuous. Finally, the most selective anticonvulsant drug for generalized absence and PTZ seizures is ethosuximide. Nevertheless, there has been no demonstration that ethosuximide enhances GABAergic synaptic transmission. This must be considered a major weakness in the general hypothesis that enhancement of GABAergic synaptic transmission is responsible for the efficacy against PTZ and generalized absence seizures of these anticonvulsant drugs.

While we have correlated two actions of these drugs with their anticonvulsant activities, by no means do we wish to imply that no other anticonvulsant mechanisms of these drugs exist. This approach must be considered to be in its preliminary stages, and all of the above hypotheses are subject to change. Nonetheless, it does appear striking that a large class of clinically useful anticonvulsant drugs can be demonstrated to have similar actions. It should be the goal of on-going studies of anticonvulsant drug mechanisms to test these hypotheses and to examine alternate hypotheses. The ultimate goal of these studies should be to develop a mechanistic classification of anticonvulsant drugs that should assist in the therapeutic management of patients with these epilepsies.

REFERENCES

1. Abdul-Ghani, A. S., Coutinho-Netto, J. Druce, D., and Bradford, H. F. (1981): Effects of anticonvulsants on the *in vivo* and *in vitro* release of GABA. *Biochem. Pharmacol.*, 30:367–368.
2. Aickin, C. C., Deisz, R. A., and Lux, H. D. (1981): On the action of the anticonvulsant 4,5-diphenylhydantoin and the convulsant picrotoxin in crayfish stretch receptor. *J. Physiol. (Lond.)*, 315:157–173.
3. Alderdice, M. T., and Trommer, B. A. (1980): Differential effects of the anticonvulsants phenobarbital, ethosuximide and carbamazepine on neuromuscular transmission. *J. Pharmcol. Exp. Ther.*, 215:92–96.
4. Anlezark, G., Horton, R. W., Meldrum, B. S., and Sawaya, C. B. (1976): Anticonvulsant action of ethanolamine-*o*-sulphate and di-*n*-prophylacetate and the metabolism of γ-aminobutyric acid (GABA) in mice with audiogenic seizures. *Biochem. Pharmacol.*, 25:413–417.
5. Asano, T., and Ogasawara, N. (1981): Chloride-dependent stimulation of GABA and benzodiazepine receptor binding by pentobarbital. *Brain Res.*, 225:212–216.
6. Ayala, G. F., Johnston, D., Lin, S., and Dichter, H. N. (1977): The mechanism of action of diphenylhydantoin on invertebrate neurons. II. Effects on synaptic mechanisms. *Brain Res.*, 121:259–270.
7. Ayala, G. F., Lin, S., and Johnston, D. (1977): The mechanism of action of diphenylhydantoin on invertebrate neurons. I. Effects on basic membrane properties. *Brain Res.*, 121:245–258.
8. Baldino, F., and Geller, H. M. (1981): Sodium valproate enhancement of gamma-amino-butyric acid (GABA) inhibition—Electrophysiological evidence for anticonvulsant activity. *J. Pharmacol. Exp. Ther.*, 217:445–450.
9. Barker, J. L., and McBurney, R. N. (1979): Phenobarbitone modulation of postsynaptic GABA receptor function on cultured mammalian neurons. *Proc. R. Soc. Lond. [Biol.]*, 206:319–327.
10. Barker, J. L., and Ransom, B. R. (1978): Pentobarbitone pharmacology of mammalian central neurones grown in tissue culture. *J. Physiol. (Lond.)*, 280:355–372.
11. Baumel, I. P., Gallagher, B. B., DiMicco, J., and Goico, H. (1973): Metabolism and anticonvulsant properties of primidone in the rat. *J. Pharmacol. Exp. Ther.*, 186:305–314.
12. Bean, B. P., Cohen, C. J., and Tsien, R. W. (1983): Lidocaine blockade of cardiac sodium channels. *J. Gen. Physiol.*, 81:613–642.
13. Blaustein, M. P. (1968): Barbiturates block sodium and potassium conductance increases in voltage-clamped lobster axons. *J. Gen. Physiol.*, 51:293–307.
14. Blaustein, M. P. (1976): Barbiturates block calcium uptake by stimulated and potassium-depolarized rat sympathetic ganglia. *J. Pharmacol. Exp. Ther.*, 196:80–86.
15. Blaustein, M. P., and Ector, A. C. (1975): Barbiturate inhibition of calcium uptake by depolarized nerve terminals in vitro. *Mol. Pharmacol.*, 11:369–378.
16. Blom, S. (1962): Trigeminal neuralgia: Its treatment with a new anticonvulsant drug (G-32883). *Lancet*, 1:839–840.
17. Bourgeois, B. F. D., Dodson, E., and Ferendelli, J. A. (1983): Primidone, phenobarbital and PEMA: I. Seizure protection, neurotoxicity and therapeutic index of individual compounds in mice. *Neurology*, 33:283–290.
18. Browne, T. R., and Penry, J. K. (1973): Benzodiazepines in the treatment of epilepsy: A review. *Epilepsia*, 14:277–310.

19. Browne, T. R., Dreifuss, F. E., Dyken, P. R., Goode, D. J., Penry, J. R., Porter, R. J., White, B. G., and White, P. T. (1975): Ethosuximide in the treatment of absence (petit mal) seizures. *Neurology*, 25:515–524.

20. Bruni, J., and Wilder, B. J. (1979): Valproic acid—Review of a new antiepileptic drug. *Arch. Neurol.*, 36:393–398.

21. Capek, R., and Esplin, B. (1977): Effects of ethosuximide on transmission of repetitive impulses and apparent rates of transmitter turnover in the spinal monosynaptic pathway. *J. Pharmacol. Exp. Ther.*, 201:320–325.

22. Carnay, L., and Grundfest, S. (1974): Excitable membrane stabilization by diphenylhydantoin and calcium. *Neuropharmacology*, 13:1097–1108.

23. Cereghino, J. J., Brock, J. T., Van Meter, J. C., Penry, J. K., Smith, L. D., and White, B. G. (1974): Carbamazepine for epilepsy. A controlled prospective evaluation. *Neurology*, 24:401–410.

24. Chapman, A., Keane, P. E., Meldrum, B. S., Simiand, J., and Vernieres, J. C. (1982): Mechanisms of anticonvulsant action of valproate. *Prog. Neurobiol.*, 19:315–359.

25. Chen, G., Weston, J. K., and Bralton, A. C., Jr. (1963): Anticonvulsant activity and toxicity of phensuximide, methsuximide and ethosuximide. *Epilepsia*, 4:66–76.

26. Choi, D. W., Farb, D. H., and Fischbach, G. D. (1977): Chlordiazepoxide selectively augments GABA action in spinal cord cell cultures. *Nature (Lond.)*, 269:342–344.

27. Choi, D. W., Farb, D. H., and Fischbach, G. D. (1981): Chlordiazepoxide selectively potentiates GABA conductance of spinal cord and sensory neurons in cell culture. *J. Neurophysiol.*, 45:621–631.

28. Connors, B. W. (1981): A comparison of the effects of pentobarbital and diphenylhydantoin on the GABA sensitivity and excitability of adult sensory ganglion cells. *Brain Res.*, 207:357–369.

29. Courtney, K. R., and Etter, E. F. (1983): Modulated anticonvulsant block of sodium sodium channels in nerve and muscle. *Eur. J. Pharmacol.*, 88:1–9.

30. Cramer, J. A., and Mattson, R. H. (1979): Valproic acid: *In vitro* plasma protein binding and interactions with phenytoin. *Ther. Drug Monit.*, 1:105–116.

31. Deisz, R. A., and Lux, H. D. (1977): Diphenylhydantoin prolongs postsynaptic inhibition and iontophoretic GABA action in the crayfish stretch receptor. *Neurosci. Lett.*, 5:199–203.

32. DeLorenzo, R. J. (1976): Calcium-dependent phosphorylation of specific synaptosomal fraction proteins: Possible role of phosphoproteins in mediating neurotransmitter release. *Biochem. Biophys. Res. Commun.*, 71:590–597.

33. Eadie, M. J., and Tyrer, J. H. (1980): *Anticonvulsant Therapy: Pharmacological Basis and Practice*. Churchill Livingstone, Edinburgh.

34. Emson, P. C. (1976): Effects of chronic treatment with amino-oxyacetic acid or sodium *n*-dipropyl-acetate on brain GABA levels and the development and regression of cobalt epileptic foci in rats. *J. Neurochem.*, 27:1489–1494.

35. Erwin, V. G., Dietrich, R. A. (1973): Inhibition of bovine brain aldehyde reductase by anticonvulsant compounds in vitro. *Biochem. Pharmacol.*, 22:2615–2624.

36. Esplin, D. (1957): Effect of diphenylhydantoin on synaptic transmission in the cat spinal cord and stellate ganglion. *J. Pharmacol. Exp. Ther.*, 120:301–323.

37. Ferrendelli, J. A., and Daniels-McQueen, S. (1982): Comparative actions of phenytoin and other anticonvulsant drugs on potassium- and veratridine-stimulated calcium uptake in synaptosomes. *J. Pharmacol. Exp. Ther.*, 220:29–34.

38. Ferrendelli, J. A., and Kinscherf, D. A. (1978): Similar effects of phenytoin and tetrodotoxin on cyclic nucleotide regulation in depolarized brain tissue. *J. Pharmacol. Exp. Ther.*, 207:787–793.

39. Ferrendelli, J. A., and Kupferberg, H. J. (1980): Succinimides. In: *Antiepileptic Drugs: Mechanisms of Action*, edited by G. H. Glaser, J. K. Penry, and D. M. Woodbury, pp. 587–596. Raven Press, New York.

40. Fincham, R. W., and Schottelius, D. D. (1982): Primidone. Interactions with other drugs. In: *Antiepileptic Drugs*, edited by D. M. Woodbury, J. K. Penry, and C. E. Pippenger, pp. 421–447. Raven Press, New York.

41. Gage, P. W., Lonergan, M., and Torda, T. A. (1980): Presynaptic and postsynaptic depressant effects of phenytoin sodium at the neuromuscular junction. *Br. J. Pharmacol.*, 69:119–121.

42. Gent, J. P., and Phillips, N. I. (1980): Sodium di-*n*-propylacetate (Valproate) potentiates responses to GABA and muscimol on single central neurones. *Brain Res.*, 197:275–278.

43. Gilbert, J. C., Buchan, P., and Scott, A. K. (1974): Effects of anticonvulsant drugs on monosaccharide transport and membrane ATPase activities of cerebral cortex. In: *Epilepsy*, edited by P. Harris and C. Maudsley, pp. 98–104. Churchill Livingstone, Edinburgh.

44. Gilbert, J. C., Scott, A. K., Wyllie, M. G. (1974): Effects of ethosuximide on adenosine triphosphatase activities of some subcellular fractions prepared from rat cerebral cortex. *Br. J. Pharmacol.*, 50:452–453.

45. Gilbert, J. C., and Wyllie M. G. (1974): The effects of the anticonvulsant ethosuximide on adenosine triphosphatase activities of synaptosomes prepared from rat cerebral cortex. *Br. J. Pharmacol.*, 52:139–140.

46. Godin, Y., Heiner, L., Mark, J., and Mandel, P. (1969): Effects of di-*n*-propylacetate, an anticonvulsant compound, on GABA metabolism. *J. Neurochem.*, 19:869–873.

47. Goldring, J. M., and Blaustein, M. P. (1976): Barbiturates block Ca spikes but not Na spikes in *Aplysia* neurons. *Soc. Neurosci. Abstr.*, 2:411.

48. Goldring, J. M., and Blaustein, M. P. (1982): Effect of pentobarbital on Na and Ca action potentials in an invertebrate neuron. *Brain Res.*, 240:273–283.

49. Goodman, L. S., Grewal, M. S., Brown, W. C., and Swinyard, A. E. (1953): Comparison of

maximal seizures evoked by pentylenetetrazol (Metrazol) and electroshock in mice, and their modification by anticonvulsants. *J. Pharmacol. Exp. Ther.*, 108:168–176.

50. Goodman, L. S., Swinyard, E. A., Brown, W. C., Schiffman, D. O., Grewal, M. S., and Bliss, E. L. (1953): Anticonvulsant properties of 5-phenyl-5-ethyl-hexahydroprimidine-4,6-dione (Mysoline), a new antiepileptic. *J. Pharmacol. Exp. Ther.*, 108:428–436.

51. Guidotti, A., Toffano, G., and Costa, E. (1978): An endogenous protein modulates the affinity of GABA and benzodiazepine receptors in rat brain. *Nature (Lond.)*, 275:553–555.

52. Hackman, J. C., Grayson, V., Davidoff, R. A. (1981): The presynaptic effects of valproic acid in the isolated frog spinal cord. *Brain Res.*, 220:269–285.

53. Haefely, W. E. (1980): GABA and the anticonvulsant action of benzodiazepines and barbiturates. *Brain Res. Bull.*, 5:873–878.

54. Handley, R., Stewart, A. S. R. (1951): Mysoline: A new drug in the treatment of epilepsy. *Lancet*, I:742–744.

55. Harrison, N. L., and Simmonds, M. A. (1982): Sodium valproate enhances responses to GABA receptor activation only at high concentrations. *Brain Res.*, 250:201–204.

56. Harvey, P. K. P., Bradford, H. F., and Davison, A. N. (1975): The inhibitory effect of sodium *n*-dipropylacetate on the degradative enzymes of the GABA shunt. *FEBS Lett.*, 52:251–254.

57. Hasbani, M., Pincus, J., and Lee, S. H. (1974): Diphenylhydantoin and calcium movement in lobster nerves. *Arch. Neurol.*, 31:250–254.

58. Hauptmann, A. (1912): Luminal bei Epilepsie. *Muenchen Med. Wochenschr.*, 59:1907–1909.

59. Hayashi, T., and Negishi, K. (1979): Suppression of retinal spike discharge by dipropylacetate (Depakene): A possible involvement of GABA. *Brain Res.*, 175:271–278.

60. Hershkowitz, N., Ayala, G. F. (1981): Effects of phenytoin on pyramidal neurons of the rat hippocampus. *Brain Res.*, 208:487–492.

61. Hershkowitz, N., Dretchen, K. L., and Raines, A. (1978): Carbamazepine suppression of posttetanic potentiation at the neuromuscular junction. *J. Pharmacol. Exp. Ther.*, 207:810–816.

62. Hershkowitz, N., and Raines, A. (1978): Effects of carbamazepine on muscle spindle discharges. *J. Pharmacol. Exp. Ther.*, 204:581–591.

63. Heyer, E. J., and Macdonald, R. L. (1982): Barbiturate reduction of calcium-dependent action potentials: Correlation with anesthetic action. *Brain Res.*, 236:157–171.

64. Hille, B. (1977): Local anesthetics: Hydrophilic and hydrophobic pathways for the drug-receptor reaction. *J. Gen. Physiol.*, 69:497–515.

65. Hondeghem, L. M., and Katzung, B. G. (1977): Time- and voltage-dependent interactions of antiarrhythmic drugs with cardiac sodium channels. *Biochim. Biophys. Acta*, 472:373–398.

66. Iadarola, M. J., and Gale, K. (1979): Dissociation between drug-induced increase in nerve terminal and non-nerve terminal pools of GABA *in vivo*. *Eur. J. Pharmacol.*, 59:125–129.

67. Iadarola, M. J., and Gale, K. (1980): Evaluation of increase in nerve terminal-dependent nerve terminal-independent compartments of GABA *in vivo*. *Brain Res. Bull.*, 5:13–19.

68. Julien, R. M., and Hollister, R. D. (1975): Carbamazepine mechanism of action. *Adv. Neurol.*, 11:263–276.

69. Kendig, J. J., Courtney, K. R., and Cohen, E. N. (1979): Anesthetics: Molecular correlates of voltage- and frequency-dependent sodium channel block in nerve. *J. Pharmacol. Exp. Ther.*, 210:446–452.

70. Kerwin, R. W., Olpe, H.-R., and Schmutz, M. (1980): The effect of sodium-*n*-dipropylacetate on γ-aminobutyric acid-dependent inhibition in the rat cortex and substantia nigra in relation to its anticonvulsant activity. *Br. J. Pharmacol.*, 71:545–551.

71. Kerwin, R. W., and Taberner, P. V. (1981): The mechanism of action of sodium valproate. *Gen. Pharmacol.*, 12:71–75.

72. Khodorov, B. I. (1981): Sodium inactivation and drug-induced immobilization of the gating charge in nerve membrane. *Prog. Biophys. Mol. Biol.*, 37:49–89.

73. Khodorov, B. I., Shishkova, L., Peganov, E., and Rovenko, S. (1976): Inhibition of sodium currents in frog Ranvier node treated with local anesthetics. Role of slow sodium inactivation. *Biochim. Biophys. Acta*, 433:409–435.

74. Killam, E. K., and Suria, A. (1980): Benzodiazepines. In: *Antiepileptic Drugs: Mechanisms of Action*, edited by G. H. Glaser, J. K. Penry, and D. M. Woodbury, pp. 597–615. Raven Press, New York.

75. Korey, S. R. (1951): Effect of dilantin and mesantoin on the giant axon of the squid. *Proc. Soc. Exp. Biol. Med.*, 76:297–299.

76. Krall, R. L., Penry, J. K., White, B. G., Kupferberg, H. J., and Swinyard, E. A. (1978): Antiepileptic drug development: II. Anticonvulsant drug screening. *Epilepsia*, 19:409–428.

77. Kupferberg, H. J. (1980): Sodium Valproate. In: *Antiepileptic Drugs: Mechanisms of Action*, edited by G. H. Glaser, J. K. Penry, and D. M. Woodbury, pp. 643–654. Raven Press, New York.

78. Lee, K. S., Hume, J. R., Giles, W., and Brown, A. M. (1981): Sodium current depression by lidocaine and quinidine in isolated ventricular cells. *Nature (Lond.)*, 291:325–327.

79. Leeb-Lundberg, F., and Olsen, R. W. (1982): Interactions of barbiturates of various pharmacological categories with benzodiazepine receptors. *Mol. Pharmacol.*, 21:320–328.

80. Leslie, S. W., Friedman, M. B., and Coleman, R. R. (1980): Effects of chlordiazepoxide on depolarization-induced calcium influx into synaptosomes. *Biochem. Pharmacol.*, 29:2439–2443.

81. Leznicki, A., and Dymecki, J. (1974): The effect of certain anticonvulsants *in vitro* and *in vivo* on enzyme activities in the rat's brain. *Neurol. Neurochir. Pol.*, 24/3:413–419.

82. Lipicky, R. J., Gilbert, D. L., and Stillman, I. M. (1971): Diphenylhydantoin inhibition of sodium conductance in squid giant axon. *Proc. Natl. Acad. Sci. U.S.A.*, 69:1758–1760.

83. Loscher, W. (1979): 3-mercaptoproprionic acid: Convulsant properties, effects on enzymes of the γ-aminobutyrate system in mouse brain and antagonism by certain anticonvulsant drugs, aminooxyacetic acid and gabaculline. *Biochem. Pharmacol.*, 28:1397–1407.

84. Loscher, W. (1980): Effect of inhibitors of GABA transaminase on the synthesis, binding, uptake and metabolism of GABA. *J. Neurochem.*, 34:1603–1608.

85. Loscher, W. (1981): Valproate induced changes in GABA metabolism at the subcellular level. *Biochem. Pharmacol.*, 30:1364–1366.

86. Loscher, W. (1981): Relationship between drug-induced changes in seizure thresholds and the GABA content of brain and brain nerve endings. *Naunyn. Schmiedbergs Arch. Pharmacol.*, 317:131–134.

87. Loscher, W., Bohme, G., Schafer, H., and Kochen, W. (1981): Effect of metabolites of valproic acid on the metabolism of GABA in brain and brain nerve endings. *Neuropharmacology*, 20:1187–1192.

88. Loscher, W., and Frey, H.-H. (1977): On the mechanism of action of valproic acid. *Arzneimittelforsch.*, 27:1081–1082.

89. Loscher, W., and Frey, H.-H. (1977): Effect of convulsant and anticonvulsant agents on level and metabolism of γ-aminobutyric acid in mouse brain. *Naunyn. Schmiedbergs Arch. Pharmacol.*, 296:263–269.

90. Lust, W. D., Kupferberg, H. J., Passonneau, J. V., and Penry, J. K. (1976): On the mechanism of action of sodium valproate: The relationship of GABA and cyclic GMP levels to anticonvulsant activity. In: *Clinical and Pharmacological Aspects of Sodium Valproate (Epilim) in the Treatment of Epilepsy*, edited by N. J. Legg, pp. 123–129. MCS Consultants, Tunbridge Wells, England.

91. Macdonald, R. L. (1983): Mechanisms of anticonvulsant drug action. In: *Recent Advances in Epilepsy I*, edited by T. A. Pedley and B. S. Meldrum, pp. 1–23. Churchill Livingstone, Edinburgh.

92. Macdonald, R. L., and Barker, J. L. (1978): Different actions of anticonvulsant and anesthetic barbiturates revealed by use of cultured mammalian neurons. *Science*, 200:775–777.

93. Macdonald, R. L., and Barker, J. L. (1978): Benzodiazepines specifically modulate GABA-mediated postsynaptic inhibition in cultured mammalian neurones. *Nature (Lond.)*, 271:563–564.

94. Macdonald, R. L., and Barker, J. L. (1979): Anticonvulsant and anesthetic barbiturates: Different postsynaptic actions on cultured mammalian neurons. *Neurology*, 29:432–447.

95. Macdonald, R. L., and Barker, J. L. (1979): Enhancement of GABA-mediated postsynaptic inhibition in cultured mammalian spinal cord neurons: A common mode of anticonvulsant action. *Brain Res.*, 167:323–336.

96. Macdonald, R. L., and Bergey, G. K. (1979): Valproic acid augments GABA-mediated postsynaptic inhibition in cultured mammaliam neurons. *Brain Res.*, 170:558–562.

97. Macdonald, R. L., and McLean, M. J. (1982): Cellular bases of barbiturate and phenytoin anticonvulsant drug action. *Epilepsia*, 23(Suppl. 1):S7–S18.

98. Werz, M. A., and Macdonald, R. L. (1985): Barbiturates decrease voltage-dependent calcium conductance of mouse neurons in dissociated cell culture. *Mol. Pharmacol.* 28:269–277.

99. Masuda, Y., Utsui, Y., Shinaishi, Y., Karasawa, T., Yoshida, K., and Shimizu, M. (1979): Relationship between plasma concentrations of diphenylhydantoin, phenobarbital, carbamazepine and 3-sulfamoylmethyl, 1,2-benisoxazole (AD-810), a new anticonvulsant agent, and their anticonvulsant or neurotoxic effects in experimental animals. *Epilepsia*, 20:623–633.

100. Matsuki, N., Quandt, F. N., Yeh, J. Z., and Ten Eick, R. (1981): Sodium channel blocking action of phenytoin in mammalian neurons in tissue cultures. *Soc. Neurosci. Abstr.*, 7:811.

101. Matthews, W. D., and Connor, J. D. (1977): Actions of iontophoretic phenytoin and medazepam on hippocampal neurons. *J. Pharmacol. Exp. Ther.*, 201:613–621.

102. McLean, M. J., and Macdonald, R. L. (1981): Phenytoin effects on action potentials of fetal mouse spinal cord neurons in cell culture. *Soc. Neurosci. Abstr.*, 7:629.

103. McLean, M. J., and Macdonald, R. L. (1983): Multiple actions of phenytoin on mouse spinal cord neurons in cell culture. *J. Pharmacol. Exp. Ther.*, 227:779–789.

104. McLean, M. J., and Macdonald, R. L. (1984): Limitation of high frequency repetitive firing of cultured mouse neurons by anticonvulsant drugs. *Neurology*, 34(suppl. 1):288.

105. McLean, M. J., Taylor, C. P., and Macdonald, R. L. (1984): Phenytoin and carbamazepine limit sustained high frequency repetitive firing of action potentials of hippocampal neurons in cell culture and tissue slices. *Soc. Neurosci. Abstr.*, 10:873.

106. Meiners, B. A., and Salama, A. I. (1982): Enhancement of benzodiazepine and GABA binding by the novel anxiolytic, tracazolate. *Eur. J. Pharmacol.*, 78:315–322.

107. Merritt, H. H., and Putnam, T. J. (1938): A new series of anticonvulsant drugs tested by experiments on animals. *Arch. Neurol. Psychiatry*, 39:1003–1015.

108. Meunier, G., Carraz, G., Meunier, Y., Eymard, P., and Aimard, M. (1963): Propriétés pharmacodynamiques de l'acide *n*-propylacetique. *Therapie*, 18:435–438.

109. Mitchell, P. R., and Martin, I. L. (1978): The effects of benzodiazepines on K+-stimulated release of GABA. *Neuropharmacology*, 17:317–320.

110. Mohler, H., and Okada, T. (1977): Benzodiazepine receptor: Demonstration in the central nervous system. *Science*, 198:849–851.

111. Morgan, K. G., and Bryant, S. H. (1977): Pentobarbital: Presynaptic effect in the squid giant synapse. *Experientia*, 33:487–488.

112. Narahashi, T. (1974): Chemicals as tools in the

study of excitable membranes. *Physiol. Rev.*, 54:813–889.

113. Narahashi, T., Frazier, D. T., Deguchi, T., Cleaves, C. A., and Ernau, M. C. (1971): The active form of pentobarbital in squid giant axon. *J. Pharmacol. Exp. Ther.*, 117:25–33.

114. Narahashi, T., Moore, J. W., and Poston, R. N. (1969): Anesthetic blocking of nerve membrane conductances by internal and external applications. *J. Neurobiol.*, 1:3–22.

115. Neuman, R. S., and Frank, G. B. (1977): Effects of dephenylhydantoin and phenobarbital on voltage clamped myelinated nerve. *Can. J. Physiol. Pharmacol.*, 55:42–47.

116. Nicoll, R. A. (1975): Pentobarbital: Action on frog motoneurons. *Brain Res.*, 96:119–123.

117. Nicoll, R. A. (1975): Presynaptic action of barbiturates in the frog spinal cord. *Proc. Natl. Acad. Sci. U.S.A.*, 72:1460–1463.

118. Nicoll, R. A. (1978): Selective actions of barbiturates on synaptic transmission. In: *Psychopharmacology: A Generation of Progress*, edited by M. A. Lipton, A. DiMascio, and K. F. Killam, pp. 1337–1348. Raven Press, New York.

119. Nicoll, R. A., Eccles, J. C., Oshima, T., and Rubia, F. (1975): Prolongation of hippocampal inhibitory postsynaptic potentials by barbiturates. *Nature (Lond.)*, 258:625–627.

120. Nicoll, R. A., and Wojtowicz, J. M. (1980): The effects of pentobarbital and related compounds on frog motoneurons. *Brain Res.*, 191:225–237.

121. Olpe, H.-R., and Jones, R. S. G. (1983): The mechanism of anticonvulsant drugs of the firing of locus coeruleus neurons: Selective activation effect of carbamazepine. *Eur. J. Pharmacol.*, 91:107–110.

122. Olsen, R. W., Lamar, E. E., and Bayless, J. D. (1977): Calcium-induced release of γ-aminobutyric acid from synaptosomes: Effects of tranquilizer drugs. *Neurochemistry*, 28:299–305.

123. Olsen, R. W., Leeb-Lundberg, F., and Napias, C. (1980): Picrotoxin and convulsant binding sites in mammalian brain. *Brain Res. Bull.*, 5(Supplement 2):217–221.

124. Olsen, R. W., and Snowman, A. M. (1982): Chloride-dependent enhancement by barbiturates of γ-aminobutyric acid receptor binding. *J. Neurosci.*, 2:1812–1823.

125. Olsen, R. W., Ticku, M. K., Van Ness, P. C. and Greenlee, D. (1978): Effects of drugs on γ-aminobutyric acid receptors, uptake, release and synthesis in vitro. *Brain Res.*, 139:277–294.

126. Ondrusek, M. G., Belknap, J. K., and Leslie, S. W. (1979): Effects of acute and chronic barbiturate administration on synaptosomal calcium accumulation. *Mol. Pharmacol.*, 15:386–395.

127. Patsalos, P. N., and Lascelles, P. T. (1981): Changes in regional brain levels of amino acid putative neurotransmitters after prolonged treatment with the anticonvulsant drugs diphenylhydantoin, phenobarbitone, sodium valproate, ethosuximide, and sulthiame in the rat. *J. Neurochem.*, 36:688–695.

128. Perry, J. G., McKinney, L., and DeWeer, P. (1978): The cellular mode of action of the anti-

epileptic drug 5,5-diphenylhydantoin. *Nature (Lond.)*, 272:271–273.

129. Pincus, J. H. (1977): Anticonvulsant actions at a neuromuscular synapse. *Neurology*, 27:374–375.

130. Pincus, J. H., and Lee, S. H. (1973): Diphenylhydantoin and calcium: Relation to norepinephrine release from brain slices. *Arch. Neurol.*, 29:239–244.

131. Pinder, R. M., Brogden, T. M., Speight, T. M., and Avery, G. S. (1977): Sodium valproate: A review of its pharmacological properties and therapeutic efficacy in epilepsy. *Drugs*, 13:81–123.

132. Polc, P., and Haefely, W. (1976): Effects of two benzodiazepines, phenobarbitone and baclofen, on synaptic transmission in cat cuneate nucleus. *Naunyn Schmiedebergs Arch. Pharmacol.*, 294:121–131.

133. Polc, P., Mohler, H., and Haefely, W. (1974): The effect of diazepam on spinal cord activities: Possible sites and mechanisms of action. *Naunyn Schmiedbergs Arch. Pharmacol.*, 284:319–337.

134. Prichard, J. W. (1980): Phenobarbital: Introduction. In: *Antiepileptic Drugs: Mechanisms of Action*, edited by G. H. Glaser, J. K. Penry, and D. M. Woodbury, pp. 473–562. Raven Press, New York.

135. Quatrone, A., and Samanin, R. (1977): Decreased anticonvulsant activity of carbamazepine in 6-hydroxydopamine-treated rats. *Eur. J. Pharmacol.*, 41:333–338.

136. Raabe, W., and Gumnit, R. J. (1977): Anticonvulsant action of diazepam: Increase of cortical postsynaptic inhibition. *Epilepsia*, 18:117–120.

137. Raines, A., and Standaert, F. G. (1966): Pre- and postjunctional effects of DPH at the cat soleus neuromuscular junction. *J. Pharmacol. Exp. Ther.*, 153:361–366.

138. Raines, A., Niner, J. M., and Pace, D. G. (1973): A comparison of the anticonvulsant, neurotoxic and lethal effects of diphenylbarbituric acid, phenobarbital and diphenylhydantoin in the mouse. *J. Pharmacol. Exp. Ther.*, 186:315–322.

139. Randall, L. O., Heise, G. A., Schallek, W., Bagdon, R. E., Banziger, R., Boris, A., and Abrams, W. B. (1961): Pharmacological and clinical studies on valium: A new psychotherapeutic agent of the benzodiazepine class. *Curr. Ther. Res.*, 3:405–425.

140. Ransom, B. R., and Barker, J. L. (1976): Pentobarbital selectively enhances GABA-mediated postsynaptic inhibition in tissue cultured mouse spinal neurons. *Brain Res.*, 114:530–535.

141. Rock, D. M., McLean, M. J., and Macdonald, R. L. (1984): Sodium valproate selectively limits sustained high frequency repetitive firing of cultured mouse neurons. *Soc. Neurosci. Abstr.*, 10:872.

142. Rosenberg, P., and Bartels, E. (1967): Drug effects on the spontaneous electrical activity of the squid giant synapse. *J. Pharmacol. Exp. Ther.*, 155:532–544.

143. Rudzik, A. D., and Mennear, J. H. (1965): The

mechanism of action of anticonvulsants. I. Diphenylhydantoin. *Life Sci.,* 4:2373–2377.

144. Sarhan, S., and Seiler, N. (1979): Metabolic inhibitors and subcellular distribution of GABA. *J. Neurosci. Res.,* 4:399–421.

145. Sastry, S. R., and Phillis, J. W. (1976): Antagonism of glutamate and acetylcholine excitation of rat cerebral cortical neurones by diphenylhydantoin. *Gen. Pharmacol.,* 7:411–413.

146. Sawaya, M. C. B., Horton, R. W., and Meldrum, B. S. (1975): Effects of anticonvulsant drugs on the cerebral enzymes metabolizing GABA. *Epilepsia,* 16:649–655.

147. Schauf, C. L., Davis, F. A., and Marder, J. (1974): Effects of carbamazepine on the ionic conductances of *Myxicola* giant axons. *J. Pharmacol. Exp. Ther.,* 189:538–543.

148. Schmidt, R. F., Vogel, M. E., and Zimmermann, M. (1967): Die wirkung von diazepam auf die präsynaptische hemmung und andere rücken marksreflexe. *Naunyn Schmiedebergs Arch. Pharmacol.,* 258:69–82.

149. Schneiderman, J. H., and Schwartzkroin, P. A. (1982): Effects of phenytoin on normal activity and on penicillin-induced bursting in the guinea pig hippocampal slice. *Neurology,* 32:730–738.

150. Schulz, D. W., and Macdonald, R. L. (1981): Barbiturate enhancement of GABA-mediated inhibition and activation of chloride ion conductance: Correlation with anticonvulsant and anesthetic actions. *Brain Res.,* 209:177–188.

151. Schwarz, J. R. (1979): The mode of action of phenobarbital on the excitable membrane of the node of Ranvier. *Eur. J. Pharmacol.,* 56:51–60.

152. Schwarz, J., and Vogel, W. (1977): Diphenylhydantoin: Excitability reducing action in single myelinated nerve fibers. *Eur. J. Pharmacol.,* 44:241–249.

153. Schwarz, J., and Spielmann, R. P. (1983): Flurazepam: Effects on sodium and potassium currents in myelinated nerve fibers. *Eur. J. Pharmacol.,* 90:359–366.

154. Seeman, P. (1972): The membrane action of anesthetics and tranquilizers. *Pharmacol. Rev.,* 24:583–655.

155. Selzer, M. E. (1979): The effect of phenytoin on the action potential of a vertebrate spinal neuron. *Brain Res.,* 171:511–521.

156. Sherwin, A. L., Eisen, A. A., and Sokolowski, C. D. (1973): Anticonvulsant drugs in human epileptogenic brain. *Arch. Neurol.,* 29:73–77.

157. Sherwin, A. K., and Robb, J. P. (1972): Ethosuximide: Relation of plasma level to clinical control. In: *Antiepileptic Drugs,* edited by D. M. Woodbury, J. K. Penry, and R. P. Schmidt, pp. 443–448. Raven Press, New York.

158. Shrager, P. (1977): Slow sodium inactivation in nerve after exposure to sulfhydryl blocking reagents. *J. Gen. Physiol.,* 69:183–202.

159. Shuto, N., and Nishigaki, T. (1970): The pharmacological studies on sodium dipropylacetate: Anticonvulsant activities and general pharmacological actions. *Pharmacokinetics,* 4:937–949.

160. Simler, S., Ziesielski, L., Maitre, M., Randrianarisoa, H., and Mandel, P. (1973): Effect of sodium di-*n*-propylacetate on audiogenic seizures and brain gamma-aminobutyric acid level. *Biochem. Pharmacol.,* 22:1701–1708.

161. Simon, D., and Penry, J. K. (1975): Sodium di-*n*-propylacetate (DPA) in the treatment of epilepsy. *Epilepsia,* 16:549–573.

162. Sironi, V. A., Cabrini, G., Porro, M. G., Ravagnati, L., and Maroserro, F. (1980): Anti-epileptic drug distribution in cerebral cortex, Ammon's horn, and amygdala. *J. Neurosurg.,* 52:686–692.

163. Skerritt, J. H., Davies, L. P., and Johnston, G. A. R. (1982): A purinergic component in the anticonvulsant action of carbamazepine. *Eur. J. Pharmacol.,* 82:195–197.

164. Skerritt, J. H., and Johnston, G. A. R. (1983): Interactions of carbamazepine with benzodiazepine receptors. *J. Pharm. Pharmacol.,* 35:464–465.

165. Skerritt, J. H., and Macdonald, R. L. (1983): Benzodiazepine Ro15-1788: Electrophysiological evidence for partial agonist activity. *Neurosci. Lett.,* 43:321–326.

166. Skerritt, J. H., and Macdonald, R. L. (1984): Diazepam enhances the action but not the binding of the GABA analog, THIP. *Brain Res.,* 297:181–186.

167. Skerritt, J. H., and Macdonald, R. L. (1984): Benzodiazepine receptor ligand actions on GABA responses: Benzodiazepines, CL 218-872, zopiclone. *Eur. J. Pharmacol.,* 101:127–134.

168. Skerritt, J. H., Werz, M. A., McLean, M. J., and Macdonald, R. L. (1974): Diazepam and its anomalous *p*-chloro-derivative Ro5-4864. Comparative effects on mouse neurons in cell culture. *Brain Res.,* 310:99–105.

169. Skerritt, J. H., Willow, M., and Johnston, G. A. R. (1982): Diazepam enhancement of low affinity GABA binding to rat brain membranes. *Neurosci. Lett.,* 29:63–66.

170. Sohn, R. S., and Ferrendelli, J. A. (1976): Anticonvulsant drug mechanisms. *Arch. Neurol.,* 33:626–629.

171. Squires, R. F., and Braestrup, C. (1977): Benzodiazepine receptors in rat brain. *Nature (Lond.),* 66:732–734.

172. Strichartz, G. R. (1973): The inhibition of sodium currents in myelinated nerve by quaternary derivatives of lidocaine. *J. Gen. Physiol.,* 62:37–57.

173. Study, R. E. (1980): Phenytoin inhibition of cyclic guanosine 3′5′-monophosphate (cGMP) accumulation in neuroblastoma cells by calcium channel blockade. *J. Pharmacol. Exp. Ther.,* 215:575–581.

174. Study, R. E., and Barker, J. L. (1981): Diazepam and (±)-pentobarbital: Fluctuation analysis reveals different mechanisms for potentiation of γ-aminobutyric acid responses in cultured central neurons. *Proc. Natl. Acad. Sci. U.S.A.,* 78:7180–7184.

175. Suria, A., and Killam, E. K. (1980): Antiepileptic drugs: Carbamazepine. In: *Antiepileptic Drugs: Mechanisms of Action,* edited by G. H. Glaser, J. K. Penry, and D. M. Woodbury, pp. 563–575. Raven Press, New York.

176. Swinyard, E. A. (1964): *The Pharmacology of*

Dipropylacetate Sodium, pp. 1–23. University of Utah, Salt Lake City.

177. Swinyard, E. A. (1972): Assay of antiepileptic drug activity in experimental animals: Standard tests. In: *Anticonvulsant Drugs, International Encyclopedia of Pharmacology and Therapeutics*, Section 19, Vol. 1, pp. 47–65. Pergamon Press, Oxford.

178. Swinyard, E. A., Brown, W. C., and Goodman, L. S. (1952): Comparative assays of antiepileptic drugs in mice and rats. *J. Pharmacol. Exp. Ther.*, 106:47–59.

179. Swinyard, E. A., and Castellion, A. W. (1966): Anticonvulsant properties of some benzodiazepines. *J. Pharmacol. Exp. Ther.*, 151:369–375.

180. Theobald, V. W., and Kunz, H. A. (1963): Pharmacology of the antiepileptic drug 5-carbamyl-5*H*-dibenzo(b,f)azepine. *Arzneimittelforsch.*, 13:122–125.

181. Ticku, M. K., and Davis, W. C. (1981): Effect of valproic acid on [³H]diazepam and [³H]-dihydropicrotoxinin binding sites at the benzodiazepine-GABA receptor-ionophore complex. *Brain Res.*, 223:218–222.

182. Ticku, M. K., and Olsen, R. W. (1978): Interaction of barbiturates with dihydropicrotoxin in binding sites related to the GABA receptor-ionophore system. *Life Sci.*, 22:1643–1651.

183. Toman, J. E. P. (1949): The neuropharmacology of antiepileptics. *Electroencephalogr. Clin. Neurophysiol.*, 1:33–44.

184. Troupin, A. S. (1983): Carbamazepine re-examined. In: *Recent Advances in Epilepsy. I.*, edited by T. A. Pedley and B. S. Meldrum, pp. 47–58. Churchill Livingstone, Edinburgh.

185. Tuttle, J. B., and Richelson, E. (1979): Phenytoin action on the excitable membrane of mouse neuroblastoma. *J. Pharmacol. Exp. Ther.*, 211:632–637.

186. Van der Kleijn, E., Guelen, P. J. M., Van Wijk, C., and Baars, I. (1975): Clinical pharmacokinetics in monitoring chronic medication with antiepileptic drugs. In: *Clinical Pharmacology of Antiepileptic Drugs*, edited by H. Schneider, D. Janz, C. Gardner-Thorpec, H. Mienardi, and A. L. Sherwin, pp. 11–13. Springer, Berlin.

187. Van der Laan, J. W., De Boer, T. H., and Bruinvels, J. (1979): Di-*n*-propylacetate and GABA degradation. Preferential inhibition of succinic semialdehyde dehydrogenase and indirect inhibition of GABA-transaminase. *J. Neurochem.*, 32:1769–1780.

188. Vyskocil, F. (1977): Diazepam blockade of repetitive action potentials in skeletal muscle fibers. A model of its membrane action. *Brain Res.*, 133:315–328.

189. Wang, C. M., and James, C. A. (1979): An analysis of the direct effect of chlordiazepoxide on mammalian cardiac tissues and crayfish and squid giant axons: Possible basis of antiarrhythmic activity. *Life Sci.*, 24:1357–1366.

190. Wilder, B. J., and Bruni, J. (1981): *Seizure Disorders: A Pharmacological Approach to Treatment*. Raven Press, New York.

191. Willow, M., and Johnston, G. A. R. (1981): Enhancement by anesthetic and convulsant barbiturates of GABA binding to rat brain synaptosomal membranes. *J. Neurosci.*, 1:364–367.

192. Wolf, P., and Haas, H. L. (1977): Effects of diazepines and barbiturates on hippocampal recurrent inhibition. *Naunyn Schmiedbergs Arch. Pharmacol.*, 299:211–218.

193. Wood, J. D. (1975): The role of γ-aminobutyric acid in the mechanism of seizures. *Prog. Neurobiol.*, 5:77–95.

194. Wood, J. D., Kurylo, E., and Tsui, S.-K. (1981): Interactions of di-*n*-propylacetate, gabacullin, and aminooxyacetic acid: Anticonvulsant activity and the γ-aminobutyrate system. *J. Neurochem.*, 37:1440–1447.

195. Woodbury, D. M. (1980): Phenytoin: Introduction and history. In: *Antiepileptic Drugs: Mechanism of Action*, edited by G. H. Glaser, J. K. Penry, and D. M. Woodbury, pp. 305–313. Raven Press, New York.

196. Woodbury, D. M., and Pippenger, C. E. (1982): Primidone. Mechanisms of action. In: *Antiepileptic Drugs*, edited by D. M. Woodbury, J. K. Penry, and C. E. Pippenger, pp. 449–452. Raven Press, New York.

197. Yaari, Y., Pincus, J. H., and Argov, Z. (1977): Depression of synaptic transmission by diphenylhydantoin. *Ann. Neurol.*, 1:334–338.

198. Yaari, Y., Pincus, J. H., and Argov, Z. (1979): Phenytoin and transmitter release at the neuromuscular junction of the frog. *Brain Res.*, 160:479–487.

199. Yeh, J. Z. (1978): Sodium inactivation mechanism modulates QX-314 block of sodium channels in squid axons. *Biophys. J.*, 24:569–574.

200. Zbicz, K. L., and Wilson, W. A. (1981): Barbiturate enhancement of spike frequency adaptation in *Aplysia* giant neurons. *J. Pharmacol. Exp. Ther.*, 217:222–227.

Section 6

NEUROCELLULAR ANATOMY AND EPILEPTIC CELL DAMAGE

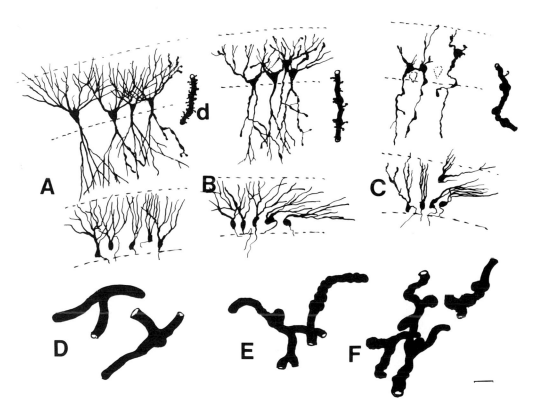

Histological changes in temporal lobe epilepsy. Three levels of alterations seen in hippocampal pyramids (*upper ensembles*) and dentate granule cells (*lower ensembles*) are indicated in **A, B,** and **C**. The "windblown" look of dentate cells is sketched in B and C; one cell with the closed parasol deformity appears in C. A length of hippocampal dendrite *d* is shown for each stage—indicating the progressive loss of spines and developing "lumpiness" or "string of beads" appearance of the dendrite shaft. Drawings **D, E,** and **F** show progressive degrees of distortion of the microvasculature. Note the tiny outpouchings, some of which may be tiny aneurysms. Calibration for D, E, F is 5 μm. From Chapter 39 in this volume by L. A. Paul and A. B. Scheibel.

Advances in Neurology, Vol. 44, edited by
A. V. Delgado-Escueta, A. A. Ward, Jr.,
D. M. Woodbury, and R. J. Porter.
Raven Press, New York © 1986.

37

Contemporary Methods in Neurocytology and Their Application to the Study of Epilepsy

Charles E. Ribak

Department of Anatomy, University of California, Irvine, California 92717

SUMMARY The contemporary neuroanatomist has a number of available methods to analyze epileptic brain tissue. Many studies have utilized Nissl- and Golgi-stained preparations to determine that gliosis and neuronal loss occur at epileptic foci as well as a decrease in the dendritic spine density. These structural changes did not reveal any specific basic mechanism that may cause epileptic activity. In contrast, the relatively newer techniques in neurocytology provide functional data that relate to the physiology and chemistry of the brain tissue. The use of immunocytochemical, histochemical, and receptor ligand-binding autoradiographic methods have aided in the understanding of cellular neurochemistry in both normal and epileptic tissue. In addition, the use of intracellular horseradish peroxidase and recording and quantitative morphological methods at both light- and electron-microscopic levels has helped gain insights into the functional state of synapses and neurons. Together, these methods have been utilized to help unravel the mystery of epilepsy.

Our laboratory has utilized immunocytochemical and quantitative light- and electron-microscopic methods to analyze four models of epilepsy; two resemble posttraumatic focal epilepsy, and the other two are genetic models of epilepsy. Our data indicate that a preferential loss of cortical GABAergic, inhibitory terminals occurs at posttraumatic epileptic foci. In contrast, the genetic models of epilepsy did not display a loss of GABAergic terminals. Instead, specific brain regions of epileptic animals had an increased number of GABAergic neurons and terminals. These data indicate that two different neuronal circuits may provide the anatomical substrate for epileptic activity: loss of inhibition and disinhibition.

METHODS IN NEUROCYTOLOGY

The neuroscientist has a number of cytological methods to analyze epileptic brain tissue. An analysis of the neuronal architecture is essential for an understanding of both normal and abnormal neuronal circuitry. Our ability to glean this knowledge of neural systems is dependent on the proper use and interpretation of methods used in neurocytology.

These methods can be divided into two general categories: classical and contemporary methods. The classical methods have been in use the longest and include Nissl, Golgi, and fiber stains as well as electron microscopy. Most studies of epileptic brains have utilized only these methods. In contrast, the contemporary methods have developed over the past decade or so, and their application to brain studies has greatly expanded our knowledge of neuroanatomy. The latter methods include immunocytochemistry, histochemistry, receptor autoradiography, intracellular labeling of physiologically identified neurons, the modern retrograde and anterograde tract-tracing methods, and quantitative computer-assisted morphometry. The following discussion of some of these methods is provided as an overview for the understanding of the type of information obtained from each method. Complete details for each of these methods can be obtained by consulting Heimer and RoBards (37), Johnson (42), or Robertson (79).

Classical Methods

The Nissl stain is utilized to demonstrate the somata or cell bodies of neurons (Fig. 1). Sections of brain tissue are placed into any one of a number of basophilic aniline dyes to stain the nucleoli and heterochromatin within the nucleus and the ribosomes and cisternae of granular endoplasmic reticulum in the perikaryal cytoplasm. All neurons and neuroglia are stained with this method, so that the distribution of somata may be determined. Numerous Nissl studies of the brain have been made to delineate the normal cytoarchitecture. These normal data for all brain regions can be utilized to compare data obtained from epileptic brains to determine if a cell loss occurs.

Another group of stains is selective for nerve fibers. Some will stain the myelin sheath of axons, while others stain the cytoskeletal core of the axons, the neurofilaments. The methods that stain myelin sheaths involve pretreatment of the tissue in a mordant such as potassium dichromate and subsequent staining of the myelin with a basic dye such as hematoxylin. Osmium tetroxide also provides an intense stain for myelin because it has a high affinity for lipids. Sections of brain tissue stained with these fiber stains reveal a unique pattern that is referred to as the myeloarchitecture. All myelinated axons will be stained with these methods. Since most of the major pathways in the brain contain myelinated axons, such stains are helpful to determine if certain pathways have degenerated as a result of a lesion. Methods that stain the neurofilaments within axons utilize silver impregnations that deposit metallic silver around mainly these structures and, to a lesser extent, nucleoli.

The Golgi method was developed over 100 years ago and has been utilized extensively because it stains selective neurons in their entirety. Since less than 1% of all neurons in a section are stained, the neurons show up very clearly against a relatively unstained background (Fig.

2). For Golgi stains, blocks of brain tissue are pretreated with potassium dichromate and then impregnated in a silver solution. Thus, silver salts are deposited throughout most of the neuron. This method has increased our knowledge about the surface structure of dendrites and their patterns and the terminal ramifications of axons in the central nervous system (Fig. 4). When combined with electron microscopy, it has the potential to demonstrate the local neuronal circuitry in a brain region (see ref. 25 and Figs. 5–8). The Golgi method has been used to study epileptic brain tissue (54,83,100). In these studies, only the most common neuron in the examined brain regions was analyzed (the pyramidal cell), because the Golgi stain is so capricious in its staining that it is unrealistic to analyze the neuronal types that are less common. Unfortunately, neurons from this latter group are the ones that appear to display major changes at epileptic foci (70). Therefore, the Golgi method provides limited data for an analysis of epileptic brain tissue.

Electron microscopy of the brain provides the fine structural details of neurons and their processes in the brain. Thus, the amount of data available is enormous and is only limited by the thinness of the section and the small area that can be examined on an individual 1 × 2 mm, Formvar-coated slot grid. Since all parts of a neuron are shown in electron microscopic preparations, they can be analyzed and described in normal preparations. Such studies have revealed many new aspects of cell structure and function (59) and provide a necessary control when epileptic brain tissue is analyzed with an electron microscope (12,28,35,70). The major differences observed in these latter studies were an increase in gliosis and a loss of terminals that form symmetric (inhibitory type) synapses (see Figs. 14–17).

Contemporary Methods

The neuroscientist became somewhat frustrated using the classical methods because they yielded primarily descriptive information without much functional significance. In the early 1970s, neuroanatomical methods became more functionally oriented when neurochemists and physiologists realized the importance of morphology. Immunocytochemistry, histochemistry, and receptor autoradiography arose as major neurocytological methods because neurochemists and pharmacologists wanted to know the exact sites within the brain where various neu-

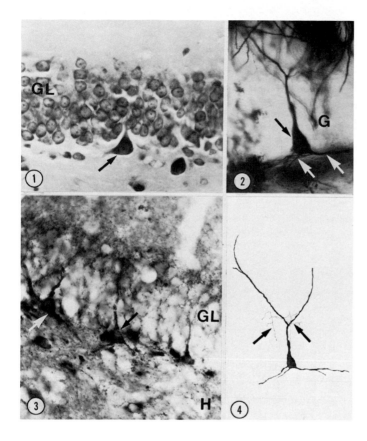

FIG. 1. Photomicrograph of a Nissl-stained preparation of the rat dentate gyrus. Small granule cell bodies in the granule cell layer (GL) and a soma of a probable horizontal basket cell (*arrow*) are stained. Cresyl violet, ×280. (From ref. 85, with permission.)

FIG. 2. Photomicrograph of a Golgi-impregnated pyramidal basket cell. The soma (*arrow*) and proximal apical dendrite are located in the granule cell layer, along with an impregnated granule cell (G) that is out of the focal plane. Two basal dendrites (*white arrows*) are the same ones shown in Fig. 5. ×300. (From ref. 75, with permission.)

FIG. 3. Photomicrograph of a section of the rat dentate gyrus immunoreacted for GAD. A pyramidal basket cell (*arrow*) with two basal dendrites and a horizontal basket cell (*white arrow*) with only one basal process are found located on the border between the granule cell layer (GL) and the hilus (H). GAD immunocytochemistry. ×240. (From ref. 85, with permission.)

FIG. 4. Drawing of the Golgi-impregnated pyramidal basket cell in Fig. 2. The axon (*arrows*) of this cell arises from the apical dendrite and sends branches into the molecular and granule cell layers. ×175. (From ref. 75, with permission.)

rotransmitters displayed their actions. In a similar way, the intracellular labeling methods were developed because physiologists needed to know the location and morphology of neurons that they had recorded. These interdisciplinary studies stimulated advancements in tract-tracing methods where various silver stains for degenerating axons were replaced almost overnight by axoplasmic transport markers such as tritiated amino acids for anterograde autoradiographic labeling of pathways and horseradish peroxidase (HRP) for retrograde and anterograde labeling. These newer methods stimulated the application of computers to analyze the data, especially the counting of silver grains that overlie tissue sections that are processed for autoradiography. Similar computer-assisted analyses have been used in other areas of descriptive anatomy to provide quantitative data that can be interpreted in a more functional way. Therefore, the contemporary methods in neurocytology provide

functional data that relate to the physiology and chemistry of the brain tissue.

Immunocytochemistry and histochemistry provide two different ways to label certain chemical substances within cells in a light- or electron-microscopic preparation. For immunocytochemistry, specific antibodies that recognize antigenic determinants of neurotransmitter synthesizing enzymes or neuroactive peptides are visualized by cross-linking them to fluorescent or HRP-labeled immunoglobulins (95). Thus, the labeling of certain types of neuronal molecules can be achieved and their distribution can be mapped in the brain and spinal cord (Figs. 3, 11, 12, 24, and 25). These studies are extremely helpful in mapping the neurons that use a particular neurotransmitter or neuroactive peptide in both normal and epileptic preparations.

Histochemical methods are similar to immunocytochemical methods in that they can lo-

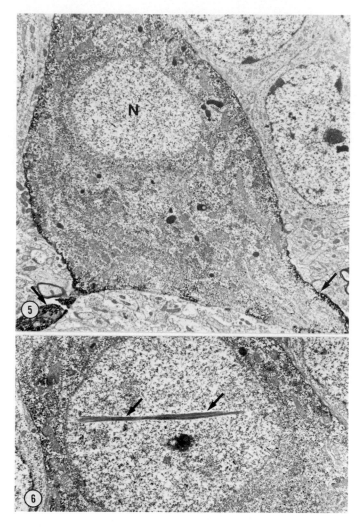

FIG. 5. Electron micrograph of the pyramidal basket cell body shown in Figs. 2 and 4. This section contains a small part of the nucleus (N) and two basal dendrites (*arrows*). Gold-toned Golgi preparation. ×5,040. (From ref. 75, with permission.)

FIG. 6. Another section from the same cell shown in Fig. 5. The nucleus displays an intranuclear rod (*arrows*) and a nucleolus. ×5,250. (From ref. 75, with permission.)

calize a specific substance to a tissue section. However, histochemistry does not provide the same level of resolution. It utilizes the normal activity of an enzyme and an added substrate to generate a light- or electron-opaque reaction product in the general vicinity of that enzyme. Enzymes specific for certain neurotransmitters, such as acetylcholinesterase, are commonly lo-

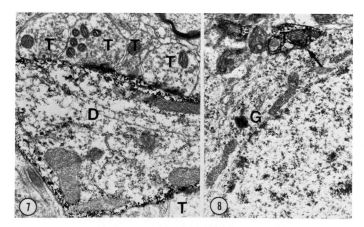

FIG. 7. Electron micrograph of a portion of a basal dendrite (D) from the same pyramidal basket cell shown in Figs. 5 and 6. This gold-labeled dendrite is contacted by numerous large axon terminals (T) that resemble mossy fiber terminals. ×13,300. (From ref. 75, with permission.)

FIG. 8. A gold-labeled axon terminal (T) from a basket cell forms a symmetric synapse (*arrow*) with the soma of a granule cell (G). ×15,600. (From ref. 75, with permission.)

calized with histochemical methods to infer that certain neurons or pathways are cholinergic even though the immunocytochemical localization of choline acetyltransferase (the synthesizing enzyme for acetylcholine) provides a more precise method (48). Histochemistry has also been used to localize the neurons that utilize monoamines as neurotransmitters. These monoamines are induced to fluoresce at a particular wavelength when excited by ultraviolet light and treated with the proper chemicals. Numerous metabolic enzymes can also be localized with histochemical methods (e.g., cytochrome oxidase, acid phosphatase, etc.).

Receptor binding autoradiography is a method that analyzes the distribution of receptors in the brain. This method relies on a radiolabeled drug (ligand) that has a high affinity for a given neurotransmitter receptor. Sections of brain tissue are incubated with ligand, washed, and coated with a photographic emulsion or tritium-sensitive films. The autoradiographs are developed and analyzed for the distribution and number of silver grains that overlie the sites of ligand–receptor binding. Many receptors in the brain have been analyzed with this method including those relevant to epileptic activity, such as gamma-aminobutyric acid (GABA), benzodiazepine (Fig. 9), glutamic acid, glycine, and cholinergic receptors.

Intracellular HRP labeling following electrophysiological recording provides a powerful method that links the function of an individual neuron with its structure. Since numerous reports of this method are available in this volume (see Chapters 12, 13, 29, and 30), only a brief description of this method is provided in this account. First, glass micropipettes are loaded with a dilute solution of HRP. Then the tips of these pipettes are inserted into neurons to obtain the intracellular electrophysiology of an individual neuron's activity. Following this recording, a small electrical current or air pressure is used to inject HRP into the neuron. The HRP is transported into all of the neuron's processes, and the neuron is visualized with a routine histochemical procedure to reveal the structure of the recorded neuron. Such recordings made in normal preparations can be compared with recordings of neurons located in an epileptic focus. These methods have provided useful data on basic mechanisms of epilepsy (see other chapters in this volume).

Tract-tracing methods that are currently used by neuroscientists involve the transport of exogenous substances that are injected into the vicinity of a neuron's soma, dendrites or its axon terminals. These regions possess the ability to pinocytose the exogenous substances and transport it in anterograde and/or retrograde directions. HRP is transported bidirectionally and can provide information about a brain region's afferents and efferents (Fig. 10). Fluorescent dyes are usually transported in a retrograde manner, and their localization is determined with a fluorescent microscope. In contrast, radiolabeled amino acids are mainly taken up by the somata of neurons, where they are incorporated into proteins that are transported in an anterograde direction. The autoradiographic method is then used to determine both the injection site that contains the labeled somata and the distribution of their axons. These various tract-tracing methods are valuable for mapping long axonal connections in the brain. Their use in the study of epilepsy has been minimal because it has been assumed that the long connections in epileptic brains are normal.

Quantitative morphometry has made substantial advances following the application of modern computers to the analysis of morphological data. Computer-assisted measurements have many advantages over the older hand counting methods, in that they provide a faster operation, more detailed analysis, and an ability to store and manipulate data for statistical analysis and three-dimensional reconstructions of structures. Many studies have applied these quantitative methods to study Nissl, Golgi, immunocytochemical, and electron-microscopic preparations so that the data can be interpreted in a more functional way than the qualitative assessment typically made for such preparations (e.g., Fig. 16). If a representative sample is taken, important comparisons can be made that have provided new insights into the basic mechanisms of epilepsy (see below).

REVIEW OF MORPHOLOGICAL STUDIES OF EPILEPSY

A thorough review of the morphological studies of epilepsy has not been made since Scheibel and Scheibel (83) provided an excellent historical account. All of the studies that were reviewed in that account utilized classical methods in neurocytology and revealed very little about basic mechanisms of the epilepsies. In fact, Spielmeyer (94), a pioneer in the field of Ammon's horn sclerosis in epilepsy, addressed this shortcoming by admitting that his "observations can tell one nothing about the essential causes of epilepsy." However, as will be shown, Spielmeyer's studies do provide a thorough neuropathological description of the epileptic brain.

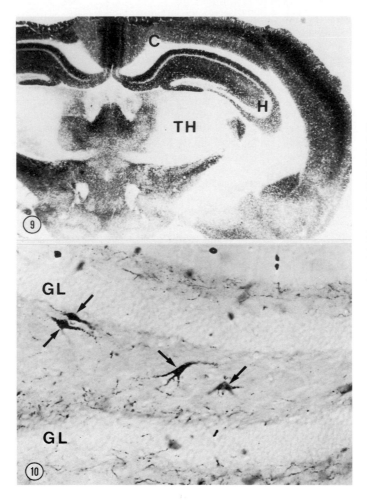

FIG. 9. Light-microscopic autoradiogram of a coronal section of a mouse (C57 BL/6J) brain that shows the distribution of benzodiazepine receptors in the cerebral cortex (C), hippocampus (H), and thalamus (TH). ^{3}H-flunitrazepam, ×14. Courtesy of Andrej Rotter.

FIG. 10. Photomicrograph of HRP-labeled neuronal somata and axon terminals in the rat dentate gyrus contralateral to the side of injection. Two bipolar and two multipolar neurons (*arrows*) are found in the hilus. Labeled commissural axons are located on both sides of the granule cell layer (GL) and occasionally within this layer. Silver intensification method for HRP, ×140. (From ref. 86, with permission.)

Numerous morphological studies of epileptic brains have been made in the past decade, and most scientists have utilized animal models in an attempt to gain a better appreciation of the functional causes of epileptic activity. When a review of the current literature is made, one is amazed at the number of different animal models that have been analyzed with neurocytological methods. It is interesting to note that a consistent finding occurs in most models of focal epilepsy: neuronal loss and gliosis. These studies are summarized in Tables 1 and 2 and are briefly discussed below. Although the descriptive studies of animal models of epilepsy with classical methods have yielded new information, most of the functionally important studies have utilized the contemporary methods.

Descriptive Studies with Classical Methods

Humans

The first analysis of epileptic tissue with a classical neurocytological method occurred over a century ago. Both Sommer (91) and Pfleger (63) used Nissl preparations of brains obtained from epileptic patients to demonstrate a neuronal loss in the hippocampus. Sommer described this loss in a specific portion of the hippocampus, the CA1 area of Ammon's horn or cornu Ammonis (CA). Thus, this CA1 area has also been referred to as Sommer's sector. This neuronal loss was observed in one third of Sommer's patients and has been described by others, including Falconer et al. (26), to be more common. Pfleger (63) also described this hardening of the hippocampus and thought it was due to a compromised circulation that occurs during a seizure. The correlation of Ammon's horn sclerosis with occlusion of the circulatory system was an important relationship referred to by Spielmeyer (94) as the vasomotor theory of epilepsy. A criticism of this theory was that not all epileptic brains displayed this sclerosis and not all ischemic incidents led to seizures. Nevertheless, sclerosis in the hippocampus had entrenched itself as an important anatomical substrate for epileptic activity. The impact of this finding is evidenced by the large number of multidisciplinary studies that have concentrated on the analysis of neuronal circuitry in the hippocampus.

Other studies from the last century provided more details about epileptic brains. For example, Alzheimer (1) and Chaslin (13) described neuronal loss and gliosis in the hippocampus and cerebral cortex, respectively. Hypertrophy of neuroglia and glial proliferation are known to occur at sites of neuronal loss in the brain. In fact, the glia are the connective tissues of the brain and may form numerous layers at sites of trauma that are called a neuroglial scar. Glial scarring in the hippocampus of epileptic brains is probably the reason why Bouchet and Cazauvieilh (9) noticed a hardening of the hippocampus in epileptic brains. The first Golgi study of epileptic brain was made by Demoor (19), who noted a diffuse spine loss and nodulated dendrites. These changes in the main receptive portion of the neuron indicated a reduction in the number of afferents.

TABLE 1. *Morphological history of human epilepsy*

Year	Investigators	Findings
1825	Bouchet and Cazauvieihl (9)	Hardening of hippocampus in epileptic brains.
1880	Sommer (91)	Extensive neuronal loss in CA1 area of hippocampus (Sommer's sector).
	Pfleger (63)	Sclerosis of hippocampus due to a circulatory embarrassment provoked during the seizure.
1891	Chaslin (13)	Neuronal loss and gliosis in cerebral cortex.
1898	Alzheimer (1)	Neuronal loss and gliosis in hippocampus.
1927	Penfield (56)	Associated the neuroglial scar as the irritative source for focal seizures.
1930	Spielmeyer (94)	Described changes in the cerebellum, including increased gliosis and loss of Purkinje cells. Linked occlusion of circulation with epilepsy in the vasomotor theory.
1930	Foerster and Penfield (29,30)	Epileptic scar contains few nerve fibers or neurons.
1940	Penfield and Humphreys (57)	Epileptic area has loss of some neurons, glial proliferation, increased number of blood vessels, and granular corpuscles.
1953	Earle et al. (20)	Molding of fetal head in birth canal causes compression of arteries in the uncus and hippocampus.
1955	Falconer et al. (26)	High incidence of hippocampal sclerosis in temporal-lobe epilepsy.
1973	Scheibel and Scheibel (83)	Golgi study reveals dendritic spine loss and nodulations for pyramidal cells with degeneration of dendritic tree. Granule cells display similar dendritic changes as well as the ''windblown'' effect.
	Brown (12)	First electron-microscopic analysis of human epileptic brain shows increased gliosis and loss of axosomatic symmetric synapses.
1975	Engel et al. (24)	Discrete lesions frequently occur in resected temporal lobes.
1977	Williams et al. (102)	Electron-microscopic study showing a loss of symmetric synapses from the perikarya and axon hillocks of pyramidal cells in neuronal ceroid lipofuscinosis
1978	Braak and Goebel (10)	Loss of pigmented stellate cells in cortical layers II and III in patients with neuronal ceroid lipofuscinosis.
1982	Engel et al. (23)	Correlated the degree of relative hypometabolism in positron computer tomography with the severity of mesial temporal sclerosis.
1983	Scheibel et al. (82)	Scanning electron microscopy showing microaneurysms in resected temporal lobes.

TABLE 2. *Neurocytology of epilepsies in experimental animals*[a]

Model	Neuronal loss	Dendritic changes	Gliosis	Symmetric (GABAergic-like) synapses
A. Genetic epilepsies				
Mongolian gerbil	(18)	Loss of spines (54)		Increase in GABAergic basket cells and synapses in hippocampal dentate gyrus that may cause disinhibition of granule cells (61,62)
Genetically epilepsy-prone rat				Increase in GABAergic neurons in the inferior colliculus (78)
B. Partial epilepsies				
Kindling	No observed loss of neurons (32)	No changes for pyramidal cell dendrites (17)	No observed gliosis (11)	
Alumina cream in monkeys	(100)	Loss of spines, reduced dendritic branching (100)	(34,35,70,100)	Preferential loss of GABAergic synapses, specifically those that arise from basket and chandelier cells (69–71)
Alumina cream in cats	(27,99)		(101)	
Isolated cortical slab in cats	(33)	Loss of dendritic spines (33)	(33,74,80)	Preferential loss of symmetric synapses at edges of slabs (74)
Cobalt in rats	(22)		(22,28)	Loss of terminals that synapse with somata of pyramidal cells (28,39)
Iron in rats	(66)	Spine loss and decrease of dendritic branching (66)	(66,103)	
Kainic acid in rats	Distant injections destroy pyramidal cells in CA3-4 (7,49); diazepam prevents this neuronal damage (8)		(49)	
Bicuculline in baboon	Specific for Sommer's sector in hippocampus (47)		(47)	
Bicuculline in rats		Swollen dendrites in distal sites, i.e., thalamus (14); sponginess to dendrites (90)	Swelling of astrocytes (90)	
Electrical stimulation of rat entorhinal cortex	CA4 and basket cells (89)	Dendritic swelling (52), dendritic nodules (89)		

[a] References are given in parentheses.

Most of the subsequent studies of human epileptic brain tissue have noted the dramatic changes that were described in these early descriptive studies. For example, Penfield (56) frequently observed the neuroglial scarring when he encountered a meningocerebral scar and suggested that it was an irritative source for focal seizures. Spielmeyer (94), like his predecessors, noted neuronal loss and thick glial proliferation in Ammon's horn sclerosis but also observed specific changes in the cerebellum where Purkinje cells were lost and glia proliferated. As already noted, he was a main proponent of the vasomotor theory of epilepsy because vasospasms and occlusions produced the same changes as those observed in epilepsy and in similar locations. The loss of neurons and proliferation of glia in temporal lobe epilepsy have also been observed by Foerster and Penfield (29,30), Penfield and Humphreys (57), Falconer et al. (26), and more recently by Engel et al. (23,24). The microscopic changes that were detected in Golgi preparations have also been confirmed in similar studies by Scheibel and Scheibel (83) and Scheibel et al. (81,82). These latter studies showed that the dendrites of pyramidal cells had a reduction in spines and possessed nodulations. In addition, the dendritic domain of pyramidal cells was decreased and granule cells of the dentate gyrus showed similar dendritic abnormalities as well as the "wind-blown look."

Electron-microscopic studies of human epileptic brain have confirmed some of these light-microscopic findings and have elucidated new data. Brown (12) has shown an increased gliosis and a loss of axosomatic symmetric synapses in temporal lobe biopsy tissue obtained from human patients with acute focal epilepsy. In another study, Williams et al. (102) noted a conspicuous loss of symmetric synapses from the perikarya and axon hillocks of pyramidal cells in a 4-year-old patient with neuronal ceroid lipofuscinosis, a disease in which the prominent feature is the occurrence of seizures. Braak and Goebel (10) reported that such patients have a decreased number of somata of aspinous stellate cells in cortical layers II and III. A reduction of these somata and of the terminals that form symmetric axosomatic synapses implies a loss of inhibitory function because (a) these structures in the rat and monkey contain glutamic acid decarboxylase (GAD), the synthesizing enzyme for the neurotransmitter GABA (67,71), and (b) evidence from physiological and pharmacological studies indicates that GABA has an inhibitory action on cortical neurons (see ref. 44).

More recently, Scheibel et al. (82) have completed a study with the scanning electron microscope of the microvasculature of surgically resected tissue blocks from patients with temporal lobe epilepsy. They observed sac-like outpouchings from blood vessels, which they refer to as microaneurysms. "Blow-outs" from such structures could introduce blood elements into the tissue which might be epileptogenic or cause the initial insult to neurons to make this brain region epileptic.

Animal Models

A large number of studies have attempted to unravel the basic mechanisms of epilepsies by analyzing the morphology of either genetic or partial epilepsies in experimental animals. The genetic models of epilepsy display seizures as young adults and mimic the human form of hereditary epilepsy. A developmental study of the brains of genetically epileptic animals can provide data about neuronal circuits both before and after seizure activity has started. The models of partial epilepsies are created by a drug or chemical administered systemically or directly applied to the brain. An analysis of the brain of an uninjected animal provides an excellent baseline to judge the changes observed after various times following drug administration and onset of seizures. These studies offer an ability to follow the full progression of seizure activity in morphological preparations. Therefore, the potential of these two categories of experimental models of epilepsies is a major resource for understanding basic mechanisms of epilepsies.

A survey of the morphological studies of epilepsies in experimental animals indicates that the partial epilepsies have been analyzed more than the genetic epilepsies (Table 2). However, the fact that more partial epilepsy studies have been made simply may indicate that the morphological changes are more striking in this model type. An investigator who has analyzed the grand mal epilepsies in baboon, *Papio papio*, has emphasized the lack of any scar or neuronal loss in this model (R. Naquet, *personal communication*). In fact, published studies on two models of genetic epilepsy have not reported gliosis in brain regions that show abnormal neuronal circuitry (Table 2A). Therefore, the types of morphological changes in genetic epilepsies are probably more subtle than those changes found in the models of partial epilepsies (see below).

Most of the models of partial epilepsies display the same features characteristic for human epilepsy. These include neuronal loss, gliosis, and dendritic spine loss and nodulation (Table 2B). The models include the direct application of alumina cream to brain tissue in monkeys and cats; isolated cortical slabs in cats; cobalt, iron, and kainic acid in rats; and bicuculline in baboons. Two other models, bicuculline and electrical stimulation in rats, do not display these characteristics but do show swollen dendrites and astrocytes. The dendritic swelling observed in electron-microscopic preparations may be the basis for the dendritic nodulation observed in other light-microscopic Golgi studies (52,89). Only one of the models of partial epilepsies stand out as having no obvious morphological changes. In kindling, neuronal loss does not occur, pyramidal cell dendrites appear normal, and gliosis has not been observed (11,17,32). However, it has been reported that a change in the density of GABAergic terminals occurs initially but appears to be a transient change because recovery occurs (4,5). Since the density of terminals was determined with a densitometer, these data may indicate changes in the GAD activity per terminal and not a reduction in the actual number of terminals. Electron-microscopic studies at similar time intervals could demonstrate such differences. Aside from the kindling model, these models of partial epilepsies for the most part are very similar in their morphology. An analysis of these models with contemporary methods in neurocytology can provide us with functionally significant data that can be used to understand basic mechanisms of epilepsies.

Studies that Utilize Contemporary Methods in Neurocytology

In contrast to the Nissl and Golgi methods, the relatively newer techniques in neurocytology provide functional data that relate to the physiology and chemistry of the brain tissue. The use of immunocytochemical, histochemical, and receptor–ligand-binding autoradiographic methods have aided in the understanding of cellular neurochemistry in both normal and epileptic tissue. Intracellular HRP and recording have increased our knowledge of physiological mechanisms at epileptic foci (see Chapters 12, 13, 29, and 30). In addition, the use of quantitative morphological methods at both light- and electron-microscopic levels has helped gain insights into the functional state of synapses and

neurons. Together, these methods have been utilized to help unravel the mystery of epilepsy.

The approach in our laboratory utilizes contemporary methods in neurocytology for the analysis of both genetic and partial epilepsies in experimental animals. The methods that are used most commonly for these studies include immunocytochemistry and quantitative morphometry at both light- and electron-microscopic levels. Studies of partial or posttraumatic focal epilepsies indicate that a preferential loss of cortical GABAergic, inhibitory terminals occurs at epileptic foci (see Table 2B). In contrast, results from studies of two genetic epilepsies display an increase of GABAergic neurons in brain regions that are linked functionally to the seizure-provoking stimulus (see Table 2A). A review of the results for these models of epilepsy is provided below, and the functional significance of these data is explained in a succeeding section.

Cortical Models of Partial Epilepsies

The initial immunocytochemical study on the morphology of cortical GABAergic neurons revealed an abundant variety of stained cell types distributed throughout all layers of neocortex (67). This study localized the synthesizing enzyme of GABA, glutamate decarboxylase (GAD). Although most of the GAD-containing neurons were classified as aspinous and sparsely spinous stellate cells, subsequent Golgi studies have revealed major subclasses of this category based on cell body shape, dendritic orientation, and axonal distribution (43,60,92,93). One cell type, the basket cell, is suggested to be GABAergic because its axonal plexus that forms pericellular nests around pyramidal cells in layer V (Fig. 11) was GAD-positive in immunocytochemical preparations (21,40,67,71). This identification was given further support from recent studies that utilized colchicine-treated immunocytochemical preparations that displayed the cell bodies of this neuronal type (38,40). Another cell type, the chandelier cell, is also considered to be GABAergic because GAD-positive reaction product has been localized to its terminals (Fig. 12) that form numerous vertical chains adjacent to axon initial segments of pyramidal cells in layers II and III where they make symmetric synapses (31,60,67). Although other GABAergic cell types have not been identified with certainty, they must exist because GAD-positive terminals contact other postsynaptic sites such as the dendritic shafts and somata of all cortical neurons, as well as a few dendritic spines (67,71). The localization of GAD within aspinous and sparsely spinous stellate neurons, together with evidence from physiological and pharmacological studies (44), strongly suggests that these neurons are responsible for GABA-mediated inhibition in the cerebral cortex. Since these neurons are found in every cortical layer and project numerous axon terminals to pyramidal cell somata and axon initial segments, they could exert a powerful inhibitory effect on cortical projection neurons. Furthermore, a decrease in the number of these inhibitory axon terminals could lead to seizure activity of pyramidal neurons.

To test the notion that a decrease of GABAergic neurons and terminals occurs at epileptic foci, we conducted a number of experiments over the past 5 years (69,70,71,73,74). In some of these studies, monkeys that received alumina gel applications and displayed seizure activity were used for GAD immunocytochemical analysis. The epileptic focus was always found around the sites of alumina gel application. In contrast, the contralateral homotopic cortex lacked independent seizure activity (36). Low-magnification light microscopy of cortex from all seizure foci revealed staining intensities for GAD that were lower than those of contralateral, nonepileptic cortices. This variation in the overall intensity of GAD-positive staining between epileptic and nonepileptic cortex indicated a difference in the number of GAD-positive terminals present in these preparations; this difference was verified by quantitative analysis at higher magnification. An assessment of the numbers of GAD-positive terminals in layers V and VI provides a measure for the relative amount of GABA-mediated synaptic inhibition of neurons that control motor behavior because pyramidal cells in these layers have major subcortical projections (43). For statistical purposes, the counts of GAD-positive terminals were averaged for layers V and VI because there were no significant differences between these two layers in either normal or epileptic cortex. For each of 5 analyzed epileptic monkeys, the mean numbers of GAD-positive axon terminals per 3,000 μm^3 at sites adjacent to alumina gel applications were at least 50% less than those in contralateral cortex (71). The former sites correspond to seizure foci, while the latter contralateral cortical sites lack independent spike activity (36). In addition, GAD-positive terminals were counted at ipsilateral sites located 0.5 to 1.0 cm away from the counting sites adjacent to

the focus. At this parafocus, there were fewer GAD-positive terminals than the contralateral cortex, and this finding was significant because the parafocus is known to display persistent seizure activity after excision of intracortical alumina granulomas and subjacent cortex.

An analysis of variance showed that significant differences occurred between the mean numbers of GAD-positive terminals in the focus, parafocus, and normal cortices ($F = 59.67$, d.f. 2,8; $p < 0.01$). Furthermore, individual comparisons of these data by the Newman–Keuls method (104) showed that the mean numbers of GAD-positive terminals at the focus were significantly less ($p < 0.01$) than those in both the parafocus and the contralateral cortex. Moreover, the mean numbers of GAD-positive terminals in the parafocus were significantly less ($p < 0.01$) than those found in the contralateral cortex. Thus, the results of this initial analysis indicate a significant decrease in the number of GABAergic axon terminals at sites of seizure foci.

This initial immunocytochemical study did not determine whether the loss of inhibitory function coincided with a degeneration of GABAergic terminals or with a loss of GAD immunoreactivity within these terminals. In addition, it was not ascertained if the loss of GABAergic terminals was selective for only this type of terminal. These issues can both be resolved at the ultrastructural level with the use of quantitative morphometric methods. Therefore, the same monkey specimens used in the immunocytochemical study were examined with the electron microscope (70). The results showed an 80% loss of terminals that form axosomatic symmetric synapses in the epileptic cortex when compared to the normal cortex (Figs. 13, 14, 16, and 17). The parafocus showed a somewhat smaller decrease than the focus, in that the parafocus had approximately 50% of the normal value. The amount of glia apposed to the cell bodies of pyramidal cells in the epileptic foci increased dramatically in comparison to the normal cortex (Figs. 13 and 14). Terminals forming symmetric synapses in the adjacent neuropil at the focus were decreased about 50%, although terminals forming asymmetric synapses in the same area were decreased by only 25%. The data from the parafocus was unexpected in that the number of symmetric synapses in the neuropil did not appear to be significantly changed from the normal, whereas the asymmetric synapses were slightly decreased, about 15%, compared to normal.

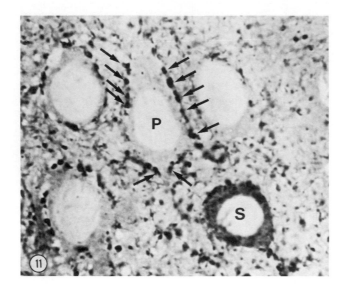

FIG. 11. Semithin, 2-μm section of colchicine-injected rat visual cortex immunoreacted for GAD. A pyramidal cell body (P) in layer V is surrounded by a pericellular basket plexus of GAD-positive terminals (*arrows*). A GAD-positive stellate cell (S) is also shown. ×1,050. (From ref. 68, with permission.)

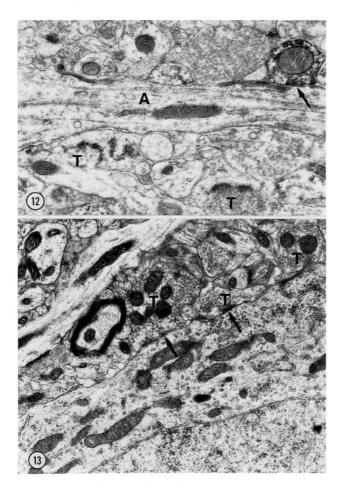

FIG. 12. Electron micrograph of a GAD-positive axon terminal that forms a symmetric synapse (*arrow*) with an axon initial segment (A) of a layer II pyramidal neuron. Such terminals probably arise from the chandelier cell, a GABAergic type of cortical neuron. Two other axon terminals (T) form asymmetric synapses in the adjacent neutropil. ×17,500. (From ref. 67, with permission.)

FIG. 13. Electron micrograph of a portion of a layer V pyramidal cell body and the associated pericellular axonal plexus that is mainly derived from GABAergic basket cells. Three terminals (T) from this plexus are adjacent to the soma and two form symmetric synapses (*arrows*) in the plane of this section. ×13,300. (From ref. 72, with permission.)

These statistically significant results indicate that the previously observed loss of GABAergic terminals at sites of focal epilepsy is caused by terminal degeneration and not a loss of GAD immunoreactivity. Also, since GABAergic terminals are more severely reduced at epileptic foci than other terminals, it appears that this selective deficit could cause seizure activity due to a loss of inhibitory function at epileptic foci. The significant loss of axosomatic synapses at parafoci, in turn, indicates that this loss may be responsible for the epileptic activity found in parafoci following the removal of the alumina gel granuloma. Together, these data indicate that a basket-cell deficit occurs at epileptic foci, and as a result the layer V pyramidal cells at such sites are probably more hyperexcitable than normal.

To determine if any other types of inhibitory, GABAergic neurons are lost in addition to the basket cell, an ultrastructural analysis of axon terminals of chandelier cells was made in the same monkey epileptic foci (69). Axon initial segments of pyramidal neurons were identified by their characteristic origin from the base of these cells and by three ultrastructural features: fascicles of microtubules, a multilayered electron-dense subaxolemmal undercoating, and numerous cisternal organelles. Some of the axon initial segments that were examined were traced for at least 40 μm in serial thin sections and beyond this point were observed to become myelinated. In single sections, 10 to 15 axon terminals were found to form symmetric synapses throughout the entire length of the axon initial segments from nonepileptic preparations. This

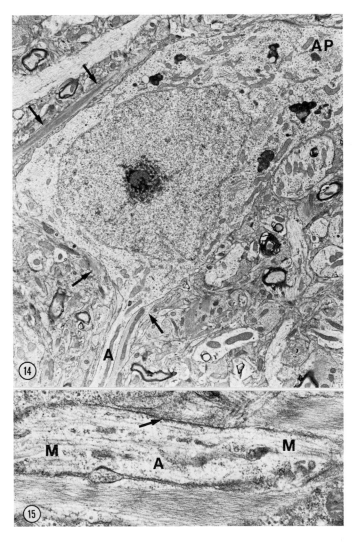

FIG. 14. Electron micrograph of a layer III pyramidal cell body, proximal apical dendrite (AP) and axon initial segment (A) from an alumina gel-treated epileptic focus in monkey sensorimotor cortex. Numerous profiles of glia are found adjacent to the soma (*arrows*) and axon hillock and initial segment. ×9,000. (From ref. 69, with permission.)

FIG. 15. Enlargement of distal portion of another axon initial segment (A) from a layer III pyramidal neuron from an epileptic focus. This axon displays fascicles of microtubules (M) and a dense coating beneath the axolemma (*arrow*). Profiles of reactive astrocytes that contain filaments lie adjacent to the initial segment. Axon terminals derived from chandelier cells are not present. ×20,000. (From ref. 69, with permission.)

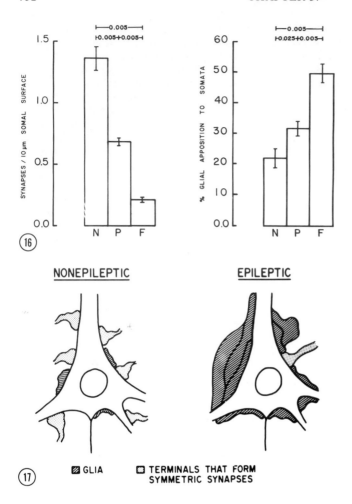

FIG. 16. Bar graphs generated from a quantitative electron-microscopic analysis of alumina gel treated monkey epileptic cortex. The bar graph on the **left** shows the number of symmetric (GABAergic-like) synapses per 10 μm of somal surface of 90 layer V pyramidal somata (10 cells from each site of each of three monkeys). The normal nonepileptic cortex (N) had the largest number, the parafocus (P) had an intermediate number, and the focus (F) had the least. The bar graph on the **right** shows the significant increases in glial apposition to layer V pyramidal neurons at the parafocus (P) and focus (F). Mean values were compared by the Student's *t*-test and significant differences are indicated by probability levels ($p <$ indicated value). The standard error of the mean appears at the top of each bar. (From ref. 70, with permission.)

FIG. 17. Schematic representation of the quantitative data shown in Fig. 16. The typical somata of layer V pyramidal cells in nonepileptic cortex **(left)** have an average of six terminals that form symmetric axosomatic synapses per section and a glial apposition of only 20% of the somal surface. In contrast, pyramidal cells from epileptic foci **(right)** display, on average, one terminal per section (an 80% loss of GABAergic-like terminals) and an increase in glial apposition. (From ref. 68, with permission.)

finding is consistent with a previous description of the axon initial segments of pyramidal neurons in primate sensorimotor cortex (88). Chandelier cell axon terminals that were reconstructed from serial sections were shown to align themselves parallel to axon initial segments and were observed to synapse with only these structures and not adjacent dendrites or spines. In epileptic cortex, the axon initial segments of pyramidal neurons were apposed by glial profiles that contained clusters of filaments typical of reactive astrocytes (Figs. 14, 15, and 18). Few if any axon terminals were observed to form symmetric synapses with these axon initial segments. Thus, the chandelier cell axons appeared to degenerate in epileptic cortex. The data from this study (69) and the previous ultrastructural study (70) indicate that at least two GABAergic neuronal types are lost at epileptic foci, basket and chandelier cells.

It was important to know if the loss of

GABAergic terminals at epileptic foci was associated with a loss of GABAergic somata. Since the terminals of both cortical basket and chandelier cells are dramatically reduced, it was predicted that this loss was due to a neuronal loss and not simply a pruning back of the axonal plexus of these GABAergic neuronal types (73). To explore this point, we utilized an anti-GAD serum that detects somal GAD in many types of neurons without the use of colchicine (51). This antiserum facilitates a better comparison of epileptic and nonepileptic tissue, because other antisera that require colchicine provide nonuniform laminar staining of GABAergic neuronal somata that is dependent on the site of colchicine injection (40). Also, the damage caused by the injection may cause nonspecific damage to the cortex that could obscure the actual data on the number of GABAergic somata. The results of this study (73) indicate that a 20 to 30% loss of small GABAergic somata is associated with the preferential loss of GABAergic terminals at epileptic foci. Therefore, the loss of GABAergic terminals at epileptic foci is due to a loss of the neuronal somata that give rise to and support these axons.

A preliminary study of the isolated cortical slab model of focal epilepsy (74) was undertaken to explore the possible loss of symmetric synapses with somata. Since the loss of inhibitory terminals was greatest adjacent to the alumina gel lesions in the monkey study (70), the possibility existed that the edges of the chronic slabs may exhibit fewer inhibitory terminals than the centers (Figs. 19 and 20). Indeed, the experimental results indicated that the number of terminals that form synapses with somata of pyramidal neurons varied depending on the location in the cortical slab. The somata located adjacent to the edges of the slabs have few if any terminals synapsing with them (Fig. 21). Instead, these somata were almost completely enveloped by layers of glia from reactive astrocytes. In contrast, somata in the center of slabs appeared to have a normal number of terminals forming symmetric axosomatic synapses. These data suggest that a loss of terminals forming symmetric synapses occurs at the edges of the cortical slabs. A subsequent quantitative study has confirmed this phenomenon. A loss of inhibitory type synapses at the edges suggests that the epileptiform activity of isolated cortical slabs arises from the pyramidal cells located at the edges and spreads into the center of the slabs via the excitatory projections of the pyramidal cells.

The two experimental models of focal epilepsy that have been analyzed with immunocytochemical and quantitative morphometric methods display a preferential loss of GABAergic neurons at epileptic foci. Data from the cobalt model of epilepsy in rats are consistent with these observations, in that Fischer (28) has shown a loss of axosomatic symmetric synapses and Hoover et al. (39) have shown a degeneration of terminals that form a dense plexus with pyramidal cell bodies. Together, these data indicate that a loss of GABAergic neurons at epileptic foci could be expected to reduce the inhibitory synaptic control over pyramidal neurons. These pyramidal neurons might display seizure activity due to a loss of feedback inhibitory circuits (Figs. 22 and 23).

Models of Genetic Epilepsies

The GABAergic neuronal system was investigated with immunocytochemical and quantitative morphometric methods in the hippocampal formation of two strains of Mongolian

NONEPILEPTIC   EPILEPTIC

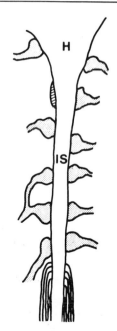
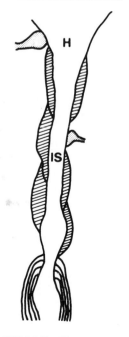

FIG. 18. Schematic diagram that summarizes the findings observed for axon hillocks (H) and initial segments (IS) from nonepileptic and epileptic preparations. The epileptic tissue displays a loss of terminals that form symmetric synapses and an increase in glial apposition as compared to nonepileptic tissue. These data indicate a loss of GABAergic chandelier cells from epileptic foci. (From ref. 69, with permission.)

(18)   ▨ GLIA   ▨ TERMINALS THAT FORM
             SYMMETRIC SYNAPSES

gerbil: a seizure-sensitive (SS) and a seizure-re-sistant (SR) strain (61,62). The SS animals exhibit seizures when exposed to a novel environment, the intensity of which is consistent for each animal over many testings. Therefore, it is possible to correlate a known history of seizure intensity with morphological observations. Since SS gerbils do not show seizure activity until approximately 50 days of age, it is also possible to compare the seizure-predisposed (SP) brains of young SS progeny with the brains of SS and SR to determine if any differences which may exist between SS and SR brains are present prior to seizure onset.

Light-microscopic counts were made of the GAD-positive neurons in the dentate gyrus and hippocampus proper (61,62). In addition, cell size and terminal density were determined. In both the hippocampus proper and dentate gyrus, more GAD-positive neurons were found in SS

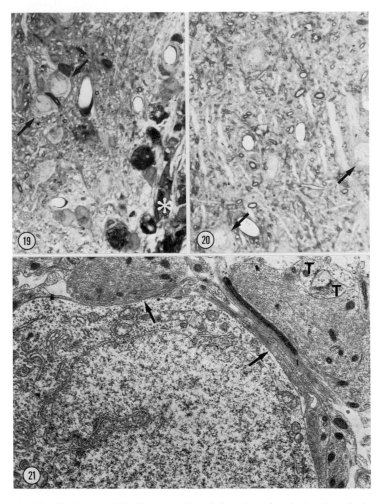

FIG. 19. Photomicrograph of a semithin, 2-μm section of the edge of an isolated cortical slab of the suprasylvian gyrus. Pyramidal cells (*arrows*) in layer III display a normal appearance even though they are close to the edge (*asterisk*) where glial proliferation has occurred. ×340.

FIG. 20. Photomicrograph obtained from the contralateral, intact suprasylvian gyrus. The somata (*arrows*) and apical dendrites of pyramidal cells in layer V are shown. ×340.

FIG. 21. Electron micrograph of a portion of a neuronal soma less than 50 μm from the edge of the slab. This soma is contacted by profiles of reactive astrocytes (*arrows*) and lacks axosomatic symmetric synapses. This loss of GABAergic-like synapses appears to be selective, because terminals (T) that form asymmetric (excitatory type) axodendritic synapses are found in the adjacent neuropil. ×7,700. (From ref. 74, with permission.)

brains than in SR. The number of these cells in SR brains was similar to that reported in normal rat. In the dentate gyrus of SS brains, the suprapyramidal blade of stratum granulosum showed a striking increase in the number of GAD-positive cells compared to the same region in SR brains (Figs. 24 and 25). This increase was most marked in the septal half of the dentate gyrus, where it amounted to nearly a 100% increase in selected brains. A similar increase in GAD-positive neurons was also found in stratum moleculare. The SP brains displayed similar increases in these two strata. Within the hippocampus, the increased number of GAD-positive somata was seen mainly in the regio inferior. The apical dendritic zone showed a 50% increase, and the strata pyramidale and oriens each showed a 20% increase. In all regions analyzed there was some variability in the number of GAD-positive neurons between animals, and this variability appeared to correlate with sei-

zure intensity. In addition, GAD-positive terminal density was also different between the two strains, with an increased density in both blades of stratum granulosum in the SS animals. The increased number of GABAergic neurons in the dentate gyrus and regio inferior of SS animals, as well as in their immature offspring (SP) that had not exhibited seizure activity, suggests a genetic aberration that may be functionally related to seizure sensitivity.

In conjunction with our light-microscopic analysis, we examined the ultrastructural appearance of the mossy tufts, the large axon terminals of the granule cells (61,62). Since the light-microscopic data indicated a substantial difference in the number and connections of inhibitory neurons within the dentate gyrus between SR and SS brains, this might be reflected in the activity and, perhaps, in the axonal morphology of the projection cells. The SR brains had mossy tufts that resembled those described

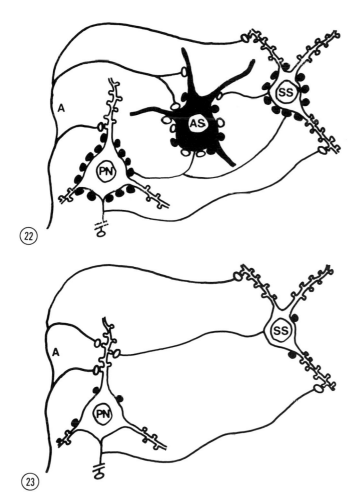

FIG. 22. Schematic diagram of the circuitry for the three major cell types in the normal cerebral cortex. GABAergic axon terminals (filled) form synapses with all cortical cells and are derived from aspinous stellate cells (AS). Spinous stellate cells (SS) are considered excitatory local circuit neurons. The pyramidal cell (PN) is shown on the **left** with its local excitatory axon collateral (clear) and subcortical projecting axon. The specific afferents (A) to the cortex are shown to terminate on all three cell types in layer IV. (From ref. 68, with permission.)

FIG. 23. Schematic diagram of the cortical cell types and circuitry found at epileptic foci (cf. Fig. 22). An 80% reduction of GABAergic axosomatic synapses is shown for both the pyramidal (PN) and spinous stellate (SS) cells and probably makes these cells hyperexcitable when excitatory thalamic afferents (A) are stimulated. These cells may generate a bursting activity because an inadequate number of inhibitory neurons is unable to control the increased activity in the excitatory feedback loop. (From ref. 68, with permission.)

in other rodent species (2,50). In contrast, the mossy tufts in the SS brains showed a depletion of synaptic vesicles and an increase in the number of cisternae of agranular reticulum (Figs. 26 and 27). Also, the mitochondria in these tufts were located close to the active zones where synaptic vesicles aggregate at synapses. The plasma membrane of SS mossy tufts was highly infolded, with some of these infoldings connected to the cisternae (Fig. 27). These observations for mossy fiber tufts are indicative of a high rate of synaptic activity among granule cells in the dentate gyrus (50). This conclusion appears to be contradictory to the light-microscopic data that indicate an increase in GABAergic inhibition in the dentate gyrus.

These light- and electron-microscopic findings may be explained by a disinhibition hypothesis (61,62). Briefly, many of the GABAergic neurons in the dentate gyrus have been shown to be the basket cells (Fig. 3; refs. 76,85), which provide feedback inhibition to the granule cells (3).

In the SS brains we have observed an increase in the number of GAD-positive terminals within the stratum granulosum. It is possible that many of these extra terminals form synapses on other basket cells, thereby disinhibiting the granule cells (Fig. 28). To test this disinhibition hypothesis for genetic models of epilepsy, we have begun to examine GAD-positive terminals in electron-microscopic preparations to determine if they form more synapses with GAD-positive basket cell somata in SS as compared to SR gerbils. Our preliminary data support this notion.

The results of this study clearly indicate a dramatic difference in the local neuronal circuitry in the hippocampus between these two strains of gerbils. A hint of a difference in circuitry was provided by the Golgi study of Paul et al. (54; also see Chapter 39) that showed a loss of dendritic spines on hippocampal pyramidal cell dendrites in region CA3 of SS gerbils. Benzodiazepine receptor binding results indicated a 30% deficit in homogenized membranes from the

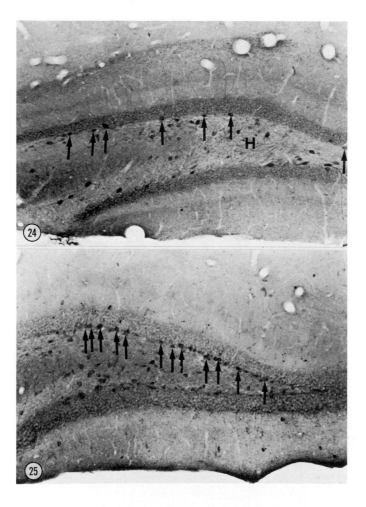

FIG. 24. Photomicrograph of a coronal section of the seizure-resistant gerbil showing the distribution of GABAergic neurons. GAD-positive pyramidal basket cells (*arrows*) are found at the dorsal border between the hilus (H) and granule cell layer. ×70.

FIG. 25. Photomicrograph of the distribution of GABAergic neurons in the seizure-sensitive gerbils' dentate gyrus. Numerous GAD-positive pyramidal basket cells (*arrows*) are found in the dorsal blade. ×70.

midbrain of SS gerbils. This deficit was localized by brain-slice receptor binding autoradiography to the substantia nigra (20% loss) and periaqueductal gray area (12% loss) by Olsen et al. (53). SS gerbils did not display lower binding in the colliculi, cerebral cortex, or hippocampus. However, only the temporal portion of the hippocampus was used in these studies, and the major increase in GABAergic neurons and terminals described in the septal half by Peterson et al. (61,62) may have evaded analysis (R. W. Olsen, *personal communication*). The findings on benzodiazepine receptors in the substantia nigra are interesting but may not relate directly

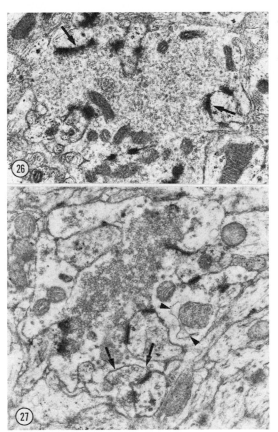

FIG. 26. Electron micrograph of a mossy tuft from a seizure-resistant gerbil hippocampus. Round synaptic vesicles fill most of this terminal, which forms typical asymmetric axospinous synapses (*arrows*). ×13,000. (From ref. 62, with permission.)

FIG. 27. Electron micrograph of a mossy tuft from a seizure-sensitive brain, showing a depletion of synaptic vesicles, membrane infoldings derived from active sites (*arrows*), and cisternae of agranular reticulum (*arrowheads*). These features are typical for "active" terminals. ×16,500. (From ref. 62, with permission.)

to the cause of the seizures because they assess only the postsynaptic structures. When the nigral GABAergic neurons in the SS and SR gerbils were counted in our preparations, we were unable to demonstrate a significant difference (*unpublished observations*). Therefore, the major deficit in the SS gerbils appears to be the nearly 100% increase in the number of GABAergic basket cells in the septal half of the dentate gyrus.

To determine if other models of genetic epilepsies display a GABAergic defect, we analyzed the genetically epilepsy-prone rat (GEPR) with immunocytochemical methods (78). The GEPR always exhibits severe generalized motor seizures in response to loud auditory stimuli. The inferior colliculus (IC) is suspected to be an important site of epileptogenesis for audiogenic seizures, based on lesion, physiological, and pharmacological studies. Therefore, the GABAergic neurons in the IC were identified and counted in four to eight light-microscopic sections throughout the rostral–caudal extent of the IC.

A dramatic increase in the number of GAD-positive neurons is seen in GEPR as compared to the nonepileptic Sprague-Dawley rat (78). This increase is most evident in the central region of the rostral–caudal axis of the IC, where it can be as much as 200 to 300%. In contrast, the number of GAD-positive neurons remains relatively constant throughout the rostral–caudal axis in the Sprague-Dawley rat. The increase in the number of GABAergic neurons in the GEPR seems to be due to a selective increase in the small and medium-size subpopulation of these neurons. This finding is significant because these neurons are considered to be the local circuit neurons in the IC whereas the large-size neurons are projection neurons. Therefore, these data for the GEPR indicate a similar GABAergic defect as observed in the SS gerbils, i.e., an increase in the number of GABAergic neurons that may result in disinhibition of the projection neurons.

FUNCTIONAL SIGNIFICANCE

Since the publication in 1969 of the last volume on basic mechanisms of epilepsies (41), two theories for epileptogenesis have been discussed. Both theories have attempted to describe the pathophysiology of focal epilepsy. The first theory involved the neuroglial impairment hypothesis put forward by Pollen and Trachtenberg (64). The second concerned the GABA deficit–hypoxia hypothesis, which de-

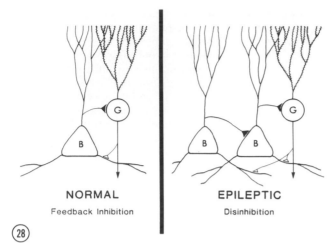

NORMAL
Feedback Inhibition

EPILEPTIC
Disinhibition

(28)

FIG. 28. Schematic diagram of the circuitry between granule and basket cells in the dentate gyrus from seizure-resistant (**left**) and seizure-sensitive (**right**) gerbils. For seizure-resistant gerbils, axon collaterals of granule cells (G) form excitatory synapses with the basal dendrites of basket cells (B), which send inhibitory axons to the soma of the granule cell (see Figs. 7 and 8). This circuitry provides a normal feedback inhibition. In contrast, the seizure-sensitive gerbils have additional basket cells (B) that inhibit other basket cells that contact granule cells (G), thereby resulting in disinhibition.

veloped from numerous pharmacological studies (see ref. 46) but was first demonstrated anatomically by our group (70,71). These two theories will be discussed, as well as a new theory to explain the GABAergic defect observed in two models of genetic epilepsies.

Gliosis and the Cellular Milieu

Based on Penfield's findings (29,30,56), the neuroglial scar was recognized for over half a century as the irritative source for focal seizures that develop after anoxic or traumatic brain damage. Pollen and Trachtenberg published two studies in 1970 (64,97) that analyzed neocortical neuroglia. It was shown that neuroglia can

buffer the extracellular space at areas of synaptic contact to protect against the increase in external potassium ions that are formed as a result of postsynaptic and spike activity. Since increases of potassium can cause seizures (105), defective neuroglia would allow for extracellular potassium accumulations that might induce seizures. Thus, Pollen and Trachtenberg (64) proposed a neuroglial impairment hypothesis as one factor in the development of focal epilepsy.

The glial impairment hypothesis was tested in several subsequent studies. It became apparent that glia have the ability to take up various transmitter products as well as potassium. However, a direct test of this hypothesis found normal potassium homeostasis in glial scar tissue (55).

TABLE 3. *The role of GABA in epilepsy*

Year	Investigators	Findings
1954	Coursin (16)	Vitamin B_6, GAD cofactor, omitted from baby formula, induces seizures
1969	Fischer (28)	Axosomatic symmetric synapses lost at cobalt epileptic foci in rats
1972	Van Gelder and Courtois (98)	GABA loss in cobalt foci in cats
1973	Brown (12)	Axosomatic symmetric synapses lost at human epileptic foci
1975	Emson and Joseph (22)	GAD activity decrease at cobalt foci in rats
	Meldrum (46)	Summary of pharmacological studies that link GABA to epilepsy
1979	Ribak, Harris, Vaughn, and Roberts (71)	Loss of GABA terminals at alumina gel foci in monkeys
1981	Bakay and Harris (6)	Loss of GAD activity, GABA levels and high-affinity GABA receptors in monkey foci
	Lloyd, Munari, Bossi, Bancaud, Talairach, and Morselli (45)	Loss of GAD activity and GABA binding in many human epileptic foci
1982	Ribak, Bradburne, and Harris (70)	Preferential loss of GABA-like symmetric synapses at alumina gel foci in monkeys

Therefore, neuroglial impairment is no longer discussed as a working hypothesis for focal epilepsy (65).

Defects in the GABAergic System

Loss of Inhibition in Focal Epilepsy

Coincident with the neuroglial impairment hypothesis, Meldrum (46) summarized a number of pharmacological studies that linked defects in the GABAergic system with epileptic activity of neurons. Indeed, Van Gelder and Courtois (98) had earlier shown a loss of GABA in cobalt foci in cats. These studies along with others (see Table 3)—including Coursin's (16), which showed infants had seizures when vitamin B_6, a GAD cofactor, was inadvertently omitted from baby formula—have demonstrated a role for GABA in epilepsy. Together, the studies that are cited in Table 3 indicate that the GABA hypothesis provides the best explanation for focal epilepsy. This hypothesis also incorporates the ischemic or hypoxia notion of Spielmeyer (94) and is based on neurocytological evidence obtained from immunocytochemical and electron microscopic data (68).

Factors that may produce epilepsy are quite numerous. Focal epilepsy in experimental models may be caused by a number of agents, such as penicillin, cobalt, alumina gel, and kainic acid. In addition, hypoxia has been implicated as a cause of human epilepsy. This notion has been investigated by Sloper et al. (87), who have shown that hypoxic monkeys display a selective degeneration of terminals which form symmetric synapses in the cerebral cortex. They indicated that these terminals are probably more sensitive to hypoxia than other terminals in the cortex because they appear to have more mitochondria per terminal. Results from our quantitative ultrastructural study (70) of epileptic monkeys are consistent with these findings, in that the mean areas of cortical terminals do not vary greatly but the mean number of mitochondria per terminal forming symmetric synapses was more than twice the number of mitochondria per terminal forming asymmetric synapses. These statistically significant data suggest that GABAergic terminals that form symmetric synapses require more energy than the other cortical terminals that form asymmetric synapses. This latter group of terminals is associated with excitatory function (15). Since most of the energy-dependent activities of axon terminals are thought to involve the exocytosis of neurotransmitter and its subsequent uptake and repackaging, the increased number of mitochondria in GABAergic terminals suggests that these terminals release neurotransmitter at more frequent intervals than the excitatory cortical terminals. Thus, GABAergic terminals may indeed provide a tonic inhibition of cortical projection neurons, as suggested by Roberts (77).

Other morphological data support this notion that GABAergic terminals are probably more active than other cortical terminals. For example, the presence of intranuclear rods (Fig. 6) within certain neurons correlates with high physiological activity (59,84). This finding is significant because the GABAergic aspinous stellate cells often display intranuclear rods within their commonly infolded nuclei, unlike pyramidal cells, which have round nuclei and lack these rods (58,60,67). The filaments that comprise these intranuclear rods may be actin filaments that could facilitate the movement of ribonucleic acid (RNA) out of the nuclei of actively synthesizing neurons. This notion is consistent with data that indicate that higher transcriptional activity occurs in neuronal nuclei with dispersed chromatin than in those with dense areas of heterochromatin (96). GABAergic cortical cells display both intranuclear rods and euchromatin. Thus, these morphological data support the hypothesis that such neurons have high metabolic rates. Since it is reasonable to expect that neurons with high metabolic rates might be more adversely affected by a compromised blood supply than those with lower metabolic requirements, it is thought that aspinous and sparsely spinous stellate neurons might be extremely vulnerable to ischemia. The data on hypoxic monkeys (87) are consistent with this notion. Thus, the death of GABAergic stellate neurons due to ischemia could be expected to reduce the inhibitory synaptic control over pyramidal neurons in the region of trauma and lead to seizure activity of pyramidal neurons.

The results from studies in our laboratory (cited above) and others are consistent with this notion in that GABAergic neurons are preferentially lost at epileptic foci. It is suggested that epileptic activity occurs at these foci as a result of this loss of inhibition (Fig. 23). Before this hypothesis is accepted as dogma, more models of partial epilepsies should be analyzed.

Disinhibition in Genetic Epilepsy

A different type of GABAergic defect occurs in models of genetic epilepsies. As already discussed, Peterson et al. (61,62) and Roberts et al. (78) both describe an increase in the number of GABAergic neurons in the seizure-sensitive gerbils and genetically epilepsy-prone rats, respectively. Since the GABA increase occurs in brain regions that are functionally linked to the specific seizure-provoking stimulus (SS gerbil hippocampus, stress-induced seizures; GEPR inferior colliculus, audiogenic seizures) and in the gerbil preliminary data indicate an exuberance of GABAergic axosomatic synapses for GABAergic basket cells, we suggest that epileptic activity occurs as a result of disinhibition in genetic epilepsy (Fig. 28).

It is apparent from the data for models of genetic epilepsies that more experimental proof is required for this point. Especially needed are neurophysiological slice experiments where granule cells can be recorded. Also, more local neuronal circuitry needs to be explored in both the gerbil hippocampus and GEPR inferior colliculus. Nevertheless, this disinhibition hypothesis is presented based on well-designed neurocytological experiments (61,62).

Our findings that show two different types of GABAergic defects in models of epilepsy should not be surprising in light of the fact that two general classes of epilepsy exist, partial and genetic. As previously reviewed, these two types of epilepsy have different morphological characteristics as described with the classical methods in neurocytology. For example, the partial epilepsies generally have a neuronal loss and gliosis at the epileptic focus. In contrast, the genetic epilepsies do not usually display these features. Furthermore, these epilepsies have different causes: partial is caused by trauma or drug injections, and genetic is caused by inherited genes. These data support the neurocytological findings from our lab that indicate two different GABAergic defects in these two types of epilepsy.

FUTURE CHALLENGES

Numerous experimental models of partial and genetic epilepsies exist. One of the major challenges in the future is to determine if some or all of them display neurocytological features common to those described in this book chapter. Specifically, do all models of partial epilepsies display a preferential loss, either anatomical or functional, of GABAergic synapses? Similarly, do all models of genetic epilepsies display an increase of GABAergic neurons that may cause disinhibition? These obvious questions will help to test the two hypotheses that are discussed as providing useful answers to the basic mechanisms of the epilepsies. Ultimately, a comparison of these experimental models must be made to the pathophysiology of human epilepsy.

The GABAergic defect in the genetic epilepsies is certainly intriguing, and future challenges will involve an analysis of the genes or other developmental factors that regulate the generation and successful development of GABAergic neurons. The results from our studies indicate that increased numbers of GABA neurons are selective for certain brain regions and subregions, and they are present prior to the onset of seizures. These changes are probably associated with a gene or group of genes that should be studied to reveal how GABA neurons are programmed in development. Are other neurotransmitter systems also defective in these genetic models of epilepsy? Finally, is there a selective advantage to having an increased number of GABAergic neurons related to phylogenetic evolution? These points need to be examined in studies planned for the next decade of epilepsy research.

ACKNOWLEDGMENTS

I am indebted to my colleagues Gary M. Peterson, Rosalinda C. Roberts, Carol A. Hunt, Kim L. Andersen, Richard M. Bradburne, Kim B. Seroogy (U. C. Irvine), László Seress (University Medical School, Pécs, Hungary), Roy A. E. Bakay (Emory University, Atlanta), Wolfgang H. Oertel (Technical University, Munich, West Germany), Rod J. Reiffenstein (University of Alberta, Edmonton), A. Basil Harris (University of Washington, Seattle), James E. Vaughn, Eugene Roberts, Robert P. Barber, and Kihachi Saito (City of Hope Research Institute, Duarte, California) for their invaluable collaborations and contributions to the work reviewed in this chapter. The author gratefully acknowledges the critical reading of the manuscript by Richard T. Robertson and the secretarial assistance of Natalie Sepion. Portions of this work were supported by grants from the National Institutes of Health (NS 15669 and NS 20228), the National Science Foundation (BNS 80-23606), the Klingenstein Foundation, and the Epilepsy Foundation of America.

REFERENCES

1. Alzheimer, A. (1898): Ein Beitrag zur pathologischen Anatomie der Epilepsie. *Monatsschr. Psychiatr. Neurol.*, 4:345–369.

2. Amaral, D. G. (1979): Synaptic extensions from the mossy fibers of the fascia dentata. *Anat. Embryol. (Berl.)*, 155:241–251.

3. Andersen, P. (1975): Organization of the hippocampal neurons and their interconnections. In: *The Hippocampus*, edited by R. L. Issacson and K. H. Pribram, pp. 155–175. Plenum, New York.

4. Babb, T. L., Brown, W. J., Feldblum, S., Pretorius, J., and Kupfer, W. (1983): Reduction of GAD-positive cells and terminals after entorhinal-dentate kindling in rats. *Soc. Neurosci. Abst.*, 9:489.

5. Babb, T. L., Brown, W. J., Pretorius, J., and Kupfer, W. (1984): Recovery of GABA recurrent inhibition in dentate gyrus after entorhinal kindling in rats. *Soc. Neurosci. Abst.*, 10:345.

6. Bakay, R. A. E., and Harris, A. B. (1981): Neurotransmitter, receptor and biochemical changes in monkey cortical epileptic foci. *Brain Res.*, 206:387–404.

7. Ben-Ari, Y., Tremblay, E., and Ottersen, O. P. (1980): Injections of kainic acid into the amygdaloid complex of the rat: An electrographic, clinical and histological study in relation to the pathology of epilepsy. *Neuroscience*, 5:515–528.

8. Ben-Ari, Y., Tremblay, E., Ottersen, O. P., and Naquet, R. (1979): Evidence suggesting secondary epileptogenic lesions after kainic acid: Pretreatment with diazepam reduces distant but not local brain damage. *Brain Res.*, 165:362–365.

9. Bouchet and Cazauvieilh (1825): De l'épilepsie considerée dans ses rapports avec l'aliénation mentale. *Arch. Gen. Med.*, 9:510–541.

10. Braak, H., and Goebel, H. H. (1978): Loss of pigment-laden stellate cells: A severe alteration of the isocortex in juvenile neuronal ceroid lipofuscinosis. *Acta Neuropathol. (Berl.)*, 42:53–57.

11. Brotchi, J., Tanaka, T., and Leviel, V. (1978): Lack of activated astrocytes in the kindling phenomena. *Exp. Neurol.*, 58:118–125.

12. Brown, W. J. (1973): Structural substrates of seizure foci in the human temporal lobe. In: *Epilepsy, Its Phenomena in Man*, edited by M. A. B. Brazier, pp. 337–374. Academic Press, New York.

13. Chaslin, P. (1891): Contribution à l'étude de la sclérose cerebrale. *Arch. Med. Exp. Anat. Pathol.*, 3:305–340.

14. Collins, R. C., and Olney, J. W. (1982): Focal cortical seizures cause distant thalamic lesions. *Science*, 218:177–179.

15. Colonnier, M. (1981): The electron-microscopic analysis of the neuronal organization of the cerebral cortex. In: *The Organization of the Cerebral Cortex*, edited by F. O. Schmidt, F. G. Worden, G. Adelman, and S. G. Dennis, pp. 125–152. MIT Press, Cambridge.

16. Coursin, D. B. (1954): Convulsive seizures in infants with pyridoxine-deficient diet. *J.A.M.A.*, 154:406–408.

17. Crandall, J. E., Bernstein, J. J., Boast, C. A., and Zornetzer, S. F. (1979): Kindling in the rat hippocampus: Absence of dendritic alterations. *Behav. Neural. Biol.*, 27:516–522.

18. Dam, A. M., Bajorek, J. C., and Lomax, P. (1981): Hippocampal neuron density and seizures in the Mongolian gerbil. *Epilepsia*, 22:667–674.

19. Demoor, J. (1898): La mécanisme et la signification de l'état moniliforme des neurones. *Ann. Soc. Roy. Sci. Med. Nat. Brux.*, 7:205–250.

20. Earle, K., Baldwin, M., and Penfield, W. (1953): Incisural sclerosis and temporal lobe seizures produced by hippocampal herniation at birth. *Arch. Neurol. Psychiatry*, 69:27–42.

21. Emson, P. C., and Hunt, S. P. (1981): Anatomical chemistry of the cerebral cortex. In: *The Organization of the Cerebral Cortex*, edited by F. O. Schmitt, F. G. Worden, G. Adelman, and S. G. Dennis, pp. 325–345. MIT Press, Cambridge.

22. Emson, P. C., and Joseph, M. H. (1975): Neurochemical and morphological changes during the development of cobalt-induced epilepsy in the rat. *Brain Res.*, 93:91–110.

23. Engel, J., Jr., Brown, W. J., Kuhl, D. E., Phelps, M. E., Mazziotta, J. C., and Crandall, P. H. (1982): Pathological findings underlying focal temporal lobe hypometabolism in partial epilepsy. *Ann. Neurol.*, 12:518–528.

24. Engel, J., Jr., Driver, M. V., and Falconer, M. A. (1975): Electrophysiological correlates of pathology and surgical results in temporal lobe epilepsy. *Brain*, 98:129–156.

25. Fairén, A., Peters, A., and Saldanha, J. (1977): A new procedure for examining Golgi impregnated neurons by light and electron microscopy. *J. Neurocytol.*, 6:311–337.

26. Falconer, M. A., Hill, D., Meyer, A., Mitchell, W., and Pond, D. A. (1955): Treatment of temporal-lobe epilepsy by temporal lobectomy: A survey of findings and results. *Lancet*, 1:827–835.

27. Feria-Velasco, A., Olivares, N., Rivas, F., Velasco, M., and Velasco, F. (1980): Alumina cream-induced focal motor epilepsy in cats. IV. Thickness and cellularity of layers in the perilesional motor cortex. *Arch. Neurol.*, 37:287–290.

28. Fischer, J. (1969): Electron microscopic alterations in the vicinity of epileptogenic cobalt-gelatine necrosis in the cerebral cortex of the rat. *Acta Neuropathol. (Berl.)*, 14:201–214.

29. Foerster, O., and Penfield, W. (1930): The structural basis of traumatic epilepsy and results of radical operation. *Brain*, 53:99–119.

30. Foerster, O., and Penfield, W. (1930): Der Narbenzug am und im Gehirn bei traumatischer Epilepsie in seiner Bedeutung für das Zustandekommen der Anfälle und für die therapeutische Bekämpfung derselben. *Z. Ges. Neurol. Psychiatr.*, 125:475–572.

31. Freund, T. F., Martin, K. A. C., Smith, A. D., and Somogyi, P. (1983): Glutamate decarboxylase immunoreactive terminals of Golgi-impregnated axoaxonic cells and of presumed basket cells in synaptic contact with pyramidal neurons of the cat's visual cortex. *J. Comp. Neurol.*, 221:263–278.

32. Goddard, G. V., McIntyre, D. C., and Leach, C. K. (1969): A permanent change in brain function resulting from daily electrical stimulation. *Exp. Neurol.*, 25:295–330.

33. Gruner, J. E., Hirsch, J. C., and Sotelo, C. (1974): Ultrastructural features of the isolated suprasylvian gyrus in the cat. *J. Comp. Neurol.*, 154:1–28.

34. Harris, A. B. (1972): Degeneration in experimental epileptic foci. *Arch. Neurol.*, 26:434–449.

35. Harris, A. B. (1975): Cortical neuroglia in experimental epilepsy. *Exp. Neurol.*, 49:691–715.

36. Harris, A. B., and Lockhard, J. S. (1981): Absence of seizures or mirror foci in experimental epilepsy after excision of alumina and astrogliotic scar. *Epilepsia*, 22:107–122.

37. Heimer, L., and RoBards, M. J., editors (1981): *Neuroanatomical Tract-Tracing Methods.* Plenum, New York.

38. Hendry, S. H. C., Houser, C. R., Jones, E. G., and Vaughn, J. E. (1983): Synaptic organization of immunocytochemically identified GABA neurons in the monkey sensory-motor cortex. *J. Neurocytol.*, 12:639–660.

39. Hoover, D. B., Culberson, J. L., and Craig, C. R. (1977): Structural changes in cerebral cortex during cobalt-induced epilepsy in the rat. *Neurosci. Lett.*, 4:275–280.

40. Houser, C. R., Hendry, S. H. C., Jones, E. G., and Vaughn, J. E. (1983): Morphological diversity of immunocytochemically identified GABA neurons in the monkey sensory-motor cortex. *J. Neurocytol.*, 12:617–638.

41. Jasper, H. H., Ward, A. A., Jr., and Pope, A., editors (1969): *Basic Mechanisms of the Epilepsies.* Little, Brown, Boston.

42. Johnson, J. E., Jr., editor (1981): *Current Trends in Morphological Techniques,* Vols. 1–3. CRC, Boca Raton, Florida.

43. Jones, E. G. (1981): Anatomy of cerebral cortex: Columnar input-output organization. In: *The Organization of the Cerebral Cortex,* edited by F. O. Schmitt, F. G. Worden, G. Adelman, and S. G. Dennis, pp. 199–235. MIT Press, Cambridge.

44. Krnjević, K. (1974): Chemical nature of synaptic transmission in vertebrates. *Physiol. Rev.*, 54:418–540.

45. Lloyd, K. G., Munari, C., Bossi, L., Bancaud, J., Talairach, J., and Morselli, P. L. (1981): Biochemical evidence for the alterations of GABA-mediated synaptic transmission in human epileptic foci. In: *Neurotransmitters, Seizures and Epilepsy,* edited by P. L. Morselli, K. G. Lloyd, W. Löscher, B. Meldrum, and E. H. Reynolds, pp. 331–354. Raven Press, New York.

46. Meldrum, B. S. (1975): Epilepsy and GABA—Mediated inhibition. *Int. Rev. Neurobiol.*, 17:1–36.

47. Meldrum, B. S., and Brierly, J. B. (1973): Prolonged epileptic seizures in primates: Ischaemic cell change and its relation to ictal physiological events. *Arch. Neurol.*, 28:10–17.

48. Mesulam, M.-M., Mufson, E. J., Levey, A. I., and Wainer, B. H. (1983): Cholinergic innervation of cortex by the basal forebrain: Cytochemistry and cortical connections of the septal area, diagonal band nuclei, nucleus basalis (substantia innominata), and hypothalamus in the rhesus monkey. *J. Comp. Neurol.*, 214:170–197.

49. Nadler, J. V., Perry, B. W., and Cotman, C. W. (1978): Intraventricular kainic acid preferentially destroys hippocampal pyramidal cells. *Nature (Lond.)*, 271:676–677.

50. Nitsch, C., and Rinne, U. (1981): Large dense-core vesicle exocytosis and membrane recycling in the mossy fibre synapses of the rabbit hippocampus during epileptiform seizures. *J. Neurocytol.*, 10:201–219.

51. Oertel, W. H., Schmechel, D. E., Mugnaini, E., Tappaz, M. L., and Kopin, I. J. (1981): Immunocytochemical localization of glutamate decarboxylase in rat cerebellum with a new antiserum. *Neuroscience*, 6:2715–2735.

52. Olney, J. W., de Gubareff, T., and Sloviter, R. S. (1983): "Epileptic" brain damage in rats induced by sustained electrical stimulation of the perforant path. II. Ultrastructural analysis of acute hippocampal pathology. *Brain Res. Bull.*, 10:699–712.

53. Olsen, R. W., Snowman, A. M., Wamsley, J. K., Lee, R., and Lomax, P. (1983): Benzodiazepine receptor binding deficit in midbrain of seizure-sensitive gerbils. *Soc. Neurosci. Abst.*, 9:399.

54. Paul, L. A., Fried, I., Watanabe, K., Forsythe, A. B., and Scheibel, A. B. (1981): Structural correlates of seizure behavior in the Mongolian gerbil. *Science*, 213:924–926.

55. Pedley, T. A., Fischer, R. S., and Prince, D. A. (1976): Focal gliosis and potassium movement in mammalian cortex. *Exp. Neurol.*, 50:346–361.

56. Penfield, W. (1927): The mechanism of cicatricial contraction in brain. *Brain*, 50:499–517.

57. Penfield, W., and Humphreys, S. (1940): Epileptogenic lesions of the brain, a histologic study. *Arch. Neurol. Psychiatry*, 43:240–261.

58. Peters, A., and Fairén, A. (1978): Smooth and sparsely-spined stellate cells in the visual cortex of the rat: A study using a combined Golgi-electron microscopic technique. *J. Comp. Neurol.*, 181:129–171.

59. Peters, A., Palay, S. L., and Webster, H. De F. (1976): *The Fine Structure of the Nervous System.* Saunders, Philadelphia.

60. Peters, A., Proskauer, C. C., and Ribak, C. E. (1982): Chandelier cells in rat visual cortex. *J. Comp. Neurol.*, 206:397–416.

61. Peterson, G. M., Ribak, C. E., and Oertel, W. H. (1984): Differences in the hippocampal GABAergic system between seizure-sensitive and seizure-resistant gerbils. *Anat. Rec.*, 208:137A.

62. Peterson, G. M., Ribak, C. E., and Oertel, W. H. (1985): A regional increase in the number of hippocampal GABAergic neurons and terminals in the seizure-sensitive gerbil. *Brain Res.*, 340:384–389.

63. Pfleger, L. (1880): Beobachtung über Schrumpfung und Sclerose des Ammonshornes bei Epilepsie. *Allg. Z. Psychiat.*, 36:359–365.

64. Pollen, D. A., and Trachtenberg, M. C. (1970):

Neuroglia: Gliosis and focal epilepsy. *Science,* 167:1252–1253.

65. Prince, D. A. (1983): Mechanisms of epileptogenesis in brain-slice model systems. In: *Epilepsy,* edited by A. A. Ward, Jr., J. K. Penry, and D. Purpura, pp. 29–52. Raven Press, New York.

66. Reid, S. A., Sypert, G. W., Boggs, W. M., and Willmore, L. J. (1979): Histopathology of the ferric-induced chronic epileptic focus in cat: A Golgi study. *Exp. Neurol.,* 66:205–219.

67. Ribak, C. E. (1978): Aspinous and sparsely-spinous stellate neurons in the visual cortex of rats contain glutamic acid decarboxylase. *J. Neurocytol.,* 7:461–478.

68. Ribak, C. E. (1983): Morphological, biochemical, and immunocytochemical changes of the cortical, GABAergic system in epileptic foci. In: *Epilepsy,* edited by A. A. Ward, Jr., J. K. Penry, and D. Purpura, pp. 109–130. Raven Press, New York.

69. Ribak, C. E. (1985): Axon terminals of GABAergic chandelier cells are lost at epileptic foci. *Brain Res.,* 326:251–260.

70. Ribak, C. E., Bradburne, R. M., and Harris, A. B. (1982): A preferential loss of GABAergic, inhibitory synapses in epileptic foci: A quantitative ultrastructural analysis of monkey neocortex. *J. Neurosci.,* 2:1725–1735.

71. Ribak, C. E., Harris, A. B., Vaughn, J. E., and Roberts, E. (1979): Inhibitory, GABAergic nerve terminals decrease at sites of focal epilepsy. *Science,* 205:211–214.

72. Ribak, C. E., Harris, A. B., Vaughn, J. E., and Roberts, E. (1981): Immunocytochemical changes in cortical GABA neurons in a monkey model of epilepsy. In: *Neurotransmitters, Seizures, and Epilepsy,* edited by P. L. Morselli, K. G. Lloyd, W. Löscher, B. Meldrum, and E. H. Reynolds, pp. 11–22. Raven Press, New York.

73. Ribak, C. E, Hunt, C. A., Bakay, R. A. E., and Oertel, W. H. (1986): A loss of small GABAergic somata is associated with the preferential loss of GABAergic terminals at epileptic foci. *Brain Res., (in press).*

74. Ribak, C. E., and Reiffenstein, R. J. (1982): Selective inhibitory synapse loss in chronic cortical slabs: A morphological basis for epileptic susceptibility. *Can. J. Physiol. Pharmacol.,* 60:864–870.

75. Ribak, C. E., and Seress, L. (1983): Five types of basket cell in the hippocampal dentate gyrus: A combined Golgi and electron microscopic study. *J. Neurocytol.,* 12:577–597.

76. Ribak, C. E., Vaughn, J. E., and Saito, K. (1978): Immunocytochemical localization of glutamic acid decarboxylase in neuronal somata following colchicine inhibition of axonal transport. *Brain Res.,* 140:315–332.

77. Roberts, E. (1980): Epilepsy and antiepileptic drugs: A speculative synthesis. In: *Antiepileptic Drugs: Mechanisms of Action,* edited by G. H. Glaser, J. K. Penry, and D. M. Woodbury, pp. 667–713. Raven Press, New York.

78. Roberts, R. C., Ribak, C. E., Peterson, G. M., and Oertel, W. H. (1984): Increased numbers of GABAergic neurons in the inferior colliculus of the genetically epilepsy prone rat. *Soc. Neurosci. Abst.,* 10:410.

79. Robertson, R. T., editor (1978): *Neuroanatomical Research Techniques.* Academic Press, New York.

80. Rutledge, L. T. (1978): The effects of denervation and stimulation upon synaptic ultrastructure. *J. Comp. Neurol.,* 178:117–128.

81. Scheibel, M., Crandall, P., and Scheibel, A. B. (1974): The hippocampal–dentate complex in temporal lobe epilepsy. *Epilepsia,* 15:55–80.

82. Scheibel, A. B., Paul, L., and Fried, I. (1983): Some structural substrates of the epileptic state. In: *Basic Mechanisms of Neuronal Hyperexcitability,* edited by H. H. Jasper and N. M. van Gelder, pp. 109–130. Alan R. Liss, New York.

83. Scheibel, M. E., and Scheibel, A. B. (1973): Hippocampal pathology in temporal lobe epilepsy. A Golgi survey. In: *Epilepsy, Its Phenomena in Man,* edited by M. A. B. Brazier, pp. 311–337, Raven Press, New York.

84. Seïte, R., Mei, N., and Couinea, S. (1971): Modification quantitative des batônnets intranucléaires des neurons sympathiques sous l'influence de la stimulation électrique. *Brain Res.,* 34:277–290.

85. Seress, L., and Ribak, C. E. (1983): GABAergic cells in the dentate gyrus appear to be local circuit and projection neurons. *Exp. Brain Res.,* 50:173–182.

86. Seroogy, K. B., Seress, L., and Ribak, C. E. (1983): Ultrastructure of commissural neurons of the hilar region in the hippocampal dentate gyrus. *Exp. Neurol.,* 82:594–608.

87. Sloper, J. J., Johnson, P., and Powell, T. P. S. (1980): Selective degeneration of interneurons in the motor cortex of infant monkeys following controlled hypoxia: A possible cause of epilepsy. *Brain Res.,* 198:204–209.

88. Sloper, J. J., and Powell, T. P. S. (1975): A study of the axon initial segment and proximal axon of neurons in the primate motor and somatic sensory cortices. *Philos. Trans. R. Soc. Lond [Biol.]* 285:173–197.

89. Sloviter, R. S. (1983): "Epileptic" brain damage in rats induced by sustained electrical stimulation of the perforant path. I. Acute electrophysiological and light microscopic studies. *Brain Res. Bull.,* 10:675–697.

90. Söderfelt, B., Kalimo, H., Olsson, Y., and Siesjö, B. (1981): Pathogenesis of brain lesions caused by experimental epilepsy. Light- and electron-microscopic changes in the rat cerebral cortex following bicuculline-induced status epilepticus. *Acta Neuropathol. (Berl.),* 54:219–231.

91. Sommer, W. (1880): Erkrankung des Ammonshorns als aetiologisches Moment der Epilepsie. *Arch. Psychiatry,* 10:631–675.

92. Somogyi, P., and Cowey, A. (1981): Combined Golgi and electron microscopic study on the synapses formed by double bouquet cells in the visual cortex of the cat and monkey. *J. Comp. Neurol.,* 195:547–566.

93. Somogyi, P., Freund, T. F., and Cowey, A. (1982): The axo-axonic interneuron in the ce-

rebral cortex of the rat, cat and monkey. *Neuroscience,* 7:2577–2609.

94. Spielmeyer, W. (1930): The anatomic substratum of the convulsive state. *Arch. Neurol. Psychiatry,* 23:869–875.

95. Sternberger, L. A., editor (1979): *Immunocytochemistry,* 2nd ed. John Wiley, New York.

96. Thomas, J. O., and Thompson, R. J. (1977): Variation in chromatin structure in two cell types from the same tissue: A short DNA repeat length in cerebral cortex neurons. *Cell,* 10:633–640.

97. Trachtenberg, M. C., and Pollen, D. A. (1970): Neuroglia: Biophysical properties and physiologic function. *Science,* 167:1248–1252.

98. Van Gelder, N. M., and Courtois, A. (1972): Close correlation between changing content of specific amino acids in epileptogenic cortex of cats, and severity of epilepsy. *Brain Res.,* 43:477–484.

99. Velasco, M., Velasco, F., and Feria-Velasco, A. (1976): Alumina cream-induced focal motor epilepsy in cats: III. Ultrastructure of the epileptogenic focus. *Arch. Invest. Med.,* 7:157–170.

100. Westrum, L. E., White, L. E., and Ward, A. A., Jr. (1964): Morphology of the experimental epileptic focus. *J. Neurosurg.,* 21:1033–1044.

101. Wilder, B. J., Schimpff, B. D., and Collins, G. H. (1972): Ultrastructure study of the chronic experimental epileptic focus. *Epilepsia,* 13:341–342.

102. Williams, R. S., Lott, I. T., Ferrante, R. J., and Caviness, V. S. (1977): The cellular pathology of neuronal ceroid lipofuscinosis. *Arch. Neurol.,* 34:298–305.

103. Willmore, L. J., Sypert, G. W., and Munson, J. B. (1978): Recurrent seizures induced by cortical iron injection: A model of posttraumatic epilepsy. *Ann. Neurol.,* 4:329–336.

104. Winer, B. J. (1962): *Statistical Principles in Experimental Design.* McGraw-Hill, New York.

105. Zuckermann, E. C., and Glaser, G. H. (1968): Hippocampal epileptic activity induced by localized ventricular perfusion with high-potassium cerebrospinal fluid. *Exp. Neurol.,* 20:87–110.

Advances in Neurology, Vol. 44, edited by
A. V. Delgado-Escueta, A. A. Ward, Jr.,
D. M. Woodbury, and R. J. Porter.
Raven Press, New York © 1986.

38

Freeze-Fracture Studies of Plasma Membranes of Astrocytes in Freezing Lesions

*Juanita J. Anders and Milton W. Brightman

Department of Anatomy, F. Edward Hébert School of Medicine, Uniformed Services University of the Health Sciences, Bethesda, Maryland 20814, and Laboratory of Neuropathology and Neuroanatomical Sciences, National Institutes of Neurological and Communicative Disorders and Stroke, National Institutes of Health, Bethesda, Maryland 20205

SUMMARY Epileptic foci are frequently associated with a proliferation and hypertrophy of fibrous astrocytes. Such proliferating astrocytes, which are involved in scar formation and are referred to as reactive, have been characterized by a number of morphological changes involving the cytoplasmic organelles and nucleus. With the development of freeze-fracture techniques, which allow for the splitting and analysis of the macromolecular structure of biological membranes, another morphological characteristic could be used to define reactive astrocytes. This characteristic is the alteration in the normal number and distribution of intramembranous particles. Specifically, there is an increase in the number of orthogonal arrays of intramembranous particles, called assemblies, in the plasma membrane of reactive astrocytes.

Besides the presence of assemblies in the plasma membranes of astrocytes, similar particle arrays are also found in the central nervous system (CNS), in cell membranes of ependymal cells, in Müller cells near the inner limiting membrane of the retina, and in satellite cells in spinal ganglia. Assemblies are concentrated in the plasma membranes of astrocytic processes that form the glia limitans at the outer surface of the brain and the perivascular sheath around parenchymal blood vessels in the adult mammalian CNS. Plasma membranes of perineuronal astrocytic processes and astrocytic cell bodies have few, if any, assemblies. The factor responsible for this polarity of assemblies in the normal CNS is unknown. However, this polarity is lost when astrocytes respond to various types of injuries to the CNS.

It has been postulated that gliosis, resulting in an epileptic scar, may be a response of cortical astrocytes to changes in the local cellular environment and that this reactivity of astrocytes may be related to plasma membrane changes. However, little is known about the initiation of the astrocytic response or the involvement of the astrocytic plasma membrane.

Because of the presence of assemblies, astrocytic plasma membranes are an ideal subject for a morphological investigation of alterations of the cell membrane. Assemblies have a distinctive structure and changes in their number and distribution can be readily identified. Also, since there is polarity of the assemblies in astrocytic plasma membranes, such that their number is greatest in subpial and perivascular areas and least in the perineuronal regions, it is easy to identify when assemblies are added or lost from the astrocytic plasma membranes of a particular brain region.

Focal cortical lesions, produced by freeze injury, were used to examine the involvement of astrocytic plasma membranes. Histopathological alterations caused by cortical freezing influenced this choice. There is an alteration of the blood-brain barrier in the region of the lesion, and a transient cortical edema is present during the initial periods when there is maximal electroencephalographic (EEG) abnormality. Therefore, many changes in the cellular environment, which may initiate the astrocytic reactivity, return to normal levels within a few hours of the injury and need not be maintained to sustain the reactive astrocytes. This makes it especially critical to examine the astrocytes during this initial period when the astrocytic reactivity is initiated.

It was found, using freeze-fracture electron-microscopic techniques, that assemblies in the astrocytic plasma membranes situated 2 to 4 mm from the lesion center are not disrupted and are normally distributed. The number of assemblies in these peripheral astrocytic processes begin to increase by 30 min after injury. This increase in number continues with time.

Astrocytes within the center of the lesion have clumped intramembranous particles, including large aggregated assemblies. Similar aggregation of assembly-with-assembly in plasma membranes of astrocytes *in vitro* occurs after treatment with protein denaturants, such as urea and guanidine HCl. Similarly, tightly clumped assemblies were found in the cell membranes of astrocytes from mature rat brain separated by differential centrifugation. This tight packing of assemblies appears to be a consistent feature of plasma membranes of damaged astrocytes both *in vivo* and *in vitro*. Progressive gliosis at the lesion site after freezing injury is characterized morphologically by increases in the number of astrocytic processes filled with glial filaments and addition of assemblies in their plasma membranes in regions of the CNS parenchyma where normally few, if any, are found.

What astrocytic function, if any, may be morphologically represented by the assemblies remains unknown. Evidence is accumulating against the suggestion that assemblies may be associated with Na^+,K^+-ATPase. More recently, it has been proposed that assemblies may represent ionic leakage sites for relocation of ions such as K^+, away from active regions. Another intriguing possibility for the function of assemblies is their relationship to the maintenance of intracellular pH. It is hoped that identification of factors responsible for maintenance of the normal polarity of assemblies in the astrocytic plasma membranes, the rapid increase of assemblies in the plasma membranes of reactive astrocytes, and the spread of reactive astrocytes in the periphery of the lesion will lead to methods for blocking astrocytic scar formation.

Astrocytes can proliferate and hypertrophy to form glial scars in response to many types of injuries to the central nervous system (CNS). Epileptic foci are frequently associated with such a proliferation of fibrous astrocytes (63). Such proliferating and scar-forming astrocytes have been primarily characterized by an increase in intermediate (8–9 nm) filaments (25,35) and glycogen, larger nuclei, an elaboration of the Golgi apparatus (46), and an increase in oxidative enzymes (1). Astrocytes with these characteristics have been referred to as reactive. With the development of the freeze-fracture technique, which allows for the splitting and analysis of the macromolecular architecture of biological membranes, another morphological characteristic can be used to define reactive astrocytes. That is, there is an increase in orthogonal arrays of intramembranous particles [referred to as assemblies by Landis and Reese (33)] in the plasma membranes of reactive astrocytes (2,3,44,65).

Orthogonal arrays of small intramembranous particles are a distinctive feature of the cytoplasmic half, or P-face, of frozen-cleaved plasma membranes from various cell types of different embryonic origins, including hepatocytes (31), epithelial cells of the intestine (56) and trachea (27), light cells of the kidney collecting tubules (26), skeletal muscle (19,49,51,53), and parietal cells of the stomach (6). In addition to astrocytes, similar arrays or assemblies are also found in the plasma membranes of certain nonneuronal cells within the nervous system, including Müller cells near the inner limiting membrane of the retina (50), ependymal cells (9,47), and satellite cells in spinal ganglia (18,45). Although the orthogonal arrays are similar in these cells, it should be kept in mind that, at this time, there is no evidence that they are a morphological representation of the same function. Assemblies are especially plentiful in the cell membranes of astrocytic processes that form the glia limitans at the outer surface of the brain and the perivascular sheath around parenchymal blood vessels in the adult mammalian central nervous system (2,15,16,24,33,34,39,41,42). As the parenchyma is approached, the number of assemblies decreases with each successive layer of astrocytic processes, so that the plasma membranes of processes and cell bodies of perineuronal satellite astrocytes have few, if any, assemblies. This polarity of the assemblies in astrocytic plasma membranes is the same in the cerebral cortical regions of both rodents and humans (Fig. 1) and is lost when astrocytes respond to various types of injuries to the CNS. However, the factor responsible for the polarity of the astrocytic plasma membranes in the normal CNS has not been found.

It has been postulated that the susceptibility of astrocytes to injury and their reactivity may be related to plasma membrane changes (60). However, little is known about the initiation of the astrocytic response or the involvement of the astrocytic plasma membrane. It has been proposed that gliosis resulting in a scar is a response of cortical astrocytes to a change in the local cellular environment caused by chronically hyperactive epileptic neurons. Besides the initiating events, Ward (63) has suggested not only that gliosis is an adaptive response to the altered local environment but also that progressive gliosis may both increase the number of epileptic neurons and augment their hyperactivity. Several years ago, we became interested in investigating what stimuli initiate astrocytes to become reactive. Experimental production of focal seizure sites can be achieved by a number of methods, including cortical application of cobalt (12,43) or alumina cream (22,23) and freezing (13,36,37). For our experiments, we chose to produce focal cortical lesions by freezing. Cobalt produces an epileptic focus that requires approximately 2 weeks for definitive electroencephalographic (EEG) epileptiform activity to appear (40). Alumina cream needs usually 35 to 60 days to produce EEG spiking, the time required being dependent upon the intensity of the alumina focus (62). Abnormal EEG discharges that follow local cortical freezing are highly variable but may occur within a few minutes to several hours after freezing. Maximal EEG abnormalities usually develop within 8 to 12 hr (37). Freeze injury produces a chronic focus and a secondary cortical focus contralateral to the primary lesion within the first 24 hr in the rat (38). The histopathological alterations caused by cortical freezing also influenced our choice. There is an alteration of the blood-brain barrier in the region of the lesion, and the cortex is edematous (29). With time, the edema fluid spreads from the cortical area and accumulates in the white matter. This transient cortical edema is present during the initial periods when there is maximal EEG abnormality (61). Therefore, changes in the cellular environment, which may initiate the astrocytic reactivity, return to normal levels within a

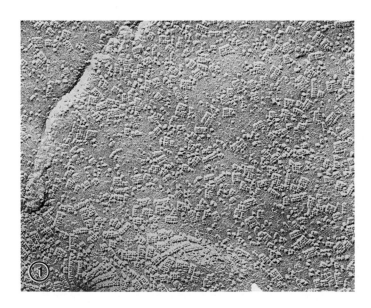

FIG. 1. Subpial astrocytic plasma membrane (P-face) with numerous assemblies. This specimen of human cerebral cortex from the frontal lobe has membrane particles comparable to those of the rat. ×116,000.

few hours of the injury and need not be maintained to sustain the reactive astrocytes (57). This transience makes it especially critical to examine astrocytes during the initial period when the astrocytic reactivity is initiated.

Based on thin-section electron-microscopic examination of freezing lesions, it is known that astrocytes undergo marked swelling during the initial 24 hr, while there is a variable amount of neuronal damage, primarily involving the dendrites (36). It has been proposed that a primary alteration of the plasma membranes of astrocytes and neurons occurs after cortical freezing and results in disorders of cation transport (59). This proposal ran parallel to the suggestion that astrocytes are involved in the transport of electrolytes between the vascular system and neurons (21,32).

Because of their content of assemblies, astrocytic plasma membranes are an ideal subject for a morphological investigation of alterations within the cell membrane. The assemblies have a distinctive structure, and changes in their number and distribution can be readily identified. Since there is polarity of the assemblies in astrocytic plasma membranes—that is, their number is greatest in subpial and perivascular areas and least in the perineuronal regions—it is also easy to recognize when assemblies are added or lost from the astrocytic plasma membranes of a particular brain region. After having established the normal number and distribution of assemblies in the plasma membranes of subpial astrocytes of the dorsal cerebral cortex of mature and developing rats (2), we examined the plasma membranes of astrocytes from the center and periphery of freezing lesions after chemically fixing and rapidly freezing the tissue within minutes of the injury (3). Nine-day-old rats were chosen for this set of experiments, since we felt that the initial changes in the astrocytic plasma membranes within minutes of freezing injury might be very subtle. There is an average of 85 assemblies/μm^2 of plasma membrane of subpial astrocytes in 9-day-old rats (Fig. 2). This mean is much lower than that of the normal adult rat (387 assemblies/μm^2 of plasma membrane) and thus makes it easier to detect increases in the number of assemblies or their rearrangement. Also, in rats of this age, the skulls are thin enough to enable thermal damage of the brain to be made directly through the cranium. The freezing injury to the brain was produced by placing a 1-mm brass rod, cooled with a mixture of dry ice and acetone, on the exposed skulls over the parietal region of the left cerebral hemisphere approximately 3 mm from the midline of anaesthetized rats for 2 sec.

Assemblies in those astrocytic plasma membranes situated 2 to 4 mm from the lesion center were not disrupted and were normally distributed, as were the other intramembranous particles. However, the number of assemblies in these peripheral astrocytes began to increase by 30 min after injury (97/μm^2, SD $\pm$ 51) (Fig. 3). This increase in number continued with time, and by 4 to 6 hr there were 167 assemblies/μm^2 of membrane (Fig. 4) (3).

Astrocytes within the center of the lesion had clumped intramembranous particles, including large aggregated assemblies (Fig. 5). This clumping characterized all samples taken from the lesion center from 15 min to 6 hr after the lesion had been made, with the more severe clumping seen after the longer time intervals (Fig. 6). Similar aggregation of assembly-with-assembly as well as clumping of the other intramembranous particles in plasma membranes of astrocytes *in vitro* was caused by the protein denaturants, urea and guanidine HCl (Fig. 7). The aggregation of assembly-with-assembly was augmented with rising concentrations of the denaturants (2). Similarly, assemblies were tightly clumped in plasma membranes of astrocytes from mature rat brain separated by differential centrifugation (4). The tight packing of assemblies would, therefore, appear to be a consistent criterion of a badly damaged astrocyte, both *in vivo* and *in vitro*.

Examination of the astrocytes with thin-section electron microscopy revealed relatively intact astrocytic processes immediately subpially. However, directly below this layer there were many swollen astrocytic processes and dendrites. There was no appreciable change in the number of glial filaments until 4 hr after freeze injury occurred (Fig. 8). Immunoperoxidase staining for glial fibrillary acidic protein (GFAP), a protein associated with glial filaments (5,20), was used to determine when the glial reaction could be determined. No such reactive astrocytes were observed in the region of the lesion until 24 hr after freezing injury (Fig. 9). Interestingly, astrocytes in the center of the lesion did not have any difference in antibody reaction when compared with the astrocytes in the control cortex, while astrocytes in the periphery of the lesion had an increased antibody reaction. The site of the epileptic focus formed by intracortical injection of alumina has been shown by EEG to be the surrounding scar tissue rather than the lesion site itself. Seizure activity in

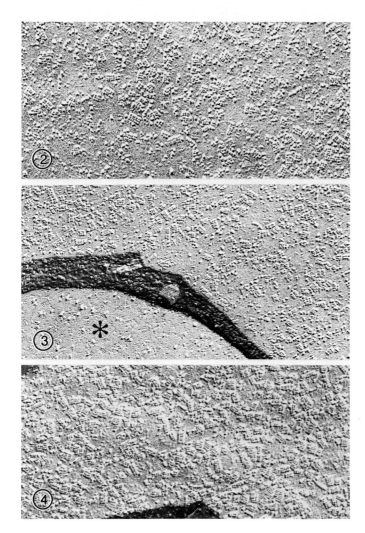

FIG. 2. P-Face of an astrocytic membrane from the glia limitans of a 9-day-old rat showing normal number and distribution of assemblies, ×116,000.

FIG. 3. The E- (*asterisk*) and P-faces of astrocytic membranes from the periphery of the lesion 30 min after cold injury. The number of assemblies is increasing. ×102,000.

FIG. 4. Assemblies continue to increase in astrocytic membranes peripheral to lesion site (9-day-old rat) 6 hr after cold injury. ×110,000.

these animals was eliminated after removal of the surrounding astrogliotic scar (23). Reactive astrocytes responding to injury of the cerebral cortex are mainly derived from proliferation and from hypertrophy of normal astrocytes at the periphery of edematous cortex. Other types of brain injury, including stab wounds in rats (5,14,35) and thermocoagulation of the motor cortex of rats (17), are also accompanied by reactive astrocytes, identified by an increased immunocytochemical staining of glial fibrillary acidic protein 24 or 48 hr after injury. There has been only one report of a rapid, intense, immunocytochemical staining of glial fibrillary acidic protein in astrocytes. This reaction occurred within 10 min of breakdown of the blood-

brain barrier in microembolization by injection of microspheres in cats (30).

The difference in the time period after injury, when changes in the number of glial filaments can be detected with thin-section electron microscopy and immunocytochemical staining, suggests that glial filaments have to be present in certain amounts before they can be detected immunocytochemically. This threshold suggests a limited sensitivity of the method. However, a strength of this technique lies not in detecting the earliest changes but in its ability to show the spread of astrocytic activity from the lesion site to other regions of the homolateral and contralateral cerebral hemispheres.

Four weeks after the freezing injury, a definite

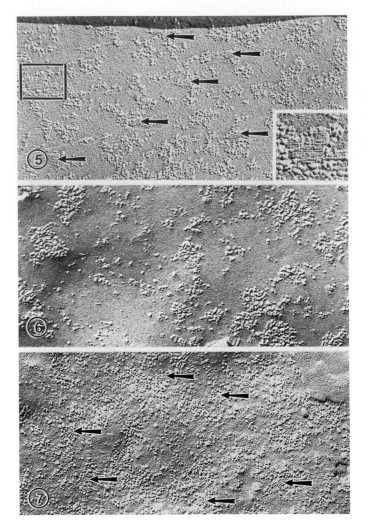

FIG. 5. Astrocytic membrane from the center of a freezing lesion 15 min after cold injury to the brain surface of a 9-day-old rat. There is an aggregation of assembly with assembly (*arrows*). ×80,500. **Inset:** A higher magnification of area delineated by the *box*. The tight packing of the assembly particles is especially striking. ×155,000.

FIG. 6. Astrocytic plasma membrane from the center of a freezing lesion (6 hr after freeze injury). Severe clumping of intramembranous particles characterizes these astrocytic plasma membranes and is believed to be a feature of membranes of badly damaged cells. ×90,000.

FIG. 7. Astrocytic membrane, 14 days *in vitro*, P-face, 30 min after addition of guanidine HCl (2 M) to the culture medium. A specific aggregation of assembly with assembly occurs (*arrows*). This aggregation of intramembranous particles is similar to that seen in plasma membranes after freezing injury (Figs. 5 and 6). ×90,000.

gliosis develops consisting of an increased number of filament-laden astrocytic processes in the glia limitans and the molecular layer of the cerebrum. When frozen and fractured, it was found that the plasma membranes of these astrocytic processes had increased numbers of assemblies and numerous gap junctions (Fig. 10). Progressive gliosis after a cold lesion is morphologically characterized by increases in the number of astrocytic processes filled with glial filaments and the maintenance of increased numbers of assemblies in astrocytic plasma membranes in the parenchyma, where normally few if any assemblies are found.

A few recent studies of astrocytic reactivity utilizing freeze-fracture techniques have also reported increases in assemblies. In the optic nerves of 2- to 4-month-old rats that had been enucleated during early postnatal life, a dense glial scar is formed. There is a threefold increment in the assemblies within the plasma membranes of intraparenchymal astrocytic processes composing this scar (65). In addition, Wujek and Reier (65) also found that these membrane alterations occurred rapidly in response to axotomy in immature rats, so that the number of assemblies at 3 hr post axotomy exceeded the values of the adult controls. In glial hypertrophy associated with hypomyelination in the murine mutant Jimpy, the density of assemblies in the reactive astrocytes doubles (44). Therefore, a wide variety of diseases and injuries that lead to neuronal damage, dysfunction, and/or loss also result in a corresponding proliferation of astro-

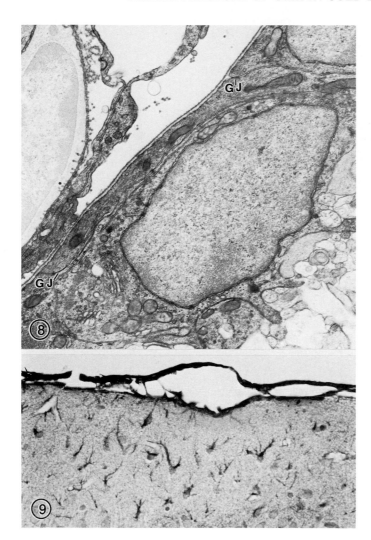

FIG. 8. Thin plastic section of the brain surface at the site of a freezing lesion 4 hr after injury. This is the earliest a subtle increase in intermediate filament bundles can be identified. Gap junctions (GJ) are present between the astrocytes forming the glia limitans. It is of interest that the astrocytes directly below the basement membrane are not swollen. However, the dendrites and glial processes directly below this outermost astrocytic layer show considerable swelling. ×21,000.

FIG. 9. Peroxidase-antiperoxidase (PAP) immunochemically stained astrocytes treated with antibody to GFAP lying in the periphery of the freezing lesion 24 hr after injury. Normally, astrocytes in the marginal layer of the dorsal cerebral cortex of 9-day-old rats show little if any staining reaction. The earliest time period after freezing injury that an increase in the GFAP staining reaction could be found was 24 hr. There was no increase in the staining reaction of the astrocytes in the center of the lesion at 24 hr post lesion. ×270.

cytes that are characterized by an increase of assemblies in their plasma membranes.

What astrocytic function, if any, may be morphologically represented by the assemblies remains unknown. The suggestion that assemblies may be associated with ion flux, such as Na^+,K^+-ATPase (18), is unlikely for several reasons. Assemblies are absent in plasma membranes where Na^+,K^+-dependent ATPase is known to be present, such as at the luminal end of epithelial cells of the choroid plexus (10) and on neurons (see Chapter 53). Further, assemblies were not demonstrated when Na^+, K^+-ATPase was isolated and functionally reconstituted in artificial liposomes (52). Finally, the electron-microscopic localization of brain

K^+-p-nitrophenylphosphatase activity, a marker for Na^+, K^+-ATPase, has shown a different distribution in the cerebral cortex from that of the assemblies (11).

It has also been proposed that assemblies represent ionic leakage sites for relocation of ions, such as K^+, away from active regions (24). This is an interesting suggestion, particularly when considered with respect to the fact that assemblies are found in plasma membranes of reactive astrocytes deep in the parenchyma in perineuronal regions.

In many types of brain injuries involving anoxia and hypercapnia there is an increase in brain CO_2 and lactic acid (7,28,48,54,55,58,64). CO_2 is membrane-permeable and can cause acid-

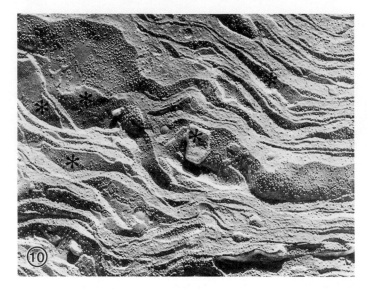

FIG. 10. The P-face and E-face (*asterisks*) of astrocytic membranes from a glial scar 4 weeks after freezing injury to the dorsal cerebral cortical surface of 9-day-old rat. These astrocytic processes extend into the molecular layer, yet they have many assemblies. ×60,000.

ification of the cellular interior (48). Evidence is increasing to suggest that intracellular pH is an important factor in cytoskeletal regulation (55). Since drugs that alter the cytoskeleton cause a redistribution of the assemblies in astrocytic plasma membranes within 20 min (3), changes in intracellular pH may affect not only the astrocytic cytoskeleton but also the plasma membrane. With respect to these findings, we have proposed that a function of the assemblies might be related to the carrier-mediated exchange of H^+ and HCO_3^- for Na^+ and Cl^- (7,28). Under normal conditions CO_2 crosses the cell membrane and is hydrated to form HCO_3^- and H^+. Since HCO_3^- is relatively impermeable, it must leave the cell by exchanging for Na^+, a mechanism that may be involved in control of intracellular pH. Identification of the factors responsible for maintenance of the normal polarity of assemblies in the astrocytic plasma membranes, the rapid increase of assemblies in reactive astrocytes, and the spread of reactive astrocytes in the periphery of the lesion may lead to future studies on ways to alter the initial response of the astrocytes and to block the formation of reactive gliosis.

ACKNOWLEDGMENTS

The authors would like to express appreciation to Pamela Sorando for her excellent technical and photographic assistance.

This investigation was supported in part by a research grant from the Epilepsy Foundation of America and Department of Defense (DoD) grant R07046. The opinions or assertions contained herein are the private ones of the author and are not to be construed as official or reflecting the views of the DoD or the Uniformed Services University of the Health Sciences. The experiments reported herein were conducted according to the principles set forth in the "Guide for Care and Use of Laboratory Animals," Institute of Laboratory Animal Resources, National Research Council.

REFERENCES

1. Al-Ali, S. Y. A., and Robinson, N. (1982): Ultrastructural study of enzymes in reactive astrocytes: Clarification of astrocytic activity. *Histochem. J.*, 14:311–321.
2. Anders, J. J., and Brightman, M. W. (1979): Assemblies of particles in the cell membranes of developing, mature and reactive astrocytes. *J. Neurocytol.*, 8:777–795.
3. Anders, J. J., and Brightman, M. W. (1982): Particle assemblies in astrocytic plasma membranes are rearranged by various agents *in vitro* and cold injury *in vivo*. *J. Neurocytol.*, 11:1009–1029.
4. Anders, J. J., Blessing, P. M., and Brightman, M. W. (1983): Freeze-fracture analyses of plasma membranes of isolated astrocytes from rat brain. *Brain Res.*, 278:81–91.
5. Bignami, A., and Dahl, D. (1976): The astrocytic response to stabbing. Immunofluorescence studies with antibodies to astrocyte-specific protein (GFA) in mammalian and submammalian vertebrates. *Neuropathol. Appl. Neurobiol.*, 2:99–110.
6. Bordi, C., and Perrelet, A. (1978): Orthogonal arrays of particles in plasma membranes of the gastric parietal cell. *Anat. Rec.*, 192:297–304.
7. Bourke, R. S., Kimelberg, H. K., and Daze, M. A. (1978): Effects of inhibitors and adenosine

on (HCO_3^-/CO_2)-stimulated swelling and Cl^- uptake in brain slices and cultured astrocytes. *Brain Res.,* 154:196–202.

8. Brightman, M. W., and Reese, T. S. (1969): Junctions between intimately opposed cell membranes in the vertebrate brain. *J. Cell Biol.,* 40:648–677.

9. Brightman, M. W., Prescott, L., and Reese, T. S. (1975): Intercellular junctions of special ependyma. In: *Brain-Endocrine Interaction II. The Ventricular System,* edited by K. M. Knigge, D. E. Scott, H. Kobyashi, and S. Ishii, pp. 146–165. Karger, Basel.

10. Brightman, M. W., Anders, J. J., Schmechel, D., and Rosenstein, J. M. (1979): The lability of the shape and content of glial cells. In: *Dynamic Properties of Glial Cells,* edited by E. Schofeniels, pp. 21–44. Pergamon, Oxford.

11. Broderson, S. H., Patton, D. L., and Stahl, W. L. (1978): Fine structural localization of potassium-stimulated *p*-nitrophenyl phosphatase activity in dendrites of the cerebral cortex. *J. Cell Biol.,* 78:R13–R17.

12. Butler, A. B., Willmore, L. J., Fuller, P. M., and Bass, N. H. (1976): Focal alterations of dendrites and astrocytes in rat cerebral cortex during initiation of cobalt-induced epileptiform activity. *Exp. Neurol.,* 51:216–228.

13. Clasen, R. A., Cooke, P. M., Pandolfi, S., Boyd, D., and Raimondi, A. J. (1962): Experimental cerebral edema produced by focal freezing. 1. An anatomic study utilizing vital dye techniques. *J. Neuropathol. Exp. Neurol.,* 21:570–595.

14. Connor, J. R., and Peters, A. (1982): Astrocytic response to CNS injury: An immunohistochemical study. *Soc. Neurosci. Abstr.,* 8:239.

15. Dermietzel, R. (1974): Junctions in the central nervous system of the cat. III. Gap junctions and membrane-associated orthogonal particle complexes (MOPC) in astrocytic membranes. *Cell Tissue Res.,* 149:121–135.

16. Dermietzel, R. (1975): Membranassoziierte orthogonale Partikelkomplexe (MOPC) in Astrozytenmembranen. Ein Beitrag zu ihrer Ultrastruktur, ihrer Verteilung und Verhalten unter verscheidenen Praparations-bedingungen. *Verhandlungen der Anatomischen Gesellschaft,* 69:607–611.

17. Duchesne, P. Y., Gheuens, J., Brotchi, J., and Gerebtzoff, M. A. (1979): Normal and reactive astrocytes: A comparative study by immunohistochemistry and by a classical histological technique. *Cell Mol. Biol.,* 24:237–239.

18. Elfvin, L. G., and Forsman, C. (1978): The ultrastructure of junctions between satellite cells in mammalian sympathetic ganglia as revealed by freeze-etching. *Ultrastruct. Res.,* 63:261–274.

19. Ellisman, M. H., and Rash, J. E. (1977): Studies of excitable membranes. III. Freeze-fracture examination of the membrane specializations at the neuromuscular junction and in the non-junctional sarcolemma after denervation. *Brain Res.,* 137:197–206.

20. Eng, L. F., and Bigbee, J. W. (1978): Immunohistochemistry of nervous system-specific antigens. In: *Advances in Neurochemistry,* Vol. 3,

edited by B. W. Agranoff and M. H. Aprison, pp. 43–98. Plenum, New York.

21. Gerschenfeld, H. M., Wald, F., Zadunaisky, J. A., and DeRobertes, E. D. P. (1959): Function of astroglia in the water-ion metabolism of the central nervous system: An electron microscope study. *Neurology,* 9:412–425.

22. Harris, H. B. (1972): Degeneration in experimental epileptic foci. *Arch. Neurol.,* 26:434–449.

23. Harris, H. B., and Lockard, J. S. (1981): Absence of seizures or mirror foci in experimental epilepsy after excision of alumina and astrogliotic scar. *Epilepsia,* 22:107–122.

24. Hatton, J. D., and Ellisman, M. H. (1981): The distribution of orthogonal arrays and their relationship to intercellular junctions in neuroglia of the freeze-fractured hypothalmo-neurohypophysial system. *Cell Tissue Res.,* 215:309–323.

25. Hirano, A. (1978): Neuronal and glial processes in neuropathology. *J. Neuropathol. Exp. Neurol.,* 37:365–374.

26. Humbert, F., Pricam, C., Perrelet, A., and Orci, L. (1975): Specific plasma membrane differentials in the cells of the kidney collecting tubule. *J. Ultrastruct. Res.,* 52:13–20.

27. Inoue, S., and Hogg, J. C. (1977): Freeze-etch study of the tracheal epithelium of normal guinea pigs with particular reference to intercellular junctions. *J. Ultrastruct. Res.,* 61:89–99.

28. Kimelberg, H. K. (1979): Glial enzymes and ion transport in brain swelling. In: *Neural Trauma,* edited by A. J. Popp, pp. 137–153. Raven Press, New York.

29. Klatzo, I., Chur, E., Fujiwara, K., and Spatz, M. (1980): Resolution of vasogenic brain edema. In: *Advances in Neurology,* Vol. 28: *Brain Edema,* edited by J. Cervos-Navarro and R. Ferszt, pp. 359–373. Raven Press, New York.

30. Klatzo, I., Laursen, H., Orze, F., Chui, E., Wilmes, F., Suzuki, R., and Horie, R. (1981): Behavior of the blood-brain barrier (BBB) in cerebrovascular disorders. In: *Cerebrovascular Diseases; New Trends in Surgical and Medical Aspects,* edited by H. Barnett, P. Paolette, E. Flamm, and G. Brambella, pp. 5–17. Elsevier-North-Holland Biomedical Press, Amsterdam.

31. Kreutziger, G. O. (1968): Freeze-etching of intercellular junctions of mouse liver. In: *Proc. 26th Mtg. Electron Microscope Society of America,* p. 234. Claitors Publishing Division, Baton Rouge.

32. Kuffler, S. W., Nicholls, J. G., and Orkland, R. K. (1966): Physiological properties of glia cells in the central nervous system of amphibia. *J. Neurophysiol.,* 29:768–787.

33. Landis, D. M. D., and Reese, T. S. (1974): Arrays of particles in freeze-fractured astrocytic membranes. *J. Cell Biol.,* 60:316–320.

34. Landis, D. M. D., and Reese, T. S. (1982): Regional organization of astrocytic membranes in cerebellar cortex. *Neuroscience,* 7:937–950.

35. Latov, N., Nilaver, G., Zimmerman, E. A., Johnson, W. A., Silverman, A.-J., Defenine, R., and Cote, L. (1979): Fibrillary astrocytes proliferate in response to brain injury. *Dev. Biol.,* 72:381–384.

36. Lee, J. C., and Bakay, L. (1966): Ultrastructural

changes in the edematous central nervous system: II. Cold induced edema. *Arch. Neurol.,* 14:36–49.

37. Lewin, E. (1972): The production of epileptogenic cortical foci in experimental animals by freezing. In: *Experimental Models of Epilepsy,* edited by D. P. Purpura, J. K. Penry, D. B. Tower, D. N. Woodbury, and R. D. Walter, pp. 37–51. Raven Press, New York.

38. Lewin, E., and McCrimmon, A. (1967): ATPase activity in discharging cortical lesions induced by freezing. *Arch. Neurol.,* 16:321–325.

39. Massa, P. T., and Mugnaini, E. (1982): Cell junctions and intramembrane particles of astrocytes and oligodendrocytes: A freeze-fracture study. *Neuroscience,* 7:523–538.

40. Mesher, R. A., Wyler, A. R., and Neafsey, E. J. (1978): The effects of chronicity on burst structure in epileptogenic foci. *Brain Res.,* 142:467–476.

41. Nabeshima, S., Reese, T. S., Landis, D. M. D., and Brightman, M. W. (1975): Junctions in the meninges and marginal glia. *J. Comp. Neurol.,* 164:127–170.

42. Nakai, Y., Kudo, J., and Hashimoto, A. (1980): Specific cell membrane differentiation in the tanycytes and glial cells of the organum vasculosum of the lamina terminales in dog. *J. Electron Microsc. (Tokyo),* 29:144–150.

43. Nakamura, I., Endo, M., Hosakawa, K., Isaki, K., Koyama, Y., and Katsukawa, K. (1981): Fine structure of experimental epileptogenic focus produced by intracerebral implantation of cobalt-gelatin stick in rabbits. *Folia Psychiatr. Neurol. Jpn.,* 35:103–111.

44. Omlin, F. X., Bischoff, A., and Moor, H. (1980): Myelin and glial membrane structures in the optic nerve of normal and Jimpy mouse. *J. Neuropathol. Exp. Neurol.,* 39:215–231.

45. Pannese, E., Luciano, L., Iurato, S., and Reale, E. (1977): Intercellular junctions and other membrane specializations in developing spinal ganglia: A freeze-fracture study. *J. Ultrastruct. Res.,* 60:169–180.

46. Peters, A., Palay, S. L., and Webster, H. de F. (1976): *The Fine Structure of the Nervous System,* pp. 233–248. W. B. Saunders Company, Philadelphia.

47. Privat, A. (1977): The ependyma and subependymal layer of the young rat: A new contribution with freeze-fracture. *Neuroscience,* 2:447–457.

48. Rapoport, S. (1976): *Blood Brain Barrier in Physiology and Medicine.* Raven Press, New York.

49. Rash, J. E., and Ellisman, M. H. (1974): Studies of excitable membranes. I: Macromolecular specializations of the neuromuscular junction and the non-junctional sarcolemma. *J. Cell Biol.,* 63:567–586.

50. Reale, E., and Luciano, L. (1974): Introduction to freeze-fracture method in retinal research. *Albrecht von Graefes Arch. Klin. Exp. Ophthalmol.,* 192:73–87.

51. Schmalbruch, H. (1979): Square arrays in the sarcolemma of human skeletal muscle fibres. *Nature (Lond.),* 281:145–146.

52. Skriver, E., Maunsbach, A. B., and Jorgensen, P. L. (1980): Ultrastructure of Na,K-transport vesicles reconstituted with purified renal Na,K-ATPase. *J. Cell Biol.,* 86:746–754.

53. Smith, D. S., Baerwald, R. J., and Hart, M. A. (1975): The distribution of orthogonal assemblies and other intercalated particles in frog sartorius and rabbit sacrospinalis muscle. *Tissue Cell,* 7:369.

54. Smith, T. G., and Purpura, D. P. (1960): Electrophysiological studies on epileptogenic lesions of cut cortex. *Electroencephalogr. Clin. Neurophysiol.,* 12:59–82.

55. Spray, D. C., Harris, A. L., and Bennett, M. V. L. (1981): Gap junctional conductance is a simple and sensitive function of intracellular pH. *Science,* 211:712–715.

56. Staehelin, L. A. (1972): Three types of gap junctions interconnecting intestinal epithelial cells visualized by freeze-etching. *Proc. Natl. Acad. Sci. U.S.A.,* 69:1318–1321.

57. Thorn, W., Scholl, H., Pfleederer, G., and Meuldener, B. (1958): Metabolic processes in the brain at normal and reduced temperatures and under anoxic and ischemic conditions. *J. Neurochem.,* 2:150–156.

58. Torack, R. M., Terry, R. D., and Zimmerman, H. M. (1959): The fine structure of cerebral fluid accumulation: Swelling secondary to cold injury. *Am. J. Pathol.,* 35:1135–1147.

59. Tower, D. B. (1960): *Neurochemistry of Epilepsy.* Charles C. Thomas, Springfield, Illinois.

60. Tower, D. B. (1978): General perspectives and conclusions of the symposium on dynamic properties of glial cells. In: *Dynamic Properties of Glia Cells,* edited by E. Schoffeniels, G. Franck, D. B. Tower, and L. Hertz, pp. 443–460. Pergamon Press, Oxford.

61. Vyskocil, F., Kriz, N., and Bures, J. (1952): Potassium-selective microelectrodes used for measuring the extracellular brain potassium during spreading depression and anoxic depolarization in rats. *Brain Res.,* 39:255–259.

62. Ward, A. A. (1972): Topical convulsant metals. In: *Experimental Models of Epilepsy,* edited by D. P. Purpura, J. K. Penry, D. B. Tower, D. M. Woodbury, and R. D. Walter, pp. 13–37. Raven Press, New York.

63. Ward, A. A. (1978): Glia and Epilepsy. In: *Dynamic Properties of Glia Cells,* edited by E. Schoffeniels, G. Franck, D. B. Tower, and L. Hertz, pp. 413–433. Pergamon Press, Oxford.

64. Withrow, C. D. (1972): Systemic carbon dioxide derangements. In: *Experimental Models of Epilepsy,* edited by D. P. Purpura, J. Keffen-Penry, D. B. Tower, D. M. Woodbury, and R. Walter, pp. 477–494. Raven Press, New York.

65. Wujek, J. R., and Reier, P. J. (1982): Changes in astrocytic plasma membranes after axotomy. *Soc. Neurosci. Abstr.,* 8:239.

Advances in Neurology, Vol. 44, edited by
A. V. Delgado-Escueta, A. A. Ward, Jr.,
D. M. Woodbury, and R. J. Porter.
Raven Press, New York © 1986.

39

Structural Substrates of Epilepsy

*L. A. Paul and **A. B. Scheibel

*Brentwood Veterans Administration Hospital, Los Angeles, California; **Department of Anatomy,
UCLA School of Medicine, Los Angeles, California 90024; and *.**Department of Neurology,
UCLA, Los Angeles, California 90024

SUMMARY   Although interest in possible structural substrates of epilepsy has
been high since anatomical abnormalities in autopsy material were first noted, a
clear pathognomic picture has yet to emerge for subtypes other than temporal
lobe epilepsy. While identification of anatomical features unique to the diseased
brain does not ensure that a cure will be found (viz. Alzheimer's disease), such
knowledge can certainly guide researchers who must search out both the necessary and sufficient etiologic agent. Such investigation is hampered by the difficulty of separating cause from effect in clinical material, where the patient may
have a history of drug use or of poorly controlled seizures. For instance, the cell-
density depletion noted in temporal-lobe epileptics could follow from, or be a
cause of, seizures.

An experimental approach to isolating the structural substrates of epilepsy
requires establishing several "levels" of epilepsy of varying duration, and observing the evolution of anatomical change. Such manipulation is, of course,
possible only when an animal model is used, and it is for this reason, among
others, that researchers have developed several of these. In general, there are
two types of animal model: one where an exogenous agent (for example, a neurotoxin) or treatment (kindling) is applied, and another that relies on a strain of
animal bred to exhibit seizures. Anatomical findings in this latter case have been
reported infrequently, although the approach, which is not confounded by central
nervous system (CNS) damage, seems promising as a model for certain types of
epilepsy. Rodents have been among the best-researched genetic preparations, and
several such reports appear in this volume.

We have investigated one such strain, the Mongolian gerbil, which has been
bred in UCLA's animal colony to exhibit seizures (the SS strain). Another strain
(SR) has been bred to be seizure-free. Our initial study compared adult SS and
SR animals with respect to two morphometric parameters in hippocampal region
CA3. We found that the SS adult gerbil had fewer dendritic spines than its nonseizuring counterpart. Dendritic spines are considered the locus of excitatory
synapses, and their density has been correlated with a variety of functional states
in other paradigms.

Our next set of questions concerned the development of these strain differences, and we accordingly set up four different age groups, bracketing the age at
which seizures first appear in the gerbil. Again, spine-density differences appeared between SS and SR animals, but in the opposite direction from the adult
case: young SS gerbils have *more* spines on CA3 dendrites than do SRs, even at
an age when seizures have not yet appeared. Thus, the brain that will have
seizures is differentiated from the brain that will not, at least with respect to this

morphologic parameter. Possible implications of these findings with respect to the development of seizures are discussed.

As highly visual creatures, we humans feel that a tangible, visible substrate ought to underlie a neuropathological condition as dramatic and complex as epilepsy. Yet the only type of epilepsy that has been reliably linked to an anatomical substrate is temporal-lobe epilepsy, characterized by partial seizures (except seizures which develop as a consequence of focal brain injury). This is true even though findings of abnormalities in patients undergoing cortical resection for intractable seizures are among the earliest reported in epilepsy research (25). DeMoor (19) was the first to suggest that identifiable morphological changes in cortical dendrites accompanied epilepsy in humans. These findings have been confirmed and extended in a series of reports over the past decade, particularly in relation to the complex partial epilepsies associated with temporal lobe dysfunction (7, 59). One of the presently best-documented areas is that of dendritic change in response to paroxysmal electrocortical activity and the ictal state. In addition, it is now suspected that there are structural alterations in the microvasculature of the areas involved in the ictal phenomena. As will be seen, all of the structural changes to be noted are, at best, correlational with the epileptic state, and little can yet be adduced as to cause or effect.

Golgi studies performed on blocks of temporal lobe tissue removed at surgery for intractable epilepsy document a series of dendritic changes in hippocampal pyramidal cells. Figure 1 presents the most significant of these. The most subtle consist of scattered loss of dendritic spines on one or more dendrites of individual cells, or on small groups of pyramidal neurons (Fig. 1, A–C). The loss may involve either apical or basilar dendrites and is usually more noticeable at dendrite tips than in more central portions of the dendritic tree. The pattern of distribution for minimal (or early) spine loss is not unexpected in light of the now-demonstrated enhanced plasticity of these areas of the dendritic tree under conditions of enrichment and aging (20) or aging (9).

More extensive alterations involve widening zones of spine loss and the appearance of periodic swellings along the denuded dendritic shaft. Dendrite branches may show changes in structure, becoming convoluted or gnarled in appearance, bearing occasional blunt protrusions or leafy excrescences. The nature and content of these enlargements remain unclear. Still more advanced alterations result in massive dying back of the dendritic tree, with swelling or pyknotic changes in the cell body culminating in cell death. Areas of neuronal loss, observed by us (58) and by others (17) are characterized by gliosis, and spotty or massive patches of fibrous astrocytic overgrowth mark the most devastated areas. The cicatrizing effect of these focal glial scars is manifest in distortions of dendritic architecture in adjacent, presumably more intact, fields. The array of changes noted here has been seen in all areas of the cornu ammonis but is noted in highest concentration among neurons of CA1 and CA2.

The dentate fascia may also be the scene of epilepsy-related cellular change, although we have seldom noted complete cell loss. Dendritic spine loss and nodulation of the dendritic shafts are fairly frequent. In addition, a group of characteristic alterations in dendritic configuration is frequently seen. In some cases, the dendritic shafts of masses of cells are deflected, usually uniformly, in one direction or another. This "windblown" appearance may conceivably represent a response to patterns of tissue tension set up by adjacent scarring foci. In other cases, the entire dendritic ensemble appears collapsed inward upon the center of axial symmetry of the individual dentate neuron, resembling a "closed parasol" (58).

Correlative studies using Golgi and scanning electron microscopic techniques have revealed other facets of tissue change which are still under analysis. We have noted at least two types of change in the vascular tree (Fig. 1, D–F). These include (a) individual swelling or extrusions from the surfaces of very small intracerebral blood vessels (capillaries, capillary arterioles, and capillary venules) and (b) irregular, lobulated lengths of vessel. In the former case, these isolated pouch-like structures ranging from 3 or 4 μm to 40 μm in diameter have been found in tissue specimens from more than one-third of two series of cases of temporal lobe epilepsy patients. The sac-like enlargements appear to occur along the course of fine vessels, at points of inflection, and at vascular bifurcations. They have been tentatively identified as "microaneurysms" (57). Some degree of support for this interpretation is obtained from the frequent presence of adjacent small pools of extravasated blood or pigments. The presumption that

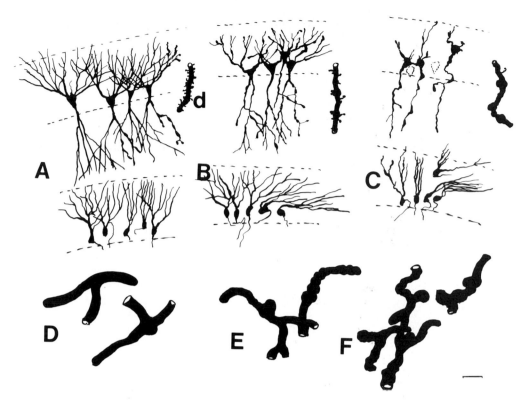

FIG. 1. An overview of histological changes found in surgically removed specimens of hippocampus from patients with temporal-lobe epilepsy. **A, B, C:** Three levels of alterations seen in hippocampal pyramids (*upper ensembles*) and dentate granule cells (*lower ensembles*). Dentate cells showing the "windblown look" are sketched in **B** and **C**; one cell with the closed parasol deformity appears in **C**. A length of hippocampal dendrite (d) is shown for each stage, indicating the progressive loss of spines and developing "lumpiness" or "string-of-beads" appearance of the dendrite shaft. **D, E, F:** Progressive degrees of distortion of the microvasculature. Note the increased lumpiness and protrusions of the vessel walls and the frequent appearance of tiny outpouchings, some of which may be tiny aneurysms. Calibration line (*lower right*) for **D, E, F** is 5 μm.

these tiny pouch-like extrusions "leak" or "blow out" periodically is an attractive one, although no other evidence is presently available to support this thesis. On the other hand, the well-documented epileptogenic capability of blood iron, hemosiderin, and other iron salts underlines a possible role of such structures in the development of neuronal hyperexcitability (33,39,61).

The lobulated lengths of vessel mentioned above may represent hyperplastic changes in the endothelial lining or pericytic involucrum of the vessel walls. The cause of such cellular overgrowth is unknown, but somewhat similar changes have been seen in very old patients and in those suffering from senile dementia, Alzheimer type (SDAT). It is worth reiterating that these vascular alterations bear an uncertain relationship to the epileptic process and to its etiology.

One reason for the difficulty in firmly establishing substrates for epilepsy may be the amorphous nature of the term itself. The International League Against Epilepsy began to publish classificatory schemes of epileptic seizures in 1964 (27). Several revisions have since appeared, reflecting increased knowledge gained from computerized tomography and telemetry monotoring to better localize the ictal and interictal activity; a discussion of some of these new classification methods is provided by Engel et al. (23). A chief distinction between the older and newer systems is that the modern approach categorizes epilepsy according to behavior and functional state, without relying on "hard" anatomical changes, an improvement since the difficulty of identifying pathognomic anatomical features is acknowledged. In addition, the problem of definition of the term "epilepsy" remains far from solved: as Gastaut and Broughton (27) state:

"At present it is still exceedingly difficult, if not impossible, to provide an acceptable classification of the epilepsies" (p. 4).

These and related reasons have encouraged many investigators to use animal models of epilepsy. A particular model may resemble one feature of human epilepsy more than others; for instance, animals that have been electrically kindled show good reproducibility of seizures and progression of seizure stages, but their seizure etiology and apparent lack of neuronal degeneration (43) limit their resemblance to human epilepsy. Or, the form of convulsions in some animal models may fail to resemble human seizures, as Nadler (46) has pointed out for the kainic acid model. Use of an animal model reflects the experimenter's interest in studying one aspect of what we have labeled "epilepsy" in humans; it need not imply that the animal is considered to be "epileptic." Such models display a range of seizure topographies and behaviors, which qualify them to greater or lesser degrees as good experimental models of epilepsy. Criteria for evaluating these models have been set forth (70), and the literature contains several comprehensive reviews (12,52).

In the area of anatomy, animal models, with their potential for experimental manipulation, offer opportunities for study that human tissue cannot provide. Obtaining material from severe epileptics can only be done when removal of tissue is clinically indicated; thus, the field of study is severely limited. Furthermore, tissue cannot be taken from anyone with a mild case of epilepsy, or when surgery is not indicated: a whole range of "epilepsies" can therefore never be studied until the patient succumbs from unrelated causes, by which time the effects of many confounding conditions, including long-term use of medication, are likely to be present.

Animal models can be divided into two types: those in which an otherwise normal animal is made to exhibit seizures through some intervention (placement of toxic substances on cortex; electrical or chemical stimulation), and specially bred strains that display the seizure phenotype. Two substances used to induce seizures are penicillin (24) and alumina cream (3) applied to exposed cortical surface. Prepared in this way, monkeys (alumina cream) (3), cats (penicillin) (8), or rats (22) develop behavioral seizures as well as epileptiform wave patterns in electroencephalograph (EEG) recordings. Another approach has been to inject "excitotoxins" (49) such as kainate (47) into the ventricles. Enkephalins have also been tested in this manner (67). The discovery that repeated subthreshold stim-

ulation of the amygdala by electric current or chemicals (28,30,31) results in an animal with EEG and behavioral seizures has generated a great deal of research. Many of the treatments that produce kindling also potentiate phenomena thought to be important in learning, such as long-term potentiation (LTP) or evoked potentials (43).

To what extent are such models similar to human epilepsy in the neuropathological picture they present? The anatomical substrates in many of the above preparations show changes similar to those found in the human. Following application of substances to cortex, neuronal loss, gliosis, changes in dendritic arborization and morphology, and spine loss [*Macacca mulatta*, intracortical alumina cream (54,73); cat, cobalt chloride injected into hippocampus (8); cat, subpial $FeCl_3$ (53)] have all been reported in the region of the focus. Brown et al. (8), at the level of the electron microscope, observed dark pyramidal cells, macrophages, and large lipid droplets. Astrocytes appeared swollen, and displayed proliferated (sic) processes, with extensive gliosis around circulatory elements. A 1984 report by Hatton and Ellisman (35) using freeze-fracture techniques on rat cortex after application of alumina gel found a redistribution in astrocytic arrays (assemblies) in brain parenchyma surrounding the lesion. Many of these changes are reminiscent of those found in humans.

Because of the manner in which these preparations were made epileptic, it is impossible to make an inference about possible causal relationships between anatomy and seizures. Also, the excitatory effect of many of the substances applied to brain cannot be separated from their toxic activity, which would make conclusions about neuroanatomical change tentative. This issue is particularly pressing with regard to the action of excitatory amino acids (glutamate, aspartate) and their analogs (kainic acid) (49).

Use of a genetically seizuring animal does not raise the problem of injury to the brain from an exogenous agent, since seizures develop without intervention as the animal matures. Several species are currently popular choices for seizure-related work. These include the photosensitive baboon (38), the epileptic beagle (74), the audiogenic mouse (36,63), and other strains of rodent (12,34,40). A variety of behavioral and electrophysiological approaches have been used in these studies. Surprisingly, however, neuroanatomical studies on a genetically seizuring animal have been few. The investigations on *Papio papio,* a well-researched preparation (45,38), did not show structural differences between seizuring and nonseizuring baboons except in those subjects which died in status epilepticus (R. Naquet, *personal communication*).

Our choice of the Mongolian gerbil for investigation of the structural substrates of seizures was motivated by a positive evaluation of the model from a behavioral point of view. Two breeding lines of gerbils, differentiated by seizure phenotype, were established at UCLA by Lomax and collaborators (41) and later maintained by A. B. Scheibel and coworkers. The SS (seizure-sensitive) gerbil reliably demonstrates seizures when placed in a novel environment (see Table 1). The SR (seizure-resistant) gerbil does not have seizures under the same conditions. Several features are advantageous when the gerbil is evaluated against criteria set forth by Wada et al. (70). Seizures in the gerbil begin to appear at about 50 days of age and stabilize to the adult pattern by the end of the third month. Although variable throughout the SS strain, seizure intensity, duration, and latency following removal from the cage (the stimulus that precipitates a seizure), once established for an individual animal, are stable for life. Gerbil seizures are precipitated by mild stress, represented by removal to the seizure testing area (10). Their seizures develop gradually, beginning at 50 days with a stereotyped increase in all parameters until the pattern stabilizes. In addition, while the seizure pattern for an individual animal seems quite invariant throughout life, there is considerable variability among animals in seizure intensity, latency following stimulation, and duration. Gerbil seizures, unlike some other rodent models [e.g., audiogenic mouse (64)], virtually never end in death. Seizure patterns in this animal span the gap from a barely detectable twitching of the vibrissae to a full-blown grand mal seizure with a long postictal depression. Our seizure scoring procedure uses a nine-point rating scale (Table 1). Thus, the species, like the human, shows a variety of "epilepsies."

Suggestions that the gerbil is a viable model have been based not only on behavioral manifestations but also on electroencephalographic

TABLE 1. *Seizure testing methods*

Gerbils are tested weekly by removal from the home cage and placement into a large plastic testing bin. The observer then monitors the animal's behavior for 5 min, measured by hand-held clock. If no seizure occurs during that time period, the animal receives 2 min of vigorous stroking on the back with an unsharpened pencil. This usually elicits a seizure if the animal has not seized in the first 5 min. Intensity (see below), duration (from time of onset), and latency (from time of placement into bin) of the seizure are noted on the animal's seizure history card. In Dr. Scheibel's laboratory we use a seizure rating scale modified after that described by Loskota et al. (42). Seizures are rated on a nine-point scale, as follows. The figure in parentheses represents the numerical rating.

(1.0) Animal continues to move about; ears flick and vibrissae twitch rapidly. Only ears and whiskers are involved.

(1.5) Ears and whiskers move. Slight tendency to bob head with minor interruption of forward movement.

(2.0) Ears flick, whiskers twitch, and head bobs up and down as animal moves forward in jerky, discontinuous fashion.

(2.5) Animal occasionally lowers head to floor of testing bin and then moves forward in repetitive pattern. Appears to be entering stage 3 seizure (below), but lifts head and moves forward.

(3.0) Animal lowers head slowly as whiskers twitch rapidly; ears flick rapidly and then flatten against head. Head stays flattened against floor and body is humped in a tense little mound. Jerky running may then occur, after which animal is quiescent for a period of time.

(3.5) Body position more extreme than in level 3.0 seizure; hind legs are pushed forward and torso back. Usually lordosis is present, followed by stereotyped forepaw movement. This level is differentiated from a level 4 seizure by the jerky running followed by quiescent period.

(4.0) Begins in same way as level 3, but usually progresses more rapidly and body position becomes much more flattened, with extreme lordosis, Straub tail, and tonic splaying of forelimbs. Levels 4.0, 4.5, and 5.0 are usually long seizures (average 5 min), while level 3.0 lasts only 2–3 min. Level 4.0 also involves eye closure, teeth chomping, tonic–clonic movements of forelimbs and sometimes hindlimbs, with pawing of the ground; blind wild running; leaps that can take animal out of the testing bin; and stereotyped forelimb movements and grooming. A quiescent phase follows and may be punctuated with head turning from side to side and forepaw movements. Position in quiescent phase more flattened than in level 3.0 seizure. Return to normal exploratory activity is sudden.

(4.5) Identical to level 4.0 with addition of *slow* falling onto side and recovery to prone posture.

(5.0) More violent seizure than 4.0 or 4.5. Animal executes one or more vigorous complete roll-overs or somersaults. Usually runs and leaps into air.

(5.5) Animal does not survive a very violent, prolonged seizure. However, only two or three such events have been noted in our colony's 5-year history.

(EEG) evidence (40). Although further work remains to be done, these authors observed paroxysmal, high-frequency, high-amplitude bursting in several neocortical regions, which was correlated with behavioral manifestations of the seizure. The location of seizure onset, while variable among animals, was consistent for an individual gerbil. Generalized seizures are paralleled by widespread EEG synchronization over a wide area of cortex, a finding confirmed by other authors (e.g., ref. 4).

Following earlier reports by Westrum et al. (73) on *Macaque* neocortex and by Scheibel et al. (58,59) on human temporal lobe, we observed (51) that certain findings of these authors appeared duplicated in gerbils. At the level of the light microscope, differences between SS and SR animals appeared in two structures: the dendritic spines located on hippocampal pyramidal cells, and in the mossy tufts, the vesicle-filled "sacs" located along dentate granule cell axons as they pass through regions CA3 and CA4. Dendritic spines on both apical and basilar dendritic segments appeared less densely distributed in SS than in SR animals, while the mossy tufts seemed more rounded, with fewer invaginations, in gerbils with seizures. Accordingly, we performed spine-density counts at the light level in both strains, and we examined as well electron micrographs of the mossy tufts in SS and SR gerbils using planimetry on randomly selected photographs (50).

Differences in mossy tuft measurements between the two strains were found. Although average tuft area was the same, the proportion of total tuft area occupied by vesicles was larger in SS than in SR animals, while the proportion of tuft taken up by dendritic spine cross-sections was smaller. Our preliminary impressions regarding spine density were further confirmed when quantitative investigations were made. In adult gerbils, SS animals had fewer spines per 45-μm CA3 dendrite segment than did SRs. This was true for both apical and basilar dendrites. Spine counts in neocortex did not reveal differences between the two strains. Thus, a pattern of spine-density decrease similar to that in human temporal lobe epileptics was found. Another change in gerbil hippocampus similar to the human has been reported: Dam et al. (18) have found reduced numbers of neurons in fields H2 and H3 for gerbils with intense seizures, as compared with animals with mild seizures or with controls.

In theory, one advantage of an animal model over studies of human tissue for establishing structure–function correlations is the opportunity to investigate the issue of causality, a matter that cannot be approached experimentally in humans. Studies that document the progressive development of seizures and concomitant anatomical changes, such as those using the kindling model, attempt to determine whether seizures are the cause or the result of anatomical abnormality. Conclusions are reached by observing temporal correlations between seizure development and anatomical change, and controls are ideally animals that have received an experimental treatment but have not displayed seizures. An equivalent approach in a genetic model such as the gerbil, where an anatomical change has been located at a certain age, is to examine the brain at various ages in development to see whether these differences precede, accompany, or follow the appearance of behavioral seizures. Since the gerbil's seizures do not begin until about 50 days of age, its brain can be studied at various times chosen with reference to initial appearance and occurrence of seizures. Gerbils of equivalent age, with few or milder seizures, can also be compared with animals with extreme ictal activity.

To approach some of these problems, we extended the dendritic spine portion of our work to include SS and SR gerbils at four ages, bracketing the age of seizure onset. The brains of 30-, 50-, 90-, and 180-day-old animals were examined for density of dendritic spines on CA3 pyramidal cells, using the same sampling protocol as in the earlier work. Since a possible explanation for our earlier findings was an interaction between strain membership and exposure to the testing situation, we added an additional control group that received minimal testing (no more than two times). Evidence shows that treatments that seem relatively minor, such as allowing a honeybee to complete one orientation flight (5), can have measurable effects on spine morphology. Loskota and coworkers (42) had found no effect of testing on the age at which seizures appeared in ontogeny but did not investigate test effects on parameters of the behavior itself. In addition to main effects of age, strain, and test frequency, interactions among these variables were also examined.

Results of our spine counts appear in Table 2 and graphically in Fig. 2. Figure 2A reveals apical spine-density differences between the two strains, as well as a contrasting trend with age in SS and SR animals. An analysis of variance of the overall effects of age and strain [BMDP8V (21)] revealed that both main effects were significant, as was the interaction between them. However, it is important to note that the *direc-*

TABLE 2. *Number of spines per 45-μm segment of apical and basilar CA3 dendrites in SS and SR gerbils by age and test condition*[a]

Gerbil type	Parameter	30 days old		50 days old			90 days old			180 days old		
		T, NT[b]	$\overline{X}$	T	NT	$\overline{X}$	T	NT	$\overline{X}$	T	NT	$\overline{X}$
SS	ASD	57.8	57.8	60.5	59.5	59.9	52.3	55.5	54.1	47.3	46.2	46.7
		(2.4)	(2.4)	(2.7)	(2.2)	(1.6)	(4.7)	(3.1)	(2.6)	(3.6)	(1.9)	(1.8)
	BSD	48.9	48.9	50.6	52.9	51.9	41.2	48.2	45.1	43.2	37.5	40.1
		(3.0)	(3.0)	(1.7)	(3.9)	(2.3)	(4.2)	(2.4)	(2.4)	(4.6)	(2.9)	(2.7)
	TSD	213.5	213.5	222.1	224.8	223.7	187.0	207.4	198.3	181.0	167.4	173.6
		(9.6)	(9.6)	(12.3)	(11.2)	(7.1)	(16.6)	(10.6)	(9.5)	(16.3)	(9.2)	(8.7)
SR	ASD	49.6	49.6	53.5	51.6	52.6	48.6	51.4	50.4	49.9	52.2	51.0
		(2.0)	(2.0)	(2.9)	(4.6)	(2.6)	(3.5)	(1.2)	(1.4)	(2.3)	(4.3)	(2.3)
	BSD	45.9	45.9	49.4	49.5	49.5	38.7	45.2	42.4	43.4	41.4	42.4
		(2.3)	(2.3)	(3.7)	(3.1)	(2.2)	(2.9)	(1.2)	(1.4)	(2.6)	(4.1)	(2.3)
	TSD	190.9	190.9	205.8	202.4	204.1	174.6	193.1	187.0	186.6	187.2	186.9
		(7.7)	(7.7)	(12.3)	(15.4)	(9.3)	(11.4)	(4.5)	(5.1)	(9.4)	(16.4)	(8.8)

[a] Total spine density (TSD), apical spine density (ASD), and basilar spine density (BSD) per 45-μm dendritic segment of hippocampal CA3 cell for all gerbils in the study, by age, strain, and test condition. Since all 30-day group animals were tested identically, values for this group are pooled. SEM given in parentheses.

[b] Test conditions: T, tested; NT, not tested; $\overline{X}$, mean.

tion of the difference between SS and SR gerbils reverses itself with age: young SS animals have *more* spines than SRs, while older SSs have fewer. Moreover, spine density declined steadily with age in SS animals and remained constant in SRs after 90 days.

While the graph for spine density is of similar shape for basilar systems (Fig. 2B), the only statistically significant effect was due to age.

No effect on spine density was found for testing frequency. While we had assumed that the only seizures the animals had were the ones they demonstrated in our testing situation, it is of course possible that they experienced other seizures in their home cages; hence, this experimental condition was a better control for exposure to the testing situation than for absolute seizure frequency. Testing frequency did affect parameters of the seizures themselves, however. Animals that had received more frequent tests showed less intense seizures than gerbils that had had only one or two tests ($p < 0.03$). (Since the seizure intensity criteria for inclusion in the study for both groups were the same, this is not due to a subject selection bias.) At the same time, more frequently tested gerbils had shorter seizures (at 90 days, animals tested frequently had seizures with an average duration of 131.5 sec; those tested less often, 351.6 sec; $p < 0.05$). The latency from the time of placement into the testing bin to the beginning of seizure, however, did not vary according to testing frequency, as one might expect if seizures are in part learned behavior.

What was the relationship between seizure intensity and spine density? If spine loss is a simple consequence of seizure intensity, we might expect to see, within the SS strain, decreased spine density in animals with more, or stronger, seizures. We were therefore surprised to find, for the 25 SS animals that had seizures, that only very low (nonsignificant) correlations existed between any seizure variable and either apical, basilar, or total spine density. This was true for the group as a whole (all ages): when similar correlations were performed for gerbils grouped by age, significant negative correlations were found between both apical and basilar spine density and seizure latency in 90-day-old gerbils. This may be of biological significance since at this age, seizures are still developing.

DISCUSSION

An important consideration in interpreting any dendritic spine study is, of course, the relationship one assumes between spines and function. Our results indicating spine decrease in adult SS animals with seizures seemed initially somewhat paradoxical: if seizures are a "consequence" of a given spine density, why should they be present in animals that demonstrate a *decrease* in structures associated with excitation? However, following the developmental study, it appeared as if the gerbil that will have seizures later in life is initially endowed with more dendritic spines than its SR counterpart. Spine density begins to diminish at about the time behavioral seizures begin, and continues to decline at a steady rate throughout the ages we have studied. During the period when seizures are beginning, however, it is an excess

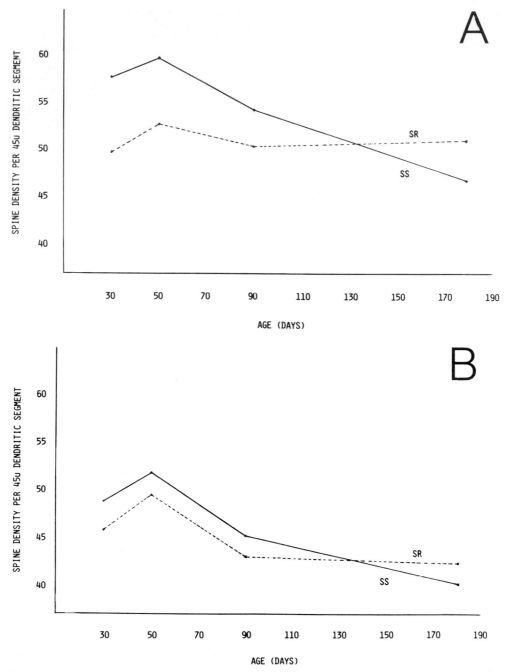

FIG. 2. Apical and basilar dendritic spine density on CA3 cells in SS (*solid line*) and SR (*broken line*) gerbils. Note that while adult SS animals have fewer spines per 45-μm segment than do SRs, young SSs have more. Note also the differing trend with age between the two strains. **A:** Apical spines. **B:** Basilar spines.

of dendritic spines, not a decrease, that is correlated with seizures.

One prevalent notion about spine density is that it reflects strength of afferentation (e.g., ref. 55). Perhaps the spine increase in apical seg-

ments of the young SS gerbil reflects increased input to that stratum, leading to a different proportion of excitatory/inhibitory input to the CA3 pyramidal cell. The stratum radiatum of CA3 receives input from a variety of sources, including the septum, dentate, brainstem, opposite hippocampus, and several additional sites (1,48), but one source that is distributed preferentially to apical, rather than to basilar, regions is the entorhinal cortex, sending its input via the perforant path (37). It would be of considerable interest to investigate the development and physiological characteristics of this pathway in SS and SR gerbils, as their seizures and spine differences develop.

An additional relationship, of central importance for understanding the contribution of abnormal neuroanatomical substrates to seizures, is the one between spines and synapses. Relatively little work has directly addressed this issue; indeed, it has often been assumed that a loss of spines must correlate with a decrease in synaptic number (e.g., ref. 60). This is not always the case, however, as several reports have shown. One such study (26) calculated several parameters of spine synapses in visual cortex of animals reared either in complete darkness, or under normal light. Light deprivation has been shown by several authors to result in reduced spine density in visual cortex (29,68). Freire's (26) study found reduced volume and surface area of spines in the dark-reared group, but did not find a significant reduction in the surface area of the synaptic zones. Cragg (16) found no difference in synaptic density in kittens deprived of light as compared with controls, but he did observe that the average number of synapses per neuron decreased in the deprivation condition. Finally, Mollgaard et al. (44) found longer, but fewer, synapses in a condition of environmental enrichment as compared to environmental deprivation. This is an experimental paradigm known to result in spine alterations (20).

In addition to changes in spine density and in synaptic profiles, a growing literature documents the modifiability of spine shape following a variety of experimental treatments. One such treatment is electrical stimulation of the perforant path (69), which resulted in increased spine head width in regions of the dentate which receive input from this pathway. Another group found similar changes in spine shape following social isolation (14) (spine stems became longer in isolated jewel fish as compared with normally reared conspecifics) and following exposure to increased environmental stimulation (13) (nurse and forager honey bees displayed wider spine heads than did newly emerged bees). A consequence of spine shape change could be an altered electrical resistance to inputs to spine synapses (69). It is of critical importance for interpreting studies such as the above to elucidate

the mechanism or mechanisms responsible for the observed plasticity. What has actually changed? Van Haareveld and Fifkova (69) speculated that spine swelling is an effect of stimulation brought about by the release of glutamate which increases the permeability of the cell membrane. Sodium entry, accompanied by Cl^- and water, results in cell (and spine) enlargement. Even more directly related to function are changes that may be taking place in the synapse itself, as reflected by alterations in various proteins that compose the postsynaptic density. The concept of the spine as an "autonomous" (i.e., independent of instructions from the nucleus) site for protein synthesis has been considered by many authors, since, if true, it could explain how new membrane could be added in response to stimulation without the need to involve the (often distant) nuclear machinery. Steward and Levy (65) found that a high proportion of the relatively few polyribosomes present in dendrites seems to be located near spine stems, and they suggest that these are present for the synthesis of proteins related to the synapse or to the spine. This position is highly suitable for regulation by synaptic activity. Westrum et al. (72) have also proposed a role for spines in protein synthesis during development.

One promising line of research pursued by others in nongenetic preparations (54) has been the idea that seizures result from a loss of inhibition, as reflected by a decrease in GAD-positive staining of nerve terminals in hippocampus of monkeys made epileptic by alumina cream. The differences we found between gerbils with and without seizures, however, were in spines and mossy tufts, structures associated with excitatory inputs to hippocampus (spines, ref. 60; tufts, ref. 6). We believe that the most parsimonious interpretation of our data is that the spine changes we noted initially in adult gerbils are a consequence of seizures. Several findings in this study argue against a particular spine density being "causal" for seizures. First, when SS gerbils begin having seizures at around 50 days of age, they have more spines in region CA3 than do SRs; as adults with seizures, they have fewer. Second, unlike Dam et al. (18), we failed to find correlations between any seizure parameter and a morphometric variable in seizuring animals. Third, a given spine density, in itself, does not always predict whether an animal is SS or SR: at 90 days of age, when seizures have been well established for at least a month, there is no difference in spine density between SS and SR. Finally, a variety of differences has been noted between SS and SR gerbils. The two strains appear to differ in their response to amygdaloid kindling (10). Seizure-sensitive gerbils have a lower afterdischarge (AD) and a longer initial AD duration than do SRs. They also required fewer ADs to develop generalized seizures than did SRs, and fewer total ADs to reach seizures of extreme intensity. Biochemical investigation, although limited in this animal, has indicated that drugs which enhance dopaminergic activity reduce seizure magnitude (15,62). Other investigators have examined the response of gerbils to commonly used anticonvulsant drugs. Some (32) reported seizure attenuation with trimethadione, phenobarbital, and diphenylhydantoin. However, Watanabe and co-workers (71) reported seizure intensification following chronic phenobarbital administration. Schonfeld and Glick (62) found seizure attenuation with diphenylhydantoin, ethosuximide, pentobarbital, and phenobarbital, but not with trimethadione. Differences in handling method, dosage, and route of injection could affect these results. Although an increase in specific binding of ³H-diazepam was shown for gerbils 10 min after seizures (2), differences between SS and SR animals have not been found (66). However, behaviors that are possibly influenced by pathways of specific chemical characteristic have appeared to be different in our strains. We observed (66) that SS and SR gerbils responded very differently to the testing situation (placement into an open field). Seizure-sensitive animals were more active and produced more fecal boli during testing; however, following the administration of flurazepam vehicle (which contains propylene glycol), they were considerably more sedated and produced fewer boli. Seizure-resistant gerbils, on the other hand, increased their production of fecal boli following the drug, and continued to increase it on subsequent flurazepam administration. Our subjective impression of the SS animal is that it is more excitable and agitated.

While it would be tempting and most flattering to our efforts, it is scarcely reasonable to assume that differences such as the above could all be accounted for by spine-density scores in one hippocampal subfield. Spine density is undoubtedly but one parameter of relevance for synaptic function, and measurable synaptic changes should be investigated in this epileptic model before functional conclusions are drawn. Unlike some other preparations, such as the monkey made epileptic by application of alumina gel to cortex (54), where changes have been seen in putatively inhibitory systems, positive results have been reported in the gerbil in structures assumed to mediate excitation. In this regard,

we believe it to be unique. We anticipate that results such as these, showing fine-structure differences between SS and SR gerbils, will stimulate other investigators to pursue this model more closely, as it is the first genetic model to yield evidence of anatomical substrate for seizures.

ACKNOWLEDGMENT

The authors gratefully acknowledge the assistance of the Hereditary Disease Foundation.

REFERENCES

1. Amaral, D. G., and Cowan, W. M. (1980): Subcortical afferents to the hippocampal formation in the monkey. *J. Comp. Neurol.*, 189:573–591.
2. Asano, T., and Mizutani, A. (1980): Brain benzodiazapine receptors and their rapid changes after seizures in the Mongolian gerbil. *Jpn. J. Pharmacol.*, 30:783–788.
3. Atkinson, J. R., and Ward, A. A., Jr. (1964): Intracellular studies of cortical neurons in chronic epileptogenic foci in the monkey. *Exp. Neurol.*, 10:285–295.
4. Bajorek, J. G., Chesarek, W., Felmer, M., and Lomax, P. (1978): Effects of met⁵-enkephalin and naloxone on spontaneous seizures in the Mongolian gerbil. *Proc. West. Pharmacol. Soc.*, 21:365–370.
5. Brandon, J. G., and Coss, R. G. (1982): Rapid dendritic spine stem shortening during one-trial learning: The honeybee's first orientation flight. *Brain Res.*, 252:51–61.
6. Brodal, A. (1981): *Neurological Anatomy in Relation to Clinical Medicine.* Oxford University Press, Oxford.
7. Brown, W. J. (1973): Structural substrates of seizure foci in the human temporal lobe. (A combined electrophysiological optical microscopic and ultrastructural study). In: *Epilepsy: Its Phenomena in Man*, edited by M. A. B. Brazier, pp. 339–374. Academic Press, New York.
8. Brown, W. J., Mitchell, A. G., Jr., Babb, T. L., and Crandall, P. H. (1980): Structural and physiologic studies in experimentally induced epilepsy. *Exp. Neurol.*, 69:543–562.
9. Buell, S. J., and Coleman, P. D. (1979): Dendritic growth in the aged human brain and failure of growth in senile dementia. *Science*, 206:854–856.
10. Cain, D. P., and Corcoran, M. E. (1980): Kindling in the seizure-prone and seizure-resistant Mongolian gerbil. *Elec. Clin. Neurol.*, 49:360–365.
11. Connor, J. R., Diamond, M. C., and Johnson, R. E. (1980): Occipital cortical morphology of the rat: Alterations with age and environment. *Exp. Neurol.*, 68:158–170.
12. Consroe, P., and Edmonds, H. L., Jr. (1979): Genetic animal models of epilepsy: Introduction. *Fed. Proc.*, 38:2397–2398.
13. Coss, R. G., Brandon, J. G., and Globus, A. (1980): Changes in morphology of dendritic spines on honeybee calycal interneurons associ-

ated with cumulative nursing and foraging experiences. *Brain Res.*, 192:49–59.

14. Coss, R. G., and Globus, A. (1978): Spine stems on tectal interneurons in jewel fish are shortened by social stimulation. *Science*, 200:787–790.

15. Cox, B., and Lomax, P. (1976): Brain amines and spontaneous epileptic seizures in the Mongolian gerbil. *Pharmacol. Biochem. Behav.*, 4:263–267.

16. Cragg, B. G. (1975): The development of synapses in kitten visual cortex during visual deprivation. *Exp. Neurol.*, 46:445–451.

17. Dam, A. M. (1980): Epilepsy and neuron loss in the hippocampus. *Epilepsia*, 21:617–629.

18. Dam, A. M., Bajorek, J. C., and Lomax, P. (1981): Hippocampal neuron density and seizures in the Mongolian gerbil. *Epilepsia*, 22:667–674.

19. DeMoor, J. (1898): La mechanisme et la signification de l'etat moniliforme des neurones. *Ann. Soc. R. Sci. Med. Nat. Brux.*, 7:205–250.

20. Diamond, M., and Connor, J., Jr. (1981): A search for the potential of the aging human brain. In: *Brain Neurotransmitters and Receptors in Aging and Age-Related Disorders*, edited by S. Enna et al., pp. 43–58. Raven Press, New York.

21. Dixon, W. J., Brown, M. B., Engelman, L., Frane, J. W., Hill, M. A., Jennrich, R. I., and Toporek, J. D., editors. (1981): *BMDP Statistical Software*. University of California Press, Los Angeles.

22. Elger, C. E., Speckman, E.-J., Prohaska, O., and Caspers, H. (1981): Pattern of intracorticalpotential distribution during focal interictal epileptiform discharges (FIED) and its relation to spinal field potentials in the rat. *Electroencephalogr. Clin. Neurophysiol.*, 51:393–402.

23. Engel, J. Jr., Troupin, A. S., Crandall, P. H., Sterman, M. B., and Wasterlain, C. G. (1982): Recent developments in the diagnosis and therapy of epilepsy. *Ann. Int. Med.*, 97:584–598.

24. Enomoto, T. F., and Marsan, C. A. (1959): Epileptic activation of single cortical neurons and their relationship with EEG discharges. *Electroencephalogr. Clin. Neurophysiol.*, 11:199–218.

25. Falconer, M. (1970): The pathological substrate of temporal lobe epilepsy. *Guy's Hosp. Rep.*, 119:47–60.

26. Freire, M. (1978): Effects of dark rearing on dendritic spines in layer IV of the mouse visual cortex. A quantitative electron microscopical study. *J. Anat.*, 126:193–201.

27. Gastaut, H., and Broughton, R. (1972): *Epileptic Seizures*. Charles C. Thomas, Springfield, Illinois.

28. Girgis, M. (1981): Electrical versus cholinergic kindling. *Electroencephalogr. Clin. Neurophysiol.*, 51:417–425.

29. Globus, A., and Scheibel, A. B. (1967): Synaptic loci on visual cortical neurons of the rabbit—The specific afferent radiation. *Exp. Neurol.*, 18:116–131.

30. Goddard, G. V. (1967): Development of epileptic seizures through brain stimulation at low intensity. *Nature (Lond.)* 214:1020–1021.

31. Goddard, G. V., and Douglas, R. N. (1976). Does the engram of kindling model the engram of normal long term memory? In: *Kindling*, edited by J. A. Wada and R. T. Ross, pp. 1–18. Raven Press, New York.

32. Goldblatt, D., Konow, A., Shoulson, I., and Macmath, T. (1971): Effect of anticonvulsants on seizures in gerbils. *Neurology*, 21:433–434.

33. Hammond, E., Ramsay, R., Villareal, H., and Wilder, B. (1980): Effects of intracortical injection of blood and blood components on the electrocorticogram. *Epilepsia*, 21:3–14.

34. Hare, J. E., and Hare, A. S. (1979). Epileptiform mice, a new neurological mutant. *J. Hered.*, 70:417–420.

35. Hatton, J. D., and Ellisman, M. H. (1984): Orthogonal arrays are redistributed in the membranes of astroglia from alumina-induced epileptic foci. *Epilepsia*, 25:145–151.

36. Henry, K. R. (1967): Audiogenic seizure susceptibility induced in C57BL/6J mice by prior auditory exposure. *Science*, 158:938–940.

37. Hjorth-Simonsen, A., and Jeune, B. (1972): Origin and termination of the hippocampal perforant path in the rat studied by silver impregnation. *J. Comp. Neurol.*, 144:215–232.

38. Killam, E. K. (1979): Photomyoclonic seizures in the baboon, *Papio papio. Fed. Proc.*, 38:2429–2433.

39. Levitt, P., Wilson, W., and Wilkins, R. (1971): The effects of subarachnoid blood on the elctrocorticogram of the cat. *J. Neurosurg.*, 35:185–191.

40. Loskota, W. J., and Lomax, P. (1975): The Mongolian gerbil (*Meriones* unguiculatus) as a model for the study of the epilepsies: EEG records of seizures. *Electroencephalogr. Clin. Neurophysiol.*, 38:597–604.

41. Loskota, W. J., Lomax, P., and Rich, S. T. (1972): The gerbil as a model for the study of epilepsy: Seizure habituation and seizure patterns. *Proc. West. Pharmacol. Soc.*, 15:189–194.

42. Loskota, W. J., Lomax, P., and Rich, S. T. (1974): The gerbil as a model for the study of the epilepsies; Seizure patterns and ontogenesis. *Epilepsia*, 15:109–119.

43. McNamara, J. O., Byrne, M. C., Dashieff, R. M., and Fitz, J. G. (1980): The kindling model of epilepsy: A review. *Prog. Neurobiol.*, 15:139–159.

44. Mollgaard, K., Diamond, M. C., Bennett, E. L., Rosenzweig, M. R., and Lindner, B. (1971): Quantitative synaptic changes with differential experience in rat brain. *Int. J. Neurosci.*, 2:113–128.

45. Naquet, R., and Meldrum, B. S. (1972): Photogenic seizures in baboon. In: *Experimental Models of Epilepsy—A Manual for the Laboratory Worker*, edited by D. Purpura et al., pp. 374–406. Raven Press, New York.

46. Nadler, J. V. (1981): Kainic acid as a tool for the study of temporal lobe epilepsy. *Life Sci.*, 29:2031–2042.

47. Nadler, J. V., Perry, B. W., and Cotman, C. W. (1978): Intraventricular kainic acid preferentially destroys hippocampal pyramidal cells. *Nature (Lond.)*, 271:676–677.

48. O'Keefe, J., and Nadel, L. (1978) *The Hippocampus as a Cognitive Map*. Clarendon Press, Oxford.

49. Olney, J. W. (1976): Brain damage and oral intake of certain amino acids. *Adv. Exp. Med. Biol.*, 69:497–506.

50. Paul, L. A., Fried, I., Watanabe, K., Forsythe, A. B., and Scheibel, A. B. (1981): Structural correlates of seizure behavior in the Mongolian gerbil. *Science,* 213:924–926.

51. Paul, L. A., Watanabe, K., Diaz, J., and Scheibel, A. B. (1978): Possible structural correlates in seizuring Mongolian gerbils. *Abstr. Soc., Neurosci.,* 4:145.

52. Purpura, D. P., Penry, J. K., Towers, D. B., Woodbury, D. M., and Walter, R. D., editors. (1972): *Experimental Models of Epilepsy—A Manual for the Laboratory Worker.* Raven Press, New York.

53. Reid, S. A., Sypert, G. W., Boggs, W. M., and Willmore, L. J. (1979): Histopathology of the ferric-induced chronic epileptic focus in cat: A Golgi study. *Exp. Neurol.,* 66:205–219.

54. Ribak, C. E., Harris, A. B., Vaughan, J. E., and Roberts, E. (1979): Inhibitory, GABAergic nerve terminals decrease at sites of focal epilepsy. *Science,* 205:211–214.

55. Ryugo, R., Ryugo, D. K., and Killackey, H. P. (1975): Differential effect of enucleation on two populations of layer V pyramidal cells. *Brain Res.,* 88:554–559.

56. Scheibel, A. B. (1980): Morphological correlates of epilepsy: Cells in the hippocampus. In: *Antiepileptic Drugs; Mechanisms of Action,* edited by G. Glaser, J. Penry, and D. Woodbury, pp. 49–61. Raven Press, New York.

57. Scheibel, A. B., Paul, L., and Fried, I. (1983): Some structural substrates of the epileptic state. In: *Basic Mechanisms of Neuronal Hyperexcitability,* edited by H. Jasper and N. van Gelder, pp. 109–130. Alan R. Liss, Inc., New York.

58. Scheibel, M. E., Crandall, P. H., and Scheibel, A. B. (1974): The hippocampal-dentate complex in temporal lobe epilepsy. *Epilepsia,* 15:55–80.

59. Scheibel, M., and Scheibel, A. B. (1973): Hippocampal pathology in temporal lobe epilepsy. A Golgi study. In: *Epilepsy, Its Phenomena in Man,* edited by M. A. B. Brazier, pp. 311–337. Raven Press, New York.

60. Scheibel, M. E., and Scheibel, A. B. (1968): On the nature of dendritic spines—Report of a workshop. *Commun. Behav. Biol. Part A Orig. Artie.,* 1:231–265.

61. Scholz, W. (1953): Selective neuronal necrosis and its topistic patterns in hypoxemia and oligemia. *J. Neuropathol. Exp. Neurol.,* 12:249–261.

62. Schonfeld, A. R., and Glick, S. D. (1980): Neuropharmacological analysis of handling-induced seizures in gerbils. *Neuropharmacology,* 19: 1009–1016.

63. Schreiber, R. A., and Graham, J. M., Jr. (1976): Audiogenic priming in DBA/2J and C57BL/6J mice; Interactions among age, prime-to-test interval, and index of seizure. *Dev. Psychobiol.,* 9:57–66.

64. Seyfried, T. N. (1979): Audiogenic seizures in mice. *Fed. Proc.,* 38:2399–2404.

65. Steward, O., and Levy, W. B. (1982): Preferential localization of polyribosomes under the base of dendritic spines in granule cells of the dentate gyrus. *J. Neurosci.,* 2:284–291.

66. Syapin, P., Duong, P. T., and Paul, L. A. (1981): Benzodiazepine activity in seizure-sensitive and seizure-resistant Mongolian gerbils. *Abstr. Soc. Neurosci.,* 7:712.

67. Urca, G., Frenk, H., Liebeskind, J. C., and Taylor, A. N. (1977): Morphine and enkephalin: Analgesic and epileptic properties. *Science,* 197:83–86.

68. Valverde, R., and Ruiz-Marcos, A. (1969): Dendritic spines in the visual cortex of the mouse: Introduction to a mathematical model. *Exp. Brain Res.,* 8:269–283.

69. Van Harreveld, A., and Fifkova, E. (1975): Swelling of dendritic spines in the fascia dentate after stimulation of the perforant fibers as a mechanism of post-tetanic potentiation. *Exp. Neurol.,* 49:736–749.

70. Wada, J. A., Osawa, T., Sato, M., Wabe, A., Corcoran, M. E., and Troupin, A. S. (1976): *Epilepsia,* 17:77–87.

71. Watanabe, K., Schain, R. J., and Bailey, B. G. (1978): Effects of phenobarbital on seizure activity in the gerbil. *Pediatr. Res.,* 12:918–922.

72. Westrum, L. E., Jones, D. H., Gray, E. G., and Barron, J. (1980): Microtubules, dendritic spines and spine apparatuses. *Cell Tissue Res.,* 208:171–181.

73. Westrum, L. E., White, L. E., Jr., and Ward, A. A., Jr. (1964): Morphology of the experimental epileptic focus. *J. Neurosurg.,* 21:1033–1046.

74. Wiederholt, W. C. (1974): Electrophysiologic analysis of epileptic beagles. *Neurology,* 24:149–155.

Advances in Neurology, Vol. 44, edited by
A. V. Delgado-Escueta, A. A. Ward, Jr.,
D. M. Woodbury, and R. J. Porter.
Raven Press, New York © 1986.

40

Epilepsy and the Blood-Brain Barrier

*,***Eain M. Cornford and **,***William H. Oldendorf

*VA Southwest Regional Epilepsy Center, Neurology and Research Services, Veterans Administration Wadsworth Medical Center, Los Angeles, California 90073; **Research Service, Veterans Administration Brentwood Medical Center, Los Angeles, California 90073; and ***Department of Neurology, Reed Neurological Research Center, UCLA School of Medicine, Los Angeles, California 90024

SUMMARY   A concern for the possible role of the blood-brain barrier (BBB) in the epilepsies was based on ultrastructural studies that demonstrated increased micropinocytosis in cerebral capillaries during seizures. Continued interest in the structure of the BBB has led to the demonstration that, in human psychomotor epilepsy, there is a thickening of the capillary basement membrane. These studies also suggest that an increase in capillary mitochondria and interendothelial tight junctions may characterize seizure-traumatized brain regions. These studies forecast an increased interest and understanding of the ultrastructural events associated with capillaries in seizure states.

Additional focus on the BBB comes from the clinical use of anticonvulsant drug levels in the control and treatment of seizures. Debate as to whether free drug levels are appropriate continues. The brain capillary is the interface between blood-borne drug and the target site, and thus an increased understanding of the events associated with brain–plasma exchange has been sought. The concept that only that fraction of drug that is freely dialyzable is available for equilibration across the BBB is not supported by recent studies, which demonstrate that protein-bound ligands are able to dissociate and gain access to the brain in the course of a single capillary transit. It has been established that albumin-bound fatty acids, steroids, and anticonvulsant drugs more readily distribute into tissues than previously believed. Thus, traditional free drug hypotheses need to be expanded to account for the fact that dissociation constants measured *in vitro* are not the same as those measured *in vivo*.

The BBB also regulates nutrient availability to the brain, and under normal conditions excess substrate is made available to the brain for metabolism. Indirect evidence is available to suggest that during seizures, BBB transport may indeed be the rate-limiting step. Specifically, glucose availability to the seizing brain may be restricted to such a degree that brain glucose utilization rates are no longer independent of plasma glucose levels. If it can be proven that BBB transport is the rate-limiting step during seizures, then it would be possible to augment brain glucose utilization rates by increasing plasma glucose levels. In addition, a depression of brain glucose utilization could be achieved by inducing hypoglycemia. It is not fully understood whether BBB rate limitation would persist postictally, nor is it known whether BBB alterations may be global or restricted to the seizure focus. Thus, future studies of the BBB in seizures will continue to investigate ultrastructural pathology, anticonvulsant drug permeability, and nutrient exchange during the ictal and postictal periods.

Almost 25 years ago, Bennett et al. (13) classified a variety of vertebrate blood capillaries and came to the conclusion that the most restrictive capillaries with the most intimate cell-to-cell connections were the brain endothelia. They constitute the blood-brain barrier. A continuous uniform basement membrane surrounds these blood-brain barrier capillaries, and cross-sectional profiles of the endothelia suggest a uniform width of 0.2 to 0.5 μm, except in the perinuclear region where the cell wall bulges. Other distinguishing characteristics are as follows:

1. The absence of fenestrations (179).

2. Few pinocytotic vesicles and pericytes surround most capillaries (69). The accumulation of foreign protein in pericytes of normal animals (42,126,213), as well as in mice (108) and rats (181), has prompted the suggestion that pericytes surrounding cerebral endothelia have phagocytic properties (36,91). This was subsequently confirmed by Broadwell and Salcman (37), and it was suggested that the pericyte served as the first line of defense if the blood-brain barrier was breached.

3. The presence of tight junctions, or "zonula occludens" (132), which are sealing cell-to-cell contacts between brain endothelia. Tight junctions are now known to be formed by the first trimester of fetal life (130), and bovine brain microvessels cultured *in vitro* also form complex tight junctions (28).

4. Some capillaries are completely tubular in profile and have been termed "seamless" endothelia by Wolff and Bar (216). These cells can be thought of as having such a prolonged intimate contact that cytoplasm has replaced the tight junctions (Fig. 1).

5. Greater numbers of mitochondria (148) and greater volumes of mitochondria are found in blood-brain barrier endothelia than in those of other tissues (149).

6. An increased electrical resistance, similar to that of tight epithelia, has been observed in frog brain capillaries (60). The increased impedance of brain capillaries (as compared to mesenteric or muscular endothelia) is consistent with a low permeability to ionic materials.

7. In mammalian brain, these capillaries are further characterized by elevated levels of enzymes, which, if present, display reduced activity in nonneural capillaries. Examples include gamma-glutamyl transpeptidase (2,153), alkaline phosphatase (27,186), aromatic amino acid decarboxylase (14,154), and nonspecific cholinesterase (34,78).

Capillaries in tissues such as muscle tend to be oriented parallel to muscle fibers and are relatively uniform in distribution. In contrast, brain capillaries are characterized by a more random three-dimensional meshwork, and the mesh is approximately uniform in any given region. However, the mesh spacing (intercapillary distance) varies with local oxygen demand, so the mean intercapillary distance is greatly reduced around nuclei in which the neuronal cell bodies are concentrated. These are coincidentally sites of high oxygen consumption (98).

The blood-brain barrier (BBB) is usually considered a basic science phenomenon, but it has importance in clinical medicine. For example, it plays an increasingly important role in modern brain-imaging methods (185). It is therefore appropriate to speculate on some of the BBB's more basic functional roles before considering its relation to clinical epilepsy and experimental seizures.

About one-fifth of the human body's tissue volume is extracellular fluid (ECF). Of this, in turn, about one-fifth (blood plasma) is pumped through the permeable-walled microvasculature to keep the composition of the entire ECF uniform. This is accomplished when the smaller, mobile fraction of ECF is brought close enough to the larger, more static interstitial ECF to permit efficient diffusional exchange. The movement occurs largely via clefts between endothelial cells. This process reduces the effective diffusional distance between any two cells in the body to a few micrometers rather than the many centimeters that may actually separate organs, with a consequent reduction in pumping energy requirements. In general, this relatively simple ECF mixing and homogenization is carried out on a nonselective basis, and the distribution of ECF solutes is the same in most regions of the body; where regional differences in the concentration of these solutes occur, a major causative mechanism appears to involve highly specific receptor sites on certain target cells.

However, in brain capillaries, there is general agreement that nonspecific routes for diffusional exchange are virtually absent and that almost all exchange of substances that occurs there is not extracellular but transcellular, requiring direct passage through the plasma membrane and cytoplasm of capillary endothelial cells. Presumably, transport of some substances such as blood gases may also involve transcellular exchange in capillary cells throughout the body, but this has not yet been studied in detail.

In more general terms, the BBB appears to

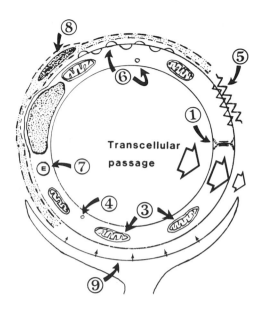
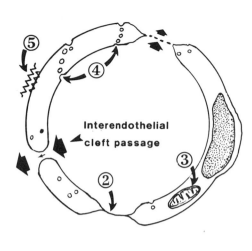

BRAIN CAPILLARY

GENERAL CAPILLARY

FIG. 1. Specific features of blood-brain barrier capillaries compared with general capillaries. Solutes must penetrate brain endothelia, gaining access to the CNS by a transcellular route. In contrast, intercellular clefts or patent fenestrations permit direct intercellular passage of plasma-borne solutes in many capillaries (46a). Other distinctive characteristics are: ① Many BBB capillaries are tubular or "seamless" (216), but cell-to-cell contacts, when observed, are characterized by the presence of tight junctions (132). ② Fenestrations, common in many capillaries, are not observed in BBB capillaries. ③ Greater numbers (148) and greater volumes (149) of mitochondria are observed in brain endothelia than in peripheral tissues. ④ Very few pinocytotic vesicles are seen in normal brain capillaries, but increased pinocytotic activity is seen in many peripheral tissues (69). Other experimental data suggest that increased pinocytotic activity is correlated with increases in capillary cyclic AMP concentrations (101,172). ⑤ Brain capillary walls have a greater electrical resistance than determined in peripheral tissues such as mesenteric and muscle capillaries. The high resistance is characteristic of epithelia with low ionic permeabilities and thus an impedance to ion diffusion (60). ⑥ Differences in both the structure (i.e., proteins) and function of the antiluminal and luminal brain capillary surfaces have been established (see text). ⑦ Histochemical studies have revealed a number of enzymes ("E") that are largely specific to BBB capillaries (30). These include alkaline phosphatase (EC 3.1.3.1), pseudocholinesterase (EC 3.1.1.8), aromatic L-amino acid decarboxylase (EC 4.1.1.28), and gamma-glutamyl transpeptidase (EC 2.3.2.2). ⑧ About one-half of mammalian brain capillaries are surrounded by a pericyte, which is in intimate contact with the antiluminal capillary surface. It is known to have phagocytic properties in normal animals (42,126,214), and these observations led to the suggestion that the pericyte serves as the first line of defense if blood-brain barrier functions are compromised (37). ⑨ While the astrocytic foot processes do not contribute to BBB function *per se,* Davson and Oldendorf (62) proposed that these glial feet communicate (*arrows*) or somehow induce the formation of barrier-type capillaries, and recent evidence supports this concept (65,198).

provide a second-order homeostatic mechanism for optimizing the neural ECF as an ultrastable subcompartment of the general ECF. Clinically it has been observed that brief abrogation of the BBB, as occurs with carotid injection of hyperosmotic solutions for cerebral angiography, is not greatly deleterious to brain function. However, it is also known that almost any significant abnormality of brain tissue results in a loss of the BBB. It might be speculated that this change results from malfunctioning as-

trocytes immediately surrounding central nervous system capillaries, which are no longer able to produce a humoral influence that maintains the BBB by inhibiting pinocytosis and fenestra formation and by causing the formation of tight interendothelial cell junctions (146).

INDUCTION OF THE BLOOD-BRAIN BARRIER

How the capillary "knows" it is in brain and should restructure itself is unknown, but these structural characteristics of brain capillaries appear to be the result of some ongoing active process in brain—perhaps mediated by astrocytes. Whatever the mechanism is, it fails in many lesions in which the normal brain histology is substantially altered. In a wide variety of brain lesions, the capillaries lose their unique structural features and develop the appearance of less restrictive general capillaries. The question as to what stimulus makes an endothelial cell develop BBB properties was addressed by Davson and Oldendorf (62). They proposed, on the basis of the paucity of pinocytotic vesicles, that the astrocyte glial foot processes somehow induced the formation of barrier-type capillaries. When iris tissue is transplanted into brain, it becomes vascularized with endothelia that do not contain DOPA decarboxylase or monoamine oxidase, enzymes that are characteristic of BBB capillaries but not those of the iris (71,202). In the reverse experiment—transplantation of embryonic central nervous system tissue into the anterior chamber of the eye—enzymatic activity was demonstrated within the "donor" central nervous system (CNS) tissue only. Such activity was not seen within the capillaries of the host iris, nor within the endothelia connecting the host iris to the donor CNS transplant (202). Glial foot induction of BBB properties was again suggested by these authors.

This concept was extended using quail-chick transplantations, where the distinctive quail nuclear morphology defined whether the endothelial cells grown were of donor or host origin. In this study, Stewart and Wiley (198) elegantly demonstrated that abdominal host vessels vascularizing grafted neural tissue formed structural, functional, and histochemical features of blood-brain barrier capillaries. In contrast, brain vessels vascularizing grafted mesodermal tissue were devoid of these characteristics (198).

In addition, fenestrated capillaries characteristic of the tissue of origin have been observed in metastatic brain tumors (94), in contrast to the typical BBB endothelia. A role for the glial feet in the synthesis of endothelial cell basement membrane has been suggested by Bar and Wolff (7), but DeBault and Cancilla's (65) study provided the best evidence for glial induction. They demonstrated that gamma-glutamyl transpeptidase could be identified in isolated brain capillaries cultured *in vitro* if glial cells were present in the media to induce this enzyme. Thus, an increasing body of information indicates that a stimulus or message originating in the glial feet processes induces the formation of barrier-type endothelial cells in the central nervous system.

DEVELOPMENT OF THE MAMMALIAN BLOOD-BRAIN BARRIER

The concept of a "leaky" or immature blood-brain barrier, which allows rather indiscriminate entry of hydrophilic solutes and small proteins, persists in the literature, but it is probably true for only the early fetal stage (59). For example, in sheep, the rate of penetration of sucrose or insulin into brain declined to the adult value by a gestational age of 130 days (74). Similar studies in the rat indicate that this decline continues postnatally, and adult rates are reached 10 to 15 days post-partum (76). During the gestational period, tight junctions between adjacent primitive capillaries are seen developing rat brain (41,68), and they are observed by the first trimester of fetal life (130). As Pardridge (160) indicates, the observation that neonatal hyperbilirubinemia often resulted in bilirubin staining of the brain was a clinical analog to experimental observations of more than 50 years ago, reporting that vital dyes more readily stained the brains of younger animals. Curiously, Broman (38) reviewed the existing literature and concluded that the blood-brain barrier of newborn animals was fully developed. However, the caricature of a leaky or immature blood-brain barrier in the developing organism gained acceptance on the basis of a model pertaining to the apparent pathogenesis of kernicterus (160). The cause of kernicterus is related to changes in albumin binding of bilirubin in the newborn (67). The elevated total protein content seen in the cerebrospinal fluid of newborns, which was originally attributed to a "leaky" BBB, is now understood to be a consequence of decreased CSF bulk flow (4). Thus, the BBB of newborn organisms is known to be almost fully developed (188), and the concept of an immature barrier in newborns must be reconsidered in the light of current data and understanding.

Bar and Wolff (8) have suggested that vascular proliferation in the developing brain is related to aerobic metabolism and that cessation of capillary branching occurs by 30 days postnatally in the rat brain. All subsequent growth occurs by endothelial cell elongation rather than cell division (8). In comparisons of suckling (14 days) and weanling (35 days) rats, it is known that the cross-sectional areas of both capillary lumens and capillary cell cytoplasmic contents are greater in sucklings (39). However, mitochondrial content was higher in the weanling animals (39). The rate of protein synthesis in rat brain microvessels is also highest in young animals, and decreases with aging (86). The (numerical) loss in cerebral capillary endothelial cells which occurs with age in rat brain is thought to be compensated for by cellular elongation (6). Thus in some respects the term "barrier" as applied to cerebral endothelia is a misnomer, since it implies a static, intransigent structure. These capillaries are, in contrast, dynamic, rather than static, and undergo continual modifications in function during progressive brain development.

Accumulating data (32,50,55) suggest blood-brain barrier transport mechanisms may operate at much higher rates in the newborn than adult brain. Transport constants for both glucose and monocarboxylic acids have been compared in anesthetized infant (suckling) and adult rat brains (54,56,59). In suckling brain, where energy is derived from monocarboxylic acid metabolism, total influx of lactate and pyruvate is greater than in adult brain. However, in the adult brain, where glucose is the primary energy source, influx of this hexose is greater than measured in the brains of sucklings.

With respect to anticonvulsant drugs, higher brain uptakes were observed in neonates than adults. The possible presence of a saturable, carrier-mediated mechanism [to account for high anticonvulsant BUIs (see Table 2) in the neonate] was empirically precluded (50). In the newborn rabbit, brain extraction of phenytoin at a trace (<0.01 μg/ml) concentration ($E = 58 \pm 6\%$) was not different from the brain extraction when the phenytoin concentration was 20 μg/ml ($E = 56 \pm 9\%$) or 100 μg/ml ($E = 55 \pm 4\%$). At a trace concentration in 70% normal rat serum, the phenytoin $E = 60 \pm 8\%$, and at a concentration of 500 μg/ml in 70% normal rat serum $E = 60 \pm 7\%$ (53). Similar studies suggest that brain uptake of valproate is not by way of a saturable mechanism (E. M. Cornford, *unpublished results*). Thus the elevated brain extraction of these two anticonvulsants (seen in Table 2) can not be attributed to a specific carrier-mediated transport mechanism in either the neonatal or adult brain. The relationship of blood flow rates (which are reduced in the neonatal brain) to anticonvulsant drug delivery in the developing brain is described elsewhere (53).

FUNCTIONAL DIFFERENCES IN THE LUMINAL AND ANTILUMINAL CAPILLARY SURFACES

Polarity of the Blood-Brain Barrier

Methods have now been established for isolating and purifying brain capillaries; a review of this information may be found elsewhere (84).

Electron-micrographic cross-sections of these isolated capillaries suggest that the capillary lumen is greatly reduced in size and that the cytoplasmic area of the capillary is thickened. Thus, the cross-sectional appearance of these isolated capillaries resembles a doughnut, wherein the surface area of the antiluminal side of the capillary greatly exceeds the surface area on the luminal side of the capillary. The isolated capillary therefore provides an excellent model for the study of transcellular transport in the brain-to-blood direction. That is to say, isolated capillaries provide information as to specific physiological traits of the antiluminal capillary surface that are not obtained in the *in vivo* studies of the movement of compounds from blood to brain. Several differences between the antiluminal surfaces of brain capillaries are now apparent and are collectively referred to as contributing to the polarity of the blood-brain barrier. Protein structures have been examined by labeling luminal capillary membranes after injection into the carotid artery and the antiluminal membranes of isolated capillaries *in vitro*. The protein composition of the luminal membrane was markedly different from that of the antiluminal surface (109).

On the luminal membrane capillary cell, for example, there are at least two sodium ion transport systems. One can be inhibited by the diuretic amiloride (the presumed Na^+ pore) and the other by furosemide (16). The furosemide-sensitive system is presumably a coupled Na^+/Cl^- cotransport system. In isolated brain capillaries neither sodium-22 nor rubidium-86 uptake could be inhibited by furosemide (15), suggesting the cotransport system is not functional at the antiluminal capillary surface. However, an Na^+/H^+ exchange system is believed to be restricted to the antiluminal side of the BBB (15). The presence of Na^+/K^+-ATPase in brain capillaries has been both demonstrated (73,83) and confirmed (21). Of more significance, however, was the demonstration that in brain capillaries Na^+/K^+-ATPase is located specifically on the antiluminal capillary surface and is not present on the luminal membrane (18). It has also been demonstrated that neutral amino acid transport across the BBB from the luminal to antiluminal side involves only a single system, which transports the large neutral amino acids such as phenylalanine, leucine, tryptophan, and methionine. This is the (leucine-preferring) L-system. There is little or no transport of the small neutral amino acids such as glycine, alanine, serine, and proline, and thus most authorities agree that the (alanine-preferring) A-system for small neutral amino acids is absent on the luminal surface of the BBB capillary. Betz and Goldstein (20) have established that the Na^+-dependent, alanine-preferring A-system is located solely on the antiluminal surface of the BBB. Furthermore, this A-system is sensitive to ouabain inhibition, suggesting this to be an energy-dependent active transport system that pumps the amino acids from the brain into the capillary lumen. It is also possible that the acidic amino acid transport system defined by Oldendorf and Szabo (151) is specifically localized on the antiluminal surface, and studies are needed to determine whether this is an active efflux mechanism.

While specific differences in luminal vs. antiluminal capillary surfaces continue to be defined in normal animals, other recent work suggests that subtle changes in polarity of the BBB can be manifested in pathological conditions. In normal mice, Vorbrodt et al. (208) determined the major location of the phosphatases alkaline phosphatase, 5'-nucleotidase nucleoside diphosphatase, and thiamine pyrophosphatase to be on the luminal plasma membrane of the endothelial cells. In contrast, in mice infected with the slow viral scrapie infection, changes in activity and distribution of these phosphatases manifested themselves in the appearance of the reaction product the antiluminal side of the vessel wall. Thus, as a result of the scrapie infection, these enzymes changed their specific localization from the luminal to the antiluminal side of the endothelial cell membranes.

Polarity of the Blood-Brain Barrier to Valproate

In single-injection, initial-rate studies, it has been determined that 43 to 44% of the saline-borne valproic acid entering the rat brain microvasculature is extracted during a single transcapillary transit (49). In contrast, 73% of the octanoic acid is extracted (144). The rate constant of valproate efflux from brain (k) is 0.744/min; thus this anticonvulsant leaves brain much more rapidly than does water ($k = 0.61$/min) (31), or by the more recent estimate of Pardridge et al. (162) ($k = 0.43$/min), isopropanol ($k = 0.63$/min) (31), or butanol ($k = 0.67$/min) (166). Since water is 85% extracted in a single capillary passage and alcohols approach 100% extraction, one would expect that valproate should be more highly extracted (i.e., similar to the 73% reported for octonoate) and/or have a lesser rate constant of efflux if the blood-brain barrier influx and efflux of this drug were equal. There-

fore these data are circumstantial evidence for a polarity of the BBB to valproic acid.

This apparent inequality of blood-to-brain versus brain-to-blood transport of valproic acid may be related to the observations that the drug may be actively transported out of cerebrospinal fluid in both dogs (80) and monkeys (117). It has been demonstrated that in dogs, valproate is pumped out of the cerebrospinal fluid (CSF) by the same anion efflux mechanism that transports gamma-aminobutyric acid (GABA) and probenecid out of the cerebrospinal fluid (120). These anion efflux mechanisms have been demonstrated in the CSF-blood barrier to be active, energy-dependent systems (175). A similar active transport of organic acids out of the brain by ATP-dependent mechanisms located on the antiluminal capillary membrane has been proposed (22). Thus, it is quite possible that valproate efflux may similarly originate on the antiluminal surface of the blood-brain barrier capillaries.

PATHOLOGICAL MODIFICATIONS OF BARRIER PROPERTIES

In almost all brain lesions, the integrity of the blood-brain barrier is compromised to some degree. This observation permitted development of traditional radioisotopic brain scanning where lesions appear as "hot spots" against a background of healthy "cold" brain; most gamma-emitting radioisotopes injected into the blood are excluded from healthy brain but can distribute from blood in a wide variety of brain lesions.

The same principle applies in contrast enhancement of lesions in computerized X-ray tomography (CT). Usually, after a scan without any injected contrast medium, 20 to 40 g of iodine is injected intravenously as a triiodinated benzoic acid derivative. Brain density increases due to the photoelectric capture of X-rays by the heavy atoms of iodine. Healthy brain shows a slight increase in radiodensity, due largely to the iodine confined to the blood in the brain. Since there is considerably more blood in gray than in white matter, the contrast between gray and white matter is increased. If a lesion is present, the capillaries are permeable to all small molecules present in the blood, and the iodine distributes out to the ECF of this region, causing the lesion's density to become much greater than the surrounding healthy brain having a normal BBB (146).

The difference between the contrasted and uncontrasted CT scan represents the distribution of isotope on a traditional ^{99m}Tc pertechnetate scan. The isotope scan shows only the abnormal region with no normal brain structure. The contrasted CT scan shows not only many normal brain structures but also regions where permeability of the BBB is increased.

Pathological alterations in the BBB capillaries have been reported in a variety of clinical situations, including inflammatory diseases, hypoxia, edema, infarction, and the trauma associated with edema (185). Typically, the alterations in permeability are secondary to damage to the CNS. It is not unexpected that differences in enzyme activities might be observed in pathological conditions, but the fact that translocations of enzymatic sites from the luminal to antiluminal capillary surfaces can occur (208) should be more closely examined in the future. Tumors of the central nervous system are characterized as having the capillary structure common to the tissue of origin (94), and many of the more malignant tumors possess fenestrated capillaries with obvious pinocytotic activity. In contrast, the new capillaries in gliomas resemble typical BBB endothelia (40). It has also been demonstrated that BBB capillaries isolated from astrocytomas (grades III–IV) averaged 55% greater total protein contents than capillaries from normal human cerebral tissues or brains of mice (133), suggesting that there are distinct differences in tumor versus BBB capillaries, even when barrier properties are operational in the tumor endothelia. For this reason, delivery of drugs to patients with gliomas has been augmented by transient osmotic disruption of the blood-brain barrier with mannitol (139).

The recent suggestion that tumor growth can be inhibited by direct inhibition of vascular growth using an angiogenesis inhibitor (111) raises the question of whether this strategy could be applied to the BBB. If brain capillary proliferation could be augmented or restricted, new forms of therapy would become feasible for neurological diseases wherein the arrest or stimulation of neovascularization would be clinically beneficial (84).

It is now well known that seizures can occur during clinical brain imaging (77,104,141,191). Other adverse effects include transient cortical blindness, brain edema, and spinal-cord injury. An underlying lesion may compromise the BBB and permit contrast media to access brain parenchyma. This may initiate seizures (191) and other sequelae. These CNS injuries have been severe enough to contribute to 22 of 69 angiography-associated deaths in one study (104). Experimental studies suggest that the angiographically induced alterations in BBB permeability of normal animals are mediated by both chemotoxicity and the hyperosmolality of the contrast medium (182). Thus, with the increased availability of brain imaging methods, the associated clinical complications have for unfortunate reasons sometimes emphasized the role of the BBB (in a very direct manner) to practicing physicians.

EXPERIMENTAL STUDY OF THE BLOOD-BRAIN BARRIER

Of the tissue-sampling single-injection methods, the Oldendorf (142) technique, first reported 14 years ago, has provided considerable information about the *in vivo* study of capillary transport processes in the brain (142,143). It has also been adapted to study both the liver (48,155), placenta (23) and uterus (112). The method requires surgical exposure of the major afferent vessel (e.g., the common carotid artery) in anesthetized laboratory animals, and the rapid (bolus) injection of a small volume (100–200 μl) of buffered saline. The injectate also contains a radiolabeled test compound (e.g., ^{14}C-drug) and a highly diffusible reference compound (^{3}H-water, or ^{14}C-butanol when a ^{3}H test drug is studied), as well as a indium-113m–

TABLE 1. *Kinetic constants of blood-brain barrier nutrient transport systems*[a]

Transport system	Representative substrate	Plasma conc. (mM)	K_m (mM)	V_{max} (nmol/min · g)	K_D (ml/min · g)	Physiological efficiency
Hexose	Glucose	5.5	11.0 ± 1.4	1420 ± 140	0.017	0.0077
MCA	Lactate	1.1	1.8 ± 0.6	91 ± 35	0.019	0.0199
Neutral aa	Phenylalanine	0.1	0.11 ± 0.01	28 ± 7	0.014	0.0039
Basic aa	Arginine	0.1	0.088 ± 0.011	7.8 ± 0.9	0.0044	0.0113
Amine	Choline	0.01	0.34 ± 0.07	11.3 ± 0.7	0.0069	0.0301
Nucleoside	Adenosine	0.001	0.025 ± 0.003	0.75 ± 0.08	0.0066	0.0333
Purine	Adenine	0.01	0.011 ± 0.003	0.50 ± 0.09	0.0024	0.0220

[a] aa, amino acid; K_m, half-saturation constant; V_{max}, maximal velocity of the transport reaction; K_D = not-saturable (diffusional) constant. Physiological efficiency = K_m/V_{max}. Modified from Pardridge (160); plasma concentrations from Cornford and Oldendorf (52a).

EDTA chelate. A short time (typically 5–10 sec) after injection, when the bolus has had time to clear the brain and prior to recirculation of isotopes, the animal is decapitated and samples of the tissue and injection solution are prepared for scintillation counting. The ratio of test to reference isotope in the brain, divided by the test/reference ratio in the injectate, represents the brain uptake index (BUI). Since the indium-113m–EDTA chelate is excluded by intact capillary endothelia, this third isotope is used to identify any small proportion of test isotope which was not washed from the circulatory space. Subtraction of this quantity provides a precise measure of corrected brain uptake.

FACILITATED
TRANSPORT MECHANISMS

The entry of metabolites utilized by the brain is carefully regulated by the presence of saturable, carrier-mediated transport mechanisms. Seven major independent carriers are recognized (168), which control brain uptake of (a) hexoses, (b) short-chain monocarboxylic acids, (c) neutral amino acids, (d) basic amino acids, (e) purine bases, (f) nucleosides, and (g) amines such as choline (Table 1). Studies with isolated brain capillaries confirm that the kinetic characteristics defined using *in vivo* methods are generally consistent with *in vitro* data (217) and unquestionably confirm the functional site of the BBB at the cerebral endothelium.

The hexose carrier has been identified and kinetically characterized *in vivo;* these data also indicate that glucose transport is symmetrical (160,167,168), suggesting the hexose carrier to be present and functional on both luminal and antiluminal surfaces of the BBB capillaries. This has been confirmed by *in vitro* studies of isolated capillaries (17). It has also been confirmed that the unnatural hexoses ^{3}O-methyl glucose and 2-deoxy-D-glucose have an affinity for the glucose carrier *in vitro* at 20°C, and the apparently elevated half-saturation constants derived were attributed to excessive leakage of the damaged endothelial cell membranes (106). The monocarboxylic acid carrier (Table 1) is also well defined *in vivo,* but definition of the kinetic parameters *in vitro* is limited to the half-saturation constant for lactate, reported to be about 2.5 mM (196) and consistent with *in vivo* data (Table 1). It is known that isolated brain capillaries use fatty acids and ketones as a source of energy (21), and that traits attributed to the developmental changes seen *in vivo* (54) are apparently demonstrable *in vitro* (21).

The large neutral amino acids exhibited stereospecificity and cross-competition for uptake in isolated microvessels. The apparent half-saturation constants for tyrosine (0.111 mM), leucine (0.133 mM), and valine (0.50 mM) *in vitro* (95) are consistent with the values reported for tyrosine (K_m = 0.15 ± 0.01 mM), leucine (0.10 ± 0.01 mM) and valine (0.51 ± 0.05 mM) *in vivo* (160). In addition, characteristics of amino acid uptake by brain endothelia isolated from rats after portacaval anastomosis (43) seem to be consistent with increases seen during *in vivo* studies (99,125).

To our knowledge, no operational demonstration of the basic amino acid transport carrier or of the purine base and choline transport systems in isolated capillaries has yet been reported. The nucleoside transport mechanism has been determined to have a half-saturation constant of 5 μM is isolated capillaries *in vitro* (12,217), confirming a previous *in vivo* demonstration (52). The apparently higher estimate of half-saturation (18 μM) obtained *in vivo* may be attributable to the lower specific activity of the ^{14}C-adenosine used in the *in vivo* studies (52). Furthermore, caution must be exercised in comparing isolated capillaries to the BBB *in vivo*. As Pardridge (160) points out, brain endothelia are invariably damaged to some degree during the isolation process; especially pertinent to comparisons of kinetic parameters is the fact that in the *in vitro* situation it is extremely difficult to separate transport *per se* from transport plus metabolism. Nonetheless, the isolated capillary system has provided, and will continue to offer, another mechanism for the study of BBB phenomena.

Blood-brain barrier nutrient transport systems may be generalized as nonconcentrative (i.e., brain levels are approximately equal to or less than plasma levels for the respective substrates). These carrier systems are typically stereospecific. The BBB selectively transports D-hexoses and the L-amino acid enantiomers (145,151, 156,168). These transport systems regulate the entry of neurotransmitter precursors (e.g., tryptophan, choline, adenine, and adenosine), while neurotransmitters or putative neurotransmitter substances tend to be excluded by the BBB. For example, the BUIs of putative neurotransmitter substances such as epinephrine (2.4 ± 0.1%), DL-norepinephrine (4.5 ± 1.3%), histamine (1.6 ± 0.4%), 5-hydroxytryptamine (2.6 ± 1.8%), 5-hydroxyindoleacetic acid (2.2 ± 0.5%), dopamine (3.8 ± 0.4%), acetylcholine (4.5 ± 0.9%), aspartate (2.8 ± 0.8%), glutamate

(3.0 ± 0.3%), adenosine triphosphate (2.3 ± 0.3%), and gamma-aminobutyric acid (0.1 ± 0.1%) are so low that they approach the background limits of measurability by the single intracarotid injection technique (52a). Furthermore, it is know that there is active metabolism of certain neurotransmitter precursors by cerebral capillaries (as indicated by the high L-DOPA decarboxylase activity), thereby inhibiting dopamine synthesis (14). This is another mechanism whereby BBB endothelia regulate neurotransmitter levels in the brain in a more indirect manner (87,110). Although cerebral capillaries exclude neurotransmitters from the brain, it has been established that receptor sites are present on BBB capillaries for a variety of compounds. Insulin, which does not cross the BBB, is known to bind to specific receptors in capillary endothelia (79,173), even though glucose transport into brain is not insulin-sensitive (122). Similarly, both adrenergic (92,135,169,219) and cholinergic (88) neurotransmitter receptors have been identified in BBB capillaries, but precise functions for all of these receptors await definition. It should also be noted that neutral amino acids are transported in most biological systems via two mechanisms, the leucine-preferring (L) and alanine-preferring (A) systems (45). The studies of Wade and Katzman (209), Schain and Watanabe (189), and Yudilevich et al. (218) convincingly indicate that the A-system does not operate on the luminal side of the BBB. In contrast, studies with isolated BBB capillaries suggest that both the A- and L-systems are operational on the antiluminal side of the BBB (see Functional Differences in Luminal and Antiluminal Capillary Surfaces, above).

RATE-LIMITING STEP

Since BBB nutrient transport systems can be likened to the first enzymatic step in metabolism of these substrates, it is sometimes important to know whether metabolism or transport across the BBB capillary is the rate-limiting step. For example, if BBB transport of glucose was found to be the rate-limiting step in a particular disease, then brain glycolysis could be accelerated simply by raising the plasma glucose concentration. Conversely, if metabolism and not transport was the rate-limiting step, then no increase in brain glycolysis could be achieved by increasing plasma glucose levels. In a study of isolated dog brains, Betz et al. (19) provided an excellent sample of a pathologically induced change from phosphorylation limitation to transport limitation of glucose. These authors measured unidirectional influx by the indicator dilution technique and simultaneously determined net glucose utilization by arterial venous sampling methods. They determined in the control state that the influx of glucose by way of the transport step was 0.75 μmol/min · g, and the glycolytic rate was 0.25 μmol/min · g. An experimental anoxic state was induced, and 1 min later glycolytic and transport rates were measured. The transport of glucose remained constant (0.75 μmol/min · g), but glycolysis was accelerated to 0.55 μmol/min · g, a rate still less than the transport rate. The increase in cerebral glycolysis results in a decrease in brain glucose levels; however, glycolysis is still under phosphorylation limitation. This acceleration of glycolysis under anoxic states is seen in a wide variety of tissues (131). Ten minutes after the anoxic state had been initiated, Betz et al. (19) again measured glycolysis and transport rates and found that glucose influx was considerably reduced (about 0.3 μmol/min · g), and glucose utilization rates had returned almost to normal (0.28 μmol/min · g). Thus the brain chooses to restrict any increases in glycolysis during anoxia by slowing the activity of the BBB transport step. In this pathological state, then, transport becomes the rate-limiting step. At 60 min postanoxia, Betz again measured glucose utilization rate and found that it had returned to normal (0.25 μmol/min · g) and that the influx rate had increased to 0.45 μmol/min · g. Thus, under these conditions of recovery, BBB transport was no longer the rate-limiting step. For a more detailed account of transport rate-limited pathways, the reader should refer to the review of Pardridge (159).

It is not clear whether transport of glucose can be the rate-limiting step in seizure states, since conclusions must be based on data obtained in different laboratories. Chapman et al. (44) demonstrated that in bicuculline-induced seizures, the rat brain glucose utilization rate (measured in whole brain) was 2.0 μmol/min · g. Since the V_{max} for BBB glucose transport is 1.4 μmol/min · g in normal rats (159), their measured glucose utilization rate in seizures exceeds the transport rate in normal animals by 30 to 40%. In a more recent study, brain glucose utilization rates were determined in a variety of brain regions of rats that had been subjected to bicuculline-induced seizures for time periods ranging from 20 to 120 min (97). These authors reported that in many regions of the brain subjected to greater than 60 min of seizure, glucose utilization rates exceeded 2.0 μmol/min · g; rates ranged up to 3.37 μmol/min − g in the auditory cortex of rats subjected to bicuculline seizures for 120 min. In contrast, Hawkins and associates (90) measured glucose influx rates into many of the same brain regions using an elegant autoradiographic technique. A detailed comparison of these two studies (90,97) again suggests that regional brain glucose utilization rates in seizure states exceed the maximal influx rates determined in comparable brain regions of normal animals (Table 2).

It has been suggested that the rate of BBB glucose transport in seizures is rapidly accelerated to accommodate the increase in cerebral demands for glucose (160). It is possible that the mechanism by which blood-brain barrier transport is rapidly activated in seizures may be the reciprocal process by which glucose transport is rapidly inactivated in studies of isolated anoxic dog brain (19). However, the evidence for rapid activation of BBB sugar transport in seizures is indirect, and studies providing confirmation of this process should be performed. In addition, studies of seizures in both rats (24) and humans (25) suggest that alterations can occur in the functional capillary surface area. This has been attributed to stretching of the endothelial cells and/or the opening up of new capillaries (i.e., ''capillary intermittency''). Capillary intermittency, which may be defined as the recruitment of additional capillary beds resulting in an in-

creased capillary surface area, is a well-accepted phenomenon in muscle tissue. The unanswered question, however, is whether or not there is a sufficient increase in brain capillary surface area during seizures to permit a 30 to 40% increase in transport. For example, in stimulated nervous activity (58) or during hypoglycemia (1), the measured rates of glucose influx were several times greater than values computed from rats anesthetized with sodium pentobarbital. Cremer (54) suggested that these higher rates can possibly be explained by capillary recruitment, a topic under investigation. The other alternative, rapid induction of BBB transport systems, is an area needing study because even if recruitment can be demonstrated, it would not necessarily preclude concomitant induction of the blood-brain barrier transport systems.

The most commonly cited example wherein BBB transport is the rate-limiting step is seen in studies of ketone-body utilization. While we are not aware of any contemporary evidence suggesting that transport by way of the amine carrier, the amino acid carriers, the purine base carrier, or the nucleoside transport system can be rate-limiting, this is not the case with monocarboxylic acids. Miller et al. (128), Cremer and Heath (57), and Ruderman et al. (184) all recognized that brain concentrations of the ketone bodies (β-hydroxybutyrate and acetoacetate) were too low to be measured, while plasma levels of these substances remained elevated.

TABLE 2. *Comparison of regional blood-brain barrier glucose influx in normal rats, and regional brain glucose utilization rates during seizures*[a]

Brain region	Glucose influx (μmol/min · g)	Brain glucose utilization (μmol/min · g)
Frontal cortex	2.12 ± 0.28	2.43 ± 0.17
Substantia nigra	1.92 ± 0.27	0.34 ± 0.06
Globus pallidus	1.44 ± 0.20	0.64 ± 0.17
Thalamus	2.38 ± 0.42	2.37 ± 0.24
Parietal cortex	2.13 ± 0.23	2.25 ± 0.11
Occipital cortex	2.09 ± 0.23	2.59 ± 0.15
Superior colliculus	2.92 ± 0.45	0.99 ± 0.15
Inferior colliculus	3.20 ± 0.40	0.62 ± 0.11
Amygdala	1.46 ± 0.17	2.37 ± 0.20
Habenula	2.85 ± 0.56	0.91 ± 0.14

[a] Influx was determined [by Hawkins et al. (90)] 10 sec after infusion of ^{14}C-glucose in 250–275 g male Long-Evans rats (mean plasma glucose level 19.8 ± 3.3 mM). Glucose consumption [Ingvar and Siesjo (97)] was measured in 310–400 g male SPF rats subjected to 60 min of bicuculline-induced seizures (mean plasma glucose levels averaged 22.3 ± 1.4 mM prior to seizures, and 17.2 ± 2.0 mM after 30 min of seizures). Note that for about half of the discrete brain regions that can be compared, the apparent maximal influx rate for glucose is less than the glucose utilization rate determined after induced seizures. Furthermore, the glucose utilization rates determined under resting conditions in normal animals by Hawkins et al. (90) are generally 30–50% greater than measured in comparable brain regions of untreated rats by Ingvar and Siesjo (97). Thus these data, despite being from different laboratories and determined by different methods, seem consistent with the suggestion that in experimental seizure states brain glucose utilization rates can exceed measured maximal glucose influx rates.

Therefore, brain utilization of these ketone bodies is limited by BBB transport in states of ketonemia. Another feature of this monocarboxylic acid transport system is that it is very sensitive to physiological changes. For example, transport capacity of this monocarboxylic acid carrier is altered in fasting states. Increased transport of β-hydroxybutyrate and acetoacetate (82) and of lactate (55) was found in adult rats fasted for several days. Furthermore, in suckling rats (15–21 days old), the influx rates for both pyruvate and lactate were determined to be twice that seen in 28-day-old weanling rats (56). Since this transport system is so responsive to physiological alterations in animal studies, it can be inferred that the same may be true in humans. Certain forms of childhood epilepsy are treated by employing a ketogenic diet regimen. It might be interesting to determine whether or not the success or failure of the ketogenic diet could be related to some form of induction of the BBB monocarboxylic acid transport system. Because transport can be expected to be rate-limiting and because ketone-body utilization rates could be conceivably measured by positron emission techniques, such a study is at least technically possible in humans.

PROTEIN BINDING

It has been established (143,164,165) that there is virtually no mixing of the injection solution with rat plasma prior to the time that the injected bolus first traverses the capillary bed. Thus, comparing the brain uptake of a drug in buffered saline with the BUI in the presence of serum (where uptake may be inhibited due to binding of the drug to plasma proteins) provides the opportunity for *in vivo* study of the effects of plasma-protein binding. This concept has

been extensively utilized to characterize the influence of plasma proteins on brain (and liver) uptake of steroid hormones (158).

Using this methodology, it is possible to test certain clinical concepts in experimental animal model situations and to make some predictions regarding factors influencing drug delivery to the brain. In the present report, brain extraction (147) of saline and serum-borne ^{14}C-phenytoin, ^{14}C-phenobarbital, ^{14}C-valproate, and ^{3}H-diazepam is reviewed in adults rats. In addition, age-related variations in brain permeability to drugs are suggested (see below).

PERMEABILITY TO ANTICONVULSANT DRUGS

Brain uptake indices, an *in vivo* measure of blood-brain barrier transfer, have been determined in experimental animals for the anticonvulsant drugs listed in Table 3. Since the brain extraction (E) of water 5 sec postinjection is 0.85 (31), then $E = \text{BUI} \times 0.85$. Thus the (saline-borne) extractions for these anticonvulsants are phenytoin, $E = 23 \pm 1\%$; phenobarbital, $E = 20 \pm 1\%$; valproic acid, $E = 32 \pm 9\%$; and diazepam, $E = 86 \pm 10\%$. With reference to the clinical situation, these E values represent that fraction of the free drug that would be cleared in a single pass through the brain. The carbonic anhydrase inhibitor acetazolamide, sometimes used in the treatment of seizure disorders, has a very low brain extraction ($E = 1 \pm 1\%$). Because intravascular markers such as mannitol and sucrose have $E = 1$ to 2%, acetazolamide may gain access via brain regions lacking BBB capillaries (e.g., choroid plexus or other circumventricular organs).

LIPID-MEDIATED BLOOD-BRAIN BARRIER PERMEABILITY

Since no selectively saturable, carrier-mediated transport of anticonvulsant drugs occurs, we sought other explanations for the increased (lipid-mediated) brain uptakes in the neonate (Table 4). Brain myelin content increases significantly during the neonatal period; hence we examined the possibility that lipophilic BBB permeability might be different in the adult and neonate (51). It was established that brain uptakes could be correlated with octanol:saline partition coefficients (an *in vitro* measure of relative lipophilic properties). Further statistical comparison of uptake data from neonatal and adult brains indicated that a functional similarity ex-

TABLE 3. *Blood-brain barrier extraction and permeability of anticonvulsant drugs after intracarotid injection*[a]

Drug	Brain extraction in saline	Permeability × surface area product (ml/min · g)
Acetazolamide	1 ± 1%	0.01
Phenytoin	23 ± 1%	0.16
Phenobarbital	20 ± 1%	0.14
Valproate	43 ± 5%	0.34
Diazepam	86 ± 10%	1.2
Paraldehyde	86 ± 24%	1.2

[a] Determined in the barbiturate-anesthetized rat. Paraldehyde data from Treiman and Chelberg (205).

ists between the two membrane systems (51). Thus the age-related variation in brain uptake of anticonvulsants could not be attributed to altered lipophilic permeability.

An alternate measure of lipophilicity has been suggested by Stein (197). The hydrogen bonding potential of a molecule (as indicated by structure) can be determined by inspection of the polar functional groups on the anticonvulsant drug. Data from this laboratory indicate that the hydrogen bond number is highly predictive of BBB permeability (Fig. 2) of anticonvulsant drugs.

EFFECT OF BLOOD FLOW RATE ON BRAIN UPTAKE

As indicated in Table 4, brain extraction of the two anticonvulsants phenytoin and phenobarbital was two to three times greater in newborn than in adult rats. Since increased BBB permeability was empirically precluded as an explanation for increased brain extraction of drugs in the newborn, the alternate possibility of decreased blood flow was examined. Owing to the larger size of newborn rabbits, quantitative measurements of cerebral blood flow could be obtained. As in the newborn rat (Table 4), elevated brain extraction of anticonvulsant drugs was observed in the newborn rabbit, but by 28 days post-partum brain extractions decreased and showed an inverse relationship to age (53). The extraction of water was determined to be 0.87 in neonate and 0.69 in 28-day-old rabbits (165), and E(drug) $=$ BUI $\times$ E(water).

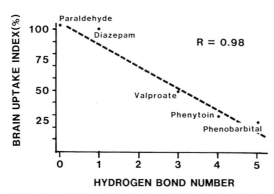

FIG. 2. Anticonvulsant permeability in the blood-brain barrier as a function of hydrogen-bonding potential. According to Stein (197), the hydrogen bond number is $N = 4$ for water, $N = 2$ for each hydroxyl group or primary amine, and $N = 1$ for carbonyl groups, secondary amines and nitriles, with $N = 0$ for ethers and other groups.

When brain extractions of anticonvulsants are corrected for age-related alterations in cerebral blood flow F, the resulting values for the permeability surface products (PS) of phenobarbital and phenytoin show no age-dependent differences. Given that $F = 0.25$ and 0.88 ml/min · g for the ether-anesthetized newborn and 28-day-old rabbit, respectively (165), then PS $= [-F$ ln$(1-E)] = 0.16$ ml/min · g for phenobarbital in the newborn rabbit and 0.13 ml/min · g in the 28-day-old rabbit (53). These values are not significantly different. Similarly, for phenytoin, PS $= 0.22$ and 0.21 ml/min · g in the newborn and 28-day-old rabbit, respectively. The PS for valproate in the neonatal rabbit (obtained from data in Table 2) can be estimated to be 0.13 ml/min · g. Valproate uptake has not been measured in the 28-day-old rabbit, but given a BUI value of 17% in the adult rabbit and assuming the flow rates to be similar to the 28-day-old rabbit, a similar estimate (PS $= 0.11$) is derived. Thus the increase in brain extraction of (saline-borne) anticonvulsants in the newborn is a function of reduced cerebral blood flow rate.

In the rat brain, comparative PS products (in milliliters per minute per gram) have been derived (from data in Table 2) for phenytoin (0.16), phenobarbital (0.14), and valproate (0.23). They are estimated with less certainty for diazepam (2.1) and acetazolamide (0.01), because these two drugs represent the extremes of permeability and exclusion.

EFFECTS OF PROTEIN BINDING ON ANTICONVULSANT PERMEABILITY

The antiepileptic drugs valproate, phenytoin, diazepam, and phenobarbital are bound (to varying degrees) by plasma protein, and it is commonly believed that only the fraction of drug that is free (dialyzable) *in vitro* is available for transport through the brain endothelial capillary *in vivo*. Initial-rate, single-injection studies from this laboratory indicate that lipid-mediated transport of both free and protein-bound phenytoin, valproate, and diazepam does indeed occur in the BBB of the adult rat. That is, a fraction of the drug entering the capillary bound to plasma protein is able to dissociate and equilibrate across the rat BBB during a single transcapillary passage.

The brain extraction measured in saline provides an estimate of maximal blood-to-brain transfer, and uptake measured in the presence of serum is representative of the *in vivo* plasma-protein binding. Comparison of brain uptake in

TABLE 4. *Permeability of anticonvulsants in the adult and newborn rat blood-brain barrier*

		Brain uptake index (%)	
Drug	Age	Saline	Serum[a]
Phenytoin	Adult	27.6 ± 1.1	12.5 ± 0.3
	Neonate	74.7 ± 6.8	72.0 ± 6.9
Phenobarbital	Adult	23.4 ± 0.9	13.9 ± 1.1
	Neonate	58.8 ± 5.8	72.3 ± 13.0
Valproate	Adult	37.5 ± 10.3	25.2 ± 8.1
	Neonate[b]	47.3 ± 8.2	17.3 ± 5.6
Diazepam	Adult	102.1 ± 7.8	40.7 ± 6.7

[a] Concentration 75–82%; each value $\overline{X}$ ± SD, N = 3–6.
[b] Newborn rabbits (less than 24 hr).

serum divided by the uptake in saline provides the fraction of the total exchangeable drug transferred from blood to brain in a single capillary passage. As indicated in Fig. 3, the similarity in exchangeable phenobarbital (in the adult rat brain *in vivo*) and the percentage of free drug *in vitro* (i.e., the dialyzable fraction) indicates that

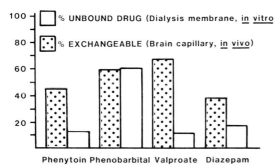

FIG. 3. Comparison of exchangeable anticonvulsant drugs measured *in vivo* (in the BBB of adult rats) and *in vitro* (by dialysis with normal human adult serum). These data demonstrate that the free fraction of a trace concentration of anticonvulsant drug, determined by equilibrium dialysis *in vitro*, does not correspond to brain extraction, as measured by single-pass, initial-rate uptake studies in experimental animals *in vivo*. The percentage of exchangeable drug *in vivo* is determined from the ratio of the BUI in human serum to the BUI in saline listed in Table 4. In the adult, 45.3% of the exchangeable diphenylhydantoin (phenytoin) is transported *in vivo*, but only 13% is freely dialyzable *in vitro;* thus a fraction of the protein-bound drug penetrates the BBB. About 60% of the phenobarbital is freely dialyzable from adult sera, and a similar quantity (59%) is exchangeable, suggesting that *in vivo* lipid-mediated transport of this drug is restricted to the free phenobarbital and no protein-bound drug is transported. Sixty-seven percent of the exchangeable valproate and 40% of the exchangeable diazepam penetrate the BBB when only 10 and 15%, respectively, is freely dialyzable. Thus, there is some dissociation and single-pass clearance of protein-bound valproate and diazepam in the rat blood-brain barrier.

in the adult brain capillary, there is little or no transport of protein-bound phenobarbital. However, the relatively higher percentages of *in vivo* exchangeable (as compared to freely dialyzable) diphenylhydantoin, valproic acid, and diazepam indicate that protein-bound anticonvulsants gain access to the brain in a single capillary passage. These data demonstrate that the free fraction of a trace concentration of anticonvulsant drug, determined by equilibrium dialysis *in vitro*, does not correspond to brain extraction, as measured by single-pass, initial-rate uptake studies in experimental animals *in vivo*. Recent studies of valproate in dogs and monkeys also indicate that drug distribution across the blood-brain barrier is not strictly dependent on the free drug concentration in plasma (121), supporting the concept suggested by our single-injection, initial-rate studies.

Eleven percent of the total serum-borne phenytoin and 23.5% of the saline-borne drug is extracted (E) by the adult rat brain. Since 13% of this drug is freely dialyzable, 13% × 0.235 = 3%, which represents the maximal extraction attributable to permeation of free drug when E is measured in the presence of serum. Since the total serum-borne E is 11%, of which only 3% is derived from the freely dialyzable drug fraction, the remaining 8% is derived from the protein-bound fraction of the phenytoin (Table 5). The BUIs of both phenytoin and phenobarbital are quite similar (comparing serum- and saline-borne drug) in the newborn brain (Table 5), suggesting brain uptake may approximate total (free plus protein-bound) serum drug concentrations.

In the presence of human serum, 12% of the total phenobarbital is extracted during a single capillary passage through the adult brain. The entire 12% can be attributed to extraction of the unbound drug, with no protein-bound phenobarbital gaining access to the rat brain. In the newborn, a BUI (serum-borne) of 70 ± 13% was measured, as compared to BUI (serum-borne) of 14 ± 1% in the adult. In further contrast, both free and protein-bound plasma phenobarbital enters the newborn brain [i.e., a fraction of the phenobarbital entering the capillary bound to plasma proteins apparently has time to dissociate and equilibrate across the endothelial cell (53)]. Considerable proportions of protein-bound valproic acid and diazepam are also extracted from human serum during a single transcapillary passage through the adult rat BBB (Table 5).

BLOOD-BRAIN BARRIER EXCLUSION OF PROTEINS AND PEPTIDES

Circulating proteins such as albumin do not gain access to brain (152), and most small peptides also do not traverse BBB capillaries (47). It may be of some significance to note that very low, but measurable uptakes ($E = 2$–3%, similar to the extraction of morphine) for methionine enkephalin and leucine enkephalin were reported (47). The similarity in brain extraction of peptides such as thyrotropin releasing hormone (TRH) to that of dextran was discussed, and the 1 to 2% extraction of these compounds was attributed to entry via specialized regions of the brain (circumventricular organs) lacking BBB capillaries (47). Subsequent studies have confirmed that the BBB excludes peptides (159); thus the entry of protein-bound anticonvulsant drugs cannot be attributed to permeation of the drug–protein complex, but rather to a stripping or release of the drug from the bound complex within the capillary. It is also possible that circulating peptides may rapidly impart signals to the CNS without traversing the brain endothelia if specific receptors exist (on the luminal surface of the BBB) and if a secondary messenger can both receive and transmit the peptide signal (161,163). Recent demonstrations of insulin

(79,173) and neurotransmitter receptors (88,92, 135,169,219) on brain capillaries would lend support to this speculative hypothesis.

ROLE OF PLASMA-PROTEIN BINDING OF ANTICONVULSANTS IN THE NEWBORN

The decreased cerebral blood flow rate in the newborn would be expected to prolong capillary transit time, since these two parameters are generally inversely related (85). Moreover, these anticonvulsants are bound to plasma proteins, and the transport of protein-bound compounds into brain is enhanced by increases in capillary transit time (157,158). Therefore we investigated the possibility that the exchangeable fraction of circulating drug may be increased in the newborn (53). As shown in Table 3, when the injected solution contained 75% serum, no alteration in neonatal brain uptake of either phenytoin or phenobarbital was observed. In contrast, the inclusion of 75% serum in studies of adult rats results in a much reduced transport of both phenobarbital and phenytoin, relative to that seen in the presence of saline.

Similar observations were also made for the newborn rabbit. Brain extraction of phenytoin in saline ($E = 59 ± 5\%$) was similar to that measured in the presence of 75% fetal ($E = 56 ± 6\%$) or adult ($E = 50 ± 3\%$) human serum. Thus, like the rat (Table 3), the newborn rabbit brain was able to maximally extract free and protein-bound phenytoin, and brain uptake was not altered by increasing plasma drug levels.

CAPILLARY TRANSPORT AND DISSOCIATION OF BOUND DRUGS

From previous work (53), it is apparent that the higher brain extraction of saline-borne anticonvulsants in the newborn is indeed a function

TABLE 5. *Relative proportion of protein-bound and free drug extracted by the blood-brain barrier in a single transit*[a]

Drug	% Bound in vitro	% Brain extraction in serum	Proportion (%) gaining access to brain from	
			Saline (free)	Serum (bound)
Phenytoin	87	11	3.6	7.4
Phenobarbital	40	12	12.0	0.0
Valproate	90	21	3.4	17.6
Diazepam	85	41	15.0	26.0

[a] *In vitro* binding measurements are slightly lower than some workers report because the only drug present in the dialysis system was the trace concentration derived from the isotopic drugs.

of reduced cerebral blood flow rate in the neonate. The data are not as simply explained, however, when brain uptakes of serum-borne drugs are measured. The similarity in exchangeable phenobarbital (in the rat brain *in vivo*) and the percentage of freely dialyzable drug *in vitro* (Fig. 3) indicates there is no transport of protein-bound phenobarbital in the adult brain. In contrast, protein-bound phenobarbital does gain access to the newborn brain (53). Protein-bound phenytoin is able to (dissociate and) traverse capillary endothelia in both the newborn (Table 3) and adult brain (Fig. 3). These results are consistent with the "free intermediate" model (Fig. 4) for the capillary transport of protein-bound substances (158).

Certain conclusions may be drawn from the single-injection studies of anticonvulsant penetration of the blood-brain barrier. It is demonstrated that greater quantities of anticonvulsant drugs may gain access to the developing, neonatal brain than measured for the adult. A possible consequence is that the potential for intoxication may be increased in newborns. Since some extraction of protein-bound phenytoin and phenobarbital occurs in newborn animals, brain levels are probably not identical to free drug concentrations; thus alternatives to the exclusive use of free drug levels in neonatal medicine might be evaluated.

The concept that only freely dialyzable anticonvulsant drugs can gain access to the brain is not consistent with the data obtained from initial-rate studies in this laboratory. It is postulated that capillary transit time is one of three major determinants influencing drug delivery to brain. (The other two determinants, rate of drug dissociation and permeation, are discussed with Fig. 4.) This information may be clinically relevant only in a situation where the precise anticonvulsant drug concentration delivered to brain is desired. However, the untoward effects of valproate upon brain development (204), the incidence of birth defects associated with phenytoin and phenobarbital treatments (123,193), and the carcinogenicity of hydantoins (192) collectively suggest that the close therapeutic monitoring of these compounds may be well justified. The precise relationship of single-injection studies to the steady-state clinical situation is not yet defined. However, information gained from the intracarotid technique in animals may assist in predicting drug delivery to brain in conditions where the steady state is not achieved. The treatment of major motor status by the rapid injection of selected phenytoin preparations is one example (207).

EPILEPSY AND THE BLOOD-BRAIN BARRIER

Experimental Seizure States

Studies employing either vital dyes or radioactive tracers have traditionally demonstrated increased (nonspecific) permeability of brain endothelia and modifications of the restrictive properties after induction of convulsions in both the BBB (11,29) and the blood-CSF barrier (115). Generally, the duration of seizure activity can be correlated with reduced barrier functions (29,172). To study the effect of experimental seizures on blood-brain barrier permeability to materials like proteins, many workers have combined the use of horseradish peroxidase with ultrastructural sectioning to examine changes in blood-brain barrier capillaries. In a variety of animal models, seizures have been evoked using drugs or electrical stimulation.

A wide variety of drugs has been employed in these studies, including dexamethasone (72) and pentylenetetrazole (91,118,119), as well as penicillin, bicuculline, methoxypyridoxine, methionine-sulfoximine, kainic acid, and pentylenetetrazole in the studies of Nitsch and Klatzo (140). The effects of electroshock seizures have been investigated by Lending et al. (115), Lee and Olszewski (114), Suzuki et al. (201), Bolwig et al. (24), Petito et al. (172), and Petito and Levy (170), as well as Westergaard et al. (215). Almost all of the studies mentioned characteristically indicate that there is an increased permeability to protein tracers in experimental seizure states. In an early study (118), it was suggested that horseradish peroxidase could pass through the capillary endothelial clefts by breaching the interendothelial tight junctions. However, in a more conclusive follow-up study, Hedley-Whyte et al. (91) indicated that the role of the endothelial vesicles as opposed to interendothelial junctions was not well defined and suggested that arteriolar and capillary vesicles might be involved. In addition, these authors concluded that increased permeability was seen initially in the arteriolar sites and that tracer molecules moved along the vessel walls into the capillaries.

In a more definitive study using electroshock seizures, Petito and Levy (170) determined that increased pinocytotic activity could be demonstrated first in arterioles and subsequently in

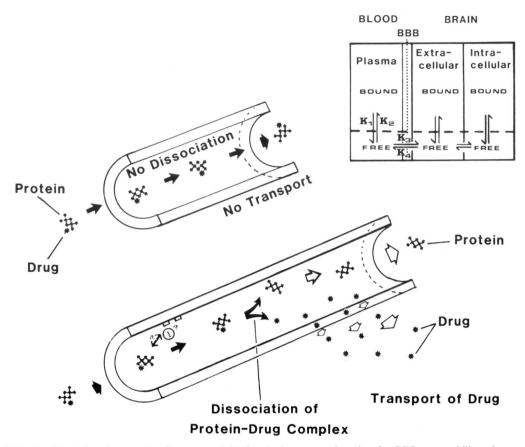

FIG. 4. The "free intermediate" concept (158) invoked as an explanation for BBB permeability of serum-bound anticonvulsant drugs (44). Three factors of importance are (a) the capillary transit time ($\gg$ the $T_{1/2}$ of k_1 and k_2) (b) the rate of unidirectional dissociation of drug from protein (= k_1), and (c) the rate of drug permeation through the endothelial membrane (= k_3). When dissociation constants are measured *in vitro* (for example by equilibrium dialysis) the $K_d = k_1/k_2$, information relative to the *in vitro* K_d can be obtained through comparative single-injection studies of brain uptakes measured in the presence or absence of serum proteins. Data from Fig. 3 indicated that the K_d measured *in vitro* for phenobarbital is unchanged *in vivo* (*upper left*). Brain uptake is exclusively attributable to diffusion of the freely dialyzable fraction of drug in the serum ($k_2 \gg k_3$, e.g., penetration of phenobarbital in the adult rat BBB). However, the K_d values for phenytoin, diazepam, and valproate are, for some unknown reason, altered in short term studies *in vivo*. Under these conditions (*lower figure*), the exchangeable drug *in vivo* will exceed the exchangeable drug *in vitro* (see Fig. 3), and drug that was bound to plasma proteins at the arteriolar–capillary junction will dissociate and gain entry to the brain (*lower figure*) during a single passage. Examples are the entry of phenytoin, valproate, and diazepam in the adult rat brain. The *in vivo* alteration of the affinity constant is apparently greater in the newborn capillary than in the adult, as suggested by the observations that a fraction of the phenobarbital which enters the newborn capillary bound to plasma proteins has time to dissociate and equilibrate across the brain endothelium (53). Membrane permeability (= k_3) is a determining factor because if the drug is relatively impermeable, protein-bound drug which dissociates in a single capillary transit will not be transported but simply reassociate (k_2 would exceed k_3) and be retained intravascularly. Furthermore, if serum proteins such as albumin have an increased transit time through the BBB capillary (1), due to some interaction of the protein with the capillary wall (W. M. Pardridge, *personal communication*) then this would also promote a net increase of drug equilibrating across the capillary into brain during a single ransit. Note that although the extracellular compartment of brain is cerebrospinal fluid, the so-called blood-CSF barrier is not represented in this diagram (*upper left*) because the BBB is some 5,000 times larger in surface area. Specific binding of anticonvulsant drugs to intracellular compartments is also known (i.e., phenytoin and benzodiazepine receptors). The possibility that for valproate uptake $k_4 > k_3$ is also discussed (see text).

capillaries, and these authors suggested that arterioles were important in maintaining and altering the blood-brain barrier. In addition, they suggested that abnormal BBB permeability, as seen in electroshock seizure states, occurred first in the arterioles. The increased pinocytotic activity observed in electroshock seizures is proportional to the number and duration of electroshocks (171,213). It has been shown that prevention of the hypertension associated with seizure states almost completely prevents BBB damage seen in experimental seizures (171), and this has been confirmed by Westergaard (213). Petito et al. (172) also observed maximal BBB pinocytosis in the thalamic area of the brain, a region characterized by high concentrations of cyclic AMP. On this basis, they suggested that cyclic adenosine monophosphate (cAMP) might be involved in micropinocytotically induced breakdown of BBB functions. Experimental data from other studies correlate rises in cAMP concentrations in capillaries with increased pinocytotic activity (101,102). Convulsive drugs also appear to induce regional changes in BBB permeability. Pentylenetetrazole seizures primarily affect the hypothalamus and preoptic area (140). The GABA-receptor blocker bicuculline induces penetration of dyes into the region of the pallidum, whereas methoxypyridoxine, the GABA-synthesis inhibitor, results in compromising BBB function in the hippocampus. Capillaries of the mammillary body are primarily affected by methionine–sulfoximine-induced convulsions, and kainic acid induces alterations in capillaries of the neocortical brain areas. These authors also indicated that loss of barrier properties was typically bilateral and confined to the anatomically limited brain areas (140).

The administration of glucocorticoids (72), pentobarbital, or the experimentally induced reduction in blood pressure (114) all appear to protect the BBB and restore barrier properties. Ultrastructural investigations confirm that there is an activation of pinocytotic activity in brain endothelia associated with seizure states that may be related to increased cerebral blood flow (171). These are temporary barrier alterations, and their extent may be influenced by factors such as relative neuronal activity (194), blood flow and blood pressure (171), and vasodilation (29). In experimental animals, it has been established that the transient increased cerebrovascular permeability to plasma proteins is reversible and occurs within 1 hr after cessation of the drug-induced seizures (119).

Clinical Observations

In a more recent study of tissues obtained from neurosurgically treated human psychomotor epilepsy, a thickening of the brain capillary basement membrane has been observed (105). Presumably this represents a chronic condition, rather than a transient alteration observed only in association with seizures. In rats, it has been suggested that the brain capillary basement membrane is thinner in immature than mature brain (68). Age-related thickening of the BBB has also been reported in humans, and it is increased in individuals with Alzheimer's disease (124). The high incidence of microvessel brain hemorrhages in infants (206) may be related to their thinner, and presumably weaker, capillary basement membrane. Thus, the observation of Kasantikul and associates (105) may represent a reinforcement of capillary basement membrane in response to seizure trauma. The latter authors also reported that capillary pericytes from sclerotic cortex were thicker than observed in control states, and the areas of capillary mitochondrial profiles tended to be greater in damaged hippocampus. Greater numbers of tight junctions were also determined in sclerotic hippocampus than in capillary profiles from normal hippocampus (105).

The clinical use of computerized tomographic brain scanning has made the imaging physician more aware of the blood-brain barrier, and a more detailed review appears elsewhere (185). This is primarily because more information can be obtained by intravenous administration of iodine contrast agents, material that is restricted from the central nervous system tissues by intact, normally functioning BBB capillaries. However, since much of the clinical brain imaging is performed on patients with a suspected neurological lesion, it is not surprising that seizures are known to be generated by contrast media (191). Particularly in the presence of metastases, the restrictive properties of the BBB endothelia seem to be compromised and permit contrast media to access brain parenchyma (77).

PATHOLOGICAL ALTERATIONS IN THE BLOOD-BRAIN BARRIER

In addition to the recognition of subtle changes in the fine structure of BBB capillaries associated with human epilepsy (105), data from animal models (hyperammonemia and portacaval anastomosis) of hepatic encephalopathy indicate that increased capillary diameter and reduced mitochondrial content characterize this condition (113). Translocation of enzymatic activities from luminal to antiluminal capillary surfaces has also been reported in viral infections of the CNS (208). It is recognized that metastatic tumors in the brain induce proliferation of non-neural capillaries (i.e., capillaries characteristic of the tissue of origin). Capillaries of cerebral metastatic lymphoma, for example, have regular endothelial cells with pinocytotic activity; fenestrations characteristic of the normal lymph gland capillaries are observed, rather than the typical cerebral capillaries (94). Because these tumors have capillaries atypical of blood-brain barrier sites, they are readily demonstrable in computerized axial tomographic (CAT) enhancement studies (185). In contrast, in low-grade gliomas, new capillaries resemble normal cerebral capillaries with maintenance of barrier properties, and therefore no CAT enhancement is demonstrated (40). In an animal study of experimentally transplanted astrocytomas, Deane and Lantos (63) studied the development of capillaries in growing tumors. They concluded that until the tumors reached a diameter of 3 to 4 mm, the ultrastructure of the developing capillaries showed no marked differences from that seen in the developing capillaries of normal embryological chick brain or rat and cat brain. In addition, capillaries of human fetal brains develop in a similar manner (3,89). Further studies (64) indicate that the number of pinocytotic vesicles found in capillaries of astrocytomas is considerably greater than that of capillaries from surrounding normal brain tissue. These workers observed a three- to sixfold increase in pinocytotic vesicles, together with minimal evidence of increased fenestrations or abnormal endothelial junctions in the tumor capillaries. It was suggested that this increased vesicle formation was related to increased transendothelial transport in these experimental astrocytomas, just as increases in vesicles had been previously reported in experimental seizure states.

Various forms of ionizing radiation are known to compromise BBB function (29). Large doses of radiation produce an acute effect on BBB function (134), whereas clinical doses typically do not have an acute effect (116). However, clinicians have been concerned that radiation initiates changes that result in compromised BBB function up to 5 years after exposure. Thus, latent pathologic effects are well documented (107,127).

It has been observed that chemotherapy has not had a significant impact upon primary brain tumors, presumably because the integrity of the BBB capillaries is retained. In animal studies, Rapoport et al. (175–177) demonstrated that it was possible to reversibly disrupt BBB function using osmotic shock. The electron microscopic studies of Brightman et al. (35) indicated that tight junctions in the endothelia were opened with this technique, and other laboratories were able to confirm the transient nature of osmotically compromised BBB function (174,200). Hypertonic arabinose was employed to deliver measles antibody into the brain of immunized monkeys (93). The possible therapeutic implications for this technique to be used in treatment of brain tumors led Neuwelt et al. (138) to develop a canine model in which the time course of mannitol-induced osmotic BBB disruption could be monitored by CAT methods. This technique has been subsequently applied in the treatment of malignant brain tumors with some significant success (137,139). It has also been suggested that the delivery of hexosaminidase-A to the brain may be achieved by this temporary osmotic disruption of BBB functions (136). The clinical relevance of this observation is that hexosaminidase-A is the enzyme deficient in Tay–Sachs disease, and at present no specific therapy for this condition is available. Delivery of some antibiotic drugs to the central nervous system is also a clinical problem when the drug does not readily cross the BBB. Strasbaugh and Brinker (199) have recently demonstrated that the delivery of gentamicin to brain can be augmented by mannitol treatment of the rabbit blood-brain barrier. Thus, the potential use of transient osmotic disruption of the BBB is currently being evaluated with optimism for use in several neuropathological conditions.

Circumventing the BBB by administering drugs directly into the cerebrospinal fluid has also been attempted with limited success. For example, antibiotics have been administered by this route in infections of the central nervous system (203,211,212). Although this route of administration is contraindicated for vincristine (70), complications have also been reported for drugs such as cytosine arabinoside (33) and methotrexate (46,81). It is well established that morphine does not penetrate the BBB, but more lipophilic analogs such as codeine (monoacetyl morphine) and heroin (diacetyl morphine) gain easy access to the brain (150). To circumvent the blood-brain barrier in clinically intractable pain, morphine has been administered intrathecally (210). This procedure has been applied with mixed results in obstetric anesthesia (10). Complications have also been reported (129), presumably because the dose must be reduced by at least one order of magnitude on the basis of plasma and CSF morphine levels compared after intrathecal and epidural administration (103). The latter study emphasizes that when a clinical decision is made to bypass the blood-brain barrier by intrathecal injection, brain endothelia prevent brain-to-blood movement, resulting in unusual pharmacokinetics. That is, the BBB may also function as a brain-to-blood barrier. The probable retention in brain of drug that otherwise would not cross the BBB must be assumed, and the dosage must be reduced to prevent undesirable side effects.

FUTURE DIRECTIONS OF STUDY

Basic science studies of the blood-brain barrier in the future are needed to focus upon the relationships between free and bound drug and on anticonvulsant delivery not only to the CNS but also to specific brain sites. Neurologists interested in the blood-brain barrier and epilepsy should be aware that the traditional free drug hypothesis needs to be expanded to account for the fact that dissociation constants measured *in vitro* are not necessarily the same *in vivo*. The observation that cerebrospinal fluid/plasma anticonvulsant levels sometimes approximate the percentage of free (unbound) drug *in vitro* is often cited in support of the free drug hypothesis. However, it is important to realize that CSF drug levels reflect permeability at the blood-CSF barrier (primarily localized to the choroid plexus), and that the blood-brain barrier is approximately 5,000 times greater in size.

The elegant methods developed by Hawkins et al. (90) in experimental animals predict that these same measurements of brain influx in specific sites will be made noninvasively in humans in the near future. As discussed by Sokoloff (195), states such as thyrotoxicosis, schizophrenia, and LSD intoxication might be considered to be accompanied by some sort of augmentation of mental activity. Early studies of oxygen and glucose consumption in these conditions, however, suggested no increment above the rate in resting, alert, idle individuals. The same phenomenon was observed in the popular prototype of brain work, the performance of arithmetic, and no increment in oxygen consumption was observed (195). The contemporary explanation was that the conscious brain operated at a sustained high level of energy demand, which was orders of magnitude higher than that accompanying a signal to induce a change in function.

More recently, autoradiographic studies in animals and positron emission tomography in humans have established that the brain is a heterogeneously functioning organ. A specific group of structures or cells displays augmented electrical and metabolic activity in response to selected stimuli. The increments may be quite large but confined to specific CNS loci. Thus, the function of the BBB in seizures needs to be evaluated for both global CNS changes as well as discrete regional responses to seizure states. This assessment must include evaluation of both luminal and antiluminal surfaces of the BBB. Direct application of the *in vitro* brain capillary model to studies of applied seizure disorders will no doubt emerge in the near future, hopefully providing information that will impact on clinical care. In addition, continuing investigations of the mechanisms responsible for alterations in BBB basement membrane are needed, as is the development of methods and techniques to reverse the alterations seen in studies of the hippocampal capillary basement membrane.

ACKNOWLEDGMENTS

We thank Dr. Antonio V. Delgado-Escueta and Dr. David M. Treiman for discussions of this work, and Dr. William M. Pardridge for critically reading this manuscript. The assistance of Samuel L. Biggers, Jr., Cynthia P. Diep, Sarah Fels, Kristin P. Landon, and Terry L. Quirk is also gratefully acknowledged. Dr. Robert S. Janicki of Abbott Laboratories, North Chicago, Illinois, kindly made ^{14}C-valproate available. This study was funded by the Department of Health, Education and Welfare under contract NO1-NS-0-2332 and was additionally supported by the Veterans Administration.

REFERENCES

1. Abdul-Rahman, A., and Siesjo, B. K. (1980): Local cerebral glucose consumption during insulin-induced hypoglycemia, and in the recovery period following glucose administration. *Acta Physiol. Scand.*, 110:149–159.
2. Albert, Z., Orlowski, M., Rzucidlo, Z., and Orlowski, J. (1966): Studies on gamma-glutamyl-transpeptidase activity and its histochemical localization in the central nervous system of man and different animal species. *Acta Histochem.*, 25:312–320.
3. Allsop, G., and Gumble, H. J. (1979): Light and

electron microscopic observations on the development of the blood vascular system of the human brain. *J. Anat.*, 128:461–477.

4. Amtorp, O. (1976): Transfer of I^{125}-albumin from blood into brain and cerebrospinal fluid in newborn and juvenile rats. *Acta Physiol. Scand.*, 96:399—406.

5. Reference deleted in proof.

6. Bar, T. H. (1978): Morphometric evaluation of capillaries in different laminae of rat cerebral cortex by automatic image analysis: Changes during development and aging. In: *Advances in Neurology, Vol. 20: Pathology of Cerebral Microcirculation*, edited by J. Cervos-Navarro, E. Betz, G. Ebhardt, R. Ferzt, and B. Wullenweber, pp. 1–9. Plenum, New York.

7. Bar, T. H., and Wolff, J. R. (1972): The formation of capillary basement membranes during internal vascularization of the rat's cerebral cortex. *Z. Zellforsch.*, 133:231–248.

8. Bar, T. H., and Wolff, J. R. (1973): Quantitative beziehungen zwischen der verzweigungsdichte und länge von capillaren im neocortex der ratte wahrend der postnatalen entwicklung. *Z. Anat. Entwicklungsgesch.*, 141:207–228.

9. Reference deleted in proof.

10. Baraka, A., Noueihid, R., and Hajj, S. (1981): Intrathecal morphine for obstetric anesthesia. *Anesthesiology*, 54:136–140.

11. Bauer, K. F. R., and Leonhardt, H. (1956): A contribution to the pathological physiology of the blood-brain barrier. *J. Comp. Neurol.*, 106:363–370.

12. Beck, D. W., Vinters, H. V., Hart, M. N., Henn, F. A., and Cancilla, P. A. (1983): Uptake of adenosine into cultured endothelium. *Brain Res.*, 271:180–183.

13. Bennett, H. S., Luft, J. H., and Hampton, J. L. (1959): Morphological classification of vertebrate blood capillaries. *Am. J. Physiol.*, 196:381–390.

14. Bertler, A., Falck, B., Owman, C., and Rosengren, E. (1966): The localization of monoaminergic mechanisms. *Pharmacol. Rev.*, 18:369–385.

15. Betz, A. L. (1983): Sodium transport in capillaries isolated from rat brain. *J. Neurochem.*, 41:1150–1157.

16. Betz, A. L. (1983): Sodium transport from blood to brain: Inhibition by furosemide and amiloride. *J. Neurochem.*, 41:1158–1164.

17. Betz, A. L., Csejtey, J., and Goldstein, G. W. (1979): Hexose transport and phosphorylation by capillaries isolated from rat brain. *Am. J. Physiol.*, 236:C96–C102.

18. Betz, A. L., Firth, J. A., and Goldstein, G. W. (1980): Polarity of the blood-brain barrier: Distribution of enzymes between the luminal and antiluminal membranes of brain capillary endothelial cells. *Brain Res.*, 192:17–28.

19. Betz, A. L., Gilboe, D. D., and Drewes, L. R. (1974): Effects of anoxia on net uptake and unidirectional transport of glucose into the isolated dog brain. *Brain Res.*, 67:307–316.

20. Betz, A. L., and Goldstein, G. W. (1978): Polarity of the blood-brain barrier: Neutral amino acid transport into isolated brain capillaries. *Science*, 202:225–227.

21. Betz, A. L., and Goldstein, G. W. (1981): Developmental changes in metabolism and transport properties of capillaries isolated from rat brain. *J. Physiol. (Lond.)*, 312:365–376.

22. Betz, A. L., and Goldstein, G. W. (1981): The basis for active transport at the blood-brain barrier. In: *Advances in Experimental Biology and Medicine*, Vol. 143, edited by H. M. Eisenberg and R. L. Suddith, pp. 5–16. Plenum, New York.

23. Bissonnette, J. M., Cronan, J. Z., Richards, L. L., and Wickman, W. K. (1979): Placental transfer of water and nonelectrolytes during a single circulatory passage. *Am. J. Physiol.*, 236:C47–C53.

24. Bolwig, T. G., Hertz, M. M., and Holm-Jensen, J. (1977): Blood-brain barrier permeability during electroshock seizures in the rat. *Eur. J. Clin. Invest.*, 7:95–100.

25. Bolwig, T. G., Hertz, M. M., Paulsen, O. B., Spotoft, H., and Rafaelsen, O. J. (1977): The permeability of the blood-brain barrier during electrically induced seizures in man. *Eur. J. Clin. Invest.*, 7:87–93.

26. Reference deleted in proof.

27. Bourne, G. H. (1958): Histochemical demonstration of phosphatases in the central nervous system of the rat. *Exp. Cell Res. [Suppl.]*, 5:101–117.

28. Bowman, P. D., Ennis, S. R., Rarey, K. E., Betz, A. L., and Goldstein, G. W. (1983): Brain microvessel endothelial cells in tissue cultures: A model for study of blood-brain barrier permeability. *Ann. Neurol.*, 14:396–402.

29. Bradbury, M. W. B. (1979): *The Concept of a Blood-Brain Barrier*. Wiley, New York.

30. Bradbury, M. W. B. (1984): The structure and function of the blood-brain barrier. *Fed. Proc.*, 43:186–190.

31. Bradbury, M. W. B., Patlak, C. S., and Oldendorf, W. H. (1975): Analysis of brain uptake and loss of radiotracers after intracarotid injection. *Am. J. Physiol.*, 229:1110–1115.

32. Braun, L. D., Cornford, E. M., and Oldendorf, W. H. (1980): Newborn blood-brain barrier is selectively permeable and differs substantially from the adult. *J. Neurochem.*, 34:147–152.

33. Breuer, A. C., Pitman, S. W., Dawson, D. M., and Schoene, W. C. (1977): Paraparesis following intrathecal cytosine arabinoside. A case report with neuropathologic findings. *Cancer*, 40:2817–2822.

34. Brightman, M. W., and Albers, R. W. (1959): Species differences in the distribution of extraneuronal cholinesterase within the vertebrate central nervous system. *J. Neurochem.*, 4:244–250.

35. Brightman, M. W., Hori, M., Rapoport, S. I., Reese, T. S., and Westergaard, E. (1973): Osmotic opening of tight junctions in cerebral endothelium. *J. Comp. Neurol.*, 128:317–326.

36. Broadwell, R. D., and Brightman, M. W. (1976): Entry of peroxidase into neurons from the central and peripheral nervous systems from

extracerebral and cerebral blood. *J. Comp. Neurol.*, 166:257–284.

37. Broadwell, R. D., and Salcman, M. (1981): Expanding the definition of the blood-brain barrier to protein. *Proc. Natl. Acad. Sci. U.S.A.*, 78:7820–7824.

38. Broman, T. (1941): The possibilities of the passage of substances from the blood to the central nervous system. (Is there a blood-brain barrier and a blood-cerebrospinal fluid barrier?). *Acta Psychiatr. Neurol.*, 16:1–25.

39. Burns, E. M., Kruckeberg, T. W., and Gaetano, P. K. (1981): Changes with age in cerebral capillary morphology. *Neurobiol. Aging*, 2:285–291.

40. Caille, J. M., Guibert-Trainer, F., Calabet, A., Billerey, J., and Piton, J. (1980): Abnormal enhancements after contrast injection. In: *Computerized Tomography*, edited by J. M. Caille and G. Salamon, pp. 166–171. Springer, Berlin.

41. Caley, D. W., and Maxwell, D. S. (1970): Development of the blood vessels and extracellular spaces during postnatal maturation of rat cerebral cortex. *J. Comp. Neurol.*, 138:31–48.

42. Cancilla, P. A., Baker, R. N., Pollock, P. S., and Frommes, S. P. (1972): The reaction of pericytes of the central nervous system to protein. *Lab. Invest.*, 26:376–383.

43. Cardelli-Cangiano, P., Cangiano, C., James, J. H., Jepson, B., Brenner, W., and Fischer, J. E. (1981): Uptake of amino acids by brain microvessels isolated from rats after portacaval anastomosis. *J. Neurochem.*, 36:627–632.

44. Chapman, A. G., Meldrum, B. S., and Siesjo, B. K. (1977): Cerebral metabolic changes during prolonged epileptic seizures in rats. *J. Neurochem.*, 28:1025–1035.

45. Christensen, H. N. (1973): On the development of amino acid transport systems. *Fed. Proc.*, 32:19–28.

46. Clark, A. W., Cohen, S. R., Nissenblatt, M. J., and Wilson, S. K. (1982): Paraplegia following intrathecal chemotherapy. Neuropathologic findings and evaluation of myelin basic protein. *Cancer*, 50:42–47.

46a. Cornford, E. M. (1984): Blood-brain barrier permeability to anticonvulsant drugs. In: *Metabolism of Antiepileptic Drugs*, edited by R. H. Levy et al., pp. 129–142. Raven Press, New York.

47. Cornford, E. M., Braun, L. D, Crane, P. D., and Oldendorf, W. H. (1978): Blood-brain barrier restriction of peptides and the low uptake of enkephalins. *Endocrinology*, 103:1297–1303.

48. Cornford, E. M., Braun, L. D., Pardridge, W. M., and Oldendorf, W. H. (1980): Blood flow rate and cellular influx of glucose and arginine in mouse liver *in vivo. Am. J. Physiol.*, 238:H553–H560.

49. Cornford, E. M., Diep, C. P., and Pardridge, W. M. (1985): Blood-brain barrier transport of valproic acid. *J. Neurochem.*, 44:1541–1550.

50. Cornford, E. M., Braun, L. D., and Oldendorf, W. H. (1982): Developmental modulations of blood-brain barrier permeability as an indicator of changing nutritional requirements in the brain. *Pediatr. Res.*, 16:324–328.

51. Cornford, E. M., Braun, L. D., Oldendorf, W. H., and Hill, M. A. (1982): Comparison of lipid-mediated blood-brain barrier penetrability in neonates and adults. *Am. J. Physiol.*, 243:C161–C168.

52. Cornford, E. M., and Oldendorf, W. H. (1975): Independent blood-brain barrier transport systems for nucleic acid precursors. *Biochim. Biophys. Acta*, 382:65–72.

52a. Cornford, E. M., and Oldendorf, W. H. (1980): Blood-brain permeability to amines and amine precursors. In: *Noncatecholic Phenylethylamines, Part 2*, edited by A. D. Mosnaim and M. E. Wolf, pp. 21–51. Marcel Dekker, New York.

53. Cornford, E. M., Pardridge, W. M., Braun, L. D., and Oldendorf, W. H. (1983): Increased blood-brain barrier transport of protein bound anticonvulsant drugs in the newborn. *J. Cereb. Blood Flow Metab.*, 3:280–286.

54. Cremer, J. E. (1982): Substrate utilization and brain development. *J. Cereb. Blood Flow Metab.*, 2:394–407.

55. Cremer, J. E., Braun, L. D., and Oldendorf, W. H. (1976): Changes during development in transport processes of the blood-brain barrier. *Biochim. Biophys. Acta*, 448:633–637.

56. Cremer, J. E., Cunningham, V. J., Pardridge, W. M., Braun, L. D., and Oldendorf, W. H. (1979): Kinetics of blood-brain barrier transport of pyruvate, lactate, and glucose in suckling, weanling and adult rats. *J. Neurochem.*, 33:439–445.

57. Cremer, J. E., and Heath, D. F. (1974): The estimation of rates of utilization of glucose and ketone bodies in the brain of the suckling rat using compartmental analysis of isotopic data. *Biochem. J.*, 142:527–544.

58. Cremer, J. E., Ray, D. E., Sarna, G. S., and Cunningham, V. J. (1981): A study of the kinetic behavior of glucose based on simultaneous estimates of influx and phosphorylation of brain regions of rats in different physiological states. *Brain Res.*, 221:331–342.

59. Cremer, J. E., Teal, H. M., and Cunningham, V. J. (1982): Inhibition, by 2-oxoacids that accumulate in maple-syrup urine disease, of lactate, pyruvate and 3-hydroxybutyrate transport across the blood-brain barrier. *J. Neurochem.*, 39:674–677.

60. Crone, C., and Oleson, S. P. (1982): Electrical resistance of brain microvascular endothelium. *Brain Res.*, 241:49–55.

61. Reference deleted in proof.

62. Davson, H., and Oldendorf, W. H. (1967): Transport in the central nervous system. *Proc. R. Soc. Med.*, 60:326–328.

63. Deane, B. R., and Lantos, P. L. (1981): The vasculature of experimental brain tumors: 1. A sequential light and electron microscope study of angiogenesis. *J. Neurol. Sci.*, 49:55–66.

64. Deane, B. R., and Lantos, P. L. (1981): The vasculature of experimental brain tumors: 2. A

quantitative assessment of morphological abnormalities. *J. Neurol. Sci.*, 49:67–77.

DeBault, L. E., and Cancilla, P. A. (1979): Gamma-glutamyl transpeptidase in isolated brain endothelial cells: Induction by glial cells *in vitro. Science*, 270:653–655.

66. Reference deleted in proof.

67. Diamond, I., and Schmid, R. (1966): Experimental bilirubin encephalopathy. The mode of entry of bilirubin-^{14}C into the central nervous system. *J. Clin. Invest.*, 45:678–689.

68. Donahue, S., and Pappas, G. D. (1961): The fine structure of capillaries in the cerebral cortex of the rat at various stages of development. *Am. J. Anat.*, 108:331–347.

69. Dunn, J. S., and Wyburn, G. M. (1972): The anatomy of the blood-brain barrier. *Scott. Med. J.*, 17:21–36.

70. Dyke, R. W. (1982): Vincristine must not be administered intrathecally. *J.A.M.A.*, 248:171–172.

71. Ehinger, B., and Falck, B. (1970): Cellular uptake of some amino acids and amines *in vitro* into rabbit and monkey anterior eye segment preparations. *Exp. Eye Res.*, 10:352–359.

72. Eisenberg, H. M., Barlow, C. F., and Lorenzo, A. V. (1970): Effect of dexamethasone on altered brain vascular permeability. *Arch. Neurol.*, 23:18–22.

73. Eisenberg, H. M., and Suddith, R. L. (1979): Cerebral vessels have the capacity to transport sodium and potassium. *Science*, 206:1083–1085.

74. Evans, C. A. N., Reynolds, J. M., Saunders, N. R., and Segal, M. B. (1974): The development of the blood-brain barrier mechanism in fetal sheep. *J. Physiol.*, 238:371–386.

75. Reference deleted in proof.

76. Ferguson, R. K., and Woodbury, D. M. (1969): Penetration of 14-C inulin and 14-C sucrose into brain, cerebrospinal fluid and skeletal muscle of developing rats. *Exp. Brain Res.*, 7:181–194.

77. Fischer, H. W. (1980): Occurrence of seizure during cranial computed tomography. *Radiology*, 137:563–564.

78. Flummerfelt, B. A., Lewis, P. R., and Gwyn, D. G. (1973): Cholinesterase activity in capillaries of the rat brain. A light and electron microscopic study. *Histochem. J.*, 5:67–77.

79. Frank, H. J. L., and Pardridge, W. M. (1981): A direct *in vitro* demonstration of insulin binding to isolated microvessels. *Diabetes*, 30:757–761.

80. Frey, H. H., and Loscher, W. (1978): Distribution of valproate across the interface between blood and cerebrospinal fluid. *Neuropharmacology*, 17:637–642.

81. Gagliano, R. G., and Costunzi, J. J. (1976): Paraplegia following intrathecal methotrexate. Report of a case and review of the literature. *Cancer*, 37:1663–1668.

82. Gjedde, A., and Crone, C. (1975): Induction processes in blood-brain barrier transfer of ketone bodies during starvation. *Am. J. Physiol.*, 229:1165–1169.

83. Goldstein, G. W. (1979): Relation of potassium transport to oxidative metabolism in isolated brain capillaries. *J. Physiol.*, 286:185–195.

84. Goldstein, G. W., and Betz, A. L. (1983): Recent advances in understanding brain capillary function. *Ann. Neurol.*, 14:389–395.

85. Goresky, C. A., and Rose, C. P. (1977): Blood-tissue exchange in the liver and heart: The influence of heterogeneity of capillary transit times. *Fed. Proc.*, 36:2629–2634.

86. Gozes, I., Cronin, B. L., and Moskowitz, M. A. (1981): Protein synthesis in rat brain microvessels decreases with aging. *J. Neurochem.*, 36:1311–1315.

87. Hardebo, J. E., and Owman, C. (1980): Barrier mechanisms for neurotransmitter amines and their precursors at the blood-brain interface. *Ann. Neurol.*, 8:1–11.

88. Harik, S. I., Sharma, V. K., Wetherbee, J. R., et al. (1981): Adrenergic and cholinergic receptors of cerebral microvessels. *J. Cereb. Blood Flow Metab.*, 1:329–338.

89. Hauw, J. J., Burger, B., and Escourolle, R. (1975): Electron microscope study of the developing capillaries of human brain. *Acta Neuropathol.*, 31:229–242.

90. Hawkins, R. A., Mans, A. M., Davis, D. W., Hibbard, L. S., and Lu, D. M. (1983): Glucose availability to individual cerebral structures is correlated to glucose metabolism. *J. Neurochem.*, 40:1013–1018.

91. Hedley-White, E. T., Lorenzo, A. V., and Hsu, D. W. (1977): Protein transport across cerebral blood vessels during metrazole-induced convulsions. *Am. J. Physiol.*, 233: C74–C85.

92. Herbst, T. J., Raichle, M. E., and Ferrendelli, J. A. (1979): Beta-adrenergic regulation of adenosine 3',5'-monophosphate concentration in brain microvessels. *Science*, 204:330–332.

93. Hicks, J. T., Albrecht, P., and Rapoport, S. I. (1976): Entry of neutralizing antibody to measles into brain and cerebrospinal fluid of immunized monkeys after osmotic opening of the blood-brain barrier. *Exp. Neurol.*, 53:768–779.

94. Hirano, A., Ghatak, N. R., Becker, N. H., and Zimmerman, H. M. (1974): A comparison of the fine structure of small blood vessels in intracranial and retroperitoneal malignant lymphomas. *Acta Neuropathol. (Berl.)*, 27:93–104.

95. Hjelle, J. T., Baird-Lambert, J., Cardinale, G., Spector, S., and Udenfriend, S. (1978): Isolated microvessels: The blood-brain barrier *in vitro. Proc. Natl. Acad. Sci. U.S.A.*, 75:4544–4548.

96. Reference deleted in proof.

97. Ingvar, M., and Siesjo, B. K. (1983): Local blood flow and glucose consumption in the rat brain during sustained bicuculline seizures. *Acta Neurol. Scand.*, 68:129–144.

98. Jacquez, J. A. (1984): Modeling exchange in capillary beds. *Fed. Proc.*, 43:148–153.

99. James, J. H., Escourrou, J., and Fischer, J. E. (1978): Blood-brain neutral amino acid transport activity is increased after portacaval anastomosis. *Science*, 200:1395–1397.

100. Reference deleted in proof.

101. Joo, F. (1979): Significance of adenylate cyclase in the regulation of the permeability of brain capillaries. In: *Pathophysiology of Cerebral Energy and Metabolism*, edited by B. B. Mrsulja, L. M. Rakie, and I. Klatzo, pp. 211–238. Plenum, New York.

102. Joo, F., Rakonczay, Z., and Wolleman, M. (1975): cAMP-mediated regulation of the permeability in the brain capillaries. *Experientia*, 31:582–584.

103. Jorgensen, B. C., Andersen, H. B., and Engquist, A. (1981): CSF and plasma morphine after epidural and intrathecal morphine. *Anesthesiology*, 55:714–715.

104. Junck, L., and Marshall, W. H. (1983): Neurotoxicity of radiological contrast agents. *Ann. Neurol.*, 13:469–484.

105. Kasantikul, V., Brown, W. J., Oldendorf, W. H., and Crandall, P. C. (1983): Ultrastructural parameters of limbic microvasculature in human psychomotor epilepsy. *Clin. Neuropathol.*, 2:171–178.

106. Kolber, A. R., Bagnell, C. R., Krigman, M. R., Hayward, J., and Morrell, P. (1979): Transport of sugars into microvessels isolated from rat brain: A model for the blood-brain barrier. *J. Neurochem.*, 33:419–432.

107. Kramer, S., and Lee, K. F. (1974): Complication of radiation therapy: The central nervous system. *Semin. Roentgenol.*, 11:75–83.

108. Kristensson, K., and Olsson, Y. (1973): Accumulation of protein tracers in pericytes of the central nervous system following systemic injection in immature mice. *Acta Neurol. Scand.*, 49:189–194.

109. Ladinsky, W. A., and Drewes, L. R. (1983): Characterization of the blood-brain barrier: Protein composition of the capillary endothelial cell membrane. *J. Neurochem.*, 41:1341–1348.

110. Lai, F. M., Udenfriend, S., and Spector, S. (1975): Presence of norepinephrine and related enzymes in isolated brain microvessels. *Proc. Natl. Acad. Sci. U.S.A.*, 72:4622–4625.

111. Langer, R., Conn, H., and Vacanti, J. (1980): Control of tumor growth in animals by infusion of an angiogenesis inhibitor. *Proc. Natl. Acad. Sci. U.S.A.*, 77:4331–4335.

112. Laufler, L. R., Gambone, J. C., Chaudhuri, G., Pardridge, W. M., and Judd, H. L. (1983): The effect of membrane permeability and binding by human serum proteins on sex steroid influx into the uterus. *J. Clin. Endocrinol. Metab.*, 56:1282–1287.

113. Laursen, H., and Diemer, N. H. (1980): Capillary size, density and ultrastructure in brain of rats with urease-induced hyperammonaemia. *Acta Neurol. Scand.*, 62:103–115.

114. Lee, J. C., and Olszewski, J. (1961): Increased cerebrovascular permeability after repeated electroshock. *Neurology*, 11:515–519.

115. Lending, M., Slobody, L. B., and Mestern, J. (1959): Effect of prolonged convulsions on the blood-cerebrospinal fluid barrier. *Am. J. Physiol.*, 197:465–468.

116. Levin, N. A., Edwards, M. S., and Byrd, A. (1979): Quantitative observations of the acute effects of x-irradiation on brain capillary permeability, Part 1. *Int. J. Oncol. Biol. Phys.*, 5:1627–1631.

117. Levy, R. (1980): CSF and plasma pharmacokinetics: Relationship to mechanisms of action as exemplified by valproic acid in the monkey. In: *Epilepsy: A Window to Brain Mechanisms*, edited by J. S. Lockard and A. A. Ward, pp. 191–200. Raven Press, New York.

118. Lorenzo, A. V., Hedley-Whyte, E. T., Eisenberg, H. M., and Hsu, D. W. (1975): Increased penetration of horseradish peroxidase across the blood-brain barrier induced by metrazole seizures. *Brain Res.*, 88:136–140.

119. Lorenzo, A. V., Shiranige, I., Liang, M., and Barlow, C. F. (1972): Temporary alteration of cerebrovascular permeability to plasma protein during drug-induced seizures. *Am. J. Physiol.*, 223:268–277.

120. Loscher, W., and Frey, H. H. (1982): Transport of GABA at the blood-CSF interface. *J. Neurochem.*, 38:1072–1079.

121. Loscher, W., and Nau, H. H. (1983): Distribution of valproic acid and its metabolites in various brain areas of dogs and rats after acute and prolonged treatment. *J. Pharmacol. Exp. Ther.*, 226:845–854.

122. Lund-Andersen, H. (1979): Transport of glucose from blood to brain. *Physiol. Rev.*, 59:305–352.

123. Mallow, D. M., Herrick, M. K., and Gathman, G. (1980): Fetal exposure to anticonvulsant drugs. Detailed pathological study of a case. *Arch. Pathol. Lab. Med.*, 104:215–218.

124. Mancardi, G. L., Perdelli, F., Rivano, C., Leonardi, A., and Bugiani, O. (1980): Thickening of the basement membrane of cortical capillaries in Alzheimer's disease. *Acta Neuropathol.*, 49:79–83.

125. Mans, A. M., Biebuyck, J. F., Saunders, S. J., Kirsch, R. E., and Hawkins, R. A. (1979): Tryptophan transport across the blood-brain barrier during acute hepatic failure. *J. Neurochem.*, 33:409–418.

126. Manz, H. J., and Robertson, D. M. (1972): Vascular permeability to horseradish peroxidase in brainstem lesions of thiamine deficient rats. *Am. J. Pathol.*, 66:565–572.

127. Mikhael, M. A. (1978): Radiation necrosis of the brain: Correlation between computed tomography pathology and dose distribution. *J. Comput. Assist. Tomogr.*, 2:71–80.

128. Miller, A. L., Hawkins, R. A., and Veech, R. L. (1973): The mitochondrial redox state of rat brain. *J. Neurochem.*, 20:1393–1400.

129. Mok, M. S., and Tsai, S. K. (1981): More experience with intrathecal morphine for obstetric anesthesia. *Anesthesiology*, 55:481.

130. Mollgard, K., and Saunders, N. R. (1975): Complex tight junctions of epithelial and endothelial cells in early foetal brain. *J. Neurocytol.*, 4:453–468.

131. Morgan, H. E., and Whitfield, C. F. (1973): Regulation of sugar transport in eukaryotic cells. *Curr. Top. Membr. Transp.*, 4:255–303.

132. Muir, A. R., and Peters, A. (1962): Quintuple-layered membrane junctions at terminal bars between endothelial cells. *J. Cell Biol.,* 12:443–447.

133. Murray, K. J., White, J. G., and Douglas, S. D. (1980): Comparative biochemical and ultrastructural studies of capillaries from normal humans, normal mice and human cerebral astrocytomas. *Surg. Neurol.,* 14:53–58.

134. Nair, V., and Roth, L. J. (1964): Effect of x-irradiation and certain other treatments on blood-brain barrier permeability. *Radiat. Res.,* 23:249–264.

135. Nathanson, J. A., and Glaser, G. M. (1979): Identification of β-adrenergic sensitive adenylate cyclase in intracranial blood vessels. *Nature (Lond.),* 278:567–569.

136. Neuwelt, E. A., Barranger, J. A., Brady, R. O., Pagel, M., Furbish, F. S., Quirk, J. M., Mook, G. E., and Frenkel, E. (1981): Delivery of hexosaminidase A to the cerebrum after osmotic modification of the blood-brain barrier. *Proc. Natl. Acad. Sci. U.S.A.,* 78:5838–5841.

137. Neuwelt, E. A., Diehl, J. T., Vu, L. H., Hill, S. A., Michael, A. J., and Frenkel, E. (1981): Monitoring of methotrexate delivery in patients with malignant brain tumors after osmotic blood-brain barrier disruption. *Ann. Int. Med.,* 94:449–454.

138. Neuwelt, E. A., Frenkel, E. P., Rapoport, S. I., and Barnett, P. (1980): Effect of osmotic blood-brain barrier disruption on methotrexate pharmacokinetics in the dog. *Neurosurgery,* 7:36–43.

139. Neuwelt, E. A., and Rapoport, S. I. (1984): Modification of the blood-brain barrier in the chemotherapy of malignant tumors. *Fed. Proc.,* 43:214–219.

140. Nitsch, C., and Klatzo, I. (1983): Regional patterns of blood-brain barrier breakdown during epileptiform seizures induced by various convulsive agents. *J. Neurol. Sci.,* 59:305–322.

141. Oakley, J., Ohemann, G. A., Ojemann, L. M., and Cromwell, L. (1979): Identifying epileptic foci on contrast-enhanced computerized tomographic scans. *Arch. Neurol.,* 36:669–671.

142. Oldendorf, W. H. (1970): Measurement of brain uptake of radiolabeled substances using a tritiated water internal standard. *Brain Res.,* 24:372–376.

143. Oldendorf, W. H. (1971): Brain uptake of radiolabeled amino acids, amines and hexoses after arterial injection. *Am. J. Physiol.,* 221:1629–1639.

144. Oldendorf, W. H. (1973): Carrier-mediated blood-brain barrier transport of short-chain monocarboxylic organic acids. *Am. J. Physiol.,* 224:1450–1453.

145. Oldendorf, W. H. (1973): Stereospecificity of blood-brain barrier permeability to amino acids. *Am. J. Physiol.,* 224:967–969.

146. Oldendorf, W. H. (1982): Some clinical aspects of the blood-brain barrier. *Hosp. Pract.* (Feb.): 143–164.

147. Oldendorf, W. H., and Braun, L. D. (1976): [3-H] Tryptamine and [3-H] water as diffusible internal standards of measuring brain extraction

of radiolabeled substances following intracarotid injection. *Brain Res.,* 113:219–224.

148. Oldendorf, W. H., and Brown, W. J. (1975): Greater number of capillary endothelial cell mitochondria in brain than muscle. *Proc. Soc. Exp. Biol. Med.,* 149:736–738.

149. Oldendorf, W. H., Cornford, E. M., and Brown, W. J. (1977); The large apparent work capability of the blood-brain barrier: A study of mitochondrial content of capillary endothelial cells in brain and other tissues of the rat. *Ann. Neurol.,* 1:409–417.

150. Oldendorf, W. H., Hyman, S. H., Braun, L. D., and Oldendorf, S. Z. (1972): Blood-brain barrier penetration of morphine, codeine, heroin and methadone after carotid injection. *Science,* 178:984–987.

151. Oldendorf, W. H., and Szabo, J. (1976): Amino acid assignment to one of three blood-brain barrier amino acid carriers. *Am. J. Physiol.,* 230:94–98.

152. Olsson, Y., Klatzo, I., Sourander, P., and Steinwall, O. (1968): Blood-brain barrier permeability to albumin in embryonic, newborn, and adult rats. *Acta Neuropathol.,* 10:117–122.

153. Orlowski, M., Sessa, G., and Green, J. P. (1974): Gamma glutamyl transpeptidase in brain capillaries: Possible site for a blood-brain barrier for amino acids. *Science,* 184:66–68.

154. Owman, C., and Rosengren, E. (1967): Dopamine formation in brain capillaries—An enzymatic blood-brain barrier mechanism. *J. Neurochem.,* 14:547–550.

155. Pardridge, W. M. (1977): Unidirectional influx of glutamine and other neutral amino acids into liver of fed and fasted rats *in vivo. Am. J. Physiol.,* 232:E492–E496.

156. Pardridge, W. M. (1977): Regulation of amino acid availability to the brain. In: *Nutrition and the Brain,* Vol. 1, edited by R. J. Wurtman and J. J. Wurtman, pp. 141–203. Raven Press, New York.

157. Pardridge, W. M. (1979): Carrier-mediated transport of thyroid hormones through the rat blood-brain barrier: Primary role of albumin-bound hormone. *Endocrinology,* 105:605–613.

158. Pardridge, W. M. (1981): Transport of protein-bound hormones into tissues *in vivo. Endocr. Rev.,* 2:103–123.

159. Pardridge, W. M. (1983): Neuropeptides and the blood-brain barrier. *Ann. Rev. Physiol.,* 45:73–82.

160. Pardridge, W. M. (1983): Brain metabolism: A perspective from the blood-brain barrier. *Physiol. Rev.,* 63:1481–1535.

161. Pardridge, W. M. (1984): Transport of nutrients and hormones through the blood-brain barrier. *Fed. Proc.,* 43:201–204.

162. Pardridge, W. M., Crane, P. D., Mietus, L. J., and Oldendorf, W. H. (1982): Kinetics of regional blood-brain barrier transport and phosphorylation of glucose and 2-deoxyglucose in the barbiturate anesthesized rat. *J. Neurochem.,* 38:560–568.

163. Pardridge, W. M., Frank, H. J. L., Cornford, E. M., Braun, L. D., Crane, P. D., and Oldendorf, W. H. (1981): Neuropeptides and the

blood-brain barrier. In: *Neurosecretion and Brain Peptides*, edited by J. B. Martin, S. Riechlin, and K. L. Bick, pp. 321–328. Raven Press, New York.

164. Pardridge, W. M., and Mietus, L. J. (1979): Transport of steroid hormones through the rat blood-brain barrier: Primary role of albumin-bound hormone. *J. Clin. Invest.*, 64:145–151.

165. Pardridge, W. M., and Mietus, L. J. (1980): Transport of thyroid and steroid hormones through the blood-brain barrier of the newborn rabbit: A primary role for protein bound hormones. *Endocrinology*, 107:1705–1710.

166. Pardridge, W. M., Moeller, T. L., Mietus, L. J., and Oldendorf, W. H. (1980): Blood-brain barrier transport and brain sequestration of the steroid hormones. *Am. J. Physiol.*, 239:L96–E103.

167. Pardridge, W. M., and Oldendorf, W. H. (1975): Kinetics of blood-brain barrier transport of hexoses. *Biochim. Biophys. Acta*, 382:377–392.

168. Pardridge, W. M., and Oldendorf, W. H. (1977): Transport of metabolic substances through the blood-brain barrier. *J. Neurochem.*, 28:5–12.

169. Peroutka, S. J., Moskowitz, M. A., Reinhard, J. F., and Snyder, S. H. (1980): Neurotransmitter receptor binding in bovine cerebral microvessels. *Science*, 208:610–612.

170. Petito, C. K., and Levy, D. E. (1980): The importance of cerebral arterioles in alterations of the blood-brain barrier. *Lab. Invest.*, 43:262–268.

171. Petito, C. K., Schaefer, J. A., and Plum, F. (1976): The blood-brain barrier in experimental seizures. In: *Dynamics of Brain Edema*, edited by H. M. Pappius and W. Feindel, pp. 38–42. Springer-Verlag, New York.

172. Petito, C. K., Schaefer, J. A., and Plum, F. (1977): Ultrastructural characteristics of the brain and blood-brain barrier in experimental seizures. *Brain Res.*, 127:251–267.

173. Pillion, D. J., Haskell, J. F., and Meezane, E. (1982): Cerebral cortical microvessels: An insulin sensitive tissue. *Biochem. Biophys. Res. Commun.*, 104:686–692.

174. Pollay, M. (1975): Effect of hypertonic solutions on the blood-brain barrier. *Neurology*, 25:852–866.

175. Rapoport, S. I. (1976): *Blood-Brain Barrier in Physiology and Medicine*. Raven Press, New York.

176. Rapoport, S. I., Bachman, D. S., and Thompson, H. K. (1972): Chronic effects of osmotic opening of the blood-brain barrier in the monkey. *Science*, 176:1243–1245.

177. Rapoport, S. I., and Thompson, H. K. (1973): Osmotic opening of the blood-brain barrier in the monkey without associated neurological deficits. *Science*, 180:971.

178. Reference deleted in proof.

179. Reese, T. S., and Karnovsky, M. J. (1967): Fine structural localization of a blood-brain barrier exogenous peroxidase. *J. Cell Biol.*, 34:207–217.

180. Reference deleted in proof.

181. Reyners, H., de Reyners, E. D., Jadin, J. M., and Masin, J. R. (1975): An ultrastructural quantitative method for the evaluation of the permeability to horseradish peroxidase of cerebral cortex endothelial cells of the rat. *Cell Tissue Res.*, 157:93–99.

182. Rosenberg, F. J., Romano, J. J., and Shaw, D. D. (1980): Metrizamide, iothalamate, and mitrizoate: Effects of internal carotid arterial injections on the blood-brain barrier of the rabbit. *Invest. Radiol.*, 15(Suppl. 6):S275–279.

183. Reference deleted in proof.

184. Ruderman, N. B., Ross, P. S., Berger, M., and Goodman, M. N. (1974): Regulation of glucose and ketone body metabolism in the brain of unanesthetized rats. *Biochem. J.*, 138:1–10.

185. Sage, M. R. (1982): Blood-brain barrier: Phenomenon of increasing importance to the imaging clinician. *A.J.R.*, 138:887–898.

186. Samorajski, T., and McLeod, J. (1961): Alkaline phosphomonoesterase and blood-brain permeability. *Lab. Invest.*, 10:492–501.

187. Reference deleted in proof.

188. Saunders, N. R. (1977): Ontogeny of the blood-brain barrier. *Exp. Eye Res.*, 25(Suppl.):523–550.

189. Schain, R. J., and Watanabe, K. S. (1972): Distinct pattern of entry of two non-metabolizable amino acids into brain and other organs of infant guinea pigs. *J. Neurochem.*, 19:2279–2288.

190. Reference deleted in proof.

191. Scott, W. R. (1980): Seizures: A reaction to contrast media for computerized tomography of the brain. *Radiology*, 137:359–361.

192. Scoville, B., and White, B. G. (1981): *Psychopharmacol. Bull.*, 17:195–197.

193. Segal, S. (1979): Editorial: Anticonvulsants and pregnancy. *Pediatrics*, 63:331–333.

194. Sokoloff, L. (1977): Relation between physiological function and energy metabolism in the central nervous system. *J. Neurochem.*, 29:13–26.

195. Sokoloff, L. (1981): Circulation and energy metabolism in the brain. In: *Basic Neurochemistry*, 3rd edition, edited by G. J. Siegel, R. W. Albers, R. Katzman, and B. W. Agranoff, pp. 471–495. Little, Brown, Boston.

196. Spatz, M., Micic, D., Mrsalja, D. B., Swink, M., and Micic, J. (1978): Changes in the capillary lactate and 2-deoxy D-glucose uptake in developing brain. *Brain Res.*, 151:619–622.

197. Stein, W. D. (1967): *The Movement of Molecules Across Cell Membranes*. Academic Press, New York.

198. Stewart, P. A., and Wiley, M. J. (1981): Developing nervous tissue induces formation of blood-brain barrier characteristics in invading endothelial cells: A study using quail-chick transplantation chimeras. *Dev. Biol.*, 84:183–192.

199. Strasbaugh, L. J., and Brinker, G. S. (1983): Effect of osmotic blood-brain barrier disruption on gentamicin penetration into the cerebrospinal fluid and brains of normal rabbits. *Antimicrob. Agents Chemother.*, 24:147–150.

200. Studer, R. K., Welch, D. M., and Siegel, B. A. (1974): Transient alteration of the blood-brain barrier: Effect of hypertonic solutions admin-

istered by carotid artery injection. *Exp. Neurol.*, 44:266–273.

201. Suzuki, O., Takanohashi, M., and Vagi, K. (1976): Protective effect of dexamethasone on enhancement of blood-brain barrier permeability caused by electroconvulsive shock. *Arzneimittelforsch.*, 26:533–535.

202. Svendgaard, N. A., Bjorklund, A., Hardebo, J. E., and Stenevi, U. (1975): Axonal degeneration associated with a defective blood-brain barrier in cerebral implants. *Nature (Lond.)*, 255:334–337.

203. Swartz, M. N. (1981): Interventricular use of aminoglycosides in the treatment of gram negative bacillary meningitis: Conflicting views. *J. Infect. Dis.*, 143:293–296.

204. Thurston, J. H., Hauhart, R. E., Shulz, D. W., Naccarato, E. F., Dodson, W. E., and Carroll, J. E. (1981): Chronic valproate administration produces hepatic dysfunction and may delay brain maturation. *Neurology*, 31:1063–1069.

205. Treiman, D. M., and Chelberg, R. D. (1983): Pharmacokinetics of paraldehyde in rat blood and brain. *Neurology*, 33(4, part 2, abstr.).

206. Volple, J. J. (1981): *Neurology of the Newborn.* Saunders, Philadelphia.

207. von Albert, H. H. (1983): A new phenytoin infusion concentrate for status epilepticus. *Adv. Neurol.*, 34:453–456.

208. Vorbrodt, A. W., Lossinsky, A. S., Wisniewski, H. M., Moretz, R. C., and Iwanoski, L. (1981): Ultrastructural cytochemical studies of cerebral microvasculature in scrapie infected mice. *Acta Neuropathol.*, 53:203–211.

209. Wade, L. A., and Katzman, R. (1975): Synthetic amino acids and the nature of L-DOPA transport at the blood-brain barrier. *J. Neurochem.*, 25:837–842.

210. Wang, J., Nauss, L., and Thomas, J. (1979): Pain relief by intrathecally applied morphine. *Anesthesiology*, 50:149–151.

211. Watanabe, I., Hodges, G. R., Dworzack, D. L., Kepes, J. J., and Duensing, G. F. (1978): Neurotoxicity of intrathecal gentamicin. A case report and experimental study. *Ann. Neurol.*, 4:564–572.

212. Weinstein, L., Goldfield, M., and Adamis, D. (1953): A study of intrathecal chemotherapy in bacterial meningitis. *Med. Clin. North Am.*, 37:1363–1376.

213. Westergaard, E. (1980): Ultrastructural permeability properties of cerebral microvasculature under normal and experimental conditions after application of tracers. *Adv. Neurol.*, 28:55–74.

214. Westergaard, E., and Brightman, M. W. (1973): Transport of proteins across normal cerebral arterioles. *J. Comp. Neurol.*, 152:17–44.

215. Westergaard, E., Hertz, M. M., and Bolwig, T. G. (1978): Increased permeability to horseradish peroxidase across cerebral vessels, evoked by electrically induced seizures in the rat. *Acta Neuropathol.*, 41:73–80.

216. Wolff, J. R., and Bar, T. (1972): "Seamless" endothelia in brain capillaries during development of the rat's cerebral cortex. *Brain Res.*, 41:17–24.

217. Wu, P. H., and Phillus, J. W. (1982): Uptake of adenosine by isolated rat brain capillaries. *J. Neurochem.*, 38:687–690.

218. Yudilevich, D. L., De Rose, N., and Sepulveda, F. V. (1972): Facilitated transport of amino acids through the blood-brain barrier of the dog studied in a single capillary circulation. *Brain Res.*, 44:569–578.

219. Zeleznikar, R. J., Jr., Quist, E. E., and Drewes, L. R. (1983): An alpha$_1$-adrenergic receptor-mediated phosphatidyl inositol effect in canine cerebral microvessels. *Mol. Pharmacol.*, 24:163–167.

Advances in Neurology, Vol. 44, edited by
A. V. Delgado-Escueta, A. A. Ward, Jr.,
D. M. Woodbury, and R. J. Porter.
Raven Press, New York © 1986.

41

Epileptic Brain Damage: Pathophysiology and Neurochemical Pathology

Bo K. Siesjö and Tadeusz Wieloch

Laboratory for Experimental Brain Research, University of Lund, Lund, Sweden S-221 85

SUMMARY   In this chapter, the pathophysiology and neurochemical pathology of epileptic brain damage is discussed on the basis of an integrative approach in which a comparison is made to cell necrosis resulting from ischemia and hypoglycemia. Two main questions are asked. First, is the brain damage resulting from these three disorders of cerebral energy metabolism similar in distribution and structural characteristics, as previously proposed? Second, is it possible to identify one or several neurochemical events, at the cellular and subcellular level, that qualify as the final common pathways leading to neuronal necrosis? A related question is, will seizures cause structural damage even if they do not critically curtail cellular oxygen supply?

A review of the literature and of recent results obtained in animals with long-term recovery following status epilepticus of known duration suggests that although brain damage caused by epilepsy shows some similarities to that incurred due to ischemic and hypoglycemic insults, it is far from identical. In well oxygenated animals with an adequate cardiovascular function, 2 hr of status epilepticus causes moderate neuronal necrosis in the cerebral cortex (layers 3–4), the hippocampus (CA4 and CA1 pyramidal cells), and the thalamus (ventromedial nuclei). In rats, status epilepticus of 30 min duration or longer invariably causes infarction of the substantia nigra (pars reticularis), with some affectation of globus pallidus as well. Notably, CA3 pyramids and dentate neurons are spared, as is the pars compacta of the substantia nigra.

Neurochemical events in ischemia, hypoglycemia, and status epilepticus show some striking dissimilarities, yet all three conditions lead to neuronal necrosis. In complete or near-complete ischemia, in which metabolic rate virtually ceases; deterioration of tissue energy state is rapid and extensive, with dramatic loss of ion homeostasis; cellular redox systems are reduced; and acidosis is marked to excessive. In hypoglycemic coma, oxygen consumption continues, albeit at a reduced rate; loss of high energy phosphates is extensive but less than complete, as is loss of ion homeostasis; cellular redox system become oxidized; and acidosis is absent. In epileptic seizures, finally, metabolic rate is markedly enhanced; perturbation of tissue energy state and of ion homeostasis is minimal to small; and acidosis is moderate. Results obtained in experimental animals suggest that neuronal necrosis, when incurred, is unrelated to energy failure and occurs in spite of adequate cellular oxygenation.

Four neurochemical events are common to all three conditions discussed. First, they all lead to an enhanced release of excitatory amino acids (i.e., glutamate and aspartate) from cellular elements to extracellular fluid. Second, they are all accompanied by Ca^{2+} influx into cells as a result of depolarization and/or interaction of agonists with cellular receptors. Third, they all lead to lipolysis with accumulation of free fatty acids. Fourth, direct or circumstantial evidence suggests that they all could be accompanied by Ca^{2+}-triggered events such as proteolysis and protein phosphorylation. It is tentatively concluded that these events constitute a final common pathway leading to cell necrosis. Loss of Ca^{2+} homeostasis may well be of crucial pathogenetic importance in this series of events. However, since the distribution of neuronal necrosis is not the same in the three conditions and since the response of different cell populations is strikingly dissimilar (e.g., CA1 versus CA3), the Ca^{2+} hypothesis of cell death becomes untenable, unless qualified. It is suggested that the vulnerability of a certain neuronal population to various insults is strongly influenced by its presynaptic inputs and by the type (and state) of its postsynaptic receptors. For example, evidence accumulates that excitotoxic mechanisms contribute to neuronal necrosis in all three conditions discussed.

Epileptic brain damage has a long scientific history. In 1825, Bouchet and Cazauvieilh (27) described atrophic changes localized to the hippocampus and uncus of brains from patients with epilepsy. Subsequently, Sommer (151) reported on loss of pyramidal cells and dense glial infiltration in a part of the hippocampus which came to be known by his name. Although the scarring constituting hippocampal (or mesial) sclerosis has remained an important entity in epileptic brain damage, subsequent work showed that neuronal loss in epileptic patients was not confined to hippocampal pyramidal cells but also encompassed small pyramidal cells in the neocortex (layers 3 and 5–6) and Purkinje cells in the cerebellum, and not infrequently also neurons in the thalamic and amygdaloid nuclei (132,151; for details and further literature, see ref. 48).

For obvious reasons, workers noting brain damage in epileptic patients enquired into its pathogenesis. Two findings seemed to provide a lead. First, a similar distribution of nerve cell damage was encountered in conditions of ischemia-hypoxia and hypoglycemia as well (30,99,151). Second, the structural damage incurred in the three conditions showed a striking resemblance. For example, in patients dying from status epilepticus, a common finding was the ischemic cell change of Spielmeyer (152), in which the shrunken cells and nuclei take on a triangular outline and stain dark (30).

It must have been natural, therefore, to suggest that epileptic brain damage occurred as a result of cellular hypoxia, especially since seizures so often compromise blood pressure and arterial oxygenation. The original proposal of Spielmeyer (153) that seizures caused cellular hypoxia by vascular spasm was soon refuted, but many subsequent workers invoked compression of nutrient arteries or drainage veins

(for literature, see ref. 48). It was early recognized, though, that consumption of oxygen by metabolically hyperactive cells would lead to the same end result (132). Furthermore, many investigators, noting the close proximity of vulnerable and resistant cells with no obvious relationship to the vascular supply, came out in favour of the Vogt and Vogt (161) theory, which explains selective vulnerability in terms of the special metabolic characteristics of affected cells. Throughout the years, proponents of these various ischemic–hypoxic hypotheses have often questioned whether epileptic discharges per se lead to neuronal damage.

Several more recent observations suggest that epileptic brain damage is unrelated to tissue hypoxia. Thus, when measurements became feasible it was demonstrated that seizures fail to reduce cerebral venous oxygen content and tension and that cellular oxygenation is upheld even in sustained seizures (for literature, see refs. 94,114,135). With the advent of techniques for assessing local metabolic rates, it emerged that two vulnerable areas (hippocampus and cerebral cortex) had markedly increased, while some resistant ones (e.g., the cerebellum and brainstem) had low metabolic rates, suggesting that the development of cell damage correlated to the enhancement of local metabolism (139). This hypothesis has received strong support from results obtained with administration of kainic acid, an excitotoxic analog of glutamic acid believed to cause cell damage, at least at distant (postsynaptic) sites, by excessive neuronal excitation (18,47,49,50,88,105,109). However, the cellular and molecular mechanisms responsible for epileptic brain damage remain largely unclarified. Furthermore, we cannot yet explain why ischemia, hypoglycemia, and epileptic seizures seem to affect neurons in the same brain areas.

It is our purpose to discuss the pathophysiology and neurochemical pathology of epileptic brain damage using an integrative approach. We begin by describing brain damage incurred following ischemia, hypoglycemia, and epileptic seizures, asking two questions. First, is the damage indeed similar in distribution and structural characteristics? Second, how does the density of cell damage relate to the duration of the insult? We proceed by considering pathophysiological conditions during ischemia, hypoglycemia, and epileptic seizures, attempting to define those that are common to the three types of insult. We then pose the question: will seizures cause structural damage even if they do not encroach upon cellular oxygen supply? We next turn to the problem of the neurochemical pathology, addressing the possibility that the cellular and molecular mechanisms of cell injury conform to a common final pathway of reactions.

NEUROPATHOLOGY OF BRAIN DAMAGE: DISTRIBUTION, DENSITY, AND STRUCTURAL CHARACTERISTICS

Until quite recently, description of cellular alterations as a result of ischemia, hypoglycemia, and status epilepticus was dominated by the terminology of workers whose armamentarium was confined to the light microscope (152). The proponents of this school consider ischemic cell change as the final common pathway by which neurons succumb to a variety of insults, including ischemia, hypoxia–ischemia, hypoglycemia, and status epilepticus (30). According to this view, the relentless series of changes, beginning with microvacuolation, due to high-amplitude swelling of mitochondria, and progressing via ischemic cell change, first without and then with "incrustation," and homogenizing cell change to the final dissolution of the cell, varies in its rate of progression only with the type of cells affected and the density of insult.

Some confusion has arisen from claims that cellular alterations observed even in properly perfusion-fixed material may be artefactual, e.g., "dark cells" and "hydropic cell change" (30). While it is clear that improper handling of tissue before or during perfusion fixation can cause artefactual changes, it now seems that the common appearance of condensed, dark-staining neurons, usually surrounded by swollen astrocytic processes, may represent a true *in vivo* event, probably reflecting movements of electrolytes and water between extracellular fluid, neurons, and glial cells (see below). What is more problematic is that these cellular alter-

ations, which may be fully reversible, are difficult to distinguish from ischemic cell change, at least when tissue is fixed by perfusion during an ongoing insult, or in the immediate postinsult period. For these reasons, we deem it justified to postpone identification of irreversibly damaged neurons until some days of recovery have been allowed. Furthermore, since the term ischemic cell change has the additional drawback of implying that ischemia is the cause of the cell death, we will use it only when referring to the findings of others. Our own groups have exploited the fact that dying or dead neurons become shrunken and avidly stainable with acid dyes. We will therefore use the term "acidophilic neurons" to denote irreversible injury (10).

In describing histopathological alterations in ischemia, hypoglycemia, and status epilepticus, we put relatively little emphasis on clinical material and derive the bulk of information from experimental studies. This is because clinical insults are usually poorly defined in terms of density and duration, and because interpretation of clinical data on hypoglycemia and convulsive states is hampered by lack of knowledge on intercurrent or terminal ischemia/hypoxia. Our discussion of ischemia (and hypoglycemia) will be confined to reversible insults of known density and duration. Thus, we will not exploit the detailed information amassed on brain damage incurred by stroke, nor will we consider changes occurring during or shortly after ischemia in models that do not allow long-term recovery.

Ischemia

The literature abounds in reports on the density and distribution of ischemic–hypoxic brain damage and in hypotheses advanced to explain its pathogenesis. Ischemia, a condition characterized by reduction or cessation of nutritional blood flow, is known to preferentially affect certain brain regions and groups of neurons. During incomplete ischemia, i.e., in conditions of reduced cerebral perfusion pressure, neuronal damage is often incurred in arterial boundary zones of the cerebral cortex and the cerebellum, i.e., in the "watershed" areas lying between the distribution territories of the major cerebral arteries (30). Ischemic insults that are uniform throughout the vascular tree, e.g., those leading to complete brain ischemia, reveal another type of selective vulnerability, one affecting discrete groups of neurons (30,152). In general, the most vulnerable ones are small pyramidal cells in layers 3 and 5 to 6 in the neocortex, pyramidal cells in the CA1 and CA3 to 4 sectors of the hippocampus, small or medium-sized neurons in the dorsolateral crest of the caudoputamen, and Purkinje cells in the cerebellum. When pronounced, the cell loss takes on the characteristics of laminar necrosis and, with dense and sustained insults, the damage is one of infarction with destruction not only of neurons but also of glial and endothelial cells, yielding cystic necrosis.

Results obtained with models of transient forebrain ischemia in gerbils and rats yield novel information on selective neuronal vulnerability. With the advent of long-term recovery models in these species it has been possible to show that short periods of ischemia cause damage, not only to CA1–CA4 pyramidal cells in the hippocampus, but also to neurons in the olfactory tubercle, lateral septum, lateral reticular nucleus of the thalamus, and entorhinal cortex (148,162). It has been emphasized that areas with such marked sensitivity to ischemia are of limbic origin, suggesting that limbic seizures in the postischemic period contribute to the final damage (162).

The most detailed information on ischemic brain damage has been obtained on the hippocampus. In discussing this information, we recall present views on the structural organization of the hippocampal formation (Fig. 1). Results

obtained following transient occlusion of one carotid artery in the gerbil showed that CA3 pyramidal cells were subjected to a reversible insult, resembling Nissl's reactive change or central chromatolysis, while CA1 neurons suffered irreversible damage, the latter progressing to fragmentation of cells after an interval whose length varied inversely with the duration of the ischemia (33,77). In a subsequent study, Kirino (76) induced 5 min ischemia by bilateral carotid artery occlusion, analyzing alterations of hippocampal neurons by light and electron microscopy after recovery periods varying between 3 hr and 21 days. His results, which were confirmed by a subsequent study (155,156), revealed three types of neuronal alterations. The first, affecting about 30% of CA4 neurons, progressed from increased stainability (after 3 hr) to ischemic cell change (after 12 hr). The second alteration, the reversible reactive change with central chromatolysis and eccentric displacement of the nucleus, was seen in CA3 neurons. The third alteration, affecting CA1 pyramidal cells, was denoted delayed neuronal death (Fig. 2). Thus, while some clumping of nuclear chromatin was seen after 1 day of recovery, and clefts appeared in the cytoplasm after 2 days, clear-cut neuronal degeneration with loss of structural integrity was not seen until after 3 to 4 days. Electron microscopy showed no abnor-

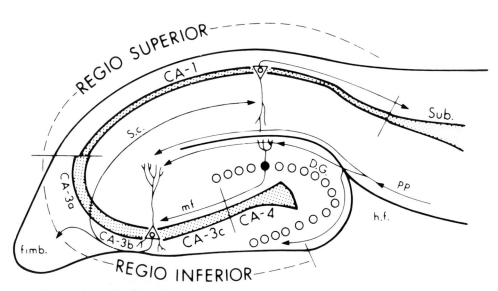

FIG. 1. Structural organization of hippocampal formation. The pyramidal cell ribbon is subdivided into the subiculum (sub.) and the CA1–CA4 sectors, the CA4 cells occupying the hilus of the dentate gyrus (D.G.). h.f. = hippocampal fissure. The sector previously designated CA2 (or h₂) is assumed to correspond to CA3a. The feed-forward excitatory circuit involves the perforant pathway (PP) axons from the entorhinal cortex, synapsing on the dentate granule cells, the mossy fibers (mf) relaying excitation to CA3 neurons, and the Schaffer collaterals (S.c.) from the latter synapsing on CA1 neurons. (From ref. 46, with permission.)

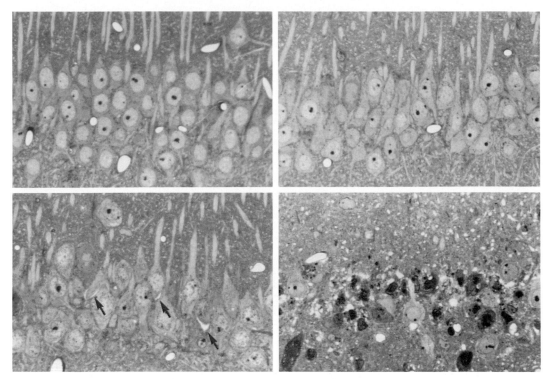

FIG. 2. Delayed neuronal death in the CA1 sector of the hippocampus of gerbils subjected to 5 min of bilateral carotid artery ligation. The figures show in succession normal controls (*top, left*), 1 day after ischemia (*top, right*), 2 days (*bottom, left*), and 4 days (*bottom, right*). After 1 day of recovery, the only abnormality was some inhomogeneity of nuclear chromatin. After 2 days, the chromatin appeared clumped and some pericaryal slits were recognized. However, clear-cell degeneration was not observed until 4 days after the ischemic episode. (From ref. 83, with permission.)

mality until after 1 day, when the amount of endoplasmic reticulum (ER) increased, the ER being arranged in parallel stacks. After 2 days, these stacks occupied a large part of the perikarya on the basal side, and the ER cisterns showed distension. After 4 days, cell destruction was obvious. Notably, mitochondrial alterations were absent at any of the times studied. The delayed nature of the death of CA1 neurons was subsequently demonstrated by electrophysiological recordings of unit activity (156). Thus, activity in both neocortical and CA1 neurons ceased within 1 min after ischemia onset, and recurred during the first 10 to 20 min of recirculation. However, although neocortical neurons retained spike activity thereafter, the CA1 neurons showed increased spike discharge for 1 day and ceased to generate spikes after 2 days.

These results lead to some important conclusions. First, rather than conforming to the relentless series of alterations collectively designated by the term ischemic cell change, hippocampal neurons injured by transient ischemia may show at least three different types of reac-

tions: (a) ischemic cell change, (b) reversible alterations of the reactive, chromatolytic type, and (c) delayed neuronal death. We note that, with this density and duration of ischemia, the two cell types suffering irreversible damage were the CA1 and CA4 neurons. Second, while some neurons show evidence of irreversible damage a few hours after the insult, others incur gross structural damage first after a delay of days. Third, the sharp transition between vulnerable CA1 and resistant CA3 neurons gives additional evidence that functional and metabolic characteristics, rather than vascular factors, are responsible for the vulnerability of some pyramidal cells (cf. also damage to CA4 neurons and lack of affectation of granule cells in the dentate gyrus).

Application of a model for reversible four-vessel occlusion in the rat to long-term recovery studies has given comparable results at the light-microscopic level and extended the analysis to other forebrain areas (118,120). Administration of graded insults (10, 20, and 30 min of ischemia) demonstrated a rank order of vulnerability with susceptibility to ischemia decreasing in the following order: CA1 > CA3 to 4 and neocortex > caudoputamen. Furthermore, although delayed neuronal damage occurred in all regions, the rate of "maturation" differed between them, being faster in the caudoputamen than in the hippocampus or neocortex. The delayed nature of the cell death was supported by metabolic data, since secondary deterioration of cellular energy state was observed in the caudoputamen and hippocampus after 48 and 72 hr, respectively (119). It should be recalled that since this model (and carotid artery occlusion in the gerbil) yields dense ischemia in forebrain structures only, hindbrain structures are usually spared. Results on models of whole-brain ischemia suggest that CA1 pyramidal neurons and Purkinje cells are equally susceptible to ischemic damage (48).

The results of Pulsinelli et al. (120) showed that some animals subjected to 10 min of ischemia did not develop brain damage, suggesting that gerbils are exceptionally susceptible to ischemic brain damage, e.g., by being seizure-prone. However, Suzuki et al. (156) failed to record clinical or electrophysiological signs of postischemic epileptic activity. Furthermore, it seems likely that the model of Pulsinelli and Brierley (108) yields higher CBF values than those published by the group (22). When forebrain ischemia was induced in the rat with a model yielding flow rates of less than 5% of control, the density of cell damage incurred was comparable to that reported in the gerbil (148,149). In fact, these results demonstrate that, even in fasted animals, some CA1 and CA4 neurons suffer irreversible damage already after 2 to 4 min of ischemia, and that longer periods (6–10 min) are required to affect neocortical or hippocampal CA3 pyramids or striatal neurons. Recent results suggest that such differences in the outcome, following similar periods of ischemia, are related to the physiological state of the animals, rather than the species. Notably, it seems that a brisk sympatho-adrenal response with high levels of circulating catecholamines ameliorates the ischemic damage (ref. 85, and Koide, Wieloch and Siesjö, *in preparation*).

Clearly, the results obtained in gerbils and rats emphasize the need to assess the final damage following ischemia, or indeed any insult leading to neuronal death, after recovery periods of several days. Ideally, this analysis should be performed at a time when dying or dead cells are easily visualized but before the neurons have disappeared. This is because ischemic cell change or intense acidophilia is easily recognized, even when affecting only a few cells,

whereas a small reduction in the number of normal cells is difficult to detect.

Hypoglycemia

Although it has been recognized for many decades that patients dying in hypoglycemic coma may show gross brain damage, the pathogenesis remained unclear until quite recently. Neuropathological examination revealed neuronal damage of varying density and localization; however, lesions were found to affect the cerebral cortex, the hippocampus, and the caudoputamen more than other structures, the vulnerable Purkinje cells usually being spared (99). The localization of lesions to selectively vulnerable areas and the appearance of neuronal alterations in the light microscope ("ischemic cell change") have inspired investigators to conclude that hypoglycemia represents one form of tissue hypoxia (30,99). However, clinical material does not allow firm conclusions to be drawn on this matter, since systemic complications such as hypotension and hypoxia must be the rule rather than the exception. For this reason, the neuropathology of hypoglycemic brain damage is best studied in animal experiments.

Several groups have addressed this problem. In the study of Brierley et al. (29), neuronal damage, mainly localized to the neocortex, was observed in 6 animals in which sensory evoked responses were extinguished for 49 to 92 min. Unfortunately, the damage was not related to the period of electroencephalographic (EEG) silence, and recovery periods were only 30 to 240 min.

In another study, Myers and Kahn (102) employed recovery periods of 11 to 270 days. Hypoglycemia of 3 to 4 hr duration did not produce brain damage, which was seen only when blood glucose concentrations were maintained below about 1 μmol/ml for 5 to 6 hr. The lesions were not related to the EEG, though, and it cannot be excluded that the lesions observed were influenced by posthypoglycemic hypotension and/or seizures.

Two crucial questions remained to be answered. First, is cell damage incurred first when the hypoglycemia is of sufficient severity to cause loss of EEG activity and/or clinical coma? Second, what is the density of cell damage incurred by hypoglycemia of varying duration? The answers had to await the advent of a recovery model, allowing the cell damage to be assessed after 1 or 2 weeks recovery following coma periods of 10 to 60 min (10,11). No cell damage occurred if insulin injection was associated with a slow wave or a burst-suppression EEG pattern. A prerequisite for injury to occur was, therefore, cell membrane failure with loss of spontaneous EEG activity ("coma"). Mild neuronal damage was incurred after 10 min, but it was regularly observed first after 30 to 40 min, and was extensive first after 60 min of hypoglycemic coma. A rank order of vulnerability was established with cell damage decreasing in the following order: subiculum, CA1 pyramidal cells, neocortical cells (layers 2–3), CA4 pyramidal cells, and neurons in the caudoputamen. A prominent lesion affected the dentate gyrus, particularly its crest, which often showed dense cellular necrosis. Damage to cerebellar cells was uncommon, and brainstem areas were spared. Localization of neuronal damage showed a striking relationship to cerebrospinal fluid (CSF) and tissue fluid pathways, suggesting that the damage was, at least in part, mediated by a fluid-borne toxin (11). A subsequent EM study confirmed and extended this observation, demonstrating cellular alterations of a type which has been considered characteristic of excitotoxic lesions (12).

Epileptic Seizures

Although patients with scizure disorders may develop brain damage, it has been difficult to relate this to the seizure discharge per se, and to accurately define conditions under which the damage is incurred. Numerous experiments have been designed to solve these problems. Unfortunately, the results are controversial, at times confusing. In discussing these results we pay particular attention to studies in which systemic variables were controlled, recovery allowed, and tissue sampled by adequate techniques for perfusion fixation.

Results obtained with single or repeated electroshock seizures appear clear-cut. Thus, loss of pyramidal cells did not occur in rats given three daily electroconvulsive seizures up to a total of 140 seizures, although recovery periods of 2 and 12 weeks were allowed (101). Obviously, longer periods of seizures are required to elicit irreversible cell damage. At first sight, results obtained in cats seem to provide information on this issue. Thus, Purpura and Gonzales-Monteguado (122) reported extensive destruction of CA1 neurons in cats when hippocampal seizures induced by methoxypyridoxine, an antimetabolite of pyridoxine, were sustained for 2 hr or longer, while others found that seizures sustained for 90 min failed to induce structural alterations in the hippocampus (133).

The interpretation is problematic for two reasons. First, Purpura and Gonzales-Monteguado (122) failed to find comparable hippocampal lesions when seizures were induced by strychnine or pentylenetetrazole. Second, none of the studies allowed a recovery period before tissue fixation.

Neuronal alterations typical of ischemic cell change have been reported in baboons after bicuculline-induced seizures lasting 82 to 299 min (95). The alterations mainly affected the neocortex (layers 3 and 5–6), the cerebellum (Purkinje and basket cells), the hippocampus (CA1 and CA3), the thalamus, and the amygdala. The animals breathed spontaneously, and all had systemic complications (arterial hypoxia, hypotension, hyperthermia, and/or hypoglycemia). When these were minimized by control of systemic variables the damage was mild to moderate and affected only the neocortex, the hippocampus, and the thalamus (97). The question arises, though, whether the lesions observed in the paralyzed animals were due to the seizure discharges *per se*. Some doubts remain, since in all animals but one the seizures were terminated by induction of anesthesia and immediate perfusion-fixation; furthermore, in the only animal allowed some recovery (seizure duration 4.5 hr), the damage was mild and confined to the neocortex. These doubts were reinforced by the results reported by Brown et al. (31), who failed to detect structural or ultrastructural damage to hippocampal (or neocortical) cells in cats in which bicuculline-induced seizures were sustained for up to 5 hr. In these animals, systemic variables were reportedly controlled and recovery periods of up to 5 hr were allowed.

Results obtained in rats highlight the problems encountered. Using bicuculline to induce sustained seizures, Blennow et al. (22) found microvacuolation and "ischemic cell change" in the neocortex and hippocampus after 2 hr of status epilepticus, and reported that moderate hypoxia, hypotension, or hypoglycemia ameliorated the lesions. When the experiments were repeated, with a different technique for perfusion fixation and with both light-microscopic (LM) and electron-microscopic (EM) analyses, the results could not be confirmed (157). Obviously, the problem was one of interpretation of histopathological alterations.

The difficulty encountered was to distinguish between ischemic cell change and the shrunken, dark-staining neurons observed when the tissue is fixed by perfusion during ongoing seizures. What was clear, though, is that the vast majority of the altered neurons disappeared from the sections when some time of recovery was allowed before perfusion-fixation. When diazepam was used to arrest the seizures for 2 hr, following 1 hr of status, very few altered cells were seen, those remaining probably reflecting irreversible cell injury (157). Similar recovery following 2 hr of status revealed many more altered cells; however, since adequate cardiovascular function could not be upheld during recovery, it seemed less likely that these alterations were due to the seizure discharge per se.

There was obviously a need for a model that allowed uneventful recovery following defined seizure periods. It proved possible to achieve this by induction of seizures with fluorothyl, which was added to the respiratory gas mixture and retained in a rebreathing system (106,107). Even when sustained for 90 min, the seizures could be terminated by a single dose of thiopental. When phentolamine was given at seizure induction, cardiovascular or respiratory problems during recovery could be obviated. As assessed after 1 week recovery, seizures sustained for 60 to 120 min caused moderate damage to py-

ramidal cells in the neocortex (layer 3) and the hippocampus (CA4 sector) and to neurons in discrete thalamic nuclei. Notably, seizures lasting 30 min or longer invariably led to infarction of the pars reticulata of the substantia nigra and of central parts of the pallidum ("pallido-reticularis") (Fig. 3). Since 1 week of recovery was allowed, cell destruction was unequivocal. In view of this, one can interpret the results of Howse (72), who sampled the rat brain at the termination of 90 min of status, to demonstrate that seizures induced by pentylenetetrazole give the same end result.

Since the neocortical and hippocampal damage resulting from 1.5 to 2 hr of status epilepticus was moderate, it is justifiable to consider models by which more localized seizure activity can be elicited. Such seizures (e.g., those that are largely confined to the limbic system) can be induced for sustained periods without causing systemic complications. The most comprehensive data exist for kainic acid (for literature, see refs. 19,49,88,105). The proposal has been made that kainic acid exerts its

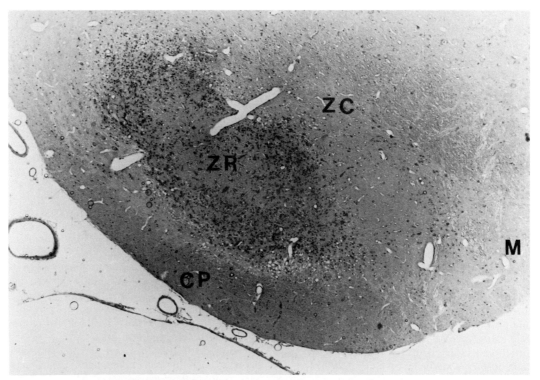

FIG. 3. Infarction of substantia nigra after 1 week of recovery, following 60 min of fluorothyl-induced status epilepticus in ventilated rats. The figure shows a hypercellular infarct affecting the zona reticulata (ZR), sparing the zona compacta (ZC). CP, cerebral peduncle; M, midline. Acid fuchsin/cresyl violet, ×40. (From ref. 106, with permission.)

toxic effects by inducing seizure discharge of affected neurons. This hypothesis finds support in results showing that local injection of kainic acid gives damage at distant sites, i.e., of neurons that are synaptically connected with those primarily affected, and that suppression of seizure activity by diazepam ameliorates the distant damage (18).

The results reported by Schwob et al. (134) and Ben Ari et al. (19), which give a detailed account of brain damage occurring as a result of systemic kainic acid administration, demonstrate that a large number of brain structures may be affected. However, these results, and those published by Lothman and Collins (88), make it clear that the limbic system is the chief target. In the hippocampus, the rank order of vulnerability was CA3 > CA4 > CA1 > dentate granule cells. With spread of the seizure discharge, the lesions also affected other structures, including the amygdala and medial thalamic nuclei, as well as the pyriform and entorhinal cortex.

Although experiments with injection of kainic acid have given much useful information on the association between seizure discharge and epileptic brain damage, they nonetheless fail to provide answers to the question: How much neuroexcitation does it take to irreversibly damage cells, and where is the damage localized? This is mainly because of the difficulty of accurately defining the duration of the effects of kainic acid, or the associated seizure discharge. For example, Schwob et al. (120) remarked that, at survival times exceeding 24 hr, the damage to CA1 pyramids could exceed that inflicted upon CA3 cells. Is this due to an ongoing cell destruction, or to "maturation" of the CA1 damage? Furthermore, Ben Ari et al. (17) found that if diazepam was given 2 hr (or more) following intraamygdaloid injection of kainic acid, the brain damage was not ameliorated. It seems, therefore, that kainic acid-induced seizures are followed by much more damage than when a comparable seizure period is induced by a systemic convulsant like fluorothyl.

Two recent articles provide hints to this problem. Using an elegant model with prior establishment of a kindled focus and subsequent amygdaloid stimulation in rats, McIntyre et al. (93) established unequivocal damage to amygdaloid and thalamic nuclei, piriform and olfactory cortex, and the CA1 sector of the dorsal hippocampus. In view of the involvement of the CA1 pyramids, it is of interest that recovery was 2 weeks. This pathology was obtained with seizure durations of 10 to 24 hr. Interruption of seizure discharge after 30 min prevented cell loss, but if the seizures were allowed to continue for 4 hr, 2 of 4 animals showed relatively extensive damage, albeit not including the CA1 sector. It would seem, therefore, that extensive cell damage may arise if seizures are sustained for longer than 2 hr. In the other study (47) the authors stimulated the cerebral cortex by focal application of convulsants and recorded neurophysiological activity in the neocortex. Seizure activity lasting for 4 to 6 hr was found to yield thalamic neuronal damage in the projection field of the stimulated area.

Density and Distribution of Cell Damage in Ischemia, Hypoglycemia, and Epileptic Seizures

At present, only data obtained in rats allow a direct comparison. It is clear from Table 1 that ischemia represents a more severe insult than hypoglycemia, and the latter a worse insult than status epilepticus. Such cell counts, and those performed on the hippocampal formation, suggest that a comparable density of damage is caused by 4 to 6 min of ischemia, 20 to 40 min of hypoglycemia, and 90 to 120 min of status epilepticus.

Our next concern is the distribution of cell damage. Table 2 shows that this is far from identical in the three conditions. In fact, the differences are large enough to suggest that little advantage is gained by considering them similar since such postulates may hamper attempts to delineate important differences in pathophysiology.

PATHOPHYSIOLOGY

Given this background information on the density and distribution of cell damage induced by ischemia, hypoglycemia, and epileptic seizures, we proceed to discuss the pathophysiology, asking two questions. First, are there common pathophysiological events which may explain why cell damage is incurred in all three conditions? Second, what factors are responsible for the differences in severity of brain damage? The discussion of pathophysiological events will be confined to those that we consider instrumental in eliciting injurious reactions at the cellular level, i.e., those leading to perturbation of cellular energy metabolism, of ion homeostasis, and of the metabolism of phospholipids and free fatty acids. Changes affecting protein constituents will be considered in a later section.

TABLE 1. *Density of cortical neuronal necrosis[a] at 1 week*

		Individual animals				
Condition	Mean	1	2	3	4	5
Ischemia 6 min.	45	12	164	22	1	
Ischemia 10 min.	2,657	3,500[c]	7,000[c]	87	43	600
Hypoglycemia 10 min.	5	19	0	33	0	0
Hypoglycemia 40 min.	635	871	40	1,007	624	1,481
Status epilepticus 30 min.	0	0	0	0	0	0
Status epilepticus 60 min.	34	70	5	26	79	2
Status epilepticus 90 min.	30	90	0	0	12	7

[a] Data from refs. 10, 107, and 149.
[b] Cells/coronal section, level of subfornical organ.
[c] Infarcted, hence estimated from neuronal counts of cortical material in identical area.

Ischemia

Pathophysiological events considered will be those occurring in reversible ischemia, i.e., a condition in which a defined period of cerebral blood flow (CBF) reduction is followed by restoration of an adequate cerebral perfusion pressure. The density of ischemia considered will be one sufficient to disrupt cerebral energy and ion homeostasis, i.e., one in which the threshold of "membrane failure" has been transgressed (8,9). We wish to recall that reversible ischemia of this type conforms to a true anaerobic–aerobic transition; in fact, since postischemic CBF is high and $CMRO_2$ is low, the immediate postischemic phase is usually characterized by cellular hyperoxia (136).

Energy Failure and Loss of Ion Homeostasis

Dense ischemia causes rapid and extensive energy failure. When the cerebral cortex is frozen through the exposed dura, it is possible to show significant decreases in phosphocreatine (PCr) and ATP concentrations, and increases in ADP and lactate concentrations, already at 5 sec after interruption of the circulation (99). Tissue ATP content decreases to zero within 5 to 7 min, while PCr, the storage form

TABLE 2. *Distribution of neuronal necrosis, and sensitivity of the rat brain to cerebral ischemia, hypoglycemia, and status epilepticus*

	Brain damage index[b]		
Brain area	Ischemia	Hypoglycemia	Status epilepticus
Cerebral cortex			
layer 1	0	0	0
layer 2	+ +	+ + + +	+
layer 3	+ + + +	+ + +	+ + + +
layer 4	+ + +	+ +	+ + + +
layer 5	+ +	+	+
layer 6	+	+	+
Caudate nucleus	+ + + +	+ + +	0
Substantia nigra	+ + +	0	+ + + +
Thalamus	+ +	+	+ +
Hippocampus CA1	+ + +	+ + +	+ + +
Hippocampus CA3	+ +	0	0
Hippocampus CA4	+ + +	+	+ + + +
Hippocampus dentate gyrus	+	+ + +	0
Hippocampus subiculum	+ + + +	+ + + +	+

[a] Data from (10,11,107,149).
[b] 0, damage not observed; +, vulnerable to maximal insult; + +, vulnerable to moderate insult; + + +, vulnerable to mild insult; and + + + +, vulnerable to minimal insult.

of ATP, vanishes from the tissue in 1 to 2 min. This rapid fall must be due to the fact that increased concentrations of ADP and H^+ shift the creatine kinase reaction (PCr + ADP + H^+ $\rightleftharpoons$ Cr + ATP) in the direction of ATP formation (142).

ATP hydrolysis is accompanied by accumulation of AMP, and the latter is deaminated and dephosphorylated to yield IMP and adenosine, respectively (84). Further dephosphorylation and deamination gives inosine, which is converted to hypoxanthine, the substrate of xanthine oxidase. Some of the nucleosides and bases formed by ischemic degradation of nucleoside monophosphates are diffusible and may be lost from the tissue during recirculation, yielding a lingering reduction in the size of the adenine nucleotide pool (ATP + ADP + AMP).

The progressive energy failure is accompanied by loss of ion homeostasis. Following cessation of blood flow, extracellular K^+ concentration (K_e^+) gradually increases over 60 to 90 sec; then K^+ suddenly floods the extracellular space and K_e^+ increases to 40 to 70 µmol/ml (62). It is tempting to conclude that the slow release of K^+ is due to shortage of ATP at the site of the membrane-bound ATPase, and that the fast release of K^+ reflects massive energy failure and/or an increase in K^+ conductance due to depolarization. Loss of ion homeostasis also leads to cellular uptake of Ca^{2+}, Na^+, Cl^-, and water, and production of acids is associated with a massive fall in pH_e (Fig. 4). Influx of Ca^{2+} occurs when K_e^+ has increased to about 13 µmol/ml, possibly because voltage-dependent Ca^{2+} gates are then opened (63). The decrease in Na^+ and Cl^- concentration is accompanied by an increase in tissue impedance corresponding to a 50% reduction in extracellular fluid (ECF) volume (71).

Perturbation of Transmitter Metabolism

Although ischemia must arrest the synthesis of many transmitters, and cause the presynaptic release of some, our interest is focussed on excitatory amino acids. Using a model of tourniquet ischemia in rats, Benveniste et al. (20) could demonstrate enhanced release of glutamate, aspartate, and taurine, the extracellular concentrations of the first two of these amino acids increasing eight- and sixfold respectively. The increased concentrations persisted for about 10 min during recirculation.

Secondary Metabolic Events

Secondary events of relevance to the present discussion are the cellular acidosis and the ac-

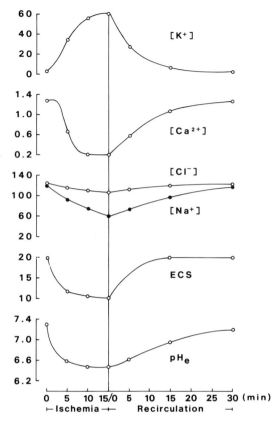

FIG. 4. Schematic diagram illustrating changes in extracellular concentrations of K^+, Ca^{2+}, Cl^-, and Na^+, as well as in extracellular fluid space (ECS) and pH_e, during and following ischemia of 15 min duration. Extracellular ion concentration in mM, ECS in percent of tissue volume. (From ref. 146, with permission.)

cumulation of free fatty acids (FFAs). During complete ischemia, and at normal tissue concentrations of glycogen and glucose, the lactic acid concentration approximates 15 µmol/g, and intracellular pH (pH_i) can be estimated to decrease from 7.0 to 6.5 (87). If a trickle of flow persists during ischemia, fasted animals show a comparable degree of lactic acidosis, but in fed animals or in those infused with glucose, the hyperglycemia can be associated with massive accumulation of lactic acid (136,137). Obviously, the nutritional state is an important determinant of the severity of the ischemic acidosis.

As originally observed by Bazan (16), ischemia is associated with accumulation of FFAs, the largest relative change affecting arachidonic acid. The amount of FFAs accumulated is proportional to the duration of the ischemia, even if this exceeds 15 to 30 min. Another important feature is that the normalization of the FFA content, following recirculation, occurs gradually over 15 to 30 min or longer (Fig. 5). We will discuss the implication of this later.

Edema

As discussed below, acidosis and accumulation of FFAs have been postulated to enhance edema formation. In this context, we recall that cell swelling may either reflect a shift of fluid from extra- to intracellular spaces, or involve net gain of electrolytes and water. When water and ion fluxes are limited to an exchange between extra- and intracellular fluids, one can envisage that some cellular elements accumulate Na^+ and Cl^-, with osmotically obliged water (90,160). Evidence exists that this is a glial event. Thus, ischemia is accompanied by gross swelling of astrocytic elements, accentuated in perineuronal and perivascular positions. Furthermore Bourke, Kimelberg, and their associates (28,81,82) have shown that an increase in K_e^+ to values exceeding 10 μmol/ml elicits astrocytic swelling, and provided hints to the mechanisms involved (see below). If the isch-

emia is of limited duration, such changes may be fully reversible, with rapid normalization of fluid spaces during recirculation. However, if less optimal conditions prevail, one encounters net flux of electrolytes and water between blood and tissue. Typically, this involves loss of K^+ to, and gain of Na^+, Cl^-, and water from, the blood (71). Progressive deterioration of ion and water homeostasis may then ensue, and involve massive accumulation of Ca^{2+} as well (171).

Hypoglycemia

Hypoglycemia jeopardizes the viability of brain cells by depriving them of glucose, their main substrate for energy production. Since the end result of hypoglycemia is failure of energy metabolism, one could argue that ischemia and hypoglycemia should affect cells similarly. However, some of the metabolic effects of hypoglycemia are indeed different from those occurring in ischemia. It is our purpose to consider events that are similar, as well as those that differ.

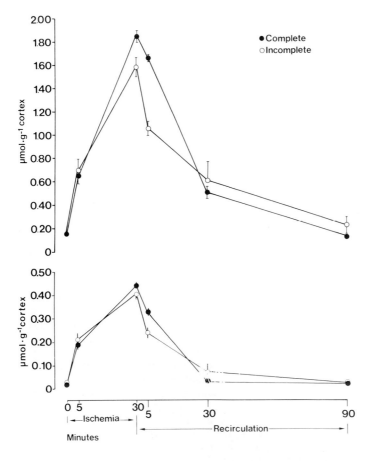

FIG. 5. Cerebral cortical concentrations of total free fatty acids (**upper panel**) and arachidonic acid (**lower panel**) during 30 min of complete and of severe, incomplete ischemia, and in the recovery period following restoration of circulation. Values are means ± SEM. Data from Rehncrona et al. (126).

Energy Failure and Loss of Ion Homeostasis

When sufficiently severe, hypoglycemia leads to extensive energy failure, with a reduction of ATP concentration to 20 to 25% of control and corresponding increases of ADP and AMP (140). Energy failure develops at blood glucose concentrations of about 1 μmol/g; however, it is less tightly correlated to blood glucose levels than to EEG activity. Thus, as long as EEG bursts persist, little change in PCr, ATP, ADP, and AMP concentrations occur, energy failure developing *pari passu* with cessation of EEG activity. The sudden perturbation of energy homeostasis involves other nucleoside triphosphates than ATP and is accompanied by accumulation of nucleosides and bases (43).

As can be expected from the depletion of energy sources, hypoglycemia of sufficient severity to abolish EEG activity leads to massive release of K^+ from cells (6,113). Subsequent work demonstrated an impedance change, reflecting a decrease in ECF volume to 50% of control (112). From this we conclude that hypoglycemia, like ischemia, leads to cellular uptake of Na^+, Cl^-, and H_2O. A recent study established that hypoglycemia causes influx of Ca^{2+} into cells, occurring as a threshold phenomenon at K_e^+ values of close to 15 μmol/ml (64,164) (Fig. 6). These experiments established that sustained breakdown of ion homeostasis is often preceded by a transient ionic shift resembling a spreading depression, and that disruption of ion and energy metabolism in one hemisphere

may precede that of the other by several minutes.

Amino Acid Transmitters

Since hypoglycemia leads to a deficient supply of exogenous glucose brain tissues are forced to utilize endogenous substrates, mainly carbohydrates and amino acids. The concerted reactions thus set in motion involve transamination/deamination reactions leading to massive depletion of glutamate, and accumulation of aspartate (4,140). A recent study has shown that hypoglycemic coma is accompanied by enhanced release of aspartate and glutamate into extracellular fluid (165). In view of the changes observed in the whole tissue contents it is interesting that more aspartate was released than glutamate (see also ref. 20).

Free Fatty Acids

Severe hypoglycemia leads to a breakdown of phospholipids and to accumulation of FFAs. Two recent studies demonstrate that, after 5 min or more of isoelectricity, close to 10% of the phospholipid pool is degraded (2,166). As Fig. 7 shows, the release of FFAs is relatively extensive. However, the amount of FFAs accumulated represents only a fraction of the loss of phospholipid-bound FFAs, suggesting that fatty acids released are either lost to the blood or oxidized in the tissue. Figure 7 shows that the total

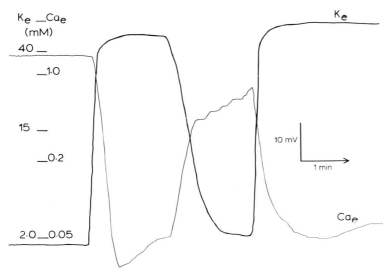

FIG. 6. Changes in extracellular potassium (K_e) and calcium (Ca_e) ion activities during hypoglycemia around the onset of isoelectricity. The measurements were made using a triple-barrelled, double-ion-sensitive microelectrode to record the activities of both ions at the same point simultaneously. (From ref. 64, with permission.)

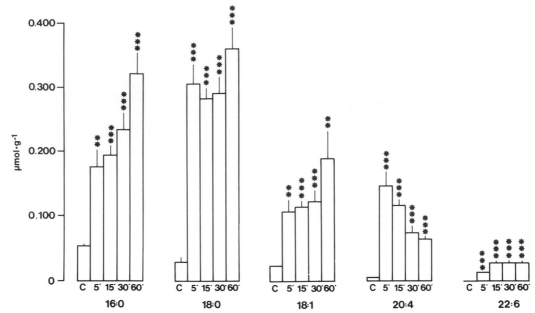

FIG. 7. Free fatty acid concentrations in cortical tissue of rats in control animals (C), during hypoglycemic coma of 5–60 min duration, and during recovery following 30 min of hypoglycemic coma. Values are means $\pm$ SEM; 16:0, palmitic acid; 18:0, stearic acid; 18:1, oleic acid; 20:4, arachidonic acid; 22:6, docosahexanoic acid; $**p < 0.01$, $***p < 0.001$ (Student's t-test). (From ref. 4, with permission.)

amount of FFAs remains relatively stable between the 5- and the 30-min "coma" period, but that the concentration of arachidonic acid falls continuously following its massive accumulation at the 5 min point.

All of the events discussed are, at least qualitatively, similar in ischemia and hypoglycemia. Two features are unique to hypoglycemia: the continued oxygen supply and the absence of tissue acidosis.

Oxygen Supply and Acid–Base Events

At increased or normal blood pressure, many regions in the brain of hypoglycemic animals show overt hyperperfusion and none is grossly underperfused (144). Accordingly, tissue oxygen tensions are maintained. The combination of substrate deficiency and continued oxygen supply has some important consequences. For example, rather than being reduced as in ischemia, cellular redox systems become oxidized (140). Furthermore, lack of exogenous substrate is compensated for by mobilization (and oxidation) of endogenous substrates, which include glycolytic metabolites, citric acid cycle intermediates, and associated amino acids.

Since many of the endogenous substrates mobilized during hypoglycemia are anions of met-abolic acids, their oxidation ought to alkalinize the cells. Data now exist to show that intracellular alkalosis does indeed arise (112). Under certain circumstances, notably a combination of hypocapnia and hypotension, the alkalosis becomes excessive in that values for pH_i approach those of the ECF, which, at the low CO_2 tensions, can exceed 7.5 (111).

Regional Metabolic and Circulatory Changes

In ischemia, the preferential localization of neuronal necrosis to certain areas is interpreted in terms of selective vulnerability, that is, it is believed that certain neurons are more vulnerable than others to the insult. Since hypoglycemia is a global insult it is puzzling that the necrotic neurons are not the same. For example, hypoglycemia damages neocortical pyramidal cells in layer 2 rather than in layers 3 or 5–6 and, in the hippocampus, the dentate crest is the most heavily affected area (10,11). To some extent, these differences can be explained by the presence, during the hypoglycemic coma, of fluid-borne toxins, probably glutamate and/or aspartate (11,12). However, some areas are largely spared during hypoglycemia (e.g., many brainstem areas and the cerebellum) (3,124). In the latter structure, only a few of the vulnerable

Purkinje cells are damaged and those are the ones in close proximity to the CSF pathways (10,11).

Estimation of glucose utilization (CMR_{gl}) in hypoglycemic coma gave the unexpected result that CMR_{gl}, which should approximate the rate of glucose delivery, was regionally heterogenous (1). Thus, many brainstem structures and the cerebellum seemed better supplied than, e.g., the neocortex, the hippocampus, and the caudoputamen. It is also notable that vascular autoregulation is better upheld in the cerebellum, and in many brainstem structures, than in neocortex and hippocampus (144). Support for the hypothesis that some regions are more resistant than others to hypoglycemia is that energy failure and depletion of endogenous substrates are considerably delayed in the cerebellum, as compared to the neocortex (3,113). Furthermore, the negative images of the protein synthesis autoradiograms of Kiessling et al. (73) showed a striking similarity to the ^{14}C-deoxyglucose autoradiograms.

In view of these results, it is tempting to conclude that the cerebellum is a resistant structure because it receives a better glucose supply than many other regions. However, since most Purkinje cells remain unaffected even after 60 min of hypoglycemic coma, and since cerebellar energy failure is extensive in the period 30 to 60 min (2), this cannot be the sole explanation. At present, the only indication that the metabolic responses may be regionally different is the finding of a lesser accumulation of FFA in the cerebellum than in the neocortex for a comparable perturbation of cellular energy state (2).

Epileptic Seizures

In terms of pathophysiology, seizures represent an entity other than ischemia and hypoglycemia. In the latter conditions, shortage of oxygen or glucose reduces oxidative metabolism and, thereby, ATP production. During seizures, increased neuronal activity augments metabolic rate, and somehow this augmentation triggers off a harmful series of reactions.

Metabolic Rate, Blood Flow, and Oxygen Supply

Epileptic seizures are associated with enhanced cerebral metabolic rates. Results obtained in cats and rats demonstrate that generalized seizures induced by pentylenetetrazole or bicuculline are accompanied by a 1.5- to 2.5-fold increase in overall or cortical metabolic rate for oxygen and glucose (25,96,114). With the advent of the deoxyglucose technique (150), it became feasible to map *local* changes in glucose utilization. The results revealed a strikingly heterogeneous metabolic response to local (46,47,88) and generalized (72,75,139) seizures. Notably, regions considered vulnerable to epileptic damage (neocortical and limbic areas) show sustained and markedly augmented metabolic rates (200–300% of control; see Fig. 8), while several resistant ones (e.g., the cerebellum in paralyzed animals) fail to participate in the hypermetabolic response. The results also showed that the development of a substantia nigra infarction is paralleled by an initially enhanced and subsequently rapidly falling metabolic rate (Fig. 8).

At present, the most extensive data on local metabolic rates exist for seizures induced by kainic acid (19,46,88). The results have given extensive information on the spread of seizure discharge, shown that CMR_{gl} correlates with locally measured neuronal activity, and confirmed that cell lesions are incurred in hypermetabolic structures. Lothman and Collins (88) concluded that limbic structures sustain a three- to six-fold rise in CMR_{gl} during seizures induced by kainic acid. Since the authors made no attempt to correct for changes in lumped constant, though, it remains to be shown whether the true increase is larger than that recorded during bicuculline-induced seizures (75,76).

The question arises whether the increased metabolic demands may outstrip oxygen (or glucose) supply. Measurements of blood flow, tissue oxygen tensions, and cellular redox state suggest that this can be the case, at least with repeated or sustained seizures. Thus, two autoradiographic studies have shown that the hyperemia is attenuated if seizures are prolonged for one hour, or longer (70,75). Furthermore, while cerebrovenous and tissue O_2 tensions often rise during seizures, indicating an abundance of cellular O_2 supply (37,54), studies of the tissue PO_2 changes suggest that *relative* hypoxia develops later on in a recurrent series of seizure discharges (37,86). *In vivo* measurements of the redox state of mitochondrial respiratory carriers (NADH and cytochrome a-a_3) gave similar results (86). These results indicate that long-lasting seizures may compromise cellular oxygenation, e.g., due to an attenuated circulatory response. However, since the measurements are qualitative they cannot reveal whether the decrease in PO_2 is sufficient to critically affect oxidative phosphorylation. Hence, it is jus-

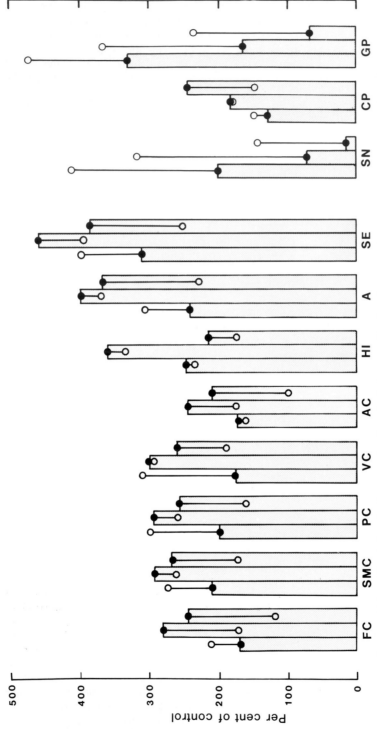

FIG. 8. Influence of bicuculline-induced seizures on local cerebral glucose utilization (*bars with filled circles*), and blood flow (*unfilled circles*). For each structure, values (percent of control) pertain to 20, 60, and 120 min of continuous seizure activity. The **left** panel (FC–SE) illustrates changes in "hypermetabolic" structures, the **right** panel (SN–GP) those in structures with time-dependent changes in metabolic rate and blood flow. FC, CMC, PC, VC, and AC denote frontal, sensorimotor, parietal, visual, and auditory cortex, respectively. HI, hippocampus; A, amygdala; SE, septal nuclei; SN, substantia nigra; CP, caudoputamen; GP, globus pallidus. (From ref. 75, with permission.)

tified to consider results bearing on the cellular energy state.

Cellular Energy State

Short-lasting seizures, especially in animals with unsupported ventilation, perturb cerebral energy state and cause accumulation of lactic acid (for literature, see ref. 135). In this context, though, we are concerned with events during sustained seizures, in animals with supported ventilation. Two studies have shown that although seizures induced by pentylenetetrazol, fluorothyl, and bicuculline lead to an initial breakdown of PCr and a decrease in the adenylate energy charge, the steady-state perturbation of cerebral (cortical) energy charge is small (42,54). Clearly, although CBF is reduced during the second hour of the status epilepticus cerebral energy state is upheld.

Results on glycolytic events are equally clearcut. Initially—i.e., soon after seizure onset— tissue concentrations of glycogen and glucose are reduced and tissue lactate content increases from control values of about 1.5 to 8 to 10 μmol/ g (42,54). Since similar lactate values were obtained after 2 hr of status epilepticus, the results reinforce the presence of a metabolic steady state.

We wish to emphasize that changes in labile cerebral metabolites show regional variations reflecting corresponding alterations in metabolic rate (56). Thus, whereas the parietal cortex and hippocampus show a similar metabolic perturbation changes in the cerebellum are slight and transient. Clearly, enhanced metabolic rate, perturbed energy metabolism, and neuronal damage are coupled events.

Since status epilepticus in rodents lead to necrosis of the substantia nigra, pars reticularis, the question arises whether metabolic perturbation in that structure is more pronounced. Recent results demonstrate that this is so. In fluorothyl-induced seizures of 20 and 60 min duration periaqueductal gray matter, tissue in close proximity to the substantia nigra, showed changes in labile phosphates and lactate very similar to those previously observed in neocortex and hippocampus (Ingvar, Folbergrová, and Siesjö, submitted). However, in substantia nigra the ATP content fell progressively (the values were 2.91 ± 0.04, 2.68 ± 0.06, and 2.18 ± 0.08 in control, 20 min seizure and 60 min seizure groups, respectively). Since the corresponding lactate concentrations were 1.57 ± 0.18, 16.1 ± 1.8, and 24.9 ± 2.4 μmol/g, respectively, the local energy failure was accompanied by progressive and massive lactic acidosis. Interruption of seizure activity caused normalization of energy state and lactate content in periaqueductal gray matter but not in substantia nigra, reflecting the irreversible damage inflicted upon the latter structure.

In theory, since relevant glycolytic metabolites, citric acid cycle intermediates, and associated amino acids were measured in these studies, it should be possible to calculate cytoplasmic and mitochondrial redox states (42,73). The results leave little doubt that the cytoplasmic $NADH/NAD^+$ system is reduced during seizures. However, a corresponding calculation of mitochondrial redox ratios from the glutamate dehydrogenase reaction yields values that are more uncertain, if not erroneous, probably due to compartmentation of the reacting species (98,135).

Changes in cerebral oxygen and glucose supply affect both glycolysis and cerebral energy state during seizures. For example, when oxygen supply is reduced by lowering of blood pressure or of arterial PO_2, the cellular lactic acidosis is enhanced (Table 3) (22). If blood pressure or arterial PO_2 is reduced even further, the seizure discharge is attenuated, and some further decline in the phosphorylation potential is observed. Similar changes—i.e., attenuation of seizure discharge and moderate deterioration of cellular energy state—are seen when blood glucose concentration falls during seizures, an event that occurs quickly if sustained seizures are induced in starved animals (23). However, under these circumstances tissue lactate concentrations fall to very low values. The lactic acidosis induced by seizure discharge is obviously critically dependent on a plentiful glucose supply. In fact, when plasma glucose levels fall towards control values during sustained seizures, signs of substrate deficiency develop, and both the adenylate energy charge and the lactate concentration are reduced (56). Thus, progressive reduction of oxygen and glucose supply has similar effects on seizure discharge and cerebral energy state but widely different effects on the accompanying acid–base changes.

In summary, structures which have markedly increased metabolic rates during seizures also show some metabolic perturbation, with moderate reduction in energy charge, increase in lactate, and raised lactate/pyruvate ratio. It follows that sparse neuronal necrosis occurs in the absence of gross energy failure. One structure, i.e., the substantia nigra, develops gross energy failure with massive accumulation of lactate during the first hour of seizure activity. In that structure, cell damage is dense and encom-

TABLE 3. *Labile cerebral metabolites in cerebral cortex of control rats, and after 2 hr of sustained bicuculline-induced epileptic seizures in standard animals (normoxic, normotensive, normothermic) and in animals with moderate hypotension (mean arterial blood pressure 75 mm Hg), or hypoxia (PaO$_2$ 44.2 ± 3.5 mm Hg)[a]*

Animals	Phosphocreatine	ATP	EC[b]	Lactate	La/Py
Control ($n = 12$)	4.47 ± 0.08	3.02 ± 0.02	0.947 ± 0.000	1.42 ± 0.10	11.5 ± 0.6
Standard ($n = 5$)	3.39 ± 0.27	2.94 ± 0.03	0.937 ± 0.002	9.14 ± 1.76	52.6 ± 7.5
Hypotension ($n = 6$)	2.65 ± 0.10*	2.94 ± 0.04	0.933 ± 0.002	16.06 ± 1.05**	92.5 ± 4.8**
Hypoxia ($n = 6$)	2.61 ± 0.30	2.80 ± 0.06	0.931 ± 0.004	23.22 ± 2.03***	143.9 ± 23.1**

[a] The values are mean ± SEM (μmol/g wet tissue). For statistical evaluation, the hypotension and hypoxia groups have been compared with the standard group. *$p < 0.05$, **$p < 0.01$, ***$p < 0.001$.
[b] EC, adenylate energy charge.
[c] La/Py, lactate/pyruvate ratio.

passes glial cells as well, suggesting a link between energy failure acidosis and necrosis.

Ion and Water Fluxes

Ion and water fluxes accompanying seizure discharges have been summarized previously (50) and are reviewed elsewhere in this handbook (see Chapters 31 and 32). In this context, we are concerned with three aspects: changes in K_e^+ during sustained seizures, the influence of added hypotension on K_e^+ levels, and the relationship between cellular efflux of K^+ and influx of Ca^{2+}.

It has been repeatedly shown that seizure discharge leads to K^+ efflux but also that K_e^+ does not rise above a ceiling value of about 10 μmol/ml (67). This is true also for sustained seizures induced by i.v. bicuculline and, when the period of burst-suppression has been reached, K_e^+ oscillates between about 4 (suppression) and 8 (burst) μmol/ml (7). If cerebral oxygenation is gradually reduced by superimposed hypotension, immediate release of K^+ does not occur; rather, K_e^+ values tend to decrease toward normal, in parallel with the attenuation of seizure discharge. It appears, therefore, that curtailment of oxygen supply affects synaptic transmission before ATP concentration is reduced, and massive efflux of K^+ does not occur until the hypotension has abolished spontaneous EEG activity (7).

The reduction in Ca_e^{2+} during induced seizures, which is unequivocal and relatively pronounced, is probably due to cellular uptake (67). This influx differs from that in ischemia and hypoglycemia, since it occurs at K_e^+ values below 10 μmol/ml. It seems likely, therefore, that factors other than K^+-coupled depolarization are responsible. One possible explanation is offered by results showing that excitatory amino acids, electrophoretically released into the tissue, reduce Ca_e^{2+} (66). We tentatively conclude that Ca^{2+} influx is at least in part due to activation by glutamate of postsynaptic Ca^{2+} gates. Studies on isolated synaptosomes have shown that such Ca^{2+} influx, and the accompanying accumulation of Na^+, can persist for some time in the postictal period, possibly reflecting a lingering increase in the membrane permeability to these ions (51).

Apart from causing fluxes of K^+ (out) and Ca^{2+} (in), seizures lead to an impedance change, suggesting that part of the ECF is imbibed by cellular elements, presumably glial (see Chapter 31). We observe that seizures lead to fluxes of ions and water of the type seen in ischemia and hypoglycemia, albeit less pronounced.

Changes in Intracellular pH

Several studies have been devoted to changes in pH$_e$ during seizures, but little information exists on how seizures alter pH$_i$. It is uncertain to what extent measurements of brain surface pH reflect pH of extracellular fluid proper (74), but those conducted with semimicro pH electrodes during bicuculline-induced seizures in rats suggest that pH$_e$ decreases by about 0.3 units (68). If one assumes that whole-tissue lactate content increases by 8 μmol/g and that the unionized form of lactic acid distributes equally in cerebral fluids one can calculate a pH shift of that magnitude (PCO$_2$ being assumed constant). Recent measurements with liquid ion-exchange microelectrodes establish that pH$_e$ is reduced by about 0.36 units after 5 and 20 min of seizures, arrest of seizure activity being followed by a surprisingly slow normalization (142). In animals made moderately hypoxic, pH$_e$ falls even further, suggesting that lactic acid formed by enhanced glycolysis is responsible. However, these data also demonstrate that lactic acid diffusion from cells cannot be the only mechanisms for acidification of ECF. Probably, transmembrane fluxes of H^+ and/or HCO_3^- via Na^+/H^+ and Cl/HCO_3^- antiporters contribute significantly, and Na^+/H^+ exchange must be responsible for the very fast initial acidification of ECF (142).

Howse et al. (74) measured total CO_2 content during short-lasting seizures and estimated the change in pH_i to be about 0.15 unit. In the absence of accurate information on pH_e and ECF volume, this remained an approximate value. However, the authors derived a similar pH change from the creatine kinase reaction. A pH shift of that magnitude was obtained in rats with bicuculline-induced status epilepticus (42). Provided that the creatine kinase equilibrium yields valid estimates of pH_i, one could conclude that, under normal conditions (tissue lactate content 8–10 μmol/g), changes in pH_i during seizures amount to about 0.2 units. This estimate has now been validated, and it has been shown that an even larger pH shift (about 0.32 units) is observed if the tissue lactic acidosis is enhanced by induced, moderate hypoxia (142). Notably, arrest of seizure activity was followed by rapid normalization of pH_i and by intracellular alkalosis. Clearly, if lactic acid production is curtailed by hypoglycemia, the pH_i change should be correspondingly smaller. On the other hand, the pronounced accumulation of lactate in the substantia nigra (see above) must be accompanied by marked extra- and intracellular acidosis. Preliminary results obtained with autoradiographic measurements of ^{14}C-DMO distribution demonstrate that this is the case, but quantification has not yet been feasible (Siesjö et al., *in preparation*).

Free Fatty Acids

Since alterations in FFA concentrations during seizures are reviewed in a separate chapter (see Chapter 44), we confine our discussion to a few points relevant to the integrative approach taken.

Since previous demonstrations of raised tissue FFA concentrations during seizures (e.g., ref. 16) pertain to animals with unassisted ventilation, the question arose whether lipolysis occurs also when arterial blood pressure and oxygenation are prevented from falling. This proved to be the case (17,143). As Fig. 9 shows, bicuculline-induced seizures were accompanied by accumulation of FFAs, mainly arachidonic and stearic acids. Total FFA content peaked at 5 min (a threefold increase), while arachidonic acid concentration was highest after 1 min (a 10-fold increase). In spite of ongoing seizures, arachi-

donic acid concentration fell continuously after its peak at 1 min, and total FFA content declined after the first 20 to 30 min. Even after 120 min, though, FFA content remained elevated at about 150% of control.

Changes in FFA concentrations in the hippocampus were similar to those observed in the neocortex (144). However, the cerebellum behaved differently, in that the only change, noted after 20 min, was a sevenfold increase in arachidonic acid concentration. Furthermore, since the control value was low, the arachidonic acid concentration in the cerebellum was only about 20% of that measured in neocortex and hippocampus.

Pathophysiological Conditions in Ischemia, Hypoglycemia, and Convulsive Disorders—An Overview

It is now possible to compare pathophysiological conditions in ischemia, hypoglycemia, and status epilepticus. Clearly, these three insults differ in terms of metabolic rate. In ischemia, metabolic rate is drastically reduced or ceases altogether due to oxygen lack. In contrast, hypoglycemia initially reduces CMR_{gl} only, and even after 30 min of isoelectricity $CMRO_2$ is upheld at values of about 50% of control, reflecting unabated delivery of oxygen (140). In convulsive states, finally, the primary insult is one of neuronal hyperactivity and, as long as blood oxygen tensions and plasma glucose concentrations are upheld, metabolic rates are markedly increased above normal.

These conditions are reflected in differences in cellular energy state and in acid–base changes (Fig. 10). Thus, whereas deterioration of energy state is extensive in ischemia, it is more moderate in hypoglycemia, and virtually absent in status epilepticus. Furthermore, whereas acidosis is marked to excessive in ischemia, it is moderate in seizures, and absent in hypoglycemia. We must conclude, therefore, that neither energy failure nor acidosis can be solely responsible for the cell damage incurred.

As Fig. 10 shows, one common metabolic event is lipolysis with accumulation of FFAs. However, scrutiny of the data discussed reveals that other factors are also common to the three conditions. These include perturbation of ion and water homeostasis, with translocation of Ca^{2+} from extra- to intracellular fluids, and accumulation of transmitters at synaptic sites, reflecting increased turnover and/or release.

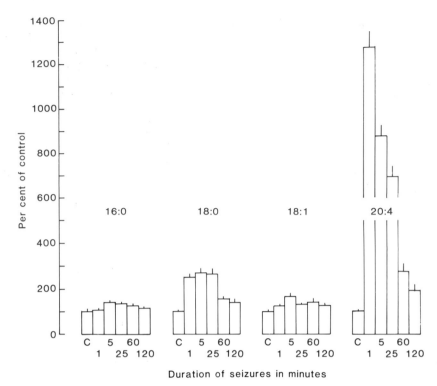

FIG. 9. Time-dependent changes in cerebral cortical concentrations of individual FFAs (16:0, 18:0, 18:1, and 20:4) during continuous bicuculline-induced seizures of 1–120 min duration. The values are means ± SEM in percent of control (C). (From ref. 144, with permission.)

NEUROCHEMICAL PATHOLOGY

Our discussion of mechanisms of cell damage is based on the fact that, for comparable insult periods, ischemia yields more damage than hypoglycemia, and the latter more damage than status epilepticus. At first sight, these differences correlate to the degree of energy failure. However, since acidosis aggravates ischemic damage in an already energy-depleted tissue, we must assume that, under those conditions, a reduction of pH_i exerts an independent, adverse effect (see below). Furthermore, it would seem that neither the perturbation of energy metabolism nor the acidosis occurring in epileptic tissue could explain why damage is incurred at all.

There is growing evidence that one initiating event in the series of reactions, the end result of which is cell death, is influx of Ca^{2+} into cells and/or its release from intracellular storage sites (65,94,136,146). However, this general hypothesis does not explain why ischemia is more harmful than hypoglycemia, nor does it account for differences in localization of cell damage in ischemia, hypoglycemia, and seizure disorders.

Furthermore, the hypothesis gives no clues to why ischemic damage often progresses to cystic infarction, with necrosis not only of neurons but also of glial cells and vascular endothelium. On the basis of this hypothesis, it is equally difficult to explain why hypoglycemia never causes cystic infarction, or why a pan-necrosis develops in the substantia nigra during seizures. For these reasons, it seems justified to consider the neurochemical pathology of excessive lactic acidosis before describing loss of Ca^{2+} homeostasis and the avalanche character of Ca^{2+}-triggered events.

Nutritional State, Lactic Acidosis, and Brain Damage

Evidence that the nutritional state significantly influences recovery from ischemia–hypoxia derives from the data of Myers (109), who emphasized the pathogenetic importance of preischemic hyperglycemia and hypothesized that it exerts its harmful effects, notably the formation of massive edema, by inducing excessive

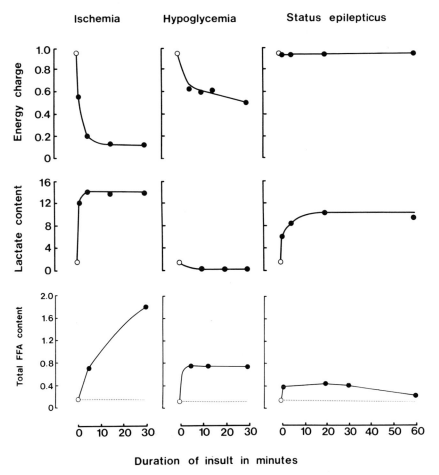

FIG. 10. Changes in cerebral cortical adenylate energy charge, lactate concentration, and total FFA content in complete ischemia, hypoglycemic coma, and bicuculline-induced status epilepticus. Lactate and FFA contents in micromoles per gram. (From ref. 146, with permission.)

lactic acidosis in brain tissues. This observation, which has been repeatedly confirmed (115,136), also provides a likely explanation for the paradoxical finding that some remaining perfusion during ischemia adversely affects recovery. A few years before this writing, this finding was controversial since other experiments indicated that the reverse was true (154). The controversy now seems resolved (136,145). Thus, if feeding or glucose infusion gives rise to preischemic hyperglycemia, the excessive acidosis caused by the enhanced glucose delivery triggers edema formation and accentuates tissue damage. In contrast, if food withdrawal prevents hyperglycemia from occurring, the remaining oxygen supply seems to ameliorate ischemic tissue damage.

Present evidence that hyperglycemia exerts its harmful effects by enhancing lactic acidosis

at tissue level is more circumstantial than conclusive, and it is not known if the effect represents a step function rather than a continuum. We will assume, though, that the degree of cellular acidosis is the decisive factor, and that gross aggravation of the brain damage requires that tissue lactate content rises to at least 15–20 μmol/g (115,136). Excessive tissue acidosis occurs under two conditions: pronounced, incomplete ischemia, and severe tissue hypoxia (135,136,146). Then, excessive acidosis only arises if the energy failure is extensive, if some perfusion persists, and if enough glucose is available to saturate the carrier translocating glucose from blood to tissue.

The evidence for a detrimental effect of acidosis is strong, and the acidosis seems somehow responsible for the development of pan-necrosis, or infarction. The evidence derived from ischemic experiments carried out on fed or glucose-infused animals receive support from other observations. For example although hypoglycemia of long duration may give extensive neuronal necrosis, and overt brain atrophy, it does not lead to pan-necrosis or infarction (10,11). Furthermore, the only area which shows gross tissue destruction in a rodent model of status epilepticus is also the only one showing marked acidosis (see above).

The mechanisms by which excessive lactic acidosis worsens the outcome of ischemia–hypoxia have not been satisfactorily clarified. It is known, though, that acidosis can prevent recovery of mitochondrial respiratory functions during recirculation (125), inhibit state 3 respiration of isolated mitochondria (69), and cause swelling and structural alterations of the microvasculature (110). Since acidosis has also been reported to inhibit Ca^{2+} uptake by mitochondria (26), it is possible that low intracellular pH compromises Ca^{2+} sequestration by these organelles. It is conceivable that one major adverse effect of acidosis is to disrupt volume regulation of glial cells. This possibility is in line with previous *in vitro* and *in vivo* results, suggesting that acidosis induces cellular edema (59,103). The mechanisms involved are not known, but the following tentative explanation can be offered, based on present knowledge of regulation of pH_i in a variety of tissues (127), of cell volume regulation (35,90,160), and of Na^+ and Cl^- fluxes in glial cells (28,81,82).

One primary effect of ATP-driven Na^+/K^+ transport is to maintain the major share of Na^+ in an extracellular position (Fig. 11). As such, Na^+ can balance impermeant intracellular anions, providing volume control by establishing a "double-Donnan" equilibrium (90,160). According to the "pump-leak" hypothesis, volume control can be upset by reduced pumping and/or increased leak, i.e., passive Na^+ entry. However, inhibition of an electroneutral Na^+/K^+ pump, i.e., one exchanging one Na^+ for one K^+, cannot by itself cause cell swelling. Swelling requires uptake of a "strong" cation (i.e., Na^+) together with a "strong" anion (i.e., Cl^-). Influx of Na^+ plus Cl^- could occur by a symport mechanism, i.e., by a membrane protein which, when binding the two ions simultaneously, translocases the ion couple inwards. Another possibility exists, though, one which links regulation of pH_i with regulation of cell volume, and which in pathological situations may cause one to be sacrificed at the expense of the other (137,138). In many cells, this leak occurs via an Na^+/H^+ antiporter. Since this achieves H^+ extrusion

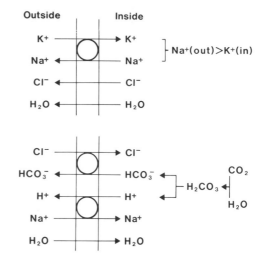

FIG. 11. Schematic diagram illustrating ion and water fluxes across glial cell membranes. **Upper** panel shows coupled Na^+/K^+ transport by an electrogenic pump, which allows outflux of Cl^-, with osmotically obliged water. **Lower** panel illustrates coupled Na^+/H^+ and Cl^-/HCO_3^- exchanges, the combined result of which is net transport of Na^+, Cl^-, and H_2O into the cells in exchange for H^+ and HCO_3^-, the source of which is metabolic H_2CO_3. Modified after Siesjö and Wieloch (146).

driven by passive Na^+ entry, it provides a means of regulating pH_i and maintains intracellular H^+ (and HCO_3^-) at nonequilibrium concentrations. In cells possessing a Cl^-/HCO_3^- antiporter, back leakage of H^+ can occur by outflux of HCO_3^-. However, if the source of H^+ and HCO_3^- is metabolic H_2CO_3, the operation of the coupled antiporters would lead to gain of Na^+, Cl^-, and osmotically obliged water, i.e., swelling. As Fig. 11 shows, this swelling tendency could be counteracted by an electrogenic Na^+/K^+ pump achieving outward translocation of Na^+, Cl^-, and water.

Obviously, in such a system cell swelling could occur if Na^+/K^+ pumping is reduced or if the activity of the Na^+/H^+ antiporter ("Na^+ permeability") is enhanced. Bourke, Kimelberg, and their associates (28,81,82), who described the presence of the two antiporters in glial cells, showed that increased K_e^+ (>10 μmol/ml) induced swelling. This could explain why astrocytic swelling occurs in ischemia and hypoglycemia, but not in epileptic seizures. However, their results showed that adenosine and noradrenaline induced comparable swelling in the absence of a rise in K_e^+, suggesting that the latter exerted its effect by depolarization-coupled release of the transmitters. If this is so, seizures could lead to astrocytic swelling by releasing adenosine, noradrenaline or other transmitters with an effect on Na$^+$ permeability (increased leak).

What, then, would be the effects of acidosis? Tentatively, we can offer the following suggestion. In cells using an Na$^+$/H$^+$ antiporter for pH$_i$ control, the rate of H$^+$ extrusion is inversely proportional to pH$_i$ (116). This means that acidosis enhances the activity of the coupled exchange, and exaggerates entry of Na$^+$ as well as the coupled influx of Cl$^-$ and water. It is then possible to outline a series of events during seizures, the end result of which is astrocytic swelling, exacerbated by acidosis (Fig. 12). In the scheme proposed, a fall in pH$_i$, if pronounced, has been assumed to have a dual effect: to accelerate Na$^+$/H$^+$ exchange (increased leak), and to retard mitochondrial production of ATP (decreased pump). It is conceivable that if the acidosis becomes pronounced, cell swelling progresses to the point where microcirculatory obstruction leads to infarction.

Excitatory Amino Acids and Neuronal Injury

The neurotoxic action of excitatory amino acids such as glutamate and aspartate is well documented, and the hypothesis has been proposed that these amino acids give characteristic neuronal lesions (109). Since similar light and electron microscopical features have been reported in studies on experimentally induced epilepsy, these acidic amino acids have been sug-

gested to be main pathogenic factors in the development of epileptic brain damage (see also refs. 46, 50).

The first experimental attempt to prove the involvement of glutamate in ischemic brain damage was performed by Jørgensen et al. (78). Since the distribution of ischemic brain damage approximates the distribution of EAA receptors, a link between these can be envisaged (see ref. 162). Thus the acute morphological changes observed following ischemia were ameliorated by local injections of a glutamate receptor (NMDA) antagonist, 2-amino-7-phosphonoheptanoic acid (AP7) (147). Furthermore, in cultured hippocampal pyramidal neurons synaptic activity and presence of glutamate enhanced neuronal death under anoxic conditions (128,129). Finally, cortical ablations leading to transection of a main excitatory input to the hippocampus significantly ameliorated ischemic brain damage, ipsilateral to the lesion (167). All these results hint that release of excitatory amino acids enhances neuronal damage. It should be emphasized, though, that removal of an inhibitory system such as the noradrenaline system originating in the locus coeruleus has an equally adverse effect (24). Thus, the balance between excitation and inhibition is of importance.

As mentioned in previous sections, one conspicuous feature of hypoglycemic brain damage is its distribution to areas facing the ventricular and subarachnoidal spaces, suggesting the formation and action of a fluid-borne neurotoxin

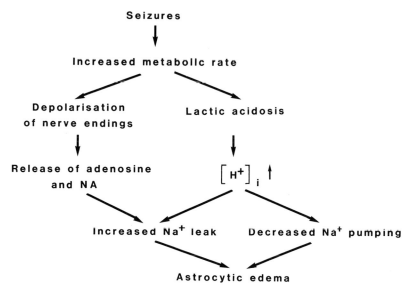

FIG. 12. Schematic diagram illustrating a tentative series of events leading to astrocytic swelling during seizures, enhanced by exaggerated lactic acidosis. For further explanation, see text.

(11). This was substantiated in an electron-microscopical study of the dentate gyrus revealing dendrosomatic degeneration with sparing of axons (12), a typical feature of excitotoxin-induced damage (109). As mentioned, a dramatic increase in the extracellular levels of glutamate and aspartate is observed during hypoglycemia (164).

The neuronal necrosis in the caudate nucleus is confined to its dorsal and lateral aspects (10,11). There is thus a neuroanatomical correlation of the damage to the glutamate containing cortico-striatal pathways (162). Transections of these pathways proved to abolish the damage in the area of the caudate nucleus shown to be innervated by these fibers (165). Moreover, blockage of the NMDA receptors in the caudate nucleus by local injections of AP7 mitigated the damage around the injection site (163), suggesting the involvement of these receptors in the development of neuronal damage.

Clearly, the localization of brain damage to certain selectively vulnerable neuronal cells, or its proximity to fluid pathways, is related to the type of postsynaptic receptors. If we conclude that neuronal necrosis is due to enhanced release of glutamate or aspartate, and their interaction with postsynaptic receptors, what are the molecular mechanisms? Two hypotheses have been advanced. According to one, Na^+ and Cl^- enter hypoxic cells, with osmotically obliged water, leading to swelling and osmolysis (129). It is not known if this hypothesis is valid for *in vivo* conditions, nor if it applies to hypoglycemia as well. The other hypothesis is that which assumes that a deranged Ca^+ metabolism forms a final common pathway. Although direct proof is lacking much circumstantial evidence suggests that excitatory amino acids exert their toxic effect by opening Ca^{2+} channels in the postsynaptic membranes. It seems justified, therefore, to consider in some detail Ca^{2+}-triggered events.

Ca²⁺ Homeostasis

Cell calcium regulation has been extensively reviewed (5,21,26,36). The following summary is based on these review articles, as well as those cited in a more recent publication (146), which gives a more detailed account of Ca^{2+} metabolism. Many cellular processes are regulated by Ca^{2+}, e.g., presynaptic release of transmitters, postsynaptic excitation by inward currents carried by Ca^{2+}, phosphorylation of proteins, and controlled degradation of structural lipids and proteins. In many of these reactions, Ca^{2+} acts as a modulator in the form of a Ca^{2+}–cal-

modulin complex. Common to all of them is that they progress in an orderly fashion only when the free, cytostolic Ca^{2+} concentration is of the order of 10^{-8} to 10^{-7} M. Thus, when this concentration increases unduly, and calmodulin is saturated, Ca^{2+}-triggered reactions are pathologically enhanced. Normally, intracellular Ca^{2+} activity is controlled by outward translocation over the plasma membrane and by intracellular sequestration mechanisms. A normal transmembrane Ca^{2+} gradient over the plasma membrane is upheld by the relative impermeability of the membrane to Ca^{2+} ions and by efficient mechanisms achieving their outward translocation. These mechanisms, which have K_m values in the nanomolar range, comprise Na^+/Ca^{2+} antiporters, probably also Ca^{2+}-dependent ATPases. Intracellular sequestration of Ca^{2+} is achieved by mitochondria and by binding to intracellular molecules such as the Ca^{2+}-binding protein (CaBP) and polyphosphoinositides (26,34,100).

Mitochondrial uptake of Ca^{2+} probably occurs electrophoretically by utilization of the transmembrane electrical gradient, and is thus an alternative to ATP formation. Release of Ca^{2+} from mitochondria, which occurs via a separate ionic channel, is supposed to be activated by Na^+ and FFAs. It is recognized that activation of the release channels can induce futile cycling of Ca^{2+} across the inner mitochondrial membrane. Re-export of Ca^{2+} sequestered by mitochondria requires translocation to the plasma membrane. Circumstantial evidence exists that the CaBP acts as a Ca^{2+} carrier in this capacity. This Ca^{2+} "buffer" has an interesting localization, since it is enriched in some of the selectively vulnerable areas in the brain, e.g., the CA1 sector of the hippocampus (13).

These relationships make it probable that severe ischemia must cause not only passive equilibration of Ca^{2+} across depolarized cell membranes but also hinder its uptake by mitochondria, leading to Ca^{2+} flooding of extramitochondrial compartments. One can also predict that reoxygenation at the termination of ischemia at least transiently should lead to sequestration of Ca^{2+} into mitochondria. However, the efficiency of this process must depend on the circumstances. For example, persistent elevations of Na^+ and FFA concentrations could maintain a constant efflux ("leak"). Furthermore, while persistent acidosis should decrease, alkalosis can be expected to enhance mitochondrial uptake of Ca^{2+}. It is equally difficult to predict whether or not reoxygenation restores Ca^{2+} transport across plasma membranes. Thus, phospholipid breakdown during ischemia may well induce an unspecific increase in Ca^{2+} permeability, which persists in the recovery period. Furthermore, specific Ca^{2+} channels could show sustained activation, e.g., by excitatory amino acids retained in the ECF, or by having developed supersensitivity to their agonists (see below). Again, we are faced with the possibility of Ca^{2+} cycling, this time across the plasma membrane. Finally, experiments with kindling-induced epilepsy suggest that the CaBP can be broken down, bereaving the cell of an important Ca^{2+} buffer (100). For all these reasons, it cannot be concluded that reoxygenation restores normal free cytosolic Ca^{2+} activities. Rather, conditions would favour increased Ca^{2+} activities sustained for some time during recirculation.

Although hypoglycemia leads to an equally extensive influx of Ca^{2+} from ECF, it seems likely that some Ca^{2+} sequestration occurs, since electron transport persists and alkalosis prevails. However, the efficiency of this sequestration is not known, since other accompaniments of the hypoglycemic state, notably influx of Na^+ and accumulation of FFA, ought to enhance release of Ca^{2+} from mitochondria.

In seizure states, finally, one could expect an even better regulation of intracellular Ca^{2+} activities, since both electron transport and ATP production are maintained, and since less Ca^{2+} enters from ECF. However, because some accumulation of FFA persists, some Na^+ enters, and moderate acidosis develops, sequestration of Ca^{2+} may be far from complete. Furthermore, as discussed below, sustained activation of Ca^{2+} gates by release of excitatory amino acids, without or with sensitization of receptor proteins, could well cause extensive Ca^{2+} influx at sites where these receptors abound, e.g., in postsynaptic domains of neocortical and limbic pyramidal neurons.

Ca^{2+}-Triggered Events

We consider four such events: proteolysis, disassembly of microtubuli, protein phosphorylation, and lipolysis. In addition, we discuss the possibility that Ca^{2+}-triggered lipolysis elicits the production and dislocation of free radicals. The major features of the cascade of events considered are schematically illustrated in Fig. 13.

Proteolysis

Brain tissues are known to contain neutral proteases (61). One proteolytic activity relevant to the present discussion is that leading to neurofilament degradation. So far, such degradation has been unequivocally shown to occur only in isolated neurofilaments, incubated in the presence of Ca^{2+}, and in intact axons incubated with the ionophore A 23187 in the presence of Ca^{2+} (130,131). The degradation was prevented by protease inhibitors. It seems likely that similar effects must be elicited when the cell is flooded with Ca^{2+} during the course of ischemia, hypoglycemia, and epileptic seizures.

Another Ca^{2+}-triggered proteolytic activity is that leading to an increased binding of glutamate to membranes from the hippocampal formation, suggesting that the number of glutamate receptors is increased. This has been shown to occur in hippocampal slices, electrically stimulated *in vitro* (89), and in plasma membranes incubated with micromolar Ca^{2+} concentrations (15). Again, these effects could be prevented by protease inhibitors (or by EDTA) (16). Probably such an increase in glutamate receptors is induced whenever Ca^{2+} activities increase. Conceivably, increased release and decreased reuptake of glutamate as well as increased receptor affinity may explain the hyperactivity of CA1 neurons in the recovery period following 5 min of ischemia in the gerbil (see above). One can envisage, therefore, that ischemia, hypoglycemia, and epileptic seizures are accompanied by activation of proteases with an ensuing, long-lasting effect on transmembrane ion traffic and neuronal excitability.

Protein Phosphorylation

Yet another type of covalent modification triggered by excessive agonist–receptor interaction and/or calcium influx/release is phosphorylation of proteins by kinases (45,60). The pathophysiological importance of such processes is that they may modulate ion permeability of membranes and excitability of neurons which may outlast the stimulation of receptors. Thus, the reactions display hysteresis: i.e., once an enzymatic process has been negatively or positively modulated by phosphorylation, the activation of the process by calcium requires several orders of magnitude less Ca^{2+} (123). For example, it has been proposed that excessive neuronal stimulation reduces presynaptic pyruvate dehydrogenase activity and that an ensuing reduction in mitochondrial Ca^{2+} sequestration enhances transmitter release (32,55). We note that such an effect could act in conjunction with postsynaptic receptor alterations to support prolonged synaptic activation. The phenomenon of

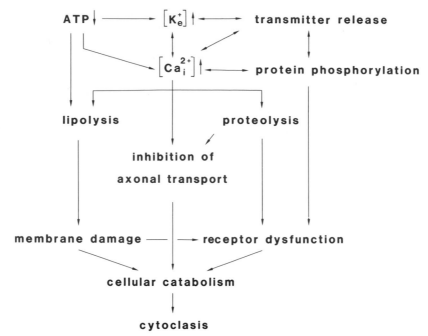

FIG. 13. Hypothetical scheme of possible events occurring during excessive neuronal activity, energy depletion, and cellular influx/release of Ca^{2+}. For further explanation, see text.

protein phosphorylation has been extensively studied in seizure conditions (see Chapters 1, 21, and 22). However, it also occurs as a result of ischemia (170), and future research may well disclose the importance of an aberrant protein phosphorylation in the pathogenesis of membrane dysfunction and cell death in general.

Disassembly of the Microtubular System

This has been proposed to occur by the formation of a complex between Ca^{2+}, calmodulin, and the tau factor necessary for tubulin polymerization, with an ensuing depolymerization and accumulation of tubulin subunits (79,91). The reaction is normally reversible. Thus, efflux/sequestration of Ca^{2+} should allow reassembly of microtubuli. However, if Ca^{2+} activities remain elevated, reassembly may be prevented or delayed. If so, and if neurofilament degradation occurs due to activation of proteases, the disruption of the cytoskeleton could have serious consequences for intracellular communication via the axonal transport system.

Lipolysis

The massive release of FFAs during ischemia is the combined result of agonist–receptor interactions, of Ca^{2+} influx/release and of deple-

tion of cellular ATP stores (Fig. 14). By the same token, the less extensive FFA accumulation in hypoglycemia could result from the persistence of some ATP production/Ca^{2+} sequestration. Similar arguments can be used to explain why lipolysis induced by seizure discharge, in itself probably mainly triggered by transmitter stimulation of membrane receptors, is moderate.

Although only hypoglycemia leads to a measurable reduction in the phospholipid pool, even small amounts of FFAs, especially the polyenoic ones, may have significant effects on cellular functions. These encompass changes in membrane fluidity and permeability, modulation of the activity of membrane-bound enzymes such as the Na^+/K^+-stimulated ATPase, and uncoupling of oxidative phosphorylation (41,146).

Oxidative modification of polyenoic FFAs, particularly arachidonic acid, occurs both enzymatically in reactions catalyzed by cyclo-oxygenase and lipooxygenase, and nonenzymatically (116,169). Although prostaglandin formation has been documented in the postischemic recirculation period and during seizures, other products may be more harmful. These include hydroxyeicosanoids, some of which cause intracellular Ca^{2+} mobilization in blood cells (104), and formation of free radical compounds (see below). An aberrant phospholipid metabolism mainly carries the risk of adversely effecting the

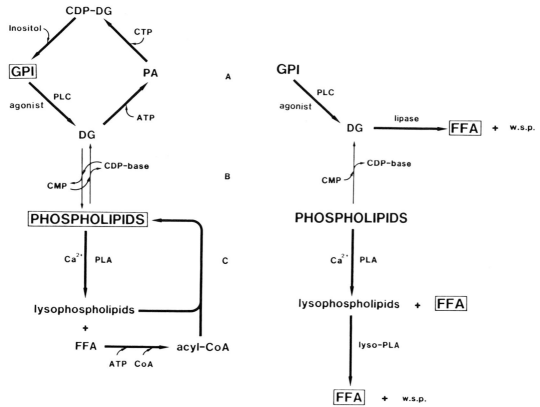

FIG. 14. The main phospholipid turnover pathways in the brain under normal (**left**) and ischemic (**right**) conditions. **Left panel, A:** The agonist-stimulated breakdown of inositol- and polyphosphoinositol glycerophospholipids (GPI) to diglyceride (DG), and its energy-dependent resynthesis by phosphorylation to phosphatidic acid (PA) and further to CDP-diglyceride (CDP-DG). **Left panel, B:** The base exchange reaction. The direction of this reaction is highly dependent on the concentrations of the reactants CMP and CMP-bases. **Left panel, C:** The Ca^{2+}-triggered breakdown, by phospholipase A (PLA), of phospholipids to lysophospholipids and FFA, and the ATP-dependent reacylation of lysophospholipids. CDP, CMP = cytidine di- and monophosphate, respectively. W.S.P. = water-soluble product. **Right panel:** Under ischemic conditions, the anabolic pathways are inhibited. The release of transmitters will trigger GPI breakdown to DG and FFA, while Ca^{2+} influx into cells causes PLA-stimulated lipolysis. Furthermore, the increased CMP levels will drive the base exchange reaction to DG and further to FFAs. Slightly modified after Wieloch and Siesjö (167).

phospholipid matrix of membranes and, thereby, of disturbing receptor function, Ca^{2+} homeostasis, and orderly ion fluxes.

Free-Radical Formation

Although formation and dislocation of free radicals are potential threats to all aerobic tissues, it has been difficult to prove that they can overwhelm the antioxidative defense. The important sites of production of free radicals, the most common of which are the superoxide and hydroxyl species and hydroperoxide radicals, are the mitochondrial electron transport chain and the sequences catalyzed by cyclo-oxygenase and lipoxygenase (52,58,117,158,159). However, radicals are also formed during syn-thesis/degradation of catecholamines, and in the xanthine oxidase reaction. It is widely held, for example, that the extreme toxicity of 6-hydroxydopamine is due to its uptake and autoxidation in dopaminergic cells (44). Furthermore, although tissues may normally contain low activities of xanthine oxidase, harmful conditions such as trauma reportedly lead to increased activities by enzymatic conversion (92).

Several events occurring in ischemia, hypoglycemia, and epileptic seizures would favour a spurt of free-radical formation, e.g., those leading to oxidation of polyenoic FFAs, release and reuptake of catecholamines, and oxidation of hypoxanthine by xanthine oxidase should conversion of xanthine dehydrogenase to xanthine oxidase occur. In theory, such formation carries the risk of radicals reacting with unsaturated acyl chains, with proteins, and with bases of nucleic acids (52). Since such reactions can cause disorder in the hydrophobic parts of membrane matrix and cross-linking of proteins, they may create molecular havoc. One property of free-radical reactions that may have devastating effects is that of self-propagation: i.e., once the reaction has been initiated, it will proceed until quenched by enzymatic reactions or endogenous free-radical scavengers. One potentially important free-radical reaction is that involving lipid peroxidation; it is self-propagating and leads to formation of lipoperoxides and hydroperoxide radicals, with these in turn reacting with polyenoic FFAs of phospholipids to form malondialdehyde. This molecule reacts with amino groups, cross-linking proteins, and phospholipids, thereby endangering the integrity of membranes and receptors (158,159).

Although free-radical production is likely to occur in disease, and although dislocation of free radicals has been proposed to contribute to tissue damage in ischemia, trauma, and epilepsy, it has been difficult to prove that it constitutes an important mechanism of damage (146). At present, the evidence is circumstantial and is derived from experiments in which a suitable prooxidant such as Fe^{2+} is injected into the tissue (168) or a radical generator is supplied. In an interesting series of experiments, one group (38–41) showed that radicals generated from the xanthine–xanthine oxidase system, or formed from added polyenoic FFAs, induced several untoward effects both *in vitro* and *in vivo*. These effects encompassed formation of cytotoxic edema, phospholipid degradation, inhibition of Na^+,K^+-ATPase activity, and reduction in reuptake of GABA and glutamate. It is clear, therefore, that free-radical formation can lead to membrane damage that can have devastating consequences. In spite of this, we still lack direct evidence that free-radical formation constitutes an important mechanism of brain damage in ischemia, hypoglycemia, and epileptic seizures. Conceivably, such evidence will be forthcoming when analyses of radical reactions are performed on areas at risk, e.g., postsynaptic domains in which Ca^{2+} influx/release is maximal.

It has been known for some time that in an *in vitro* system in which free radical formation is promoted by iron salts, a lowering of pH enhances malondialdehyde formation. Such results were recently confirmed and extended, and it was shown that a pH fall of only 0.5 units markedly accelerated malondialdehyde formation, reduction in the contents of polyunsaturated, phospholipid-bound FFAs, and disappearance of α-tocopherol from tissue constitutents (141). Possibly, the detrimental effect of low pH involves the release of pro-oxidant iron, normally bound to proteins (121,141). Whatever the mechanism, it seems possible that ischemia aggravates damage by enhancing free radical reactions.

SYNTHESIS AND CONCLUSION

It has remained an enigma that ischemia and hypoglycemia, two global insults, preferentially affect certain selectively vulnerable neurons, with sparing of others, often in close proximity to the necrotic ones. It now seems likely that this electively in response is, at least in part, related to the release of excitatory amino acids at the postsynaptic membranes of vulnerable neurons.

Circumstantial evidence thus exists that the initiating event in the cascade of reactions leading to ischemic and hypoglycemic damage is influx of Ca^{2+} across plasma membranes and/ or its release from intracellular sequestration sites. In both conditions, Ca^{2+} influx is extensive and indicative of passive equilibration across depolarized plasma membranes. Why, then, is damage due to hypoglycemia less extensive than that to ischemia? Tentatively, two factors contribute. First, there is clear evidence that ischemic brain damage is exaggerated by the concomitant acidosis. Second, since oxygen supply is maintained and part of the ATP stores are retained in hypoglycemia, the tissue is not in a completely catabolic state. Thus, conditions are at hand for continued sequestration of Ca^{2+} and/or resynthesis of phospholipids with an ensuing removal of free fatty acids.

How, then, is it possible to fit epileptic brain damage into the scheme? We submit that although ATP stores are upheld, activation of Ca^{2+} gates by excitatory transmitters leads to influx of Ca^{2+} into cellular elements that are densely innervated and possess a high density of Ca^{2+} channels, and that intracellular Ca^{2+} homeostasis is deranged to such an extent that lipolysis and proteolysis are induced. Evidently, this assumption also provides a tentative explanation for the phenomenon of selective neuronal vulnerability, since vulnerable cells (e.g., limbic and neocortical pyramids) seem to possess high Ca^{2+} conductances in dendritic domains. This explanation does not suffice, though, since graded insults of the type discussed may cause extensive damage to cells in the CA1 sector without affecting those in the CA3 sector or in the dentate gyrus. Furthermore, we lack a satisfactory explanation for the damage to the pallidoreticularis system. Thus, provided we adhere to the Ca^{2+} hypothesis of cell death, we must assume that cells differ, not only in terms of density of Ca^{2+} gates but also in efficacy of intracellular Ca^{2+} sequestration. As another possibility, cells may differ in their ability to control Ca^{2+}-triggered reactions or to quench the products of such reactions. Alternatively, they might be resistant to such damage due to an efficient antioxidative defense system.

In summary, by using this integrative approach we must conclude that one likely initiating event in the causation of ischemic, hypoglycemic, and epileptic brain damage is receptor activation and increased intracellular Ca^{2+} concentration, triggering a series of reactions, the end result of which is membrane damage and death. Probably, such reactions elicit structural alterations of the lipid and protein components of cellular membranes; free-radical reactions with lipid peroxidation and cross-linking of proteins; sustained modification of key enzymes, receptor proteins, and ion gates by protein phosphorylation; and proteolytic degradation of the cytoskeleton required for intracellular transport and information transfer. In ischemia, and possibly also in epileptic seizures, acidosis aggravates the damage.

ACKNOWLEDGMENTS

Work from the authors' own laboratory was supported by grants from the Swedish Medical Research Council (project 14X-263), and from the U.S. Public Health Service (grant 5 R01 NS-07838). The authors wish to acknowledge the skilled secretarial work of Erna Björkengren and Yvonne Hagberg.

REFERENCES

1. Abdul-Rahman, A., and Siesjö, B. K. (1980): Local cerebral glucose consumption during insulin-induced hypoglycemia, and in the recovery period following glucose administration. *Acta Physiol. Scand.*, 110:149–159.
2. Agardh C.-D., and Siesjö, B. K. (1981): Hypoglycemic brain injury: Phospholipids, free fatty acids, and cyclic nucleotides in the cerebellum of the rat after 30 and 60 minutes of severe insulin-induced hypoglycemia. *J. Cereb. Blood Flow Metab.*, 1:267–275.
3. Agardh, C.-D., Kalimo, H., Olsson, Y., and Siesjö, B. K. (1981): Hypoglycemic brain injury: Metabolic and structural findings in rat cerebellar cortex during profound insulin-induced hypoglycemia and in the recovery period following glucose administration. *J. Cereb. Blood Flow Metab.*, 1:71–84.
4. Agardh, C.-D., Chapman, A. G., Nilsson, B., and Siesjö, B. K. (1981): Endogenous substrates utilized by rat brain in severe insulin-induced hypoglycemia. *J. Neurochem.*, 36:490–500.
5. Akerman, K. E. O., and Nicholls, D. G. (1983): Physiological and bioenergetic aspects of mitochondrial calcium transport. *Rev. Physiol. Biochem.*, 95:149–201.
6. Astrup, J., and Norberg, K. (1976): Potassium activity in cerebral cortex in rats during progressive severe hypoglycemia. *Brain Res.*, 103:418–423.
7. Astrup, J., Blennow, G., and Nilsson, B. (1979): Effects of reduced cerebral blood flow upon EEG pattern, cerebral extracellular potassium, and energy metabolism in the rat cortex during bicuculline-induced seizures. *Brain Res.*, 177:115–126.
8. Astrup, J., Siesjö, B. K., and Symon, L. (1981): Thresholds in cerebral ischemia—The ischemic penumbra. *Stroke*, 12:723–725.
9. Astrup, J. (1982): Energy-requiring cell functions in the ischemic brain. *J. Neurosurg.*, 56:482–497.
10. Auer, R. N., Olsson, Y., and Siesjö, B. K. (1984): Hypoglycemic brain damage: Correlation with EEG isoelectric time. A quantitative study. *Diabetes*, 33:1090–1098.
11. Auer, R. N., Wieloch, T., Olsson, Y., and Siesjö, B. K. (1984): Distribution of hypoglycemic brain damage: Relationship to white matter and cerebrospinal fluid pathways. *Acta Neuropathol. (Berl.)*, 64:177–191.
12. Auer, R., Kalimo, H., Olsson, Y., and Wieloch, T. (1985): The dentate gyrus in hypoglycemia: Pathology implicating excitotoxin mediated neuronal necrosis. *Acta Neuropathol (Berl.)* (*in press*).
13. Baimbridge, K. G., and Miller, J. J. (1982): Immunochemical localization of calcium-binding protein in the cerebellum, hippocampal formation and olfactory bulb of the rat. *Brain Res.*, 245:223–229.
14. Baudry, M., and Lynch, G. (1980): Regulation of hippocampal glutamate receptors: Evidence for the involvement of a calcium-activated protease. *Proc. Natl. Acad. Sci. U.S.A.*, 77:2298–2302.
15. Baudry, M., Kramer, K., and Lynch, G. (1983): Irreversibility and time course of calcium stimulated ^{3}H-glutamate binding to rat hippocampal membranes. *Brain Res.*, 270:142–145.
16. Bazan, N. G. (1970): Effects of ischemia and electroconvulsive shock on free fatty acid pool in the brain. *Biochim. Biophys. Acta*, 218:1–10.
17. Bazán, N. G., Morelli de Liberti, S. A., and Rodriguez de Turco, E. B. (1982): Arachidonic acid and arachidonoyl-diglycerols increase in rat cerebrum during bicuculline-induced status epilepticus. *Neurochem. Res.*, 7:839–843.
18. Ben-Ari, Y., Tremblay, E., Ottersen, O. P., and Meldrum, B. S. (1980): The role of epileptic ac-

tivity in hippocampal and "remote" cerebral lesions induced by kainic acid. *Brain Res.*, 191:79–97.

19. Ben-Ari, Y., Tremblay, E., Riche, E., Ghilini, G., and Naquet, R. (1981): Electrographical, clinical, and pathological alterations following systemic administration of kainic acid, bicuculline, or pentetrazole: Metabolic mapping using the deoxyglucose method with special reference to the pathology of epilepsy. *Neuroscience*, 6:1361–1391.

20. Benveniste, H., Drejer, J., Schousboe, A., and Diemer, N. H. (1984): Elevation of the extracellular concentrations of glutamate and aspartate in rat hippocampus during transient cerebral ischemia monitored by intracerebral microdialysis. *J. Neurochem.*, 43:1369–1374.

21. Berridge, M. J. (1979): Modulation of nervous activity by cyclic nucleotides and calcium. In: *The Neurosciences: Fourth Study Program*, edited by F. O. Schmitt and F. G. Worden, pp. 873–889. MIT Press, Cambridge, Massachusetts.

22. Blennow, G., Brierly, J. B., Meldrum, B. S., and Siesjö, B. K. (1978): Epileptic brain damage. The role of systematic factors that modify cerebral energy metabolism. *Brain*, 101:687–700.

23. Blennow, G., Folbergrová, J., Nilsson, B., and Siesjö, B. (1979): Effects of bicuculline-induced seizures on cerebral metabolism and circulation of rats rendered hypoglycemic by starvation. *Ann. Neurol.*, 5:139–151.

24. Blomqvist, P., Lindvall, O., and Wieloch, T. (1985): Lesions of the locus coeruleus system aggravate ischemic damage in the rat brain. *Neurosci. Lett.*, 58:353–358.

25. Borgström, L., Chapman, A. G., and Siesjö, B. K. (1976): Glucose consumption in the cerebral cortex of the rat during bicuculline induced status epilepticus. *J. Neurochem.*, 27:971–973.

26. Borle, A. B. (1981): Control, modulation, and regulation of cell calcium. *Rev. Physiol. Biochem. Pharmacol.*, 90:13–164.

27. Bouchet, C., and Cazauvieilh, A. (1825): De l'épilepsie considéré dans ses rapport avec l'aliénation mentale. *Archives Générales de Medicine (Paris)*, 9:519–542.

28. Bourke, R. S., Waldman, J. B., Kimelberg, H. K., Barron, K. D., San Filippo, B. D., Popp, A. J., and Nelson, L. R. (1981): Adenosine-stimulated astroglial swelling in cat cerebral cortex *in vivo* with total inhibition by a nondiuretic acylaryloxyacid derivative. *J. Neurosurg.*, 55:364–370.

29. Brierley, J. B., Brown, A. W., and Meldrum, B. S. (1971): The nature and time course of the neuronal alterations resulting from oligaemia and hypoglycemia in the brain of *Macaca mulatta. Brain Res.*, 25:483–499.

30. Brierley, J. B. (1976): Cerebral Hypoxia. In: *Greenfield's Neuropathology*, 3rd ed., edited by W. Blackwood and J. A. N. Corsellis, pp. 43–85. Arnold, London.

31. Brown, W. J., Mitchell, A. G., Jr., Babb, T. L.,

and Crandall, P. H. (1980): Structural and physiologic studies in experimentally induced epilepsy. *Exp. Neurol.*, 69:543–562.

32. Browning, M., Dunwiddie, T., Bennett, W., Cispen, W., and Lynch, G. (1979): Synaptic phosphoproteins: Specific changes after repetitive stimulation of the hippocampal slice. *Science*, 203:60–62.

33. Bubis, J. J., Fukimoto, T., Ito, U., Mrsulja, B., Spatz, M., and Klatzo, I. (1976): Experimental cerebral ischemia in Mongolian gerbils. V. Ultrastructural changes in H3 sector of the hippocampus. *Acta Neuropathol. (Berl.)*, 36:285–294.

34. Buckley, J. T., and Hawthorne, J. N. (1972): Erythrocyte membrane polyphosphoinositide metabolism and the regulation of calcium binding. *J. Biol. Chem.*, 247:7218–7223.

35. Cala, P. M. (1983): Volume regulation by red blood cells: mechanisms of ion transport. *Mol. Physiol.*, 4:33–52.

36. Carafoli, F., and Crompton, M. (1978): The regulation of intracellular calcium: In: *Membrane Properties: Mechanical Aspects, Receptors, Energetics and Calcium Dependence of Transport, Vol. 10*, edited by F. Bronner and A. Kleinzeller, pp. 151–216. Academic, New York.

37. Caspers, H., and Speckmann, F.-J. (1972): Cerebral pO_2, pCO_2 and pH: Changes during convulsive activity and their significance for spontaneous arrest of seizures. *Epilepsia*, 13:699–725.

38. Chan, P. H., and Fishman, R. A. (1980): Transient formation of superoxide radicals in polyunsaturated fatty acid-induced brain swelling. *J. Neurochem.*, 35:1004–1007.

39. Chan, P. H., Kerlan, R., and Fishman, R. A. (1983): Reductions of γ-aminobutyric acid and glutamate uptake and $(Na^+ + K^+)$-ATPase activity in brain slices and synaptosomes by arachidonic acid. *J. Neurochem.*, 40:309–316.

40. Chan, P. H., Fishman, R. A., Caronna, J., Schmidley, J. W., Prioleau, G., and Lee, J. (1983): Induction of brain edema following intracerebral injection of arachidonic acid. *Ann. Neurol.*, 13:625–632.

41. Chan, P. H., and Fishman, R. A. (1985): Brain edema. In: *Handbook of Neurochemistry, Vol. 10*, edited by A. Lajtha, pp. 153–174. Plenum Publishing Corp., New York.

42. Chapman, A. G., Meldrum, B. S., and Siesjö, B. K. (1977): Cerebral metabolic changes during prolonged epileptic seizures in rats. *J. Neurochem.*, 28:1025–1035.

43. Chapman, A. G., Westerberg, E., and Siesjö, B. K. (1981): The metabolism of purine and pyrimidine nucleotides in rat cortex during insulin-induced hypoglycemia and recovery. *J. Neurochem.*, 36:179–189.

44. Cohen, G. (1978): The generation of hydroxyl radicals in biologic systems: Toxicological aspects. *Photochem. Photobiol.*, 28:669–675.

45. Cohen, P. (1982): The role of protein phosphorylation in neural and hormonal control of cellular activity. *Nature (Lond.)*, 296:613–620.

46. Collins, R. C., Lothman, E. W., and Olney, J. W. (1983): Status epilepticus in the limbic system: Biochemical and pathological changes. In: *Advances in Neurology, Vol. 34: Status Epilepticus,* edited by A. V. Delgado-Escueta, C. G. Wasterlain, D. M. Treiman, and R. J. Porter, pp. 277–288. Raven Press, New York.

47. Collins, R. C., and Olney, J. W. (1982): Focal cortical seizures cause distant thalamic lesions. *Science,* 218:177–179.

48. Corsellis, J. A. N., and Meldrum, B. S. (1976): The pathology of epilepsy. In: *Greenfields Neuropathology,* edited by W. Blackwood and J. A. N. Corsellis, pp. 771–795. Arnold, London.

49. Coyle, J. T. (1983): Neurotoxic action of kainic acid. *J. Neurochem.,* 41:1–11.

50. Coyle, J. T., Bird, S. J., Evans, R. H., Gulley, R. L., Nadler, J. V., Nicklas, W. J., and Olney, J. W. (1981): Excitatory amino acid neurotoxins; selectivity, specificity, and mechanism of action. *Neurosci. Res. Progr.,* 19:330–427.

51. Delgado-Escueta, A., and Horan, M. P. (1980): Brain synapses in epilepsy. In: *Mechanisms of Action of Antiepileptic Drugs,* edited by G. H. Glaser, J. K. Penry, and D. M. Woodbury, pp. 85–126. Raven Press, New York.

52. Demopoulos, H. B., Flamm, E. S., Pietronigro, D. D., and Seligman, M. L. (1980): The free radical pathology and the microcirculation in the major central nervous system disorders. *Acta Physiol. Scand. [Suppl.],* 492:91–119.

53. Diemer, N. H., and Siemkowicz, E. (1981): Regional neurone damage after cerebral ischemia in the normo- and hypoglycemic rat. *Neuropathol. Appl. Neurobiol.,* 7:217–227.

54. Duffy, T. F., Howse, D. C., and Plum, F. (1975): Cerebral energy metabolism during experimental status epilepticus. *J. Neurochem.,* 24:925–934.

55. Erulkar, S. D. (1983): The modulation of neurotransmitter release at synaptic junctions. *Rev. Physiol. Biochem. Pharmacol.,* 98:64–175.

56. Folbergrová, J., Ingvar, M., and Siesjö, B. K. (1981): Metabolic changes in cerebral cortex, hippocampus, and cerebellum during sustained bicuculline-induced seizures. *J. Neurochem.,* 37:1228–1238.

57. Folbergrová, J., Ingvar, M., Nevander, G., and Siesjö, B. K. (1985): Cerebral metabolic changes during and following fluorothyl-induced seizures in ventilated rats. *J. Neurochem.,* 44:1419–1426.

58. Fridovich, I. (1978): The biology of oxygen radicals. The superoxide radical is an agent of oxygen toxicity: Superoxide dismutases provide an important defense. *Science,* 201:875–880.

59. Friede, R. L., and van Houten, W. H. (1961): Relations between post-mortem alterations and glycolytic metabolism in the brain. *Exp. Neurol.,* 4:197–204.

60. Greengard, P. (1979): Cyclic nucleotides, phosphorylated proteins, and the nervous system. *Fed. Proc.,* 38:2208–2217.

61. Guroff, G. (1964): A neutral calcium activated proteinase from the soluble fraction of rat brain. *J. Biol. Chem.,* 239:149–155.

62. Hansen, A. J., and Zeuthen, T. (1981): Extracellular ion concentrations during spreading depression and ischemia in the rat brain cortex. *Acta Physiol. Scand.,* 113:437–445.

63. Harris, R. J., Symon, L., Branston, N. M., and Bayhan, M. (1981): Changes in extracellular calcium activity in cerebral ischemia. *J. Cereb. Blood Flow Metab.,* 1:203–209.

64. Harris, R. J., Wieloch, T., Symon, L., and Siesjö, B. K. (1984): Cerebral extracellular calcium activity in severe hypoglycemia: Relation to extracellular potassium and energy charge. *J. Cereb. Blood Flow Metab.,* 4:187–193.

65. Hass, W. K. (1981): Beyond cerebral blood flow, metabolism and ischemic thresholds: Examination of the role of calcium in the initiation of cerebral infarction. In: *Cerebral Vascular Disease, Proc. 10th Salzburg Conf. Cerebral Vascular Disease, Vol. 3,* edited by J. S. Meyer, H. Lechner, M. Reivich, E. O. Ott, and A. Arabinar, pp. 3–17. Exerpta Medica, Amsterdam.

66. Heinemann, U., and Pumain, R. (1980): Extracellular calcium activity changes in cat sensorimotor cortex induced by iontophoretic application of amino acids. *Exp. Brain Res.,* 40:247–250.

67. Heinemann, U., Lux, H. D., and Gutnick, M. J. (1977): Extracellular free calcium and potassium during paroxysmal activity in the cerebral cortex of the cat. *Exp. Brain Res.,* 27:237–243.

68. Heuser, D. (1978): The significance of cortical extracellular H^+, K^+ and Ca^{2+} activities for regulation of local cerebral blood flow under conditions of enhanced neuronal activity. In: *Cerebral Vascular Smooth Muscle and Its Control,* edited by M. J. Purves, pp. 339–349. Elsevier, Amsterdam.

69. Hillered, L., Ernster, L., and Siesjö, B. K. (1984): Influence of in vitro lactic acidosis and hypercapnia on respiratory activity of isolated rat brain mitochondria. *J. CBF Metabol.,* 4:430–437.

70. Horton, R. W., Meldrum, B. S., Pedley, T. A., and McWilliam, J. R. (1980): Regional cerebral blood flow in the rat during prolonged seizure activity. *Brain Res.,* 192:399–412.

71. Hossmann, K.-A. (1982): Treatment of experimental cerebral ischemia. *J. Cereb. Blood Flow Metab.,* 2:275–297.

72. Howse, D. C. (1983): Cerebral energy metabolism during experimental status epilepticus. In: *Advances in Neurology, Vol. 34: Status Epilepticus,* edited by A. V. Delgado-Escueta, C. G. Wasterlain, D. M. Treiman, and R. J. Porter, pp. 209–216. Raven Press, New York.

73. Howse, D. C., and Duffy, T. E. (1975): Control of the redox state of the pyridine nucleotides in the rat cerebral cortex. Effect of electroshock-induced seizures. *J. Neurochem.,* 24:935–940.

74. Howse, D. C., Caronna, J. J., Duffy, T. E., and Plum, F. (1974): Cerebral energy metabolism, pH, and blood flow during seizures in the cat. *Am. J. Physiol.,* 227:1444–1451.

75. Ingvar, M., and Siesjö, B. K. (1983): Local blood flow and glucose consumption in the rat

brain during sustained bicuculline-induced seizures. *Acta Neurol. Scand.*, 68:129–144.

76. Ingvar, M., and Siesjö, B. K. (1985): Measurements of brain glucose utilization in pathological states: Problems and pitfalls. In: *The Metabolism of the Human Brain Studied with Positron Emission Tomography*, edited by T. Greitz et al., pp. 195–205. Raven Press, New York.

77. Ito, U., Spatz, M., Walker, J. T., Jr., and Klatzo, I. (1975): Experimental cerebral ischemia in Mongolian gerbils. I. Light microscopic observations. *Acta Neuropathol. (Berl.)*, 32: 209–223.

78. Jørgensen, M. B., and Diemer, N. H. (1982): Selective neuron loss after cerebral ischemia in the rat: Possible role of transmitter glutamate. *Acta Neurol. Scand.* 66:536–546.

79. Kakiuchi, S., and Sobue, K. (1981): Ca^{2+} and calmodulin dependent flip-flop mechanism in microtubule assembly-dissassembly. *FEBS Lett.*, 132:141–148.

80. Kiessling, M., Weigel, K., Gartzen, D., and Kleihues, P. (1982): Regional heterogeneity of L-[3-^{3}H]-tyrosine incorporation into rat brain proteins during severe hypoglycemia. *J. Cereb. Blood Flow Metab.*, 2:249–253.

81. Kimelberg, H. K., and Bourke, R. S. (1984): Mechanisms of astrocytic swelling. In: *Cerebral Ischemia*, edited by A. Bes, P. Braquet, R. Paoletti, and B. K. Siesjö, pp. 131–146. Elsevier, Amsterdam.

82. Kimelberg, H. K., Bourke, R. S., and Stieg, P. E. (1982): Swelling of astroglia after injury to the central nervous system. In: *Head Injury: Basic and Clinical Aspects*, edited by R. G. Grossman and P. L. Gildenberg, pp. 31–44. Raven Press, New York.

83. Kirino, T. (1982): Delayed neuronal death in the gerbil hippocampus following ischemia. *Brain Res.*, 239:57–69.

84. Kleihues, P., Kobayashi, K., and Hossmann, K. A. (1974): Purine nucleotide metabolism in the cat brain after one hour of complete ischemia. *J. Neurochem.*, 23:417–425.

85. Koide, T., Wieloch, T., and Siesjö, B. K. (1985): Circulating catecholamines modulate ischemic brain damage. *Acta Neurol. Scand.*, 72(Suppl.):265–266.

86. Kreisman, N. R., Lamanna, J. C., Rosenthal, M., and Sick, T. J. (1981): Oxidative metabolic responses with recurrent seizures in rat cerebral cortex: Role of systemic factors. *Brain Res.*, 218:175–188.

87. Ljunggren, B., Norberg, K., and Siesjö, B. K. (1974): Influence of tissue acidosis upon restitution of brain energy metabolism following total ischemia. *Brain Res.*, 77:173–186.

88. Lothman, E. W., and Collins, R. C. (1981): Kainic acid induced limbic seizures: Metabolic, behavioural, electroencephalographic, and neuropathological correlates. *Brain Res.*, 218:299– 318.

89. Lynch, G., and Baudry, M. (1984): The biochemistry of memory: A new and specific hypothesis. *Science*, 224:1057–1063.

90. MacKnight, A. D. C., and Leaf, A. (1977): Regulation of cellular volume. *Physiol. Rev.*, 57:510–573.

91. Marcum, J. M., Dedman, J. R., Brinkley, B. R., and Means, A. R. (1978): Control of microtubule assembly-disassembly by calcium dependent regulator protein. *Proc. Natl. Acad. Sci. U.S.A.*, 75:3771–3775.

92. McCord, J. M., and Roy, R. S. (1982): The pathophysiology of superoxide: Roles in inflamation and ischemia. *Can. J. Physiol. Pharmacol.*, 60:1346–1352.

93. McIntyre, D. C., Nathanson, D., and Edson, N. (1982): A new model of partial status epilepticus based on kindling. *Brain Res.*, 250:53–63.

94. Meldrum, B. S. (1983): Metabolic factors during prolonged seizures and their relation to nerve cell death. In: *Advances in Neurology, Vol. 34: Status Epilepticus*, edited by A. V. Delgado-Escueta, C. G. Wasterlain, D. M. Treiman, and R. J. Porter, pp. 261–275. Raven Press, New York.

95. Meldrum, B. S., and Brierley, J. B. (1973): Prolonged epileptic seizures in primates. Ischemic cell change and its relation to ictal physiological events. *Arch. Neurol.*, 28:10–17.

96. Meldrum, B. S., and Nilsson, B. (1976): Cerebral blood flow and metabolic rate early and late in prolonged epileptic seizures induced in rats by bicuculline. *Brain*, 99:523–542.

97. Meldrum, B. S., Vigoroux, R. A., and Brierley, J. B. (1973): Systemic factors and epileptic brain damage. Prolonged seizures in paralysed, artificially ventilated baboons. *Arch. Neurol.*, 29:82–87.

98. Merrill, D. K., and Guynn, R. W. (1981): The calculation of the mitochondrial free NAD^+ NADH H$^+$ ratio in brain: Effect of electroconvulsive seizure. *Brain Res.*, 239:71–80.

99. Meyer, A. (1963): Intoxications. In: *Greenfield's Neuropathology*, edited by W. Blackwood, W. H. McMenemey, A. Meyer, R. M. Norman, and D. S. Russel, pp. 235–287. Arnold, London.

100. Miller, J. J., and Baimbridge, K. G. (1983): Biochemical and immunohistochemical correlates of kindling-induced epilepsy: Role of calcium binding protein. *Brain Res.*, 278:322–326.

101. Mouritzen Dam, A. (1982): Hippocampal neuron loss in epilepsy and after experimental seizures. *Acta Neurol. Scand.*, 66:601–642.

102. Myers, R. E., and Kahn, K. J. (1971): Insulin-induced hypoglycemia in the non-human primate. II. Long-term neuropathological consequences. In: *Brain Hypoxia*, edited by J. B. Brierley and B. S. Meldrum, pp. 195–206. William Heinemann Medical Books, London.

103. Myers, R. E. (1979): Lactic acid accumulation as a cause of brain edema and cerebral necrosis resulting from oxygen deprivation. In: *Advances in Perinatal Neurology*, edited by R. Korobkin, and G. Guilleminault, pp. 85–114. Spectrum, New York.

104. Naccache, P. H., Shaafi, R. I., Borgeat, P., and Goetzl, F. J. (1981): Mono- and dihydroxyeicosatetraenoic acids alter calcium homeostasis in rabbit neurophils. *J. Clin. Invest.*, 67:1584– 1587.

105. Nadler, J. V. (1981): Kainic acid as a tool for the study of temporal lobe epilepsy. *Life Sci.,* 29:2031–2042.

106. Nevander, G., Ingvar, M., Auer, R., and Siesjö, B. K. (1984): Irreversible brain cell damage after short periods of status epilepticus. *Acta Physiol. Scand.,* 120:155–157.

107. Nevander, G., Ingvar, M., Auer, R., and Siesjö, B. K. (1985): Status epilepticus in well-oxygenated rats causes neuronal necrosis. *Ann Neurol.* (*in press*).

108. Nilsson, B., Norberg, K., Nordström, C.-H., and Siesjö, B. K. (1975): Rate of energy utilization in the cerebral cortex of rats. *Acta Physiol. Scand.,* 93:569–571.

109. Olney, J. (1978): Neurotoxicity of excitatory amino acids. In: *Kainic as a Tool in Neurobiology,* edited by E. G. McGeer, J. W. Olney, and P. L. McGeer, pp. 95–121. Raven Press, New York.

110. Paljärvi, L., Rehncrona, S., Söderfeldt, B., Olsson, Y., and Kalimo, H. (1983): Brain lactic acidosis and ischemic cell damage: Quantitative ultrastructural changes in capillaries of rat cerebral cortex. *Acta Neuropathol. (Berl.),* 60:23–240.

111. Pelligrino, D., and Siesjö, B. K. (1981): Regulation of extra- and intracellular pH in the brain in severe hypoglycemia. *J. Cereb. Blood Flow Metab.,* 1:85–96.

112. Pelligrino, D., Almquist, L.-O., and Siesjö, B. K. (1981): Effects of insulin-induced hypoglycemia on intracellular pH and impedance in the cerebral cortex of the rat. *Brain Res.,* 221:129–147.

113. Pelligrino, D., Yokoyama, H., Ingvar, M., and Siesjö, B. K. (1982): Moderate arterial hypotension reduces cerebral cortical blood flow and enhances cellular release of potassium in severe hypoglycemia. *Acta Physiol. Scand.,* 115:511–513.

114. Plum, F., Howse, D. C., and Duffy, T. E. (1974): Metabolic effects of seizures. In: *Brain Dysfunction in Metabolic Disorders,* edited by F. Plum, *Res. Publ. Assoc. Nerv. Ment. Dis.,* Vol. 53, pp. 141–157. Raven Press, New York.

115. Plum, F. (1983): What causes infarction in ischemic brain?: The Robert Wartenberg Lecture. *Neurology,* 33:222–233.

116. Porter, N. A., Wolf, R. A., Yarbro, E. M., and Weenen, H. (1979): The autooxidation of arachidonic acid: Formation of the proposed SRS-A intermediate. *Biochem. Biophys. Res. Commun.,* 89:1058–1064.

117. Pryor, W. A. (1978): The formation of free radicals and the consequences of their reactions in vivo. *Photochem. Photobiol.,* 28:787–801.

118. Pulsinelli, W. A., and Brierley, J. B. (1979): A new model of bilateral hemispheric ischemia in the unanesthetized rat. *Stroke* 10(3):267–272.

119. Pulsinelli, W. A., and Duffy, T. E. (1983): Regional energy balance in rat brain after transient forebrain ischemia. *J. Neurochem.,* 40:1500–1503.

120. Pulsinelli, W. A., Brierley, J. B., and Plum, F.

(1982): Temporal profile of neuronal damage in a model of transient forebrain ischemia. *Ann. Neurol.,* 11:491–498.

121. Pulsinelli, W. A., Kraig, R. P., and Plum, F. (1985): Hyperglycemia, cerebral acidosis, and ischemic brain damage. In: *Cerebrovascular Diseases,* edited by F. Plum and W. Pulsinelli, pp. 201–205. Raven Press, New York.

122. Purpura, D. P., and Gonzales-Monteagudo, M. D. (1960): Acute effects of methoxypyridoxine on hippocampal end-blade neurons; An experimental study of "special pathoclisis" in the cerebral cortex. *J. Neuropathol. Exp. Neurol.,* 19:421–432.

123. Rasmussen, H., and Waisman, D. M. (1983): Modulation of cell function in the calcium messenger system. *Rev. Physiol. Biochem. Pharmacol.,* 95:111–148.

124. Ratcheson, R., Blank, A. C., and Ferrendelli, J. A. (1981): Regionally selective metabolic effects of hypoglycemia in brain. *J. Neurochem.,* 36:1952–1958.

125. Rehncrona, S., Mela, L., and Siesjö, B. K. (1979): Recovery of brain mitochondrial function in the rat after complete and incomplete cerebral ischemia. *Stroke,* 10:437–446.

126. Rehncrona, S., Westerberg, E., Åkesson, B., and Siesjö, B. K. (1982): Brain cortical fatty acids and phospholipids during and following complete and severe incomplete ischemia. *J. Neurochem.,* 38:84–93.

127. Roos, A., and Boron, W. F. (1981): Intracellular pH. *Physiol. Rev.,* 61:296–434.

128. Rothman, S. M. (1983): Synaptic activity mediates death of hypoxic neurons. *Science,* 220:536–537.

129. Rothman, S. M. (1985): The neurotoxicity of excitatory amino acids is produced by passive chloride influx. *J Neuroscience,* 5:1483–1489.

130. Schlaepfer, W. W., and Hasler, M. B. (1979): Characterization of the calcium-induced disruption of neurofilaments in rat peripheral nerve. *Brain Res.,* 168:299–309.

131. Schlaepfer, W. W., and Zimmerman, U. P. (1985): Mechanisms underlying the neuronal response to ischemic injury. Calcium-activated proteolysis of neurofilaments. *Progr. Brain Res.,* 63 (*in press*).

132. Scholz, W. (1959): The contribution of pathoanatomical research to the problem of epilepsy. *Epilepsia (Amsterdam),* 1:36–55.

133. Schwartz, I. R., Broggi, G., and Pappas, G. D. (1970): Fine structure of cat hippocampus during sustained seizure. *Brain Res.,* 18:176–180.

134. Schwob, J. E., Fuller, T., Price, J. L., and Olney, J. W. (1980): Widespread patterns of neuronal damage following systemic or intracerebral injections of kainic acid: A histological study. *Neuroscience,* 5:991–1014.

135. Siesjö, B. K. (1978): *Brain Energy Metabolism.* Wiley, Chichester, New York.

136. Siesjö, B. K. (1981): Cell damage in the brain: A speculative synthesis. *J. Cereb. Blood Flow Metab.,* 1:155–185.

137. Siesjö, B. K. (1984): Cerebral circulation and metabolism. *J. Neurosurg.,* 60:883–908.

138. Siesjö, B. K. (1985): Acid-base homeostasis in the brain: Physiology, chemistry, and neuro-chemical pathology. *Prog. Brain Res.*, 63 (*in press*).

139. Siesjö, B. K. and Abdul-Rahman, A. (1979): A metabolic basis for the selective vulnerability of neurons in status epilepticus. *Acta Physiol. Scand.*, 106:377–378.

140. Siesjö, B. K., and Agardh, C.-D. (1983): Hypoglycemia. In: *Handbook of Neurochemistry, Vol. 3*, edited by A. Lahjta, pp. 353–381. Plenum, New York.

141. Siesjö, B. K., Bendek, G., Koide, T., Westerberg, E., and Wieloch, T. (1985): Influence of acidosis on lipid peroxidation in brain tissues in vitro. *J CBF Metabol.*, 5:253–258.

142. Siesjö, B. K., von Hanwehr, R., Nergelius, G., Nevander, G., and Ingvar, M. (1984): Extra-and intracellular pH in the brain during seizures and in the recovery period following arrest of seizure activity. *J. Cereb. Blood Flow Metab.*, 5:47–57.

143. Siesjö, B. K., Folbergrová, J., and MacMillan, V. (1972): The effect of hypercapnia upon intra-cellular pH in the brain, evaluated by the bicarbonate-carbonic acid method and from the creatine phosphokinase equilibrium. *J. Neurochem.*, 19:2483–2495.

144. Siesjö, B. K., Ingvar, M., and Westerberg, E. (1982): The influence of bicuculline-induced seizures on free fatty acid concentrations in cerebral cortex, hippocampus, and cerebellum. *J. Neurochem.*, 39:796–802.

145. Siesjö, B. K., Ingvar, M., and Pellegrino, D. (1983): Regional differences in vascular auto-regulation in the rat brain in severe insulin-induced hypoglycemia. *J. Cereb. Blood Flow Metab.*, 2:478–485.

146. Siesjö, B. K., and Wieloch, T. (1985): Brain Injury: Neurochemical aspects. In: *Central Nervous System Trauma—Status Report*, edited by D. Becker, and J. Povlishock, pp. 513–532. Williaum Byrk Press Inc., Richmond, Virginia.

147. Simon, R. P., Swan, J. H., Griffith, T., and Meldrum, B. S. (1984): Blockade of N-methyl-D-aspartate receptors may protect against ischemic damage in the brain. *Science*, 226:850–852.

148. Smith, M.-L., Béndek, G., Dahlgren, N., Rosén, I., Wieloch, T., and Siesjö, B. K. (1984): Models for studying long-term recovery following forebrain ischemia in the rat. 2. A two vessel occlusion model. *Acta Neurol. Scand.*, 69:385–401.

149. Smith, M.-L., Auer, R. N., and Siesjö, B. K. (1984): The density and distribution of ischemic brain injury in the rat following two to ten minutes of forebrain ischemia. *Acta Neuropathol.* (*Berlin*), 64:319–332.

150. Sokoloff, L., Reivich, M., Kennedy, C., Des Rosiers, M. H., Patlack, C. S., Pettigrew, K. D., Sakurada, O., and Shinohara, M. (1977): The 14-C-Deoxyglucose Method for the measurement of local cerebral glucose utilization: Theory, procedure, and normal values in the conscious and anesthetized albino rat. *J. Neurochem.*, 28:897–916.

151. Sommer, W. (1880): Erkrankung des Ammonshornes als aetiologisches Moment der Epilepsie. *Archiv für Psychiatrie und Nervenkrankheiten*, 10:631–675.

152. Spielmeyer, W. (1922): *Histopathologie des Nervensystems*, pp. 74–79. Springer, Berlin.

153. Spielmeyer, W. (1927): Die Pathogenese des epileptischen Krampfes. *Zeitschrift für die gesamte Neurologie und Psychiatrie*, 109:501–520.

154. Steen, P. A., Michenfelder, J. D., and Milde, J. H. (1979): Incomplete versus complete cerebral ischemia: Improved outcome with a minimal blood flow. *Ann. Neurol.*, 6:389–398.

155. Suzuki, R., Yamaguchi, T., Kirino, T., Orzi, F., and Klatzo, I. (1983): The effects of 5-minute ischemia in mongolian gerbils: I. Blood-brain barrier, cerebral blood flow, and local cerebral glucose utilization changes. *Acta Neuropathol. (Berl.)*, 60:207–216.

156. Suzuki, R., Yamaguchi, T., Choh-Luh, L., and Klatzo, I. (1983): The effects of 5-minute ischemia in Mongolian gerbils: II. Changes of spontaneous neuronal activity in cerebral cortex and CA1 sector of hippocampus. *Acta Neuropathol. (Berl.)*, 60:217–222.

157. Söderfeldt, B., Kalimo, H., Olsson, Y., and Siesjö, B. K. (1983): Bicuculline-induced epileptic brain injury. Transient and persistent cell changes in rat cerebral cortex in the early recovery period. *Acta Neuropathol.*, 62:87–95.

158. Tappel, A. L. (1975): Lipid peroxidation and fluorescent molecular damage to membranes. In: *Pathobiology of Cell Membranes, Vol. 1*, edited by B. F. Trump and A. V. Arstila, pp. 145–170. Academic, New York.

159. Tappel, A. L. (1980): Measurement of and protection from in vivo lipid peroxidation. In: *Free Radicals in Biology, Vol. 4*, edited by W. A. Pryor, pp. 1–47. Academic, New York.

160. Tosteson, D. C., and Hoffman, J. F. (1960): Regulation of cell volume by active cation transport in high and low potassium sheep red cells. *J. Gen. Physiol.*, 44:169–194.

161. Vogt, C., and Vogt, O. (1937): Sitz und Wesen der Krankheiten im Lichte der topistischen Hirnforschung und des Variierens der Tiere. *Journal für Psychologie und Neurologie (Leipzig)*, 47:237–457.

162. Wieloch, T. (1985): Neurochemical correlates to selective neuronal vulnerability. *Progr. Brain Res.*, 63 (*in press*).

163. Wieloch, T. (1985): Hypoglycemia-induced neuronal damage is prevented by a N-methyl-D-aspartate receptor antagonist. *Science* (*in press*).

164. Wieloch, T., Auer, R. N., Westerberg, E., Tossman, U., Ungersted, U., and Engelsen, B. (1985): Hypoglycemic brain damage is mediated by excitotoxins. In: *Excitatory Amino Acids*, edited by P. Roberts. Macmillan Press, London. (*in press*.)

165. Wieloch, T., Engelsen, B., Westerberg, E., and Auer, R. (1985): Lesions of the glutamatergic cortico-striatal projections ameliorate hypoglycemic brain damage in the striatum. *Neurosci. Lett.*, 58:25–30.

166. Wieloch, T., Harris, R. J., Symon, L., and

Siesjö, B. K. (1984): Influence of severe hypoglycemia on brain extracellular calcium and potassium activities, energy and phospholipid metabolism. *J. Neurochem.,* 43:160–168.

167. Wieloch, T., and Siesjö, B. K. (1982): Ischemic brain injury: The importance of calcium lipolytic activities, and free fatty acids. *Path. Biol.,* 30:269–277.

168. Willmore, L. J., and Rubin, J. J. (1981): Antiperoxidant pretreatment and iron-induced epileptiform discharges in the rat: EEG and histopathologic studies. *Neurology (N.Y.),* 31:63–69.

169. Wolfe, L. S. (1982): Eicosanoids: Prostaglandins, thromboxanes, leukotrienes, and other derivatives of carbon-20 unsaturated fatty acids. *J. Neurochem.,* 38:1–14.

170. Yanagihara, T. (1980): Phosphorylation of chromatin proteins in cerebral anoxia and ischemia. *J. Neurochem.,* 35:1209–1215.

171. Yanagihara, T., and McCall, J. T. (1982): Ionic shift in cerebral ischemia. *Life Sci.,* 30:1921–1925.

Advances in Neurology, Vol. 44, edited by
A. V. Delgado-Escueta, A. A. Ward, Jr.,
D. M. Woodbury, and R. J. Porter.
Raven Press, New York © 1986.

42

Cell Damage in Epilepsy and the Role of Calcium in Cytotoxicity

Brian S. Meldrum

Department of Neurology, Institute of Psychiatry, De Crespigny Park, London, SE5 8AF, United Kingdom

SUMMARY Status epilepticus may be followed by the loss of selectively vulnerable neurons in the hippocampus and neocortex. The acute cytopathology preceding cell loss is that of "ischemic cell change" or "dark cell change." In the hippocampus, selectively vulnerable neurons (CA3 and CA1 pyramidal neurons, hilar polymorphic neurons) show swelling of mitochondria in the perikaryon and dendrites after 30 to 120 min of seizure activity. Electron-microscopic studies with the combined oxalate/pyroantimonate technique reveal dense calcium pyroantimonate deposits in the swollen mitochondria. Suppression of seizure activity for 30 to 60 min is sufficient to allow recovery of normal mitochondrial morphology and calcium load. A small proportion of vulnerable neurons develop ischemic cell change with multiple vacuoles containing calcium pyroantimonate deposits.

Neurons prone to burst firing accumulate calcium during seizures, and eventually show massive "overloading" of mitochondria. Although by analogy with studies in muscle a cytotoxic role for raised cytosolic calcium concentration has been proposed, the link between increased $[Ca^{2+}]$ activation of phospholipases and proteinases and ichemic cell change remains uncertain.

Atrophy of the hippocampus, neocortex, and cerebellum in the brains of patients with chronic epilepsy was first described by Bouchet and Cazauvieilh (5). A detailed description of the selective neuronal loss in the hippocampus was first given by Sommer (38). In the same year (1880), it was proposed by Pfleger (30) that the lesions found in patients with epilepsy were the consequence of local vascular or metabolic disturbance associated with the seizures. The similarity in the type of cellular change observed acutely after ischemia and after status epilepticus and the overall similarity in the pattern of selective vulnerability in the two circumstances led Spielmeyer (39), Scholz (34,35), and Peiffer (27) to conclude that focal ischemia and local metabolic insufficiency (as implied, for example,

in the concept of "consumptive hypoxia") during or directly after seizure activity were the causes of the pathology (24).

Measurements of cerebral metabolic rate ($CMRO_2$ and CMR_{glu}) during seizures in animals and man [reviewed by Chapman (7)] show that $CMRO_2$ increases up to two- to threefold. CMR_{glu} increases in parallel to, or in excess of, $CMRO_2$, so that lactate and pyruvate accumulate. Cerebral blood flow (CBF) commonly increases proportionately more than the increase in metabolism, so that there is an "arterialization" of venous blood, as originally described by Penfield during direct observation of focal cortical seizures (28). However, as a consequence of (a) arterial hypotension occurring late in prolonged status epilepticus or (b) the devel-

opment of focal edema, CBF may be locally insufficient relative to the increased cerebral metabolism. Such phenomena contribute to focal
pathology occurring in the cerebral and cerebellar cortex along the arterial boundary zones
(e.g., the junction in the cerebellar cortex of the
territories supplied by the anterior cerebellar artery and the posterior superior cerebellar artery). However, experimental studies in rats and
baboons show that acute neuronal cytopathology and subsequent neuronal loss can occur in
selectively vulnerable neurons in relation to seizures in which there is no overall or regional
impairment of CBF (9,22). The acute neuronal
pathology appears to be directly linked to the
excessive neuronal activity and is not dependent
on systemic physiological changes. The pattern
and evolution of the cellular changes is closely
similar to that induced by excitotoxins (such as
kainate, ibotenate, and folate) (see Chapter 43).
A characteristic feature of the cytopathology is
swelling of mitochondria in dendrites and soma
associated with accumulation of calcium in the
mitochondria (see below). The substantial evidence that an increase in cytosolic calcium contributes to cell death in cardiac and vascular
smooth muscle in ischemia (11,23,44) has led to
the suggestion that the increase in cytosolic calcium during seizure activity could be the critical
mechanism leading to the appearances of ischemic cell change and subsequent nerve cell loss
(21,22). This chapter describes the accumulation
of calcium in selectively vulnerable neurons
during seizures, the reversibility of this accumulation, and the possible role of calcium in determining the appearances of ischemic cell
change and neuronal loss.

INTRACELLULAR [Ca²⁺] AND ITS REGULATION

Extracellular $[Ca^{2+}]$ is approximately 1.3 mM,
as determined by ion-sensitive electrodes (see
Chapter 32). Intracellular $[Ca^{2+}]$ can be estimated by a variety of indirect and direct
means, including fluorescent indicators such as
aequorin and Quin-2 (2), and more recently by
intracellular microelectrodes (1). These indicate
a basal $[Ca]_i$ near 100 nM. Ca^{2+} thus passively
enters the cell down gradients of concentration
and potential.

At resting membrane potential there is only
a small Ca^{2+} entry (leakage Ca^{2+} current),
but with depolarization, voltage-sensitive Ca^{2+}
channels open, producing a depolarizing action
and, if the density of Ca^{2+} channels is sufficient,
creating a regenerative calcium spike.

To balance this entry, an outward Ca^{2+} pump
operates, with ATP providing the energy to
transport Ca^{2+} against the electrochemical gradient. Inside the cell there are numerous Ca^{2+}
buffering systems. These include proteins that
can bind Ca^{2+}, most notably calmodulin and calcium-binding protein. The latter has a regional
distribution in the hippocampus that may be significant for events in epilepsy (high in dentate
granule cells, low in CA3 neurons) (3,16). Various organelles can take up calcium. These include the endoplasmic reticulum, vesicular
structures, the nucleus, and the mitochondria.

Intracellular calcium (not bound to protein)
can be visualized at the electron-microscopic
(EM) level by a combined oxalate/pyroanti-
monate method (4,42). In control material
(12,13), the most prominent calcium pyroantimonate deposits occur in the synaptic vesicles
(Fig. 1). Presynaptic vesicles apparently provide
an important regulatory system, because with
increased synaptic activity the exocytotic delivery of Ca^{2+} is increased.

Mitochondrial calcium entry and efflux has
been extensively studied *in vitro* (26). Ca^{2+} uptake is influenced by $[Ca^{2+}]$ and pH and is dependent on mitochondrial respiration. Ca^{2+} efflux is also related to $[Ca^{2+}]$ and to $[Na^+]_o$. The
$[Ca^{2+}]$ at which influx and efflux are equal provides a set point. This set point tends to be situated above the local $[Ca^{2+}]_i$ for neurons, so that
at rest the mitochondria are not accumulating
Ca^{2+}.

SEIZURE ACTIVITY AND THE INTRACELLULAR ACCUMULATION OF CALCIUM

Measurements of extracellular $[Ca^{2+}]$ using
ion-sensitive electrodes in cortex or hippocampus (see Chapter 32) show that a decrease
in $[Ca^{2+}]_o$ occurs at or before the onset of burst
firing and that it becomes maximal within a few
seconds, reaching a stable level at one- to two-
thirds of control level in the presence of sustained seizure activity. In neurons showing burst
firing, there is a massive influx of Ca^{2+} associated with the paroxysmal depolarizing shift and
the slower spikes occurring later in the bursts
(18,43).

This influx exceeds the capacity of the plasma
membranes to transport Ca^{2+} outward, so that
Ca^{2+} progressively accumulates. $[Ca^{2+}]_o$ is
maintained constant (at a reduced level) by the
entry of Ca^{2+} from plasma.

Studies with the oxalate/pyroantimonate procedure in animals exposed to sustained seizures

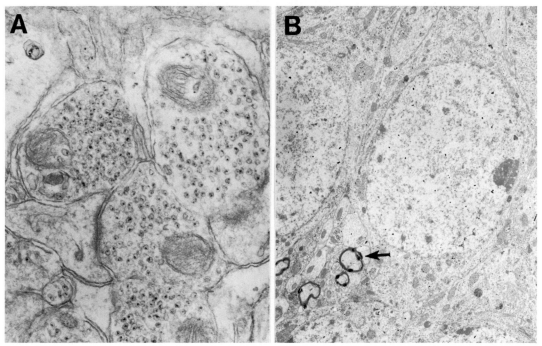

FIG. 1. Control rat hippocampus perfused with Karnovsky's fixative containing potassium oxalate and subsequently treated with osmium tetroxide–pyroantimonate, producing electron-dense calcium pyroantimonate deposits. **A:** Neuropil in CA1, showing calcium deposits in synaptic vesicles. ×50,400. (From ref. 13, with permission.) **B:** Dentate granule cells, with fine calcium deposits in the nuclei. *Arrow* indicates splitting of myelin lamellae, with deposits in the splits. ×6,300.

induced with bicuculline, allylglycine, or kainic acid (10–14) show increased calcium pyroantimonate deposits predominantly in those neurons that show burst firing. These deposits are most marked in swollen mitochondria in the cell bodies of CA3 neurons but are also evident in CA1 pyramidal neurons and in some hilar polymorphic neurons. They are not seen in dentate granule cells. In some pyramidal neurons, dilation of the endoplasmic reticulum and of the Golgi apparatus occurs, often with calcium pyroantimonate deposits in the swollen spaces.

Swollen perineuronal astrocytic processes occur throughout the pyramidal cell layer and also subjacent to the dentate granule cells. These swollen processes often contain calcium pyroantimonate deposits.

In the neuropil, the deposits in synaptic vesicles are relatively less prominent than in control material, and there is a tendency for the vesicles to clump together. However, in particular laminae of the basal and apical dendrites there are focal swellings that contain grossly distended mitochondria, filled with dense pyroantimonate deposits. The focal swellings are usually spher-

ical or ovoid, and it is sometimes possible to identify in one section two focal swellings separated by a dendritic branch with normal appearances (see Fig. 4B in ref. 25). Excitatory synapses are commonly identifiable (as asymmetric synaptic junctions) on the focal swellings (see Fig. 3).

With the exception of the severest form of dark cell change (shown in Fig. 2B), all the above appearances are acutely reversible. Thus if after 60 or 90 min of seizure activity sufficient diazepam is administered to suppress cortical paroxysmal activity and the brain is perfused subsequently, then the time course of recovery of each of the types of change can be followed (10,14).

Swelling of perineuronal astrocytic processes is largely absent after 30 min of seizure suppression but persists slightly longer in the hilar region. Mitochondrial swelling and the associated calcium pyroantimonate deposits disappear after 30 to 60 min (both in pyramidal cell soma and in focal swellings on basal dendrites). The only abnormality still seen after 1 or 4 hr is dark cell change (including vacuoles with calcium de-

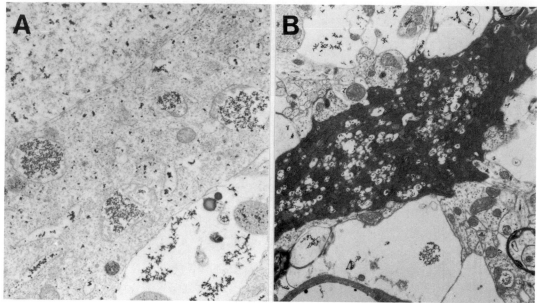

FIG. 2. Rat hippocampus perfusion fixed (oxalate/pyroantimonate technique) after 2 hr of seizure activity induced by L-allylglycine. **A:** Calcium pyroantimonate deposits are prominent in the nucleus, in swollen mitochondria and dilated endoplasmic reticulum of a CA3 pyramidal neuron, and in the adjacent swollen astrocytic process. ×21,600. **B:** A shrunken electron-dense pyramidal neuron ("dark cell change," "ischemic cell change") is surrounded by grossly swollen astrocytic processes. Calcium pyroantimonate deposits are evident in the neuron within microvacuoles, whose fine structural origin is uncertain. Deposits occur free within the astrocytic processes. ×9,900.

posits) involving a small number of neurons in the hilar region and scattered in the CA3 and CA1 zones.

CALCIUM ENTRY AND ISCHEMIC BRAIN DAMAGE

During acute hypoxia or ischemia, $[Ca^{2+}]_o$ in cortex or hippocampus falls rapidly at the time of cessation of electrical activity (due to opening of voltage-sensitive Ca^{2+} channels) (15). The increase in intracellular $[Ca^{2+}]$ is apparently buffered by binding to protein; no increase in calcium pyroantimonate deposits is seen (36). However, during the reperfusion phase after moderately prolonged forebrain ischemia there is accumulation of Ca^{2+} in neurons that is initially (at 30 min) nonselective, involving dentate granule cells and pyramidal neurons.

Subsequently, once electrical activity is returning, a selective pattern emerges, with granule cells appearing normal, and pyramidal neurons in CA3 and CA1 showing a progressive accumulation of calcium. This can probably be attributed to burst firing occurring in these pyramidal neurons, with initial repolarization.

Thus, the common factor leading to similar patterns of acute neuronal change and similar selective vulnerability in the hippocampus may be the occurrence of burst firing with high Ca^{2+} entry.

An important role for excitatory neurotransmitters in the induction of ischemic brain damage is indicated by recent experiments showing that 2-amino-7-phosphonoheptanoate, an antagonist of excitation at the N-methyl-D-aspartate-preferring receptor, protects against acute neuronal changes induced by forebrain ischemia (37).

There is a type of delayed neuronal death after transient ischemia, which affects the CA1 pyramidal neurons in gerbils and rats, that in terms of the sequence of morphological change is totally unlike ischemic cell change. It exhibits a different physiopathogenesis in which cell death is preceded by proliferation of endoplasmic reticulum and by peripheral chromatolysis and not by mitochondrial swelling (17,29).

CALCIUM CYTOTOXICITY AND ISCHEMIC CELL CHANGE

There is substantial experimental evidence indicating a role for calcium cytotoxicity in myo-

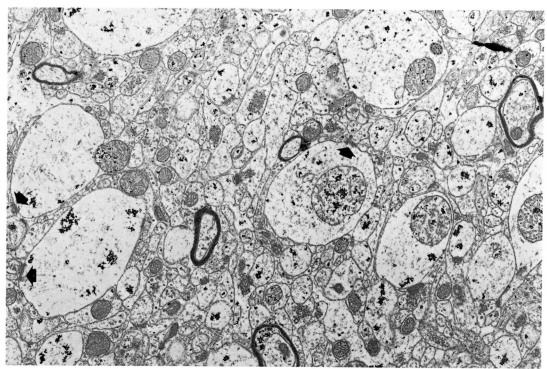

FIG. 3. Neuropil in the outer part of the stratum oriens in the CA3 region of the hippocampus after 2 hr of seizure activity induced by L-allylglycine. Calcium pyroantimonate deposits are prominent within swollen mitochondria and free in focal swellings on basal dendritic branches. Asymmetric (excitatory) synaptic terminals (*arrows*) are identifiable in the focal swellings. × 12,800.

pathic changes associated with ischemia or toxic myopathies. Thus, in *in vitro* experiments, low $[Ca^{2+}]$ or calcium entry blockers protect against ischemic damage in cardiac muscle and experimental myopathies. Enhancement of calcium entry by the ionophore A 23187 causes mitochondrial swelling and myofibrillar degeneration in muscle fibers (31). Myopathic changes induced by glutamate and other excitatory agonists are also calcium-dependent (8,19,20).

Activation of phospholipase A_2, of phosphokinases, and of various proteinases by raised $[Ca^{2+}]$ can be demonstrated in *in vitro* assays. Among peptidases and proteinases, some are activated by "low $[Ca^{2+}]$" (equivalent to 50 μM, or several hundred times basal cytosolic $[Ca^{2+}]$) and some are activated by "high $[Ca^{2+}]$" (>0.5 mM, i.e., equivalent to extracellular $[Ca^{2+}]$). The calcium-activated protease responsible for degradation of neurofilaments requires high $[Ca^{2+}]$ (>0.5 mM) (33). Activation of phospholipase A_2 by increased Ca^{2+} is presumably responsible for the progressive accumulation of free fatty acids during seizures (6). These enzyme activations could account for the loss of structural detail and the specific staining reac-

tions observed during "coagulative necrosis" or ischemic cell change (e.g., the enhanced eosinophilia relate to the increase in free fatty acids). However, direct proof that an increase in cytosolic $[Ca^{2+}]$ is a necessary and sufficient cause for ischemic cell change in neurons is lacking. The experiments illustrated here demonstrate a correlation between calcium accumulation in mitochondria (in vulnerable neurons) and the occurrence of ischemic cell change (in a proportion of the affected neurons). However, the two phenomena could be parallel but independent consequences of burst firing. Experiments that show protection of the brain against hypoxia or ischemia by calcium entry blockers (40,41) do not establish a critical involvement of calcium entry in neuronal pathology as many other effects are significantly involved (e.g., on blood viscosity, vascular smooth muscle, etc.) (23). A recent study employing dissociated hippocampal neurons in culture suggests that excitotoxin damage is dependent on external $[Cl^-]$ but not on external $[Ca^{2+}]$ (32).

In summary, a massive entry of calcium into selectively vulnerable neurons occurs during seizure activity. Within the first few minutes, enhanced cytosolic $[Ca^{2+}]$ activates phospholipase A_2 (6), and within 30 to 60 min mitochondria become distended and progressively loaded with calcium. However, as long as the cell is capable of generating ATP by oxidative metabolism, then the cytopathology is reversible. The critical event determining irreversibility in the progression to ischemic cell change remains unknown.

ACKNOWLEDGMENTS

I thank my colleagues Dr. T. Griffiths, Dr. M. C. Evans, and Dr. A. G. Chapman for their collaboration and the Wellcome Trust for financial support.

REFERENCES

1. Alvarez-Leefmans, F. J., Rink, T. J., and Tsien, R. Y. (1981): Free calcium ions in neurones of *Helix aspersa* measured with ion-selective microelectrodes. *J. Physiol.*, 315:531–548.
2. Ashley, R. H., Brammer, M. J., and Marchbanks, R. (1984): Measurement of intrasynaptosomal free calcium by using the fluorescent indicator quin-2. *Biochem. J.*, 219:149–158.
3. Baimbridge, K. G., Miller, J. J., and Parkes, C. O. (1982): Calcium-binding protein distribution in the rat brain. *Brain Res.*, 239:519–525.
4. Borgers, M., Thorné, F., and van Neuten, J. M. (1981): Subcellular distribution of calcium and the effects of calcium-antagonists as evaluated with a combined oxalate–pyroantimonate technique. *Acta Histochem. [Suppl.] (Jena)*, 24:327–332.
5. Bouchet, C., and Cazauvieilh, P. (1825): De l'épilepsie considerée dans ses rapports avec l'aliénation mentale. *Archives Générales de Médecine (Paris)*, 9:510–542.
6. Chapman, A. G. (1981): Free fatty acid release and metabolism of adenosine and cyclic nucleotides during prolonged seizures. In: *Neurotransmitters, Seizures and Epilepsy,* edited by P. L. Morselli, K. G. Lloyd, W. Löscher, B. Meldrum, and E. H. Reynolds, pp. 165–173. Raven Press, New York.
7. Chapman, A. G. (1984): Cerebral energy metabolism and seizures. In: *Recent Advances in Epilepsy.* II, edited by T. Pedley and B. S. Meldrum, pp. 19–63. Churchill Livingstone, Edinburgh.
8. Donaldson, P. L., Duce, I. R., and Usherwood, P. N. R. (1983): Calcium accumulation precedes the degenerative effects of L-glutamate on locust muscle fibres. *Brain Res.*, 274:261–265.
9. Evans, M. C., Griffiths, T., and Meldrum, B. S. (1983): Early hippocampal changes in the rat following bicuculline and L-allylglycine-induced seizures: A light and electron microscope study. *Neuropathol. Appl. Neurobiol.*, 9:39–52.
10. Evans, M. C., Griffiths, T., and Meldrum, B. S. (1984): Kainic acid seizures and the reversibility of calcium loading in vulnerable neurons in the hippocampus. *Neuropathol. Appl. Neurobiol.*, 10:285–302.

11. Farber, J. L. (1981): The role of calcium in cell death. *Life Sci.*, 29:1289–1295.
12. Griffiths, T., Evans, M. C., and Meldrum, B. S. (1982): Intracellular sites of early calcium accumulation in the rat hippocampus during status epilepticus. *Neurosci. Lett.*, 30:329–334.
13. Griffiths, T., Evans, M. C., and Meldrum, B. S. (1983): Intracellular calcium accumulation in rat hippocampus during seizures induced by bicuculline or L-allylglycine. *Neuroscience*, 10:385–395.
14. Griffiths, T., Evans, M. C., and Meldrum, B. S. (1984): Status epilepticus: The reversibility of calcium loading and acute neuronal pathological changes in the rat hippocampus. *Neuroscience*, 12:557–567.
15. Harris, R. J., Symon, L., Branston, N. M., and Bayhan, M. (1981): Changes in extracellular calcium activity in cerebral ischemia. *J. Cereb. Blood Flow Metab.*, 1:203–210.
16. Jande, S. S., Maber, L., and Lawson, D. E. M. (1981): Immunohistochemical mapping of vitamin-D-dependent calcium-binding protein in brain. *Nature (Lond.)*, 294:765–767.
17. Kirino, T., and Sano, K. (1984): Fine structural nature of delayed neuronal death following ischemic in the gerbin hippocampus. *Acta Neuropathol. (Berl.)*, 62:209–218.
18. Krnjević, K., Morris, M. E., and Reifenstein, R. J. (1980): Changes in extracellular Ca^{2+} and K^+ activity accompanying hippocampal discharges. *Can. J. Physiol. Pharmacol.*, 58:579–583.
19. Leonard, J. P., and Salpeter, M. M. (1979): Agonist induced myopathy at the neuromuscular junction is mediated by calcium. *J. Cell Biol.*, 82:811–819.
20. Leonard, J. P., and Salpeter, M. M. (1982): Calcium-mediated myopathy at neuromuscular junctions of normal and dystrophic muscle. *Exp. Neurol.*, 76:121–138.
21. Meldrum, B. S. (1981): Metabolic effects of prolonged epileptic seizures and the causation of epileptic brain damage. In: *Metabolic Disorders of the Nervous System,* edited by F. C. Rose, pp. 175–187. Pitman Medical Press, London.
22. Meldrum, B. S. (1983): Metabolic factors during prolonged seizures and their relation to nerve cell death. In: *Advances in Neurology, Vol. 34: Status Epilepticus: Mechanisms of Brain Damage and Treatment,* edited by A. V. Delgado-Escueta, C. G. Wasterlain, D. M. Treiman, and R. J. Porter, pp. 261–276. Raven Press, New York.
23. Meldrum, B. S. (1984): Calcium entry blockers and cerebral function: Introduction. In: *Calcium Entry Blockers in Cardiovascular and Cerebral Dysfunctions,* edited by T. Godfraind, A. Hermann, and D. Wellens, pp. 207–219. Raven Press, New York.
24. Meldrum, B. S., and Corsellis, J. A. N. (1984): Epilepsy. In: *Greenfield's Neuropathology, 4th ed.,* edited by W. Blackwood and J. A. N. Corsellis, pp. 921–950. Arnold, London.
25. Meldrum B., Griffiths, T., and Evans, M. (1982): Hypoxia and neuronal hyperexcitability—A clue

to mechanisms of brain protection. In: *Protection of Tissues Against Hypoxia,* edited by A. Wauquier, M. Borgers, and W. K. Amery, pp. 275–286. Elsevier North Holland, Amsterdam.

26. Nicholls, D., and Akerman, K. (1982): Mitochondrial calcium transport. *Biochim. Biophys. Acta,* 683:57–88.

27. Peiffer, J. (1963): *Morphologische Aspekte der Epilepsien.* Springer, Berlin.

28. Penfield, W., von Santha, K., and Cipriani, A. (1939): Cerebral blood flow during induced epileptiform seizures in animals and man. *J. Neurophysiol.,* 2:257–267.

29. Petito, C. K., and Pulsinelli, W. A. (1984): Delayed neuronal recovery and neuronal death in rat hippocampus following severe cerebral ischemia: Possible relationship to abnormalities in neuronal processes. *J. Cereb. Blood Flow Metab.,* 4:194–205.

30. Pfleger, L. (1880): Beobachtungen über schrumpfung und sklerose des ammonshorns bei epilepsie. *Allgemeine Zeitschrift für Psychiatrie,* 36:359–365.

31. Publicover, S. J., Duncan, C. J., and Smith, J. L. (1978): The use of A23187 to demonstrate the role of intracellular calcium in causing ultrastructural damage in mammalian muscle. *J. Neuropathol. Exp. Neurol.,* 37:554–557.

32. Rothman, S. (1984): Synaptic release of excitatory amino acid neurotransmitter mediates anoxic neuronal death. *J. Neurosci.,* 4:1884–1891.

33. Schlaepfer, W. W., and Freeman, L. A. (1980): Calcium-dependent degradation of mammalian neurofilaments by soluble tissue factor(s) from rat spinal cord. *Neuroscience,* 5:2305–2314.

34. Scholz, W. (1951): *Die Krampfschadigungen des Gehirns.* Springer, Berlin.

35. Scholz, W. (1959): The contribution of patho-anatomical research to the problem of epilepsy. *Epilepsia (Amsterdam),* 1:36–55.

36. Simon, R. P., Griffiths, T., Evans, M. C., Swan, J. H., and Meldrum, B. S. (1984): Calcium overload in selectively vulnerable neurons of the hippocampus during and after ischemia: An EM study in the rat. *J. Cereb. Blood Flow Metab.,* 4:350–361.

37. Simon, R. P., Swan, J. H., Griffiths, T., and Meldrum, B. S. (1984): Blockade of N-methyl-D-aspartate receptors may protect against ischemic damage in the brain. *Science,* 226:850–852.

38. Sommer, W. (1980): Erkrankung des ammonshornes als aetiologisches moment der epilepsie. *Archiv für Psychiatrie und Nervenkrankheiten,* 10:631–675.

39. Spielmeyer, W. (1927): Die pathogenese des epileptischen krampfes. *Zeitschrift für die gesamte Neurologie und Psychiatrie,* 109:501–520.

40. Steen, P. A., Newberg, L. A., Milde, J. H., and Michenfelder, J. D. (1984): Cerebral blood flow and neurologic outcome when nimodipine is given after complete cerebral ischaemia in the dog. *J. Cereb. Blood Flow Metab.,* 4:82–87.

41. Van Reempts, J., and Borgers, M. (1982): Morphological assessment of pharmacological brain protection. In: *Protection of Tissues against Hypoxia,* edited by A. Wauquier, M. Borgers, and W. K. Amery, pp. 263–274. Elsevier Biomedical, Amsterdam.

42. Wick, S. M., and Kepler, P. K. (1982): Selective localization of intracellular Ca^{2+} with potassium antimonate. *J. Histochem. Cytochem.,* 30:1190–1204.

43. Wong, R. K. S., and Prince, D. A. (1978): Participation of calcium spikes during intrinsic burst firing in hippocampal neurons. *Brain Res.,* 159:385–390.

44. Wrogemann, K., and Pena, S. D. J. (1976): Mitochondrial calcium overload: A general mechanism for cell-necrosis in muscle diseases. *Lancet,* i:672–674.

Advances in Neurology, Vol. 44, edited by
A. V. Delgado-Escueta, A. A. Ward, Jr.,
D. M. Woodbury, and R. J. Porter.
Raven Press, New York © 1986.

43

Excitotoxic Mechanisms of Epileptic Brain Damage

*John W. Olney, *Robert C. Collins, and **Robert S. Sloviter

*Departments of Psychiatry, Pathology and Neurology, Washington University, St. Louis, Missouri 63110; and **Neurology Center, Helen Hayes Hospital, West Haverstraw, New York, and College of Physicians and Surgeons, Columbia University, New York, New York 10032*

SUMMARY It is well established that the putative excitatory neurotransmitters, glutamate (Glu) and aspartate (Asp), are neurotoxins that have the potential of destroying central neurons by an excitatory mechanism. Kainic acid (KA), a rigid structural analog of Glu, powerfully reproduces the excitatory neurotoxic (excitotoxic) action of Glu on central neurons and, in addition, causes sustained limbic seizures and a pattern of seizure-linked brain damage in rats that closely resembles that observed in human epilepsy. In the course of studying the seizure-related brain damage syndrome induced by KA, we observed that a similar type of brain damage occurs as a consequence of sustained seizure activity induced by any of a variety of methods. These included intraamygdaloid or supradural administration of known convulsants such as bicuculline, picrotoxin and folic acid, or systemic administration of lithium and cholinergic agonists or cholinesterase inhibitors that have not commonly been viewed as convulsants. We have further observed that this type of brain damage can be reproduced in the hippocampus by persistent electrical stimulation of the perforant path, a major excitatory input to the hippocampus that is thought to use Glu as transmitter. It is a common feature of all such neurotoxic processes that the acute cytopathology resembles the excitotoxic type of damage induced by Glu or Asp, which is acute swelling of dendrites and vacuolar degeneration of neuronal soma, without acute changes in axons or axon terminals. We have found that the seizure–brain damage syndrome induced by cholinergic agents can be prevented by pretreatment with atropine and that the syndrome induced by any of the above methods, cholinergic or noncholinergic, can be either prevented or aborted respectively by either pre- or posttreatment with diazepam.

Our findings in experimental animals may be summarized in terms of their potential relevance to human epilepsy as follows. Sustained complex partial seizure activity consistently results in cellular damage if allowed to continue for longer than 1 hr. Hippocampal, or Ammon's horn, sclerosis is the primary pathological result. It may be a priority goal, therefore, in the management of human epilepsy to control such seizure activity within very narrow limits. This proposal is discussed in terms of three major transmitter systems that may be involved: cholinergic, GABAergic, and glutamergic/aspartergic.

The cholinergic system may play a role in generating or maintaining this type of seizure activity, and anticholinergics may protect against it provided they are given prior to commencement of behavioral seizures.

We propose that GABAergic circuits, as a result of excessive Glu/Asp bombardment, may be impaired early in the course of limbic complex partial seizures, and that by disinhibiting seizure circuits this may contribute importantly to the maintenance of seizure activity and severity of brain damage. Pharmaceutical approaches that promote GABAergic inhibition are quite promising prophylactically, since by suppressing seizure activity they also reduce the exposure of GABAergic neurons to Glu/Asp excitotoxic bombardment and, in general, decrease the chances that excitotoxic brain damage will occur.

In addition to such roles as Glu and Asp may play in epileptogenesis, we propose that the excitotoxic activity of these endogenous transmitters is responsible for much of the cellular damage associated with sustained seizures. It is possible that specific antagonists of excitatory amino acid receptors might protect against seizure-mediated brain damage. Recent evidence suggests that such antagonists suppress certain types of seizures in rats and prevent excitotoxins from destroying neurons in the rodent hypothalamus.

Excitatory transmission in the mammalian central nervous system is thought to be mediated primarily by the acidic amino acids, glutamate and aspartate, and these agents are probably the only central nervous system transmitters that have an exclusively excitatory action. Acetylcholine, also a major central nervous system transmitter candidate, is predominantly an excitant, but exerts inhibitory action at some synapses. It has been known for years that glutamate and aspartate, in addition to being neuronal excitants, have excitotoxic properties (i.e., excitation-related neurotoxicity). We have shown that either systemic or intraamygdaloid administration of cholinergic agonists or cholinesterase inhibitors results in sustained seizure activity and a pattern of acute brain damage resembling that known to occur in human epilepsy. We have also observed that a similar pattern of brain damage occurs as a consequence of sustained seizures induced by any of several methods, and in each case the cytopathological changes resemble the excitotoxin type of cellular damage induced by glutamate or aspartate. On the basis of these and related findings, we propose that both of these major excitatory transmitter systems may participate in the pathogenesis of epilepsy-related brain damage, the cholinergic system contributing to initiation and/or maintenance of seizure activity and the glutamate/aspartate system being uniquely responsible for the excitotoxic destruction of central neurons. Here we review evidence supporting this hypothesis.

FOUNDATIONS OF THE EXCITOTOXIC CONCEPT

The excitatory properties of acidic amino acids were first explored systematically in the 1960s by Curtis and Watkins (10), who found that glutamate, aspartate, and certain of their structural analogs excite neuronal firing when administered microiontophoretically onto the dendrosomal surfaces of spinal neurons. Whereas glutamate and aspartate were moderately (and equally) potent as neuronal excitants, some of their neuroactive analogs were substantially more potent. In subsequent studies the excitatory actions of glutamate and aspartate have been demonstrated in nearly every region of the central nervous system, and additional analogs with glutamate/aspartate-like excitatory properties have been found, as have agents that specifically antagonize these properties (59). Several classes of excitatory amino acid receptors have now been described based primarily on electrophysiological responses of single neurons to agonists and/or antagonists (11); ligand-binding experiments have further contributed to an understanding of glutamate/aspartate receptor systems (7). Absence of an extracellular enzyme system for inactivating the excitatory actions of glutamate or aspartate caused early researchers to discount a transmitter role for these agents, but the discovery in brain of special uptake mechanisms capable of rapid removal of glutamate or aspartate from the synaptic cleft (25) eliminated this objection and rendered tenable the now widely held belief that glutamate and aspartate may be the transmitters released at the majority of excitatory synapses in the mammalian central nervous system (for recent reviews, see ref. 11,60).

In 1957, Lucas and Newhouse reported (26) that subcutaneous administration of glutamate to suckling mice results in acute degeneration of neurons in the inner layers of the retina. In a series of studies (reviewed in refs. 34,36), Olney and colleagues confirmed this finding and observed, in addition, that either oral or subcutaneous administration of glutamate to animals of various species causes acute necrosis of neurons in or near certain brain regions that lack blood-brain barriers (circumventricular organs). In molecular specificity studies (44), these authors found that the specific glutamate analogs identified by Curtis and Watkins (10,60) as neuroexcitants reproduce the neurotoxic effects of glutamate on circumventricular organs when administered systemically to immature mice, that these analogs display a parallel order of potencies for their excitatory and toxic actions, that analogs lacking excitatory activity also lack neurotoxicity, and that specific antagonists of the excitatory activity of glutamate and its analogs effectively protect against their neurotoxicity (46). In ultrastructural studies (33,44), it was observed that the toxic action of glutamate and its analogs impinge selectively upon dendrosomal portions of the neuron which house the excitatory receptors through which the depolarizing effects of glutamate putatively are mediated (Fig. 1). These initial observations led to the "excitotoxic" hypothesis (34,44,49) that a depolarization mechanism underlies glutamate

neurotoxicity and that the toxic action may be mediated through dendrosomal synaptic receptors specialized for glutamergic or aspartergic neurotransmission.

THE DENDROSOMATOTOXIC/ AXON-SPARING NATURE OF AN EXCITOTOXIN LESION

The type of brain damage induced by excitotoxins has been termed "dendrosomatotoxic/ axon-sparing" because of the striking early changes that occur in dendrosomal components, while axons passing through or terminating in the lesioned area (Fig. 1) remain quite normal in appearance (34). This description accurately depicts the cytopathological changes observed either in retina (32) or circumventricular organ brain regions (33,44) following systemic excitotoxin administration or in any region of the central nervous system following direct injection of an excitotoxin (Fig. 2). The latter point was first documented in a 1975 report (47) describing this type of lesion induced in rat brain by direct intradiencephalic injection of cysteine-*S*-sulfonic acid, an excitotoxin that accumulates in body

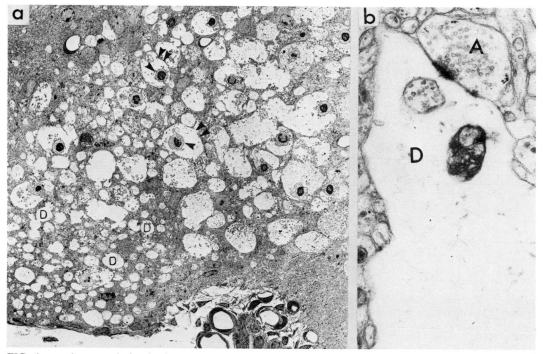

FIG. 1. **a:** An acute lesion in the arcuate nucleus of the hypothalamus resulting from oral administration of glutamate to an infant mouse 5 hr previously. Note endematous swelling of dendrites (D) and neuronal cell bodies (*double arrows*) and pyknotic nuclear changes (*single arrow*). ×500. **b:** A magnified view from mouse hypothalamus of a normal axon (A) in synaptic contact with a swollen degenerating dendrite (D) 30 min after systemic glutamate injection. ×20,000. (From ref. 36, with permission.)

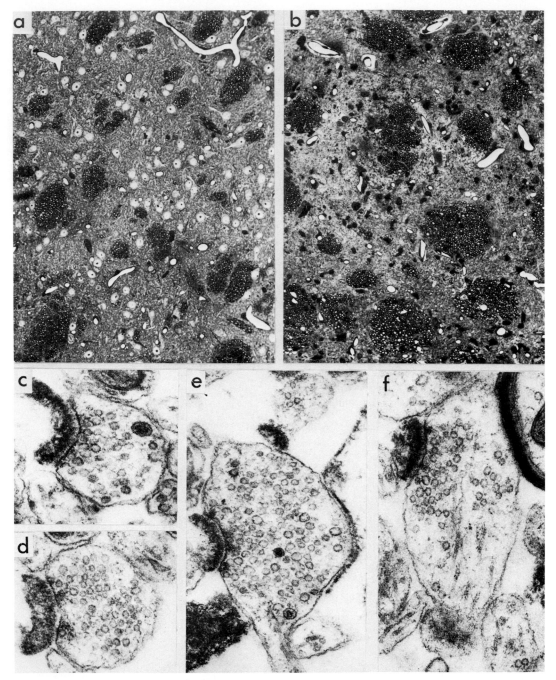

FIG. 2. **a:** Light-microscopic view of the adult rat neostriatum 21 days following microinjection of GABA (1 µmol). Note the normal appearance of neuronal cell bodies and all other tissue components. ×250. **b:** Adult rat neostriatum 21 days following microinjection of glutamate (1 µmol). Note the absence of neuronal cell bodies and presence of numerous dark cells, most of which are glia. Note also the preservation of axonal bundles. ×250. **c–f:** These synaptic complexes are characteristic of those abundantly present in the striatum up to 3 wk after excitotoxin injection, in this case kainic acid (10 nmol). The presynaptic axon terminals appear quite normal and remain attached to postsynaptic receptor fragments severed from dendrosomal plasma membranes of striatal neurons, which have degenerated and disappeared from the scene. ×50,000. Modified from Olney (35).

tissues as an aberrant metabolite implicated in the human neurodegenerative condition, sulfite oxidase deficiency. It was then shown (35,49) that glutamate itself and several of its more potent excitotoxic analogs (homocysteic acid, *N*-methylaspartic acid, and kainic acid), when injected into the brain, induce a local dendrosomatotoxic/axon-sparing lesion (Fig. 2), with each agent displaying a toxic potency proportional to its known excitatory potency. Because of the dendrosomatotoxic/axon-sparing character of the excitotoxin lesion, several of the more potent excitotoxins—especially kainic acid, ibotenic acid, and *N*-methylaspartic acid—have been widely used in recent years as axon-sparing lesioning agents for removing neuronal groups from a given brain region without disturbing axons passing through or terminating in the region (8,13).

KAINIC ACID: AN ENIGMATIC EXCITOTOXIN

Although kainic acid, a particularly powerful excitant (53) and neurotoxin (48), resembles other excitotoxins in producing a dendrosomatotoxic/axon-sparing local lesion when injected directly into brain, this agent is a unique excitotoxin, especially with regard to its convulsant properties and tendency to induce an apparently seizure-linked pattern of disseminated lesions in brain regions distant from the injection site (1,16,43,52). Following injection of kainic acid either systemically (10–12 mg/kg s.c.) or intracranially (1–3 nmol), adult rats display seizures that are primarily referrable to the limbic system and that behaviorally resemble fully kindled amygdaloid seizures. Staring, head bobbing, and wet dog shakes occur early, and these behaviors correlate with electrographic discharge activity recorded from depth electrodes in the ventral hippocampus (3). This is followed by episodes of rearing on hindlimbs with peroral frothing and head and forepaw clonus. These "rearing, praying, salivating" episodes recur repetitively with increasing frequency until there is little or no respite between seizure episodes (limbic status epilepticus).

Predictably, after approximately 1 hr of such seizure activity, histological examination of the brain reveals acute cytopathological changes in various limbic and closely related brain regions (piriform and entorhinal cortices, hippocampus, lateral septum, and several thalamic and amygdaloid nuclei). In each of these regions, the acute neuropathological reaction has similar ultrastructural characteristics—it consists of massive edematous swelling of neuronal dendrites (see Fig. 14) and either swelling or dark cell degeneration of neuronal cell bodies, while axon terminals in synaptic contact with these degenerating dendrosomal elements retain a normal appearance (3,43,52). Clearly, there is a resemblance between these neuronal changes and the excitotoxin-type dendrosomatotoxic/axon-sparing cytopathology described above. These changes are accompanied by dramatic edematous swelling of glial cells that lie in the immediate vicinity of the specific neuronal elements undergoing degeneration (17,35,52).

As several authors have noted (1,3,30,31), the pattern of damage induced by kainic acid closely resembles that associated with human temporal-lobe epilepsy (6). This is true for the pattern of damage induced by either systemic or intracranial application of kainic acid, with the important exception that direct injection of kainic acid into brain causes damage at the local injection site in addition to the seizure-linked pattern of disseminated lesions. Diazepam prevents both the seizures and the brain damage induced by systemic kainic acid (17) and prevents the seizures and disseminated but not local damage induced by intraamygdaloid kainic acid (1). In addition to these observations made in rats, it has been demonstrated in baboons that intracranial administration of kainic acid results not only in local damage but in sustained seizures and a disseminated distant pattern of brain damage (30).

tool in epilepsy research, its apparent ability to induce brain damage both directly by an excitotoxic mechanism and indirectly by a seizure mechanism poses interpretational problems. Since both the local lesions and disseminated seizure-related lesions induced by kainic acid have the same dendrosomatotoxic/axon-sparing character (compare Figs. 2 and 3), it might be argued that the disseminated lesions are not seizure-mediated, but rather result from kainic acid migrating to the distant site and destroying neurons by its direct excitotoxic action. Assuming that the disseminated lesions are indeed seizure-mediated, as the bulk of evidence suggests (36), it is puzzling that they have the same cytopathological characteristics as a lesion induced by direct exposure to an excitotoxin. To resolve the interpretational conundrum presented by the kainic acid model and to further explore the relationship between sustained seizures and disseminated lesions, we have pursued several alternate approaches for inducing seizure-related brain damage.

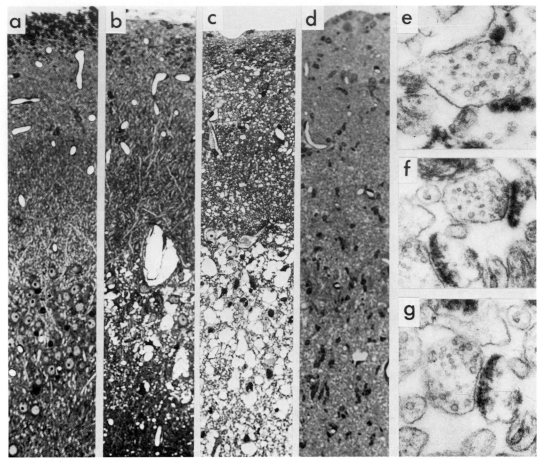

FIG. 3. Characteristics of a typical distant lesion induced in the rat piriform cortex by kainic acid injection into the diencephalon. **a:** Saline control. **b:** Early changes (primarily swelling of dendrites and glia) 4 hr after kainic acid. **c:** More advanced degenerative changes, including necrosis of piriform cortical neurons, 24 hr after intradiencephalic injection of kainic acid. **d:** Absence of piriform cortical neurons and replacement by glia 1 week after kainic acid. **e–g:** Electron micrographs from the piriform cortical region 1 week after intradiencephalic injection of kainic acid showing intact axon terminals which have adherent postsynaptic receptor densities, but absent from the scene are the dendrosomal elements that previously housed these receptors. Magnification: **a–d,** ×280; **e–g,** ×50,000. Modified from Olney (36).

TREATMENT CONDITIONS THAT RESULT IN SUSTAINED SEIZURES AND EXCITOTOXIN-LIKE DISSEMINATED LESIONS

Intraamygdaloid or Intrastriatal Folic Acid

Prompted by the report of Ruck et al. (50) that methyltetrahydrofolate competes powerfully for kainic acid binding, we injected several folate compounds into the rat amygdala or striatum and found that although methyltetrahydrofolate was rather weak, certain other folates, including folic acid itself, were very effective in causing sustained limbic seizure activity and a dissemi-nated pattern of seizure-related brain damage without inducing local damage (41,42) (Fig. 4). The ability of folic acid to induce seizure-related distant lesions without damage at the local injection site has been confirmed by McGeer et al. (28). Diazepam pretreatment blocks the seizures and seizure-related brain damage induced by folic acid (18), just as it blocks the seizure-related brain damage syndrome induced by kainic acid (17). Folic acid thus exemplifies a convulsant that, like kainic acid, induces sustained seizures and distant brain damage but that lacks the kainic acid property of destroying neurons by a direct (local) toxic action; it follows that the distant toxicity of folic acid cannot readily be explained by its diffusion to distant vulnerable sites, since once having diffused there, it lacks direct toxic action.

Whether a common receptor mediates the actions of kainic acid and folic acid, as postulated by Ruck et al., has been disputed. Others (14) have been unable to confirm that methyltetrahydrofolate competes for kainic acid binding. Our findings do not support the proposal that a folate receptor mediates the excitotoxic (direct) neurodestructive action of kainic acid, but it remains to be clarified whether common mechanisms might underlie the sustained seizure activity and disseminated lesions that both agents induce. Clifford and colleagues (2) and McLennan et al. (29) recently reported that folates and kainic acid have similar excitatory effects in hippocampal slice preparations, and in an earlier study Davies and Watkins (12) demonstrated microiontophoretically that folic acid augments the excitatory actions of either glutamate or acetylcholine on rat cerebrocortical neurons. The convulsant properties of folic acid, first reported by Hommes and Obbens (22), and associated brain damage that we now demonstrate, are of potential clinical interest in view of evidence that the administration of folic acid to epilepsy patients sometimes results in an increase in seizure frequency (57).

Systemic Dipiperidinoethane or Intraamygdaloid DPE-di-*N*-oxide

In other studies related to seizure-related brain damage phenomena, we have reexamined and expanded upon our previous observation (40) that dipiperidinoethane (DPE), an agent not structurally related to kainic acid, mimics the seizure-related brain damage effects of kainic acid when administered subcutaneously to adult rats. Since DPE did not reproduce this syndrome when injected in very high doses into the amygdala, we initially proposed that a metabolite generated peripherally might be responsible for the central toxicity. Synthesis of several DPE analogs by J. F. Collins recently permitted an investigation of this possibility. We found (37) that an oxidized derivative, DPE-di-*N*-oxide, which structurally resembles the cholinergic agonist oxotremorine, does induce a kainic acid-like seizure-related brain damage syndrome when injected into the amygdala (Fig. 5).

Intraamygdaloid Cholinergic Agonists or Cholinesterase Inhibitors

Pursuing the suggestion in our DPE-di-*N*-oxide findings that a cholinergic mechanism might underlie the seizure-related brain damage induced by DPE, we injected several cholinergic agonists and cholinesterase inhibitors into the rat amygdala (basolateral nucleus) and found that each class of agent caused a seizure-related brain damage syndrome (38) (Fig. 6). By preliminary analysis, the syndrome induced by DPE-di-*N*-oxide or known cholinomimetics appears to be folate-like, rather than kainic acid-like, in that it consists of seizures and a distant dissem-

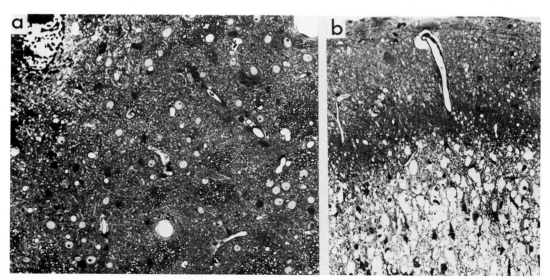

FIG. 4. Distant lesion in the rat piriform cortex (**b**) 22 hr after injection of folic acid (150 nmol) into the striatum (**a**). Note that striatal neurons in **a** close to the injection site (**upper left corner**) appear normal, whereas piriform cortical neurons in **b** are acutely necrotic. ×240. (From ref. 36, with permission.)

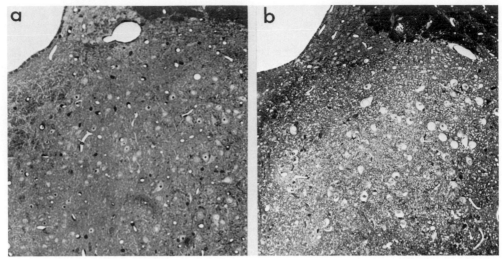

FIG. 5. Light-micrographic scene from the mediodorsal nucleus of the thalamus of adult rat brain 4 hr following intraamygdaloid administration of saline (a) or DPE-di-*N*-oxide (b). Note that mediodorsal neurons appear swollen with pyknotic nuclei in **b** compared to their normal appearance in **a**. This thalamic nucleus receives fiber projections from the site of DPE-di-*N*-oxide injection (basolateral amygdaloid nucleus) and from nearby olfactory cortical structures, which are activated in this seizure brain-damage syndrome. The saline-treated animal remained behaviorally normal, whereas the DPE-di-*N*-oxide-treated animal displayed repetitive rearing, praying seizures for several hours prior to sacrifice. ×200. (From ref. 37, with permission.)

inated pattern of brain damage in the absence of local damage at the injection site. The most consistently effective and potent cholinergic agent we have tested is the cholinesterase inhibitor neostigmine, which causes a well developed seizure-related brain damage syndrome in 100% of animals receiving 4 nmol by microinjection into the basolateral amygdala. Thus, neostigmine has approximately the same potency as kainic acid for inducing the seizure-related brain damage component of kainic acid neurotoxicity, and it achieves this without inducing local damage at the injection site. Of the cholinergic agonists tested, carbachol was the most consistently effective, and we found that atropine blocks the seizure-related brain damage syndrome induced by carbachol. It should be mentioned that Wasterlain et al. (59) have used intraamygdaloid carbachol successfully in the rat to produce a model of amygdaloid kindling, and the convulsant properties of carbachol have been known for years (20,27).

Systemic Cholinergic Agonists or Cholinesterase Inhibitors in Lithium-Pretreated Rats

Honchar, Olney, and Sherman (23) recently demonstrated that certain cholinergic agonists or cholinesterase inhibitors, when administered

subcutaneously, induce a seizure-related brain-damage syndrome closely resembling the one that kainic acid induces by subcutaneous administration, provided the rat is pretreated with lithium (Fig. 7). The role of lithium in this syndrome remains to be elucidated; if rats are pretreated with lithium chloride (2–3 meq/kg s.c.) and 24 hr later given pilocarpine (20–30 mg/kg s.c.), a severe seizure-related brain-damage syndrome develops, which, if not interrupted by diazepam treatment, is uniformly lethal after 5 to 10 hr of status epilepticus. By comparison, Turski et al. reported very recently (58), and we have confirmed (J. W. Olney and J. Labruyere, *unpublished results*), that a seizure-related brain damage syndrome can be induced in rats by intraperitoneal treatment with pilocarpine alone (Fig. 8), but it requires a dose of 400 mg/kg and the syndrome is not uniformly lethal. Thus, by an unknown mechanism lithium permits pilocarpine to induce a severe seizure-related brain-damage syndrome at approximately one-twentieth the dose that would be required in the absence of lithium pretreatment. The lithium/cholinotoxic syndrome is prevented by either atropine or diazepam pretreatment. After the seizure activity is well established, atropine does not influence either the seizures or the brain-damage process, but diazepam arrests the seizures and attenuates the brain damage (45).

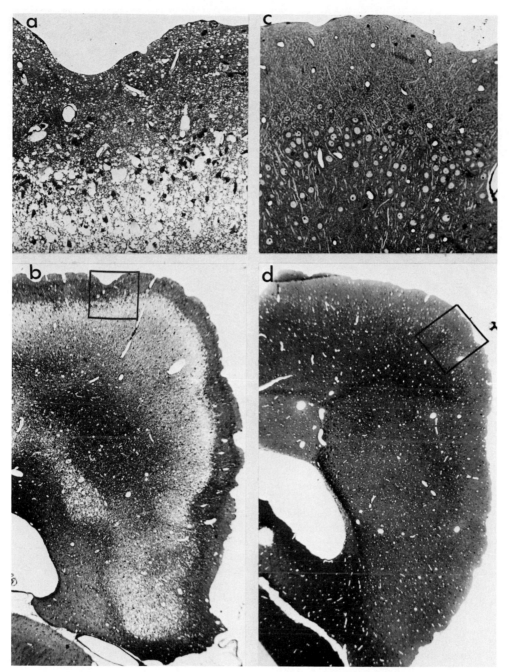

FIG. 6. The entorhinal–subicular region of adult rat brain 24 hr following intraamygdaloid injection of physostigmine, 25 nmol (**a** and **b**) or saline (**c** and **d**). Views **a** and **c** are magnified from the boxed regions in **b** and **d**, respectively. The agents were injected approximately 2 mm rostral to the scenes shown here. The pattern of acute brain damage in **b** resembles that associated with seizures induced by systemic administration of kainic acid, DPE or the cholinergic agonist pilocarpine (see Fig. 8). The rat in **b** had sustained limbic seizures for approximately 5 hr. Magnification: **a** and **c**, ×220; **b** and **d**, ×40. Modified from Olney et al. (38,45).

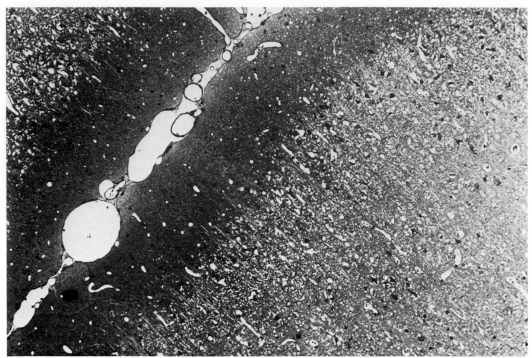

FIG. 7. Cingulate cortex of an adult rat treated with lithium chloride (3 meq/kg s.c.) and pilocarpine (30 mg/ kg s.c.) 30 hr and 6 hr prior to sacrifice, respectively. Superficial portions of the cortex, primarily layer I, are spared while layers II, III, and IV are diffusely involved in the toxic reaction. The acute reaction consists primarily of massive swelling of glial cells and neuronal dendrites with dark cell changes in neuronal somata. This rat displayed sustained complex partial seizure activity for 5 hr prior to sacrifice. ×100. (From ref. 45, with permission.)

Administering the cholinesterase inhibitor, physostigmine (0.4 mg/kg s.c.) to lithium-pretreated rats results in a seizure-related brain-damage syndrome that appears similar if not identical to that induced by lithium/pilocarpine treatment.

How closely the pattern of disseminated brain damage induced by systemic lithium/pilocarpine treatment resembles that induced by systemic kainic acid warrants further careful evaluation. Our preliminary observations suggest that the patterns are remarkably similar in general, but certain differences can be discerned. For example, although systemic kainic acid is known to damage the frontoparietal cerebral cortex (52,61) and substantia nigra (52), cellular degeneration in these regions is more consistently and more dramatically present following lithium/pilocarpine treatment. Conversely although the lithium/pilocarpine lesion pattern usually includes hippocampal damage, this is more consistently and dramatically a feature of kainic acid treatment. It is our impression that these differences are most clearly evident in animals

that have been examined after only 1 to 2 hr of seizure activity, whereas after 4 to 6 hr the patterns become indistinguishable. Thus, it is possible that some of the circuits activated initially in one syndrome are different from those activated initially in the other, but as either syndrome progresses to an advanced stage of status epilepticus, many if not all of the same limbic and related circuits become involved and the resulting patterns of brain damage become increasingly similar.

Our findings with cholinergic compounds signify that excessive stimulation of central cholinergic receptors, either by exogenous agonist or endogenous acetylcholine, is sufficient in itself to cause a seizure-related brain-damage syndrome resembling that caused by experimental convulsants such as kainic acid, folates, and DPE. Thus, the possibility that cholinergic mechanisms might play a contributory role in the seizure-related brain damage syndromes induced by these agents warrants consideration, as does the possibility that cholinergic mechanisms could play a role in human epileptogenesis, particularly genesis of the type of seizures that results in brain damage.

Convulsants Applied Topically to the Sensorimotor Cortex

Collins and Olney (5) recently reported that persistent focal motor seizure activity induced by topical (supradural) application of various convulsants (penicillin, folic acid, bicuculline, picrotoxin, or physostigmine) over the rat sensorimotor cortex results in glutamate-type (dendrosomatotoxic/axon-sparing) local lesions in specific thalamic nuclei that receive glutamergic innervation from cortical neurons involved in the seizure process (Fig. 9). We chose this particular preparation as an alternative to the limbic seizure model in an effort to facilitate interpretation of results: i.e., the system is anatomically simple and it is relatively well established that a specific neuronal pathway (cortico–thalamic) being primarily activated (Fig. 10) uses glutamate as transmitter (15). Our finding that persistent discharge activity in a glutamergic

pathway causes acute glutamate-type damage, localized to distant neurons being fired upon, strongly supports the hypothesis that endogenous glutamate may play a role in the cellular damage associated with seizures.

Reduced oxygen supply to the brain is an unlikely explanation for the thalamic lesions, since the focal seizure activity is restricted behaviorally to repetitive unilateral forearm jerking, which does not compromise respiratory function. Moreover, a relative oxygen or energy deficit at the local site of damage due to failure of energy resources to keep up with metabolic demand is also an unlikely explanation, since it does not account for the dendrosomatotoxic/axon-sparing nature of the lesion—i.e., why should a focal energy deficit spare metabolically active presynaptic terminals while destroying postsynaptic dendrosomal structures?

Sustained Perforant Path Stimulation

In recent studies (54,55), Solviter has demonstrated that persistent electrical stimulation of the perforant path (putative glutamergic excita-

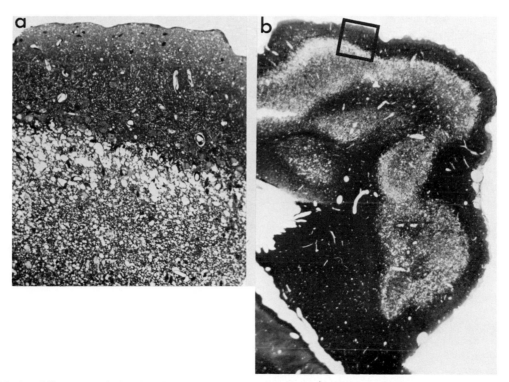

FIG. 8. Olfactory cortical and subicular region of adult rat brain 24 hr following subcutaneous administration of pilocarpine 400 mg/kg. The boxed region in **b** is shown at higher magnification in **a**. This rat displayed status limbic seizure activity for 6 hr following pilocarpine treatment. Magnification: **a**, ×180; **b**, ×30. (From J. W. Olney and J. Labruyere, *unpublished results.*)

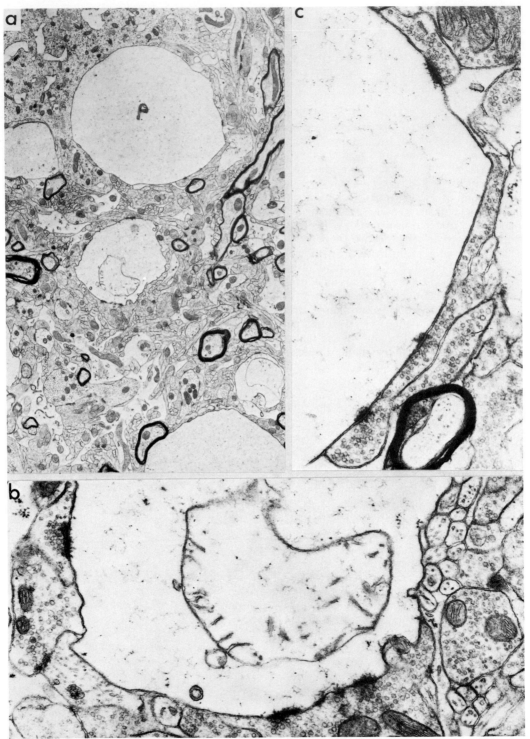

FIG. 9. **a:** Survey electron-microscopic view showing swollen processes in the ventrolateral nucleus of the thalamus after 2 hr of focal motor seizure activity induced by supradural application of folic acid over the sensorimotor cortex. ×2,000. **b, c:** Magnified views that reveal the dilated processes to be degenerating dendrites, which are in contact with normal appearing presynaptic axon terminals. These changes are indistinguishable from the dendrosomatotoxic reaction that characterizes glutamate neurotoxicity. ×32,000. (From ref. 5, with permission.)

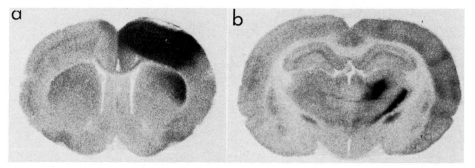

FIG. 10. When focal motor seizures are induced in the rat by instilling convulsants in a supradural well over the sensorimotor cortex, ^{14}C-deoxyglucose metabolism becomes greatly increased in the cortical focus and the pathways of seizure spread. **a:** This autoradiogram illustrates metabolic activation in the forelimb region of the rat sensorimotor cortex during intense penicillin-induced focal motor seizures expressed behaviorally as repetitive jerking of the contralateral forelimb. A slight increase in metabolism can also be seen in ipsilateral projections into dorsolateral caudate and in callosal pathways to contralateral cortex and caudate. **b:** There is increased metabolism in two ipsilateral thalamic nuclei, the ventrolateral nucleus, and the forelimb sector of the ventral basal complex. These are the same nuclei that show glutamate-type excitotoxic changes after several hours of focal motor seizures (see Fig. 9). (From ref. 5, with permission.)

tory input to the hippocampus) causes kainic acid-like electrophysiological and light-microscopic histopathological changes in the rat hippocampus (Fig. 11). By the twin pulse technique, Sloviter established (Fig. 12) that before epileptiform activity is recordable in the hippocampus of either kainic acid-treated (56) or perforant path-stimulated rats (54,55), there is a measurable loss of the recurrent inhibitory action that dentate granule neurons, through inhibitory interneurons, normally exert over their own firing. Impairment of this inhibitory mechanism may play a crucial role in status seizure phenomena, as it leads to disinhibited burst firing of dentate granule cells (in response to excitatory input that normally would not induce such firing), which in turn generates epileptiform activity that spreads in a relatively unimpeded manner throughout hippocampal and related limbic circuits. Collins and colleagues (4), using ^{14}C-deoxyglucose autoradiographic methods, have corroborated that the dentate gyrus initially restricts entry of seizures from entorhinal cortex into the rest of the hippocampus and that with persistent excitatory input this resistance is overcome (Fig. 13). Olney et al. have shown (39) by electron microscopy that the acute hippocampal cytopathology induced by perforant path stimulation is indistinguishable from the seizure-linked cytopathology induced in the hippocampus by kainic acid, folates, or cholinergic agents (Figs. 14 and 15), which in turn has the dendrosomatotoxic/axon-sparing characteristics of the lesions that any excitotoxin, including glutamate or aspartate, induces locally when injected into brain. An explanation for these sev-

eral correlations is suggested by the fact that persistent hippocampal discharge activity, a common denominator linking perforant path stimulation with kainic acid, folate, or cholinergic drug treatment, probably entails excessive release of endogenous excitotoxins (glutamate or aspartate) at many hippocampal synapses. The pattern of dendrosomal damage in each case (Fig. 15) follows a laminar distribution corresponding closely with putative glutamate/aspartate innervation patterns in the hippocampus (36,39,43).

DISCUSSION

In these studies we employed a wide variety of methods of inducing sustained seizure activity, a major goal being to ascertain to what extent seizure-related cytopathology occurs as an inevitable consequence of sustained seizures per se as opposed to other toxic mechanisms peculiar to a given method of inducing seizure activity. Some experiments were designed to clarify the possible involvement of specific transmitter systems in seizure-related brain damage phenomena. Since we were able to demonstrate that a specific type of cytopathological reaction—namely, an excitotoxic type of reaction—results from sustained seizures regardless of the inductory method employed, this type of reaction can reasonably be interpreted as a seizure-mediated phenomenon.

Whether the disseminated lesions induced by kainic acid are entirely seizure-mediated or are partially due to a direct toxic action of kainic acid is now a moot issue, since a similar if not

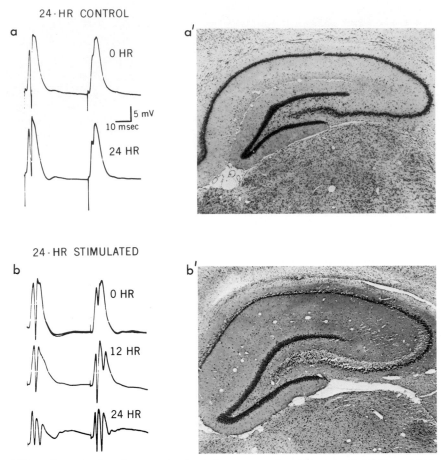

FIG. 11. Effect of sustained perforant path stimulation on granule cell recurrent inhibition and hippocampal structure. **a, a′**: Granule-cell-evoked potentials, recurrent inhibition and hippocampal structure of a "stimulated control" rat. Urethane anesthesia and electrical stimulation above the perforant path for 24 hr did not alter inhibition (ability of first granule-cell spike to inhibit the second spike) or structure. **b, b′**: The 24-hr-stimulated rat showing loss of recurrent inhibition and the selective pattern of morphological changes in the ipsilateral hippocampus. Dentate granule cells and CA2 pyramidal cells are relatively unaffected. ×30. (From ref. 54, with permission.)

identical brain damage syndrome can be induced by systemic convulsants that lack the kainic acid property of exerting a direct toxic action. Moreover, the kainic acid pattern of hippocampal damage is induced in its entirety by electrical stimulation of the perforant path, i.e., without exposing the hippocampus either to kainic acid or any other convulsant chemical. In addition, we have shown by two separate approaches, one employing chemical convulsants and the other electrical stimulation, that when excessive discharge activity is induced in a fiber path that uses glutamate as transmitter, it results in acute glutamate-type degeneration of the dendrosomal structures innervated by the glutamate fibers. Since the glutamate/aspartate type of cytopathology is a prominent feature of each seizure-re-

lated brain-damage syndrome we have examined, and the distribution of this pathology in each syndrome tends to conform to putative glutamate/aspartate innervation patterns (to the extent that these patterns are known), we propose that much of the cellular pathology associated with sustained seizure activity, regardless of the method of seizure induction, can be explained by seizure-mediated release (and inefficient reuptake) of either glutamate or aspartate at excitatory synapses.

It may be questioned whether excessive release of glutamate or aspartate would destroy postsynaptic neurons, considering the exceedingly efficient uptake processes in axon terminals and glia for inactivating glutamate or aspartate (21,25). We propose that continuous discharge activity through glutamate/aspartate axon terminals may represent a condition that compromises these homeostatic mechanisms— i.e., repetitive depolarization and repolarization of the axonal membrane may consume so much energy from the terminal that its reuptake process fails for want of energy to drive it. This might impair the uptake capacity enough to allow toxic concentrations of glutamate to accumulate in the synaptic cleft. While uptake of glutamate into glia might be expected to function as an auxiliary protective mechanism, glial uptake may also be impaired, since glia in the region of injury are grossly edematous and swollen—a pathological state possibly reflecting the deleterious effects of large amounts of potassium released by repetitively firing neurons (24).

If glutamate/aspartate excitatory receptors play a major role in seizure-related brain damage syndromes, as we propose, it follows that antagonists (11,60) that block synaptic transmis-

sion at these receptors may be useful in the prophylactic or therapeutic management of such syndromes. The most abundant glutamate/aspartate-type receptor in the central nervous system is thought to be the N-methylaspartate receptor. Croucher et al. (9) have shown that antagonists that preferentially block this receptor effectively suppress pentylenetetrazole or audiogenic seizures. Similarly, we have shown (46) that these antagonists protect circumventricular organ neurons against the direct neurotoxic actions of N-methylaspartate or glutamate. Thus, these glutamate/aspartate antagonists might protect against seizure-mediated brain damage by either or both of two mechanisms. They might act as anticonvulsants that suppress the contribution made by glutamate/aspartate transmission to the seizure process, or as antitoxins that, by blocking glutamate/aspartate receptors, prevent the excessive glutamate/aspartate released by persistent seizure activity from inducing receptor-mediated excitotoxic de-

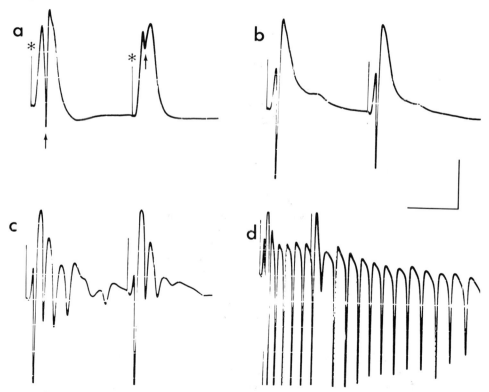

FIG. 12. Effect of kainic acid on recurrent inhibition and hippocampal granule-cell activity. Potentials recorded in the inner (or suprapyramidal) granule-cell layer were evoked by continuous twin stimuli (20 V, 0.1 msec duration, 2 Hz, 40 msec apart) to perforant path. **a:** Pre-drug control. *Asterisks* denote stimulus artifacts. Note that the second of the two granule cell population spikes (*arrows*) is smaller than the first, reflecting recurrent inhibition. **b:** At 50 min after the injection of kainic acid (10 mg/kg, i.v.). Note increased granule-cell spike amplitude and decreased recurrent inhibition. **c:** At 58 min. **d:** At 66 min after kainic acid. Note large amplitude, repetitive spikes. Also note reduced timebase in **d.** Calibration bars: 20 msec in **a, b,** and **c**; 40 msec in **d**; 10 mV in **a, b, c,** and **d.** Positivity upward. (From ref. 56, with permission.)

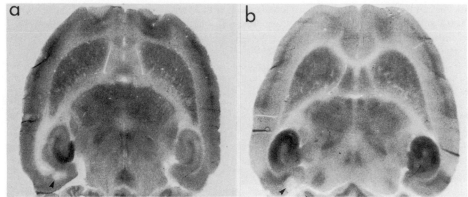

FIG. 13. **a**: A weak seizure focus in the entorhinal cortex (*arrow, left*) causes activation of the perforant path and increased metabolism confined to the ipsilateral dentate gyrus (compare with normal pattern on the right side). **b**: Strong electrical stimulation of the perforant path (*arrow*) induces prolonged seizures and intense activation of metabolism throughout bilateral limbic pathways, including the hippocampus major, septum, and midline thalamic nuclei (compare with **a**). (From ref. 4, with permission.)

generation of the postsynaptic neuron. Unfortunately, the unavailability of these antagonists in amounts necessary for *in vivo* animal testing has hampered their evaluation as clinically useful anticonvulsant/antitoxins.

Our emphasis on the glutamate-type excitotoxic mechanism does not rule out the participation of other mechanisms in the cell damage associated with seizures. Our aim is to identify those features of the cellular pathology that can readily be explained on this basis and single out for separate study those features that cannot. For example, the selective dendritic swelling with axonal sparing that we observed in the thalamus of rats undergoing focal cortical seizures is precisely the type of cytopathology observed in any excitotoxin-induced lesion, whereas a laminar pattern of axonal swelling detected in layer IV of sensory cortex in the same animals appears to be a different type of cytopathology (5).

Meldrum and colleagues (19; also see Chapter 42) have demonstrated that allylglycine induces a seizure-related brain-damage syndrome closely resembling the syndromes we describe here, and they attribute the cytopathological changes to an abnormal influx of calcium into postsynaptic dendrites and cell bodies. Schanne and associates (51) have exposed cultured hepatocytes to 10 different membrane-active cytotoxic agents in the presence or absence of calcium and have shown that these toxins are lethal to hepatocytes only in the presence of calcium. They postulate that regardless of the specific mechanism by which a toxin disrupts the integrity of the plasma membrane, an influx of cal-

cium across the damaged membrane, aided by a steep concentration gradient, is the final common pathway for toxic cell death.

As explanations for seizure-linked cell death, the calcium influx and excitotoxic proposals are not mutually exclusive hypotheses. When excessive glutamate is iontophoresed upon the surface of a central neuron, it leads first to accelerated firing, then transiently to a state of reversible depolarization block and finally (if application of glutamate is continued) to irreversible block and permanent electrical silence (10). It is not unlikely that these events entail pathological changes in plasma membrane permeability to various ions, including calcium. Thus, it is quite conceivable that an intrasynaptic accumulation of glutamate might trigger an abnormal dendrosomal influx of calcium, in which case both mechanisms would be operative as separate steps in the pathophysiology of this type of cell damage, the excitotoxic process as the primary membrane-toxic mechanism and calcium influx as a secondary mechanism, which either alone or together with other undetermined mechanisms destroys the cell.

Our demonstration of seizure-linked brain damage induced by cholinergic agonists raises the question of whether the cholinergic transmitter system has excitotoxic properties similar to those of glutamate, i.e., the property of destroying the postsynaptic neurons that house the transmitter's own receptor system. This intriguing question certainly warrants investigation. However, in view of our preliminary impression that cholinergic agonists when injected directly into brain induce distant damage without destroying local neurons, we tentatively suspect that cholinoceptive neurons serve as conduits of this toxic process without themselves undergoing degeneration. Since hyperstimulation of cholinoceptive neurons may secondarily lead to excessive activation of glutamergic (or aspartergic) neurons, this may explain the neuronal degeneration associated with cholinergically induced seizures. Indeed it seems quite likely that cholinoceptive neurons in some cases use glutamate or aspartate as

transmitter. This would represent the simplest mechanism by which persistent stimulation of cholinergic receptors might result in excessive release of glutamate or aspartate.

Concerning the role of cholinergic mechanisms either in experimental or human seizure-related brain damage syndromes, it is an interesting possibility that cholinergic circuits contribute to the pathophysiology in a manner that glutamate/aspartate circuits cannot; i.e., if excessive synaptic release of glutamate or aspar-

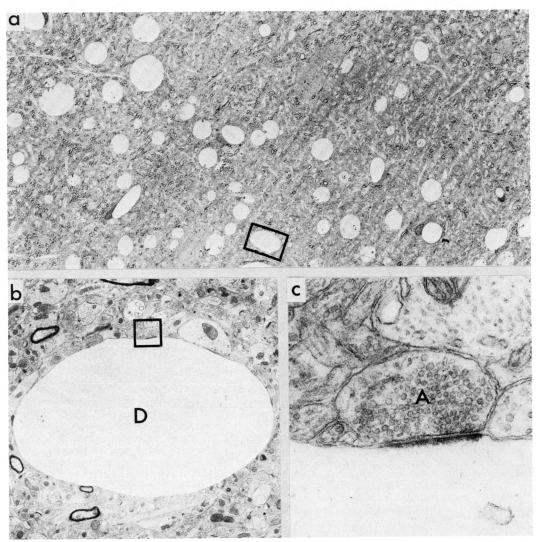

FIG. 14.   a: Survey view of the distal apical CA3 dendritic field showing numerous massively dilated dendritic segments after repetitive electrical stimulation of the perforant path. One of the swollen dendrites (D) in the boxed region is progressively magnified in **b** and **c** to show the normal appearance of an axon terminal (A) that makes asymmetric synaptic contact with the abnormal dendritic process. The pathological reaction in this region is entirely confined to specific dendritic structures that receive synaptic contacts such as the one shown in **c**, which we postulate are excitatory, glutamergic, and of perforant path origin. The surrounding neuropil is well preserved and shows no degenerative changes. Magnification: **a**, ×500; **b**, ×4,000; **c**, ×32,000. (From ref. 39, with permission.)

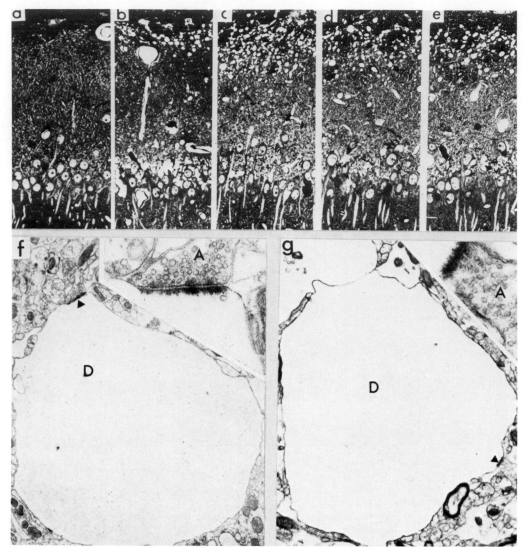

FIG. 15. Panels **a–e** are from the CA1 region of rat hippocampus; the pyramidal cells are at **bottom**, alveus at **top**, and stratum oriens (basilar dendritic field) in **between**. Treatment conditions were: **a**, control; **b**, kainic acid (12 mg/kg sc) 4 hr previously; **c**, perforant path stimulation for 2 hr; **d**, intraamygdaloid folic acid (25 nmol) 4 hr previously; **e**, lithium chloride (3 meq/kg s.c.) 1 day previously, then physostigmine (40 mg/kg sc) 4 hr prior to sacrifice. A characteristic acute seizure related brain damage reaction consisting of two laminar bands of edematous swollen structures is evident. Swollen elements in the pyramidal cell layer are glia, and those in the stratum oriens are massively dilated distal dendrites of CA1 pyramids. The swollen dendrites in the electron micrographs (**f** and **g**) are from the CA1 distal basilar dendritic field of the brains shown in **b** and **c** following kainic acid and perforant path stimulation, respectively. In each case, the postsynaptic dendrite (D) displays conspicuous edematous degenerative changes while the presynaptic axon (A) appears normal. Magnification: **a–e**, ×200; **f** and **g** ×8,000; **insets**, ×45,000. (From refs. 39, 41, 43, and 45, with permission.)

tate progresses rapidly to depolarization block, circuits employing these transmitters are an unlikely source of the sustained drive that keeps neurons firing for hours in status epilepticus. A neuron that has succumbed to depolarization block and electrical silence cannot serve as generator for continued seizure activity. If it were

an intrinsic characteristic of the cholinergic transmitter system to support discharge activity for hours without either the pre- or postsynaptic membrane breaking down, this system might play a crucial role in seizure-related brain damage phenomena—it might provide the sustained drive that keeps glutamate/aspartate neurons firing upon their postsynaptic members long enough to have pathological consequences. To increase the explanatory power of this hypothesis, one need only include the ubiquitous GABAergic inhibitory system and consider what the consequences would be if, early in the seizure process, GABAergic neurons lying postsynaptic to glutamate neurons are relentlessly fired upon and damaged such that their inhibitory functions are silenced. This would disinhibit the cholinergic drive mechanism and contribute powerfully to maintenance of sustained seizure activity.

Our findings in experimental animals may be summarized in terms of their potential relevance to human epilepsy as follows. Sustained complex partial seizure activity consistently results in cellular damage if allowed to continue for more than 1 hr. It may be a priority goal, therefore, in the management of human epilepsy to control such seizure activity within very narrow limits. We have discussed this proposal in terms of three major transmitter systems that may be involved.

Cholinergic system. This system may play a role in generating or maintaining this type of seizure activity, and anticholinergics may protect against it provided they are given prior to commencement of behavioral seizures. Thus, while anticholinergics may not be useful for arresting such seizures they conceivably could be employed in prevention.

GABAergic system. We postulate that GABAergic circuits, as a result of excessive glutamate/aspartate bombardment, may be impaired early in the course of limbic complex partial seizures and that this may contribute importantly to the maintenance of seizure activity. Consistent with this, we found diazepam, a potentiator of GABA's effects, highly effective in either preventing or arresting such seizures and, more importantly, in preventing seizure-linked brain damage. This confirms clinical experience regarding the efficacy of diazepam in arresting status epilepticus and suggests its potential value in preventing seizure-linked brain damage.

Glutamate/aspartate system. In addition to such roles as glutamate and aspartate may play in epileptogenesis, we propose that the excitotoxic activity of these agents is responsible for much of the cellular damage associated with sustained seizures. Whether specific antagonists of excitatory amino acid receptors might protect against seizure-linked brain damage warrants exploration in view of evidence that such antagonists are effective anticonvulsants against pentylenetetrazole or audiogenic seizures in rats (9)

and prevent excitotoxins from destroying neurons in the rodent hypothalamus (46).

ACKNOWLEDGMENTS

This work was supported in part by MH37967 and Research Scientist Award MH38894 (to J.W.O.), NS-14834 (to R.C.C.), and a grant from the Epilepsy Foundation of America (to R.S.S.).

REFERENCES

1. Ben-Ari, Y., Tremblay, E., Ottersen, O. P., and Naquet, R. (1979): Evidence suggesting secondary epileptogenic lesions after kainic acid: Pretreatment with diazepam reduces distant but not local brain damage. *Brain Res.,* 165:362–365.
2. Clifford, D. B., Lothman, E. W., and Ferrendelli, J. A. (1982): Effects of amino acid antagonists on epileptiform burst induced by folic acid and *N*-methyl-D,L-aspartic acid, in vitro. *Neurosci. Abst.,* 8:882.
3. Collins, R.C., Lothman, E. W., and Olney, J. W. (1983): Status epilepticus in the limbic system— Biochemical and pathological changes. In: *Advances in Neurology, Vol. 34: Status Epilepticus,* edited by A. V. Delgado-Escueta et al., pp. 277–288. Raven Press, New York.
4. Collins, R. C., Tearse, R. G., and Lothman, E. W. (1983): Functional anatomy of limbic seizures: Focal discharges from medial entorhinal cortex in rat. *Brain Res.,* 280:25–40.
5. Collins, R. C., and Olney, J. W. (1982): Focal cortical seizures cause distant thalamic lesions. *Science,* 218:177–179.
6. Corsellis, J. A. N., and Meldrum, B. S. (1976): Epilepsy. In: *Greenfield's Neuropathology, 3rd ed.,* edited by W. Blackwood and J. A. N. Corsellis, pp. 771–795. Arnold, London.
7. Coyle, J. T., Ferkany, J., Zaczek, R., Slevin, J., and Retz, K. (1983): Kainic acid: Insight into its receptor-mediated neurotoxic mechanisms. In: *Excitotoxins,* edited by K. Fuxe, P. Roberts, and R. Schwarcz, pp. 112–121. Macmillan, London.
8. Coyle, J. T., McGeer, E. G., McGeer, P. L., and Schwarcz, R. (1978): Neostriatal injections: A model for Huntington's chorea. In: *Kainic Acid As a Tool in Neurobiology,* edited by E. G. McGeer, J. W. Olney, and P. L. McGeer, pp. 139–159. Raven Press, New York.
9. Croucher, M. J., Collins, J. F., and Meldrum, B. S. (1982): Anticonvulsant action of excitatory amino acid antagonists. *Science,* 216:899–901.
10. Curtis, D. R., and Watkins, J. C. (1960): The excitation and depression of spinal neurons by structurally related amino acids. *J. Neurochem.,* 6:117–141.
11. Davies, J., Evans, R. H., Jones, A. W., Mewett, K. N., Smith, D. A. S., and Watkins, J. C. (1983): Recent advances in the pharmacology of excitatory amino acids in the mammalian central nervous system. In: *Excitotoxins,* edited by K. Fuxe, P. Roberts, and R. Schwarcz, pp. 43–54. Macmillan, London.

12. Davies, J., and Watkins, J. C. (1978): Facilitatory and direct excitatory effects of folate and folinate on single neurones of cat cerebral cortex. *Biochem. Pharmacol.*, 22:1667–1668.

13. Fuxe, K., Roberts, P., and Schwarcz, R. (editors). (1983): *Excitotoxins.* Macmillan, London.

14. Ferkany, J. W., Slevin, J. T., Zaczek, R., and Coyle, J. T. (1982): Failure of folic acid derivatives to mimic the actions of kainic acid in brain in vitro or in vivo. *Neurobehav. Toxicol. Teratol.*, 4:573–579.

15. Fonnum, F., Storm-Mathiesen, J., and Divac, I. (1981): Biochemical evidence for glutamate as neurotransmitter in corticostriatal and corticothalamic fibres in rat brain. *Neuroscience*, 6:863–873.

16. Fuller, T. A., and Olney, J. W. (1979): Effects of morphine or naloxone on kainic acid neurotoxicity. *Life Sci.*, 24:1793–1798.

17. Fuller, T. A., and Olney, J. W. (1981): Only certain anticonvulsants protect against kainate neurotoxicity. *Neurobehav. Toxicol. Teratol.*, 3:355–361.

18. Fuller, T. A., Olney, J. W., and Conboy, V. T. (1981): Diazepam markedly attenuates the neurotoxicity of folic acid. *Neurosci. Abst.*, 7:811.

19. Griffiths, T., Evans, M. C., and Meldrum, B. S. (1982): Intracellular sites of early calcium accumulation in the rat hippocampus during status epilepticus. *Neurosci. Lett.*, 30:329–334.

20. Grossman, S. P. (1963): Chemically induced epileptiform seizures in the cat. *Science*, 142:409–411.

21. Henn, F. A., Goldstein, M., and Hamberger, A. (1974): Uptake of the neurotransmitter candidate glutamate by glia. *Nature (Lond.)*, 249:663–664.

22. Hommes, O. R., and Obbens, E. A. M. T. (1972): The epileptogenic action of Na-folate in the rat. *J. Neurol. Sci.*, 16:271–281.

23. Honchar, M. P., Olney, J. W., and Sherman, W. R. (1983): Systemic cholinergic agents induce seizures and brain damage in lithium-treated rats. *Science*, 220:323–325.

24. Hosli, L., Andres, P. E., and Hosli, E. (1979): Depolarization of cultured astrocytes by glutamate and aspartate. *Neuroscience*, 4:1593–1598.

25. Logan, W. J., and Snyder, S. H. (1972): High affinity uptake systems for glycine, glutamic and aspartic acids in synaptosomes of rat central nervous tissues. *Brain Res.*, 42:413–431.

26. Lucas, D. R., and Newhouse, J. P. (1957): The toxic effect of sodium L-glutamate on the inner layers of the retina. *Arch. Ophthalmol.* 58:193–201.

27. MacLean, P. D., and Delgado, J. M. R. (1953): Electrical and chemical stimulation of frontotemporal portion of limbic system in the waking animal. *Electroencephalogr. Clin. Neurophysiol.*, 5:91–100.

28. McGeer, P. L., McGeer, E. G., and Nagai, T. (1983): GABAergic and cholinergic indices in various regions of rat brain after intracerebral injections of folic acid. *Brain Res.*, 260:107–116.

29. McLennan, H., Collingride, G. L., and Kehl, S. J. (1983): Electrophysiological actions of kainate and other excitatory amino acids, and the structure of their receptors. In: *Excitotoxins,*

edited by K. Fuxe, P. Roberts, and R. Schwarcz, pp. 19–32. Macmillan, London.

30. Menini, C., Meldrum, B. S., Riche, D., Silva-Comte, C., and Stutzmann, J. M. (1979): Sustained limbic seizures induced by intraamygdaloid kainic acid in the baboon: Symptomatology and neuropathological consequences. *Ann. Neurol.*, 8:501–509.

31. Nadler, J. V., Perry, B. W., and Cotman, C. W. (1978): Preferential vulnerability of hippocampus to intraventricular kainic acid. In: *Kainic Acid as a Tool in Neurobiology,* edited by E. G. McGeer, J. W. Olney, and P. L. McGeer, pp. 219–237. Raven Press, New York.

32. Olney, J. W. (1969): Glutamate-induced retinal degeneration in neonatal mice. Electron microscopy of the acutely evolving lesion. *J. Neuropathol. Exp. Neurol.*, 28:455–474.

33. Olney, J. W. (1971): Glutamate-induced neuronal necrosis in the infant mouse hypothalamus: An electron microscopic study. *J. Neuropathol. Exp. Neurol.*, 30:75–90.

34. Olney, J. W. (1978): Neurotoxicity of excitatory amino acids. In: *Kainic Acid as a Tool in Neurobiology,* edited by E. McGeer, J. W. Olney, and P. McGeer, Raven Press, New York.

35. Olney, J. W. (1979): Excitotoxic amino acids and Huntington's disease. In: *Advances in Neurology, Vol. 23: Huntington's Disease,* edited by T. N. Chase, A. Wexler, and A. Barbeau, pp. 609–624. Raven Press, New York.

36. Olney, J. W. (1983): Excitotoxins: An overview. In: *Excitotoxins,* edited by K. Fuxe, P. Roberts, and R. Schwarcz, pp. 82–96. Macmillan, London.

37. Olney, J. W., Collins, J. F., and deGubareff, T. (1982): Dipiperidinoethane neurotoxicity clarified. *Brain Res.*, 249:195–197.

38. Olney, J. W., deGubareff, T., and Labruyere, J. (1983): Seizure-related brain damage induced by cholinergic agents. *Nature (Lond.)*, 301:520–522.

39. Olney, J. W., deGubareff, T., and Sloviter, R. S. (1983): "Epileptic" brain damage in rats induced by sustained electrical stimulation of the perforant path. II. Ultrastructural analysis of acute hippocampal pathology. *Brain Res. Bull.*, 10:699–712.

40. Olney, J. W., Fuller, T. A., Collins, R. C., and deGubareff, T. (1980): Systemic dipiperidinoethane mimics the convulsant and neurotoxic actions of kainic acid. *Brain Res.*, 200:231–235.

41. Olney, J. W., Fuller, T. A., and deGubareff, T. (1981): Kainate-like neurotoxicity of folates. *Nature (Lond.)*, 292:165–167.

42. Olney, J. W., Fuller, T. A., deGubareff, T., and Labruyere, J. (1981): Intrastriatal folic acid mimics the distant but not local brain damaging properties of kainic acid. *Neurosci. Lett.*, 25:207–210.

43. Olney, J. W., Fuller, T., and deGubareff, T. (1979): Acute dendrotoxic changes in the hippocampus of kainate treated rats. *Brain Res.*, 176:91–100.

44. Olney, J. W., Ho, O. L., and Rhee, V. (1971): Cytotoxic effects of acidic and sulphur-containing

amino acids on the infant mouse central nervous system. *Exp. Brain Res.*, 14:61–76.

45. Olney, J. W., Honchar, M. P., and Sherman, W. R. (1983): Diazepam prevents lithium-pilocarpine neurotoxicity in rats. *Neurosci. Abst.*, 9:401.

46. Olney, J. W., Labruyere, J., Collins, J. F., and Curry, K. (1981): D-Aminophosphonovalerate is 100-fold more powerful than D-alpha-aminoadipate in blocking *N*-methylaspartate neurotoxicity. *Brain Res.*, 221:207–210.

47. Olney, J. W., Misra, C. H., and deGubareff, T. (1975): Cysteine-*S*-sulfate: Brain damaging metabolite in sulfite oxidase deficiency. *J. Neuropathol. Exp. Neurol.*, 34:167–176.

48. Olney, J. W., Rhee, V., and Ho, O. L. (1974): Kainic acid: A powerful neurotoxic analogue of glutamate. *Brain Res.*, 77:507–512.

49. Olney, J. W., Sharpe, L. G., and deGubareff, T. (1975): Excitotoxic amino acids. *Neurosci. Abst.*, 1:371.

50. Ruck, A., Kramer, S., Metz, J., and Brennan, M. J. W. (1980): Methyltetrahydrofolate is a potent and selective agonist for kainic acid receptors. *Nature (Lond.)* 287:852–853.

51. Schanne, F. A. X., Kane, A. B., Young, E. E., and Farber, J. L. (1979): Calcium dependence of toxic cell death: A final common pathway. *Science*, 206:700–702.

52. Schwob, J. E., Fuller, T., Price, J. L., and Olney, J. W. (1980): Widespread patterns of neuronal damage following systemic or intracerebral injections of kainic acid: A histological study. *Neuroscience*, 5:991–1014.

53. Shinozaki, H., and Konishi, S. (1970): Action of several anthelmintics and insecticides on rat cortical neurons. *Brain Res.*, 24:368–371.

54. Sloviter, R. S. (1983): "Epileptic" brain damage in rats induced by sustained electrical stimulation of the perforant path. I. Acute electrophysiological and light microscopic studies. *Brain Res. Bull.*, 10:675–697.

55. Sloviter, R. S., and Damiano, B. P. (1981): Sustained electrical stimulation of the perforant path duplicates kainate-induced electrophysiological effects and hippocampal damage in rats. *Neurosci. Lett.* 24:279–284.

56. Sloviter, R. S., and Damiano, B. P. (1981): On the relationship between kainic acid-induced epileptiform activity and hippocampal neuronal damage. *Neuropharmacology*, 20:1003–1014.

57. Smith, D. B., and Obbens, E. A. M. T. (1979): Antifolate-antiepileptic relationships. In: *Folic Acid in Neurology, Psychiatry, and Internal Medicine*, edited by M. I. Botez and E. H. Reynolds, pp. 267–283. Raven Press, New York.

58. Turski, W. A., Cavalheiro, E. A., Schwarz, M., Czuczwar, S. J., Kleinrok, Z., and Turski, L. (1983): Limbic seizures produced by pilocarpine in rats: Behavioural, electroencephalographic and neuropathological study. *Behav. Brain Res.*, 9:315–336.

59. Wasterlain, C. G., Masuoka, D., and Jonec, V. (1981): Chemical kindling: A study of synaptic pharmacology. In: *Kindling 2*, edited by J. A. Wada, pp. 315–329. Raven Press, New York.

60. Watkins, J. C. (1978): Excitatory amino acids. In: *Kainic Acid As a Tool in Neurobiology*, edited by E. McGeer, J. W. Olney, and P. McGeer, pp. 37–69. Raven Press, New York.

61. Zucker, D. K., Wooten, G. F., Lothman, E. W., and Olney, J. W. (1981): Neuropathological changes associated with intravenous kainic acid. *J. Neuropathol. Exp. Neurol.*, 40:324.

Advances in Neurology, Vol. 44, edited by
A. V. Delgado-Escueta, A. A. Ward, Jr.,
D. M. Woodbury, and R. J. Porter.
Raven Press, New York © 1986

44

The Accumulation of Free Arachidonic Acid, Diacylglycerols, Prostaglandins, and Lipoxygenase Reaction Products in the Brain During Experimental Epilepsy

Nicolas G. Bazan, Dale L. Birkle, Wilson Tang, and T. Sanjeeva Reddy

Louisiana State University Medical Center, LSU Eye Center, New Orleans, Louisiana 70112

SUMMARY   There has been increasing biochemical evidence since 1970 that one of the targets for convulsion-induced changes is the cell membrane of neurons. This is partly based on the observation that following seizures, there are increased levels of diacylglycerols and free fatty acids, which are products of the degradation of the major component of cell membranes, phospholipids. In addition, the production of prostaglandins from the free fatty acid, arachidonic acid, is activated after convulsions. This implies that alterations in the metabolism of lipids in brain are a major effect of seizures, and that the further study of these biochemical pathways may reveal important information pertinent to defining the basic mechanism of seizures and seizure-related pathology and may help in the development of potentially effective treatments.

   The effects of seizures on brain lipid metabolism and some recent studies from our laboratory are described in this chapter. Our results demonstrate that (a) in rat brain, dexamethasone—a phospholipase A_2 inhibitor—attenuates bicuculline-induced free fatty acid accumulation in a dose-dependent manner; (b) bicuculline-induced status epilepticus does not alter the activation (synthesis of arachidonoyl coenzyme A) or acylation of fatty acids as assayed *in vitro,* indicating that the availability of high-energy cofactors (ATP) may be the critical factor responsible for decreased fatty acid acylation *in vivo;* (c) bicuculline-induced fatty acid accumulation is localized mainly in the synaptosomal fraction of the rat brain; (d) induction of seizures in the rat by bicuculline treatment produces a marked stimulation of lipoxygenase activity in synaptosomes that, in turn, results in a large increase in the synthesis of hydroxyeicosatetraenoic acids (HETEs). This effect is also observed following membrane depolarization with 45 mM K^+, and (e) bicuculline-induced status epilepticus stimulates the synthesis of prostaglandin D_2. Possible mechanisms and consequences of alterations in specific lipids are described. Also, the possible involvement of a stimulated arachidonic acid cascade, particularly of hydroxylated products, in the release of neurotransmitters is discussed. Other aspects of the interaction between neurotransmission and the production of eicosanoids are reviewed.

   The metabolic pathways leading to the "lipid effect"—i.e., the production of free fatty acids, diacylglycerols, and arachidonic acid metabolites (eicosanoids)— are numerous and involve a wide variety of enzymes. The mechanism of this "lipid effect" may involve a seizure-induced overstimulation of normal lipid pathways that operate in neurotransmission. The physiological significance of phospholipids, diacylglycerols, and eicosanoids in neurotransmission is not well defined. However, overstimulation by convulsions may lead to receptor-mediated alterations in membrane lipids, membrane perturbation and/or changes in the lipid environmemt of key enzymes, and consequently, the production from lipid precursors of potential second messengers (e.g., eicosanoids, diacylglycerols, inositol 1,4,5-*tris*-phosphate). The synthesis and release of prostaglandins is stimulated by a variety of neurotransmitters and by nerve stimulation and has been localized to the neuronal and synaptosomal fraction of brain. A particular class of putative second messengers (diacylglycerols and inositol 1,4,5-*tris*-phosphate) are derived from phosphoinositides, a group of membrane phospholipids with active metabolism linked to receptor activation and cell signaling.

The release and accumulation of free fatty acids has characteristics of a specific, receptor-mediated process, but the mechanism of this effect is still unknown. The primary event, resulting in the "lipid effect," remains to be ascertained, as does the role of the "lipid effect" as a possible cause or effect of seizures. The profile of accumulated free fatty acids suggests that activation of phospholipase A_2 may be a key event. Alternatively, diacylglycerol lipase may release free fatty acids from diacylglycerol produced by a phospholipase C. The phosphoinositides may be the source of diacylglycerol and free arachidonic acid through either of these pathways. Diacylglycerol is a modulator of phospholipid- and calcium-dependent protein kinase C, and the other product, inositol 1,4,5-*tris*-phosphate, may serve as a signal for calcium mobilization from nonmitochondrial stores. Alterations as a consequence of changes in protein kinase C may lead to impaired function of specific phosphoproteins of excitable membranes. This is an area of exploration for the future. Close study of the "lipid effect" of seizures may provide information on possible endogenous pro- and anticonvulsants. While there remains a number of unanswered questions regarding the "lipid effect" of seizures, investigation of this problem should result in a better understanding of the role of the cell membrane and lipids in neurotransmission and the pathophysiology of convulsions.

The "lipid effect" of convulsions has opened new avenues for investigation into the basic mechanisms of epilepsy including:

1. Unraveling "in-membrane" events in molecular terms. Is the release of free fatty acids, particularly arachidonic acid, engaged in a selective receptor-mediated sequence of events in epilepsy?

2. Studies about the mechanism and consequences of the free fatty acid changes in various models of epilepsy. Is the released arachidonic acid a direct modulator of excitable membrane properties? Is the loss of the arachidonic acid from membrane phospholipids the "effector" in epilepsy or do the oxygenated metabolites (prostaglandins, hydroxyeicosatetraenoic acids, leukotrienes) play that role?

3. Role of prostaglandins and lipoxygenase leukotriene pathways in epilepsy. What is the role of the prostaglandins and lipoxygenase–leukotriene pathways in epilepsy? Are these changes the consequence of other central events or are they themselves the "mainstream" events?

4. Why are diacylglycerols enriched in stearate arachidonate accumulated in the brain of experimental animals undergoing convulsions? Is this a lipid effect related to the free fatty acid accumulation or is it independent? Is this change involved in the activation of modulators such as protein kinase C? Are polyphosphoinositides involved? Is a failure of cell signaling in molecular events the trigger mechanism for seizures?

5. Investigation into the endogenous promoters of epilepsy. Because the changes in brain free fatty acids and diacylglycerol are early events in experimental epilepsy and localized in the synapses, these experimental models may provide us with an unusual opportunity to investigate endogenous promoters of epilepsy and the formation of endogenous antiepileptics. In addition, the design and development of pharmacological substances more specific and effective for the treatment of epilepsy may be helped by these studies.

Research into the effects of seizures on lipid metabolism in the brain is relatively new. In 1970 it was observed that electroconvulsive shock elevates the level of free fatty acids, particularly arachidonic acid, in rat brain (12,21). Later it was shown that diacylglycerols enriched in the 1-stearoyl-2-arachidonoyl molecular species also accumulate during seizures (6,20). In addition, various convulsive stimuli increase the synthesis of the potent autocoids, prostaglandins, from arachidonic acid (64,104,148, 166,171). This chapter describes the effects of convulsions on lipid metabolism in the brain. The possible metabolic pathways and mechanisms involved in the accumulation of free arachidonic acid and diacylglycerols and the enzymatic oxygenation of arachidonic acid are discussed.

LIPIDS OF EXCITABLE MEMBRANES

The synaptic plasma membrane is composed of proteins, cholesterol and glycerolipids, as is the plasma membrane of all cells. However, the synaptic plasma membrane is unique in that it contains phospholipids highly enriched in polyunsaturated fatty acids, particularly arachidonic acid (20:4, *n*-6) and docosahexaenoic acid (22:6, *n*-3) (151,153). The synaptic plasma membrane participates in frequent exocytotic events, and polyunsaturated fatty acids may facilitate these processes by conferring a high degree of membrane fluidity. The occurrence of highly fluid membrane domains may be critical for receptor binding, lateral diffusion and internalization of proteins, and the transmission of signals from the exterior to the interior of the synaptic terminal or the postsynaptic effector cell (37,53, 92,93).

The lipid milieu of protein components of membranes is extremely important in the control of protein functions. For example, the lipid environment of receptors, ionic channels, and transport proteins can modify the degree of affinity and the number of binding sites (30, 127,128). Lipids, in addition to proteins, may form pores through the cell membrane. Polar lipids, such as phospholipids, have a strongly hydrophobic component (the fatty acyl chains) and a hydrophilic phosphate-base group. Different base groups have differing hydrophilicity; choline is extremely polar by virtue of its tertiary amine structure, while serine is less polar. Phospholipids are soluble in aqueous media by the formation of micelles; the nonpolar part of these molecules is oriented towards the interior of the micelle and the polar moieties face out-

ward in surface interaction with dipolar water. Inverted micelles are formed in nonpolar media. Ionic pores through the plasma membrane may be inverted micelles, stacked in a cylindrical fashion, with the polar groups acting as the "lumen" of the pore and the nonpolar groups providing the appropriate interaction with the membrane in which the pore resides (the hexagonal or H_{II} structure) (53). This hypothesis suggests that lipid composition plays an important role in the control of ion fluxes, because small alterations of either the polar or nonpolar part of phospholipids would result in changes in the structure and affinity of ionic pores.

The lipids of excitable membranes are metabolically active. Alterations in the content and composition of lipids may modulate the release, uptake, and postsynaptic effects of neurotransmitters. One example of this is the role that 20:4 and its oxygenated metabolites may play as regulators of neurotransmitter release and second messengers for the postsynaptic actions of neurotransmitters (13,16a,31,49,76,79,115, 140,143,163–165).

Very recently, it has been shown that nervous tissue is capable of synthesizing docosanoids, lipoxygenase-like metabolites, from docosahexaenoic acid (16a). Because electroconvulsive shock (12) and bicuculline-induced convulsions (20,24,130,142) promote the accumulation of free docosahexaenoic acid in the brain, docosanoids may be generated. Also, because lipoxygenase products from arachidonic acid are biologically very potent substances (see below), it is likely that the docosanoids may play physiological roles in excitable membranes, thereby showing specific functions for polyunsaturated fatty acids, as opposed to just playing a role in membrane fluidity. A critical issue is how oxygenated metabolites are produced by enzyme-mediated steps and the free radical peroxidation reactions. Perhaps when there is an overstimulation of the former and the latter is triggered, the onset of irreversible neuronal damage occurs.

FREE FATTY ACIDS AND
ACYL CHAINS OF
MEMBRANE PHOSPHOLIPIDS

In brain, most 20:4 is esterified at the second carbon of the glycerol backbone of glycerolipids (85). The esterified pool of 20:4 is 5 to 6 μmol/ g wet weight (10), while the endogenous pool of free 20:4 is estimated to be nearly 1,000-fold lower, i.e., 20 to 30 nmol/g wet weight (12). The distribution of 20:4 in phospholipids of different membrane fractions exhibits some degree of specificity. Synaptic membranes are highly enriched in 20:4, as compared to glial and axodendritic membranes (9,44,65). In synaptosomes, phosphatidylethanolamine, phosphatidylserine, phosphatidylinositol and phosphatidylcholine contribute 52, 2.6, 18 and 27.6%, respectively, of the total 20:4 esterified in phospholipids (152). Because the total mass of phosphatidylcholine and phosphatidylethanolamine is much larger than other phospholipids, these lipids contribute the largest amount of 20:4. However, phosphatidylinositol is highly enriched in 20:4, which accounts for 30 to 40% of the total esterified fatty acids in this phospholipid. In contrast, 20:4 represents only 14% of the total fatty acids in phosphatidylethanolamine and only 6% of the total fatty acids in phosphatidylcholine (10). Arachidonic acid (20:4) contributes to the maintenance of a highly fluid membrane, particularly in domains rich in phospholipids containing this acyl group. In addition, 20:4 serves as the precursor for the potent autocoids, prostaglandins (PGs), hydroxyeicosatetraenoic acids (HETEs), and leukotrienes (LTs).

Free fatty acids are rapidly accumulated in brain during convulsions. A single electroconvulsive shock induces the release of 20:4, stearic acid (18:0), 22:6, and palmitic acid (16:0), with 20:4 liberated at the fastest rate (12,21). A twofold increase in free 20:4 is observed after a single electroconvulsive shock; repeated electroshock over several days does not cause a further increase (13,17). Diethyl ether anesthesia suppresses the electroshock-induced production of free fatty acids, but pentobarbital exerts only a small reduction (13). A convulsion-induced release of fatty acids is also observed in mechanically ventilated animals; therefore, it is not merely the result of hypoxia. In bicuculline-induced status epilepticus, a twofold increase in free fatty acids occurs with the first tonic–clonic seizure with a maximal 17-fold increase observed during the status epilepticus (20,24, 130,142). Free 20:4, 22:6, 18:0, 16:0, and oleic acid (18:1, *n*-9) are increased in the cerebrum, while there is a predominant increase of 22:6 in the cerebellum (130). Free 20:4 and 18:0 are the fatty acids most rapidly accumulated; regional studies indicate that fatty acid release is more active in the hippocampus and cerebral cortex than in the cerebellum (130,142).

DIACYLGLYCEROLS

Diacylglycerols are a key intermediate in glycerolipid metabolism and play the role of second messenger by activating phospholipid-dependent, calcium-dependent protein kinase C (89). Their concentration in brain is low due to rapid turnover. Diacylglycerols arise from the cleavage of the polar head group from phospholipids by phospholipase C, by the deacylation of triacylglycerols by triacylglycerol lipase, by the phosphodiesteratic cleavage of phosphoinositides (90,91,96) and by the back reaction of the choline and ethanolamine-phosphotransferases (85).

During seizures, diglycerols accumulate concomitant with the release of free fatty acids. This effect occurs after electroconvulsive shock (6), bicuculline-induced status epilepticus (20,130), carbamylcholine-induced seizures (150,154), and ischemia (5,11,12). The accumulation of diacylglycerols reflects an increase in the 1-stearoyl-2-arachidonoyl molecular species and a slight increase in diacylglycerols containing 22:6; there is no change in diacylglycerols containing 16:0 or 18:1 (6). There are regional differences in diacylglycerol accumulation during bicuculline-induced seizures, with a greater increase in total diacylglycerols in the cerebrum as compared to the cerebellum (20,130).

ENZYMATIC OXYGENATION OF FREE ARACHIDONIC ACID: PROSTAGLANDINS, HYDROXYEICOSATETRAENOIC ACIDS, AND LEUKOTRIENES

In addition to an increase in free fatty acids and diacylglycerols, the synthesis of prostaglandins also is stimulated during convulsions (64,104,148,166,171). Free 20:4 can be metabolized by two distinct dioxygenases: cyclooxygenase, which catalyzes the formation of prostaglandins (PGs), and lipoxygenase, which catalyzes the formation of hydroxyeicosatetraenoic acids (HETEs) and leukotrienes (78,95). An epoxygenation pathway also exists (113, 114). All require the presence of free 20:4; esterified 20:4 is not a substrate (61,98). Indeed, the release of 20:4 is thought to be the rate-limiting step in the synthesis of these oxygenated metabolites, termed eicosanoids (164). Conversely, the normally very low level of free 20:4 in a tissue results in a low basal level of eicosanoids. Cyclooxygenase and lipoxygenase introduce molecular oxygen into 20:4 through the formation of peroxide intermediates, so total anoxia in a tissue would inhibit eicosanoid synthesis. However, the enzymes require only 5 to 10 μM O_2, so hypoxic conditions that induce the release of 20:4 generally permit the synthesis of eicosanoids (95).

The activity of lipoxygenase has not been well characterized in brain, although there have been reports of the occurrence of hydroxylated derivatives of 20:4 in mouse brain (2a), rat cerebral cortex (136), and gerbil brain (147), and one recent report of the presence of 5-HETE in the cerebrospinal fluid from humans with subarachnoid hemorrhage (155). In addition, the presence of lipoxygenase reaction products in the rat (31,33), canine (34), and bovine retina (32) has been reported. Lipoxygenases found in leukocytes and platelets have been studied extensively, and most of the knowledge concerning mammalian lipoxygenases is derived from this work (8). Lipoxygenases catalyze the addition of molecular oxygen to a methylene carbon in a long-chain polyunsaturated fatty acid (78,134). Most investigators have focused on the lipoxygenases that act on 20:4, but other unsaturated fatty acids and hydroxy-fatty acids will serve as substrates as well (7,16a,170).

The biosynthesis of leukotrienes from 20:4 is shown in Fig. 1. In this scheme, addition of oxygen occurs at carbon-5 via the 5-lipoxygenase, resulting in the formation of 5-hydroperoxy-6-cis-8,11-14-trans-eicosatetraenoic acid (5-HPETE). This compound can be reduced to form the corresponding hydroxy derivatives (5-HETE). Alternatively, a dehydrase converts the peroxy-group to the epoxide, 5,6-oxido-7,9,11-trans-14-cis-eicosatetraenoic acid, a short-lived intermediate (leukotriene A$_4$). This compound is enzymatically hydrolyzed to produce 5,12-dihydroxy-6-cis-8,10-trans-14-cis-eicosatetraenoic acid (leukotriene B$_4$). Nonenzymatic hydrolysis of leukotriene A$_4$ yields diHETEs of differing stereochemistry [6-trans- and 6-trans-12-epi-leukotriene B$_4$ and the epimers (at C-6) of 5,6-dihydroxy-7,9,11,14-eicosatetraenoic acid]. Leukotriene A$_4$ is converted to leukotriene C$_4$ by the addition of a cysteinylglycinyl gamma-glutamyl moiety by glutathione-S-transferase. The peptide chain is modified by glutamyl transpeptidase and gamma-glutamyl transpeptidase, and by hydrolysis and aminolysis to yield leukotrienes D$_4$, E$_4$, and F$_4$ (Fig. 1). Leukotrienes C$_4$, D$_4$, E$_4$, and F$_4$ comprise the potent biological mediator, slow-reacting substance of anaphylaxis (SRS-A) (134). These compounds have been identified in a number of cell types, most notably leukocytes, macrophages, and lung. In addition to the metabolites shown in Fig. 1, initial oxygenation of 20:4 can occur at carbon 8, carbon 12, or carbon 15, resulting in the formation of 8,9-leukotriene A$_4$, 11,12-leukotriene A$_4$, or 14,15-leukotriene A$_4$. It has been proposed that these oxygenations occur via lipoxygenases specific for particular carbons. The re-

sulting epoxide intermediates can be converted to leukotrienes B and C, i.e., 8,9-leukotriene B$_4$, 11,12-leukotriene B$_4$, 14,15-leukotriene C$_4$, etc., although the occurrence of this wide variety of metabolites has been shown in only a few isolated systems (78).

The control of lipoxygenase-mediated 20:4 metabolism is under active investigation. Aside from the requirements for molecular oxygen, free 20:4, and glutathione, the factors that modulate lipoxygenase activity are largely unknown. Compounds that increase intracellular calcium, such as the ionophore A23187, stimulate production of lipoxygenase reaction products (8). In the rat, neutrophil lipoxygenase activity has been shown to be calcium-dependent (141). Also, inflammatory stimuli and pathological insult increase the formation of leukotrienes (134). Recently, it was shown that potassium-induced depolarization of the rat retina increases the conversion of radiolabeled 20:4 to hydroxy derivatives (31). Increased lipoxygenase activity has been demonstrated in pancreatic islets stimulated with glucose (106) and in human granulocytes stimulated with the chemotactic peptide, N-formyl-Nle-Leu-Phe-Nle-Tyr-Lys (36). Lipoxygenase can be inhibited by a number of antioxidants, such as vitamin E, butylated hydroxytoluene (BHT), and nordihydroguaiaretic acid (NDGA) (8).

Prostaglandin biosynthesis is also a multistep process that begins with the addition of molecular oxygen, resulting in the formation of the cyclic endoperoxide intermediate, prostaglandin G$_2$ (PGG$_2$) (Fig. 2). The peroxide group of PGG$_2$, at carbon 15, is converted to a hydroxyl group by peroxidase activity that appears to be inherent in the cyclooxygenase enzyme (112). This results in the formation of PGH$_2$, which is further metabolized through the conversion of the endoperoxide moiety by various reductases and isomerases (95). The conversion of PGG$_2$ to PGH$_2$ causes the production of an oxygen free radical, the nature of which is still undetermined (80). This free radical can oxidize organic materials, including the cyclooxygenase enzyme, and is thought to be responsible for the phenomenon of self-deactivation that is observed during prostaglandin synthesis (95). Hydrogen donors, such as the catecholamines, hydroquinone, and other antioxidants, can inhibit self-deactivation of cyclooxygenase, by virtue of their free-radical-scavenging properties, and thereby stimulate the synthesis of prostaglandins. Prostaglandin synthesis can be inhibited by a wide variety of drugs known as nonsteroidal antiinflammatory agents (95).

The synthesis of prostaglandins in the central

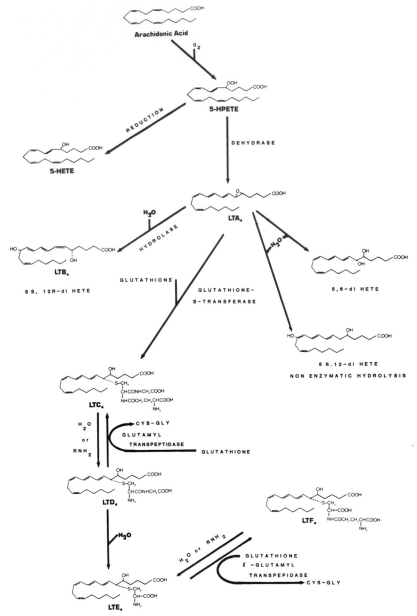

FIG. 1. Lipoxygenation of arachidonic acid (20:4). Initial addition of O_2 can occur at C-5 (shown), C-8, C-12, or C-15. LT, leukotriene.

nervous system has been verified by a number of techniques (1,2,51,86,167). The relative proportions of one prostaglandin to another vary depending on the brain area and the species; however, all species examined to date show the capacity for synthesis of these compounds (1,2,164). The quantitation of prostaglandins in brain tissue from heads decapitated into liquid nitrogen (167) or from animals sacrificed by

head-focused microwave irradiation (3.5 kW) (4) has shown that the *in vivo* level of these compounds is extremely low, because of the low level of available free 20:4 (12,38,103,167). If samples are taken a few seconds post-mortem, the levels of prostaglandins rise dramatically, as do the levels of the precursor, free 20:4 (12). The rapid and large postmortem increase in prostaglandins, coupled with the phenomenon of self-

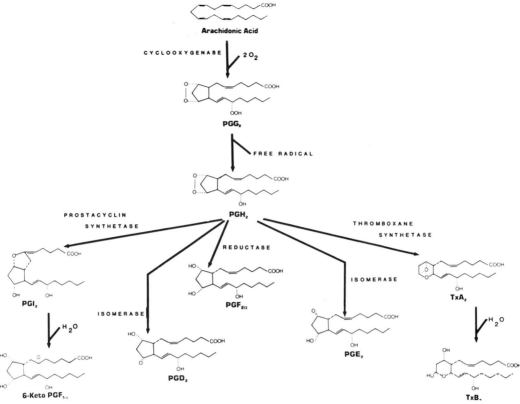

FIG. 2. Cyclooxygenation of arachidonic acid (20:4). PG, prostaglandin; Tx, thromboxane.

deactivation of cyclooxygenase, has made the *in vitro* study of brain prostaglandin synthesis a difficult undertaking. In addition, the techniques used in processing the tissue, such as the rapidity of extraction, have contributed substantially to reports of erroneously high levels of prostaglandins in the brain.

Several factors aside from postmortem ischemia have been shown to stimulate the synthesis of prostaglandins in the brain. A relationship between increased neuronal activity and increased prostaglandin synthesis was suggested (13,40, 50,83,122). These and other studies indicate that electrical stimulation of the brain, either directly or through afferent stimulation, causes an increase in the level of prostaglandins. The intraventricular administration of some neurotransmitters also has this effect (83,163–165). In addition, stimulation of the central nervous system by convulsant drugs causes increased prostaglandin synthesis. The first confirmation of convulsion-induced stimulation of prostaglandin synthesis by the more specific methods of thin-layer chromatography and radioim-

munoassay was reported by Zatz and Roth (171). They demonstrated that electroconvulsive shock or administration of pentylenetetrazol caused a rapid increase in PGF and PGE. This effect was inhibited by pretreatment with the cyclooxygenase inhibitor, indomethacin. The rise in prostaglandin synthesis had a delayed and more prolonged time course than the seizure activity, and the authors proposed that the seizure caused the stimulation of prostaglandin synthesis, rather than increased prostaglandin synthesis resulting in seizures. In agreement with this, indomethacin did not alter electroshock-induced convulsions as measured by observation of the animals, despite a nearly complete inhibition of prostaglandin synthesis.

Convulsion-induced increases in prostaglandin synthesis have been quantitated by a number of methods (104,148), including gas chromatography–mass spectrometry, which is considered to be the most sensitive and specific. $PGF_{2\alpha}$ increases from basal levels of 126 pg/mg protein to 1425 pg/mg protein in the cortex of rats treated with pentylenetetrazol (64). PGE_2

also increases, but to a much lesser extent (approximately fourfold). Even subconvulsant doses of pentylenetetrazol cause a threefold increase in $PGF_{2\alpha}$ levels. Interestingly, these changes were not observed in the cerebellum. Increased prostaglandin levels also have been measured in the cerebrospinal fluid in epilepsy or febrile convulsions (156,166).

POSSIBLE MECHANISMS FOR ALTERATIONS IN MEMBRANE LIPIDS

Accumulation of free fatty acids and diacylglycerols during convulsions may result from the activation of several enzymes (16,23) (Fig. 3): (a) phospholipases A_1 and A_2, (b) phospholipase C, (c) diacylglycerol lipase, and (d) triacylglycerol lipase. In addition, inhibition of the fatty acid activation–acylation pathway could contribute to the accumulation of free fatty acids. Phospholipases degrade glycerolipids, by the cleavage of glyceryl–acyl or phosphoryl–ester bonds (96). Phospholipases A_1 and A_2 remove the fatty acid at the first and second carbon of the glycerol backbone. Phospholipase C removes the phosphate-base group from phospholipids, generating diacylglycerol. Phosphoinositide-specific phosphodiesterase is a phospholipase C specific for phosphoinositides. In addition, monoacylglycerol, diacylglycerol and triacylglycerol can be deacylated by specific lipases (45).

The endogenous concentration of free fatty acids is maintained at a level that is approximately 1,000-fold lower than esterified fatty acids. Various convulsive stimuli will induce up to a 15-fold increase in free fatty acids. This increase is highly significant in terms of the free fatty acid pool; however, it represents a slight change in terms of the total esterified pool of fatty acids. For this reason, the source of the seizure-induced accumulation of fatty acids has been difficult to determine. Because very little triacylglycerol is degraded during electroconvulsive shock, triacylglycerol lipase activation does not seem to be a prevalent response to convulsions (12). Hence, phospholipids appear to be the major source of free fatty acids. The free fatty acids accumulated in brain are 20:4, 18:0, 16:0, 22:6, and palmitoleic acid (16:1, *n*-9); therefore, more than one enzyme may be involved in the effect. However, due to the predominant accumulation of 20:4 and the enrichment of this fatty acid at the second carbon of phospholipids, it was suggested that the activation of a phospholipase A_2 is involved in the free fatty acid release mechanism (12,13,21). Phospholipase A_2 is distributed widely in various subcellular fractions of the brain including nerve-ending membranes and synaptic vesicles (15,162). Studies about the regulatory events that govern phospholipase A_2 activity have not been conclusive. Occurrence of phospholipase A_2 in a zymogen form has been demon-

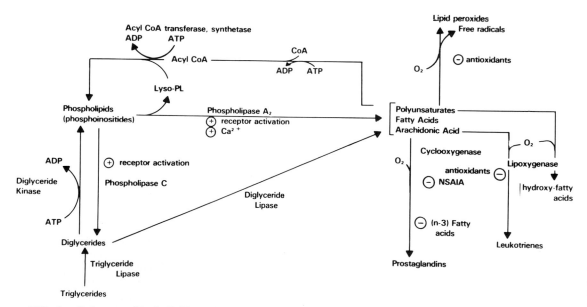

FIG. 3. Pathways of brain lipid metabolism. NSAIA, nonsteroidal antiinflammatory agents; Lyso-PL, lysophospholipids.

lipase A_2 in a zymogen form has been demonstrated in porcine pancreas (56), and proteolytic action by thrombin and trypsin can activate phospholipase A_2 in platelets, suggesting the existence of a phospholipase macromolecular precursor (120). Phospholipase A_2 activity is influenced by calcium and by cAMP, which regulates calcium flux and storage (39,108). Hormonal and neurotransmitter regulation of phospholipase A_2 activity may occur indirectly through the regulation of cAMP levels or other second messengers; this has been suggested as the mechanism underlying free fatty acid release in brain (13,18,21). Membrane fluidity changes or membrane perturbation also can affect phospholipase A_2 activity by alteration of the accessibility of the substrate to the active site or by alteration of the enzyme conformation. Consequently, with the onset of increased neuronal activity, phospholipase A_2 can be activated through various mechanisms, including changes in cAMP levels, alteration in the availability of calcium, changes in the ionic environment, and changes in membrane fluidity or structure.

Steroids and Convulsions

A protein inhibitor, lipomodulin, also called lipocortin or macrocortin, that regulates phospholipase A_2 has been described (62,82). Corticosteroids induce the synthesis in lung of a protein that inactivates phospholipase A_2 (62); conversely, stimulation of phospholipase activity in transformed mouse fibroblasts depends on protein synthesis (75,116).

To date, the inhibitory effect of corticosteroids on phospholipase A_2 activity has not been directly demonstrated in brain, although steroids have been employed therapeutically in the treatment of edema and head injury (60). Recently, our laboratory has investigated the effect of dexamethasone treatment on the release of free fatty acids caused by bicuculline-induced status epilepticus (157) and following cryogenic brain edema (26). Dexamethasone pretreatment (1.25, 1.6 or 2 mg/kg for 2 days) caused a slight decrease in the endogenous basal levels of free fatty acids. Pretreatment with dexamethasone at all doses attenuated bicuculline-induced accumulation of free fatty acids. Dexamethasone appeared to provide some degree of specificity towards suppressing the increase in certain fatty acids, depending on the dose given. At the lowest dose, the release of all fatty acids was lowered by approximately 30%, except 18:0,

which decreased only 17%. When the dose of dexamethasone was increased, there was a specific, but incomplete, inhibition of the release of 20:4 and 18:0. With a dose of 1.6 mg/kg, the increase in 18:0 and 20:4 was suppressed by 35 and 45%, respectively. With a dose of 2 mg/kg, the release of 18:0 was reduced 42%, while the increase in 20:4 was lowered 48%. The attenuation of the increase in the other fatty acids remained at 30%. The increase in total fatty acid level was reduced 40% at a dose of 1.6 mg/kg and 46% at a dose of 2.0 mg/kg.

These results indicate that pretreatment with low doses of dexamethasone causes a generalized suppression of seizure-induced fatty acid release. Dexamethasone-induced attenuation of the release of specific fatty acids (18:0 and 20:4) is seen only with higher doses of the drug. In any case, pretreatment with the steroid did not cause a complete inhibition of the seizure-induced fatty acid release. One possible explanation is that in addition to dexamethasone mediated inhibition of phospholipase A_2, there are other factors affecting deacylation of brain phospholipids such as membrane perturbation (see Fig. 4). Therefore, phospholipase A_2-mediated release of fatty acids may be only one of the mechanisms by which fatty acids are accumulated during convulsions. Alternatively, in bicuculline-induced status epilepticus, it is conceivable that a derangement of phospholipase A_2 controlling mechanisms may take place.

Hence, we conclude from these studies that glucocorticoids likely promote an inhibition of phospholipase A_2 in brain. Brain function and pathology have been related to steroids and to convulsions. In depressive illness, there is an increased content of cortisol (135) and electroconvulsive therapy is useful. However, dexamethasone treatment interferes in the efficacy of this regimen (87). Moreover, steroids are known to be present in relatively high concentrations in brain and to appear in the systemic circulation in a circadian rhythm. We have shown that in cryogenic brain edema (26) and in bicuculline-induced status epilepticus (157) glucocorticoids inhibit the release of free arachidonic acid by inhibiting phospholipase A_2; therefore, the following may be altered at different times of the day: a) epileptic convulsions may lead to brain damage when they occur in the evening, because of the lower steroid content; b) the same may be true with head and spinal cord injury; c) a higher convulsive threshold may exist in the morning because of the known elevated levels of brain steroids.

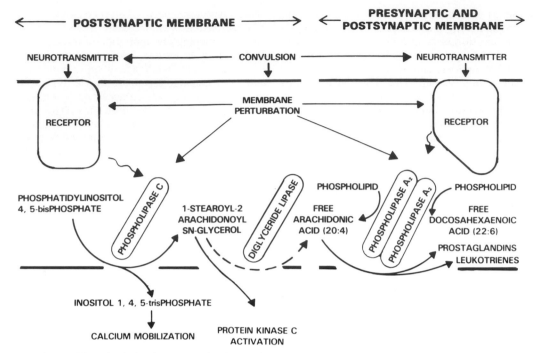

FIG. 4. Hypothetical scheme showing interaction of convulsive stimuli and brain lipid metabolism.

Another important issue is how the fate of arachidonic acid to oxygenated metabolites is affected at different times of the day and the role of these metabolites in the functions and pathological conditions discussed here. Although studies on how circadian rhythms affect the lipids discussed in this chapter are not available, very recently the effect of a circannual rhythm has been described in brain free fatty acids and diacylglycerols in a pentylenetetrazoyl-induced convulsion model (109).

Our hypothesis correlating phospholipids containing arachidonic acid from excitable membranes, steroids and convulsions has a bearing on a number of neurological and psychiatric disorders, such as epilepsy, injury and effectiveness of electroconvulsive therapy in endogenous depression.

Fatty Acid Activation-Acylation and Inositol Lipids

Another mechanism proposed for the control of the free fatty acid pool is rapid activation–acylation reactions catalyzed by acyl coenzyme A (CoA) synthetase (ligase) and acyl CoA transferase (21,129). These enzymes are localized mainly in microsomes, although activity has been measured in brain mitochondria, nuclei,

and synaptosomes (152,154). Acyl CoA synthetase converts free fatty acid to fatty acyl CoA and requires the presence of magnesium and ATP. An arachidonoyl CoA synthetase recently has been shown in human platelets (161) and in other tissues, including brain (74,111,123). Fatty acyl CoA is esterified to lysophospholipids or glycerol 3-phosphate by acyl CoA transferase. Saturated species of fatty acyl CoA are acylated at C-1 and unsaturated species at C-2 of glycerol 3-phosphate. Recently, the preferential utilization of arachidonoyl CoA by 1-acyl-*SN*-glycerol-3-phosphocholine acyltransferase in liver microsomes was reported (97).

In vivo experiments have indicated that electroconvulsive shock, bicuculline-induced status epilepticus, and acute hypoxia alter the uptake of 20:4 in brain, resulting in the slow removal of labeled 20:4 from the free fatty acid pool and a decreased acylation of phospholipids (6,25,55, 118,119,149). We have investigated whether bicuculline-induced status epilepticus alters the activation and acylation of 20:4 and 22:6 in microsomal and/or synaptic plasma membrane fractions of rat brain.

The activation of 20:4 and 22:6 in microsomes and synaptic plasma membrane was measured by quantitation of the conversion of radiolabeled fatty acids to their respective acyl CoA. Activation of 20:4 was four- to fivefold higher than that of 22:6 in microsomes; in the synaptic plasma membranes the difference was less than twofold (Table 1). The substrate affinity, as measured by the apparent K_m values, was twofold higher for 20:4 than for 22:6 in both microsomes and synaptic plasma membranes. Although there are no previous studies on the activation of these polyunsaturated fatty acids in neuronal membranes, the values are similar to those obtained with other fatty acids (46,57,58). Subcellular fractions made from brains of bicuculline-treated (10 mg/kg i.p.) rats did not differ in terms of the acyl CoA synthetase activity.

The activity of acyltransferase was measured in the synaptic plasma membranes isolated from cerebrum of control and bicuculline-treated rats using radiolabeled 20:4 (Fig. 5) or 22:6 (Fig. 6) as substrates, and was assayed *in vitro* in the presence of exogenous lysophospholipids. The activity of acyl transferase was four- to fivefold higher for 20:4 than for 22:6. The activity of acyltransferase for polyunsaturated fatty acids was lower than that previously reported for 18:1 and 16:0 in synaptic plasma membranes (58). Bicuculline-induced status epilepticus did not alter the activity of acyltransferase under our experimental conditions.

Since the uptake of radiolabeled 20:4 into brain lipids is decreased by hypoxia, treatment with bicuculline, or electroconvulsive shock in the intact animal (25,118,119,149), the lack of an effect with bicuculline on the activation–acylation reactions in these studies may be due to the fact that the reactions were assayed *in vitro* under optimal conditions, including the ad-

dition of exogenous cofactors. Therefore, the differences between the availability of endogenous cofactors in control and drug-treated groups may have been overcome. If that was the case, treatment with bicuculline did not cause any alteration in the basic functioning of acyl CoA synthetase and transferase. These results indicate that the availability of substrates and cofactors are critical considerations. In this context, it is known that in bicuculline-induced status epilepticus the levels of endogenous ATP are reduced within 30 sec (47,48,63,125).

An alternative pathway for the release of fatty acids is via the action of diacylglycerol lipase. The major diacylglycerol produced during seizures is the 1-stearoyl-2-arachidonoyl species, and this is also the major molecular species of the phosphoinositides, phosphatidylinositol, phosphatidylinositol 4-phosphate, and phosphatidylinositol 4,5-bis-phosphate (10,90). The phosphoinositides are a small pool of phospholipids that are rapidly hydrolyzed in many cells in response to a variety of hormones and neurotransmitters (59,107). Enzymes specific for phosphodiesteratic cleavage of these lipids, resulting in the formation of diacylglycerol and inositol 1-phosphate, inositol 1,4-*bis*-phosphate, or inositol 1,4,5-*tris*-phosphate occur in brain (28,54,59). We proposed that the diacylglycerols accumulated in brain during convulsions or early ischemia may represent the lipid-soluble product of the cleavage of phosphoinositides (Fig. 4) (5,14,24,158). This hypothesis also is supported by recent reports of a rapid receptor-mediated activation of phosphatidylinositol 4,5-*bis*-phosphate degradation, leading to the production of

TABLE 1. *Effect of bicuculline on the apparent* K_m *and* V_{max} *for the synthesis of arachidonoyl CoA and docosahexaenoyl CoA in synaptic plasma membrane (SPM) and microsomes*[a]

Location	K_m (μM)		V_{max} (nmol/min · mg protein)	
	20:4, $n - 6$	22:6, $n - 3$	20:4, $n - 6$	22:6, $n - 3$
Microsomes				
Control	16 ± 0.4	8.3 ± 0.7	27 ± 1.0	6.0 ± 0.2
Bicuculline-treated	17 ± 2.1	8.0 ± 0.4	28 ± 1.7	5.7 ± 0.3
SPM				
Control	11 ± 0.1	6.1 ± 0.7	2.7 ± 0.2	1.5 ± 0.1
Bicuculline-treated	11 ± 0.2	5.1 ± 0.2	2.4 ± 0.2	1.3 ± 0.1

[a] Ventilated rats were treated with bicuculline (10 mg/kg, i.p.) and sacrificed 6 min later. Synaptic plasma membranes and microsomes were isolated by density-gradient centrifugation (44). Long-chain acyl CoA synthetase was assayed under optimal conditions as described previously (123). The assay mixture contained: 30 μmol Tris-HCl (pH 8.0), 200 nmol ATP, 50 nmol coenzyme A, 200 nmol dithiothreitol, 4 μmol MgCl$_2$, 0.5–8 nmol [1–^{14}C]arachidonate (58 μCi/μmol) or [U-^{14}C]docosahexaenoate (40 μCi/μmol), and 40–60 μg microsomal or synaptic plasma membrane protein in a final volume of 200 μl. Each value represents mean ± SE ($n = 3$ triplicates).

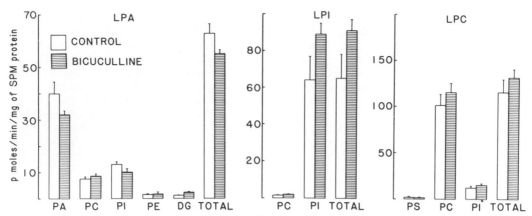

FIG. 5. Effect of bicuculline on acylation of [1-¹⁴C]20:4 in synaptic plasma membrane (SPM). The assay system contained: 100 μM phosphate buffer, pH 7.4; 200 μM coenzymeA; 25 mM ATP; 100 μM MgCl₂; 100 μM lysophosphatidic acid (LPA), lysophosphatidylinositol (LPI) or lysophosphatidylcholine (LPC); 0.6 nmol [1-¹⁴C]20:4 (900,000 cpm); and 150 μg of synaptic plasma membrane protein, in a final volume of 50 μl. The incubation was carried out at 37°C for 10 min, and stopped by extraction with chloroform:methanol. Lipids were separated by thin-layer chromatography (132,133) and quantitated by liquid scintillation counting. Blanks were treated in the same manner, with boiled enzyme used as the enzyme source. PA, phosphatidic acid; PC, phosphatidylcholine; PI, phosphatidylinositol; PE, phosphatidylethanolamine; DG, diacylglycerol.

diacylglycerol and inositol 1,4,5-*tris*-phosphate in brain (28,29,54,77,146). Diacylglycerols can be degraded by the action of diacylglycerol lipase resulting in the release of fatty acids. The coupling of these two effects, the release of 20:4 and the accumulation of diglyceride, occurs in platelets during stimulation by thrombin (27,41,99).

Convulsion-induced stimulation of prostaglandin synthesis may result from cerebral hypoxia, as hypoxia is a stimulus for both fatty acid release and subsequent prostaglandin synthesis

(69). Alternatively, the drugs used to induce seizures could have direct effects on cyclooxygenase. A third possible mechanism is that increased prostaglandin synthesis is the result of increased neuronal activity. Prostaglandin synthesis has been localized in the synaptosomal fraction of the brain (121). The synthesis of PGI₂ occurs in the cerebral vasculature (1,2), but other brain prostaglandins appear to be produced by neurons (163–168). The activity of PGD₂ synthetase in rat brain is highest in the nerve cell fraction, as compared to glial cells and

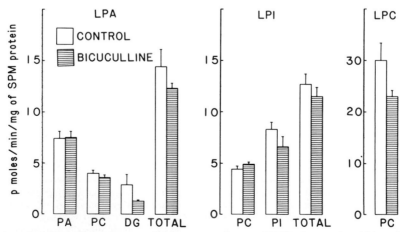

FIG. 6. Activity of acyltransferase in synaptic plasma membranes (SPM) of control and bicuculline-treated rats using [U-¹⁴C]22:6. Details of the assay conditions are described under Fig. 5, except 3 nmol [U-¹⁴C]22:6 (600,000 cpm) was used. PA, phosphatidic acid; PC, phosphatidylcholine; DG, diacylglycerol; PI, phosphatidylinositol.

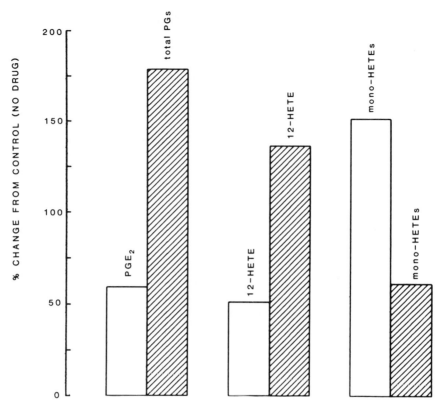

FIG. 7. Effect of bicuculline on eicosanoid synthesis in synaptosomes and microsomes isolated from prelabeled rat brains. Rat brain was prelabeled *in vivo* by bilateral intraventricular injection of 1 μCi [1-^{14}C]20:4 (Na$^+$ salt). At 1 hr later, ventilated rats were treated with bicuculline (10 mg/kg, i.p.) and sacrificed 6 min later. Synaptosomes and microsomes were isolated by density gradient centrifugation (52). Lipid extracts were prepared immediately after isolation of subcellular fractions. Radiolabeled products of [1-^{14}C]20:4 were isolated and quantitated by high-performance liquid chromatography (32). *Open bars,* synaptosomes; *hatched bars,* microsomes. Mono-HETE indicates the sum of 5-HETE and 15-HETE.

microvessels (140). In addition, a PGD$_2$-binding protein has been identified in the rat brain (168). This protein appears to be a receptor for PGD$_2$ and occurs in discrete and well-defined neuronal tracts that correlate with some of the central effects of this prostaglandin. Prostaglandin synthesis in brain can be increased by the stimulation of the cortex or reticular formation and can be evoked by the stimulation of the hindpaw (40,83,122). The results of various studies suggest that stimulation of prostaglandin synthesis during convulsions is dependent on increased neuronal activity. The evidence for this includes the observation that convulsive drugs, such as picrotoxin and pentylenetetrazol, are ineffective in increasing prostaglandin synthesis in isolated synaptosomes, thus ruling out a direct effect of the drugs on either cyclooxygenase or the release of precursor, 20:4 (148). Convulsion-stimulated prostaglandin synthesis probably is not due to hypoxia, as it has been shown that after

decapitation ischemia, the level of PGF$_{2\alpha}$ is 10-fold lower that that measured after treatment with pentylenetetrazol or picrotoxin (67). In addition, pentylenetetrazol induces a large increase in prostaglandin synthesis in ventilated animals (67). A demonstration of seizure-induced stimulation of fatty acid release directly resulting in an increased prostaglandin synthesis has remained elusive; however, some experiments strongly suggest this to be the case (103,105). Treatment of rats with convulsive doses of pentylenetetrazol or carbachol results in a preferential release of 20:4 and a large increase in PGF$_{2\alpha}$ levels (104). It is noteworthy that the amount of accumulated free 20:4 is about 100 times greater than that of the total prostaglandins; therefore, the synthesis of prostaglandins has no appreciable effect on the pool size of free 20:4.

Recently, our laboratory has been concerned with the effect of bicuculline-induced status epilepticus on the metabolism of 20:4 in glycero-lipids and via the lipoxygenase and cyclooxygenase pathways. In addition, an effort has been made to discern the subcellular localization of changes in 20:4 metabolism by comparing microsomal and synaptosomal fractions. Rat brain was prelabeled *in vivo* by intraventricular injection of [1-^{14}C]20:4; ventilated rats then were treated with bicuculline, and the synaptosomal and microsomal fractions were isolated by differential centrifugation. This paradigm provided subcellular fractions with [1-^{14}C]20:4-labeled glycerolipids. After isolation, these fractions were incubated *in vitro* with a low or high potassium concentration. Measurement of the changes in the labeled pool of arachidonate, production of eicosanoids, and alterations in endogenous free fatty acids were quantitated. The analyses uncovered several interesting points. Synaptosomes produced eicosanoids most actively, as compared to microsomes, cytosol, and total homogenate. All major prostaglandins were detected and 5-HETE, 12-HETE, and LTB$_4$ were formed. Treatment with bicuculline induced a 30% increase in total endogenous free fatty acids of the synaptosomal fraction (Table 2). In microsomes, no changes in free fatty acids were evident as a result of bicuculline treatment. Bicuculline treatment also caused an increase in the production of eicosanoids (Fig. 7). During the *in vitro* incubation of synaptosomes and microsomes, there was a further release of both endogenous and labeled 20:4 (Fig. 8). Potassium-induced depolarization enhanced the release of [1-^{14}C]20:4 only in the synaptosomal fraction; there was a specific decrease in the labeling of phosphatidylinositol. Also, potassium depolarization resulted in an increase in HETE synthesis specific to synaptosomes (Fig. 9). Interestingly, potassium-induced depolarization

had a more pronounced effect in synaptosomes from bicuculline-treated rats compared to synaptosomes from untreated animals (data not shown).

The results from this study indicate that the subcellular source of fatty acids released during bicuculline-induced seizures is the synaptosomes. It further supports the hypothesis that free fatty acid release is the consequence of mechanisms triggered by increased neuronal activity. As observed by others (101,102), potassium-stimulated release of 20:4, which occurred only in the synaptosomal fraction in our experiments, provides additional evidence for this hypothesis. In addition, this is the first evidence of a seizure-induced stimulation of brain lipoxygenase activity. The observation that HETE synthesis is stimulated both by bicuculline (*in vivo*) and by potassium depolarization, and that these changes are localized in the synaptosomal fraction, provides strong evidence for an association of lipoxygenase activation with increased neuronal activity.

Despite all that has been learned about the interactions of brain lipid metabolism and convulsions, there are several basic questions that remain unanswered. First, are free fatty acid, diacylglycerol, and eicosanoid accumulation-independent, or related phenomena? The interdependency and cyclic nature of glycerolipid metabolism (Fig. 3) indicate that the effects of convulsions are related in some way, although identical changes have not been observed for all types of convulsive stimuli. A second crucial question is whether changes in lipid metabolism are the result of the specific—i.e., receptor-mediated—effects of increased neuronal activity or rather a response to membrane perturbation (Fig. 4). The profile of changes with the preferential accumulation of polyunsaturated fatty acids and diacylglycerols points to an overstimulation of a set of specific pathways of glycerolipid metabolism.

In an effort to further define the particular metabolic steps that are altered by convulsions, pharmacological manipulation of various pathways has been attempted. Pretreatment of rats with α-methyl-*p*-tyrosine, an inhibitor of norepinephrine and dopamine synthesis, causes an inhibition of the electroshock-induced release of fatty acids (6) and the bicuculline-induced accumulation of diacylglycerols, and a potentiation of the bicuculline-induced release of fatty acids (130). Pretreatment with *p*-chlorophenylalanine, an inhibitor of serotonin synthesis, increases the basal level of free fatty acids, but has no effect on bicuculline-induced fatty acid

TABLE 2. *Effect of bicuculline on endogenous free fatty acids*[a]

Location	Free arachidonic acid (% control)	Total free fatty acids (% control)
Synaptosomes	139.9	118.9
Microsomes	98.6	93.9

[a] Ventilated rats were treated with bicuculline (10 mg/kg, i.p.), sacrificed, and the subcellular fractions were isolated (52). Free fatty acids were separated from total lipid extracts by gradient-thickness thin-layer chromatography and quantitated by gas chromatography, using nonodecanoic acid as an internal standard (19).

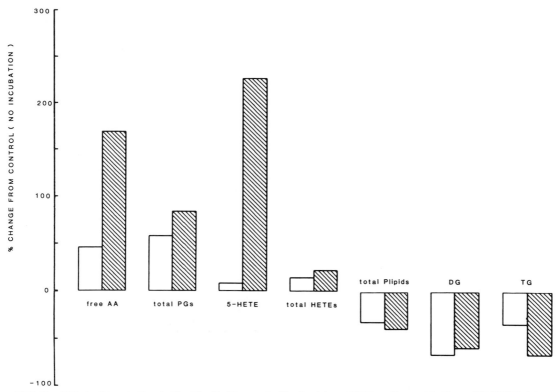

FIG. 8. Effect of incubation in Bradford's Ringers buffer for 1 hr at 37°C on the metabolism of [1-^{14}C]20:4 in synaptosomes from untreated (*open bars*) and bicuculline-treated (*hatched bars*) rat brain. AA, arachidonic acid; Plipids, phospholipids; DG, diacylglycerol; TG, triacylglycerol.

release (130). Pretreatment of rats with some antiepileptic drugs (diazepam, trimethadione, and diphenylhydantoin) has been shown to attenuate the free fatty acid release induced by bemegrid, an analeptic similar to pentylenetetrazol (144). These results indicate that specific mechanisms, possibly involving catecholamine mediators, are responsible for seizure-induced fatty acid and diacylglycerol accumulation. There have been conflicting reports concerning the direct interaction of neurotransmitters and prostaglandin synthesis. Some groups have demonstrated a stimulation of prostaglandin production in perfused brain, brain slices, homogenates, and synaptosomes, after addition of catecholamines or indoleamines (35,81,137,167). In some studies, the effects of norepinephrine were inhibited by β-adrenergic receptor antagonists (81). Other investigators have concluded from their experiments that catecholamine-stimulated prostaglandin synthesis either does not occur or can be attributed to the antioxidant properties of the catechol structure (71). Support for this hypothesis comes from data showing that cate-

cholamines are active only at concentrations above 100 μM and that stimulatory effects can be seen with compounds that have hydrogen donor properties, but no receptor agonist activity (35,167). In light of recent reports of excitatory amino acid and peptide neurotransmitters in the brain, more work must be done to define the interactions of neurotransmitters and lipid metabolism.

POSSIBLE CONSEQUENCES OF ALTERED MEMBRANE LIPID METABOLISM

An additional aspect of convulsion-induced changes in lipid metabolism is the possible effects of the catabolism of membrane lipids and the transient accumulation of the products, free fatty acids and diacylglycerols (23). The loss of key fatty acids from lipids produces alterations in membrane fluidity and the function of membrane-bound enzymes and ion channels (145). The production of lysophospholipids, as a con-

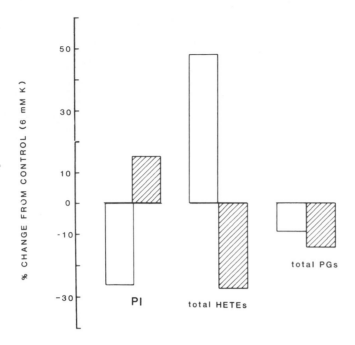

FIG. 9. Effect of incubation in depolarizing media (45 mM K$^+$) on [1-^{14}C]20:4 metabolism in synaptosomes (*open bars*) and microsomes *hatched bars*) from untreated rat brain. PI, phosphatidylinositol; PG, prostaglandin.

sequence of phospholipase A$_2$-mediated fatty acid release, results in detergent-like effects on lipid membranes. The hydrolysis of the functionally important, although minor, lipids of excitable membranes, the phosphoinositides, results in the production of putative second messengers, diacylglycerol and inositol 1,4,5-*tris*-phosphate (Fig. 4). Diacylglycerol has been shown to activate protein kinase C, a cAMP-independent, calcium- and phospholipid-dependent enzyme (89). Inositol 1,4,5-*tris*-phosphate acts as an intracellular messenger in the liver, causing the release of non-mitochondrial stores of calcium (88). The accumulation of this compound in brain during seizures has been demonstrated, and inositol 1,4,5-*tris*-phosphate and inositol 1,4-*bis*-phosphate are produced in rat brain stimulated with cholinergic agonists (28,29), and inositol phosphates display increased incorporation of ^{32}P during bicuculline-induced status epilepticus (158). Treatment *in vivo* with lithium, an inhibitor of the dephosphorylation of inositol phosphates, induces an accumulation of inositol 1-monophosphate in rat brain and exacerbates tissue damage and convulsions due to cholinergic agents (84,138). An enhanced turnover of brain polyphosphoinositides during bicuculline-induced convulsions was also detected (158).

Aside from the effects mentioned above, stimulated production of prostaglandins could have an important role in the response of the brain to seizures. The data describing the modulation of neuronal activity by prostaglandins are almost as confusing as those concerned with the alteration of prostaglandin synthesis by neurotransmitters. PGE$_2$ and PGF$_{2\alpha}$, when administered intraventricularly in the cat, cause an inhibition of acetylcholinesterase, thereby potentiating the gross behavioral changes induced by cholinomimetic agents (72,73). In conflict with this, PGF$_{2\alpha}$ blocks the stimulatory effect of acetylcholine in the rabbit cortex (139). PGE$_2$ reduces the inhibitory effect of norepinephrine in the cortex (139) and in the Purkinje neurons of the cerebellum (143). PGE$_2$ has been shown to be a presynaptic inhibitor of norepinephrine release in rat brain slices (126) and to modulate cAMP synthesis in response to norepinephrine (117). Pharmacological studies into the action of PGF$_{2\alpha}$ in brain have shown that this prostaglandin has an amphetamine-like action on the metabolism, uptake, and release of dopamine (110). The central nervous system effects of PGF$_{2\alpha}$ (hypertension, tachycardia, and increased body temperature) can be antagonized by the alpha-adrenergic blocker, phenoxybenzamine, and stimulated by the dopaminergic antagonist, fluspirilene (43). With regard to interactions between prostaglandins and the effects of seizure-inducing stimuli, PGE$_2$ and PGD$_2$ have been suggested to decrease convulsions and to act as feedback inhibitors (42,66–68), while PGF$_{2\alpha}$ increases convulsions (131). This effect has been observed with drug-induced seizures, but the administration of prostaglandins or treatment with cyclooxygenase inhibitors appears to have no substantial effect on convulsions caused by electroshock (100,171).

The alternate pathway of 20:4 metabolism—i.e., oxygenation catalyzed by lipoxygenase—has been unexplored with regard to its role in the effects of seizures. In fact, the study of the enzymatic production of 20:4 hydroperoxides and hydroxides in the brain has only been pursued recently. It is well known that cerebral ischemia, followed by restoration of blood flow induces the formation of lipid peroxides, and it has been postulated that these compounds play an important role in ischemia-induced tissue damage (169). During cerebral ischemia, a decrease in ATP production and an increase in intracellular calcium are early events (160). These effects can be attributed to a decrease in the activity of Na^+/K^+-ATPase, resulting in depolarization of neurons, and accumulation of NADH, leading to a loss of calcium from the mitochondria. Increased influx of calcium through the plasma membrane also may occur and may be important in the activation of lipolytic enzymes, partcularly phospholipases. In addition, the lack of ATP can lead to an inhibition of the reacylation of fatty acids. The net result is a large increase in the level of free fatty acids, particularly 20:4. Upon reperfusion and the resumption of an adequate oxygen supply, 20:4 is autooxidized to form hydroperoxides and enzymatically oxygenated to form the endoperoxide precursors of prostaglandins or the hydroperoxide precursors of leukotrienes. These reactions generate free radicals and have been proposed to lead to the cellular damage observed in percussion-induced head injury and other edema-producing insults (94,159). Another source of free radicals is mitochondria, where degradation of the mitochondrial membrane causes the uncoupling of oxidation–phosphorylation reactions. These free radicals can induce further lipid peroxidation, exacerbating damage to cell membranes. Similar events may take place during seizures, which also results in the depolarization of neurons and an increased calcium influx. In addition to free-radical-induced peroxidation of 20:4, alterations in the production of leukotrienes via lipoxgenase could have significant effects on seizure-related phenomena. These extremely potent autocoids have been shown to act as calcium ionophores, to modulate cyclic nucleotide levels, to stimulate chemotaxis and lysosomal enzyme release, to induce vasospasm, and to increase capillary permeability (8,78,134). Leukotrienes C_4 and D_4, applied by micropressure injection to rat cerebeller Purkinje cells, cause a prolonged excitation as measured by an increased firing rate (115). This effect is similar to that of PGE_1, which also causes stimulation of Purkinje cell firing when applied by microiontophoresis (143). Aside from the production of leukotrienes from 20:4, lipoxygenase-mediated metabolism of other polyunsaturated fatty acids may occur during seizures. The production of hydroxy derivatives of 22:6 has been shown in platelets (7), trout gill (70), and canine retina and pigment epithelium (16a,124). There is a large accumulation of 22.6 during seizures; therefore, metabolism of this fatty acid by lipoxygenase would result in the synthesis of yet another group of possible endogenous mediators. The production of lipoxygenase products of 20:4 and 22:6 by the retina (16a,34,124), an integral part of the central nervous system (3,22), supports the hypothesis that these products may be modulators of neuronal activity. It is possible that some of these compounds, prostaglandins, leukotrienes, and other lipoxygease-reaction products, are endogenous modulators of convulsions. These autocoids could affect ion fluxes, pre- and postsynaptic responses, neurotransmitter release, and blood flow.

The identification of endogenous substances in the brain with anticonvulsant and proconvulsant activity will be an important step toward the design of more effective antiepileptic drugs. New knowledge on the biochemical mechanisms involved in the generation of endogenous substances such as these will lead to an understanding of how to mobilize them and/or slow their synthesis.

CONCLUDING REMARKS

Seizures cause selective alterations in brain lipid metabolism, resulting in an accumulation of free fatty acids, diacylglycerides, and the oxygenated products of arachidonic acid, prostaglandins, and leukotrienes. The mechanisms for these effects are still unknown but seem to be linked to an increase in neuronal activity and neurotransmitter release. It is likely that several mechanisms are responsible and that presynaptic and postsynaptic membranes are involved. Early and reversible alterations in lipid metabolism may reflect an overstimulation of the metabolic pathways that normally operate during neurotransmission, such as the remodeling of the fatty acid composition of membrane glycerolipids and the production from membrane lipids of second messengers, like diacylglycerols, inositol 1,4,5-*tris*-phosphate, and eicosanoids. Subsequent pathological changes in membrane lipids are likely due to the generalized breakdown of cell membranes, perhaps triggered by an overstimulation of the normal metabolic pathways or by the production of highly reactive free radicals. The prevention of severe alterations in brain lipid metabolism could have therapeutic value in the treatment of epilepsy; however, there still is much to be learned about the effects of seizures on membrane lipids.

Among these challenges are the resolution of the "in-membrane" events in molecular terms. Is the release of fatty acids due to selective, receptor-mediated events? What is the primary event? Are second messengers or signals such as protein phosphorylation involved?

Second, further studies of the consequences of free fatty acid release are needed. Is arachidonic acid a direct modulator of the properties of excitable membranes? Is the loss of arachidonic acid a signaling mechanism?

Related to this last point is the question of the role of the oxygenated metabolites of arachidonic acid, prostaglandins and leukotrienes, in the response to seizures. Are the changes seen in this metabolic pathway the consequence of other events or part of the primary event? Another important question is why 1-stearoyl-2-arachidonoyldiacylglycerol accumulates in brain during convulsions. Is this related to or independent of fatty acid accumulation? Are these diacylglycerols involved in the activation of modulators such as protein kinase C? Are polyphosphoinositides the source of accumulated diacylglycerols by way of a failure in cell signaling events?

Finally, because alterations in free fatty acids, eicosanoids, and diacylglycerols are very early responses to experimental epilepsy, these models provide an opportunity to study endogenous promotors of seizures, and the formation of endogenous antiepileptics. In addition, an understanding of the changes in lipid metabolism that occur during convulsions will provide us with important insight into the role membrane lipids play in the fundamental operation of the central nervous system.

ACKNOWLEDGMENTS

The support of the Esther A. and Joseph Klingenstein Fund, Inc., New York and the Epilepsy Foundation of America is gratefully acknowledged.

REFERENCES

1. Abdel-Halim, M. S., Lunden, I., Cseh, G., and Anggard, E. (1980): Prostaglandin profiles in nervous tissue and blood vessels of the brain of various animals. *Prostaglandins,* 19:249–258.
2. Abdel-Halim, M. S., vonHolst, H., Meyerson, B., Sachs, C., and Anggard, E. (1980): Prostaglandin profiles in tissue and blood vessels from human brain. *J. Neurochem.,* 34:1331–1333.
2a. Adesuyi, S. A., Cockrell, C. S., Gamache, D. A., and Ellis, E. F. (1985): Lipoxygenase metabolism of arachidonic acid in brain. *J. Neurochem.,* 45:770–776.
3. Ames, A., and Nesbett, F. B. (1981): *In vitro* retina as an experimental model of the central nervous system. *J. Neurochem.,* 37:867–877.
4. Anton, R. F., Wallis, C., Randall, C. L. (1983): In vivo regional levels of PGE and thromboxane in mouse brain: Effect of decapitation, focused microwave fixation, and indomethacin. *Prostaglandins,* 26:421–429.
5. Aveldano, M. I., and Bazan, N. G. (1975): Rapid production of diacylglycerols enriched in arachidonate and stearate during early brain ischemia. *J. Neurochem.,* 25:919–920.
6. Aveldano, M. I., and Bazan, N. G. (1979): Alpha-methyl-*p*-tyrosine inhibits the production of free arachidonic acid and diacylglycerols in brain after a single electroconvulsive shock. *Neurochem. Res.,* 4:213–221.
7. Aveldano, M. I., and Sprecher, H. (1983): Synthesis of hydroxy fatty acids from 4,7,10,13,16,19-[1-^{14}C]docosahexaenoic acid by human platelets. *J. Biol. Chem.,* 258:9339–9343.
8. Bailey, D., and Chakrin, L. (1981): Arachidonate lipoxygenase. *Annu. Rep. Med. Chem.,* 16:213–227.
9. Baker, R. R. (1979): The fatty acids composition of phosphoglycerides of nerve cell bodies isolated in bulk from rabbit cerebral cortex: Changes during development and positional distribution. *Can. J. Biochem.,* 57:378–384.
10. Baker, R., and Thompson, W. (1972): Positional distribution and turnover of fatty acids in phosphatidic acid, phosphoinositides, phosphatidylcholine and phosphatidylethanolamine in rat brain *in vivo. Biochim. Biophys. Acta,* 270:489–503.
11. Banschbach, M. W., and Geison, R. L. (1974): Post-mortem increase in rat cerebral hemisphere diglyceride pool size. *J. Neurochem.,* 23:875–877.
12. Bazan, N. (1970): Effects of ischemia and electroconvulsive shock on free fatty acid pool in the brain. *Biochim. Biophys. Acta,* 218:1–10.
13. Bazan, N. G. (1971): Changes in free fatty acids of brain by drug induced convulsions, electroshock and anaesthesia. *J. Neurochem.,* 18:1379–1385.
14. Bazan, N. G. (1976): Free arachidonic acid and other lipids in the nervous system during early ischemia and after electroshock. *Adv. Exp. Med. Biol.,* 72:317–335.

15. Bazan, N. G. (1971): Phospholipases A_1, and A_2 in brain subcellular fractions. *Acta Physiol. Lat. Am.*, 21:101–106.

16. Bazan, N. G., Aveldano de Caldironi, M. I., Cascone de Suarez, G. D., and Rodriguez de Turco, G. B. (1980): Transient modifications in brain free arachidonic acid in experimental animals during convulsions. In: *Neurochemistry and Clinical Neurology*, edited by L. Batistin, G. Hashim, and A. Lajtha, pp. 167–179. Alan R. Liss, New York.

16a. Bazan, N. G., Birkle, D. L., and Reddy, T. S. (1984): Docosahexaenoic acid (22:6, n-3) is metabolized to lipoxygenase reaction products in the retina. *Biochem. Biophys. Res. Comm.*, 125:741–747.

17. Bazan, N. G., Aveldano de Caldironi, M. I., and Rodriguez de Turco, E. B. (1982): Rapid release of free arachidonic acid in the central nervous system due to stimulation. *Prog. Lipid Res.*, 20:523–529.

18. Bazan, N., Bazan, H. E. P., Kennedy, W., and Joel, C. (1971): Regional distribution and rate of production of free fatty acids in rat brain. *J. Neurochem.*, 18:1387–1393.

19. Bazan, N. G., and Joel, C. D. (1970): Gradient-thickness thin-layer chromatography for the isolation and analysis of trace amounts of free fatty acids in large lipid samples. *J. Lipid Res.*, 11:42–47.

20. Bazan, N., Morelli de Liberti, S., and Rodriguez de Turco, E. (1982): Arachidonic acid and arachidonoyl-diglyceroles increase in rat cerebrum during bicuculline-induced status epilepticus. *Neurochem. Res.*, 7:839–843.

21. Bazan, N. G., and Rakowski, H. (1970): Increased levels of brain free fatty acids after electroconvulsive shock. *Life Sci.*, 9:501–507.

22. Bazan, N. G., and Reddy, T. S. (1985): Retina. In: *Handbook of Neurochemistry, Vol. 8: Neural Membranes*, edited by A. Lajtha, pp. 507–575. Plenum Publishing Company, New York.

23. Bazan, N. G., and Rodriguez de Turco, E. B. (1980): Membrane lipids in the pathogenesis of brain edema: Phospholipids and arachidonic acid, the earliest membrane components changed at the onset of ischemia. *Adv. Neurol.*, 28:197–205.

24. Bazan, N. G., and Rodriguez de Turco, E. B. (1983): Seizures promote breakdown of membrane phospholipids in the brain. In: *Neural Transmission, Learning and Memory.*, edited by R. Caputto and C. Ajmone Marsan, pp. 187–194. Raven Press, New York.

25. Bazan, N. G., Rodriguez de Turco, E. B., and Morelli de Liberti, S. A. (1983): Free arachidonic acid and membrane lipids in the central nervous system during bicuculline induced status epilepticus. *Adv. Neurol.*, 34:305–310.

26. Bazan, N. G., Turco, E. B. R., and Politi, E. (1984): Dexamethasone Inhibits the Production of Free AA in Cryogenic Brain Edema. *Trans. Am. Soc. Neurochem.*, 15:105.

27. Bell, R., Kennerly, D., Stanford, N., and Majerus, P. (1979): Diglyceride lipase: A pathway for arachidonate release from human platelets. *Proc. Natl. Acad. Sci. U.S.A.*, 76:3238–3241.

28. Berridge, M. J., Dawson, R. M. C., Downes, C. P., Heslop, J. P., and Irvine, R. F. (1983): Changes in the levels of inositol phosphates after agonist-dependent hydrolysis of membrane phosphoinsitides. *Biochem. J.*, 212:473–482.

29. Berridge, M. J., Downes, C. P., and Hanley, M. R. (1982): Lithium amplifies agonist-dependent phosphatidylinositol responses in brain and salivary glands. *Biochem. J.*, 206:587–595.

30. Bidard, J. N., Rossi, B., Renaud, J. F., and Lazdunski, M. (1984): A search for an 'ouabain-like' substance from the electric organ of electrophorus electricus which led to arachidonic acid and related fatty acids. *Biochim. Biophys. Acta*, 769:245–252.

31. Birkle, D. L., and Bazan, N. G. (1984): Effects of K^+ depolarization on the synthesis of prostaglandins and hydroxyeicosatetra(5,8,11,14)-enoic acids (HETE) in the rat retina. Evidence for esterification of 12-HETE in lipids. *Biochim. Biophys. Acta*, 795:564–573.

32. Birkle, D. L., and Bazan, N. G. (1984): Lipoxygenase- and cyclooxygenase-reaction products and incorporation into glycerolipids of radiolabeled arachidonic acid in the bovine retina. *Prostaglandins*, 27:203–216.

33. Birkle, D. L., and Bazan, N. G. (1985): Metabolism of arachidonic acid in the central nervous system. The enzymatic cyclooxygenation and lipoxygenation of arachidonic acid in the mammalian retina. In: *Phospholipids in the Nervous System, Vol. 2. Physiological Roles*, edited by L. Horrocks, J. Kanfer, and G. Porcellati, pp. 193–208. Raven Press, New York.

34. Birkle, D. L., Reddy, T. S., Armstrong, D., Koppang, N., and Bazan, N. G. (1984): Arachidonic acid metabolism and its conversion to eicosanoids in retina and pigment epithelium in canine ceroid lipofuscinosis. *Invest. Ophthal. Vis. Sci.*, 25:62.

35. Birkle, D., Wright, K., Ellis, C., and Ellis, E. (1981): Prostaglandin levels in isolated brain microvessels and in normal and norepinephrine-stimulated cat brain homogenates. *Prostaglandins*, 21:865–877.

36. Bonser, R., Siegel, M., McConnell, R., and Cuatrecasas, P. (1981): Chemotactic peptide stimulated endogenous arachidonic acid metabolism in HL60 granulocytes. *Biochem. Biophys. Res. Commun.*, 102:1269–1275.

37. Boonstra, J., Nelemans, S. A., Feijen, A., Bierman, A., Van Zoelen, E. J. J., Van Der Saag, P. T., and De Laat, S. W. (1982): Effect of fatty acids on plasma membrane lipid dynamics and cation permeability in neuroblastoma cells. *Biochim. Biophys. Acta*, 692:321–329.

38. Bosisio, E., Galli, C., Galli, G., Nicosia, S., Spangnuolo, C., and Tosi, L. (1976): Correlation between release of free arachidonic acid and prostaglandin formation in brain cortex and cerebellum. *Prostaglandins*, 11:773–781.

39. Bradford, P. G., Marinetti, G. V., and Abood, L. G. (1983): Stimulation of phospholipase A_2

and secretion of catecholamines from brain synaptosomes by potassium and A23187. *J. Neurochem.*, 41:1684–1693.

40. Bradley, P. B., Samuels, G. M. R., and Shaw, J. E. (1969): Correlation of prostaglandin release from the cerebral cortex of cats with the electrocorticogram, following stimulation of the reticular formation. *Br. J. Pharmacol.*, 37:151–157.

41. Broekman, M. J., Ward, J. W., and Marcus, A. J. (1981): Fatty acid composition of phosphatidylinositol and phosphatidic acid in stimulated platelets. *J. Biol. Chem.*, 256:5037–5040.

42. Brus, R., Herman, Z., and Szkilnik, R. (1980): Central effects of prostaglandin D_2. *Pol. J. Pharmacol. Pharm.*, 32:681–684.

43. Brus, R. (1981): Effect of the blockade of adrenergic, serotoninergic and cholinergic receptors of the central nervous system on the action of prostaglandin $F_{2\alpha}$ in rat. *Acta Med. Pol.*, 22:1–6.

44. Butler, M., and Abood, C. G. (1982): Use of phospholipase A to compare phospholipid organization in synaptic membranes, myelin and liposomes. *J. Membr. Biol.*, 66:1–7.

45. Cabot, M. C., and Gatt, S (1977): Hydrolysis of endogenous diacylglycerol and monoacylglycerol by lipases in rat brain microsomes. *Biochemistry*, 16:2330–2334.

46. Caintrill, R. C., and Carey, E. M. (1975): Changes in the activities of de novo fatty acid and synthesis and palmitoyl CoA synthesis in relation to myelination in rabbit brain. *Biochim. Biophys Acta*, 380:661–669.

47. Chapman, A. G. (1981): Free fatty acid release and metabolism of adenosine and cyclic nucleotides during prolonged seizures. In: *Neurotransmitters, Seizures and Epilepsy*, edited by P. L. Morselli, pp. 165–173. Raven Press, New York.

48. Chapman, A. G., Meldrum, B. S., and Siesjö, B. K. (1977): Cerebral metabolic changes during prolonged epileptic seizures in rats. *J. Neurochem.*, 28:1025–1035.

49. Clarenbach, P., Raffel, G., Meyer, D., and Hertting, G. (1976): Inhibition of indomethacin and niflumic acid of catecholamine-uptake into rat hypothalamic and striatal synaptosomes. *Arch. Int. Pharmacodyn. Ther.*, 219:79–86.

50. Coceani, F., Pace-Asciak, C., Volta, F., and Wolfe, L. S. (1967): Effect of nerve stimulation on prostaglandin formation and release from the rat stomach. *Am. J. Physiol.*, 213:1056–1064.

51. Coceani, F., and Wolfe, L. S. (1965): Prostaglandins in the brain and the release of prostaglandin-like compounds from the cat cerebellar cortex. *Can. J. Physiol. Pharmacol.*, 43:445–450.

52. Cotman, C. W. (1974): Isolation of synaptosomal and synaptic plasma membrane fractions. *Methods Enzymol.*, 31:445–452.

53. Cullis, P. R., De Kruijff, B., Hope, M. J., Nayar, R., and Schmid, S. L. (1980): Phospholipids and membrane transport. *Can. J. Biochem.*, 58:1091–1100.

54. Dawson, R. M. C., Irvine, R. T., and Hira-

sawa, K. (1982): The hydrolysis of phosphatidylinositol in nervous tissue. In: *Phospholipids in the Nervous System, Vol. 1*, edited by L. A. Horrock, G. B. Ansell, and G. Porcellati, pp. 241–249. Raven Press, New York.

55. Der, O. M., and Sun, G. Y. (1981): Degradation of arachidonoyl-labeled phosphatidylinositols by brain synaptosomes. *J. Neurochem.*, 36:355–362.

56. Detters, G. H., Postema, N. M., Nieumenhuizen, W., and Van Deenan, L. L. M. (1968): Purification and properties of an anionic zymogen of phospholipase A from porcin pancreas. *Biochim. Biophys. Acta*, 159:118–129.

57. Fisher, S. K., Doherty, F. J., and Rowe, C. E. (1982): Deacylation and acylation of phospholipids in nervous tissue. In: *Phospholipids in the Nervous System, Vol. 1*, edited by L. A. Horrocks, G. B. Ansell, and G. Porcellati, pp. 63–74. Raven Press, New York.

58. Fisher, S. K., and Rowe, C. E. (1980): The acylation of lysophosphatidylcholine by subcellular fractions of guinea-pig cerebral cortex. *Biochim. Biophys. Acta*, 618:231–241.

59. Fisher, S. K., Van Rooijen, L. A. A., and Agranoff, B. W. (1984): Renewed interest in the polyphosphoinositides. *Trends Biochem. Sci.*, 9:53–56.

60. Fishman, R. A. (1982): Steroids in the treatment of brain edema. *N. Engl. J. Med.*, 306:359–360.

61. Flower, R., and Blackwell, G. J. (1976): The importance of phospholipase-A_2 in prostaglandin biosynthesis. *Biochem. Pharmacol.*, 25:285–291.

62. Flower, R. J., and Blackwell, G. J. (1979): Anti-inflammatory steroids induce biosynthesis of a phospholipase A_2 inhibitor which prevents prostaglandin generation. *Nature (Lond.)*, 278:456–459.

63. Folbergrovà, J., Ingvar, M., and Siesjö, B. K. (1981): Metabolic changes in cerebral cortex, hippocampus, and cerebellum during sustained bicuculline-induced seizures. *J. Neurochem.*, 37(5):1228–1238.

64. Folco, G. C., Longiave, D., and Bosisio, E. (1977): Relations between prostaglandin E_2, $F_{2\alpha}$ and cyclic nucleotides levels in rat brain and induction of convulsions. *Prostaglandins*, 13:893–900.

65. Fontaine, R. N., Harris, R. A., and Schroeder, F. (1980): Amino phospholipid asymmetry in murine synaptosomal plasma membrane. *J. Neurochem.*, 34:269–277.

66. Forstermann, U., Heldt, R., Friedhelm, K., and Hertting, G. (1982): Potential anticonvulsive properties of endogenous prostaglandins formed in mouse brain. *Brain Res.*, 240:303–310.

67. Forstermann, U., Heldt, R., and Hertting, G. (1983): Increase in brain prostaglandins during convulsions is due to increased neuronal activity and not to hypoxia. *Arch. Int. Pharmacodyn. Ther.*, 263:180–188.

68. Forstermann, U., Heldt, R., and Hertting, G. (1983): Effects of intracerebroventricular administration of prostaglandin D_2 on behaviour,

blood pressure and body temperature as compared to prostaglandins E_2 and $F_{2\alpha}$. *Psychopharmacology (Berlin)*, 80:365–370.

69. Gaudet, R., Alam, I., and Levin, L. (1980): Accumulation of cyclooxygenase products of arachidonic acid metabolism in gerbil brain during reperfusion after bilateral common carotid artery occlusion. *J. Neurochem.*, 35:653–658.

70. German, B., Bruckner, G., and Kinsella, J. (1983): Evidence against a $PGF_{4\alpha}$ prostaglandin structure in trout tissue—A correction. *Prostaglandins*, 26:207–210.

71. Gilbert, J. C., Davison, D. V., and Wyllie, M. G. (1978): Studies of the physiological roles of prostaglandins in the central nervous system. *Neuropharmacology*, 17:417–419.

72. Grbovic, L., and Radmanovic, B. Z. (1979): Prostaglandins E_2 and $F_{2\alpha}$ and gross behavioural effects of cholinomimetic substances injected into the cerebral ventricles of unanaesthetized cats. *Neuropharmacology*, 18:667–671.

73. Grbovic, L., and Radmanovic, B. Z. (1981): Prostaglandins E_2 and $F_{2\alpha}$ and acetylcholinesterase activity in the slices of some structures in the cat's brain. *Arch. Int. Physiol. Biochim.*, 89:379–383.

74. Groot, P. H. E., Scholte, H. R., and Hulsmann, W. (1976): Fatty acid activation: Specificity, localization and function. *Adv. Lipid Res.*, 14:75–126.

75. Gryglewski, R. J., Panczenko, B., Korbut, R., Grodzinska, L., and Ocetkiewicz, A. (1975): Corticosteroids inhibit prostaglandin release from perfused mesenteric blood vessels of rabbit and from perfused lungs of sensitized guinea pig. *Prostaglandins*, 10:343–355.

76. Gullner, H. G. (1983): Endogenously synthesized prostaglandins stimulate sympathetic nervous system activity. *Prostaglandins Leukotrienes Med.*, 10:345–348.

77. Hallcher, L. M., and Sherman, W. R. (1980): The effects of lithium ion and other agents on the activity of myo-inositol-1-phosphatase from bovine brain. *J. Biol. Chem.*, 225:10896–10901.

78. Hammarstrom, S. (1983): Leukotrienes. *Annu. Rev. Biochem.*, 52:355–377.

79. Hedqvist, P. (1973): Prostaglandin mediated control of sympathetic neuroeffector transmission. *Adv. Biosci.*, 9:461–473.

80. Hemler, M., and Lands, W. (1980): Evidence for a peroxide-initiated free radical mechanism of prostaglandin biosynthesis. *J. Biol. Chem.*, 255:6253–6261.

81. Hillier, K., and Templeton, W. W. (1982): Stimulation of prostaglandin synthesis in rat cerebral cortex via a beta-adrenoceptor. *Gen. Pharmacol.*, 13:21–25.

82. Hirata, F., and Iwata, M. (1983): Role of lipomodulin, a phospholipase inhibitory protein, in immunoregulation by thymocytes. *J. Immunol.*, 130:1930–1936.

83. Holmes, S. (1970): The spontaneous release of prostaglandins into the cerebral ventricles of the dog and the effect of external factors on this release. *Br. J. Pharmacol.*, 37:653–658.

84. Honchar, M. P., Olney, J. W., and Sherman, W. R. (1983): Systemic cholinergic agents induce seizures and brain damage in lithium-treated rats. *Science*, 30:323–325.

85. Horrocks, L., and Harder, H. (1983): Fatty acids and cholesterol. In: *Handbook of Neurochemistry, Vol. 3*, edited by A. Lajtha, pp. 1–16. Plenum, New York.

86. Horton, E. W., and Main, I. H. M. (1967): Identification of prostaglandins in central nervous tissues of the cat and chicken. *Br. J. Pharmacol.*, 30:582–602.

87. Horne, R. L., Pettinati, H. M., Menken, M., Sugerman, A. A., Varga, E., and Wilson, G. F. (1984): Dexamethasone in electroconvulsive therapy: efficacy for depression and post-ECT amnesia. *Biol. Psych.*, 19:13–27.

88. Joseph, S. K., Thomas, A. P., Williams, R. J., Irvine, R. F., and Williamson, J. R. (1984): myo-Inositol 1,4,5-trisphosphate. A second messenger for the hormonal mobilization of intracellular Ca^{2+} in liver. *J. Biol. Chem.*, 259:3077–3081.

89. Kawahara, Y., Takai, Y., Minakuchi, R., Sano, K., and Nishizuka, Y. (1980): Phospholipid turnover as a possible transmembrane signal for protein phosphorylation during human platelet activation by thrombin. *Biochem. Biophys. Res. Commun.*, 97:309–317.

90. Keough, K. M. W., MacDonald, G., and Thompson, W. (1972): A possible relation between phosphoinositides and the diglyceride pool in rat brain. *Biochim. Biophys. Acta*, 270:337–347.

91. Keough, K. M. W., and Thompson, W. (1972): Soluble and particulate forms of phosphoinositide phosphodiesterase in ox brain. *Biochim. Biophys. Acta*, 270:324–336.

92. Kimelberg, H. K., and Paphadjopoulos, D. (1971): Phospholipid protein interactions: Membrane permeability correlated with monolayer "penetration." *Biochim. Biophys. Acta*, 223:205–209.

93. Kondo, K., Shimizu, T., and Hayaishi, O. (1981): Effects of prostaglandin D_2 on membrane potential in neuroblastoma × glioma hybrid cells as determined with a cyanine dye. *Biochem. Biophys. Res. Commun.*, 98:648–655.

94. Kontos, H., Wei, E., Povlishock, J., Dietrich, D., Magiera, C., and Ellis, E. (1980): Cerebral anteriolar damage by arachidonic acid and prostaglandin G_2. *Science*, 209:1242–1245.

95. Lands, W. (1979): The biosynthesis and metabolism of prostaglandins. *Annu. Rev. Physiol.*, 41:633–652.

96. Lands, W., and Crawford, C. (1976): Enzymes of membrane phospholipid metabolism in animals. In: *The Enzymes of Biological Membranes, Vol. 2*, edited by A. Martonosi, pp. 3–85. Plenum, New York.

97. Lands, W. E. M., Inove, M., Sugiura, Y., and Okuyama, H. (1982): Selective incorporation of polyunsaturated fatty acids into phosphatidylcholine by rat liver microsomes. *J. Biol. Chem.*, 257:14968–14972.

98. Lands, W., and Samuelsson, B. (1968): Phos-

pholipid precursor of prostaglandins. *Biochim. Biophys. Acta*, 164:426–429.

99. Lapetina, E. G., Billah, M., and Cuatrecasas, P. (1981): The initial action of thrombin on platelets. *J. Biol. Chem.*, 256:5032–5040.

100. Laychock, S., Johnson, D., and Harris, L. (1980): PGD$_2$ effects on rodent behavior and EEG patterns in cats. *Pharmacol. Biochem. Behav.*, 12:747–754.

101. Lazarewicz, J. W., Leu, V., Sun, G. Y., and Sun, A. Y. (1983): Arachidonic acid release from K$^+$-evoked depolarization of brain synaptosomes. *Neurochem. Int.*, 5:471–478.

102. Majewska, M. D., and Sun, G. Y. (1982): Activation of arachidonyl-phosphatidylinositol and phosphatidylcholine turnover by K$^+$-evoked stimulation of brain synaptosomes. *Neurochem. Int.*, 4:427–433.

103. Marion, J., Pappius, H. M., and Wolfe, L. S. (1979): Evidence for the use of a pool of the free arachidonic acid in rat cerebral cortex tissue for prostaglandin F$_{2\alpha}$ synthesis in vitro. *Biochim. Biophys. Acta*, 573:229–237.

104. Marion, J., and Wolfe, L. (1978): Increase *in vivo* of unesterified fatty acids, prostaglandin F$_{2\alpha}$ but not thromboxane B$_2$ in rat brain during drug-induced convulsions. *Prostaglandins*, 16: 99–110.

105. Marion, J., and Wolfe, L. S. (1979): Origin of the arachidonic acid released post-mortem in rat forebrain. *Biochim. Biophys. Acta*, 574:25–32.

106. Metz, S. A., Fujimoto, W. F., and Robertson, R. P. (1982): Lipoxygenation of arachidonic acid: A pivotal step in stimulus-secretion coupling in the pancreatic beta cell. *Endocrinology*, 111:2141–2143.

107. Michell, R. H. (1975): Inositol phospholipids and cell surface receptor function. *Biochim. Biophys. Acta*, 415:81–145.

108. Moskowitz, N., Puszkin, S., and Schook, W. (1983): Characterization of brain synaptic vesicle phospholipase A$_2$ activity and its modulation by calmodulin, prostaglandin E$_2$, prostaglandin F$_{2\alpha}$, cyclic AMP and ATP. *J. Neurochem.*, 41(6):1576–1586.

109. Morelli de Liberti, S. A., de Los Santos de Schaub, E. B., and Rodriguez de Turco, E. G. (1985): Circannual rhythm of free fatty acids and diacylglycerols in 5-day-old rat cerebrum during pentylenetetrazol-induced convulsions. *J. Neurochem.*, 45:1055–1061.

110. Nielsen, J., Fossum, L., and Sparber, S. (1980): Metabolism of ^{3}H-dopamine continuously perfused through push-pull cannulas in rats' brain: Modification by amphetamine or prostaglandin F$_{2\alpha}$. *Pharmacol. Biochem. Behav.*, 13:235–242.

111. Normann, P. T., Thomassen, M. S., Christiansen, E. N., and Flatmark, T. (1981): Acyl CoA synthetase activity of rat liver microsomes. *Biochim. Biophys. Acta*, 664:416–427.

112. Ohki, S., Ogino, N., Yamamoto, S., and Hayaishi, O. (1979): Prostaglandin hydroperoxidase, an integral part of prostaglandin endoperoxide synthetase from bovine vesicular gland microsomes. *J. Biol. Chem.*, 254:829–836.

113. Oliw, E. H., Lawson, J. A., Brash, A. R., and Oates, J. A. (1981): Arachidonic acid metabolism in rabbit renal cortex. *J. Biol. Chem.*, 256:9924–9931.

114. Oliw, E. H., and Oates, J. A. (1981): Oxygenation of arachidonic acid by hepatic microsomes of the rabbit mechanism of biosynthesis of two vicinal dihydroxyeicosatrienoic acids. *Biochim. Biophys. Acta*, 666:327–340.

115. Palmer, M. R., Mathews, R., Hoffer, B. J., and Murphy, R. C. (1980): Electrophysiological response of cerebellar purkinje neurons to leukotriene D$_4$ and B$_4$. *J. Pharmacol. Exp. Ther.*, 219:91–96.

116. Pang, S. S., Hong, S. L., and Levine, L. (1977): Prostaglandin production by methylcholanthrene-transformed mouse BALB/3T3. *J. Biol. Chem.*, 252:1408–1413.

117. Partington, C., Edwards, M., and Daly, J. (1980): Regulation of cyclic AMP formation in brain tissue by α-adrenergic receptors: Requisite intermediacy of prostaglandins of the E series. *Proc. Natl. Acad. Sci. U.S.A.*, 77:3024–3028.

118. Pediconi, M. F., Rodriguez de Turco, E. B., and Bazan, N. G. (1982): Diffusion of intracerebrally injected (1-^{14}C) arachidonic acid and (2-^{3}H)glycerol in the mouse brain. Effects of ischemia and electroconvulsion shock. *Neurochem. Res.*, 7:1453–1463.

119. Pediconi, M. F., Rodriguez de Turco, E. B., and Bazan, N. G. (1983): Effects of postdecapitation ischemia on the metabolism of (^{14}C) arachidonic acid and (^{14}C) palmitic acid in the mouse brain. *Neurochem. Res.*, 8:835–845.

120. Pickett, W. C., Jesse, R. J., and Cohen, P. (1976): Trypsin-induced phospholipase activity in human platelets. *Biochem. J.*, 160:405–408.

121. Raffel, G., Clarenbach, P., Peskar, B. A., and Hertting, G. (1976): Synthesis and release of prostaglandins by rat brain synaptosomal fractions. *J. Neurochem.*, 26:493–498.

122. Ramwell, P., and Shaw, J. (1966): Spontaneous and evoked release of prostaglandins from cerebral cortex of anesthesized cats. *Am. J. Physiol.*, 211:125–134.

123. Reddy, T. S., and Bazan, N. G. (1983): Kinetic properties of arachidonoyl coenzyme A synthetase in rat brain microsomes. *Arch. Biochem. Biophys.*, 226:125–133.

124. Reddy, T. S., Birkle, D. L., Armstrong, D., and Bazan, N. G. (1985): Change in content, incorporation and lipoxygenation of docosahexaenoic acid in retina and retinal pigment epithelium in canine ceroid lipofuscinosis. *Neurosci. Lett.*, 59:67–72.

125. Rehncoona, S., Siesjö, B. K., and Westerberg, E. (1978): Adenosine and cyclic AMP in cerebral cortex of rats in hypoxia, status epilepticus and hypercapnia. *Acta Physiol. Scand.*, 104: 453–463.

126. Reimann, W., Steinhauer, H., Hedler, L., Starke, K., and Hertting, G. (1981): Effect of prostaglandins D$_2$, E$_2$, F$_2$ on catecholamine release from slices of rat and rabbit brain. *Eur. J. Pharmacol.*, 69:421–427.

127. Rhoads, D. E., Ockner, R. K., Peterson, N. A., and Raghupathy, E. (1983): Modulation of membrane transport by free fatty acids: Inhibition of

synaptosomal sodium-dependent amino acid uptake. *Biochemistry*, 22:1965–1970.

128. Rhoads, D. E., Osburn, L. D., Peterson, N. A., and Raghupathy, E. (1983): Release of neurotransmitter amino acids from synaptosomes: Enhancement of calcium-independent efflux by oleic and arachidonic acids. *J. Neurochem.*, 41:531–537.

129. Rodriguez de Turco, E. B., Cascone, G. D., Pediconi, M. F., and Bazan, N. G. (1977): Phosphatidate, phosphatidylinositol, diacylglycerols and free fatty acids in the brain following electroshock, anoxia, or ischemia. *Adv. Exp. Med. Biol.*, 83:389–396.

130. Rodriguez de Turco, E. B., Morelli de Liberti, S., and Bazan, N. G. (1983): Stimulation of free fatty acid and diacylglycerol accumulation in cerebrum and cerebellum during bicuculline-induced status epilepticus. Effect of pretreatment with α-methyl-*p*-tyrosine and *p*-chlorophenylalanine. *J. Neurochem.*, 40:252–259.

131. Rosenkranz, R. P., and Killam, K. F. (1979): Potentiation of pentylenetetrazole and electroshock induced seizures by prostaglandin $F_{2\alpha}$. *Proc. West. Pharmacol. Soc.*, 22:43–45.

132. Roughan, P., Holland, R., and Slack, C. (1979): On the control of long chain fatty acid synthesis in isolated intact spinach (*Spinacia oleracea*) chloroplasts. *Biochem. J.*, 184:193–202.

133. Rouser, G., Fleisher, S., and Yamamoto, A. (1976): Two-dimensional thin layer chromatographic separation of polar lipids and determination of phospholipids by phosphorus analysis of spots. *Lipids*, 5:494–496.

134. Samuelsson, B. (1983): Leukotrienes: Mediators of immediate hypersensitivity reactions and inflammation. *Science*, 220:568–575.

135. Sachar, E. J., Asnis, G., Halbreich, U., Nathan, R. S., and Halpern, F. (1980): Recent studies in the neuroendocrinology of major depressive disorders. *Psych. Clin. North Am.*, 3:313–326.

136. Sautebin, L., Spagnuolo, C., Galli, C., and Galli, G. (1978): A mass fragmentographic procedure for the simultaneous determination of HETE and $PGF_{2\alpha}$ in the central nervous system. *Prostaglandins*, 16:985–988.

137. Schaeffer, A., Komlos, M., and Seregi, A. (1978): Effects of biogenic amines and psychotropic drugs on endogenous prostaglandin biosynthesis in the rat brain homogenates. *Biochem. Pharmacol.*, 27:213–218.

138. Sherman, W. R., Leavitt, A. L., Honchar, M. P., Hallcher, L. M., and Phillips, B. E. (1981): Evidence that lithium alters phosphoinositide metabolism: Chronic administration elevates primarily *d-myo*-inositol-1-phosphate in cerebral cortex of the rat. *J. Neurochem.*, 36:1947–1951.

139. Sherstnev, V., and Gromov, A. (1980): Effect of prostaglandin $F_{2\alpha}$ and E_2 on sensitivity of rabbit cortical neurons to acetylcholine and noradrenalin. *Neirofiziologiya*, 12:239–245.

140. Shimizu, T., Mizuno, N., Amano, T., and Hayaishi, O. (1979): Prostaglandin D_2, a neuromodulator. *Proc. Natl. Acad. Sci. U.S.A.*, 76:6231–6234.

141. Siegel, M. I., McConnell, R. T., Bonser, R. W., and Cuatrecasas, P. (1981): The production of 5-HETE and leukotriene B in rat neutrophils from carrageenan pleural exudates. *Prostaglandins*, 21(1):123–132.

142. Siesjö, B. K., Ingvar, M., and Westerberg, E. (1982): The influence of bicuculline-induced seizures on free fatty acid concentrations in cerebral cortex, hippocampus and cerebellum. *J. Neurochem.*, 39:796–802.

143. Siggins, G., Hoffer, B., and Bloom, F. (1971): Prostaglandin-norepinephrine interactions in brain: Microelectrophoretic and histochemical correlates. *Ann. N.Y. Acad. Sci.*, 180:302–323.

144. Sklenovsky, A., and Chmela, Z. (1982): Effect of antiepileptic drugs on free fatty acids in the brain during seizure state. *Activ. Nerv. Sup.*, 24:282–283.

145. Solomon, L. P., Leipkalns, V. A., and Spector, A. A. (1976): Changes in $(Na^+ + K^+)$-ATPase activity of Ehrlich ascites tumor cells produced by alteration of membrane fatty acid composition. *Biochemistry*, 15:982–987.

146. Soukup, J. F., Friedel, R. O., and Schanberg, S. M. (1978): Cholinergic stimulation of polyphosphoinositide metabolism in brain in vivo. *Biochem. Pharmacol.*, 27:1239–1243.

147. Spagnuolo, C., Sautebin, L., Galli, G., Racagni, G., Galli, C., Mazzari, S., and Finesso, M. (1979): $PGF_{2\alpha}$, Thromboxane B_2 and HETE levels in gerbil brain cortex after ligation of common carotid arteries and decapitation. *Prostaglandins*, 18:53–61.

148. Steinhauer, H., Anhut, H., and Hertting, G. (1979): The synthesis of prostaglandins and thromboxane in the mouse brain in vivo: Influence of drug induced convulsions, hypoxia and the anticonvulsants trimethadione and diazepam. *Naunyn-Schmiedebergs Arch. Pharmacol.*, 310:53–58.

149. Strosznajder, J., and Sun, G. Y. (1981): Effects of acute hypoxia on incorporation of [1-^{14}C]arachidonic acid into glycerolipids of rat brain. *Neurochem. Res.*, 6:767–774.

150. Su, K., and Sun, G. (1977): The effects of carbamylcholine on incorporation *in vivo* of [1-^{14}C] arachidonic acid into glycerolipids of mouse brain. *J. Neurochem.*, 29:1059–1063.

151. Su, K. L., and Sun, G. Y. 1978): Acyl group composition of metabolically active lipids in brain: Variances among subcellular fractions and during postnatal development. *J. Neurochem.*, 31:1043–1047.

152. Sun, G. Y., and Su, K. L. (1979): Metabolism of arachidonyl phosphoglycerides in mouse brain subcellular fractions. *J. Neurochem.*, 32:1053–1059.

153. Sun, G. Y., and Sun, A. Y. (1972): Phospholipids and acyl groups of synaptosomal and myeline membranes isolated from the cerebral cortex of squirrel monkey (*Saimiri Sciureus*). *Biochim. Biophys. Acta*, 280:306–315.

154. Sun, G. Y., Tang, W., Majewska, M. D., Halett, D. W., Foudin, L., and Huang, S. (1983): Involvement of phospholipid metabolism in neural membrane functions. In: *Neural Membranes*, edited by G. Y. Sun, N. G. Bazan, J. Y. Wu, G.

Porcellati, and A. Y. Sun, pp. 67–95. Humana, Clifton, New Jersey.

155. Suzuki, N., Nakamura, T., Sukehiro, I., Ishikawa, Y., Sasaki, T., and Takao, A. (1983): Identification of 5-hydroxyeicosatetraenoic acid in cerebrospinal fluid after subarachnoid hemorrhage. *J. Neurochem.*, 41:1186–1189.

156. Tamai, I., Takei, T., Maekawa, K., and Ohta, H. (1983): Prostaglandin $F_{2\alpha}$ concentrations in the cerebrospinal fluid of children with febrile convulsions, epilepsy and meningitis. *Brain Dev.*, 5:357–362.

157. Tang, W., and Bazan, N. G. (1984): Dexamethasone Decreases Bicuculline-induced Accumulation of Brain FFA. *Trans. Am. Soc. Neurochem.*, 15:152.

158. Vadnal, R., Van Rooijen, L. A. A., and Bazan, N. G. (1985): Enhanced inositide turnover during bicuculline-induced status epilepticus. *Trans. Am. Soc. Neurochem.*, 16:311.

159. Wei, E., Kontos, H., Dietrich, D., Povlishock, J., and Ellis, E. (1981): Inhibition by free radical scavengers and by cyclooxygenase inhibitors of pial arteriolar abnormalities from concussive brain injury in cats. *Circ. Res.*, 48:95–103.

160. Wieloch, T., and Siesjö, B. K. (1982): Ischemic brain injury: The importance of calcium, lipolytic activities, and free fatty acids. *Pathol. Biol. (Paris)*, 30:269–277.

161. Wilson, D. B., Prescott, S. M., and Majerus, P. W. (1982): Discovery of an arachidonoyl coenzyme A synthetase in human platelets. *J. Biol. Chem.*, 257:3510–3515.

162. Woelk, N., Peiler-Ichikawa, K., Bingalia, L., Goralli, G., and Porcellati, G. (1974): Distribution and properties of phospholipases A_1 and A_2 in synaptosomes and subsynaptosomal fractions of rat brain. *Hoppe-Seyler's Z. Physiol. Chem.*, 555:1535–1542.

163. Wolfe, L. (1975): Possible roles of prostaglandins in the nervous system. *Adv. Neurochem.*, 1:1–49.

164. Wolfe, L. S. (1982): Eicosanoids: Prostaglandins, thromboxanes, leukotrienes, and other derivatives of carbon-20 unsaturated fatty acids. *J. Neurochem.*, 38:1–13.

165. Wolfe, L. S., and Coceani, F. (1979): The role of prostaglandins in the central nervous system. *Annu. Rev. Physiol.*, 41:669–684.

166. Wolfe, L., and Mamer, O. (1975): Measurement of prostaglandin $F_{2\alpha}$ levels in human cerebrospinal fluid in normal and pathological conditions. *Prostaglandins*, 9:183–192.

167. Wolfe, L., Pappius, H., and Marion, J. (1976): The biosynthesis of prostaglandins by brain tissue *in vitro*. *Adv. Prostaglandin Thromboxane Leukotriene Res.*, 1:345–355.

168. Yamashita, A., Watanabe, T., and Hayashi, O. (1983): Autoradiographic localization of a binding protein(s) specific for prostaglandin D_2 in rat brain. *Proc. Natl. Acad. Sci. U.S.A.*, 80:6114–6118.

169. Yoshida, S., Inoh, S., Asano, T., Sano, K., Kubota, M., Shimazaki, H., and Ueta, N. (1980): Effect of transient ischemia on free fatty acids and phospholipids in the gerbil brain: Lipid peroxidation as a possible cause of postischemic injury. *J. Neurosurg.*, 53:323–331.

170. Yoshimoto, T., Miyamoto, Y., Ochi, K., and Yamamoto, S. (1982): Arachidonate 12-lipoxygenase of porcine leukocyte with activity for 5-hydroxyeicosatetraenoic acid. *Biochim. Biophys. Acta*, 713:638–646.

171. Zatz, M., and Roth, R. (1975): Electroconvulsive shock raises prostaglandins F in rat cerebral cortex. *Biochem. Pharmacol.*, 24:2101–2103.

Advances in Neurology, Vol. 44, edited by
A. V. Delgado-Escueta, A. A. Ward, Jr.,
D. M. Woodbury, and R. J. Porter.
Raven Press, New York © 1986.

45

Brain Protein Metabolism in Epilepsy

*,†Barney E. Dwyer, *,†Claude G. Wasterlain, *,†Denson G. Fujikawa,
and **Leslie Yamada

*Epilepsy Research Laboratory and **Department of Pharmacy, Veterans Administration Medical Center,
Sepulveda, California 91343; and †Department of Neurology and Brain Research Institute, UCLA School of
Medicine, Los Angeles, California 90024*

SUMMARY   Both generalized and focal seizures dissociate brain polyribosomes
and severely inhibit brain protein synthesis. This effect is found in freely convulsing animals and in animals that have been paralyzed and oxygen-ventilated
in order to prevent hypoxemia, cerebral hypoxia, and other systemic changes
associated with convulsions.

Recent autoradiographic studies have shown that generalized seizures can result in striking focal inhibition of brain protein synthesis in adult rats and newborn
marmoset monkeys. Local cerebral glucose metabolism and local cerebral blood
flow were also studied in newborn marmosets by autoradiography. Although
flow and metabolism are closely matched in control marmosets, seizures result in
large local increases in 2-deoxyglucose metabolism, with lesser or no increases in
local cerebral blood flow resulting in a relative mismatch. Those regions in which
protein synthesis was most severely inhibited were those in which the relative
mismatch between blood flow and metabolism was most marked.

The molecular mechanisms regulating protein biosynthesis are not known.
Translational regulation during seizures appears to be exerted, in large part, at
the initiation step. A likely mechanism is the inhibition of ternary complex formation, one of the early steps in the initiation process, by increases in the intracellular ratio of [GDP]:[GTP]. This ratio is related to the cells' energy charge.
Reduced levels of ATP during seizures can lead to an increased ratio of
[GDP]:[GTP] via the enzyme nucleoside diphosphate kinase (E.C. 2.7.4.6) and
to inhibition of protein synthesis initiation. Regulation of protein biosynthesis
during seizures is likely to be complex and exerted at many sites; some of these
possibilities are discussed.

Protein metabolism is essential for normal cell function and during development for normal brain growth and maturation. Several experimental studies have shown that epileptic seizures disrupt brain protein synthesis (23). We outline the results of these studies and suggest mechanisms by which protein synthesis may be regulated both during epileptic seizures and in the postictal period. We also comment on the possible relationship of altered protein metabolism to epileptic brain injury.

The discussion has been limited to the effect of generalized seizures on brain protein synthesis and does not include recent work on focal seizures (see, e.g., ref. 6), since regulatory mechanisms are likely to be similar. Finally, the scope of this chapter is limited to the effect of seizures on brain protein synthesis. It does not explore the important role protein synthesis may play in the development of epilepsy, a role suggested by studies in the kindling model of epileptogenesis (4,34).

SINGLE SEIZURES AND THE INHIBITION OF BRAIN PROTEIN SYNTHESIS

Many studies of protein synthesis in animals given electroshock seizures were an outgrowth of efforts to understand the relationship between macromolecule synthesis and behavior. It was known that agents that induced retrograde amnesia in animal models inhibited brain protein synthesis. Because electroconvulsive shock (ECS) could also induce retrograde amnesia, the relationship between ECS and brain protein synthesis was studied in several laboratories. Vesco and Giuditta (53) found that if adult rabbits were subjected to six consecutive electroshocks applied to the head at intervals of 12 to 15 min between shocks, the number of free polyribosomes in brain was decreased while the number of monoribosomes increased. The ability of ECS to dissociate brain polyribosomes was confirmed after the administration of only a single ECS to mice (19,40) and rabbits (48) but not rats that were paralyzed and ventilated with 100% O_2 (59). Popoli and Giuditta (48) found that the ratio of monoribosomes to polyribosomes was significantly increased even 60 min after ECS, while MacInnes et al. (40) found that recovery of normal polyribosome profiles was faster, possibly reflecting species differences. Some doubt has been cast on the results of these studies by recently reported experiments that show that reduced rates of protein synthesis (amino acid incorporation in a gel-filtered, postmitochondrial supernatant system from rabbit brain) could be accounted for by ECS-induced hyperthermia lasting up to 30 min after a single ECS (47).

Protein synthesis measured *in vivo* followed a course similar to polyribosome disaggregation. Table 1 shows the incorporation of ^{14}C- and ^{3}H-labeled amino acids into brain protein after ECS. Results were variable, ranging from 24% inhibition (8) to 80% inhibition (18) immediately after ECS. Since precursor specific activity was not measured, these studies do not provide a true measure of protein synthesis. The large variability probably reflects, at least in part, the different strains of mice used and the choice of precursor. Furthermore, these studies employed tracer quantities of radioactive amino acid injected either intraperitoneally or intravenously so that absorption, metabolism, and the extent of cerebral uptake of the precursor amino acid are quite different and may vary in unexpected ways during seizures.

Initially depressed by ECS, amino acid incorporation into brain protein began to return toward control levels almost immediately and by 15 min had recovered to pre-ECS levels (16,18). Inhibition was not associated with any particular subcellular fraction (17). Protein synthesis measured *in vitro* was reduced by about 50% in a postmitochondrial supernatant system derived from rabbit brain when animals were killed 10 min after ECS (42). Reduced protein synthesis could not be attributed to impaired ribosomal function after ECS, and the authors concluded

TABLE 1. *Effect of single seizures on the incorporation of radioactive amino acids into brain protein* in vivo

Species	ECS	Precursor amino acid	Protein synthesis (% of control)[b]	References
Mouse	TCE[a], 12 mA, 0.2-sec pulse	L-[1-^{14}C]Leucine i.v.	76 (2 min)	(8)
Mouse	TCE, 40 V a.c., 0.1 sec	L-[4,5-^{3}H]Leucine i.p.	20 (2.5 min)	(18)
Mouse	TCE, 40 V a.c., 0.1 sec	L-[4,5-^{3}H]Leucine i.p.	N.S. (15 min)	(18)
Mouse	TCE, 0.1 sec, 17 mA	L-[U-^{14}C]Leucine i.p.	50 (0–5 min)	(16)
Mouse	TCE, 0.1 msec, 17 mA	L-[U-^{14}C]Leucine i.p.	N.S. (15–20 min)	(16)
Mouse	TCE, 12.5–15 mA, 0.2 sec	L-[4,5-^{3}H]Lysine i.p.	47 (5 min)	(16)
Mouse	TCE, 12.5–15 mA, 0.2 sec	L-[1-^{14}C]Leucine i.p.	29 (5 min)	(17)

[a] Current applied through transcorneal electrodes.
[b] Time of sacrifice I after electroshock given in parentheses.
[c] N.S., not significant.

that protein synthesis initiation was defective. However, in light of the data of Nowak and Passonneau (47), caution should be exercised in interpreting the results of these studies.

BRAIN PROTEIN SYNTHESIS DURING CONTINUOUS EPILEPTIC SEIZURES IN A PHYSIOLOGICALLY CONTROLLED RAT MODEL

Status epilepticus is a clinical term to describe a prolonged series of epileptic seizures during which the subject does not regain consciousness between seizures. Experimental models of status epilepticus have been used to advance our understanding of the way prolonged paroxysmal central nervous system (CNS) activity may damage the brain and the role that altered protein metabolism may play in this process. Brain protein synthesis has been studied during repetitive ECS in rats that were paralyzed to prevent muscle contractions and that were artificially ventilated with 100% oxygen to prevent hypoxemia and cerebral hypoxia (55,56,59). The results are shown in Fig. 1. Adult rats, paralyzed and ventilated with 100% O_2, were given an electroconvulsive shock every 30 sec for up to 50 min, after which animals were killed and brain polyribosome profiles were measured. After 50 min of seizures, but not after 15 min, brain polyribosomes had disaggregated. Polyribosome profiles were unaffected by either the surgical preparation, the electrical current, or the artificial ventilation. Anesthesia (2% halothane) that prevented electrical seizures in the electroencephalograph (EEG) also prevented polyribosome disaggregation.

The structural integrity of cerebral ribosomes appeared unaffected by 50 min of status epilepticus. Ribosomes from convulsing rats incorporated [³H]phenylalanine into acid precipitable material in the presence of polyuridylic acid (poly-U) template as well as control ribosomes (Table 2). There was no evidence that polyribosome disaggregation was caused by activation of ribonuclease. Ribonuclease activity was assayed by measuring the extent of degradation of [¹⁴C]poly-U in postmitochondrial supernatant systems derived from brain. Table 3 shows that the extent of [¹⁴C]poly-U degradation in these brain systems was unaffected by seizures. As further proof, monoribosomes and disomes that accumulated during status epilepticus were found to be dissociable into subunits in buffers containing 0.5 M potassium salts (Fig. 2). Monoribosomes produced by ribonuclease action are bound to small strands of mRNA. These ribosomes will not dissociate into subunits buffers containing high salt concentrations, but the monosomes and disomes found during SE did. One last line of evidence for the lack of ribonuclease activation during seizures was that polyribosomes were found to be reassociated 1 hr after the end of seizures. This occurred even after administration of actinomycin D, an inhibitor of DNA-dependent RNA polymerase (Fig.

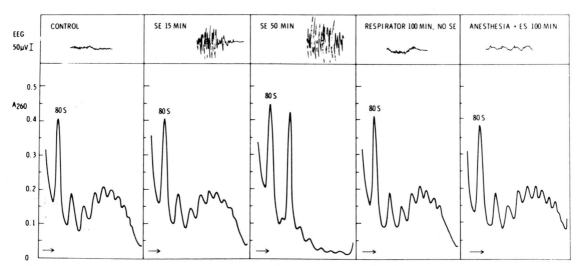

FIG. 1. Effect of status epilepticus on rat brain polysomal profiles. Rats were paralyzed with succinylcholine, tracheotomized, and ventilated with 100% O_2. In status epilepticus (SE) animals, seizures were induced electrically every 30 sec. The anesthesia plus electrical stimulation (ES) group received the same electrical stimulation as SE rats plus 2% halothane anesthesia. The EEGs shown were recorded immediately before killing. For further details see ref. 59. (From ref. 59, with permission.)

TABLE 2. *Radioactivity incorporated into acid-precipitable material by cell-free systems from control and status epilepticus brains*[a]

Group	5 min	10 min	15 min
Control	1290	2075	2622
SE 50 min	681	1046	1112
Control + poly-U	1625	2591	3014
SE + poly-U	1816	2760	3311

[a] Radioactivity incorporated into TCA-precipitable material by brain postmitochondrial supernatant. Final concentrations of the assay system were: 50 mM Tris HCl, pH 7.4 at 0°C, 25 mM KCl, 12 mM $MgCl_2$, 0.25 mM sucrose, 2 mM creatine phosphate, 1 mM ATP, 1 mM GTP, 0.1 mg creatine kinase/ml, 1 mg ribosomes, 2 mg pH 5 enzymes, 1 μCi [^{3}H]phenylalanine (specific activity 2 Ci/mmol), and 0.5 A_{260} unit of poly-U where indicated. Values represent the means of five experiments (each done in triplicate). See ref. 59 for further details.

3). Thus reaggregation of polyribosomes may not require synthesis of new mRNA, suggesting that the functional integrity of mRNA in brain was preserved during seizures. These data taken together suggested that the initiation step of protein synthesis was a major site of translational regulation during prolonged seizures (59). However, Wasterlain (56) also showed that the incorporation of [^{3}H]leucine into brain protein was reduced by about 30% during the first 5 min of seizure activity in the same animal model (Table 4). At 5 min there was little evidence of polyribosome disaggregation. Thus it appears that the rate of elongation of polypeptide chains is also reduced during status epilepticus. Protein synthesis is a complex and highly coordinated process, and it is reasonable to expect that translational regulation would be expressed at several sites.

TABLE 3. *Effect of status epilepticus on brain ribonuclease activity*[a]

Group	Activity (cpm/mg protein · hr)
Control	1422 ± 126
SE 15 min	1389 ± 76
SE 25 min	1481 ± 91
SE 50 min	1457 ± 142

[a] Effect of seizures on [^{14}C]poly-U degradation by brain postmitochondrial supernatants. Forebrains were homogenized in buffer containing 0.25 M sucrose, 12 mM $MgCl_2$, 100 mM KCl, 50 mM Tris HCl (pH 7.6). For each sample, values from duplicate aliquots taken after 15, 30, and 60 min of incubation at 37°C were averaged. Values represent the means ± SEM of five experiments. For further details see ref. 59.

Recovery of brain protein synthesis after seizures depends on the number of seizures administered. Reaggregation of brain ribosomes was more rapid when the duration of seizures was shorter (Fig. 4). When seizures were administered for 25 min, substantial reaggregation of brain ribosomes had occurred within 1 hr of seizure cessation. After 3 hr of recovery, polyribosome profiles were normal (Fig. 4). When seizures were extended to 50 min, some evidence of polyribosome accumulation was present after a 3-hr recovery period, but profiles were obviously abnormal and no ribosome reaggregation was evident within 1 hr of seizure cessation. The abnormal polyribosome profiles found at 1 and 3 hr after 50 min of seizure activity may reflect abnormal cerebral activity in these animals. This is suggested by EEG recordings, which showed that epileptiform activity continued spontaneously after cessation of electroshocks when the latter were administered frequently for greater than 25 min. Little polyribosome reassociation was found even after a 3-hr recovery period when electroshock seizures were continued for 100 min. After termination of ECS, these animals often convulsed spontaneously until death ensued.

We can conclude from these studies that even though the effects of muscle contractions can be prevented and adequate cerebral oxygenation can be maintained, prolonged epileptic seizures can result in a severe reduction of brain protein synthesis. While protein synthesis inhibition in these animals could be attributed to continued seizure activity, it is quite possible that prolonged inhibition of protein synthesis during seizures may also contribute to the development of subsequent brain damage and death.

STATUS EPILEPTICUS IN THE NEONATE: THE EFFECT OF SEIZURES ON PROTEIN SYNTHESIS IN THE DEVELOPING BRAIN

Protein synthesis is essential for normal brain growth and development. Many developmental processes that occur postnatally, including cell division, cell migration and differentiation, the outgrowth of axons and dendrites, and myelination, require the synthesis of new protein. Anything that interferes with protein synthesis during critical developmental periods may also impair brain maturation. Seizures in the immature rat severely reduce brain protein synthesis in both forebrain and hindbrain (25). In rats 4 and 11 days old, bicuculline-induced seizures resulted in protein synthesis inhibition to about 40 and 25% of control values, respectively. Cere-

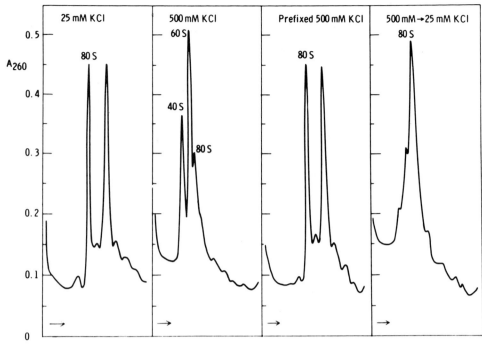

FIG. 2. Instability in high ionic strength buffers. Free polysomal profiles from rats subjected to 25 min of status epilepticus. Brain ribosomes (0.5 mg) were centrifuged at 234,000 *g* for 90 min over 15–35% sucrose density gradient. The final KCl concentration is indicated on top of the gradient. $MgCl_2$ concentration was 5 mM in all cases. Prefixation was carried out by adding 0.1% formaldehyde to the ribosomal suspension immediately before layering on sucrose gradients. In this figure, all tracings are from the same (representative) brain. For further details see ref. 59. (From ref. 59, with permission.)

bral protein synthesis was also significantly reduced when seizures were induced by repeatedly exposing rats to the vapors of the convulsant flurothyl (hexafluorodiethyl ether, Indoklon®) for 2 hr (25). Furthermore, protein synthesis, which transiently returned to near-control levels in both forebrain and hindbrain 1 hr after the end of seizures, was significantly reduced after 5 and 24 hr (Fig. 5). It is possible that reduced rates of protein synthesis both during and after seizures are responsible for the impaired brain development (58) and for the delayed appearance of behavioral milestones (60) found in this experimental model of neonatal seizures. The inhibitory effect of seizures on brain protein synthesis was confirmed in a primate. Epileptic seizures induced with bicuculline in newborn marmoset monkeys reduced the rate of protein synthesis in forebrain (frontal pole) by 52% (24).

AUTORADIOGRAPHIC STUDIES OF BRAIN PROTEIN SYNTHESIS DURING EXPERIMENTAL EPILEPSY

It is clear from the preceding sections that brain protein synthesis is severely inhibited during epileptic seizures. The results cited above were obtained from analysis of whole brain and grossly dissected brain regions; most *in vitro* studies utilized protein synthesizing systems prepared from whole brain or cortex. Autoradiographic techniques, however, have also revealed striking local effects of seizures on brain protein synthesis in both the adult (35) and the neonate (24).

In adult rats, convulsive status epilepticus produced local effects on brain protein synthesis that were quite different from those seen in the newborn marmoset. Kiessling and Kleihues (35) injected [³H]tyrosine intravenously and used stripping film so that they could assess ³H incorporation into protein at the cellular level. Tyrosine incorporation was reduced in neurons of cortical layers 2 and 5, resulting in a "pseudolaminar" pattern of cell labeling (Fig. 6), quite unlike the "columnar" appearance found in the newborn marmoset. Tyrosine incorporation was also markedly reduced in the pyramidal neurons of the hippocampus and in granule cells of the dentate gyrus. Other local effects, including preferential inhibition of protein synthesis in cells in the mediodorsal thalamic nuclei and ap-

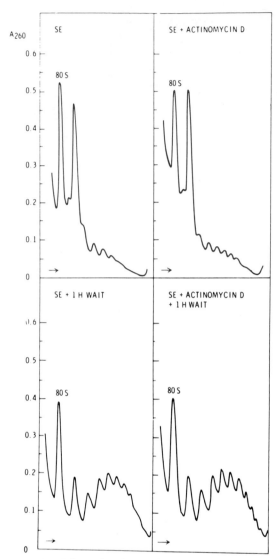

FIG. 3. Effect of actinomycin D on recovery. Rats pretreated with intracerebral actinomycin D or artificial cerebrospinal fluid (CSF) alone were subjected to SE. Actinomycin D inhibited [³H]uridine incorporation into acid-precipitable material over 80% (data not shown) but did not prevent reaggregation of brain polysomes. For further details see ref. 59. (From ref. 59, with permission.)

parent sparing of the cerebellum, have been described and discussed in greater detail (35). However, these authors employed tracer amounts of [³H]tyrosine and did not measure the specific activity of tyrosine in their study. Caution must be exercised when interpreting these results, since the autoradiographic images may reflect not only rates of protein synthesis but

also seizure-related effects on amino acid transport and precursor pool specific activity.

We have recently developed a quantitative autoradiographic method for measuring local rates of brain protein synthesis (20) and have used it to study the effects of convulsive status epilepticus on brain protein synthesis in newborn marmoset monkeys (24). Seizures were induced by the intramuscular injection of bicuculline (5 mg/ kg). A strong tonic seizure occurred within 3 min after injection, followed by tonic–clonic convulsions for the duration of the experiment. Protein synthesis in the cerebral cortex and hippocampus was profoundly inhibited during seizures (Figs. 7 and 8; Table 5). In the cortex, regions in which protein synthesis was severely inhibited alternated with regions in which protein synthesis was relatively maintained, creating a "columnar" pattern. These columns were irregular in appearance, were often distributed asymmetrically, and penetrated the cortical mantle to varying depths. In the hippocampus, protein synthesis inhibition was also strikingly focal; severe inhibition was found in some groups of neurons, while adjacent groups of neurons were less affected. In some subcortical gray-matter structures such as the thalamus, protein synthesis was less affected during seizures than in the cortex and hippocampus (Fig. 7, Table 5), but in other areas (e.g., caudate) it was severely inhibited. Particularly striking was the finding that protein synthesis in the lateral geniculate nuclei was unaffected during seizure activity. In the proliferating external granular layer of the cerebellum, protein synthesis appeared little affected during convulsions (Fig. 8). However, protein synthesis was markedly inhibited in other neuronal populations in the same cerebellum, particularly in the internal granular layer. It is not known why rates of protein synthesis in certain neuronal populations are differentially affected during seizure activity. Our results in newborn marmoset are not likely to be caused by alteration of precursor specific activity in local brain regions. Our method uses a "flooding" amount of [¹⁴C]valine, as described by Dunlop et al. (15), which expands the pool of free valine in the brain 10- to 20-fold and maintains the specific activity of brain acid-soluble valine at a constant level for at least 2 hr. We found that brain acid-soluble valine specific activity was the same in seizure and control marmosets, so we feel that our autoradiographs accurately reflect local rates of brain protein synthesis during seizures.

It is quite likely that those regions in which protein synthesis inhibition is greatest are those

TABLE 4. *Brain protein synthesis in status epilepticus*[a]

| | 0–5 min of seizures | | 25–30 min of seizures | | 55–60 min of seizures | |
| | Leucine (cpm/μM) | Protein (cpm/mg) | Leucine (cpm/μM) | Protein (cpm/mg) | Leucine (cpm/μM) | Protein (cpm/mg) |
Group						
Control group ± SEM	3,786 ± 137	654 ± 41	3,792 ± 147	699 ± 18	3,838 ± 172	666 ± 36
Electroconvulsive shock group ± SEM	6,278 ± 218	471 ± 11	6,264 ± 199	424 ± 14	6,093 ± 204	338 ± 36
p	<0.001	<0.001	<0.001	<0.001	<0.001	

[a] [³H]Leucine incorporation into cerebral proteins after 5-min pulses (500 μCi) injected during repetitive electroconvulsive seizures in paralyzed, oxygen-ventilated rats. See ref. 56 for further details.

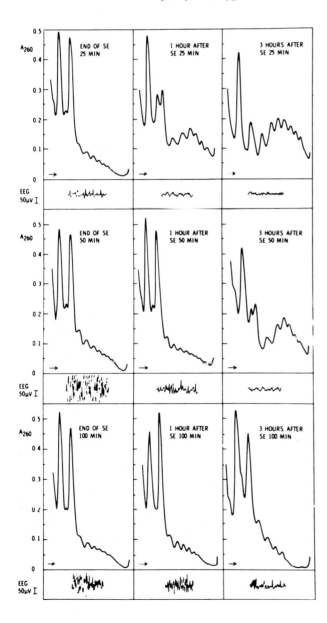

FIG. 4. Recovery from status epilepticus. The EEGs shown were recorded immediately before sacrifice. The *horizontal arrow* indicates the direction of centrifugation. In all tracings, the first large peak on the left represents 80-S ribosomes. For further details see ref. 59. (From ref. 59, with permission.)

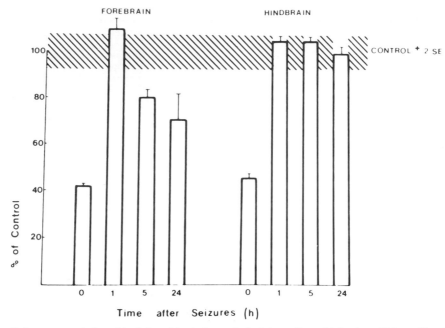

FIG. 5. Seizures were induced in 4-day-old rats by a single intraperitoneal injection of bicuculline (8 mg/kg). [3H]Lysine (1 μCi/μmol) was injected i.p. 60 min before killing. The value of time 0 (60 min after bicuculline injection) depicts the rate of protein synthesis during seizures. Bars represent the means ± SE of experimental rats, expressed as percentage of control values. The hatched area represents mean control values ± SE. For further details see ref. 25. (From ref. 25, with permission.)

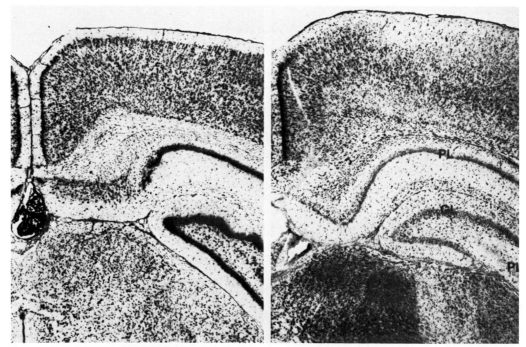

FIG. 6. Parasagittal region of the cerebral hemisphere demonstrating marked focal reduction of [3H]tyrosine incorporation into neurons of the cortex and of the pyramidal layer (PL) and granular layer (GL) of the hippocampus. In addition, note the irregular extent of incorporation within the adjacent midbrain structures. **Left:** control rat. **Right:** status epilepticus. Unstained autoradiographs (×30). For further details and discussion see ref. 35. (From ref. 35, with permission.)

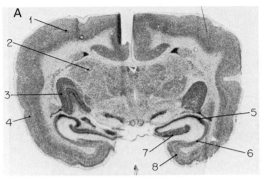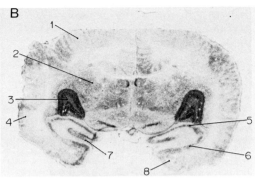

FIG. 7. Quantitative autoradiography of brain protein synthesis. Local forebrain protein synthesis during bicuculline-induced seizures in newborn marmosets. Marmoset monkeys (5–7 days old) were injected with 150 mM [1-^{14}C]-L-valine (10 μmol/g, 0.1 μCi/μmol, i.p.), followed immediately by bicuculline (5 mg/kg, i.m.) or 0.9% NaCl in controls. Animals were killed up to 1 hr after seizure onset. Brains were removed frozen and cut into 20-μm coronal sections and exposed to Kodak SB-5 X-ray film as previously described (20). Rates of protein synthesis were measured in the brain regions indicated in the figure and representative autoradiographs from **(A)** control and **(B)** convulsing marmosets are shown. Areas designated in the figure are: 1, parietal cortex; 2, thalamus; 3, lateral geniculate nucleus; 4, temporal cortex; 5, hippocampus CA3 subregion; 6, hippocampus CA1 subregion; 7, dentate gyrus; 8, entorhinal cortex. Rates of protein synthesis were measured in these regions and are shown in Table 5. (From ref. 24, with permission.)

that are actively involved in seizure activity and incur the greatest metabolic stress. We have studied the effects of seizures on cerebral glucose utilization and on blood flow by autoradiography (Figs. 9 and 10). During seizures in ketamine-anesthesized marmosets, relative 2-deoxyglucose (2DG) uptake was dramatically increased in several structures, including cerebral cortex, hippocampus, and basal ganglia, while other regions such as the lateral geniculate nuclei were not affected. Relative cerebral blood flow was not significantly changed during seizure activity. A highly significant correlation was found between increased uptake of 2DG and

inhibition of protein synthesis during seizures, but an even higher correlation existed between the ratios of increases in 2DG and isopropyl-iodoamphetamine (IMP) uptake and the degree of inhibition of protein synthesis (Fig. 11).

Some aspects of the methodology used for these studies should be considered. First, it is assumed that the kinetic and lumped constants described by Sokoloff et al. (52) are invariant between control and seizure states. While this assumption appears true under several physiological conditions (51), it is not valid under certain pathological conditions (29,62). Crane et al. (9) have shown that when the transport of glu-

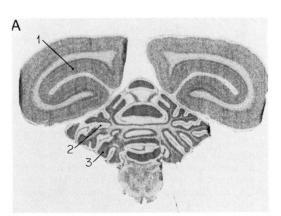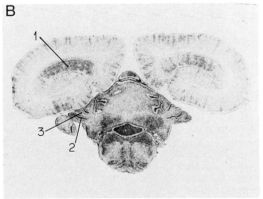

FIG. 8. Quantitative autoradiography of brain protein synthesis during bicuculline-induced seizures in newborn marmosets. Experimental procedures were the same as described in the legend of Fig. 6. Representative autoradiographs from **(A)** control and **(B)** convulsing marmosets are shown. Areas designated in the figure are: 1, striate cortex; 2, external granular layer; 3, internal granular layer. (From ref. 24, with permission.)

TABLE 5. *Rates of local brain protein synthesis (LBPS) in newborn marmoset monkeys during bicuculline-induced status epilepticus[a]*

Brain region	LBPS (%/hr)		
	Control	Seizure	% of Control
Cortex			
Striate	1.69 ± 0.16	0.59 ± 0.17	35[b]
Parietal	1.60 ± 0.07	0.52 ± 0.11	33[b]
Temporal	1.53 ± 0.05	0.54 ± 0.07	35[b]
Entorhinal	1.38 ± 0.06	0.68 ± 0.20	49[b]
Hippocampus			
CA1	1.68 ± 0.15	0.65 ± 0.08	39[b]
CA3	2.26 ± 0.11	0.90 ± 0.13	40[b]
Dentate	1.87 ± 0.04	0.77 ± 0.04	41[b]
Thalamus	1.31 ± 0.08	1.02 ± 0.28	78[c]
Lateral geniculate	2.04 ± 0.12	1.89 ± 0.46	93[c]

[a] Marmoset monkeys (5–7 days old) were injected with 150 mM [1-14C]-L-valine (10 μmol/g, 0.1 μCi/μmol, i.p.), followed immediately by bicuculline (5 mg/kg, i.m.) or 0.9% NaCl in controls. Animals were killed up to 1 hr after seizures had started. Each measurement is the mean ± SD for 3 animals.
[b] $p < 0.001$.
[c] Not significantly different from control.

a serious overestimate of the cerebral metabolic rate of glucose by the deoxyglucose method.

We have used [3H]-3-*O*-methyl-D-glucose (30) to estimate local cerebral glucose concentrations during seizures in ketamine anesthetized marmosets, and our preliminary results suggest that brain glucose is not depleted in this model. Furthermore, this, coupled with the fact that blood glucose concentrations are normal or elevated, suggests that the effects of seizures on the value of the lumped constant (relative to that of control animals) is minimal, and that 14C content in brain regions visualized by autoradiography reflects in large part the relative rate of glucose utilization in these structures during seizures. However, a serious difficulty in the interpretation of double-label autoradiographs using deoxyglucose and iodoantipyrine or iodoamphetamine is the difference in the time of injection of the two tracers. [14C]Deoxyglucose is injected at the onset of the experiment, resulting in higher blood levels at early times and in a deoxyglucose uptake that undoubtedly is skewed toward the early events in the course of prolonged seizures. On the other hand, the uptake of iodoamphetamine and iodoantipyrine reflects events occurring during the last minute of the half-hour experiment. While the animals have continuous seizure activity, the increasing duration of the periods between tonic–clonic movements suggests they are not in a true met-

cose from blood to brain becomes rate-limiting for cerebral glucose utilization (rather than glucose phosphorylation, which is usually the case), the value for the lumped constant may increase significantly. If a correction is not made for this "lumped constant effect," it can lead to

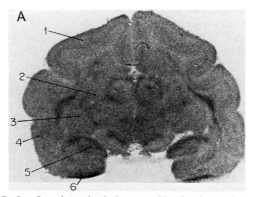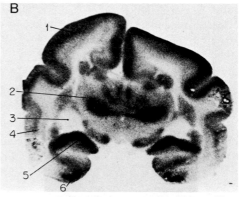

FIG. 9.   Local cerebral glucose utilization in newborn marmoset monkeys during generalized bicuculline seizures. Marmoset monkeys were anesthetized with ketamine (50 mg/kg, i.p.) and the jugular vein was exposed for isotope injection. Epileptic seizures were induced with bicuculline (10 mg/kg, i.m.). [1-14C]-2-Deoxy-D-glucose (2DG) was injected at the time of the first tonic seizure and animals were killed by decapitation 45 min later. Brains were frozen and cut in 20-μm coronal sections. When animals were injected with both *N*-isopropyl-[123I]-*p*-iodoamphetamine (IMP), a cerebral blood flow tracer (see Fig. 10), and 2DG, tissue sections were exposed to Kodak SB-5 X-ray film for 13 hr to obtain a 123I image, and after waiting 7 half-lives for 123I to decay (123I $T_{1/2}$ = 13 hr) the tissue sections were reexposed to SB-5 film to obtain a 14C image (38). The optical density of autoradiographs was measured with a Sargent Welch model PPD densitometer with a 0.25-mm light aperture. Representative autoradiographs from **(A)** control and **(B)** convulsing marmosets are shown. Areas designated in the figure are: 1, parietal cortex; 2, thalamus; 3, lateral geniculate nucleus; 4, temporal cortex; 5, hippocampus; 6, entorhinal cortex.

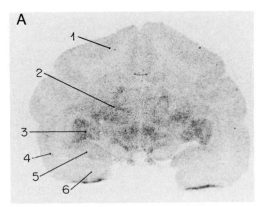 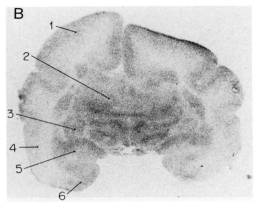

FIG. 10. Local cerebral blood flow in newborn marmoset monkeys during generalized bicuculline seizures. Local cerebral blood flow was measured using N-isopropyl-$[^{123}I]$-p-iodoamphetamine (IMP) (37,64). Blood flow was measured in the same animals in which 2-deoxyglucose metabolism was studied (Fig. 9). The $[^{123}I]$IMP was injected during the last minute of the experiment. Following decapitation, brain tissue was processed for autoradiography as described in Fig. 9. Representative autoradiographs from (A) control and (B) convulsing marmosets are shown. Areas designated are: 1, parietal cortex; 2, thalamus; 3, lateral geniculate nuclei; 4, temporal cortex; 5, hippocampus; 6, entorhinal cortex.

abolic steady state, and it is possible that some of the differences observed between the blood flow images and the metabolic images reflects differences between early and late seizures rather than a true mismatch between metabolism and blood flow.

Despite the qualitative nature of these studies, the large increases in 2DG uptake and/or mismatch between 2DG and IMP uptake in brain regions which show severe protein synthesis inhibition suggest that a local mismatch between blood flow and metabolism may be a factor in the effect of seizures on brain protein synthesis in immature marmosets.

SEIZURES AND THE REGULATION OF BRAIN PROTEIN SYNTHESIS

Role of Brain Energy Metabolism

The translation of mRNA into protein involves a series of steps by which mRNA is bound to ribosomes, forming a competent 80-S ribosome initiation complex (initiation), synthesis of the polypeptide chain by the energy-dependent polymerization of amino acids coded for by the mRNA (elongation), and release of the completed polypeptide chain (termination). One of the first steps in protein synthesis initiation is the formation of a ternary complex between initiation factor eIF-2, the initiator species of methionyl-tRNA and GTP, which subsequently binds to a 40-S ribosomal subunit in one of the several steps in the initiation process.

Walton and Gill (54) have shown in a reticulocyte system that the formation of initiation complexes is sensitive to changes in the ratio of GTP/GDP and suggested that this ratio and thus the rate of protein synthesis could be regulated by the adenylate energy charge potential of the cell. This is defined by Atkinson (1) as

$$ECP = \frac{[ATP] + \frac{1}{2}[ADP]}{[ATP] + [ADP] + [AMP]}$$

and is a measure of the availability of high-energy phosphate bonds for performing cell work.

Ternary complex formation *in vitro* in a brain system is inhibited when the ratio of [GDP]:[GTP] increases (21). This is true over at least a 30-fold concentration range of GTP (Table 6); GMP has little effect on ternary complex formation (Fig. 12), as have ADP, AMP, UDP, UMP, CDP, and CMP.

On the basis of these data we have described a mechanism by which the adenylate energy charge of the cell may regulate brain protein synthesis during seizures (21). Epileptic seizures place severe demands on cerebral energy metabolism. Rates of cerebral energy utilization have been estimated to increase three- to fivefold during the seizure discharge (6,27,36,50), and significant reductions of brain high-energy phosphate compounds are found shortly after seizure onset. While most of the reduction in high-energy phosphates can be prevented by paralyzing and oxygen-ventilating animals (7), there is still a small but significant fall in the brain adenylate energy charge potential

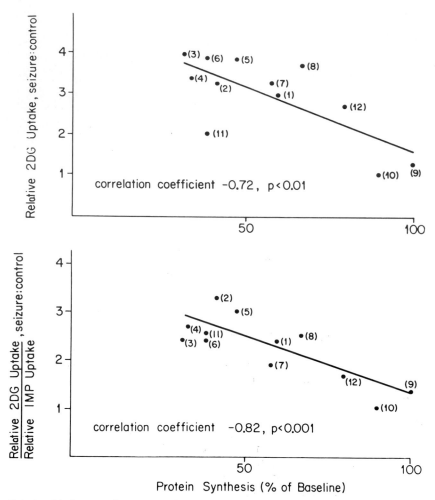

FIG. 11. Relationship between local rates of brain protein synthesis during bicuculline-induced seizures and local 2-deoxyglucose and IMP uptake. Local 2-deoxyglucose and IMP uptake were expressed relative to that in optic tract, a structure in which the rate of protein synthesis was unaffected during bicuculline seizures (24). Best fit straight lines were determined by linear regression analysis and drawn through the data points. The numbered points correspond to the following brain structures: 1, frontal cortex; 2, striate cortex; 3, parietal cortex; 4, temporal cortex; 5, entorhinal cortex; 6, hippocampus; 7, caudate nucleus; 8, putamen; 9, lateral geniculate nuclei; 10, optic tract; 11, frontal white matter; 12, substantia nigra.

(5,14,28,32). A small increase in the ratio of [ADP]:[ATP] presumably results in an increased ratio of [GDP]:[GTP] sufficient to inhibit protein synthesis initiation. This is unlikely to be the whole explanation for protein synthesis inhibition during seizures. One prominent mechanism for the regulation of protein synthesis initiation involving the phosphorylation of initiation factor eIF-2 is well established in the reticulocyte and is a distinct possibility in the brain.

Protein synthesis initiation is a highly regulated process (2,31,33), and regulation may be exerted at several sites during seizures.

Role of Ionic Equilibrium

Massive membrane depolarization during a seizure discharge can disturb ionic equilibrium in brain. Moody et al. (44) found that the extracellular potassium concentration rose to 10 mM in penicillin epileptogenic foci in cat cortex (baseline value 3.4 mM). Disturbed ionic equilibrium may lead to altered rates of protein synthesis. Lipton and Heimbach (39) showed that lysine incorporation into hippocampal slices was sensitive to the intracellular ratio of [K$^+$]:[Na$^+$]. The restoration of normal extracellular [K$^+$] oc-

TABLE 6. *Effect of added GDP on ternary complex formation*[a]

[GDP]:[GTP]	[GTP] (mM)				
	0.1	0.3	0.5	1.5	3.0
0	100	100	100	100	100
1:10	62	63	57	57	52
1:2	31	31	27	23	22

[a] Ternary complex formation was assayed by retention of radioactivity on nitrocellulose filters at the GTP concentrations indicated. GDP was added in molar ratios of 0 (complete system without added GDP), 1:10, and 1:2 with GTP over the range of concentrations employed. GTP-independent binding was subtracted from all determinations. The results are expressed as percent of control.

curs very quickly in the interictal period (44). However, it may contribute in part to the inhibition of protein synthesis during seizures, possibly by the regulation of ternary complex formation during the initiation process (21) or by a direct effect on the elongation of polypeptide chains (26,67).

Role of Physiological Changes during Seizures

Status epilepticus in freely convulsing adult animals produces dramatic physiological effects,

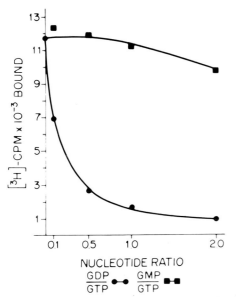

FIG. 12. Effect of GDP and GMP on GTP-dependent ternary complex formation. Ternary complex formation was assayed by retention of radioactivity on nitrocellulose filters (21). GTP was present in the assay mixture at 1.5 mM and various amounts of GDP or GMP were added to give the desired concentration ratio. GTP-independent binding was subtracted from all measurements.

including hypoxemia and cerebral hypoxia, metabolic and respiratory acidosis, and hyperthermia (41,57). In the neonate the brain may also become depleted of glucose in spite of normal blood glucose concentrations (22,61). Several studies suggest that all of these factors are associated with reduced brain protein synthesis. Protein synthesis was significantly reduced *in vivo* in rat brain during hypoxia (43) and *in vitro* in rabbit cortex slices obtained from animals breathing 8% oxygen (3). Lactic acidosis during seizures may be partially responsible for protein synthesis inhibition (43,45). Hypoglycemia also results in reduced brain protein synthesis *in vivo* (43). In hypoglycemia, lactic acid does not accumulate in the brain. It is more likely that inhibition is related to energy failure and falling high-energy phosphate concentrations. Hyperthermia is also known to inhibit brain protein synthesis in some species. Little is known about mechanisms that regulate protein synthesis under these pathological conditions, and specific local effects on rates of brain protein synthesis have not been investigated.

Role of RNA Metabolism

Several studies suggest that RNA processing was inhibited in rat brain following a single flurothyl-induced seizure (66) or in cat cortex during status epilepticus induced by the topical application of cobalt powder (10). This effect was found in rabbit brain in the poly-A-containing RNA species immediately following electroshock (11) and persisted 30 min postictally at a time when the EEG pattern had returned to normal (12). Later studies showed that abnormal RNA metabolism could persist in the postictal recovery period for at least 12 hr (13,65). The meaning of altered RNA metabolism with respect to normal cell function is not clear. Protein synthesis returns to control levels shortly after a single electroconvulsive shock at a time when abnormal RNA metabolism is reported in the brain.

CONCLUSIONS

Epileptic seizures severely inhibit brain protein synthesis in both the immature and the adult rat. This has been confirmed in newborn marmoset monkeys. Autoradiographic studies have demonstrated that inhibition of protein synthesis is not uniform throughout the brain but instead shows striking focality, possibly reflecting active involvement in seizure activity by those neurons. Furthermore, these studies show striking differences between adult and newborn animals. The mechanisms by which brain protein synthesis is regulated are not known in detail. Protein synthesis is a highly energy-dependent process, and its inhibition under conditions of severe cellular metabolic stress might be expected. This may have survival value by reducing the cell energy requirements during a period of increased energy demand. However, prolonged epileptic seizures can lead to brain injury and death. The role of prolonged protein synthesis inhibition in this process is not clear, but it may reduce cell viability by altering the synthesis of key enzymes or structural proteins necessary for cell survival. In the developing brain, protein synthesis inhibition may result in reduced brain cell growth and differentiation, leading to reduced cell number and cell size, aberrant growth of axons and dendrites, abnormal synaptic organization, and ultimately in permanent morphological and behavioral abnormalities.

ACKNOWLEDGMENTS

This work was supported by Research Grant NS13515 from National Institute of Neurological and Communicative Diseases and Stroke (NINCDS) and by the Research Service of the Veterans Administration. We wish to thank Susan L. Mailheau for her help in the preparation of this manuscript.

REFERENCES

1. Atkinson, D. E. (1968): The energy charge of the adenylate pool as a regulatory parameter. Interaction with biofeedback modifiers. *Biochemistry*, 7:4030–4034.
2. Austin, S. A., and Clemens, M. J. (1980): Control of the initiation of protein synthesis in mammalian cells. *FEBS Lett.*, 110:1–7.
3. Blomstrand, C. (1970): Effect of hypoxia on protein metabolism in neuron- and neuroglia cell-enriched fractions from rabbit brain. *Exp. Neurol.*, 29:175–188.
4. Cain, D. P., Corcoran, M. E., and Staines, W. A. (1980): Effects of protein synthesis inhibition on kindling in the mouse. *Exp. Neurol.*, 68:409–419.
5. Chapman, A. G., Meldrum, B. S., Siesjö, B. K. (1977): Cerebral metabolic changes during prolonged epileptic seizures in rats. *J. Neurochem.*, 28:1025–1035.
6. Collins, R. C., and Nandi, N. (1982): Focal seizures disrupt protein synthesis in seizure pathways: An autoradiographic study using [1-14C]-leucine. *Brain Res.*, 248:109–119.
7. Collins, R. C., Posner, J. B., and Plum, F. (1970): Cerebral energy metabolism during electroshock seizures in mice. *Am. J. Physiol.*, 218:943–950.
8. Cotman, C. W., Banker, G., Zornetzer, S. F., and McGaugh, J. L. (1971): Electroshock effects on brain protein synthesis: Relation to brain seizures and retrograde amnesia. *Science*, 173:454–456.
9. Crane, P. D., Pardridge, W. M., Braun, L. D., Nyerges, A. M., and Oldendorf, W. H. (1981): The interaction of transport and metabolism on brain glucose utilization: A reevaluation of the lumped constant. *J. Neurochem.*, 36:1601–1604.
10. Cupello, A., Ferrillo, F., Lazzarini, G., and Rosadini, G. (1976): Effect of experimental status epilepticus on the pattern of RNA synthesis in cerebral cortex. *Exp. Neurol.*, 53:601–609.
11. Cupello, A., Ferrillo, F., and Rosadini, G. (1979): Pattern of labeling of rabbit brain cortex poly(A)-associated RNA after a single electroconvulsive shock. *Exp. Neurol.*, 673:451–457.
12. Cupello, A., Ferrillo, F., and Rosadini, G. (1980): Altered pattern of brain cortex poly(A)-RNA synthesis persisting after post-convulsive EEG recovery. *Exp. Neurol.*, 69:247–252.
13. Cupello, A., Ferrillo, F., and Rosadini, G. (1981): Long-lasting effects of electroconvulsive shock on the pattern of poly(A)-RNA synthesis in rabbit cerebral cortex. *Neurochem. Res.*, 6:175–182.
14. Duffy, T. E., Howse, D. C., and Plum, F. (1975): Cerebral energy metabolism during experimental status epilepticus. *J. Neurochem.*, 24:925–934.
15. Dunlop, D. S., van Elden, W., and Lajtha, A. (1975): A method for measuring brain protein synthesis rates in young and adult rats. *J. Neurochem.*, 24:337–344.
16. Dunn, A. (1971): Brain protein synthesis after electroshock. *Brain Res.*, 35:254–259.
17. Dunn, A. J., and Bergert, B. J. (1976): Effects of electroconvulsive shock and cycloheximide on the incorporation of amino acids into proteins of mouse brain subcellular fractions. *J. Neurochem.*, 26:369–375.
18. Dunn, A., Giuditta, A., and Pagliuca, N. (1971): The effect of electroconvulsive shock on protein synthesis in mouse brain. *J. Neurochem.*, 18:2093–2099.
19. Dunn, A., Giuditta, A., Wilson, J. E., and Glassman, E. (1974): The effect of electroshock on brain RNA and protein synthesis and its possible relationship to behavioral effects. In: *Psychobiology of Convulsive Therapy*, edited by M. Fink, S. Kety, J. McGaugh, and T. A. Williams, pp. 185–197. V. H. Winston, Washington, D.C.
20. Dwyer, B. E., Donatoni, P., and Wasterlain, C. G. (1982): A quantitative autoradiographic method for the measurement of local rates of brain protein synthesis. *Neurochem. Res.*, 7:563–576.
21. Dwyer, B., and Wasterlain, C. G. (1980): Regulation of the first step of the initiation of brain protein synthesis by guanosine diphosphate. *J. Neurochem.*, 34:1639–1647.
22. Dwyer, B. E., and Wasterlain, C. G. (1981): Prolonged seizures deplete brain glucose in normoglycemic neonates. *Neurology (Minn.)*, 31:162.
23. Dwyer, B. E., and Wasterlain, C. G. (1981): Regulation of brain protein synthesis during status epilepticus. In: *Status Epilepticus: Mechanisms of Brain Damage and Treatment*, edited by A. V. Delgado-Esueta, C. G. Wasterlain, D. M. Trei-

man, and R. J. Porter, pp. 299–306. Raven Press, New York.

24. Dwyer, B. E., and Wasterlain, C. G. (1984): Selective focal inhibition of brain protein synthesis during generalized bicuculline seizures in newborn marmoset monkeys. *Brain Res.*, 309:109–121.

25. Fando, J. L., Conn, M., and Wasterlain, C. G. (1979): Brain protein synthesis during neonatal seizures: An experimental study. *Exp. Neurol.*, 63:220–228.

26. Fando, J. L., and Wasterlain, C. G. (1980): A simple reproducible cell-free system for measuring brain protein synthesis. *Neurochem. Res.*, 5:197–207.

27. Ferrendelli, J. A., and McDougal, D. B., Jr. (1971): The effect of electroshock on regional CNS energy reserves in mice. *J. Neurochem.*, 18:1197–1205.

28. Folbergrová, J., Ingvar, M., and Siesjo, B. K. (1981): Metabolic changes in cerebral cortex, hippocampus, and cerebellum during sustained bicuculline-induced seizures. *J. Neurochem.*, 37:1228–1238.

29. Ginsberg, M. D., and Reivich, M. (1979): Use of the 2-deoxy-D-glucose method of local cerebral glucose utilization in the abnormal brain: Evaluation of the lumped constant during ischemia. *Acta Neurol. Scand.*, 60(Suppl. 72):226–227.

30. Gjedde, A., and Diemer, N. H. (1983): Autoradiographic determination of regional brain glucose content. *J. Cereb. Blood Flow Metab.*, 3:303–310.

31. Gross, M. (1980): The control of protein synthesis by hemin in rabbit reticulocytes. *Mol. Cell. Biochem.*, 31:25–36.

32. Howse, D. C. N. (1979): Metabolic responses to status epilepticus in the rat, cat and mouse. *Can. J. Physiol. Pharmacol.*, 57:205–212.

33. Hunt, T. (1980): The initiation of protein synthesis. *Trends Biochem. Sci.*, 5:178–181.

34. Jonec, V., and Wasterlain, C. G. (1979): Effect of inhibitors of protein synthesis on the development of kindled seizures in rats. *Exp. Neurol.*, 66:524–532.

35. Kiessling, M., and Kleihues, P. (1981): Regional protein synthesis in the rat brain during bicuculline-induced epileptic seizures. *Acta Neuropathol.*, 55:157–162.

36. King, L. J., Lowry, O. H., Passonneau, J., and Venson, V. (1967): Effects of convulsants on energy reserves in the cerebral cortex. *J. Neurochem.*, 14:599–611.

37. Lear, J. L., Ackermann, R. F., Kameyama, M., and Kuhl, D. E. (1982): Evaluation of [123I] isopropyliodoamphetamine as a tracer for local cerebral blood flow using direct autoradiographic comparison. *J. Cereb. Blood Flow Metab.*, 2:179–185.

38. Lear, J. L., Jones, S. C., Greenberg, J. H., Fedora, T. J., and Reivich, M. (1981): Use of 123I and 14C in a double radionuclide autoradiographic technique for simultaneous measurement of LCBF and LCMRgl: Theory and method. *Stroke*, 12:589–597.

39. Lipton, P., and Heimbach, C. J. (1978): Mechanism of extracellular potassium stimulation of protein synthesis in the *in vitro* hippocampus. *J. Neurochem.*, 31:1299–1307.

40. MacInnes, J. W., McConkey, E. H., and Schlesinger, K. (1970): Changes in brain polyribosomes following an electro-convulsive seizure. *J. Neurochem.*, 17:457–460.

41. Meldrum, B. S., and Horton, R. W. (1973): Physiology of status epilepticus in primates. *Arch. Neurol.*, 28:1–9.

42. Metafora, S., Persico, M., Felsani, A., Ferraiuolo, R., and Giuditta, A. (1977): On the mechanism of electroshock-induced inhibition of protein synthesis in rabbit cerebral cortex. *J. Neurochem.*, 28:1335–1346.

43. Metter, E. J., and Yanagihara, T. (1979): Protein synthesis in rat brain in hypoxia, anoxia and hyperglycemia. *Brain Res.*, 161:481–492.

44. Moody, W. J., Jr., Futamachi, K. J., and Prince, D. A. (1974): Extracellular potassium activity during epileptogenesis. *Exp. Neurol.*, 42:248–263.

45. Morimoto, K., Brengman, J., and Yanagihara, T. (1978): Further evaluation of polypeptide synthesis in cerebral anoxia, hypoxia and ischemia. *J. Neurochem.*, 31:1277–1282.

46. Myer, J. S., Gotoh, F., and Favale, E. (1966): Cerebral metabolism during epileptic seizures in man. *Electroencephalogr. Clin. Neurophysiol.*, 21:10–22.

47. Nowak, T. S., Jr., and Passoneau, J. V. (1984): Hyperthermia and reduced protein synthesis after electroconvulsive shock. *Trans. Am. Soc. Neurochem.*, 15:165.

48. Popoli, M., and Giuditta, A. (1980): Effect of electroconvulsive shock on polysomes of rabbit brain, liver and kidney. *J. Neurochem.*, 35:1319–1322.

49. Posner, J. B., Plum, F., and Poznak, A. V. (1969): Cerebral metabolism during electrically induced seizures in man. *Arch. Neurol.*, 20:388–395.

50. Saktor, B., Wilson, J. E., and Tiekert, C. G. (1966): Regulation of glycolysis in brain, in situ, during convulsions. *J. Biol. Chem.*, 241:5071–5075.

51. Sokoloff, L. (1979): The (14C) deoxyglucose method: Four years later. *Acta Neurol. Scand.*, 60(Suppl. 72):640–649.

52. Sokoloff, L., Reivich, M., Kennedy, C., Des Rosiers, M. H., Patlak, C. S., Pettigrew, O., Sakurada, O., and Shinohara, M. (1977): The [14C] deoxyglucose method for the measurement of local cerebral glucose utilization: Theory, procedure, and normal values in the conscious and anesthetized albino rat. *J. Neurochem.*, 28:897–916.

53. Vesco, C., and Giuditta, A. (1968): Disaggregation of brain polysomes induced by electroconvulsive treatments. *J. Neurochem.*, 15:81–85.

54. Walton, G. M., and Gill, G. N. (1976): Preferential regulation of protein synthesis initiation complex formation by purine nucleotides. *Biochim. Biophys. Acta*, 447:11–19.

55. Wasterlain, C. G. (1972): Breakdown of brain polysomes in status epilepcus. *Brain Res.*, 39:278–284.

56. Wasterlain, C. G. (1974): Inhibition of cerebral protein synthesis by epileptic seizures without

motor manifestations. *Neurology, (Minn.)*, 24:175–180.

57. Wasterlain, C. G. (1974): Mortality and morbidity from serial seizures. An experimental study. *Epilepsia*, 15:155–176.

58. Wasterlain, C. G. (1976): Effects of neonatal status epilepticus on rat brain development. *Neurology, (Minn.)*, 26:975–986.

59. Wasterlain, C. G. (1977): Effects of epileptic seizures on brain ribosomes: Mechanism and relationship to cerebral energy metabolism. *J. Neurochem.*, 29:707–716.

60. Wasterlain, C. G. (1977): Effects of neonatal seizures on ontogeny of reflexes and behavior. An experimental study in the rat. *Eur. Neurol.*, 15:9–19.

61. Wasterlain, C. G., and Duffy, T. E. (1976): Status epilepticus in immature rats. Protective effects of glucose on survival and brain development. *Arch. Neurol.*, 33:821–827.

62. Welsh, F. A., Greenberg, J. H., Jones, S. C., Ginsberg, M. D., and Reivich, M. (1979): Correlation between glucose utilization and metabolite levels following middle cerebral artery occlusion in the cat. *Acta Neurol. Scand.*, 60 (Suppl. 72):270–271.

63. White, P. T., Grant, P., Mosier, J., and Craig, A. (1961): Changes in cerebral dynamics associated with seizures. *Neurology, (Minn.)*, 11:354–361.

64. Winchell, H. S., Horst, W. W., Braun, L., Oldendorf, W. H., Hattner, R., and Parker, H. (1980): N-isopropyl [^{123}I] p-iodoamphetamine: Single pass brain uptake and washout; Binding to brain synaptosomes; And localization in dog and monkey brains. *J. Nucl. Med.*, 21:947–952.

65. Wynter, C. V. A. (1981): Persistence of altered RNA synthesis in rat cerebral cortex 12 h after a single electroconvulsive shock. *J. Neurochem.*, 32:495–504.

66. Wynter, C. V. A., Ioannow, P., and Mathias, A. P. (1975): The effect of convulsions induced by flurothyl on ribonucleic acid synthesis in rat cerebral cortex during the recovery phase. *Biochem. J.*, 152:449–467.

67. Zomzely, C. E., Roberts, S., and Rapaport, D. (1964): Characteristics of amino acid incorporation into proteins of microsomal and ribosomal preparations of rat cerebral cortex. *J. Neurochem.*, 11:567–582.

Section 7

BASIC MECHANISMS
OF EPILEPSY IN MAN

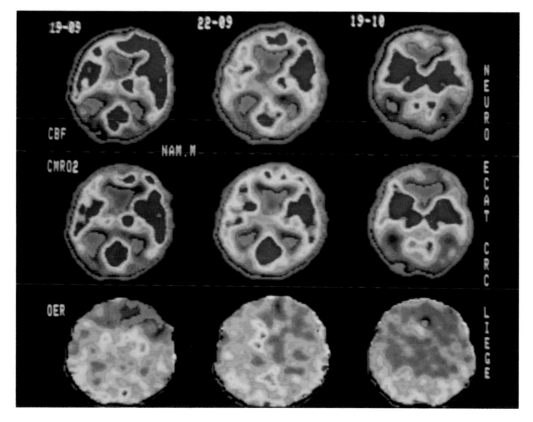

Ictal positron emission tomography scan demonstrates increased cerebral blood flow (CBF) and cerebral metabolic rate for O_2 or $CMRO_2$ on the right cortical regions and in the homolateral basal ganglia and thalamus contrasting with decreased oxygen extraction ratio (OER) observed on the right frontal region. Three days later, the patient was free of seizures, increased CBF and $CMRO_2$ is less marked; OER returns to normal values in the right frontal area; 1 month later, there is no longer asymmetry for CBF, OER, or $CMRO_2$. From Chapter 47 in this volume by G. Franck, B. Sadzot, E. Salmon, J. C. Depresseux, T. Grisar, J. M. Peters, M. Guillaume, and D. Lamotte.

Advances in Neurology, Vol. 44, edited by
A. V. Delgado-Escueta, A. A. Ward, Jr.,
D. M. Woodbury, and R. J. Porter.
Raven Press, New York © 1986.

46

Identification of Seizure-Mediating Brain Structures with the Deoxyglucose Method: Studies of Human Epilepsy with Positron Emission Tomography, and Animal Seizure Models with Contact Autoradiography

*,**,†,§Robert F. Ackermann, **,†,‡,§Jerome Engel, Jr., and
*,**Michael E. Phelps

*Division of Nuclear Medicine and Biophysics, Department of Radiological Sciences, **Laboratory of
Biomedical and Environmental Sciences, †Department of Neurology, ‡Department of Anatomy, and
§Brain Research Institute, UCLA School of Medicine, Los Angeles, California 90024

SUMMARY This chapter describes tomographic and autoradiographic studies
of human and animal seizure syndromes employing Sokoloff's deoxyglucose
method.

The method's rationale rests on two principal facts: that adult brains normally
utilize glucose almost exclusively as their exogenous energy source, and that
deoxyglucose, a glucose analog, accumulates in brain cells in proportion to their
activity level. Thus, computed tomography or contact autoradiography allows
visualization and indirect measurement of changes in the activity of different brain
structures under specified conditions, such as between, during, or immediately
following seizures.

In humans, partial seizures have been the most extensively studied, with ^{18}F-
fluorodeoxyglucose and positron emission tomography. Interictally, the brains of
patients with partial seizures are characterized by hypometabolism that is particularly severe in the vicinity of seizure foci. In many cases, these focal hypometabolic zones become hypermetabolic ictally. Other brain areas may also become
hypermetabolic ictally, or they may instead become hypometabolic. Often the
physical extent of interictal hypometabolic zones is substantially greater than the
extent of overt pathology. This indicates that hypometabolism can result from
subtle, presently undescribed, structural or functional derangements, as well as
from frank neuronal loss.

A variety of animal seizure "models" have also been studied, with ^{14}C-2-deoxy-
glucose and contact autoradiography. Each model has produced a unique deoxyglucose utilization pattern, but thus far none that closely resembles any of the
human seizure patterns. This probably reflects true differences between the mechanisms mediating different types of animal seizures and those mediating human
seizures.

Although in widespread use for only a few years, the Sokoloff method has
already demonstrated its ability to distinguish among a variety of seizure types

in both humans and animals, and to correctly identify those structures most involved in focal seizures. Thus, the method can be of great aid in narrowing the search for seizure-mediating mechanisms.

METHODOLOGY

From Hughlings Jackson's time, epileptologists have attempted to discover the extent to which different brain areas participate in seizures. Until 1977, the inherent sampling limitations of neurophysiological and neurochemical techniques made this goal difficult to achieve. However, the advent of the Sokoloff method for estimating brain glucose utilization (71), which allows epileptologists to survey the entire brain in a single observation, promises to be of great aid in uncovering the mechanisms of seizure initiation and propagation. Application of this method to human seizures by means of positron emission tomography (PET) (41,59) and animal seizures by means of contact autoradiography (71) has already begun to reveal the neuronal constellations that characterize each focal or generalized seizure type.

The Sokoloff method exploits several well-established facts about brain metabolism. First, under normal conditions the adult brain utilizes glucose almost exclusively for obtaining metabolic energy (i.e., ATP production). Second, the hexose facilitated-transport system and hexokinase accept not only glucose but also several deoxyglucose analogs, among them 2-fluorodeoxyglucose (FDG) and 2-deoxyglucose (2DG). The structures of FDG and 2DG differ from glucose only in that the OH group at the C-2 position of glucose is replaced by either a fluorine atom or a hydrogen atom, respectively. Thus, both FDG and 2DG are transported across the blood-brain barrier (BBB) by the facilitated transport system, and are phosphorylated by hexokinase to form FDG 6-phosphate or 2DG 6-phosphate. However, the structures of FDG and 2DG 6-phosphates do not resemble sufficiently that of glucose 6-phosphate to be metabolized any further by glucose-oxidative enzymes, nor are they substrates for the pentose shunt or for glycogen production. Consequently, phosphorylated FDG or 2DG accumulates within brain cells in proportion to their rate of exogenous glucose utilization, which in turn is proportional to the magnitude of their energy requirements (for detailed discussions, see refs. 41, 59, 66, and 71).

Metabolically derived energy is required by both neurons and glia for normal "housekeeping" functions common to all living cells.

Beyond that, neuronal firing imposes its own additional energy demands, the primary one that of reversing the ion fluxes that mediate excitatory or inhibitory postsynaptic potentials, and also action potentials (50). Other ATP-requiring mechanisms linked to neuronal firing, such as transmitter synthesis, release, and reuptake, add to the metabolic burden imposed by neuronal activity. Such considerations lead to a third premise of the Sokoloff technique: that increased 2DG accumulation results from the direct and indirect effects of increased neuronal activity, and decreased 2DG accumulation from decreased activity.

2DG and FDG Methods

Animal studies employ 2DG labeled with ^{14}C, or occasionally ^{3}H or ^{18}F. The labeled 2DG is administered during the seizure condition of interest and is later detected by sectioning the brain and placing the sections in direct contact with photographic film. The labeling isotope's ability to expose the film is proportional to its concentration: the greater the concentration of labeled 2DG within any given structure, the greater the optical density of its image on the developed film. The local metabolic rate within a given brain structure can then be calculated if, in addition to its 2DG accumulation, blood 2DG and glucose levels (measured from timed arterial samples) are also determined (for details, see ref. 71).

Human studies employ FDG labeled with ^{18}F (or less commonly ^{11}C-2DG). As each ^{18}F nucleus decays, it produces a positron that is annihilated by an ambient electron. Each annihilation results in two gamma rays that travel in opposite directions and, having sufficient energy to exit the brain, register on detectors surrounding the head (58) (Fig. 1). The principles of computed tomography are employed to reconstruct the cross-sectional distribution of the tissue ^{18}F concentration. From this distribution, which is analogous to an animal autoradiogram, local metabolic rate is then calculated in a manner similar to that of the animal experiments (for details, see refs. 58, 60).

"Steady-State" Assumption

Like all tracer methods, the 2DG/FDG method assumes that the process being mea-

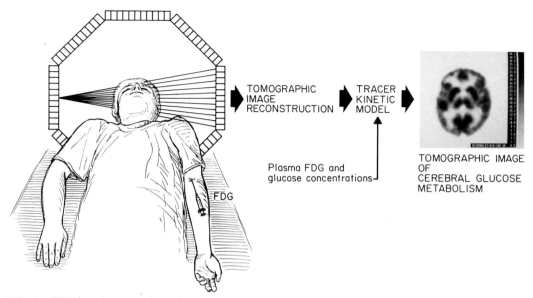

FIG. 1. PET imaging procedure. Gamma rays from annihilated positrons register on detectors surrounding the head **(left)**. A computer (*arrows*) then combines these data with blood FDG and glucose levels to construct an image of local glucose metabolic rate **(right)**. (From ref. 61, with permission.)

sured remains unchanging throughout the course of the measurement. This is called a "steady-state" condition. Under "steady-state" conditions, several inferences can be drawn concerning the nature of an integrated sequence of enzymatic reactions such as those involved in glucose oxidation. One is that all the enzymatic reactions of an integrated sequence occur at the same rate, equal to the sequence's slowest reaction (i.e., the rate-determining step). Therefore, if the rate of any one of the sequence's reactions is determined, the rate of the entire sequence will then also be known. With regard to the 2DG method specifically, this means that under "steady-state" conditions the rate of glucose phosphorylation is the same as the overall rate of glycolysis, given the absence of significant breakdown or synthesis of glycogen. Although the rate of glucose phosphorylation is difficult to measure directly, it can be estimated accurately by measuring the rate at which phosphorylated FDG or 2DG accumulates. However, although FDG and 2DG are very similar in structure to glucose and to each other, they are not identical. Consequently, all three have somewhat different affinities for the hexose facilitated-transport system and are therefore transported across the BBB at somewhat different rates. They also have different affinities for hexokinase, and are therefore phosphorylated at different rates (72). These differences between glucose and its analogs are taken into account

by inclusion of a term called the "lumped constant" (LC) in the denominator of Sokoloff's equation. For rats under normal metabolic conditions, the value of the LC is approximately 0.5, indicating that 2DG is normally phosphorylated at about half the rate of glucose.

The LC and Metabolism

Frequently, the question has arisen as to whether the LC value remains the same under unusual metabolic conditions, such as may occur during and immediately following seizures (69). Crane et al. (18) showed that under conditions of severe insulin-induced hypoglycemia the LC may exceed a value of 1.0 (see also ref. 57). This change in the LC value occurs because under severe hypoglycemia (in which by definition the supply of glucose is less than the demand) the rate-limiting step for 2DG phosphorylation shifts from the rate of the phosphorylation reaction itself to the rate of transport across the BBB. Hexokinase has greater affinity for glucose than for 2DG by a factor of approximately 3 (54), while the hexose transport carrier has greater affinity for 2DG than for glucose by a factor of approximately 1.4. The same shift from phosphorylation to BBB transport as the rate-limiting step can also occur in the presence of normal plasma glucose levels if there is sudden increase in cellular glucose demand that is sufficiently large to exceed the BBB's transport capacity (18). Such sudden large increases in glucose demand may occur with prolonged severe seizures (status epilepticus) (20,30,33, 42). Obviously, if the usual 0.5 value for the LC is used under the conditions just described, for which larger LC values would be more appropriate, the calculated metabolic rate will overestimate the true rate (for detailed discussions, see refs. 30, 42).

However, although it is easy to imagine how it might vary under a variety of pathological conditions including seizures, the LC has thus far proven to be remarkably stable under all but the most extreme metabolic conditions (30,38,42, 43,55,57,68,73). A possible reason for this is that simple theoretical predictions do not take into account the many, presently poorly understood, compensatory mechanisms (e.g., increased blood flow, transport reserve, or increased transport via increased capillary permeability and surface area) that can act to restore falling substrate levels (34). Therefore, whether or not seizures change the LC value by generating energy demands beyond the brain's ability to increase glucose supply remains an empirical question to be answered experimentally for each structure of interest in each seizure state (interictal, ictal, postictal) of each seizure syndrome (30). It cannot be simply assumed *a priori* that any seizure necessarily alters significantly the LC value.

Similar arguments apply to the values of the various transport and enzymatic reaction kinetic (*k*) constants in the Sokoloff equation. These constants are known to vary from normal values when the metabolic rate or substrate levels are either extremely high or extremely low (69,70). However, the range of these constants' values is small over a wide range of plasma glucose values (67). Moreover, the structural similarity between glucose and deoxyglucose results in their *k* values' changing in parallel under any given metabolic condition, thus stabilizing the values of any ratio terms in the Sokoloff equation that comprise these constants (38,69).

Seizures and the "Steady State"

Undoubtedly, the most serious problem with FDG studies of epilepsy is that the episodic nature of seizures clearly violates the assumption of metabolic "steady state." Most seizures last 30 to 120 sec (7) and are usually followed by postictal depression that lasts at least several minutes. The brain's metabolic rate increases sharply during seizures (see below); by contrast, metabolism decreases to subnormal levels during postictal depression (22,44). Under such conditions of varying metabolism during the course of measurement, the calculated metabolic rate represents the average rate over all conditions occurring within the 40- to 45-min measurement period (40). However, it must be noted that this average is weighted in correspondence with plasma 2DG levels, which are highest immediately after a bolus infusion and thereafter fall off precipitously with time, resulting in an approximately exponential weighting that favors events that occur immediately after the infusion (40) (Fig. 2). Consequently, if a single seizure occurs shortly after a 2DG or FDG infusion bolus, the resulting 2DG autoradiogram or FDG computed tomographic scan will represent glucose utilization during both the ictal and the immediate postictal period.

These considerations thus reveal several problems for valid interpretation of seizure-related FDG scans or 2DG autoradiograms. First, we cannot be sure precisely when (ictally or postictally) regions of abnormally high or abnormally low glucose utilization were hyper- or hypometabolic. For example, it cannot be assumed that all hypermetabolic structures necessarily became so during ictus; some may have become hypermetabolic postictally. Second, since brief epochs of generally increased metabolism (ictus) are almost invariably paired with substantially longer epochs of generally decreased metabolism (postictus), the calculated metabolic rate of any particular area will necessarily be normalized. That is, extreme hyper- or hypometabolism will tend to be underestimated in those structures that are hyperactive ictally and hypoactive postictally, or vice versa. Such problems can be partially circumvented by appropriate experimental design strategies and

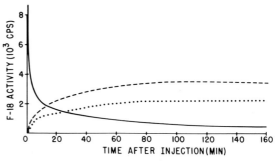

FIG. 2. Typical blood FDG function (*solid line*) following a bolus infusion. The *upper dotted function* represents gray matter accumulation of ^{18}F activity, and the *lower dotted function* the white matter activity.

by use of complementary positron tracer paradigms such as the blood flow and ^{15}O oxygen utilization methods that allow briefer sampling epochs (40–150 sec) (39,51,65). However, it must be kept in mind that although glucose and oxygen metabolism normally are linked, and that blood flow normally is regulated by metabolic demand, the usual relationships among these parameters may change under pathological conditions such as seizures. For example, stressed brain regions may metabolize glucose anaerobically (47), or they may switch to ketones and amino acids as alternate energy-yielding substrates. Also, the normally tight coupling between metabolism and blood flow may break down (1,2,42,77). Therefore, these other indicators of brain metabolism must be interpreted cautiously and in concert with glucose metabolic data, not merely substituted for them.

In summary, although epileptic phenomena present some methodological difficulties with respect to obtaining precise estimates of metabolic rate and with respect to determining the precise temporal sequencing of observed deviations from normal metabolism, seizures are at the same time ideally suited to the greatest single strength of the Sokoloff method: its ability to reveal, with a single procedure, discrete regions of normal and abnormal metabolic activity throughout the entire brain. Epilepsy is the consequence of, and in turn provokes, abnormal brain activity; the Sokoloff method has thus far proven effective in identifying those structures involved in different kinds of seizures and in tracking the changing energy states of those structures through changing seizure states.

HUMAN SEIZURE STUDIES

Thus far, the human seizure type most extensively studied with PET has been complex partial epilepsy, particularly in patients with temporal lobe foci. This has been due primarily to the method's value in localizing and differentiating unilateral seizure "foci" in candidates for temporal lobe resection as therapy for otherwise intractable seizures (28).

Complex Partial Epilepsy and Hypometabolism

Interictal FDG scans of patients with partial epilepsy obtained by Engel and co-workers revealed that the temporal lobe containing the focus had decreased glucose utilization and decreased perfusion compared to its contralateral homolog (21,48) (Fig. 3). In many cases, the rest of the brain, including the contralateral temporal

lobe, also had abnormally low metabolic rates, but not as low as the "epileptic" temporal lobe (24). Although no relationship was found between the degree of metabolic abnormality and the frequency of interictal spikes (24), PET's ability to correctly identify unilateral temporal foci was established by its agreement with localizations derived from a battery of electrophysiological and behavioral tests (27), by the high proportion of favorable clinical outcomes when the more hypometabolic lobe was excised (23), and by the correspondingly high incidence of overt pathology subsequently observed in the removed temporal lobes (21). Invariably, the frank pathological lesion was found to occupy only a small portion of the interictal hypometabolic zone. Thus, interictal hypometabolism can indicate not only frank neuronal loss but also more subtle anatomical or functional derangements in tissue that otherwise appears to be structurally normal using routine histological methods (21).

It is important to note, however, that the relationship between hypometabolism and pathology was not perfect. In some cases, lesions were subsequently found in temporal lobes that had been judged to be metabolically normal. In other cases, no lesions were noted in temporal lobes that had been judged to be hypometabolic. In most of the latter cases, however, there was a plausible explanation for this lack of correspondence (23,24). The PET data were found to be most helpful in identifying the site of the seizure focus when used in conjunction with other, complementary, indicators of epileptogenic pathology (23,24).

Theodore et al. (75) also used PET to study temporal lobe epilepsy. Their study confirmed that interictally the temporal lobe containing the epileptic focus tends to be more hypometabolic than its contralateral counterpart; that the hypometabolic region extends well beyond the focus, sometimes into frontal and parietal regions; and that there is no relation between either the degree or the extent of interictal hypometabolism and the frequency of interictal scalp spiking.

One of their patients had a postictal scan 18 min after a secondarily generalized tonic–clonic seizure. In this case there was bilaterally decreased metabolism, with reduced temporal-lobe asymmetry as compared to the previous interictal scan, and the relatively hypometabolic region extending into the frontal lobe.

Recently, the FDG studies described above were confirmed and extended in another interictal study of temporal-lobe epileptics. Using ^{15}O

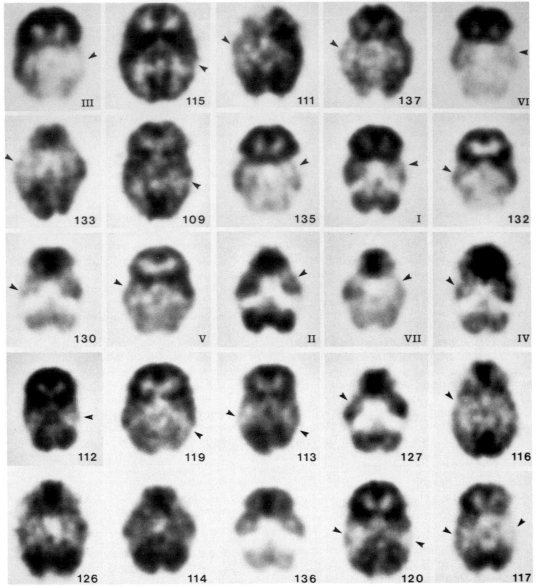

FIG. 3. Typical interictal FDG scans from patients with partial seizures. *Arrows* indicate temporal-lobe hypometabolism (From ref. 21, with permission.)

positron labeling techniques that allow estimation of oxygen metabolic rate, blood flow, and oxygen extraction (32), Bernardi et al. (6) confirmed that interictally temporal-lobe epileptics have global decreases in both metabolism and blood flow compared to controls. Reduced oxygen utilization and blood flow were seen in both cortical and basal ganglia regions; both temporal lobes were hypometabolic compared to controls, but oxygen utilization and blood flow were more reduced in that temporal lobe judged to contain the seizure focus (see also refs. 19, 81). An important novel finding was

that, together with its reduced oxygen utilization, the ''epileptic'' temporal lobe had a significantly elevated oxygen extraction fraction, suggesting that its oxygen supply is only marginally adequate interictally. Bernardi et al. speculated that the epileptic temporal lobe may therefore be vulnerable to further neuronal damage during and immediately following seizures, when oxygen demands are greater.

Considered together, the interictal studies described above indicate that (a) in partial epilepsy there are global reductions in both brain metabolism and blood flow; (b) superimposed on these are disturbances specific to the region that hosts the seizure focus; (c) the anatomical extent of these disturbances far exceeds the bounds of any frank structural lesion; and (d) so far, there is no readily apparent relationship between the severity of the observed metabolic disturbances and any of the commonly measured epileptic parameters.

Complex Partial Seizures and Hypermetabolism

Both Engel et al. (22,25) and Theodore et al. (75) obtained spontaneous ictal scans from some of their partial epilepsy patients. The occurrence of a seizure during an FDG scan frequently resulted in globally increased metabolism, with particularly increased metabolism in the presumed seizure foci and projection areas. This is to say that temporal regions that were hypometabolic interictally became hypermetabolic ictally (Fig. 4). However, the occurrence of a seizure during a scan did not invariably lead exclusively to increased metabolism. In several cases, except for the hypermetabolic epileptic focus and its projection areas, there was globally decreased metabolism, and there was one case in which the hippocampus, the presumed seizure focus, had normal metabolism ictally while the remainder of the temporal lobe was hypometabolic (24,25,48).

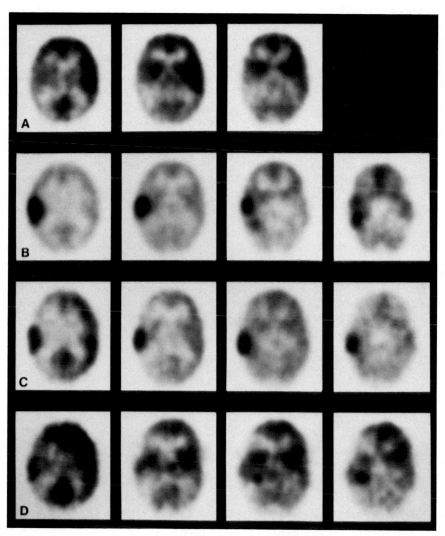

FIG. 4. Interictal (rows **A** and **D**), and ictal (rows **B** and **C**) FDG scans from a patient with partial motor seizures. Note that the hypermetabolic regions in the ictal scans are hypometabolic interictally. (From ref. 25, with permission.)

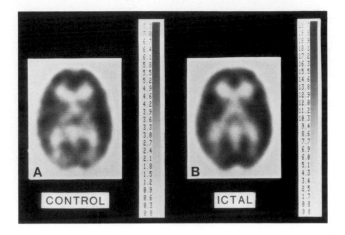

FIG. 5. (A) Control and (B) ictal FDG scans from a petit mal patient. Note that the great ictal hypermetabolism required that each of the two scans be displayed with its own gray scale for each to be discerned. Note also that although ictal metabolism is greatly increased, there is no change in utilization pattern. (From ref. 22, with permission.)

FDG and Generalized Seizures

Besides the studies of partial epilepsy described above, there have been preliminary FDG studies of generalized human seizures. For example, Engel et al. (26) studied four petit mal patients. Each patient had two FDG scans, one in which petit mal absences were induced by hyperventilation, and a second when the seizures had subsequently been brought under anticonvulsant control. In contrast to scans from temporal lobe patients, neither ictal nor interictal petit mal scans had distinguishing patterns of glucose utilization (Fig. 5). Rather, there was a global two- to threefold increase in glucose utilization when petit mal seizures occurred during a scan. This is the greatest increase in glucose utilization reported thus far in the human seizure literature, despite the fact that petit mal seizures appear to be milder than other kinds of seizures. A possible reason for this disparity between apparent seizure severity and glucose utilization is that unlike other types of

seizures, petit mal attacks do not lead to behavioral or electrographic postictal depression. Therefore, it may be that ictal petit mal FDG scans reflect only elevated (ictal) and normal (postictal) metabolism, without a period of postictally decreased metabolism to counterbalance ictal increases. This latter point was perhaps illustrated by another preliminary study by Engel et al. (22), who infused FDG immediately before or immediately following electroconvulsive therapy (ECT). In contrast to petit mal scans, the ictal ECT scans showed only moderately increased metabolism throughout the brain compared to control scans. By contrast, the same patient's postictal ECT scans showed decreased metabolism throughout the brain, compared to the control scans (Fig. 6). ECT-induced seizures generally last no more than 60 sec, and they are followed immediately by profound postictal behavioral and EEG depression lasting up to 10 min (presumably the consequence of greatly reduced neuronal activity). Therefore, "ictal" ECT scans comprise a significant postictal com-

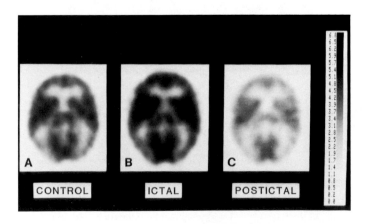

FIG. 6. (A) Control, (B) ictal, and (C) postictal FDG scans of a patient undergoing electroconvulsive therapy (ECT). Note the general ictal hypermetabolism and postictal hypometabolism. (From ref. 22, with permission.)

ponent, and this postictal component may account both for the observed postictal decreases and for the only moderate increases in metabolism seen on "ictal" ECT scans.

Finally, there have been several preliminary FDG studies of Lennox–Gastaut syndrome. Gur et al. (36) reported two cases in which there was marked interictal hypometabolism in one temporal lobe, similar to partial-seizure patients. However, Chugani et al. (9), in a study comprising many more patients, have found in different patients varying patterns of hypometabolism, ranging from unilaterally focal to bilaterally diffuse. Thus, it appears that the 2 patients of the former study formed a subset from a much larger population of patients whose symptoms, although similar in many respects, are caused by a variety of pathologies.

ANIMAL STUDIES

A variety of animal seizure "models" have been studied with 2DG: genetic seizures (53,74), convulsant-induced seizures (5,8,14,15,30,49, 56,76) and stimulation-induced seizures (29,37, 46,78). Thus far, 2DG utilization patterns obtained from studies of animal seizure models have not closely resembled those observed in any human studies. A reason for this lack of congruence between animal and human studies may be "artifactual" in that the resolution of most extant tomographs limits meaningful observations to cortical regions and only the larger subcortical structures, while the resolution of autoradiograms, which approaches 100 μm (35), allows visualization of many smaller subcortical structures. More likely, this discrepancy reflects actual differences between humans and animals in the degree of neocortical development and functional specialization, or inherent differences in the epileptogenic processes under study. In any case, the animal studies have in their own right yielded important insights into the nature of seizure-mediating mechanisms.

For example, Engel et al. (29) studied a "model" of temporal-lobe epilepsy, amygdala-kindled limbic seizures, in rats. They found that partial seizures increased 2DG uptake in the nearby direct projection areas of the amygdala. However, with fully kindled seizures, the increased 2DG uptake extended to more "distant" or diffuse projection areas such as the hippocampus and substantia nigra (see also refs. 7, 45). Ackermann et al. (3) studied amygdala kindling in rat pups (52) and found that 2DG uptake in limbic structures was proportional to the number of kindling stimulations administered

prior to the 2DG experiment. Notably, this was true even of those animals that had been kindled beyond the first appearance of generalized motor seizures. These results reinforce the earlier findings of Pinel and Rovner (62,63), who found that further administration of afterdischarge-evoking stimulations, beyond that necessary for seizure generalization, continued to promote the kindling process toward the eventual emergence of spontaneous seizures.

Such results support the intuitively appealing notion that the severity of overt seizure signs generally reflects the intensity of the underlying seizure-causing neuronal activity. Other 2DG studies suggest further that both the anatomical extent and magnitude of seizure-induced 2DG uptake depend directly on the intensity of activity within the seizure "focus." For example, Collins et al. (10,15) found that the greater the concentration of penicillin administered to rat cortex, the larger was the volume of 2DG uptake surrounding the injection site, the more intense was that uptake, the more extensive was uptake in the projection areas of the seizure focus, and the more severe and varied were the seizure manifestations. Thus, the larger the focus and the greater the intensity of activity within it, the greater its ability to organize and drive "downstream" structures (see also refs. 13, 17, 46). Moreover, these and other 2DG studies (37, 78,79) demonstrate that seizures propagate along normal neuroanatomical pathways; no new or unusual pathways are created by the seizure-initiating process.

Each animal seizure model studied thus far has produced a unique, model-specific 2DG pattern. Together with the human findings, such an outcome indicates that each seizure syndrome is a unique physiological entity and therefore cannot be perfectly "modeled" by another seizure syndrome. On the other hand, it is equally apparent that the seizures within certain classes—e.g., generalized tonic–clonic (5), or limbic-kindled (16), or interictal cortical focus (14)—are clearly related to each other in that they have common involved structures and, consequently, common overt behavioral signs.

PHYSIOLOGICAL INTERPRETATION OF FDG SCANS AND 2DG AUTORADIOGRAMS

The two most striking and consistent FDG and 2DG findings reported thus far have been that seizures result in greatly increased glucose utilization, particularly in the structures that can be presumed on the basis of electrophysiological

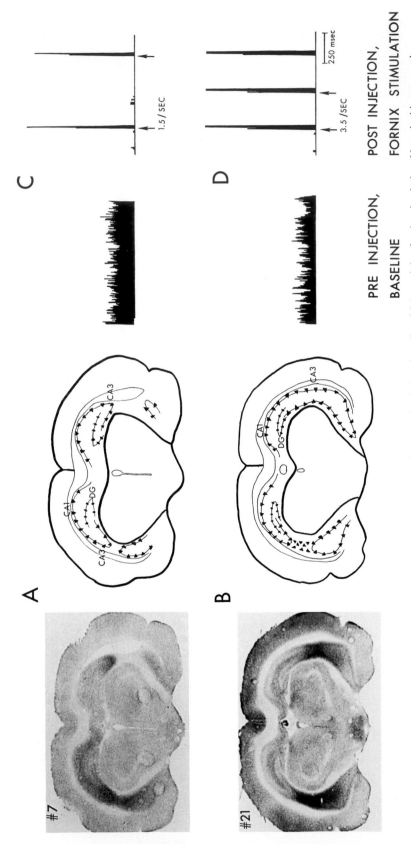

FIG. 7. A, B: 2DG autoradiograms and corresponding diagrams for two animals (numbers 7 and 21) receiving fornix stimulation. Note the hippocampal hypermetabolism. **C, D:** Poststimulation time histograms of multiple pyramidal unit activity in the same two animals, before (**left**) and during (**right**) fornix stimulation. *Arrows* indicate occurrence of stimulations. The activity seen immediately after each stimulation represents a combination of stimulus artifact, evoked potentials, and invasion of action potentials into some pyramidal cell bodies. Note the almost complete cessation of unit activity between stimulations. (From ref. 4, with permission.)

data to mediate the seizures, and that many human epileptic brains are hypometabolic interictally, particularly in the vicinity of seizure foci.

Hypermetabolism is easily interpretable as representing increased neuronal activity in seizure-participating nuclei.

Hypometabolism, on the other hand, is not so easily interpreted. It has frequently been suggested that hypometabolism represents "inhibition" (12,80), the idea being that the decreased metabolism results from decreased activity of a given area's principal neurons. However, decreased firing of principal neurons is the consequence of increased firing by inhibitory neurons (31,64), which typically fire at a much higher rate than principal neurons (4). Therefore, any region in which there is profoundly increased surround inhibition should evince increased, not decreased, glucose utilization; this has been shown to be true for hippocampal inhibition (4) (Fig. 7). Rather, decreased metabolism might be expected in the projection areas of inhibited principal neurons because of their reduced terminal activity; to date this latter possibility has not been confirmed experimentally.

A second, more plausible, explanation for hypometabolism is that it represents reduced activity of both principal neurons and interneurons within the hypometabolic region (cf. ref. 11). This could be due to reduced excitatory input into the hypometabolic region from distant structures that are themselves inhibited, or in the case of human interictal hypometabolism it could be due to subtle, presently undiscovered abnormalities of local neuronal circuitry.

CONCLUSION

There is now a substantial body of evidence that the 2DG method can correctly identify those structures most directly involved in a wide variety of neurophysiological and neuropharmacological phenomena (70). As discussed here, the extended range of metabolic perturbations presented by interictal, ictal, and postictal states makes seizures particularly suitable for study with the Sokoloff method, despite the difficulties they present for calculating precisely the absolute metabolic rate. Rather than precisely quantifying epilepsy-induced metabolic changes, the method's primary value is that of correctly identifying those structures most directly involved in various seizure states. This will allow epileptologists interested in particular seizure syndromes to narrow their search for underlying neurochemical and neurophysiological seizure-inducing derangements to specific subsets of

structures, thereby accelerating significantly the rate at which data necessary for understanding seizure-causing, seizure-propagating, and seizure-ending mechanisms are acquired.

ACKNOWLEDGMENT

Supported by DOE contract #DE-AC03-76-SF00012 and NIH grant #NS-15654.

REFERENCES

1. Abdul-Rahman, A., and Siesjö, B. K. (1980): Local cerebral glucose consumption during insulin-induced hypoglycemia, and in the recovery period following glucose administration. *Acta. Physiol. Scand.*, 110:149–159.

2. Ackermann, R. F., Chugani, H. T., Finch, D. M., Babb, T. L., Lear, J. L., and Engel, J., Jr. (1983): Autoradiographic studies of stimulation-induced changes in rat hippocampal metabolism and blood flow. *J. Cereb. Blood Flow Metab.*, 3(Suppl. 1):S238–S239.

3. Ackermann, R. F., Chugani, H. T., Handforth, A., Moshé, S., Caldecott-Hazard, S., and Engel, J., Jr. (1986): Autoradiographic studies of cerebral metabolism and blood flow in rat amygdala kindling. In: *Kindling 3*, edited by J. A. Wada. Raven Press, New York. (*In press.*)

4. Ackermann, R. F., Finch, D. M., Babb, T. L., and Engel, J., Jr. (1984): Increased glucose metabolism during long-duration recurrent inhibition of hippocampal pyramidal cells. *J. Neurosci.*, 4:251–264.

5. Ben-Ari, Y., Tremblay, E., Riche, D., Ghilini, G., and Naquet, R. (1981): Electrographic, clinical and pathological alterations following systemic administration of kainic acid, bicuculline or pentetrazole: Metabolic mapping using the deoxyglucose method with special reference to the pathology of epilepsy. *Neuroscience*, 6:1361–1391.

6. Bernardi, S., Trimble, M. R., Frackowiak, R. S. J., Wise, R. J. S., and Jones, T. (1983): An interictal study of partial epilepsy using positron emission tomography and the oxygen-15 inhalation technique. *J. Neurol. Neurosurg. Psychiatry*, 46:473–477.

7. Blackwood, D. H. R., Kapoor, V., and Martin, M. J. (1981): Regional changes in cerebral glucose utilization associated with amygdaloid kindling and electroshock in the rat. *Brain Res.*, 224:204–208.

8. Chugani, H. T., Ackermann, R. F., Chugani, D. C., and Engel, J., Jr. (1984): Opioid-induced epileptogenic phenomena: Anatomical, behavioral, and electroencephalographic features. *Ann. Neurol.*, 15:361–368.

9. Chugani, H. T., Engel, J., Jr., Mazziotta, J. C., and Phelps, M. E. (1984): 18F-2-fluorodeoxyglucose positron emission tomography in medically refractory childhood epilepsy. *Neurology*, 34 (Suppl. 1):107(abstr.).

10. Collins, R. C. (1976): Metabolic response to focal penicillin seizures in the rat: Spike discharge vs. afterdischarge. *J. Neurochem.*, 27:1473–1482.

11. Collins, R. C. (1978): Use of cortical circuits during focal penicillin seizures: An autoradiographic study with [14C] deoxyglucose. *Brain Res.*, 150:487–501.

12. Collins, R. C. (1980): Intracortical localization of 2-deoxyglucose metabolism: On-off metabolic columns. In: *Cerebral Metabolism and Neural Function*, edited by J. V. Passoneau, R. A. Hawkins, W. D. Lust, and F. A. Welsh, pp. 338–351. Williams and Wilkins, Baltimore.

13. Collins, R. C., and Caston, T. V. (1979): Functional anatomy of occipital lobe seizures: An experimental study in rats. *Neurology*, 29:705–716.

14. Collins, R. C., and Caston, T. V. (1979): Activation of cortical circuits during interictal spikes. *Ann. Neurol.*, 6:117–125.

15. Collins, R. C., Kennedy, C., Sokoloff, L., and Plum, F. (1976): Metabolic anatomy of focal motor seizures. *Arch. Neurol.*, 33:536–542.

16. Collins, R. C., Lothman, E. W., and Olney, J. W. (1983): Status epilepticus in the limbic system: Biochemical and pathological changes. *Adv. Neurol.*, 34:277–288.

17. Collins, R. C., Tearse, R. G., and Lothman, E. W. (1983): Functional anatomy of limbic seizures: Focal discharges from medial entorhinal cortex in rat. *Brain Res.*, 280:25–40.

18. Crane, P. D., Pardridge, W. M., Braun, L. D., Nyerges, A. M., and Oldendorf, W. H. (1981): The interaction of transport and metabolism on brain glucose utilization: A re-evaluation of the lumped constant. *J. Neurochem.*, 36:1601–1604.

19. Depresseux, J. C., Franck, G., and Sadzot, B. (1983): Regional cerebral blood flow and oxygen uptake in human focal epilepsy. In: *Current Problems in Epilepsy I: Cerebral Blood Flow and Metabolism*, edited by M. Baldy-Moulinier, D. H. Ingvar, and B. S. Meldrum, pp. 76–81. J. Libbey, London.

20. Diemer, N. H., and Gjedde, A. (1983): Autoradiographic determination of brain glucose content and visualization of the regional lumped constant. *J. Cereb. Blood Flow Metab.*, 3(Suppl. 1):S79–S80.

21. Engel, J., Jr., Brown, W. J., Kuhl, D. E., Phelps, M. E., Mazziotta, J. C., and Crandall, P. H. (1982): Pathological findings underlying focal temporal lobe hypometabolism in partial epilepsy. *Ann. Neurol.*, 12:518–528.

22. Engel, J., Jr., Kuhl, D. E., and Phelps, M. E. (1982): Patterns of human local cerebral glucose metabolism during epileptic seizures. *Science*, 218:64–66.

23. Engel, J., Jr., Kuhl, D. E., Phelps, M. E., and Crandall, P. H. (1982): Comparative localization of epileptic foci in partial epilepsy by PCT and EEG. *Ann. Neurol.*, 12:529–537.

24. Engel, J., Jr., Kuhl, D. E., Phelps, M. E., and Mazziotta, J. C. (1982): Interictal cerebral glucose metabolism in partial epilepsy and its relation to EEG changes. *Ann. Neurol.*, 12:510–517.

25. Engel, J., Jr., Kuhl, D. E., Phelps, M. E., Rausch, R., and Nuwer, M. (1983): Local cerebral metabolism during partial seizures. *Neurology*, 33:400–413.

26. Engel, J., Jr., Lubens, P., Kuhl, D. E., and Phelps, M. E. (1985): Local cerebral metabolic rate for glucose during petit mal absences. *Ann. Neurol.*, 17:121–128.

27. Engel, J., Jr., Rausch, R., Lieb, J. P., Kuhl, D. E., and Crandall, P. H. (1981): Correlation of criteria used for localizing epileptic foci in patients considered for surgical therapy of epilepsy. *Ann. Neurol.*, 9:215–224.

28. Engel, J., Jr., Sutherling, W. W., Cahan, L., Crandall, P. H., Kuhl, D. E., and Phelps, M. E. (1984): The role of emission tomography in the surgical therapy of epilepsy. In: *Advances in Epileptology: XVth Epilepsy International Symposium*, edited by R. J. Porter, R. H. Mattson, A. A. Ward, and M. Dam, pp. 427–432. Raven Press, New York.

29. Engel, J., Jr., Wolfson, L., and Brown, L. (1978): Anatomical correlates of electrical and behavioral events related to amygdaloid kindling. *Ann. Neurol.*, 3:538–544.

30. Evans, M. C., and Meldrum, B. S. (1984): Regional brain glucose metabolism in chemically-induced seizures in the rat. *Brain Res.*, 297:235–245.

31. Finch, D. M., and Babb, T. L. (1977): Response decrement in a hippocampal basket cell. *Brain Res.*, 130:354–359.

32. Frackowiak, R. S. J., Lenzi, G.-L., Jones, T., and Heather, J. D. (1980): Quantitative measurement of regional cerebral blood flow and oxygen metabolism in man using 15O and positron emission tomography: Theory, procedure, and normal values. *J. Comput. Assist. Tomogr.*, 4:727–736.

33. Gjedde, A. (1982): Calculation of cerebral glucose phosphorylation from brain uptake of glucose analogs *in vivo*: A re-examination. *Brain Res. Rev.*, 4:237–274.

34. Gjedde, A. (1983): Modulation of substrate transport to the brain. *Acta Neurol. Scand.*, 67:3–25.

35. Goochee, C., Rasband, W., and Sokoloff, L. (1980): Computerized densitometry and color coding of [14C] deoxyglucose autoradiographs. *Ann. Neurol.*, 7:359–370.

36. Gur, R. C., Sussman, N. M., Alavi, A., Gur, R. E., Rosen, A. D., O'Connor, M., Goldberg, H. I., Greenberg, J. H., and Reivich, M. (1982): Positron emission tomography in two cases of childhood epileptic encephalopathy (Lennox–Gastaut syndrome). *Neurology*, 32:1191–1194.

37. Handforth, A., and Ackermann, R. (1985): Functional 2-deoxyglucose mapping of progressive states of status epilepticus induced by amygdala stimulation in rat. *Soc. Neurosci. Abstr.*, 11:1318.

38. Hawkins, R. A., Phelps, M. E., Huang, S.-C., and Kuhl, D. E. (1981): Effect of ischemia on quantification of local cerebral glucose metabolic rate in man. *J. Cereb. Blood Flow Metab.*, 1:37–51.

39. Huang, S.-C., Carson, R. E., Hoffman, E. J., Carson, J., MacDonald, N., Barrio, J. R., and Phelps, M. E. (1983): Quantitative measurement of local cerebral blood flow in humans by positron computed tomography and 15O-water. *J. Cereb. Blood Flow Metab.*, 3:141–153.

40. Huang, S.-C., Phelps, M. E., Hoffman, E. J., and Kuhl, D. E. (1981): Error sensitivity of fluo-

rodeoxyglucose method for measurement of cerebral metabolic rate of glucose. *J. Cereb. Blood Flow Metab.*, 1:391–401.

41. Huang, S.-C., Phelps, M. E., Hoffman, E. J., Sideris, K., Selin, C. J., and Kuhl, D. E. (1980): Noninvasive determination of local cerebral metabolic rate of glucose in man. *Am. J. Physiol.*, 238:E69–E82.

42. Ingvar, M., and Siesjö, B. K. (1983): Local blood flow and glucose consumption in the rat brain during sustained bicuculline-induced seizures. *Acta Neurol. Scand.*, 68:129–144.

43. Kato, A., Diksic, M., Yamamoto, L., and Feindel, W. (1985): Quantification of glucose utilization in an experimental brain tumor model by the deoxyglucose method. *J. Cereb. Blood Flow Metab.*, 5:108–114.

44. Kety, S. S., Woodford, R. B., Harmel, M. H., Freyhan, F. A., Appel, K. E., and Schmidt, C. F. (1947–1948): Cerebral blood flow and metabolism in schizophrenia: The effect of barbiturate semi-narcosis, insulin coma and electroshock. *Am. J. Psychiatry*, 104:765–770.

45. Kimura, H., and Wada, J. (1980): Metabolic exploration of amygdaloid kindled seizure using ^{14}C-2-deoxyglucose method. *Epilepsia*, 21:186 (abstr.).

46. Kliot, M., and Poletti, C. E. (1979): Hippocampal afterdischarges: Differential spread of activity shown by the [^{14}C] deoxyglucose technique. *Science*, 204:641–643.

47. Kreisman, N. R., Rosenthal, M., Sick, T. J., and LaManna, J. C. (1983): Oxidative metabolic responses during recurrent seizures are independent of convulsant, anesthetic, or species. *Neurology*, 33:861–867.

48. Kuhl, D. E., Engel, J., Jr., Phelps, M. E., and Selin, C. (1980): Epileptic patterns of local cerebral metabolism and perfusion in humans determined by emission computed tomography of ^{18}FDG and ^{13}NH$_3$. *Ann. Neurol.*, 8:348–360.

49. Lothman, E. W., and Collins, R. C. (1981): Kainic acid induced limbic seizures: Metabolic, behavioral, electroencephalographic and neuropathological correlates. *Brain Res.*, 218:299–318.

50. Mata, M., Fink, D. J., Gainer, H., Smith, C. B., Davidsen, L., Savaki, H., Schwartz, W. J., and Sokoloff, L. (1980): Activity-dependent energy metabolism in rat posterior pituitary reflects sodium pump activity. *J. Neurochem.*, 34:213–215.

51. Mintun, M. A., Raichle, M. E., Martin, W. R. W., and Herscovitch, P. (1984): Brain oxygen utilization measured with O-15 radiotracers and positron emission tomography. *J. Nucl. Med.*, 25:177–187.

52. Moshé, S. L. (1981): The kindling phenomenon and its possible relevance to febrile seizures. In: *Febrile Seizures*, edited by K. B. Nelson and J. H. Ellenberg, pp. 59–63. Raven Press, New York.

53. Noebels, J. L., and Sidman, R. L. (1979): Inherited epilepsy: Spike-wave focal motor seizures in the mutant mouse tottering. *Science*, 204:1334–1336.

54. Pardridge, W. M., Crane, P. D., Mietus, L. J., and Oldendorf, W. H. (1982): Kinetics of regional blood-brain barrier transport and brain phosphorylation of glucose and 2-deoxyglucose in the barbiturate-anesthetized rat. *J. Neurochem.*, 38:560–568.

55. Pardridge, W. M., Crane, P. D., Mietus, L. J., and Oldendorf, W. H. (1982): Nomogram for 2-deoxyglucose lumped constant for rat brain cortex. *J. Cereb. Blood Flow Metab.*, 2:197–202.

56. Pazdernik, T. L., Cross, R. S., Giesler, M., Samson, F. E., and Nelson, S. R. (1985): Changes in local cerebral glucose utilization induced by convulsants. *Neuroscience*, 14:823–835.

57. Pettigrew, K. D., Sokoloff, L., and Patlak, C. S. (1983): A theoretical derivation of the lumped constant for the 2-deoxyglucose method for measuring local cerebral metabolism in the brain. *J. Cereb. Blood Flow Metab.*, 3(Suppl. 1):S89–S90.

58. Phelps, M. E., Hoffman, E. J., Mullani, N. A., and Ter-Pogossian, M. H. (1975): Application of annihilation coincidence detection to transaxial reconstruction tomography. *J. Nucl. Med.*, 16:210–224.

59. Phelps, M. E., Huang, S.-C., Hoffman, E. J., Selin, C., Sokoloff, L., and Kuhl, D. E. (1979): Tomographic measurement of local cerebral glucose metabolic rate in humans with (F-18)-fluorodeoxy-d-glucose: Validation of method. *Ann. Neurol.*, 6:371–388.

60. Phelps, M. E., Mazziotta, J. C., and Huang, S.-C. (1982): Study of cerebral function with positron computed tomography. *J. Cereb. Blood Flow Metab.*, 2:113–162.

61. Phelps, M. E., Shelbert, H. R., and Mazziotta, J. C. (1983): Positron computed tomography for studies of myocardial and cerebral function. *Ann. Int. Med.*, 98:339–359.

62. Pinel, J. P. J., and Rovner, L. I. (1978): Experimental epileptogenesis: Kindling-induced epilepsy in rats. *Exp. Neurol.*, 58:190–202.

63. Pinel, J. P., and Rovner, L. I. (1978): Electrode placement and kindling-induced experimental epilepsy. *Exp. Neurol.*, 58:335–346.

64. Prince, D. A., and Wilder, B. J. (1967): Control mechanisms in cortical epileptogenic foci: "Surround" inhibition. *Arch. Neurol.*, 16:194–202.

65. Raichle, M. E., Martin, W. R. W., Herscovitch, P., Mintun, M. A., and Markham, J. (1983): Brain blood flow measured with intravenous H$_2$^{15}O. II. Implementation and validation. *J. Nucl. Med.*, 24:790–798.

66. Reivich, M., Kuhl, D., Wolf, A., Greenberg, J., Phelps, M., Ido, T., Casella, V., Fowler, J., Hoffman, E., Alavi, A., Som, P., and Sokoloff, L. (1979): The [^{18}F] fluorodeoxyglucose method for the measurement of local cerebral glucose utilization in man. *Circ. Res.*, 44:127–137.

67. Savaki, H. E., Davidsen, L., Smith, C., and Sokoloff, L. (1980): Measurement of free glucose turnover in brain. *J. Neurochem.*, 35:495–502.

68. Schuier, F., Orzi, F., Suda, S., Kennedy, C., and Sokoloff, L. (1983): The lumped constant for the [^{14}C]deoxyglucose method in hyperglycemic rats. *J. Cereb. Blood Flow Metab.*, 1(Suppl. 1):S63.

69. Sokoloff, L. (1979): The [^{14}C] deoxyglucose method: Four years later. *Acta Neurol. Scand.*, 60(Suppl. 72):640–649.

70. Sokoloff, L. (1981): Localization of functional activity in the central nervous system by measurement of glucose utilization with radioactive deoxyglucose. *J. Cereb. Blood Flow Metab.*, 1:7–26.

71. Sokoloff, L., Reivich, M., Kennedy, C., Des Rosiers, H., Patlak, C. S., Pettigrew, K. D., Sakurada, O., and Shinohara, M. (1977): The [^{14}C] deoxyglucose method for the measurement of local cerebral glucose utilization: Theory, procedure, and normal values in the conscious and anesthetized albino rat. *J. Neurochem.*, 28:897–916.

72. Sols, A., and Crane, R. K. (1954): Substrate specificity of brain hexokinase. *J. Biol. Chem.*, 210:581–595.

73. Suda, S., Shinohara, M., Miyaoka, M., Kennedy, C., and Sokoloff, L. (1983): Local cerebral glucose utilization in hypoglycemia. *J. Cereb. Blood Flow Metab.*, 1(Suppl. 1):S62.

74. Suzuki, J., Nakamoto, Y., and Shinkawa, Y. (1983): Local cerebral glucose utilization in epileptic seizures of the mutant E1 mouse. *Brain Res.*, 266:359–363.

75. Theodore, W. H., Newmark, M. E., Sato, S., Brooks, R., Patronas, N. De La Paz, R., DiChiro, G., Kessler, R. M., Margolin, R., Manning, R. G., Channing, M., and Porter, R. J. (1983): [^{18}F] Fluorodeoxyglucose positron emission tomography in refractory complex partial seizures. *Ann. Neurol.*, 14:429–437.

76. Torbati, D., and Lambertsen, C. J. (1983): Regional cerebral metabolic rate for glucose during hyperbaric oxygen-induced convulsions. *Brain Res.*, 279:382–386.

77. Wasterlain, C. G., Dwyer, B. E., and Fujikawa, D. (1983): Metabolic studies of neonatal seizures in newborn marmaset monkeys: A possible role in the pathogenesis of brain damage for mismatch between flow and metabolism. In: *Current Problems in Epilepsy; 1: Cerebral Blood Flow, Metabolism and Epilepsy*, edited by M. Baldy-Mouliniere, D. H. Ingvar, and B. S. Meldrum, pp. 121–129. John Libbey, London.

78. Watson, R. E., Jr., Edinger, H. M., and Siegel, A. A. (1983): [^{14}C]2-Deoxyglucose analysis of the functional neural pathways of the limbic forebrain in the rat. III. The hippocampal formation. *Brain Res. Rev.*, 5:133–176.

79. Watson, R. E., Jr., Troiano, R., Poulakos, J., Weiner, S., Black, C. H., and Siegel, A. (1983): A [^{14}C] 2-deoxyglucose analysis of the functional neural pathways of the limbic forebrain in the rat. I. The amygdala. *Brain Res. Rev.*, 5:1–44.

80. Webster, W. R., Servière, J., and Brown, M. (1984): Inhibitory contours in the inferior colliculus as revealed by the 2-deoxyglucose method. *Exp. Brain Res.*, 56:577–581.

81. Yamamoto, Y. L., Ochs, R., Gloor, P., Ammann, W., Meyer, E., Evans, A. C., Cooke, B., Sako, K., Gotman, J., Feindel, Witt, Diksic, M., Thompson, C. J., and Robitalle, Y. (1983): Patterns of rCBF and focal energy metabolic changes in relation to electroencephalic abnormality in the inter-ictal phase of partial epilepsy. In: *Current Problems in Epilepsy; 1: Cerebral Blood Flow, Metabolism and Epilepsy*, edited by M. Baldy-Mouliniere, D. H. Ingvar, and B. S. Meldrum, pp. 51–62. John Libbey, London.

Advances in Neurology, Vol. 44, edited by
A. V. Delgado-Escueta, A. A. Ward, Jr.,
D. M. Woodbury, and R. J. Porter.
Raven Press, New York © 1986

47

Regional Cerebral Blood Flow and Metabolic Rates in Human Focal Epilepsy and Status Epilepticus

*G. Franck, *B. Sadzot, *E. Salmon, **J. C. Depresseux, *T. Grisar,
**J. M. Peters, **M. Guillaume, **L. Quaglia, **G. Delfiore, and
**D. Lamotte

*Department of Neurology, University of Liege, CHU Sart Tilman, 4000 Liege, Belgium; and
**Cyclotron Research Center, B_{30}, Sart Tilman, 4000 Liege, Belgium

SUMMARY   Positron emission tomography with the oxygen-15 steady state or bolus inhalation technique was used to provide quantitative values of regional cerebral blood flow (CBF), oxygen extraction ratio (OER) and oxygen consumption (CMRO$_2$) in 25 patients with partial complex seizures during the interictal state and in 5 patients during status epilepticus. Glucose utilization (CMRglu) was also studied in one case of status epilepticus with the ^{18}F-fluorodeoxyglucose technique (^{18}FDG). Interictal scans showed zone(s) of hypoperfusion and hypometabolism without significant variation of the OER in approximately 80% of patients. In 62%, there was a strong correlation between the overall EEG localization and the area(s) of hypoperfusion and hypometabolism. In all cases, ictal scans revealed a focal or multifocal increase in CBF and CMRO$_2$. The localization of the most affected regions correlated well with the spatial distribution of the electroencephalograph (EEG) abnormalities. Comparison of the different values of CBF, CMRO$_2$, and OER showed that the increase in perfusion always exceeded that of oxygen consumption and hence was accompanied by a significant decrease of OER; the latter was always the most prominent in the region of the epileptic focus determined by serial EEG recordings. These results showed that the supply of oxygen by blood flow is large enough to meet metabolic demand. When comparing these values with CMRglu, it appeared that the relative changes in CMRglu and CBF were very similar, indicating that the increase in blood flow correlated with the enhancement in glucose utilization. The observed imbalance between blood flow, glucose utilization, and oxygen consumption could suggest that an impairment of oxygen utilization by the mitochondria could occur in the epileptic focus during prolonged status epilepticus.

The possibilities offered by positron emission tomography (PET) for the investigation of human cerebral metabolism and haemodynamics have been recently used to get new insights into the pathogenesis of focal and generalized human epilepsies.

The fluorine-18-labeled 2-fluorodeoxyglucose (^{18}FDG) method has been the most frequently used. Interictal ^{18}FDG scans of patients with partial epilepsy but without radiologically evident structural damage showed one or more regions of focal or lateralized hypometabolism (20,24,25,48,69,70,75). The hypometabolic zone correlates well with the location of the epileptic focus determined electrophysiologically and with the presence of structural pathology observed following surgical resection (21,70,75).

In contrast, ^{18}FDG scans during partial seizures (20,22,23,24,48,70) show hypermetabolism in the areas of ictal onset and spread. In some patients, however, focal or diffuse decrease in metabolism was also seen (22,26).

In order to better characterize the aerobic metabolism of the human epileptic brain and the coupling between metabolism and circulation in ictal and interictal states, the techniques of oxygen-15 steady-state (28,44,51,68) or bolus inhalation (14,15,34,39,40,62) were used to provide quantitative values of regional cerebral blood flow (CBF), oxygen extraction ratio (OER: the fraction of oxygen extracted from the arterial blood), and oxygen utilization ($CMRO_2$). The preliminary results available in the literature (4,75) showed a similar tendency towards reduced CBF and $CMRO_2$ in the hemisphere ipsilateral to the EEG focus during the interictal state; bilateral changes in basal ganglia and cerebellum were also detected (4). It was also demonstrated (4) that the decreased CBF and $CMRO_2$ at the site of the epileptic focus was accompanied by an increase in the OER, suggesting that the reserve of oxygen supply was diminished and that the tissue metabolic requirements were high, even interictally. However, no data are available about the relationship between blood flow and metabolism in human brain during status epilepticus.

We report a PET study of 25 patients with partial complex seizures during the interictal state and of 5 patients during status epilepticus; we analyze our results for CBF, $CMRO_2$, OER, and glucose utilization (CMRglu) (in one case, during status epilepticus) in relation to electroencephalographic (EEG) abnormalities.

METHODS FOR CBF, OER, $CMRO_2$, AND CMRglu DETERMINATIONS

Theory

Cerebral Blood Flow

Radiolabeled water can be administered for evaluating CBF either by intravenous injection of $H_2^{15}O$ (62) or by inhalation of $C^{15}O_2$, leading to an almost instantaneous labeling of $H_2^{15}O$ in the pulmonary capillary bed (72).

As $C^{15}O_2$ is inhaled by the subject at a constant rate, the concentration of $H_2^{15}O$ goes up in blood and tissues, where it reaches a steady-state equilibrium after 8 to 10 min delay. CBF can thus be computed from properly calibrated PET image contents and equilibrium blood concentrations (28,44). This ''equilibrium'' approach has the advantage of simple and rapid data processing.

A number of drawbacks have nonetheless

been stressed in that approach. Sensitivity of determinations decreases with increasing CBF, while propagated errors increase (43). The partial volume effect results in inaccuracies in computed values for CBF (2,12,34,51). The operational procedure leads to a one-parameter evaluation of CBF, and a predetermined value has to be allotted to the volume of distribution of radiolabeled water, with a difficult-to-control systematic error on blood flow (13). Furthermore, there are controversies concerning the significance and value to be attributed to the volume of distribution of radiolabeled water (11,15,40).

These drawbacks of the continuous inhalation technique stimulated search for other strategies of tracer administration (14,15,33,39,40,62). Some of our patients were thus investigated in parallel using a bolus inhalation of $^{15}O_2$ and $C^{15}O_2$.

Cerebral Oxygen Uptake Rate

Despite limitations due to the blood flow-dependent permeability of water through the blood-brain barrier (19), the use of radiolabeled water as a CBF tracer is useful in supplying flow and volume parameters for the computation of the kinetics of water of metabolism within cerebral tissue.

In order to measure $CMRO_2$ after the administration of $^{15}O_2$, it is necessary to determine the respective concentrations of $^{15}O_2$, and $H_2^{15}O$ in the arterial blood (16). In addition, it is important to model local tissue kinetics of $^{15}O_2$ and the recirculating radiolabeled water within cerebral tissue.

The most commonly used method for determining $CMRO_2$ utilizes continuous administration of $^{15}O_2$ to the subject, with PET detection performed when the radioactive concentrations of ^{15}O and radiolabeled water of metabolism have reached a steady state within blood and tissues (28,44,68). The extraction coefficient is computed as a linear function of the ratio between the respective local image contents detected during the continuous inhalation of $^{15}O_2$ and $C^{15}O_2$. Oxygen uptake rate, $CMRO_2$, is then computed as the product of CBF, OER, and arterial blood oxygen content.

Neglecting the contribution of ^{15}O in that approach led to overestimation of OER in cases where local blood volume was increased (49). Correction for this contribution is possible in the equilibrium approach, using a subsequent determination of local blood volume with the inhalation of ^{11}CO (49) or $C^{15}O$ (56).

The complete sequence of the equilibrium method for evaluating CBF, OER, and $CMRO_2$ comprises, therefore, the successive continuous inhalation of $C^{15}O_2$ and $^{15}O_2$ and a short breath of ^{11}CO or $C^{15}O$. The shortcomings are the high doses of radiation to the patient (45) and the errors linked to movements of the patient during (and between) the three successive time-consuming data-collection efforts.

These considerations led us to design other approaches, using bolus rather than continuous administration of ^{15}O (14,56). We developed a method for the two-parameter assessment of $CMRO_2$ and Vox (volume of distribution of oxygen), including correction for the contribution of the local intravascular ^{15}O (14).

Glucose Uptake Rate

Utilization of ^{18}F-2-fluoro-2-deoxyglucose with PET detection has proved its potential for determinating local glucose uptake rate in the human brain. Phelps et al. (58) developed a computional procedure based on the three-compartment model of Sokoloff et al. (67) for the evaluation of kinetic constants of FDG tissue uptake and for computing local CMRglu, taking into account corrections for hydrolysis of phosphorylated FDG within brain tissue. Uncertainties about the lumped constant in the equations limit quantitative interpretation of data, especially in diseased tissues.

Methods

In the present study, CBF, OER, and $CMRO_2$ were evaluated using the steady-state method and the bolus administration of tracers. Local radioactive concentrations in the brain were measured with an ECAT IV (Ortec & EG) tomograph; slices were adjusted parallel to the orbito–meatal reference plane (levels +2.2 to +6.2 cm above the orbito–meatal plane); data were collected and reconstructed in the medium resolution mode (FWHM = 8.4 mm in the main section).

The equilibrium determinations were performed using a radioactive flow rate of about 0.5 mCi/ml to the patient's airmask and 1,200,000-count images. The bolus inhalation utilized a single breath from an airbag containing 80 mCi; a sequence of two scans was performed 30 to 120 and 130 to 220 sec after inhalation.

Radioactive concentrations in the arterial blood were measured by catheterization of one humeral artery and by counting and gravimetry of blood samples.

The algorithm for computing CBF, $CMRO_2$, and OER from the steady-state method was based on previously published equations (28).

The data obtained using the bolus approach were processed using the ratio between two time-integrated PET image contents as obtained 30 to 120 and 130 to 220 sec after administration of $C^{15}O_2$ and $^{15}O_2$. That procedure allows a two-parameter analysis for concomitantly determining CBF and $CMRO_2$, taking into account necessary corrections for local volume of distribution of radiolabeled water and local blood volume. Using a precalibrated computing procedure allows us to proceed with functional images on a pixel-by-pixel basis.

The CMRglu determinations were performed with 5 to 10 mCi of FDG, injected intravenously; the radioactive concentration of FDG was measured by well-counting and gravimetry of arterial plasma samples. Scans were performed at the same levels as with $^{15}O_2$ studies. CMRglu were determined, using equations published by Phelps et al. (58).

The quantitative processing of data was performed for each pixel value, minimizing errors due to the partial volume effect. The values were tested for normality and for symmetry on a basis of 4.8-cm^2 regions.

RESULTS

Interictal State

$^{15}O_2$ PET studies and conventional X-ray computed tomography (CT) scans were performed on 25 patients with partial complex epilepsy during the interictal state. Quantitative determinations of CBF, $CMRO_2$, and OER values were first made in each region of the entire brain. Then the values of regions of interest (ROI) showing very significant side-to-side asymmetry according to Engel's procedure (24) were chosen. The available EEG recordings were reviewed for each patient.

Of the 21 patients with normal X-ray CT scans (Fig. 1), 17 (81%) showed region(s) of hypoperfusion (−22.5%) and hypometabolism (−20.9%); in contrast there was no significant variation in the OER (Table 1). Asymmetries were more pronounced in patients with abnormal X-ray CT scans ($n = 4$): CBF, −68.6%; $CMRO_2$, −78% (Table 2).

Among the patients with normal X-ray CT scans, 13 (61.9%) showed a focal or lateralized hypoperfused and hypometabolic region that corresponded to the overall EEG localization (Table 3). Preoperative corticography and ster-

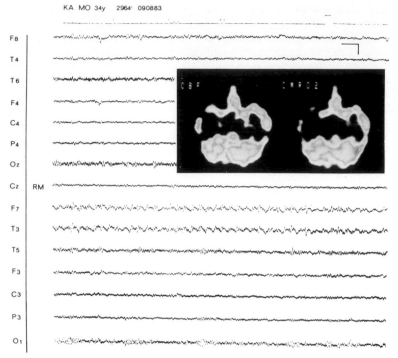

FIG. 1.   KA. M. A 34-year-old woman with uncontrolled complex partial seizures of unknown etiology since the age of 12 years. Left, carotid arteriogram and X-ray CT scan were normal. Monopolar EEG recording showed a left temporal epileptic focus (F7 and T3). PET scan ($^{15}O_2$ steady-state inhalation technique; level plus 3 cm above the orbitomeatal line) displayed a left temporal area with equally decreased CBF and $CMRO_2$.

eoelectroencephalography (SEEG) in 2 cases showed discharges more closely related to the anatomical distribution of the PET findings than the surface EEG. However, no correlation was found between the PET findings and the frequency of interictal epileptiform discharges or seizures prior to scanning. Two patients (9.5%) whose EEGs failed to reveal an epileptic focus

TABLE 1. *Interictal studies in patients with normal X-ray CT scan[a]*

	Temporal area ($n = 17/21$)			Cerebellum ($n = 9/13$)		
Parameter	A	B	%	A'	B'	%
CBF (ml/100 g · min)	34.8 ± 7.05	44.9 ± 9.1	−22.5[b]	41.4 ± 6.3	49.4 ± 7.4	−16.2[b]
OER (%)	49.3 ± 4.5	48.4 ± 3.3	−1.9[c]	49.8 ± 4.6	49.6 ± 3.7	−0.4[c]
$CMRO_2$ (μmol/100 g · min)	136.8 ± 25.8	173.0 ± 33.4	−20.9[b]	165.6 ± 27.5	195.3 ± 29	−15.2[b]

[a] Mean values and SD for the region of maximum interest selected in epileptic patients on their numerical printout (64 pixels cortical). For temporal area: A, affected side on visual analysis; B, contralateral side. For cerebellum: A', cerebellar lobe homolateral to the temporal area of low flow and metabolism; B', contralateral cerebellar lobe. CBF, cerebral blood flow; OER, oxygen extraction rate; $CMRO_2$, cerebral metabolic rate of oxygen. Percentage (%) of asymmetry expressed as

$$\frac{\text{affected side} - \text{contralateral side}}{\text{contralateral side}} \times 100$$

[b] Statistical significance by paired Student's *t*-test (also significant with unpaired two-tailed Student's *t*-test), $p < 0.001$.

[c] Not significantly different.

TABLE 2. *Interictal studies in patients with abnormal X-ray CT scan[a]*

Parameter	Contralateral	Ipsilateral	%
CBF (ml/100 g · min)	44.4 ± 13.7	26.3 ± 10.2	−68.6[b]
OER (%)	52.1 ± 4.8	46.9 ± 6.1	−11.1[c]
CMRO$_2$ (μmol/100 g · min)	183.9 ± 69.8	103.3 ± 42.4	−78.0[d]

[a] Mean values and standard deviation in 4 patients with abnormal CT scan (interictal state). ROI are selected in the same way as for patients with normal CT scan. Asymmetry (%) is expressed as

$$\frac{\text{affected side} - \text{contralateral side}}{\text{contralateral side}} \times 100$$

[b] Statistical significance by paired two-tailed Student's t-test, $p < 0.02$.
[c] $p < 0.2$.
[d] $p < 0.05$.

displayed a lateralized region of hypoperfusion and hypometabolism. However, patients with bilateral EEG abnormalities usually showed more widespread hypoperfused and hypometabolic regions, mostly in the parietal and frontal areas, than those with a localized EEG focus. Three patients (14.3%) with focal EEG discharges did not show any significant PET modifications. Two other patients (9.6%) showed no congruent foci, but unfortunately no SEEG were available for these patients. These results are in agreement with those reported by Engel (24) and Theodore (69) using the [18]FDG technique (Table 3).

Since it has been suggested by Bernardi et al. (4) that marked disturbances of flow and metabolism could be observed in the cerebellum, we have compared, when available, the values of CBF, CMRO$_2$, and OER in the cerebellar hemispheres (Table 1). We found a slight but statistically significant decrease, but only in the cerebellar hemisphere homolateral to the affected temporal area. The discrepancy could result from a difference in the data analysis, since these authors always compared the value of each measurement with those obtained in the same anatomical region in age-matched normal volunteers.

Ictal Studies and Status Epilepticus

Kuhl et al. (48) reported the first measurements of brain metabolism and flow in human epilepsy by ^{18}F-deoxyglucose and ^{13}N-ammonia positron emission tomography. Their data (three studies in 2 patients) clearly showed foci of increased glucose utilization (82–130%) and blood flow that correlated both temporally and anatomically with ictal EEG spike foci. However, further studies by Engel et al. (20,22,23,26) showed that the ictal [18]FDG scan patterns, especially in partial epilepsies, were unique to each patient. Focal as well as generalized increases or decreases in metabolism were observed. According to these authors, ictal hypermetabolism could represent activation of excitatory or inhibitory synapses in the epileptogenic region and its projection fields—ictal hypometabolism

TABLE 3. *Results in 21 interictal studies[a]*

Result	Franck et al. (unpublished results) n = 21 (O$_2$–CO$_2$) Number of patients	%	Engel et al. (24) n = 50 (FDG) Number of patients	%	Theodore et al. (69) n = 28 (FDG) Number of patients	%
PET, EEG localization agree	13	61.9	28	56	15	53.6
EEG nonlocalized, PET shows hypometabolic region	2	9.5	4	8	6	21.4
PET normal, EEG shows focal discharges	3	14.3	5	10	2	7.1
Both studies nonlocalizing	1	4.7	10	20	4	14.3
Studies show noncongruent foci	2	9.6	3	6	1	3.6

[a] EEG and interictal PET results in 21 patients with CPS and normal CT scan. Classification from Theodore et al. (69).

most likely reflects postictal depression. These authors could not, however, demonstrate any quantitative relationship between alterations in metabolism and EEG or behavioral patterns of ictal events. Indeed, the [18]FDG technique is based on achievement of steady-state conditions, and quantitative studies are not possible for transient events, such as seizures. The patterns obtained represent a weighted average of local metabolism data associated with ictal, postictal, and interictal states that occur during the scanning procedure. In order to obtain steady-state ictal conditions, we selected 4 patients (NAM. M.; BOL. M.; REI. G.; DAIS. M.) who had a common electroclinical pattern, clinically characterized by confusion and generalized and/or partial seizures (2 with epilepsia partialis continua), and electroencephalographically characterized (Fig. 2) by continuous periodic lateralized epileptic discharges [PLEDs, according to Chatrian et al. (10)]. These patients were not known to be epileptic prior to this illness; their status epilepticus was the result of aminophylline intoxication (BOL. M.), diazepam withdrawal (NAM. M.), and hepatic (DAIS. M.) or hypertensive encephalopathy (REI. G.). Two of them (BOL. M. and NAM.

M.) were recorded at three different periods during and after their status epilepticus. We also compared the results with those in a fifth patient (REN. V.), who had recurrent electrical fits starting in the left temporal area and occurring spontaneously (10 fits) during the course of the PET scanning procedure. In these 5 cases, X-ray CT scans and carotid angiograms were normal. The EEG and behavior were carefully monitored.

Blood Flow and Oxygen Consumption

Ictal scans obtained with the [15]O_2 technique (Fig. 3) revealed—in all cases—a focal or multifocal increase in cortical blood flow and oxygen consumption. The localization of the most affected regions correlated with the spatial distribution of the epileptic EEG abnormalities (Figs. 2 and 3: 1 = NAM. M.). Basal ganglia and thalamus (which represents projection fields) also showed increased CBF and $CMRO_2$ on the same side as the epileptic focus (Fig. 3), except in one patient (Fig. 3: 2 = REIN. G.), who was suffering from severe hypertension.

Quantitative data from regions of interest (ROI) selected on numerical printouts (64 pixels)

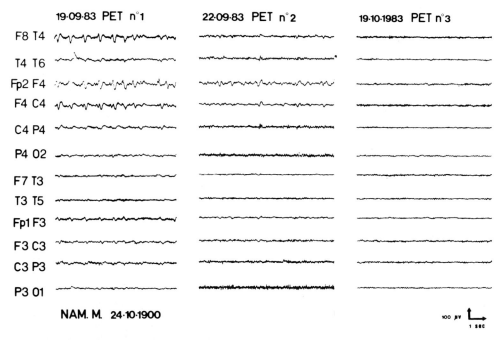

FIG. 2. NAM. M. An 83-year-old woman. After acute diazepine withdrawal, she began to show left-sided focal motor attacks followed by generalized seizure. The patient was confuse with mild left hemiparesis when the first EEG was recorded (September 9, 1983). It showed continuous PLEDs on the right frontal area. Three days later, there was only a focus of slow waves on the same region and the EEG returned to normal one month later. Representative sections of her PET scan are represented in Fig. 3 (region 1) and Fig. 6.

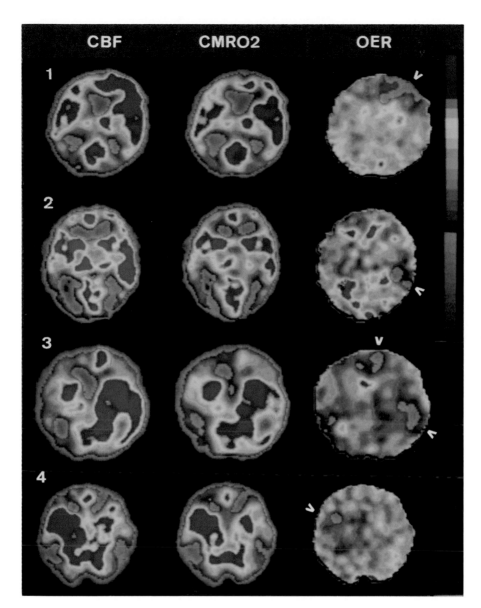

FIG. 3. Selected sections from $^{15}O_2$ scans (steady-state inhalation technique) of four patients (1, NAM. M.; 2, REI. G.; 3, DAIS. M.; 4, REN. V.) with electrical (PLEDs: patients 1, 2) or electroclinical status epilepticus (PLEDs and epilepsia partialis continua, patient 3; left temporal fits, patient 4). These scans demonstrate focal (1, 2, 4) or multifocal (3) increase in CBF and CMRO$_2$ on the side corresponding to the EEG focus. The regions of decreased OER (*arrows*) closely correspond to the spike focus determined in the EEGs recorded during and after the status epilepticus.

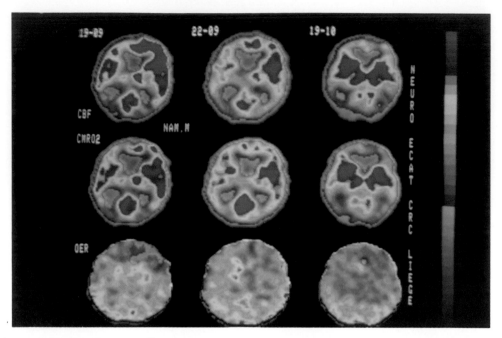

FIG. 6. NAM. M. PET scans ($^{15}O_2$ steady-state inhalation technique) performed at 4.6 cm above the orbito–meatal line at three different periods corresponding to the EEG records given in Fig. 2. Ictal PET scan (September 19, 1983) demonstrates an increased CBF (*top line*) and $CMRO_2$ (*middle*) on the right cortical regions and in the homolateral basal ganglia and thalamus, contrasting with a decreased OER (*bottom*) observed on the right frontal region. Three days later (September 22, 1983), the patient being seizure-free, the increased CBF and $CMRO_2$ are less marked; OER returns to normal values in right frontal area; 1 month later (October 19, 1983) there is no longer asymmetry for CBF, OER, or $CMRO_2$.

are given in Table 4 and confirm this increased CBF and $CMRO_2$. The most striking feature is the significant decrease in the oxygen extraction rate (OER) in the cortical area(s) involved by the epileptic phenomenon (Fig. 3: 1–4). The OER represents the fraction of oxygen extracted from arterial blood (oxygen arteriovenous difference) and thus expresses the relationship between cerebral blood flow (or oxygen supply) and cerebral consumption (or oxygen utilization rate). The decrease in OER during status epilepticus means (a) that the increase in perfusion proportionally exceeds that of oxygen consumption and consequently (b) that oxygen supply by blood flow is sufficient to meet metabolic demand.

In addition, the lowest values for OER, as selected with a computed ROI program (51 pixels) and shown in Table 5, were always observed in cortical regions which closely corresponded to the spike focus; the latter was determined by the EEG, recorded during and after the status epilepticus. An example is patient NAM. M., in whom the major abnormalities were observed in the frontal areas (Fig. 2 and Fig. 3: 1). In 2 patients (BOL. M. and NAM. M.), serial PET scans and EEG were recorded during and after the status epilepticus until complete EEG and clinical recovery occurred.

Quantitative values for CBF, $CMRO_2$, and OER obtained in the patient BOL. M. at three different periods from three selected regions of interest are shown in Fig. 4. The corresponding EEG is presented in Fig. 5. During the status epilepticus (epilepsia partialis continua), the EEG recordings revealed continuous spikes, spike and wave complexes, and sharp waves in the right hemisphere. Five days later, the patient was seizure-free and the spikes were restricted to the right frontal areas. Two weeks later, the EEG showed slight diffuse slowing in the right hemisphere, with some slow waves in the right frontal region.

The PET scans obtained during status epilepticus showed a marked increase in CBF and $CMRO_2$ in the entire right hemisphere, which was most prominent in the right frontal area (Fig. 4, regions 1 and 2). The contralateral regions were also affected, but to a lesser degree. These modifications persisted but were diminished during the second PET; finally, the values obtained from the third PET no longer showed interhemispheric asymmetry.

The modifications of the OER are more interesting because there is a marked contrast between the frontal areas (Fig. 4; regions 1 and 2) and other regions distant from the epilepticus

focus (Fig. 4: 3). The values obtained in regions 1 and 2 are significantly decreased during the status epilepticus in comparison with those observed subsequently in the same regions during the second and third PET when the patient was seizure-free. In region 3, remote from the epileptic focus, values during these three periods did not vary significantly and were very close to those measured during the second and third PET scan in the frontal areas. The same evolution was observed in the case NAM. M. (Figs. 2 and 6).

These data are in partial agreement with those in one case of epilepsia partialis continua reported by Engel et al. (20,22,23,26), who showed an increased ictal metabolism (^{18}FDG) in the entire brain. However, these authors reported that the area of the "suspected" focus was not as active as other brain regions in the contralateral hemisphere, whereas our results clearly indicate that the highest CBF and $CMRO_2$ increases were observed in the suspected epileptic focus (by EEG), although the best marker is represented by the decreased OER (Fig. 3: 1–4).

Blood Flow, Glucose Utilization, and Oxygen Consumption

In order to compare consumption rates of oxygen and glucose with blood flow, we obtained CBF, $CMRO_2$, and OER sequentially with the $^{15}O_2$ equilibrium technique and CMRglu with the ^{18}FDG technique in the patient REIN. G. The quantitative data selected in the more active region and the contralateral area at three different levels above the orbito-meatal line are given in Table 6, together with other parameters, such as the metabolic rate (MR), and the glucose extraction rate (GER) ratio, as described by Baron et al. (3) and Wise et al. (73). It can be seen that the increases in blood flow and glucose uptake are very similar. These results indicate that there is no mismatch between glucose supply and utilization, since the glucose extraction rate (GER) is not modified. In contrast, the metabolic rate (MR) is significantly decreased in the area of decreased OER, i.e., in the epileptic focus. These results seem to indicate that glucose utilization is more important than oxygen consumption.

DISCUSSION

Interictal State

Our study clearly shows a significant decrease in $CMRO_2$ in the temporal areas corresponding

TABLE 4. Ictal studies[a]

ROI	NAM. M. (n = 7)			REI. G. (n = 18)			DAIS. M. (n = 13)		
	L	R	%	L	R	%	L	R	%
CBF (ml/100 g · min)	33.7 ± 3.6	49.2 ± 2.8	+45.9	29.5 ± 7.3	53.1 ± 17.8	+80	34.4 ± 7.8	51.3 ± 12.5	+49.3
OER (%)	50.25 ± 2.5	39.8 ± 3.5	−20.75	54.9 ± 4.3	43.2 ± 3.9	−21.3	48.4 ± 4.2	43.1 ± 3.8	−10.7
CMRO$_2$ (μmol/100 g · min)	136.2 ± 15.7	155.1 ± 12.3	+13.9	130.8 ± 30.9	179.5 ± 52.9	+37.23	138.9 ± 32.3	175.9 ± 44.2	+27.4

[a] Mean values and standard deviations for different ROI of 64 pixels selected on the numerical printouts in cortical areas involved by the augmented flow and metabolism (at three or four different levels above the orbito–meatal line). L, left; R, right. Asymmetry (%) is expressed as

$$\frac{\text{affected side} - \text{contralateral side}}{\text{contralateral side}} \times 100$$

This approach was not possible for patient REN. V., for which the abnormal area was too limited and for BOL. M., for which only one level was scanned. All the difference are significant at $p < 0.001$ by the paired Student's t-test and are also significant ($p \leq 0.05$) by the unpaired t-test.

TABLE 5. *Ictal studies*[a]

ROI	NAM. M., frontal			REI. G., postcentral and parietal			DAIS. M., mid-temporal			REN. V., anterior temporal			BOL. M., anterior temporal		
	L	R	%	L	R	%	L	R	%	L	R	%	L	R	%
CBF (ml/100 g · min)	35	57	+62.9	37	104	+181.1	39	65	+66.7	102	52	+96.2	73	135	+83.4
OER (%)	48	35	−27.1	59	37	−37.3	50	38	−24	38	52	−26.9	40	34	−15.0
CMRO$_2$ (μmol/100 g · min)	142	161	+13.3	180	319	+77.2	156	202	+29.5	318	220	+44.5	229	355	+55.0

[a] Values taken in the cortical region of maximum interest, i.e., showing the maximum uncoupling (always corresponding to the EEG focus) and the contralateral area. These values are selected using a region-of-interest program (except for patient BOL. M., on a numerical printout). Asymmetry (%) is expressed as

$$\frac{\text{affected side } - \text{ contralateral side}}{\text{contralateral side}} \times 100$$

L, left; R, right.

to the epileptic focus determined by conventional and SEEG recordings. These results agree with other reports (4,7,20,24,25,48,69,70,71,75) and suggest that such localized (or more diffuse) hypometabolism is characteristic of the epileptic area in patients with partial complex epilepsy during the interictal state. The modifications of CBF and CMRO$_2$ are always coupled, indicating that this hypometabolism is accompanied by a concomitant hypoperfusion. These results give a final answer to the controversy concerning whether or not the CBF of patients with partial seizures is increased (36,63) or decreased (41,42,50,71) during the interictal period, as suggested earlier with the use of the ^{133}Xe technique.

There are some discrepancies in the literature about the values of the OER. According to Bernardi et al. (4), the OER is higher in the epileptic focus, suggesting that at the site of, or surrounding, the focus, reserves of oxygen are decreased interictally. The opposite observation is made by Yamamoto et al. (75), who found a pattern of reduced CBF, CMRO$_2$, and OER in their patients. In our population, we have observed a significant decrease in the OER only in those patients with pathological X-ray CT scans. The significance of this decreased blood flow and metabolism is not yet understood. It could result from neuronal loss and vascular changes (21,48) or from the severity of the astrocytic reaction (75). The debate remains open, and further studies are clearly needed.

The small but significant decrease in CBF and CMRO$_2$ we have observed in the cerebellar hemisphere homolateral to the hypoperfused

and hypometabolic cerebral area(s) is even more difficult to explain. Bernardi et al. (4) have found a decrease in these parameters in both cerebellar hemispheres. Again, further studies are needed to understand the involvement of the cerebellum in epilepsy.

Ictal Patterns and Status Epilepticus

Blood Flow and Oxygen Consumption

Measurements in man of local CBF and CMRO$_2$ with positron emission tomography and the ^{15}O$_2$ technique confirm and extend previous data showing that focal ictal states are characterized by a large increase in CBF and metabolism (8,18,22,26,29,35,48,55,57,61,69,70). However, it clearly appears, in all our patients, that the increase in perfusion always exceeds that in oxygen consumption and hence is accompanied by a significant decrease in OER. This later phenomenon is always the most prominent in those cortical regions that correspond to the spiking focus as determined by EEG recordings and, as shown in serial studies, it is reversible when the patient becomes seizure-free.

Thus, these results are the first demonstration in humans—confirming previous experimental data in animals (6,9,17,25,35,37,38,54,59,60)—that (a) the supply of oxygen by blood flow is large enough to meet the metabolic demands of status epilepticus and (b) consequently there is no mismatch between blood flow and metabolic rate, as suggested by others (1,27,32,46,47), to explain the neuronal cell damage occurring in selectively vulnerable regions of the brain during

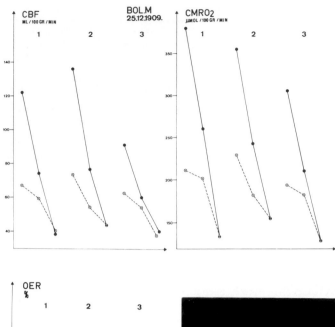

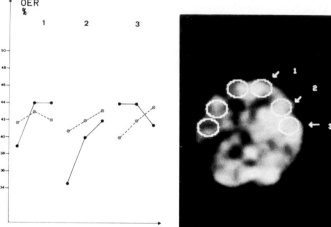

FIG. 4. BOL. M. ($^{15}O_2$ bolus inhalation technique). Quantitative values for CBF (ml/100 g · min), CMRO$_2$ (μmol/100 g · min) and OER (%) selected in three regions of interest (1, 2, 3, bottom right; ●——● homolateral to the EEG focus; ○– – –○ contralateral) at three different periods corresponding to the dates given in Fig. 5 (EEG recordings). For further explanation, see the text.

status epilepticus (for a general review, see ref. 65).

Blood Flow, Glucose Utilization, and Oxygen Consumption

The relative changes in CMRglu (^{18}FDG technique) and CBF values obtained in one of our patients are very similar, indicating that the increase in blood flow correlates with the enhancement in glucose utilization. Moreover, the rate of glucose consumption—in comparison to availability as defined by the GER values—was similar in the epileptic focus and in the contralateral brain area, suggesting a normal glucose supply to the focus in contrast with the oversupply of oxygen. However, the metabolic ratio (MR)—i.e., the balance between oxygen and glucose consumption—is significantly decreased in the epileptic focus. This index has a value of approximately 0.67 ml oxygen/mg glucose in normal tissue as determined from global measurements of CMRO$_2$ and CMRglu (64). A fall in this index, as shown in the epileptic focus, indicates a relative increase in the nonoxidative metabolism of glucose. However, an overestimation of CMRglu cannot be ruled out. Indeed, it has been assumed that the "lumped constant" used for calculation of CMRglu is not influenced by the pathologically enhanced glucose utilization. Unfortunately, this assumption seems to be unfounded (66), and in the absence of a method for measuring it regionally in humans, the necessity of assuming a constant value is potentially the major source of error in the interpretation of the results of CMRglu, GER, and MR.

The observed imbalance between blood flow and oxygen consumption, as shown quantita-

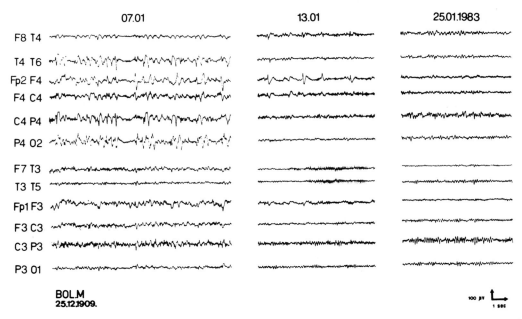

F8 T4

T4 T6

Fp2 F4

F4 C4

C4 P4

P4 O2

F7 T3

T3 T5

Fp1 F3

F3 C3

C3 P3

P3 O1

07.01   13.01   25.01.1983

BOL.M
25.12.1909.

100 μV
1 sec

FIG. 5. BOL. M. A 74-year-old woman with a history of asthma and aminophylline intoxication (55.4 mg/l). She was hospitalized because of a generalized seizure followed by confusion. The first EEG (January 7, 1983), recorded 6 hr after the onset of the disease, while she was confused, with mild left hemiparesis and continuous clonic movements of the left hand, showed spikes, spike and wave complexes, and sharp waves on her right hemisphere. Five days later, spikes were localized on right frontal areas (patient being seizure-free). Right carotid arteriogram and X-ray CT scan were normal. Three weeks later, she was alert and physical examination was normal.

tively by the decreased OER values, could suggest that an impairment of oxygen utilization by the mitochondria occurs in the epileptic focus during prolonged status epilepticus. Recent experimental studies (59) seem to indicate that the neuronal cell damage observed in status epilepticus would result from an excessive influx of CA^{2+} into selective brain cells, associated with paroxysmal activity during status epilepticus. Ultrastructural observations (30,31) showing a marked increase in the amount of calcium deposits, particularly in swollen and disrupted mitochondria, favor this hypothesis. This Ca^{2+} accumulation (66) could then activate various hy-

TABLE 6. *Ictal studies: Patient REI. G.*[a]

Parameter	L	R	%
CBF (ml/100 g · min)	34.3 ± 5.8	61.7 ± 17.2	+79.6
OER [CMRO$_2$/CBF × CaO$_2$) × 100]	54.7 ± 3.5	42.7 ± 3.5	−21.9
CMRO$_2$ (ml/100 g · min)	3.36 ± 0.44	4.69 ± 1.24	+39.6
CMRglu (mg/100 g · min)	5.03 ± 0.3	9.15 ± 0.98	+81.9
MR CMRO$_2$/CMRglu	0.66 ± 0.05	0.5 ± 0.1	−24.9
GER (CMRglu/CBF × Cpglu) × 100	10.3 ± 0.1	10.6 ± 0.2	+2.9

[a] Mean values and standard deviations for different parameters, in the more active region (post central and parietal) and the contralateral area, at three different levels [OM + 3.8 − 4.6 − 5.4 above the orbitomeatal (OM) line]. L, left; R, right. Asymmetry (%) is expressed as

$$\frac{\text{affected side} - \text{contralateral side}}{\text{contralateral side}} \times 100$$

CMRglu, cerebral metabolic rate of glucose; MR, metabolic rate; GER, glucose extraction rate; Cpglu, glucose plasmatic concentration.

drolases, including phospholipase A_2, leading, among other things, to accumulation of free fatty acids (65,66). Such accumulation might then inhibit or uncouple mitochondria (5,74) and, because oxygen is present, activate cyclooxygenase and lipoxygenase, resulting in the production of hydroperoxides and related free compounds that are toxic to the cells (65,66). In other words, all these experiments, in humans and in animals, seem to confirm that excessive enhancement of local metabolic rates per se would be the cause of the neuronal damage (52,53,65,66).

ACKNOWLEDGMENTS

This research was supported by a grant from Belgian National Fund for scientific research (1.4.647.84F) to G. Franck, J. C. Depresseux, and M. Guillaume.

REFERENCES

1. Ackermann, R. F., Chugani, H. T., Finch, D. M., Babb, T. L., Lear, J. L., and Engel, J. (1983): Autoradiographic studies of stimulation-induced changes in rat hippocampal metabolism and blood flow. *J. Cereb. Blood Flow Metab.*, 3:S238–S239.
2. Baron, J. C., Bousser, M. G., Comar, D., Soussaline, F., and Castaigne, P. (1981): Non invasive tomographic study of cerebral blood flow and metabolism in vivo. *Eur. Neurol.*, 20:273–284.
3. Baron, J. C., Lebrun-Grandie, Ph., Collard, Ph., Crouzel, C., Mestelan, G., and Bousser, M. G. (1982): Noninvasive measurement of blood flow, oxygen consumption, and glucose utilization in the same brain regions in man by positron emission tomography: Concise communication. *J. Nucl. Med.*, 23:391–399.
4. Bernardi, S., Trimble, M. R., Frackowiak, R. S., Wise, R. J., and Jones, T. (1983): An interictal study of partial epilepsy using positron emission tomography and the oxygen-15 inhalation technique. *J. Neurol. Neurosurg. Psychiatry*, 46:473–477.
5. Björntorp, P., Ellis, H. A., and Bradford, R. H. (1964): Albumin antagonism of fatty acid effects on oxidation and phosphorylation reactions in rat liver mitochondria. *J. Biol. Chem.*, 239:339–344.
6. Blennow, G., Nelsson, B., and Siesjö, B. K. (1977): Sustained epileptic seizures complicated by hypoxia, arterial hypotension or hyperthermia: Effects on cerebral energy state. *Acta Physiol. Scand.*, 100:126–128.
7. Bonte, F. J., Stokely, E. M., Devous, M. D., and Homan, R. W. (1983): Single-photon tomographic study of regional cerebral blood flow in epilepsy. A preliminary report. *Arch. Neurol.*, 40:267–270.
8. Brodersen, P., Paulson, O. B., Bolwig, T. G., Rogon, Z. E., Rafaelsen, O. J., and Lassen, N. A. (1973): Cerebral hyperemia in electrically induced epileptic seizures. *Arch. Neurol.*, 28:334–338.
9. Chapman, A. G., Meldrum, B. S., and Siesjö, B. K. (1977): Cerebral metabolic changes during prolonged epileptic seizures in rats. *J. Neurochem.*, 28:1025–1035.
10. Chatrian, G. E., Shaw, C. M., and Leffman, H. (1964): The significance of periodic lateralized epileptiform discharges in EEG: An electrographic, clinical and pathological study. *Electroencephalogr. Clin. Neurophysiol.*, 17:177–193.
11. Depresseux, J. C. (1983): A method for the local evaluation of the volume of rapidly exchangeable water in the human brain. In: *Positron Emission Tomography of the Brain*, edited by W. Heiss and M. E. Phelps, pp. 95–102. Springer, Berlin.
12. Depresseux, J. C. (1984): La biocinétique des indicateurs radioactifs: Réexamen de quelques notions à la lumière de la tomographie démission positronique. *Ann. Radio.*, 27:702–707.
13. Depresseux, J. C. (1984): Le volume effectif de distribution de l'indicateur: le "second paramètre" dans l'évaluation de débits sanguins par indicateurs inerts et diffusibles. *J. Biophys. Med. Nucl.*, 9:254–269.
14. Depresseux, J. C., Cheslet, J. P., and Franck, G. (1983): An original method for the concomitant tomographic assessment of cerebral blood flow, oxygen extraction rate and exchangeable water volume in man. *J. Cereb. Blood Flow Metab.*, 3:152–153.
15. Depresseux, J. C., Cheslet, J. P., and Hodiaumont, J. (1982): Evaluation tomographique chez l'homme du débit sanguin cérébral et du volume cérébral d'eau rapidement échangeable. *J. Biophys. Med. Nucl.*, 6:173–177.
16. Depresseux, J. C., Raichle, M. E., Larson, K. B., Markham, J., and Ter Pogossian, M. M. (1981): An introduction to the measurement of the cerebral oxygen uptake rate by inhalation of $^{15}O_2$: Analysis of the contributions of $^{15}O_2$ and $H_2^{15}O$ in the brain radioactivity. *Eur. Neurol.*, 20:207–214.
17. Duffy, T. E., Howse, D. C., and Plum, F. (1975): Cerebral energy metabolism during experimental status epilepticus. *J. Neurochem.*, 24:925–934.
18. Dymond, A. M., and Crandall, P. H. (1976): Oxygen availability and blood flow in the temporal lobes during spontaneous epileptic seizures in man. *Brain Res.*, 102:191–196.
19. Eichling, J. O., Raichle, M. E., Grubb, R. L., and Ter Pogossian, M. M. (1974): Evidence of the limitations of water as a freely diffusible tracer in the brain of the rhesus monkey. *Circ. Res.*, 35:358–364.
20. Engel, J. (1984): The use of positron emission tomographic scanning in epilepsy. *Ann. Neurol.*, 15:S180–S191.
21. Engel, J., Brown, W. J., Kuhl, D. E., Phelps, M. E., Mazziotta, J. C., and Crandall, P. H. (1982): Pathological findings underlying focal temporal lobe hypometabolism in partial epilepsy. *Ann. Neurol.*, 12:518–528.
22. Engel, J., Kuhl, D. E., and Phelps, M. E. (1982): Patterns of human local cerebral glucose metab-

olism during epileptic seizures. *Sciences,* 218:64–66.

23. Engel, J., Kuhl, D. E., and Phelps, M. E. (1983): Regional brain metabolism during seizures in humans. In: *Advances in Neurology: Status Epilepticus,* edited by A. V. Delgado-Escueta, C. G. Wasterlain, D. M. Treiman, and R. J. Porter, pp. 141–148. Raven Press, New York.

24. Engel, J., Kuhl, D. E., Phelps, M. E., and Crandall, P. H. (1982): Comparative localization of epileptic foci in partial epilepsy by PCT and EEG. *Ann. Neurol.,* 12:529–537.

25. Engel, J., Kuhl, D. E., Phelps, M. E., and Mazziotta, J. C. (1982): Interictal cerebral glucose metabolism in partial epilepsy and its relation to EEG changes. *Ann. Neurol.,* 12:510–517.

26. Engel, J., Kuhl, D. E., Phelps, M. E., Rausch, R., and Nuwer, M. (1983): Local cerebral metabolism during partial seizures. *Neurology,* 33:400–413.

27. Folbergrovà, J., Ingvar, M., and Siesjö, B. K. (1981): Metabolic changes in cerebral cortex, hippocampus, and cerebellum during sustained bicuculline-induced seizures. *J. Neurochem.,* 37:1228–1238.

28. Frackowiak, R. S. J., Lenzi, G.-L., Jones, T., and Heather, J. D. (1980): Quantitative measurement of regional cerebral blood flow and oxygen metabolism in man using ^{15}O and positron emission tomography: Theory, procedure, and normal values. *J. Comput. Assist. Tomogr.,* 4:727–736.

29. Gibbs, F. A., Lennon, W. G., and Gibbs, E. L. (1934): Cerebral blood flow preceding and accompanying epileptic seizures in man. *Arch. Neurol. Psychiatry,* 32:257–272.

30. Griffiths, T., Evans, M. C., and Meldrum, B. S. (1983): Intracellular calcium accumulation associated with early pathology of the rat hippocampus following drug-induced seizures. *J. Cereb. Blood Flow Metab.,* 3:S274–S275.

31. Griffiths, T., Evans, M. C., and Meldrum, B. S. (1983): The role of calcium in selective neuronal loss in status epilepticus: An experimental study in the rat hippocampus. In: *Current Problems in Epilepsy: Cerebral Blood Flow, Metabolism and Epilepsy,* edited by M. Baldy-Moulinier, D. H. Ingvar, and B. S. Meldrum, pp. 285–291. John Libbey, London.

32. Heiss, W. D., Turnheim, M., Vollmer, R., and Rappelsberger, P. (1979): Coupling between neuronal activity and focal blood flow in experimental seizures. *Electroencephalogr. Clin. Neurophysiol.,* 27:396–403.

33. Herscovitch, P., Markham, J., and Raichle, M. E. (1983): Brain blood flow measurement with intravenous $H_2^{15}O$. Theory and error analysis. *J. Nucl. Med.,* 24:782–789.

34. Herscovitch, P., and Raichle, M. E. (1983): Effect of tissue heterogeneity on the measurement of cerebral blood flow with the equilibrium $C^{15}O_2$ inhalation technique. *J. Cereb. Blood Flow Metab.,* 3:407–415.

35. Horton, R. W., Meldrum, B. S., Pedley, T. A., and McWilliam, J. R. (1980): Regional cerebral blood flow in the rat during prolonged seizure activity. *Brain Res.,* 192:399–412.

36. Hougaard, K., Oikawa, T., Sveinsdottir, E., Skinhøj, E., Ingvar, D. H., and Lassen, N. A. (1976): Regional cerebral blood flow in focal cortical epilepsy. *Arch. Neurol.,* 33:527–535.

37. Howse, D. C. (1978): Metabolic response to status epilepticus in the rat, cat and mouse. *Can. J. Physiol. Pharmacol.,* 57:205–212.

38. Howse, D. C. (1983): Cerebral energy metabolism during experimental status epilepticus. In: *Advances in Neurology: Status Epilepticus,* edited by A. V. Delgado-Escueta, C. G. Wasterlain, D. M. Treiman, and R. J. Porter, pp. 209–216. Raven Press, New York.

39. Huang, S. C., Carson, R., Hoffman, E. J., Carson, J., MacDonald, N., Barrio, J. R., and Phelps, M. E. (1983): Quantitative measurement of local cerebral blood flow in humans by positron computed tomography and ^{15}O-water. *J. Cereb. Blood Flow Metab.,* 3:141–153.

40. Huang, S. C., Carson, R., and Phelps, M. E. (1982): Measurement of local blood flow and distribution volume with short-lived isotopes. *J. Cereb. Blood Flow Metab.,* 2:99–108.

41. Ingvar, D. H. (1973): Regional cerebral blood flow in focal cortical epilepsy. *Stroke,* 4:359–360.

42. Ingvar, D. H. (1975): rCBF in focal cortical epilepsy. In: *Cerebral Circulation and Metabolism,* edited by T. W. Langfitt, L. C. McHenry, Jr., M. Reivich, and H. Wollman, pp. 361–364. Springer-Verlag, New York.

43. Jones, S. C., Greenberg, J. H., and Reivich, M. (1982): Error analysis for the determination of cerebral blood flow with the continuous inhalation of ^{15}O-labeled carbon dioxide and positron emission tomography. *J. Comput. Assist. Tomogr.,* 6:116–124.

44. Jones, T., Chesler, D. A., and Ter-Pogossian, M. M. (1976): The continuous inhalation of oxygen-15 for assessing regional oxygen extraction in the brain of man. *Br. J. Radiol.,* 49:339–343.

45. Kearfott, K. K. (1982): Absorbed dose estimates for positron emission tomography (PET): $C^{15}O$, ^{11}CO and $CO^{15}O$. *J. Nucl. Med.,* 23:1031–1037.

46. Kreisman, N. R., Rosenthal, M., LaManna, J. C., and Sick, T. J. (1983): Cerebral oxygenation during recurrent seizures. In: *Advances in Neurology: Status Epilepticus,* edited by A. V. Delgado-Escueta, C. G. Wasterlain, D. M. Treiman, and R. J. Porter, pp. 231–239. Raven Press, New York.

47. Kreisman, N. R., Rosenthal, M., Sick, J., and LaManna, J. C. (1983): Oxidative metabolic responses during recurrent seizures are independent of convulsant, anesthetic, or species. *Neurology,* 33:861–867.

48. Kuhl, D. E., Engel, J., Phelps, M. E., and Selin, C. (1980): Epileptic patterns of local cerebral metabolism and perfusion in humans determined by emission computed tomography of ^{18}FDG and $^{13}NH_3$. *Ann. Neurol.,* 8:348–360.

49. Lammertsma, A. A., and Jones, T. (1983): Correction for the presence of intravascular oxygen-15 in the steady-state technique for measuring regional oxygen extraction ration in the brain: 1. Description of the method. *J. Cereb. Blood Flow Metab.,* 3:416–424.

50. Lavy, S., Melamed, E., Portnoy, Z., and

Carmon, A. (1976): Interictal regional cerebral blood flow in patients with partial seizures. *Neurology*, 26:418–422.

51. Lebrun-Grandié, Ph., Baron, J. C., Soussaline, F., Loch'h, C., Sastre, J., and Bousser, M.-G. (1983): Coupling between regional blood flow and oxygen utilization in the normal human brain. A study with positron tomography and oxygen 15. *Arch. Neurol.*, 40:230–236.

52. Meldrum, B. S. (1981): Metabolic effects of prolonged epileptic seizures and the causation of epileptic brain damage. In: *Metabolic Disorders of the Nervous System*, edited by F. C. Rose, pp. 175–187. Pitman Medical, London.

53. Meldrum, B. S. (1983): Metabolic factors during prolonged seizures and their relation to nerve cell death. In: *Advances in Neurology: Status Epilepticus*, edited by A. V.-Delgado-Escueta, C. G. Wasterlain, D. M. Treiman, and R. J. Porter, pp. 261–275. Raven Press, New York.

54. Meldrum, B. S., and Nilsson, B. (1976): Cerebral blood flow and metabolic rate early and late in prolonged epileptic seizures induced in rats by bicuculline. *Brain*, 99:523–542.

55. Meyer, J. S., Gotoh, F., and Favale, E. (1966): Cerebral metabolism during epileptic seizures in man. *Electroencephalogr. Clin. Neurophysiol.*, 21:10–22.

56. Mintun, M. A., Raichle, M. E., Martin, W. R. W., and Herscovitch, P. (1984): Brain oxygen utilization measured with O-15 radiotracers and positron emission tomography. *J. Nucl. Med.*, 25:177–187.

57. Penfield, W., Von Santha, K., and Cipriani, A. (1939): Cerebral blood flow during induced epileptiform seizures in animals and man. *J. Neurophysiol.*, 2:257–267.

58. Phelps, M. E., Huang, S. C., Hoffman, E. J., Salin, C., Sokoloff, L., and Kuhl, D. E. (1979): Tomographic measurement of local cerebral glucose metabolic rate in humans with (F-18)2-fluoro-2-deoxy-D-glucose: Validation of method. *Ann. Neurol.*, 6:371–388.

59. Pinard, E., Ben-Ari, Y., Tremblay, E., and Seylaz, J. (1983): Is intratissue hypoxia responsible for hippocampal lesions during seizures induced by kainic acid? In: *Current Problems in Epilepsy: Cerebral Blood Flow Metabolism and Epilepsy*, edited by M. Baldy-Moulinier, D. H. Ingvar, and B. S. Meldrum, pp. 252–257. John Libbey, London.

60. Plum, F., Howse, D. C., and Troy, B. (1968): Metabolic effects of seizures. In: *Brain Dysfunction in Metabolic Disorders*, edited by F. Plum, pp. 141–157. Raven Press, New York.

61. Posner, J. B., Plum, F., and Van Poznak, A. (1969): Cerebral metabolism during electrically induced seizures in man. *Arch. Neurol.*, 20:388–395.

62. Raichle, M. E., Martin, W. R. W., Herscovitch, P., Mintun, M. A., and Markham, J. (1983): Brain blood flow measured with intravenous $H_2^{15}O$. II. Implementation and validation. *J. Nucl. Med.*, 24:790–798.

63. Sakai, F., Meyer, J., Naritomi, M., and Hsu, M. C. (1978): Regional cerebral blood flow and EEG in patients with epilepsy. *Arch. Neurol.*, 35:648–657.

64. Siesjö, B. K. (1978): Utilization of substrate by brain tissues. In: *Brain Energy Metabolism*, edited by B. K. Siesjö, pp. 101–130. John Wiley, New York.

65. Siesjö, B. K. (1981): Cell damage in the brain: A speculative synthesis. *J. Cereb. Blood Flow Metab.*, 1:155–185.

66. Siesjö, B. K., Ingvar, M., Folbergrova, J., and Chapman, A. G. (1983): Local cerebral circulation and metabolism in biculline-induced status epilepticus: Relevance for development of cell damage. In: *Advances in Neurology: Status Epilepticus*, edited by A. V. Delgado-Escueta, C. G. Wasterlain, D. M. Treiman, and R. J. Porter, pp. 217–230. Raven Press, New York.

67. Sokoloff, L., Reivich, M., Kennedy, C., Des Rosiers, H., Patlak, C. S., Pettigrew, K. D., Sakurada, O., and Shinohara, M. (1977): The (^{14}C) deoxyglucose method for the measurement of local cerebral glucose utilization: Theory, procedure and normal values in the conscious and anesthetized albino rat. *J. Neurochem.*, 28:897–916.

68. Subramanyam, R., Alpert, N. M., Hoop, B., Brownell, G. L., and Taveras, J. M. (1978): A model for regional cerebral oxygen distribution during continuous inhalation of $^{15}O_2$, $C^{15}O$ and $C^{15}O_2$. *J. Nucl. Med.*, 19:48–53.

69. Theodore, W. H., Brooks, R., Sato, S., Patronas, N., Margolin, R., Di Chiro, G., and Porter, R. J. (1984): The role of positron emission tomography in the evaluation of seizure disorders. *Ann. Neurol.*, 15:S176–S179.

70. Theodore, W. H., Newmark, M. E., Sato, S., Brooks, R., Patronas, N., De la Paz, R., DiChiro, G., Kessler, R. M., Margolin, R., Manning, R. G., Channing, M., and Porter, R. J. (1983): ^{18}F-Fluorodeoxyglucose positron emission tomography in refractory complex partial seizures. *Ann. Neurol.*, 14:429–437.

71. Touchon, J., Valmier, J., and Baldy-Moulinier, M. (1983): Regional cerebral blood flow in temporal lobe epilepsy: Interictal studies. In: *Current Problems in Epilepsy: Cerebral Blood Flow, Metabolism and Epilepsy*, edited by M. Baldy-Moulinier, D. H. Ingvar, and B. S. Meldrum, pp. 33–38. John Libbey, London.

72. West, J. B., and Dollery, C. T. (1962): Uptake of oxygen-15 labeled CO_2 compared with carbon-11 labeled CO_2 in the lung. *J. Appl. Physiol.*, 17:9–13.

73. Wise, R. J., Rhodes, C. G., Gibbs, J. M., Hatazawa, J., Palmer, T., Frackowiak, R. S., and Jones, T. (1983): Disturbance of oxidative metabolism of glucose in recent human cerebral infarcts. *Ann. Neurol.*, 14:627–637.

74. Wojtczak, L. (1976): Effect of long-chain fatty acids and acyl-CoA on mitochondrial permeability transport and energy-coupling processes. *J. Bioenerg. Biomembr.*, 8:293–311.

75. Yamamoto, Y. L., Ochs, R., and Gloor, P. (1983): Patterns of rCBF and focal energy metabolic changes in relation to electroencephalographic abnormality in the interictal phase of partial epilepsy. In: *Current Problems in Epilepsy: Cerebral Blood Flow, Metabolism and Epilepsy*, edited by M. Baldy-Moulinier, D. H. Ingvar, and B. S. Meldrum, pp. 51–62. John Libbey, London.

Advances in Neurology, Vol. 44, edited by
A. V. Delgado-Escueta, A. A. Ward, Jr.,
D. M. Woodbury, and R. J. Porter.
Raven Press, New York © 1986.

48

Neuronal, Dendritic, and Vascular Profiles of Human Temporal Lobe Epilepsy Correlated with Cellular Physiology *in Vivo*

*T. L. Babb and **W. J. Brown

Departments of *Neurology and **Pathology, UCLA School of Medicine, Los Angeles, California 90024

SUMMARY   Partial complex seizures are known to arise from abnormal firing of neurons in cortex that has histologic abnormalities associated with tumors, infarcts, or neuron loss. The latter pathology of sclerosis is most frequently found in the hippocampus, and partial seizures from this region are focalized by direct electrical recordings and treated by anterior temporal lobectomy. Although we can link this hippocampal sclerosis to nearby hyperexcitability, the synaptic mechanisms involved in hippocampal seizure genesis are not yet known. We have used *in vivo* microelectrode recordings from hippocampal neurons and found rare instances of anomalous bursting patterns as well as coupled firing. Postinhibitory "rebound excitation" has also been recorded, supporting the concept that synchronized hippocampal outputs are important for seizure genesis. Immunocytochemistry of GAD-positive inhibitory interneurons indicates no significant loss in inhibition in the sclerotic hippocampus and a normal number of inhibitory interneurons in its output target, the presubiculum. The presubiculum, with its multi-layered cortex, may amplify and propagate seizures to other cortices. Golgi and electron microscopy of epileptic neurons have shown pre- and postsynaptic alterations that may contribute to seizure genesis. Finally, ultrastructural analysis of capillaries in sclerotic hippocampus indicates deficient plasma–tissue transport that may contribute to cell loss or may alter neuronal excitability.

HISTORY OF PATHOLOGY IN TEMPORAL LOBE EPILEPSY

Studies on Temporal Lobe Seizures

Although the localization of focal motor seizures to lesions or infarcts of the frontal cortex had been reported by Hughlings Jackson as early as 1872 (29), the localization of complex partial seizures to temporal lobe structures developed later and has continued to be controversial. In 1888, Jackson described notes supplied to him by various physicians on over 50 cases, all of whom had the classic symptoms of complex partial epilepsy in that there was evidence of an "intellectual aura" (*déjà vu* or crude sensations), only slight movements, and a defect of consciousness ("dreamy state") (30). These symptoms had been recognized earlier as much different from those seizures associated with sensory or motor cortex; however, Jackson's inference that these "dreamy state" seizures were "localized" to the temporal lobe came from two necropsy reports: one of a tumor in the temporo–sphenoidal lobe (32) and another with softening of the uncinate gyrus (33). These clinicopathologic descriptions confirmed several previous case reports that linked complex partial seizures (usually olfactory sensations) to tumors of the olfactory tract (46), to degeneration of uncinate gyrus (26), and to a basal anterior temporal-lobe tumor (2).

Electrographic Studies of Temporal Lobe Epilepsy

From these early clinical observations, Jackson (31) proposed that the physiological basis of focal seizures was excessive discharge from neurons adjacent to focal cerebral lesions. This view has remained undisputed to the present day; however, there was no means to verify this hypothesis before the use of electro-encephalography (EEG). In 1937, Gibbs, Gibbs, and Lennox (24) described a generalized 6-Hz rhythm associated with clinical signs of clouding of consciousness or amnesia as well as simple motor and emotional changes. Although this "cerebral dysrhythmia" was associated with psychomotor or temporal-lobe seizures, the EEG did not provide specific cerebral localization of the pathology, nor did it support Jackson's concept of focal neuronal discharge. In 1941, Jasper and Kershman (34) published their attempt to confirm this EEG classification of Gibbs et al. (24), and they demonstrated clearly that for temporal-lobe epilepsy the patterns of the EEG were not as important as the localization of the abnormal EEG. This paper was a key advance in the use of the EEG for classifying generalized and partial complex seizures. Based on interseizure scalp EEG recordings, they concluded (34, pp. 923–924) that

> Patients with clearly focal cortical seizures have a localized electroencephalographic pattern, those with pure petit mal seizures the bilaterally synchronous wave and spike pattern and those with only psychomotor episodes usually sharp waves and 6 per second rhythms, often bilaterally synchronous but sometimes localized.

They further concluded (34, p. 932) that

> It seems clear from the nature of these disturbances that the temporal lobe and subjacent structures, probably in the archipallium, are the regions primarily involved. This is in accord with the electrographic localization, which so frequently seems to be deep to the temporal lobes (e.g. the hippocampus) near the midline.

Although these studies suggested that the focus of epileptic excitability may be in mesial as well as lateral temporal lobe, it would take a decade before surgery for psychomotor seizures was specifically designed to include the hippocampus and hippocampal gyrus.

Surgery for Temporal Lobe Epilepsy

In 1950, Penfield and Flanigin (43) reported on the results of 10 years of temporal lobe excisions to relieve temporal-lobe seizures. In a footnote (43, p. 497) they commented:

> One of us (W.P.) operated on a patient with temporal lobe epilepsy in 1928 and occasionally carried out similar procedures during the next 11 years, but it was not until the introduction of electroencephalography into clinical practice that the importance and frequency of this type of focal seizure became evident.

Ironically, the electrocorticographic studies were carried out by Dr. Jasper, who had earlier (1941) suggested that epileptic foci may reside in the hippocampus (34); however, in only 2 of 51 cases was the hippocampus removed. Only 52.9% of these surgeries were considered a "success":

51 Excisions of the Temporal Lobe 1 to 10 Years after Operation

Success ("Cured")	52.9%
Worthwhile ("Improved 50% or more")	25.4%
Failure (No or slight improvement)	21.5%

The following year, Bailey and Gibbs (9) reported their surgical results where they had emphasized that EEG analysis of low temporal spiking correlated with a psychomotor seizure type. Of 1,250 patients studied with scalp EEG exhibiting an anterior temporal spiking focus, 98% had a psychomotor seizure type. "It has been concluded that psychomotor epilepsy is caused by a discharging lesion in the anterior temporal lobe and that anterior temporal lobe epilepsy is the commonest type of focal epilepsy" (9, p. 365). In 25 patients, they removed varying extents of temporal neocortex but never the hippocampus and reported "success" in 48%:

Therapeutic Effect on Psychomotor Seizures

Success [Great (20%) or Moderate (28%)]	48%
Slight	28%
None	24%

These results did not differ significantly from Penfield and Flanigin (43), and the authors offered several explanations (43, pp. 368–369) for failing to localize and remove the epileptic tissue:

> Microscopic study of the cortex removed at operation has not revealed frequent pathological alterations, but it must be remembered that only the superficial parts of the first and second convolutions were removed for study; the rest of the extirpation was made by suction. When looked at in detail from electrodes on the exposed surface of the brain, an epileptic focus is found to be not a point or an area but a constellation of points or a number of areas. A focus must be thought of in much the same terms as a contusion of the brain.

The authors did not suggest that these EEG spikes may be propagated to the lateral temporal cortex from the hippocampus, as suggested 10 years earlier by Jasper and Kershman (34).

Penfield and Baldwin (42) reanalyzed the tissue from 157 temporal lobectomies and found that in 100 cases the lesion was atrophic and nonneoplastic. In the majority of the cases the sclerosis was found in the uncus and hippocampus. Finally, they concluded that ". . . these changes are ischemic in origin. But we also find evidence that once established, there is further progressive destructive change over the course of many years" (42, p. 633). They proposed an ontogenetic model of the cause of mesial temporal sclerosis, which they called "incisural sclerosis" [see also Earle et al. (19)], which specified that the arteries supplying this region were compressed against the incisura of the tentorium during birth, high intracranial pressure, or other conditions. Although temporal herniation may occur in some cases, this mechanism for damage has not been fully supported because (a) mesial temporal sclerosis is rarely accompanied by damage to the calcarine cortex, which is also supplied by the posterior cerebral artery; (b) there is similar damage to cerebellum and other structures not directly supplied by any arteries near the tentorial opening; and (c) it is now known that over 80% of the granule cells of the hippocampus develop after birth (1,3), and dividing neuroblasts would be destroyed by perinatal anoxia. However, in human hippocampal sclerosis the granule-cell layer is less affected than pyramidal neurons, and there is no evidence that stratum granulosum is disorganized, as would be expected if neuroblasts were damaged during migration. Despite the inadequacy of "incisural sclerosis" as

a unitary etiology of hippocampal sclerosis, this concept led Penfield and Baldwin (42) to an important conceptual breakthrough. They concluded (42, pp. 633–634) that

> In nearly every one of these cases the distribution of abnormality was that which would have been produced by temporal herniation of the tentorium. The abnormality is therefore called incisural sclerosis and *the technic of surgical excision must be planned to include the hippocampal region* [italics ours].

In a discussion at the end of this paper, Dr. W. J. Mixter commented (42, p. 634):

> . . . I think most of us have had the feeling—I know I did—up to a short time ago that the lesion lay much more on the surface of the temporal lobe rather than deeply, and that it could be picked up by electroencephalography in the absence of any appearance of scar tissue. That is important, because partial operations in this region, with removal of the surface focus— I know from my own experience—do not give relief.

In the decades that have followed, surgery for temporal-lobe seizures have included the hippocampal formation, and the benefit from surgery has improved. Green and Scheetz (25) reported that temporal-lobe excisions that included the hippocampus and hippocampal gyrus in 60 psychomotor epileptics resulted in 68.3% "success":

Seizure Control in 60 Patients

No seizures, auras or medication	11.7%
Reduction of seizures auras and medication	56.6%
No significant change	31.7%

Although several nonstandard means of assessing seizure relief have been published in reporting "success" with temporal lobectomies including the hippocampus, the median is 70 to 75%. For example, Falconer et al. (22) report 86%; Talairach and Bancaud (57) report 77%; Van Buren et al. (59) report 80% with large resections and 50% with small resections; and Crandall (15) reports 71%. For a review and discussion of the present status of temporal-lobe surgery, see Spencer (52). These papers clearly show that seizure relief is likely in about 75% of psychomotor epileptics if the hippocampal formation is removed, but only about 50% are relieved if it is not. This very strongly indicates that the primary epileptic tissue generating psychomotor seizures is usually located in the archicortex (hippocampal formation) of the mesial temporal lobe, and that this epileptic tissue can be "localized" by direct recordings from the hippocampus.

In 1963, Crandall et al. (16) reported on 8 psychomotor epileptics whose seizure foci could not be determined using scalp EEGs. Direct chronic intracerebral recordings of hippocampal seizure activity was sufficiently clear in 6 patients to recommend unilateral temporal lobectomy. Mesial temporal pathology was found in all the resected specimens and all patients had seizure relief. Direct recordings from suspected hippocampal foci during the onset of spontaneous seizures have proved to be the most reliable diagnostic technique. Further (15, p. 272),

> Depth electrode studies were indispensable to subsequent surgical treatment. . . . In summary, depth electrode studies with recordings made during the ictus were successful in verifying a single seizure focus in approximately three-fourths of our patients.

These technical advances in EEG localization increased the number of psychomotor epileptics treated by anterior temporal-lobe resection. The availability of this physiologically identified epileptic tissue supplemented enormously the descriptions of the pathological substrates of temporal-lobe epilepsy, which had previously been studied by fortuitous postmortem brain examinations or by examination of resected superficial temporal cortex.

Neuropathology Studies in Temporal Lobe Epilepsy

As described earlier, Jackson and Beevor (32) related the presence of mesial temporal lesions to "dreamy state" seizures preceded by an aura, which we now know are temporal lobe seizures. Other postmortem studies in epileptics showed a variety of pathologies, with the most common being sclerosis of the hippocampus. In 1880, Sommer (51) reported detailed microscopic studies of losses of pyramidal cells in the prosubiculum (Rose's H1, now called Sommer's sector) of epileptics. Bratz (10) emphasized that not only were prosubicular neurons damaged, but also the pyramids of CA4 or the hilus of the fascia dentata (Rose's H4 and H5). He also noted the resistant sector of spared CA2 pyramidal cells (Rose's H2–3). However, these hippocampal lesions were found not exclusively in temporal lobe epileptics but also in patients with

general convulsive disorders. Second, in postmortem studies of patients with well-documented temporal lobe epilepsy, "hypoxic" damage or sclerosis was found in thalamus (25% of 55 cases studied), amygdala (27%), and cerebellum (45%) when the incidence of hippocampal sclerosis was 65% (39). This notion that diffuse hippocampal sclerosis was due to anoxia or ischemia was a recurrent theme expressed by the German pathologists, such as Spielmeyer (55) and Scholz (49). They concluded that the sclerosis was the result of repeated seizures or "ictal damage" (50).

In 1935, Stauder (56) noted the hippocampal or Ammon's horn sclerosis in 33 of 36 postmortem cases where the patients had a history of clinical seizures typical of temporal-lobe epilepsy. His paper took the position that this type of sclerosis was significantly more likely than with other epilepsies and such damage may be the cause rather than the result of temporal lobe seizures. This notion gained more support from (a) therapeutic temporal-lobe resections, especially in the 1950s, when the mesial temporal lobe (hippocampus) was found to be epileptogenic (see earlier section) and (b) the fact that when these lobes were examined, sclerosis was the most common pathology. For example, Meyer et al. (40) reported definitive hippocampal sclerosis in seven of 14 (50%) resected temporal lobes and marginal gliosis in four hippocampi (29%). They concluded (40, pp. 282–283) that

> The fact that following temporal lobectomy the clinical features were so frequently improved strongly suggests that the pathological changes were somehow responsible for the epilepsy, which had improved as a consequence of their removal. This is in keeping with the general clinical observation that the mechanisms responsible for epilepsy are dependent not so much on the nature of the pathological change as on its site.

Although an incidence of clear hippocampal sclerosis as a diffuse pathology was shown to be about the same for temporal lobe epileptics as for other chronic epileptics (50%) (40,47), more recent studies have shown that hippocampal sclerosis is more likely to be found in clearly defined temporal lobe epilepsy. For example, when the clinical signs of a temporal-lobe seizure were preceded by an *aura*, mesial temporal sclerosis was present in 90% of the resected lobes (21), which suggests again that the epileptogenic tissue giving rise to typical psychomotor seizures is usually near sclerotic mesial temporal-lobe structures. This conclusion seems even more compelling in conjunction with other reports that surgical benefit from temporal lobectomy may be as high as 92% when the resected lobe contains mesial temporal sclerosis but only 64% success when the pathological lesions are "equivocal" (23).

As indicated earlier, in 1961 a group of researchers (16) at the University of California at Los Angeles initiated a program to define epileptic hyperexcitability directly by the use of electrodes chronically implanted in the mesial temporal lobe structures, which have been reported as commonly sclerotic in patients with psychomotor seizures, and then to evaluate the type and extent of pathology observed after anterior temporal lobectomy. This combined physiology and pathology approach offers the best opportunity to define the structural substrates of temporal lobe seizures. In 1973, Brown (11) reported the results of pathological alterations observed in physiologically identified epileptic tissue located in 29 resected temporal lobes. He concluded that in 65% of the cases hippocampal sclerosis was the only major pathology found in the standard 6-cm block of temporal lobe. Seventy-three percent of these cases had seizure relief. In 18% of the cases there were glial hamartomas outside the hippocampus proper but within the temporal lobe, and all these patients had seizure relief. One patient had a malignant astrocytoma in the resected temporal lobe and became seizure-free. In 14% of the cases, no pathology could be found in the temporal-lobe specimen. Of these, only one benefited from temporal lobectomy, and Brown suggested that ". . . there could be a small lesion posterior to the lobectomy resection line" (11, p. 370).

These latter studies are of great significance because they confirm in greater detail that focal or anatomically restricted neuropathology is a sufficient cause of temporal lobe seizures. When these local lesions are removed, the psychomotor seizures are relieved or significantly altered. Hence, although there may be a process of neuron loss in the hippocampus due to ischemia or anoxia that occurs with repeated seizures, it is not true that such passive neuronal destruction is the sole source of hippocampal sclerosis. Rather, it appears that hippocampal sclerosis is a pathological substrate adjacent to active epileptogenic neurons, analogous to hyperexcitable neurons surrounding tumors or infarcts.

The association between hippocampal sclerosis and hippocampal hyperexcitability is the final link that needs to be established in order to confirm that temporal lobe seizures arise from abnormal circuitry near a focus of observable pathology. The microanatomical basis for this abnormal circuitry has not yet been established; however, ongoing studies relating specific seizure foci to abnormal neuronal discharges (4) coupled with sophisticated anatomical studies in human temporal lobe (11) offer the basis for postulating and testing several epileptogenic mechanisms responsible for temporal lobe epilepsy.

The remainder of this chapter will fully describe the type and extent of abnormalities found in physiologically verified epileptic temporal lobe in order to distinguish synaptic abnormalities that may be considered primarily epileptogenic and not merely ischemic cell loss. This question has remained a problem that is not well understood by epileptologists. In all these cases, we have postlobectomy follow-up of seizure benefit to confirm that after this epileptic tissue was excised the typical temporal lobe seizures were eliminated or altered.

Hence, our strategy as described in this chapter has been to use electrophysiological techniques to define the seizure "focus" and then use postlobectomy microanatomical techniques to test a variety of proposed synaptic mechanisms that may contribute to seizure genesis. We have limited our patient population to those with hippocampal sclerosis and contrasted such findings to those where the temporal-lobe seizures arise from lateral temporal neocortex, adjacent to such pathologies as angiomas, heterotopias or hamartomas. Such lesions have virtually no hippocampal damage and can serve as a type of "control."

PATHOPHYSIOLOGY AND MICROANATOMY OF TEMPORAL LOBE EPILEPSY

Microelectrode Recordings of Neurons in Epileptic Hippocampus

In 1972 we developed a technique for long-term *in vivo* recordings of neurons in the hippocampal formation of psychomotor epileptics (5). Because these microelectrode bundles (see Fig. 1) (4) were inserted bilaterally along the axis of the pes and gyrus hippocampi, we were able to evaluate interictal and ictal firing patterns of "nonepileptic" and "primary" epileptic neurons, i.e., neurons in the hippocampus where stereoelectroencephalograph (SEEG) seizures started and where seizure relief followed hippocampal removal. Finally, these prelobectomy

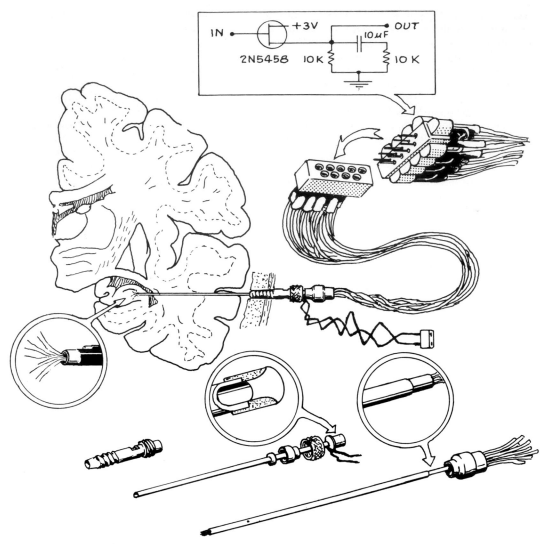

FIG. 1. Schematic drawing of the technique used for chronically implanted fine-wire microelectrodes (40 μm diameter each). Only one cannula (bipolar recording and/or stimulating macro-electrode) plus one bundle of nine fine wires is shown here. Typically, these cannulae plus microelectrodes are implanted bilaterally in amygdala; anterior, middle, and posterior hippocampus; anterior, middle, and posterior gyrus hippocampi; and anterior or middle presubiculum. This array allows us to test various physiological properties of anterior to posterior hippocampal formation for later comparison with postlobectomy microanatomical studies. (from ref. 4, with permission.)

neuronal recordings were studied with various techniques and related to the pathological/anatomical alterations as a strategy for defining the microanatomical bases for neuronal epileptogenesis.

Approximately 300 single neurons in "primary" or independently identified epileptic hippocampal formation have been analyzed for anomalous burst firing (4) that would be significantly different from the patterns found in normal hippocampal neurons (5). Although there

have been reports of "epileptic bursting" in human and monkey (13) epileptic neocortex, others (28,44) have not confirmed this concept of "trigger" or pacemaker cells in human epileptic cortex. Our own visual and computer analysis (for details see ref. 4) have revealed a variety of bursting patterns in both normal and epileptic hippocampus. These bursts are typical of Ammon's horn pyramidal cells in that there is a clear "inactivation response," i.e., spikes of decreasing amplitude (35). Interspike interval analyses of these neurons have demonstrated that only 4% of the cells in human epileptic hippocampus have the structured or stereotyped (invariant) intraburst firing pattern (see Fig. 2) (4) first described by Calvin et al. (13). Such results do not support the concept of pacemaker cells in epileptic hippocampus. Rather, it appears that the majority of neurons in epileptic hippocampus have "regular" bursts, and the "triggering" of seizures must involve some additional mechanisms such as synchrony.

We have studied the prevalence of "coupled firing" or synchronized bursts in only those instances where we were able to have simultaneous recordings of neurons by two microelectrodes in the same epileptic hippocampus (see Fig. 3). Because of this sampling problem, it is unlikely that we will be able to accurately test whether or not synchronous bursts are signifi-

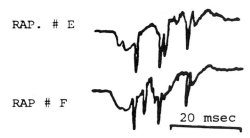

RAP. # E

RAP # F

20 msec

FIG. 3. Waveforms from two hippocampal neurons within 5 mm of each other, recorded from different fine wires in the same bundle in anterior hippocampus, adjacent to the onsets of all electrographic seizures. Note that although the bursts are not identical, several discharges are coincident between the two neurons, suggesting that they would have synchronized outputs to target regions such as the presubiculum.

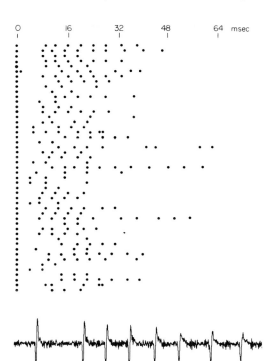

FIG. 2. Dot display of an "anomalous" burst pattern recorded from a neuron in the anterior hippocampus, the region where macroelectrodes recorded focal seizure onsets. Note that the first intervals in most of the bursts are longer than the succeeding intervals. This burst pattern was very stable throughout the day (waking) and throughout a sleep study with all sleep stages (e.g., SWS and REM). At the bottom is a digitized plot of the waveforms of this bursting pattern, with the decreasing spike amplitudes ("inactivation response") typical of hippocampal pyramidal cells. (From ref. 4, with permission.)

cantly more prevalent in epileptic than in nonepileptic hippocampus. In order to test for synchrony, we have utilized focal electrical stimulation and measured durations and recovery from recurrent inhibition. By analyzing both evoked field potentials (population excitatory presynaptic potentials and population spikes) and evoked firing, we have observed long recurrent inhibition in epileptic hippocampus (60) and, most importantly, there is a rebound excitation that appears to synchronize neuronal firing. By contrast, in normal hippocampus there appears to be shorter recurrent inhibition (60) and less rebound excitation. These are at present only preliminary results that require further confirmation. However, the concept of release from inhibition as a mechanism for seizure-triggering is very attractive because it would provide a synchronous output from cell-sparse hippocampus to drive monosynaptic targets that could propagate seizures.

The model described above of "synchronous inhibition" and "rebound excitation" as mechanisms for recruitment of neurons for seizure genesis is well supported by physiological studies in animal hippocampus. For example, intracellular studies of *in vitro* hippocampal slices made epileptogenic by penicillin (14) exhibit epileptic membrane phenomena (paroxysmal depolarization shifts and bursts); however, "ictal" events appear to depend on larger populations of neurons. The importance of recruiting epileptic neuronal aggregates has been emphasized using hippocampal slices (61), and one important mechanism for this recruitment has been synchrony. Although many investigators assume that synchronous bursting occurs exclusively through direct excitatory connections, it is well known that optimal synchrony of hippocampal firing occurs immediately at the end of synchronous recurrent inhibition (see "rebound excitation" in ref. 53 and "late excitation and repetitive firing" in ref. 54). In support of this notion that recurrent inhibition is an important mechanism for synchronizing the larger number of neurons needed to generate a seizure, several studies have demonstrated evoked prolonged inhibition in an epileptic focus (20,58). Our preliminary results in human epileptic hippocampus clearly demonstrate long recurrent inhibition and rebound excitation. These direct neuronal recordings provide strong support for a model of postinhibitory synchronized outputs as a mechanism for human hippocampal formation seizure genesis. Further preliminary results suggest that these hippocampal neurons may drive an even larger number of neurons in the presubicular complex, thereby providing seizure propagation to many other cortical regions. In summary, then, we suggest that synchronous firing from hippocampal neurons followed by uninhibited excitation of retrohippocampal (presubiculum) neurons is needed for typical hippocampal seizures. The microanatomical studies described next provide direct tests of this proposed synaptic organization of human epileptic hippocampal formation.

Distribution of Neuron Loss and Epileptogenicity

The typical pattern of hippocampal sclerosis in "primary" temporal-lobe epilepsy (i.e., cured by anterior temporal lobectomy) is shown in Fig. 4. The most important findings are that most cell loss is in anterior hippocampus, especially Ammon's horn. Posterior hippocampus is also damaged significantly; however, the cell loss is less than in anterior hippocampus (7,51). We have found a direct link between the extent of cell loss in Ammon's horn and nearby seizure genesis. In patients whose SEEG seizures originate exclusively from anterior hippocampus, there is significant anterior cell loss and no statistically significant pyramidal cell loss in posterior Ammon's horn (8). Figure 5 shows this quantitative relationship between anterior damage and anterior focal seizure genesis. These results strongly support a model of hippocampal damage as a prerequisite for synaptic reorganization.

We next asked the question, if there are so few neurons in Ammon's horn, how can sufficient numbers of neurons be recruited to generate seizures? As can be seen from Figs. 4 and 5, the transitional subicular complex is *not* damaged, even when it is only one synapse away from severe Ammon's horn sclerosis in the anterior sector of the hippocampus. Figure 4 is a comparison of primary epileptic and control anterior mesial temporal lobe to show clearly that subiculum and presubiculum (even more so) are cytologically normal while dentate gyrus and Ammon's horn are severely damaged. The importance of this profile of spared target neurons in the subicular complex is that they may serve to amplify or propagate the relatively few excitatory outputs from sclerotic hippocampus proper. Hence, this cytology supports a "dual-focus" model of focal seizure genesis whereby only a few synchronized Ammon's-horn outputs would trigger a large number of presubicular neurons and thereby provide widespread excitatory, epileptic propagation to other cortical areas.

Inhibitory Interneurons in Human Epileptic Hippocampus and Presubiculum

In the preceding sections we have hypothesized that Ammon's-horn cells are *not* "epileptic" because they lack GABA-mediated recurrent inhibition. Rather, we have proposed that hippocampal neurons have ample recurrent inhibition, exhibit "rebound excitation" in order to synchronously fire hippocampal neurons, which in turn recruit the large population of spared presubicular neurons. We have additionally hypothesized that local recurrent inhibition is decreased in "epileptic" presubiculum, which would enhance the epileptogenic propagation by the presubiculum. We have directly tested this model by quantification of GABA interneurons and terminals as detected by immunocytochemistry of glutamic acid decarboxylase (GAD), the synthesizing enzyme for the inhibitory transmitter gamma-aminobutyric acid (GABA).

Unilateral hippocampal seizure foci were identified by intracerebral recordings during typical clinical seizures in patients with drug-resistant complex partial epilepsy. Resection of the anterior temporal lobe, including the entire hippocampal formation, allowed us to quantify the anatomical distribution of GAD-positive inhibitory interneurons and terminals. Alternate sections were processed for routine cytology. The GAD antibody (41) and the avidin-biotin conjugate (ABC)–horseradish peroxidase (HRP) (27) were used on tissue from 24 human hippocampal epileptics and 2 normal monkeys (as controls). In the control monkey hippocampi, GAD-positive interneuron counts in all seven subfields (fascia dentata, CA4, CA3, CA2, CA2,

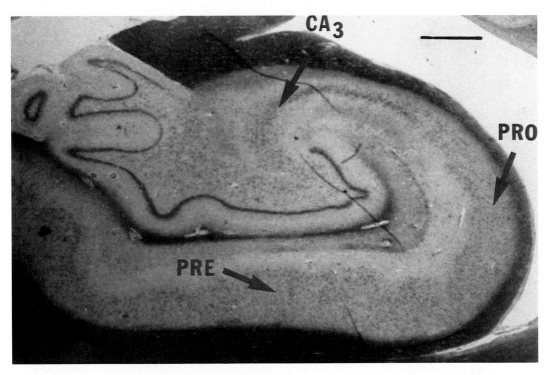

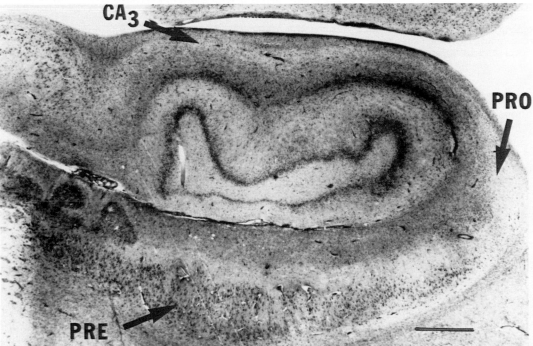

FIG. 4. Low-power photomicrograph of normal **(top)** and epileptic **(bottom)** anterior hippocampal formation. Note the loss of neurons in the enclosed dentate gyrus and all Ammon's-horn subfields. *Arrow* pointing to CA3 **(bottom)** indicates severe loss of pyramidal cells extending around to the prosubiculum (PRO), where sclerosis is typically greatest. Hence, it is clear that there are very few hippocampal output neurons in typical hippocampal epilepsy. By contrast, note that in the presubiculum (PRE) there is normal layering and normal numbers of neurons in epileptic hippocampal formation **(bottom)** when compared to autopsy control PRE **(top)**. Calibration bar 1 mm.

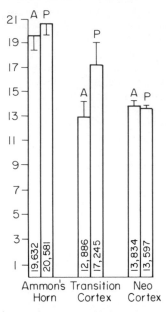

FIG. 5. Comparison of the regional distribution of cell loss in anterior temporal lobe, where 100% of electrographic seizures had a focal onset (**left** histogram) and control cell densities (**right** histogram). Note that for the epileptic Ammon's horn only the anterior region shows cell loss statistically lower than anterior control hippocampus. Furthermore, the posterior Ammon's-horn cell densities were not significantly different between the epileptic temporal lobe and control, presumably because no focal seizures were generated from posterior hippocampus. These data strongly support the concept that cell loss is necessary for the adjacent tissue to generate focal seizures. Finally, note that neither the transitional cortex (subiculum and presubiculum) nor the temporal neocortices are damaged in primary focal anterior hippocampal epilepsy.

prosubiculum, presubiculum) were similar to those of normal rats (6) and also were not significantly greater than in human epileptics (except for CA3, where there was a 50% loss of GAD cells). In other words, despite severe Ammon's-horn sclerosis or loss of pyramids, there was little loss of recurrent inhibitory interneurons. This finding does not support the concept of "disinhibition" in the Ammon's horn as a mechanism for seizure genesis. Similarly, the number of GAD-positive interneurons in the monkey presubiculum were numerically identical to those in human hippocampal epileptics. In other words, there were normal densities of pyramidal cells in presubiculum and normal densities of inhibitory interneurons in presubiculum of temporal lobe epileptics.

Further studies of Ammon's horn and presubicular neurons are necessary in order to provide better statistical relationships between electrical excitability, physiological evidence for recurrent inhibition and the density of GABA-secreting interneurons and terminals in CA fields and presubiculum of "epileptic" human hippocampus. It must be emphasized that these

preliminary studies only suggest that disinhibition cannot account for seizure genesis in either Ammon's horn or presubiculum. These studies of inhibitory circuitry have encouraged us to use many other microanatomical techniques to test the "dual-focus" model described above.

Golgi-Impregnated Neurons and Dendrites in Human Hippocampal Formation

One of the earliest methods for studying the structure of the mammalian hippocampal formation was the Golgi and Cox reduced silver techniques (12,37). These methods reveal only a few neurons and their processes; hence it is possible to visualize entire neurons "typical" of epileptic or nonepileptic control tissue. Obviously this approach is potentially very valuable in comparing postsynaptic dendrites and spines, which may be morphologically unique to epileptic hippocampus. Using the rapid Golgi method, Scheibel and Scheibel (48) published qualitative descriptions of "epileptic" hippocampal neurons that included a variety of dendritic profiles. However, they were unable to relate these profiles to clinical, electrographic, or other cytologic indices of focal hippocampal epilepsy. More recently, we have routinely studied "epileptic" hippocampal neurons and quantitatively compared various dendritic parameters to control hippocampus. As expected, in control Ammon's-horn neurons the shapes, branching patterns, and spines of dendrites were similar to those of normal subhuman mammals. Figure 6 (left side) shows a camera lucida drawing of a normal (control) CA2 pyramidal cell. This hippocampus had no cytological abnormalities, based on an adjacent hematoxylin–eosin stain. The Golgi-impregnated basilar dendrites have typical spines, and the primary apical dendrite has typical secondary branches with clear spines very close to the apex of the cell body. This is typical of CA2 pyramids, as described earlier by Lorente de No (37) and Scheibel and Scheibel (48): "In CA2 pyramids, the principal apical shaft is very short or non-existent. The apical dendritic bouquet accordingly starts virtually at the neck of the soma (48, p. 315)." When we quantified the average length from the soma to the first apical branch the distance was 16.5 μm

(see Fig. 6, control). In contrast, this primary apical shaft in epileptic CA2 neurons was over twice as long (34 μm, Fig. 6, epileptic). Because these long primary dendrites did not have spines, it is very likely that this membrane would be reinnervated not by typical excitatory synapses, which terminate on spines, but rather by inhibitory synapses that typically surround the soma. Such available membrane could receive direct inhibitory input, since axo–somatic inhibitory synapses would be nearby, and inhibitory axons might migrate to synapse on noninnervated membrane in a manner similar to "sprouting" and reinnervation of denervated dendritic zones in hippocampus of mammals (38). This hypothesis of "sprouted" inhibitory axons on proximal dendrites of epileptic Ammon's-horn cells would support the concept presented earlier that there is increased inhibition that contributes to synchronous hippocampal rebound excitatory output.

In evaluating the architecture of distal "excitatory" dendrites, it is clear (Fig 6, epileptic) that there are significantly fewer branches in epileptic (mean 5.75) compared to control (mean

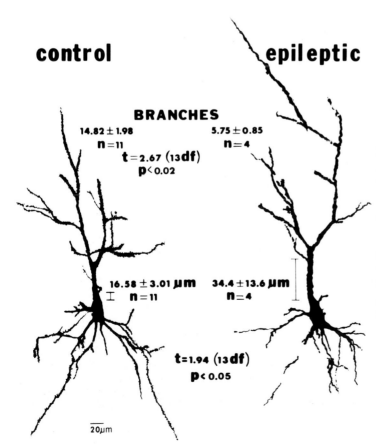

control   **epileptic**

BRANCHES

14.82 ± 1.98   5.75 ± 0.85
n = 11   n = 4

t = 2.67 (13 df)
p < 0.02

16.58 ± 3.01 μm   34.4 ± 13.6 μm
n = 11   n = 4

t = 1.94 (13 df)
p < 0.05

20 μm

FIG. 6. Camera lucida drawings of typical cells used for quantitative analysis of nonepileptic (control) and epileptic Golgi-filled neurons in CA2. Significantly fewer branches and spines were counted in epileptic neurons, suggesting inefficient excitatory synapses in epileptic CA2. The proximal dendritic zone, which is branch-free and spine-free, was significantly longer (soma to first branch) in epileptic CA2, suggesting that this membrane may be reinnervated by recurrent inhibitory axons "sprouting" from their nearby axosomatic sites.

14.82) dendrites. Furthermore, there are fewer spines in "epileptic" pyramidal dendrites. Hence, it is very possible that excitatory inputs to epileptic hippocampal neurons are less effective. This may sound paradoxical if we try to view "epileptic" tissue as "hyperexcitable" at a single cell. However, our thesis is that seizures can only be generated by synchronous firing of neurons. Perhaps this "high threshold" for firing created by loss of spines would assist synchrony, because only clearly suprathreshold inputs would fire such spine-deficient neurons and in turn would fire a larger population of hippocampal neurons. The following studies of dendritic ultrastructure confirm that the pre- and postsynaptic apposition is abnormally "insulated" by glia in the excitatory dendritic zone of "epileptic" CA2 pyramids.

Ultrastructure of Synapses in Normal and Epileptic Hippocampal Neurons

In order to study the axosomatic (inhibitory) and axodendritic (excitatory) synapses on normal and epileptic human pyramidal cells, electron micrographs were made of selected regions. This technique allowed us to visualize, with the highest possible resolution, presynaptic boutons and vesicles and postsynaptic receptor densities.

Thin cross-sections of the hippocampus were fixed by rapid immersion in cold buffered glutaraldehyde mixtures. Blocks of various CA subfields were easily made under the dissecting microscope without staining. These blocks were embedded in Epon 812, cut tilted to get an optimal view of cell lines. Thin sections were then made, and serial electron micrographs were reconstructed as a montage to identify a complete view of the soma and apical dendrite. Figure 7 shows one such montage, with the cell body at the upper left (soma), the proximal dendrite extending left to right, and the more distal dendrite, coursing through stratum radiatum, shown from right to left on the bottom. The importance of this low-magnification montage reconstruction is that synaptic profiles at the soma (which are inhibitory synapses) and on distal dendrites (which are excitatory synapses) can be restudied with higher magnifications. For example, we can visualize the extent to which axons might be "insulated" from the soma or dendritic spines in epileptic tissue compared to nonsclerotic normal pyramidal cells. Ribak et al. (45) reported extensive glial sheaths between "inhibitory" symmetric synapses in monkey alumina gel epileptic neocortical foci, and they

postulated that this would reduce recurrent inhibition and contribute to epileptogenicity. They further reported glial invasions of the asymmetric excitatory synapses, but indicated that the "insulation" of excitatory synapses was probably less than that for the inhibition. Although we have not yet quantified the "loss" or "separation" of synapses in our electron micrographs, we can easily find sheaths of glia intertwined with the vesicle–receptor appositions for both axosomatic (inhibitory) and axodendritic (excitatory) synapses. At the same time, despite nearby glia, there are normal-appearing pre- and postsynaptic densities. Hence, at the present time we feel our ultrastructural analyses require better quantification before we can estimate the relative "loss" of inhibitory versus excitatory efficacy.

Figure 8 is a comparison of axodendritic excitatory synapses in normal (top) and epileptic (bottom) human hippocampus. It is clear that in the normal stratum radiatum (excitatory synapse zone) there are many clearly defined asymmetric synapses (see arrows) around the dendrite. By contrast, in the "epileptic" stratum radiatum, glial sheaths (G) are adjacent to the dendrite at several points. However, next to this glia there are well-defined asymmetric excitatory synapses (see arrows). Hence, this is a clear example of intact excitatory synapses in the midst of gliosis. Similar findings are numerous with axosomatic synapses, suggesting that neurons in epileptic hippocampus have "decreased" synaptic efficacy but not providing strong evidence of how that might contribute to seizure-sensitivity. Clearly, these ultrastructural synaptic studies will require a major systematic quantitative effort to answer questions that cannot be resolved by the coarser cytochemical or immunocytochemical techniques described previously.

Ultrastructural Studies of Microcirculation in Epileptic Human Hippocampus

Electron microscopy is useful not only for studies of synapses but also for the quantitative study of capillaries in epileptic tissue. There has been a long-standing and still unresolved debate as to whether or not neuron loss in hippocampus is caused by ischemia, either chronic alteration in vessels or repeated seizure-triggered vasoconstriction. For example, Spielmeyer (55) suggested that neuron loss in hippocampus resulted from vascular insufficiency either before the hippocampus developed a seizure focus or afterward with each seizure. In 1933 Scholz (50) ex-

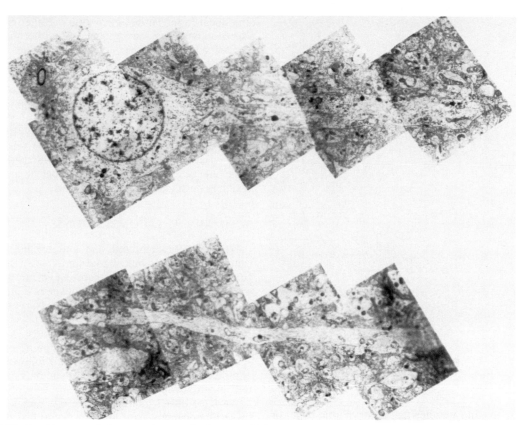

FIG. 7. Montage of electron micrograph of a pyramidal neuron from the presubiculum. The soma at the **upper left** can be studied in greater detail by reexposing that ultrathin section at higher magnification to evaluate axo–somatic (inhibitory) synapses. Axo–dendritic synapses that are excitatory to distal dendrites (**bottom,** right to left) may be magnified similarly. ×2,630. (Modified from ref. 11.)

tended this interpretation and coined the term "ictal damage" to refer to angiospasms or ictal ischemic cell loss. Our recent correlational studies of hippocampal neuron loss and seizure history have not found strong evidence that each seizure causes more cell loss (7). These results can be interpreted in several ways. First of all, there must be a distinction drawn separating focal, partial seizures from severe generalized tonic–clonic seizures, where it is well known that systemic and pulmonary circulation may be compromised. In mild partial hippocampal seizures in humans, local blood flow to hippocampal gyrus was found to increase (17,18). This finding by itself would suggest that in partial complex seizures hippocampal cell loss is not caused by ischemic episodes. However, Dymond and Crandall (18) also recorded local oxygen availability and found that despite the increased flow, there was a selective unilateral decrease in oxygen availability in the region of the hippocampal focus during a severe hippocampal seizure. This finding does support the notion of a metabolic insufficiency coincident with seizures, but the question remaining is whether or not the lowered oxygen availability is capable of killing cells.

As already indicated, ultrastructural analysis of capillaries would provide one test of a possible plasma–tissue exchange deficiency in an epileptic focus. For example, although blood flow may increase, the capillary permeability may be inadequate to provide appropriate metabolic exchange needed for neurons firing at high rates. To test this, Kasantikul et al. (36) reported that in human sclerotic or epileptic hippocampus the basal lamina are three times thicker than normal, are surrounded by a thick perithelial cell, and have significantly fewer areas of mitochondria in either the endothelium or perithelium (see Fig. 9). This means that it is very unlikely that this "thick" blood-brain barrier could be overcome by increased transport mechanisms, because there are too few mito-

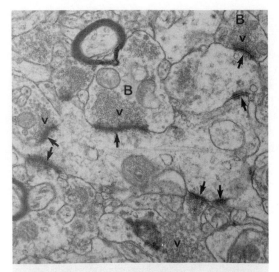

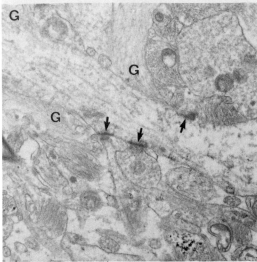

FIG. 8. Electron micrographs of axo–dendritic excitatory synapses in stratum radiatum of CA2 for comparison of normal **(top)** with epileptic **(bottom)** human hippocampal synaptic ultrastructure. Note that in the epileptic tissue many synaptic appositions have apparently been replaced by glial slips (G). However, adjacent to this glia are some intact synapses (*arrows*). In contrast, in normal tissue large vesicle-filled (V) boutons (B) line the surface of the dendrite, and normal dendritic spine synapses are numerous.

chondria per area to provide the energy needed for normal plasma–tissue exchange. Hence, this analysis of "epileptic" hippocampus microvasculature lends support to the notion that during seizures there may be abnormal metabolism of neurons which may result in hypoxia or ionic imbalances. Such circulatory alterations may contribute to cell death or possibly even may

alter focal hippocampal excitability. Either the altered excitability may enhance firing because of a mechanism such as decreased buffering, or it may decrease firing by similar mechanisms or others that may help to terminate focal discharges. In either case, although ultrastructural analysis of capillaries cannot predict the physiology of adjacent neurons, nevertheless the structure of altered microvasculature contributes to our understanding of focal epilepsy when these vascular profiles are compared with all the other microanatomical and physiological data available on human hippocampal foci.

SUMMARY AND CONCLUSIONS

We have demonstrated that anterior hippocampal sclerosis is linked to anterior focal seizures, which suggests that there is synaptic reorganization following focal hippocampal injury. This synaptic reorganization is necessary for focal seizure genesis.

This model of hippocampal damage and "plasticity" as essential for focal temporal lobe seizures is supported by the fact that following anterior temporal lobectomy these complex partial seizures stop occurring.

We have direct microelectrode recordings of these hippocampal neurons in order to test the synaptic physiology of "epileptic" hippocampus. While there is a small percentage of neurons that fire in an "abnormal" burst pattern, the number is so small that these could not be considered sufficient to "trigger" seizures without other epileptogenic mechanisms of "abnormal" circuitry.

One such mechanism, synchronization of firing, has been observed with paired microelectrode recordings in "epileptic" hippocampus. In addition, long-lasting recurrent inhibition in hippocampus has been found to be followed by "rebound excitation." Hence, it is possible the inhibitory mechanisms in hippocampus contribute to the probability of joint or synchronous firing of the few neurons remaining in sclerotic hippocampus. In turn, these synchronous discharges may monosynaptically drive the cytologically intact presubiculum, which would propagate seizure discharges. The presubiculum, then, would constitute the "hyperexcitable fringe" with a population of neurons sufficient to generate a clinical seizure.

Microanatomical studies of the distribution of inhibitory interneurons and terminals in epileptic hippocampus and presubiculum using GAD immunocytochemistry have supported the concept that there is ample recurrent inhibition

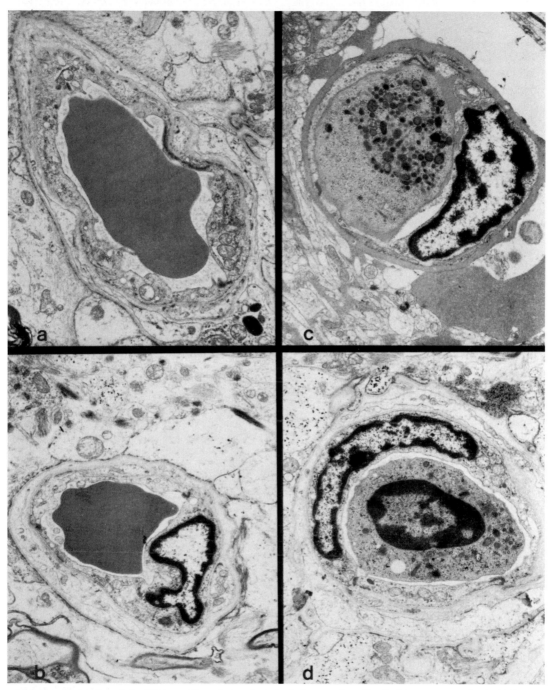

FIG. 9. Examples of the thick capillary network typical of sclerotic epileptic hippocampus. Such thick capillary "walls" and inadequate mitochrondria areas strongly indicate impaired plasma–tissue transport that may contribute to cell loss or altered neuronal excitability. **a–d**: Capillary prototypes from areas CA1, 2, 3, and 4, respectively, of human sclerotic cortex. The basal lamina are roughly two to three times normal thickness. Immersion-fixed hippocampal cortex. Although **a** is not through the endothelial nucleus, it is similar in every other respect. ×7,225. (From ref. 36, with permission.)

in epileptic hippocampus despite the severe loss of output neurons. This direct evidence of inhibitory circuits supports our physiological conclusions that inhibition may help to synchronize hippocampal outputs to presubiculum. Furthermore, our quantification has shown normal inhibitory interneurons in the presubiculum adjacent to epileptic hippocampus. This would not support the concept that either Ammon's horn or presubicular neurons are disinhibited.

Microanatomical studies of Golgi-embedded postsynaptic sites in epileptic hippocampus have revealed long portions of the apical shaft denuded of spines and therefore potentially reinnervated. Electron microscopy of pre- and postsynaptic profiles have revealed synaptic sites "insulated" by glia but also other sites with typical synaptic appositions. Neither the Golgi nor the ultrastructural analysis have been quantified in sufficient detail to demonstrate a preferential loss of inhibitory versus excitatory communication. Such detailed studies are under way, and they will provide important supporting information for the other physiologic and microanatomic techniques being studied concurrently.

Comparisons of normal and "epileptic" (sclerotic) microvasculature have revealed thicker basal lamina in epileptic tissue, increased thickness of perithelial cells, and significantly smaller areas of mitochondria that normally would provide the energy necessary for transport across capillary walls. Such apparently decreased capillary permeability may contribute to cell loss in epileptic hippocampus, may compromise ion-exchange mechanisms that contribute to neuron membrane stability, and may contribute to altered firing or termination of firing in nearby neurons. Such alterations in microvasculature may be merely a reflection of early damage or ongoing damage and may not actually affect the synaptic mechanisms of epileptic hippocampus. However, as we continue to combine the results from all these various techniques, we will develop a fuller understanding of mechanisms essential to focal seizure genesis in hippocampal cortex with its well-defined input–output circuits. The models and mechanisms may, in turn, help to explain some of the other partial seizures arising in other cortical areas.

ACKNOWLEDGMENTS

The authors wish to thank all the professional and technical assistance that was essential in completing this work. The research has been supported by National Institutes of Health (NIH) grant NS02808 and the UCLA Department of Neurology and Pathology. Scientists and technicians working with the Clinical Neurophysiology Project (NS 02808) deserve special thanks for their generous collaborative efforts in all the cellular neurophysiology studies. These studies have been made possible only through the joint efforts of Dr. Paul Crandall, Dr. Charles Wilson, and Dr. Masako Isokawa-Akesson. The microanatomical studies were possible because of the great neurosurgical skill of Dr. Paul Crandall, who provided intact *en bloc* temporal lobectomies. The various microanatomical analyses were possible because of the expert work of James Pretorius, M.S. and many others in the Division of Neuropathology.

REFERENCES

1. Altman, J., and Bayer, S. (1975): Postnatal development of the hippocampal dentate gyrus under normal and experimental conditions. In: *The Hippocampus, Vol. 1,* edited by R. Isaacson and K. Pribram, pp. 95–122. Plenum, New York.
2. Anderson, J. (1887): On sensory epilepsy: A case of basal tumour, affecting the left temporosphenoidal lobe, and giving rise to paroxysmal taste-sensation and dreamy state. *Brain,* 9:385.
3. Angevine, J. B. (1965): Time of neuron origin in the hippocampal region: An autoradiographic study in the mouse. *Exp. Neurol. Suppl.,* 2:1–70.
4. Babb, T. L., and Crandall, P. H. (1976): Epileptogenesis of human limbic neurons in psychomotor epileptics. *Electroencephalogr. Clin. Neurophysiol.,* 40:225–243.
5. Babb, T. L., Carr, E., and Crandall, P. H. (1973): Analysis of extracellular firing patterns of deep temporal lobe structures in man. *Electroencephalogr. Clin. Neurophysiol.,* 34:247–257.
6. Babb, T. L., Brown, W. J., Pretorius, J., and Kufper, W. (1984): Recovery of GABA recurrent inhibition in dentate gyrus after entorhinal kindling in rats. *Neurosci. Abst.,* 10:345.
7. Babb, T. L., Brown, W. J., Pretorius, J., Davenport, C., Lieb, J. P., and Crandall, P. H. (1984): Temporal lobe volumetric cell densities in temporal lobe epilepsy. *Epilepsia,* 25:729–740.
8. Babb, T. L., Lieb, J. P., Brown, W. J., Pretorius, J., and Crandall, P. H. (1984): Distribution of pyramidal cell density and hyperexcitability in the epileptic human hippocampal formation. *Epilepsia,* 25:721–728.
9. Bailey, P., and Gibbs, A. (1951): The surgical treatment of psychomotor epilepsy. *J. A. M. A.,* 145:365–370.
10. Bratz, E. (1899): E. Ammonshornbefunde der epileptischen. *Arch. Psychiatr. Nervenkr.,* 31:820–836.
11. Brown, W. J. (1973): Structural substrates of seizure foci in the human temporal lobe. In: *Epilepsy: Its Phenomena in Man* edited by M. A. B. Brazier, pp. 339–374. Academic, New York.

12. Cajal, S. R. y (1968): *The Structure of Ammon's Horn*, C. C. Thomas, Springfield, Illinois. Translated by L. M. Kraft.

13. Calvin, W. H., Ojemann, G. A., and Ward, A. A., Jr. (1973): Human cortical neurons in epileptogenic foci: Comparison of inter-ictal firing patterns to those of "epileptic" neurons in animals. *Electroencephalogr. Clin. Neurophysiol.*, 34:337–351.

14. Courtney, K. R., and Prince, D. A. (1977): Epileptogenesis in neocortical slices. *Brain Res.*, 127:191–196.

15. Crandall, P. H. (1975): Postoperative management and criteria for evaluation. In: *Neurosurgical Management of the Epilepsies*, edited by Purpura et al., pp. 265–280. Raven Press, New York.

16. Crandall, P. H., Walter, R. D., and Rand, R. W. (1963): Clinical applications of studies on stereotactically implanted electrodes in temporal-lobe epilepsy. *J. Neurosurg.*, 20:827–840.

17. Dymond, A. M., and Crandall, P. H. (1973): Intracerebral temperature changes in patients during spontaneous epileptic seizures. *Brain Res.*, 60:249–254.

18. Dymond, A. M., and Crandall, P. H. (1976): Oxygen availability and blood flow in the temporal lobes during spontaneous epileptic seizures in man. *Brain Res.*, 102:191–196.

19. Earle, K. M., Baldwin, M., and Penfield, W. (1953): Incisural sclerosis and temporal lobe seizures produced by hippocampal herniation at birth. *A.M.A. Arch. Neurol. Psychiatr.*, 69:27–42.

20. Ebersol, J. S. (1977): Initial abnormalities of neuronal responses during epileptogenesis in visual cortex. *J. Neurophysiol.*, 40:514–526.

21. Falconer, M. A., and Cavanagh, J. B. (1959): Clinicopathological considerations of temporal lobe epilepsy due to small focal lesions. *Brain*, 82:483–504.

22. Falconer, M. A., Hill, D., Meyer, A., Mitchell, W., and Pond, D. A. (1955): Treatment of temporal-lobe epilepsy by temporal lobectomy. A survey of findings and results. *Lancet*, 1:827–835.

23. Falconer, M. A., Serafetinides, E. A., and Corsellis, J. A. N. (1964): Etiology and pathogenesis of temporal lobe epilepsy. *Arch. Neurol.*, 10:233–248.

24. Gibbs, F. A., Gibbs, E. L., and Lennox, W. G. (1937): Epilepsy; A paroxysmal cerebral dysrhythmia. *Brain*, 60:377–388.

25. Green, J. R., and Scheetz, D. G. (1964): Surgery of epileptogenic lesions of the temporal lobe. *Arch. Neurol.*, 10:135–148.

26. Hamilton, A. M. (1882): On cortical sensory discharging lesions (sensory epilepsy). *New York Medical Journal and Obstetrical Review*, 36:575.

27. Hsu, S. M., Raine, L., and Fanger, H. (1981): The use of avidin-biotin-peroxidase complex (ABC) in immunoperoxidase techniques: A comparison between ABC and unlabeled antibody (PAP) procedures. *J. Histochem. Cytochem.*, 29:577–580.

28. Ishijima, B., Hori, T., Yoshimasu, N., Fukushima, T., Hirakawa, K., and Sekino, H. (1975): Neuronal activities in human epileptic foci and surrounding areas. *Electroencephalogr. Clin. Neurophysiol.*, 39:643–650.

29. Jackson, J. H. (1931): On the anatomical and physiological localisation of movements in the brain. In: *Selected Writings of John Hughlings Jackson*, edited by James Taylor, pp. 37–76. Hodder and Stoughton, London.

30. Jackson, J. H. (1931): On a particular variety of epilepsy ("intellectual aura"), one case with symptoms of organic brain disease. In: *Selected Writings of John Hughlings Jackson*, edited by James Taylor, pp. 385–405. Hodder and Stoughton, London.

31. Jackson, J. H. (1931): On convulsive seizures. In: *Selected Writings of John Hughlings Jackson*, edited by James Taylor, pp. 412–457. Hodder and Stoughton, London.

32. Jackson, J. H., and Beevor, C. E. (1890): Case of tumour of the right temporo-sphenoidal lobe bearing on the localisation of the sense of smell and on the interpretation of a particular variety of epilepsy. *Brain*, 12:346–357.

33. Jackson, J. H., and Coleman, W. S. (1931): Case of epilepsy with tasting movements and "dreamy state"—very small patch of softening in the left uncinate gyrus. In: *Selected Writings of John Hughlings Jackson*, edited by James Taylor, pp. 458–463. Hodder and Stoughton, London.

34. Jasper, H. H., and Kershman, J. (1941): Electroencephalographic classification of the epilepsies. *Arch. Neurol. Psychiatr.*, 45:903–943.

35. Kandel, E. R., and Spencer, W. A. (1961): Electrophysiology of hippocampal neurons. II. After-potentials and repetitive firing. *J. Neurophysiol.*, 24:243–259.

36. Kasantikul, V., Brown, W. J., Oldendorf, W. H., and Crandall, P. H. (1983): Ultrastructural parameters and limbic microvasculature in human psychomotor epilepsy. *Clin. Neuropathol.*, 2:171–178.

37. Lorente de No, R. (1934): Studies on the structure of the cerebral cortex. II. Continuation of the study of the Ammonic system. *J. für Psychologie und Neurologie*, 46:113–177.

38. Lynch, G., and Cotman, C. W. (1975): The hippocampus as a model for studying anatomical plasticity in the adult brain. In: *The Hippocampus, Vol. 1: Structure and Development*, edited by R. L. Isaacson and K. L. Pribram, pp. 123–154. Plenum, New York.

39. Margerison, J. H., and Corsellis, J. A. N. (1966): Epilepsy and the temporal lobes. *Brain*, 89:499–530.

40. Meyer, A., Falconer, M. A., and Beck, E. (1954): Pathological findings in temporal lobe epilepsy. *J. Neurol. Neurosurg. Psychiatry*, 17:276–285.

41. Oertel, W. H., Schmechel, D. E., Mugnaini, E., Tappaz, M. L., and Kopin, I. H. (1981): Immunocytochemical localization of glutamate decarboxylase in rat cerebellum with anti-serum. *Neuroscience*, 6:2715–2735.

42. Penfield, W., and Baldwin, M. (1952): Temporal lobe seizures and the technic of subtotal temporal lobectomy. *Ann. Surg.*, 136:625–634.

43. Penfield, W., and Flanigin, H. (1950): Surgical therapy of temporal lobe seizures. *A.M.A. Arch. Neurol. Psychiatr.*, 64:491–500.

44. Rayport, M., and Waller, H. J. (1967): Technique and results of micro-electrode recording in human epileptogenic foci. *Electroencephalogr. Clin. Neurophysiol. [Suppl.]*, 25:143–151.

45. Ribak, C. E., Bradburne, R. M., and Harris, A. B. (1982): A preferential loss of GABAergic, symmetric synapses in epileptic foci: A quantitative ultrastructural analysis of monkey neocortex. *J. Neurosci.*, 2:1725–1735.

46. Sanders, W. (1874): Epileptische anfälle mit gehruchs-empindungen bei zerstörung des linken tractus olfactorius durch einen tumor. *Arch. Psychiatr. Nervenkr.*, 4:234.

47. Sano, K., and Malamud, N. (1953): Clinical significance of sclerosis of the cornu ammonis. *Arch. Neurol. Psychiatr.*, 70:40–53.

48. Scheibel, M. E., and Scheibel, A. B. (1973): Hippocampal pathology in temporal lobe epilepsy. A Golgi survey. In: *Epilepsy, Its Phenomena in Man*, edited by M. A. Brazier, pp. 311–337. Academic, New York.

49. Scholz, W. (1933): Uber die entstehung des hirnbefundes bei der epilepsie. *Z. qes. Neurol. Psychiat.*, 145:471.

50. Scholz, W. (1959): The contribution of patho-anatomical research to the problem of epilepsy. *Epilepsia*, 1:36–55.

51. Sommer, W. (1880): Erkrankung des Ammonshorns als aetiologisches moment der epilepsie. *Arch. Psychiatr. Nervenkr.*, 10:631–675.

52. Spencer, S. S. (1981): Depth electroencephalography in selection of refractory epilepsy for surgery. *Ann. Neurol.*, 9:207–214.

53. Spencer, W. A., and Kandel, E. R. (1961): Hippocampal neuron response to selective activation of recurrent collaterals of hippocampofugal axons. *Exp. Neurol.*, 4:149–161.

54. Spencer, W. A., and Kandel, E. R. (1962): Hippocampal neuron responses in relation to normal and abnormal functin. In: *Physiologie de L'Hippocampe*, pp. 71–104, C.N.R.S., Paris.

55. Spielmeyer, W. (1927): Die pathogenese des epileptischen krampfes. *Zeitschift für die gesamte Neurologie und Psychiatrie*, 109:501–520.

56. Stauder, K. H. (1935): Epilepsie und schlafenlappen. *Arch. Psychiatr. Nervenkr.*, 104:181–211.

57. Talairach, J., and Bancaud, J. (1974): Stereotaxic exploration and therapy in epilepsy. In: *Handbook of Clinical Neurology, Vol. 15: The Epilepsies,* edited by P. J. Vinken and C. W. Bruyn, pp. 758–782. North Holland, Amsterdam.

58. Tuff, L. P., Racine, R. J., and Adamec, R. (1983): The effects of kindling on GABA-mediated inhibition in the dentate gyrus of the rat. I. Paired-pulse depression. *Brain Res.*, 277:79–90.

59. Van Buren, J. M., Ajmone-Marsan, C., Mutsuga, N., and Sadowsky, D. (1975): Surgery of temporal lobe epilepsy. In: *Neurosurgical Management of the Epilepsies*, edited by D. P. Purpura et al., pp. 155–196. Raven, New York.

60. Wilson, C. L., Isokawa-Akesson, M., Babb, T. L., Wang, M. L., and Engel, J. E. (1985): Temporal lobe neuronal excitability in complex partial epilepsy. In: *Proceedings of the 16th Epilepsy International Congress.*

61. Wong, R. K. S., and Traub, R. D. (1983): Synchronized burst discharge in disinhibited hippocampal slice. I. Initiation in CA2 and CA3 regions. *J. Neurophysiol.*, 49:442–458.

Advances in Neurology, Vol. 44, edited by
A. V. Delgado-Escueta, A. A. Ward, Jr.,
D. M. Woodbury, and R. J. Porter.
Raven Press, New York © 1986.

49

Neuronal Firing Patterns from Epileptogenic Foci of Monkey and Human

Allen R. Wyler and Arthur A. Ward, Jr.

Department of Neurological Surgery, University of Washington, Seattle, Washington 98195

SUMMARY   The chronic, recurrent seizures induced in the monkey by cortical scarring occur spontaneously for years and share much of the phenomenology of spontaneous seizures of focal cortical onset in the human.

Chronic extracellular recording in the focus of the chronic epileptic monkey reveals:

1. A spectrum of abnormalities of unit firing ranging from grossly abnormal firing patterns to normal activity.

2. Group I (highly epileptic) neurons fire exclusively in bursts, which are invariant during different behavioral states and during operant conditioning. Although firing within the bursts is not easily modified, the interburst interval can be modified indicating that these apparently denervated cells still have some synaptic input. All group I cells are pyramidal neurons.

3. Group II (weakly epileptic) neurons exhibit variable burst firing, which may be intermixed with normal unit firing. The firing patterns of these cells can be modified by synaptic inputs. During operant conditioning, burst firing can decrease; during drowsiness or when inattentive, burst firing can approach that characteristic of group I cells.

There is a direct relationship between the number of group I epileptic (pacemaker) neurons in the focus and the epileptogenicity of that focus as measured by frequency of spontaneous seizures in that monkey.

The distribution of neurons encountered in the focus varies. On average, approximately 10% are group I (pacemaker) neurons; group II constitute 40%; and 50% of cells encountered exhibit normal firing patterns.

In addition to firing in unstructured bursts, an unusual burst structure termed the long-first-interval (LFI) burst has been described that appears to be unique to the chronic focus. It is so named because the first interspike interval is longer than the remaining interspike intervals in the burst. The long first interval is extraordinarily invariant.

There is little relationship between unit firing in bursts and the interictal EEG. During early parts of a spontaneous seizure, the two events become time-locked. During seizures, unit firing is synchronous with surrounding neurons and the spike portion of the EEG (as in penicillin foci). Firing of group I neurons does not change significantly preceding a spontaneous seizure.

Thus, group I neurons appear to act as pacemakers to the focus and group II cells provide the critical mass that, when synchronized to the burst firing of the pacemakers, is capable of initiating the ictal event.

Experiences with extracellular recording of neurons in human cortical foci over the past 25 years are summarized. Burst firing, long-first-interval bursts, and other features of the data recorded in the primate model have been confirmed. Further characterization is not possible in the clinical setting because of the ambiguity regarding the focus, limited recording time, and inability to manipulate inputs.

To best understand the neuronal mechanisms that make up the phenomenon of focal epilepsy in human, it would be ideal to study neurons from human brain. Although such opportunities may occasionally arise during surgery to remove cortical foci, the questions that may be addressed in the operating room are limited. In addition, our ability to point to a specific region of cortex and have confidence that it is "the epileptogenic focus" is most often tenuous except for the occasional well-defined cortical cicatrix. Although brain may be resected and taken to the laboratory for study using the "slice" preparation, this has obvious limitations (32). The most obvious problem is that epilepsy is a very comlex disorder that is modified by a host of endogenous and exogenous factors and cannot be studied in a preparation devoid of the influence of the remainder of the central nervous system. Because of these considerations, we have invested the majority of our research efforts into one specific model of focal cortical epilepsy: the chronic alumina-gel monkey model.

This model was discovered serendipitously by Kopeloff (22) during a series of experiments that were not even directed at epilepsy. As with many chance findings, this one has yielded the most accurate laboratory model of focal epilepsy available (15). The factors which make this preparation so valuable are: (a) it is a primate model; (b) it generates chronic, spontaneous seizures; (c) its histopathology is remarkably similar to what is seen from human foci (29,36); (d) much of its natural history is identical to the human disorder. This includes some similarities, which are often subtle. For example, biologic perturbations such as menstruation, stress, and sleep deprivation may effect the occurrence of seizures in monkeys just as they do in humans (19,20). After an initial period, the frequency of seizures stabilizes and thereafter the monkey continues to exhibit spontaneous seizures at roughly the same frequency for many years, as is often true of seizures of focal origin in humans.

In spite of the similarities noted above, this model has been criticized for harboring an alumina granuloma, a finding not present in humans. However, the presence of alumina is not essential for the induced focus to generate sei-

zures. In Kopeloff's original experiments, epileptogenic foci were produced by applying disks containing alumina to the pial surface, not intracortically. However, it may be argued that he had not shown conclusively that alumina did not cross the pial barrier. Harris (11,12) demonstrated that severe seizure foci could be produced by injecting alumina hydroxide into the subarachnoid space over the central fissure. He then showed that the alumina is incorporated into macrophages and occasional glia in layer I. The deeper layers where the epileptic activity is generated are devoid of alumina, as judged by histochemical and electron-microscopic criteria. In another group of monkeys made epileptic by the intracortical injection of alumina, Harris and Lockard (13) microsurgically removed the granulomas but left the surrounding gliosis. These monkeys continued having seizures as frequently as before the granuloma removal. In a second series of surgeries, a larger area of gliosis was then resected, and only after this operation did the seizures stop. Therefore, it is clear that it is not the alumina granuloma that is intimately associated with the clinical manifestation of seizures; rather it is the surrounding cortical gliotic scar.

The aluminum hydroxide gel obviously induces the development of a highly epileptic scar. Why other heavy metals are not as successful in generating chronic epilepsy is not at all clear. The cortical scar surrounding the granuloma is in itself an interesting and still unfinished area of investigation. First, the neurons are reduced in number, and those present have abnormal dendrites: they are deformed, have varicosities, and there is a reduction in dendritic branching. There can be a dramatic reduction in dendritic spines in both monkey and human foci (28,29,36). It is interesting that such "sick-looking" neurons are presumed to be involved in the epileptic process yet there is no unequivocal evidence that these are the neurons generating the bursts of APs so commonly associated with the epileptic process or, indeed, that they are capable of generating even a single action potential.

The glia are also of interest in that certain abnormalities are noted. First, unlike nonepileptic gliosis in cortex, glia surrounding alumina foci show specific alterations in histochemical properties particularly with respect to dehydrogenases (4; W. A. Meyer, *unpublished data*). Such glia have been termed "activated astrocytes" by Brotchi (4), who has described such histochemical changes in experimental animals as well as in gliotic human cortex associated with seizures. His data indicated that the histochemical changes are characteristic only of gliosis associated with seizures; areas of apparently equivalent reactive gliosis in the absence of seizures do not show these histochemical changes. The development of "activated" astrocytes appears to be related to the development of epileptic electrical activity but precedes the occurrence of clinical seizures. Thus these histochemical characteristics of glia in the focus are not the result of occurrence of clinical seizures: they appear to be related to mechanisms responsible for the epileptogenesis. In addition to the presence of activated astrocytes, the distribution of gliosis in the focus of the chronic monkey is somewhat laminar with a dense band in the deeper cortical layers (layers IV and V) (11). These peculiarities appear to be characteristic only of epileptogenic cortex. W. A. Meyer and A. R. Wyler (*unpublished data*) examined precentral cortex of non-epileptic monkeys that had repeated microelectrode penetrations over a period of months. The cortex had developed a dense gliosis, but this was neither laminar nor did it contain "activated" astrocytes. These monkeys had been monitored for seizures using the same techniques as for epileptic monkeys (17), and no spontaneous seizures were observed.

In the work to be described, alumina-induced epileptogenic foci were specifically placed in sensorimotor cortex. This produces focal motor seizures that can be easily monitored by computerized techniques 24 hr/day, 7 days/week (17). This region of cortex has been studied extensively in nonepileptic monkeys, thereby yielding a host of normative data against which to judge abnormal neuronal behavior.

NEURONAL FIRING PATTERNS IN THE CHRONIC MONKEY MODEL

Until Evarts (7) pioneered techniques for extracellular recordings from single neurons in the awake behaving monkey, the majority of neurophysiologic studies of the chronic monkey model were done on acute preparations which means the animals were paralyzed and under local anesthesia. Calvin, Sypert, and Ward (5) were the first to utilize Evarts' techniques to study the firing patterns of single neurons from nonanesthetized epileptic monkeys. In addition to finding neurons that fired in unstructured bursts, they reported an extremely interesting burst structure that they termed the long-first-interval (LFI) burst because the first interspike interval (ISI) of the burst was longer than the remaining ISIs of the burst (Fig. 1). While only a fraction of the neurons they encountered fired in LFI bursts, those units exhibiting it did so consistently. Of special interest were those neurons that generated LFI bursts in which the variance of the long first interval was less than 2% of the mean. Such precision of the timing pattern is highly unusual and is difficult to explain on the sole basis of hypersynchronous synaptic input. This was the first clue that neurons may generate bursts from intrinsic mechanisms. Later Calvin et al. (6) were able to record LFI bursts from epileptogenic cortex of humans (Fig. 2), further increasing the interest in the mechanism by which this particular structured burst pattern in produced and also further strengthening the link between the monkey model and human focal epilepsy. Moreover, the ability to record from undrugged, awake monkeys provided a major advance in understanding the dynamics of neuronal activity within chronic epileptogenic cortex of a physiologically intact primate.

Epilepsy in humans can be influenced by various behavioral states and, in many cases, by the patients' level of arousal. That is the reason both sleep and waking EEGs are needed in evaluating many seizure disorders. This relationship is also true for the monkey model. Thus, to

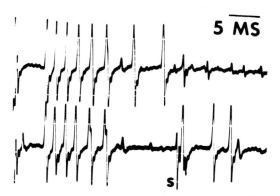

FIG. 1. **Top** trace is an antidromically evoked LFI burst from a pyramidal tract neuron recorded from precentral focus of monkey. **Bottom** trace is two antidromically evoked LFI bursts in response to paired stimuli spaced 28 msec apart. Note that the duration of the second burst is considerably less than the preceding burst, a finding consistently seen with such burst firing units.

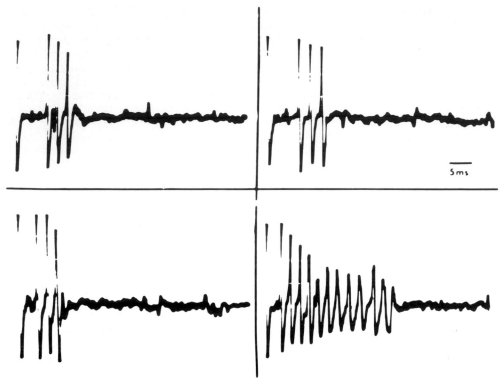

FIG. 2.   Four examples of LFI bursts recorded from human cortex. Note that these burst samples are virtually identical to what has been recorded from alumina foci of monkey.

better quantify differences between normal and abnormal neuronal firing patterns, a method for controlling the monkeys level of attention was sought. In 1969, Fetz (8) developed a paradigm by which monkeys could be operantly conditioned to control the firing rates of single neurons recorded within precentral cortex. By applying Fetz's techniques to chronic epileptic monkeys, two advantages over previous recordings were gained: (a) the monkeys' behavioral state could be controlled for specified periods of time thus allowing a comparison of firing behavior at different levels of consciousness; and (b) the neurons to be studied could be manipulated physiologically through their own synaptic pathways thereby providing observations of neuronal firing during various synaptic biases. However, to better understand the data generated in this way, it is necessary to know just how it is that monkeys can alter the firing of cortical neurons during the process of operant conditioning. From a large series of experiments (41,42), it was determined that monkeys operantly control precentral neurons by making peripheral movements that alter afferent activity

fed back to the cortical neurons. Indirect evidence suggests that the majority of afferent activity is from muscle spindles.

In 1973, Fetz and Wyler (9) operantly conditioned an epileptic monkey to control the firing rates of several single pyramidal-tract neurons (PTN) that fired in the LFI burst mode. Using their operant conditioning techniques, they were able to show that such neurons could be manipulated by the monkey in the following ways. (a) The firing rates could be increased, and this was accomplished by shortening the interval between bursts (Fig. 3). (b) However, the firing rates could not be significantly inhibited because the bursts appeared to recur in a modestly rhythmic pattern even though single APs between bursts would be suppressed. (c) To a small degree the interval between bursts could be decreased transiently for periods of 200 to 300 msec, but this was not consistent enough to lower the firing rates significantly and (d) in a few cases, the monkeys could be reinforced to preferentially increase the incidence of single APs so that bursts occurred less frequently (Fig. 3).

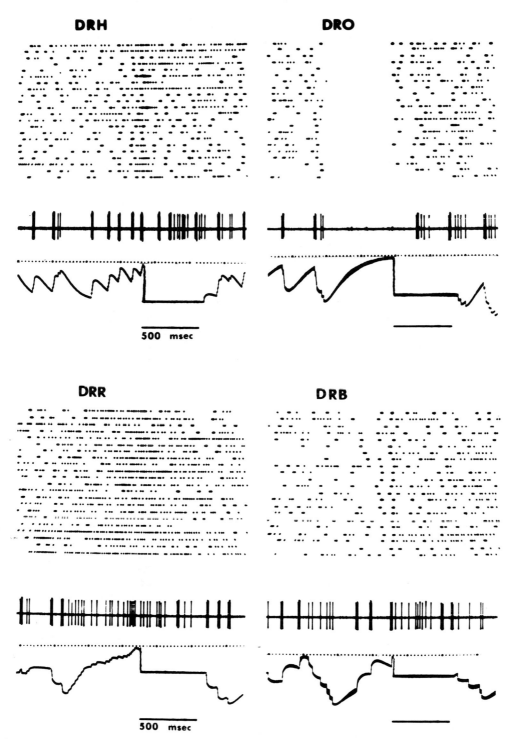

FIG. 3. Dot rasters and samples of unit activity during four different operant schedules centered around the point at which the neuron met reinforcement criteria (**bottom** trace for each shows the analog output of the voltage integrator, with the *dotted line* representing threshold for reinforcement). DRH reinforced the monkey to produce higher rates of firing, DRO reinforced for low firing rates, DRR reinforced for regular (i.e., nonburst) firing, and DRB reinforced for burst firing. The unit was a pyramidal-tract neuron firing LFI bursts.

Those experiments provided three important results. The neurons were identified (by antidromic latencies) as "fast" PTNs, thereby providing a morphologic correlate (i.e., pyramidal shaped neurons within the deeper layers of cortex) to the physiological data. It provided evidence that the burst generating mechanism could be synaptically triggered, and it provided a strong inference that these "epileptic" neurons were not totally deafferented.

Although the LFI burst pattern is distinctive, it is not characteristic of most neurons within an epileptic focus and is often not found in many alumina foci. Therefore, a more quantitative method was needed by which single neurons from these foci could be objectively identified. From early studies of normal precentral neurons, Evarts (7) had found that during wakefulness, most PTNs had modal ISIs between 30 and 60 msec. In contrast, ISIs within the high-frequency bursts that characterize epileptic activity are usually less than 5 msec and commonly about 2 msec (Fig. 4). Therefore, a measure termed the burst index (BI) was devised for the purpose of discriminating abnormal from normal firing patterns within precentral cortex, and this was defined as the percentage of ISIs less than 5 msec to all ISIs per 15 sec epocs. After each 5 min of recording, the mean and standard deviation of the BI was computed. After applying this measure to a large sample of neurons within alumina-induced foci, a classification of abnormalities could be defined based on the magnitude and variability of the neurons' BI during periods in which monkeys were awake but not active. Normal neurons have a mean BI less than 10. Epileptic neurons have BIs greater than 10 and are divided into two classes. Group 2 epileptic neurons have very labile BIs that are usually greater than 10 and have a variability of greater than ±10. Group 1 epileptic neurons have mean BIs greater than 10, but have a variability less than ±10. In addition, group 1 epileptic pyramidal-tract neurons will often respond to an antidromically evoked (juxtathreshold) action potential (AP) with a burst that is structurally identical to those which occur spontaneously. Both groups of epileptic neurons are found to reside in cortex that surrounds the alumina granuloma (Fig. 5). Because the BI (burst firing) of group 1 epileptic neurons is so invariant during different behavioral states and during operant conditioning, it has been proposed that these units be viewed as "pacemakers" of the epileptogenic focus. The validity of the BI as an objective measure of abnormal unit firing in chronic precentral foci was subsequently confirmed by Schmidt et al. (30).

The classification of epileptic neurons into two groups was based primarily on the observations that some neurons (the group 2 epileptic neurons) decreased their burst firing when the monkey was placed on an operant schedule whereas the group 1 epileptic neurons did not change their burst firing significantly under similar shifts in the monkeys' behavioral state. This observation could be more precisely quantified through the use of the burst index. In many cases, group 2 neurons fired with modestly high BIs during nonoperant periods, in which the monkeys would often become drowsy or inattentive. When monkeys were placed on an operant schedule, many of these same neurons decreased burst firing and their BIs approached normal values. The electroencephalographic (EEG) correlate to this observation was that during operant periods, the background rhythms became more desynchronized and the voltage decreased in amplitude. In addition, during operant periods, many monkeys had fewer epileptiform spikes in the EEG than during nonoperant periods. These EEG observations are not too dissimilar to what is observed in some human epileptics who have frontal foci. Thus, it was felt that a more in-depth investigation of the neuronal firing changes that occur during these behavioral states would lend insight into the dynamics of focal epilepsy.

To maximize the information that operant conditioning studies might yield, a more quantitative paradigm was needed than originally designed by Fetz. Fetz' paradigm required monkeys to increase and decrease neuronal firing rates from baseline values. To better quantify operant control, the task was changed to require monkeys to alter the neurons' firing pattern rather than firing rate. This was done by reinforcing the monkey to generate sequential ISIs that were within a specific range. This resulted not only in altering firing rate (since it is a function of ISIs) but also in changing firing pattern from phasic to tonic. Because Evarts had shown many precentral neurons to have modal ISIs near 45 msec, a 30- to 60-msec ISI range was chosen. As a consequence, the data analysis was directed toward the distribution of ISIs rather than firing rates.

OPERANT CONTROL OF NORMAL AND EPILEPTIC NEURONS

Normal Neurons

Normal precentral neurons from nonepileptic monkeys were studied first to obtain control data. When given the task to fire neurons toni-

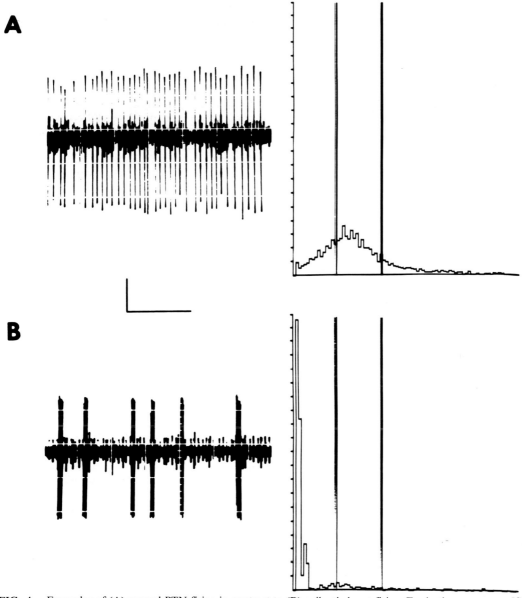

FIG. 4. Examples of **(A)** normal PTN firing in contrast to **(B)** epileptic burst firing. For both neurons, an ISI histogram is to their right with the cursors at 30 and 60 msec. At the slow sweep speed the individual APs comprising the bursts in **B** can not be resolved. Calibration bars are 100 μV and 200 msec. (From ref. 45, with permission.)

cally with ISIs between 30 and 60 msec, monkeys can do so for over 80% of neurons (47). During the preconditioning period, it is common for the modal ISI of the unit to be near the 30- to 60-msec range (Fig. 6A), and if the monkey gains control of the neuron, the ISI histograms show an increase of ISIs within or just adjacent to the 30- to 60-msec target range. In the majority of cases, as the monkey is placed on the first operant period, the modal ISI shortens to-

wards the 30-msec boundary. As the monkey gains further control over the neuron, the modal ISI remains fixed and only the ISI histogram's distribution decreases its variance, so that it becomes more gaussian around the modal ISI. In effect, this means that the numbers of longer ISIs decrease as the numbers of 30- to 60-msec ISIs increase, and this in turn will result in an increase in the unit's firing rate.

However, it became apparent that the modal

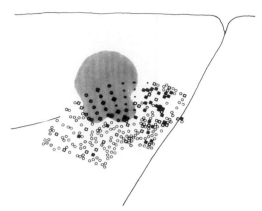

FIG. 5. Two hundred thirty-eight PTN and non-PTNs unequivocally isolated from 142 radially oriented electrode penetrations within the epileptogenic left precentral cortex of one monkey. The alumina injection granuloma is indicated by the *shaded area.* Neurons are classified as normal (*open circles*), group 2 (*open rectangles*), or group 1 (*solid rectangles*). Note the relative focality of group 1 neurons along the perimeter of the alumina granuloma. (From ref. 45, with permission.)

ISIs were relatively fixed and did not change significantly even if outside of the target range, as shown in Fig. 6. Figure 6A is the ISI histogram of the preconditioning period and shows a modal ISI of 25 msec. Figure 6B is of the second operant period and demonstrates that although there is an increase of ISIs near the 30 msec boundary, the modal ISI is 26 msec. To determine if this propensity for neurons to fire with a modal ISI near 30 msec was a peculiarity of the operant task or a more general property of precentral neurons, the firing of similar neurons was recorded from a nonepileptic monkey during the performance of repetitive movements against a minimum load (45). These neurons also fired with modal ISIs near 30 msec (Fig. 7). The data indicate that when the neurons are driven by a modest proprioceptive bias (such as used in the operant conditioning paradigm), they fire with a modal interval that is "physiologic" for the neuron, and that for the majority the modal ISI across a large group of normal precentral neurons is near 30 msec.

The same results were obtained for normal neurons recorded within chronic epileptogenic foci. It was also noted that normal neurons from chronic foci also had relatively fixed modal ISIs when the monkey was controlling them, as is the case for nonepileptic monkeys. Moreover, in subsequent work it was found that the modal ISI was relatively refractory to being operantly controlled by the monkey. Figure 6, C through I, illustrates that point. Initially, the monkey was

conditioned to fire the neuron within a 30- to 60-msec range, but in subsequent periods the range was moved first to 40 to 70 msec and then to 45 to 75 msec. The modal ISI moved only from 26 to 28 msec. The ISI target range was then lowered to 0 to 20 msec, but the neuron's ISI distribution remained fairly gaussian and very short ISIs were not generated.

The above data allow several conclusions to be made. First, it appears that a neuron's discharge pattern (under the conditions of this paradigm) is synaptically initiated but is centered around a modal ISI, which appears physiologic for that neuron. The physiologic output of the neuron is relatively fixed and not easily manipulated by the monkey. Finally, monkeys cannot be reinforced to generate the very short ISIs that characterize epileptic neurons; i.e., they cannot generate significant BIs through normal synaptic drive.

The accuracy with which monkeys could control precentral PTNs was compared among three groups of neurons (41,43): (a) from nonepileptic monkeys, (b) from cortex contralateral to a chronic focus, and (c) from normal PTNs within a chronic focus. The accuracy of control among these three groups was not significantly different, meaning that epileptic monkeys can control normal precentral PTNs as well as nonepileptic monkeys. However, the length of time the monkeys needed to gain control over the PTNs recorded within the focus was significantly longer than what was needed to control analogous PTNs contralateral to the focus.

Because the data analysis had been directed at studying the ISI distribution of neurons, a subtle abnormal pattern began to emerge. Many of the neurons recorded within the epileptic focus but considered normal by the BI criteria had decidedly abnormal ISI distributions, in that their modal ISI were between 5 and 18 msec (Fig. 8) (21,46). As is the case with other precentral neurons, these units can not be made to shift significantly their modal ISI. From evaluation of the actual spike trains, it was apparent that these neurons were firing repetitive doublets, and the ISIs of the doublets were between 5 and 18 msec. This firing pattern is not commonly recorded from precentral cortex of nonepileptic monkeys and therefore is considered abnormal, but not clearly epileptic because of the absence of obvious burst firing.

Group 1 Epileptic Neurons

As was the case with normal neurons, the monkeys can bring the majority of these neurons under operant control. However, there are some

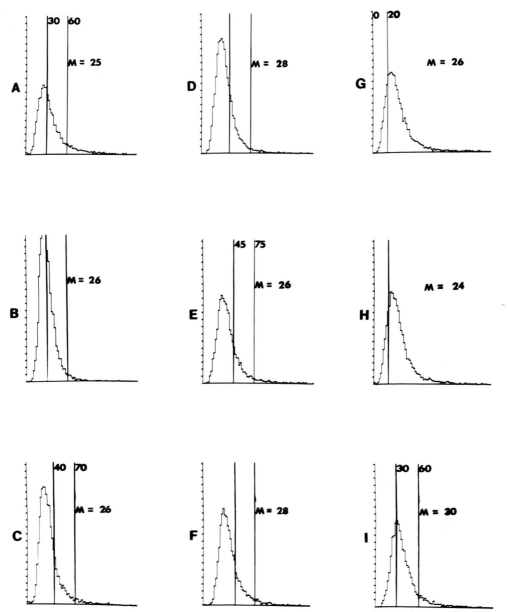

FIG. 6. A series of ISI histograms from 5-min periods during one experiment. All histograms are constructed from all ISIs between 1 and 150 msec during each 5-min period. **A:** Preconditioning period. All other histograms are from sequential operant periods. Shifts in the target ISI range are given at the top of the cursors and the units' modal ISI is to the right of the cursors. Bin width is 2 msec.

very major differences between the two types of neurons as well as some similarities. The most striking difference is that when the monkey attempts to gain operant control of these neurons, only the interval between bursts changes, and the net result is that the interburst interval (not the interspike interval) moves towards the 30- to 60-msec target range. Thus, only if the bursts themselves are equated to single APs of normal neurons are the two groups similar. In other words, the burst response of the neuron appears to be a unitary event that is synaptically initiated. The similarity between normal and group 1 epileptic neurons is that both increase the occurrence of the neurons' modal ISI when operantly controlled. Whereas a modal ISI near 30 msec is "physiologic" for normal neurons, a modal ISI near 2 msec is normal for epileptic

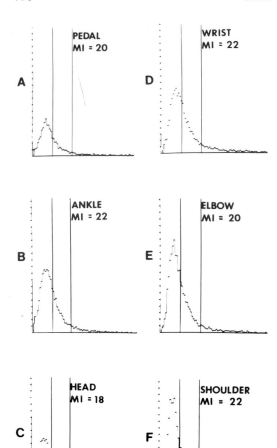

FIG. 7. ISI histograms from a precentral neuron during a monkey's participation in several different tasks that required repetitive movements at several different areas under minimal load. For example, pedal was a task similar to a bicycle. Note that although this unit is most strongly activated by contralateral shoulder and elbow movements, the unit's modal ISI does not change significantly between tasks. For comparison to previous histograms, the cursors are set at 30 and 60 msec.

lets that have very short ISIs. This is presumed to be due to a combination of factors that include the synchronization of synaptic activity, in addition to a mild depolarization of the soma because of less tonic inhibition. During sleep, the bursts from group 1 epileptic neurons may become more intense in that more APs per burst occur (49).

Group 2 Epileptic Neurons

The firing pattern of group 2 neurons during operant conditioning is more complex than seen in the previous two groups. However, one facet of their firing behavior remains similar within all three groups: if monkeys are reinforced to fire these neurons within a 30- to 60-msec ISI range, the neurons' physiological modal ISI predominates. Unlike normal neurons, which fire a modal ISI near 30 msec, or group 1 epileptic neurons, which fire modal ISIs near 2 msec, group 2 epileptic neurons have modal ISIs between 6 and 18 msec. What makes the firing behavior of these units more complex than the others is the shifts in ISIs that occur during nonoperant periods. As noted earlier, initial distinction between group 1 and group 2 neurons was based on the fact that the latter had a more variable BI, especially during nonoperant periods. Many group 2 neurons will have BIs within the range of normal during the monkey's participation in an operant task, but the BI will become abnormal when the monkey is on a nonoperant period. For other group 2 neurons, the BI will never become normal but will drop significantly during operant conditioning. Further, as was the case for normal and group 1 epileptic neurons, burst firing becomes more intense during slow-wave sleep.

The effect that the monkey's level of consciousness has upon the neurons' burst firing could be due to either a nonspecific (e.g., reticular thalamic projections) or direct afferent activity used in mediating the operant response. To sort out these two possibilities, experiments were conducted with epileptic monkeys with bilateral recording mounts. Neurons were recorded simultaneously from the focus and the contralateral, homotopic cortex. For the first five operant periods the monkey was reinforced to control one of the two neurons; then for the next five operant periods the contingencies were reversed and the monkey was reinforced to control the opposite unit (Fig. 8). Thus, the neurons' firing behavior could be observed as the monkey was alert and participating in the operant task but under two conditions: with and without di-

neurons. Further, even though the monkeys can be successfully reinforced to increase 30- to 60-msec ISIs from these units, they are only decreasing the interval between bursts, and hence the BI does not decrease.

Another parallel between normal and epileptic neurons (both group 1 and group 2) can be seen during the transition between wakefulness and sleep (39,49). During slow-wave sleep events such as spindles, there is a tendency for normal neurons to fire in doublets and occasional trip-

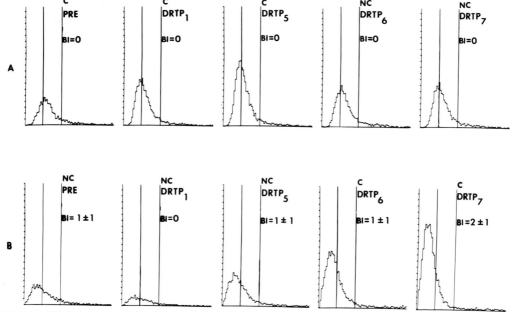

FIG. 8. ISI histograms of 5-min periods in which normal neurons were recorded simultaneously from precentral cortex contralateral **(upper row)** to and from within an epileptogenic focus **(lower row)**. PRE, preconditioning period; DRTP, operant periods and the subscript note the number of the period; C, denotes which neuron was the one the monkey was reinforced to control; NC, the noncontingent neuron. Histogram cursors mark 30 and 60 msec.

rected afferent drive to the neuron. For most normal neurons, the mean modal ISI shortened as it became the neuron the monkey was reinforced to control: the modal ISI dropped from a mean of 38 when noncontingent to near 30 when contingent. If the same units' activity was compared to nonoperant periods, the ISI histogram had less variance during operant periods. Thus two effects were noted. First, simply attending to the operant task decreased the variance of the ISI histogram. Second, if the neuron was being operantly controlled, the modal ISI shortened towards 30 msec and the ISI histogram variance decreased further. The first effect correlates primarily with the nonspecific effect of "alerting," and the second effect appears due to increasing afferent drive to the neurons.

When one of the two neurons is an epileptic unit, the results are very similar except that epileptic neurons always generate shorter ISIs than normal neurons. The changes in variance and modal ISI are not noticeable for the group 1 neurons (Fig. 9), but the interval between bursts becomes shorter during alerting only, and shorter yet during attempts to operantly control the neurons. For group 2 neurons, the very short (2–5 msec) ISIs decrease with alerting alone and the modal ISI shifts towards the range of 6 to 18 msec (Fig. 10). With attempts by the monkey to

control the unit, the modal ISI becomes shorter. The interesting point is that the group 2 neurons can have their burst firing significantly modified by the nonspecific effects of alerting whereas the group 1 neurons are relative refractory to this same effect.

INTERACTIONS BETWEEN NEURONS

In many experiments, two neurons were recorded simultaneously through the same electrode with their APs well enough isolated that their firing behaviors could be compared. Most commonly, the neuron pairs have consisted of two normal neurons or a group 2 and normal neuron. However, on a few occasions, a group 1 and group 2 unit have been recorded simultaneously. It is of interest that in no case have two group 1 epileptic neurons been recorded simultaneously. If the firing of neuron pairs is analyzed using a cross correlation histogram, it is common to find that pairs of normal neurons will fire within one msec of each other. This has been previously described by Allum et al. (1) from studies of precentral PTNs recorded from nonepileptic monkeys. This relationship has been interpreted as indicating a commonality of synaptic projections to the two neurons. Because the neurons are recorded from the same elec-

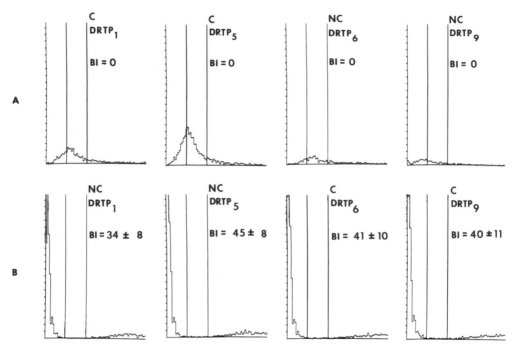

FIG. 9.   ISI histograms of 5-min periods in which a normal neuron (**upper row**) was recorded from right precentral cortex, and a group 2 neuron was recorded from left (**lower row**) precentral cortex. DRTP, operant period. NC means the neuron was not the one the monkey was reinforced to control, whereas C means it was the neuron the monkey was reinforced to control.

trode, it can be presumed they are likely to reside in the same cortical column. This presumed commonality of synaptic input has also been observed between a group 1 epileptic and normal neuron (Fig. 11). What is of interest is that neurons with such decidedly different firing patterns can be recorded from what is presumed to be the same cortical column. That also suggests that the burst firing of the group 1 epileptic neuron is not due primarily to hypersynchronous synaptic input, since the normal neuron fires normally. Moreover, it suggests that during the interictal periods whatever process that results in burst firing from the group 1 neuron is likely to be intrinsic, rather than a generalized process that should affect surrounding neurons (for example, the more generalized response of neurons to the application of penicillin).

THE RELATIONSHIP BETWEEN EPILEPTIC NEURONS AND SEIZURES

Although burst-firing neurons have always been thought to represent the single cell hallmark of epileptogenic cortex, this assumption has always been empirical. For example, one can record neurons from normal cortex, then apply penicillin to that cortex, and the neurons will begin to fire bursts and EEG seizures will develop. However, a more direct correlation between abnormal burst firing and the occurrence of spontaneous seizures was not described until recently. Wyler et al. (46) recorded 1,600 neurons from 13 monkeys. Since each monkey had been monitored by polygraph and videotape and all seizures had been recorded, a correlation could be tested between the monkeys' daily seizure frequencies and the numbers of epileptic neurons recorded from their respective foci. To normalize the sampling differences between subjects, the ratio of group 1 neurons to the sum of group 1 plus group 2 neurons was used as a measure of the single-neuron epileptogenicity of each focus. This ratio was then plotted against the mean number of seizures per day for each monkey. The result was a highly significant logarithmic correlation of 0.95. Since then, additional data from five other epileptic monkeys have been added to this correlation and the correlation coefficient has not changed (Fig. 12). These data imply a direct relationship between the number of group 1 epileptic (pacemaker) neurons in a focus and the epileptogenicity of the focus.

Because of the similarities between the

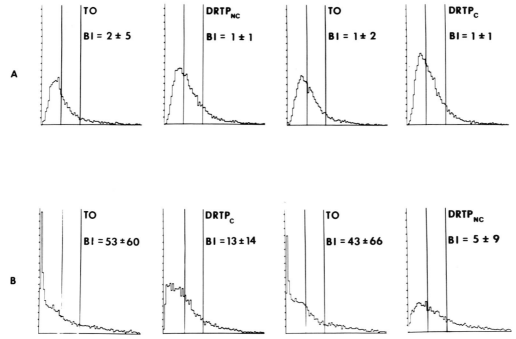

FIG. 10. As in the previous two illustrations, this is from an experiment in which a normal and a group 1 epileptic neuron were recorded simultaneously. TO = time out or nonoperant period. C denotes which neuron the monkey was reinforced to control, and NC is the neuron that was noncontingent. Other abbreviations are as given in Fig. 9.

monkey model and human focal epilepsy, these findings also help explain many of the perplexing results of epilepsy surgery. For example, often patients who have undergone such surgery have a significant reduction in the number of their clinical seizures, yet are not seizure-free. It could be hypothesized that the surgery removed only enough group 1 neurons so that the seizures were markedly reduced but not eliminated. Because the relationship between epileptic neurons and seizures is logarithmic rather than linear, it would take only a relatively small reduction of group 1 neurons to produce a marked reduction of seizures. Most of all, this relationship confirms that burst firing neurons are intimately associated with the phenomenon of spontaneous seizures.

CORRELATIONS BETWEEN NEURONAL AND EEG SPIKES

The relationship between unit firing and EEG epileptiform spikes has not been studied as extensively in the human and the chronic monkey model as it has in acute preparations such as the penicillin model. Prince and Futamachi (24) studied the relationship in anesthetized monkey and found a loose correlation between EEG

spiking and burst firing. In another series of recordings from awake behaving monkeys, Wyler and Burchiel (41) found no consistent relationship between EEG spikes and neuronal firing when both were recorded through a tungsten microelectrode. These findings relate only to the activity of an interictal focus.

Wyler (40) has studied a series of 44 neurons from awake monkeys before, during, and after spontaneous seizures. During the interictal periods there was little relationship between EEG spikes and unit firing. However, during the earlier parts of a focal seizure the two events became time-locked and more pronounced as the seizure progressed into the clonic phase (Fig. 13). During the seizure, unit burst firing became synchronous with surrounding neurons and with the spike portion of the EEG. Unit silence would most often accompany the slow wave portion of the spike and wave complex. Thus, the two events (burst firing from either normal or epileptic neurons and EEG spikes) became synchronous only during ictal events. These ictal data may help explain some of the differences between chronic alumina and acute penicillin foci. The relationship between spikes and unit firing is much tighter in penicillin foci than in alumina foci. However, the penicillin focus is

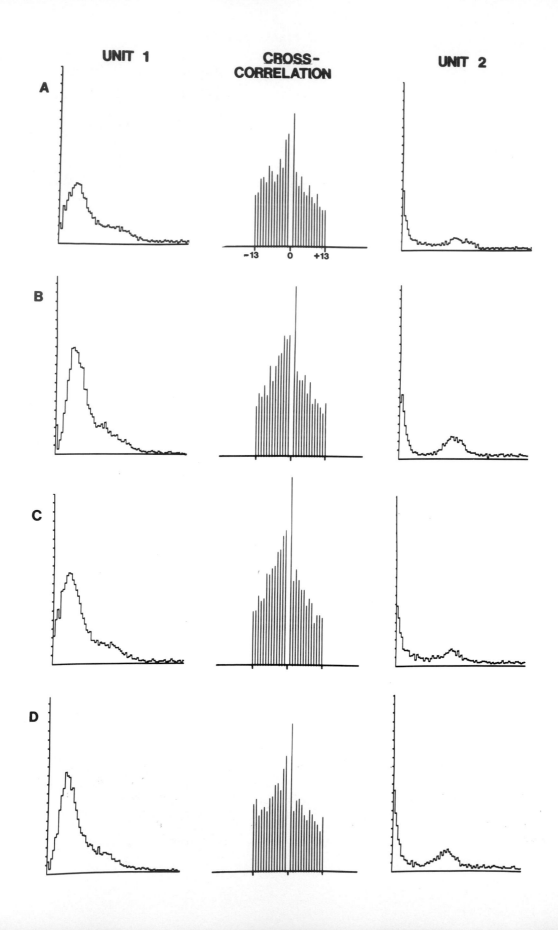

UNIT 1   CROSS-CORRELATION   UNIT 2

A

B

C

D

−13   0   +13

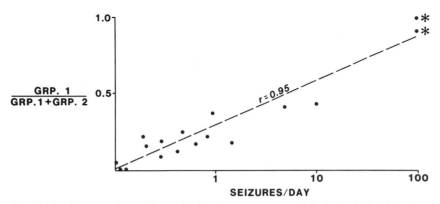

FIG. 12. Correlation between the numbers of epileptic neurons recorded within foci of 17 epileptic monkeys and the number of spontaneous daily seizures those monkeys had documented. The asterisk denotes two monkeys that had epilepsia partialis continuua.

more like an ictal focus than an interictal focus, and thus a stronger relationship between unit firing and EEG spikes would be expected from that model.

During the onset of seizures, not every neuron began firing synchronously with field potential spikes. Normal neurons had one of three responses: (a) they would begin to fire synchronously with background multiunit activity but continued to fire single APs or an occasional doublet, but not full bursts; (b) a few normal neurons synchronized with background activity and fired unstructured bursts; (c) for some neurons outside the focus, the spontaneous activity would stop abruptly and remain silent until the seizure began to spread clinically, at which time the unit would begin to fire in synchrony with the EEG spikes. At the termination of the seizure, all unit activity would cease. During this period of electrical silence the monkeys would often display a focal paralysis. At the same time as the paralysis was present, PTNs could still be invaded by an antidromic AP. This last finding is of considerable interest, since it may suggest that the clinical postictal paralysis may not be due entirely to a depolarization of cortical neurons.

The response of epileptic units was similar, and group 2 neurons increased their BI in the seconds before the seizure became evident clinically and their bursts became synchronous with background activity. However, the bursts of the group 1 neurons did not change significantly in the moments immediately preceding the seizure. Both group 1 and group 2 neurons were also silent at the termination of the seizure and for several seconds thereafter. When both groups of neurons resumed firing, it was noted that initial firing was always single APs and not bursts. This "normal" firing continued for several seconds before burst firing resumed. It is of additional interest that during the postictal period, group 1 PTNs responded to antidromic invasion with a single AP, whereas preictally they had responded with a burst. Schmidt et al. (30) had previously noted that burst firing neurons resumed firing with normal patterns immediately after an ictal event.

The general lack of correlation between EEG spikes and unit firing in this model is similar to what has been recorded in human epileptics' brain. In a recent study (50), a total of 90 neurons were recorded from 17 awake patients during the course of surgery. Although 40 neurons fired APs in some relation to electrocorticograph (ECoG) spikes, the relationships were variable between units and often for the same unit (Fig. 14). For many units, APs were more consistently related to one phase of the local field potential recorded through the microelectrode than to the ECoG recorded from the overlying surface. As with the data from monkeys, synchronous firing between single units recorded simultaneously by the same microelectrode was rarely seen except at the onset of an ictal event.

FIG. 11. ISI and cross-correlation histograms from an experiment in which a normal and an epileptic neuron were recorded simultaneously through the same extracellular microelectrode. The cross-correlation histogram looks for APs of unit 2 that occur within ±13 msec of the firing of unit 1. The scales on the two type of histograms are not similar.

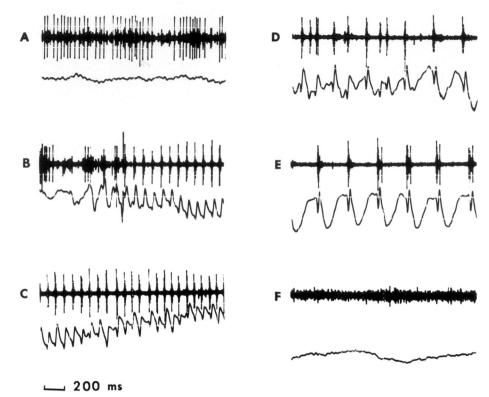

FIG. 13. Traces of unit activity (band pass 300 hz- 10 khz) and EEG (A) before, (B) at the start of a seizure, (C–E) during the seizure, and (F) during the postictal period. Note that during the seizure, there is a good correlation between the onset of spikes in the EEG and the synchronous firing of multiunit activity.

SUMMARY OF THE INTERICTAL FOCUS

From the preceding sections it is clear that the neuronal composition of the average interictal alumina-induced epileptogenic focus is not binary—e.g., normal and epileptic neurons. Rather, it is a complex admixture of neurons that span a continuum of abnormalities that ends with the group 1 pacemaker epileptic neurons. The spectrum begins with neurons that are normal as judged by (a) the distribution of their ISIs, (b) their modal ISI when under operant control, and (c) the degree to which they can be operantly controlled. These neurons do not differ from normal neurons recorded from similar regions of nonepileptic monkeys. The gradation into abnormality begins very subtly and is demonstrable only in the neurons' ISI distribution: the modal ISI is between 5 and 18 msec, and the distribution is obviously skewed toward shorter intervals. That this group of neurons is abnormal is purely based on statistical inference in that their presence is more obvious in epileptogenic cortex than in normal cortex. The next gradation along the spectrum are the group 2 epileptic neurons: neurons that have a pro-

pensity to burst fire when the monkeys are inattentive and not participating in an operant task. The distinction between these group 2 neurons and the group 1 epileptic neurons is purely arbitrary and was based on the variability of the neurons' BI. The group 1 neurons are the most obviously abnormal, because they tend to fire bursts regardless of the monkey's behavioral state or level of attention. One hypothesis to account for the differences in firing behavior between these groups of neurons is that their $F–I$ curves (the firing frequency the neuron generates to a given amount of current injected into it) are different and more steep than normal neurons. The further along the spectrum towards group 1 a neuron is, the steeper the neuron's $F–I$ curve.

Data indicate that the average active focus of monkey contains approximately 10% (or less) group 1 epileptic neurons, 40% group 2, and 50% nonepileptic neurons (38). However, these percentages are variable from focus to focus, with the highest percentage of group 1 epileptic neurons recorded from monkeys with epilepsia partialis continua. That group 1 epileptic neurons are closely associated with the phenomenon of

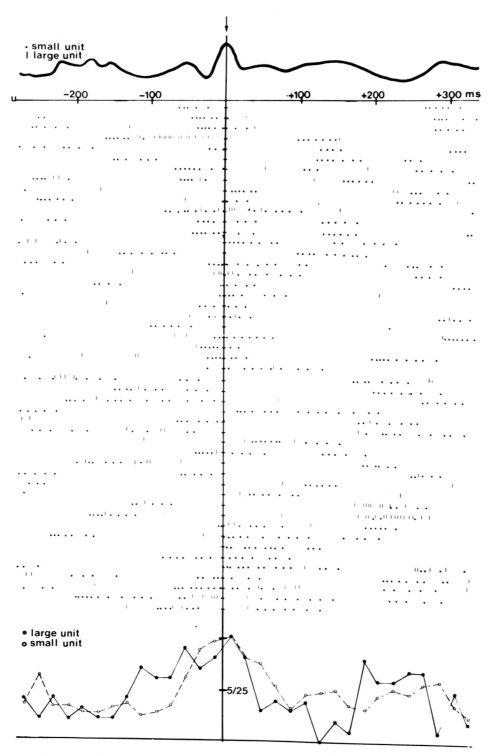

FIG. 14. Dot raster of two simultaneously recorded neurons recorded from human cortex and their relationship to the surface EEG spike **(upper trace).** At the bottom is an incidence histogram, showing the relative occurrence of both units from 300 msec before to 300 msec after the surface spike. (From ref. 49, with permission.)

spontaneous seizures was dramatically illustrated by the surprisingly high correlation between their presence in foci and the number of siezures the foci generate. Moreover, from the limited observations of neuronal firing during the transition between interictal to ictal foci, it appears that unit activity synchronizes to the group 1 neurons before the onset of the clinical seizure. The multiunit activity then becomes tightly associated with EEG spikes as the seizure begins. Thus, the group 1 neurons are viewed as pacemakers to the focus and the group 2 neurons are thought to provide a "critical mass" of neurons that, when synchronized to the burst firing of the pacemakers, is capable of initiating an ictal event.

The fact that the neurons within chronic foci really define a gradation of abnormalities is also compatible with the theory that epileptic neurons are abnormal because they have lost normal regulatory mechanisms that, if present, would not allow burst firing (31). The observation that group 2 neurons can have their burst firing influenced so strongly by level of arousal would also imply that the inhibiting mechanism is to a large degree synaptically mediated. Perhaps the only difference between group 1 and group 2 neurons is the degree of this synaptic loss. This would be compatible with the histologic observation that many of the neurons within chronic foci have lost synaptic spines, yet would still be compatible with the fact that even the group 1 epileptic neurons can, to some degree, be operantly controlled by the monkeys. These observations can also be compatible with the finding that GABA is decreased in the focus.

ABSENCE OF AN "INHIBITORY SURROUND"

If a small cotton pledget is soaked in penicillin and then applied to the surface of cortex, an intense epileptogenic focus is produced. If one then records the activity of neurons in the immediately surrounding area, one can find many units that are inhibited during active ECoG spiking within the focus. This inhibition of neural activities peripheral to the focus has been termed the "inhibitory surround" (37). The role this phenomenon may play in modulating ictal events has been speculative. However, a similar type of surround has not been found adjacent to alumina foci. The most convincing data again come from single-unit operant conditioning experiments. If neurons are recorded in the regions near an active, spike-producing focus, monkeys can be reinforced successfully to fire those neu-

rons tonically with no apparent inhibition. The accuracy with which these neurons can be controlled is not significantly different from that of normal neurons within nonepileptic cortex.

This lack of a "surround inhibition" in interictal alumina foci when compared to penicillin foci may be a function of several differences between the two models. First, the surround inhibition was originally recorded from cortex of paralyzed, anesthetized cats, and under these conditions cortical activity may be considerably more synchronized than in the awake behaving monkey. Second, the penicillin focus is "hotter" than the interictal alumina focus, meaning that it can generate sequential ictal events whereas the alumina focus may generate only a few seizures per week. Therefore, the penicillin model is more a model of an ictal than in interictal focus. The recordings from human and monkey cortex indicated that as a seizure becomes imminent, neurons within the focus begin to become more synchronized. Thus, it would seem that neurons within a penicillin focus should be more synchronized than neurons within alumina foci. A significant increase in synchronization would have a more profound effect on projected activity that will affect surrounding pools of neurons. This may account for the absence of an inhibitory surround in the alumina focus. Furthermore, the findings from monkey also suggest that the inhibitory surround is unlikely to exist near the interictal focus of humans.

MIRROR FOCUS

Mirror foci are understood to be independent epileptic foci that develop secondarily as a result of persistent transsynaptic activation from chronic, primary foci (23). This is in distinction to areas of cortex that demonstrate "projected" epileptiform EEG spikes. When fully evolved, these mirror foci are thought to be capable of continued epileptic activity if the primary focus has been removed. If this is the case, then it would be expected that the mirror focus should contain neurons that exhibit the same characteristics ascribed to epileptic neurons recorded from primary foci: i.e., one should be able to record neurons that fire in bursts and have epileptiform ISI histogram distributions.

Over 300 neurons have been studied from precentral cortex contralateral to chronic foci in six monkeys, and all neurons were the subject of operant conditioning experiments and recorded for periods in excess of 30 min each (43). In all cases, the neurons were recorded from cortex that demonstrated spontaneous epileptiform spikes (Fig. 15). In no case did the neurons demonstrate BIs characteristic of epileptic neurons, nor were their ISI histograms abnormal. Although many PTNs fired in synchrony with EEG spikes during periods when the monkeys were inattentive, as soon as they were placed on an operant schedule to control neurons either contralateral or ipsilateral to the chronic focus, the neurons became dissociated from the spikes. As stated in an earlier section, these neurons were operantly controlled to the same degree of accuracy as comparable neurons recorded from nonepileptic monkeys. Thus, evidence for single-unit epileptic activity was not seen in cortex contralateral to chronic epileptogenic foci. If "mirror foci" are understood to be secondarily independent epileptic foci that have developed as a result of persistent transsynaptic activation from chronic, primary foci, then on a single-neuron level, evidence of a truly independent mirror focus in monkey precentral cortex is lacking. These data are compatible with those of Harris and Lockard (13), who showed that when the primary focus is removed surgically, spiking from contralateral cortex ceases. Thus, if one is to demonstrate convincingly that a true mirror focus has developed, then is must be shown that after removal of the initial focus, seizures that originate from the contralateral focus persist. Much of the support for the mirror focus concept is derived from EEG data only and has not involved either single-neuron recordings nor seizure monitoring. Just because two areas of cortex show nonsynchronous EEG spiking does not provide compelling evidence that a mirror focus exists.

The inability to provide single neuronal data to support the concept of mirror foci in monkey may be explained by the following possibilities. First, the most conclusive reports supporting the existence of mirror foci have utilized animals with lissencephalic cortex. Second, the data have been based primarily on the persistence of EEG spiking rather than continued spontaneous seizures after the removal of the primary focus. The implication of the concept of mirror foci to humans is that a chronic focus, for example, in one temporal lobe will over time generate a second focus in the contralateral temporal lobe. However, this does not seem to be the case, because neurosurgeons have been removing temporal lobe foci that have been present for years without seizures arising from the other lobe. It is true that some epileptics have bilateral temporal foci; however, these patients usually have bilateral structural damage. Thus, the overwhelming evidence is that the phenomenon of mirror foci is not present within the primate cortex.

STUDIES OF NEURONS IN HUMAN BRAIN

Neurosurgeons have used the opportunity that the surgery for epilepsy offers to study the behavior of neurons within the human brain. Most often this has been during craniotomies (6,14,16,27,34) but Babb et al. (2,3) have also implanted fine wire electrodes for prolonged recordings during the course of the patients' evaluation with depth electrodes. Most recently, Prince and Wong (26) and Schwartzkroin et al. (32) have used the *in vitro* slice preparation to study human neurons with intracellular recordings.

The results from human recording are confusing and have not yet yielded a great deal of insight toward understanding the basic mechanisms of the epilepsies. The reasons are many. First, the conditions under which most recordings were made were variable and often effected by various anticonvulsant and other drugs. Second, although there are now highly accurate criteria for defining what constitutes normal and "epileptic" activity from precentral cortex of monkey, such standardization of firing patterns from human cortex is not possible. This is because there has been no systematic quantification of the ISI distribution of normal neurons from nonepileptic human cortex. Although "normal" neurons recorded from the amygdala and hippocampus of humans have been shown to produce burst firing (34), this has not been recorded for neurons in nonepileptogenic lateral temporal cortex. Third, there is little security at the time of recording that one is studying the actual epileptogenic focus. In many instances, recordings are made from the lateral temporal lobe and the focus is actually within mesial temporal lobe. In addition to the vagueness of not knowing if the lateral or mesial temporal regions harbor the focus, one can not be sure the focus has been removed until sufficient time has passed to say that the patient no longer suffers spontaneous seizures. Finally, the size of epileptogenic foci is ambiguous in most cases.

Because of the problems just mentioned, future studies of human brain must be very carefully designed to yield meaningful data. This also means that the patients' outcome from surgery also needs to be considered before data can be fully interpreted. However, with the advent of newer diagnostic tools, such as the positron emission tomography (PET) and nuclear magnetic resonance (NMR) scanners, more accuracy in defining the location of epileptic foci will be available. This in turn will surely increase our ability to interpret data derived from biopsies of

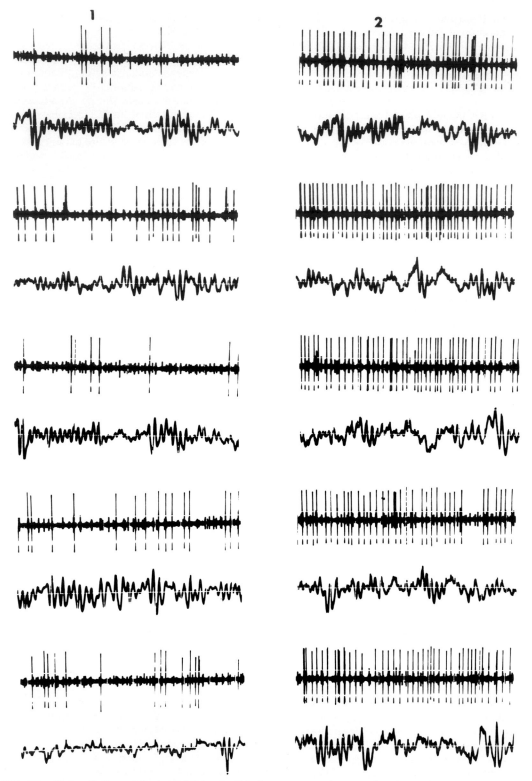

FIG. 15. Unit activity and the local field potentials from precentral cortex directly contralateral to an active chronic epileptogenic focus. Column 1 is activity-sampled during a time-out period, whereas Column 2 is sampled during an operant period. This unit's firing is little affected by the presence of spikes in the local field potential.

human brain and will ultimately increase our understanding of the basic mechanisms of the epilepsies.

CONCLUSION

It is abundantly clear from the rather large body of data that has been generated over recent years that the phenomenon of clinical epilepsy is not the consequence of a pathological alteration in a single, isolated property of the nervous system. A host of alterations in the physiology, morphology, and neurochemistry of brain has been shown to be associated with the epileptic process.

In seizures of focal cortical origin, there is general agreement that the essential feature involves the abnormal discharge of neurons. For that reason, the major thrust of this chapter has been to describe some of the electrophysiological properties of neurons in the epileptic focus. The first problem to be defined is those features which uniquely set the focus apart from the rest of the cortex. As has been pointed out, this is difficult to accomplish in the human. However, the primate model of chronic epilepsy of focal cortical origin does provide such an opportunity. Topical application of convulsant drugs or other activating agents provides similar strategies for the study of other activating aspects of the epileptic process.

In the focus, the next step is the study of those properties that characterize the interictal pathophysiology. In the absence of an interictal focus, propagating seizures do not occur. Thus, the experimental preparation should be one that most closely approximates the human interictal focus. The chronic monkey model appears to satisfy these criteria, while many other experimental models may be more effective surrogates for the ictal phenomena.

It is now clear that, in both monkey and human, the epileptogenic focus is populated by a spectrum of neurons. These range from neurons whose firing patterns are, under all circumstances, normal. There is an intermediate group of neurons whose firing patterns vary and show fluctuating degrees of normal activity. Some of these weakly epileptic neurons may, under most circumstances, be normal, only rarely exhibiting abnormal patterns of firing. Others may, under most circumstances, show varying degrees of normal burst firing and only rarely be captured back into normal patterns of firing. Finally, there are highly epileptic, group 1 or pacemaker neurons that fire almost exclusively in high-frequency bursts. These patterns of burst firing may themselves be subdivided into nonstereotyped and stereotyped bursts. Their activity is not easily modified by changes in behavioral state or operant conditioning. Thus they do appear to serve as pacemakers to the focus. Their essential role is further supported by the observation that the frequency of clinical seizures in monkeys is logarithmically related to the density of pacemaker neurons in the focus. It comes as somewhat of a surprise that the pacemaker neurons are relatively infrequent in the focus of those monkeys having spontaneous seizures at frequencies that approximate those seen in the average clinical setting. The weakly epileptic cells are more numerous, while usually about half the neurons appear to be functionally normal neurons.

The sequence of events during the onset of a seizure is less well understood. It appears that, at certain times, synaptic relationships are such that the burst firing of the pacemaker cells is able to recruit an enlarging number of the weakly epileptic cells into the bursting mode of firing. When this reaches a critical level, the activity of normal neurons is entrained and a regenerative, propagating seizure results that spreads through the brain over normal synaptic pathways.

The details of those factors that set the stage for the transition from the interictal to the ictal state are poorly understood. Some of these factors must be synaptic to account for the relationship between behavioral state (stress, sleep) with the occurrence of seizures in both the monkey and humans. Other factors probably involve local ionic mechanisms and possibly alterations of local microcirculation.

All the elements that are responsible for the maintenance of the interictal focus are also incompletely known. It appears that there are significant alterations of neuronal membranes of cells in the focus, which may be associated with the burst firing. Some of these changes may be structural; others may involve ectopic sites of spike initiation. Abnormalities of the neuronal environment exist, characterized by the intense astroglial gliosis that appears to be a ubiquitous property of chronic epileptic foci. Alterations of extracellular space may have profound consequences on ionic fluxes in association with the high-frequency burst firing. The local synaptic wiring appears to be a major factor. It is well documented in both monkey and human that all regions of cortex are not equally epileptogenic. The sensorimotor cortex is highly epileptogenic in both primate species, as are those cortical regions of the medial temporal lobe. The properties of such cortical areas that bestow such high epileptogenicity upon them are completely unknown. These constitute some of the many challenges for the future.

REFERENCES

1. Allum, J. H. J., Hepp-Reymond, M. C., and Gysin, R. (1982): Cross-correlation analysis of interneuronal connectivity in the motor cortex of the monkey. *Brain Res.*, 231:325–334.
2. Babb, T. L., Carr, E., and Crandall, P. H. (1973): Analysis of extracellular firing patterns of deep temporal lobe structures in man. *EEG Clin. Neurophysiol.*, 34:247–257.
3. Babb, T. L., and Crandall, P. H. (1976): Epileptogenesis of human limbic neurons in psychomotor epileptics. *Electroencephalogr. Clin. Neurophysiol.*, 40:225–243.
4. Brotchi, J. (1978): The activated astrocyte—A histochemical approach to the epileptic focus. In: *Dynamic Properties of Glia Cells*, edited by E. Schoffeniels, G. Frank, D. B. Towers, and L. Hertz, pp. 429–433. Pergamon, Oxford.
5. Calvin, W. H., Sypert, G. W., and Ward, A. A., Jr. (1968): Structured timing patterns within bursts from epileptic neurons on undrugged monkey cortex. *Exp. Neurol.*, 21:535–541.
6. Calvin, W. H., Ojemann, G. A., and Ward, A. A., Jr. (1973): Human cortical neurons in epileptogenic foci: Comparison of interictal firing patterns to those of "epileptic" neurons in animals. *Electroencephalogr. Clin. Neurophysiol.*, 34:337–351.
7. Evarts, E. V. (1964): Temporal patterns of discharge of pyramidal tract neurons during sleep and waking in the monkey. *J. Neurophysiol.*, 27:152–171.
8. Fetz, E. E. (1969): Operant conditioning of cortical unit activity. *Science*, 163:955–958.
9. Fetz, E. E., and Wyler, A. R. (1973): Operantly conditioned firing patterns of epileptic neurons in the monkey motor cortex. *Exp. Neurol.*, 40:586–607.
10. Harris, A. B. (1972): Degeneration in experimental epileptic foci. *Arch. Neurol.*, 26:434–449.
11. Harris, A. B. (1973): Ultrastructure and histochemistry of alumina in cortex. *Exp. Neurol.*, 38:33–63.
12. Harris, A. B. (1975): Cortical neuroglia in experimental epilepsy. *Exp. Neurol.*, 49:691–715.
13. Harris, A. B., and Lockard, J. S. (1981): Absence of seizures or mirror foci in experimental epilepsy after excision of alumina and astrogliotic scar. *Epilepsia*, 22:107–122.
14. Ishijimia, B., Hori, T., Yoshimasu, N., Fukushima, T., et al. (1975): Neuronal activities in human epileptic foci and surrounding areas. *Electroencephalogr. Clin. Neurophysiol.*, 39:643–650.
15. Jasper, A. H. (1972): Application of experimental models to human epilepsy. In: *Experimental Models of Epilepsy*, edited by D. P. Purpura, J. K. Penry, D. Towers, D. M. Woodbury, and R. Walter, pp. 585–602. Raven, New York.
16. Li, C. L., and Van Buren, J. M. (1972): Microelectrode recordings in the brain of man with particular reference to epilepsy and dyskinesia. In: *Neurophysiology Studied in Man*, edited by G. G. Somjen, pp. 49–63. Excerpta Medica, Amsterdam.
17. Lockard, J. S., and Barensten, R. I. (1967): Behavioral experimental epilepsy in monkeys. I. Clinical seizure recording apparatus and initial data. *Electroencephalogr. Clin. Neurophysiol.*, 22:482–486.
18. Lockard, J. S., and Wyler, A. R. (1974): The influence of attending on seizure activity in a monkey model. *Epilepsia*, 20:157–168.
19. Lockard, J. S. (1980): Social primate model of epilepsy. In: *Epilepsy: A Window to Brain Mechanisms*, edited by J. S. Lockard, and A. A. Ward, Jr., pp. 165–190. Raven, New York.
20. Lockard, J. S. (1975): Motor seizure telemetry and initial data in free-roaming monkey model with spontaneous seizures. *Epilepsia*, 16:199–207.
21. Klein, S., and Wyler, A. R. (1980): Operant control of precentral neurons: An inability to produce burst firing from normal cells in chronic epileptogenic foci. *Brain Res.*, 185:419–422.
22. Kopeloff, L. M., Chusid, J. G., and Kopeloff, N. (1942): Recurrent convulsive seizures in animals produced by immunological and chemical means. *Am. J. Psychiatry*, 98:881–902.
23. Morrell, F. (1969): Physiology and histochemistry of the mirror focus. In: *Basic Mechanisms of the Epilepsies*, edited by H. H. Jasper, A. A. Ward, Jr., and A. Pope, pp. 357–376. Little, Brown, Boston.
24. Prince, D. A., and Futamachi, K. J. (1970): Intracellular recordings from chronic epileptogenic foci in the monkey. *Electroencephalogr. Clin. Neurophysiol.*, 29:496–510.
25. Prince, D. A., and Wilder, B. J. (1967): Control mechanisms in cortical epileptogenic foci 'surround inhibition'. *Arch. Neurol.*, 16:194–202.
26. Prince, D. A., and Wong, R. K. S. (1981): Human epileptic neurons studied in vitro. *Brain Res.*, 210:323–333.
27. Rayport, M., and Waller, H. J. (1967): Technique and results of microelectrode recording in human epileptogenic foci. *Electroencephalogr. Clin. Neurophysiol. [Suppl.]*, 25:143–151.
28. Scheibel, M. E., and Scheibel, A. B. (1973): Hippocampal pathology in temporal lobe epilepsy. A Golgi study. In: *Epilepsy: Its Phenomena in Man*, edited by M. A. B. Braizer, pp. 315–335. Academic, New York.
29. Scheibel, M. E., Crandall, P. H., and Scheibel, A. B. (1974): The hippocampaldentate complex in temporal lobe epilepsy. A golgi study. *Epilepsia*, 15:55–80.
30. Schmidt, E. M., Mutsuga, N., and McIntosh, J. S. (1976): Chronic recording of neurons in epileptogenic foci of monkeys during seizures. *Exp. Neurol.*, 52:459–466.
31. Schwartzkroin, P. A., and Wyler, A. R. (1980): Mechanism underlying epileptiform burst discharge. *Ann. Neurol.*, 7:95–107.

32. Schwartzkroin, P. A., Turner, D. A., Knowles, W. D., and Wyler, A. R. (1983): Studies of human and monkey "epileptic" neocortex in the in vitro slice preparation. *Ann. Neurol.*, 13:249–257.

33. Sypert, G. W., and Ward, A. A. Jr. (1967): The hyperexcitable neuron: Microelectrode studies of the chronic epileptic focus in the intact, awake monkey. *Exp. Neurol.*, 19:104–114.

34. Verzeano M., Crandall, P. H., and Dymond A. (1971): Neuronal activity in the amygdala in patients with psychomotor epilepsy. *Neurophychologia*, 9:331–344.

35. Ward, A. A., Jr. (1969): The epileptic neuron: Chronic foci in animals and man. In: *Basic Mechanisms of the Epilepsies*, edited by H. H. Jasper, A. A. Ward, Jr., and A. Pope, pp. 263–288. Little, Brown, Boston.

36. Westrum, L. E., White, L. E., and Ward, A. A., Jr. (1964): Morphology of the experimental epileptic focus. *J. Neurosurg.*, 21:1033–1046.

37. Wilder, B. J. (1972): Projection phenomena and secondary epileptogenesis mirror foci. In: *Experimental Models of Epilepsy*, edited by D. P. Purpura, J. K. Penry, D. Tower, D. M. Woodbury, and R. Walter, pp. 85–109. Raven Press, New York.

38. Wyler, A. R., and Fetz, E. E. (1974): Behavioral control of firing patterns of normal and abnormal neurons in chronic epileptic cortex. *Exp. Neurol.*, 42:448–464.

39. Wyler, A. R., Fetz, E. E., and Ward, A. A., Jr. (1973): Spontaneous firing patterns of epileptic neurons in the monkey motor cortex. *Exp. Neurol.*, 40:567–585.

40. Wyler, A. R. (1982): Neuronal activity during seizures in monkeys. *Exp. Neurol.*, 76:574–585.

41. Wyler, A. R., and Burchiel, K. J. (1981): Operant control of epileptic neurons in chronic foci of monkeys. *Brain Res.*, 212:309–329.

42. Wyler, A. R., Burchiel, K. J., and Robbins, C. A. (1979): Operant control of precentral neurons in monkeys: Evidence against open loop control. *Brain Res.*, 171:29–39.

43. Wyler, A. R., and Burchiel, K. J. (1978): Effects of chronic epileptic foci on control of pyramidal tract neurons in monkeys. *Epilepsia*, 19:547–554.

44. Wyler, A. R. (1978): Single unit analysis of 'mirror foci' in chronic epileptic monkeys. *Brain Res.*, 150:201–204.

45. Wyler, A. R., Lange, S. C., Neafsey, E. J., and Robbins, C. A. (1980): Operant control of precentral neurons: Control of modal interspike intervals. *Brain Res.*, 190:29–38.

46. Wyler, A. R., Burchiel, K. J., and Ward, A. A., Jr. (1978): Chronic epileptic foci in monkeys: Correlation between seizure frequency and proportion of pacemaker epileptic neurons. *Epilepsia*, 19:475–483.

47. Wyler, A. R., Robbins, C. A., and Klein, S. (1979): Non-burst epileptic firing patterns of neurons in chronic epileptic foci. *Brain Res.*, 169:173–177.

48. Wyler, A. R., Finch, C. A., and Burchiel, K. J. (1978): Epileptic and normal neurons in monkey neocortex: A quantitative study of operant control. *Brain Res.*, 151:269–281.

49. Wyler, A. R. (1974): Epileptic neurons during sleep and wakefulness. *Exp. Neurol.*, 42:593–608.

50. Wyler, A. R., Ojemann, G. A., and Ward, A. A., Jr. (1982): Neurons in human epileptic cortex: Correlation between unit and EEG activity. *Ann. Neurol.*, 11:301–308.

Advances in Neurology, Vol. 44, edited by
A. V. Delgado-Escueta, A. A. Ward, Jr.,
D. M. Woodbury, and R. J. Porter.
Raven Press, New York © 1986.

50

Hippocampal Slices in Experimental and Human Epilepsy

Philip A. Schwartzkroin

Departments of Neurological Surgery and Physiology and Biophysics, University of Washington, Seattle, Washington 98195

SUMMARY Many models of epileptiform activity have been developed using *in vitro* slices, particularly the *in vitro* hippocampal slice preparation. Using this preparation, investigators have elucidated some of the intrinsic neuronal and synaptic properties that appear to be involved in the generation of burst activity and hyperexcitability typical of epileptic brain. A variety of potassium and calcium conductances, in dendritic as well as somatic membrane, have been found in hippocampal neurons that produce burst discharges; appropriate channel blockers can modulate the firing patterns of these neurons. Receptor antagonists, particularly those which interact with the gamma-aminobutyric acid (GABA) receptor–chloride channel complex, have also been found to be very effective in producing epileptiform activity in the reduced central nervous system (CNS) slice preparation. In most acutely produced epileptogenic slice tissues, it appears that blockade of inhibition, intrinsic mechanisms of excitability, and recurrent excitatory synaptic connections interact to synchronize the cell population.

Slice preparations of brain tissue taken from epileptic foci induced in chronic animals have been studied. The kainic acid model, kindling model, and other chronic models of epileptiform activity (alumina gel, freeze lesions) have been studied *in vitro;* results of these studies suggest that in these tissues there is an alteration in PSP efficacy. Seizure sensitivity in immature CNS tissue may also be produced, in part, by a late development of inhibitory postsynaptic potentials (IPSPs).

Studies of cortical slices taken from human epileptic brain during surgery for intractable seizures have begun to reveal some interesting clues about cellular mechanisms underlying discharge in abnormal tissue. Spontaneous, rhythmic post-synaptic potential (PSP) activity has been recorded particularly in slices taken from mesial temporal lobe structures involved in epileptic foci. It is still unclear, however, whether such activity is a reflection of epileptogenicity of this tissue, or is rather characteristic of even normal tissue from mesial temporal cortex.

We have learned much about the cellular and synaptic properties of CNS neurons using the *in vitro* slice preparation and have developed a variety of animal preparations in which we can model epileptiform activity. However, it is still unclear if any of these preparations accurately model human epileptiform abnormalities. A major challenge for modern epilepsy research is to build a bridge between experimental animal models of epilepsy and the epilepsies that occur in the clinical human population.

There is a wide variety of models of epileptiform activity that can be developed using the *in vitro* slice preparation and, in particular, preparations of hippocampus. Because both intrinsic cell properties and synaptic circuitry have been well studied in the hippocampal slice, it has been possible to assess the epileptogenic effects of a variety of treatments on cell and synaptic characteristics. This chapter summarizes some of the *in vitro* models in which such analyses have been carried out, and also briefly describes a few of the *in vivo* models that can be studied using the *in vitro* hippocampal slice method. With these model systems as background, we may then consider the data from studies of slice preparations of human cortical and hippocampal tissue taken during surgery on patients with medically intractable epilepsy.

Because there are a large number of models presently employed to study epilepsy, and because a wide range of epileptiform phenomenology has been described in these models, it is worthwhile to begin to assess the degree to which these models actually shed light on aspects of the human epileptic condition. It should be emphasized that human epilepsy comes in a great variety of forms. Unfortunately, it has often been unclear which forms or features of epilepsy a given model attempts to address. It would be useful for the reader to continually examine the relevance of these particular models as the data are summarized.

EXPERIMENTAL EPILEPSY PRODUCED IN THE *IN VITRO* HIPPOCAMPAL SLICE

There are numerous methods for producing epileptiform activity in hippocampal slices, just as there are a variety of means of inducing epileptic discharge in the intact brain. In slice work, the most common technique has been to add an agent that blocks inhibitory postsynaptic potentials (IPSPs) to the bathing medium. Such blockers as penicillin or bicuculline (14,30, 75,77), which presumably block the gamma-aminobutyric acid (GABA) receptor, or picrotoxin (3,30), which reportedly blocks the chloride channel, induce bursting activity and afterdischarge when added to the slice bathing medium. This activity may be spontaneous, or triggered by electrical stimulation in the appropriate afferent pathways. In form, this epileptiform activity appears to be analogous to interictal "spikes" seen in *in vivo* experiments on hippocampus. These antagonist agents produce subtly different discharge patterns (Fig. 1), probably because of differences in their means and

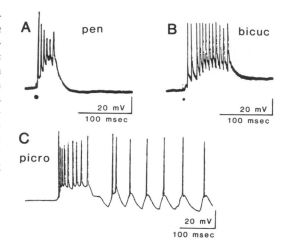

FIG. 1. Examples of hippocampal pyramidal cell burst discharges following slice treatment with three commonly used epileptogenic agents. Drugs were included in the bathing medium. A: Penicillin, 3.4 × 10^{-3} M. B: Bicuculline, 10^{-5} M. C: Picrotoxin, 10^{-5} M. Bursts were elicited by orthodromic stimulation (at dots) in A and B and occurred spontaneously in C. Note the longer duration of the bicuculline and picrotoxin bursts compared to the penicillin discharge; the latter is followed by an afterhyperpolarization which curtails the burst. Picrotoxin often gave rise to burst–afterdischarge sequences.

efficacies in blocking synaptic inhibition. Penicillin can induce spontaneous, rhythmic bursts. The bursts triggered by electrical stimulation in penicillin-containing solution are of relatively brief duration (50–100 msec) and followed by long afterhyperpolarizations (AHPs) (75,79). Several studies have shown that these penicillin burst AHPs are complex and not simply a reflection of a calcium-dependent potassium conductance such as follows normal bursting activity in hippocampal neurons (29,30,79). Bicuculline and picrotoxin produce epileptiform activity at far lower concentrations than penicillin. They, too, produce bursts of action potentials, but these bursts tend to be somewhat longer. In the case of picrotoxin, the initial burst is often followed by a flurry of afterdischarge depolarizations (43). Both bicuculline and picrotoxin bursts are also followed by long afterhyperpolarizations, probably due to a calcium-dependent potassium conductance (3,30). A variety of authors have termed the burst discharge produced by these agents a "paroxysmal depolarization shift" (PDS), taking that term from the *in vivo* literature dealing with epileptiform activity produced acutely by topical application of epileptogenic agents (13,49,50,62).

Potassium channel blocking agents have also

been shown to produce hyperexcitability and epileptiform bursting in hippocampal slice preparations (Fig. 2). Whether applied in the bathing medium, in small droplets directly to the slice, or intracellularly, these agents tend to produce prolonged cell depolarizations with concurrent rhythmic bursting activity. Tetraethylammonium (TEA), which presumably blocks the "inward rectifier" potassium current, effectively broadens action potentials and produces a voltage-dependent cell depolarization (76). Application of TEA to hippocampal tissue enhances the calcium potentials produced in hippocampal neurons and blocks cell repolarization either following normal sodium action potentials or after broader calcium bursts. Another potassium blocker, 4-aminopyridine (4-AP), has been shown to act specifically on the potassium A-current (28). It is thought that the A-current normally mediates spike firing adaptation, so that blockade of this conductance leads to more efficient repetitive firing. Further, 4-AP dramatically increases the efficacy of excitatory synaptic transmission (11). Application of 4-AP in the bathing medium also results in dramatic depolarizations and cell bursting activity. One other substance with apparent potassium channel effect has been frequently employed in studies of hippocampal cell characteristics: barium. The barium ion has a complex effect,

efficiently substituting for calcium in carrying positive charge through the calcium channel into the cell, but also blocking (or at least not activating) a variety of potassium conductances; for example, the calcium-dependent conductance is not activated by Ba^{2+}. Barium-treated tissue produces long burst discharges, which include plateau depolarizations lasting for several seconds (35). These effects can be offset by hyperpolarizing influences such as IPSPs or intracellular injection of hyperpolarizing current.

Unlike blockers of the GABA–chloride channel complex, the potassium blocking agents do not directly affect the IPSP. Given the exploding catalog of potassium channels found in mammalian central nervous system (CNS) neurons, it appears there is ample opportunity for abnormalities in these conductances to lead to cell hyperexcitability and bursting. Analysis of membrane channels in mutants of lower species (for instance, the fruit fly) have shown that there is specific gene control of these channels (68); thus, there seems to be a clear mechanism by which genetics can influence the development of hyperexcitability in these neuronal elements.

Since blockade of outward current carried by potassium ions seems to have an epileptogenic effect on hippocampal neurons, one might assume that increases in extracellular potassium concentration would have similar effects.

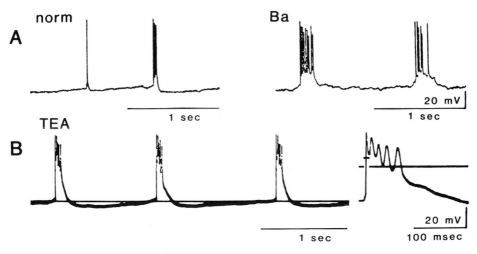

FIG. 2. Effects of two different potassium antagonists, barium (Ba) **(A)** and tetraethylammonium (TEA) **(B)**. A: The first trace shows spontaneous bursting in a normal CA3 pyramidal cell; bursts are relatively short and followed by AHPs. Addition of 10^{-3} M barium to the bathing medium led to prolonged bursts and blockade of the AHP. (Traces provided by J. Schneiderman.) **B:** Intracellular infusion of TEA (leakage from an intracellular electrode containing 0.5 M TEA) into a CA1 pyramidal cell produced spontaneous rhythmic bursting. Bursts were of long duration, with broad spikes and a very slow repolarization phase. Marked hyperpolarizations occurred between bursts. The morphology of a single burst is shown in the faster sweep speed trace to the right; this burst was elicited by a brief injection (10 msec, 0.5 nA) of depolarizing current (current monitor above recording trace).

Studies have indeed shown that increasing the extracellular potassium concentration (from a normal resting level of 3–5 mM to 10–12 mM) increases cell excitability (60,63) and, in fact, induces spontaneous burst discharge in many hippocampal neurons. *In vivo* measurements of extracellular potassium concentration, using ion-sensitive electrodes (23), have shown that extracellular potassium rises to a level of 10 to 12 mM during seizure activity. However, in hippocampal slices, one cannot produce seizures simply by increasing extracellular potassium concentration to these levels. At best, these heightened potassium levels increase the rate of interictal burst discharge. As seems to be the case for GABA-blocking agents, increasing extracellular potassium concentration produces only interictal-like activity (Fig. 3B). In contrast, reduction of extracellular chloride can have dramatic effects on cell excitability, which may extend to ictal episodes (59). Reduction of normal chloride concentration (133 mM in most bathing medium solutions) to 20 to 30 mM produces a slice condition in which seizure-like episodes and spreading depression occur spontaneously and can be quite easily triggered by appropriate electrical stimulation (Fig. 3A). Simultaneous increases in potassium and decreases in chloride do have interactive effects in hippocampal slice tissue, but raising extracellular potassium does not seem to affect the frequency or magnitude of ictal episodes.

Such data are especially interesting if one is interested in basic mechanisms of cellular hyperexcitability in hippocampus, but it may be somewhat unclear what the relevance of these manipulations is to real epileptic activity. Certainly, it is rare to find a potassium channel blocker like TEA or a GABA blocker like bicuculline within the human brain. The connection, however, is real and potentially important. One major hypothesis regarding development of epileptic activity in human brain suggests that hyperexcitability is a result of loss of inhibition (for instance, death of inhibitory interneurons) in the affected structures. Blockade of GABAergic inhibition is one method of modeling this hypothesis. The model is, in some respects, self-fulfilling, since one can reliably produce hyperexcitability by blocking inhibition in hippocampal tissue. However, loss of inhibition can also be mediated via a variety of manipulations that may more closely mimic naturally occurring epileptogenic trauma. For instance, studies have shown that inhibition is particularly vulnerable to periods of hypoxia. When hippocampal slices are exposed to low-oxygen environments, it is the IPSP that is reduced early in the hypoxic period (18). This IPSP decrement is followed by a period of transient hyperexcitability, which is also correlated with a demonstrable increase in extracellular potassium (33,41). Both these features, blockade of inhibition and increasing extracellular potassium concentration, can be induced in the slice preparation. Interestingly, the hyperexcitability that occurs transiently early in the hypoxic period is inevitably followed by periods of relative neuronal silence. We have found that this silence may reflect long periods of spreading depression, in which neurons are dramatically depolarized, their membrane resistances shunted, and their ability to generate action potentials completely abolished. Degree of recovery from such hypoxic episodes depends on the duration of the hypoxic period.

The mechanisms responsible for the burst discharges seen when hippocampal tissue is treated with epileptogenic agents such as penicillin seem to deal both with intrinsic cell properties (Fig. 4) and with synaptic connectivities (Fig. 5). Studies of bursting activity, particularly studies of PDS generation, have been carried out primarily with GABA-blocking agents. These studies have been facilitated by the finding (in *in vitro* slice preparations) that hippocampal pyramidal cells have a significant intrinsic calcium conductance (78,90). The calcium conductance is present in normal hippocampal neurons, par-

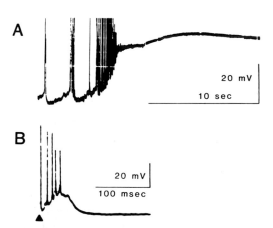

FIG. 3. **A:** Intracellular recording from CA1 pyramidal cell, showing spontaneous bursting and onset of a spreading depression. The slice had been exposed to a bathing medium with a low chloride concentration (20 mM as compared to 133 mM in normal medium). **B:** High potassium concentration in the bathing medium (10 mM as compared to 5 mM in normal solution) gave rise to "interictal" burst discharge (here triggered by an orthodromic stimulus at the *arrowhead*).

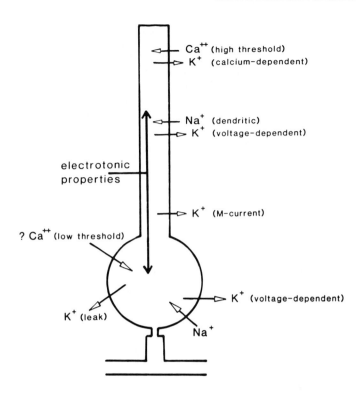

FIG. 4. Schematic showing some of the intrinsic cellular phenomena that have been investigated in the *in vitro* hippocampal slice preparation. Membrane conductances to various ions (voltage- and drug-dependent) as well as cellular electrotonic properties all contribute to the balance of excitability in pyramidal neurons.

ticularly in the CA3 cells, which show spontaneous burst discharges even in their normal state (92). Several investigators have suggested that a calcium conductance underlies the generation of depolarizing afterpotentials (DAPs) that are characteristic of hippocampal pyramidal neurons (91). It has been shown that summation of these DAPs can be the generator of at least part of the paroxysmal depolarization shift, thus indicating that at least one component of the PDS is an intrinsically generated potential. When sufficiently depolarized, pyramidal neurons can also generate all-or-none calcium spikes (78). These spikes may be triggered during some stages of epileptiform activity, and help drive neurons to highly depolarized levels for significant periods of time. One particularly interesting aspect of calcium spike electrogenesis (or cellular depolarization mediated by a more gradual calcium influx) has been the implication of dendritic membrane in these processes (94). Studies have shown that hippocampal calcium conductances are located largely on pyramidal cell dendrites (10). This localization appears to confer an amplifier function on the dendrite. Synaptic inputs that trigger calcium influx may be amplified by the action of calcium mediated depolarization and/or spikes, and thus produce somatic–axon hillock currents far greater than

produced if the PSP were electrotonically conducted to the cell body. In addition, several studies have suggested that hippocampal dendrites contain "hot spots" of high-density sodium channels (70,94). Such regions could function as independent spike generators, serving to amplify incoming synaptic activity and to confer a great degree of independence upon the dendrites. Initiation of dendritic action potentials in one branch of a dendrite could make it unnecessary for the cell to integrate large numbers of synaptic inputs at the cell soma or initial segment.

These various mechanisms that increase cell excitability and amplify excitatory synaptic input appear to render individual hippocampal neurons intrinsically hyperexcitable. Why do we not find them in a tonic state of bursting or high frequency discharge? Normal hippocampal neurons are also endowed with a variety of hyperpolarizing inhibitory mechanisms. In fact, a large number of hippocampal potassium conductances have recently been described using the *in vitro* slice preparation. These potassium conductances have an inhibitory function by virtue of their hyperpolarizing the neuron to the potassium equilibrium potential; this potential is negative to cell resting potential and spike threshold. Perhaps the most interesting of these

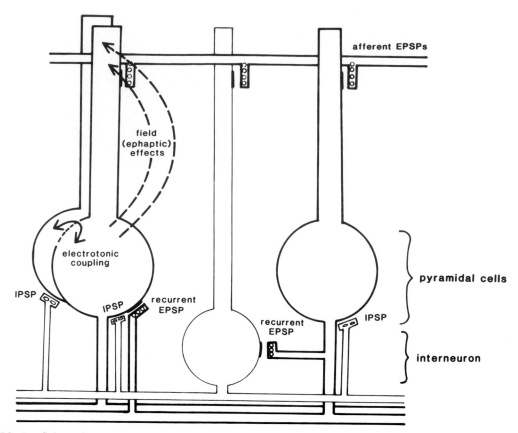

FIG. 5. Schematic of local synaptic and interactive influences that impinge upon individual hippocampal cells and help determine their outputs. Afferent EPSPs, recurrent and feed-forward inhibition from interneurons, electrotonic coupling, and ephaptic effects have been studied in the hippocampal slices. They represent only a partial list of factors that, when considered with intrinsic cellular properties, contribute to cellular excitability patterns.

potassium conductances for epilepsy research is the calcium-dependent potassium conductance, which is activated by increases in intracellular calcium concentration (36). Calcium influx (in the dendrites), which induces burst activation, is immediately followed by the hyperpolarizing calcium-dependent potassium efflux (Fig. 4). This efficient coupling of calcium and potassium conductances allows individual bursts to occur but provides an effective means of terminating the burst and preventing the cell from becoming tonically depolarized. Other potassium conductances, such as the cholinergic M-current (32), are modulated by synaptic influences (see below).

For the individual hippocampal neuron, it is clear that there is a delicate balance between the depolarizing excitatory intrinsic conductances and hyperpolarizing inhibitory conductances. An imbalance in these conductances can lead to abnormal activity (80). It is important to note that such changes in an individual neuron are not epileptic per se. The intrinsic mechanisms are important primarily in giving these hippocampal neurons a *capability* for abnormal activity.

To better understand how these intrinsic cell properties might be involved in epileptiform discharge, it is important to study synaptic interactions leading to hyperexcitability and cell synchronization. This has been the focus of a variety of studies using the hippocampal slice preparation. Not surprisingly, the initial experiments in this area focused on changes in IPSP activity that resulted from applying epileptogenic agents (such as penicillin, bicuculline, and picrotoxin) to the slice. As already mentioned, treatment of slices with these agents effectively blocks GABA-mediated inhibition, and leads directly to burst activity in hippocampal pyramidal cells (Fig. 6). With the decrease in IPSP, one can record an apparently larger excitatory PSP

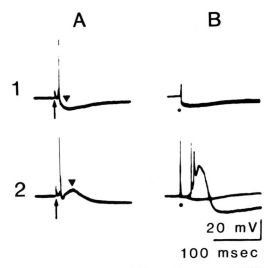

A　　　　**B**

1

2

20 mV

100 msec

FIG. 6. Effects of penicillin on hippocampal IPSPs. Penicillin was added to the bathing medium (3.4 × 10^{-3} M) and intracellular recordings were obtained from CA1 pyramidal cells. Cells were activated by orthodromic stimulation (*arrow* in **A**, *dot* in **B**). The usual IPSP elicited by orthodromic stimulation (**A1**, **B1**) was blocked by penicillin (**A2**), leading to burst discharge (**B2**).

(EPSP) (15,77). It is presently unclear whether this increase in EPSP amplitude is strictly a result of IPSP blockade (that is, a larger EPSP results from removing the usual IPSP which normally subtracts from the EPSP), or whether there is an actual increase in the synaptic excitatory drive to these cells. One popularly held hypothesis is that removal of IPSP activity releases dendritic excitability produced by cationic influx through the various sodium and calcium channels.

Although in most slice experiments the IPSP has been manipulated with GABA blockers, it is possible that GABA-induced inhibition in intact brain can be affected by a variety of traumas such as hypoxia, by induction of high extracellular potassium, or even by genetic conditions. Recent immunocytochemical studies of epileptic brain have given support to the hypothesis that destruction of sensitive inhibitory interneurons may lead to epileptic activity (66). These investigations have shown a clear reduction of GAD-staining interneurons, a loss that can be shown to occur experimentally even before onset of epileptiform spiking.

Although loss of inhibition is unquestionably an effective means of increasing the excitability of individual neurons, it does not explain the mechanism of synchronization that is characteristic of epileptiform discharge. Studies of synchronization mechanisms in hippocampal slices have indicated that there is a population of pacemaker-like cells in the CA2–CA3 region of hippocampus that appears to initiate discharge during epileptiform activity (93), and that the build-up of synchronized activity within this pacemaker region is based on a low frequency of excitatory interactions within the pyramidal-cell population (46,85). Excitatory interaction (which may be direct from pyramidal cell to pyramidal cell, or even mediated by excitatory interneurons) is normally overwhelmed by the strong inhibitory influences of the IPSP. However, when IPSPs are blocked, this excitatory synaptic interaction is sufficient to provide a build-up of synchronized synaptic activity. Although such synchronization may not necessarily depend on the intrinsic excitatory capabilities (e.g., calcium spiking) of individual pyramidal cells (39), it seems likely that the propensity of individual hippocampal neurons to burst facilitates the synchronization of the population. Because the intrinsic burst amplifies the synaptic efficacy of a given neuron, fewer and/or less strong synaptic interactions need be postulated. Recent studies have shown that activity in a single CA2 pyramidal cell can directly recruit the discharge frequency of a large CA2 population (54).

Along with this excitatory interaction mediated by conventional chemical synaptic interaction, there appears to be some degree of electrotonic coupling among pyramidal cells (48). Such coupling occurs within small groups of cells (two to five neurons). Lucifer yellow injections into hippocampal neurons show strong dye coupling within such a population (42,47). Electrophysiological studies, however, suggest that the coupling ratio among such cells is probably low, and that the effects of such electrotonic coupling are modulatory rather than a primary means for synchronization (16). Such electronic coupling may serve to amplify excitatory inputs; modeling studies have shown that the electrotonic influences combine with conventional excitatory synaptic interactions to modify the degree of synchronization established by the chemical synaptic interaction (84).

Both intrinsic cellular mechanisms and synaptic activities can be further modulated by a variety of factors in the cellular environment. One strong candidate for such a modulatory role is the acetylcholine (ACh) released by the septal input to hippocampal neurons. ACh seems to have a complex effect in hippocampus. Acetylcholine blocks the potassium M-current via muscarinic synapses on postsynaptic cells, thus increasing cell input resistance, depolarizing the cells slightly, and increasing the effectiveness of synaptic inputs to the cell (8,32). These excitatory effects on the postsynaptic cell are apparently coupled with other ACh actions. Investigators working in the slice preparation have also reported that acetylcholine has a presynaptic inhibitory effect on both excitatory and inhibitory inputs (88). Finally, it has been suggested that acetylcholine produces a disinhibition, perhaps by acting directly on inhibitory interneurons (7). Another putative neurotransmitter, dopamine, has similarly been implicated as a modulator that can affect the excitability of pyramidal neurons. Studies have shown that dopamine tends to *decrease* cell excitability by increasing the calcium-dependent potassium current that hyperpolarizes these cells (9). Investigators have suggested that this action is an effect on intracellular calcium concentration itself rather than on potassium channels. Classical neurotransmitters such as norepinephrine may have a predominantly neuromodulatory role, rather than producing primary effects on pyramidal cells (55). Similarly, adenosine (17) and even dynorphin (19,51) may act in a modulatory capacity. These drugs can increase or decrease cellular excitability and/or increase or decrease the effectiveness of primary synaptic inputs (probably mediated by excitatory amino acids and by GABA). Slice experiments have shown that even GABA may have modulatory effects. Studies have shown that GABA applied to the dendrites of pyramidal cells produces a depolarization rather than the classical IPSP hyperpolarization (2,5,83). Since there are few inhibitory symmetric synapses in the dendrites of pyramidal cells (26,73), it is likely that the GABA effect on dendrites is on extrasynaptic receptors (4,56). Although the function of such extrasynaptically mediated depolarization is presently unclear, one can imagine that these receptors become activated when there is a superabundance of GABA released at the normal synapse zones. Alternatively, there may be GABA interneurons that release their transmitter in the dendritic region of hippocampal neurons, producing the primary depolarization without the need for synaptic specializations (a humoral effect).

A host of non-synaptic influences have also been identified in recent hippocampal slice studies. There is evidence that decreased function of an electrogenic sodium/potassium ATPase pump may give rise to cellular depolarization in these cells (1). Although it is unclear that such a pump effect makes the cells more excitable per se, it is clear that decreased pump action makes it more difficult for cells to repolarize after they are depolarized, and thus would add to influences that tend to maintain cells in a depolarized state. The role of calcium and other divalent cations in maintaining cell stability has also been investigated. It has long been accepted that cells require a minimum extracellular divalent cation concentration for membrane stability (25); reduction of calcium or of other divalent cations extracellularly leads to leaky cell membranes and cell hyperexcitability. Some of this effect is undoubtedly due to loss of the "screening" effect of the divalent cation, but calcium may have a more specific role. Calcium actions intracellularly, such as maintenance of cellular pH, or as "second messenger," have also been suggested in a variety of studies. Effects of lowered divalent cation concentration are clearly illustrated in studies that revealed spontaneous synchronized activity in hippocampal slices in which synaptic activity was completely blocked by omitting calcium (37,82,96). Investigators have attributed the development of such synchronized discharge to ephaptic influences, products of the fields so prominent in hippocampus. Indeed, studies in the normal hippocampal slice have indicated that, because extracellular fields are so large, they can have important effects on cell transmembrane potential (86). Thus, such ephaptic effects may be important in even normal cellular activity, but must certainly become a factor when large cell populations discharge synchronously and produce field potentials of 20 or 30 mV. Changes in the efficacy of such ephaptic influences may be mediated by changes in extracellular space and resistance, which in turn may be secondary to increases in extracellular potassium concentration or chloride concentration.

Studies of cellular tissue hyperexcitability using the *in vitro* slice preparation have identified a large variety of mechanisms and influences that can account for changes in cell discharge properties. These studies have given us a large library of possibilities from which to choose in considering what mechanisms may be involved in development of epileptogenesis *in vivo*. Because of the limitations of this acute slice preparation, however, it is unclear which, if any, of these mechanisms are involved in the production of epileptiform activity in the intact animal. To gain a better understanding of these more chronic situations, it is necessary to try to relate the insights gained from acute studies in the *in vitro* preparation to chronic models of epilepsy.

MODELS OF EPILEPSY PRODUCED *IN VIVO* BUT STUDIED *IN VITRO*

Recently, a number of laboratories have tried to attack the mechanisms underlying chronic epileptiform activity *in vivo* by studying these mechanisms in the *in vitro* slice preparation. In such experiments, a chronic epileptic focus is first established in the intact animal. Animals are then sacrificed at various times following the induction of epileptogenesis, the brains removed and sliced, and experiments conducted on *in vitro* tissue similar to those carried out on slices prepared for acute studies of epileptogenesis (as already described). This approach has the apparent advantage that abnormalities observed in tissue from epileptic animals can be related to a chronic form of epileptiform activity. The disadvantage to this approach is that the tissue has been radically disconnected from the intact circuitry that is responsible for generation of the abnormal activity. Thus, even if abnormal cell and/or synaptic properties are observed, there is still a problem in relating those abnormalities to the changes responsible for epileptogenesis in the chronic "intact" state. Despite this objection, however, the approach does bring us one step closer to "real" epilepsy, and therefore these studies are of considerable interest.

One chronic model that has received considerable attention both *in vivo* and *in vitro* is that produced by injection of the neurotoxin, kainic acid, into the hippocampus (or into the ventricle overlying hippocampus) (57,58,69). These studies have shown that such injection preferentially destroys the CA3 pyramidal cells of hippocampus, thus producing a deafferentation model similar to that seen in some forms of human epilepsy. Other investigators have studied the effects of kainic acid on pyramidal cells when the drug is added directly to the bathing medium of the slice preparation (22,67). Kainate administered in such an acute manner has a depressive effect on IPSP activity and also directly depolarizes the cells of the CA3 population. The results of intraventricular injection of kainate in the intact animal have been followed at various periods after the intact animal has been injected. We and others (24,44) have come to similar conclusions about the effect of this treatment (Fig. 7). At relatively short intervals between injection and the time at which the

hippocampus is studied in the slice preparation (that is, at 2–3 weeks postinjection), the primary findings are: (a) a general decrease in synaptic activity, manifest in both excitatory and inhibitory input; (b) decrease or loss of the hyperpolarizing afterpotentials (the calcium-dependent potassium-mediated AHPs) in CA1 neurons following repetitive spiking due to depolarizing current injection (such AHPs are characteristic of normal CA1 pyramidal cells); (c) prolonged and exaggerated depolarizing afterpotentials (DAPs) that can trigger repetitive discharge; and (d) tendency of the population to emit synchronous burst discharge (multi-peaked field potentials) in response to orthodromic input (in the normal slice, only one population spike is seen in CA1 in response to orthodromic stimulation). Interestingly, this pattern of alteration in the kainate-treated animal is not consistent over time. If one waits until 3 months following the kainate injection before carrying out the analysis *in vitro,* the experimenter will see a somewhat different pattern of cellular/synaptic alterations in the hippocampal slice. In these preparations, the AHPs of the remaining CA1 cells seem to be quite normal, but the synaptic pattern is radically different. IPSPs are selectively smaller and fewer, while EPSPs are particularly large. It is unclear what is responsible for the reduction in IPSPs, for recordings in the slice still suggest the presence of an interneuron population. It has been suggested, however, that the number of GAD reactive neurons in kainate-treated tissue is reduced from normal, so kainate injections may indeed reduce the inhibitory interneuron population. The cells remaining in the slices at 2 to 3 months following kainate injection have also been found to have somewhat increased input resistance. This change could, in part, account for the large EPSPs, and certainly could provide one mechanism by which the cell population might become more responsive to excitatory input. As at the shorter survival times, the population within hippocampus responds to stimulation with burst discharges (as seen in multiple population spikes); however, this tendency seems to be somewhat stronger than at the shorter survival times and includes some spontaneous field potential bursting. The mechanisms responsible for such increases in tissue excitability are certainly not yet apparent. One interesting suggestion is that there is a growth of recurrent excitatory collaterals within the cell population that has been denervated by removal of the CA3 neurons. Such collateral reinnervation could provide a circuitry for hyperexcita-

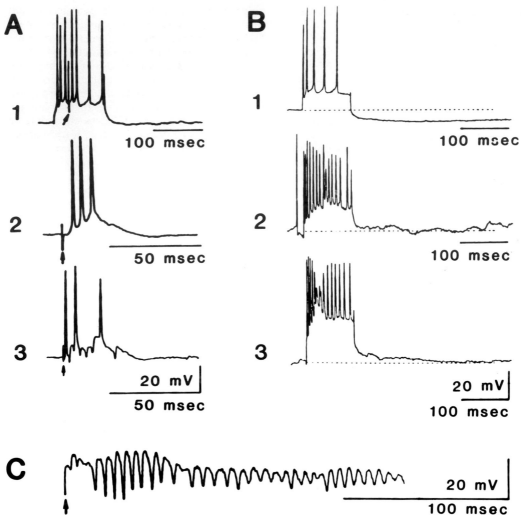

FIG. 7. Effects of chronic kainic acid injections on hippocampal electrophysiology *in vitro*. Intraventricular injections of kainate (0.5 μg in 1 μl) were made in rats to destroy CA3 pyramidal neurons. Three weeks or 3 months later, the animals were sacrificed and the hippocampus was examined *in vitro*. **A:** IPSPs were selectively attenuated at 3 months survival. Orthodromic stimulation (*arrow*) produced no obvious IPSP, even when the stimulus was superimposed in a depolarizing current pulse (**A1**). The same orthodromic stimulus did trigger a burst response (**A2**), often correlated with visible field potential population spikes (**A3**). **B:** At shorter survivals (3 weeks), the most striking selective effect was loss of the postburst AHP. In normal tissue, repetitive firing produced by depolarizing current injection (**B1**) is followed by a calcium-dependent, potassium-mediated after-hyperpolarization. In kainate-treated tissue, current-induced firing was followed by no such AHP (**B2, B3**). **C:** At both early and late survival times, field potential afterdischarge could be elicited by orthodromic stimulation. This effect was most prominent in tissue from animals given bilateral kainate injections.

tion and synchronization of excitatory input to the remaining pyramidal neurons. Another possibility is that there is a development of denervation supersensitivity to excitatory neurotransmitters. These possibilities have also been considered as possible mechanisms for development of epileptogenic activity in the human brain.

Another well-studied approach to epileptogenesis, recently employed in slice labora-

tories, is the kindling model (53,65). Experimenters have tried to find alterations in hippocampal neurons in slices taken from animals that have been kindled *in vivo*. These attempts have been rather unsuccessful when recordings have been made exclusively from the pyramidal cell populations (40). Recently, however, Oliver and Miller (61) have reported changes in the granule cell population (in response to input from per-

forant path stimulation) in tissue taken from animals kindled to stage 5 seizures. They reported
that the input resistance of granule cells is increased significantly in the kindled animals and
that there is an apparent increase in IPSP efficacy (Fig. 8A). This latter, seemingly paradoxical, effect is seen in experiments involving
paired-pulse stimulation. In normal hippocampal
dentate recording, paired-pulse stimulation at
short intervals results in an early inhibition of
the test pulse; at longer intervals (from 40-msec
to several-hundred-millisecond intervals) the
test pulse is normally potentiated. In kindled
hippocampus, this later potentiation effect was
absent, suggesting that a long-lasting component
of the IPSP was increased in these animals. It is
somewhat difficult to provide a rationale for
such increases in inhibition in a tissue that has
been rendered *more* excitable by the kindling

paradigm. One explanation is that the inhibition
increase is a reaction by the dentate (which
serves as a "gateway" to hippocampus) against
the development of hyperexcitability: that is,
this region develops the IPSP as a protective
mechanism. Such an explanation has also been
offered with regard to the apparent increase in
benzodiazepine receptor binding in dentate following kindling (87). Because kindling-induced
changes in hippocampus have been so difficult
to identify, investigators have started to look at
other regions that might be involved by the kindling stimulation. One such study investigated
the responses of pyriform cortex neurons to
amygdala kindling. McIntyre et al. (52) reported
that cells in pyriform cortex from kindled rats
show a marked increase in their burst tendency
as compared to normal pyriform neurons (Fig.
8B). Kindling also produced a tendency for af-

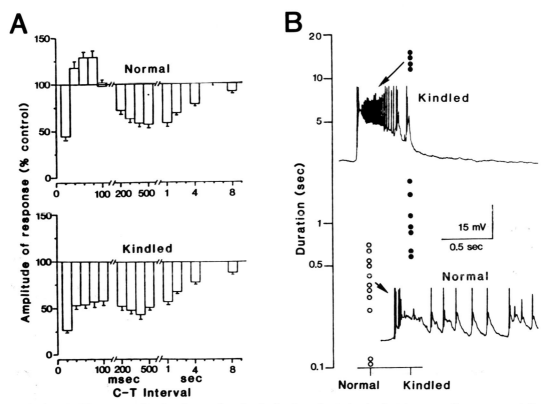

FIG. 8.   A: Histograms showing the results of paired-pulse stimulation in dentate gyrus. *Bars* represent the
amplitude of the response to the second pulse (test or "T") compared to the response to the first pulse (control
or "C"). In normal tissue (**top** histogram), there is an early inhibition (test response less than control at 20-
msec C–T interval) followed by facilitation (at 40- to 80-msec C–T interval). In commissural-kindled animals
(**lower** histogram), the facilitation is absent and inhibition extends for several seconds. (Figure courtesy of
M. W. Oliver and J. J. Miller.) **B:** Graph of burst durations as recorded in slices of pyriform cortex from normal
(*open circles*) and amygdala-kindled (*closed circles*) rats. Trace insets exemplify the longer duration bursts in
kindled (**top** trace) compared to normal (**lower** trace) tissue. (Figure courtesy of D. C. McIntyre and R. K. S.
Wong.)

terdischarge in this pyriform region, a tendency that was suppressed by treatment of the tissue by norepinephrine.

Other chronic models of epilepsy have also been examined in the *in vitro* preparation, some of which involve examination of neocortical rather than hippocampal slices. Two such examples are the alumina foci from monkey and the freeze lesions from guinea pig. Examination of monkey cortex surrounding the region of alumina injection was carried out in our laboratories (81) (Fig. 9). Alumina foci (as described in many publications previously; e.g., ref. 89) have been studied with a large number of intra- and extracellular recording techniques *in vivo*. The tissue examined in our slices was taken from regions shown to generate high amplitude epileptiform activity, as determined by electrocorticograph (ECoG) monitoring in the intact animal. Small pieces of cortex were removed from the anesthetized animal, sliced, and examined in the *in vitro* incubation chamber. The results from this study were inconclusive. The equivocal results were due, in part, to the fact that tissue taken from the center of an active alumina focus tended to be gliotic, making intracellular recording difficult. Extracellular monitoring of the tissue failed to reveal any epileptiform field potential discharge; intracellular recordings from individual cells showed very little spontaneous activity and no spontaneous burst discharges. However, cells could be synaptically driven by stimulation in white matter or at the pial surface. There was a tendency in this "alumina tissue" for IPSPs to be smaller and less effective than in normal tissue (although IPSPs from normal tissue *in vitro* were more rare than would have been expected in *in vivo* cortex). In some situations, orthodromic stimulation of neurons initiated burst discharge, but these bursts were always of a graded nature,

quite different from the all-or-none PDS that is typical of epileptiform discharge in acute models of epilepsy. Perhaps significant was our observation that action potentials often appeared to fractionate in alumina tissue. Such a tendency towards fractionation has also been seen in recordings from alumina foci *in vivo,* but the reason for such a change in action potential generation is still to be determined.

In contrast to our findings in the alumina cortical slices, Lighthall and Prince (45) have recently reported that cortical cells from chronic freeze lesion foci exhibit abnormal bursting activity. Their examination of these neurons revealed no obvious changes in the intrinsic cellular properties of these neurons, only an increased tendency for cells to discharge PDS-like depolarizations. Such bursts could occur at variable latencies from the stimulus and were unlike the intrinsic bursts characteristic of some normal pyramidal cells in guinea pig neocortex. The authors suggest that the bursts are the result of a modified synaptic input to these cells, since neither intrinsic properties nor cell structure (as seen at the light microscopic level with intracellular horseradish peroxidase injections) were altered. Similar burst discharges, all-or-none depolarizations with variable latency (onset from stimulus), have also been reported by Prince and Wong (64) in recordings from slices of human epileptic neocortex.

A variety of animal preparations show epileptiform-like activity without the need for introducing epileptogenic agents into the tissue, or subjecting the tissue to a traumatizing treatment. A variety of such preparations has just begun to be studied in our laboratory. For instance, rats experiencing febrile seizures as young pups (34) (1–2 weeks postnatal) have been studied *in vitro* when they mature. Recordings from hippocampus from these animals suggest that there is a change in the degree of inhibition in the mature animal, perhaps as a result of loss of inhibitory interneurons produced by the hypoxia/ischemia associated with the febrile seizure. Consistent with this explanation are the subtle morphological abnormalities seen in hippocampus of these febrile-seizure animals. A decrease in IPSP efficacy and/or occurrence has also been seen in preliminary studies of rats with a genetic predisposition toward seizure activity (38). These animals are predisposed to seizures produced by a variety of stimuli (including auditory stimulation, pentylenetetrazol injection, and hyperthermia). Although it is unclear that the abnormality in the brain of these animals is localized to hippocampus, the fact that hippocampus is

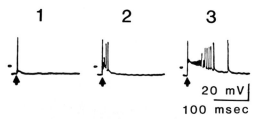

1   **2**   **3**

20 mV

100 msec

FIG. 9. Recording from a cortical slice taken from an alumina focus in monkey. No spontaneous bursting was seen in such tissue, but orthodromic stimulation (*arrow*) could trigger long-duration bursts. These burst responses were graded with the intensity of the stimulus (increasing intensity from 1 to 3); fractionated spikes were often seen as components of the bursts.

normally a site of low-threshold seizure generation suggested it as a structure in which changes might be sought.

Unlike the condition of these epileptic animals, we have found that in normal immature rabbit hippocampus, there is a tendency toward spontaneous seizure discharge and seizure-like spreading depression (31). Such spontaneous events have been recorded at both the extracellular and intracellular level in hippocampal slices from immature animals (ages 8–10 days postnatal) (Fig. 10). The seizure-like spreading depression episodes are most prominent in the CA1 region of hippocampus, occurring spontaneously in CA1 at a time when no such events can be seen in CA3. In fact, it is relatively rare for spreading depression to invade the CA3 region. One possible explanation for this difference of sensitivity is the differential development of inhibition in these two pyramidal cell regions. Previous studies (72) showed that IPSPs develop quite early in the CA3 region (at prenatal time) but rather late in the CA1 area (starting at 10–14 days postnatal); thus, the hyperpolarizing IPSP might "protect" the CA3 cells (but not CA1 cells) against increases in excitation. Another possible factor involved is the ability of the tissue to regulate extracellular potassium. Using potassium sensitive microelectrodes, we have seen large rises in extracellular potassium levels correlated with the development of these spreading depression episodes. Further, blockade of sodium potassium ATPase by ouabain interferes with the ability of pyramidal neurons to repolarize following seizure-dependent depolarization. Interestingly, these spontaneous spreading depression events in immature tissue are similar in form to comparable events seen in mature tissue when extracellular

chloride is removed or lowered. Such events can also be produced in mature tissue with appropriate hypoxia treatment (33). It appears from these studies of immature rabbit hippocampus that there are critical periods of development during which hippocampal tissue is particularly seizure-prone. The causes for this critical period sensitivity may be numerous, depending on a variety of maturing systems.

These studies *in vitro* of chronic epileptiform phenomena have shown us a variety of different aspects of epileptogenesis. Certainly, the different forms of epileptiform activity manifest *in vivo* may have different reflections in the *in vitro* preparation. This observation, although perhaps obvious, is exceedingly important when we try to determine the underlying mechanisms of human epileptiform activity. These various experimental approaches may model different aspects of the various forms of human epileptiform activity. Given this possibility, what specifics can we take from the studies of various animal models that will shed light on the epileptiform activities we see in human brain? How can we make the bridge between animal models of epilepsy and the human epileptic activity?

HUMAN EPILEPTIC TISSUE STUDIED *IN VITRO*

One approach to this problem is simply to study the human epileptic tissue in the same experimental context as used for studies of animal models. This approach has been used *in vivo*, with several attempts made to examine epileptiform activity *in situ* in the human brain. Such studies have been limited primarily to recordings of extracellular activity (12) but have indeed provided a basis for evaluating activities seen in animal models. However, the extracellular recordings cannot provide us with an understanding of what basic mechanisms are responsible for the abnormal epileptic patterns. An alternative approach to the *in situ* recording is to remove epileptic tissue, slice it, and study it *in vitro*, much as has been done for the various animal models already described. That this approach is feasible was demonstrated several years ago (74), but the question of whether such an approach can, in fact, give us important information about epileptogenesis has still to be resolved. This section presents data from our studies of human epileptogenic cortex and hippocampus. Finally, I ask some questions (but do not answer them) about how these findings and the findings from animal models may be related to give us insights into underlying mechanisms of epileptogenesis.

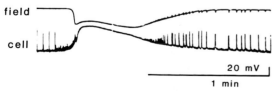

field

cell

20 mV

1 min

FIG. 10. Spontaneous spreading depression episode in a hippocampal slice from immature (10 days postnatal) rabbit. Simultaneous field and intracellular records were obtained in the CA1 region of the slice. A large (30–40 mV) DC negative shift was seen in the field recording during cellular depolarization. These spontaneous events were preceded by a brief period of increased cellular excitability and rise in extracellular potassium (not shown). The recovery phase was characterized by "clonic" burst discharges, which occurred synchronously among cells in the affected slice.

In attempting to study epileptiform activity *in vitro,* it is important that we are able to study tissue in which we are confident that epileptic activity exists. Such confidence implies that we must, in the *in vivo* situation, be able to localize an epileptic focus. It is, of course, important for the neurosurgeon as well as for the experimentalist to be able to make such a determination, for accurate identification of a focus will be a major factor in determination of the outcome of neurosurgery for intractable epilepsy. A variety of clinical techniques have been used to determine whether a particular region of cortex is "epileptic." Electroencephalograph (EEG) and ECoG criteria have perhaps been most commonly used in determining the sites of high-amplitude "epileptic" spiking. The usual surface recordings have been supplemented in various centers by implanted depth and strip electrodes which monitor activity from deeper temporal lobe regions (6). New methods for monitoring regions of abnormal activity include the computed tomography (CT) and positron emission tomography (PET) scans, nuclear magnetic resonance (NMR), and magnetic encephalograms (20). These more recent techniques, rather than clarifying the issue of the origin of epileptogenic activity, have suggested that most epilepsies, even the so-called "focal" epilepsies, involve multiple foci.

Much evidence has suggested that temporal-lobe foci are relatively common, and it is the temporal "partial complex" epilepsies that appear to be most difficult to treat with medication. Thus, it is the temporal-lobe focus that is most usually removed during neurosurgical procedures. Even with localization of the focus to the temporal lobe, however, a number of localization questions remain. For instance, are the mesial temporal structures (including hippocampus) usually the sites of seizure initiation? Experimental studies have certainly indicated that these structures have lower seizure thresholds than lateral neocortical sites, and histological examination of epileptic temporal lobe tissue has revealed pathologies localized primarily to mesial tissue (21,27). CT analysis has also indicated that mesial temporal structures are often sclerotic and herniated (95).

The question remains, however, as to whether we can identify generator or pacemaker sites in the temporal lobe and distinguish them from the sites that receive projected activity. Both types of activity (pacemaker and projected) may be reflected in high-amplitude electroencephalographic spikes; in fact, spikes in a "projected" region may be of even higher amplitude than

seen at a "generation" site, for pathological changes may severely deplete a generator region of neurons. Histologic procedures that identify regions of reactive gliosis and regions of activated astrocytes (via the hydrogenase staining) are helpful indicators of focus localization, but are *post facto* and thus do not really help either the surgeon or the electrophysiologist in determining which regions to remove and study.

Our experimental concern with the accurate identification of the focus stems from the equivocal results from our initial investigations of neocortical temporal tissue (81). Neocortical tissue from surgical procedures for intractable epilepsy was obtained, cut into 500-μm-thick slices, and maintained *in vitro* as has been done for tissue from experimental animals. Recordings were made with intracellular micropipettes, and stimulation of the tissue was carried out with electrodes placed in the underlying white matter and/or at the pial surface. Aside from confirming that such tissue could be maintained *in vitro,* and that we could record intracellularly from neurons of human brain, the results of these experiments were rather disappointing. Our major findings (Fig. 11) from slices of human neocortex can be summarized as follows.

1. There was little spontaneous activity in these slices. That is, neither intracellular nor extracellular recordings showed that cells were normally spontaneously active. Although recordings from animal tissue *in vitro* normally show a reduced level of spontaneous activity

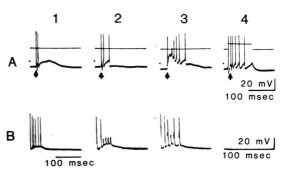

FIG. 11. Recordings from human "epileptic" neocortex maintained *in vitro.* There was little spontaneous activity in this tissue, but bursts could be evoked by orthodromic stimulation of some cells (stimulus at *arrow* in **A**, at beginning of trace in **B**). Bursts were graded with stimulus intensity (increasing intensity from **A1** to **A3**) and often included fractionated spikes (**A3, B2, B3**). Inhibition was weak in these slices, with no IPSP apparent even when the stimulus was superimposed in a depolarizing current pulse (**A4**) (0.5 nA for 100 msec). Note that the time scale for **B1** is different from that of **B2** and **B3**.

compared to *in vivo* controls, the absence of spontaneous activity in these human slices was striking.

2. There was no spontaneous burst discharge that might reflect underlying epileptiform abnormalities. The absence of such activity was particularly discouraging, since examination of mechanisms underlying epileptiform events required that the tissue display epileptiform activity. In some cells, stimulation evoked bursts of action potentials initiated from graded EPSPs. Such bursts were relatively rare, and never of an all-or-none nature. This result is in striking contrast to the results reported by Prince and Wong (64), who showed that neocortical cells from human epileptic foci could, in fact, discharge in abnormal burst patterns when stimulated. As in the tissue from the alumina monkey, we found that the action potentials driven by these graded EPSPs sometimes fractionated in an abnormal manner.

3. The intrinsic cellular properties of neurons from such tissue (resting potential, input resistance, time constant, etc.) were relatively normal (as far as we could determine without "controls").

4. In many neurons, IPSPs appeared to be reduced or absent, with a resultant prolongation of the EPSP. This effect was not strong, and given our difficulties of eliciting normal IPSPs from normal cortical tissue from monkey, we were somewhat reluctant to interpret this decrease in IPSP as a function of the epileptic nature of the tissue; rather, it seemed to be a product of the slice preparation itself.

5. Neurons that were intracellularly stained with Lucifer yellow (so that we could relate cell structure with electrophysiological characteristics) did not show any striking morphological abnormalities (as examined at the light-microscopic level). We could not, on the basis of morphology, differentiate between neurons that generated burst discharge as opposed to those that responded to stimulation with a single action potential.

Interpretation of all the above findings was, of course, made difficult by the fact that these data could not be compared with comparable results gathered in normal control tissue. This problem was particularly serious, since most studies using the *in vitro* preparation report a considerable degree of variability, even in normal tissue. To develop some means of evaluating pathological activity in our samples, we divided our tissue samples into two separate groups. One group was clearly from the center of an actively discharging region of cortex, as determined *in situ* with ECoG recording; the other region was of more questionable relationship to the center of the so-called "focus." Dividing our tissue in this manner, and reexamining our data, we found little to correlate with epileptic activity. Burst discharges, in fact, appeared to be somewhat more frequent in the tissue of questionable relationship to the focus. Proper controls, however, for evaluation of this tissue are still to be obtained.

Because of these somewhat disappointing results and because of our concern that epileptogenic activity was generated in mesial rather than lateral neocortical structures, we approached another series of studies in a slightly different way. Tissue samples were obtained both from lateral neocortex, and from deep temporal structures (sometimes including hippocampus) when surgical treatment for the epileptic condition involved temporal lobectomy. We could thus compare activity in lateral and mesial tissue obtained from the same patient. Both neocortical and mesial temporal tissue were cut into somewhat thicker slices than those used in previous studies; slices were made approximately 700 μm thick rather than 500 μm thick. This latter modification was carried out in hopes that the thicker slice would maintain more cortical circuitry and thus enable the tissue to generate spontaneous events that were "cut away" in our previous studies.

The results from this later series of experiments (71) were rather provocative and unanticipated. Our recordings were unlike anything we had observed in recordings from a variety of animal models (acute or chronic) of epileptiform activity. The striking activity consisted of spontaneous rhythmic PSP-like events, which could be seen in a large percentage of impaled neurons (Fig. 12). This activity was superimposed on a normal level of spontaneous activity in the slice, although a spontaneous background devoid of epileptiform burst discharges. The rhythmic PSP-like activity was found more frequently in tissue from mesial than from lateral temporal cortex (approximately 77% of neurons from mesial structures, as opposed to only 25% of neurons from lateral neocortical structures). These potentials appeared to be synaptic potentials mediated by conventional chemical transmission, based on the observations that (a) current manipulation of the membrane potential produced appropriate alterations of event amplitude, and even reversed various components of the event; (b) similar current manipulations of membrane potential during stimulus-evoked

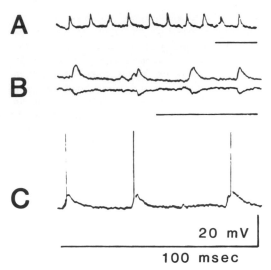

FIG. 12. Intracellular recordings from mesial temporal lobe slices. **A:** A large proportion of neurons in mesial tissue from human epileptic brain displayed spontaneous, rhythmic, PSP-like events. **B:** When simultaneous recordings were obtained from two neurons, near-synchronous activity was observed. However, the PSP varied considerably from cell to cell, and included both depolarizing and hyperpolarizing components. **C:** Depolarizing events could trigger action potential discharge in some cells. Note the change in time scale (100-msec bars) for **A, B,** and **C.**

synaptic activation produced parallel changes in the orthodromically triggered PSP; (c) current manipulation of cell membrane did not affect the frequency of occurrence of these events, suggesting that the driver for these potentials was not affected by the injected current; and (d) these events were blocked by application of tetrodotoxin (TTX) in the dendritic regions of the cell (TTX presumably blocked action potential generation in the fibers mediating input to these neurons). These rhythmic spontaneous PSPs were extremely complex, composed of depolarizing and hyperpolarizing components, each of which had a different reversal potential. The depolarizing components were large enough to trigger action potentials in some neurons.

These observations of unusual synaptic input to the mesial cortical neurons need not be considered reflections of epileptic activity. However, the spontaneous rhythmic nature of the events was intriguing. Simultaneous intracellular recordings from two neurons within a slice (with the electrodes spaced at distances ranging from 200 to 1500 μm apart) showed that the spontaneous events occurred approximately synchronously throughout a given slice. These events then reflected at least two aspects of

what might be considered epileptiform activity: increased excitatory synaptic input, and synchronous rhythmic discharge. Interpretation of these events as epileptic, of course, cannot be made definitively at this time. It is certainly possible that such events are relatively normal features of tissue from mesial temporal structures. This interpretation seems somewhat unlikely, however, since the spontaneous PSPs were occasionally recorded in neocortical slice tissue, and were sometimes absent in tissue from mesial regions. The source of generation of these events is certainly unclear at the present time. In our recordings it appeared that these events were synaptically generated, and it is possible that generation of such activity is entirely a synaptic phenomenon, a product of the peculiarities of the population circuitry. It is also possible that a small number of pacemaker neurons, abnormal in their discharge characteristics and not seen in our recorded sample, were responsible for driving the rhythmic activity throughout the rest of the slice. The question of which or how much of each of these alternative explanations is involved in generating these rhythmic PSPs brings us back to the matter of whether epileptic activity (even that seen in a variety of animal models) is a result of activity in a few abnormal neurons, or an expression of some circuitry abnormality. The mechanisms remain to be elucidated.

CRITICAL QUESTIONS

The results of our studies on human epileptic tissue suggest that studies of epileptogenesis may be carried out in the *in vitro* slice preparation. Certainly the occurrence of spontaneous rhythmic PSPs in our own studies, and the Prince and Wong (64) observation of stimulus-evoked PDS-like events warrant further investigation. Our studies also reinforce the suspicion that mesial temporal tissue is primarily involved in generation of epileptiform activity, at least in a large majority of cases. Our data have not, however, given us any answers about the special characteristics of human epileptic neurons or epileptic circuitry. These studies have also not provided clear bridges or links between human epileptogenesis and the models so often studied. In fact, our data from these human tissue slices, and the results from slice studies of various chronic animal models of epileptiform activity, highlight a number of questions critical to our continued electrophysiological analysis of epileptic foci. These questions will undoubtedly determine the course of much of our future experimental work.

1. Given what we know about human epileptogenesis, which animal models are appropriate for study? What do each of these model? Can they be profitably studied using the *in vitro* slice preparation?

2. Are there, in fact, *in vitro* models of a variety of forms of epilepsy, or are the *in vitro* phenomena focused on one limited form of epileptogenesis? For instance, are all our *in vitro* data relevant only to focal epilepsies, or can generalized epilepsy be studied in slices?

3. Is the paroxysmal depolarization shift (the PDS) really the "hallmark" of epileptic activity? Is this type of activity seen in all forms of epilepsy, *in vivo* and *in vitro*? Is it characteristic of the focus itself, or more often seen in regions receiving abnormal input? Is it prominent only within regions in which cells have peculiar intrinsic characteristics?

4. What is the role and the fate of inhibitory interneurons in epileptic foci? Is loss of inhibition characteristic of all forms of epilepsy? Of all models?

5. Do morphologically abnormal neurons produce abnormal physiology? Is there a correlation between bursting neurons and neurons seen to have identifiable pathologies (for instance, loss of spines and fine dendrites seen in Golgi studies)?

6. Is there still an "epileptic neuron" versus "epileptic aggregate" controversy? What is meant by these opposing views in light of our recent understanding of how burst generation is carried out? What are the data supporting each point of view?

These are just some of the questions that must be answered in our future studies. At present, I do not believe there are any definitive answers to any of the questions. Our challenge for the future is to transform our opinions about the answers into experimentally testable hypotheses.

ACKNOWLEDGMENTS

The author's research is supported by National Institutes of Health grants NS 15317, NS 00413, NS 18895, and NS 17111, and by National Science Foundation grant BNS 8209906.

REFERENCES

1. Alger, B. E. (1984): Characteristics of a slow hyperpolarizing synaptic potential in rat hippocampal neurons. *J. Neurophysiol.*, 52:892–910.

2. Alger, B. E., and Nicoll, R. A. (1979): GABA-mediated biphasic inhibitory responses in hippocampus. *Nature (Lond.)*, 281:315–317.

3. Alger, B. E., and Nicoll, R. A. (1980): Epileptiform burst hyperpolarization: Calcium-dependent potassium potential in hippocampal CA1 pyramidal cells. *Science*, 210:1122–1124.

4. Alger, B. E., and Nicoll, R. A. (1982): Pharmacological evidence for two kinds of GABA receptor on rat hippocampal pyramidal cells studied in vitro. *J. Physiol.*, 328:125–141.

5. Andersen, P., Dingledine, R., Gjerstad, L., Langmoen, I. A., and Mosfeldt-Laursen, A. (1980): Two different responses of hippocampal pyramidal cells to application of gamma-aminobutyric acid. *J. Physiol.*, 305:279–296.

6. Babb, T. L., Carr, E., and Crandall, P. D. (1973): Analysis of extracellular firing patterns of deep temporal lobe structures in man. *Electroencephalogr. Clin. Neurophysiol.*, 34:247–257.

7. Ben-Ari, Y., Krnjevic, K., Reinhardt, W., and Ropert, N. (1981): Intracellular observations on the disinhibitory action of acetylcholine in the hippocampus. *Neuroscience*, 6:2475–2484.

8. Benardo, L. S., and Prince, D. A. (1982): Cholinergic excitation of mammalian hippocampal pyramidal cells. *Brain Res.*, 249:315–331.

9. Benardo, L. S., and Prince, D. A. (1982): Dopamine modulates a Ca^{++}-activated potassium conductance in mammalian hippocampal pyramidal cells. *Nature (Lond.)*, 297:76–79.

10. Benardo, L. S., Masukawa, L. M., and Prince, D. A. (1982): Electrophysiology of isolated hippocampal pyramidal dendrites. *J. Neurosci.*, 2:1614–1622.

11. Buckle, P. J., and Haas, H. L. (1982): Enhancement of synaptic transmission by 4-aminopyridine in hippocampal slices of the rat. *J. Physiol.*, 326:109–122.

12. Calvin, W. H., Ojemann, G. A., and Ward, A. A., Jr. (1973): Human cortical neurons in epileptogenic foci: Comparison of interictal firing patterns to those of "epileptic" neurons in animals. *Electroencephalogr. Clin. Neurophysiol.*, 34:337–351.

13. Dichter, M., and Spencer, W. A. (1969): Penicillin-induced interictal discharges from the cat hippocampus. I. Characteristics and topographical features. *J. Neurophysiol.*, 32:649–662.

14. Dingledine, R., and Gjerstad, L. (1979): Penicillin blocks hippocampal IPSPs, unmasking prolonged EPSPs. *Brain Res.*, 168:205–209.

15. Dingledine, R., and Gjerstad, L. (1980): Reduced inhibition during epileptiform activity in the in vitro hippocampal slice. *J. Physiol.*, 305:297–313.

16. Dudek, F. E., Andrew, R. D., MacVicar, B. A., Snow, R. W., and Taylor, C. P. (1983): Recent evidence for and possible significance of gap junctions and electrotonic synapses in the mammalian brain. In: *Basic Mechanisms of Neuronal Hyperexcitability*, edited by H. H. Jasper and N. M. Van Gelder, pp. 31–73. Alan R. Liss, New York.

17. Dunwiddie, T. V. (1980): Endogenously released

adenosine regulates excitability in the in vitro hippocampus. *Epilepsia*, 21:541–548.

18. Dunwiddie, T. V. (1981): Age-related differences in the in vitro rat hippocampus. *Dev. Neurosci.*, 4:165–175.

19. Dunwiddie, T., Mueller, A., Palmer, M., Stewart, J., and Hoffer, B. (1980): Electrophysiological interactions of enkephalins with neuronal circuitry in the rat hippocampus. I. Effects on pyramidal cell activity. *Brain Res.*, 184:311–330.

20. Engel, J., Jr., Kuhl, D. E., Phelps, M. E., and Crandall, P. H. (1982): Comparative localization of epileptic foci in partial epilepsy by PCT and EEG. *Ann. Neurol.*, 12:529–537.

21. Falconer, M. A. (1974): Mesial temporal (Ammon's horn) sclerosis as a common cause of epilepsy. Etiology, treatment and prevention. *Lancet*, 1:767–770.

22. Fisher, R. S., and Alger, B. E. (1983): Electrophysiology of kainic acid (KA) induced epileptiform activity in the rat hippocampal slice. *Soc. Neurosci. Abstr.*, 9:908.

23. Fisher, R. S., Pedley, T. A., Moody, W. J., Jr., and Prince, D. A. (1976): The role of extracellular potassium in hippocampal epilepsy. *Arch. Neurol.*, 33:76–83.

24. Franck, J. E., and Schwartzkroin, P. A. (1983): Kainate lesioned hippocampi become epileptogenic. *Soc. Neurosci. Abstr.*, 9:908.

25. Frankenhaeuser, B., and Hodgkin, A. L. (1957): The action of calcium on the electrical properties of squid axons. *J. Physiol.*, 137:218–244.

26. Gottlieb, D. I., and Cowan, W. M. (1972): On the distribution of axon terminals containing spheroidal and flattened synaptic vesicles in the hippocampus and dentate gyrus of the rat and cat. *Z. Zellforsch.*, 129:413–429.

27. Green, J. D., and Petsche, H. (1961): Hippocampal electrical activity. IV. Abnormal electrical activity. *Electroencephalogr. Clin. Neurophysiol.*, 13:868–879.

28. Gustafsson, B., Galvan, M., Grafe, P., and Wigstrom, H. (1982): A transient outward current in a mammalian central neurone blocked by 4-aminopyridine. *Nature (Lond.)*, 299:252–254.

29. Hablitz, J. J. (1981): Altered burst responses in hippocampal CA3 neurons injected with EGTA. *Exp. Brain Res.*, 42:483–485.

30. Hablitz, J. J. (1981): Effects of intracellular injections of chloride and EGTA on postepileptiform-burst hyperpolarizations in hippocampal neurons. *Neurosci. Lett.*, 22:159–163.

31. Haglund, M. M., and Schwartzkroin, P. A. (1984): Seizure-like spreading depression in immature rabbit hippocampus in vitro. *Develop. Brain Res.*, 14:51–59.

32. Halliwell, J. V., and Adams, P. R. (1982): Voltage-clamp analysis of muscarinic excitation in hippocampal neurons. *Brain Res.*, 250:71–92.

33. Hansen, A. J., Hounsgaard, J., and Jahnsen, H. (1982): Anoxia increases potassium conductance in hippocampal nerve cells. *Acta Physiol. Scand.*, 115:301–310.

34. Holtzman, D., Obana, K., and Olson, J. (1981): Hyperthermia-induced seizures in rat pup: A model for febrile convulsions in children. *Science*, 213:1034–1036.

35. Hotson, J. R., and Prince, D. A. (1981): Penicillin- and barium-induced epileptiform bursting in hippocampal neurons: Actions on Ca^{++} and K^+ potentials. *Ann. Neurol.*, 10:11–17.

36. Hotson, J. R., Prince, D. A., and Schwartzkroin, P. A. (1979): Anomalous inward rectification in hippocampal neurons. *J. Neurophysiol.*, 42:889–895.

37. Jefferys, J. G. R., and Haas, H. L. (1982): Synchronized bursting of CA1 hippocampal pyramidal cells in the absence of synaptic transmission. *Nature (Lond.)*, 300:448–450.

38. Jobe, P. C., Woods, T. W., McNatt, N. E., Kearns, G. L., Wilson, J. T., and Dailey, J. W. (1982): Genetically epilepsy-prone rats (GEPR), a model for febrile seizures? *Fed. Proc.*, 41:1560.

39. Johnston, D., and Brown, T. H. (1984): Mechanisms of neuronal burst generation. In: *Electrophysiology of Epilepsy*, edited by P. A. Schwartzkroin and H. V. Wheal, pp. 277–301. Academic, London.

40. Kairiss, E. W., Smith, G. K., and Racine, R. J. (1983): Intracellular observations in *in vitro* hippocampus of kindled rats. *Soc. Neurosci. Abstr.*, 9:489.

41. Kass, I. S., and Lipton, P. (1982): Mechanisms involved in irreversible anoxic damage to the in vitro rat hippocampal slice. *J. Physiol.*, 332:459–472.

42. Knowles, W. D., Funch, P. G., and Schwartzkroin, P. A. (1982): Electrotonic and dye coupling in hippocampal CA1 pyramidal cells in vitro. *Neuroscience*, 7:1713–1722.

43. Knowles, W. D., Miles, R., Wong, R. K. S., and Linsker, R. (1983): Simulation of in vitro epileptiform multiple bursts. *Soc. Neurosci. Abstr.*, 9:909.

44. Lancaster, B., Wheal, H. V., and Ashwood, T. J. (1983): Hippocampal electrophysiology after kainic acid treatment: A chronic model of focal epilepsy. *Soc. Neurosci. Abstr.*, 9:908.

45. Lighthall, J. W., and Prince, D. A. (1983): Neuronal activity in areas of chronic cortical injury. *Soc. Neurosci. Abstr.*, 9:907.

46. MacVicar, B. A., and Dudek, F. E. (1980): Local synaptic circuits in rat hippocampus: Interaction between pyramidal cells. *Brain Res.*, 184:220–223.

47. MacVicar, B. A., and Dudek, F. E. (1980): Dye-coupling between CA3 pyramidal cells in slices of rat hippocampus. *Brain Res.*, 196:494–497.

48. MacVicar, B. A., and Dudek, F. E. (1981): Electrotonic coupling between pyramidal cells: A direct demonstration in rat hippocampal slices. *Science*, 213:782–785.

49. Matsumoto, H., and Ajmone-Marsan, C. (1964): Cortical cellular phenomena in experimental epilepsy: Interictal manifestations. *Exp. Neurol.*, 9:286–304.

50. Matsumoto, H., Ayala, G. F., and Gumnit, R. J., (1969): Neuronal behavior and triggering mechanisms in cortical epileptic focus. *J. Neurophysiol.*, 32:688–703.

51. McGinty, J. F., Henriksen, S. J., Goldstein, A., Terenius, L., and Bloom, F. E. (1983): Dynorphin is contained within hippocampal mossy fibers: Immunochemical alterations after kainic

acid administration and cholchicine-induced neurotoxicity. *Proc. Natl. Acad. Sci.*, 80:589–593.

52. McIntyre, D. C., Wong, R. K. S., and Miles, R. (1983): Effect of amygdala kindling of pyriform cortex response: Intracellular studies with in vitro slice. *Soc. Neurosci. Abstr.*, 9:764.

53. McNamara, J. O., Byrne, M. C., Dasheiff, R. M., and Fitz, J. G. (1980): The kindling model of epilepsy: A review. *Prog. Neurobiol.*, 15:139–159.

54. Miles, R., and Wong, R. K. S. (1983): Single neurones can influence synchronized population discharge in the CA3 region of the guinea pig hippocampus. *Nature (Lond.)*, 306:371–373.

55. Mueller, A. L., and Dunwiddie, T. V. (1983): Anticonvulsant and proconvulsant actions of alpha- and beta-noradrenergic agonists on epileptiform activity in rat hippocampus *in vitro. Epilepsia*, 24:57–64.

56. Mueller, A. L., Chesnut, R. M., and Schwartzkroin, P. A. (1983): Actions of GABA in developing rabbit hippocampus: An in vitro study. *Neurosci. Lett.*, 39:193–198.

57. Nadler, J. V. (1981): Kainic acid as a tool for the study of temporal lobe epilepsy. *Life Sci.*, 29:2031–2042.

58. Nadler, J. V., Perry, B. W., Gentry, C., and Cotman, C. W. (1980): Degeneration of hippocampal CA3 pyramidal cells induced by intraventricular kainic acid. *J. Comp. Neurol.*, 192:333–359.

59. Ogata, N. (1978): Possible explanation for interictal-ictal transition: Evolution of epileptiform activity in hippocampal slice by chloride depletion. *Experientia*, 34:1035–1036.

60. Ogata, N., Hori, N., and Katsuda, N. (1976): The correlation between extracellular potassium concentration and hippocampal epileptic activity in vitro. *Brain Res.*, 110:371–375.

61. Oliver, M. W., and Miller, J. J. (1983): Characteristics of inhibitory processes in the dentate gyrus following kindling-induced epilepsy. *Soc. Neurosci. Abstr.*, 9:484.

62. Prince, D. A. (1968): The depolarization shift in "epileptic" neurons. *Exp. Neurol.*, 21:467–485.

63. Prince, D. A., and Schwartzkroin, P. A. (1978): Non-synaptic mechanisms in epileptogenesis. In: *Abnormal Neuronal Discharge*, edited by N. Chalazonitis and M. Boisson, pp. 1–12. Raven Press, New York.

64. Prince, D. A., and Wong, R. K. S. (1981): Human epileptic neurons studied in vitro. *Brain Res.*, 210:323–333.

65. Racine, R. (1978): Kindling: The first decade. *Neurosurgery*, 3:234–252.

66. Ribak, C. E., Bradburne, R. M., and Harris, A. B. (1982): A preferential loss of GABAergic symmetric synapses in epileptic foci: A quantitative ultrastructural analysis of monkey neocortex. *J. Neurosci.*, 2:1725–1735.

67. Robinson, J. H., and Deadwyler, S. A. (1981): Kainic acid produces depolarization of CA3 pyramidal cells in the in vitro hippocampal slice. *Brain Res.*, 221:117–127.

68. Salkoff, L., and Wyman, R. (1981): Genetic modification of potassium channels in *Drosophila Shaker* mutants. *Nature (Lond.)*, 293:228–230.

69. Schwarcz, R., Zaczek, R., and Coyle, J. T. (1978): Microinjection of kainic acid into the rat hippocampus. *Eur. J. Pharmacol.*, 50:209–220.

70. Schwartzkroin, P. A. (1977): Further characteristics of hippocampal CA1 cells in vitro. *Brain Res.*, 128:53–68.

71. Schwartzkroin, P. A., and Knowles, W. D. (1984): Intracellular study of human epileptic cortex: In vitro maintainance of epileptiform activity? *Science*, 223:709–712.

72. Schwartzkroin, P. A., and Kunkel, D. D. (1982): Electrophysiology and morphology of the developing hippocampus of fetal rabbit. *J. Neurosci.*, 2:448–462.

73. Schwartzkroin, P. A., Kunkel, D. D., and Mathers, L. H. (1982): Development of rabbit hippocampus: Anatomy. *Dev. Brain Res.*, 2:453–468.

74. Schwartzkroin, P. A., and Prince, D. A. (1976): Microphysiology of human cerebral cortex studied in vitro. *Brain Res.*, 115:497–500.

75. Schwartzkroin, P. A., and Prince, D. A. (1977): Penicillin-induced epileptiform activity in the hippocampal in vitro preparation. *Ann. Neurol.*, 1:463–469.

76. Schwartzkroin, P. A., and Prince, D. A. (1980): Effects of TEA on hippocampal neurons. *Brain Res.*, 185:169–181.

77. Schwartzkroin, P. A., and Prince, D. A. (1980): Changes in excitatory and inhibitory synaptic potentials leading to epileptogenic activity. *Brain Res.*, 183:61–76.

78. Schwartzkroin, P. A., and Slawsky, M. (1977): Probable calcium spike in hippocampal neurons. *Brain Res.*, 135:157–161.

79. Schwartzkroin, P. A., and Stafstrom, C. E. (1980): Effects of EGTA on the calcium-activated afterhyperpolarization in hippocampal CA3 pyramidal cells. *Science*, 210:1125–1126.

80. Schwartzkroin, P. A., and Wyler, A. R. (1980): Mechanisms underlying epileptiform burst discharge. *Ann. Neurol.*, 7:95–107.

81. Schwartzkroin, P. A., Turner, D. A., Knowles, W. D., and Wyler, A. R. (1983): Studies of human and monkey "epileptic" neocortex in the in vitro slice preparation. *Ann. Neurol.*, 13:249–257.

82. Taylor, C. P., and Dudek, E. E. (1982): Synchronous neural afterdischarges in rat hippocampal slices without active chemical synapses. *Science*, 218:810–812.

83. Thalmann, R. H., Peck, E. J., and Ayala, G. F. (1981): Biphasic response of hippocampal pyramidal neurons to GABA. *Neurosci. Lett.*, 21:319–234.

84. Traub, R. D., and Wong, R. K. S. (1983): Synaptic mechanisms underlying interictal spike initiation in a hippocampal network. *Neurology*, 33:257–266.

85. Traub, R. D., and Wong, R. K. S. (1983): Synchronized burst discharge in disinhibited hippocampal slice: II. Model of cellular mechanism. *J. Neurophysiol.*, 49:459–471.

86. Turner, R. W., Richardson, T. L., and Miller, J. J. (1984): Ephaptic interactions contribute to paired pulse and frequency potentiation of hip-

pocampal field potentials. *Exp. Brain Res.,* 54:567–570.

87. Valdes, F., Dashieff, R. M., Birmingham, F., Crutcher, K., and McNamara, J. O. (1982): Benzodiazepine receptor increases following repeated seizures: Evidence for localization to dentate granule cells. *Proc. Natl. Acad. Sci.,* 79:193–197.

88. Valentino, R. J., and Dingledine, R. (1981): Presynaptic inhibitory effect of acetylcholine in the hippocampus. *J. Neurosci.,* 1:784–792.

89. Ward, A. A., Jr. (1972): Topical convulsant metals. In: *Experimental Models of Epilepsy,* edited by D. P. Purpura, J. K. Penry, D. B. Tower, D. M. Woodbury, and R. D. Walter, pp. 13–35. Raven Press, New York.

90. Wong, R. K. S., and Prince, D. A. (1978): Participation of calcium spikes during intrinsic burst firing in hippocampal neurons. *Brain Res.,* 159:385–390.

91. Wong, R. K. S., and Prince, D. A. (1981): Afterpotential generation in hippocampal pyramidal cells. *J. Neurophysiol.,* 45:86–97.

92. Wong, R. K. S., and Schwartzkroin, P. A. (1982): Pacemaker neurons in the mammalian brain: Mechanisms and function. In: *Cellular Pacemakers. Vol. 1: Mechanisms of Pacemaker Generation,* edited by D. O. Carpenter, pp. 237–254. Wiley, New York.

93. Wong, R. K. S., and Traub, R. D. (1983): Synchronized burst discharge in disinhibited hippocampal slice. I. Initiation in CA2–CA3 region. *J. Neurophysiol.,* 49:442–458.

94. Wong, R. K. S., Prince, D. A., and Basbaum, A. I. (1979): Intradendritic recordings from hippocampal neurons. *Proc. Natl. Acad. Sci.,* 76:986–990.

95. Wyler, A. R., and Bolender, N.-F. (1983): Preoperative CT diagnosis of mesial temporal sclerosis for surgical treatment of epilepsy. *Ann. Neurol.,* 13:59–64.

96. Yaari, Y., Konnerth, A., and Heinemann, U. (1983): Spontaneous epileptiform activity of CA1 hippocampal neurons in low extracellular calcium solutions. *Exp. Brain Res.,* 51:153–156.

Advances in Neurology, Vol. 44, edited by
A. V. Delgado-Escueta, A. A. Ward, Jr.,
D. M. Woodbury, and R. J. Porter.
Raven Press, New York © 1986.

51

Amino Acid and Catecholamine Markers of Metabolic Abnormalities in Human Focal Epilepsy

*Allan L. Sherwin and **Nico M. van Gelder

*Neuropharmacology Department, Montreal Neurological Institute, Montreal, Quebec, Canada H3A 2B4; and **Centre de Recherche en Sciences Neurologiques, Département de Physiologie, Faculté de Médecine, Université de Montréal, Montréal, Quebec, Canada H3C 3J7*

SUMMARY Studies of various parameters of amino acid and catecholamine metabolism in human cerebral cortex have provided a number of biochemical markers that appear to delineate areas of focal epileptic activity. These observations have been consolidated further by investigations of a number of experimental models of epilepsy in animals. In appraising this data, it is important to take into consideration whether the tissue samples were obtained during an actual seizure state or in an interictal period. It is also important when possible to assess the extent of astrogliosis and neuronal loss. Sites of spontaneously active epileptic spiking in the cerebral neocortex have a somewhat different amino acid profile when compared to gray matter obtained from surrounding nonspiking gyri several centimeters away. There is an elevation in glycine content, a relative diminution in taurine, and a trend towards lowered glutamic acid levels. However, the concentrations of the eight amino acids measured appear in both the foci and surround to still be within the general range for normal tissue.

Measurements of key enzymes involved in the synthesis and regulation of neurotransmitters provide a complementary method of evaluating functional changes in epileptic brain as they are generally less labile than their substrates. There is a moderate increase in the activity of glutamic acid dehydrogenase, an enzyme that plays an important role in the synthesis of glutamic acid from glucose. In some patients a decrease in glutamic acid decarboxylase has also been reported: this enzyme forms gamma-aminobutyric acid (GABA) from glutamic acid and is thus important for inhibition in the central nervous system. Moreover, there is a striking increase in the activity of tyrosine hydroxylase, the rate-limiting enzyme responsible for catecholamine synthesis. The possibility of a focal abnormality in catecholamine metabolism is reinforced by the simultaneous finding of a relative decrease in the number of alpha-1 postsynaptic receptor sites. An important marker of energy metabolism in neural tissue, Na^+,K^+-ATPase activity, has also been found to be decreased in actively spiking human cerebral cortex.

Data from experimental animal foci produced by topical application of convulsant agents show a consistent drop in glutamic acid tissue content. This can be matched to an efflux of glutamic acid from the cortical surface, which in turn is proportional to the electrographic activity of the spike focus. In addition, there is often also a decrease in taurine and GABA in such foci, as well as an increase in the levels of a number of neutral amino acids. Generalized seizures induced by the systemic administration of convulsants to animals were preceded by or coincided with a diminution in cerebral glutamic acid content. Following the onset of seizures, taurine levels tended to decrease in contrast to the gradual elevation observed in the GABA content. With respect to regulatory enzymes, the activity of tyrosine hydroxylase in cerebral cortex is elevated following repeated generalized electroconvulsive seizures, and this is associated with an increase in the turnover of norepinephrine and a decrease in the density of adrenergic receptor sites.

These findings point to the presence of an interrelated disturbance of energy, amino acid and catecholamine metabolism in epileptic cerebral cortex. None of these findings so far have been demonstrated unequivocally to be the direct cause for the development of epilepsy, but they are likely to contribute to the imbalance between excitation and inhibition that marks this dysfunction.

Human focal epilepsy has numerous etiologies, including anoxia, brain injury, infection, vascular lesions, and tumors, particularly teratomas and low-grade gliomas. The common denominator in all these lesions is the long latent period before the onset of epilepsy; during this period there is a gradual maturation of the lesion prior to the appearance of clinical seizures. Medial temporal (hippocampal) sclerosis is found in the majority of patients with temporal-lobe epilepsy (15). The histopathological findings in the neocortex of the convexity of the temporal lobe in the majority of patients with neurosurgically treatable focal epilepsy are surprisingly subtle, the most consistent finding being mild to moderate astrogliosis, with evidence of some neuronal loss (66). Biochemical abnormalities in human epilepsy as revealed by means of positron emission tomography (PET) with ^{18}F-fluorodeoxyglucose (FDG) (68) or oxygen-15 (145) include hypermetabolism during focal seizures but hypometabolism in the interictal period. The size of the zone of impaired glucose metabolism in temporal-lobe epilepsy is generally larger than the surgical pathological lesion but correlates well with the severity of the damage (68).

CHARACTERIZATION OF SURGICAL SPECIMENS

The description of tissues derived from neurosurgical treatment should always include observations of the appearance and consistency of the brain at the time of operation and the detailed histopathology of the immediately adjacent areas. It is also important if possible to indicate whether the region sampled was or was not the site of either electrographic or clinical seizure activity just prior to the time of the excision. Epileptiform discharges are activated by partial or complete withdrawal of antiepileptic drugs and electrical or pharmacological stimulation. Numerous important parameters of metabolic activity are considerably altered during or immediately following electrographic or behavioral seizures (11,68). Such activity will be significantly suppressed during general anesthesia especially if therapeutic levels of antiepileptic agents are maintained. Following phenobarbital withdrawal there is a significant increase in peak cerebral glucose metabolic rate, as demonstrated by means of FDG–PET (119).

The neuroanatomical features of the hippocampus, the amygdala, and the various regions of the neocortex must be taken into consideration in the selection of both test and control samples. Biochemical studies of gray matter will require meticulous dissection to remove the pia, superficial blood vessels and underlying white matter. Harvey et al. (48,111) found a substantial difference in the relative distribution of various antiepileptic drugs between cerebral cortex, subcortical white matter, and plasma at the time of operation. There is a good correlation between the actual brain antiepileptic drug content and seizure control, with phenobarbital and phenytoin having an additive effect (58,112). It is imperative to recognize and take cognizance of the many subtle differences in tissues derived from various forms of neurosurgical therapy. Ward (138) has recently summarized the principles of neurosurgical management of epilepsy. Technical factors, including the period of ischemia during surgery, may have both qualitative and quantitative effects on biochemical and morphological parameters depending on the stability of the substances being measured. The criteria for the classification and selection of patients for neurosurgical treatment have been reviewed by McNaughton and Rasmussen (70,71). A brief overview of some of the procedures utilized to identify and excise epileptogenic human tissues has been provided in Table 1 to illustrate some of the physiological and pharmacological variables that must be considered in evaluating biochemical data. Cooperative efforts between the various research groups involved in the study of neurosurgically derived tissue samples should help to reconcile certain differences in data. Experimental animal models designed to mimic neurosurgical conditions may also prove helpful, particularly in differentiating the effects of seizure activity and tissue damage. Studies of human epileptic tissues require a team approach to ensure quality control, and published work should include as many clinical and laboratory details as possible.

OVERALL ENERGY METABOLISM

Efforts to establish a causal relationship between biochemical changes in brain and epilepsy have included a number of direct measurements of metabolic conditions in tissues excised during the course of neurosurgical treatment. Elliott and Penfield (34) showed that the respiratory and glycolytic abilities of epileptogenic tissue were not abnormal. As samples of definitely normal tissue became available only rarely, they also carried out similar determinations on cerebral cortex from various mammalian species. The resulting biochemical data was plotted against body weight or brain weight on an appropriate scale, to derive by extrapolation or interpolation a probable average value for normal human brain. The variability found in other species provided an indication of the probable variability of average values for human tissue. Later studies by Pappius and Elliott (86) showed no significant difference in the total acetylcholine levels, sodium and potassium content, or magnesium-activated Na^+,K^+-ATPase. The latter enzyme is essential in the regulation of univalent cation transport in brain. Sherwin et al. (109) found a normal distribution of lactic dehydrogenase isoenzymes in human epileptic tissue even in areas of gliosis in contrast to malignant glial tumors, where there was a shift towards anaerobic glycolysis. The latter finding is consistent with the phenomenon of increased production of lactic acid by neoplastic tissues. Many radioisotope studies, culminating most recently in the PET technique, suggest an increase of glucose utilization in epileptic regions when these exhibit seizure activity, but suggest that apart from these periods such sites may be somewhat hypometabolic. The vast and growing literature on this subject may be fairly summarized by stating

TABLE 1. *Comparison of EEG, anesthetic, and neurosurgical techniques*[a]

1. (a) Extensive preoperative EEG videomonitoring with scalp and sphenoidal electrodes after reducing antiepileptic drug therapy. Operation under local anesthesia with neuroleptic drugs (fentanyl). Electocorticography (ECoG) using surface and depth electrodes acutely inserted into amygdaloid and/or hippocampal regions. Electrical stimulation of cortex and deep medial temporal structures. Methohexital activation often employed. Antiepileptic drugs discontinued just before operation. Subpial resection and partial *en bloc* excision (41,87,97,143).
   (b) Stereotaxic implantation of chronic depth electrodes under general anesthesia. Prolonged EEG videomonitoring following reduction in antiepileptic drug therapy including limited electrical stimulation. Operation after an interval of several weeks as described above (82,83).
   (c) Deviations from technique include general anesthesia with nitrous oxide in some cases, but this is discontinued 10 min before ECoG recording, relaxants allowed to wear off for stimulation of motor cortex. Supplemented by bolus injections of fentanyl (39,40).

2. EEG video investigation using stereotaxically implanted chronic depth electrodes with diminution of antiepileptic drug therapy. Operation later with full antiepileptic drug therapy and general anesthesia. ECoG occasionally employed. Block resection of temporal lobe with ligation of pial vessels (26,30,136).

3. Stereo EEG employing numerous stereotaxically implanted electrodes acutely over the course of part of a day or prolonged recording with chronically implanted electrodes. Recording of seizures enhanced by reduction of antiepileptic drug therapy. Electrical and pharmacological stimulation often employed. Operation several weeks later with full antiepileptic drug therapy and general anesthesia. Localized excision of epileptic foci or more extensive removal (3,10,106,118).

4. Subdural strip electrodes inserted under general anesthesia followed by prolonged EEG videomonitoring under reduced antiepileptic drug therapy. Operation after an interval as described in 1(a) (9,62,144).

5. Epidural electrodes placed at craniotomy under general anesthesia followed by prolonged recording extended by electrical stimulation following reduction of drug therapy. Second stage of operation under general anesthesia without further recording (43).

[a] This table is intended as an overview only; as techniques are frequently modified without further publication, precise details must be obtained directly from the individual neurosurgical centers.

that most indices of brain metabolism, including mitochondrial respiration, blood and oxygen supplies, energy substrate delivery, and pH, appear to be quite adequate and responsive to enhanced energy requirements during seizures.

AMINO ACID CHANGES IN HUMAN FOCAL EPILEPSY

The first study on the subject was by Tower (120,121), who observed that tissue levels of glutamic acid fell during incubation of brain slices from human epileptic cortex, in contrast to the increase observed in slices from normal cortex. The development of the automated amino acid analyzer enabled the authors (131) to carry out a more detailed survey of amino acid patterns in a series of patients with well localized foci in the temporal or frontal lobes [Table 1, method 1(a)]. These regions of active epileptic spiking could be clearly differentiated from a surrounding non-

spiking region, which by therapeutic necessity was also included in the excision (Figs. 1 and 2). Neither chronic depth electrode implantation nor preexcision methohexital activation of the ECoG were employed in this particular group of patients. Samples obtained from the surrounding nonspiking cerebral cortex served as a "disease" control in an effort to minimize the effects of previous drug therapy or operative conditions. The nonspiking areas selected were from the most peripheral available surrounding cortex and were only utilized if they had histopathologic findings similar to the spiking region. Samples for analysis were obtained immediately following complete excision of entire portions of the affected tissue; however, in some cases selected areas were removed early in the operation and frozen immediately. Both procedures yielded essentially similar results. Following excision of the biochemical samples, the immediately adjacent regions of cortex and white matter

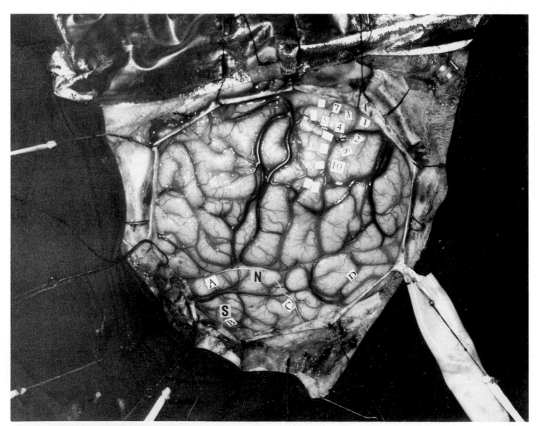

FIG. 1. Operative field for left temporal-lobe excision in a patient with partial seizures. Specimen from spiking cortex obtained at region marked S; nonspiking sample from area marked N. Histopathologic study of the cerebral cortex adjacent to both of these regions revealed a similar degree of mild astroglial proliferation with a few scattered clusters of reactive astrocytes without evidence of neuronal loss. (From ref. 114, with permission.)

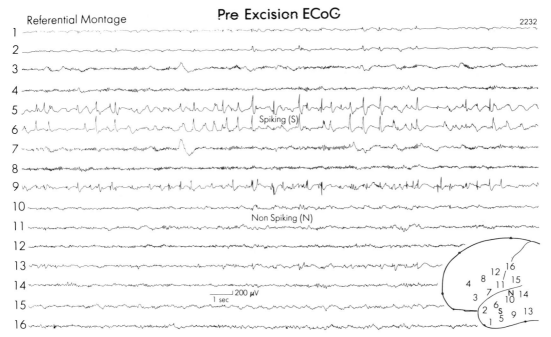

FIG. 2. Electrocorticogram (ECoG) of patient depicted in Fig. 1 showing active spiking at electrodes 5 and 6 in comparison to a nonspiking region at electrode 10. Operation under local anesthesia 17 days after antiepileptic drugs had been temporarily discontinued [Table 1, Method 1(a)]. (From ref. 114, with permission.)

werc submitted for histopathological study. Possible effects of the neurosurgical procedure on amino acid content were controlled by performing sham operations in monkeys, using electrocautery and suction.

The sites of spontaneously active epileptic spiking in the superficial cerebral cortex had a somewhat different amino acid profile when compared to gray matter obtained from surrounding nonspiking gyri several centimeters away. The differences were marked by the presence of an increase in glycine content, a relative diminution in taurine, and a trend towards lowered glutamic acid levels. Although these results supported the concept that actively spiking human epileptic cortex could be biochemically distinguished from the nonspiking surround, the lack of nonepileptic control tissue limited this study. The concentrations of the eight amino acids measured in ref. 131 and an additional report (132) appeared, in both the foci and surround, to be within the general range for normal tissue. The range of amino acid levels that might be anticipated in normal human cortex was estimated by extrapolation of the values quoted in the literature for humans and a number of other species (14,17).

Perry et al. (88,90) also determined the amino

acid content of actively spiking epileptic cortex, although the operative technique and drug therapy employed at the time of sampling differed considerably from the above study. Their patients were under general anesthesia with 0.5 percent halothane and the electrocorticographic (ECoG) epileptic discharges were activated by methohexital [Table 1; method 1(c) modified]. Cerebral cortex obtained from a group of nonepileptic patients (deep-brain tumors or head trauma), rather than an individually paired sample from the same patient, served as controls. A comparison between spike foci and nonspiking areas in epileptic patients exposed to the same drugs and operative conditions was thus not possible (32). These investigators also noted an elevated glycine level in some patients, but no significant abnormality in the tissue content of the other amino acids was found except for glutamic acid. They considered the concentration of this amino acid to be increased relative to their mean control value of 7.58 μmol/g. The latter value appears unusually low for normal tissue in view of the fact that the literature shows the range of glutamic acid levels in mammalian cortex to vary on the average between 10 to 12 μmol/g fresh tissue. Postmortem changes or anoxia cannot account for such a low level, as the same authors have shown that glutamic acid levels remain quite constant for long periods after death (89).

AMINO ACIDS AND CATECHOLAMINES IN EPILEPSY MODELS

The Glutamic Acid Cycle

Among the large number of substances and metabolic processes that have been found altered during various seizure conditions, few have so consistently been asociated with as many different forms of epilepsy as glutamic acid (135). The biological characteristics of this amino acid certainly fulfill many of the criteria to be anticipated if it were to participate in the epileptic process. Glutamic acid concentrations are among the highest of all free amino acids present in most cells, including neurons (soma, axo–dendritic extensions, as well as terminals). It represents an endogenous product of metabolism in most organs, especially brain, and a base-line quantity of glutamic acid is continuously released from the brain (11,127). Moreover, natural metabolic or physiological activation enhances its release. Upon external application to most mammalian neurons, glutamic acid causes rapid depolarization, which is sustained until application is discontinued, whereupon the membrane abruptly repolarizes (11). When introduced intracellularly or when applied externally, the amino acid appears to alter in *Aplysia* the discharge patterns of autonomously firing neurons (17), a process also known to be associated with intracellular calcium movement and affected by pentylenetetrazol (116). The physiological modifications of discharge patterns by the glutamate ion in some respects bear a striking resemblance to those demonstrated by Ward (137,142) to occur in discharging neurons of an epileptic region.

A complex metabolic cycle (Fig. 3) is present in the central nervous system that rapidly removes glutamic acid upon release by uptake into the glia, where it is converted by an energy-dependent reaction involving a nitrogenous donor group (NH_4R) to glutamine (neutralized). Glutamine in turn is transported back into neuronal elements where it is reconverted to glutamic acid, which may then give rise to the related amino acids aspartic acid and gamma-aminobutyric acid (GABA). It appears that this cycle of glutamic acid detoxification is limited either by the amount of glutamic acid that can be transformed into glutamine in glial elements and/or

by the rate at which glutamine can be processed out of the glia to give rise to GABA and a preferentially released small pool of glutamic acid (108,133). An excess of free glutamic acid (which is usually very small) and glutamine is transferred to the cerebrospinal fluid (CSF) via the interstitial fluid. Glutamine is by far the most abundant amino acid in the CSF, and hence the glutamate/glutamine ratio is very low. Woodbury and Esplin (141) were the first to demonstrate a significant relationship between brain GABA, the glutamate/glutamine concentration ratio, and seizure threshold. Later, Jasper et al. (51) showed that the rate of release of GABA and glutamic acid from the surface of the cerebral cortex in the cat exhibited systematic variations with the state of activation of the ECoG. The rate of release of glutamic acid was observed to be lower in sleeping cats than in aroused animals; the GABA release was reciprocal to that of glutamate, low in aroused and high in sleeping animals.

Koyama (55) found that the most pronounced decrease in glutamic acid and GABA occurred in the area adjacent to the application of cobalt that had induced the epileptic focus. This abnormality became progressively less with increasing distance from the lesion. Similar changes were observed in the endogenous amino acid content of chronically undercut cortex in the cat, but only when focal epileptogenicity developed (57). On superfusion of the exposed cortex with artificial CSF *in vivo*, both the cobalt focus and undercut cortex exhibited either no change or a small increase in the rates of release of aspartic acid and GABA. In contrast, these preparations consistently exhibited a marked (three- to fourfold) increase in the release rate of glutamic acid as compared with similarly superfused contralateral intact cortex (57). The diminution in glutamic acid content and its enhanced efflux from the cortical surface exhibited a temporal relationship to the onset of focal spiking in the EEG.

Dodd et al. (31), in a series of elegant experiments, showed that glutamic acid release is proportional to the activity of the epileptic discharge (Fig. 4). Cobalt lesions, which are very epileptogenic and produce clinical partial motor seizures, release approximately twofold more glutamic acid into the superfusate than the milder nickel foci, which induce EEG spikes but no behavioral attacks. This amount was in turn still higher than the release from a damaged but nonepileptic cobalt site. No release of GABA was observed from the epileptic foci in these

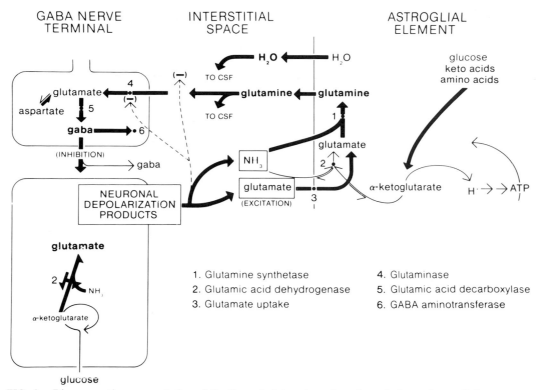

FIG. 3. Diagrammatic representation of the flow of glutamate carbon through the various cellular compartments of the CNS. During neuronal discharge ammonia generation increases, glucose metabolism accelerates and release of glutamate occurs. A combination of factors therefore promotes enhanced GDH activity during seizures. Glutamine synthesis in glia supplies a large part of the glutamate in nerve terminals where it serves as the substrate for GABA. (From ref. 134, with permission.)

models, perhaps due to its active reuptake while traversing the relatively long path of diffusion from the deeper cortical layers (e.g., layer 4). Another explanation may be that there is indeed some type of failure in GABA release mechanisms in seizure disorders as suggested by reports of low GABA levels in the CSF (46,63). Other changes in the CSF in epilepsy include an increase in the level of the brain isoenzyme of creatine phosphokinase (110), as well as alterations in taurine and glutamic acid (76). Dodd et al. (31) also noted a reduction in glutamine release from these active foci. This reduction is likely to reflect disturbed glutamine metabolism, which mainly takes place in the glia (see Fig. 3). The lower glutamine efflux and the absence of glycine release also helped rule out the possibility that the enhanced rate of glutamic acid efflux from the foci was merely due to local damage of the blood brain barrier, since glutamine and glycine levels are both very high in blood. The temporal coincidence of these events

is striking. The results, moreover, are complemented by data from a different but similarly conceived study (130) in which the amino acid content of the underlying cortex was measured. The reduction in the actual tissue glutamate content during the course of cobalt-induced epilepsy was also proportional to the severity of the seizure activity generated and the distance of the sampled site from the focus (130). Specific antagonists of excitation caused by glutamic and aspartic acids have an anticonvulsant action (28).

Amino Acids in Brain Tissue and Body Fluids

Some of the changes reported in the levels of various other amino acids in epileptic cortex can be attributed to a direct linkage of their metabolism to that of glutamic acid (glutamine, GABA, aspartic acid). For other amino acids, such a connection is either nonexistent (e.g., taurine, threonine) or tenuous at best (e.g., gly-

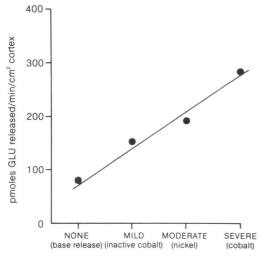

FIG. 4. Glutamic acid (GLU) release into cortical superfusate of 6-7 day-old epileptic foci in rats. This graph is plotted from data presented by Dodd et al. (31) to demonstrate a clear correlation between the relative intensity of the epileptic discharge (spiking) as shown by electrocorticography and the amount of glutamic acid released from the tissue. The "severe" spiking lesions were accompanied by behavioral seizures.

cine). With respect to certain nutritionally essential amino acids—for example, phenylalanine or threonine—the body fluid concentrations and tissue content are intimately dependent on sodium-stimulated transport and tissue-exchange mechanisms, which are also used by other nonessential neutral amino acids (e.g., tyrosine, serine, glycine). The alterations in the tissue levels of taurine are of considerable importance, since this amino acid is only to a small extent synthesized or metabolized in most mammals (128). Moreover, the transport (exchange) mechanisms responsible for maintaining the tissue content are not utilized by any other amino acid, with the exception perhaps of GABA or beta-alanine. Hence, a change of the tissue taurine levels implies, for the most part, an alteration in the ability of such tissues to sequester the amino acid within the cells. A loss of taurine from cells thus might be reflected by changes of body-fluid taurine concentrations (CSF and blood). Edmonds et al. (33) have carried out detailed studies of a strain of beagle dogs with a genetic predisposition to spontaneous tonic–clonic seizures. Biochemical studies performed in collaboration with van Gelder et al. (128) revealed that affected animals sampled in the nonseizure state exhibited both an enhanced loss of taurine from the cerebral

cortex and altered taurine concentrations in the blood. Anomalies in the ratios of the concentrations of these same amino acids have been reported by Aslam et al. (1) and Huxtable et al. (50) in studies of blood samples from patients with generalized epilepsy.

Catecholamines and the Seizure Threshold

Lesions of the dorsal noradrenergic bundle in rats lowers their threshold for pentylene tetrazol or maximal electroconvulsive seizures and also facilitates the production of seizures by kindling (23,65). These lesions result in a depletion of norepinephrine in the cortex and an increase in the alpha-1 receptor density (B_{max}), as can be demonstrated with labeled prazosin (72, 101). This may be an example of an increase in receptor sites as a consequence of a relative deficiency of neurotransmitter. Increasing central catecholamine levels significantly reduces the severity of seizures in spontaneously epileptic gerbils (24) or rats (54). The potential significance of the monoamines in the basic mechanisms of the epilepsies was first established by the purely clinical observations of the adverse effects of high-dose reserpine treatment employed some years ago for a variety of serious mental illnesses (4,92). Preparations from the roots of *Rauwolfia serpentina* had been used for centuries for the treatment of mental disorders (67). We now know that the mechanism underlying its sedative and antipsychotic effects includes a depletion of brain catecholamine stores. Among their actions, this group of neurotransmitters modulates the activity of neuronal networks, with norepinephrine exerting a predominantly inhibitory effect in the cerebral cortex. Reader et al. (98–100) have demonstrated electrophysiologically *in vivo* that norepinephrine also interacts with various other neurotransmitters, including the important inhibitory factor GABA, to enhance their effectiveness. In retrospect it is not surprising that reserpine was found to lower the threshold of patients for electroshock therapy and to cause some patients to have grand mal seizures for the first time (4). Epileptiform abnormalities were noted in the electroencephalograms (EEGs) of previously normal subjects. Patients with a past history of trauma or previous neurosurgical scars (topectomy, prefrontal lobotomy) were more prone to seizures. Patients with previously controlled epilepsy had a marked increase in frequency of both convulsive and petit mal attacks. The increased incidence of seizures did not persist beyond the first 6 weeks of reserpine therapy, even though high doses continued to be administered, suggesting an effect on seizure threshold which could be readily overcome by increasing antiepileptic drug dosage. Chen et al. (22) later observed that anticonvulsants such as phenytoin reversibly antagonize the effects of reserpine in a competitive fashion. Higher brain monoamine levels reduce seizure susceptibility, as shown by early observations of the anticonvulsant effect of monoamine oxidase inhibitors that block their metabolism (94). Experiments employing either an alpha-2 agonist (clonidine) or a beta antagonist (propanolol) ligands in animal models have revealed that these drugs have antiepileptic properties both *in vivo* (61,84,85) and *in vitro* (74). A good correlation between alterations in noradrenergic afferents and focal epileptic discharges has been demonstrated by Chauvel and colleagues in studies of cobalt epilepsy in the rat (12,20,122,123).

ENZYME DETERMINATIONS IN HUMAN EPILEPTIC FOCI

Glutamic Acid and Energy Metabolism

Measurement of enzymes associated with amino acid and neurotransmitter metabolism or activity-dependent energy utilization and cation transport is a complementary method of evaluating functional changes in epileptic brain. Enzymic activities are generally less labile than changes in their substrates, because protein synthesis plays a role. Rapport et al. (96), in a study of actively spiking human epileptic cortex, observed a localized reduction in Na$^+$,K$^+$-ATPase but not cholinesterase activity, in comparison to an adjacent nonspiking gyrus or control tissue from nonepileptic patients. These particular epileptic foci exhibited considerable astrogliosis on histological examination, which along with the observed neuronal loss may account for the discrepancy from the results of Pappius and Elliott (86) cited above. McGeer et al. (69) measured the activity of glutamic acid decarboxylase (GAD), the enzyme that decarboxylates glutamic acid to form GABA, in biopsies from epileptic foci obtained during neurosurgical therapy. Two patients exhibited normal enzymatic activity, while the third case was found to have somewhat low activity. The controls were cortex obtained at autopsy under conditions to ensure adequate preservation of enzyme activity. Tursky et al. (124) found no difference in the GAD activity of stereotaxic biopsy samples of human hippocampus as compared to nonep-

ileptic tissues removed during other types of neurosurgery. This report of normal GAD activity in epileptic hippocampus is supported by the detailed immunohistochemical studies of Babb et al. (see Chapter 48) who investigated patients undergoing temporal lobectomy at UCLA. They too could not detect a significant change. Tursky et al. (124) also noted no difference in the activity of pyridoxal kinase, which catalyzes the formation of the GAD cofactor, pyridoxal phosphate, or in oxygen consumption. They did find evidence of abnormal glial metabolism, as indicated by a lower incorporation of radioactively labeled carbon from acetate into glutamine. This suggests that epileptic tissue may have less ability to transform glutamate to glutamine, which is compatible with the notion that there is a localized disturbance in astroglial metabolism.

A recent survey by Sherwin et al. (114) of enzymic activities in human epileptic cortex (Table 2 and Fig. 5) also failed to find a significant increase in the mean activity of GAD in actively spiking cortical foci. All patients (51 cases) were operated upon following complete or partial withdrawal of antiepileptic drugs to activate the epileptic process, and except for 5 cases local anesthesia was employed. None had received valproic acid, which is a GABA aminotransferase (GABA-T) inhibitor and also exhibits prolonged pharmacologic effects. Approximately half the patients also received intravenous methohexital towards the end of the preexcision ECoG, in efforts to activate additional epileptic activity (Table 1; Method 1). It should be noted that most of the cortical tissues assayed in these studies, both spiking and nonspiking, were found to have only mild to moderate histopathological changes which were similar in specimens selected from both areas (Table 3 and Fig. 6). Medial temporal structures, which invariably show considerable astrogliosis and neuronal loss (15), had to be excluded from this study because the protocol required a suitably paired anatomically similar control.

Lloyd et al. (see Chapter 52), in contrast, observed a diminution of GAD activity in human epileptic foci. Such foci were identified by a stereo-EEG and followed by operation about 1 month later under general anesthesia with steady state antiepileptic drug therapy (Table 1; Method 3). The samples were obtained adjacent to sites of depth electrode implantation, and medial temporal structures were not excluded. The penetration of the cortex by a depth electrode results in localized necrosis with neuronal loss, which is known to stimulate the migration of

TABLE 2. *Comparison of enzymic activities in paired samples of focal spiking and peripheral nonspiking human epileptic neocortex each obtained from the same patient[a]*

Enzyme		Spiking	Nonspiking
Glutamic acid dehydrogenase	17	135.77 ± 10.22	118.58 ± 9.42[b]
Glutamic acid decarboxylase	13	10.63 ± 0.95	9.96 ± 1.10
GABA aminotransferase	12	36.49 ± 1.05	36.46 ± 1.48
Glutamine synthetase	20	96.94 ± 3.81	96.52 ± 4.10
Tyrosine hydroxylase	14	16.23 ± 2.39	10.67 ± 1.95[b]

[a] Values are micromole per hour per gram wet weight ± standard error, except for tyrosine hydroxylase, given in nanomoles per hour per gram wet weight.
[b] Significant at $p < 0.001$ (*t*-paired statistics).

astroglia from considerable distances toward the electrode tract. The dilution of neuronal structures by the glial proliferations could lower the total GAD activity in small samples from these regions. However, in all human studies of GAD activity there does appear to be a certain number of cases that demonstrate low enzyme activity. It may be possible therefore that in certain individuals a failure of GABA-mediated inhibition will contribute to seizure activity (36). In the data of Lloyd et al. (60), this phenomenon appears to be much more evident in various tumoral lesions where neuronal replacement by neoplastic glia would be expected.

Sherwin et al. (114) also examined the related enzyme GABA-T, which is responsible for the destruction of GABA; this enzyme exhibited somewhat less variability than GAD (Fig. 5). In agreement with Lloyd et al. (60), no difference in the activity of GABA-T was found in spiking cerebral cortex. Glutamine synthetase (GS),

which plays an important role in the detoxification of ammonia (27) by forming glutamine (Fig. 3), was also not altered in the foci. This enzyme is mainly localized in the glial cells and is being considered as a candidate for an astrocyte-specific marker (80). Posttraumatic astrogliosis and low-grade astrocytomas are both long known to give rise to epileptic discharges (66). Following experimental trauma to rat cortex, increased GS activity can be seen at the edge of the lesions within 15 min, reaching a maximum in 2 to 3 weeks, then subsiding to only a slight increase at 5 months (81). High-affinity uptake of beta-alanine is also increased in the margins of epileptogenic scars induced by the injection of ferric chloride in rat cortex (105). The absence of differences in GS activity between spiking and nonspiking cortex are not unexpected, since the majority of specimens exhibited only mild to moderated gliosis which was scattered and affected the two regions fairly equally. More re-

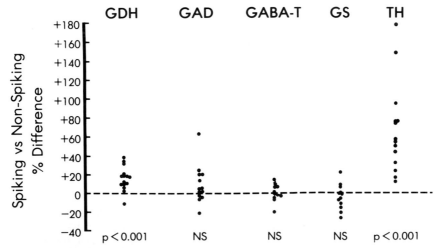

FIG. 5. A comparison between spiking epileptic human cerebral cortex and nonspiking surrounding cortex with respect to the activities of glutamic acid dehydrogenase (GDH), glutamic acid decarboxylase (GAD), GABA aminotransferase (GABA-T), glutamine synthetase (GS), and tyrosine hydroxylase (TH). Data refer to the percentage by which the enzyme activity of spiking cortex differs from its matching nonspiking control sample, [(spiking − nonspiking)/nonspiking] × 100. (From ref. 114, with permission.)

TABLE 3. *Distribution of neuropathological diagnoses in regions of human cerebral cortex sampled for enzymic analysis*

Group	Number of patients	Neocortical histopathology[a]
1	23	Very mild astroglial proliferation with a few clusters of reactive astrocytes scattered in the cortical neurophil without evidence of neuronal loss.
2	21	Mild to moderate astrogliosis with multiple cortical extensions of subpial or white matter and slight neuronal loss.
3	7	Marked proliferation of fibrous astrocytes with neuronal loss involving all cortical lamina in at least one convolutional segment.

[a] Histopathologic changes in hippocampus, amygdala, and other medial temporal structures were evaluated separately.

cently, a two- to threefold increase in GS activity in epileptic tissue with dense astrogliosis was noted in 3 ganglioglioma tumors and in 2 patients with very severe focal seizures due to tuberous sclerosis (113). The lesions in the latter 5 patients were all characterized by a striking proliferation of well-differentiated astrocytes. Increased amounts of GS and glial fibrillary acidic protein have also been demonstrated in astrocytomas by immunohistochemical techniques (91). The data suggest that increased GS activity may serve as a marker of astrocytic proliferation in certain types of epileptogenic lesions.

The spiking versus nonspiking investigative approach to delineate differences in human focal epilepsy has been validated further by the results of determinations of glutamic acid dehydrogenase (GDH) and tyrosine hydroxylase (TH) (114). GDH, the enzyme responsible for the incorporation of glucose carbon into glutamic acid via alpha-ketoglutarate, was elevated in all but one of 17 actively spiking foci (Table 2, Fig. 5). As this enzyme is allosterically regulated by adenosine 5'-diphosphate and guanosine 5'-triphosphate (7), it is conceivable that some change in its properties could accrue from the secondary effects of repeated neuronal discharge, as has been documented to occur in the case of TH (see below). During development and growth, brain levels of glutamic acid and GDH increase in a parallel manner so that activity of GDH becomes quite high in adult brain. Glucose supplies at least 10 times as much glutamic acid by synthesis in situ as from the blood (104). The reactions involved include transamination or reductive amination of alpha-ketoglutaric acid, the latter is catalyzed by GDH. Moreover, GDH is likely to play a role in detoxifying ammonia known to be released as the result of epileptic activity. A kinetic analysis of GDH enzymic activity in actively spiking human cerebral cortex (114) demonstrates that the ami-

nating reaction involving the condensation of ammonia and alpha-ketoglutaric acid is much more likely to occur than the degradation of glutamic acid (21). This is further corroborated by the high levels of glutamic acid present in neural tissue.

Tyrosine Hydroxylase and Adrenoceptors

A most striking finding in our study was the observation that regions of focal epileptic spiking were marked by a significant increase (52.1%) in the activity of TH, which is the rate-controlling enzyme in catecholamine biosynthesis (Table 2, Fig. 5). This increase was associated with spontaneous epileptic activity, as it was also found in cases where neither electrical stimulation nor methohexital activation were employed. The activity of this enzyme reflects neuronal excitability, in that depolarization of the central or peripheral sympathetic nervous system stimulates TH activity and catecholamine production (107). This abnormality, which hints at altered monoaminergic function in epileptic tissue, has been reinforced by a subsequent study of adrenoceptor-binding sites in membranes prepared from spiking and nonspiking cortex (13). The radioligands employed were ^{3}H-prazosin (for alpha-1 sites), ^{3}H-p-aminoclonidine (for alpha-2 sites), and ^{3}H-dihydroalprenolol (for beta sites). In regions of active spiking, there was a significant reduction in the number (B_{max}) of alpha-1 postsynaptic receptor binding sites without any change in their affinity (K_d). The density and affinity of the alpha-2 and beta receptors, in contrast, were not altered. The combination of an increase in TH activity and a diminution in the number of receptor sites suggests a subsensitivity of postsynaptic alpha-1 adrenoceptors (37). The adrenoceptors are potentially useful markers of the diverse processes involved in the development of

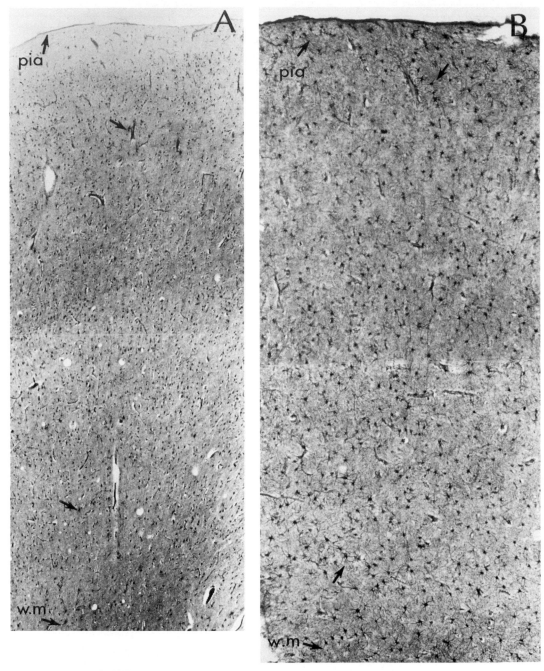

FIG. 6. Neocortical histopathology. **A:** Transverse cortical section of anterior temporal lobe showing mild gliosis in the form of scattered hypertrophic astrocytes. *Arrows* point toward two reactive astrocytic clusters. **B:** Transverse section of slightly atrophic temporal cortex with severe gliosis involving all lamina. *Arrows* point toward clusters of hypertrophic astrocytes. Cajal gold chloride sublimate stain; **A** × 21, **B** × 34. (From author's unpublished data, courtesy of Dr. Yvon Robitaille.)

focal neuronal hyperexcitability. They are composed of proteins that are firmly lodged in cellular membranes and thus have both a structural identity and a physiological function.

ENZYME CHANGES IN EPILEPSY MODELS

Glutamate and Energy Metabolism

Histochemical studies of cortex from cobalt epilepsy in rat and some human foci have shown increased GDH activity (14). Similar results were obtained in experimental portal–systemic encephalopathy in the rat, a condition in which hepatic coma is often preceded by hyperexcitability (79). Also in rat, GDH activity was found increased just prior to and during certain types of seizures (140). On the other hand, two reports describe decreased GDH activities, one associated with topical mescaline application to the cortex (73), the other involving a circumscribed cobalt focus (126). These discrepancies once more underline that animal models of epilepsy can only serve as approximations of the condition encountered in humans. In the majority of GAD studies in animals, the region assayed was clearly associated with an extensive area of tissue injury. Ribak et al. (102) have shown that epileptic foci induced by the application of alumina cream to monkey neocortex are characterized by astrogliosis along with a significant decrease in the number of axon terminals that contain immunoreactive GAD. There is also a reduction in the number of symmetrical synapses (103), which is similar to abnormalities observed in neuropathological studies of human focal epilepsy (15). This would suggest a functional loss of GABAergic inhibitory synapses in astroglial scars. Bakay and Harris (2) in similar studies in the monkey found that epileptic cortex demonstrated markedly reduced GABA–receptor binding. When the epileptic condition did not involve damage to the CNS, such as in various strains of animals genetically predisposed to epilepsy, no evident deficiencies of GAD or GABA have been detected (1). The other two enzymes directly implicated in GABA metabolism, GS and GABA-T, have not been reported altered in most studies.

Tyrosine Hydroxylase and Adrenoceptors

Tyrosine hydroxylase activity is significantly elevated in the midbrain of the epilepsy prone rat (29). In normal rats, a single electroconvulsive seizure (ECS) leads to a transient increase in the activity of TH in the striatum; the change is attributed to a conformational change in the enzyme, resulting in an augmented affinity of the apoenzyme for its pteridine cofactor (64). Repeated daily ECS treatment leads to a long lasting increase in TH activity as a consequence of increased new enzyme synthesis. These changes are first observed in the locus coeruleus, followed 1 to 4 days later by certain other brain areas. This does not appear to be a generalized response of all catecholaminergic neurons within the brain, and the change may be restricted to noradrenergic neurons. The delay observed for changes in immunoreactive TH is in keeping with the transport of enzyme from its production site in the locus coeruleus to nerve terminals in such structures as the hippocampus, cerebellum, and frontal lobe. Changes in TH activity resulting from repeated ECS (75) or direct stimulation of the locus coruleus (59) are accompanied by an increased turnover of norepinephrine (53,67,107). There is a concomitant decrease in the number of adrenoceptor binding sites (B_{max}) without any alteration in their affinity (52,115). Such alterations have been postulated to be part of the mechanism responsible for the therapeutic efficacy of electroshock therapy in depressive illness, as similar changes can be observed in animals receiving repeated ECS or the antidepressant drug imipramine (8). The enhanced TH activity accompanied by decreased adrenoceptor site density is also compatible with the observation that a similar increase in TH activity in frontal cortex occurs when the alpha-1 postsynaptic receptors are blocked following the administration of the specific antagonist drug prazosin to rats (37).

BIOCHEMICAL CHANGES IN EPILEPTOGENESIS

Biochemical changes found in experimental or spontaneous epileptic conditions may or may not be significant etiologically. Physical injury by itself can induce similar although less dramatic alterations in amino acids, catecholamines, or enzymes. Moreover, since such injuries, combined with a genetic predisposition, may be a trigger for the onset of a chronic seizure state, the biochemical correlates of brain injury and epilepsy may partially overlap. An appraisal of findings such as those reported above must thus take into consideration whether the changes are not only coincident with seizures but also evolve in temporal relationship with the development of epilepsy. Finally, as has been emphasized by Gloor (42), a distinction has to be made between the biochemical characteristics of a central nervous system chronically predisposed towards the development of epilepsy (genetic and/or environmental) and acute changes associated with actual seizures.

In an attempt to address some of these issues, data from a number of studies have been compiled as shown in Tables 4 and 5. Amino acid changes in cortex actually exhibiting seizure activity at the time of removal can be subdivided into data from cerebral cortex subjected to physical injury and tissue removed from previously normal animals injected with a convulsant agent (Table 4). In Table 5, the data is derived from studies of conditions where there is a spontaneously occurring epileptic predisposition but where the brain was not necessarily in a seizure state at the time of sampling. One can draw several conclusions from these results, subject to debate, but the one outstanding consistency is the invariable deficiency of glutamic acid, combined with a tendency for an increase among several neutral amino acids: glycine, alanine, threonine, and serine (129,130). Taurine, despite its apparent implication in the epileptic process, shows far less consistent changes, although when an alteration does occur it usually is in the direction of a decrease. GABA levels are almost always decreased in damaged epileptic cortex, either because of the damage or because the tissues were in a seizure condition at the time of removal.

A recent study attempted to trace the course of amino acid alterations accompanying epileptic events in the cerebral cortex (134). Cats were injected intramuscularly with a large dose of penicillin, and the removal of tissue samples was matched to the electrophysiological signs of generalized spike-and-wave epilepsy (Fig. 7). If specific amino acid changes are indeed to be considered as being part of the pathogenesis of the epileptic discharge, they should precede the electrographic manifestations. Such a temporal sequence is demonstrated in the preepileptic state before the onset of the epileptic discharge that coincides with the decrease in the cortical content of glutamic acid (IIB, Fig. 7). This change occurred when an increased amplitude of visual evoked potentials in association cortex heralds the gradual onset of spike-and-wave epileptic activity. The decrease of glutamic acid and that of aspartic acid occur in parallel with an almost stoichiometric increase of glutamine, GABA, or both, while taurine levels in the preepileptic state remain near normal. As the preepileptic state progresses to an epileptic condition, characterized by absence seizures and generalized 4- to 5-Hz spike-and-wave discharges, a failure of glial capture mechanisms for taurine and glutamate appears to occur, since both

TABLE 4. *Changes in brain amino acid content in animal models of epilepsy*[a]

Convulsant	Species	Tau	Asp	Glu	Gln	GABA	Thr	Ser	Gly	Ala	Reference
Topical (brain damage)											
Cobalt	Cat	↑	↓	↓		↓	↑	↑	↑		(55)
Cobalt	Cat	—	↓	↓	↑	↓		↑	↑	↑	(125)
Cobalt	Mouse	↓	—	↓		↓		↑	↑	↑	(125)
Penicillin	Cat			↓		↓					(44)
Cobalt	Rat	↓	↓	↓	—		—	—	—	↑	(25)
Cobalt	Rat		↓	↓	—	↓			—		(35)
Penicillin	Cat	↓	—	—	—	↓	—	—	—	↑	(76)
Cobalt	Cat	↓	↓	↓	↓	↓	↑	↑	↑	↑	(76)
Cobalt	Mouse	↓	↓	↓		↓		—	↑		(16)
Systemic (no damage)											
Pentylenetetrazol	Mouse								↑		(5)
Bicuculline	Rat		↓	↓	↑	↑				↑	(18)
Penicillin	Cat	—									(38)
Pentylenetetrazol	Mouse	—									(6)
Pentylenetetrazol	Rabbit	—									(6)
Penicillin	Cat	↓	↓	↓	—	↑	—	—	—	—	(134)
L-Allyl glycine	Rat	—	—	—	↑	↓					(19)
Bicuculline	Rat	↑	—	—	—	↑					(19)
Kainic acid	Rat	↓	↓	↓	↓	↑					(19)

[a] Modified from ref. 1, with permission.
[b] Increased (↑) or decreased (↓) significantly as compared to controls, or unchanged (—).

TABLE 5. *Changes in brain amino acid content in spontaneously occurring human and animal epilepsy*

Reference	Species investigated	Damage	Amino acids analyzed[a]					
			Tau	Asp	Glu	Gln	GABA	Gly
(121)	Human	Yes			↓			
(125)	Human	Yes	↓	—	↓	—	—	↑
(88)	Human	Yes	—	—	↑	—	↑	↑
(56)	Cat	Yes	↓	↓	↓	↓	↓	↑
(47)	Baboon	No	—	—	—	—	—	—
(33)	Dog	No	—	—	—	—	—	—
(49)	Rat	No	—	—	—	—	—	—
(77)	Mouse	No			↓	↓	↑	

[a] Increased (↑) or decreased (↓) significantly as compared to controls, or unchanged (—).

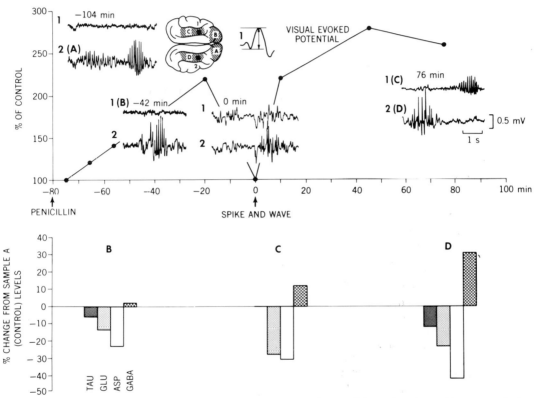

FIG. 7. Illustration of parallel changes in EEG, visual evoked potentials, and amino acid content during development of generalized penicillin epilepsy in the cat. **Top:** Selected EEG samples are shown along with the evolution of the visual evoked potentials. Penicillin was injected 80 min before the first appearance of spike-and-wave discharge (0 min). Insets show the recording points (1 and 2), areas sampled (**A–D**, *shaded*), and the measured visual potential (from point 1). **Bottom:** Changes in brain tissue content of taurine (TAU), glutamic acid (GLU), aspartic acid (ASP), and GABA are expressed in percentage of control values (sample A). After sample A had been taken, 24 min before penicillin injection, spindles appeared homolaterally. At 38 min after penicillin injection, when the EEG had not changed appreciably but the visual evoked potentials had increased to 175% of control value, sample B was taken. There is a significant diminution of GLU and ASP and a minor decrease of TAU. Spike-and-wave discharge started 42 min later. At the time when samples C and D were removed, a left–right asymmetry in epileptic activity was noted. While the right cortex [trace 2 (D)] continued to exhibit spike-and-wave bursts, the left cortex [trace 1(C)] showed only spindles for more than 15 min. This difference is reflected in the biochemical findings with respect to differences of TAU and GABA between samples C and D. Note that despite the absence of epileptic discharge in sample C, the evoked potential at 76 min, monitored from point 1, was still increased, indicating a persistent enhanced responsiveness to visual stimuli. (From ref. 134, with permission.)

amino acids are lost from the tissue. Glutamine levels fall while GABA concentrations are maintained or become elevated, but increasingly at the expense of aspartic acid. A plausible explanation for the increasing excitability during the development of epilepsy in this model may be a presumed increase in interstitial glutamic acid concentration, possibly in combination with subsequent failure of GABA inhibition. These findings closely parallel the amino acid changes observed by Chapman et al. (19) following systemic bicucullin-induced seizure development and are compatible with previous findings in experimental and spontaneous forms of epilepsy in animals and humans. Quite evidently, this type of combined electrophysiological and biochemical approach aimed at elucidating the specific causes of epilepsy is a promising method for future research.

The catecholamines have also been shown to influence the metabolism of amino acids (139), cyclic nucleotides (45), and other neurotransmitters (116). Stimulation of glucose metabolism and glucose entry by catecholamines has been associated with a more rapid turnover of glutamic acid (78), and this association provides the possibility of a functional interrelation between the observed increase in the activities of GDH and TH. The data obtained this far suggest that there may be a localized defect in catecholamine metabolism and the adrenoceptors at sites of active focal epileptic discharge in human epileptic cortex. This may impair the action of GABA as well as diminishing the activities of certain key enzymes such as Na^+,K^+-ATPase (Na^+/K^+ exchange pump) and adenylate cyclase, which are stimulated by the binding of norepinephrine to adrenoceptors (117). The findings thus complement the earlier report from the University of Washington of a localized decrease in the activity of Na^+,K^+-ATPase in actively spiking cortex as compared to an adjacent gyrus (95). Grisar et al. (see Chapter 53) recently found alterations in this enzyme in astroglial cells isolated from human epileptic brain. These enzymes are essential in the regulation of univalent cation transport and activity-dependent energy utilization in nervous tissue. Repeated noradrenergic stimulation increases base-line Na^+,K^+-ATPase activity, an effect that can be inhibited by blocking the adrenoceptors receptors with the alpha-1 antagonist prazosin (117). This receptor-mediated stimulation is also reduced, to a lesser extent, by the beta-receptor antagonist propranolol. An interaction between both alpha- and beta-receptors may be involved, as has been shown to occur for catecholamine-stimulated adenylate cyclase. The stimulation of the Na^+,K^+-ATPase by norepinephrine is consistent with many of its physiological effects, including ouabain-inhibited hyperpolarization *in vitro* and *in vivo* and alterations in the sensitivity to other neurotransmitters.

A FINAL APPRAISAL

None of the metabolic alterations found so far in human focal epileptic brain can be clearly associated with the origin of the epileptic state but may merely reflect the end result of enhanced discharge activity. This appears to be the case, for example, with respect to the localized elevation of TH activity in regions of active focal spiking. The diminution in the density of alpha-1 postsynaptic receptor sites, however, may prove to be marker of a localized deficit in local cortical inhibitory mechanisms responsible for preventing the spread of the epileptiform activity (93). Moreover, when all the data obtained by the various investigative groups are taken together, they point to a partial "uncoupling" of the integrated series of metabolic mechanisms that normally assure a smooth redistribution of the glucose carbon and free ammonia among various cellular compartments of the CNS (78). In the process, glutamic acid, a strongly excitatory substance, is formed but is then transformed into glutamine, which represents an easily diffusible and electrophysiologically neutral form of glutamic acid. Glutamine in turn gives rise eventually to the potent inhibitory agent GABA and, to a lesser extent, the excitatory amino acid aspartate. An excessive efflux of glutamic and aspartic acid could pose difficulties in maintaining normal GABA-mediated inhibition, aside from the possibility that the process will cause excessive excitation because of the depolarizing action on neurons in the vicinity of excessive release. It is more likely that the two phenomena are never entirely separable, and it may be a moot debate to argue that epilepsy represents a specific failure of inhibition or a uniquely excessive excitation process.

One point nevertheless needs to be emphasized when contemplating new therapeutic approaches to the treatment of epilepsy. It is quite obvious that the glial elements play a crucial role in balancing glutamic acid-mediated excitation and inhibition modulated by GABA. These cells represent a "buffer" by transforming glutamic acid into glutamine to provide the substrate for GABA synthesis at inhibitory synapses. The process is complex, energy-requiring, and ammonia- and pH-regulated. Other modulatory influences include the levels of calcium (116), zinc, and taurine, and the effects of important osmotic adjustments. Yet, unlike neurons, glial function appears to be far more plastic. These cells can and do proliferate even in adulthood; their energy substrates are far less selective and more versatile, while their capacity to capture extraneous substances is prodigious. For all these reasons it would appear that even if epilepsy might not represent a direct malfunction of glia per se, therapeutic manipulation to enhance the metabolic buffering capacity of these cells may offer some promise of alleviating this disorder. Furthermore, the possibility exists for an enhancement of the natural inhibitory mechanisms by the use of appropriate adrenoceptor agonist or antagonist ligands as adjuncts in the treatment of certain epilepsies. This may be particularly appropriate when an already abnormal seizure threshold is reduced further by sleep deprivation or hormonal changes during the menstrual cycle.

ACKNOWLEDGMENTS

We thank Dr. A. Olivier (Neurosurgery), Dr. Y. Robitaille (Neuropathology), Dr. F. Quesney (Electrocorticography), Dr. M. Abou-Madi (Neuroanesthesiology), and Ms. N. Isaacs (Nursing) for their expert assistance and advice. The submission of this manuscript coincided with the fiftieth anniversary of the Montreal Neurological Institute. The authors also wish to express their appreciation to Dr. T. Rasmussen, Dr. H. H. Jasper, Dr. K. A. C. Elliott, Dr. J. P. Robb, and Dr. W. Feindel for their interest in our collaborative research during the latter third of this period. This work was supported by the Medical Research Council of Canada (grant MT1451, to A. L. Sherwin).

This chapter is dedicated to Dr. Francis L. McNaughton, former neurologist-in-chief of the Montreal Neurological Institute and the first full professor of neurology at McGill University. A gifted diagnostician and dedicated teacher of both neuroanatomy and clinical neurology, he has made fundamental contributions to the International Classification of the Epilepsies through his detailed studies of the functional anatomy of the human cerebral cortex.

REFERENCES

1. Aslam-Janjua, N., Metrakos, J. D. and van Gelder, N. M. (1982): Plasma amino acids in epilepsy. In: *Genetic Basis of the Epilepsies,* edited by V. E. Anderson, W. A. Hauser, J. K. Penry, and C. F. Sing, pp. 181–197. Raven Press, New York.

2. Bakay, R. A. E., and Harris, A. B. (1981): Neurotransmitter, receptor and biochemical changes in monkey cortical epileptic foci. *Brain Res.,* 206:387–404.

3. Bancaud, J., Talairach, J., Waltregny, P., Bresson, M., and Morel, P. (1968): L'Activation par la mégimide dans le diagnostic topographique des épilepsies corticales focales (étude clinique, EEG at SEEG). *Rev. Neurol.,* 119:320–325.

4. Barsa, J. A., and Kline, N. S. (1955): Treatment of two hundred disturbed psychotics with reserpine. *J.A.M.A.,* 158:110–113.

5. Battistin, L., Varotto, M., and De Lorenzi, A. (1975): Amino acid uptake in vivo by the mouse brain and by various regions of the rabbit brain after drug-induced convulsions. *Brain Res.,* 89:215–224.

6. Battistin, L., Varotto, M., Tezzon, F., and Pistollato, L. (1979): Levels and uptake of taurine in various brain regions after drug induced generalized convulsions. *Neurochem. Res.,* 4:457–464.

7. Bayley, P. M., and Radda, G. K. (1966): Conformational changes and the regulation of glutamate dehydrogenase activity. *J. Biochem.,* 98:105–111.

8. Bergstrom, D. A., and Kellar, K. J. (1979): Adrenergic and serotonergic receptor binding in rat brain after chronic desmethylimipramine treatment. *J. Pharmacol. Exp. Ther.,* 209:256–261.

9. Blume, W. T., Girvin, J. P., McLachlan, R. S., and Jones, D. C. (1984): Use of subdural electroencephalography in candidates for surgical relief of uncontrolled partial epileptic seizures. *Can. J. Neurosci.,* 11:333.

10. Bouvier, G., Saint-Hilaire, J. M., Vezina, J. L., Béique, R., and Picard, R. (1976): La chirurgie fonctionnelle de l'épilepsie. *Union Med. Can.,* 105:1483–1485.

11. Bradford, H. F., and Dodd, P. R. (1976): Biochemistry and basic mechanisms in epilepsy. In: *Biochemistry and Neurological Disease,* edited by A. N. Davison, pp. 114–167. Blackwell Scientific, Oxford.

12. Bregman, B., Dedek, J., Nassif, S., Trottier, S., and Chauvel, P. (1983): Noradrenergic mechanisms control propagation of chronic cobalt activities in the rat. In: *Current Problems in Epilepsy, Vol. 1: Cerebral Blood Flow, Metabolism and Epilepsy,* edited by M. Baldy-Moulinier, D. H. Ingvar, and B. S. Meldrum, pp. 351–356. Libbey, London.

13. Brière, R., Sherwin, A. L., Robitaille, Y., Olivier, A., Quesney, F., and Reader, T. (1986): Alpha-1 adrenoceptors are decreased in human epileptic foci. *Ann. Neurol.,* 19 (*in press*).

14. Brotchi, J. (1978): The activated astrocyte: A histochemical approach to the epileptic focus. In: *Dynamic Properties of Glia Cells,* edited by E. Schoffeniels, G. Franck, L. Hertz, and D. B. Tower, pp. 429–433. Pergamon, Oxford.

15. Brown, W. J. (1973): Structural substrates of seizure foci in the human temporal lobe. In: *Epi-*

lepsy, its Phenomena in Man, edited by M. A. B. Brazier, pp. 339–374. Academic, New York.

16. Carruthers-Jones, D. I., and van Gelder, N. M. (1978): Influence of taurine dosage on cobalt epilepsy in mice. *Neurochem. Res.* 3:115–123.

17. Chaplaia, R. A., and Kraner, G. (1976): The effect of glutamate on heating pacemaker neurons isolated from the abdominal ganglion of *Aphysia californica. Brain Res.,* 101:141–147.

18. Chapman, A. G., Meldrum, B. S., and Siesjö, B. K. (1977): Cerebral metabolic changes during prolonged epileptic seizures in rats. *J. Neurochem,* 28:1025–1035.

19. Chapman, A. G., Westerberg, E., Premachandra, M., and Meldrum, B. S. (1984): Changes in regional neurotransmitter amino acid levels in rat brain during seizures induced by L-allyglycine, bicuculline and kainic acid. *J. Neurochem.,* 43:62–70.

20. Chauvel, P., Trottier, S., Nassif, S., and Dedek, Jr. (1982): Une alteration des afferences noradrenergiques est-elle en cause dans les epilepsies focales? *Ref. Electroencephalogr. Neurophysio. Clin.,* 12:1–7.

21. Chee, P. Y., Dahl, J. L., and Fabien, L. A. (1979): The purification and properties of rat brain glutamate dehydrogenase. *J. Neurochem.,* 33:53–60.

22. Chen, G., Ensor, C. R., and Bohner, B. (1954): A facilitation action of reserpine on the central nervous system. *Proc. Soc. Exp. Biol. Med.,* 86:507–510.

23. Corcoran, M. E., and Mason, S. T. (1980): Role of forebrain catecholamines in amygdaloid kindling. *Brain Res.,* 190:473–484.

24. Cox, B., and Lomax, P. (1976): Brain amines and spontaneous epileptic seizures in the mongolian gerbil. *Pharmacol. Biochem. Behav.,* 4:263–267.

25. Craig, C. R., and Hartman, E. R. (1973): Concentration of amino acids in the brain of cobalt-epileptic rat. *Epilepsia,* 14:409–414.

26. Crandall, P. H. (1973): Developments in direct recordings from epileptogenic regions in the surgical treatment of partial epilepsies. In: *Epilepsy: Its Phenomena in Man,* edited by M. A. B. Brazier, pp. 287–310. Academic, New York.

27. Cremer, J. E. (1964): Amino acid metabolism in rat brain studied with ^{14}C-labelled glucose. *J. Neurochem.,* 11:165–168.

28. Croucher, M. J., Collins, J. F., and Meldrum, B. S. (1982): Anticonvulsant action of excitatory amino acid antagonists. *Science,* 26:899–901.

29. Dailey, J. W., Battarbee, H. D., and Jobe, P.C. (1982): Enzyme activities in the central nervous system of the epilepsy-prone rat. *Brain Res.,* 231:225–230.

30. Delgado-Escueta, A. V., and Walsh, G. D. (1983): The selection process for surgery of intractable complex partial seizures: Surface EEG and depth electrography. In: *Epilepsy,* edited by A. A. Ward, Jr., J. K. Penry, and D. Purpura, pp. 295–326. Raven Press, New York.

31. Dodd, P. R., Bradford, H. F., Abdul-Ghani, A. S., Cox, D. W. G., and Continho-Netto, J. (1980): Release of amino acids from chronic epileptic and subepileptic foci in vivo. *Brain Res.,* 193:505–517.

32. Durelli, L., and Mutani, R. (1983): The current status of taurine in epilepsy. *Clin. Neuropharmacol.,* 6:37–48.

33. Edmonds, H. L., Hegreberg, C. C., van Gelder, N. M., Sylvester, D. M., Clemmons, R. M., and Chatburn, C. C. (1979): Spontaneous convulsions in beagle dogs. In: *Animal Models of Epilepsy (Symp.),* Fed. Proc., 38:2424–2428.

34. Elliott, K. A. C., and Penfield W. (1948): Respiration and glycolysis of focal epileptogenic human brain tissue. *J. Neurophysiol.,* 11:485–490.

35. Emson, P. C., and Joseph M. H. (1975): Neurochemical and morphological changes during the development of cobalt-induced epilepsy in the rat. *Brain Res.,* 93:91–110.

36. Fariello, R. G. (1985): Perspectives in the development of antiepileptic drugs: The importance of the GABA and glutamate systems. In: *Epilepsy,* edited by P. Morselli and R. J. Porter. Butterworth, London (*in press*).

37. French, T. A., Masserano, J. M., and Weiner, N. (1983): Activation of tyrosine hydroxylase in the frontal cortex by phentolamine and prazosin. *J. Pharm. Pharmacol.,* 35:618–620.

38. Frigyesi, T. L., and Lombardini, J. B. (1978): Lack of correlation between taurine levels in 16 brain regions and paroxysmal discharges in the thalamocortical circuit. *Neurosci. Lett.,* 7:213–217.

39. Geevarghese, K. P., and Garretson, H. D. (1977): "Alert" anesthesia in craniotomy. In: *Anesthesia for Neurological Surgery (International Anesthesiology Clinics),* edited by K. P. Geevarghese, pp. 231–251. Little, Brown, Boston.

40. Gilbert, R. G. B., and Brindle, G. F. (1966): Anesthetic management for surgery of temporal lobe epilepsy. In: *Anesthesia for Neurosurgery,* edited by R. G. B. Gilbert, G. F. Brindle, and A. Galindo, pp. 842–847. Little, Brown, Boston.

41. Gloor, P. (1975): Contributions of electroencephalography and electrocortiography to the neurosurgical treatment of the epilepsies. In: *Advances in Neurology, Vol. 8: Neurosurgical Management of the Epilepsies,* edited by D. P. Purpura, J. K. Penry, and R. D. Walter, pp. 59–105. Raven Press, New York.

42. Gloor, P. (1982): Toward a unifying concept of epileptogenesis. In: *Advances in Epileptology: XIIIth. Epilepsy International Symposium,* edited by H. Akimoto, H. Kazamatsuri, M. Seino, and A. A. Ward, Jr., pp. 83–86. Raven Press, New York.

43. Goldring, S. (1978): A method for surgical management of focal epilepsy, especially as it relates to children. *J. Neurosurg.,* 49:344–356.

44. Gottesfeld, Z., and Elazar, Z. (1972): GABA and glutamate in different EEG stages of the penicillin focus. *Nature (Lond.),* 240:478–479.

45. Gross, R. A., and Ferrendelli, J. A. (1982): Re-

lationships between norepinephrine and cyclic nucleotides in brain and seizure activity. *Neuropharmacol.*, 21:655–661.

46. Hagenfeldt, L., Bjerkenstedt, L., Edman, G., Sedvall, G., and Wiesel, F. A. (1984): Amino acids in plasma and CSF and monamine metabolites in CSF: Interrelationship in healthy subjects. *J. Neurochem.*, 42:833–837.

47. Hansen, S., Perry, T. L., Wada, J. A., and Sokol, M. (1973): Brain amino acids in baboon with light-induced epilepsy. *Brain Res.*, 50:480–483.

48. Harvey, C. D., Sherwin, A. L., and van der Klein, E. (1977): Distribution of anticonvulsant drugs in gray and white matter of human brain. *Can. J. Neurosci.*, 4:89–92.

49. Huxtable, R. J., and Laird, H. E. (1978): Are amino acid patterns necessarily abnormal in epileptic brains? Studies on the genetically seizure-susceptible rat. *Neurosci. Lett.*, 10:341–345.

50. Huxtable, R. J., Laird, H., Lippincott, S. E., and Watson, P. (1983): Epilepsy and the concentration of plasma amino acids in humans. *Neurochem. Int.*, 5:125–135.

51. Jasper, H. H., Khan, R. T., and Elliott, K. A. C. (1965): Amino acids released from the cerebral cortex in relation to its state of activation. *Science*, 147:1448–1449.

52. Kellar, K. J., Cascio, C. S., Bergstrom, D. A., Butler, J. A., and Iadarola, P. (1981): Electroconvulsive shock and reserpine: Effects on β-adrenergic receptors in rat brain. *J. Neurochem.*, 37:830–836.

53. Kety, S. S., Javoy, F., Thierry, A. M., Julou, L., and Glowinski, J. (1967): A sustained effect of electroconvulsive shock on the turnover of norepinephrine in the central nervous system of the rat. *Proc. Natl. Acad. Sci. U.S.A.*, 58:1249–1254.

54. Ko, H. K., Dailey, J. W., and Jobe, P. C. (1982): Effect of increments in norepinephrine concentrations on seizure intensity in the genetically epilepsy-prone rat. *J. Pharmacol. Exp. Ther.*, 222:662–669.

55. Koyama, I. (1972): Amino acids in the cobalt induced epileptogenic and nonepileptogenic cat's cortex. *Can. J. Physiol. Pharmacol.*, 50:740–752.

56. Koyama, I. (1978): Amino acid concentration in the brain of a cat with spontaneous chronic epilepsy. *J. Tokyo Women's Med. Coll.*, 48:428–431.

57. Koyama, I., and Jasper, H. (1977): Amino acid content of chronic undercut cortex of the cat in relation to electrical after discharge: Comparison with cobalt epileptogenic lesions. *Can. J. Physiol. Pharmacol.*, 55:523–536.

58. Leppik, I. E., and Sherwin, A. L. (1977): Anticonvulsant activity of phenobarbital and phenytoin in combination. *J. Pharmacol. Exp. Ther.*, 200:570–575.

59. Libet, B., Gleason, C. A., Wright, E. W., and Feinstein, B. (1977): Suppression of an epileptiform type of electrocortical activity in the rat by stimulation in the vicinity of locus coeruleus. *Epilepsia*, 18:451–462.

60. Lloyd, K. G., Munari,C., Worms, P., Bossi, L., and Morselli, P. L. (1983): Indications for the use of gamma-aminobutyric acid (GABA)-agonists in convulsant disorders. In: *Progress in Clinical and Biological Research, Vol. 124: Epilepsy: An Update on Research and Therapy*, edited by G. Nistico, R. Di Perry, and H. Meinardi, pp. 285–297. Liss, New York.

61. Louis, W. J., Papanicolaou, J., Summers, R. J., and Vajda, F. J. E. (1982): Role of central β-adrenoceptors in the control of pentylenetetrazol-induced convulsions in rats. *Br. J. Pharmacol.*, 75:441–446.

62. Lueders, H., Hahn, J., Lesser, R. P., Dinner, D. S., Rothner, D., and Erenberg, G. (1982): Localization of epileptogenic spike foci: Comparative study of closely spaced scalp electrodes, nasopharyngeal, sphenoidal, subdural and depth electrodes. In: *Advances in Epileptology: XIIIth Epilepsy International Symposium*, edited by H. Akimoto, H. Kazamatsuri, M. Seino, and A. A. Ward, Jr., pp. 185–189. Raven Press, New York.

63. Manyam, B. V., and Hare, T. A. (1983): Cerebrospinal fluid GABA measurements: Basic and clinical considerations. *Clin. Neuropharmacol.*, 6:25–36.

64. Masserano, J. M., Takimoto, G. S., and Weiner, N. (1981): Electroconvulsive shock increases tyrosine hydroxylase activity in the brain and adrenal gland of the rat. *Science*, 214:662–665.

65. Mason, S. T., and Corcoran, M. E. (1978): Forebrain noradrenaline and metrazol-induced seizures. *Life Sci.*, 23:167–172.

66. Mathieson, G. (1975): Pathologic aspects of epilepsy with special reference to the surgical pathology of focal cerebral seizures. In: *Advances in Neurology, Vol. 8: Neurosurgical Management of the Epilepsies*, edited by D. P. Purpura, J. K. Penry, and R. D. Walter, pp. 107–138. Raven Press, New York.

67. Maynert, E. W., Marczynski, T. J., and Browning, R. A. (1975): The role of the neurotransmitters in the epilepsies. In: *Advances in Neurology, Vol. 13: Current Reviews*, edited by W. J. Friedlander, pp. 79–147. Raven Press, New York.

68. Mazziotta, J. C., and Engel, Jr., J. (1984): The use and impact of positron computed tomography scanning in epilepsy. *Epilepsia*, 25(Suppl):S86–S104.

69. McGeer, P. L., McGeer, E. G., and Wada, J. A. (1971): Glutamic acid decarboxylase in Parkinson's disease and epilepsy. *Neurology*, 21:1000–1007.

70. McNaughton, F. L. (1952): The classification of the epilepsies. *Epilepsia*, 1:1–10.

71. McNaughton, F. L., and Rusmussen, T. (1975): Criteria for selection of patients for neurosurgical treatment. In: *Advances in Neurology, Vol. 8: Neurosurgical Management of the Epilepsies*, edited by D. P. Purpura, J. K. Penry, and R. D. Walter, pp. 37–48. Raven Press, New York.

72. Miach, P. J., Dausse, J. P., Cardot, A., and Meyer, P. (1980): ^{3}H-Prazosin binds specifically to "alpha 1"-adrenoceptors in rat brain.

Naunyn-Schmiedebergs Arch. Pharmacol., 312:23–26.

73. Mison-Crighel, N., and Badiu, G. H. (1971): Enzymic pattern changes in the cat neocortex produced by a mescaline epileptogenic focus. *Rev. Roum. Neurol.*, 8:55–60.

74. Mueller, A. L., Hoffer, B. J., and Dunwiddie, T. V. (1981): Noradrenergic responses in rat hippocampus: Evidence for mediation by alpha and β receptors in the *in vitro* slice. *Brain Res.*, 214:113–126.

75. Musacchio, J. M., Julou, L., Kety, S. S., and Glowinski, J. (1969): Increase in rat brain tyrosine hydroxylase activity produced by electroconvulsive shock. *Proc. Natl. Acad. Sci. U.S.A.*, 63:1117–1119.

76. Mutani, R., Durelli, L., Mazzarion, M., Valentini, C., Monaco, F., Fumero, S., and Mondino, A. (1977): Longitudinal changes of brain amino acid content occurring before, during and after epileptic activity. *Brain Res.*, 122:513–521.

77. Naruse, H., Kato, M., Kurokawa, M., Haba, R., and Yabe, T. (1960): Metabolic defects in a convulsive strain of mouse. *J. Neurochem.*, 5:339–369.

78. Nicklas, W. J., Berl, S., and Clarke, D. D. (1975): Relationship between amino acid and catecholamine metabolism in brain. In: *Metabolic Compartmentation and Neurotransmission: Relation to Brain Structure and Function*, edited by S. Berl, D. D. Clarke, and D. Schneider, pp. 497–513. Plenum, New York.

79. Norenberg, M. D. (1976): Histochemical studies in experimental portal–systemic encephalopathy. I. Glutamic dehydrogenase. *Arch. Neurol.*, 33:265–269.

80. Norenberg, M. D. (1979): The distribution of glutamine synthetase in the rat central nervous system. *J. Histochem. Cytochem.*, 27:756–762.

81. Norenberg, M. D. (1982): Immunohistochemical study of glutamine synthetase in brain trauma. *Proc. 58th Annu. Meet. Am. Assoc. Neuropathol.*, Philadelphia, p. 347 (abst).

82. Olivier, A. (1983): Surgical management of complex-partial seizures. In: *Progress in Clinical and Biological Research, Vol. 124: Epilepsy: An Update on Research and Therapy*, edited by G. Nistico, R. Di Perri, and H. Meinardi, pp. 309–334. Alan R. Liss, New York.

83. Olivier, A., and Bertrand, G. (1982): *Stereotaxic Implantation of Depth Electrodes for Seizure Recording: Surgical Technique Used at the Montreal Neurological Hospital*, p. 59. MNI Publications, Montreal.

84. Papanicolaou, J., Summers, R. J., Vajda, F. J. E., and Louis, W. J. (1982): Anticonvulsant effects of clonidine mediated through central alpha 2-adrenoceptors. *Eur. J. Pharmacol.*, 77:163–166.

85. Papanicolaou, J., Summers, R. J., Vajda, F. J. E., and Louis, W. J. (1982): The relationship between alpha-2 adrenoceptor selectivity and anticonvulsant effect in a series of clonidine-like drugs. *Brain Res.*, 241:393–397.

86. Pappius, J., and Elliott, K. A. C. (1954): Adenosine triphosphate, electrolytes and oxygen uptake rates of human normal and epileptogenic cerebral cortex. *Can. J. Biochem. Physiol.*, 32:484–490.

87. Penfield, W., and Jasper, H. (1954): *Epilepsy and the Functional Anatomy of the Human Brain*, edited by W. Penfield and H. Jasper. Little, Brown, Boston.

88. Perry, T. L., and Hansen, S. (1981): Amino acid abnormalities in epileptogenic foci. *Neurology*, 31:872–876.

89. Perry, T. L., Hansen, S., and Gandlham, S. S. (1981): Postmortem changes of amino compounds in human and rat brain. *J. Neurochem.*, 36:406–412.

90. Perry, T. L., Hansen, S., Kennedy, J., Wada, J. A., and Thompson, G. B. (1975): Amino acids in human epileptogenic foci. *Arch. Neurol.*, 32:752–754.

91. Pilkington, G. J., and Lantos, P. L. (1982): The role of glutamine synthetase in the diagnosis of cerebral tumors. *Neuropathol. Appl. Neurobiol.*, 8:227–236.

92. Post, R. M., and Uhde, T. W. (1983): Treatment of mood disorders with antiepileptic medications: Clinical and theoretical implications. *Epilepsia*, 24 (Suppl. 2):S97–S108.

93. Prince, D. A., and Wilder, B. J. (1967): Control mechanisms in cortical epileptogenic foci: "Surround inhibition." *Arch. Neurol.*, 16:194–202.

94. Prockop, D. J., Shore, P. A., and Brodie, B. B. (1959): An anticonvulsant effect of monoamine oxidase inhibitors. *Experientia*, 15:145–147.

95. Rapport, R. L., Harris, A. B., Friel, P. N., and Ojemann, G. A. (1975): Human epileptic brain: Na,K ATPase activity and phenytoin concentrations. *Arch. Neurol.*, 32:549–554.

96. Rapport, R. L., Harris, A. B., Lockard, J. S., and Clark, A.F. (1981): Na K ATPase in serially excised segments of epileptic monkey cortex. *Epilepsia*, 22:123–127.

97. Rasmussen, T. (1982): Localizational aspects of epileptic seizure phenomenon. In: *New Perspectives in Cerebral Localization*, edited by R. A. Thompson and J. R. Green, pp. 177–203. Raven Press, New York.

98. Reader, T. A. (1983): The role of the catecholamines in neuronal excitability. In: *Neurology and Neurobiology, Vol. 2: Basic Mechanisms of Neuronal Hyperexcitability*, edited by H. Jasper and N. van Gelder, pp. 281–321. Liss, New York.

99. Reader, T. A., and Jasper, H. H. (1984): Interactions between monoamines and other transmitters in cerebral cortex. In: *Neurology and Neurobiology, Vol. 10: Monoamine Innervation of Cerebral Cortex*, edited by L. Descarries, T. A. Reader, and H. H. Jasper, pp. 195–225. Liss, New York.

100. Reader, T. A., Ferron, A., Descarries, L., and Jasper, H. H. (1979): Modulatory role for biogenic amines in the cerebral cortex. Microiontophoretic studies. *Brain Res.*, 160:217–229.

101. Reader, T.A., and Brière, R. (1983): Long-term unilateral noradrenergic denervation: Monoamine content and ^{3}H-prazosin binding sites in rat neocortex. *Brain Res. Bull.*, 11:687–692.

102. Ribak, C. E., Harris, A. B., Vaughn, J. E., and Roberts, E. (1979): Inhibitory, GABAergic nerve terminals decrease at sites of focal epilepsy. *Science*, 205:211–214.

103. Ribak, C. E., Bradburne, R. M., and Harris, A. B. (1982): A preferential loss of GABAergic, symmetric synapses in epileptic foci: A quantitative ultrastructural analysis of monkey neocortex. *J. Neurosci.*, 2:1725–1735.

104. Roberts, R. B., Flexner, J. B., and Flexner, L. B. (1959): Biochemical and physiological differentiation during morphogenesis—XXIII: Further observations relating to the synthesis of amino acids and proteins by the cerebral cortex and liver of the mouse. *J. Neurochem.*, 4:78–90.

105. Robitaille, Y., and Sherwin, A. L. (1984): High affinity (^{3}H) B-alanine uptake by scar margins of ferric chloride-induced epileptogenic foci in rat isocortex. *J. Neuropathol. Exp. Neurol.*, 43:376–383.

106. Saint-Hilaire, J. M., Bouvier, G., Lymburner, J., et al. (1976): La stereoélectroencephalographie synchronisee avec l'enregistrement visuel et sonore dans l'exploration chronique de l'épilepsie. *Union Med. Can.*, 105:1538–1541.

107. Salzman, P. M., and Roth, R. H. (1980): Poststimulation catecholamine synthesis and tyrosine hydroxylase activation in central noradrenergic neurons. 1. In-vivo stimulation of the locus coeruleus. *J. Pharmacol. Exp. Ther.*, 212:64–73.

108. Schousboe, A., and Hertz, L. (1981): Role of astroglial cells in glutamate homeostasis. In: *Advances in Biochemical Psychopharmacology, Vol 27: Glutamate as a Neurotransmitter*, edited by G. Dichiara and G. L. Gessa, pp. 103–108. Raven Press, New York.

109. Sherwin, A. L., Leblanc, F. E., and McCann, W. P. (1968): Altered LDH isoenzymes in brain tumors. *Arch. Neurol.*, 18:311–316.

110. Sherwin, A. L., Norris, J. W., and Bulcke, J. A. (1969): Spinal fluid creatine kinase in neurologic disease. *Neurology*, 19:993–999.

111. Sherwin, A. L., and Sokolowski, C. D. (1975): Phenytoin and phenobarbitone levels in human brain and cerebrospinal fluid. In: *Clinical Pharmacology of Anti-Epileptic Drugs*, edited by H. Schneider, D. Janz, C. Gardner-Horpe, H. Meinardi, and A. L. Sherwin, pp. 274–280. Springer-Verlag, Berlin.

112. Sherwin, A. L., Harvey, C. D., and Leppik, I. E. (1977): Antiepileptic drugs in human cerebral cortex: Clinical relevance of cortex: Plasma ratios. In: *Epilepsy, The Eighth International Symposium*, edited by J. K. Penry, pp.103–108. Raven Press, New York.

113. Sherwin, A. L., Robitaille, Y., and Olivier, A. (1982): Comparative study of glutamine synthetase activity in human seizure foci and primary brain tumors. *Proc. Can. Assoc. Neuropathol.* (abstr.), Montreal.

114. Sherwin, A. L., Quesney, F., Gauthier, S., Olivier, A., Robitaille, Y., McQuaid, P., Harvey, C., and van Gelder, N. (1984): Enzyme changes in actively spiking areas of human epileptic cerebral cortex. *Neurology*, 34:927–933.

115. Standford, S. C., and Nutt, D. J. (1982): Comparison of the effects of repeated electroconvulsive shock on alpha 2- and beta adrenoceptors in different regions of rat brain. *Neuroscience*, 7:1753–1757.

116. Sugaya, E., and Onozuka, M. (1978): Intracellular calcium: Its movement during pentylenetetrazole-induced bursting activity. *Science*, 200:797–799.

117. Swann, A. C. (1983): Stimulation of brain Na, K-ATPase by norepinephrine in vivo: Prevention by receptor antagonists and enhancement by repeated stimulation. *Brain Res.*, 260:338–341.

118. Talairach, J., and Bancaud, J. (1974): Stereotaxic exploration and therapy in epilepsy. In: *Handbook of Clinical Neurology, Vol. 15: The Epilepsies*, edited by P. J. Vinken and G. Bruyn, pp. 758–782. North-Holland, Amsterdam.

119. Theodore, W. H., Brooks, R. D., Patronas, Margolin, R., Sato, S., Porter, R. J., and Di-Chiro, G. (1984): The effect of phenobarbital and phenytoin on cerebral glucose metabolism measured by positron emission tomography. *Neurology*, 342 (Suppl. 1):118 (abst).

120. Tower, D. B. (1953): Biochemical abnormalities in epileptogenic cerebral cortex. *XIX Int. Physiol. Congr. Abstr. Commun.*, pp. 834–835.

121. Tower, D. B. (1960): *Neurochemistry of Epilepsy*. Charles C. Thomas, Springfield, Illinois.

122. Trottier, S., Berger, B., Chauvel, P., Dedek, J., and Gay, M. (1981): Alterations of the cortical noradrenergic system in chronic cobalt epileptogenic foci in the rat: A histofluorescent and biochemical study. *Neuroscience*, 6:1069–1080.

123. Trottier, S., Claustre, Y., Caboche, J., Dedek, J., Chauvel, P., Nassif, S., and Scatton, B. (1983): Alterations of noradrenaline and seratonin uptake and metabolism in chronic cobalt-induced epilepsy in the rat. *Brain Res.*, 272:255–262.

124. Tursky, T., Lassanova, M., Sramka, M., and Nadvornik, P. (1976): Formation of glutamate and GABA in epileptogenic tissue from human hippocampus in vitro. *Acta Neurochir. [Suppl.]* (Wien), 23:111–118.

125. Van Gelder, N. M. (1972): Antagonism by taurine of cobalt induced epilepsy in cat and mouse. *Brain Res.*, 47:157–165.

126. Van Gelder, N. M. (1974): Glutamate dehydrogenase, glutamic acid decarboxylase and GABA amino transferase in epileptic mouse cortex. *Can. J. Physiol. Pharmacol.*, 52:952–959.

127. Van Gelder, N. M. (1980): Glutamic acid metabolism and epilepsy (review). *Neurosciences*, 6 (Suppl.): 163–177.

128. Van Gelder, N. M. (1981): The role of taurine and glutamic acid in the epileptic process: A genetic predisposition. *Rev. Pure Appl. Pharmacol. Sci.*, 2:293–316.

129. Van Gelder, N. M. (1982): Glutamic acid in chronically hyperirritable nervous tissue. In: *Advances in Epileptology: XIIIth Epilepsy International Symposium*, edited by H. Akimoto, H. Kazamatsuri, M. Seino, and A. A. Ward, Jr., pp. 323–329. Raven Press, New York.

130. Van Gelder, N. M., and Courtois, A. (1972): Close correlation between changing content of specific amino acids in epileptogenic cortex of cats, and severity of epilepsy. *Brain Res.,* 43:477–484.

131. Van Gelder, N. M., Sherwin, A. L., and Rasmussen, T. (1972): Amino acid content of epileptogenic human brain: Focal versus surrounding regions. *Brain Res.,* 40:385–393.

132. Van Gelder, N. M., Sherwin, A. L., Sacks, C., and Andermann, F. (1975): Biochemical observations following administration of taurine to patients with epilepsy. *Brain Res.,* 94:297–306.

133. Van Gelder, N. M., and Drujan, B. D. (1980): Alterations in the compartmentalized metabolism of glutamic acid with changed cerebral conditions. *Brain Res.,* 200:443–455.

134. Van Gelder, N. M., Siatitsas, I., Menini, C., and Gloor, P. (1983): Feline generalized penicillin epilepsy: Changes of glutamic acid and taurine parallel the progressive increase in excitability of the cortex. *Epilepsia,* 24:200–213.

135. Waelsch, H. (1949): The metabolism of glutamic acid. *Lancet,* 257:1–5.

136. Walter, R. D. (1973): Tactical considerations leading to surgical treatment of limbic epilepsy. In: *Epilepsy, Its Phenomena in Man,* edited by M. A. B. Brazier, pp. 99–119. Academic, New York.

137. Ward, A. A., Jr. (1969): The epileptic neuron: Chronic foci in animals and man. In: *The Basic Mechanisms of the Epilepsies,* edited by H. H. Jasper, A. A. Ward, Jr., and A. Pope, pp. 263–288. Little, Brown, Boston.

138. Ward, A. A., Jr. (1983): Surgical management of epilepsy. In: *Epilepsy: Diagnosis and Management,* edited by T. R. Browne and R. G. Feldman, pp. 281–296. Little, Brown, Boston.

139. Waszezak, B. L., and Walters, J. R. (1983): Dopamine modulation of the effects of gamma-aminobutyric acid on substantia nigra pars reticulata neurons. *Science,* 220:218:221.

140. Weichert, P., and Gollnitz, G. (1969): The activity of glutaminase and glutamine synthetase acid ammonia metabolism before, during and after convulsions. *J. Neurochem.,* 16:689–693.

141. Woodbury, D. M., and Esplin, D. W. (1959): Neuropharmacology and neurochemistry of anticonvulsant drugs. In: *The Effect of Pharmacological Agents on the Nervous System, Proc. Association for Research in Nervous and Mental Dis., Vol. 37,* edited by F. J. Braceland, pp. 24–56. Williams & Wilkins, Baltimore.

142. Wyler, A. R., and Ward, A. A., Jr. (1980): Epileptic neurons. In: *Epilepsy: A Window to Brain Mechanisms,* edited by J. S. Lockard and A. A. Ward, Jr., pp. 51–68. Raven Press, New York.

143. Wyler, A. R., Ojemann, G. A., and Ward, A. A., Jr. (1981): Neurons in human epileptic cortex. Correlation between unit and EEG activity. *Ann. Neurol.,* 11:301–308.

144. Wyler, A. R., Ojemann, G. A., Lettich, E., and Ward, A. A., Jr. (1984): Subdural strip electrodes for localizing epileptogenic foci. *J. Neurosurg.,* 60:1195–1200.

145. Yamamoto, Y. L., Ochs, R., Gloor, P., Ammann, W., Meyer, E., Evans, A. C., Cooke, B., Sako, K., Gotman, J., Feindel, W. H., Diksic, M., Thompson, C. J., and Robitaille, Y. (1983): Patterns of rCBF and focal energy metabolic changes in relation to electroencephalographic abnormality in the interictal phase of partial epilepsy. In: *Current Problems in Epilepsy, Vol. 1: Cerebral Blood Flow, Metabolism and Epilepsy,* edited by J. Baldy-Moulinier, D. H. Ingvar, and B. S. Meldrum, pp. 51–62. Libbey, London.

Advances in Neurology, Vol. 44, edited by
A. V. Delgado-Escueta, A. A. Ward, Jr.,
D. M. Woodbury, and R. J. Porter.
Raven Press, New York © 1986.

52

Alterations of GABA-Mediated Synaptic Transmission in Human Epilepsy

*K. G. Lloyd, *L. Bossi, *P. L. Morselli, **C. Munari, †M. Rougier, and †H. Loiseau

Research Department, L.E.R.S.–Synthélabo, 75013 Paris, France; INSERM Unit, Centre P. Brocca, 75014 Paris, France; and Faculty of Medicine, University of Bordeaux, 33076 Bordeaux, France

SUMMARY   Although animal models consistently indicate that gamma-amino-butyric acid (GABA) synaptic function (GABA levels, synthesis, uptake and/or receptors) is decreased in seizure states, there is little evidence to date in support of such a hypothesis for human epilepsy. This chapter presents the results of an in-depth study of the activity of the GABA-synthesizing enzyme L-glutamic acid decarboxylase (GAD) in brain tissue removed during neurosurgical resection for intractable epilepsy. The tissue studied is unique in that identified (by stereo EEG) foci were excised (rather than large blocks of tissue containing mixtures of foci and nonepileptic material) and compared with nonepileptic (stereo EEG and morphological definitions) tissue from the same patients.

In patients in which there was no indication of a tumor, GAD activity in the foci was low in more than 50% of the patients examined. Furthermore, when the population distribution of GAD was compared in epileptic versus nonepileptic tissue fragments from all patients, the peak distribution of epileptic tissue fragments occurred at much lower GAD activities than for the nonepileptic fragments (0–20 versus 41–80 nmol CO_2/mg protein · hr, respectively). A small subgroup of epileptic fragments occurred with a normal GAD distribution, indicating that the presence of an epileptic focus was not invariably associated with low GAD activity.

When the low levels of GABA "A" binding sites in these epileptic tissue fragments are taken into consideration in combination with the low GAD levels, then it can be estimated that 60 to 70% of the present patient population had deficient GABAergic transmission in epileptic foci as compared to nonepileptic brain tissue from the same patients.

It follows that the GABA hypothesis of human epilepsy is not an exclusive or unitary hypothesis, and some patients appear to have normally functioning GABA synapses (as assessed biochemically) in epileptogenic areas. Thus, other neurotransmitter and neurohumoral systems certainly play a role in the epileptic process.

In a large number of epileptic patients, the clinical symptoms appear to be related to the existence of a primary focus, which can be localized and studied by different electroencephalographic (EEG) techniques. It is also commonly accepted that in certain patients, who are unresponsive to currently available pharmacological treatment, the stereoencephalographic identification of an epileptogenic area and its removal by neurosurgery may lead to the complete remission of the clinical syndrome. The removed brain material can subsequently be studied by available biochemical, pharmacological, and neuroanatomical techniques in an attempt to understand whether or not there are common pathological processes or biochemical alterations underlying the syndrome. In other words, independently from the etiopathogenesis, we have today the possibility of studying human brain samples that have been characterized by various EEG techniques and directly linked with the genesis, the spreading, or the maintaining of the epileptic discharge.

What could one study in such precious material? There are literally dozens of known and putative neurotransmitters and neuromodulators in the brain. In this regard, epilepsy has been suggested to be due to either an excess of excitatory mechanisms or to a loss of inhibitory neurotransmission (for further discussion of this subject see Chapters 15, 43, and others).

The major inhibitory neurotransmitter in the brain is gamma-aminobutyric acid (GABA), and it is known from animal models that any means of severely diminishing GABA synaptic activity (e.g., inhibition of synthesis, direct block of the receptor) or blocking GABA receptor-mediated events (the entry of chloride ions via the chloride ionophore) immediately induces seizures (23). This does not constitute proof that a similar mechanism exists in human epilepsy, but it provides a basis for the investigation of seizure phenomena, both in animal models and in humans.

The assessment of dynamic changes in GABA synaptic activity is not a simple procedure. GABA itself is relatively easy to measure, and highly specific and sensitive methods exist. However, GABA levels alter rapidly postmortem (27), making it very difficult to evaluate their meaning when the postmortem time differs from one sample to another (6). Furthermore, even when this parameter can be reliably controlled, the meaning of GABA levels per se is still open to question, as it has been shown that considerable changes can occur in GABA turnover without altering steady-state GABA levels (29).

The assay of L-glutamatic acid decarboxylase (GAD), the enzyme converting L-glutamic acid to GABA, poses fewer pitfalls than the assay of GABA, GAD being quite stable in postmortem and excised tissue. However, antemortem conditions may affect GAD activity, especially in the case of relatively prolonged hypoxia (18). This may create a problem when comparing epileptic versus nonepileptic patients, but is not a problem when an epileptogenic area is compared to normal tissue taken from the same patient.

The postsynaptic GABA macromolecular receptor complex (GABA, benzodiazepine receptors, and chloride ion channel) is not known to be labile under normal ante- or postmortem conditions. However, this may indicate that the proper control studies have not yet been performed.

The present review is intended to evaluate those studies performed on biochemical indices of GABA synaptic function in epileptic foci in humans with a comparison to similar studies in laboratory animal models.

LITERATURE REVIEW

Brain Tissue from Epileptic Patients

There are relatively few studies that have directly attacked the problem of a possible dysfunction of GABA synaptic function in human epileptic tissue. This is in spite of the potential availability of tissue from the surgical resection of uncontrolled temporal-lobe epilepsy. The reports on this type of material encompass fewer than a dozen papers over a span of two decades.

The parameter most commonly studied is the concentration of GABA in the tissue. However, before consideration of the findings themselves, an editorial comment is due.

As already stated, GABA levels are very susceptible to postmortem changes (6,27) and although the immediate freezing of neurosurgical material as soon as it is removed reduces this problem, this does not eliminate the problem. Furthermore, the distribution of GABA is not strictly confined to neurons, as there exists an efficient glial GABA uptake system (17), and glial GABA is not involved in synaptic transmission or its dysfunction. Finally, a large number of different GABA neurons exist, and in the cortex a minimum of 25% of all axon terminals appear to be GABAergic (8). Even if a dysfunction of GABA neurons exists in epilepsy, it is not to be expected that all GABA neurons or pathways are involved. Thus, a loss of activity in a subpopulation of GABA neurons could well be masked by the remainder of normal (or even hyperactive) GABA neurons.

With the above comments in mind, it is not surprising that the changes observed in GABA levels have not been reproducible from one study to another (Table 1). Perry and collaborators (30,31) have consistently observed an increase in GABA levels in cortical tissue. However, in the initial report (31), there was a lack of specificity for the changes in GABA as the concentrations of five of the six amino acids studied were increased, whereas in the subsequent report (30), which includes the material from the earlier publication, the changes seen in the GABA levels were more specific. For these studies, the control tissue was taken from nonepileptic patients, posing a problem in terms of drug therapy, anesthesia, and related methodological questions.

Van Gelder and collaborators (39) studied tissue from 18 patients, using electrocorticograms (ECoGs) to determine the regions of maximal EEG abnormality. This technique does not really define a true focus, and the control tissue, while coming from the same patients, still exhibited ECoG abnormalities. No overall changes in GABA levels were noted in the epileptic regions, and no subgrouping of patients was readily evident (6 below control, 6 equal to control, and 6 above control levels).

In one case of vitamin B6-dependent seizures, cortical material was removed after death occurred during status epilepticus (26). Although GABA levels were markedly decreased, the reference (control) material was not well age-matched, and any differences in postmortem time between the patient and the controls is not indicated.

In some studies an effort was made to assess the dynamics of GABA synaptic activity in tissue taken from epileptic patients (Table 2). In the earliest investigations of GABAergic mechanisms in epileptic tissue, Tower (37) noted that slices of epileptic brain tissue were unable to maintain the synthesis of GABA, whereas adjacent nonepileptic tissue from the same patient was able to continue synthesis of the neurotransmitter. Subsequently, McGeer et al. (28) reported on GAD levels in "electrophysiologically abnormal" cortical regions (however, not identified as foci) removed neurosurgically from epileptic patients. Two of these patients exhibited GAD values well within the range of similar material removed from the brains of nonepileptic patients. The third patient had GAD activities below or in the very low normal range.

In a more recent investigation, we have studied a larger number of tumoral and nontumoral epileptic patients (21). In the latter cases the origin of the seizures was defined by stereo EEG using depth electrodes. Control tissue was taken from the same patients and was normal both in terms of stereo EEG and histopathology. In this study, GAD activity, ^{3}H-GABA binding and GABA-T activity were evaluated (Table 2, Fig. 1). An update on GAD activity is presented in the next section.

Although the means for ^{3}H-GABA binding were not significantly different between control, nontumoral epileptic and tumoral epileptic tissues, definite subpopulations of epileptic tissues could be identified that were deficient in ^{3}H-GABA binding. Thus, 10 of 18 nontumoral cases had ^{3}H-GABA binding values in the epileptogenic areas below the values of control tissues [< mean − 2(SEM)], whereas only 4 were above the controls [> mean + 2(SEM)]. For the tumor cases, 5 of 7 cases had low ^{3}H-GABA binding in the pathological tissue, and none exhibited an enhanced binding. In those cases in which there was sufficient tissue to perform a kinetic analysis, the alteration was due to a change in B_{max}, not in the K_d.

GABA-T activity was normal, or even tended to be elevated, in the epileptic tissue from both nontumoral and tumoral epilepsy patients.

The general observation from this study was that if those patients with a severe deficit in either GAD activity and/or ^{3}H-GABA binding are considered together, then about 60 to 70% of the cases in this patient group have a dysfunctional GABA synapse. No deficit in GABAergic function was observed in about 30% of the cases.

Thus, the available data from the literature do not, in general, offer a strong support for the GABA hypothesis of epilepsy. However, the majority of these studies did not use well-identified epileptic foci in comparison to normal tissue taken from the same patients. Those studies that did investigate such tissue [e.g., Tower (37) and Lloyd et al. (21)] provide a basis for further investigation of the GABA hypothesis.

UPDATE OF STUDIES ON GAD ACTIVITY IN EPILEPTIC TISSUE

In this study, three patient groups have been analyzed: two groups of epileptic patients where no tumor was discernible (one from Bordeaux, one from Paris) and one group (from Paris) for which the epilepsy was associated with the presence of a tumor.

TABLE 1. *Alterations of GABA levels in regions removed neurosurgically or post-mortem from epileptic human brains*

Study	Regions	EEG definition of focus	GABA levels		Comments
Van Gelder et al. (39)	Focal versus peripheral cortex (neurosurg.)	ECoG to determine maximal abnormality	3 cases ↓	25–50%	No overall change or evident subgrouping
			3 cases ↓	15–25%	Uncertain definition of focus
			6 cases ↓	2–10%	"Peripheral" tissue still abnormal (ECoG)
			4 cases ↑	20–30%	
			2 cases ↑	40–50%	
Perry and Hansen (30)	Temporal and frontal cortex (neurosurg.)	Cortical and depth electrodes	130% Of normal tissue ($p <$ 0.05)		Control tissue not from the same patients but from nonepileptic patients on different medications
					No significant alterations in homocarnosine (114%)
Perry et al. (31)	Temporal and frontal cortex (neurosurg.)	Cortical and depth electrodes	149% Of normal tissue ($p <$ 0.05)		Control tissue not from the same patients but from nonepileptic patients with different medications
					Five of six amino acids measured were increased
					Specificity for GABA
					Homocarnosine also increased (150%)
Lott et al. (26)	Frontal cortex, occipital cortex (post-mortem)	Died in status epilepticus	30–40% Of control tissue		Vitamin B6-dependent seizures
					Poorly age-matched controls

TABLE 2. *Studies of GABA synthesis, binding, and metabolism on tissue removed from human epileptic patients*

Study	EEG definition of focus	Parameters studied	Comments
Cortex (37)	Electrocorticogram direct stimulation (neurosurgery)	Ability to maintain GABA levels in brain slices Nonepileptic: 4.75 $\xrightarrow[\text{incubation}]{\text{1 hr}}$ 6.1 μmol/g tissue Epileptic: 4.35 $\xrightarrow[\text{incubation}]{\text{1 hr}}$ 3.3 μmol/g tissue	Patients served as their own control
Cortex (28)	"Electrophysiologically abnormal" (biopsy)	GAD activity (μmol/g · hr in cortex) Normal range: 5.6–16.0 Patient I: 5.1–7.3 Patient II: 9.6–11.5 Patient III: 8.8	Material not identified as focus Controls from nonepileptic patients with different medication, etc.
Cortex, hippo-campus (21)	Stereo EEG from depth electrodes, nontumor (neurosurgery)	^{3}H-GABA binding (fmol/mg protein) Control: 129 ± 19 Epileptic: 116 ± 21 10/19 With GABA binding below control (2 × SEM) 4/19 With GABA binding above control (2 × SEM) GABA-T activity (nmol/mg protein · 15 min) Control: 1.61 ± 0.22 Epileptic: 1.91 ± 0.23 3/15 With GABA-T below control (2 × SEM) 3/15 With GABA-T above control (2 × SEM)	EEG-normal tissue from the same patient served as control tissue Mixture of cortical and hippocampal tissue Definite subgroup of patients with low GAD and/or ^{3}H-GABA binding levels

Na⁺ INDEPENDENT ³H-GABA BINDING (25 nm)   GABA-TRANSAMINASE ACTIVITY

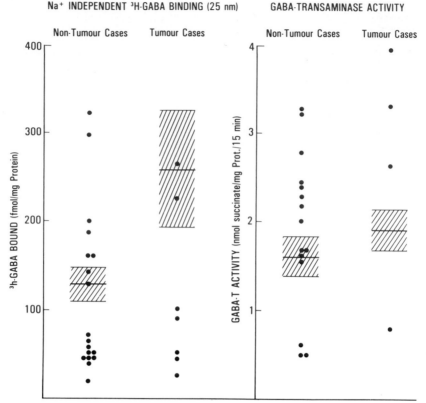

FIG. 1. Na⁺-independent ³H-GABA binding and GABA-transaminase activity in the epileptic foci of individual epileptic patients. The points represent the activity in the foci of individual patients with epilepsy of either tumoral or nontumoral origin. The shaded area represents the activity (mean ± SEM) for normal tissue from the same patients.

The material included in the Paris studies was obtained from 45 patients undergoing neurosurgical intervention for intractable epilepsy. Fourteen cases were associated with the presence of a tumor (tumor cases), and in the remaining 31 there was no indication of a tumor (nontumor cases). For the Bordeaux study (ongoing), material from 9 patients was available, none of which were associated with the presence of a tumor. The timing of the various phases of the procedure is indicated in Fig. 2. For the nontumor cases, the focus was previously (1 month prior to surgery) identified by stereo EEG taken from 8 to 10 in-depth electrodes (5). The recordings normally were made during at least three epileptic attacks. Control tissue from nontumor cases demonstrated a normal stereo EEG and was removed due to its presence in the surgical approach to the abnormal tissue. Pathological tissue consisted of both zones of epileptogenic tissue (ZE) and associated severely lesioned zones (lesional zone, ZL) as previously defined (5,21). For the tumor cases, the pathological

tissue was defined by morphological (and in some cases also electrophysiological) means. Normal (N) tissue was without morphological abnormalities. GAD activity was measured according to Bird and Iversen (7).

For the two groups of patients with epilepsy without the presence of a tumor, the results were very similar. If the data from all of the patients are considered (i.e., from patients from whom no normal tissue was available in addition to those patients from whom both normal tissue and epileptogenic tissue were excised), the epileptogenic zones (ZE) exhibited considerably less GAD activity than did the normal tissue (Fig. 3). This was highly significant ($p < 0.01$) for both groups of patients.

Not only were those findings qualitatively similar, but the quantitative results were also very comparable in terms of GAD activity in both control and epileptogenic tissue (Fig. 3).

When only those cases supplying both epileptogenic and normal tissues were analyzed, the results parallel those found with the entire pa-

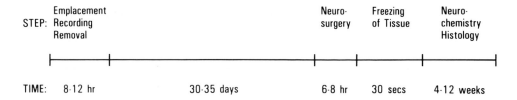

IE. ACUTE ELECTRODE EMPLACEMENT ONLY

FIG. 2. Temporal sequence of the electrode emplacement, neurosurgery, freezing of tissue, and biochemical analysis for the study of epileptic (nontumor) patients.

tient population. Thus, when the epileptogenic tissue fragments from the two patient groups are divided into subpopulations of low GAD activity [less than mean of N − 2(SEM)], within the normal variation [mean of N ± 2(SEM)] and high GAD activity [greater than mean of N + 2(SEM)] in the Paris group, a deficit in GAD activity was found in 54% (7/13) of the cases with both normal and epileptogenic tissue, whereas 70% (19/27) was the value obtained when all cases were induced. In the Bordeaux group, GAD activity in the epileptogenic zone was low in all (3) cases with both normal and epileptogenic tissue, whereas 88% (7/8) of the

total population had low GAD activity in the epileptogenic zone.

These results are reflected in the population-distribution curves for the individual normal or epileptogenic tissue fragments. For the Paris study (Fig. 4), 36 tissue fragments of normal (N) tissue, 62 tissue fragments from epileptogenic zones from patients who also had normal tissue removed, and 171 fragments of epileptogenic tissue from the entire group were available. GAD activity in the normal tissue fragments followed a normal distribution pattern, with almost all tissue fragments having an activity between 40 and 100 nmol CO_2/mg protein · hr.

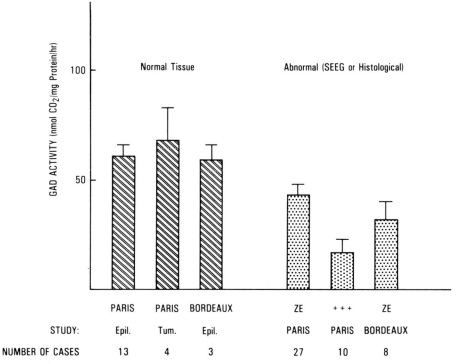

FIG. 3. GAD activity in normal and epileptogenic tissue from the different patient groups. Results are expressed as the mean with SEM. The data from all patients (with and without normal tissue) are included. In each group the GAD activity in the pathological tissue (ZE or + + +) is significantly ($p < 0.01$) lower than that of the corresponding normal tissue. SEEG, stereoencephalography.

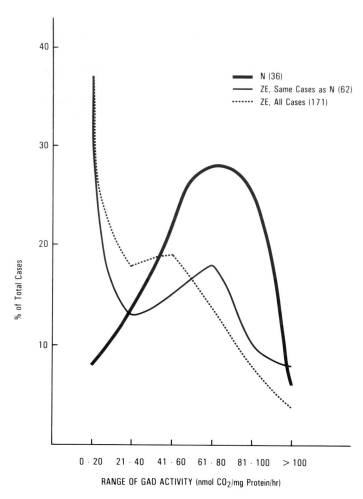

FIG. 4. Population distribution of GAD activity in normal and epileptogenic tissue fragments from the Paris study. The number of tissue fragments occurring within each range of GAD activity is expressed as a percent of the total number of tissue fragments examined in each group (N = normal; ZE = epileptogenic). The number of tissue fragments available in each group is indicated in parentheses.

In contrast, the distribution of GAD activity in epileptogenic tissue, from both those patients having normal and epileptogenic tissue and also from all patients, was shifted very much to lower GAD activities. In fact, most of the tissue fragments exhibited GAD activity between 0 and 40 nmol CO_2/mg protein · hr. A minor peak of GAD activity occurred within the range of the normal tissue fragments. This suggests that the epileptogenic tissue fragments can be divided into two distinct populations with respect to GAD activity: the major population with a very low activity, and the other with GAD activity within the normal range.

The distribution of GAD activity in the tissue fragments from the Bordeaux study very closely parallels the distribution described above. Thus, almost all (80%) of normal tissue fragments exhibited GAD activity in the range of 40 to 80 nmol CO_2/mg protein · hr, whereas 80% of the epileptogenic tissue fragments (grouped as either from patients with both epileptogenic and

normal tissue or from the whole population) exhibited GAD activity less than 40 nmol CO_2/mg protein · hr. In this smaller group of patients there did not appear to be a subpopulation of epileptogenic tissue fragments with GAD activity within the range of the normal tissue fragments.

The group of patients for whom the epilepsy was associated with the presence of a tumor demonstrated alterations qualitatively similar to the two nontumor epileptic groups, but the changes were of a greater magnitude. The mean GAD activity in the normal tissue of these tumor patients was similar to that from the two other patient groups (Fig. 3). However, the pathological tissue exhibited mean GAD activity much lower than that in the epileptogenic tissue from the nontumor patients (Fig. 3).

The level of GAD activity appeared to be correlated to the degree of pathology of the tissue. Thus, as seen in Fig. 5, the lowest mean GAD activity was in the most pathologically altered

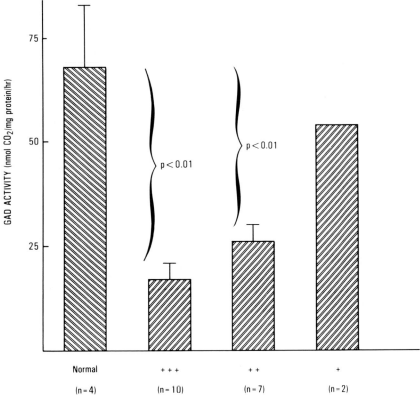

FIG. 5.   GAD activity in pathological tissue: patients from epilepsy–tumor group. Results are expressed as the mean with SEM, with the number of patients in parentheses. The tissue was rated histologically as severely pathological (+ + +, severe infiltration and gliosis), moderately pathological (+ +), and minimal pathological alterations (+).

tissue (+ + +), with progressively higher GAD activity in only moderately (+ +) or minimally (+) affected tissue.

When these tumor patients were examined on an individual basis, all 3 cases with both normal and pathological tissue (+ + +) and 9 of the 10 cases studied with or without normal tissue exhibited very low GAD activity [less than the mean of normal tissue − 2(SEM)].

The population distribution of the normal-tissue fragments from these tumor patients was similar to that exhibited for similar material from nontumoral epileptic patients, except for the occurrence of a "tail" of high GAD activity (23% of fragments having a GAD activity > 100 nmol CO_2/mg protein · hr). However, most (55%) of the normal tissue fragments possessed a GAD activity between 40 and 80 nmol CO_2/mg protein · hr. The distribution of GAD activity in the pathological (+ + +) tissue fragments was, as could be predicted from the mean values, very different from that of the normal fragments. Most of these tissue fragments (65% for cases with both normal and + + + tissue; 60% for

tissue from all patients) had GAD activities less than 20 nmol CO_2/mg protein · hr.

The overall results from these studies offer a strong basis for the GABA hypothesis of epilepsy, at least for those patients who present for neurosurgical resection. It is implicit that this patient population is either refractory or unresponsive to antiepileptic medication. As many of the presently used antiepileptic drugs are proposed to exert their activity by potentiating the action of endogenous GABAergic transmission (cf. ref. 20), a loss of the ability to synthesize GABA together with a loss of receptor responsiveness (35) would be likely not only to explain the poor response to medication, but also to suggest that this loss of inhibitory synaptic activity is at least partially responsible for the creation of the focus.

As noted in the discussion of the literature, previous support for the GABA hypothesis of epilepsy has been limited. Why then does the present study provide such striking support? At least part of the answer is methodological in nature. Thus, in the present study the foci (in the nontumoral patients) were carefully defined by depth electrodes and stereoencephalography. As the electrodes were only in place for 6 to 8 hr, it is highly unlikely that a necrotic reaction to the foreign material could account for the results. This is supported by (a) the lack of necrotic features upon histological examination of the tissue (half of each tissue fragment being taken for biochemistry, the other for histology), (b) the fact that the electrodes penetrated both normal and epileptogenic tissue to an equal extent, and (c) the observation that a similar electrode emplacement in the cat amygdala or hippocampus does not result in reduced GAD activity (K. G. Lloyd, *unpublished data*).

Another important advantage to this study is the use of control and epileptogenic tissue from the same patients. This avoids problems such as differences in drug regime, freezing time, associated disease states, etc.

The parameter studied (GAD activity) is one that does not undergo rapid alterations after removal from the brain, although the clinical status of the patient is highly relevant (18). We have also measured GABA levels in some of these patients. For those epileptogenic fragments not related to the presence of a tumor, GABA levels were not different from the non-epileptogenic normal tissue; however, in those pathological regions associated with the presence of a tumor, GABA levels were significantly decreased (57% of control, $p < 0.01$). The data in the nontumoral epileptic tissue are in good agreement with the literature (see above) and, together with the decreases seen in tumoral areas, suggest that GABA levels are a poor reflection of the functional state of GABA synapses and are only altered under the most severe conditions.

RELEVANCE OF ANIMAL MODELS TO HUMAN BIOCHEMISTRY

Numerous animal models for epilepsy exist with a pharmacological, neuroanatomical, or genetic basis. Any manipulation provoking a diminution in GABA synaptic function results in seizures. Thus, inhibition of GABA synthesis by GAD inhibitors (e.g., allylglycine, aminooxyacetic acid, or hydrazine derivatives of pyridoxal phosphate) (35,40,41) or blockade of GABA receptors or receptor-mediated chloride ion channels (e.g., by bicuculline or picrotoxin) (41) rapidly provoke convulsions. Two groups (35,40) have determined that the onset of seizures after GAD inhibition is highly correlated with the decreased availability of newly synthesized GABA. Although such findings are consistent with the GABA hypothesis of epilepsy, they do not provide direct support for the suggestion that either a genetic state or a neuropathological condition (e.g., cell necrosis, glial infiltration) produces GABA neuron loss, which can be related in a causal manner to the onset of seizures.

An alteration of GABA neuron function is observed in diverse models of seizure disorders which do not *a priori* depend on inhibition of GABA receptors or synthesis. Thus, in the cobalt focus in the rat cortex, the penicillin focus in the cat cortex, and the alumina gel focus in the monkey cortex (Table 3), there are large losses in GAD activity, GABA levels, and GABA uptake. The latter finding is indicative that GABA neurons are probably destroyed under these conditions. In the monkey and rat, the changes in GABA synaptic function paralleled the onset and severity of seizures.

A dysfunctional GABA synapse may well also be related to the proconvulsant condition in genetically sound-sensitive mice (DBA/2) strain. In these mice there is a decreased ability to synthesize GABA as well as a deficient GABA receptor binding and GABA release (in response to potassium) mechanisms (2,15,16,36).

It should be noted that not all seizure conditions are associated with an apparently dysfunctional GABA synapse. Thus, from the available data, amygdaloid kindling does not alter GABA synaptic activity (GABA levels and recognition sites) (11,19). Also, epileptic cerebral tissue from dogs (38) or photosensitive *Papio papio* (14) has normal GABA levels. However, more recent studies demonstrate that a decrease in CSF GABA levels parallels the degree of photosensitivity (23a).

An interesting and practical corollary to the GABA hypothesis of epilepsy is that the GABA deficiency state should respond to GABA replacement therapy, in a parallel manner to the response of Parkinson's disease patients to L-DOPA or dopamine agonist therapy. The available evidence is in strong support of this, as GABA agonists exert a broad-spectrum antiepileptic activity in animal models (9,24,41). Furthermore, progabide, a nontoxic GABA agonist available for use in clinical trials (22), exhibits an antiepileptic action in different types of human epilepsies (1,25).

It should be noted that the human data presented in this review suggest that some severe forms of epilepsy, which have a severe loss of both GABA synthesis and GABA receptors, will be relatively unresponsive to treatment based on augmenting GABA synaptic activity and/or efficacy.

TABLE 3. *Alterations in GABA synaptic function in experimental seizure models*

Animal model	Alteration in GABA synaptic activity		Reference
	Component	Alteration	
Cobalt focus, rat cortex	GAD	↓ 45–90%	(4)
	GABA uptake	↓ 60–65%	(3)
	GABA	↓ 40–70%	(10,33,34)
Penicillin focus, cat cortex	GAD	↓ 20%	(12)
	GABA uptake	↓ 50–60%	(13)
	GABA	↓ 30–40%	
Aluminal gel, monkey cortex	GAD	↓ 60%	(32)
	GABA uptake	↓ 50–70%	
	GABA	↓ 45–55%	
	GABA "A"	↓ 50–55%	

SUMMARY AND CONCLUSIONS

The GABA hypothesis of epilepsy has been examined in different types of tissue originating from epileptic patients. Only in those studies where the epileptogenic area has been precisely defined (e.g., using stereoelectroencephalography from depth electrodes) and compared to nonepileptic tissue from the same patients has it been possible to demonstrate a dysfunction of GABA synaptic activity in the epileptogenic areas in a large subpopulation of epileptic patients. Furthermore, except in cases of extremely low GAD activity (e.g., in certain tumor regions), GABA levels are within the normal range. This combination of factors is likely to explain the lack of support for the GABA hypothesis in studies not using these criteria.

These studies with human tissue, together with data from relevant animal models, suggest that in epileptic patients presenting for neurosurgical intervention (no indication of a tumor), about 50 to 70% have a decreased ability to synthesize and/or respond to GABA in the epileptogenic regions. When a tumor is present, almost all severely pathological regions demonstrate a greatly reduced GAD activity as compared to normal tissue from the same patients.

It follows from these data that the GABA hypothesis is not an exclusive or unitary hypothesis, as some patients appear to have normally functioning GABA synapses (as assessed biochemically) in epileptogenic areas. Thus, other neurotransmitter and neurohumoral systems certainly play a role in the epileptic process.

REFERENCES

1. Abstracts, 15th Epilepsy International Symposium (1983), edited by R. J. Porter, R. H. Mattson, A. A. Ward, Jr., and M. Dam. Raven Press, New York.

2. Al-Ani, A. T., Tunnicliff, G., Rick, J. T., and Kohut, G. A. (1970): GABA production, acetylcholinesterase activity and biogenic amine levels in brain for mouse strains differing in spontaneous activity and reactivity. *Life Sci.,* 9 (I): 21–27.

3. Altamura, A. C., Bonati, M., Brunello, N., Giordano, P. L., and Algeri, S. (1978): The activity of some neurotransmitter-synthetizing enzymes in experimental cobalt epilepsy. *Neurosci. Lett.,* 7:83–87.

4. Balcar, V. J., Pumain, R., Mark, J., Borg, J., and Mandel, P. (1978): GABA-mediated inhibition in the epileptogenic focus, a process which may be involved in the mechanism of the cobalt-induced epilepsy. *Brain Res.,* 154:182–185.

5. Bancaud, J., Talairach, J., Bonis, A., Schaub, E., Szikla, G., Morel, P., and Bordas-Ferrer, M. (1966): *La Stereo-Electroencéphalographie de l'Epilepsie.* Masson, Paris.

6. Baxter, C. F. (1970): The nature of γ-aminobutyric acid. In: *The Handbook of Neurochemistry, Vol. IV.,* edited by A. Lajtha, pp. 289–353. Plenum, New York.

7. Bird, E. D., and Iversen, L. L. (1974): Huntington's chorea. Post mortem measurement of glutamic acid decarboxylase, choline acetyl transferse and dopamine in basal ganglia. *Brain,* 97:457–472.

8. Bloom, F. E., and Iversen, L. L. (1971): Localizing ³H-GABA in nerve terminals of rat cerebral cortex by electron microscope autoradiography. *Nature (Lond.),* 229:628–633.

9. Cepeda, C., Worms, P., Lloyd, K. G., and Naquet, R. S. (1982): Action of progabide in the photosensitive baboon, *Papio papio. Epilepsia,* 23:463–470.

10. Emson, P. C., and Joseph, M. H. (1975): Neurochemical and morphological changes during the development of cobalt-induced epilepsy in the rat. *Brain Res.,* 93:91–110.

11. Fabisiak, J. P., and Schwartz, W. S. (1982): Cerebral free amino-acids in the amygdaloid kindling model of epilepsy. *Neuropharmacology,* 21:179–182.

12. Gottesfeld, Z., and Elazar, Z. (1972): GABA and glutamate in different EEG stages of the penicillin focus. *Nature (Lond.),* 240:478–479.

13. Gottesfeld, Z., and Elazar, Z. (1975): GABA syn-

thesis and uptake in penicillin focus. *Brain Res.*, 84:346–350.

14. Hansen, S., Perry, T. L., Wada, J. A., and Sokol, M. (1973): Brain amino acids in baboons with light-induced epilepsy. *Brain Res.*, 50:480–483.

15. Hertz, L., Schousboe, A., Fornby, B., and Lennox-Buchthal, M. (1974): Some age-dependent biochemical changes in mice susceptible to seizures. *Epilepsia*, 15:619–631.

16. Horton, R. W., Prestwick, S. A., and Meldrum, B. S. (1982): γ-Aminobutyric acid and benzodiazepine binding sites in audiogenic seizure-susceptible mice. *J. Neurochem.*, 39:864–870.

17. Iversen, L. L. (1978): Biochemical psychopharmacology of GABA. In: *Psychopharmacology, A Generation of Progress*, edited by M. A. Lipton, A. DiMascio, and K. F. Killam, pp. 25–38. Raven Press, New York.

18. Iversen, L. L., Bird, E. D., Spokes, E., Nicholson, S. H., and Suckling, C. J. (1979): Agonist specificity of GABA binding sites in human brain and GABA in Huntington's disease and schizophrenia. In: *GABA-Neurotransmitters*, edited by P. Krogsgaard-Larsen, J. Scheel-Kruger, and H. Kofod, pp.179–190. Munksgaard, Copenhagen.

19. Kalichman, M. W. (1982): Neurochemical correlates of the kindling-model of epilepsy. *Neurosci. Biobehav. Rev.*, 6:165–181.

20. Lloyd, K. G. (1983): Role of GABAergic systems in the mechanism of action of antiepileptic drugs. *Thérapie*, 38:355–362.

21. Lloyd, K. G., Munari, C., Bossi, L., Stoeffels, C., Talairach, J., and Morselli, P. (1981): Biochemical evidence for the alteration of GABA-mediated synaptic transmission in pathological brain tissue (stereo-EEG or morphological definition) from epileptic patients. In: *Neurotransmitters, Seizures and Epilepsy*, edited by P. L. Morselli, K. G. Lloyd, W. Löscher, B. S. Meldrum, and E. Reynolds, pp. 325–338. Raven Press, New York.

22. Lloyd, K. G., Morselli, P. L., Depoortere, H., Fournier, V., Zivkovic, B., Scatton, B., Broekkamp, C. L. E., Worms, P., and Bartholini, G. (1983): The potential use of GABA agonists in psychiatric disorders: Evidence from studies with progabide in animal models and clinical trials. *Pharmacol. Biochem. Behav.*, 18:957–966.

23. Lloyd, K. G., Zivkovic, B., Scatton, B., and Bartholini, G. (1984): Evidence for functional roles of GABA pathways in the mammalian brain. In: *Actions and Interactions of GABA and Benzodiazepines*, edited by N. G. Bowery, pp. 59–79. Raven Press, New York.

23a. Lloyd, K. G., Scatton, B., Voltz, C., Bryere, P., Valin, A., and Naquet, R. (1985): Cerebrospinal fluid amino acid and monoamine metabolite levels of *Papio papio*: Correlation with photosensitivity. *Brain Res.* (*in press*).

24. Löscher, W. (1982): Comparative assay of anticonvulsant and toxic potencies of sixteen GABAmimetic drugs. *Neuropharmacology*, 21: 803–810.

25. Loiseau, P., Bossi, L., Guyot, M., Orofiamima, B., and Morselli, P. L. (1983): Double-blind crossover trial of progabide versus placebo in severe epilepsies. *Epilepsia*, 24:703–715.

26. Lott, I. T., Coulombe, T., Di Paolo, R. V., Richardson, E. P., and Levy, H. L. (1978): Vitamin B₆-dependent seizure: Pathology and chemical findings in brain. *Neurology*, 28:47–54.

27. Lovell, R. A., Elliot, S. J., and Elliott, K. A. C. (1963): The γ-aminobutyric acid and factor I content of brain. *J. Neurochem.*, 10:479–488.

28. McGeer, P. L., McGeer, E. G., and Wada, J. A. (1971): Glutamic acid decarboxylase in Parkinson's disease and epilepsy. *Neurology*, 21:1000–1007.

29. Mao, C. C., and Costa, E. (1978): Biochemical pharmacology of GABAergic transmission. In: *Psychopharmacology: A Generation of Progress*, edited by M. A. Lipton, A. DiMascio, and K. F. Killam, pp. 307–318. Raven Press, New York.

30. Perry, T. L., and Hansen, S. (1981): Amino acid abnormalities in epileptogenic foci. *Neurology*, 31:872–876.

31. Perry, T. L., Hansen, S., Kennedy, J., Wada, J. A., and Thompson, G. B. (1975): Amino acids in human epileptogenic foci. *Arch. Neurol.*, 32:752–754.

32. Ribak, C. E., Harris, A. B., Vaughn, J. E., and Roberts, E. (1979): Inhibitory GABAergic nerve terminals decrease at sites of focal epilepsy. *Science*, 205:211–214.

33. Ross, S. M., and Craig, C. R. (1981): Studies on γ-aminobutyric acid transport in cobalt experimental epilepsy in the rat. *J. Neurochem.*, 36:1006–1011.

34. Ross, S. M., and Craig, C. R. (1981): γ-Aminobutyric acid concentration, L-glutamic L-decarboxylase activity and properties of the γ-aminobutyric receptor in cobalt epilepsy in the rat. *J. Neurosci.*, 1:1388–1396.

35. Tapia, R. (1974): The role of γ-aminobutyric acid metabolism in the regulation of cerebral excitability. In: *Neurohumoral Coding of Brain Function*, edited by R. D. Mejers and R. R. Drucker, pp. 3–26. Plenum, New York.

36. Ticku, M. (1979): Differences in γ-aminobutyric acid receptor sensitivity in inbred strains of mice. *J. Neurochem.*, 33:1135–1138.

37. Tower, D. B. (1960): *Neurochemistry of Epilepsy*. Charles C Thomas, Springfield, Illinois.

38. Van Gelder, N. M., Edmonds, H. C., Hegerberg, G. A., Chatburn, C. C., Clemmons, M. R., and Sylvester, D. M. (1980): Amino acid changes in a genetic strain of epileptic beagle dogs. *J. Neurochem.*, 35:1087–1091.

39. Van Gelder, N. M., Sherwin, A. L., and Rasmussen, R. (1972): Amino-acid content of epileptogenic human brain: Focal versus surrounding regions. *Brain Res.*, 40:385–393.

40. Wood, J. D., and Peesker, S. J. (1973): The role of GABA metabolism in the convulsant and anticonvulsant actions of amino-oxyacetic acid. *J. Neurochem.*, 20:379–387.

41. Worms, P., and Lloyd, K. G. (1981): Functional alterations of GABA synapses in relation to seizures. In: *Neurotransmitters, Seizures and Epilepsy*, edited by P. L. Morselli, K. G. Lloyd, W. Löscher, B. S. Meldrum, and E. Reynolds, pp. 37–48. Raven Press, New York.

Advances in Neurology, Vol. 44, edited by
A. V. Delgado-Escueta, A. A. Ward, Jr.,
D. M. Woodbury, and R. J. Porter.
Raven Press, New York © 1986.

53

Neuron-Glia Relationships in Human and Experimental Epilepsy: A Biochemical Point of View

Thierry M. Grisar

Laboratory of Neurochemistry, University of Liège, 4020 Liège, Belgium

SUMMARY   The generation of focal cortical epilepsy as observed in human partial complex seizures is presumably due to enhanced physiologic responses or paroxysmal depolarization shifts (PDSs). However, the molecular mechanism that underlies these phenomena remains unknown. It could be due to a genetically determined error in a structural or regulatory protein or to posttranslational events that modulate membrane excitability. Since neither neuronal PDSs or interictal EEG spikes are sufficient to produce clinical epilepsy, the clinical expression of epilepsy may need the breakdown of neuronal or glial mechanisms that limit the spread of seizures. Hence, biochemical membrane studies of neurons and glia are necessary to understand the expression of human and experimental epilepsy.

This chapter will review the role of glia in controlling neuronal excitability and neuron–glia relationships in experimental and human epilepsy. Data exploring the hypothesis that glial control of extracellular K^+ or $(K^+)_o$ is deficient in focal epilepsy induced by cold lesions will be reviewed. The role of glial carbonic anhydrase (CA) and glial control of putative amino acid transmitters in audiogenic epilepsy will be discussed.

In the cold lesion, $(K^+)_o$ activation constants of synaptosomal (Na^+,K^+)-ATPase are significantly decreased in the actively firing chronic focus, suggesting that the apparent affinity of the synaptosomal enzyme for K^+ was increased within epileptic tissue that was actively firing. Interestingly, while sustained focal paroxysms could raise synaptosomal (Na^+,K^+)-ATPase, glial (Na^+,K^+)-ATPase and its activation by $(K^+)_o$ remained decreased during sustained paroxysms in both acute and chronic lesions. Moreover, while the decrease of the absolute level of glial enzyme activity was less evident 45 days after lesion production, the poor response of glial enzyme to $(K^+)_o$ never reversed to "normal" values. Hence, these experiments provided new information that glial (Na^+,K^+)-ATPase responds to K^+ in a different manner when compared to synaptic enzyme. Glial ATPase and its activation by $(K^+)_o$ remain decreased in either actively discharging acute lesions or in the indolent chronic foci. This could mean a reduction in the ability of glial membranes to maintain $(K^+)_o$ homeostasis. As already suggested by Dichter (27), the impairment in glial control of elevated $(K^+)_o$ could be mainly responsible for the transition of interictal discharges to ictal episodes, within the primary and the secondary foci. The inverse interpretation could be proposed for normal or perifocal areas (PF) where the physiological efficiency of glial enzyme remained optimal even at high K^+ concentrations, thus indicating an increase rather than a reduction of the protective ability of glial membranes.

Since abnormal ATPase activities were found in an experimental model of focal epilepsies, we attempted to determine whether abnormalities in K^+-activation mechanisms of (Na^+,K^+)-ATPase in glial and synaptosomes enriched fractions were present in human temporal-lobe epilepsy.

Our experiments used highly enriched glial cell fractions isolated from the temporal neocortices of 15 patients suffering from partial complex epilepsy and who have well-identified hippocampal–amygdalar or medial temporal and hippocampal sclerosis. They demonstrate that glial (Na^+,K^+)-ATPase decreased its total activities and lost or decreased its response to a range of K^+ concentrations previously shown to activate (i.e., between 3 and 18 mm K^+). Although synaptosomal (Na^+,K^+)-ATPase also decreased in total activities, no significant changes in its reactivity to external K^+ were observed. Using a different technique for preparing glial cells, a similar loss of reactivity by glial (Na^+,K^+)-ATPase was recently reported in human cerebral epileptogenic foci produced by brain tumors (75). These authors also reported a high degree of correlation between the degree of epileptogenesis of cortical areas with the decreased sensitivity of glial (Na^+,K^+)-ATPase to K^+.

We also analyzed CA activity in gliotic and epileptogenic cortical tissues from cats with cortical freeze lesions. The results were compared with a genetic model of epilepsy, namely, audiogenic seizure DBA/2J mice, as a function of age and severity of seizure activity.

In the cold lesions, no significant modifications in CA activities were seen in the primary (F) and secondary (M) focus in comparison to sham-operated animals (control) and to the perifocal areas (PF).

In audiogenic mice, CA activities increased with age in both audiogenic (DBA/2J) and nonepileptic (C57/BL) controls. During the first 30 days of life, CA activities always measured higher in DBA/2J mice, and more particularly from days 23 and 24, i.e., 1 to 3 days following the peak of maximal severity score of seizure. A steep decrease of the severity score of seizure together with a decrease in brain CA activity was seen after a single intraperitoneal injection of acetazolamide (150 mg/kg). The anticonvulsant effect of this drug decreased with the age of the DBA/2J mice in parallel with the increase of CA activities mentioned above.

Whether or not these differences in CA activity are species-related or have something to do with cortical hyperexcitability has yet to be resolved. However, if one supposes that these modifications of CA activity are a biochemical change associated with seizure, the hypothesis that enhanced CA activity in glial cells of epileptogenic cortex is an adaptive mechanism to overcome the eventual defect in anion transport has only been verified, in our experience, in genetic models. In the cat with freeze lesions, astrogliosis is not accompanied by enhanced CA activity.

Although a considerable amount of data have emphasized the role of glial cells in controlling neurotransmitter substances at the synaptic cleft, the integrity of such glial property had not been investigated in epileptogenic tissue. Theoretically, one can imagine that a glial defect in regulating extracellular glutamate or gamma-aminobutyric acid (GABA), for instance, might have deep influence on the adjacent neurons. This hypothesis had been poorly tested. We performed some experiments using glutamate uptake in astrocytes cultivated from both normal C57/BL mice versus audiogenic DBA/2J prone mice. The uptake (V_{max}) is much higher in the cultivated astrocytes from the seizure-susceptible mice. This might be related either to a simple species difference or to the epileptic features of the DBA/2J prone mice. In this latter hypothesis, a genetically determined potential of these astrocytes to accumulate with higher efficiency the extracellular glutamate, at the synaptic cleft, diminishes the amount of glutamate excitation and could be considered a protective mechanism against the seizure susceptibility. Similar protective properties have recently been ascribed to CA.

On the other hand, we recently found that the glutamate content of the audiogenic mice cerebral cortex is higher than in C57/BL normal mice, particularly so at an age where the seizure susceptibility is high. The ratio of glutamate to GABA is higher in the DBA/2J mice and decreases with age after day 20. This supports the view that the glutamatergic synapses are either more active or increased in number in the epileptogenic cortex of the audiogenic seizure susceptible mice.

Recent results seem to indicate that this surplus of glutamate in the DBA/2J mice might be produced by an accelerated rate of the catabolism of putrescine. This might be of major interest, since polyamines are known to influence protein synthesis and the subsequent development and maturation of nerve cells. This polyamines–GABA/glutamate shunt could, therefore, be one of the biochemical links between development and seizure susceptibility.

Since 1965, one of the major conceptual advances in the neurosciences has been the emergence of glial cells in the control of neuronal excitability. Excellent reviews touching on the biochemistry, physiology, and histochemistry of glial cells have been published by several authors (63,128).

In 1846, Virchow introduced the term "neuroglia" (158) for all interstitial substances other than neurons in the walls of the ventricle and spinal cord. By 1873, the Golgi staining technique (48) distinguished neurons and glia, while through 1909 to 1911, Cajal established the ectodermal origins of neuroglial cells (16) in his classic work on the spinal cord of the chick embryo. Cajal noted three cell types: neuroblasts, astrocytes, and a third cell type that was identified later by Del Rio Hortega in 1919 (124) as a cell type distinct from macroglia and known as microglia. Del Rio Hortega thus separated the third cell type of Cajal into oligodendrocytes and microglia. Today, the complete developmental history of neuroglial cells remains unknown. In 1976, Sturrock (147) proposed the existence of four distinct glial cell types: (a) the early glioblast will give either (b) a small glioblast or (c) a large glioblast. The former will provide (d) the young astrocyte and then the mature astrocyte; the latter will give the lineage of light, medium, and dark oligodendrocyte. Microglia could derive either from pericytes or from small glioblasts (see ref. 13 for review).

Quantitative relationships between neurons and glia in mammalian cortex have been established by several authors (68,117,139) for proper understanding of their spatial configurations, functional interactions, and relative contributions to biochemical structure and metabolism. In cat striate cortex, Sholl (139) calculated that about 55% of the volume was occupied by neuronal perikarya and dendrites combined. A reasonable estimate for the neuronal compartment of human eulaminate and eugranular isocortex would be 35 to 40% of the fresh volume; the next largest contribution (20 to 25%) was visualized as voluminous expansions of protoplasmic astrocytes (139). Since the extracellular space is in general estimated as a volume fraction on the order of 20%, this leaves another 20% of the fresh volume for oligodendroglia, myelin sheaths, and mesodermal derivatives (microglia and blood vessels).

This cellular heterogeneity of the central nervous system imposes upon neurobiology the task of establishing clear qualitative relationships between these complex cytological constituents. Cajal recognized the importance of glia as early as 1895; he attributed two roles to the cortical glia, namely, the control of the flow of "nervous currents" and the flow of blood. These aspects of neuron–glia relationships in the central nervous system (CNS), however, were largely neglected until 1965. Understandably, more attention was focused first on neuronal cells in view of their extraordinary electrical properties and their fabulous power to transfer information through the nervous system. Thus, until the 1970s it was tacitly assumed that biochemical properties of nervous tissues reflected events occurring in neuronal cells. The main function of glial cells was to "glue neurons together." Some pioneers like Lugaro in 1907 (90) or Holmgren in 1904 (71) and Geren (44), following Cajal in 1895 (16), recognized some more dynamic roles for glial cells, such as removing "toxic" substances from the extracellular space (ECS), providing neuronal "nutrition," and finally forming myelin. Modern morphological, biochemical, and physiological techniques allowed new dynamic approaches towards glial cell functions in both the peripheral and the central nervous systems. This major change started with the work of Kuffler and Nicholls (82) on the electrophysiology of glial cells membranes. This was followed by the introduction of techniques using cell separation either by gradient centrifugation or tissue culture techniques (24,63,128 for review). Tower (152) wrote in 1978:

> Clearly both of the major classes of glial cells are important partners with neurons in

the structural and functional integrity of the nervous system: the oligodendroglia and Schwann cells interacting with axons to function as a unit in impulse conduction and transmission from one neuronal element to another or to effector organs; and the astrocytes interacting with neurons in metabolic and modulatory fashions.

From this considerable amount of work, glial cells have progressively acquired the status of a major control system for brain excitability. This regulatory role occurs by maintaining either extracellular ions and neurotransmitter homeostasis or by forming and sustaining the myelin sheath on axons of the CNS. The purpose of this chapter is first to review the recent progress that has been achieved in these areas.

In 1970, Trachtenberg and Pollen (153) and Franck (36) independently proposed that a significant factor in the development of focal epilepsy could be a degradation of the spatial buffering function of the glial cells. Indeed, a striking astroglial gliosis is very often present in epileptic foci in both experimental and human epilepsy. These authors hypothesized that the reactive astroglia investing the epileptogenic neurons may be incapable of "spatially buffering" ions like K^+ released by firing neurons. Histoenzymological abnormalities of astrocytes have also been described in focal epilepsy, and a causal relationship with epileptogenicity in man as well as in animal has been suggested (14). The conversion of proteoplasmic astrocytes in large numbers would indeed intuitively be consistent with changes in their above mentioned function, possibly characterized by an abnormal handling of ions and/or the metabolism of neurotransmitter substances, such as glutamate and GABA. Since this time, however, several electrophysiological and biochemical observations have both supported and contradicted this view, and accordingly expressed some differences in the meaning of neuron–glia relationships in epilepsy. Hence, the present chapter also reviews the contributions of glial cells to seizure phenomena both in human and experimental epilepsy.

GLIAL CONTROL OF NEURONAL EXCITABILITY

From their pioneer work on the electrophysiology of the leech ganglia, Kuffler and Nicholls (82) concluded the glial cells were not essential for neuronal signaling over a period of a few hours.

On the other hand, in 1960, using biochemical methods, Hyden proposed the concept that the neuron and its satellite cells form a functional unit (73).

In fact, glial cells interfere with neuronal excitability in at least two major ways: (a) the oligodendrocytes interact with axons to furnish them with their myelin sheath but also probably by some metabolic interactions, and (b) the astrocytes are mainly known to control the microenvironment of surrounding neurons but could also be capable of providing them with important metabolic substrates.

Most of what we know about the biochemistry of oligodendroglia has been derived from studies of myelin and myelination and is beyond the scope of this chapter, since virtually nothing is known about epilepsy and myelination. In contrast, there have been a considerable number of studies concerned with the astrocytic control of the composition of the extra cellular space (ECS) and its influence on neuronal excitability. This role can be played either by controlling the ionic composition of the ECS or by removing (inactivating) putative neurotransmitter substances from the ECS.

Ion Homeostasis

Potassium

Repetitive action potentials result in accumulation of potassium ions in the extracellular space adjacent to neurons (37,149). From a resting level of 3 mM, K^+ can increase to 10 or 20 mM during intense nerve activity, whereas values as high as 30, 50, or 80 mM have been seen in spreading depression, anoxia, or hypoglycemia (37,145,149).

Increases of $(K^+)_o$ would have an excitatory effect on neurons, since K^+ depolarizes neuronal membranes and evokes repetitive firing of isolated axons. Also, the amplitude of spike potentials and excitatory postsynaptic potentials (EPSPs) of motor neurons shows a linear relationship to the resting potential versus external potassium (94).

Evidence supporting the view that K^+ is involved in the so-called "primary afferent depolarization" and in transmitter release from primary afferent terminals has also been reviewed by Sykova (149). However, increased $(K^+)_o$ can have a dual effect according to the level of this elevation: low increases in general facilitate neuronal excitability and synaptic transmission, while higher elevations (greater than 6–8 mM) can lead to neuronal depression (149). Moreover, Weight and Erulkar (167) illustrated how the modulation of transmitter release by K^+ accumulation induced by postsynaptic impulse activity can function as a direct negative feedback, supporting many results showing that the frequency of impulses in some firing neurons increases first as a "burst" and then the neurons stop firing (167).

Therefore the mechanisms by which accumulated K^+ is cleared from the ECS are of major importance when discussing the control systems of neuronal excitability under both normal and pathological conditions. Although many observations support the conclusion that excessive changes in $(K^+)_o$ are cleared by active transport across neuronal membranes, the fluctuations in $(K^+)_o$ are probably also compensated by other transports across glial membranes, blood-brain barrier, and diffusion in the extracellular space.

The possible involvement of glial cells in this regulatory process has been proposed by several authors (37,38), but opinions remain divided about the nature (i.e., active or passive) by which glial cells (mainly astrocytes) could limit the rise of K^+. Electrophysiological results in general favor the concept of passive spatial buffering system as proposed by Orkand (103), whereas biochemical observations support the idea of an active accumulation of K^+ mediated by the (Na^+,K^+)-ATPase (37,38).

K^+ transport in glial cells

According to the "spatial buffer mechanism" (103), K^+ enters the glial cells in the region with a high $(K^+)_o$ and leaves it elsewhere in regions where the $(K^+)_o$ is lower. This local buildup of extracellular K^+ and the consequent glial cell membrane depolarization cause current to flow through the so-called "glial syncitium." This purely passive process only requires that the local glial cell membrane is permeable to K^+. Two facts from electrophysiological studies were the ingredients of this theory.

1. Glial cells function as highly selective K^+ electrodes, membrane potential varying with changes of $(K^+)_o$, according to the Nernst Law ("Nernstian behavior"). Moreover, only a single K^+ channel has been recently recorded with oligodendroglial membrane patches (76). Accordingly, most investigators agree that glial membranes are almost exclusively permeable to K^+ (see also ref. 164).

2. Glial cells are electrically coupled both *in vivo* (82,120) and *in vitro* (97,98) with evidence of the existence of low-resistance interconnections between astrocytes (gap junctions).

A school opposite to the "spatial buffering function" of glial cells contends that extracellular K^+ is cleared by active transport mechanisms and that glial membranes, in fact, do not behave as a perfect K^+ electrode (Table 1). Although this may be due to nonnegligible Na^+ and Cl^- conductance (163), this non-Nernstian behavior of glial cells is more likely the consequence of increased intracellular K^+ concentration when the extracellular K^+ is raised (22).

In fact, several investigators found K^+ accumulation in glial structures when exposed to elevated external K^+ concentrations (37,38,56). Early slice experiments by Franck (37,56) have clearly shown that an increase of the external potassium from 3 to 20 mM led to a step increase in intracellular K^+ concentration in a cellular compartment identified as the glial cells (56).

The ability of isolated glial cells to accumulate potassium efficiently was then demonstrated with either bulk isolated (60) or cultured astrocytes (66). Moreover, faster accumulation of labeled K^+ into the glial compartment of brain slices (36), as well as into astrocytes of primary cultures (66,98), than into corresponding neuronal structures also suggested that the main uptake of K^+ occurs in glia cells. The correlation between rates of $^{43}K^+$ uptake and potassium concentration indicated a K_m value of 10 to 15 mM for K^+ transport into cultured astrocytes (38), suggesting a major activation of this process when the extracellular concentration is increased well above the resting level (37,40). Walz et al. (164) confirmed that membrane potential characteristics of astrocytes in primary culture reveal exclusive potassium conductance and potassium accumulator properties.

Several mechanisms have been proposed to explain this specific glial K^+ accumulation: (a) the passive entrance of the "spatial buffer mechanism," (b) a K^+–Cl^- exchange, (c) a net active uptake of K^+, and (d) an Na^+–K^+ exchange through the Na^+,K^+ pump.

As recalled by Gardner-Medwin (41), the spatial buffer mechanism is a purely passive process, a form of facilitated K^+ diffusion. This transport, however, would require that K^+ passively cross the glial membrane against an important electrochemical gradient in such a manner that $(K^+)_i$ does not vary significantly. This is no longer supported by experiments cited above, and recent evidence shows that a large change in intraglial K^+ concentration does exist in "glia elements" of the retina of the drone honeybee when light is flashed to activate surrounding photoreceptors ("neuronal elements") (22).

TABLE 1. *Relation between glial membrane potential* (in vitro *and* in vivo) *and the decimal logarithm of external potassium*[a]

Material	Slope of the Nernst diagram (mV)	$(K^+)_o$ range (mM)	Reference
Optic nerve of *Necturus maculosus*	59	1.5–75	Kuffler and Nicholls (1966) (82)
Rat optic nerve	42	3–45	Dennis and Gerschenfeld, (1969) (26)
Rabbit cerebellar explants	27	14.2–114	Wardell (1966) (166)
	27	5.7–14.2	
C_6 glioma cells	31	4.5–80	Kukes et al., (1976) (81)
Human TC 526 glioblastoma	54	2.5–5.3	Manuelidis et al.
	25	5.3–16.5	(1975) (91)
Cat cerebral cortex	"Less than would be predicted by the Nernst equation"	2.9–40	Pape and Katzman, (1972) (104)
Cat cerebral cortex	38	3–40	Ransom and Goldring, (1973) (120)
Cat cerebral cortex (penicillin focus)	"Several discrepancies between rises in $(K^+)_o$ and glial"	Single interictal discharges (3.6 mM)	Futamachi and Pedley, (1976) (41)
	61	Ictal episodes	
	30 (once)	7 mM	
Cat spinal cord	61, 65	5 mM	Lothman and Somjen, (1975) (89)
Cultured rat astrocytes	52	3–50	Moonen et al. (1980) (98)
	51	1.5–100	Walz et al. (1984) (164)
Cultured mouse oligodendrocytes	51		Kettenman et al. (1983) (76)

[a] Compiled from ref. 98.

Moreover, one must keep in mind that the cellular membrane is a phospholipid bilayer with embedded active proteins, undergoing constant modifications of their tridimensional structures. Energy sources like ATP and other phosphate donors are constantly used, maintaining the membranous system far from the thermodynamic equilibrium. In other words, the cellular membranes have to be thought in terms of "open thermodynamic systems." This is particularly true as far as cation movements are concerned, since (Na^+,K^+)-ATPase exists and is a specific energy-dependent molecular machinery for cation transport (see below). Hence, from this theoretical point of view, we feel that uptake of K^+ within the glial cells, as in any other cells, must be an active process.

In fact, a potassium-induced stimulation of oxygen uptake in glial cells has been illustrated in brain slices (64), in isolated glial cells (64), and in subventricular white matter that is known to be highly enriched in glial cells. Its virtual absence in jimpy mice (63,64), which are deficient in glial cells, also supports this notion.

Similarly, a potassium-induced reduction of ATP content observed in brain slices seems to occur predominantly in astrocytes (64). Although these experiments on K^+-enhanced O_2 uptake only provide indirect arguments and were most often observed in high-potassium media (± 50 mM), these observations further support the concept that the metabolic effects of increased extracellular potassium concentrations are exerted mainly on glial cells.

A K^+-dependent uptake of chloride into glia has also been described under circumstances requiring elevated (and pathological) extracellular levels of potassium (10–12). This involves both passive and carrier-mediated transport of cations with Cl^-, and transfer of an osmotic equivalent of water. Carbonic anhydrase was shown to be implicated in this process (11). As discussed by us elsewhere (56), a crucial K^+ concentration (i.e., ± 20 mM) seems to demarcate the border between the so-called "physiological" and "pathological" biochemical events observed in brain tissue incubated *in vitro*. In our opinion, this Cl^-,K^+-dependent water uptake probably corresponds to a model of brain edema, as recently discussed by Kimelberg (81) and Walz and Hertz (163). An ouabain-resistant net uptake of potassium into cultured astrocytes over and above that caused by diffusion has been shown to be much more intense than in neurons, where the mechanism appears to be stimulated by elevated potassium concentrations (162). Finally, that glial cells contain a potassium-dependent, ouabain-sensitive, hyperpolarizing electrogenic pump has also been shown by several electrophysiological studies (97,98). Its significance in K^+ homeostasis versus axonal pump has been questioned, however (145). Walz et al. (164) also claimed that an ouabain effect on the glial membrane potential does not rule out the possibility of an impairment of the only K^+ accumulation, rather than an impairment in the electrogenic exchange of Na^+ and K^+.

The potassium–sodium exchange observed in brain slices when external potassium increases from 3.7 to 20 mM is presumably mediated by the Na^+,K^+ pump (37,38). Because this exchange occurs essentially in a glial compartment, the concept of a specific activation of the glial Na^+,K^+ pump in K^+-enriched media has recently been favored (38). Until now, the key experiments, calculating simultaneous fluxes (both outfluxes and influxes) of Na^+ and K^+ in isolated glial versus neuronal cells in progressive K^+-enriched media, both *in vitro* and *in vivo*, are still missing.

The recent discovery of a specific K^+-activated glial (Na^+,K^+)-ATPase has supported the idea of a special role of glial cells in an active control of external K^+ concentration mediated by the Na^+,K^+ pump (50,55).

Brain (Na^+,K^+)-ATPase

Another way to illustrate a key role of astrocytes in active control of extracellular K^+ in the CNS would be to demonstrate that these cells do in fact have a specific molecular machinery to actively pump K^+ in K^+-enriched media. This approach, however, is very often neglected by most electrophysiological studies, which underestimate the significance of the molecular pathways used by almost all the cellular membranes along the phylogenetic tree (from *Escherichia coli* to human brain) to carry K^+ inside the cells, i.e., the Na^+,K^+ pump, enzymatically controlled by the (Na^+,K^+)-ATPase.

In 1957, Skou (142) demonstrated that a microsomial fraction of crab (*Carcinus maenas*) leg nerve was able to hydrolyze ATP in the presence of Mg^{2+}, Na^+, and K^+ ions. The K^+ activated

ATP hydrolysis only in the presence of both Mg^{2+} and Na^+. That this system was in fact the enzymatic support of the Na^+,K^+ pump was further demonstrated by the fact that the same low concentrations of cardiac glycosides (ouabain–strophantidin) inhibited both the activity of this microsomial fraction and Na^+ outflux (1,47).

This sodium and potassium ion-stimulated adenosine triphosphatase, a membrane-embedded protein, was then shown to be the enzyme responsible for the active transport of Na^+ and K^+ ions in most animal cells (1). Since this discovery, several reviews and symposia have been dedicated to this fundamental enzyme (1,47).

The evolutionary significance of this enzyme is to maintain an osmotic equilibrium in the intracellular compartment, and it is important to remember that up to 30% of the total energy supplied by the mitochondrial respiratory chain is devoted to this Na^+,K^+ pump in a large variety of mammalian cells (1). The enzyme consists of a large subunit (MW 92,000–120,000), designated alpha, and a smaller glycosylated subunit (MW 35,000–55,000) designated beta (47). The alpha subunit is the catalytic site which is phosphorylated by ATP in the presence of Mg^{2+} and Na^+ (47). It might also be in part a binding site for cardiac glycosides.

The sequence of the enzymatic reaction can be written as follows:

$$E_1 + ATP \cdot Mg^{2-} \rightleftharpoons E_1 \cdot ATP \cdot Mg \tag{1}$$

$$E_1 \cdot ATP \cdot Mg \overset{3Na^+_i}{\rightleftharpoons} E_1 \sim P + ADP \cdot Mg^{2-} \tag{2}$$

$$E_1 \sim P \rightleftharpoons E_2 - P + 3Na^+_o \tag{3}$$
$$3Na^+_i$$

$$E_2 - P \overset{2K^+_o}{\underset{\text{cardiac}}{\rightleftharpoons}} E_2 + P_i$$
$$\text{glycosides } 2K^+_o \tag{4}$$

$$E_2 \rightleftharpoons E_1 + 2K^+_i$$
$$2K^+_o \tag{5}$$

where E_1 and E_2 correspond to two different three-dimensional structural conformations of the enzyme and Na^+_i, Na^+_o, K^+_i, and K^+_o represent, respectively, internal and external Na^+ and K^+ ions. According to this model (1), the reaction involved essentially a phosphorylation step that leads to phosphorylated intermediary compound ($E_1 - P$), which binds Na^+_i, and a dephosphorylation step that produced an E_2 form, which binds external K^+, the latter step being specifically inhibited by cardiac glycosides. Different models have also been proposed (47).

This enzyme is present in high concentrations in the brain and other nervous tissue (ref. 143, Chapter 34). Since it is usually thought that the (Na^+,K^+)-ATPase is responsible for transporting three Na^+ ions for every two K^+ ions, its activity can hyperpolarize a nerve cell, thus maintaining the ion gradients of Na^+ and K^+ that are the energy source of the nerve impulse. The relationships between (Na^+,K^+)-ATPase and neurotransmission have also been investigated, the enzyme being considered as a trigger for neurotransmitter release at the synaptic cleft (159). Activating neurotransmitters showed a biphasic effect on (Na^+,K^+)-ATPase: activation at low concentrations, followed by inhibition at high concentrations. The first phase was prevented by addition of ethyleneglycol-bis-(2-aminoethyl)-tetraacetic acid (EGTA), i.e., calcium-free media (79). These data could indicate an evolutionary significance of the effect of neurotransmitters on the synaptosomal (Na^+,K^+)-ATPase.

For these reasons the (Na^+,K^+)-ATPase activities have been determined in brain tissue under many circumstances (ref. 143, Chapter 34). Several authors have assumed that the absolute value of enzyme activity in brain tissue is an accurate indicator of the Na^+,K^+ pump efficiency in exchanging Na^+ and K^+ ions across the plasma membranes (55,143). In fact, several reviews (55,63,143) showed that the absolute values of enzyme specific activities vary extensively from author to author, from preparation to preparation, and from one technical procedure to another. Moreover, some preparations of nervous systems, such as cultured astrocytes (98), neuroblastoma cells (77), or dorsal-root ganglia (141), often exhibit low levels of enzyme activity, while actively pumping Na^+ and K^+ at high capacities.

Our early experiments (36,37,56) showed a sodium–potassium exchange in mammalian brain slices when increasing the external potassium concentrations from 3 to 20 mM. We concluded that this was probably due to the activation of the Na^+,K^+ pump described above. These conclusions prompted us to investigate the catalytic properties of both glial and neuronal (Na^+,K^+)-ATPase. However, when we started to investigate the relative contribution of glial cells and neurons in the clearance of external K^+, studies on the K^+ activation mechanisms of the enzyme within neuronal, synaptic, and glial fractions provided more information on their membranous physiological characteristics than the absolute levels of (Na^+,K^+)-ATPase.

We utilized tissue fractionation on sucrose–Ficoll gradients for preparing whole glial or neuronal cells, synaptosomes, and plasma membranes from different mammalian species such as rabbit, cat, and human. Obviously the purity and integrity of these different fractions are important factors in determining the validity of conclusions based on results obtained in this type of study. Since 1969, this problem has been extensively discussed elsewhere (9,50, 51,55,59,60,63).

ATPase activities were first determined by a conventional technique (detecting the amount of inorganic phosphate produced by the enzymatic reaction) and later by a kinetic method determining the initial velocity (measuring the rate of liberation of protons in low-buffered media) (50,52 for review).

As shown in Fig. 1, sensitivity to potassium differed between glial and neuronal enzymes supporting data previously shown by Henn et al. (60). Neuronal enzymes reached maximal activities at 3 to 5 mM K^+. Similar results were observed with the K^+-pNPase (38,55). This was further confirmed by Moonen and Franck (96) on pure mature cultured astrocytes. Like the Na^+,K^+ exchange observed in rat brain slices, this glial enzyme characteristic is dependent on a process of maturation, since it cannot be observed either in bulk isolated glial cells from young animals (37,53) or in immature cultured astrocytes (96) where neuronal and glial enzyme exhibited similar kinetics in response to K^+. More recently, Atterwill et al. (2) showed that optimal activity by K^+ ions was observed in 1 mM K^+ media in immature cultured astrocytes from rat cerebella, while it was detected only at 8 to 10 mM K^+ in corresponding neuronal cultures. Although no statistical conclusions can be drawn from this latter study, these discrepancies (as otherwise pointed out by the authors) might be related to the immaturity of the preparation.

More interestingly, our kinetic approach measures an accurate initial velocity of the enzymatic reaction (52), as demonstrated from Lineweaver–Burke diagrams. The apparent affinity of the glial enzyme for the substrate ($ATP \cdot Mg^{2+}$) is considerably increased by high K^+ ion concentrations (i.e., 20 mM). Accordingly, the so-called "physiological efficiency" (i.e., V_{max}/K_{mapp} ratio) of the glial (Na^+,K^+)-ATPase is specifically enhanced in K^+-enriched media, while this phenomenon is absent in neu-

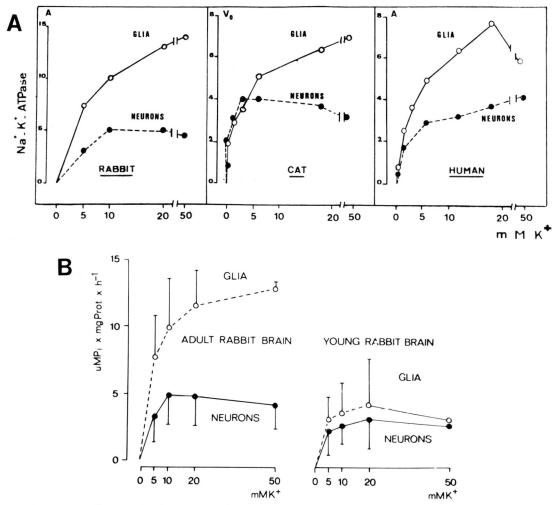

FIG. 1. A: Influence of K$^+$ on the (Na$^+$,K$^+$)-ATPase activities of glia cells and neuronal cells enriched fractions from different mammalian brain. Note the differences between neuronal and glial enzymes in response to elevated K$^+$ concentrations (37,38,53). B: Influence of age on the K$^+$ activation of glial and neuronal (Na$^+$,K$^+$)-ATPase (37).

ronal preparations (50,51,55). Regardless of the kinetic models used to explain (Na$^+$,K$^+$)-ATPase activities, glial and neuronal ATPases must be two different molecular entities based on their different affinities to (K$^+$)$_o$. This only occurred in adult or mature neural preparations.

Sweadner (148) confirmed the presence of two molecular forms of brain (Na$^+$,K$^+$)-ATPase by resolving on gel electrophoresis in sodium dodecylsulfate two subspecies of the enzyme catalytic alpha subunit, so-called alpha$^+$ and alpha subunits. The pure form of alpha$^+$ was only seen in rat brain axolemma, whereas alpha was isolated in pure cultured astrocytes. Hence, it was hypothesized that alpha$^+$ might be the neuronal

form while alpha would be more specific for glial cells. Other brain structures (microsomes, synaptosomes) exhibited both alpha$^+$ and alpha subspecies. Alpha$^+$ and alpha subspecies are different in affinity to strophantidin, in sensitivity to digestion by trypsin, and in the number or reactivity of sulfhydryl groups. The differences observed in affinity to strophantidin (i.e., high affinity for alpha$^+$, low affinity for alpha$^-$) are of particular interest, since the glycosidic site of the enzymatic protein has traditionally been considered to be similar to the catalytic site of external K$^+$.

Specific inactivation of the alpha$^+$ but not the alpha molecular form of (Na$^+$,K$^+$)-ATPase by pyrithiamin (93) further support the idea of two functionally distinct molecular forms of the enzyme. These subspecies of (Na^+,K^+)-ATPase catalytic unit may be found, however, in rat cervical ganglia (148) as well as in neural, muscle, and secretory tissues using immunoblots with polyclonal antisera (140). This could question whether there is cellular specificity for $alpha^+$ and $alpha^-$ subunits in the brain. Studying the relative proportion of high- and low-affinity ouabain sites in both immature cultured astrocyte and neuronal cells from rat cerebella, Atterwill et al. (2) found both subunits in astrocytes, although the low-affinity site $(alpha^-)$ was more represented in glial structures. Again, they were dealing with immature cultured astrocytes. That $alpha^-$ subspecies might be a glial subunit is also favored by its increased affinity for ATP in K^+-enriched media, as observed when using NaI-treated glial enzyme (50). This latter phenomenon is not observed with the $alpha^+$ subspecies (K. J. Sweadner, *personal communication,* ISN Meeting, Vancouver, 1983). Putting together all this experimental information, it is reasonable to conclude, as we previously proposed in 1978 (55), that glial and neuronal enzyme are two different molecular enzymes.

More recently, we confirmed the presence of the $alpha^+$ and $alpha^-$ subspecies of (Na^+,K^+)-ATPase in mice, in the baboon *Papio papio,* and in human brains (Fig. 2).

We feel that the relative proportion of $alpha^+$ and $alpha^-$ in a neural membrane could determine both ouabain and K^+ sensitivity of (Na^+,K^+)-ATPase and accordingly of the Na^+,K^+ pump. For example, high concentrations of the alpha subunit in mature glial cells could explain their specific abilities to pump external K^+ when it reaches higher concentrations (up to 20 mM). If only $alpha^+$ or higher concentrations of $alpha^+$ are present as in axolemma (148), the membrane would pump K^+_o on higher yield, but in the presence of more physiological variations of K^+_o, i.e., between 3 and 6 mM.

Experiments comparing ion fluxes measurements and relative proportion of $alpha^+$ and $alpha^-$ (Na^+,K^+)-ATPase subspecies in both glial and neuronal structures are needed to verify this hypothesis.

Chloride, bicarbonate, and protons

External chloride, bicarbonate, and proton homeostasis in the central nervous system and its relation to K^+ homeostasis, as well as the role of glial structures in these functions, has been extensively studied in the last 20 years by the Albany Medical College group, starting with the work of R. S. Bourke and D. B. Tower in 1966 (10) and followed by a considerable amount of work on brain slices and on bulk isolated and cultured cells by R. S. Bourke, H. K. Kimelberg, and S. Narumi. Excellent reviews have focused on this topic (11,12,78,80), which continues to provide many intriguing problems. This chapter does not cover these areas of glial function, since they are discussed elsewhere in this volume (see Chapter 35).

Termination of Neurotransmitter Activity by Glial Cells

A research area that has also been opened recently concerns the interactions between neurons and glial cells involving putative amino acid transmitters (65). Astrocytes, by accumulating these neuroactive substances at the same synaptic level, may therefore be of major importance for termination of the activity of certain transmitters in a way similar to the already discussed K^+ homeostasis mechanism (65). This illustrates a very important neuron–glial relationship that could be crucial in the regulation of nerve activity.

Two putative amino acid transmitters, glutamate and aspartate, are taken up very efficiently by astrocytes, while other neuroactive substances such as GABA, taurine, and adenosine (67) are also efficiently accumulated by astrocytes, though not at a rate corresponding to the glutamate uptake. Less information is available on the subsequent fate of these latter compounds, but glutamate is converted to glutamine by an enzyme specific to glial cells, namely, glutamine synthetase. GABA metabolizing enzymes are present and active in both glial cells and neurons.

The Glial Glutamate–Glutamine Cycle

About 20 years ago, Waelsch and his co-workers (161) introduced the concept of metabolic compartmentation in brain tissue, by demonstrating that incorporation of ^{14}C-acetate into glutamine exceeded the peak specific activity of its precursor, glutamate. Since this pioneer work, a large amount of information suggested that adult mammalian brain exhibits at least two different compartments: i.e., a "large pool" containing most of the glutamate, and a "small pool" containing the smaller fraction of glutamate, which is rapidly transformed into glutamine (20,42,65,157). Although still controversial, the idea that nerve endings and neuronal perikarya are found in a large, GABA-releasing

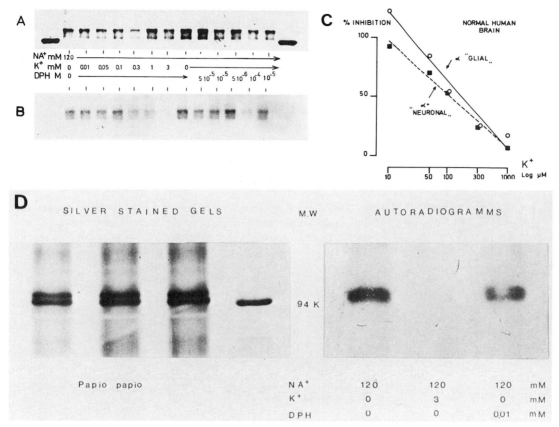

FIG. 2. Subspecies of alpha-catalytic subunit of the (Na⁺,K⁺)-ATPase as found on sodium dodecyl sulfate gel electrophoresis and corresponding autoradiograms. Notice the decrease of phosphorylation both in K⁺-enriched media and in the presence of 10^{-4} phenytoin (From D. Guillaume, T. Grisar, and A. V. Delgado-Escueta, *unpublished observations.*) Human brain (normal cortectomy): **A,** SDS-page gel electrophoresis; **B,** autoradiogram; **C,** diagram of decreased level of phosphorylation (in percent inhibition) in progressive K⁺-enriched media (100% corresponds to a K⁺-free medium). **D,** The photosensitive baboon *Papio papio.*

pool and glial cells in a small, GABA-accumulating pool, was proposed by several authors (3,105,156). A transfer of GABA from one compartment to the other and a transfer of glutamine in the opposite direction then have been envisaged, maintaining the constituents of the tricarboxylic acid cycles in each compartment (4). On the basis of pharmacological experiments on brain slices, Benjamin and Quastel (7,8) proposed that glutamate released from neurons at the synaptic cleft could be taken up by glial cells and converted to glutamine, which is then returned to presynaptic nerve endings, where it is transformed to glutamate and ammonia. In this context, an efficient, high-affinity uptake of glutamic acid is one of the most spectacular characteristics of glial cells and more particularly astrocytes. This has been demonstrated autoradiographically (29,70,86,99,129), using bulk isolated glial cells (5,59,62,114) and glial cell-line

astrocytoma (144), Muler cells (15), satellite cells in peripheral ganglia (122), and astrocytes in primary cultures (6,61,131) (Fig. 3).

In connection with the termination of transmitter activity by net accumulation into adjacent astrocytes, it is interesting to point out that increasing extracellular potassium concentration (which follows nerve activity *in vivo*) enhances the uptake of glutamate (131) (Fig. 3).

A net uptake of glutamate also occurs in synaptosomes under certain conditions (146,168). However, as recalled by Hertz (65):

In view of the extraordinarily high uptake rates for glutamate into glial cells and the known contamination of synaptosomal preparations with glial cell membranes, great caution should, however, be exerted in ascertaining an uptake of glutamate into nerve endings . . . high affinity uptake [of glutamate] in hippocampus (168) or in

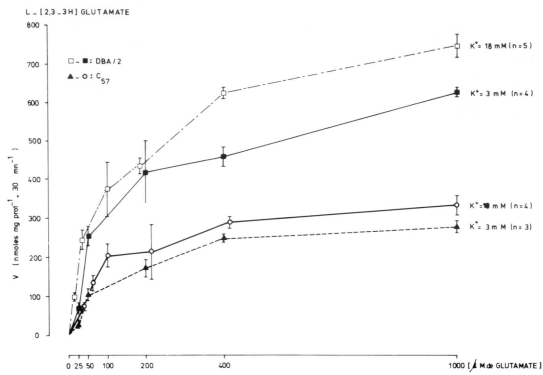

FIG. 3. Glutamate uptake in cultured glial cells in primary cultures of varying external glutamate concentrations. (From R. Perot and T. Grisar, *unpublished observations*.)

striatum (100) is reduced after surgically or chemically induced lesions of presumably glutaminergic pathways.

These findings indicate that nerve endings take up glutamate partly at the synaptic cleft, as otherwise demonstrated in different preparations of cultured neurons (6,72).

Therefore, neurons in general seem to have a much less efficient glutamate uptake than astrocytes, although glutamate concentrations in both cells should be approximately identical, since both cells also incorporate labeled glucose into glutamate.

It is now generally accepted that glutamine-synthetase (Glu-S; EC 6.3.1.2) is a glial and more specifically astrocytic enzyme (92,130, 132,155), whereas glutamate decarboxylase (GAD; EC 4.1.1.15) is found at a higher specific activity in nerve endings (see Chapters 15 and 37).

Consequently, it is generally thought that glutamine is predominantly formed by glial cells, whereas GABA is preferentially synthesized in nerve endings.

Meister (95) has recently reviewed the mechanisms of action of glutamine synthetase from

glutamate, which catalyzes the reversible formation of glutamine and ammonia at the expense of cleavage of ATP to ADP and inorganic phosphate. Patel et al. (105,106) related the regional development of this enzyme to differentiation rather than acquisition of astrocytes in agreement with Norenberg's demonstration (102) of glutamine synthetase in long radial fibers and processes of astroglial cells. On the other hand, Lacoste et al. (84) studied the regulation of the biosynthesis of glutamine synthetase in neuroblastoma cells and demonstrated that removal of glutamine from the culture medium resulted in a 10-fold increase in enzyme activity. This led to the concept of derepression of neuronal glutamine synthetase at low concentrations of glutamine. This phenomenon of derepression may be less important in astrocytes where a more powerful biosynthetic pathway for glutamine synthetase exists, possibly as a result of their differentiation in primary cultures. A regulatory mechanism, where astrocyte depolarization and repolarization would channel a flux of glutamine toward the neurons subsequent to a glutamate flux in the opposite direction, has been proposed by Ramaharobandro et al. (119) in their comparison of glutamine and glutamate transport in cultured neuronal and glial cells. Recently, Drejer et al. (28) showed that conditioned medium from different cultured neurons produces a specific effect on GABA and L-glutamate uptake in cultured astrocytes, indicating that this development of astrocytic amino acid uptake might depend upon both brain ontogenesis, regional origin of the astrocytes, and surrounding neuronal cell types. The development profile of enzymes involved in the glutamate and GABA metabolism in cultured neurons and astroctyes has also been established by comparison with the profile of these enzymes in the brain *in vivo* (134).

That glutamine formed in astrocytes is further released in extracellular space appears obvious from several experiments (123). However, ". . . no high affinity uptake of glutamine has been demonstrated with certainty into any cell type of the central nervous system" (65).

GABA Metabolism in Glial Cells

There is no doubt that GABA is a major inhibitory neurotransmitter released from GABA-ergic synapses and that glutamate decarboxylase is highly concentrated within inhibitory nerve terminals (see Chapters 15 and 37). Both potassium-induced, calcium-dependent and calcium-independent release of GABA have been found in many neuronal structures (65).

A more disputed problem is to what extent GABA is also released from glial structures, in a non-transmitter-related role but with some consequences on the adjacent pre- or postsynaptic cells (135,136).

The action of extracellular GABA must be terminated by uptake into adjacent cellular structure, since GABA transaminase, the only GABA catabolizing enzyme, is an intracellular enzyme. A large amount of experiments have proved that this GABA uptake *in vivo* occurs in both neuronal and glial structures (see refs. 65 and 135 for review). However, only a cellular high affinity uptake of GABA, rather than a one-to-one homoexchange, can be of major importance for transmitter inactivation at the synaptic level. There is little doubt, however, that such GABA uptake occurs into synaptosomes and into cerebral astrocytes in primary cultures (62,65,137). Interestingly enough, this glial uptake of GABA is drastically diminished in Na^+-free or low-Na^+ media (135,137), while the effect of $(K^+)_o$ withdrawal is still controversial (65).

Thus, the intracellular GABA content in astrocytes *in vivo* is mainly acquired by this uptake from extracellular fluid, since no GAD activity was found in glial structures (138,171), while relatively high activity of the GABA transaminase was found (125), thus explaining very low contents of GABA measured in glial structures (172).

Glial Control of Other Putative Amino Acids Transmitters

Some uptake of glycine, taurine (133), and aspartate (65) has been shown into glial cells in primary culture. Aspartate may be of specific interest, since a high-affinity uptake in astrocytes has been found to be much more intense than the GABA uptake (65). Accordingly, a flow of aspartate from neurons to glial cells might therefore constitute another link between these two cellular metabolisms. Since evidence was accumulated showing that aspartate may be a transmitter (74) released from synaptosomes by electrical pulses of high-K^+ media, this glial property could add a new important functional role of glial structures in inactivating transmitter substances at the synaptic cleft.

Glial Control of Neuronal Metabolism

More indirect control of nerve function by glial cells could be exerted through glial regulation of neuronal metabolism. We have briefly reviewed the importance of the removal of the excess extracellular potassium released during nerve activity. In fact, the removal of the excess extracellular potassium released during nerve activity might be of great importance not only in terms of neuronal membrane excitability but also in terms of intracellular glial metabolism. As first suggested by Kuffler and Nicholls (82) and recently emphasized by Pentreath and Kai-Kai (111,113), the leakage of K^+ ions by neurons and its subsequent entry within the glial syncithium could act as a signal stimulating metabolic pathways within the glial cells, which can in turn produce metabolic support for adjacent neurons. For instance, antidromic stimulation of nerves entering the leech or snail ganglia increased incorporation of radioactively labeled 2-deoxyglucose (^{3}H-DG) into glycogen in glial cells surrounding activated neurons (112). The constant physical relationship between neurons and glia in the evolution of the nervous system suggests that these two cell types are functionally interrelated. Glia may support neurons by supplying metabolites such as glucose (82) or lipid precursors (49). We have described above the concept of an intracellular transport of glutamate and glutamine. Glial cells have also been suspected to furnish adjacent neurons with amino acids for neuronal protein synthesis (59). Associated with release of K^+ during neuronal firing, the glycogen synthesis in glial cells increases; increased intracellular K^+ in glial cells in turn produces metabolic support for adjacent neurons (11). A detailed study of the regulation of glycogen metabolism in primary and transformed astrocytes *in vivo* confirmed the existence of regulatory enzymes for synthesis and degradation of glycogen within glial cells (23). Glial cells are also responsible for an increased production of somatostatin in cultured sensory neurons of the dorsal-root ganglion (101). Direct evidence for transfer of molecules from glia to the neuron was provided by Lasek and Tytell (85), who showed macromolecular proteins being transferred from glia to the axon in the form of a particle that includes actin in its structure. Another example is the recent work of Yu et al. (173), who found that pyruvate carboxylase, which catalyzes the formation of oxaloacetate from pyruvate and thus leads to a net synthesis of tricarboxylic acid (TCA) cycle constituents, was not detectable in cerebral cortex neurons or granule cells, while the enzyme was present both in brain homogenates and cultured astrocytes. The transfer of alpha-ketoglutarate from astrocytes to neurons was postulated to explain the replenishment of neuronal TCA cycle constituents.

NEURON–GLIA RELATIONSHIPS IN EPILEPSY

Experimental Models

C. Fere (34) wrote in 1890 that

L'examen microscopique de la region cérébrale alterée montra qu'aux endroits où les membranes s'étaient fusionees avec l'écorce il s'était developpé dans cette dernière du tissu conjonctif aux dépens des elements nerveux.

For almost a century now, gliosis has been described to mean "astrogliosis in as much as oligodendroglia was recognized as a cell group long after gliosis was a well known sequel to a wide variety of pathological conditions" (109,110). Histological examination of human material from 12 cases of epilepsy provided, as early as 1930, eloquent evidence of a long-continued cicatricial traction ["cicatricial contraction" of Penfield (109)] with astroglial gliosis deeper in the brain cortex (109). Since then, striking astroglial gliosis has been often de-

scribed in epileptic foci of humans and animals (14,17,165).

The conversion of protoplasmic astrocytes in the epileptic cortex into fibrous astrocytes in large numbers could intuitively change their function, and also could dramatically modify their metabolic interactions with adjacent neurons (165). The theory of simple mechanical stimulation of neurons by glial fibrous scar has recently lost favor in the face of all their presently known dynamic properties. From histoenzymological studies in 161 human biopsies, reactive astrocytes with a high level of dehydrogenase activities (the so-called "activated astrocytes") have been shown to be related to focal epilepsy. This was also verified in the cobalt lesion model in rats (14). Microscopic gliosis, although nonspecific, might affect an heterogeneous population of glial cells according to different biochemical alterations following different types of injuries. Such pathological alterations of glial metabolism could therefore consist of either abnormal control of extracellular microenvironment, and more precisely abnormal handling of $(K^+)_o$, or abnormal amino acid transmitters inactivation, or disturbances in the control of neuronal intermediary metabolism. This could conceivably lead to either paroxysmal depolarization shifts or spread of seizures. On the other hand, glial function might be modified in a direction in which they reduce the spread of epileptic discharges, acting as a protective or adaptive mechanism against seizures rather than being the source of the initial abnormal neuronal discharges.

Epilepsy as a Deficiency of Glial Control of $(K^+)_o$

K^+ movement in epileptogenic cortex

In 1970, Pollen and Trachtenberg (116,153) and Franck (36) independently proposed that a significant factor in the development of focal epilepsy could be a degradation of the spatial buffering function of the glial cells. In fact, extrusion of K^+ from "normal" glial cells induced by intracellular injection of Na^+ and Li^+ was found to provoke high-frequency discharges of neighboring neurons (57,58) during the period of glial depolarization. Therefore, it is a reality that poor "spatial buffering" of $(K^+)_o$ by glia can induce neuronal discharges.

However, the principal test for answering this question would be testing whether "abnormal" glia in regions of gliosis is deficient in its capacity to spatially buffer $(K^+)_o$. Transmembrane potentials of inexcitable cells in gliotic cortex of epileptogenic freezing lesions were first found to be similar to those reported in normal cortex (107,108). As pointed out by Ward (165), epileptic activity would release, in gliotic cortex, 45×10^{13} K^+ ions/sec $\cdot$ cm^2. In normal glia, the glial current would carry away only 31×10^{13} K^+ ions/sec $\cdot$ cm^2, and K^+ would accumulate in the extracellular space. The membrane properties of these glia in the chronic focus indicate, however, that they can carry away at least 62×10^{13} K^+ ions/sec $\cdot$ cm^2, which is clearly an adequate safety factor. From this point of view, glia in the epileptic focus would be more, rather than less, effective than normal glia in removing interstitial K^+.

Experiments performed further in this area with K^+-specific microelectrodes produced some essential information. Fairly good agreement seems to exist that the unstimulated baseline of $(K^+)_o$ is not higher in a gliotic and epileptogenic cortex scar than in normal cortical tissue (145). There is also little doubt that change in $(K^+)_o$ follows rather than leads to convulsive activity (145) (see Chapters 31, 32, 33). Equally good agreement is not found, however, with respect to the rate of clearing K^+ from gliotic and epileptogenic scar tissue. It was not measurably different from that in normal tissue in animals with a small chronic cold lesion (107,108), whereas Lewis et al. (87) showed that dense gliosis in alumina gel epileptogenic foci of monkeys was associated with slowed potassium clearance. In addition, studies of potassium kinetics in the chronic alumina lesion (46) showed there are significant differences in the properties of normal glia as compared to the glia of epileptogenic foci. A large reduction in specific membrane resistance of gliotic tissue was observed. This has been recently confirmed in slices from human gliotic and epileptogenic cortex incubated *in vitro* (115), leading again to the conclusion that the glia in the epileptic focus is more effective than glia in normal brains in removing interstitial K^+. One must keep in mind, however, that a decrease in specific membrane resistance can only be interpreted as an increase of K^+ permeability assuming that glial membranes act as perfect K^+ electrodes, which is no longer as well established as is tacitly assumed in most of the reviews on this subject (Table 1).

It is also important to point out a possible flaw in studies that use K^+-sensitive microelectrodes. The thickness of such electrodes remains very large by comparison with the extracellular space size (100–200 Å). A small dead space is then created, allowing errors in the determination of both baseline and movements of $(K^+)_o$ (149). If adjacent glial cells are recorded in the same time, however, this error can be minimized (145), although the determination of the fine and fast tuning of extracellular $(K^+)_o$ by active process at the synaptic cleft might be underestimated.

Therefore, most but not all electrophysiological studies would tend to discredit the Pollen and Trachtenberg and Franck theory of epileptic discharges being caused by a failure of K^+ spatial buffering of glial cells. None of them, however, have been able to measure the rate of decay of epileptic-evoked K^+ transients in the presence of an afterdischarge.

Biochemical approach

As early as 1965, D. B. Tower (150) demonstrated the inability of cortical slices excised from human epileptic neocortex to accumulate external K^+ at the same magnitude as normal human brain. He further concluded "the crucial experiments designed to evaluate (Na^+,K^+)-ATPase and fluxes of sodium and potassium between extracellular and intracellular compartments of human samples taken from epileptogenic foci remain to be done" (151).

Furthermore, Escueta et al. (31) demonstrated an abnormal decrease in the pump flux of K^+ and Na^+ and an abnormal increase in the downhill movement of ions (32,33) in synaptosomes isolated by discontinuous Ficoll ultracentrifugation from epileptogenic foci of cold lesions in cat. In the primary and mirror epileptogenic foci, no significant changes in base-line K^+ and Na^+ were observed within synaptosomes, but total accumulation of K^+ and total extrusion of Na^+ and ouabain inhibition of such processes were profoundly decreased within synaptosomes of the epileptogenic foci. These results prompted several laboratories to investigate the variations of (Na^+,K^+)-ATPase-specific activities in the epileptic foci. Changes in (Na^+,K^+)-ATPase activities within the whole-brain fraction have been reported to be either increased (86) or decreased (118), and various interpretations have been given to explain these observations. In whole-brain fractions of acute freezing lesions, total (Na^+,K^+)-ATPase activity increased with total brain sodium. Total-brain potassium decreased (33). The increase of (Na^+,K^+)-ATPase activity was considered to be a compensatory change resulting from increased total brain sodium. Consequently, the Na^+,K^+ pump was considered to change as an effect of and not as a cause of epileptogenic discharges. A second explanation proposed for these observations was that all the observed findings were the result of cerebral edema, which is quite prominent in an 8-hr-old lesion (33). In chronic lesions, reduced enzyme activities had been suspected to be the result mainly of lesion production, but similar decreases in the mirror focus argued in favor of reduced enzyme activity being linked to epileptogenesis. Thus, epileptogenic discharges, cerebral edema, and tissue destruction have all been considered important variables that determine (Na^+,K^+)-ATPase activity. However, the relative importance of these processes, as well as the specific contribution of neurons, synapses, and glia to the observed (Na^+,K^+)-ATPase changes, remained uncertain.

Further experiments had examined (Na^+,K^+)-ATPase activities in synaptosomes isolated from both acute and chronic freezing lesions (33). In the epileptogenic acute lesion (8-, 18-, and 24-hr-old lesions with marked cerebral edema), (Na^+,K^+)-ATPase increased activities within synapses by 55 to 100%. Acute freezing lesions that did not have epileptogenic discharges also exhibited elevated (Na^+,K^+)-ATPase activities (by 60%), indicating a significant contribution of cerebral edema in enhancing enzyme levels (33). In the indolent lesion, (Na^+,K^+)-ATPase decreased activities by 20 to 35% during the interictal state. When focal discharges became sustained, (Na^+,K^+)-ATPase activities measured similar to controls. When focal ictal paroxysms in the chronic focus secondarily generalized, (Na^+,K^+)-ATPase raised activities above "normal" levels (30% increase compared to control tissues). In chronic lesions, therefore, the enhancement of (Na^+,K^+)-ATPase activities by secondarily generalized ictal paroxysms was clearly demonstrated while the significance of the decreased Na^+,K^+ activity in the indolent focus remained to be clarified (33).

To approach this problem more critically, some experimental modifications were carried out (54). Larger freezing lesions and thus more astrogliosis were produced, which allowed the successful harvest of glial fractions. The rate of ATP hydrolysis was measured by the rate of liberation of H^+ ions, and the method of Grisar et al. (52) was used for the kinetic analysis of (Na^+,K^+)-ATPase. In particular, $(K^+)_o$ activitation of the enzyme was analyzed (54), and the focal gliotic lesion site was studied separately from the surrounding region or the perifocal site and mirror focus. Biochemical analysis was carried out during continuous and sustained 3-sec focal epileptogenic discharges in the primary and mirror focus (Fig. 4).

Using the hysteretic model for analyzing (Na^+,K^+)-ATPase, the increase in synaptosomal enzyme activities in the acute cold lesion and their decrease in the subacute and chronic epileptogenic states were verified (54). Several differences were noticeable, however; the enzyme shifts were not as marked, and 45 days after lesion production, activities increased toward normal levels. No significant changes were observed in the secondary focus during the acute and chronic epileptogenic states, whereas a slight decrease in enzyme activities was seen in the perifocal area.

Striking changes in the glial (Na^+,K^+)-ATPase activities occurred; enzyme activities dramatically decreased in both the primary and secondary foci of acute and chronic lesions. The $(K^+)_o$ activation of the glial enzyme in the primary and secondary foci of acute and chronic lesions was absent 3, 6, and up to 45 days after lesion production.

Reaction velocities of the glial enzyme between 3 and 18 mM K^+ decreased. Both V_{max} and K_{mapp} were significantly decreased compared to both control animals and the perifocal area (54).

In the perifocal area, glial (Na^+,K^+)-ATPase was also decreased 1 to 13 days after lesion production, but in subsequent weeks these activities returned to normal levels. The K^+ activation of enzyme activities even increased in the perifocal areas after 45 days of seizure activity (54).

Studies on K^+ activation mechanisms in synaptosomes from the actively firing chronic epileptogenic foci revealed further important observations. The K^+ activation constant of synaptosomal (Na^+,K^+)-ATPase was significantly decreased in the actively firing chronic focus. The apparent affinity of the synaptosomal enzyme for K^+, therefore, appeared to be increased within epileptic tissue that was actively firing. Interestingly, while sustained focal paroxysms could raise synaptosomal (Na^+,K^+)-ATPase, glial (Na^+,K^+)-ATPase and its activation by $(K^+)_o$ remained decreased during sustained paroxysms in acute chronic lesions. Moreover, while the decrease of the absolute level of glial enzyme activity was less evident after 45 days, the poor response of glial enzyme to $(K^+)_o$ never reversed to "normal" values (54). Hence, these experiments provided new information that glial (Na^+,K^+)-ATPase responds to K^+ in a different manner when compared to

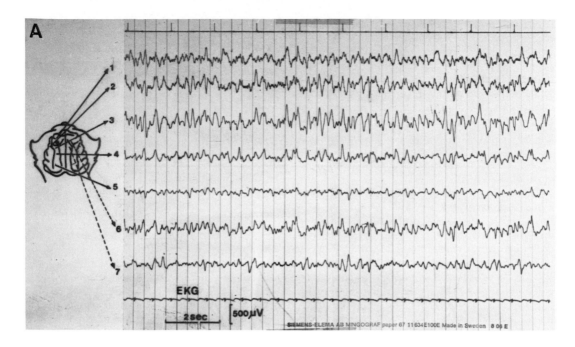

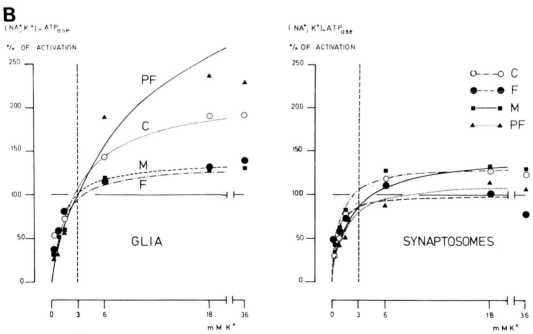

FIG. 4. A: The freeze lesion on the anterior suprasylvian gyrus of the cat produced spike-and-wave complexes in the primary focus F (channels 1, 2, 3 on ECoG) and in the secondary focus M (channel 6), while a perifocal (PF) area (channel 5) is normal. B: K$^+$ influence on the (Na$^+$,K$^+$)-ATPase activities of bulk isolated glia cells and synaptosomes from F, M, and PF as compared with sham-operated cats (C). (From ref. 54, with permission.)

synaptic enzyme. Glial ATPase and its activation by $(K^+)_o$ remain decreased in either actively discharging acute lesions or in the indolent chronic foci. This might indicate a reduction of

the protective ability of glial membranes in $(K^+)_o$ homeostasis. As already suggested by Dichter (27), the impairment in glial control of elevated $(K^+)_o$ could be mainly responsible for the transition of discharges to total episodes, within the primary and the secondary foci. Interestingly enough, the inverse interpretation could be proposed for the normal or perifocal area (PF), where the physiological efficiency of glial enzyme remained optimal even at high K^+ concentrations, thus indicating an increase rather than a reduction of the protective ability of glial membranes (Fig. 4B).

Epilepsy associated with modifications of glial carbonic anhydrase

Carbonic anhydrase (CA; EC4.2.1.1) is an enzyme that catalyzes the hydration of CO_2 to form HCO_3^- for anion intracellular transport and for CO_2 fixation reactions involving synthesis of several vital compounds in the CNS. It is known to be associated with glial cells (45). Whether or not this enzyme is preferentially located in oligodendroglia or astroglia still remains controversial (19,21,25,83,126). On the other hand, acetazolamide (5-acetamido-1,3,4-thiadiazole 2-sulfonamide, Diamox®), a specific inhibitor of CA, has been shown to have anticonvulsant properties in experimental animals (169) and to be a useful antiepileptic drug in human beings (169). Hence, the role of glial CA in the generation and/or arrest of seizure has been investigated. Woodbury and Kemp (170) and White and Woodbury (see Chapter 35) showed that the cobalt-induced focal epileptogenic lesions in the frontal cortex of rats were associated with an increase in glial-cell CA in the regions of increased polyspike activity in the electroencephalograph (EEG). This was accompanied by a decrease in total brain CO_2 and an increase in CO_2 fixation. This suggested that the glial enzyme response to increased neuronal firing enhances the capability of glial cells to handle the increased neuronal metabolic production of CO_2. Hence, the glial CA response would be a protective mechanism to the increased neuronal activity.

We have analyzed CA activity in a model of epilepsy with both gliotic and epileptogenic cortical tissue, namely, the cat with cortical freeze lesion. The results were also compared with a genetically determined model of audiogenic seizure (DBA/2J mice) as a function of age and severity score of seizure activity. In cat (Table 2), no significant modifications were seen in the primary (F) and secondary (M) foci in comparison to sham-operated animals (control) and to the perifocal areas (PF). No epileptogenic activities are recorded in the perifocal areas of the cold lesion.

In mice (Fig. 5), CA activities increased with

TABLE 2. *Carbonic anhydrase (CA) activity in epileptogenic brain of the cat with freeze lesion[a]*

Age of lesions (days)	Primary focus (F)	Secondary focus (M)	Perifocus (PF)
1	0.33	0.76	0.75
3	0.56	0.37	0.51
30	0.39 ± 0.06	0.38 ± 0.17	0.47 ± 0.15
	(n = 6)	(n = 6)	(n = 6)

[a] Data are given in U/mg protein. Epileptogenic brain tissue exhibiting ECoG discharges (F, M) is compared with the perifocus (PF) where no discharges were recorded. Control value in nonepileptogenic tissue (sham-operated animals): 0.40 ± 0.05 (n = 6).

age in both audiogenic (DBA/2J) and nonepileptic (C57/BL) controls. During the first 30 days of life, CA activities always measured higher in DBA/2J mice, and more particularly at days 23 and 24, i.e., 1 to 3 days following the peak of maximal severity score of seizure. A step decrease of the severity score of seizure together with a decrease in brain CA activity were seen after a single i.p. injection of acetazolamide (150 mg/kg). The anticonvulsant effect of this drug decreased with the age of the DBA/2J mice, in parallel with the increase of CA activities (data not shown).

Whether or not these differences in CA activity are species related or have something to do with cortical hyperexcitability now must be resolved. If one supposes, however, that these modifications of CA activity are a biochemical change associated with seizure, the hypothesis that enhanced CA activity in glial cells of epileptogenic cortex is an adaptive mechanism to overcome the eventual defect in anion transport has only been verified, in our experiences, in genetic models. In the cat with freeze lesions, astrogliosis is not accompanied by enhanced CA activity.

Epilepsy and the deficiency of glial control of putative amino acid transmitters

Although a considerable amount of data emphasized the role of glial cells in controlling neurotransmitter substances at the synaptic cleft (see above), the integrity of such glial property had not been investigated in epileptogenic tissue. Theoretically, one can imagine that a glial defect in regulating extracellular glutamate or GABA, for instance, might have deep influence on the adjacent neurons. This hypothesis had been poorly tested. We recently performed some

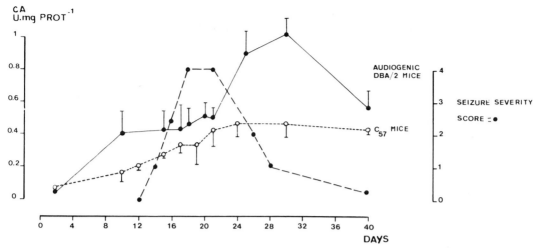

FIG. 5. Carbonic anhydrase activities in whole homogenized cortex of DBA/2J audiogenic and C57/BL normal mice as a function of age.

experiments using glutamate uptake in astrocytes cultivated from both normal C57/BL mice versus audiogenic DBA/2J prone mice. As shown in Fig. 3, the uptake (V_{max}) is much higher in the cultivated astrocytes from the seizure-susceptible mice. This might be related either to a simple species difference or to the epileptic features of the DBA/2J prone mice. In this latter hypothesis, a genetically determined potential of these astrocytes to accumulate with higher efficiency the extracellular glutamate at the synaptic cleft diminishes the amount of glutamate excitation and could be considered a protective mechanism against the seizure susceptibility. Similarly, protective properties have recently been ascribed to carbonic anhydrase.

On the other hand, we recently found that the glutamate content of the audiogenic mice cerebral cortex is higher than in C57/BL normal mice, and more particularly at an age where the seizure susceptibility is high (Fig. 3). The ratio of glutamate to GABA is higher in the DBA/2J mice and decreases with age after day 20. This supports the view that the glutamatergic synapses are either more active or increased in number in the epileptogenic cortex of the audiogenic seizure susceptible mice.

Recent results (not shown) seem to indicate that this surplus of glutamate in the DBA/2J mice might be produced by an accelerated rate of the catabolism of putrescine. This might be of major interest, since polyamines are known to influence protein synthesis and the subsequent development and maturation of nerve cells. This polyamines–GABA/glutamate shunt could therefore be one of the biochemical links between development and seizure susceptibility.

Human Temporal-Lobe Epilepsy

Tissue Sources

The elucidation of basic phenomena underlying epileptogenesis in animals has added little to the understanding, diagnosis, and even treatment of human epilepsies. The relationships between experimental data and human partial epilepsies still remain to be understood. There are various reasons why information on basic mechanisms of human partial epilepsies remains meager.

First, it is difficult to obtain brain tissues from humans with epilepsy. These tissues have to be suitably fresh and obtained in amounts sufficient for biochemical investigations. Also, there are at least two neurosurgical techniques used to excise the epileptogenic foci in patients with intractable partial complex seizures, namely "*en bloc*" anterior temporal lobectomy, developed by Falconer, and selective corticectomies, routinely used by Talairach's and Penfield's school. The former provides larger samples of both temporal neocortex and hippocampus (very often the site of the epileptogenic foci and the gliotic sclerosis) available in amounts sufficient for large-scale biochemical and *in vitro* physiological experiments. Corticectomy samples are probably more interesting, although the specimens are very small (from 20 to 200 mg). They are dissected from cortex areas, defined in terms of epileptogenic, irritative, and pathologic zones. However, experiments performed on both kinds of surgical samples must be interpreted carefully, taking into account the presence of antiepileptic drugs, anesthesia (halothane and artificial ventilation), and possible hypoxia during surgery (e.g., hypoxia following pial-vessel ligations). An important improvement developed by Sherwin and the Montreal School is the performance of selective corticectomies on "nonspiking" cortex and "spiking" brain areas under local anesthesia and after complete withdrawal of antiepileptic drugs.

Second, it is also difficult to obtain brain tissues from normal humans that can serve as controls. Two types of control samples can be used. Human brain tissue can be dissected quickly after death in patients without neurological diseases. This will always raise the question of whether the brain tissue can be extracted fast enough without appreciable alterations of the metabolism of brain cells. There is a need, therefore, for many "control" experiments in animals, evaluating the influence of the delay between death and autopsy on the biochemical parameter being studied. Alternatively, a more adequate control consists of normal cerebral cortical samples dissected by neurosurgeons when removing deep tumors, cysts, or aneurysms. These samples are especially suitable for comparison, since anesthetic and surgical techniques used are similar to those used during lobectomy or corticectomy.

We have now used all these brain samples (neocortex or hippocampus from anterior temporal lobectomies, selective corticectomies, postmortem tissue and cerebral corticectomies removed during neurosurgical excision of tumors or cysts) in the process of analyzing neuron–glia relationships in human temporal lobe epilepsy. We present here some of our recent results in the field.

(Na+,K+)-ATPase in Human Temporal Lobe Epilepsy

Since abnormal ATPase activities were found in experimental models of epilepsies (see above), we attempted to determine if the K^+-activation mechanisms of (Na^+,K^+)-ATPase in glial and synaptosomes enriched fractions isolated from human temporal lobe that contained a well-identified epileptogenic focus.

Our experiments, using highly enriched glial cell fractions isolated from the temporal neocortices of 15 patients suffering of partial complex epilepsy and who have well-identified hip-

pocampal–amygdalar or medial temporal and hippocampal sclerosis, successfully demonstrate that glial (Na^+,K^+)-ATPase decreased its total activities and lost or decreased its response to a range of K^+ concentrations previously shown to activate (i.e., between 3 and 18 mM K^+) (Fig. 6A). Although synaptosomal (Na^+,K^+)-ATPase also decreased total activities, no significant changes in its reactivity to external K^+ were observed (Fig. 6B). Using a different technique for preparing glial cells, a similar loss of reactivity by glial (Na^+,K^+)-ATPase was recently reported in human cerebral epileptogenic foci produced by brain tumors (75). These authors also reported a high degree of correlation between the degree of epileptogenesis of cortical areas with the decreased sensitivity of glial (Na^+,K^+)-ATPase to K^+.

Several possibilities could explain the abnormal (Na^+,K^+)-ATPase observed in these cellular fractions.

1. The antiepileptic drug that patients were receiving or halothane anaesthesia used during surgery could inhibit the enzyme or alter its regulation by K^+ ions. Although further experimental data are needed before definite and final conclusions can be made, our observations from two additional cases suggest the high probability that these factors are not responsible for the altered glial enzyme property. Both cases had normal neuropathological findings, were receiving antiepileptic drugs, and underwent halothane, endotracheal intubation, and the same surgical procedure used in the 15 patients who had abnormal rate reactions for glial (Na^+,K^+)-ATPase. Those cases, in spite of the antiepileptic drugs, halothane anaesthesia, and anterior temporal lobectomy, exhibited K^+ activation mechanisms of glial (Na^+,K^+)-ATPase similar to those reported in normal cats and rabbit brain and in autopsy brains of neurologically normal patients.

2. Ischemic hypoxia induced by surgical interruption of pial arterial blood supply prior to *en bloc* resection could also impair (Na^+,K^+)-ATPase activity. This possibility is also unlikely, because glial enzyme had already decreased the total level of glial enzyme activities and its sensitivity to K^+ ions in the temporal neocortex excised before ligation of arterioles and anterior temporal lobectomy (data not shown).

3. The third and most likely explanation is that glial and synaptosomal (Na^+,K^+)-ATPase activities are both decreased within the temporal neocortices of human anterior temporal lobes that contained both hippocampal amygdalar epileptogenic foci and hippocampal sclerosis.

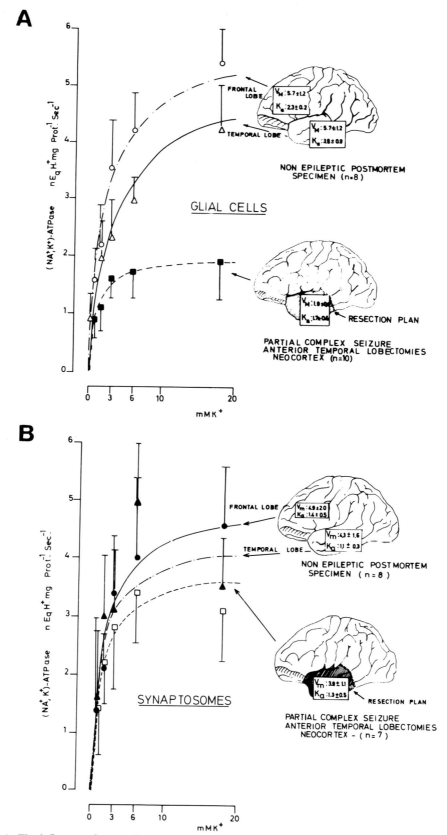

FIG. 6. **A:** The influence of external potassium on the (Na^+, K^+)-ATPase activities of bulk isolated glial cells from human postmortem brain cortex as compared with temporal lobe specimen from patients suffering from intractable complex partial seizures (see text for details). **B:** Synaptosomal fractions.

Most important, perhaps, glial (Na^+,K^+)-ATPase lost its sensitivity to extracellular K^+. These observed abnormalities in enzyme activities are probably part of the biochemical lesions of the underlying disease process. According to our previous model (50,51) and as discussed for data obtained in animals (54), these findings suggest that glial membranes in human temporal neocortex from patients with partial complex seizures of temporal origin have reduced their capacities to actively control elevated concentrations of external potassium during epileptiform paroxysms. This may be of great importance in the spread of seizures and accordingly in clinical manifestations of epilepsy. An unresolved issue is whether these biochemical lesions cause epilepsy or are the result of the epileptogenic paroxysms. Our previous experiments on the epileptogenic foci of freezing lesions in cats (54; also see above) showing the close relations of ictal epileptogenic activities and impaired glial (Na^+,K^+)-ATPase favor the concept that impaired glial functions play a role in the genesis of epilepsy.

However, the epileptogenic process and its neuropathological (127) accompaniments may be more complex and quite different in human temporal lobe. Positron emission tomography (PET) and single photon emission tomography (SPECT) most recently have both shown that local cerebral metabolic rates for glucose and oxygen and regional cerebral blood flow are decreased in the cerebral hemisphere ipsilateral to the define focus (30,39). Both studies show that the abnormal biochemical regions are more extensive than the EEG focus would have predicted. Our experiments did not address the issue of whether the impaired glial (Na^+,K^+)-ATPase functions caused the impaired cerebral metabolic rates for glucose and oxygen or whether the latter caused the abnormal rate reactions for glial (Na^+,K^+)-ATPase. Decreased regional cerebral blood flow and hypoperfusion of the temporal lobe could conceivably explain both the abnormal rate reactions for glial (Na^+,K^+)-ATPase and the drop in cerebral metabolic rates for glucose and oxygen.

Alternatively, a variety of more subtle mechanisms regulating (Na^+,K^+)-ATPase functions could be operational. A diminution of the density of norepinephrine (NE) or NE-containing terminals, of cortical NE content, of tyrosine hydroxylase activity, and of the high-affinity uptake of NE has been observed in chronic cobalt epilepsy and perhaps in human partial cortical epilepsies (18,154).

Pharmacologic concentrations of NE stimulate (Na^+,K^+)-ATPase in crude brain homogenates (69), and it is conceivable that decreased NE could produce a drop in glial (Na^+,K^+)-ATPase activities. Decreased GAD activity, GABA binding sites (88), and GAD-containing nerve terminals (121) have also been described in human partial epilepsies. Their relations to our observed abnormalities in glial (Na^+,K^+)-ATPase are not known. Future experiments addressing these issues and relating *in vitro* biochemical processes with the metabolic functions assessed by PET and SPECT in the epileptic brain *in situ* are necessary.

An impaired (Na^+,K^+)-ATPase function within glial membranes is particularly significant since it may explain why anterior temporal lobectomies have been necessary as a surgical form of treatment for medically intractable temporal-lobe epilepsy. Theoretically, the excision of the focal epileptogenic lesion should be sufficient to cure focal epilepsy. On this basis, cortical resection has earned a secure role in the surgical treatment of focal cortical epilepsy since it was pioneered by Foerster and Penfield (35). However, amygdalectomies, hippocampectomies, and even focal excisions of local temporal regions have proven ineffective in curing or significantly controlling temporal-lobe epilepsy. Instead, resection of the anterior 5 to 6 cm of the anterior temporal lobe or wider zones of epileptogenic areas has proven necessary. Continuing analysis of patients operated on since 1928 by Penfield et al. (35) has revealed that a greater and wider zone of epileptogenicity with multiple epileptogenic cortical areas exists in these temporal lobes with the region of lowest threshold, giving the local sign of the habitual usual seizure. Follow-up studies have further indicated that success in stopping seizures correlated with the completeness of the removal of the widely epileptogenic cortex. Excisions limited to restricted foci of lowest seizure threshold usually failed to provide a satisfactory reduction in seizures. Discovering biochemical lesions in a wider region of the anterior temporal lobe synaptically linked and surrounding the epileptogenic foci of lowest threshold could explain why focal excisions have failed to control seizures and thus provide one further rationale for anterior temporal lobectomy.

CONCLUSIONS ON RESPECTIVE ROLES OF GLIA AND NEURON IN EPILEPTOGENESIS

At the neuronal level, the generation of focal cortical epilepsy is generally attributed either to enhanced physiological responses or to paroxysmal depolarization shifts (160) that lead to the formation of interictal electroencephalographic spikes. The molecular events that underlie these phenomena remain unknown.

Physiologists hypothesized that paroxysmal depolarization shifts may result either from prolonged and enhanced synaptic drive, generated by increased excitatory feedback (utilizing interneurons of synaptic pathways within the focus), or from a primary membrane disease of neurons and synapses. Hypothetically, the production by neurons of initially enhanced responses and their subsequent production of such large and paroxysmal transmembrane depolarization shifts might result from abnormal behavior of certain molecular components (probably some abnormal proteins) of the neuronal plasma membrane.

The fundamental biochemical lesion in epilepsy could be of genetic origin. Experimental models of genetic epilepsy and studies of human genetic epidemiology show that single genes can exert major effects on cellular excitability within discrete central neural pathways. In addition, single-locus mutations are now known to produce abnormal gene products in neurons that subsequently generate interictal EEG spikes.

Neither neuronal paroxysmal depolarization shifts nor intcrictal EEG spikes are sufficient to produce epilepsy, however. The clinical expression of epilepsy necessitates recruitment of the surrounding normal neurons, utilization of pathways prepared for the propagation of seizures, and breakdown of mechanisms that limit the spread of seizures. From our experiments, we feel that abnormal glial cells, which contain a defect in their active spatial buffering function, could trigger the transition from the interictal to the ictal state.

Our results suggest that glial (Na^+,K^+)-ATPase is unable to clear elevated concentrations of K^+_o optimally during sustained epileptiform paroxysms. In brain tissue surrounding the seizure focus, however, the physiological efficiency of glial cells is maintained at optimal levels. Such impairment in glial control of elevated K^+_o (to 10–20 mM) could be mainly responsible for the transition of interictal discharges to ictal episodes rather than for the development of paroxysmal depolarization shifts. It is possible that the clinical expression of partial seizures involves two interacting factors:

1. A genetically determined susceptibility of the cortical neurons to produce paroxysmal depolarization shifts (low epileptogenic threshold)—as yet unidentified biochemically—clinically known as the epilepsy susceptibility gene.

2. An acquired cerebral cortical lesion that produces abnormal glial cells in the seizure focus with definite or reversibly impaired spatial buffering function, causing sustained elevations of K^+_o and triggering ictal transitions.

As recalled by Gastaut (43):

> The existence of a predisposition to epilepsy was postulated for the first time by Tissot in 1772, who wrote in his Treatise of Epilepsy: To produce epilepsy, two conditions must be met: (1) a disposition of the brain to enter into seizures more easily than in the healthy state (i.e., a genetic defect of neuronal membrane metabolism); and (2) a cause for initiation which activates this disposition (i.e., an acquired lesion such as abnormal glial cells).

This working hypothesis must now be verified in genetic models of focal and generalized epilepsies.

ACKNOWLEDGMENTS

I express my gratitude to Professors G. Franck, E. Schoffeniels, and A. V. Delgado-Escueta for their constant enthusiasm and scientific support.

I thank A. Minet and M. Vergniolles-Burette for their excellent technical work and I am grateful to C. Elias, Mrs. Gillet, and R. Mitchell for secretarial and word-processing assistance.

This work was also supported by the Belgian Rotary Foundation and Department of Health and Human Services contract N01-NS-0-2332 (U.S.A.).

REFERENCES

1. Albers, R. W. (1976): The (sodium plus potassium)-transport ATPase. In: *The Enzymes of Biological Membranes*, edited by A. N. Martonosi, pp. 283. Plenum, New York.
2. Atterwill, C. K., Cunningham, V. J., and Balazs, R. (1984): Characterization of Na^+,K^+-ATPase in cultured and separated neuronal and glial cells from rat cerebellum. *J. Neurochem.*, 43:8–18.
3. Balazs, R., Patel, A. J., and Richter, D. (1972): Metabolism of amino acids and ammonia in rat brain cortex slices *in vitro:* A possible role of ammonia in brain function. *J. Neurochem.*, 25:197–206.
   pp. 167–184. MacMillan, London.
4. Balazs, R., Machiyama, Y., Hammond, B. J., Julian, T., and Richter, D. (1970): The operation of the tricarboxylic acid cycles in brain tissue *in vitro. Biochem. J.*, 116:445–467.

5. Balcar, V. J., Roth-Schechter, B. F., and Mandel, P. (1978): Effect of chronic pentobarbitol treatment on high affinity uptake of L-glutamate by cultured glial cells. *Biochem. Pharmacol.*, 27:2955–2956.

6. Balcar, V. J., and Hauser, K. L. (1978): Transport of (^{3}H)-L-glutamate and (^{3}H)-L-glutamine by dissociated glial and neuronal cells in primary culture. *Proc. Eur. Soc. Neurochem.*, 1:498.

7. Benjamin, A. M., and Quastel, J. H. (1972): Locations of amino acids in brain slices from rat. *Biochem. J.*, 128:631–646.

8. Benjamin, A. M., and Quastel, J. H. (1975): Metabolism of amino acids and ammonia in rat brain cortex slices *in vitro:* A possible role of ammonia in brain function. *J. Neurochem.*, 25:197–206.

9. Blomstrand, C., and Hamberger, A. (1969): Protein turnover in cell-enriched fractions from rabbit brain. *J. Neurochem.*, 16:1401–1407.

10. Bourke, R. S., and Tower, D. B. (1966): Fluid compartmentation and electrolytes of cat cerebral cortex in vitro. II. Sodium, potassium and chloride of nature cerebral cortex. *J. Neurochem.*, 13:1099.

11. Bourke, R. S., and Nelson, K. M. (1972): Further studies on the K^+ dependent swelling to primate cerebral cortex *in vivo.* The enzymatic basis of the K^+ dependent transport of chloride. *J. Neurochem.*, 19:663.

12. Bourke, R. S., Daze, M. A., and Kimelberg, H. K. (1978): Chloride transport in mammalian astroglia. In: *Dynamic Properties of Glia Cells,* edited by E. Schoffeniels, G. Franck, L. Hertz, and D. B. Tower, p. 337. Pergamon, Oxford.

13. Bondar, R. L. (1978): Development of glia. In: *Dynamic Properties of Glia Cells,* edited by E. Schoffeniels, G. Franck, D. B. Tower, and L. Hertz, pp. 3–12. Pergamon, London.

14. Brotchi, J. (1978): The activated astrocyte: A histochemical approach to the epileptic focus. In: *Dynamic Properties of Glia Cells,* edited by E. Schoffeniels, G. Franck, L. Hertz, and D. B. Tower, pp. 429–433. Pergamon, New York.

15. Bruun, A., and Ehinger, B. (1974): Uptake of certain possible neurotransmitters into retinal neurons of some mammals. *Exp. Eye Res.*, 19:435–447.

16. Cajal, S. R. (1909–1911): *Histologie du Système Nerveux de l'Homme et des Vertébrés.* Maloine, Paris.

17. Cavanagh, J. B., Falconer, M. A., and Meyer, A. (1958): Some pathogenic problems of temporal lobe epilepsy. In: *Temporal Lobe Epilepsy,* edited by M. Baldwin, and P. Bailey, pp. 140–148. Thomas, Springfield, Illinois.

18. Chauvel, P., Trottier, S., Nass, F. S., and Bregman, B. (1982): Alterations of cortical noradrenergic mechanisms in cobalt foci. In: *Advances in Epileptology: XIIIth Epilepsy International Symposium,* edited by H. Akimoto, H. Kazamatsuri, M. Seino, and A. Ward, pp. 531–535. Raven Press, New York.

19. Church, G. A., Kimelberg, H. K., and Sapirstein, V. S. (1980): Stimulation of carbonic anhydrase activity and phosphorylation in primary astroglial cultures by norepinephrine. *J. Neurochem.*, 34:873–879.

20. Clarke, D. D., Ronan, E. J., Dicker, E., and Tirri, L. (1974): Ethanol and its relation to amino acid metabolism in brain. In: *Metabolic Compartmentation and Neurotransmission,* edited by S. Berl, D. D. Clarke, and D. Schneider, pp. 449–460. Plenum, New York.

21. Clos, J., Legrand, C., Legrand, J., Ghandour, M. S., Labourdette, G., Vincendon, G., and Gombas, G. (1982): Effect of thyroid state and undernutrition on S-100 protein and astroglia development in rat cerebellum. *Dev. Neurosci.*, 5:285–292.

22. Coles, J. A., and Tsacopoulos, M. (1979): Potassium activity in photoreceptor, glial cells and extracellular space in the drone retina. Changes during photostimulation. *J. Physiol. (Lond.)*, 290:525–549.

23. Cummins, C. J., Lust, W. D., and Passoneau, J. V. (1983): Regulation of glycogenolysis in transformed astrocytes *in vitro. J. Neurochem.*, 40:137–144.

24. De Belleroche, J. S., and Bradford, H. F. (1973): The synaptosome: An isolated working neuronal compartment. *Prog. Neurobiol.*, 1:275–298.

25. Delaunoy, J. P., Hog, F., Devilliers, G., Bansart, M., Mandel, P., and Sensenbrenner, M. (1980): Developmental changes and localization of carbonic anhydrase in cerebral hemispheres of the rat and in rat glial cell cultures. *Cell. Mol. Biol.*, 26:235–240.

26. Dennis, M. J., and Gerschenfeld, H. M. (1969): Some physiological properties of identified neuroglial cells. *J. Physiol.*, 203:211–222.

27. Dichter, M. A., Herman, C. J., and Selzer, M. (1972): Silent cells during interictal discharges and seizures in hippocampal penicillin foci. Evidence for the role of extracellular K^+ in the transition from the interictal state to seizures. *Brain Res.*, 48:173–183.

28. Drejer, J., Meier, E., and Schousboe, A. (1983): Novel neuron-related regulatory mechanisms for astrocytic glutamate and GABA high affinity uptake. *Neurosci. Lett.*, 37:301–306.

29. Ehinger, B. (1972): Cellular location of the uptake of some amino acids into the rabbit retina. *Brain Res.*, 46:297–311.

30. Engel, J., Jr., Kuhl, D. E., and Phelps, M. E. (1981): Patterns of local metabolism during partial seizures in man. *Neurology,* 31:130–145.

31. Delgado-Escueta, A. V., Davidson, D., and Reilly, E. L. (1974): Potassium transport within synaptosomes isolated from epileptogenic foci. *Brain Res.*, 78:223–237.

32. Delgado-Escueta, A. V., and Appel, S. H. (1972): The effects of electroshock seizures on potassium transport within synaptosomes from rat brain. *J. Neurochem.*, 19:1625–1638.

33. Delgado-Escueta, A. V., and Horan, M. P. (1980): Brain synaptosomes in epilepsy: Organization of ionic channels and the Na^+-K^+ pump. In: *Antiepileptic Drugs: Mechanisms of Action,* edited by G. H. Glaser, J. K. Penry, and D. M. Woodbury, pp. 85–126. Raven Press, New York.

34. Fere, C. (1890): *Les Epilepsies et les Epilep-tiques,* pp. 1–636. F. Alcan, Paris.

35. Foerster, O., and Penfield, W. (1930): The structural basis of traumatic epilepsy and results of radical operations. *Brain,* 53:99–139.

36. Franck, G. (1970): Echanges cationiques au niveau des neurones et des cellules gliales du cerveau. *Arch. Int. Physiol. Biochim.,* 78:613–720.

37. Franck, G., Grisar, T., Moonen, G., and Schoffeniels, E. (1978): Potassium transport in mammalian astroglia. In: *Dynamic Properties of Glia Cells,* edited by E. Schoffeniels, G. Franck, L. Hertz, and D. B. Tower, pp. 315–325. Pergamon, Oxford.

38. Franck, G., Grisar, T., and Moonen, G. (1983): Glial and neuronal Na^+K^+ pump. *Adv. Cell. Neurobiol.,* 4:133–159.

39. Franck, G., Depresseux, J. C., Sadzot, B., Cheslet, J. P., Salmon, E., Grisar, T., Guillaume, M., and Lamotte, D. (1983): Regional cerebral blood flow and oxygen uptake rate in human focal epilepsy and status epilepticus. *Int. Symposium on Basic Mechanisms of the Epilepsies,* San Diego, Calif., pp. 163.

40. Futamachi, K. J., and Pedley, T. A. (1976): Glial cells and extracellular potassium: Their relationship in mammalian cortex. *Brain Res.,* 109:311–322.

41. Gardner-Medwin, A. R. (1983): A study of the mechanisms by which potassium moves through brain tissue in the rat. *J. Physiol.,* 335:353–374.

42. Garfinkel, D. (1972): Possible correlations between morphological structures in the brain and the compartmentations indicated by stimulation. In: *Metabolic Compartmentation in the Brain,* edited by R. Balazs and J. E. Cremer, pp. 129–136. MacMillan, London.

43. Gastaut, H. (1982): "Benign" or "functional" (versus "organic") epilepsies in different stages of life: An analysis of the corresponding age-related variations in the predisposition to epilepsy. Henri Gastaut and the Marseille School's contribution to the neurosciences. *Electroencephalogr. Clin. Neurophysiol.* 35(Suppl.):17–44.

44. Geren, B. B. (1954): The formation from the Schwann cells surface of myelin in the peripheral nerves of chick embryos. *Exp. Cell Res.,* 7:558–562.

45. Giacobini, E. (1962): A cytochemical study of the localization of carbonic anhydrase in the nervous system. *J. Neurochem.,* 9:169–177.

46. Glotzner, F. L. (1973): Membrane properties of neuroglia in epileptogenic gliosis. *Brain Res.,* 55:159–171.

47. Glynn, I. M., and Karlish, S. J. D. (1975): The sodium pump. *Annu. Rev. Physiol.,* 37:13.

48. Golgi, C. (1873): Sulla struttura della sostanza grigia dell cervello. *Gazz. Med. Ital. Lombarda,* 33:244–246.

49. Gould, R. M., Pant, H., Gainer, H., and Tylett, M. (1983): Phospholipid synthesis in the squid giant axon: Incorporation of lipid precursors. *J. Neurochem.,* 40:1293–1299.

50. Grisar, T., Frere, J. M., and Franck, G. (1979): Effects of K^+ ions on kinetic properties of the Na^+K^+ATPase (EC 3.6.1.3) of bulk isolated glial cells, perikaria and synaptosomes from rabbit brain cortex. *Brain Research,* 165:87–103.

51. Grisar, T., Franck, G., and Schoffeniels, E. (1980): Glial control of neuronal excitability in mammals. II. Enzymatic evidence: Two molecular forms of the Na^+K^+-ATPase in brain. *Neurochem. Int.,* 2:311–320.

52. Grisar, T., Frere, J. M., Charlier-Grisar, J., Franck, G., and Schoffeniels, E. (1978): Synaptosomal Na^+K^+ATPase is a hysteretic enzyme. *FEBS Lett.,* 89:173–176.

53. Grisar, T., and Franck, G. (1975): Glial cell control of extracellular K^+ content in the CNS. *Abstr. of the 5th Int. Mtg. of the Int. Soc. for Neurochem. (Barcelona),* 160:228.

54. Grisar, T., Franck, G., and Delgado-Escueta, A. V. (1982): Glial contribution to seizures: K^+ activation of Na^+K^+ATPase in bulk isolated glial cells and synaptosomes of epileptogenic cortex. *Brain Res.,* 261:75–84.

55. Grisar, T., Franck, G., and Schoffeniels, E. (1978): K^+ activation mechanisms of the Na^+K^+ATPase of bulk isolated glia cells and neurons. In: *Dynamic Properties of Glia Cells,* edited by E. Schoffeniels, G. Franck, L. Hertz, and D. B. Tower, pp. 353–363. Pergamon, Oxford.

56. Grisar, T., and Franck, G. (1981): Effect of changing K^+ ion on rat cerebral cortex slices in vitro. A study during development. *J. Neurochem.,* 36:1853.

57. Grossman, R. G., and Rosman, L. J. (1971): Intracellular potentials of inexcitable cells in epileptogenic cortex undergoing fibrillary gliosis after local injury. *Brain Res.,* 55:159–171.

58. Grossman, R. G., and Seregin, L. (1977): Glial–neural interaction demonstrated by the injection of Na^+ and Li^+ into cortical glia. *Science,* 195:196–198.

59. Hamberger, A. (1971): Amino acid uptake in neuronal and glial cell fractions from rabbit cerebral cortex. *Brain Res.,* 31:169–178.

60. Henn, F. A., Haljamme, M., and Hamberger, A. (1972): Glial cell function: Active control of extracellular K^+ concentration. *Brain Res.,* 43:437–443.

61. Henn, F. A., and Hamberger, A. (1971): Glial cell function: Uptake of transmitter substances. *Proc. Natl. Acad. Sci. U.S.A.,* 68:2686–2690.

62. Henn, F. A., Goldstein, M. N., and Hamberger, A. (1974): Uptake of the neurotransmitter candidate glutamate by glia. *Nature (Lond.),* 249:663–664.

63. Hertz, L. (1977): Biochemistry of glial cells. In: *Cell, Tissue and Organ Cultures in Neurobiology,* edited by S. Fedoroff and L. Hertz, pp. 39–71. Academic, New York.

64. Hertz, L. (1978): Energy metabolism in glial cells. In: *Dynamic Properties of Glial Cells,* edited by E. Schoffeniels, G. Franck, L. Hertz, and D. B. Tower, pp. 121–132. Pergamon, Oxford.

65. Hertz, L. (1979): Functional interactions between neurons and astrocytes. I. Turnover and

metabolism of putative amino acid transmitters. *Prog. Neurobiol.*, 13:277–323.

66. Hertz, L. (1979): Functional interactions between neurons and astrocytes. II. Potassium homeostasis at the cellular level. *Prog. Neurobiol.*, 13:324–368.

67. Hertz, L. (1979): Kinetics of adenosine uptake into astrocytes. *J. Neurochem.*, 31:55–62.

68. Hess, H. H., and Pope, A. (1972): Quantitative neurochemical histology. In: *Handbook of Neurochemistry*, edited by A. Lajtha, pp. 289–327. Plenum, New York.

69. Hexum, T. D. (1977): The effect of catecholamines on transport of (Na,K)-adenosine triphosphatase. *Biochem. Pharmacol.*, 26:1221–1227.

70. Hökfelt, T., and Ljungdahl, A. (1972): Application of cytochemical techniques to the study of suspected transmitter substances in the nervous system. In: *Advances in Biochemical Psychopharmacology*, edited by E. Costa and P. Greengard, pp. 1–36. Raven Press, New York.

71. Holmgren E. (1904): Über die trophospongien der nerverzellen. *Anat. Anz.*, 24:225–244.

72. Hosli, L., and Hosli, E. (1978): Action and uptake of neurotransmitters in CNS tissue culture. *Rev. Physiol. Biochem. Pharmacol.*, 81:136–188.

73. Hyden, H. (1967): Dynamic aspects on the neuron-glia relationship. A study with microchemical methods. In: *The Neuron*, edited by H. Hyden, pp. 179–219. Elsevier, Amsterdam.

74. Johnson, J. L. (1978): The excitant amino acids glutamic and aspartic acid as transmitter candidate in the dorsal sensory neuron: Reconsiderations. *Life Sci.*, 20:1637–1644.

75. Kawano, T., Kurihara, M., and Mori, K. (1983): Na-K-ATPase activity of the human glioma. Abstract of the 9th Meeting of the International Society for Neurochemistry, Vancouver. *J. Neurochem.*, 41:5152B.

76. Kettenmann, H., Sonnhof, U., and Schachner, M. (1983): Exclusive potassium dependence of the membrane potential in cultured mouse oligodendrocytes. *J. Neurosci.*, 3:500–505.

77. Kimelberg, H. K. (1974): Active potassium transport and $(Na^+ + K^+)$-ATPase activity in cultured glioma and nemoblastoma cells. *J. Neurochem.*, 22:971.

78. Kimelberg, H. K., Bowman, C., Biddlecome, S., and Bourke, R. S. (1979): Cation transport and membrane potential properties of primary astroglial cultures from neonatal rat brains. *Brain Res.*, 177:533–550.

79. Kometiani, Z. P., Tsakadze, L. G., and Jariashvili, T. Y. (1984): Functional significance of the effect of nemotransmitters on the Na^+,K^+-ATPase system. *J. Neurochem.*, 1246.

80. Kimelberg, H. K., Biddlecome, S., and Bourke, R. S. (1979): SITS-inhibitable Cl^- transport and Na^+ dependent H^+ production in primary astroglial cultures. *Brain Res.*, 173:111.

81. Kukes, G., Elul, R., and De Vellis, J. (1976): The ionic basis of the membrane potential in a rat glial cell line. *Brain Res.*, 104:71–92.

82. Kuffler, S. W., and Nicholls, J. G. (1966): The physiology of neuroglia cells. *Ergeb. Physiol.*, 57:1–90.

83. Kumpulainent, N. T., and Nystrom, S. H. M. (1981): Immunohistochemical localization of carbonic anhydrase isozyme C in human brain. *Brain Res.*, 220:220–225.

84. Lacoste, L., Chaudmary, K. D., and Lapoynt, J. (1982): Derepression of the glutamine synthetase in neuroblastoma cells at low concentrations of glutamine. *J. Neurochem.*, 39:78–85.

85. Lasek, R. J., and Tytell, M. A. (1981): Macromolecular transfer from glia to the axon. *J. Exp. Biol.*, 95:153–165.

86. Lewin, E., and McCrimon, A. (1967): ATPase activity in discharging cortical lesions induced by freezing. *Arch. Neurol.*, 16:321–325.

87. Lewis, D. V., Mutsuga, N., Schuette, W. H., and VanBuren, J. (1977): Potassium clearance and reactive gliosis in the alumina gel lesion. *Epilepsia*, 18:132–136.

88. Lloyd, K. G., Munari, C., Bossi, L., Stoeffels, C., Talairac, N. J., and Morselli, P. L. (1981): Biochemical evidence for the alterations of GABA-mediated synaptic transmission in pathological brain tissue (stereo EEG or morphological definition) from epileptic patient. In: *Neurotransmitters Seizures, and Epilepsy*, edited by R. L. Morselli et al., pp. 325–338. Raven Press, New York.

89. Lothman, E. W., and Somjen, G. G. (1975): Extracellular potassium activity, intracellular and extracellular potential responses in the spinal cord. *J. Physiol.*, 252:115–136.

90. Lugaro, E. (1907): Sulle funzioni delle neuroglia. *Riv. Patol. Nerv. Ment.*, 12:225–233.

91. Manuelidis, L., Manuelidis, E. E., and Prichard, J. (1975): Relationship between membrane potential and external potassium in human glioblastoma cells in tissue culture. *J. Cell. Physiol.*, 87:179–188.

92. Martinez-Hernandez, A., Bell, K. P., and Norenberg, M. D. (1977): Glutamine synthetase: Glial localization in brain. *Science*, 195:1356–1358.

93. Matsuda, T., Iwata, H., and Cooper, J. R. (1984): Specific inactivation of $\alpha(+)$ molecular form of (Na^+K^+)-ATPase by pyrithiamin. *J. Biol. Chem.*, 259:3858–3863.

94. Matsuura, S. (1969): Effects of changes in extracellular K^+ concentration on resting and action potentials of the toad spinal Motoneuron. *Osaka City Med. J.*, 15:29–45.

95. Meister, A., Griffith, O. W., Novogrodsky, A., and Tate, S. S. (1979): New aspects of glutathione metabolism and translocation in mammals. *Ciba Found. Symp.*, 72:135–161.

96. Moonen, G., and Franck, G. (1977): Potassium effect on (Na^+,K^+)-ATPase activity of cultured new-born rat astroblasts during differentiation *Neurosci. Lett.*, 4:263.

97. Moonen, G., and Nelson, P. G. (1978): Some physiological properties in astrocytes in primary cultures. In: *Dynamic Properties of Glial Cells*, edited by E. Schoffeniels, G. Franck, D. B. Tower, and L. Hertz, pp. 389–393. Pergamon, New York.

98. Moonen, G., Franck, G., and Schoffeniels, E. (1980): Glial control of neuronal excitability in mammals: 1. Electrophysiological and isotopic evidence in culture. *Neurochem. Int.*, 2:299.

99. McLennan, H. (1976): The autoradiographic localization of L-(^{3}H)-glutamate in rat brain tissue. *Brain Res.*, 115:139–144.

100. McGeer, E. G., and McGeer, P. L. (1979): Biochemical mapping of specific neuronal pathways. In: *Advances in Cellular Neurobiology*, edited by S. Fedoroff and L. Hertz. Academic, New York.

101. Mudge, A. W. (1981): Effect of chemical environment on levels of substance P and somatostatin in cultured sensory neurons. *Nature (Lond.)*, 292:764–767.

102. Norenberg, M. D., and Lapham, L. W. (1974): The astrocyte response in experimental portal encephalopathy: An electron microscopy study. *J. Neuropathol. Exp. Neurol.*, 33:422–435.

103. Orkand, R. K. (1969): Neuroglial-neuronal interactions. In: *Basic Mechanisms of the Epilepsies*, edited by H. H. Jasper, A. Ward, and A. Pope, pp. 737–746. Little, Brown, Boston.

104. Pape, L. G., and Katzman, R. (1972): Response of glia in cat sensorimotor cortex to increased extracellular potassium. *Brain Res.*, 38:71–92.

105. Patel, A. J., and Balazs, R. (1974): Factors affecting the development of metabolic compartmentation in the brain. In: *Metabolic Compartmentation and Neurotransmission*, edited by S. Berl, D. D. Carke, and D. Schneider, pp. 363–383. Plenum, New York.

106. Patel, A. J., Regan, C. M., Annunzata, P., Meier, E., and Balazs, R. (1982): Biochemical characterization and interaction of neuronal and glial cells in culture. *Biochem. Soc. Trans.*, 10:413–421.

107. Pedley, T. A., Fisher, R. S., and Prince, D. A. (1976): Focal gliosis and potassium movement in mammalian cortex. *Exp. Neurol.*, 50:346–361.

108. Pedley, T. A., Fisher, R. S., Futanachi, K. J., and Prince, D. A. (1976): Regulation of extracellular potassium concentration in epileptogenesis. *Fed. Proc.*, 35:1254–1259.

109. Penfield, W. (1927): The mechanism of cicatricial contraction in the brain. *Brain*, 50:499–517.

110. Penfield, W. (1932): Neuroglia: Normal and pathological. In: *Cytology and Cellular Pathology of the Nervous System, Vol. 2*, edited by W. Penfield, pp. 423–472. P.B. Hoeber, New York.

111. Pentreath, V. W. (1982): Potassium signalling of metabolic interactions between neuron and glia cells. *Trends Neurosci.*, 5:339–344.

112. Pentreath, V. W., Seul, L. H., and Kai-Kai, M. A. (1982): Incorporation of (^{3}H)2-deoxyglucose into glycogen in nervous tissues. *Neurosciences*, 7:159–767.

113. Pentreath, V. W., and Kai-Kai, M. A. (1982): Significance of the potassium signal from neurons to glia cells. *Nature (Lond.)*, 295:59–61.

114. Pfeiffer, S. E., Betschart, B., Cook, J., Mancinci, P., and Morris, R. (1977): Glial cell lines. In: *Cell, Tissue and Organ Cultures in Neurobiology*, edited by S. Fedoroff and L. Hertz, pp. 278–346. Academic, New York.

115. Picker, S., and Goldring, S. (1982): Electrophysiological properties of human glia. *Trends Neurosci.*, 5:73–76.

116. Pollen, D. A., and Trachtenberg, M. C. (1970): Neuroglia: Gliosis and focal epilepsy. *Science*, 167:1252–1253.

117. Pope, A. (1978): Neuroglia: Quantitative aspects. In: *Dynamic Properties of Glia Cells*, edited by E. Schoffeniels, G. Franck, D. B. Tower, and L. Hertz, pp. 13–20. Pergamon, New York.

118. Rapport, R. L., Harris, A. B., Friel, P. N., and Ojemann, G. A. (1975): Human epileptic brain NaKATPase activity and phenytoin. *Arch. Neurol.*, 32:549–554.

119. Ramaharobandro, N., Borg, J., Mandel, P., and Mark, J. (1982): Glutamine and glutamate transport in cultured neuronal and glial cells. *Brain Res.*, 244:113–121.

120. Ransom, B. R., and Goldring, S. (1973): Ionic determinants of membrane potential of cells presumed to be glia in cerebral cortex of cat. *J. Neurophysiol.*, 36:855–868.

121. Riback, C. E., Harris, A. B., Vaughn, J. E., and Robertz, E. (1981): Immunocytochemical changes in cortical neurons in a monkey model of epilepsy. In: *Neurotransmitters, Seizures, and Epilepsy*, edited by P. L. Morselli et al., pp. 11–22. Raven Press, New York.

122. Roberts, P. J., and Keen, P. (1974): (^{14}C) glutamate uptake and compartmentation in glia of rat dorsal sensory ganglion. *J. Neurochem.*, 23:201–209.

123. Riepe, R. E., and Norenberg, M. D. (1977): Muller cell localization of glutamine synthetase in rat retina. *Nature (Lond.)*, 268:654–655.

124. Del Rio Hortega, P. (1919): El tercer alemento de los centros nerviosos. *Bol. Soc. Esp. Biol.*, :69–120.

125. Robinson, N., and Wells, F. (1973): Distribution and localization of sites of gamma aminobutyric acid metabolism in the adult rat brain. *J. Anat.*, 114:365–378.

126. Roussel, G., Delaunoy, J. P., Nussbaum, J. L., and Mandel, P. (1979): Demonstration of a specific localization of carbonic anhydrase C in the glial cells of rat CNS by an immunohistochemical method. *Brain Res.*, 160:47–55.

127. Scheibel, A. B. (1980): Morphological correlates of epilepsy: Cells in the hippocampus. In: *Antiepileptic Drugs: Mechanisms of Action*, edited by G. H. Glaser, J. K. Penry, and D. M. Woodbury, pp. 49–61. Raven Press, New York.

128. Schoffeniels, E., Franck, G., Tower, D. B., and Hertz, L. (1978): *Dynamic Properties of Glia Cells*, pp. 1–467. Pergamon, London.

129. Schon, F., and Kelly, J. S. (1974): Autoradiographic localization of (^{3}H)GABA and (^{3}H)-glutamate over satellite glial cells. *Brain Res.*, 66:275–288.

130. Schousboe, A., Hertz, L., Svenneby, G., and Kvamme, E. (1979): Phosphate activated glutaminase activity and glutamine uptake in astro-

cytes in primary cultures. *J. Neurochem.,* 32:943–950.

131. Schousboe, A., Hertz, L., and Svenneby, G. (1977): Uptake and metabolism of GABA in astrocytes cultured from dissociated mouse brain hemispheres. *Neurochem. Res.,* 2:217–229.

132. Schousboe, A., Svenneby, G., and Hertz, L. (1977): Uptake and metabolism of glutamate in astrocytes cultured from dissociated mouse brain hemispheres. *J. Neurochem.,* 29:999–1005.

133. Schousboe, A. (1978): Glutamate, GABA and taurine in cultured normal glial cells. In: *Dynamic Properties of Glia Cells,* edited by E. Schoffeniels, G. Franck, L. Hertz, D. B. Tower, pp. 173–182. Pergamon, Oxford.

134. Schousboe, A., Larsson, O. M., Wood, J. D., and Krogsgaard-Larsen, P. (1983): Transport and metabolism of GABA in neurons and glia: Implications for epilepsy. *Epilepsia,* 24:533–538.

135. Schrier, B. K. (1977): Transmitter, putative transmitter-related enzymes studied in cultured cells systems. In: *Cell, Tissue and Organ Cultures in Neurobiology,* edited by S. Fedoroff and L. Hertz, pp. 423–439. Academic, New York.

136. Sellstrom, A., and Hamberger, A. (1977): Potassium-stimulated γ-aminobutyric acid release from neurons and glia. *Brain Res.,* 119:189–198.

137. Sellstrom, A., and Hamberger, A. (1975): Neuronal and glial systems for γ-aminobutyric acid transport. *J. Neurochem.,* 24:847–852.

138. Sellström, A., Sjösberg, L. B., Hamberger, A. (1975): Neuronal and glial systems for γ-aminobutyric acid metabolism. *J. Neurochem.,* 25:393–398.

139. Sholl, D. A. (1953): Dendritic organization in the neurons of the visual and motor cortices of the cat. *J. Anat.,* 87:387–406.

140. Siegel, G. J., Desmond, T. J., and Ernst, A. (1984): Immunoreactive subspecies of (Na⁺K⁺)-ATPase catalytic subunit. *Abst. 15th Annu. Meet. of the American Society for Neurochemistry,* Portland, Oregon, March 11–16.

141. Skaper, S. D., and Varon, S. (1981): Na⁺,K⁺-ATPase and ouabain binding activities of nerve, growth-factor-supported acid deprived chick embryo dorsal root ganglia. *J. Neurosci. Res.,* 6:133.

142. Skou, J. C. (1957): The influence of some cations on an adenosine triphosphatase from peripheral nerves. *Biochim. Biophys. Acta,* 23:394.

143. Stahl, W. L., and Brodekson, S. H. (1976): Localization of Na⁺,K⁺-ATPase in brain. *Fed. Proc.,* 35:1260–1264.

144. Snodgrass, S. R., and Iversen, L. L. (1974): Amino acid uptake in human brain tumors. *Brain Res.,* 76:95–107.

145. Somjen, G. G. (1980): Influence of potassium and neuroglia in the generation of seizures and their treatment. In: *Antiepileptic Drugs: Mechanisms of Action,* edited by G. M. Glaser, K. F. Penry, and D. M. Woodbury, pp. 155–167. Raven Press, New York.

146. Storm-Mathisen, J. (1977): Glutamic acid and excitatory nerve endings. Reduction of glutamic acid uptake after axotomy. *Brain Res.,* 120:379–386.

147. Sturrock, R. R. (1976): Light microscopic identification of immature glial cells in semithin sections of the developing mouse corpus callosum. *J. Anat.,* 122:521–537.

148. Sweadner, K. J. (1979): Two molecular forms of (Na⁺K⁺)-stimulated ATPase in brain: Separation and difference in affinity for strophantidin. *J. Biol. Chem.,* 254:6060–6067.

149. Sykova, E. (1983): Extracellular K⁺ accumulation in the central nervous system. *Prog. Biophys. Mol. Biol.,* 42:135–189.

150. Tower, D. B. (1965): Problems associated with studies of electrolyte metabolism in normal and epileptogenic cerebral cortex. *Epilepsia,* 6:183.

151. Tower, D. B. (1969): Neurochemical mechanisms. In: *Basic Mechanisms of the Epilepsies,* edited by H. H. Jasper, A. A. Ward, Jr., and A. Pope. Little, Brown, Boston.

152. Tower, D. B. (1978): General perspectives and conclusions of the symposium on dynamic properties of glial cells. In: *Dynamic Properties of Glia Cells,* edited by E. Schoffeniels, G. Franck, L. Hertz, and D. B. Tower, pp. 443–460. Pergamon, Oxford.

153. Trachtenberg, M. C., and Pollen, D. A. (1970): Neuroglia: Biophysical properties and physiologic function. *Science,* 167:1248–1252.

154. Trottier, S., Claustre, Y., Caboche, J., Dedek, J., Chauvel, P., Nassif, S., and Scatton, B. (1983): Alterations of noradrenaline and serotonin uptake and metabolism in chronic cobalt-induced epilepsy in the rat. *Brain Res.,* 272:255–262.

155. Utley, J. D. (1963): Gamma aminobutyric acid and 5-hydroxytryptamine concentrations in neurons and glial cells in the medial geniculate body of the cat. *Biochem. Pharmacol.,* 12:1228–1230.

156. Van De Berg, C. J. (1972): A model of compartmentation in mouse brain based on glucose and acetate metabolism. In: *Metabolic Compartmentation in the Brain,* edited by R. Balazs and J. E. Cremer, pp. 137–166. McMillan, London.

157. Van De Berg, C. J., Matheson, D. F., and Ronda, G. (1974): A model of glutamate metabolism in brain or biochemical analysis of a heterogeneous structure. In: *Metabolic Compartmentation and Neurotransmission,* edited by S. Berl, D. D. Clarke, and D. Schneider, pp. 515–540. Plenum, New York.

158. Virchow, R. (1846): Über das granulierte anschen der wandungen der gehirnventrikel. *Allg. Z. Psychiat.,* 3:424–450.

159. Vizi, E. S. (1978): Na⁺K⁺-activated adenosine-triphosphatase as a trigger in transmitter release. *Neuroscience,* 3:367–384.

160. Ward, A. (1961): The epileptic neuron. *Epilepsia,* 2:70–79.

161. Waelsch, H., Berl, S., Rossi, C. A., Clarke, D. D., and Purpura, D. P. (1964): Quantitative aspects of CO₂ fixation in mammalian brain in vivo. *J. Neurochem.,* 11:717–728.

162. Walz, W., and Hertz, L. (1982): Ouabain-sensitive and ouabain resistant net uptake of potassium into astrocytes and neurons in primary cultures. *J. Neurochem.*, 39:70–77.

163. Walz, W., and Hertz, L. (1985): Comparison between fluxes of potassium and of chloride in astrocytes in primary cultures. *Brain Res.*, *(in press)*.

164. Walz, W., Wuttke, W., and Hertz, L. (1985): Astrocytes in primary cultures: Membrane potential characteristics reveal exclusive potassium conductance and potassium accumulator properties. *Brain Res.*, *(in press)*.

165. Ward, A. (1978): Glia and epilepsy. In: *Dynamic Properties of Glia Cells*, edited by E. Schoffeniels, G. Franck, L. Hertz, and D. B. Tower, pp. 413–427. Pergamon, Oxford.

166. Wardell, W. M. (1966): Electrical and pharmacological properties of mammalian neuroglial cells in tissue culture. *Proc. R. Soc. Lond.* *[Biol.]*, 165:326–361.

167. Weight, F. F., and Erulkar, S. D. (1976): Modulation of synaptic transmitter release by repetitive postsynaptic action potentials. *Science*, 193:1023–1025.

168. Wofsey, A. R., Kuhar, M. J., and Snyder, S. H. (1971): A unique synaptosomal population which accumulates glutamic and aspartic acids in brain tissue. *Proc. Natl. Acad. Sci. U.S.A.*, 68:1102–1106.

169. Woodbury, D. M. (1980): Antiepileptic drugs. Carbonic anhydrase inhibitors. In: *Antiepileptic Drugs: Mechanisms of Action*, edited by G. H. Glaser, J. K. Penry, and D. M. Woodbury, pp. 617–633. Raven Press, New York.

170. Woodbury, D. M., and Kemp, J. W. (1979): Initiation, propagation and arrest of seizures. In: *Pathophysiology of Cerebral Energy Metabolism*, edited by B. B. Marsulja, L. M. Rakie, S. Klatzoi, and M. Spatz, pp. 313–351. Plenum, New York.

171. Wu, J. Y., Wong, E., Saito, K., Roberts, E., and Schousboe, A. (1976): Properties of L-glutamate decarboxylase from brains of adult and newborn mice. *J. Neurochem.*, 27:653–659.

172. Wu, P. H., Burden, D. A., and Hertz, L. (1979): Net production of aminobutyric acid in astrocytes in primary cultures determined by a sensitive mass spectrometric method. *J. Neurochem.*, 32:379–390.

173. Yu, A. C., Drejer, J., Hertz, L., and Schousboe, A. (1983): Pyruvate carboxylase activity in primary cultures of astrocytes and neurons. *J. Neurochem.*, 41:1484–1487.

Subject Index

Cl⁻ and, 626–627,1049,1050
conductance, 21,137,198–200,283,641–642,1049
currents, 141–153,226–227,251–252
depolarization and, 664
in epilepsies, 18,282,620,622–625,
    641–655,684,699,1048–1052
epileptogenesis and, 18,282,413,620
in ES, 252–253,619,622–625,631–632,652–653
GABA and, 992–994
in glial cells, 619,624,626–627,629–631,
    683,699,700,708–710,1045,
    1048–1051,1058–1063
hyperpolarization and, 244,622
in interstitial fluid, 664–665
in kindling, 650
laminar changes in, 622–624,628–629
Na⁺ and, 625–627
Na⁺,K⁺-ATPase and,
    681,683–684,696,705–710,1045–1046,1065
in PTZ seizures, 632
reuptake of, 625
seizure arrest and, 697
in seizures, 622–625,632–633,641–655,663
SOC and, 240,251,252–254
synaptic, 664–665
synchrony and, 610–611
translocation of, 198–200,683–684
Picrotoxin
    binding sites, 366
    BZ binding and, 366–367
    electrical field effects, 610–611
    as GABA antagonist, 366
    ³H DHP binding and, 366
    hippocampus and, 589,610–611
    PTZ and, 366
    ³⁵S TBPS binding and, 368
Plasma membranes
    assemblies of, 765–766,768–772
    of astrocytes, 765
    freeze-fracture studies of, 765–772
Polyamines
    glutamate and, 1047,1063
    SAM and, 469–470
Positron emission tomography, (PET)
    in epilepsies, 39,922
    methods, 922–924
    ¹⁵O in, 935
    in partial epilepsy, 925–927,937–939
    radionuclides for, 23
Postactivation hyperpolarization, (PAH), mechanisms
    of, 19–20
Postsynaptic potential, (PSP), in hippocampal slices,
    991
Posttetanic potential, (PTP)
    PHT action on, 448–449
    seizures and, 448–449
Primidone
    as anticonvulsant, 721,729
    mechanism of action, 721
    MES seizure and, 721
Pro-dynorphin peptides
    Ca⁺⁺ and, 503
    of hippocampus, 501,502,505–508
Prostaglandins, (PGs)
    convulsions and, 879,882,885,890—891,894

metabolism of, 882–886,890–891
neurotransmission and, 880
Proteinases
    Ca⁺⁺ dependent, 405
    glutamate receptors and, 405–406
    substrates, 405
Protein synthesis
    autoradiography and, 907–913
    bicuculline effect, 906–907,908,910–911,914
    in brain, 903–916
    in developing brain, 906–907
    energy needs of, 903,913–914
    in epilepsy, 903–916
    GTP/GDP and, 913–914
    inhibition of, 904–905
    mRNA and, 905–906,913,915
    polyribosomes in, 905–906,909
    regulation of, 905,915
    in seizures, 903–916
    in status epilepticus, 905–906
    tyrosine incorporation and, 907–908,910
Proteolysis
    Ca⁺⁺ and, 837,854
    in neuronal injury, 837
Psychology
    of frontal lobe epilepsies, 16
    of temporal lobe epilepsies, 14–15
Purkinji cells
    GABA and, 291
    seizures and, 100
Pyramidal cells
    AHP of, 164
    basket cells of, 742
    bursting in, 992
    Ca⁺⁺ currents of, 161,652
    cable structure of, 159–160
    of cortex, 277–278,549–550
    currents of, 157–160
    EM of, 740,742,750–751
    GABA and, 748,749–750,752
    of hippocampus, 156–164,185,270–271,279,
        504,506–507,584–586,607–608,959,992,997
    inward currents of, 161–162
    in ischemia, 815–816
    kainic acid and, 999–1000
    K⁺ currents of, 163–164
    kainic acid and, 999–1000
    outward currents of, 162–164
    opioid peptides and, 491,501,503–504,509–510
    seizures and, 819
    tracts of, 972,974
    voltage clamp studies of, 156–157
Pyramidal-tract neurons, (PTN)
    in epileptogenic cortex, 972,974
    LFI bursts and, 970
Pyrethroids
    action of, 211,215
    Na⁺ channel and, 215

Quinuclidinylbenzylate, (QNB), carbachol and,
    416,417
Quisqualate, Ca⁺⁺ and, 642

Rat
    2DG studies of, 929